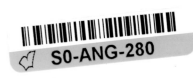

Diagnostic Surgical Pathology of the Head and Neck

Diagnostic Surgical Pathology of the Head and Neck

Edited by

Douglas R. Gnepp, M.D.

Professor of Pathology
Brown University School of Medicine
Senior Surgical Pathologist
Rhode Island Hospital
Providence, Rhode Island

W.B. SAUNDERS COMPANY
A Harcourt Health Sciences Company
Philadelphia London New York St. Louis Sydney Toronto

W.B. SAUNDERS COMPANY
A Harcourt Health Sciences Company

The Curtis Center
Independence Square West
Philadelphia, Pennsylvania 19106

Library of Congress Cataloging-in-Publication Data

Diagnostic surgical pathology of the head and neck / edited by Douglas R. Gnepp.—1st ed.

p. cm.

ISBN 0–7216–6856–9

1. Head—Diseases—Diagnosis.   2. Neck—Diseases—Diagnosis.
   3. Pathology, Surgical.   I. Gnepp, Douglas R.
   [DNLM: 1. Head—pathology.   2. Diagnostic Techniques, Surgical.
   3. Head—surgery.   4. Neck—pathology.   5. Neck—surgery.   WE 705 D536 2000]

RC936.D53   2000   617.5′ 1075—dc21

DNLM/DLC   99-22687

Acquisitions Editor: Marc Strauss
Developmental Editor: Cathy Carroll
Project Manager: Agnes Hunt Byrne
Production Manager: Linda Garber
Illustration Specialist: Peg Shaw

DIAGNOSTIC SURGICAL PATHOLOGY OF THE HEAD AND NECK   ISBN 0–7216–6856–9

Printed in the United States of America.

Last digit is the print number: 9   8   7   6   5   4   3   2   1

*This book is dedicated to the memory of
Fred and Ethel Gnepp, Harry Schneider, Julius Raden,
Charles "Chuck" Waldron, Zina Fleet, Jan Tyler, and Portia LeFebvre.*

Contributors ▪
▪
▪

CARL M. ALLEN, D.D.S., M.S.D.

Professor and Director, Oral and Maxillofacial Pathology, The Ohio State University, College of Dentistry; Professor, Department of Pathology, The Ohio State University, College of Medicine and Public Health, Columbus, Ohio
Odontogenic Cysts and Tumors

DANIEL A. ARBER, M.D.

Director of Hematopathology, City of Hope National Medical Center, Duarte, California
Hematopoietic Lesions

JERRY E. BOUQUOT, D.D.S., M.S.D.

Director of Research, The Maxillofacial Center for Diagnostics and Research, Morgantown, West Virginia; Consultant in Oral Pathology, New York Eye and Ear Infirmary, New York, New York; Consultant in Pediatric Oral Pathology, Pittsburgh Children's Hospital, Pittsburgh, Pennsylvania
Lesions of the Oral Cavity

MARGARET S. BRANDWEIN, M.D.

Associate Professor of Pathology and Otolaryngology, Mount Sinai School of Medicine of New York University; Attending Pathologist, Mount Sinai–New York Hospital Medical Center, New York, New York
Nonsquamous Pathology of the Larynx, Hypopharynx, and Trachea
Salivary and Lacrimal Glands

JOHN D. CRISSMAN, M.D.

Professor of Pathology and Dean, School of Medicine, Wayne State University, Detroit, Michigan
Squamous Intraepithelial Neoplasia of the Upper Aerodigestive Tract

DOUGLAS D. DAMM, D.D.S.

Professor of Oral Pathology, University of Kentucky, College of Dentistry, and University of Kentucky Hospital, Lexington, Kentucky
Odontogenic Cysts and Tumors

GUSTAVE L. DAVIS, M.D.

Clinical Professor of Pathology, Yale University School of Medicine, New Haven; Senior Pathologist, Department of Pathology and Laboratory Medicine, Bridgeport Hospital, Yale-New Haven Health Center; Bridgeport Pathology Consultants P.C., Bridgeport, Connecticut
Ear: External, Middle, and Temporal Bone

RONALD A. DeLELLIS, M.D.

Professor of Pathology, Joan and Sanford I. Weill Medical College of Cornell University; Vice-Chairman for Anatomic Pathology, New York Presbyterian Hospital/New York Weill Cornell Center, New York, New York
Pathology of the Thyroid and Parathyroid Glands

SAMIR K. EL-MOFTY, D.M.D., Ph.D.

Associate Professor of Pathology, Otolaryngology, and Head and Neck Surgery and Professor of Oral Pathology, Washington University School of Medicine; Attending Medical Staff, Barnes Hospital, Jewish Hospital, and St. Louis Children's Hospital; Consultant Pathologist, Veterans Administration Hospital, St. Louis, Missouri
Soft Tissue and Bone Lesions

DOUGLAS R. GNEPP, M.D.

Professor of Pathology, Brown University School of Medicine; Senior Surgical Pathologist, Rhode Island Hospital, Providence, Rhode Island
Nonsquamous Pathology of the Larynx, Hypopharynx, and Trachea; Salivary and Lacrimal Glands

GERARDO GUITER, M.D.

Assistant Professor of Pathology, Joan and Sanford I. Weill Medical College of Cornell University; Attending Pathologist, New York Presbyterian Hospital/New York Weill Cornell Center, New York, New York
Pathology of the Thyroid and Parathyroid Glands

JOHN D. HENLEY, M.D.

Assistant Professor of Pathology, Indiana University School of Medicine, Indianapolis, Indiana
Salivary and Lacrimal Glands

ANDREW G. HUVOS, M.D.

Professor of Pathology, Cornell University Medical College; Attending Pathologist, Memorial Sloan-Kettering Cancer Center, New York, New York
Nonsquamous Lesions of Nasal Cavity, Paranasal Sinuses, and Nasopharynx

SILLOO B. KAPADIA, M.D.

Professor of Pathology and Surgery, Pennsylvania State University College of Medicine; Director of Surgical Pathology, Department of Anatomic Pathology, The Milton S. Hershey Medical Center, Hershey, Pennsylvania
Nonsquamous Pathology of the Larynx, Hypopharynx, and Trachea

MICHAEL KYRIAKOS, M.D.

Professor of Surgical Pathology, Washington University School of Medicine; Senior Surgical Pathologist, Barnes Hospital, St. Louis, Missouri
Soft Tissue and Bone Lesions

MARIO A. LUNA, M.D.

Professor of Pathology and Oral Pathology, University of Texas M.D. Anderson Cancer Center and Dental School; Pathologist, University of Texas M.D. Anderson Cancer Center, Houston, Texas
Cysts of the Neck, Unknown Primary Tumor, and Neck Dissection

L. JEFFREY MEDEIROS, M.D.

Professor of Pathology, University of Texas M.D. Anderson Cancer Center; Chief, Lymphoma Section, Department of Hematopathology, University of Texas M.D. Anderson Cancer Center, Houston, Texas
Hematopoietic Lesions

STEPHEN P. NABER, M.D., Ph.D.

Associate Professor of Pathology, Tufts University School of Medicine, Boston; Chief, Molecular Pathology and Genetics, Baystate Medical Center, Springfield, Massachusetts
Molecular Biology and Genetics of Head and Neck Tumors

BRAD W. NEVILLE, D.D.S.

Professor and Director, Division of Oral Pathology, Department of Stomatology, College of Dental Medicine, Medical University of South Carolina, Charleston, South Carolina
Odontogenic Cysts and Tumors

HIROMASA NIKAI, D.D.S., Ph.D.

Professor, Faculty of Dentistry, Hiroshima University, Hiroshima, Japan
Lesions of the Oral Cavity

BAYARDO PEREZ-ORDÓÑEZ, M.D.

Assistant Professor, Department of Pathobiology and Laboratory Medicine, University of Toronto; Director of Surgical Pathology, Sunnybrook and Women's College Health Sciences Center, Sunnybrook Site, Toronto, Ontario, Canada
Nonsquamous Lesions of Nasal Cavity, Paranasal Sinuses, and Nasopharynx

MADELEINE PFALTZ, M.D.

Staff Member and Staff Pathologist, Institute of Clinical Pathology, University of Zurich, Zurich, Switzerland
Cysts of the Neck, Unknown Primary Tumor, and Neck Dissection

MARY RICHARDSON, D.D.S., M.D.

Associate Professor of Pathology, Medical University of South Carolina, College of Medicine, Charleston, South Carolina
Squamous Cell Carcinoma of the Upper Aerodigestive System

WAEL A. SAKR, M.D.

Professor of Pathology and Oncology, Wayne State University School of Medicine and Carmanos Cancer Institute; Director of Anatomic Pathology, Harper Hospital, Detroit, Michigan
Squamous Intraepithelial Neoplasia of the Upper Aerodigestive Tract

PIETER J. SLOOTWEG, M.D., D.M.D., Ph.D.

Professor of Oral Pathology, Department of Pathology, University Medical Center Utrecht, Utrecht, Netherlands
Squamous Cell Carcinoma of the Upper Aerodigestive System

BARBARA J. WEINSTEIN, M.D.

Assistant Clinical Professor, Tufts University School of Medicine; Director of Cytology Laboratory, New England Medical Center, Boston, Massachusetts
Pathology of the Thyroid and Parathyroid Glands

MARK R. WICK, M.D.

Professor of Pathology, Associate Director of Surgical Pathology, University of Virginia School of Medicine; Staff Pathologist, University of Virginia Medical Center, Charlottesville, Virginia
Cutaneous Tumors and Pseudotumors of the Head and Neck

HUBERT J. WOLFE, M.D.

Professor of Pathology, Tufts University School of Medicine; Director, Molecular Pathology Laboratory, New England Medical Center, Boston, Massachusetts
Molecular Biology and Genetics of Head and Neck Tumors

Preface ■
■
■

It has been more than 10 years since the last comprehensive head and neck pathology textbook was published. During this period there have been many changes and advances in the field of head and neck pathology. The region of the head and neck is one of the most complex areas of the body from an anatomic and pathologic perspective, with a variety of different organ systems and tissue types within its domain.

My purpose is to provide a comprehensive textbook for the surgical pathologist, the otolaryngologist, and the head and neck or oral surgeon to use when diagnosing a difficult case or for anyone interested in reviewing head and neck pathology. Special emphasis is given to diagnostic surgical pathology and differential diagnosis. Straightforward, common lesions are covered in an appropriate fashion with greater emphasis given to more difficult problematic areas.

To minimize redundancy throughout the various chapters, I have elected to include the precancerous lesions from all mucosal sites in a single chapter, the mucosal squamous carcinomas in a single chapter, and the nonsquamous cancers and other lesions on a regional basis in individual chapters. Also, because of the increasing importance of staging information as part of the surgical pathology report, I have included the current head and neck tumor staging system in an appendix. In addition, there are separate chapters covering bone and soft tissue lesions and skin tumors that have a predilection for the head and neck. I have also reviewed lacrimal gland and sac lesions to better round out the text to make it more useful for the reader.

All photomicrographs are of hematoxylin-eosin stained glass slides except where otherwise indicated.

I would like to thank all the authors for their scholarly contributions. I also would like to thank Ms. Robin Kiernan for her excellent secretarial assistance; Dr. Irving Dardick for digitizing the color images; Drs. Hongwei Bai, Sally Chai, Li Juan Wang, and Monique DePaepe for help in translation; and Dr. Shamlal Mangray for help with proofreading. I would also like to express my appreciation for all the help and assistance that Cathy Carroll and Marc Strauss of W.B. Saunders have given me throughout this project. Lastly, I would especially like to thank my wife, Diane, and my sons, Ari and Ethan, for their understanding and support.

DOUGLAS R. GNEPP

Contents ■
■
■

Squamous Intraepithelial Neoplasia of the Upper Aerodigestive Tract

John D. Crissman and Wael A. Sakr

BACKGROUND AND SCOPE OF THE PROBLEM

The epidemiology, clinicopathologic classification, and natural history of squamous cell carcinoma of the upper aerodigestive tract (UADT) has been extensively investigated. These observations have led to better definitions of precursor and in situ neoplastic changes that have, in turn, contributed to a more comprehensive understanding of the etiologic factors and the pathobiology of the development of this common cancer. Although there is general agreement that epithelial precursors for invasive squamous cell carcinoma exist, agreement about diagnostic schema of classification has not been reached. The histologic definitions for dysplasia or squamous intraepithelial neoplasia (SIN) in UADT mucosa has not achieved consensus;[1, 2] for several reasons.

Historically, most patients with squamous neoplasia of the head and neck present during the invasive phase of the disease, often with advanced tumors and many with regional (and/or systemic) metastases. Accordingly, there are limited series of patients in which the histologic changes preceding squamous carcinoma have been sampled. The main bodies of literature documenting the progression of squamous mucosa precursors to invasive cancer are in the laryngeal glottis.[3, 4] The same observations in the oral cavity are described primarily in the oral pathology literature.[5–7] These two bodies of investigative literature have often used different terminology and histologic definitions.

The clinical terms used to describe lesions representing early neoplasia by oral surgeons, dentists, and otolaryngologists, such as *leukoplakia* and *erythroplakia,* have an imperfect correlation with the variety of histologic definitions associated with these gross mucosal appearances. The classic example is *leukoplakia,* a term used to describe white lesions in the oral cavity and, by some authors, in the larynx. This clinical, "gross" description, however, translates most often to a histologically benign, nondysplastic but hyperplastic squamous epithelium that is covered by a variably thick layer of keratin.[5–8] Conversely, the clinical observation of erythroplakia is invariably associated with a thin, nonkeratinizing epithelium that is characterized by loss of maturation and significant nuclear atypia.[9]

At the microscopic level, the criteria used to establish the diagnosis of squamous intraepithelial neoplasia in the upper aerodigestive tract have suffered from "extrapolating" of those histologic definitions learned from the long experience with intraepithelial neoplasia of the uterine cervix. Although both anatomic sites are primarily lined by squamous mucosa, the most common site of cancer development in the cervix is usually composed of metaplastic squamous mucosa. Clearly, dysplasia/SIN arising in metaplastic squamous epithelium does not have the propensity to contain or form cytoplasmic or surface keratin, which is the norm for dysplasia/SIN arising in normally keratinized mucosa. Dysplasia/SIN arising in the head and neck mucosa are invariably composed of epithelial hyperplasia, usually with prominent keratinization, a phenomenon that is uncommon in the uterine cervix.[10] Furthermore, numerous classification systems are proposed to characterize these early histologic changes in the UADT; more than 20 classifications can be found for such lesions in the larynx.[11] This complicates the comparison of gross and microscopic definitions in published series, making delineation of conclusions difficult.

Finally, the different anatomic regions within the UADT manifest wide variations in the thickness of the lining mucosa. The buccal mucosa, alveolar ridge, dorsal tongue, and laryngeal glottis all have thickened mucosa to provide mechanical protection from mastication, phonation and other normal activity. Sites such as the pharynx, palatine arch, floor of mouth, ventral tongue, and supraglottic larynx have a thin, more fragile squamous lining (Fig. 1–1). The response of these different areas of the epithelium to both carcinogenic and noncarcinogenic injuries results in alterations with variable gross appearances and histologic presentations. In general, the most common response to mucosal injury is cell proliferation or hyperplasia, often with development of surface keratinization (Fig. 1–2). However, carcinogenic influences can result in keratinizing hyperplasia without evidence of dysplasia/SIN. At this early phase, recognition of neoplastic transformation cannot be ascertained.

The etiologic factors associated with the development of invasive squamous cell carcinoma of the UADT include the use of tobacco, smokeless tobacco, and alcohol, which are the major known carcinogens associated with SIN in Western civilization.[12–15] During recent years, there has been increasing awareness of the importance of detecting squamous neoplasia during its preinvasive stages. Multiple studies have emphasized the beneficial effects of better coordination between dentists, general practitioners, and histopathologists regarding the recognition, early detection, and diagnosis of intraepithelial neoplasia, particularly of the oral cavity.[16, 17] In addition to the efforts aimed at characterizing the clinicopathologic profile of intraepithelial neoplasia, recent reports have focused on exploring the molecular events associated with the early neoplastic transformation. Detection of molecular abnormalities include immunohistochemical expression of mutated genes (i.e., *p53, k-ras,* and retinoblastoma gene), markers of proliferation and apoptosis, integrins, and other cell adhesion molecules.[18–20] Recently there has been increasing interest in measuring dysplasia/SIN using biologic markers in an attempt to quantitate the progression (and potential reversal) of the neoplastic intraepithelial changes by cessation of carcinogens (smoking and alcohol) and by exploring the potential chemopreventive effects of agents such as vitamin compounds, retinoic acid, and fenretinide.[21, 22]

The purpose of this review is to summarize the pertinent studies and observations dealing with the diagnostic criteria and the natural history of squamous intraepithelial neoplasia of the UADT and incorporate them in the framework of the authors' experiences. Although the morphologic criteria of dysplasia/SIN and the detailed microscopic parameters by which this lesion is evaluated are common to different locations of the UADT, we have attempted to follow the somewhat arbitrary "anatomical" divisions of the head and neck region, addressing (1) the nasal cavity, paranasal sinuses, and nasopharynx; (2) the oral cavity; and (3) the larynx. The detailed morphologic description of preinvasive neoplasia (dysplasia/SIN) of the oral cavity and the larynx and their clinical correlation and pertinent marker studies are addressed jointly at the end of the chapter. Finally, we have adopted an approach to the grading of squamous intraepithelial neoplasia that classifies the lesion into low-grade and

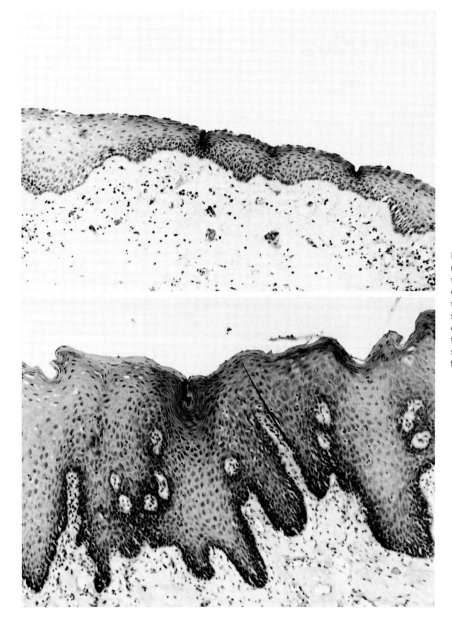

Figure 1–1. Squamous epithelium within the "normal" morphologic range. The thickness of the squamous epithelial lining of the upper aerodigestive tract differs according to the anatomic region. Marked variations in the number of the cell layers exist depending on the source of the biopsy (floor of mouth [top], or dorsum of the tongue [bottom]). In both samples, the architectural and cytologic features of maturation are preserved. A thin layer of acellular keratin covers the surface.

high-grade categories. This is somewhat different from the three-grade system previously used by the authors and other investigators. We believe a two-grade classification is a more reproducible system. The reduction of the grading system to two categories may help in better stratifying patients for clinical protocols, chemoprevention trials, and follow-up studies. This is also in accordance with the changing philosophy of simplifying the grading schema used for intraepithelial neoplasia in other organ systems (e.g., uterine cervix, prostate).[23, 24]

NOSE, PARANASAL SINUSES, AND NASOPHARYNX

Clinical and Epidemiologic Aspects

The literature dealing with histologic definitions of preinvasive neoplasia of the upper respiratory portion of the UADT is extremely limited. The few studies that address intraepithelial neoplasia in the nasopharynx are in association with invasive carcinoma. Most of the interest in preinvasive and invasive carcinomas have focused on investigating "molecular" or immunohistochemical alterations of the spectrum of neoplasia. Examples of intraepithelial neoplasia can be found in reports investigating the role of Epstein-Barr virus or other molecular changes in nasopharyngeal carcinoma. These studies have, for the most part, investigated markers in the "dysplastic" epithelium adjacent to invasive carcinoma.[25–27]

Exposure to wood manufacturing products and adenocarcinoma of the nasal cavity and paranasal sinuses has been well documented.[28] However, identification of precursor mucosal changes is not documented for woodworkers. The spectrum of hyperplastic, metaplastic, and neoplastic changes within the nasal epithelial lining has been well described in workers exposed to nickel fumes.[29] In a longitudinal study designed to investigate the effects of reduced exposure to nickel fumes on nasal mucosal alterations, Boysen et al.[29] reported a reduction in dysplasia in workers who had lowered their exposure to nickel over the study period. Sinonasal papillomas, primarily inverted papilloma, can harbor areas of dysplasia/neoplasia. Barnes and Bedetti[30] reported dysplasia and carcinoma in situ in 6% and 3%, respectively, in a series of 61 inverted papillomas. It is conceivable that these preinvasive changes are the precursors of the invasive squamous cell carcinoma reported to be discovered in 4% to

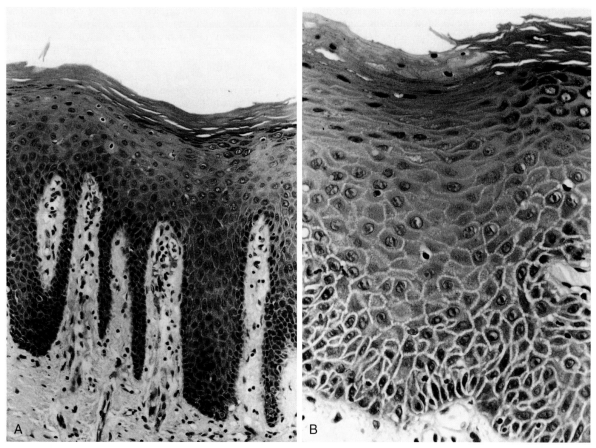

Figure 1–2. Squamous epithelial hyperplasia without squamous intraepithelial neoplasia (SIN) and keratinizing squamous epithelium without SIN. *A,* Moderately thickened epithelium with elongated and focally anastomosing rete ridges (pseudoepitheliomatous pattern). The maturation is maintained without nuclear atypia or abnormal keratinization. The surface is covered by a layer of acellular keratin *(left). B,* Higher magnification of benign, keratinizing squamous epithelium showing expansion of the parabasal cell layer with normal maturation and preserved nuclear orientation. There is surface keratinization with a layer of parakeratotic cells and acellular keratin *(right).*

6% of cases of resected papillomas.[31] In general, dysplastic changes are diagnosed using criteria similar to those used for other squamous mucosa.

Morphologic Features and Differential Diagnosis

The gross appearance of intraepithelial neoplasia in the nasopharynx is that of a "bulging" or thickened mucosa that is usually adjacent to the mass of invasive malignancy. Pathmanathan et al.[32] reported 11 cases of isolated dysplasia or carcinoma in situ originating from the nasopharynx from a pool of 1811 patients (0.6%). In this study, designed primarily to investigate the role of the Epstein-Barr virus in the pathogenesis of nasopharyngeal carcinoma, the authors described isolated preinvasive mucosal changes in a small fraction of cases identified via a large screening program. The alterations were described as thickened epithelium with loss of normal stratification and nuclear pleomorphism. These mucosal changes involve the full thickness of the nonkeratinizing surface epithelium. The dysplastic changes can also result in "thinned" epithelium with few cell layers, which exhibit both architectural and cytologic abnormalities similar to erythroplasia in the oral cavity.

Molecular and Biomarker Studies

Sheu et al.[33] studied the immunohistochemical expression of *p53* and *bcl-2* in normal, inflamed, dysplastic, and invasive nasopharyn-

geal carcinoma. The authors reported that 80% of dysplastic epithelium adjacent to invasive nasopharyngeal carcinoma had detectable expression of *p53* protein. They also found overexpression of *p53* and increased expression of *bcl-2* in the dysplastic epithelium. Both this study and the previously mentioned report by Pathmanathan et al.[32] have indirectly implicated dysplastic epithelium as the precursor of invasive carcinoma in the nasopharynx by virtue of the intermediate position it occupied between normal mucosa and invasive carcinoma. In addition, the expression of the viral genome *p53* and *bcl-2* molecular markers in these areas of transition from normal to dysplastic to invasive cancer argue for these intermediate preinvasive mucosal changes leading to invasive carcinoma.

ORAL CAVITY

Clinical and Epidemiologic Aspects

There is extensive literature dealing with the spectrum of early neoplastic changes in the mucosa of the oral cavity.[34] As previously mentioned, two major types of intraepithelial neoplastic changes are found in the oral cavity: thin erythroplakic mucosa with dysplasia/SIN and keratinizing hyperplastic (leukoplakic) mucosa that may or may not have the histologic changes of dysplasia/SIN. In spite of a resurgence of interest in the early detection and the potential for reversal of preinvasive changes by chemoprevention, there are persisting difficulties in terms of reproducibility of diagnoses, especially for hyperplastic keratinizing epithelium with minimal evidence of maturation abnormalities on histologic examination. These discrepancies are due to variability in the terminology and diagnostic criteria, especially in the keratinizing hyperplastic mucosal lesions. Unfortunately, few studies have addressed the prevalence of oral cavity dysplasia/SIN with documented histologic confirmation.[35] Only a fraction of the gross mucosal changes of white or leukoplakic mucosal appearance will contain histologic changes of dysplasia/SIN.[34, 35] These observations are confirmed by several studies originating from different geographic areas where tobacco consumption is prevalent.[36] Studies of clinical leukoplakia reported a wide range of prevalence in the study populations and varied from 0.6% to 10%, of which 0.2% to 1% were reported to harbor dysplasia/SIN on histologic examination.[35, 36] The overlapping and variable terminology makes drawing conclusions from these studies difficult. Most studies were able to establish a higher prevalence of a variety of white oral lesions with the use of tobacco, smokeless tobacco, and alcohol. Recognizing the need to address these issues of terminology and histologic definition, a symposium dealing with the detection, clinical staging, and histologic definition of oral leukoplakia was held in 1994.[36] The results of the consensus conference are integrated into the following discussion.

Morphologic Features and Differential Diagnosis

Gross Mucosal Changes of Injury

Two major mucosal alterations occur in response to carcinogenic exposures of the UADT: (1) thickened keratotic hyperplastic mucosa with a dull or whitish gross appearance (clinical leukoplakia) (Fig. 1–3), and (2) thin, friable atrophic mucosa with a red gross appearance (clinical erythroplakia) (Fig. 1–4).

Leukoplakia

Leukoplakia is a clinical term used to describe a white-appearing mucosal change that usually occurs in response to some form of injury.[2] Leukoplakia *IS NOT* a histologic term and its use as a specific histopathologic entity is discouraged. Nevertheless, the clinical leukoplakia appearance results from an injury inducing hyperplasia, usually with prominent surface keratinization.[34, 37–40] These thick hyperplastic lesions can develop in response to injury, including by carcinogens, and the resulting hyperplasia is occasionally accompanied by cytologic atypia and epithelial changes of dysplasia.[38, 41] Because surface keratin formation associated with hyperplasia progresses to invasive cancer more often when dysplasia/SIN is present, these histologic terms need careful definition.[42]

Thick white squamous mucosal patches are more common on the buccal mucosa, alveolar ridge, and dorsal tongue.[42, 43] Leukoplakic changes occurring in this mucosa may be the result of numerous types of injuries and can be associated with dysplasia/SIN.[41, 44] Leukoplakic mucosal changes found in the normally thin mucosa of the ventral tongue, tonsil, retromolar trigone, and hypopharynx are usually the result of carcinogenic exposure and should be viewed with heightened suspicion for harboring dysplasia/SIN.[36, 42] When all etiologies suspected to cause gross appearance of leukoplakia are considered, the prevalence of those caused by carcinogens becomes exceedingly high at approximately 25%, whereas the prevalence of leukoplakia attributed to tobacco use only was estimated to be 4.3%.[36]

Erythroplakia

Erythroplakia is also a lesion with a distinct gross appearance; it presents as a red, hyperemic-appearing mucosal surface with variably distinct borders.[45, 46] This alteration invariably represents the result of UADT carcinogens, typically resulting from the effects of tobacco or alcohol, or both. Erythroplakia is most commonly observed in thin squamous mucosa such as is found in the ventral tongue, floor of mouth, palatine arch, and retromolar trigone.[45, 46]

Erythroplakia is characterized by a thin or atrophic mucosa, usually with little or no histologic evidence of epithelial maturation, typically underlined by a richly vascular, often inflamed, lamina propria. The thin mucosa is usually composed of atypical cells without significant keratinization, resulting in weakened epithelial surface integrity and a propensity for mechanical trauma.

The overwhelming majority of clinical erythroplakic mucosal changes have histologic alterations of high grade or severe dysplasia/SIN high grade.[45, 46] The histologic changes of dysplasia/SIN in these thin mucosa are similar to those described in the "classic" dysplasia/carcinoma in situ (CIS) sequence of the uterine cervix. Not surprising is the frequent observation of concurrent invasive carcinoma in surgical specimens from mucosa with the clinical appearance of erythroplakia.[45, 46]

Speckled Mucosa

After the recognition that essentially all erythroplakia and some leukoplakia represent intraepithelial neoplasia, commonly severe in the former and variable in the latter, the observation that admixtures of the two can co-exist was made (Fig. 1–5).[45] These "combined" mucosal changes were commonly referred to as "speckled" lesions and, in our opinion, were classified under leukoplakia in the older literature because of the predominantly whitish appearance.[47] It is important to recognize that clinical erythroplakia is invariably associated with the histologic changes of severe dysplasia/CIS, and that "speckled lesions" have a prognosis more akin to their most ominous erythroplakic component. Accordingly, speckled lesions behave in a similar manner to pure erythroplakic mucosal alterations. The observation that many of the speckled leukoplakias may have been classified as a leukoplakia may explain why some observers in the past found such a high frequency of subsequent carcinoma in what was erroneously classified as pure leukoplakia. The frequency with which clinical leukoplakia becomes neoplastic varies greatly depending on the study population (Table 1–1), but a fivefold higher risk of neoplastic development has been calculated to be conservative. Causative agents include carcinogens such as tobacco and alcohol, friction on the mucosal surface, and microscopic organisms such as *Candida albicans*.[47] It was recently proposed that the term *leukoplakia* be restricted in use to nondefinable lesions that are not premalignant in nature,[36] as has been done in this discourse. Lesions that are easily definable and therefore not discussed herein include tobacco-induced white lesions (although some may subsequently develop into cancerous lesions) with the exception of those found in reverse-smokers; hairy leukoplakias, now referred to as Greenspan lesions; and *Candida*-associated lesions that respond to treatment.

Leukoplakias have been shown to be accompanied by cytologic atypia and epithelial changes of dysplasia.[38, 41] Because surface keratin formation associated with hyperplasia progresses to invasive cancer more often when dysplasia/SIN is present, these histologic terms need careful definition.[42] Some have also argued that dysplasia be graded, as moderate to severe dysplasia progresses to cancer more often than does mild dysplasia.[47] Dysplasia/SIN can be associated with leukoplakic changes in the oral mucosa, alveolar ridge, and dorsal tongue,[41, 44] where the thick white squamous mucosa patches are more common[42, 43] and may be the result of numerous

Text continued on page 10

Table 1–1. Frequency of Subsequent Carcinoma in Oral Leukoplakia

Mucosal Alteration and Reference	Percent of Patients Progressing to Carcinoma
Leukoplakia	
Gupta et al.[65]	3%
Silverman et al.[43]	6%
Shibuya et al.[62]	17%

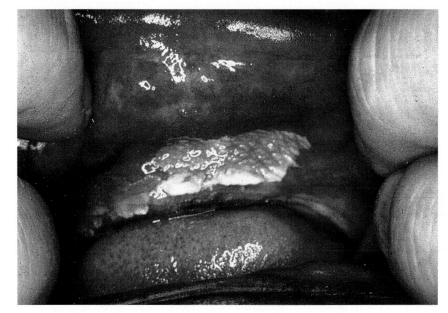

Figure 1–3. Leukoplakia. This term should not be used as a histologic or microscopic diagnosis. Clinically, it characterizes a mucosal surface with a white, keratotic appearance translating most often to a hyperplastic, histologically benign mucosa—that is, without squamous intraepithelial neoplasia.

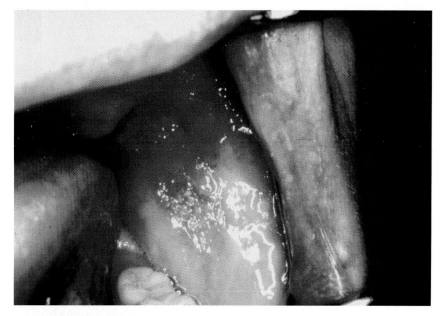

Figure 1–4. Erythroplakia. Characteristically thinned, severely reddened and congested mucosal surface with variably defined borders.

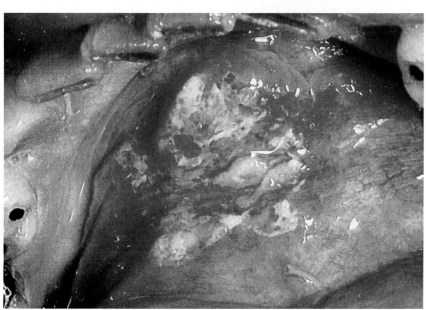

Figure 1–5. Speckled lesions. Variable combinations of a red mucosal surface and a white keratotic appearance, often with ill-defined borders between the two components.

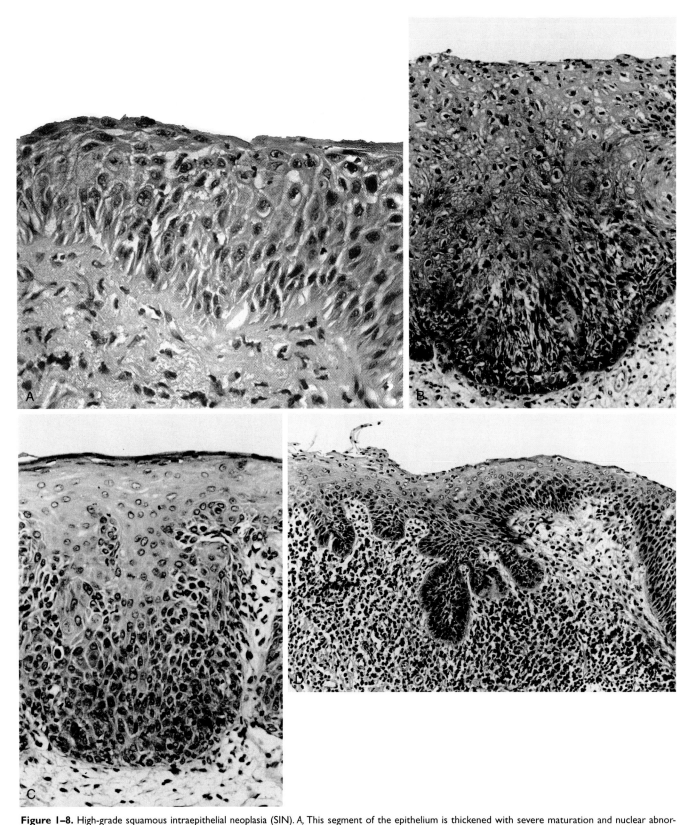

Figure 1–8. High-grade squamous intraepithelial neoplasia (SIN). A, This segment of the epithelium is thickened with severe maturation and nuclear abnormalities qualifying for a diagnosis of high-grade SIN. Although there is no evidence of surface keratinization (no layer of acellular keratin), the top layers of the epithelium show cellular (intracytoplasmic) keratinization. B, A more elaborate cellular keratinization is evident in this biopsy sample. There is no surface keratinization, but the upper two thirds of the lining is composed of atypical, large cells with abundant intracytoplasmic keratinization. C, The significant architectural and nuclear abnormalities are limited to the lower half of the epithelium. There is a combination of surface keratinization with thin-layer parakeratosis and intracytoplasmic keratinization in the upper layers of the lining. D, This segment of squamous epithelium is of variable thickness but with similar, severe architectural and nuclear abnormalities evident in the lower half of the lining. There is a combination of surface and intracytoplasmic keratinization.

Figures 1–9 through 1–11. Keratinizing squamous epithelium from gross lesions of leukoplakia. The spectrum of microscopic changes of tissue samples from lesions characterized clinically as leukoplakia is wide ranging, from benign squamous epithelium to high-grade squamous intraepithelial neoplasia and in situ squamous cell carcinoma.

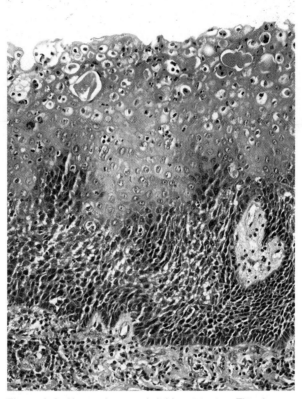

Figure 1–9. Abnormal intraepithelial keratinization. This phenomenon is an indication of altered maturation and signifies neoplastic transformation. This photomicrograph illustrates diffuse keratinization with large cells containing abundant intracytoplasmic keratin.

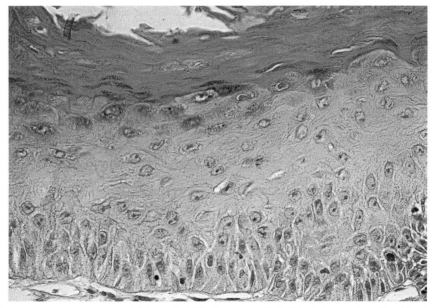

Figure 1–10. Low-grade keratinizing squamous intraepithelial neoplasia. The lower one third of the lining contains cells with enlarged, atypical nuclei and occasional mitotic figures. The upper layers of the lining show normal maturation and are covered by a layer of keratin and parakeratotic cells.

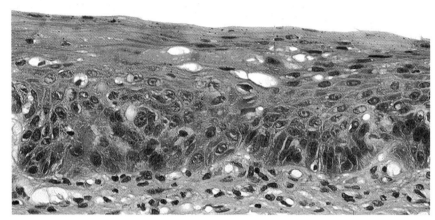

Figure 1–11. High-grade keratinizing squamous intraepithelial neoplasia (SIN). The extent of cytologic abnormalities is more pronounced with significant nuclear pleomorphism and anaplasia. As emphasized in the text, the diagnosis of keratinizing high-grade SIN does not require full-thickness cytologic changes.

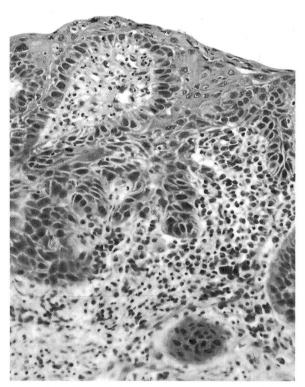

Figure 1–12. High-grade keratinizing squamous intraepithelial neoplasia (SIN). Full-thickness abnormal architectural and cytologic changes of SIN can be associated with surface keratinization. The changes illustrated in this photomicrograph qualify for keratinizing high-grade SIN and can be encountered as a component of speckled mucosa.

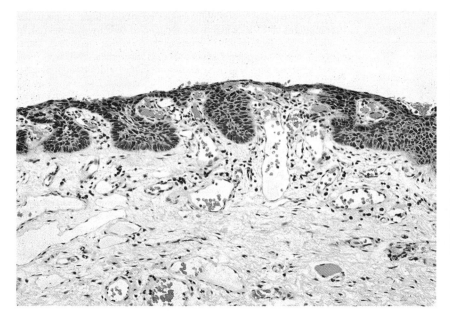

Figure 1–13. High-grade nonkeratinizing squamous intraepithelia neoplasia (SIN). Severe dysplastic mucosal changes of nonkeratinizing high-grade SIN usually involve a thinned lining. The few cell layers of this biopsy sample show architectural and cytologic changes typical of SIN III or in situ squamous cell carcinoma. This is the typical microscopic finding of the clinical erythroplakia pictured in Figure 1–4. The rich vascularity in the lamina propria accounts for the red appearance. The microscopic changes of nonkeratinizing SIN correlate with a gross or clinical appearance of an erythroplakic or a speckled mucosa. The criteria used to diagnose and grade this form of SIN are similar to those applied in the uterine cervix, by assessing the proportional thickness of the architectural and cytologic changes of dysplasia.

Figure 1–14. High-grade squamous intraepithelial neoplasia. This biopsy sample shows full-thickness architectural change with loss of normal maturation and disarray of orientation. Cytologically, nuclear enlargement, pleomorphism, anaplasia, and increased mitotic activity are all evident. The segment of the lining with a more pronounced surface keratin correlates with the white mucosal change as shown in Figure 1–5.

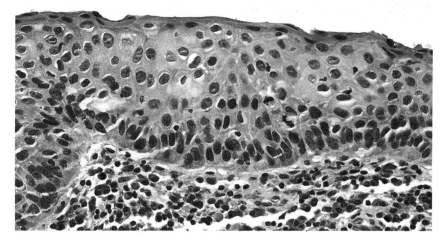

Table 1–2. Risk Factors Associated with Malignant Transformation of Leukoplakia

1. Long duration of leukoplakia
2. Gender (women are at greater risk than men)
3. Idiopathic leukoplakia (i.e., occurring in nonsmokers)
4. Presence of epithelial dysplasia
5. Location on the tongue or the floor of the mouth
6. Presence of *Candida albicans*
7. Nonhomogeneous leukoplakia defined as a white and red lesion (herein included in the class speckled mucosa)

types of injury. Leukoplakic mucosal changes found in the normally thin mucosa of the ventral tongue, tonsil, retromolar trigone, and hypopharynx are usually the result of carcinogenic exposure and should be viewed with heightened suspicion of harboring dysplasia/SIN.[36, 42] Risk factors for the progression of leukoplakia, including dysplasia, are listed in Table 1–2.

Leukoplakia has been categorized by some as either homogeneous or nonhomogeneous. Homogeneous leukoplakia is a large category and includes leukoplakic lesions that are thin, uniformly flat in appearance, of constant texture, and of a predominantly white color. The surface of such a lesion may be smooth, corrugated, or wrinkled. Dysplasia is usually not evident in homogeneous leukoplakias, and progression to malignancy is rare. Nonhomogeneous leukoplakias, which often cause mild localized discomfort, may have mixed color and texture. White and red nonhomogeneous leukoplakias are considered to be speckled mucosa in this treatise and are discussed subsequently. Textures may be considered papillary, exophytic, or verrucous in nature. A particular form of oral leukoplakia recently termed *proliferative verrucous leukoplakia* (PVL) has been shown to have a higher tendency to progress to squamous cell carcinoma.[48–52] The most common sites of occurrence for PVL are the buccal mucosa (63%), gingiva (56%), and tongue (47%) in females and the tongue (82%) and gingiva (45%) in males.[48] The lesion is more prevalent in females (ratio of 4 : 1). Only 31% of patients had a history of tobacco use.[48] This aggressive form often starts as a unifocal lesion, predominantly in mandibular or alveolar locations and buccal mucosa, with gross appearance of a warty, somewhat papillary surface. The lesion tends to rapidly become multifocal with a propensity to harbor significant degrees of dysplastic epithelial alterations. Silverman and Gorsky[5] studied 54 patients with PVL, 17 of whom were included in the original report by Hansen et al.[52] Seventy percent of patients developed carcinoma (mean 7.7 years from initial diagnosis, range 1–27 years); a second malignancy developed in another PVL site in 31.5% of the cases. In the original report by Hansen et al.,[52] 87% of their 30 patients developed squamous cell carcinoma within a follow-up period that extended to 20 years in some patients. More than 40% of this cohort died of their tumors.[52] If these data are combined with data from Silverman and Gorsky's series, the PVL-associated deaths is 50%.[48] This entity is often diagnosed retrospectively as the lesions are found to persist, become more numerous, and resist treatment.

Patients who are later diagnosed with PVL may present with hyperkeratosis and leukoplakic lesions described as homogeneous in nature. Over time, the lesions become exophytic and wartlike and begin to appear nodular. Erythematous regions also begin to emerge in the white plaques. Dysplasia often occurs late in the progression of this disease, placing importance on the treatment of hyperplastic lesions. With progression, additional white lesions, often bilateral, appear in PVL patients. Regional lymph node involvement and metastases may also be a late feature of PVL progression in patients developing squamous carcinoma. These patients should be treated with an aggressive surgical approach; adding radiation has offered no additional survival benefit.[48] Recently, Brennan et al.[53] showed that leukoplakia that have *p53* mutations in cells near the surgical margin have a greater risk of localized recurrence than those that do not harbor mutations of this tumor suppressor gene.

Hansen et al.[52] originally suggested 10 histologic stages in the continuum of PVL, which were reduced to four by Suarez et al.[49]: clinical flat leukoplakia, verrucous hyperplasia, verrucous carcinoma, and conventional squamous cell carcinoma. PVL may have any of these stages as well as intermediates and any combination during its course.

Treatment of PVL has proven complicated, primarily owing to its propensity to recur at the treatment site and spread to additional areas in the oral cavity. Surgical excision, carbon dioxide laser treatment, cryosurgery, chemotherapy, and photodynamic therapy have all been used to treat PVL. Zakrzewska et al.[51] have shown that the lowest recurrence rates were found with photodynamic therapy. This modality, however, is a recent addition to the battery of weapons used by the oncologist, and follow-up times for patients undergoing this treatment are shorter than those for other modalities. Thus, additional studies with longer periods of follow-up will determine the true usefulness of this method of treatment. In all cases, rigorous follow-up is required for PVL patients with the continued biopsy of both old and new lesions. In many cases, several rounds of treatment may be required to contain the disease, although no treatments have proven effective curatively.

Verrucous hyperplasia, on the other hand, originally termed oral florid papillomatosis,[50] is a diagnosis that should be used only following microscopic evaluation. In addition to the oral cavity where it is most frequently seen, this lesion could be encountered in the sinuses, where it may be associated with scheiderian papillomas that show evidence of keratinization, and in the larynx.[49] This lesion was first described by Shear and Pindborg in 1980.[50] It is slightly more common in females and is most frequently found in the sixth to eighth decades. The gingival and alveolar mucosa are the most frequent sites of involvement, followed, in decreasing order, by buccal mucosa, tongue, floor of mouth, lip, and palate.[49] In Shear and Pindborg's initial report, 53% of patients had an associated leukoplakia. In 29% of patients there was an associated verrucous carcinoma, in 66% of patients there was epithelial dysplasia, and in 10% of patients there was typical squamous cell carcinoma.[49, 50] The major differential diagnosis is with verrucous carcinoma, as both lesions exhibit florid papillary and verrucoid growth, and some authors consider verrucous hyperplasia to represent a precursor of verrucous carcinoma. Suarez et al.[49] emphasize the exophytic growth pattern of verrucous hyperplasia contrasted to that of the downward invasive growth exhibited by verrucous carcinoma. This differential clearly requires careful gross and microscopic correlation.

Clinicopathologic Correlation

The recognition that these two major types of squamous mucosal response to injury represent two ends of a spectrum of gross and histologic appearance is an important step in understanding intraepithelial neoplasia. The major problem in developing a balanced set of rules to diagnosing dysplasia/SIN of the UADT is that many examples combine features from both ends of the diagnostic spectrum. The most common mucosal reaction to any type of injury is characterized by epithelial proliferation and hyperkeratosis (clinical leukoplakia). This process may or may not be in response to carcinogenic injury. The frequency of clinical leukoplakia becoming neoplastic varies greatly. Establishing neoplasia is greatly dependent on the presence (or absence) of cellular atypia that reflect "genetic" changes, which can now be documented using a wide range of recently described molecular techniques. These observations regarding clinical mucosal appearance, their histologic correlates, and their clinical course are critical to our understanding of intraepithelial neoplasia and the progression to invasive carcinoma.

The observation that persisting erythroplakic or speckled mucosa is commonly associated with dysplasia/SIN is also critical in understanding the spectrum of SIN occurring with UADT. This typical erythroplakic-appearing mucosa invariably has a paucity (or absence) of surface maturation and a prominence of "uncommitted" basal-like cells with nuclear pleomorphism constituting the full thickness of the thin epithelium. Erythroplakic change is ominous and almost always represents high-grade SIN. In contrast, leukoplakia may or may not represent irreversible neoplastic injury. Neoplastic change can only be absolutely confirmed by the histologic changes of dysplasia/SIN.

LARYNX AND HYPOPHARYNX

Clinical and Epidemiologic Aspects

The normal histology of squamous mucosa lining the larynx, pyriform sinus, and hypopharynx vary in degrees of normal thickness, similar to the oral cavity. However, only the laryngeal glottis has a thick epithelium with surface keratinization. The remaining mucosa of the supraglottic larynx, adjacent pyriform sinus, and hypopharynx are thin with little or no surface keratinization. The common explanation for the thicker keratinized epithelium of the glottis is to protect the mucosa because of the mechanical trauma of phonation. The laryngeal glottis is the most common site for the development of squamous cancer for this anatomic region.

The major carcinogens affecting the larynx and associated mucosal structures are cigarette smoke and alcohol.[12] Use of oral tobacco has not been incriminated as a cause of squamous cancer in the larynx. Nutrition becomes an important element in the development of squamous and other cancers, primarily as a preventative component. Poor nutrition appears to result in a susceptibility to develop cancers.[15]

The role of cigarette smoke is well recognized as a causative agent in the etiology of laryngeal cancers, especially of the glottis.[54] However, the amount of alcohol ingestion also correlates with the development of squamous cancer in both the supraglottic larynx and the glottis.[55] The relative contribution of alcohol and tobacco in the development of laryngeal cancers is more than additive as the two carcinogens appear to potentiate each other in a multiplicative manner.[56]

Morphologic Features and Differential Diagnosis

In the literature, the mucosal appearances, by the clinical observation, of the larynx are not as well documented as they are in the oral cavity. Although both red and white mucosal alterations are recognized by laryngologists as abnormal, consensus as to their relative importance has not been achieved. Part of the summary of Workshop No. 2 of the Centennial Conference of Laryngeal Cancer includes the following: "The pathologists insisted in the majority that the appearance of a reddish, edematous, sometimes granular lesion is most character-

istic of pure CIS. However, all of the laryngologists insisted that more often than not, this type of base for CIS had a whitish or keratotic covering, either thick, punctate, thin, or even friable."[2]

Laryngologists use the term *keratosis* for thick white mucosal plaques, and *red* for the thin erythematous-appearing epithelial changes.[57, 58] The term *keratosis with and without atypia* has historical support and has been used for a number of years.[57] Keratosis usually refers to hyperplasia with prominent surface keratinization. It is the authors' impression that most glottic mucosal changes are of the keratinizing hyperplasia variety and are analogous to oral "leukoplakia with atypia." The presence of epithelial dysplasia/SIN is relatively uncommon in this anatomic site but represents the epithelial changes most likely to progress to invasive cancer.[60] Red thin mucosal alterations of the true cords are rare and correlate with the exceedingly rare "classic" CIS of the true cord. However, thin reddish changes occur in the supraglottis and adjacent mucosa with a speckled pattern or with white thickened plaques and are invariably associated with dysplasia/SIN/invasive carcinoma on biopsy and histologic examination.

Clinicopathologic Studies

In general, a review of the literature reveals numerous terms for what are interpreted as similar approaches for the grading of dysplasia/SIN.[57, 58, 60] We feel, as do others,[59] that the minor variations between keratosis without atypia and keratosis with mild atypia are difficult to separate with reproducible certainty and are likely to represent neoplastic transformation and should be viewed as a single entity. Although the subclassification of epithelial dysplasia/SIN of the UADT into histologic grades analogous to other organ systems has not been well defined, there is a growing body of evidence demonstrating that various grading systems have biologic significance in predicting the probability of progression.[60] One of the first classification systems was reported by Kleinsasser, who separated abnormal laryngeal biopsies into three subgroups:[61]

Grade 1, or simple hyperplasia, consists of hyperplasia with normal cell maturation. Only a small number of patients with this biopsy interpretation progress to invasive cancer.

Grade 2 represents a "small group" of biopsies that show atypical nuclei and disturbances of differentiation. For these patients, observation is recommended.

Grade 3, or precancerous epithelium, is referred to as carcinoma in situ by some pathologists. The epithelium contains all the changes observed in squamous cancer except invasion.

The division of the continuous spectrum of histopathologic alterations defining squamous intraepithelial neoplasia is, at best, arbi-

Table I–3. Frequency of Progression to Invasive Squamous Carcinoma in the Larynx

Progression to Invasive Cancer	Total Number of Patients	Number Progressing	Percent	Reference
Keratosis without atypia or with minor atypia	362	5	1.4	60*
	808	33	4.1	59
	98	2	2.0	57
Total	**1268**	**40**	**3.2**	
Keratosis with moderate atypia	230	31	13.5	60*
	23	4	17.4	59
	24	3	12.5	57
Total	**277**	**38**	**13.7**	
Keratosis with severe atypia/carcinoma in situ	367	42	11.4	60*
	90	25	27.8	59
	39	9	23.1	57
Total	**496**	**76**	**15.3**	

*This data was compiled from references 67–75 as cited in reference 60.

Table 1–4. Frequency of Subsequent Carcinoma in Laryngeal Keratosis

Reference	Number of Patients	Number Progressing to Carcinoma (%)
McGavran, Bauer, & Ogura[72]	84	3 (3.57)
Gabiel & Jones[66]	30	1 (3.33)
Norris & Peale[74]	116	5 (4.31)
Total	230	9 (3.90)

trary. Review of the literature supports this position (Table 1–3).[57, 59–61, 63–75] With 1268 biopsies interpreted as keratosis without atypia or with mild atypia, 40 cases (3.2%) progressed to invasive squamous carcinoma. These observations are derived from a diverse group of studies, many of which are primarily clinically oriented, many with less than stringent histopathologic definitions. Nevertheless, the 3.2% is remarkably similar to the results of several smaller series with careful pathology review, resulting in a low frequency of progression to invasive cancer for these keratinizing hyperplastic epithelial alterations with little or no dysplasia/SIN (Table 1–4).[58, 72, 74]

The summary data from Table 1–3 reviewing the pertinent literature contain very few biopsies graded as moderate atypia, and those classified as such have a frequency of progression to invasive carcinoma of 13.7%. This figure is not significantly different from the 15.3% reported for biopsies classified as severe atypia/CIS. We know that the "classic" atrophic forms of severe dysplasia/CIS are a relatively rare adjunct to invasive carcinomas or an isolated event.[76] Our interpretation of these seemingly anomalous observations is that the small group of intermediate SIN II (keratosis with moderate atypia) were biopsies with some nuclear/cytoplasmic alterations but with prominent surface or epithelial keratinization and, as a result, were "undergraded."[77] Although the frequency of DNA aneuploidy and, more importantly, the rate of progression to invasive cancer are similar for those "intermediate" lesions and high-grade SIN, the former group are commonly downgraded into a lower grade of dysplasia/SIN.[61, 67, 78, 79] This would account for the similar frequency of progression to invasive carcinoma between the historical groups of "intermediate SIN" and high-grade SIN categories (see Table 1–3). This observation is confirmed in the excellent study of Hellquist[77] in which the dysplasia he called "well differentiated" had

the highest rate of progression to invasive squamous cancer. His examples of this well-differentiated group of SIN demonstrate extensive cytoplasmic keratinization at all levels in the epithelium with little if any nuclear pleomorphism. In our experience, this lesion, characterized by extensive epithelial keratinization, is often "undergraded" and represents an epithelial dysplasia with a high frequency of progression to invasive carcinoma.

The second important prognostic observation reported by Hellquist et al.[67] was that keratosis/SIN that persisted or recurred was ominous, an observation not commonly stressed in the clinical or pathology literature. A high-grade dysplasia/SIN is usually characterized by proliferation of immature cells in the lower and middle layers and a degree of superficial keratinization. This morphologic profile is recognized by most experienced pathologists as a prominent feature of high-grade SIN but is "undergraded" by some observers and placed in lower grade SIN because of the evidence of maturation as reflected by surface keratinization. Unfortunately, many of the "clinicopathologic" studies include pathology descriptions with little or no detail of the histologic criteria for classification of the epithelial alterations.

CLASSIFICATION OF INTRAEPITHELIAL NEOPLASIA

The histologic changes representing dysplasia/SIN in the UADT encompass a continuum with two distinct appearances at the two opposite ends of this spectrum:

1. Hyperplastic squamous mucosa with prominent surface keratinization (leukoplakic appearance); these lesions have a rate of progression to a higher grade of dysplasia/SIN or invasive carcinoma proportional to the degree of "cytoplasmic and nuclear atypia." One form of cytologic atypia not usually stressed as abnormal is the presence of premature keratinization (Fig. 1–6), which is characterized by prominent cytoplasmic keratin formation in the lower or middle portions of the epithelium, either as focal (pearls) or diffuse cytoplasmic keratinization. A classification scheme defining grades of keratinizing dysplasia has been found predictive of the risk for persisting dysplasia/SIN and/or subsequent invasive cancer.

2. Thin or atrophic squamous mucosa with little or no cellular maturation and prominent "nuclear atypia" (erythroplakic appearance) invariably have a histologic diagnosis of the "classic" form of severe dysplasia/CIS as originally described in the uterine cervix. This "classic" form of intraepithelial neoplasia is uniformly recog-

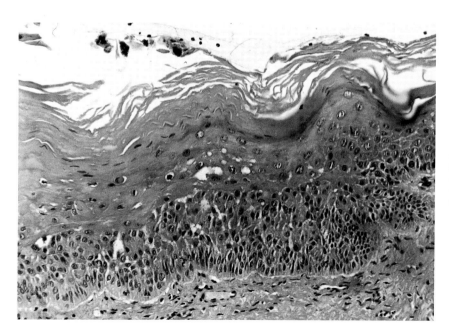

Figure 1–6. High-grade keratinizing squamous intraepithelial neoplasia (SIN). The epithelium is thickened and shows nuclear crowding and atypia in the lower one half to one third of the lining. Despite some evidence of maturation in the upper layers, the changes in this segment qualify for high-grade SIN.

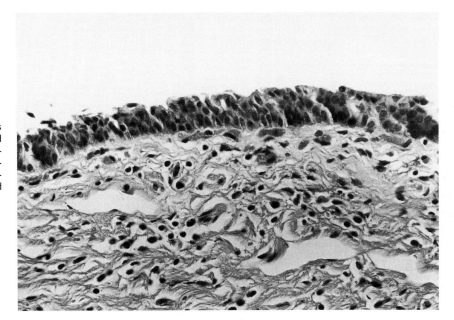

Figure 1–7. High-grade nonkeratinizing squamous intraepithelial neoplasia. The lining mucosa is thinned and limited to a few layers of highly atypical "immature" cells that persist to the top layer of the epithelium with no evidence of cellular or surface keratinization. The underlying lamina propria is inflamed and richly vascularized.

nized by the pathology community and has a high rate of transformation or progression to invasive cancer (Fig. 1–7).

Defining the histologic criteria for intraepithelial neoplasia remains relatively straightforward for the two ends of this histologic spectrum but is problematic when overlapping features of these extremes coexist. The two ends of the spectrum described in the previous section, atrophic dysplasia/SIN and hyperplastic keratinizing dysplasia/SIN, are relatively easy to recognize, especially the former. However, when admixtures of these two ends occur, the definition of grades of SIN becomes less well defined. Histologic changes of intraepithelial neoplasia combining features from the two ends of the spectrum–normal thickness mucosa with a proliferation of immature basal-like cells in the lower regions of the epithelium and variable degrees of surface keratinization–are commonly underdiagnosed and may not be recognized as high-grade epithelial dysplasia/SIN (Fig. 1–8, see p. 6). Any evidence of surface maturation in the uterine cervical SIN grading scheme results in a lower grade assigned. This is clearly *not* the case in intraepithelial neoplasia of the UADT mucosa. Surface keratinization is commonplace in UADT SIN and must be recognized as such. Epithelial hyperplasia with or without prominent surface keratinization will require a different set of guidelines than thin mucosa with little or no evidence of surface maturation. The remaining portion of this chapter is devoted to expressing the rules we have found helpful and our interpretation of the literature in supporting our conclusions. General guidelines to the important features in gauging grades of SIN are given in Tables 1–5 and 1–6.

Table 1–5. WHO Classification of Precancerous Epithelial Changes and Histopathologic Parameters

1. Loss of polarity of the basal cells
2. Proliferation of the basal cells
3. Increased nuclear:cytoplasmic ratios
4. Epithelial hyperplasia with papillary submucosal extension
5. Irregular epithelial stratification and cellular pleomorphism
6. Keratinization of single cells (dyskeratosis) or cell groups in the prickle layer
7. Increased mitotic figures, especially in the prickle layer
8. Presence of abnormal mitotic figures
9. Nuclear pleomorphism and hyperchromatism
10. Enlarged, prominent nucleoli

Definition and Classification of Squamous Intraepithelial Neoplasia

1. Orderly or normal maturation with and without hyperplasia is defined by the relative relationship of basal and parabasal (immature and normal proliferating cells) to maturing keratinocytes of the intermediate zone and the superficial protective keratotic layers. The determination of hyperplasia is relative and depends on the extent of proliferation compared with the normal thickness of the mucosa for its anatomic site. Hyperplasia that maintains normal maturation characteristics is often reversible when the offending agent is removed. Carcinogens result in genetic damage that, if not repaired, persist or progress, and the resulting phenotypic expression of the damage may be but is not always expressed by dysplasia/SIN in either hyperplastic or thin mucosa. When carcinogens result in altered phenotypic histologic expression, invariably abnormal maturation of the epithelium will result. In effect, genetic alterations produce an "uncoupling" of normal maturation, and these maturation abnormalities are invariably associated with nuclear and cytologic aberrations.[56] Normal maturation results in an orderly mosaic-like pattern with similar-sized nuclei maintaining an equidistant relationship. The distance is defined by the gradual increasing of cell cytoplasm volume (often with keratinization) and nuclear shrinkage and condensation as epithelial maturation develops during the cellular migration toward the epithelial surface. The nuclei gradually undergo either pyknosis or karyorrhexis as a final step in the maturation process. Concurrent with epithelial maturation is an increase in cytoplasmic volume accompanied by an increase in keratin intermediate filaments, which provide surface mechanical protection by the development of hyaline-keratin cytoplasmic bundles.

2. Nuclear pleomorphism, usually with hyperchromasia, is invariably associated with cellular disorganization and epithelial dysplasia characterized by the loss of normal cellular maturation. Abnormal maturation is commonly associated with:

   a. Premature or early cytoplasmic keratinization (dyskeratosis) in the lower one third to two thirds of the epithelium, a common but not often stressed sign of dysplasia.

   b. Excessive cytoplasmic keratinization in all levels of the epithelium, another change that is seldom recognized as a significant maturation abnormality (Fig. 1–9, see p. 7).

   c. Abnormal proliferation of immature cells in the lower and middle portions of the epithelium but with evidence of surface maturation and keratinization. This may repre-

Table 1–6. Classification of Squamous Intraepithelial Neoplasia (SIN)

Grade	Hyperplastic Form	Atrophic Form
Hyperplasia/keratosis	Thickened, hyperplastic epithelium Rare mitosis confined to suprabasal layer Normal maturation Surface keratinization common No nuclear pleomorphism	Atrophy Thin mucosa Normal mucosal maturation No nuclear pleomorphism
SIN I (low-grade)	Epithelial hyperplasia Increased mitoses common (1–2/high-power field) Three or more layers of basal-like cells Minor nuclear pleomorphism Cytoplasmic keratinization in the surface layers	Some proliferation of basal-like cells Increased mitoses (1–2/high-power field) Minor nuclear pleomorphism Surface maturation still evident
SIN II (high-grade)	Epithelial hyperplasia Mitoses in all layers common, including abnormal forms Marked epithelial maturation abnormalities with immature "basal-like" cells constituting inner and middle one third or in combination with premature keratinization, including presence of "pearls" Prominent nuclear pleomorphism Increased chromatin staining	Proliferation of "basal-like" cells involving the full thickness Prominent submucosal changes similar to SIN II Numerous mitoses at all levels—may have abnormal forms Prominent nuclear pleomorphism Little or no evidence of maturation or keratinization

sent the most common expression of the hyperplastic form of epithelial dysplasia occurring in the UADT.

d. Loss of the normal development of cytoplasmic keratinization resulting in a thin epithelium with little or no evidence of cellular maturation. This form represents the "classic" form of CIS with immature or uncommitted cells constituting the full thickness of the nonproliferative or atrophic epithelium and is associated with an erythroplakic mucosal appearance.

Histopathologic Classification of Squamous Intraepithelial Neoplasia

It is important to develop an objective system to define the degree of morphologic alterations with specific and hopefully reproducible criteria to help the clinician assessing the biologic potential of a SIN lesion for persisting or progression to invasive cancer (see Tables 1–5 and 1–6). The observations that seem most applicable to define degrees of abnormality or dysplasia/SIN include the following[61]:

1. *Hyperplasia.* Classic CIS presenting grossly as erythroplakia is usually a thin mucosa without hyperplasia. Most dysplasia/SIN have a thickened hypercellular epithelium, which must be judged to have normal or abnormal maturation. This assessment is crucial in determining grade (Fig. 1–10, see p. 7).

2. *Keratinization.* Most, but not all, hyperplastic epithelia have evidence of cytoplasmic keratin formation. Probably one of the most important issues in grading dysplasia/SIN of the UADT is recognizing that the development of cytoplasmic keratin near the surface invariably represents normal epithelium.

   a. Surface keratinization in the form of acellular keratin with or without parakeratosis is the usual form of keratinizing dysplasia/SIN. Generally, the proliferation of immature cells or abnormal sized nuclei into the upper epithelium define this form of dysplasia/SIN (Fig. 1–11, see p. 8).

   b. Cytoplasmic keratin in the upper portion of the epithelium signifies epithelial maturation, but, similar to 2a, proliferation of abnormal cells into the upper epithelium defines dysplasia/SIN (Fig. 1–12, see p. 8).

   c. Hyperkeratinization with excessive cytoplasmic keratin accumulation into the lower epithelium is also distinctly abnormal. Either diffuse accumulation or keratin with or without nuclear abnormalities is pathologic and represents high-grade dysplasia/SIN. Focal areas of keratin formation in the lower epithelium also represent a matu-

ration abnormality and usually are associated with high-grade dysplasia/SIN.

3. *Epithelial maturation.* This observation is the most variable and the most difficult to define. It is an attempt to assess the nuclear and cytoplasmic volume (area) ratios with the development of keratinization evident in the expanding cytoplasm of the cells in the middle and especially the upper one third of the epithelium.

Deviation from the expected pattern of maturation in hyperplastic epithelium can take many forms: (1) proliferation of basal-like cells above the suprabasal region; (2) extension of intermediate cells to the surface, especially without evidence of expansion of the cytoplasm, usually with evidence of keratin formation; (3) enlarged hyperchromatic nuclei in the outer epithelium (Figs. 1–13 and 1–14, see p. 9); and (4) excessive cytoplasmic keratin formation in the lower epithelium.

In general, epithelial maturation is the orderly progression of basal cells to intermediate cells with expanding cytoplasm as the cells migrate toward the surface. The nuclei are initially small (basal cells), become larger (intermediate), and are gradually lost (keratinization). The nuclei always maintain a pattern of equidistance, with the distance between nuclei becoming greater as the cytoplasmic volume increases. We refer to this nuclear pattern as "mosaic," and it is critical in the histologic definition of normal maturation.

4. *Mitoses.* One could expect increased mitoses (0 to 1 per high-power field) in a hyperproliferative hyperplastic epithelium. In reactive hyperplastic processes, morphologically normal mitoses are confined to the basal/suprabasal layers of the epithelium and the presence of mitoses above this level is pathologic. Abnormal mitoses invariably reflect neoplastic transformation.

5. *Nuclear pleomorphism* for the purpose of this discussion refers to variation in nuclear size, shape, and chromatin staining in adjacent cells. Normally the nuclei become smaller as they migrate toward the surface with a predictable maturation process, eventually disappearing in hyperkeratosis or remaining as pyknotic remnants in parakeratosis. Mild nuclear pleomorphism can be seen in low-grade lesions, while appreciable variation in nuclear size, shape, and staining characteristics is invariably found in high grade SIN.

▪ BIOMARKERS OF EPITHELIAL MATURATION AND INTRAEPITHELIAL MATURATION

Numerous investigators have diligently searched for markers of maturation or abnormal expression of markers indicative of loss of maturation. The resurgence of interest in chemoprevention and reversal of oral mucosal changes such as leukoplakia has resulted in attempts to identify biomarkers that can be used to monitor epithelial maturation.[80] One of the first markers to be carefully investigated was the expression of cytokeratins with the hope that expression of abnormal cytokeratins would signify abnormal epithelium.[81] Unfortunately, cytokeratins vary greatly within dysplastic epithelium, as does the phenotypic expression (morphology) reflecting genetic alterations.[81] In general, simple or low molecular weight keratins are expressed in "classic" or atrophic forms of CIS but not in those demonstrating normal surface maturation with hematoxylin-eosin identifiable surface cytoplasmic keratin, usually of high molecular weight.[82] However, not all studies have been able to confirm these observations.[83, 84] Attempts at identifying "marker" chromosome or genetic changes signaling neoplastic transformation have resulted in a number of important observations. Cell DNA content has repeatedly demonstrated increased or abnormal DNA content in most severe dysplasia/SIN. Measurements confirming abnormal DNA nuclear content have been performed by image analysis.[78, 79] Almost all high-grade dysplasia/SIN have abnormal DNA nuclear content. In addition, some dysplasia/SIN with prominent keratinization are also aneuploid, despite having less obviously abnormal nuclear alterations. This seems a surprising observation from a morphologic perspective but reinforces what we have learned, namely that "excessive" keratinization in an abnormal pattern also signifies expression of neoplastic change. Similar but more sophisticated observations documenting individual chromosomal polysomy in preinvasive epithelial changes have also been reported.[85] Subsequent molecular-oriented studies have identified a number of abnormalities in dysplasia/SIN; however, the two most commonly reported analyzed gene products are overexpression of epidermal growth factor receptor (EGFR) and *p53* oncogene. These studies found increased EGFR expression with high grades of SIN.[86, 87] Both increased p53 gene product and *p53* mutations have been identified in noninvasive SIN and have been noted to increase in invasive carcinomas.[87, 88] p53 gene product expression, measured by immunohistochemistry, is also increased in SIN adjacent to invasive cancers[89] and is thought by some to represent a potential marker of recurrence when present in surgical margins.[74]

Several recent studies provide strong evidence in support of augmenting traditional histopathologic examination with genetic testing. Mao and coworkers[90] correlated loss of heterozygosity (LOH) in a significant number of oral leukoplakias at 9p21 and 3p14 with a greater probability of progression to head and neck squamous cell carcinoma. This finding suggests the potential of microsatellite analysis in predicting cancer risk of oral leukoplakia.[91] Rosin et al.[92] also used this technique in studying the progression of oral lesions initially diagnosed as epithelial hyperplasia or mild/moderate dysplasia. They found that almost all lesions progressing to squamous cell carcinoma exhibiting LOH at these two sites did not progress. Five other regions (4q, 8p, 11q, 13q, and 17p) were examined. Loss of any of these additional chromosomes, in addition to 3p and/or 9p, provided better predictive value of developing squamous carcinoma, with nearly 60% of the hyperplastic or dysplastic lesions exhibiting LOH at 3p and/or 9p plus LOH at an additional site developing carcinoma. These data are preliminary and additional prospective studies are necessary to better understand their importance. Since microsatellite analysis can be done noninvasively on exfoliative cells collected by scraping the lesion surface, this technique may provide additional data relevant to patient care.

▌ REFERENCES

Background and Scope

1. Miller AH: Premalignant laryngeal lesions, carcinoma in situ, superficial carcinoma—definition and management. In: Alberti DW, Bryce DP, eds. *Summation Workshop #2. Centennial Conference on Laryngeal Cancer.* New York City, Appleton-Century-Crofts, 1976:167.

2. WHO Collaborating Center for Oral Precancerous Lesions: Definition of leukoplakia and related lesions: An aid to studies on oral precancer. *Oral Surg Oral Med Oral Pathol* 1978;46:518–539.

3. Goldman NC: Problems in outpatients with laryngeal hyperplastic lesions. *Acta Otolayngol Suppl (Stockh)* 1997;527:70–73.

4. Fiorella R, Di Nicola V, Resta L: Epidemiological and clinical relief on hyperplastic lesions of the larynx. *Acta Otolaryngol Suppl (Stockh)* 1997;527:77–81.

5. Abbey LM, Augars GE, Gunsolley JC, et al: Intraexaminer and interexaminer reliability in the diagnosis of oral epithelial dysplasia. *Oral Surg Oral Med Oral Pathol* 1995;80:188–191.

6. Scala M, Moresco L, Comandini D, et al: The role of the general practitioner and dentist in the early diagnosis of preneoplastic and neoplastic lesions of the oral cavity. *Minerva Stomatol* 1997;46(3):133–137.

7. Colella G, DeLuca F, Lanza A, Tartaro GP: The malignant transformation of leukoplakia of the oral cavity. A review of the literature and clinical case reports. *Minerva Stomatol* 1995;44(6):291–300.

8. Onofre MA, Sposto MR, Navarro CM, et al: Potentially malignant epithelial oral lesions: Discrepancies between clinical and histological diagnosis. *Oral Dis* 1997;3(3):148–152.

9. Bouquot JE, Ephros H: Erythroplakia: The dangerous red mucosa. *Pract Periodontics Aesthet Dent* 1995;7(6):59–67, quiz 68.

10. Lumerman H, Freedman P, Kerpel S: Oral epithelial dysplasia and the development of invasive squamous cell carcinoma. *Oral Surg Oral Med Oral Pathol* 1995;79:323–329.

11. Blackwell KE, Fu YS, Calcaterra TC: Laryngeal dysplasia: A clinicopathologic study. *Cancer* 1995;75(2):457–463.

12. Rothman KJ, Keller AZ: The effect of joint exposure to alcohol and tobacco on risk of the mouth and pharynx. *J Chron Dis* 1972;25:711–716.

13. Grasscr JA, Childers E: Prevalence of smokeless tobacco use and clinical oral leukoplakia in a military population. *Mil Med* 1997;162(6):401–404.

14. Tomar SL, Winn DM, Swango PA, et al: Oral mucosal smokeless tobacco lesions among adolescents in the United States. *J Dent Res* 1997;76(6):1277–1286.

15. Winn DM: Diet and nutrition in the etiology of oral cancer. *Am J Clin Nutrition* 1995;61(2):437S–445S.

16. Cowan CG, Gregg TA, Kee F: Prevention and detection of oral cancer: The views of primary care dentists in Northern Ireland. *Br Dent J* 1995;179(9):338–342.

17. Peters E, McGaw WT: Detection of premalignant oral lesions: A 10-year retrospective study in Alberta. *J Can Dent Assoc* 1995;61(9):775–778.

18. Mao L, Lee JS, Fan YH, et al: Telomerase activity in head and neck squamous cell carcinoma and adjacent tissues. *Nat Med* 1996;2(6):682–685.

19. Gopalakrishnan R, Weghorst CM, Lehman TA, et al: Mutated and wide-type expression and HPV integration in proliferative verrucous leukoplakia and oral squamous cell carcinoma. *Oral Surg Oral Med Oral Pathol Oral Radio Endod* 1997;83(4):471–477.

20. Wood MW, Medina JE, Thompson GC, et al: Accumulation of the p53 tumor-suppressor gene product in oral leukoplakia. *Otolaryngol Head Neck Surg* 1994;11(6):758–763.

21. Kaugars GE, Silverman S Jr, Lovas JGL, et al: Use of antioxidant supplements in the treatment of human oral leukoplakia. Review of the literature and current studies. *Oral Surg Oral Med Oral Pathol* 1996;81:5–14.

22. Lippman SM, Shin DM, Lee JJ, et al: p53 and retinoid chemoprevention of oral carcinogenesis. *Cancer Res* 1995;55:16–19.

23. Bostwick DG, Montironi R: Prostatic intraepithelial neoplasia and the origins of prostatic carcinoma. *Pathol Res Pract* 1995;191(9):828–832.

24. Lonky NM, Navarre GL, Saunders S, et al: Low-grade Papanicolaou smears and the Bethesda system: A prospective cytohistopathologic analysis. *Obstet Gynecol* 1995;85(5 Pt 1):716–720.

Nose, Paranasal Sinuses, and Nasopharynx

25. Bouvier G, Hergenhahn M, Polack A, et al: Characterization of macromolecular lignins as Epstein-Barr virus inducer in foodstuff associated with nasopharyngeal carcinoma risk. *Carcinogenesis* 1995;16(8):1879–1885.

26. Liebowitz D: Nasopharyngeal carcinoma: The Epstein-Barr virus association. *Semin Oncol* 1994;21(3):376–381.

27. Hildesheim A, Levine PH: Etiology of nasopharyngeal carcinoma: A review. *Epidemiol Rev* 1993;15(2):466–485.

28. Boysen M, Voss R, Solberg A: The nasal mucosa in softwood exposed furniture workers. *Acta Otolaryngol (Stockh)* 1986;101:501–508.

29. Duffus JH: Epidemiology and the identification of metals as human carcinogens. *Sci Prog* 1996;79(Pt 4):311–326.

30. Barnes L, Bedetti C: Oncocytic schneiderian papilloma: A reappraisal of cylindrical cell papilloma of the sinonasal tract. *Hum Pathol* 1984; 15(4):344–351.

31. Christensen WN, Smith RR: Scheiderian papillomas: A clinicopathological study of 67 cases. *Hum Pathol* 1986;15:393–400.

32. Pathmanathan R, Prasad U, Sadler R, et al: Clonal proliferations of cells infected with Epstein-Barr virus in preinvasive lesions related to nasopharyngeal carcinoma. *N Engl J Med* 1995;333(11):693–698.

33. Sheu L-F, Chen A, Meng C-L, et al: Analysis of *bcl-2* expression in normal, inflamed, dysplastic nasopharyngeal epithelia, and nasopharyngeal carcinoma: Association with *p53* expression. *Hum Pathol* 1997;28(5): 556–562.

Oral Cavity

34. Shafer WG, Waldron CA: A clinical and histopathologic study of oral leukoplakia. *Surg Gynecol Obstet* 1991;112:411–420.

35. Schepman KP, van der Meij EH, Smeele LE, et al: Prevalence study of oral white lesions with special reference to a new definition of oral leukoplakia. *Eur J Cancer B Oral Oncol* 1996;32B(6):416–419.

36. Axell T, Pindborg JJ, Smith CJ, van der Waal, and the International Collaborative Group on Oral White Lesions: Oral white lesions with special reference to precancerous and tobacco-related lesions: Conclusions of an international symposium held in Uppsala, Sweden, May 18–21, 1994. *J Oral Pathol Med* 1996;25(2):49–54.

37. Shklar G: Patterns of keratinization in oral leukoplakia. *Arch Otolaryngol* 1968;87:92–96.

38. Silverman S, Gorsky M, Lozada F: Oral leukoplakia and malignant transformation. *Cancer* 1984;53:563–568.

39. Einhorn J, Wersall J: Incidence of oral carcinoma in patients with leukoplakia of the oral mucosa. *Cancer* 1967;20:2189–2193.

40. Banoczy J: Follow-up studies in oral leukoplakia. *J Maxillofac Surg* 1977;5:69–75.

41. Banoczy J, Ceiba A: Occurrence of epithelial dysplasia in oral leukoplakia. *Oral Surg Oral Med Oral Pathol* 1976;42:766–774.

42. Waldron CA, Shafer WG: Leukoplakia revised: A clinicopathologic study of 3256 oral leukoplakias. *Cancer* 1975;36:1386–1392.

43. Silverman S, Rozen RD: Observations on the clinical characteristics and natural history of oral leukoplakia. *J Am Dent Assoc* 1968;76:772–777.

44. Pindborg JJ, Renstrup G, Poulsen HE, et al: Studies in oral leukoplakias v. clinical and histological signs of malignancy. *Acta Odontol Scand* 1963;21:404–414.

45. Mashberg A: Erythroplasia: The earliest sign of asymptomatic oral cancer. *J Am Dent Assoc* 1978;96:615–620.

46. Shafer WG, Waldron CA: Erythroplakia of the oral cavity. *Cancer* 1975;36:1021–1028.

47. van der Waal I, Schepman KP, van der Meij EH, Smeele LE: Oral leukoplakia: A clinicopathological review. *Oral Oncol* 1997;33:291–301.

48. Silverman S Jr, Gorsky M: Proliferative verrucous leukoplakia: A follow-up study of 54 cases. *Oral Surg Oral Med Oral Pathol Oral Radiol Endod* 1997;84:154–157.

49. Suarez P, Batsakis JG, el-Naggar AK: Leukoplakia still a gallimaufry or is progress being made? A review. *Adv Anat Pathol* 1998;5:137–155.

50. Shear M, Pindborg J: Verrucous hyperplasia of the oral mucosa. *Cancer* 1980;46:1855–1862.

51. Zakrzewska JM, Lopes V, Speight P, Hopper C: Proliferative verrucous leukoplakia a report of ten cases. *Oral Surg Oral Med Oral Pathol* 1996;82:396–401.

52. Hansen LS, Olson JA, Silverman S Jr: Proliferative verrucous leukoplakia. A long-term study of thirty patients. *Oral Surg Oral Med Oral Pathol* 1985;60:285–298.

53. Brennan JA, Mao L, Hruban RH, et al: Molecular assessment of histopathological staging in squamous cell carcinoma of the head and neck. *N Engl J Med* 1995;332:429–435.

Larynx and Hypopharynx

54. Brugere J, Guenel P, LeClerc A, et al: Differential effects of tobacco and alcohol in cancers of the larynx, pharynx and mouth. *Cancer* 1986; 57:391–395.

55. De Stefani E, Correa P, Oreggia F, et al: Risk factors for laryngeal cancer. *Cancer* 1987;60:3087–3091.

56. Guenel P, Chastang JF, Luce D, et al: A study of the interaction of alcohol drinking and tobacco smoking among French cases of laryngeal cancer. *J Epidemiol Comm Health* 1988;42:350–354.

57. Crissman JD: Laryngeal keratosis and subsequent carcinoma. *Head Neck Surg* 1979;1:386–391.

58. Crissman JD, Visscher DW, Sakr W: Premalignant lesions of the upper aerodigestive tract: Pathologic classification. *J Cell Biochem* 1993; (Suppl 17F):49–56.

59. Sllamniku B, Bauer W, Painter C, et al: The transformation of laryngeal keratosis into invasive carcinoma. *Am J Otolaryngol* 1989;10:42–54.

60. Crissman JD, Zarbo RJ: Dysplasia, in-situ carcinoma and progression in squamous cell carcinoma of the upper aerodigestive tract. *Am J Surg Pathol* 1989;13(Suppl 1):5–16.

61. Kleinsasser O: Cancer of the larynx: A study of development and early growth. *J Otolaryngol Soc Aust* 1968;2:8–12.

62. Shibuya H, Amagasa T, Seto K-I, et al: Leukoplakia-associated multiple carcinomas in patients with tongue carcinoma. *Cancer* 1986;57:843–846.

63. Doyle PJ, Flores A, Douglas GS: Carcinoma in-situ of the larynx. *Laryngoscope* 1977;87:310–316.

64. Elman AJ, Goodman M, Wang CC, et al: In-situ carcinoma of the vocal cords. *Cancer* 1979;43:2422–2428.

65. Gupta PC, Mehta FS, Daftary DK, et al: Incidence rates of oral cancer and natural history of oral precancerous lesions in a 10-year follow-up study of Indian villagers. *Community Dent Oral Epidemiol* 1980;8:283–333.

66. Gabriel CE, Jones DG: Hyperkeratosis of the larynx. *J Laryngol Otol* 1973;87:129–134.

67. Hellquist H, Lundgren J, Olofsson J: Hyperplasia, keratosis, dysplasia and carcinoma in-situ of the vocal cords: A follow-up study. *Clin Otolaryngol* 1982;7:11–27.

68. Henry RC: The transformation of laryngeal leukoplakia to cancer. *J Laryngol Otol* 1979;93:447–459.

69. Holinger PH, Schild JA: Carcinoma in-situ of the larynx. *Laryngoscope* 1995;85:1707–1708.

70. Kaimbic V: Difficulties in management of vocal cord precancerous lesions. *J Laryngol Otol* 1978;92:305–315.

71. Maran AGD, MacKenzie IJ, Stanley RE: Carcinoma in-situ of the larynx. *Head Neck Surg* 1984,7.28–31.

72. McGavran MH, Bauer WC, Ogura JH: Isolated laryngeal keratosis: Its relation to carcinoma of the larynx based on a clinicopathologic study of 87 consecutive cases with long term follow-up. *Laryngoscope* 1960;70:932–950.

73. Miller AH, Fisher HR: Clues to the life history of carcinoma in-situ of the larynx. *Laryngoscope* 1971;81:1475–1480.

74. Norris CM, Peale AR: Keratosis of the larynx. *J Laryngol Otol* 1963;77:635–647.

75. Pene F, Fletcher GH: Results in irradiation of the in-situ carcinomas of the vocal cords. *Cancer* 1976;37:2586–2590.

76. Bauer WC, McGavran MH: Carcinoma in-situ and evaluation of epithelial changes in laryngopharyngeal biopsies. *JAMA* 1972;221:72–74.

77. Hellquist H, Olofsson J, Grontoft O: Carcinoma in-situ and severe dysplasia of the vocal cords. *Acta Otolaryngol* 1981;92:543–555.

78. Crissman JD, Zarbo RJ: Quantitation of DNA ploidy in squamous intraepithelial neoplasia of the laryngeal glottis. *Arch Otolaryngol Head Neck Surg* 1991;117:182–188.

79. Grontoft O, Hellquist H, Olofsson J, et al: The DNA content and nuclear size in normal, dysplastic and carcinomatous laryngeal epithelium. *Acta Otolaryngol* 1978;86:473–479.

Biomarkers of Epithelial Maturation and Intraepithelial Maturation

80. Lee JS, Lippman SM, Hong WK, et al: Determination of biomarkers for intermediate end points in chemoprevention trials. *Cancer Res* 1992;(Suppl)52:2707–2710.

81. Lindberg K, Rheinwald JG: Suprabasal 40kd keratin (k19) expression as an immunohistologic marker of premalignancy in oral epithelium. *Am J Pathol* 1989;134:89–98.

82. Smedts F, Ramaekers F, Robben H, et al: Changing patterns of keratin expression during progression of cervical intraepithelial neoplasia. *Am J Pathol* 1990;136:657–668.

83. Cotrera MD, Zarbo RJ, Sakr WA, et al: Markers for dysplasia of the upper aerodigestive tract. *Am J Pathol* 1992;141:817–825.

84. Ogden GR, Chisholm DM, Adi M: Cytokeratin expression in oral cancer

and its relationship to tumor differentiation. *J Oral Pathol Med* 1993;22:82–86.

85. Hittleman WN, Voravud N, Shin DM, et al: Early genetic changes during upper aerodigestive tract tumorigenesis. *J Cell Biochem* 1996;(Suppl 17F):233–236.

86. Miyaguchi M, Olofsson J, Hellquist HB: Immunohistochemical study of epidermal growth factor receptors in severe dysplasia and carcinoma insitu of the vocal cords. *Acta Otolaryngol* 1991;(1):149–152.

87. Shin DM, Ro JY, Hong WK, et al: Dysregulation of epidermal growth factor receptor expression in premalignant lesions during head and neck tumorigenesis. *Cancer Res* 1994;54:3153–3159.

88. Boyle JD, Hakim J, Koch W, et al: The incidence of p53 mutations increases with progression of head and neck cancer. *Cancer Res* 1993; 53:4477–4480.

89. Shin DM, Kim J, Ro JY, et al: Activation of p53 gene expression in premalignant lesions during head and neck tumorigenesis. *Cancer Res* 1994;54:321–326.

90. Mao L, Lee JS, Fan YH, et al: Frequent microsatellite alterations at chromosomes 9p21 and 3p14 in oral premalignant lesions and their value in carcinoma risk assessment. *Nat Med* 1996;2:682–685.

91. Mao L: Can molecular assessment improve classification of head and neck premalignancy? [Editorial.] *Clin Cancer Res* 2000;6:321–322.

92. Rosin MP, Cheng X, Poh C, et al: Use of allelic loss to predict malignant risk for low-grade oral epithelial dysplasia. *Clin Cancer Res* 2000; 6:357–362.

2 : Squamous Cell Carcinoma of the Upper Aerodigestive System

Pieter J. Slootweg and Mary Richardson

INTRODUCTION

Squamous cell carcinoma (SCC) of the upper aerodigestive tract (UADT) is the most common malignant neoplasm of the mucosal lining of the upper food and air passages.[1, 2] In the Netherlands in 1994, 2034 new cases were registered as part of approximately 63,500 new malignancies arising in a population of 15.4 million inhabitants.[3] Worldwide statistics mention 412,000 new cases annually.[4] It is evident that this tumor, which carries an overall death risk of 40%,[3] represents a major health problem in the head and neck area, and a large proportion of the workload of people working in a head and neck oncologic care setting will come from patients suffering from this disease.

GENERAL COMMENTS

Epidemiology and Risk Factors

Geographic variations in the occurrence of cancer have been recognized for many years. The estimates are not uniformly based on incidence data gathered by cancer registries but are also extrapolated from mortality data. With that caveat, it is likely that the gathered international information represents relative cancer burden and site-specific patterns for many areas of the world.[5]

Head and neck cancer is an important contributor to the worldwide cancer burden. Globally, head and neck cancer ranks as the sixth most common cancer. Among developing countries, head and neck cancer ranks third, and it is the fourth most common cancer for men worldwide.[4, 5] Greater than 90% of all UADT cancers are SCC occurring in the fifth and sixth decade of life, with rates progressing with age. Furthermore, with a few exceptions, the incidence is higher in men than in women.[6] Pertinent epidemiologic data are briefly mentioned here for the various UADT sites.

Lip

The highest rates of lip cancer are in men from South Australia (13.5 per 100,000) and Canada (11.0 per 100,000; Newfoundland fishermen).[5, 7] The lowest rates occur in Asia (0.9 per 100,000). The incidence in the black population of the United States is very low to nil.[5] Lip cancer is uncommon in women. The risk of lip cancer seems to be decreasing.[5]

Oral Cavity and Pharynx

Cancer of the oral cavity and pharynx consists of a diverse group of tumors with a large geographic variation. The largest contribution to the world total of oral cavity and pharynx cancers is from Southern Asia (34.6%), where they are mainly cancers of the mouth and tongue, and from China (15.7%), where they are mainly cancers of the nasopharynx.[4] Within the European community, oral cancer constitutes approximately 4.2% of all cancers.[8] The highest incidence among males (primary tumors of the pharynx) is reported from France (Bas-Rhin and Calvados), with annual rates of 40 per 100,000.[7, 8] The highest rates among women occur in parts of India. In India there is a more equal sex distribution of oral cancer.[7, 9]

In their overview of the worldwide incidence of cancers, Parkin et al.[4] reported the female incidence of cancer of the mouth and pharynx to be the highest in Southern Asia (female incidence being 10.1 per 100,000) and in Melanesia (14.1 per 100,000). In the United States, cancer of the UADT represents approximately 4% of all malignancies. Oral cavity and pharynx cancer constitute about 50% of these UADT cancers. In the United States it ranks seventh among blacks and 12th among whites.[7]

Mapping of cancer mortality in the United States from 1950 to 1969 showed elevated rates among urban Northern males. This pattern was consistent with available major risk factors: tobacco use and drinking alcohol. Among females, mortality was highest in the rural South. The major risk identified was the longstanding use of smokeless tobacco products (snuff). Recent updates (1970–1989) among U.S. females reveal a decrease in the high-risk Southeast and several new high-risk areas along the Pacific and Florida coasts.[7]

Tumors of the postcricoid region have historically been seen in Northern European women, especially those from rural Sweden, but also in those from the United Kingdom and Asia.[10, 11] In these regions, Plummer-Vinson syndrome (Patterson-Kelly syndrome, sideropenic dysphagia) was prevalent.[11, 12] The syndrome is characterized by dysphagia, glossitis, iron-deficient anemia, cheilitis, and achlorhydria. Mucosal webs frequently develop along the anterior esophageal wall, and when carcinoma arises in these patients, the lesion is usually proximal to the web. Approximately 30% to 70% of patients with postcricoid carcinoma have Plummer-Vinson syndrome; however, only 3% to 10% of patients with Plummer-Vinson syndrome will develop carcinoma. The time of peak incidence of carcinoma occurs about 15 years after the onset of Plummer-Vinson syndrome.[11]

Larynx

Laryngeal cancer throughout the world has a higher incidence in men than in women. It occurs most frequently in the sixth and seventh decade of life. Within the United States, the male:female ratio is 5:1, and this ratio is similar and reasonably consistent worldwide.[13, 14] The incidence is higher among black residents than white residents in the same geographic region.[15] The highest incidence rates in men are reported for Southern Europe (annual incidence, 14.7 per 100,000), with Western Europe having the second highest rates (annual incidence, 11.4 per 100,000).[4] Coleman et al.[16] observed a three- to fourfold differential between Mediterranean and English populations that has remained constant over the past 20 years.

Tobacco use and alcohol consumption are strongly associated with laryngeal cancer. Users of dark tobacco have a higher risk for laryngeal cancer than users of light (flue-cured) tobacco.[17] In a large multicenter study evaluating alcohol consumption and tobacco use, the risk associated with cigarette smoking was approximately 10 for all subsites within the larynx and hypopharynx. The risk from alcohol varied by site but was highest for the epilarynx and hypopharynx. This study also found the combined exposure to alcohol and tobacco to be consistent with a multiplicative relative risk model.[18] A nonalcoholic drink, maté, has been associated with an increased risk for laryngeal cancer in studies from Latin American countries. This drink is a tea-like infusion of the herb *Ilex paraguariensis.* DeStefani et al.[19] have hypothesized that a phenolic compound in the drink may act as a promoter.

Sinonasal Cavities

Cancer of the nasal and paranasal sinuses is infrequent. Within the United States, the incidence is 0.75 per 100,000 persons. The most common site of occurrence is the maxillary sinus, which is affected twice as often as the nasal cavity. The least frequent areas involved are the ethmoid and sphenoid sinuses. The male:female ratio is 2:1.[20] The age of onset is around the sixth decade of life. Globally, these cancers are far more common in Japanese (incidence per 100,000, 2.6 to 2.2 for males and 1.4 to 1.2 for females), and in certain African populations (2.5 in males, 1.8 in females).[21]

Sinonasal cancers have a multifactorial etiology: sinonasal squamous cell cancers may develop from exposure to nickel, softwood dust, and mustard gas production, whereas adenocarcinomas may develop from exposure to hardwood, chrome pigment, and leather dust.[22–26] Another agent frequently cited as being involved with cancer of the nasal cavity is thorotrast.[20] Moreover, Epstein-Barr virus, well known within the context of nasopharyngeal carcinoma, appears to play a role in the pathogenesis of a diverse spectrum of sinonasal carcinomas.[27]

Nasopharynx

The epidemiology of nasopharyngeal carcinoma suggests the interaction of several variables: diet, viral agents, and genetic susceptibility. The endemic areas include Southern China and Northern Africa. The incidence in China increases from North to South, 2 to 3 per 100,000 to 25 to 40 per 100,000, respectively.[28] Kadanos of Malaysia, Eskimos, and other Arctic region populations have high rates approaching those of Southern China. Intermediate rates (3 to 6 per 100,000) are present in Southeast Asia, including Thais, Vietnamese, Malays, and Filipinos. In North Africa, it appears that nasopharyngeal carcinoma is elevated mainly in the Arab populations.

Regarding age and gender, in all populations the rates are higher in men than in women. Age distribution, however, does show variation between populations. In high-risk areas (e.g., Southern China), the peak age is between 45 and 54, with a declining incidence in older persons. In areas with low to moderate risk, an adolescent age peak has been noted.[28] The consumption of salt-cured fish (Chinese style) has been implicated in studies of the Tanka culture, which has one of the highest incidences of nasopharyngeal carcinoma. The Epstein-Barr virus has been found in all forms of nasopharyngeal carcinoma.[28]

Trachea

Squamous cell carcinoma of the trachea has shown a strong male predominance of four times as many men as women.[29] There is a strong association with cigarette smoking.[30] Two of the largest series documented that between 33% and 37% of patients with SCC of the trachea have another malignancy of the respiratory tract or subsequently will develop one.[29]

Analytic Epidemiology

The study of the epidemiology of head and neck cancer has identified alcohol use and tobacco use as independent risk factors, and combined they have a multiplicative risk.[1, 8, 17] Tobacco products such as cigarettes, cigars, snuff, and chews (e.g., betel quid that consists of the leaf of the betel vine *[Piper betel],* areca nut, lime, and tobacco) are risk factors for head and neck cancer.[9, 31] Factors such as dietary deficiencies, after correcting for alcohol and tobacco use,

particularly of vitamins A and C, iron, and certain trace elements, are thought to predispose to oral cancers.[9, 31] Other risks include previous irradiation; work in furniture, asbestos-related, and nickel industries; poor oral hygiene; and infection with the Epstein-Barr virus.[1, 14] The association between either lichen planus or marijuana smoking and risk for oral cancer is still controversial.[31]

Exposure to alcohol and tobacco affects various sites. With cigarette smoking, the gradient of the dose response and the magnitude of the risk show differences by gender and by primary site. Some studies have found women to have a greater risk than men per pack-year stratum.[8, 17] The subsites within the UADT that exhibit the greatest risk associated with alcohol exposure are the floor of the mouth, the hypopharynx, and the supraglottis.[32] Higher smoking-associated risk estimates have been reported for subsites of the larynx (glottis) and hypopharynx. Smokeless tobacco has a high risk for the oral cavity.[17]

Case reports of head and neck cancer occurring within the first two decades are rare, with the exception of nasopharyngeal cancers within the intermediate risk areas. Other patients with cancers in the first two decades may be individuals with genetic disorders or children with laryngeal papillomatosis.[33]

Syndromes

Family occurrences of head and neck cancer have given credence to the role of inheritance in this particular neoplastic process. Few disorders have been associated with increased incidence of head and neck cancers; laryngeal cancers have been described as part of the multiple cancers in Lynch-II syndrome.[34]

Bloom's syndrome is an autosomal recessive disorder characterized by a high incidence of cancer at a young age. Twenty-eight of the initial 103 identified as Bloom's syndrome patients developed cancer, and 5 of these cancers were head and neck carcinomas (epiglottis, pyriform sinus, larynx, and two base of tongue; age range 26–34 years).[35]

Fanconi's anemia is a recessively inherited disorder associated with increased risk for malignancies, including head and neck tumors.[36] The reported cases of carcinoma in this area include nine on the tongue (dorsal, lateral, and base), two on the pyriform sinus, one in the postcricoid area, and three on the gingiva and buccal mucosa.[37] Although the ratio of male to female in Fanconi's anemia is 2:1, the ratio is reversed among these patients with SCC.[37]

Xeroderma pigmentosum is an autosomal recessive disease characterized by a DNA excision repair deficit. Damage to the chromosome is elicited by exposure to ultraviolet light. SCC on the anterior third of the tongue is frequent within the first two decades of life. These patients in the first two decades have an estimated 10,000 times greater frequency of tongue tumors than expected for that age group. SCC of the gingiva and palate also occur with increased frequency in these patients.[38]

Ataxia-telangiectasia is cytogenetically characterized by an increased number of spontaneously induced chromosomal aberrations. There are two separate clinical patterns of malignancy in these patients. In one, the patients developed solid tumors, which include malignancies of the oral cavity within its spectrum.[39]

One autosomally dominant disorder known as Li-Fraumeni syndrome is characterized by an early onset of tumors. Among these tumors, laryngeal carcinomas have been reported. These patients also have a high incidence of second primary tumors.[40]

Within the immunologically compromised population, which would include organ transplant patients as well as patients with human immunodeficiency virus infection, there is known to be an increase in oral tumors. A recent report of increased oral SCC in patients infected with human immunodeficiency virus has been noted.[41] Those cases of head and neck cancers occurring in organ transplant patients are predominantly seen along the vermilion border of the lip and are frequently associated with renal transplantion.[42]

Etiology

As outlined previously, the most important risk factors for SCC are alcohol and tobacco use,[1, 8, 43–46] but there is also increasing evidence that viruses are implicated in at least some cases of SCC.[1, 8, 47–49] The viruses that are considered to be of interest in this area are human papilloma virus (HPV), herpes simplex virus (HSV), and Epstein-Barr virus (EBV). EBV has already been mentioned as being associated with nasopharyngeal carcinomas, not only in the undifferentiated and nonkeratinizing tumors[50] but also in keratinizing squamous carcinomas.[51] Proof that herpes simplex virus is implicated in head and neck carcinogenesis is still lacking, although herpes simplex virus antigens have been observed in some oral cancers.[47] DNA from HPV has been detected in head and neck tumor tissue, but, as it also has been detected in apparently normal mucosa, the role of HPV in the initiation of tumor development in the mucosal linings of the UADT is not well understood.

Recently, some evidence was presented that genetic predisposition also plays a role in the origin of SCC,[52, 53] although it has also been reported that environmental factors may contribute to familial aggregation of SCC.[54, 55]

Because cancer development implies damage to genetic material, it is important to analyze the genetic aberrations occurring in SCC and to try to relate these changes to the above-mentioned risk factors. Indeed, several investigations report multiple genetic abnormalities to be present in SCC, resulting in inappropriate activation of oncogenes or abrogation of tumor suppressor gene functions.[56–58] One of the most extensively investigated genetic abnormalities is that of the p53 gene. This gene serves as a control in cellular proliferation by coding for a protein that prevents cells with damaged DNA to proceed through the cell cycle, thus allowing time for DNA repair or, if repair does not occur, causing apoptosis.[59] In this way, cells with abnormal DNA cannot proliferate, and the importance of a normally functioning p53 gene is exemplified by the observation that in many tumors, SCC included, p53 gene mutations are present.[60, 61]

The significance of p53 dysfunction in SCC initiation and development is supported by its association with the epidemiologic risk factor of smoking; there is evidence that tobacco products may induce p53 gene mutations,[62] and an association between p53 mutations and smoking has been observed.[60, 61] Moreover, HPV-coded proteins may block the functions of the p53 protein, and therefore a causative role of HPV in SCC development, although not yet formally established, may also operate by disturbing the normal function of p53.[48, 49]

Multiple Primary Tumors

As the entire mucosal lining of the UADT is exposed to the same carcinogenic agents, the occurrence of multiple primary tumors is not surprising and has indeed been documented extensively, their incidence varying from 10% to 35%,[63–75] whereas the risk of developing a second malignancy from treatment to death has been reported as 4% to 6% per year.[76, 77] Such tumors are considered synchronous if they are diagnosed at the same time as or within a 6-month period of identification of the primary lesion; if second cancers are diagnosed 6 months or more after the diagnosis of the primary cancers, they are metachronous neoplasms.[64]

To qualify as multiple primary tumors, lesions have to satisfy the following requirements: both lesions have to be malignant as determined by histology, the lesions should be separated by normal-appearing mucosa (if the intervening mucosa demonstrates dysplasia, it is considered a multicentric primary[74]), and the possibility that the second neoplasm represents a metastasis should be excluded.[64] Those second primary cancers are observed not only in the UADT but also in the lungs, the latter especially in case of laryngeal SCC[65, 67, 68] or in other body sites. Two independent variables in head and neck carcinomas have been found to influence the occur-

rence of second metachronous cancer: anatomic site of the original primary tumor and age.[74] Second primary tumors in the head and neck area are more often seen when the first SCC is located in the oral cavity, oropharynx, or hypopharynx.[67] Within the oral cavity, patients with their primary tumor in the floor of the mouth, retromolar area, or lower alveolar process seem to be more at risk for a second primary SCC than patients with tumors at other intraoral sites.[73] The oropharyngeal and hypopharyngeal sites associated with frequent second primary tumors are the base of the tongue (46%) and the pyriform sinus (34%), respectively.[74]

Most second primary tumors are metachronous, although sometimes an unusually high proportion of synchronously occurring SCCs is found.[74] There also appears to be a genetic background for developing multiple SCCs of the UADT, as demonstrated by an increased sensitivity for mutagens in this group of patients.[78, 79] Second primary tumors adversely influence the prognosis of UADT-SCC patients. Conditional on surviving for 2 years, the survival at 5 years was under 50% and nearly 70%, respectively, for those with versus those without a second cancer in the first 2 years.[71] Prevention and detection of these second primary tumors may play the most important role in improving overall survival rates in the future.[68]

Local and Distant Metastasis

Squamous cell carcinoma of the UADT predominantly metastasizes to the lymph nodes of the neck, the site of the involved nodes being dependent on the localization of the primary tumor (see Chapter 10).[80, 81] The adverse influence of metastatic neck node deposits on patient survival is firmly established, the prognosis being diminished roughly by half if lymph node metastases are present at presentation or during follow-up.[82–87] Prognosis further worsens if the tumor spreads beyond the lymph node into the soft tissues of the neck; this growth pattern is known as extracapsular spread.[82, 83, 85, 88–92] Whether there is any prognostic difference between gross extracapsular spread and microscopic extracapsular extension is controversial. Two studies identified macroscopic transcapsular spread as the major prognostic factor,[89, 90] whereas others found this prognostic significance also for histologically observed capsular penetration.[91, 92] Extracapsular spread is only slightly correlated with nodal size; nodes less than 1 cm may already exhibit this feature.[89]

Not only extracapsular spread but also the presence of a desmoplastic stromal response in tumor-positive lymph nodes has been shown to worsen prognosis.[92] The prognostic significance of neck node disease justifies a very meticulous examination of neck dissection specimens, as a high incidence of micrometastases (size <3 mm) has been found in patients without clinically manifest neck node disease.[93] Therefore, one should realize that, although pretreatment evaluation of nodal status in many institutions is based on palpation, depending on palpation for detection or exclusion of nodal involvement has proven unreliable; nevertheless, it remains part of the initial staging.[93]

Neck node disease also correlates with an increased risk for development of distant metastases.[94–96] Patients with disease in the neck had twice as many distant metastases as those without (13.6% versus 6.9%), whereas the presence of extranodal spread meant a threefold increase in the incidence of distant metastases, compared with patients without this feature (19.1% versus 6.7%).[95] Originally, distant metastases defined as metastatic SCC at sites below the clavicle were considered to be rare.[97] However, since this report in the early 1920s, the occurrence of distant metastases of UADT-SCC, predominantly occurring in the lungs, has been extensively demonstrated in clinical as well as autopsy studies (Figs. 2–1, see p. 35, and 2–2).[96, 98–112] As the lungs are also the most common site of second primary tumors in patients with UADT-SCC, it has not always been possible to answer the question as to whether a lung lesion is a second primary tumor or a metastasis from a UADT-SCC.[107, 113–115] Demonstrating origin from a bronchus supports the

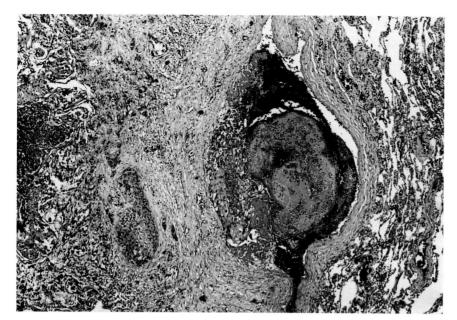

Figure 2–2. Photomicrograph shows tumor in a thrombosed lung blood vessel as well as tumor growing elsewhere in the lung. In this way head and neck tumors may spread to the lung.

diagnosis of a second primary tumor, but the small size of endobronchial biopsies does not always allow evaluation of this feature.

Histology and Prognosis

A UADT-SCC is a malignant epithelial tumor with squamous differentiation characterized by the formation of keratin or the presence of intercellular bridges or both.[116] This diagnosis is usually not difficult to make, the most significant diagnostic problem being very marked pseudoepitheliomatous hyperplasia of the mucosa, often overlying a granular cell tumor or an infectious process that may be mistaken for SCC.[117] However, when trying to infer data with prognostic significance from the histology, one enters an area replete with difficulties and uncertainties. In fact, tumor size and stage still represent the most significant prognostic factors for a patient with a UADT-SCC,[118] and whether careful assessment of histomorphologic features adds anything of relevance to the prognosis other than at a statistical level is doubtful.

Nevertheless, for over 70 years pathologists have been trying to obtain information regarding prognosis by scrutinizing their histologic slides. When briefly reviewing this area, studies aimed at establishing associations between histology and survival as well as between histology and neck node disease will be taken into account. Different approaches have been followed to obtain prognostically relevant data from histologic examination. The first attempts were done by Broders.[119] His classification system was based on the proportion of the neoplasm resembling normal squamous epithelium. Although some authors report histologic grade to have prognostic significance,[120] UADT-SCC in most instances exhibits a heterogeneous cell population with differences in the degree of differentiation, which may lead to a high degree of intraobserver and interobserver differences in the histologic grading of a tumor. Furthermore, in practice, most of the UADT-SCC are graded as moderately differentiated, which may explain the poor correlation between patient outcome and histologic grading based on degree of differentiation.[121, 122] In an extensive multicenter study on more than 3000 patients, it was concluded that grading of UADT-SCC, although a common practice, has not evolved as an important factor in treatment planning, this being due to the modest differences in survival rates between well and poorly differentiated tumors.[123]

To obtain a more detailed morphologic evaluation of the growth potential of a UADT-SCC, Jakobsson et al.[124] developed a multifactorial grading system, thereby paying attention not only to

tumor features but also to the relationship of the tumor to the surrounding host tissue. This system has been used for SCC at various locations in the UADT with varying results, as reviewed by Anneroth et al.[125] Some studies indicate that the value of this multifactorial grading system may improve when only the deeply invasive margins of the tumor are evaluated.[126–134] Tumor features that are assessed in this multifactorial grading system are degree of keratinization, nuclear pleomorphism, and number of mitotic figures. Features related with tumor-host relationship are pattern of invasion, stage of invasion, and extent of peritumoral lymphoplasmacytic infiltration. Each assessed feature is scored from 1 to 4 and the scores for each morphologic feature are added together into a total malignancy score.[125]

As not all morphologic features are necessarily of equal prognostic importance, however, attention also has been paid to the importance of individual histologic parameters. The most important appears to be the pattern of invasion, tumors invading with pushing borders being less aggressive than tumors exhibiting diffuse spread with tiny strands or single cells (Fig. 2–3).[126, 130–132, 135–147] Data on the specific significance of other parameters from the multifactorial grading system are less extensive. The importance of the number of mitoses has been demonstrated in two studies.[130, 136] Moreover, a grading system based on the presence or absence of keratin (Fig. 2–4) as the only parameter to divide between well-differentiated and poorly differentiated cases was shown to make an independent statistically significant contribution to the prediction of prognosis.[140]

When looking at the peritumoral lymphocytic infiltrate, one study mentions an inverse correlation between extent of infiltrate and incidence of neck node metastasis[148]; no prognostic significance for this feature was found in other investigations.[138, 143, 146] However, when analyzing the significance of individual cellular components, the number of T-lymphocytes appeared to have some relevance.[130, 132, 149–152] The host's reaction to an SCC may be visible not only as a peritumoral lymphocytic infiltrate but also as tumor-associated tissue eosinophilia, a feature of uncertain prognostic significance.[153–156]

Other histologic items that are not included in this multifactorial grading system[125] but nevertheless are considered to be prognostically important are tumor thickness,[126, 138, 146, 148, 157–171] perineural growth (Fig. 2–5),[126, 135, 159, 164, 171–175] and vascular invasion (Fig. 2–6).[138, 144, 147, 159, 164, 170, 176, 177] The significance of the density of tumor vessels in the stroma adjacent to the tumor is controversial.[178–187] Concerning perineural invasion, one should be aware of the fact that in and around the oral cavity, intraneural and perineural epithelial structures are present that are not associated with malignant growth but probably are persisting epithelial embryologic structures.[188–193] Those structures are found at the medial surface of the mandible in the area where the mandibular raphe is present[188] and are known as Chievitz's organ,[189, 191–193] or they may be present in association with intrabony nerves, probably representing odontogenic epithelial nests[190, 193] (Fig. 2–7), as well as in the anterior maxilla, probably representing a nasopalatine duct remnant.[193] The intimate relationship between these islands of epithelium and peripheral nerves could be erroneously interpreted to represent perineural and intraneural invasion.[193]

Aside from the evaluation of the aforementioned tumor features that could be prognostically significant, the pathologist contributes to an additional significant prognostic parameter by evaluating the completeness of primary excision.[121] Almost all authors who have investigated the significance of tumor at the surgical margins agree that this finding is associated with an increase in local recurrence and in mortality. Some authors observed this association only in patients with invasive tumor at the margins[166, 194–196]; others found the same negative influence in the event of tumor close to the margins (<5 mm)[144, 197] or with patients having dysplasia or carcinoma in situ at the surgical margins.[198–201] Probably, the negative influence

of positive surgical margins is due, at least partly, to its close association with other tumor factors that have an adverse effect on prognosis, especially T-stage.[202, 203] In a series of small intraoral cancers, completeness of excision turned out to be the only factor of prognostic relevance, other histologic variables being irrelevant in predicting recurrence at the primary site.[204] In this study, definition of completeness of excision was dependent on tumor features. In the event of invasive growth in tiny nests and strands of tumor cells, the distance between individual tumor nests had to be less than the distance between the resection margin and the tumor nest closest to this margin. Thus, if the distance between tumor nests was greater than the margin–tumor distance, resection was considered not to be sufficiently radical, and hence the surgery was tabulated as incomplete.

It is obvious from the foregoing that, when dealing with an UADT-SCC specimen, the pathologist should pay attention to all tumor features that may assist the clinician in assessing the need for further treatment. Therefore, the pathology report should at least include data on tumor size and thickness, growth pattern, perineural and vasoinvasive growth, degree of differentiation, and evaluation of the margins. If a neck dissection is included, the size, number, site, side relative to the primary tumor, and presence or absence of extracapsular spread should be stated because of prognostic signifi-

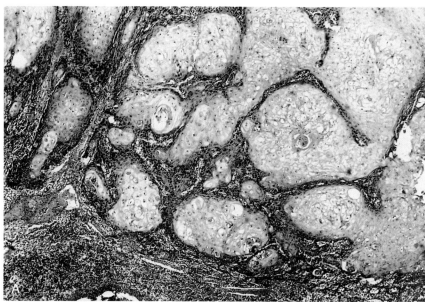
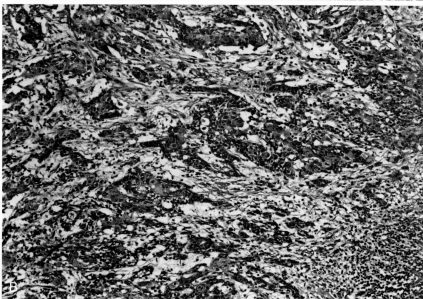

Figure 2–3. *A,* Squamous cell carcinoma growing in large cohesive fields. *B,* Squamous cell carcinoma growing in tiny strands.

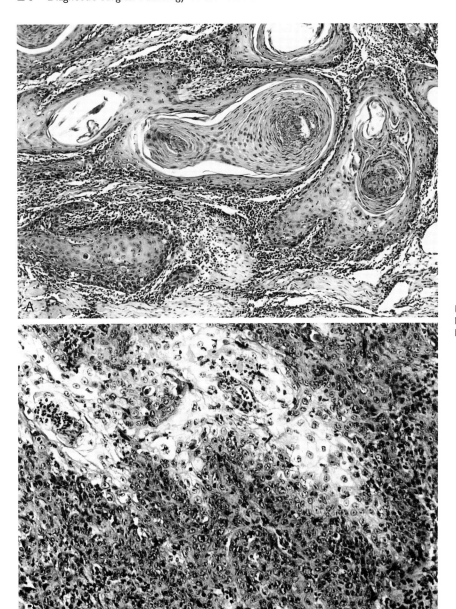

Figure 2–4. *A,* Squamous cell carcinoma with large keratin masses. *B,* Squamous cell carcinoma lacking keratin; only spinous differentiation can be observed.

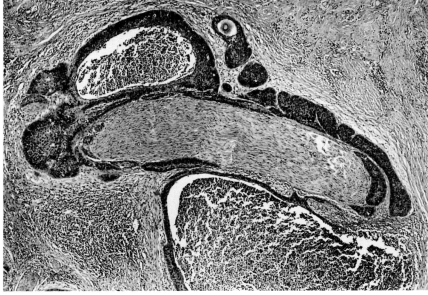

Figure 2–5. Photomicrograph showing squamous cell carcinoma growing perineurally.

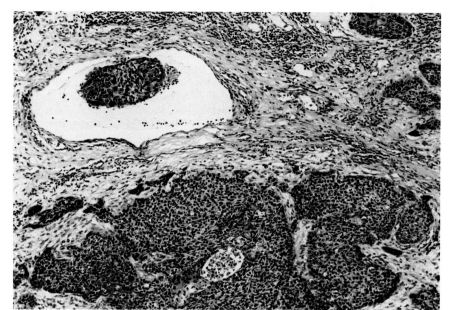

Figure 2–6. Photomicrograph showing squamous cell carcinoma with intravascular tumor embolus.

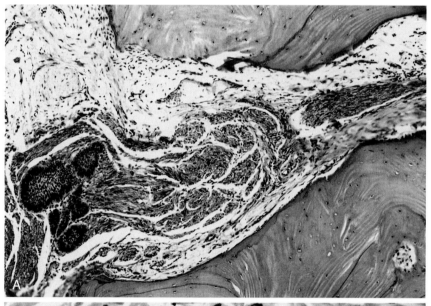

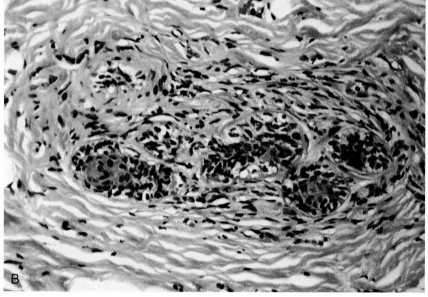

Figure 2–7. *A,* Odontogenic epithelial nests may be associated with nerves passing through the jaw bone. This feature should not be mistaken for perineural spread. *B,* Juxaoral organ of Chievitz (Chievitz's organ). Note nests of epithelial cells rest with peripheral polarization of some of the basal cells. These nests should not be misinterpreted as malignant.

cance.[205] A standard form may be helpful and will facilitate computer-based analysis when performing retrospective studies. A suggestion for standardization of surgical pathology reporting for larynx malignancies was recently published.[206]

In addition to studying conventional histopathologic aspects that could have prognostic significance, attempts have been made to obtain data with predictive value in other ways.[122, 207] Some authors have tried to obtain more objective data for features also assessed in routine histologic sections. This especially applies to rate of proliferation, originally measured by counting mitoses but nowadays analyzed by employing proliferation markers, antibodies directed at cellular proteins that are only expressed by cycling cells.[122] Until now, few studies have provided objective evidence for an association with number of proliferatively active tumor cells and patient outcome.[122, 130, 134, 208–213] The same applies for measuring proliferation by DNA flow cytometry.[214] Also, authors have tried to obtain more objective criteria for nuclear morphology by applying morphometric techniques, either singly[215–217] or in combination with cytophotometric DNA measuring.[141]

Whether p53 protein overexpression is of predictive value, either positive or negative, has been investigated extensively.[218] p53 protein overexpression has been reported to be predictive of shorter survival because of its association with earlier development of both tumor recurrence and second primary tumors.[219] Moreover, detection of cells harboring p53 gene mutations in lymph nodes and at surgical margins has been reported to improve the prediction of local tumor recurrence by demonstrating the presence of tumor cells at sites judged to be tumor-free by conventional histopathologic assessment.[220]

SITE-SPECIFIC FEATURES

Nasopharynx

The endodermally derived pharynx is traditionally divided into three functional and structural sections: the nasopharynx, the oropharynx, and the hypopharynx. The most cephalad of these divisions is a cuboidal structure, the nasopharynx. Anteriorly, the nasopharynx communicates with the nasal cavity via the choanae, laterally with the middle ears via the eustachian tubes, and inferiorly with the oropharynx. On the roof of the nasopharynx is the pharyngeal tonsil, which overlies the occipital bone and posterior portion of the body of the sphenoid bone. The floor of the nasopharynx is an imaginary horizontal line from the level of the palate to the posterior pharyngeal wall.

The distribution and frequency of occurrence of stratified squamous epithelium, intermediate epithelium (transitional), and ciliated epithelium within the nasopharynx has been mapped and outlined by Ali[221] and appears to be fairly constant between the ages of 10 and 50 years. Approximately 40% of the anterior wall and approximately 20% of the posterior wall are covered by ciliated epithelium. Occasional mucus-secreting cells may be seen in the posterior aspect of the nasopharynx.

One of the most important areas from a pathologic standpoint is the lateral wall of the nasopharynx. The lateral wall contains the site of the opening of the eustachian tube, which forms a triangular prominence, the torus tubarius. The fossa of Rosenmüller (pharyngeal recess, sinus of Morgagni, nasopharyngeal fossa) is a depression posterior to the torus tubarius. The fossa is formed by a herniation of the nasopharyngeal mucosa through a deficiency between the skull base and the most superior fibers of the superior constrictor muscle. The fossa also overlies the foramen lacerum. In an imaging study, the extent of the depth of the fossa of Rosenmüller was calculated to be greater than 10 mm and the orifice narrower than 5 mm in over 50% of the cases studied.[221] This increased depth may hinder accessibility to biopsy and would be clinically significant because the fossa of Rosenmüller is the most common site of origin for nasopharyngeal carcinoma.[222–224]

An extensive network of lymphatics drains the nasopharynx. Those from the roof and posterior wall join in the midline, pass through the pharyngeal fascia, and drain to the right and left retropharyngeal lymph nodes (nodes of Rouviére). The other two chains frequently receiving drainage from the nasopharynx are the cervical chain and the spinal accessory nodes. A well-recognized initial presentation for nasopharyngeal carcinoma (NPC) is a metastatic lymph node deposit within jugular or supraclavicular areas of the neck.[80] Presentation in the apex of the posterior triangle of the neck is a noteworthy characteristic of nasopharyngeal carcinoma. Other common sites of metastasis from the nasopharynx are the lymph nodes of the retropharyngeal space.[225]

Etiology. The etiology of nasopharyngeal carcinoma is a multifactorial interaction of race, genetics, environment, and EBV.[226] Reports of familial clusters suggest a genetic component.[226–228] Genetic susceptibility in Chinese people has been noted with HLA-A2 and other additional loci at B (HLA-B17, HLA-Bw46, HLA-Bsin2).[229, 230] Dietary factors have been proposed, such as nitrosamine-rich salted fish (Chinese style) in Southeast China, which has one of the highest incidences, particularly among the seafaring Tankas, for whom salted fish is a prominent dietary component.[231, 232] The dietary factors, however, have not explained the male:female ratio of 3:1 (which is seen in both endemic and nonendemic areas) or the ubiquitous association with EBV.[226, 233]

Presence of EBV within the epithelial cells and not the lymphoid infiltrate has been demonstrated by various methodologies, including karyotyping, electron microscopy, in situ hybridization, polymerase chain reaction (PCR), and immunohistochemistry.[226, 230, 234, 235, 236–238] Serologic association of EBV with nasopharyngeal carcinoma was first noted by Old et al.[239] and subsequently verified by Henle et al.[240] High titers of IgA antibodies to EBV-specific antigens, viral capsulated antigen, and early antigen have been reported to correlate with tumor-burden, relapse, and clinical progression.[226, 233]

Cytogenetic studies have shown a consistent loss of genetic material at two defined loci (RAF-1 and D3 S3) on the short arm of chromosome 3 in Chinese patients with nasopharyngeal carcinoma.[236] Both the loss of genetic material and EBV genome have been found in the same tumor.[236] Loss of genetic material was observed at early stages of disease.[226] Further studies will be needed to confirm the significance of these cytogenetic findings.

Clinical Features. Nasopharyngeal carcinoma occurs in all age groups, most commonly in those 40 to 60 years old.[229] It is most common in males, by a 3:1 ratio, in contrast to SCC of other head and neck sites, which show an even higher male incidence of 9:1.[233] In some intermediate and low-risk areas, there is a bimodal age distribution, with peaks in the second and sixth decades.[241, 242] In the United States among blacks, there is a peak in 10 to 19 year olds.[243] In areas of Africa, nasopharyngeal carcinoma accounts for approximately 10% to 20% of childhood malignancies[235]; and in the Sudan, it is the most common pediatric cancer.[244] In the high incidence region of Southern China, however, nasopharyngeal carcinoma is only rarely seen in children.[235]

The most common site of origin for nasopharyngeal carcinoma is on the lateral wall at the fossa of Rosenmüller. In a study of 342 cases of nasopharyngeal carcinoma, 82% occurred in the lateral pharynx and 12% in the midline, and in the remaining 6% the nasopharyngeal mucosa appeared normal.[245] Patients may present with a variety of symptoms: serous otitis media, nasal obstruction, epistaxis, or cervical adenopathy commonly seen in the apex of the posterior cervical triangle. The majority of patients (60–72%) will present with unilateral or bilateral cervical adenopathy.[233] The site of the primary tumor may be occult.

More advanced disease is usually present if the patient is presenting with hearing loss, otalgia, headache, or evidence of cranial nerve involvement (10–12% of the cases).[229] The cranial nerve involvement is easily explained by the proximity of the nasopharynx to the foramen lacerum and the contents of the most commonly involved region in nasopharyngeal carcinoma extension, the paranaso-

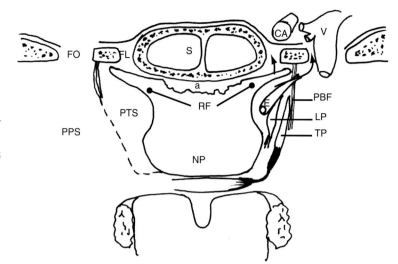

Figure 2–8. Schematic horizontal section through the nasopharynx (NP). a, adenoids; CA, carotid artery; E, eustachian tube; FL, foramen lacerum; FO, foramen ovale; LP, levator palati; PBF, pharyngobasilar fascia; PPS, parapharyngeal space; PTS, paratubal space, RF, Rosenmüller's fossa; S, sphenoid sinus; TP, tensor palati; V, trigeminal ganglion.

pharyngeal space that contains branches of the trigeminal nerve (Fig. 2–8).[246, 247] In one computed tomography (CT) study of 262 patients with nasopharyngeal carcinoma, cranial nerve palsy of the third through the sixth cranial nerves had evidence of erosion of the base of the skull; however, the reverse was not found.[248] Other presentations or evidence of relapse of tumor may be paraneoplastic syndromes such as hypertrophic osteoarthropathy syndrome (Pierre-Marie syndrome), leukemoid reaction, and fever of unknown origin.[249]

One of the unique clinical features of nasopharyngeal carcinoma is the propensity for distant metastasis. At the time of presentation, 5% to 11% of patients have distant metastases.[250] During the course of the disease, 50% to 60% of patients develop distant metastases.[249] Autopsy series report the overall metastasis incidence to be 87%, with the common sites being bone, lung, and liver.[233, 251, 252] The natural history of disease progression is short, with 78% of metastases occurring within 18 months of the first symptoms.[233] After detection of systemic metastases, median survival is only about 6 months.[253] The frequency of distant metastatic sites for nasopharyngeal carcinoma as compared with those of other UADT-SCC is the following: bone (65% versus 25% UADT-SCC); liver (29% versus 23% UADT-SCC); and lung (18% versus 84% UADT-SCC).[249] Approximately 25% of patients with evidence of metastatic disease will have involvement of the bone marrow.[249]

A number of different staging systems for nasopharyngeal carcinoma have been developed in different parts of the world. Among the most important are the Ho,[224] the Kyoto,[254] and the American Joint Committee on Cancer/Union Internationale Contre le Cancer (AJCC/UICC)[255, 256] tumor, node, and metastasis (TNM) classifications. The most recent TNM classification proposed by the AJCC[255] and UICC[256] can be found in the Appendix on Head and Neck Tumors: TNM staging. The original staging system proposed by Ho, developed in an area with one of the highest incidences of nasopharyngeal carcinoma, has undergone some modification,[257] which has reduced the number of stages without reducing the accuracy of predicting prognosis. Some advocate that the modified classification of Ho's system shows a more even distribution of patients among stages, with a greater power of predicting prognosis, than other classification systems (Table 2–1).[254] Unfortunately, there has not been one single generally accepted classification for comparison of treatment of nasopharyngeal carcinoma between centers.

Pathology. Cancer of the nasopharynx accounts for 3.7% of the UADT.[14] All forms of nasopharyngeal carcinoma are derived from the surface epithelium of the nasopharynx, having ultrastructural features such as tonofilaments and desmosomes of SCC.[258, 259] Tumors with glandular differentiation do not form part of the histologic spectrum shown by nasopharyngeal carcinoma.

When comparing the revised World Health Organization (WHO) classification (1991) with the first one (1978) there are significant alterations, as shown in Table 2–2.[116, 260] The second edition of the WHO histologic typing of UADT tumors divides nasopharyngeal carcinoma into two broad histologic types, keratinizing SCC and nonkeratinizing carcinomas. This dichotomy is based on the observation that both nonkeratinizing types of nasopharyngeal carcinoma are associated with a marked propensity for cervical lymph node metastasis and radiosensitivity; they have clinical evidence of metastasis ranging from 80% to 90%, and bilateral neck nodes are present in about 40% of patients.[245] Irrespective of their histologic subtypes, almost 100% of cases of nasopharyngeal carcinoma have demonstrable EBV-encoded small RNAs in the nuclei of their tumor cells, as demonstrated by in situ hybridization,[234, 250] although the positive hybridization signal in keratinizing nasopharyngeal carcinoma was less in proportion to malignant cells, usually limited to basal cells, than in other histologic types of nasopharyngeal carcinoma.[250]

Keratinizing nasopharyngeal carcinoma exhibits the features of a conventional SCC as occurs anywhere in the UADT. These keratinizing tumors (1) are infrequently seen in high incidence areas (less than 5%),[226] (2) represent one quarter to one half of nasopharyngeal carcinoma in low-incidence populations,[226, 229] (3) are less often associated with lymph node or distant metastases,[233] (4) are usually not radiosensitive,[226] (5) occur primarily in adults, and (6) have been associated with cigarette smoking.[226, 261]

The nonkeratinizing carcinoma group is subclassified into differentiated and undifferentiated subtypes.[116] As mentioned earlier, these two subclassified groups have overlapping histologic features and similar epidemiologic and biologic characteristics (frequent lymph node involvement and distant metastases). Nasopharyngeal carcinoma nonkeratinizing, differentiated consists of cells in which squamous differentiation is not evident on light microscopy; these cells have distinct margins and usually form plexiform masses and papillary structures. Some find this pavement-like arrangement of cells with well-defined borders reminiscent of urothelial transitional cell carcinoma[229] and thus this type of NPC may mimic cylindrical cell carcinoma, an SCC type occurring in the sinonasal cavities and discussed under that heading.

Undifferentiated carcinoma consists of cells with oval or round vesicular nuclei and prominent nucleoli. The cell margins are indistinct, imparting a characteristic syncytial growth pattern, and the cells may be arranged in irregular masses or as loosely connected cells in a lymphoid stroma.[116] When associated with a lymphoid stroma, these tumors may be referred to as the lymphoepithelial type of undifferentiated carcinoma or as lymphoepithelioma, an entity to be discussed under a separate heading.

Table 2–1. Ho's Classification and Modified Ho's Classification

Stage Classification		Ho's Classification (1978) (224)	Stage Classification		Modified Ho's Classification 1989
T stage	T1	Tumor confined to the nasopharynx (space behind choanal orifices and nasal septum and above the posterior margin of the soft palate in the resting position)	T stage	T1 and T3	Same as those of Ho's classification (1978)
	T2	Extension to the nasal fossa, oropharynx, or adjacent muscles or nerves below the base of the skull		T2N	Nasal fossa(e) involvement without parapharyngeal involvement or T3 features
	T3	Beyond T2 limits			
		T3a Bone involvement below the base of the skull; this includes floor of the sphenoid sinus			
		T3b Involvement of the base of the skull			
		T3c Involvement of the cranial nerve(s)			
		T3d Involvement of the orbits, laryngopharynx, or infratemporal fossa			
N stage	N0	No cervical lymph nodes palpable	N stage	N0, N1, N2, N3	Same as those of Ho's classification (1978)
	N1	Node(s) wholly in the upper cervical level bounded below by the skin crease extending laterally and backward from or just below the thyroid notch (laryngeal eminence)			
	N2	Node(s) palpable between the crease and the supraclavicular fossa, the upper limit being a line joining the upper margin of the sternal end of the clavicle and the apex of an angle formed by the lateral surface of the neck and the superior margin of the trapezius			
	N3	Node(s) palpable in the supraclavicular fossa and/or skin involvement in the form of carcinoma on cuirasse (with diffuse skin involvement) or satellite nodules above the clavicles			
M stage	M0	No hematogenous metastases	M stage	M0, M1	Same as those of Ho's classification (1978)
	M1	Hematogenous metastases present, and/or lymph nodal metastases below the clavicle			
Stage grouping	I	T1 N0	Stage grouping	I	(T1, T2N, T20) N0 M0
	II	T2 and/or N1		IIa	(T1, T2N, T20) (N1 N2) M0
	III	T3 and/or N2		IIb	(T2p, T3, T3p) N0 M0
	IV	N3 (any T)		IIIa	(T2p, T3, T3p) (N1, N2) M0
	V	M1		IIIb	(T1, T2n, T2p) N3 M0
				IVa	(T2p, T3, T3p) N3 M0
				IVb	M1 (any T, any N)

Modified from Teo PM, Leung SF, Yu P, et al: A comparison of the Ho's, International Union Against Cancer, and American Joint Committee stage classifications for nasopharyngeal carcinoma. Cancer 1991;67:434–439.

The distinction between these three histologic types—squamous cell carcinoma, differentiated nonkeratinizing carcinoma, and undifferentiated carcinoma—is not always sharp. In one study, 26% of 363 nasopharyngeal carcinomas examined had more than one histologic type.[259] In biopsies with more than one histologic type, the tumor is classified by the predominant histologic type.[259] Some have found the demarcation between the subtypes of nonkeratinizing carcinoma to be the most problematic.[262, 263] A practical approach is to classify nasopharyngeal carcinoma as differentiated nonkeratinizing if there is evidence of maturation (flattening or spindling) within the tumor cords. The distinction between the differentiated nonkeratinizing carcinoma and the undifferentiated carcinoma may be more academic than real when considering prognosis; however, knowledge of the histologic features may prove useful when confronted with subsequent metastatic disease.

Differential Diagnosis. Keratinizing nasopharyngeal carcinoma should not give origin to differential diagnostic problems other than for SCC at other UADT sites. Differentiated nonkeratinizing nasopharyngeal carcinoma may resemble, as already mentioned, cylindrical cell carcinoma of the paranasal sinuses. Further details on differential diagnosis of the nasopharyngeal carcinoma, undifferentiated type will be mentioned when lymphoepithelioma is discussed.

Treatment and Prognosis. For treatment of nasopharyngeal carcinoma, irradiation is usually the first choice. The survival of nasopharyngeal carcinoma patients is influenced by age, sex, T and N stage, and histologic type, undifferentiated nasopharyngeal carcinoma being more radiosensitive than SCC.[229] For patients treated with radiotherapy, 5- and 10-year survival rates have been reported to be 58% and 47%, respectively.[264] The treatment modality for nasopharyngeal carcinoma is based on the histologic type, keratinizing versus nonkeratinizing carcinoma. The nonkeratinizing histologic types are radiosensitive. External beam-supervoltage radiotherapy is the standard treatment of locoregionally confined nasopharyngeal carcinoma.[226] The keratinizing types of NPC have poor response to irradiation and are, therefore, more amenable to surgical resec-

Table 2–2. Classification of Nasopharyngeal Carcinoma (116, 260)

World Health Organization (1978)

1. Squamous cell carcinoma (WHO type I)
2. Nonkeratinizing carcinoma (WHO type II)
3. Undifferentiated carcinoma (WHO type III)

World Health Organization (1991)

1. Squamous cell carcinoma
2. Nonkeratinizing carcinoma
   A. Differentiated nonkeratinizing carcinoma
   B. Undifferentiated carcinoma

Data from Shanmugaratnam K: Histological Typing of Tumours of the Upper Respiratory Tract and Ear, 2nd ed. Berlin: Springer, 1991:28–33; Shanmugaratnam K: Histologic Typing of Upper Respiratory Tract Tumours. International Typing of Tumours, No. 19. Geneva: World Health Organization, 1978:32–33.

tion.[229] Although improvements in radiation technique have occurred, both local control and distant failure remain a problem. Neoadjuvant chemotherapy studies have shown nasopharyngeal carcinoma to be sensitive to pre-irradiation chemotherapy.[226] In one matched cohort study of 61 patients with locoregional stage IV nasopharyngeal carcinoma, induction chemotherapy (cisplatin-5FU) followed by radiotherapy improved rates of 5-year cumulative incidence of distant metastasis ($19\pm5\%$ versus $34\pm6\%$), 5-year actuarial disease-free survival ($64\pm6\%$ versus $42\pm7\%$), and 5-year actuarial overall survival ($69\pm6\%$ versus $48\pm7\%$), as compared with radiotherapy alone.[265] The patients were matched for T classification, N classification, histology, and level of cervical lymph node metastases.

Several features have prognostic significance in nasopharyngeal carcinoma. Those features associated with a favorable outcome are (1) female gender, (2) younger than 40 years of age at onset, and (3) lymphoepithelioma histology.[230] Those features associated with unfavorable prognosis are (1) symptoms for more than 1 year, (2) keratinizing carcinoma histology, (3) positive lymph nodes in the lower neck, (4) cranial nerve involvement, and (5) distant metasta-

ses.[230] Those features not appearing to have an impact on prognosis are (1) unilateral or bilateral lymph nodes in the upper neck, (2) fixed nodes, and (3) involvement of bone at the base skull base.[230]

Sinonasal Cavities

The sinonasal region is located in the mid-portion of the face and is composed of the centrally located paired nasal cavities surrounded by paired paranasal sinuses. The paranasal sinuses comprise the maxillary, frontal, ethmoidal, and sphenoidal sinuses. This maze of cavities abuts the base of the skull and lies adjacent to vital structures (Fig. 2–9).

The nasal cavity has a roof, floor, lateral wall, and septum. It is divided anteriorly into the nasal vestibule and posteriorly into the nasal antrum with turbinates. The nasal vestibule is bordered inferiorly by the palatine process of the maxilla and medially by the septal cartilage, and the superior and lateral walls are composed by the soft tissue of the nasal ala. The soft tissue lining of the vestibule is an extension of integument, with its keratinizing stratified squamous epithelium and secondary appendages. This lining extends for approximately 1 to 2 cm from the external rim of the nose into the nares. Just beyond the limen nasi (which is a ridge across the roof of the nasal cavity formed by a border of the upper lateral cartilage) is roughly the location of the mucocutaneous junction. This junction demarcates the beginning of the respiratory mucosa of ectodermal origin, which is referred to as the schneiderian membrane. This membrane lines the nasal antrum with turbinates and paranasal sinuses. The superior, middle, and inferior turbinates (conchae), which have associated meatuses, hang into the nasal lumen along the lateral walls of the nasal cavity. The roof is formed by the cribriform plate, the sphenoid bone, and the frontal bone. Posteriorly, the conchae end approximately 1 cm anterior to the choanal orifice, which is a continuum of the posterior aspect of the nasal cavity into the anterior opening of the nasopharynx.

The ethmoid labyrinth in the adult is a completely pneumonized lattice of approximately 3 to 18 cells per side. The roof of the labyrinth is adjacent to the anterior cranial fossa. The lateral wall of the ethmoid is the medial wall (lamina papyracea) of the orbit, and the medial wall of the ethmoid sinus forms the lateral wall of the

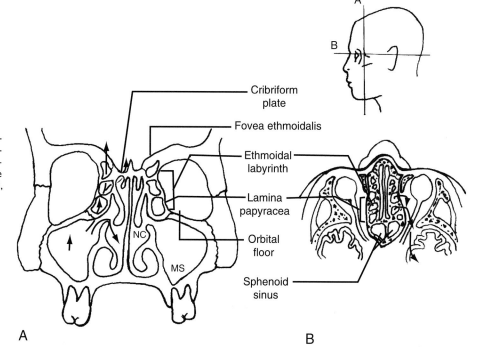

Figure 2–9. Sinus schematic with a *(A)* horizontal and *(B)* coronal section. The arrows indicate pathways of tumor spread into adjacent structures and sinuses via the intricate sinonasal labyrinth. MS, maxillary sinus; NC, nasal cavity.

Cribriform plate
Fovea ethmoidalis
Ethmoidal labyrinth
Lamina papyracea
Orbital floor
Sphenoid sinus

NC
MS

A

B

nose and attachment for the middle turbinate. Owing to the close proximity of the adjacent nasal passages and sinuses, the ethmoid sinus is the second most frequently involved sinus by tumor extension, after the maxillary sinus.

The maxillary sinus (antrum of Highmore) is the largest of the sinuses and encompasses the majority of the corpus of the maxilla. The walls of the maxillary sinus abutting the nasal cavity and orbit are thin, whereas those of the anterior and posterior walls are relatively thick. The apices of the premolars and molars of the maxilla protrude into the maxillary sinus and are covered by a thin plate of bone. The ostium from the maxillary sinus leads into an area within the middle meatus and is situated at the superior aspect of the maxillary sinus. The location of this ostium causes drainage of the sinus while in an upright position to be unfavorable.

Clinical Features. Malignancy of the sinonasal region represents 0.2% to 0.8% of all malignancies and approximately 3% of all those of the UADT.[20] SCC represents approximately 65% of the malignancies in the sinonasal region.[14, 266] The distribution of carcinoma by anatomic site is maxillary sinus (55–60%), nasal cavity (19–35%), ethmoid sinus (9–15%), nasal vestibule (4%), and frontal and sphenoid sinuses (1% each).[14, 267]

The majority of the tumors in this region present in a late stage, T3 and T4, as the initial presenting signs are usually nonspecific. The nonspecific findings have been noted to delay diagnoses from 3 to 14 months in one series.[268] Extent of tumor at the time of diagnosis best correlates with prognosis rather than degree of differentiation, with the exception of anaplastic carcinoma.[269]

Regional metastases from sinonasal neoplasms are uncommon (9–14% for SCC).[20] Metastasis from these tumors usually implies soft tissue extension (antral tumors, cheek and soft palate; ethmoid tumors, medial canthal skin and nasopharyngeal extension).[20] The maxillary sinus drains primarily to the submandibular nodes. The lymphatic drainage of the ethmoid labyrinth is to the superior cervical nodes, and some drain directly posteriorly to the retropharyngeal nodes.[270] With recent advances in imaging, assessment of retropharyngeal lymph nodes is possible.[225]

Although site-specific systems have been proposed,[271] the only internationally recognized staging system is for maxillary and ethmoid tumors. In 1938, Ohngren[272] proposed a theoretical plane from the medial canthus of the eye to the angle of the mandible, which created an anterior inferior infrastructure and a superior posterior suprastructure to the maxillary sinus area. This hypothetical division has clinical relevance, as the anterior inferior tumors present early, whereas the superior posterior tumors usually present after extensive tumor growth has occurred. The AJCC[273] and the UICC[274] have adopted a T classification for maxillary sinus and ethmoid as noted in the Appendix on TNM staging for Head and Neck Tumors.

Pathology. Within the histologic classification of the nasal cavity and paranasal sinuses, there is some confusing and controversial terminology. The majority of the carcinomas are of the keratinizing squamous variety, but most of the controversy revolves around the use of the terms cylindrical cell carcinoma (Ringertz' carcinoma), transitional cell carcinoma, and schneiderian carcinoma. Cylindrical cell carcinoma can be found in the literature since 1900 as a histologic type of nasal carcinoma but was fully described by Ringertz in 1938.[275] The histologic description given by Ringertz was of a sometimes papillary nonkeratinizing epithelial tumor that invaginated into the stroma. The invaginating epithelial growths had a palisading basal layer forming a crisp demarcation at the epithelial-stromal interface and forming a ribbon or garland-like pattern with zones of necrosis.

In the American literature over a decade earlier, Quick and Cutle[276] introduced the James Ewing term transitional cell carcinoma for a category of upper airway tumors that "exhibited transitional epithelial characteristics with cylindrical or cuboidal cells free of keratosis." While investigating the effects of irradiation on tumors of the upper airway, Ewing found that patients with transitional cell carcinoma survived longer and the tumors were more radiosensitive than the conventional SCC, hence justification for the entity. Ew-

ing's histologic description was similar to Ringertz' description. Ewing, however, attributed the necrosis to the effects of irradiation on the tumor. Schneiderian carcinoma was also a term coined by James Ewing. This term referred to poorly differentiated carcinomas originating from the schneiderian membrane and was never clearly defined as an entity.[275, 277] The term is infrequently used.

The term transitional carcinoma was used by later investigators to describe malignant transformation in transitional papillomas of the nasal cavity. "Transitional" was chosen because of the histologic resemblance of the malignant epithelium to that of transitional epithelium of the urogenital tract.[278, 279] Recent articles may be found that equate all three terms, transitional, schneiderian, and cylindrical cell carcinomas.[280]

Clinical justification for the separate classification of cylindrical cell carcinoma and transitional cell carcinoma was proposed by Friedmann and Osborn in 1982.[279] They observed cylindrical cell carcinoma to have a lesser tendency to spread via the lymphatics. Others, however, have reported cylindrical cell carcinoma to have a clinical course similar to that of SCC.[266, 281, 282] The current WHO classification recognizes cylindrical cell carcinoma in the sense as defined by Ringertz[275] as one of the histologic types of sinonasal carcinomas but does not use the term transitional carcinoma anymore.[262]

Within current American literature, the terms cylindrical cell carcinoma and transitional cell carcinoma are infrequently used. Some authors employ these designations to denote lesions also categorized as nonkeratinizing SCC of the nasal cavity and paranasal sinuses[283, 284] and consider them to be similar to nonkeratinizing nasopharyngeal carcinoma[284]; others use the term cylindrical cell carcinoma to identify a variant of sinonasal SCC that may exhibit intracellular mucin production and sometimes has a growth pattern similar to a papilloma, making stromal invasion not immediately apparent.[285] To end this discussion on semantics and nosology, we advocate usage of the WHO approach, recognizing cylindrical cell carcinoma as one of the variants of sinonasal SCC and recognizable by features as originally outlined by Ringertz—a papillary lesion composed of invaginating ribbons of pleomorphic nonkeratinizing cells that are mainly cylindrical and often arranged perpendicularly to the underlying basement membrane. The lesion invades with a pushing border, which makes stromal infiltration not immediately apparent when evaluating small biopsies (Fig. 2–10). The tumor may exhibit squamous metaplasia which, if extensive, makes cylindrical cell carcinoma indistinguishable from conventional SCC. Sometimes cylindrical cell carcinoma contains foci of less well differentiated tumors such as small cell carcinoma or high grade adenocarcinoma.[116, 275] Scarcity of data prevents assessment of the significance of this observation. To facilitate future studies, it is wise to diagnose these cases as cylindrical cell carcinoma while recording that other histologic features are also observed.

Differential Diagnosis. Cylindrical cell carcinoma should not be confused with papillary squamous cell carcinoma (PSCC), a lesion to be discussed more extensively in the section devoted to specific variants of SCC. Distinctive features are the lack of cylindrical cells in PSCC and the presence of papillary protrusions covered with an epithelial lining with the features of carcinoma in situ found in PSCC but absent in cylindrical cell carcinoma. Moreover, the histology of cylindrical cell carcinoma may mimic that of inverted papilloma. However, the presence of numerous microcysts in the multilayered epithelial ribbons in some parts of the material is valuable in confirming the diagnosis of inverted papilloma, whereas their absence in conjunction with cellular atypia should cause concern that the diagnosis might be SCC.[286]

Treatment and Prognosis. The probability of 5-year survival for patients with carcinoma of the sinonasal area is approximately 50%.[14] Within the nasal cavity, malignancy of the nasal vestibule and septum has a better prognosis, perhaps because of earlier diagnosis[266, 287, 288] than in the remainder of the nasal cavity and paranasal sinuses. For patients with antral and ethmoidal disease, the probability of surviving 5 years is 48% and 68%, respectively.[267] The

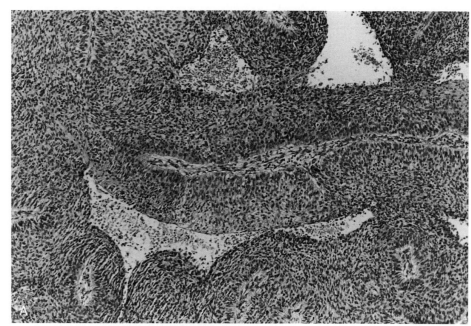

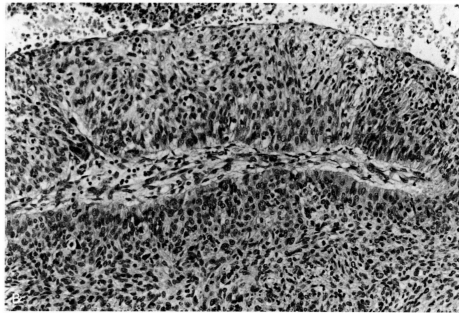

Figure 2–10. *A,* Low power micrograph of cylindrical cell carcinoma. The strands of polymorphic cells that make up the tumor show a well-defined interface with the adjacent stroma. *B,* At higher magnification, the polymorphous nature of the cells and the cylindrical aspect of basal and suprabasal cells are clearly shown.

5-year survival rate for patients with T2, T3, and T4 cancers of the antrum was 73%, 41%, and 15%, respectively.[268] There does not appear to be a significant correlation of survival with patient's sex or age at time of presentation.[268] Although multimodality therapy does not seem to change the 5-year survival rate, it appears to have improved the local control of tumor.[268] Factors limiting patient survival are related to local recurrence, nodal metastasis, soft tissue extension to the palate or nasopharynx, proptosis, and orbital symptoms, as metastases account for approximately 10% of deaths.[20, 289]

Larynx and Hypopharynx

The hypopharynx and larynx are anatomically intimately associated and constitute the division point between the digestive tract and the lower respiratory tract. Owing to the nature of their anatomic proximity, accurate identification of a primary tumor site may be difficult; however, identification of the primary site has prognostic significance. Malignancy of the hypopharynx/larynx in the United States represents approximately 34% of all UADT cancer; the larynx being the most common at 28% and the hypopharynx representing 6.6% of UADT.[14] Globally, tumors of the larynx are the second most common tumor of the respiratory tract and the 11th most common cancer in men.[15]

Hypopharynx

The conically shaped hypopharynx is the most caudate portion of the endodermally derived pharynx. It communicates superiorly with the oropharynx and inferiorly with the larynx and esophagus. The superior border of the hypopharynx is an imaginary horizontal line drawn across at the level of the tip of the epiglottis. The inferior boundary is defined anteriorly by the aryepiglottic folds, which lead to the endolarynx and posteriorly by the inlet to the cervical esophagus.

The hypopharynx is divided into three regions: the paired pyriform sinuses or recesses, the posterior pharyngeal wall, and the postcricoid region. The pyriform sinuses are bilaterally elongated, pear-shaped, three-walled gutters that open into the hypopharyngeal cavity and extend anteriorly and laterally on either side of the larynx. The borders of the pyriform sinus are formed superiorly by glossoepiglottic folds and medially by the hypopharyngeal surface of the aryepiglottic folds and the arytenoid and cricoid cartilages. The medial wall of the pyriform sinus is separated from the ventricle of the larynx and outer aspect of the cricoid cartilage by a thin submucosal layer of muscle.[290] The lateral wall of the pyriform sinus lies against the thyroid cartilage and blends into the posterior pharyngeal wall. Inferiorly, the pyriform sinus is in continuum with the entryway into the esophagus.

The posterior pharyngeal wall joins the lateral limits of the pyriform sinus and inferiorly with the cervical esophagus. The postcricoid region is a funnel-shaped area extending from the level of the arytenoid cartilages to the inferior border of the cricoid cartilage. Lateral borders of the postcricoid region blend with the pyriform sinus.

Stratified squamous epithelium lines the hypopharynx. The epithelium is nonkeratinizing; however, when subjected to chronic irritation, orthokeratinization or parakeratinization may be found. Within the submucosa are seromucinous glands, scattered lymphoid aggregates, and a rich anastomosing network of lymphatics.

Within the United States and Canada, the frequency of involvement within the hypopharynx by cancer is the pyriform sinus (65–85%), the posterior pharyngeal wall (10–20%), and the postcricoid area (5–15%).[291] Carcinoma of this region, with the exception of the postcricoid area, occurs predominantly in men and is associated with alcohol use and smoking.

Carcinomas of the hypopharynx generally have a poor prognosis, primarily because of a combination of unrestricted area for tumor growth, multifocality, and extensive lymphatic network. These tumors are notorious for submucosal spread beneath an intact mucosa, early lymph node metastasis, and a high rate of systemic metastases (20–40%).[291] There appears to be no relationship between the degree of differentiation and the invasiveness of hypopharyngeal SCC, which means that their clinical aggressiveness cannot be explained by a higher percentage of poorly differentiated cancers at this site.[292] Some investigators have estimated the extent of submucosal spread to be anywhere from 1.0 to 0.5 cm for pyriform sinus and postcricoid area, respectively.[293] This characteristic submucosal spread may not be accurately assessed clinically or by radiographic modalities (CT or MRI).[294, 295]

Because of the paucity of early presenting symptoms, most patients present with advanced disease. In a recent study of 408 patients with tumors of the pyriform sinus, 67% had T3 or T4 lesions and 87% were stage III or IV at presentation.[294] Approximately one fourth of these patients will present with a mass in the neck and 70% will have lymph node disease at presentation.[294, 296] Upper and middle cervical nodes of levels II and III are most commonly involved.[297]

Tumors of the pyriform sinus, particularly those involving the medial wall, frequently secondarily involve the larynx.[294, 298] The posterior hypopharyngeal wall tumors are usually exophytic and also frequently large at presentation (80% >5 cm).[291] Tumors of the posterior hypopharyngeal wall metastasize to upper and middle cervical nodes, and in over 40% of patients, the retropharyngeal nodes are involved.[291]

Carcinomas of the postcricoid area have shown a marked geographic variation in incidence. They are associated with Plummer-Vinson syndrome and nutritional deficiencies (see section on Epidemiology). Carcinoma of this area may extend inferiorly, involving the esophagus and trachea and thus necessitating the removal of a portion of the trachea. The lymphatics drain to the middle and lower cervical and paratracheal nodes. Eighteen percent will have bilateral cervical node metastases and most local recurrences are due to unrecognized involvement of the paratracheal nodes.[291]

The staging for the hypopharynx is primarily directed for tumors of the pyriform sinus. Within the former TNM classification system, a 4 to 5 cm posterior pharyngeal wall tumor without laryngeal fixation would remain a T1 lesion. The lesion, however, would have a prognosis similar to a T3 lesion.[299] The most recent AJCC/UICC[255, 256] staging for hypopharyngeal cancer recognizes tumor size as an additional issue in staging, as is mentioned in the Appendix on staging Head and Neck Tumors.

Treatment and Prognosis. Treatment for the hypopharynx is the combined use of radiation and surgery. The majority of lesions involve the pyriform sinus and combined therapy is recommended, with the exception of T1 and T2 lesions (single modality therapy).[294] In one large study of tumors of the pyriform sinus, the overall 5-year disease-free survival rate for combined therapy is 65.2%.[294] A drop in survival after 2 years is primarily due to distant metastasis and to second primary malignancies.[10] The value of adjunctive chemotherapy in pyriform sinus malignancy is still unclear.[10]

Larynx

The larynx is divided traditionally into three subsites: supraglottic, glottic, and subglottic regions (Fig. 2–11). Embryologically, the supraglottic region is derived from the third and fourth branchial arches (buccopharyngeal anlage), and the glottic and subglottic regions originate from the sixth branchial arch (pulmonary anlage). These two regions fuse somewhere at the level of the ventricle.[300]

Because of the embryologic derivation and independent lymphatic circulation, there is a unique compartmentalization of the larynx. The supraglottic region is one compartment and the glottic and subglottic regions make up the other compartment. The anatomic barriers have been demonstrated by dye studies and histology.[300] These anatomic barriers and the site of origin influence the growth and spread of laryngeal carcinoma.[301] The supraglottic area extends from the tip of the epiglottis superiorly to the ventricle inferiorly.

Encompassed within the supraglottic area is the epiglottis (lingual and laryngeal aspects), the laryngeal aspect of the aryepiglottic folds, the arytenoids, the false vocal cords, and the ventricles. The supraglottic area has frequently been subdivided into the suprahyoid and infrahyoid areas. Those carcinomas in the suprahyoid area (tip of epiglottic rim of aryepiglottic folds and arytenoids) tend to have a worse prognosis than infrahyoid tumors and behave similarly to hypopharyngeal tumors.[291] The inferior border of the supraglottis is an imaginary horizontal line drawn across the apex of the ventricle. The supraglottic larynx lymphatics drain laterally and superiorly through the thyrohyoid membrane and drain into the subdigastric and superior jugular nodes.

The glottis includes the paired true vocal cords and the anterior and posterior commissure. Lymphatics of the true vocal cords are sparse to nonexistent. The anterior commissure tendon (Broyles' ligament) is an important band of fibrous tissue that contains certain lymphatics and blood vessels and attaches to the thyroid cartilage devoid of the tumor-resistant perichondrium.[291] Tumors of the anterior commissure may grow upward to the epiglottis or may penetrate the thyroid cartilage, particularly if the thyroid cartilage has ossified. The inferior border of the glottic area is 1 cm below the apex of the ventricle. The subglottic area is from the lower edge of the glottis to the inferior aspect of the cricoid cartilage. The lymphatic drainage from these two areas is lateral and inferior through the cricothyroid membrane to the paratracheal nodes, deep cervical nodes, and prelaryngeal (Delphian) node.

Both lingual and superior portions of the laryngeal aspects of the epiglottis are covered by nonkeratinized stratified squamous epithelium. The stratified squamous epithelium on the inferior laryngeal aspect of the epiglottis merges with respiratory-type epithelium. Respiratory epithelium lines the false vocal cords, ventricle, and subglottis. The vibratory edge of the true vocal cord is lined by a nonkeratinizing stratified squamous epithelium. The interface between the ciliated columnar epithelium of the ventricle and the stratified squamous epithelium of the true vocal cord is often abrupt. There may be a "transitional" zone where the epithelium may appear "disorganized" and thickened and the cells may have enlarged basaloid features but mitotic figures are confined to the basal cell

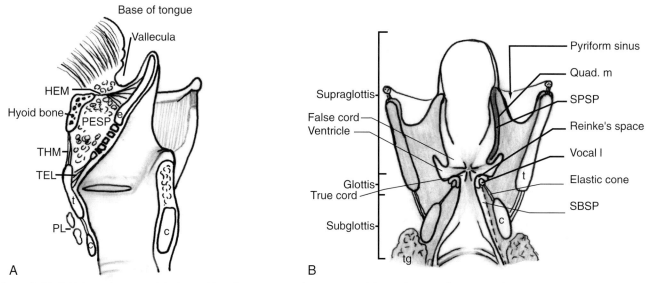

Figure 2–11. *A,* Midsagittal section of the larynx. Note fenestrations in lower aspect of the epiglottic cartilage. c, cricoid cartilage; e, epiglottis; HEM, hyoepiglottic membrane; PESP, pre-epiglottic space; PL, pre-laryngeal (Delphian) lymph nodes; t, thyroid cartilage; TEL, thyroepiglottic ligament; THM, thyrohyoid membrane. *B,* Coronal section of the larynx. c, cricoid; Quad. m, quadrangular membrane; SBSP, subglottic space; SPSP, supraglottic space; t, thyroid cartilage; tg, thyroid gland; Vocal l, vocal ligament.

layer.[302] This transitional zone is a metaplastic area and should not be mistaken for dysplasia or carcinoma in situ (Fig. 2–12, see p. 35).

A spatial subdivision within the larynx has been demonstrated through pathohistologic study of serial sections of the larynx (see Fig. 2–11). The majority of SCCs of the larynx have been observed to respect the limitations of the fibroelastic membranes and skeletal structures for an extended period of time.[303] This intralaryngeal compartmentalization has been the anatomic basis for various surgical procedures.[300] The first spatial area is known as the supraglottic space (not to be confused with the supraglottic region). This space extends from subjacent to the supraglottic mucosal surface to the quadrangular membrane and inferiorly to the lower edge of the vestibular ligaments and petiole. The space is bordered laterally by the quadrangular membrane and the laryngeal surface of the epiglottic cartilage.

The pre-epiglottic space is triangular and bounded superiorly by the hyoepiglottic ligament, anteriorly by the thyrohyoid membrane, and posteriorly by the epiglottis. There are foramina in the infrahyoid epiglottic cartilage that allow tumor spread from the laryngeal side of the epiglottis into this space and thus outside of the larynx. This space communicates in its inferior aspect with the paraglottic space.

The paraglottic space is the largest connecting spatial structure within the laryngeal soft tissues. This space surrounds the whole of the ventricles lateral to the quadrangular membrane and medial to perichondrium of the thyroid cartilage and is limited inferiorly by the elastic conus and the cricothyroid membrane. Recently described are elastic and fibroelastic membranes that are subjacent to ventricular mucosa and in continuity with the elastic conus and quadrangular membrane,[304] thus providing a continuous elastic membrane that bridges the supraglottis and glottic areas. Lesions from the pyriform sinus may involve this space. Tumors entering this space have the potential for spread to the pre-epiglottic space; thus, a glottic or subglottic lesion could gain access to the supraglottic region.

Reinke's space is of particular interest in that it is the smallest space to be described and lies between the vocal cord fold epithelium and the vocal ligament. This region is composed of a few blood vessels and very poor lymphatic drainage. Its widest extent is in the craniocaudal direction within the middle third of the vocal folds. The space narrows toward the anterior commissure.

The subglottic space is the most inferior space. The upper boundary is made up of the vocal ligament and elastic conus (fibers from the vocal ligament), which reaches the lower edge of the cricoid cartilage and extends into the submucosal region of the trachea. With this information, it should be noted that there is no vertical separation of the lymphatic drainage of the larynx into a left and right side and, therefore, as clinically observed, contralateral metastasis may be seen.

Clinical Features. In discussing the spread of laryngeal carcinoma, it should be noted that traditionally the tumors have been divided by site: supraglottic, glottic, transglottic, and subglottic. The supraglottic tumors involve the false vocal cord, the ventricle, and the epiglottis (laryngeal or lingual aspects) and represent about 30% to 35% of laryngeal tumors.[305] These tumors have a marked propensity to spread to the pre-epiglottic space primarily through fenestrations within the epiglottic cartilage. Approximately 1% of these supraglottic tumors invade the glottis. Invasion of cartilage is exceedingly rare, restricted only to those cases in which the cartilage has undergone osseous metaplasia. The incidence of lymph node metastasis averages about 40%. The tumors are primarily treated by irradiation or laryngectomy.

Tumors of the glottic area are the most frequent, accounting for approximately 60% to 65% of laryngeal carcinomas.[270] Glottic tumors arise from the true vocal cords, primarily from the anterior third of the vocal cord and frequently produce hoarseness. Because of early symptoms, tumors of the glottis may be found in an early stage. Five-year disease-free rates for T1 carcinomas (localized to the vocal cord) have been reported as high as 90%[306] and therefore these sites have a better prognosis than other laryngeal sites. The degree of anterior commissure involvement appears to have prognostic significance, patients with a progressively heavier involvement of the anterior commissure subsite having a progressively worse outcome.[307] The incidence of lymph node metastasis in T1 through T4 tumors is 1.9%, 16.7%, 25%, and 65%, respectively.[291] Lesions of the glottis tend to be localized for an extended period of time, primarily due to paucity of lymphatic vessels within Reinke's space and the cartilaginous walls. Early cases are usually treated by irradiation. Irradiation failures can be subsequently treated by salvage surgery.

The concept of a "transglottic lesion" was first presented in 1961 by McGavran.[135] The term *transglottic* does not refer to an anatomic site within the larynx but to a pattern of glottic tumor spread that crossed the laryngeal ventricle, therefore involving the supraglottis and glottis with paraglottic space involvement. This particular pattern of involvement appeared to have an aggressive clinical course with a high incidence of lymph node metastasis (52%).[135] Transglottic carcinomas are treated primarily by laryngectomy and lymph node dissections. They are fortunately less than 5% of all cases of laryngeal carcinoma.[305] With time and imprecise usage, there has been deviation from the original 1961 concept of transglottic tumor (supraglottic/glottic as well as glottic /infraglottic). Therefore, it is better to specify tumor extension by recording the defined anatomic subsites involved and refrain from the term *transglottic.*

The infraglottic or subglottic tumors are also rare, representing less than 5% of all the cases.[305] Tumors included within this category are tumors that involve the region between the lower edge of the true vocal cord (where the squamous epithelium ends) and the first tracheal cartilage[308] or extending 1 cm below the edge of the true cord.[305] Other investigators have defined the subglottis as extending from the lower boundary of the glottis to the lower margin of the cricoid cartilage.[206] The tumors limited to the subglottic area are exceedingly rare. This particular tumor frequently shows extension into the trachea. Metastasis to cervical lymph nodes is approximately 15% to 20% and the involvement of paratracheal lymph nodes is approximately 50%. These tumors are treated primarily by surgical excision and neck dissection, including the paratracheal lymph nodes.

The staging system for laryngeal carcinomas is mentioned in the Appendix on TNM staging for Head and Neck Tumors.[309] Several suggestions for alteration of the TNM classification system have been proposed.[310, 311] It has been argued that there are embryologic, anatomic, functional, and oncologic reasons to divide the larynx into two main areas only, the supraglottis and the glottis (vocal folds), without any further subsites and to abandon a separate group of subglottic tumors.[310] Moreover, it has been proposed that the T size of a tumor should not be assessed according to the extent of an anatomic region, but measured in millimeters of greatest surface extent only.[310] Furthermore, the T2 category of vocal cord tumors should not contain those that lead to an inhibited mobility of the fold. All tumors with reduced vocal fold mobility or fixation should be classified as T3 or T4.[310] Finally, the N status should include number, size, site of metastasis, and presence of extracapsular spread.[310] Other investigators found that the addition of clinical information—presence and intensity of local symptoms attributable to the tumor, perilocal symptoms attributable to the inflammation surrounding the tumor at its primary site, extralocal symptoms due to interference of the tumor with normal function within the upper aerodigestive tract or in the body as a whole, and distant symptoms implying that the tumor has spread beyond the primary locus—to the TNM classification had an impact on prognostic estimations.[311]

Treatment and Prognosis. In addition to the inverse relationship of primary tumor size with prognosis, lymph node metastasis is another extremely important prognostic factor in laryngeal cancer.[312] Both cervical metastasis and disease-free survival have been shown to be related to depth of invasion; for tumors with a thickness greater than or equal to 3.25 mm, an elective neck dissection is recommended.[313]

In advanced laryngeal carcinoma, cervical metastasis has been shown to be the most important prognostic variable for survival. A study with 159 patients (supraglottic 97, glottic 60, and subglottic 2) found disease-free survival rates to be 87% in patients with no regional metastasis, 82% in patients with one to two positive lymph nodes and 33% in patients with three or more positive lymph nodes ($P < .001$).[314] Risk of distant metastasis was 5% in node-negative patients and 36% in node-positive patients. Patients with three or more positive lymph nodes had decreased survival rates (at 48 months, for node-negative patients, 68%; for patients with one to two nodes, 62%; and for patients with three or more nodes, 20%). Distant metastasis was found to be more common in patients with involvement of lower jugular and supraclavicular lymph nodes.[314]

Extracapsular spread of carcinoma has significant impact on survival, a factor that is still ignored in the TNM staging, which does not include this issue as a separate item worthy of being recorded.[309]

In one series of patients, extracapsular spread was present in 31% of N1 nodes and the 5-year survival rate of patients without extracapsular spread was 76%, whereas for patients with nodal metastases showing this phenomenon it was only 17%.[312] The presence of extracapsular spread, no matter the size of the lymph node, should be included in the surgical pathology report. The prognostic significance of micrometastases is still being assessed.[93]

Differential Diagnosis. One of the more problematic areas of diagnosis in the larynx is in the evaluation of postirradiation persistence of SCC. Often dysplasia or atypia may be limited to the mucosa. Owing to the difficulty in distinguishing between tumor recurrence and postirradiation atypia, most pathologists would prefer to err on the side of conservatism. Pseudomalignant tissue reactions are well documented after irradiation. Full-thickness mucosal atypia that is histologically identical to dysplasia or carcinoma in situ may be observed. The distinction between benign and malignant can be very difficult with the diagnosis of malignancy based on stromal invasion. The histology of these radiation-induced lesions may show increased mitotic activity and even atypical mitotic figures. Grossly, the growths may be flat or broad-based polypoid lesions with ulceration and radiating vascular connective tissue. An indistinct border between the pleomorphic stromal cells and pleomorphic endothelial cells is a useful finding in radiation-induced atypia. The tinctorial quality of the cytoplasm may be gray-blue on hematoxylin-eosin stained sections. Immunohistochemistry and flow cytometry findings are nonspecific. When the examiner is trying to make the distinction between recurrent tumor and tissue reaction, finding low power granulation tissue architecture and similar degrees of cytologic atypia in both the endothelial cells and stroma aid in establishing the benign nature of the lesion.[315]

"Early" cancer of the larynx is a term that has been used to describe malignant lesions limited to the mucosa similar to a variety of other sites, including stomach, esophagus, cervix, and so on.[316] The "early" cancers of the larynx are usually located in the glottis. Unfortunately, the term has been used by clinicians and pathologists to convey different ideas. The clinical definition of early glottic cancer implies a Tcis or T1 lesion, with full chordal motility and no risk of neck metastasis. The pathologic definition describes a microscopically invasive carcinoma that transgresses the basement membrane but is confined to the lamina propria and has metastatic potential.[317] The pathologic description does not include extension into adjacent muscle or cartilage. Mucosal lesions of the glottis composed of carcinoma in situ with a microscopic focus of invasion or a "superficial extending" carcinoma (confined to the lamina propria)[318] represent early glottic cancer. Biologically, invasion is present, as is the potential for metastasis.[316]

Trachea

The trachea is a hollow tube beginning at the lower border of the cricoid cartilage, at the level of the sixth cervical vertebra, extending inferiorly via the thoracic inlet to the mediastinum and ending at the bifurcation into the left and right bronchi. The lining is a ciliated pseudostratified columnar epithelium. Within the underlying connective tissue are numerous minor seromucous glands. The walls are formed by hyaline cartilage rings that are incomplete posteriorly.

Neoplasms of the trachea are extremely rare. Malignancies of the trachea represent less than 0.2% of all malignancies within the respiratory tract and 0.04% of all malignant neoplasms.[319] Carcinoma is the most common malignant tumor occurring in the trachea and accounts for approximately 80% to 90% of all malignant tracheal neoplasms.[320, 321] Owing to the rarity of the tracheal carcinomas, there is limited knowledge of these neoplasms.

Clinical Features. The most frequent tumor site within the trachea is not well established. Some reports have placed the most frequent site within 4 cm of the carina,[322] while others have reported

Text continued on page 47

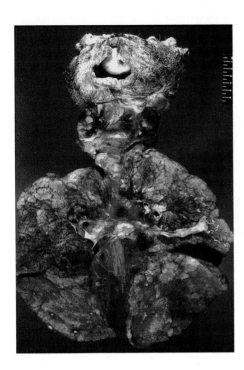

Figure 2–1. Autopsy specimen. A tumor originating in the floor of the mouth has perforated the skin of the chin (this is not the mouth). Pleural nodules indicative of distant metastasis are present in both lungs.

Figure 2–12. *A*, A section through the junction of the ventricular epithelium (right), true cord epithelium (left), and intermediate epithelium present between the two. *B*, Histologic section shows the presence of ventricular epithelium (left) and an extensive area of intermediate epithelium (right). Note extensive chronic inflammation within the underlying connective tissue and goblet cell formation within the ventricular epithelium. The transitional zone of intermediate epithelium has a slightly disordered appearance and immature squamous metaplasia. These may be misinterpreted as dysplasia.

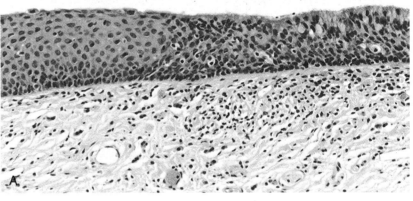

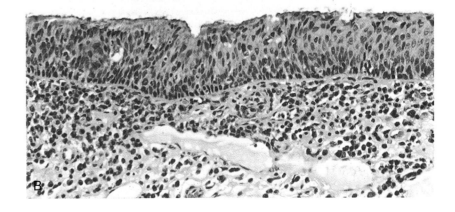

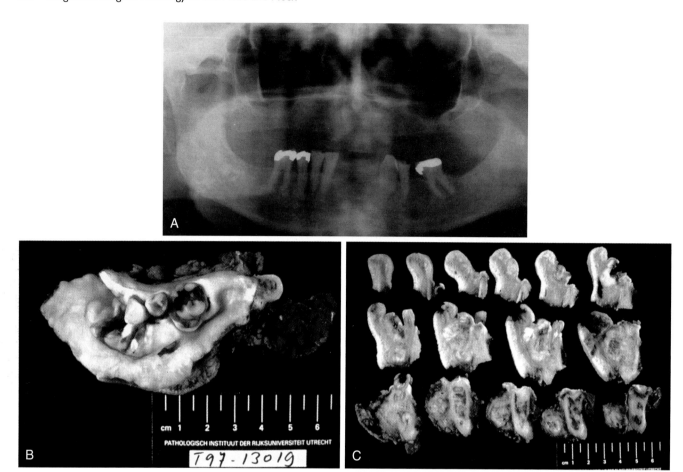

Figure 2–13. Radiologic and macroscopic presentation of lip cancer showing perineural spread into the mandible. *A,* Radiograph showing bone loss in left premolar area. *B,* Occlusal view of specimen showing tumor lying buccally to the cuspid-premolar area. *C,* Surgical specimen sliced buccolingually to display tumor extension into jaw and soft tissues.

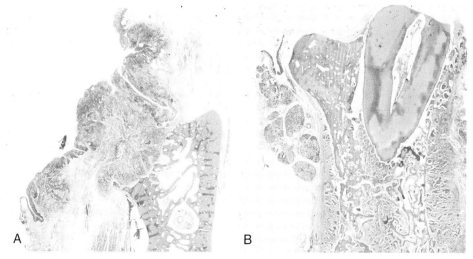

Figure 2–16. *A,* Squamous cell carcinoma destroying mandibular bone by erosion. The marrow spaces of the mandible are still uninvolved. *B,* Squamous cell carcinoma showing diffuse invasion of the mandibular bone and the perimandibular periosteum.

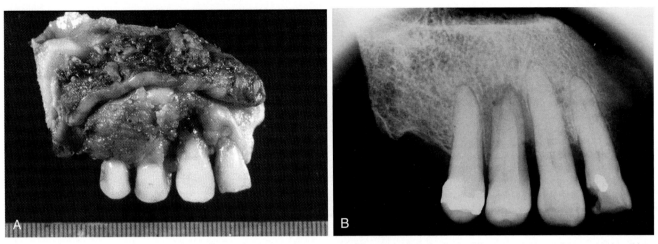

Figure 2–17. *A,* Surgical specimen of squamous cell carcinoma occurring at the maxillary gingiva. *B,* Radiograph of the same specimen shows periodontal bone loss around the first premolar tooth, which indicates tumor growth in the periodontal ligament space.

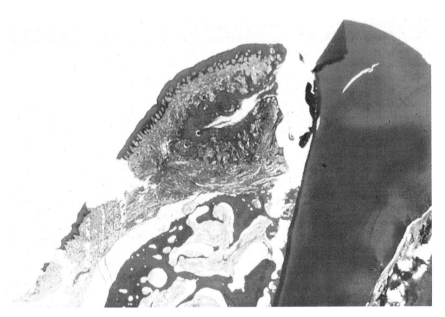

Figure 2–18. Photomicrograph shows squamous cell carcinoma growing in a periodontal pocket and underneath an apparently healthy gingiva. In this way, the tumor may remain unnoticed for some time.

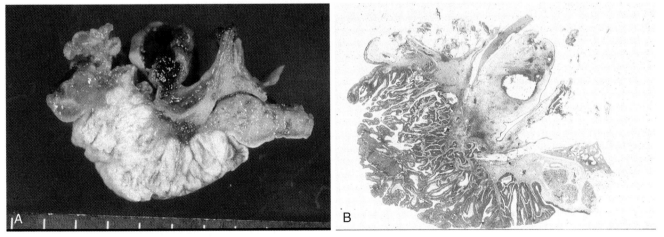

Figure 2–21. *A,* Surgical specimen of a squamous cell carcinoma of the upper alveolar ridge. The tumor has eroded away the maxillary bone. In the antral mucosal lining, polyp formation (middle top) has occurred. *B,* Hematoxylin-eosin stained slide of the same specimen. The polypoid, non-neoplastic changes in the antral mucosa are clearly visible.

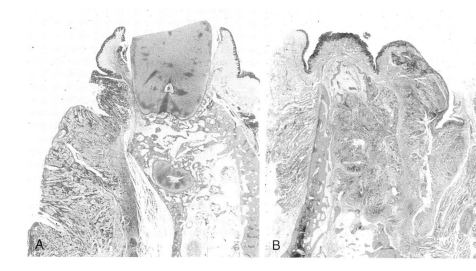

Figure 2–23. *A,* The tumor merely touches the mandible by growing into the gingiva. Although these tumors clinically may be adherent to the mandible, actual bone involvement is not present. *B,* Squamous cell carcinoma located lateral to the mandible may spread into the bone by perforating the lingual as well as the buccal cortical bone. Thus, the alveolar ridge is not the only way of entrance for a tumor to invade the mandible.

Figure 2–25. *A,* Photomicrograph shows cystic tumor in neck node. *B,* Higher magnification shows the pleomorphic epithelium lining the cysts. This presentation of metastatic tumor suggests the oropharynx as primary site.

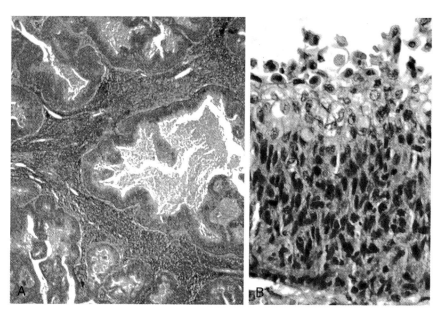

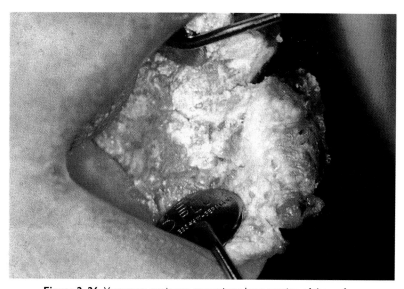

Figure 2–26. Verrucous carcinoma occupying a large portion of the surface of the right cheek and corner of the mouth. The lesion exhibits a heavily keratinized and irregular surface.

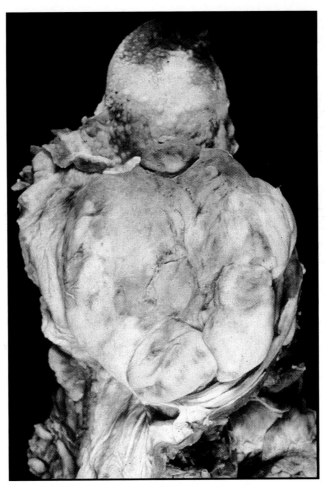

Figure 2–28. Autopsy specimen. Spindle cell carcinoma presenting itself as a large polypoid mass in the right pyriform sinus.

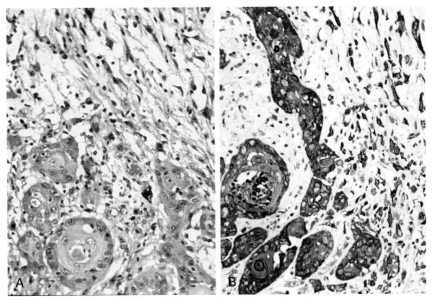

Figure 2–29. Spindle cell carcinoma. *A,* Hematoxylin-eosin stained section shows conventional squamous cell carcinoma in association with pleomorphic spindle cells. *B,* Both cell populations exhibit keratin positivity.

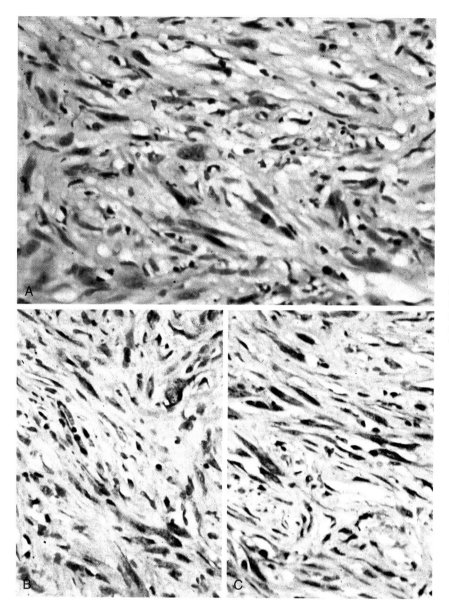

Figure 2–32. Photomicrographs show an intraosseous spindle cell carcinoma. A, Pure spindle cell component. B, Positivity for keratin indicating epithelial character. C, Positivity for desmin that should not be mistaken as an indication for a sarcoma with myogenic differentiation.

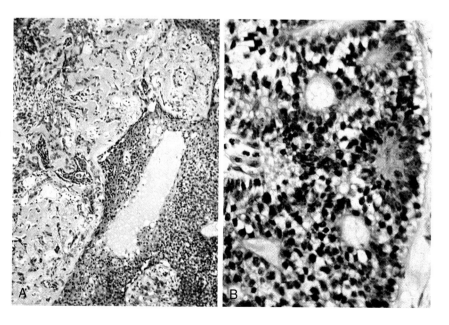

Figure 2–34. A, Photomicrograph shows a variety of patterns in teratocarcinosarcoma. In the mesenchymal component, osteoid is present. B, In the epithelial areas, rosette formation indicates neuroectodermal differentiation.

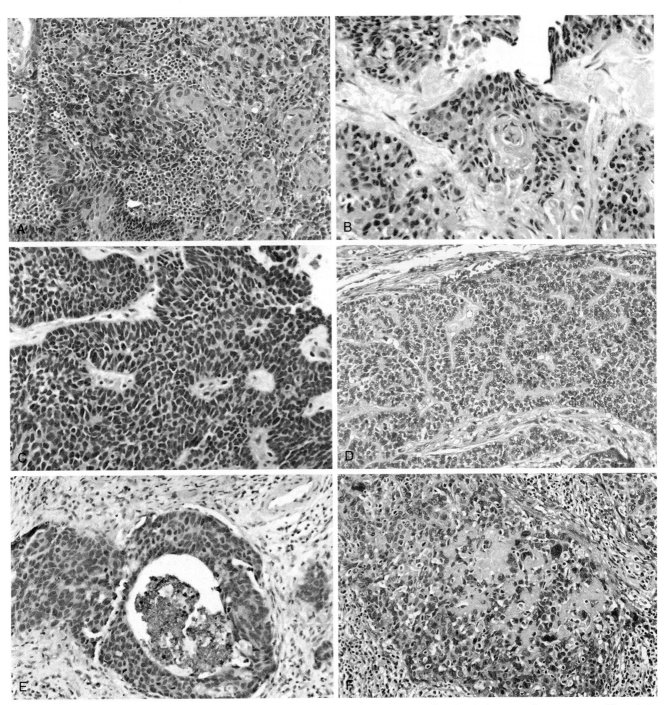

Figure 2–35. *A*, Photomicrograph of basaloid squamous cell carcinoma with the abrupt transition from basaloid tumor cells to squamous differentiation. *B*, Note the abrupt keratin pearl within the island of basaloid tumor cells in basaloid squamous cell carcinoma. *C*, Basaloid tumor cells of basaloid squamous cell carcinoma illustrating nuclear pleomorphism and slight basal cell palisading. *D*, Section of basaloid squamous cell carcinoma within a background of myxoid-appearing stroma. *E*, Photomicrograph demonstrating comedo necrosis within an island of basaloid squamous cell carcinoma. *F*, An island of basaloid squamous cell carcinoma illustrating nuclear pleomorphism and prominent hyalinization of stroma, which is frequently associated with microcyst formation.

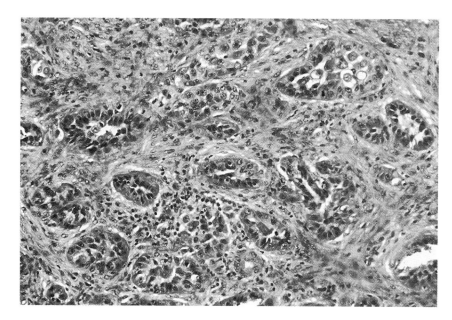

Figure 2–39. Histologic section of adenoid squamous cell carcinoma shows pseudoglandular formation lined by a basilar layer of polygonal cells containing a central lumen of detached "glassy" keratinocytes.

Figure 2–40. Photomicrograph showing adenoid squamous cell carcinoma with prominent keratin pearl formation and pseudoglandular alveolar areas.

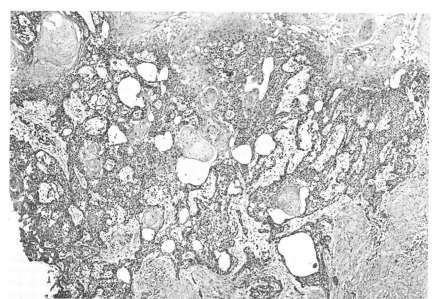

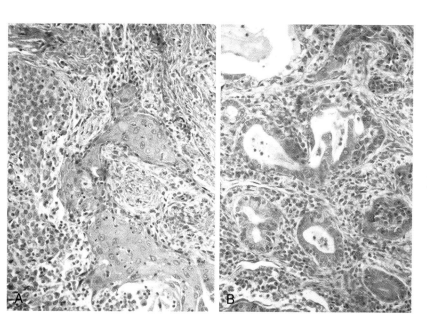

Figure 2–42. A, Photomicrograph showing an area of squamous differentiation within an adenosquamous cell carcinoma. B, Presence of adenocarcinoma component within an adenosquamous cell carcinoma.

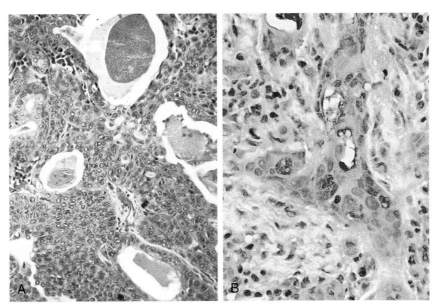

Figure 2–43. *A,* A section of adenosquamous cell carcinoma illustrating adenocarcinoma with well-formed ductal structures and no mucocytes. *B,* Photomicrograph of mucin within the glandular elements of adenosquamous cell carcinoma. (Mucicarmine stain.)

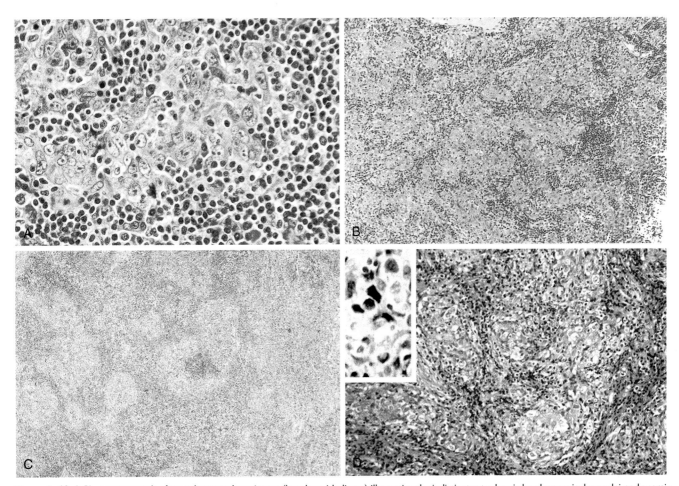

Figure 2–46. *A,* Photomicrograph of nasopharyngeal carcinoma (lymphoepithelioma) illustrating the indistinct cytoplasmic borders, vesicular nuclei, and prominent nucleolus. Note the mixed inflammatory background. *B,* Photomicrograph of lymphoepithelioma with a syncytial growth pattern of the epithelium within a background of lymphocytes. *C,* Photomicrograph demonstrates the sinusoidal pattern of spread of a lymphoepithelioma metastatic to a lymph node. *D,* Photomicrograph showing lymphoepithelioma. *Inset,* Same tumor subjected to in situ hybridization for detecting Epstein-Barr virus RNA transcripts (EBERs). Nuclear positivity is clearly visible.

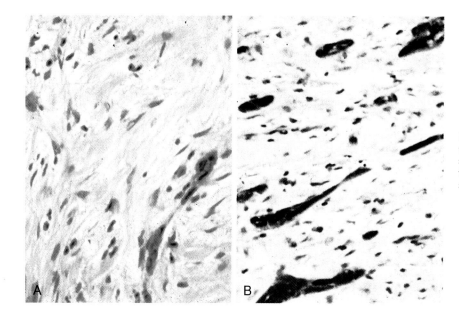

Figure 2–48. *A*, Photomicrograph shows desmoplastic epidermoid carcinoma; pleomorphic epithelial cells are present in tiny nests, surrounded by a prominent fibrous stroma. *B*, Staining with antikeratin antibody serves to highlight the neoplastic epithelium.

Figure 2–49. *A*, Photomicrograph shows fibro-osseous tissue resembling fibrous dysplasia. Only a few epithelial nests are present in this area from a squamous cell carcinoma that invades bone and has evoked an osteoblastic reaction. *B*, By immunohistochemical staining for keratin, the invading epithelial nests are more clearly displayed.

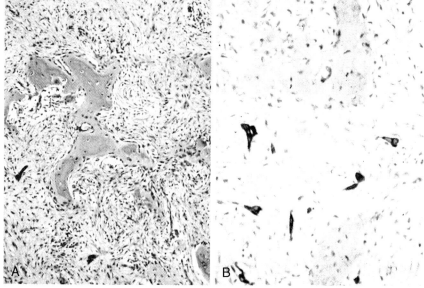

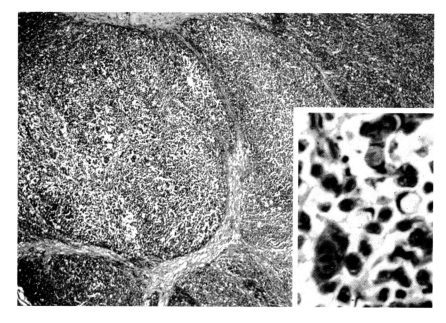

Figure 2–51. Low power photomicrograph showing large tumor areas with intervening fibrous septa mimicking malignant lymphoma. *Inset,* At high power, clusters of cells with eosinophilic cytoplasm indicate the epithelial nature of this lesion.

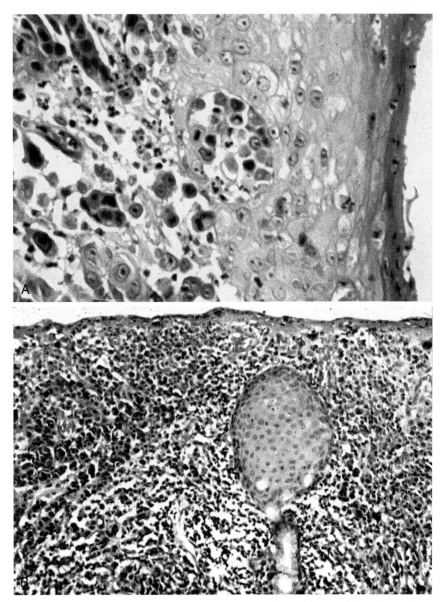

Figure 2–52. *A,* Photomicrograph showing poorly differentiating squamous cell cancer invading overlying healthy epithelium, thus mimicking melanoma. *B,* Elsewhere, the tumor surrounds a squamous epithelial nest that represents squamous metaplasia in salivary tissue; this should not be mistaken for squamous differentiation of the tumor cells.

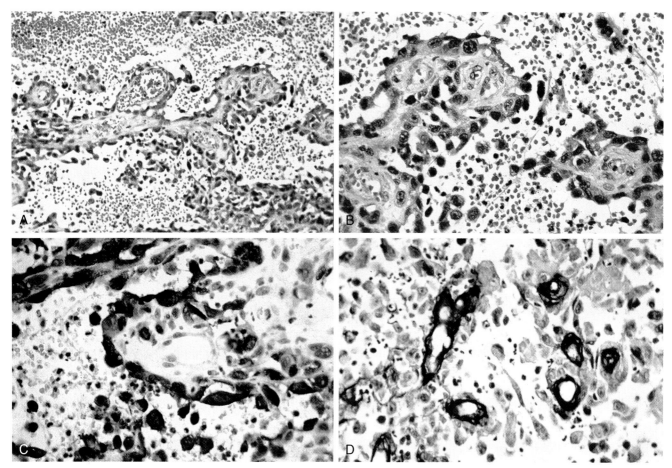

Figure 2–53. *A,* Low power photomicrograph showing blood lakes surrounded by pleomorphic cells. *B,* At higher magnification, the nuclear pleomorphism of the cells that cover fibrous stalks is clearly visible. *C,* Keratin immunohistochemistry reveals the epithelial nature of the cells that line the blood lakes. *D,* Factor VIII immunohistochemistry only stains the endothelial cells that line the vessels in the fibrous stalks. This histologic and immunohistochemical picture is typical for pseudoangiosarcomatous squamous cell carcinoma with blood lakes originating through acantholysis and intratumoral hemorrhage.

that 40% to 45% are seen in the upper third of the trachea and only 30% to 35% in the lower third.[323] There are also reports of carcinoma developing in scars after tracheotomy.[324] The tumor growth is often sessile and obstructive in nature, producing asymmetric narrowing within the tracheal lumen. Approximately 10% of cases are shown to have a circumferential growth pattern.[321]

Two histomorphologies, adenoid cystic carcinoma and SCC, constitute approximately 85% of the carcinomas.[321, 325] In the North American surgical literature, adenoid cystic carcinoma predominates, whereas in radiotherapy series, SCC is more common.[326]

Treatment and Prognosis. A review of the literature containing 321 cases found a 5-year survival rate of approximately 25% for SCC and 80% for adenoid cystic carcinomas.[326] Approximately 17% to 40% of the patients at the time of surgery for tracheal malignancies show extension into the mediastinum.[321] The status of surgical margins and positive lymph nodes have an adverse effect in SCC.[325] In Grillo and Mathiesen's series,[325] 35 patients had SCC. Thirteen patients died with cancer and 6 of these 13 patients had positive nodes and 4 had invasive tumor at the surgical margins. In contrast, within the group of 22 patients alive without cancer, 2 had positive lymph nodes, 1 had invasive carcinoma, and 6 had carcinoma in situ at the surgical margins. Almost all these patients had postoperative irradiation. The treatment for tracheal malignancies has involved both surgical resection and irradiation. The current information suggests that surgery, with or without radiation, appears to be the most effective therapy.[325] In patients who cannot undergo surgery, curative radiation treatment may be given, resulting in overall 1-, 2-, and 5-year survival rates of 46%, 21%, and 8%, respectively. The dose of radiation appears to be of influence, the 5-year survival rate dropping from 12% for patients receiving doses greater than 56 Gy to 5% for lower doses.[327] Currently, no TNM classification exists for the trachea.

Lip

Clinical Features. Squamous cell carcinoma of the lip represents 12% of UADT-SCCs.[328] In the Netherlands, they represent 19.8% of all oral cavity cancers.[3] Most of these tumors occur in men. The predilection site is the vermilion border of the lower lip, which is the mucosal strip between the mucocutaneous junction and the point of contact between the lips. Sun exposure appears to represent the most significant etiologic factor.[329, 330] Clinically, these tumors manifest themselves either as exophytic or ulcerating lesions. Sometimes they are heavily keratinized, thus showing an irregular whitish-brown surface.

Squamous cell carcinoma of the lip is staged according to size: T1, tumors not exceeding 2 cm diameter; T2, tumors more than 2 cm but not more than 4 cm; and T3, tumors larger than 4 cm. T4 tumors invade adjacent structures such as facial skin, mandibular bone, or tongue.[329, 331]

Treatment and Prognosis. Tumors are treated by surgery, irradiation, or a combination of both modalities. An overall survival rate of 83% has been reported: 87% for cases without metastasis as opposed to only 20% for cases with lymph node involvement.[330] Incidence of lymph node metastasis varied from 5% for T1,T2 tumors to 67% for T3,T4 cases; submental or submandibular nodes are the ones involved.[328, 329]

The incidence of metastasis has also been related to tumor thickness, invasion pattern, and perineural invasion. When comparing lip cancers that had metastasized with those that had not, the following differences were observed. The mean thickness was 2.5 mm for N0 cases and 7.5 mm for N+ cases. Seventy-six percent of the N0 tumors were 3 mm thick or less, whereas only one N+ lesion (3%) was less than 3 mm thick. Five percent of the N0 lesions, compared with 77% of the N+ cases, were at least 6 mm thick. Three percent of the N0 cases had a diffusely invading tumor, compared with 57% of N+ cases. Perineural invasion was seen in 5% of the

N0 cases and 41% of the N+ cases.[332] Perineural invasion may lead to tumor spread along the mental nerve into the mandible. This may become manifest by sensory disturbances and widening of the mandibular canal.[333] Therefore, radiographs of the mandible are mandatory in preoperative staging and during follow-up to detect this insidious way of spread shown by SCC of the lip. As intramandibular tumor spread may occur a considerable time after treatment of the lip, these patients may inadvertently be considered to suffer from a primary intramandibular tumor (Fig. 2–13, see p. 36).

Oral Cavity

Within the oral cavity, SCC may occur at various sites including the following: maxillary and mandibular alveolar ridge, the floor of the mouth, the retromolar trigone, the tongue, the cheek, and the hard palate. In the Dutch cancer registry, cancer at these locations represented 0.9% of all new cancers and 27.1% of all UADT cancers registered in 1994.[3] Because site-specific characteristics and clinicopathologic features for each site vary, they will be discussed separately for the various locations.

Tongue

The tongue is subdivided into the mobile tongue, which belongs to the oral cavity, and the base of the tongue, which belongs to the oropharynx, the line demarcated by the circumvallate papillae separating both parts.[331] SCC of the tongue represents 50% of all intraoral cancers, two thirds of these being located at the mobile tongue.[328] SCC is most often located at the lateral border, from which it may extend into the adjacent floor of the mouth. SCC at the dorsal surface of the tongue is extremely rare, and if present is most frequently a verrucous carcinoma. Most SCCs in the tongue grow as ulcerating, deeply invasive tumors, and their frequency of metastatic disease is the highest of all intraoral SCCs: 20% to 40% for T1 tumors, 40% for T2 tumors, and 75% for T3 tumors.[329] However, metastatic rates for the base of the tongue that belongs to the oropharynx are even higher: 70% for T1 cases.[329] The lymph nodes mostly involved are those that lie in the jugulodigastric area.[329]

Pathology. When examining surgical specimens from the mobile tongue with SCC, one should realize that the tumor may penetrate deeply into the tongue muscle, often by skipping uninvolved areas. Moreover, the possibility of perineural spread requires identification and histologic examination of the lingual nerve at the dorsal margin of the surgical specimen.

A lesion occurring at the dorsum of the tongue that may simulate SCC is the granular cell myoblastoma with its pseudoepitheliomatous hyperplasia of the covering epithelium.[117] Finding granular cells in the submucosa will allow proper classification.

Treatment and Prognosis. Tongue SCCs are staged according to their size and depending on spread beyond the tongue: T1, less than 2 cm; T2, greater than 2 cm to 4 cm; T3, greater than 4 cm; and T4 in the event of spread into extrinsic tongue musculature such as hyoglossus, styloglossus, genioglossus, and palatoglossus muscles.[331] The influence of size and stage on survival is as follows: Patients with T1N0 and T2N0 lesions have similar 3- and 5-year survival statistics (48% and 44% for the former and 56% and 44% for the latter group).[202] Patients with T3N0 cancer had a 50% rate of death due to cancer.[202] The T1N1 group had a 3-year survival rate of 80%, and the T2N1 group had a rate of 44%.[202] The T3N1 rate for 3-year tumor-free survival was 13%. These findings indicate that increasing size of the tumor by T stage and the presence of nodal disease both significantly decreased survival.[202] The discrepancy in survival rates between the T1N0 and T1N1 groups could possibly be explained by the small sample size of the latter group. In more general terms, in other series, 5-year survival ranges from 70% to 15% depending on the size of the tumor and the presence of nodal metastasis.[8, 329]

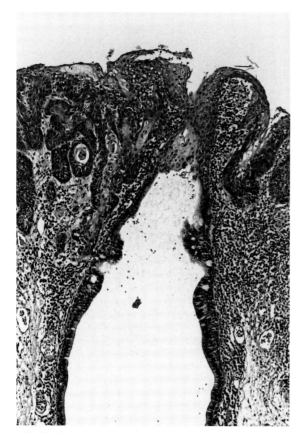

Figure 2–14. Squamous cell carcinoma in the floor of the mouth at the orifice of the submandibular duct may cause obstruction and dilatation of the duct.

T1 or T2 tumors may be cured by surgery or radiotherapy. More extensive lesions usually are treated using both modalities. Owing to the high incidence of nodal metastasis, treatment of tongue cancer includes either irradiation or surgery of the neck; the choice between these depends on the method chosen for treatment of the primary tumor.[8, 329]

Floor of the Mouth

The floor of the mouth is a horseshoe-shaped mucosal area between the lateral border of the tongue medially and the gingiva of the lower alveolar ridge laterally or, in its anterior part, ventrally. Dorsally, it extends to left and right tonsillar areas. SCC at the floor of the mouth represents 9% of all UADT-SCC and 15% to 20% of oral cavity cancers.[328]

Anteriorly in the floor of the mouth, ducts of the bilaterally located submandibular salivary glands open into the oral cavity. SCC at this site may obstruct salivary flow, leading to enlargement of these glands, which may simulate submandibular lymph node metastasis (Fig. 2–14). This feature possibly is responsible for a 24% to 56% false-positive (clinically positive but histologically negative) error in assessing lymph nodes in patients with floor-of-the-mouth cancer.[291] Moreover, SCC may extend along these ducts.[334]

Squamous cell carcinoma of the floor of the mouth is staged similarly to SCC of the tongue; T1, T2, and T3 according to size and T4 when the tumor invades adjacent structures either by horizontal spread to involve the mandibular bone or the lateral border of the tongue or by vertical growth into the deep muscles of the floor of the mouth.

Treatment and Prognosis. Approximately 12% of T1 lesions are associated with occult metastatic disease. Metastasis to lymph nodes occurs in 30%, 47%, and 53% of T2, T3, and T4 cancers, respectively.[328] The submandibular lymph nodes represent the first echelon involved. Five-year survival rate is also related to tumor size and drops from 85% to 32% across the various tumor stages.[8, 328] One recent study mentions that in cancer of the floor of the mouth, the patients with the best 3-year tumor-free survival rates were those with cancer staged as T1N0 (70%) and T1N1 (62%), the relationship between T stage and survival being highly significant but the relationship between N status and survival not being significant.[202]

Treatment of SCC of the floor of the mouth is mainly surgical, sometimes including a small rim of the mandibular alveolar bone if the tumor extends to less than 1 cm from the bone. If the tumor is fixed to the alveolar bone, treatment is the same as for tumors primarily occurring on the lower alveolar ridge; this is discussed elsewhere. Whether or not to treat the neck in cases of floor-of-the-mouth SCC without clinically manifested neck node disease is controversial.[328]

At the floor of the mouth, the close association between the invading SCC and the sublingual gland may result in malignant squamous cells intermingled with mucus-containing cells (Fig. 2–15).

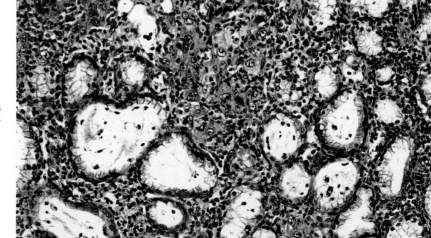

Figure 2–15. By invading mucous glands, squamous cell carcinoma may mimic mucoepidermoid carcinoma.

This should not lead to an inappropriate diagnosis of mucoepidermoid carcinoma but should be recognized as a site-related phenomenon.

Cheek

The cheek is covered by the buccal mucosa, which extends from the retromolar trigone posteriorly to the lips anteriorly. Its upper and lower borders are formed by the junction with the buccal side of the maxillary and mandibular alveolar mucosa. SCC at this site accounts for 8% of oral cavity cancers.[329] The tumor may spread diffusely into the underlying tissues, initially without causing symptoms that alarm the patient into seeking medical advice. The tumor may penetrate into the cheek musculature or extend into the maxillary or mandibular bone when growing upward or downward.

Treatment and Prognosis. Tumors are staged according to size, and this staging has proved to be prognostically significant by a drop in 5-year survival rates from 60% to 5% for T1 compared with T4 tumors. Lymph node metastases are observed in 10% of presenting patients; mostly they are located in the submandibular or upper cervical area.[329] Treatment consists of either surgery or radiotherapy or both, depending on the size of the lesions, and may sometimes include a full-thickness resection including mucosal lining as well as skin and intervening tissue layers. In T1 or T2 tumors without clinically detectable nodal metastasis, treatment of the neck is optional. In T3 and T4 tumors, it is required.[329]

Alveolar Ridge

The mucosa covering the alveolar ridge of upper and lower jaw is firmly attached to the underlying bone and, in dentate individuals, to the root surface of the teeth. In the lower jaw, it extends from left to right retromolar area, bordered lingually by the floor of the mouth and buccally by the buccal mucosa. In the upper jaw, its lateral border is the transition to the buccal mucosa; at its palatal side, no sharp anatomic border is present, the alveolar mucosa merging into the mucosal lining covering the hard palate. Dorsally the mucosal lining of the upper alveolar ridge is also bordered by the retromolar area.

Squamous cell carcinoma of the alveolar ridge constitutes from 7% to 18% of all intraoral cancers, including cancer of the lip.[291] Tumors at this site may be ulcerating or exophytic. As they occur at sites naturally firmly connected to bone, tumors at this location are always fixed to the bone. Radiographs are needed to assess the extent of bone involvement, which may be either by erosion, resorbing bone over a broad front, or by penetration through haversian canals and marrow spaces, the former growth pattern known as expansive and the latter as infiltrative (Fig. 2–16, see p. 36).[335–339] There are some indications that initially, when only the alveolar ridge is involved, SCC exhibits an expansive growth pattern, whereas the infiltrative pattern is associated with growth of the tumor into the basal bone, which is less easily resorbed.[338] The variation in patterns of bone involvement have until now not be shown to have any relationship with metastatic rate or other established clinicopathologic parameters. However, recognizing the variation in bone involvement by tumor is necessary to correlate histologic findings with preoperative radiographs. In cases with an expansive growth pattern, the radiographs will give a reliable picture of the extent of bone involvement, whereas in cases with an infiltrative pattern of bone involvement, the real tumor size will be underestimated as the tumor penetrates into bone with an initially undisturbed architecture.

In case of dentate patients, tumor may invade the periodontal ligament space, causing loose teeth (Fig. 2–17, see p. 37). Gingival bleeding also may occur. As these symptoms also may be seen in cases of inflammatory periodontal disease, SCC of the alveolar ridge may be confused with this affliction, causing delay in diagnosis. This occurs especially in cases in which the tumor is located at the inner side of the gingiva in the mucosal area that faces the tooth surface while leaving the outer gingival surface uninvolved, giving the impression of a healthy gingival margin while the carcinoma is lurking in an invisible site (Fig. 2–18, see p. 37).

Histologically, SCC invading the periodontal ligament spaces should not be confused with gingival mucosal lining exhibiting pseudoepitheliomatous hyperplasia (Fig. 2–19). Moreover, one should keep in mind that the gingival tissues may contain numerous intraepithelial nests and strands, either dental lamina rests or tangentially cut elongated rete pegs extending from the overlying epithelium (Fig. 2–20). These structures may mimic intragingival subepithelial tumor extension but can be recognized because they lack cytonuclear atypia. On the other hand, intragingival tumor extension may be mistaken for non-neoplastic intragingival epithelial structures.

In the upper jaw, SCC may penetrate through the bone into the maxillary sinus, followed by spread into this paranasal cavity. Owing to concomitant edematous thickening of the antral mucosal lining or even polyp formation, the actual tumor size may be overestimated when the extent of tumor involvement of the jaw is assessed in the radiographs (Fig. 2–21, see p. 37). In the lower jaw, tumor may not only spread into the body of the mandible but also may exhibit perimandibular spread. As this growth pattern may not be apparent on radiographs, the size of the tumor may be underestimated (Fig. 2–22).

Treatment and Prognosis. Squamous cell carcinoma of the lower alveolar ridge is second to SCC of the tongue in its frequency of lymph node metastasis; an average number of 30% is mentioned; the nodes mostly involved are the submandibular and the upper jugular nodes.[329] Owing to this high frequency of metastasis, elective treatment of the neck should be considered for patients with primary tumors that overlie the symphysis, are moderately or poorly differentiated, or display radiographic or histologic evidence of mandibular invasion.[340] Five-year survival rate varies from 70% to 30% depending on the T stage.[8] Staging is done based on tumor size for T1 to T3 stages, just as for the other sites. Staging a tumor as T4

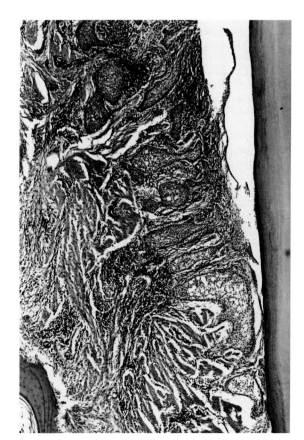

Figure 2–19. The epithelium that lines the gingival pocket may show reactive hyperplasia. These changes should not be interpreted as neoplastic.

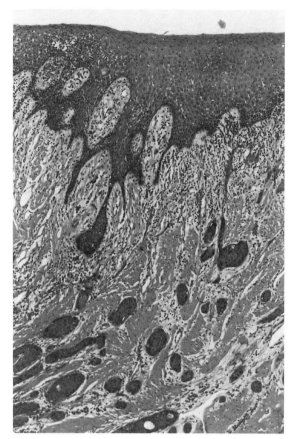

Figure 2–20. Photomicrograph shows odontogenic epithelial nests underneath normal gingival mucosa. This situation should not be mistaken for submucosal tumor extension.

requires demonstration of tumor growth through the cortical bone into the medullary cavity; merely superficial erosion of the cortical bone and some periosteal remodeling do not justify classification as T4 (Fig. 2–23, see p. 38).

Treatment of alveolar ridge SCC is by surgery. In the maxilla, this usually means a total or subtotal hemimaxillectomy. In the lower jaw a mandibulectomy should be performed, usually in combination with some type of neck-node dissection.[329] In the last few years, many papers have been published concerning the feasibility of jaw bone–preserving surgery. The common opinion is that in patients with SCC of the lower alveolar ridge, a complete resection of the jaw is not necessary, provided that sufficient mandibular bone is uninvolved to enable the surgeon to remain at a safe distance from the tumor.[341, 342] In cases of atrophic edentulous jaws, this will almost always be impossible. If the tumor involves dentate jaw areas, a rim mandibulectomy may be performed.[335–339, 341, 342] It should be stressed, however, that the decision to perform a rim mandibulectomy needs to be based on a very thorough assessment of the extent of bone involvement by tumor, which includes technically superb radiographs, including the use of intraoral dental films.

It has been reported that in the case of tumors involving bone by expansive growth, radiographs are quite reliable in indicating the real extent of bone loss due to tumor.[335, 336] However, in cases of more diffuse tumor spread in cancellous bone, the radiographs may not be in accordance with the histologic extent of bone involvement by tumor, and sometimes additional surgery to obtain free bone margins will be necessary. Also, spread along the inferior alveolar nerve may give origin to tumor at the margins, and therefore, histologic examination of this nerve at the ventral as well as at the dorsal bone margin is required.[343–345] In case of more extended mandibulectomies, these nerve ends are situated at the mental foramen ventrally and the mandibular foramen dorsally. When more limited surgery is

performed, the cut nerve ends should be identified within the mandibular canal.

In cases of previous irradiation, radiation-induced bone changes that allow diffuse tumor spread within the mandible make any preoperative assessment of bone involvement by tumor unreliable; in these instances, bone-preserving surgery, therefore, is not possible.[346]

Although the majority of SCCs have been reported to invade the jaw at the occlusal ridge, at least in the mandibles not previously irradiated,[341, 346] it has also been observed that the route of entry by which the tumor invades the jaw is dependent on the tumor's position relative to the bony surface and that penetration of the lingual as well as the buccal cortical plate may occur (see Fig. 2–23)[335]; this finding implies that not only horizontal rim mandibulectomies but also sagittal or oblique osteotomy planes may be chosen to perform bone-preserving surgery.[342] The ultimate decision on how to handle an SCC approaching or involving the mandible should be based on a combination of imaging techniques and good clinical judgment.[347]

Retromolar Trigone

The retromolar trigone or retromolar area consists of a triangular mucosal surface that lines the ventral surface of the ascending mandibular ramus. It is bordered ventrocaudally by the gingiva posterior to the last molar tooth in the mandible, mostly the third, and ventrocranially by the mucosa covering the maxillary tuberosity; its lateral and medial borders are respectively the buccal mucosa and the anterior tonsillar pillar. As tumors of the retromolar area are predominantly classified together with those occurring in one of the adjacent mucosal areas, no data on frequency of involvement of this site are available.

Clinical Features. Tumors of the retromolar trigone do not differ substantially from those of the lower alveolar ridge in clinical behavior and type of metastases. They may spread into the buccal mucosa but more often spread into the tonsillar area. Moreover, tumors involving the retromolar area may penetrate deep into the parapharyngeal soft tissue and exhibit spread along lingual as well mandibular nerves, sometimes as distant as the site where both nerves join to enter the base of the skull. Lateral growth of SCC at this site involves the medial side of the ascending mandibular ramus (Fig. 2–24).

Treatment and Differential Diagnosis. Treatment will usually be surgical, followed by irradiation for more extensive tumors.[329] It should also be noted that SCC at the retromolar trigone may mimic ameloblastoma by pronounced palisading of the carcinoma cells at the tumor-stroma interface and the development of intercellular edema in the tumor nests. This point is more extensively discussed in the section on specific SCC subtypes and diagnostic pitfalls.

Hard Palate

The mucosal lining covering the hard palate is enclosed laterally and ventrally within the horseshoe-shaped upper alveolar ridge mucosa, from which it cannot be demarcated because both consist of mucosa firmly attached to underlying bony tissue. Dorsally, the hard palate mucosa is bordered by the mucosal surface of the soft palate that belongs to the oropharynx.

Clinical Features. Incidence data for palatal SCC range from a low of 0.8% to a high of 62% of oral SCC, the latter figure being from countries where people smoke cigarettes with the burning end within the mouth. This habit of "reverse smoking" has been reported from South India, the Philippines, Sardinia, Jamaica, Venezuela, Colombia, Panama, and some islands of the South Caribbean.[348] In an area in India where the habit of smoking cigars with the lighted end inside the mouth is prevalent, palatal cancer accounts for 45% of all oral cancers.[349] Reverse smoking is done to keep the ashes from falling in food or on clothes and to extend the burning time of the cigar or cigarette.[348] Incidence data include cases from soft as well as

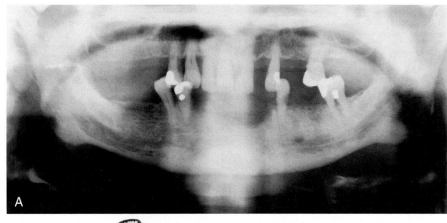

Figure 2–22. *A,* Radiograph shows a reduction in the height of the mandibular bone in the left premolar area due to squamous cell carcinoma in the same area. *B,* On histologic examination, the tumor can be seen not only to have hollowed out the alveolar ridge but also to have spread alongside the lingual periosteum. This latter mode of spread cannot be detected in the radiograph.

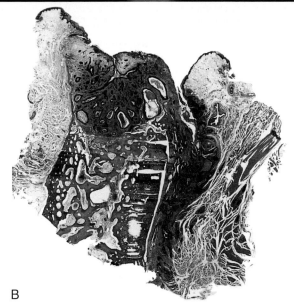

B

hard palate, one quarter of SCCs being located at the hard palate and the remaining ones occurring in the soft palate or uvula.[328]

Treatment and Prognosis. Tumors of the hard palate behave as tumors of the upper alveolar ridge and are staged and treated accordingly; surgery is the preferred treatment modality. Elective treatment of the neck generally is not required except in cases with more extensive tumors.[8]

Oropharynx

The oropharynx is situated between the nasopharynx cranially and the hypopharynx caudally. It is subdivided in the following anatomic regions: base of the tongue, tonsil and tonsillar fossa, soft palate, and posterior pharyngeal wall. Incidence data on SCC for the various subsites within the oropharynx are not available. Taken together, oropharyngeal SCC equals cancer of the lip in frequency of occurrence.[328, 329]

Base of the Tongue

Anteriorly, a line demarcated by the circumvallate papillae separates the base of the tongue from the mobile tongue. Posteriorly it ends at the base of the epiglottis. The lateral borders are both sulci glossopalatini, the tonsils and the tonsillar fossae as well as the faucial pillars.

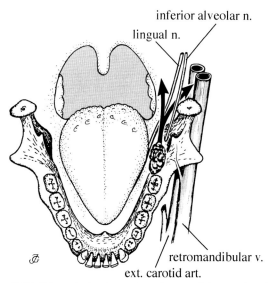

inferior alveolar n.

lingual n.

retromandibular v.

ext. carotid art.

Figure 2–24. Schematic drawing to show the spread that may be taken by squamous cell carcinoma of the retromolar trigone. Growth may be submucosally toward soft palate or infratemporal space in a cranial direction or laterally toward the parapharyngeal space and the large vessels of the neck.

Clinical Features. An SCC at the base of the tongue may attain considerable size before being recognized, pain and dysphagia being the most frequent presenting symptoms. Staging is done based on size for stages 1 through 3 as for the other previously mentioned locations. Tumors are classified as stage 4 when they invade mandibular bone, soft tissues of the neck, or extrinsic tongue muscles. Tumors located laterally may spread into the retromolar trigone, anterior faucial pillar, and tonsil. Medially situated tumors invade the extrinsic tongue musculature and may extend posteriorly to the epiglottis and pre-epiglottic space.

Treatment and Prognosis. Treatment mostly is by a combination of surgery and irradiation. As SCC of the base of the tongue has a high frequency of neck node metastasis, up to 70% with T1 tumors, elective treatment of the neck is indicated.[329] Mostly, the metastases are located in upper and middle cervical nodes. Contralateral or bilateral nodal metastases occur in 20% to 30% of cases.[291]

The prognosis for SCC occurring at the base of the tongue varies from 60% to 15% 5-year survival depending on tumor stage.[329]

Tonsillar Area and Soft Palate

The tonsillar area is bordered by the anterior and posterior faucial pillar and glossopalatine sulcus. Cranially this area is continuous with the inferior surface of the soft palate. Tumors in this area may involve the faucial pillars, the tonsillar area proper, and the soft palate. Tumors arising in different sites in this area may vary in their clinical aspects and behavior. In cases of SCC of the tonsil, the tumor usually exhibits deep penetration into underlying tissues or may extend into the base of the tongue or the lateral pharyngeal wall. Moreover, the tumor is notorious for its tendency to grow submucosally in a cranial direction into the nasopharynx, which may not be recognized at preoperative tumor staging. Tumors of the faucial pillars and the soft palate tend to grow more superficially, involving large mucosal areas without penetrating deeply.

Pathology. Histologically, these lesions exhibit severe epithelial dysplasia or carcinoma in situ in which invasive growth occurs multifocally. In the palate, the invading SCC may penetrate into the seromucinous palatal glands and in this way the tumor may mimic mucoepidermoid carcinoma histologically (see Fig. 2–15).

A lesion occurring at the soft and hard palate that may simulate SCC clinically as well as histopathologically is necrotizing sialometaplasia.[350] Recognition of the lobular architecture of the squamous epithelial islands and necrotic remnants of salivary gland tissue are distinctive features helpful in distinguishing this lesion from SCC.

Treatment and Prognosis. Tumor staging in this area is not different from staging in other sites: T1, T2, or T3 depending on size and T4 when the tumor invades mandibular bone or soft tissues of the neck such as the parapharyngeal space,[255, 256] a site also at risk with SCC of the retromolar area.

The different behaviors of tumors of the tonsillar area proper and of the faucial pillars and soft palate are also demonstrated by a lower frequency of metastasis shown by tumors at the latter site: 38% for T2 faucial pillar cancers, compared with 68% for T2 tonsillar cancers.[328] The lymph nodes most frequently involved are the cervical ones.[81] Sometimes, these metastases exhibit cystic degeneration (Fig. 2–25, see p. 38), and, in case of a yet undiscovered oropharyngeal primary SCC, these metastases may be mistaken for branchiogenic carcinoma.[351, 352] From analysis of a series of 136 cases with cystic squamous cell carcinoma in the neck, it was concluded that in most of these cases, the origin of the primary site will be in faucial or lingual tonsillar crypt epithelium. None of these cases was a branchiogenic carcinoma.[353]

Treatment of tonsillar as well as faucial or palatal SCC is surgery or irradiation for small lesions and a combination of both modalities for larger ones. Treatment includes the neck nodes in case of tonsillar tumors of any size. For palatal and faucial tumors, the value of elective treatment of a clinically negative neck is debatable. The prognosis for SCC in the tonsillar area as well as the palate varies

from an approximately 90% to a 20% 5-year survival rate, depending on tumor stage.[329]

Pharyngeal Wall

The superior border of the pharyngeal wall is at the level of the soft palate; the lower border is at the level of the vallecula. Tumors at this site usually have attained a large size before being discovered, as they are relatively symptom-free, which may be responsible for the fact that 60% to 80% of the tumors at this site are T3 or T4.[291] Tumors may extend cranially into the nasopharynx, posteriorly into the prevertebral fascia, and caudally into the hypopharynx and pyriform sinuses. Neck node metastasis is present in 50% to 60% of cases, sometimes bilaterally in cases of tumor at or near the midline.[291] Treatment usually is by irradiation, as surgery is technically difficult in this area and includes the neck nodes. Local control varies from 71% to 37%, depending on tumor stage.[329]

■ SQUAMOUS CELL CARCINOMA: UNUSUAL VARIANTS

Verrucous Carcinoma

Clinical Features. Verrucous carcinoma (VC) is defined as a warty variant of SCC characterized by a predominantly exophytic overgrowth of well-differentiated keratinizing epithelium with locally aggressive pushing margins.[116] Since its first description by Ackerman in 1948,[354] this tumor has been the subject of a continuous debate concerning diagnostic features as well as mode of treatment.[355–373]

Its occurrence originally was related to the use of chewing tobacco or snuff, although this was never substantiated by controlled epidemiologic investigations. Moreover, HPV appears to be of etiologic significance[374–380] although not supported universally.[381]

Verrucous carcinoma predominantly occurs in older people, the majority of cases being observed in patients in their sixth decade or older, and it has a predilection for males.[382] Preferred sites at which VC does occur in the head and neck area are the oral cavity (75% of all VC), in which they account for 3% to 4% of all SCC, and the larynx (15% of all VC), in which they constitute 3% of all SCC.[383, 384] Within the oral cavity, buccal mucosa and gingiva are the most frequently involved sites.[367–369] VC is a rare oral carcinoma with an annual incidence rate of one to three cases for every million persons.[384] When occurring in the larynx, the second most frequently involved head and neck site, the vocal cords are the preferred location.[364] VC may also arise, in order of decreasing frequency, in nasal fossa, sinonasal tract, and nasopharynx.

Clinically, the tumor manifests itself as a broadly implanted papillary nonulcerating soft tissue mass lacking induration and exhibiting a red, white, or red and white surface, depending on the amount of surface keratinization.[364] It often occupies large surface areas (Fig. 2–26, see p. 38). When located in the vicinity of the jaw, radiographs may reveal erosion of bony tissue.

Pathology. Histologically, VC is broadly based and invasive, with plump papillary invaginations of thickened and infolding epithelium that lack the usual cytologic criteria of malignancy.[366] Mitoses are rare, and, when observed, they are located in a suprabasal position immediately above the basal cell layer where they normally occur, a feature that may be helpful in recognizing VC.[360] Clefts within the infolding epithelium may contain cellular debris and keratin plugs, but keratin may also be absent.[359]

At the junction between the normal epithelium and the lesion, VC normally exhibits an abrupt transition (Fig. 2–27). The history of this border zone has been described in detail by Jacobson and Shear,[359] who noted that in VC the inwardly projecting epithelial folds often cause a margin of normal epithelium to retract down with them into the underlying connective tissue, a feature that may be helpful in distinguishing VC from reactive inflammatory epithelial

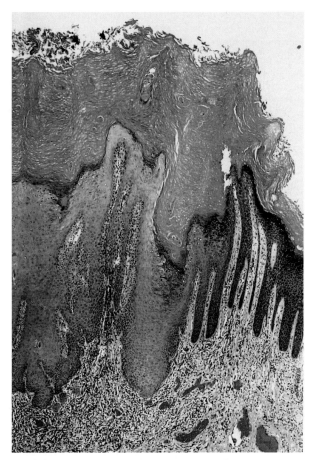

Figure 2–27. Photomicrograph shows the junction of verrucous carcinoma with normal epithelium. The difference between the blunt epithelial invagination of the tumor (left side) and the sharply pointed rete pegs of the adjacent epithelium (right side) are clearly visible.

hyperplasia. The stroma adjacent to the tumor almost always exhibits a chronic lymphoplasmacytic infiltrate. When the surgical specimen contains bone, osteoclasts may be present at the bony surface, indicating resorption due to tumor invasion. Sometimes, keratin masses in the stroma may evoke a foreign body giant cell reaction. Perineural invasion and vascular invasion are not features of a VC. Sometimes, lesions with the overall morphology of a VC may contain areas of ordinary SCC of varying grade.[359, 366, 368, 385] For these lesions, which accounted for 20% in a series of 104 VC cases, the designation *hybrid tumor* has been employed.[368] These hybrid tumors did not have any distinctive clinical characteristics but they were shown to have a higher tendency to recur locally: 6 of 20 (30%) for hybrid tumors versus 15 of 84 (17.9%) for VC in its strictest sense.[368] The quantity of SCC within a VC required for a lesion to qualify as hybrid tumor has not been defined. In line with the axiom that the course of a tumor is determined by its less-differentiated component, a wise approach is to diagnose all VCs with areas of SCC as a hybrid tumor and to treat them as SCC.

Differential Diagnosis. Histologically, VC has to be distinguished from reactive inflammatory epithelial hyperplasia, squamous papilloma, conventional SCC, and papillary SCC.[116, 366, 382] Lack of cellular atypia serves to rule out conventional SCC and papillary SCC, the latter lesion to be discussed more extensively under that specific heading.[386] Distinguishing VC from squamous papilloma and reactive inflammatory epithelial hyperplasia may be more problematic. Determining the DNA content by nuclear extinction cytometry on Feulgen stained histologic sections has been reported to be diagnostically useful in detecting cells with abnormal DNA content in VC, which may be helpful in differentiating between VC and benign lesions.[387] Recording nuclear size with image analysis has

been suggested to be helpful in differentiating between VC and squamous papilloma, as the cells in VC are, in general, larger (>300 μm) than in papillomas (<250 μm).[388]

The major problem is to distinguish between reactive inflammatory epithelial hyperplasia and VC, as both are composed of thickened epithelium lacking cellular atypia and a stromal component densely infiltrated by lymphocytes and plasma cells. It may be helpful to realize that in reactive inflammatory hyperplasia, the rete pegs in most instances form an anastomosing network and exhibit slender extensions, whereas in VC, the rete pegs are blunt.[382] Moreover, suprabasal mitoses typically seen in VC are absent in inflammatory epithelial hyperplasia. Nevertheless, excluding or confirming VC usually requires close cooperation between clinician and pathologist.

Other real or purported entities that may give origin to diagnostic confusion are verrucous hyperplasia[385, 389–391] and proliferative verrucous hyperplasia.[391, 392] Verrucous hyperplasia was described first by Shear and Pindborg in 1980[389] as a lesion resembling VC both clinically and histologically, but different from VC in exhibiting an exophytic growth pattern without submucosal invasion in contrast with the endophytic broad-based invasive growth pattern shown by VC. Therefore, in verrucous hyperplasia, the lesion lies above the level determined by a connecting line drawn between the border between lesion and uninvolved epithelium at either side, whereas in VC, the bulk of the lesion lies below such a line. However, this feature may be difficult to evaluate. Moreover, parts of an individual lesion may be situated above the level of the normal mucosa and other parts below, and therefore, the view has been proposed that verrucous hyperplasia and VC are in fact one and the same lesion.[366, 382, 385, 390, 391] Possibly the site of occurrence determines whether a VC grows predominantly exophytically or endophytically. This assumption was inferred from a comparative study in which it was shown that exophytic verrucous proliferations occurred in a minor proportion of cases (26%) on mucosal areas tightly bound down to underlying bone, the so-called mucoperiosteum (alveolar process and palate), whereas the endophytic verrucous proliferations did so in a larger proportion of cases (53%).[385] These site-related differences in growth pattern of verrucous proliferations may be explained as follows: An exophytic lesion may form when a loosely textured lamina propria is able to follow the extensive epithelial folding that occurs when, in a localized area, epithelium proliferates in a horizontal as well as in a vertical direction. In contrast, if the supporting tissue is tightly bound to the periosteum, as in cases occurring at the palate or alveolar process, the epithelial rete pegs cannot heap up into an exophytic mass but proliferate in a downward direction. In this way, the presence of an endophytic or an exophytic growth pattern of the verrucous lesion is a result of the different texture of the supporting connective tissue and thus site-dependent.

Alternatively, verrucous hyperplasia could be a precursor lesion that may progress to either VC or conventional SCC.[393] Irrespective of whether one considers verrucous hyperplasia to be an entity in its own right, a superficially growing form of VC, or a pre-neoplastic lesion, the lesion has to be removed entirely by surgical excision, going through a tissue level deep enough to ensure complete removal. As this approach is adequate for VC as well, discussion on where to put verrucous hyperplasia is somewhat academic.

Proliferative verrucous leukoplakia is a lesion first described by Hansen et al.[392] The lesion begins as a simple hyperkeratosis that in time becomes exophytic and wart-like, and, finally, malignant degeneration into SCC may occur. Some stages in this continuum may be histologically similar to VC and one has to rely on clinical data, especially a long history of flat thickened keratoses that have changed in clinical appearance by becoming more exophytic.[391–394]

Treatment and Prognosis. Although some authors consider radiotherapy to be as effective as surgery in treating VC,[361, 370–373] most others mention surgery as the most effective mode of treatment for VC.[366, 369, 395, 396] If one combines several studies on treatment of VC, the initial control rate for radiation treatment of VC of the oral cavity was 59% with a final salvage rate of almost 80%, and it was concluded that radiation as well as surgery can be used to treat VC but that, because of superior cure rates, surgical therapy should remain the mainstay of treatment.[393] Ferlito et al.[397] collected 148 cases of VC from the head and neck treated primarily with irradiation, the majority of which exhibited a treatment failure (persistence/recurrence), the overall local control rate being 64 of 148 (43.2%), which they consider ample support for the theory that irradiation is far less effective than surgery because VC, although not radioresistant, is less radiosensitive than conventional SCC. Nevertheless, radiotherapy is recommended for cases of laryngeal VC that cannot be resected with preservation of laryngeal function[398]

As the VC does not give origin to neck node metastasis, neck dissection does not form part of the treatment of VC.[116, 356, 357, 360, 366, 368, 369, 374] However, one should exclude coexistent conventional SCC by extensive histologic sampling from any case of surgically excised VC to be sure that there is no risk for neck node metastasis. These hybrid tumors have been shown to have a higher tendency to recur locally.[368]

In the past, radiotherapy was considered to be strictly contraindicated as treatment of VC because of the supposed risk for transformation of VC to a far more aggressively behaving SCC, the so-called anaplastic transformation,[356, 357, 364, 369, 374, 399–401] which has been attributed to interaction between HPV and irradiation.[374] However, critical analysis of these data has shown that radiation therapy probably plays no role in this malignant transformation of VC, as it has also been shown to occur independently of the employed treatment.[366–368, 382, 402]

Verrucous carcinoma is notorious for its association with other UADT mucosal (pre-)malignancies. These lesions may be part of the VC or may occur elsewhere in the mucosal lining of the UADT either synchronously or metachronously.[354–357, 359, 364, 368, 370, 385, 390] Because of the frequent association of VC with metachronous and synchronous UADT-SCC that may be as high as 37%,[368, 385] every patient with VC must be considered at high risk and be subjected to close follow-up.

Spindle Cell Carcinoma

Spindle cell carcinoma (SpCC), also called pseudosarcoma, sarcomatoid SCC, "collision" tumor, or sarcomatoid carcinoma, is a biphasic tumor composed of SCC cells and pleomorphic spindle-shaped cells.[116] Since its original description, several theories have been forwarded regarding the significance of the pleomorphic cells,[403–407] these cells representing either non-neoplastic bizarre stromal areas,[408–411] metaplastically altered SCC cells,[412–424] or cells forming a separate mesenchymal neoplasm that forms a collision tumor with the SCC component, for which the term *carcinosarcoma* is employed.[425–430] There is ample evidence, however, that SCC cells can exhibit differentiation toward cells with a mesenchymal phenotype, histologically as well as ultrastructurally,[413, 414, 417, 421, 423, 431–434] and immunohistochemically[420–423, 432–437] and therefore it appears to be most appropriate to consider these neoplasms as a variant of SCC in which the pleomorphic component originates through dedifferentiation of the SCC component.[406] Metastasis is to the cervical lymph nodes; the deposits may exhibit conventional SCC, SpCC, or both together.[411, 412, 414, 416, 418, 419, 421, 422, 425, 426, 437–439]

Clinical Features. An SpCC typically occurs in the oral cavity and the larynx[418, 439]; less frequently, it may arise in the sinonasal area and pharynx. In the larynx, SpCC constitutes 1.3% of all SCC[383]; concerning age and sex, no differences between SpCC and conventional SCC have been reported. Similar to conventional SCC, there is a strong association with a history of cigarette smoking. Macroscopically, the SpCC may be a polypoid tissue mass or a fungating or ulcerated lesion not different from conventional SCC (Fig. 2–28, see p. 39).[419]

Pathology. Histologically, SpCC typically exhibits areas of SCC and areas of pleomorphic spindle cells. The former component

may be very scant or limited to noninvasive areas of epithelial dysplasia or carcinoma in situ located at the surface of the tumor, and its identification may require extensive sampling for histologic examination. Often, the overlying epithelium may be ulcerated, and, because of this, the squamous component may not be seen. The pleomorphic spindle cells usually form the bulk of the lesion; they are arranged in fascicles or whorls. Storiform, myxoid, microcystic, or giant cell areas may also be present.[405] Moreover, foci of osteoblastic or chondroblastic differentiation (both benign and malignant) sometimes are observed.[405, 411, 414, 418, 421, 439, 440] There may be sharp borders between SCC areas and the spindle cell component, but a gradual transition, SCC-cells "dropping off" from the epithelial nests or overlying squamous epithelium into the pleomorphic spindle cell areas frequently may also be observed.[411, 441]

Ultrastructural examination may reveal epithelial features such as desmosomes or tonofilaments in the spindle cells.[413, 421, 423, 431–435] More easy to employ is immunohistochemistry, by which expression of epithelial markers can be analyzed. It has been demonstrated that the spindle cells in SpCC may exhibit keratin positivity in proportions varying from 40% to 78% of cases in reported series when employing broad-spectrum antikeratin antibodies (Fig. 2–29, see p. 39).[420–423, 432–437] When extending the antikeratin antibody panel by using different antibodies against various keratin subtypes in the weight range of 44 to 60 kDa, positivity for keratin could be demonstrated in six of seven cases (85.7%).[423] Moreover, double-labeling has indicated keratin as well as vimentin in individual spindle cells,[421, 432] thereby illustrating the versatility of the intermediate filament phenotype.

As SpCCs may in their spindle cell component exhibit not only vimentin expression but also other mesenchymal filaments, especially myogenic markers,[435, 437, 442] positivity for this marker does not rule out a diagnosis of SpCC. Even the absence of keratin positivity cannot be considered evidence against a diagnosis of SpCC, as this may be due to loss of reactivity for antikeratin antibodies due to fixation or embedding procedures or to a phenotypic change of the tumor cells. Tumors purely composed of pleomorphic spindle cells without any expression of keratin have been observed to recur as conventional SCC and serve to illustrate the profound divergence in differentiation morphologically as well as immunohistochemically shown by SCC cells.[422]

Sometimes SpCC exhibits acantholysis; in this way spaces lined by pleomorphic cells are formed that may mimic angiosarcoma (Fig. 2–30). At other body sites, the label *pseudoangiosarcomatous carcinoma* has been employed for lesions with this histomorphology.[443] It has also to be mentioned that conventional SCC sometimes contains myxoid areas with enlarged stromal cells exhibiting swollen vesicular nuclei, sometimes showing mitoses. However, these cells are dispersed among a non-neoplastic background and not densely packed in whorls of fascicles as in SpCC, which identifies them as part of a stromal reaction. Therefore, in these cases, a diagnosis of SpCC does not apply. Moreover, the observation that stromal fibroblasts as well as endothelial cells may both show these atypical changes may be helpful in distinguishing between SpCC and SCC with atypical stromal features (Fig. 2–31).

Differential Diagnosis. When SCC and spindle cells are both observed, the diagnosis of SpCC is easily made. In the absence of the SCC component, diagnosis is more difficult, because in these instances one has to distinguish between the so-called monophasic SpCC and a possible medley of mesenchymal spindle cell lesions, either benign or malignant, such as various types of spindle cell sarcomas and nodular fasciitis.[405, 406, 441]

Nodular fasciitis may exhibit mitotic figures, but they are not atypical; moreover, no cellular pleomorphism is present. Therefore, discerning this lesion from SpCC should not be too problematic. Distinguishing between monophasic SpCC and spindle cell sarcomas such as fibrosarcoma and leiomyosarcoma may be more difficult. However, sarcomas in the head and neck area located at mucosal surfaces are extremely rare, and, when they do occur, an intervening fibrous layer usually separates the lesion from the over-

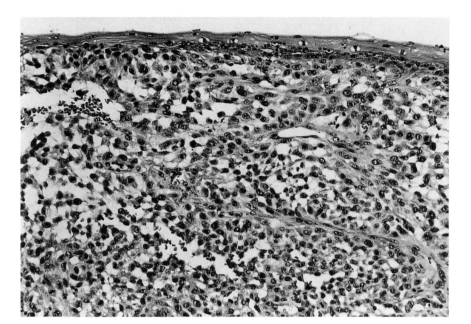

Figure 2–30. Spindle cell carcinoma exhibiting pronounced acantholysis. Covering squamous epithelium lacks atypical features.

lying epithelium. In the case of SpCC, just as in conventional SCC, the tumor is either ulcerating or directly abutting onto the overlying epithelium without an intervening uninvolved stroma. This feature may be helpful in making the appropriate diagnosis. However, if SpCC occurs intraosseously,[444] its distinction from sarcomas with a spindle cell appearance may be extremely difficult or even impossible if immunohistochemistry or electron microscopy fail to reveal epithelial characteristics (Fig. 2–32, see p. 40).

When occurring in the larynx, the differential diagnosis of SpCC also includes the recently recognized benign proliferative lesion that has been labeled inflammatory myofibroblastic tumor. This lesion shares a lot of overlapping features with SpCC, such as clinical presentation as a polypoid or pedunculated mass and histologic features such as spindle cells displaying mitotic figures lying in a myxoid or fibrous stroma; its differentiation from SpCC may prove to be extremely difficult. Key features assisting in differentiating SpCC from the inflammatory myofibroblastic tumor are the absence of dysplastic or carcinomatous epithelial components and no atypical mitotic figures.[445]

Sometimes, UADT mucosal melanomas may present as polypoid masses composed of pleomorphic spindle cells. When keeping this possibility in mind, immunohistochemistry with the appropriate antibodies (S100, HMB45) serves to confirm or rule out this diagnosis if melanin is not found in the primary tumor. For a more extensive discussion of the histologic features of nodular fasciitis, inflammatory myofibroblastic tumor of the larynx, melanoma, and spindle cell sarcoma that may be helpful in the differential diagnosis, the reader is referred to their descriptions elsewhere in this book. For practical purposes, it is advisable to consider a pleomorphic spindle cell lesion occurring at the mucosal surfaces at the UADT to be a SpCC.[406]

This discussion on SpCC and its differential diagnosis will be finalized by remarking that SpCC sometimes may assume the appearance of an innocuous granulation tissue polyp. Although it has been mentioned that reactive growths may mimic SpCC,[408] the converse may also be true and has gained far less attention.[416] Nevertheless, sometimes SpCC may exhibit a very edematous or densely collagenous stroma with only dispersed, slightly

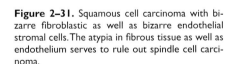

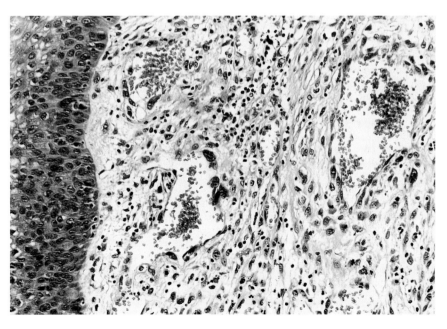

Figure 2–31. Squamous cell carcinoma with bizarre fibroblastic as well as bizarre endothelial stromal cells. The atypia in fibrous tissue as well as endothelium serves to rule out spindle cell carcinoma.

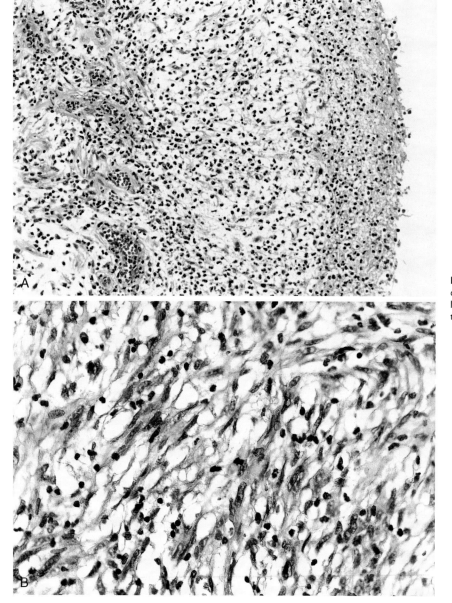

Figure 2–33. A, Photomicrograph shows spindle cell carcinoma masquerading as an innocuous granulation polyp. B, In the recurrent lesion, the real nature of the lesion became apparent.

pleomorphic spindle cells and an ulcerated surface, and therefore the true neoplastic nature of the lesion is easily overlooked. Only after several recurrences, the lesion may reveal the more characteristic appearance of an SpCC (Fig. 2–33). The converse situation, granulation tissue mimicking SpCC, may occur following ionizing-radiation exposure. After radiation exposure, bizarre granulation tissue–containing pleomorphic spindle cells and atypical mitotic figures may develop that should not be misinterpreted as tumor recurrences displaying the histomorphology of SpCC[315]; this was discussed previously in the section on laryngeal SCC.

An SpCC should not be confused with the so-called teratocarcinosarcoma.[446, 447] This neoplasm typically occurs in the nasal cavity and the paranasal sinuses, sites at which SpCC rarely occurs, and is characterized by an extremely diverse histologic pattern with mature and immature glands; benign squamous and malignant poorly differentiated epithelia; and rhabdomyosarcomatous, chondrosarcomatous, and neuroepithelial differentiation (Fig. 2–34, see p. 40). Although this tumor is considered by some authors to be part of the spectrum exhibited by SpCC,[406] its far more complex histology and

different predilection site make its classification as a distinct entity separate from SpCC more appropriate.

Treatment and Prognosis. Treatment of SpCC is the same as for conventional SCC. The assumption that SpCCs growing as polypoid masses have a better prognosis than SpCCs growing invasively[405, 419] has not been supported by other studies.[415, 418, 439, 448, 449] Batsakis et al.[441] reviewed the lethality of SpCC in the head and neck and correlated their findings by anatomic site. Sixty percent of 53 patients with tumors of the oral cavity died within 1 month to 6 years, 77% of 13 patients with tumors of the sinonasal tract died within 6 months to 2.5 years, and 34% of 65 patients with tumors of the larynx died within 4 months to 2 years. Polypoid glottic tumors appeared to have the most favorable prognosis (90% 3-year survival), whereas supraglottic, hypopharyngeal, sinonasal, and oral SpCCs did poorly regardless of their gross appearance. Batsakis et al. concluded that SpCCs manifest a biologic behavior that is more aggressive than most conventional SCCs.[441] However, in a series of early stage (T1–T2) glottic tumors, patients with SpCC treated with irradiation had similar control rates to irradiated patients with disease of similar volume with the more typical SCC.[450]

Basaloid Squamous Carcinoma

Basaloid squamous carcinoma (BSC), a rare histologic variant of SCC, was first characterized in the UADT in 1986 by Wain et al.[451] Although identical basaloid tumors have been described in a variety of body sites[452, 453] including the esophagus[454, 455] and lung,[456] this variant has a marked predilection for the base of the tongue, supraglottic larynx, and hypopharynx (pyriform sinus). Clinically it is considered an aggressive tumor with a propensity for regional lymph nodal (80%) and systemic metastases (60%).[451]

Clinical Features. Since the original report of UADT-BSC, over 100 cases have appeared in the English literature. The most common sites still remain the base of the tongue, hypopharynx (pyriform sinus), and supraglottic larynx.[451, 455, 457–473] Among the most common complaints at patient presentation are a neck mass, dysphagia, hoarseness, weight loss, otalgia, sore throat, cough, and hemoptysis. This tumor has a high prevalence in the older population, with a median age of 63 years (range 27–88 years); a male predominance (82%), and presentation at a high stage (stage III-IV).[470]

The aggressive biologic nature of BSC is manifest by frequent lymph node metastasis (64%) and distant metastasis (44%) to lung, liver, bones, brain, and skin, frequent local recurrence, and a mortality rate of 38% (at 17 months median follow-up).[470] The justification for distinction of this variant of SCC appears to be at least twofold: (1) recognition of the tumor's tendency to present at a high clinical stage (stage III and IV, although the sites of predilection may significantly contribute to this feature) and (2) to prevent the diagnostic confusion of this variant with another entity having a different prognosis (e.g., adenoid cystic carcinoma) or requiring a different treatment modality (neuroendocrine carcinoma).

Basaloid squamous carcinoma may be related to tobacco and alcohol abuse and possibly other risk factors. In a review of 90 reported cases, 42 of the 90 patients were known to have smoked tobacco or consumed alcohol or both.[470] There has also been one case of BSC arising in a patient after radiotherapy for a prior neoplasm.[466] Second primary tumors have also been reported in patients with BSC.[467, 471, 473]

The macroscopic descriptions of BSC have been those of an exophytic mass[461, 467, 468] as well as a flat lesion[462, 466] with central ulceration and marginal submucosal induration.[468] The size of the lesions have ranged from 1 to 6 cm.[470] A tendency for prominent deep and lateral submucosal soft tissue infiltration has been noted.[467, 476]

Pathology. As the name implies, this tumor is biphasic with distinct histologic findings. Perhaps the most salient feature of this tumor is the intimate and often abrupt association of the basaloid component with the squamous component (Fig. 2–35A and B, see p. 41). The basaloid component of the tumor is defined by four features: (1) solid growth of cells in a lobular configuration, closely apposed to surface mucosa; (2) small, crowded cells with scant cytoplasm; (3) dark, hyperchromatic nuclei without nucleoli; and (4) small cystic spaces containing material resembling mucin that stains with periodic acid-Schiff or alcian blue (Fig. 2–35C and D). Ancillary features include small and large foci of necrosis within central areas of tumor lobules (comedonecrosis) (Fig. 2–35E) and hyalinization of the stroma, often in association with microcyst formation (Figs. 2–35E and 2–36). Wain[451] required the associated squamous component to be among the following: invasive SCC that usually has a superficial location (usually well or moderately differentiated), overlying surface epithelium with dysplasia (usually severe dysplasia or carcinoma in situ) (Fig. 2–37), or focal squamous differentiation within basaloid tumor islands. Criteria used to identify the squamous epithelium required the presence of two or more of the following: (1) individual cell keratinization, (2) intercellular bridging, (3) keratin pearl formation, and (4) cells arranged in a mosaic pattern.

Since the initial description, other histologic features have been described. Among these are prominent festoon, cribriform, pseudoglandular, or trabecular growth pattern of the basaloid cells,[455, 457, 466] individual cell necrosis, large vesicular nuclei, nucleoli, prominent mitotic activity,[457, 474] with some containing abnormal mitotic figures,[455] and a focal spindle cell component.[468]

Perineural invasion has not been a consistent finding.[455, 460, 462, 470] Moreover, lymphovascular infiltration has been observed in four of nine cases (44.4%).[455] Nodal metastases may show either basaloid cells, basaloid cells with conventional SCC, or the presence of only conventional SCC. In two series, extracapsular extension within the lymph node metastasis was present in over 50% of the patients with nodal involvement.[462, 470]

Ultrastructurally, the basaloid cells were described as polygonal and the chromatin was finely dispersed within pale nuclei. The cytoplasm was found to contain desmosomes, rare tonofilaments, and free ribosomes. On electron microscopy of the cyst-like spaces identified on light microscopy, they were found to be lined by basement membrane material and filled with loose stellate granules or replicated basal lamina arranged in parallel stacks or globular masses. Squamous components contained well-formed desmosomes and

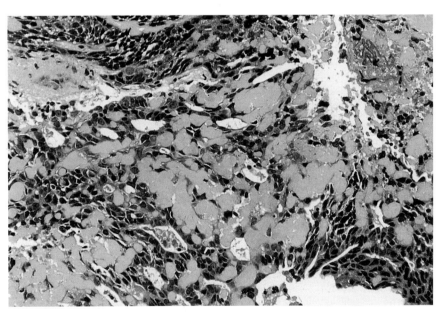

Figure 2–36. Photomicrograph of basaloid squamous cell carcinoma showing prominent hyalinized stroma with the beginnings of microcyst formation.

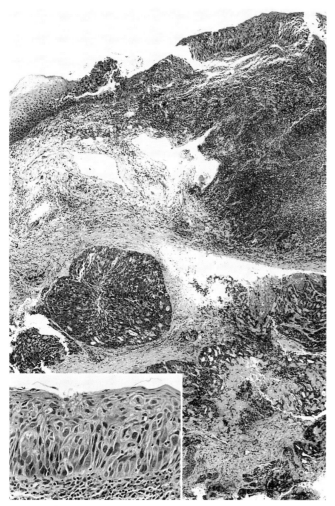

Figure 2–37. Photomicrograph of a basaloid squamous cell carcinoma with the overlying mucosa demonstrating carcinoma in situ, as shown in inset.

clumps of tonofilaments. None of the following were observed: neurosecretory granules, myofilaments with dense bodies, secretory granules, cytoplasmic organization, or cellular polarity.[451]

Immunohistochemical staining features were investigated on 40 cases of BSC reported by Banks et al.[457] Their findings were as follows: 100% keratin staining with 34βE12 antibody, 79% with a AE1/AE3, 83% for low molecular weight keratin 8/18 (CAM 5.2), 83% for epithelial membrane antigen, 53% for carcinoembryonic antigen, 39% for S100 protein; 75% stained diffusely but weakly with neuron-specific enolase. None of the tumors were positive for chromogranin, synaptophysin, muscle-specific actin, or glial-fibrillary acid protein.

The keratin staining pattern in general has been observed to be limited to the cells with eosinophilic cytoplasm. The basaloid cells specifically have shown weak to absent staining.[455, 457] The carcinoembryonic antigen has been found to be limited primarily to the squamous component of the tumor, but rare ductal cell staining has been observed.[455] Staining for actin has also had variable reports of positivity.[455, 457, 464] Ferlito et al.[475] summarized their immunohistochemical findings in a series of 15 patients as follows: reactivity for cytokeratin, epithelial membrane antigen, carcinoembryonic antigen, and vimentin (vimentin immunostaining being displayed as a delicate perinuclear ring or perinuclear dot and being found only in the basaloid cells but not in the squamous component). Positivity is focally observed for S100 protein, muscle-specific actin, and collagen IV.

Two studies have evaluated the DNA ploidy of BSC. In one report it was concluded that patients with an aneuploid BSC had a bet-

ter survival rate than those with a diploid BSC.[455] However, in another study, the better survival for aneuploid BSC tumors could not be confirmed: patients with aneuploid and diploid tumors both had unfavorable outcomes manifest by local recurrence or distant metastasis or both.[470]

Differential Diagnosis. Because of the heterogeneous nature of BSC, there is potential for diagnostic error. Biopsies not representative of the whole lesion may be devoid of the biphenotypic expression required to make the correct diagnosis. Absence of the squamous component may suggest the diagnosis of adenoid cystic carcinoma or a neuroendocrine carcinoma,[474] whereas the possibility of a basal cell adenocarcinoma also should be taken into account.[475]

Adenoid cystic carcinoma of the solid variant is the major consideration in the differential diagnosis. Both tumors may have areas with a cribriform growth pattern. Among the most useful distinguishing characteristics of BSC from adenoid cystic carcinoma is that the prior has continuity with an overlying epithelium, which has carcinoma in situ, severe dysplasia, or SCC. Other helpful characteristics are the fact that the BSC has greater nuclear pleomorphism, evidence of squamous differentiation, and more frequent mitotic figures than adenoid cystic carcinoma and more prominent necrosis.[477] The clinical features separating these two neoplasms are fairly distinct. Adenoid cystic carcinoma rarely presents with frequent lymph node metastasis and has a longer, more protracted course than BSC. BSC also has a different site of predilection than adenoid cystic carcinoma, as indicated earlier. The immunohistochemical staining patterns of adenoid cystic carcinoma and BSC may have some utility in separating these two neoplasms in small biopsies. Carcinoembryonic antigen shows ductal positivity within adenoid cystic carcinoma while being limited primarily to the squamous component in BSC. S100 is not particularly useful in distinguishing these two neoplasms. Also, muscle-specific actin has been found to be positive in about 60% of the cases of adenoid cystic carcinoma that have a cribriform pattern.[455] In one series, no BSC with a cribriform pattern reacted with muscle-specific actin.[457]

Another consideration in the differential diagnosis is small cell (neuroendocrine) carcinoma (SCEC), which is composed, on histologic examination, of sheets of small hyperchromatic cells showing nuclear molding and may occur in the same sites.[478] This tumor lacks stromal mucin or pseudoglandular cribriform patterns and rarely is connected to the surface mucosa.[479] Immunohistochemistry may be useful in differentiating BSC from SCEC. Neuron-specific enolase may be positive in both tumors; however, unlike SCEC, BSC lacks positivity for chromogranin and synaptophysin.[457] Positivity for chromogranin or synaptophysin would exclude BSC.[457, 479] The keratin staining patterns are different in these two neoplasms as well; SCEC frequently shows a globular-appearing perinuclear staining pattern that is not observed in BSC.[479] It has also been reported that BSC reacts with the high molecular weight cytokeratin antibody 34E12, which failed to show any reactivity with SCEC.[480] Ultrastructurally, BSC lacks neuroendocrine differentiation. SCEC, even poorly differentiated, frequently contains dense core granules, supporting this line of differentiation.

Basal cell adenocarcinoma can be distinguished from BSC by its predominant location in major salivary gland tissue, a site where BSC does not occur, and a far lesser degree of aggressiveness, which is exemplified by a blander histology.[475]

Metastatic basal cell carcinoma of the skin, although uncommon, may enter the differential diagnosis when the initial presentation is a lymph node metastasis.[481–483] The frequency of metastatic basal cell carcinoma in large series ranges from 0.0028% to 0.55%.[482, 483] The size of the basal cell carcinoma has also been correlated with metastasis (3 cm in diameter had a 1.9% incidence of metastasis).[483] In most cases of metastatic basal cell carcinoma, the primary tumor is present when the metastasis is detected[481] or the patient has a history of frequent recurrence.[481] Clinical detection of a skin lesion and biopsy confirmation of a primary tumor should aid in resolving this dilemma. Finally, it should be kept in mind that

BSC occurring at other sites, such as the lung, may metastasize to the neck nodes.

Treatment and Prognosis. There has been some question of the proposed aggressive nature of BSC. The sites of predilection for this SCC variant may contribute to the perceived advanced stage at presentation. Banks et al.[457] thought that, stage-for-stage, the BSC treatment and behavior were similar to those of conventional SCC. Luna et al.[466] in their series of nine patients compared age, sex, clinical stage, site, date of diagnosis, and treatment of BSCs to those patients with conventional SCC. Although the series was small and needs confirmation, they found the biologic behavior of BSC similar to that of conventional SCC. Another report has come to a similar conclusion.[462] Coppola et al.[460] suggested that perhaps the percentage of basaloid component in tumors may correlate with prognosis and explain conflicts in results. In the series by Coppola et al., the basaloid component represented 50% to 80% of the tumor, for each case. The treatment still remains primarily radical surgery in combination with radiotherapy or chemotherapy. Owing to the fact that more than 50% of the cases present with lymph node metastasis at the time of diagnosis, systemic adjunctive chemotherapy should be investigated.[484] Because of these clinical and histologic features, BSC should be recognized as a distinct variant of SCC.

Adenoid Squamous Cell Carcinoma

In 1947, Lever[485] first described a variant of SCC of the skin that he called *adenoacanthoma.* He postulated that the tumor arose from the eccrine sweat ducts and glands. The tumor was composed of a combination of glandular and squamous differentiation. Several years later Lever modified his concept, and others concurred, that the gland-like spaces were the result of acantholysis of solid nests of SCC.[486, 487] Muller[487] suggested the name *adenoid squamous cell carcinoma* (ASCC) to avoid confusion with adenoacanthoma of the endometrium. Other synonyms include pseudoglandular squamous cell carcinoma, acantholytic squamous cell carcinoma, and squamous cell carcinoma with gland-like features.[488–492]

The largest series on ASCC of skin showed the lesion to present most often as an ulcer or nodule on sun-exposed areas of the head and neck region, predominantly in elderly men.[488] There was often an associated adenoid actinic keratosis and therefore sun exposure was considered an important factor. About 2% to 3% of these patients with lesions over 2 cm had evidence of deep invasion with metastasis, both lymph node and visceral.[488] A later series with 55

cutaneous cases of ASCC from 49 patients found that 19% of the patients died of metastatic or recurrent disease. This clinical behavior was somewhat more aggressive than conventional SCC of the skin, and prognosis seemed to correlate with lesion size; a size greater than 1.5 cm means an unfavorable course.[492]

Clinical Features. A recent review of the literature of ASCC collected 26 cases involving the oral cavity and one in the nasopharynx. Twenty-two of the cases were described on the vermilion border of the upper or lower lip, with the lower lip being the most common oral site of occurrence, accounting for 17 of 26 cases.[493] The mean age of occurrence was 54.5 years (range 41–75 years). Tumor size, when reported, was 2 cm or smaller. One patient with a lip lesion was immunocompromised.[493] The largest single series of oral ASCC[494] contained 15 cases on the lip with a mean patient age of 56.1 years (range 41–57) and a male predominance. All 15 patients were alive and disease free after 27.6 months of follow-up. Just over one third of these patients developed a subsequent lesion on the vermilion area of the lip several years after diagnosis of the initial lesion.

In contrast to the indolent course of the ASCC of the skin and lip, cases involving mucosal surfaces of the head and neck devoid of sun exposure may behave more aggressively. The first reported intraoral case was in 1977[495] and involved a lesion of the posterior lateral aspect of the tongue in a 61-year-old man. The tumor recurred 4 months after treatment and the patient died of sepsis 8 months after initial diagnosis. That same year, Takagi et al.[496] reported two cases. Both patients experienced local recurrence and died of their disease (38 months and 46 months after diagnosis). The remaining cases are from nasopharynx[497] and floor of mouth.[493] Both patients were male and aged 42 and 58 years with no evidence of disease. Others have observed cases in the supraglottic larynx,[498] the hypopharynx, and the sinonasal tract.[499]

Pathology. Adenoid squamous cell carcinoma is included in the World Health Organization (WHO) classification of upper respiratory tract tumors and defined as an SCC in which pseudoglandular spaces or lumina result from acantholysis of tumor cells.[116] On gross examination, the majority of these lesions appear as either ulcerations, hyperkeratotic surfaces, or exophytic, warty-appearing lesions and range in size from 0.4 to 12 cm.[492]

Microscopically, the tumor is characterized by a lobular growth pattern of keratinizing SCC that shows central regions containing rounded spaces (pseudoglandular alveolar areas that are lined by a basal layer of polygonal cells with the central lumina containing detached dyskeratotic acantholytic neoplastic cells, "glassy" keratinocytes) (Figs. 2–38 and 2–39, see p. 42).[489] Prominent keratin pearl

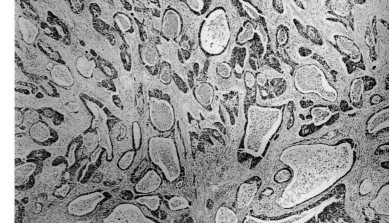

Figure 2–38. Invasive adenoid squamous cell carcinoma showing extensive acantholysis of pseudoglandular structures.

formation is usually present (Fig. 2–40, see p. 42). In some instances, this acantholysis is sufficient to mimic a neoplastic angiomatous proliferation,[500] similar to the one observed in SpCC.[443] No true glandular formations are seen. No intracellular mucin is present in these lesions. ASCC may exhibit limited focal communication between the submucosal or dermal tumor and the overlying surface epithelium.[487, 492] Numerous sections may be required to demonstrate this relationship.

Specific cytologic features,[501] histochemical staining characteristics,[488] and ultrastructure[497] of this variant have been reported. Immunohistochemistry has demonstrated these tumors to be positive for cytokeratins (AE1/AE3) and epithelial membrane antigen and negative for carcinoembryonic antigen, S100, CD34, and Factor VIII–related antigen.[492, 500] The ultrastructural findings have supported the squamous origin with a few hemidesmosomes and attached tonofilaments and no glandular features (e.g., intracytoplasmic microvilli or secretory granules).[497]

Differential Diagnosis. The differential diagnosis includes adenosquamous carcinoma (ASC, the next variant of SCC to be discussed) and mucoepidermoid carcinoma. On morphology alone, the presence of abundant keratin pearl formation and lack of mucocytes may eliminate mucoepidermoid carcinoma. The absence of intracytoplasmic mucin and no true glandular component (adenocarcinoma) separates this lesion from ASC.[499]

Treatment and Prognosis. The clinical behavior described in the WHO classification is that of a low-grade malignancy. Others have concluded, however, that ASC within the head and neck region has a worse prognosis than conventional SCC, although numbers of patients reported until now are too small to support this assumption.[497, 499, 502] Treatment of these lesions is similar to treatment of conventional SCC.[502]

Adenosquamous Carcinoma

Adenosquamous carcinoma is a rare and controversial neoplasm that, as the name implies, possesses histomorphologic features of an adenocarcinoma and SCC. It has been described in a variety of body sites, including the uterine cervix, lung, and pancreas.[503–505] ASC in the upper respiratory tract was defined in 1968 by Gerughty et al.[506] with a series of 10 patients. This investigation showed the neoplasm to be extremely aggressive, with 80% of the patients having proven metastasis.

Clinical Features. Around 100 cases of ASC in the upper respiratory tract have been reported in the English-language literature.[506–516] Over 50 unreported cases of oral ASC are present in the files of the Armed Forces Institute of Pathology (AFIP) (Dr. Gary Ellis, personal communication, 1996). Eighty-five percent of AFIP cases arose from the tongue, floor of the mouth, and tonsillar-palatine region.[517] The most common site of the cases in the literature is the larynx (in decreasing frequency: supraglottic, transglottic, glottic) of which there are 20 reported cases.[507] Other reported sites include the nose and paranasal sinuses,[506, 508, 509] tongue,[506] maxillary alveolus,[510] floor of mouth,[506] upper lip,[511] nasopharynx,[511] oropharynx,[511] and hypopharynx.[511–515]

There is a marked male predominance. The most frequent age of occurrence is the sixth and seventh decade of life (range 39–76 years). Symptoms are similar to those of SCC occurring in the respective sites. In the reported laryngeal cases, the ratio of male to female is 19:1, the average patient age is 60.8 years; 25% had cervical lymph node metastasis, and 5-year survival rate was 22% (two of nine patients).[509]

Etiology has not been defined. Unfortunately, in many reports, tumor staging was not included and, therefore, direct comparisons by site, stage, and treatment are difficult. Evidence of the aggressive biologic nature of ASC is best supported with the reported occurrence of lymph node metastasis (25–80%),[506, 507] distant metastatic sites including lung, liver, bone marrow, kidney, adrenal, colon,[507, 514] and the 5-year survival rates of 25%[506] and 22%.[507] Owing to the lack of staging information in the reported

cases, however, no comparison to 5-year survival rates of SCC can be made.

In the series by Gerughty et al.[506] (three tongue, two floor of mouth, two nose, and three in larynx), the tumor size ranged from 0.2 cm to 1.0 cm, half of the cases had perineural invasion, 80% of the cases had cervical lymph node metastasis, and 5-year survival rate was 25%. In another study, 21 cases of mucoepidermoid/ASC carcinoma involving the larynx and hypopharynx were evaluated.[512] Nine of the 21 cases were deemed compatible with Gerughty's description of ASC. In nine patients (patients per stage: I, two; II, two; III, three; IV, three), the rate of metastasis was 33% and a 3-year survival rate by actuarial methods was 53%. These ASCs did not appear to act as aggressively as those described by Gerughty. Other associated findings described with ASC have been pulmonary lymphangitic carcinomatosis[514] and possibly a radiation-induced lesion.[516] ASC may be included in some classifications of salivary gland neoplasms[517] or as a variant of SCC[511] and by others under mucoepidermoid carcinoma.[518]

Pathology. The gross description of these lesions has been of an erythroplakic ulcerated area to a polypoid broad-based mass.[506, 515] Tumor size has ranged from 0.2 cm to 5 cm in greatest dimension. The histologic criteria defined by Gerughty[506] required a neoplasm to be composed of an admixture or separate areas of SCC and adenocarcinoma. Four basic components were observed: ductal carcinoma in situ, adenocarcinoma, SCC, and a mixed carcinoma. The squamous epithelium required two or more of the following features: (1) intercellular bridging, (2) keratin pearl formation, (3) parakeratotic differentiation, (4) individual cell keratinization, and (5) cellular arrangements showing pavement or mosaic patterns (Figs. 2–41 to 2–44 [see Figs. 2–42 and 2–43 on pp. 42, 43]). The glandular epithelium required the demonstration of intracytoplasmic sialomucin by (preferably) high iron diamine–alcian blue or periodic acid-Schiff stain retention after diastase digestion and Mayer's mucicarmine (see Fig. 2–43B p. 43). The tumor cells were of three basic types: basaloid cells, squamous cells, and undifferentiated cells. All cell types were represented in the tumors even though one cell type may predominate.

In Gerughty's series,[506] early lesions were observed to show only ductal carcinoma in situ, which was frequently multifocal and, in one case, confluent with the overlying surface epithelium. Since Gerughty's description,[506] some modifications have been made. First, the strict requirement for intracytoplasmic mucin has not been a requisite for some examiners to make this diagnosis.[517] This is reflected in the WHO classification description of ASC.[116] The adenocarcinoma component has well-formed ductal structures usually without mucocytes. In the vast majority of cases, overlying mucosa has a carcinoma in situ or superficial SCC. The deeply invasive submucosal aspect of the tumors frequently displays transformation from SCC to adenocarcinoma.[519] Reports in the literature have suggested this arrangement by reporting the initial biopsy containing SCC and subsequent resection showing ASC.[507, 514]

Histogenesis of ASC is debatable. Gerughty considered the neoplasm to be from totipotential cells from the excretory duct of minor salivary glands.[506] Other investigators have included mucosal lining of the upper respiratory tract as a source.[518] The original series cited the presence of the ductal carcinoma in situ preceding the fully developed characteristic ASC, the presence of intracytoplasmic mucin, and the prominence of ductal components in nodal metastasis as grounds for supporting a glandular origin.[506]

Immunocytochemistry studies have shown positive staining for the high molecular weight cytokeratins (LKL1) in both the squamous and glandular components. All glandular components stained positive for carcinoembryonic antigen and low molecular weight cytokeratins (19KD) while the squamous component was negative for both.[511]

Differential Diagnosis. The differential diagnosis of ASC includes ASCC, mucoepidermoid carcinoma, nonkeratinizing SCC, and necrotizing sialometaplasia.

The first entity in the differential diagnosis is ASCC, which is exceedingly rare in this region and considered to be of nonglan-

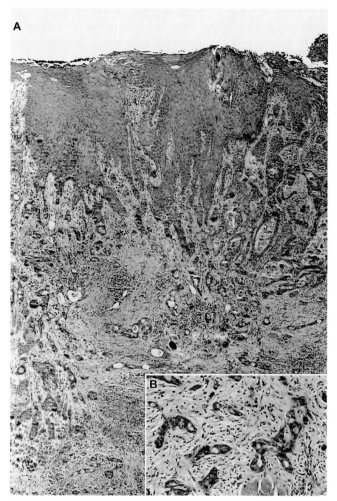

Figure 2–41. *A,* Low power view of an adenosquamous carcinoma, demonstrating surface squamous cell carcinoma blending into a deeply invasive adenocarcinoma. *B,* Close-up of the atypical ductal structures.

dular origin. This tumor is, as previously discussed, a variant of SCC with pseudoglandular formations or an alveolar appearance because of central acantholysis. There is no intracytoplasmic mucin production in these tumors or well-formed areas of ductal adenocarcinoma.

Distinguishing ASC from mucoepidermoid carcinoma is more difficult. Both neoplasms may be of ductal or surface mucosa origin and share some similar cell types. Mucoepidermoid carcinoma does not usually exhibit anaplastic nuclear features and is not associated with carcinoma in situ of the overlying mucosa. ASC, in contrast to mucoepidermoid carcinoma (1) has a tendency for demonstrable intercellular bridges, (2) demonstrates keratin pearl formation and dyskeratosis, and 3) has distinct areas of adenocarcinoma.[511, 520]

The third differential diagnosis, nonkeratinizing SCC, may have rare mucin-containing pseudoglandular structures; however, no areas of definitive adenocarcinoma or keratinization are present.[511] This lesion is more extensively discussed in the section on sinonasal carcinoma.

The fourth differential diagnosis is that of a benign entity, necrotizing sialometaplasia, which may be confused with mucoepidermoid carcinoma or SCC. This lesion is most frequently associated with minor salivary or seromucinous glands. The overlying surface is usually ulcerated. Within the subjacent minor glands there may be intraductal proliferation of metaplastic squamous cells, partial necrosis of salivary seromucinous glands, and vascular proliferation. The overall lobular configuration of the lesion is an important distinguishing characteristic.[520] Necrotizing sialometaplasia is discussed in more detail in the chapter on salivary glands. Coexistence of ASC with a salivary gland tumor has also been observed.[521]

Treatment and Prognosis. ASC is considered to have an aggressive behavior in comparison to standard SCC and mucoepidermoid carcinoma.[506, 522–524] As mentioned earlier, owing to limited numbers for comparison, it is difficult to determine whether the aggressiveness is site-related[517] or inherent to the tumor.[506, 522, 523] The primary mode of recommended treatment is surgical.[515, 523] Radiation alone overall has had poor results[507, 515] with a rare exception.[513] Radiation combined with radical surgery, however, has been reported to improve local control.[513]

Papillary Squamous Cell Carcinoma

In a 1988 article discussing squamous papillary neoplasms of the UADT, Crissman et al.[525] proposed the term *papillary carcinoma* for a rare variant of SCC. This lesion, named papillary squamous cell carcinoma (PSCC) in the current WHO classification[116] has also been described in other parts of the body such as skin,[526] uterine cervix,[527] conjunctiva of the eye,[528] and the thymus.[529] Within the UADT, PSCC has been mentioned as making up part of the histologic spectrum shown by the clinical entity proliferative verrucous leukoplakia,[386, 391, 392] a condition more extensively discussed within the context of VC.

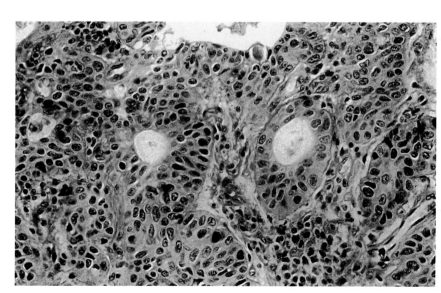

Figure 2–44. Adenosquamous cell carcinoma with duct carcinoma in situ formation.

In the study on papillary neoplasia within the adult UADT, Crissman et al. presented six cases of PSCC. These patients had an average age of 63.3 years, with the onset of disease ranging from 46 to 79 years, and did not have a history of recurrent papillomatosis. The architectural features were those of an exophytic neoplasm with a papillary configuration. The epithelium lining the fibrovascular cores showed either carcinoma in situ or pronounced cellular pleomorphism with surface keratinization. Lesions without an invasive component were called noninvasive papillary carcinoma to distinguish them from invasive papillary carcinoma that had foci of SCC in association with the superficial papillary component. The invasion was usually found within the vascular cores or in the base of the stalks. Five of the six patients were male; three lesions were present in the larynx, one in the nasopharynx, one in the pyriform sinus, and one in the oropharynx.[525] Data on HPV involvement are conflicting.[525, 530–532]

Clinical Features. Clinical features of PSCC in general are unknown. More details are available for PSCC occurring in the larynx than in other anatomic areas. In a series of 104 cases identified in the files of the Otorhinolaryngic—Head & Neck Pathology Tumor Registry of the AFIP, there were 25 females and 79 males, aged 27 to 89 years, with a mean age at presentation of 60.7 years. Clinical presentation was generally hoarseness. A large number of patients were smokers or used alcohol, or both. Tumor size varied from 0.3 cm to 6 cm in greatest dimension, and the larger tumors were frequently associated with vocal cord impairment or fixation.[530]

Pathology. The histologic features of PSCC are a papillary display of fibrovascular cores lined by markedly dysplastic epithelium of normal or increased thickness. The malignant-appearing squamous epithelium may be composed entirely of immature basal-like cells or have prominent nuclear and cellular pleomorphism in the lower portion of the epithelium with varying degrees of surface keratinization.[525] If no invasion of the atypical epithelium is observed, lesions are called noninvasive PSCC or *papillary dysplasia*[531] and represent part of the spectrum of verrucous hyperplasia. The invasive form of PSCC has the above findings with an associated invasive SCC. Frequently squamous neoplasms with papillary components contain predominantly noninvasive areas and it may require extensive histologic sampling to find areas of invasion.[393, 525]

In the invasive type of PSCC, both typical keratinizing cord-like and nonkeratinizing ribbon-like patterns of invasive SCC have been found.[531] Two histologic patterns have been identified in PSCC: papillary-frond or broad-based exophytic growth (Fig. 2–45). The papillary pattern consisted of multiple, thin, delicate filiform, finger-like papillary projections. The papillae contained a delicate fibrovascular core surrounded by the neoplastic epithelium. Tangential sectioning would yield commonly one or occasionally a number of central fibrovascular cores, but would appear more like a bunch of celery cut across the stalk. The exophytic pattern consisted of a broad-based, bulbous to exophytic growth of the squamous epithelium. The projections were rounded and cauliflower-like in growth pattern. Tangential sectioning would yield a number of central fibrovascular cores, but the outer aspect was lobular, not papillary (see Fig. 2–45).[530]

Differential Diagnosis. The growth pattern of this neoplasm evokes a clinical and histologic differential diagnosis ranging from solitary papilloma to VC. Applying the criterion of invasion to diagnose PSCC simplifies the diagnostic process when considering a solitary papilloma with atypia. The diagnosis of noninvasive PSCC in contrast to papilloma requires the epithelium to be severely dysplastic or carcinoma in situ, not just focal areas of atypia. PSCC is not associated with recurrent papillomatosis or inverting papillomas.[393, 525] The history of a recurrent adult or juvenile papillomatosis with marked dysplasia having a rapid rate of recurrence has been well documented. Malignant transformation in these lesions, however, is very rare.[533–535] Moreover, PSCCs occur in older patients.

Verrucous carcinoma is another differential diagnostic consideration. The fronded fibrovascular-based epithelial growth pattern as well as the presence of the significant cytologic atypia distinguishes PSCC from the bland cytologic character of VC. VC has a more sessile base with a confluent downward "pushing border" rather than exhibiting features of an infiltrative cell process[393] and is usually associated with a greater degree of hyperkeratosis.

Finally, PSCC has to be distinguished from nonkeratinizing or cylindrical cell carcinoma, this latter lesion being characterized by ribbons of cylindrical epidermoid cells and lacking the papillae covered with a layer of epidermoid cells exhibiting severe atypia and disturbed maturation (for more detail, see the section on sinonasal SCC).

Treatment and Prognosis. The clinical course of the noninvasive PSCC is not known. Whether this lesion has a high frequency of progression to an invasive neoplasm is unclear. It is currently recommended that papillary dysplasia or noninvasive PSCC be treated by complete surgical excision. The treatment of an invasive PSCC is based on the stage of the invasive component.[531] In the series of 104 laryngeal PSCCs, patients were treated with excisional biopsy, vocal cord stripping, and laryngectomy in conjunction with radiation. Eighty-seven patients had no evidence of disease at the time of last follow-up. Of the 92 patients with an exophytic pattern, 10 died with widely metastatic disease, and 7 patients died with locally recurrent disease. Four of 12 patients with the papillary pattern developed local recurrence, but none died of disease. The authors conclude that the group of papillary and exophytic SCCs generally has a better prognosis than usual SCCs and that the papillary histologic variant appears to have an even better prognosis than the exophytic type.[530]

Lymphoepithelioma

Lymphoepithelioma, also called lymphoepithelial carcinoma, is a histologic variant of SCC that was first reported by Regaud and Reverchon[536] and independently by Schmincke.[537] At present it is defined by the occurrence of a distinctive intermingling of undifferentiated carcinoma cells with a prominent lymphoid stroma.[116] Lymphoepithelioma mainly occurs in the nasopharynx; occasionally, tumors with the same histomorphologic features have been described in the oropharynx (Waldeyer's ring region), salivary glands, tonsils, tongue, soft palate, uvula, floor of the mouth, sinonasal tract, larynx, trachea, hypopharynx, lung, thymus, stomach, skin, breast, uterine cervix, vagina, and urinary bladder under a variety of terms: undifferentiated carcinoma of nasopharyngeal type, undifferentiated carcinoma with lymphoid stroma, lymphoepithelioma, lymphoepithelial-like carcinoma, and lymphoepithelial carcinoma. Unlike lymphoepithelioma of the nasopharynx, lymphoepithelioma arising at these other sites, with the exception of the major salivary glands, does not exhibit a close association with EBV.[234, 250, 538–542]

As the majority of cases of lymphoepithelioma involve the nasopharynx, clinical, epidemiologic, and other data are mainly based on tumor series at this location, and therefore discussion of these characteristics will be based on lymphoepithelioma in the nasopharynx unless explicitly stated otherwise; lymphoepithelioma of the salivary glands is discussed in Chapter 6.

Clinical Features. Lymphoepithelioma has its highest worldwide incidence in people of Southeast China, Southeast Asia, the Arctic Regions, and Malaysia.[543–545] Regions of occurrence have been designated as high incidence (e.g., South China province of Kwantung and Hong Kong), intermediate incidence (e.g., North Africa), and low incidence (e.g., Europe and the United States). Lymphoepithelioma represents the majority of nasopharyngeal cancer in regions where nasopharyngeal cancer is endemic.[233] Within the United States, where nasopharyngeal cancer represents only 0.2% of all cancers, 60% of these are lymphoepithelioma.[229] In contrast, in Chinese regions where nasopharyngeal cancer represents 18% to 25% of all cancers, lymphoepithelioma accounts for more than 90% of these.[51, 229] Moreover, lymphoepithelioma is the most common type of nasopharyngeal cancer in young people (greater than 90%).[235] Other features specific for lymphoepithelioma are occur-

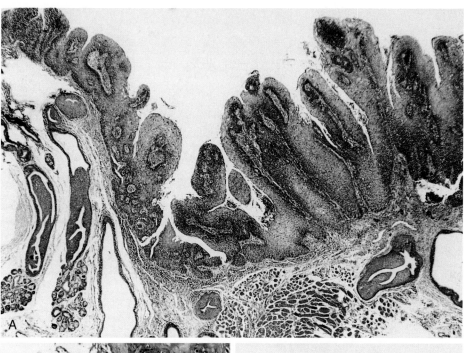

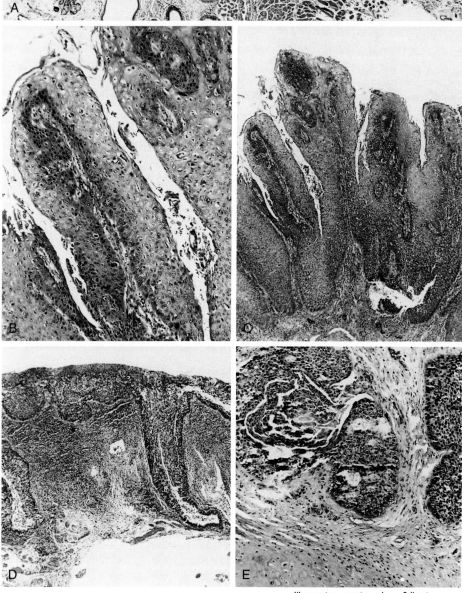

Figure 2–45. Papillary squamous cell carcinoma. *A, B,* & *C,* Papillary frond-like type: Note delicate finger-like extensions of tumor extending up from and along the surface, composed of dysplastic epithelium lining delicate, simple, fibrovascular cores. *D,* Dysplastic epithelium extending into adjacent seromucinous gland duct. *E,* A small focus of invasive squamous carcinoma from an adjacent area, which extends almost down to the cartilage.

Illustration continued on following page

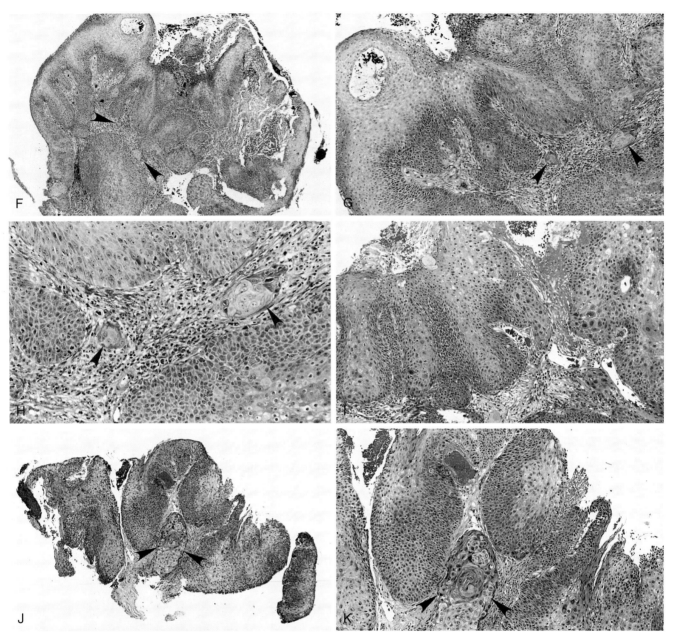

Figure 2–45 *Continued. F–K,* Broad-based exophytic growth type. Note polypoid, broad-based, exophytic growth with complex fibrovascular cores lined, at least focally, by dysplastic epithelium (*H*). Areas of invasion were noted in this biopsy specimen in two of the biopsy fragments (*F, H, J, K;* arrowheads).

rence at a younger age than other head and neck SCCs; absence of a strong alcohol or tobacco etiologic relationship; lack of substantial risk for a second primary tumor (1.3%)[221]; and very high rate of systemic dissemination.[233]

Similar to nasopharyngeal cancer in general, lymphoepithelioma usually arises on the lateral or posterior-superior wall of the nasopharynx. The clinical appearance of the tumor may be exophytic, infiltrative, or ulcerative. Dickson found the gross appearance of tumor in the nasopharynx to be exophytic in 74.2% of lesions, infiltrative in 14.4% of lesions, and ulcerative in 6.7% of lesions; in 4.8%, the appearance of the lesion was not well documented.[223]

Pathology. Microscopically, lymphoepithelioma is composed of cells containing large, round or oval, vesicular nuclei with a smooth, thin nuclear membrane and one to three prominent eosinophilic nucleoli.[546] The borders of the amphophilic cytoplasm are indistinct (Fig. 2–46*A,* see p. 43). Frequently, spindle-shaped tumor cells with hyperchromatic nuclei are present.[259] The associated infiltrate is mixed and composed of T-lymphocytes and may contain plasma cells, follicular dendritic cells, or abundant eosinophils.[230] Individual tumor cells may be surrounded by the mixed infiltrate, resembling Hodgkin's disease.[547] The presence of noncaseating granulomas negative for acid-fast bacilli, sarcoid-like granulomas, and localized amyloid has been reported in the adjacent stroma.[263]

Historically, but inaccurately, lymphoepithelioma was subdivided into two histologic types: Regaud's type (clusters, nests, or aggregates of neoplastic epithelial cells with lymphoid elements), and Schmincke's type (dispersed tumor cells forming a syncytial net beneath an inflammatory infiltrate) (Fig. 2–46*B,* see p. 43).[233, 548, 549] These two types were essentially descriptions of two growth patterns of an undifferentiated carcinoma. Familiarity with these variations in the histomorphology of undifferentiated carcinoma is useful, particularly when the examiner is confronted with a small biopsy of the primary tumor or when evaluating a metastatic deposit in a cervical lymph node with an occult primary tumor (Fig. 2–46*C,* see p. 43). Designation of lymphoepithelioma as a Regaud or a Schmincke type does not have prognostic significance.

Various histologic findings are reported to have an impact on the prognosis. The presence of a high density of follicular dendritic cells (S100 positive),[550] and eosinophils[551] has been associated with a good prognosis. The presence of a spindle cell phenotype or "cord-like" arrangement and increased nuclear anaplasia has been reported to indicate a poor prognosis.[263]

Confirming the presence of the EBV within tumor cells of diagnostic tissue has proven to be useful. The expression of EBV-encoded RNA-1(EBER-1) detected by in situ hybridization technique in primary lymphoepithelioma and in metastatic cells of lymphoepithelioma has been found to be helpful in specimens in which this diagnosis is suspected (Fig. 2–46D, see p. 43).[250] Others have used polymerase chain reaction for detecting EBV in paraffin-embedded tissue and tissue from fine needle aspiration in patients with unknown primary tumors.[237, 238] The usefulness of tumor ploidy determination remains controversial.[230]

Differential Diagnosis. Because of the frequently inconspicuous epithelial nature of undifferentiated carcinoma including lymphoepithelioma and because its most common presentation is metastases to cervical lymph nodes, the differential diagnosis is diverse. Included in the differential diagnosis are Hodgkin's disease, large cell lymphoma, lymphoid hyperplasia, melanoma, and sinonasal undifferentiated carcinoma.

Hodgkin's disease as a differential diagnosis presents the most deceptive pitfall, particularly if the initial histologic diagnosis is based on a cervical lymph node in a young patient with adenopathy.[546, 552] Lymph nodes containing undifferentiated carcinoma exhibit varying degrees of nodal replacement by tumor. Capsular fibrosis and dense bands of collagen entrapping discohesive tumor cells are histologic findings that may be common to Hodgkin's disease and lymphoepithelioma.[546, 547, 552] The carcinoma cells may have vesicular nuclei with prominent eosinophilic nucleoli reminiscent of the mononuclear variants of Reed-Sternberg cells.[547] Immunohistochemical stains are very helpful in this dilemma. The undifferentiated carcinoma cells will be positive for cytokeratin and negative for leukocyte common antigen, LeuM1, L26, and UCHL1.[547]

Undifferentiated carcinoma is morphologically easily mistaken for a large cell lymphoma (Fig. 2–47). Again, the immunohistochemical stains for cytokeratins (AE1/AE3) can be useful. The majority (97%)[553] of nasopharyngeal cancer will be positive for cytokeratins, with the caveat that cytokeratin positivity has been reported in rare lymphomas.[554] Leukocyte common antigen positivity in undifferentiated carcinoma has not yet been reported in the epithelial component.

Lymphoid hyperplasia is a common finding in nasopharyngeal biopsies and should be included in the differential diagnosis of the lymphoepithelioma type of undifferentiated carcinoma when nasopharyngeal lymphoid hyperplasia accompanies cervical adenopathy in a patient who tests positive for human immunodeficiency virus type 1.[555] Cytokeratin stains again should resolve this question. An increase incidence of lymphoepithelioma in patients with acquired immunodeficiency syndrome (AIDS) has not been observed.[556]

Melanoma is rare in the nasopharynx. The nuclear features of undifferentiated carcinoma and melanoma may be similar. The immunohistochemical staining patterns for undifferentiated carcinoma are the reverse for melanoma. In undifferentiated carcinoma, HMB45 and S100 are negative while cytokeratin is positive.[263]

Sinonasal undifferentiated carcinoma is similar histomorphologically to lymphoepithelioma. Cells of sinonasal undifferentiated carcinoma, however, are smaller, are frequently associated with large areas of necrosis, do not usually contain spindle-shaped cells, are not associated with a positive serology for EBV, and are frequently positive, by immunohistochemical staining, for neural markers (e.g., neuron specific enolase).[263]

Treatment and Prognosis. Treatment and prognosis were discussed previously under the discussion of nasopharyngeal carcinoma.

Other Unusual Features and Diagnostic Pitfalls in Squamous Cell Carcinomas

Squamous cell carcinoma variants such as SpCC, VC, and other entities discussed previously are not rare and have obtained recognition as a specific subtype of UADT-SCC. There are, however, other, less frequently observed morphologic variants of SCC that have gained less attention. The first to be discussed is the so-called *desmoplastic squamous cell carcinoma* (DSCC).[557] Clinically, this lesion presents itself as a firm submucosal mass. Histologic examination demonstrates a fibrous lesion in which clumps of vesiculated nuclei are observed. Immunohistochemistry of these latter cells demonstrates cytoplasmic positivity for keratin (Fig. 2–48, see p. 44). Ultrastructural examination also reveals epithelial features such as tonofilaments and desmosomes. Because of the preponderance of fibrous tissue, the lesion may be mistaken for a benign spindle cell lesion, such as proliferative myositis or nodular fasciitis.[557] If DSCC invades bone, extensive bony remodeling may occur, leading to a histomorphology suggesting fibrous dysplasia with the invading tumor being present as only tiny strands (Fig. 2–49, see p. 44).

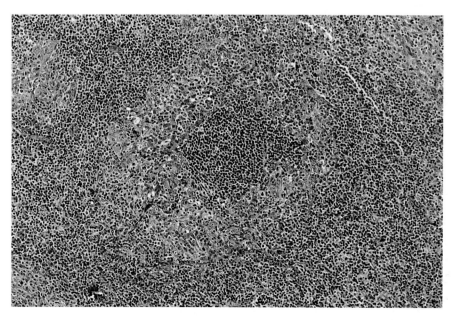

Figure 2–47. Note the poorly differentiated carcinoma cells of lymphoepithelioma mimicking a lymphoma.

A DSCC should not be confused with SpCC, because, in that SCC type, the malignant nature is obvious and the lesion exhibits sarcomatous features, whereas in DSCC, the major part of the lesion consists of desmoplastic stroma simulating a benign mesenchymal proliferation. As only two cases of DSCC have been published, one at the right lateral aspect of the posterior mobile tongue and the other in the right base of the tongue,[557] it is not known whether this SCC subtype behaves differently from conventional SCC. In the gingiva, DSCC may be confused with odontogenic epithelial nests, a feature mentioned in the discussion of alveolar ridge SCC.

Another SCC variant not widely recognized is the so-called *superficial extending carcinoma* (SEC), primarily occurring in larynx and hypopharynx.[318] SEC is a poorly or moderately differentiated infiltrating SCC showing an entirely or predominantly superficial type of growth. In spite of its intramucosal site, lymph node metastases may be present.[318] SEC is notorious for its association with multiple synchronous and metachronous neoplasms in the UADT. SEC should not be confused with microinvasive SCC. The latter lesion is basically an intraepithelial lesion with tiny foci of penetration through the epithelial basement membrane, whereas SEC occupies the mucosal lining extending to underlying glands or muscle; in other words, the entire lamina propria is involved. To date, the prognostic significance of distinguishing between conventional SCC and SEC is unclear.[318]

An SCC may also mimic odontogenic epithelial tumors, in particular the acanthomatous ameloblastoma by exhibiting palisading of the basal cell layer facing the stroma and by showing epithelial spindle cell areas with extensive intercellular edema that display an abrupt transition to distinctly circumscribed keratin pearls (Fig. 2–50). The lack of "reverse polarization" of the nucleus from the basement membrane within the palisaded layer and no evidence of collagen condensation in the subjacent connective tissue should aid in preventing the erroneous diagnosis of ameloblastoma for a lesion that is an SCC. (Refer to Chapter 9 for more detail.) For some unknown reasons, SCCs that mimic some microscopic features of ameloblastomas are frequently observed in the retromolar area.

Poorly differentiated SCC may exhibit a nodular growth pattern with intervening fibrous bands, thus simulating malignant lymphoma. Occasional cells with eosinophilic cytoplasm and cells arranged in clusters will reveal the epithelial nature of such a lesion, and immunohistochemistry with appropriately selected markers (broad-spectrum keratin and panleukocytic markers) will confirm the diagnosis of poorly differentiated SCC (Fig. 2–51, see p. 44). Moreover, poorly differentiated SCC may invade an overlying uninvolved epithelial lining and in this way mimic the intraepithelial extension of a malignant melanoma (Fig. 2–52, see p. 45). Also in this case, individual cells or cell clusters showing more classic SCC features can be found as evidence against a diagnosis of malignant melanoma. However, in small biopsy specimens, the unwary observer may be lead astray by this growth pattern. Immunohistochemistry can also be helpful in this situation, with broad-spectrum keratin stains being positive in the former and S100 and HMB45 staining positively in the latter.

If SCC exhibits extensive acantholysis, lumina occur lined by cells with pleomorphic nuclei, a growth pattern closely mimicking angiosarcoma. This feature may occur in SpCC[443] as well as in ASCC,[500] but angiosarcoma-like areas may also be part of more conventional SCC. Immunohistochemistry will reveal that the pleomorphic cells lining the lumina are positive for keratin and negative for endothelial markers, thus confirming their epithelial nature (Fig. 2–53, see p. 46)

TREATMENT

Although surgery is most often the mode of treating SCC of the head and neck, radiotherapy and chemotherapy, either alone or in combination, play an important role in therapy. Their value is discussed briefly.

Radiotherapy

Radiotherapy plays a central role in the treatment of head and neck tumors. The combination of high locoregional cure rates and a good functional outcome may be reached by radiotherapy, with salvage surgery in reserve. Radiotherapy may be given as primary treatment for head and neck tumors, eventually in combination with induction chemotherapy for very advanced cases. Combined surgery and radiotherapy as a treatment modality is used for advanced head and neck tumors.

Primary Radiotherapy with Salvage Surgery in Reserve

Radiotherapy is accepted as the primary treatment for T1 and T2 laryngeal cancer because of the obvious advantage of voice preservation and voice quality.[558, 559] Local control rates may be 90% or more for T1 glottic tumors and around 80% for T1 supraglottic and

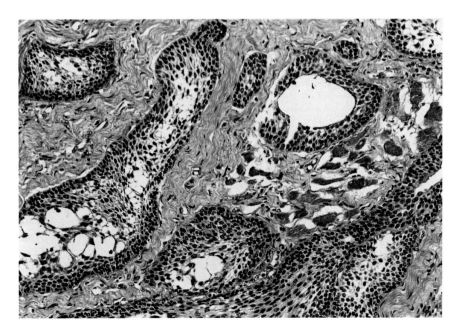

Figure 2–50. Sometimes, squamous cell carcinoma may mimic ameloblastoma by acantholysis and peripheral palisading.

T2 tumors with normal mobility of the vocal cord.[558, 559] Impairment of vocal cord mobility may result in decreased local control rates of around 70%, which decrease even further to around 50% for vocal cord fixation.[559, 560] Salvage surgery in cases of local recurrence is successfully applied in two of three patients. Extension of the tumor beyond the larynx results in local cure rates with conventional radiotherapy of 30% to 40%.

Prognostic factors for local control in radiotherapy for laryngeal cancer are patient factors like sex (woman fare better) and continuation of smoking, tumor factors like size and impairment of vocal cord mobility, and treatment factors such as radiation dose.[558–560] A conventional fractionation schedule for radiotherapy of head and neck tumors consists of 33 to 35 fractions of 2 Gy given five times weekly to the primary tumor. Increasing the tumor dose beyond 70 Gy in fractions of 2 Gy will result in an unacceptable increased rate of complications.[561] To improve the results for advanced tumors, unconventional radiation schedules may be used.[562] The use of smaller doses per fraction, and using two fractions a day (hyperfractionation), will allow a higher total dose in the same overall treatment time without risk of increase of late complications.

In a randomized trial conducted under supervision of the European Organization for Research and Treatment of Cancer (EORTC), a significant increase in local regional control in oropharyngeal cancer is shown with a fractionation schedule of 70 fractions of 1.15 Gy in 7 weeks.[563] Fowler showed that reduction of overall treatment time from 7 to 5 weeks may result in 20% to 25% improvement in local control in cancer of the tonsillar region.[564] After a lag period of 3 to 4 weeks, accelerated clonogenic repopulation of tumor cells during radiotherapy is noted, likely caused by reoxygenation and reduced tissue pressure by reduced tumor volume.[565] To counteract this accelerated repopulation, an increase in the daily fraction 3 to 4 weeks after the start of radiotherapy is necessary. With an accelerated hyperfractionation schedule, a total dose of about 70 Gy may be given in 5 weeks. In weeks 4 and 5, two daily fractions may be given with a concomitant boost to the primary tumor region as the second daily fraction.[562]

Adjuvant Radiotherapy

Adjuvant radiotherapy is mostly used as postoperative treatment based on histologic parameters: resection margins not free of tumor; growth pattern (spidery growth), perineural growth, tumor thickness, and bone invasion.[144] In postoperative radiotherapy, fast-proliferating tumors may be treated more successfully with accelerated fractionation, as compared with conventional fractionation of 50 to 60 Gy in 5 to 6 weeks.[566]

Radiotherapy for Positive Neck Nodes

Patients with a single positive neck node or a neck node smaller than 3 cm may be cured in 90% of cases with primary radiotherapy.[567] For undifferentiated tumors in neck nodes, regional control with radiotherapy is high, even for neck nodes larger than 3 cm. For all other nodes larger than 3 cm, a combination of neck dissection with radiotherapy is preferable to gain higher regional control rates.

Chemotherapy

Chemotherapy may be given as part of the primary treatment of patients with squamous cell cancer as follows[568]:

- Prior to radiotherapy or surgery (neoadjuvant or induction chemotherapy)
- After radiotherapy or surgery (adjuvant chemotherapy)
- Synchronous with radiotherapy (chemoradiotherapy)

Despite high response rates, neoadjuvant chemotherapy has not been shown to improve survival in many randomized trials.[569] A few recent trials have suggested a clinical benefit for chemoradiotherapy.[570–572] A recent meta-analysis suggested that chemotherapy may increase absolute survival by 6.5% (95% confidence interval 3.1–9.9%).[573] The benefit of neoadjuvant chemotherapy was much less than that of chemoradiotherapy (3.7% versus 12.1%). Currently, however, chemotherapy cannot yet be considered to be a part of standard primary treatment.

Neoadjuvant chemotherapy, followed by radiotherapy, may play a role in organ preservation in patients with advanced laryngeal cancer,[574] in those with hypopharyngeal cancer,[575] and in patients with bulky, unresectable tumors, in whom radiotherapy alone is not expected to result in significant tumor reduction. The combination of cisplatinum and 5-fluorouracil is often used in this setting.

Chemotherapy may also be given as palliative treatment to patients with locally recurrent disease, which cannot be cured with surgery or radiotherapy, or to patients with distant metastases.[576] The median survival of these patients is 5 to 6 months and is not improved by chemotherapy. Its aim is to relieve symptoms and to improve quality of life. It may be considered in symptomatic patients with a good performance status, measurable disease, and normal renal function. In view of its low toxicity, weekly administration of methotrexate is considered standard treatment in recurrent or metastatic disease by many centers. Although cisplatin monotherapy and cisplatin-containing combinations result in higher response rates, this seems to be outweighed by increased toxicity.

CONCLUDING REMARKS

Squamous cell carcinoma is the most common head and neck malignancy. Usually, the diagnosis is easily made, although there are diagnostic pitfalls, as mentioned in this chapter. The major diagnostic responsibility for the pathologist dealing with head and neck specimens coming from patients suffering from this tumor is the identification of either macroscopic or microscopic features having prognostic significance and necessitating additional treatment. An adequate anatomic knowledge of the various head and neck sites from which tumor resection specimens are submitted is required in performing this task. A histologic section can be sent anywhere for additional consultation; however, overlooking macroscopic features because of lack of anatomic expertise may cause irreparable loss of clinically relevant information and thus negatively influence optimal patient care.

REFERENCES

Introduction

1. Vokes EE, Weichselbaum RR, Lippman SM, et al: Head and neck cancer. N Engl J Med 1993;328:184–194.
2. Tobias JS: Cancer of the head and neck. Br Med J 1994;308:961–966.
3. Visser O, Coebergh JWW, Schouten LJ, van Dijck JAAM (eds): Incidence of cancer in the Netherlands 1994. Sixth Report of the Netherlands Cancer Registry. Utrecht: Vereniging van Integrale Kankercentra, 1997.
4. Parkin DM, Pisani P, Ferlay J: Estimates of the worldwide incidence of eighteen major cancers in 1985. Int J Cancer 1993;54:594–606.

Epidemiology and Risk Factors

5. Muir CS, Nectoux J: International patterns of cancer. In Schottenfeld D, Fraumeni JF (eds): Cancer Epidemiology and Prevention, 2nd ed. New York: Oxford University Press, 1996:141–167.
6. Parkin DM, Muir CS, Whelan SW, et al (eds): Cancer Incidence in Five Continents, Vol VI. IARC Sci Publ. no. 120. Lyon: International Agency for Research on Cancer, 1992.
7. Blot WJ, McLaughlin JK, Devesa SS, Fraumeni JF: Cancers of the oral cavity and pharynx. In Schottenfeld D, Fraumeni JF (eds): Cancer Epidemiology and Prevention, 2nd ed. New York: Oxford University Press, 1996:666–680.
8. Boyle P, Macfarlane GJ, Blot WJ, et al: Review. European School of Oncology advisory report to the European Commission for the Europe

Against Cancer Programme: Oral carcinogenesis in Europe. Oral Oncol Eur J Cancer 1995;31b:75–85.

9. Paterson IC, Eveson JW, Prime SS: Molecular changes in oral cancer may reflect aetiology and ethnic origin. Oral Oncol Eur J Cancer 1996;32b:150–153.

10. Elias MM, Hilgers FJM, Keus RB, et al: Carcinoma of the pyriform sinus: A retrospective analysis of treatment results over a 20-year period. Clin Otolaryngol 1995;20:249–253.

11. Hoffman RM, Jaffe PE: Plummer-Vinson syndrome. A case report and literature review. Arch Intern Med 1995;155:2008–2011.

12. Ferguson MM, Dagg JH: Nutritional disorders. In Jones JH, Mason DK (eds): Oral Manifestations of Systemic Diseases. Philadelphia: W.B. Saunders, 1980:211–228.

13. Austin DF, Reynold P: Laryngeal cancer. In Schottenfeld D, Fraumeni JF (eds): Cancer Epidemiology and Prevention, 2nd ed. New York: Oxford University Press, 1996:618–636.

14. Muir C, Weiland L: Upper aerodigestive tract cancers. Cancer 1995;75:147–153.

15. Cattaruzza MS, Maisonneuve P, Boyle P: Epidemiology of laryngeal cancer. Oral Oncol Eur J Cancer 1996;32b:293–305.

16. Coleman MP, Estève J, Damiecki J, et al: Trends in cancer incidence and mortality. IARC Sci Publ. no. 121. Lyon: International Agency for Research in Cancer, 1993.

17. Spitz MR: Epidemiology and risk factors for head and neck cancer. Sem Oncol 1994;21:281–288.

18. Tuyns AJ, Esteve J, Raymond L, et al: Cancer of the larynx/hypopharynx, tobacco and alcohol. IARC International Case Control Study in Turin and Varese (Italy), Zaragoza and Navarra (Spain), Geneva (Switzerland) and Calvados (France). Int J Cancer 1988;41:483–491.

19. DeStefani E, Correa D, Oreggia F: Risk factors for laryngeal cancer. Cancer 1987;60:308–309.

20. Osguthorpe JD: Sinus neoplasia. Arch Otolaryngol Head Neck Surg 1994;120:19–25.

21. Muir CS, Nectoux J: Descriptive epidemiology of malignant neoplasms of nose, nasal cavities, middle ear and accessory sinuses. Clin Otolaryngol 1980;5:195–211.

22. Doll R, Morgan IG, Speizer FE: Cancer of the lung and sinuses in nickel workers. Br J Cancer 1970;24:623–632.

23. Vaughan TL, Davis S: Wood dust exposure and squamous cell cancers of the upper respiratory tract. Am J Epidemiol 1991;133:560–564.

24. Merler E, Baldasseroni A, Laria R, et al: On the causal association between exposure to leather dust and nasal cancer: Further evidence from a case-control study. Br J Indust Med 1986;43:91–95.

25. Davies JM, Easton DF, Birdstrup PL: Mortality from respiratory cancer and other causes in United Kingdom chromate production workers. Brit J Indust Med 1991;48:299–313.

26. Wada S, Miyanishi P, Nishimoto Y: Mustard gas as a cause of neoplasia in man. Lancet 1968;1:1161–1163.

27. Leung SI, Yuen ST, Chung LP, et al:. Epstein-Barr virus is present in a wide histological spectrum of sinonasal carcinomas. Am J Surg Pathol 1995;19:994–1001.

28. Yu MC, Henderson BE: Nasopharyngeal Cancer. In Schottenfeld D, Fraumeni JF (eds): Cancer Epidemiology and Prevention, 2nd ed. New York: Oxford University Press, 1996:603–18.

29. Houston HE, Payne WS, Harrison EG Jr, et al: Primary tracheal tumors in the infant and adult. Arch Otolaryngol 1953;58:1–9.

30. Baraka ME: Malignant tumours of the trachea. Ann R Col Surg Engl 1984;66:27–29.

31. Boyle P, Macfarlane GJ, Zheng T, et al: Recent advances in epidemiology of head and neck cancer. Curr Opin Oncol 1992;4:471–477.

32. Blot WJ, McLaughlin JK, Winn DM, et al: Smoking and drinking in relation to oral pharyngeal cancer. Cancer Res 1988;48:3282–3287.

33. Gindhart TD, Johnston WH, Chism SE, et al: Carcinoma of the larynx in childhood. Cancer 1980;46:1683–1687.

34. Trizna Z, Schantz SP: Hereditary and environmental factors associated with risk and progression of head and neck cancer. Otolaryngol Clin North Am 1992;25:1089–1103.

35. Berkower AS, Biller HF: Head and neck cancer associated with Bloom's syndrome. Laryngoscope 1988;98:746–748.

36. Snow DG, Campbell JB, Smallman LA: Fanconi's anaemia and postcricoid carcinoma. J Laryngol Otol 1991;105:125–127.

37. Lustig JP, Lugassy G, Neder A, Sigler E: Head and neck carcinoma in Fanconi's anaemia: Report of a case and review of the literature. Oral Oncol Eur J Cancer 1995;31b:68–72.

38. Patton LL, Valdez IH: Xeroderma pigmentosum: Review and report of a case. Oral Surg Oral Med Oral Pathol 1991;71:297–300.

39. Hecht F, Hecht BK: Cancer in ataxia-telangiectasia patients. Cancer Genet Cytogenet 1990;46:9–12.

40. Gardner GM, Steiniger JR: Family cancer syndrome: A study of the kindred of a man with osteogenic sarcoma of the mandible. Laryngoscope 1990;100:1259–1263.

41. Flaitz CM, Nichols CM, Adler-Storthz K, et al: Intraoral squamous cell carcinoma in human immunodeficiency virus infection. Oral Surg Oral Med Oral Pathol Oral Radiol Endod 1995;80:55–62.

42. Mullen DL, Silverberg SG, Penn I, Hammond WS: Squamous cell carcinoma of the skin and lip in renal homograft recipients. Cancer 1976;37:729–734.

Etiology

43. Elwood JM, Pearson JCG, Skippen DH, et al: Alcohol, smoking, social and occupational factors in the etiology of cancer of the oral cavity, pharynx and larynx. Int J Cancer 1984;34:603–612.

44. Brugere J, Guenel P, Leclerc A, et al: Differential effects of tobacco and alcohol in cancer of the larynx, pharynx and mouth. Cancer 1986;57:391–395.

45. Macfarlane GJ, Zheng T, Marshall JR, et al: Alcohol, tobacco, diet and the risk of oral cancer: A pooled analysis of three case-control studies. Eur J Cancer 1995;31b:181–187.

46. Scully C: Oral precancer: Preventive and medical approaches to management. Eur J Cancer 1995;31b:16–26.

47. Scully C: Viruses and oral squamous carcinoma. Eur J Cancer 1992;28b:57–59.

48. Yeudall WA: Human papillomaviruses and oral neoplasia. Eur J Cancer 1992;28b:61–66.

49. Brachman DG: Molecular biology of head and neck cancer. Semin Oncol 1994;21:320–329.

50. Hording U, Nielsen HW, Albeck H, et al: Nasopharyngeal carcinoma: Histopathological types and association with Epstein-Barr virus. Eur J Cancer 1993;29b:137–139.

51. Pathmanathan R, Prasad U, Chandrika G, et al: Undifferentiated, non-keratinizing and squamous cell carcinoma of the nasopharynx. Variants of Epstein Barr virus-infected neoplasia. Am J Pathol 1995;146:1355–1367.

52. Vries N de, Drexhage HA, Waal LP de, et al: Human leukocyte antigens and immunoglobulin allotypes in head and neck cancer patients with and without multiple primary tumors. Cancer 1987;60:957–961.

53. Copper MP, Jovanovic A, Nauta JJP, et al: Role of genetic factors in the etiology of squamous cell carcinoma of the head and neck. Arch Otolaryngol Head Neck Surg 1995;121:157–160.

54. Goldstein AM, Blot JW, Greenberg RS, et al: Familial risk in oral and pharyngeal cancer. Eur J Cancer 1994;30b:319–322.

55. Cloos J, Reid CBA, Snow GB, Braakhuis BJM: Review. Mutagen sensitivity. Enhanced risk assessment of squamous cell carcinoma. Eur J Cancer 1996;32b:367–372.

56. Field JK: Oncogenes and tumour-suppressor genes in squamous cell carcinoma of the head and neck. Eur J Cancer 1992;28b:67–76.

57. Schantz SP: Carcinogenesis, markers, staging and prognosis of head and neck cancer. Current Opinion Oncol 1993;5:483–490.

58. Scully C: Oncogenes, tumour suppressor genes and viruses in oral squamous cell carcinoma. J Oral Pathol Med 1993;22:337–347.

59. Carey TE: Genetic mechanisms in the development and progression of head and neck cancer. Curr Opin Otolaryngol Head Neck Surg 1995;3:75–83.

60. Field JK, Pavelic ZP, Spandidos DA, et al: The role of the p53 tumor suppressor gene in squamous cell carcinoma of the head and neck. Arch Otolaryngol Head Neck Surg 1993;119:1118–1122.

61. Brennan JA, Boyle JO, Koch WM, et al: Association between cigarette smoking and mutation of the p53 gene in squamous cell carcinoma of the head and neck. N Engl J Med 1995;332:712–717.

62. Denissenko MF, Pao A, Tang M, Pfeifer GP: Preferential formation of benzo(a)pyrene adducts at lung cancer mutational hot spots in p53. Science 1996;274:430–432.

Multiple Primary Tumors

63. Slaughter DP, Southwick HW, Smejhel W: Field cancerization in oral stratified epithelium. Cancer 1953;6:963–968.

64. Gluckman JL, Crissman JD, Donegan JO: Multicentric squamous cell carcinoma of the upper aerodigestive tract. Head Neck Surg 1980;3:90–96.

65. Hordijk GJ, de Jong JM: Synchronous and metachronous tumours in patients with head and neck cancer. J Laryngol Otol 1983;97:619–621.

66. Day GL, Blot WJ: Second primary tumors in patients with oral cancer. Cancer 1992;70:14–19.

67. Haughey BH, Arfken CL, Gates GA, et al: Meta-analysis of second malignant tumors in head and neck cancer: The case for an endoscopic screening protocol. Ann Otol Rhinol Laryngol 1992;101:105–112.

68. Terhaard CJ, Hordijk GJ, van den Broek P, et al: T3 laryngeal cancer: A retrospective study of the Dutch Head and Neck Oncology Cooperative Group: Study design and general results. Clin Otolaryngol 1992;17:393–402.

69. Robinson E, Zauber A, Fuks Z, et al: Clinical characteristics of patients with epidermoid carcinoma of the upper aerodigestive tract who develop second malignant tumors. Cancer Detection Prevent 1992; 16:297–303.

70. Boysen M, Loven JO: Second malignant neoplasms in patients with head and neck squamous cell carcinomas. Acta Oncol 1993;32:283–288.

71. Day GL, Blot WJ, Shore RE, et al: Second cancers following oral and pharyngeal cancer: Patient's characteristics and survival patterns. Eur J Cancer 1994;30b:381–386.

72. Söderholm AL, Pukkala E, Lindqvist C, et al: Risk of new primary cancer in patients with oropharyngeal cancer. Br J Cancer 1994;69:784–787.

73. Jovanovic A, van der Tol IGH, Kostense PJ, et al: Second respiratory and upper digestive tract cancer following oral squamous cell carcinoma. Eur J Cancer 1994;30b:225–229.

74. Schwartz LH, Ozsahin M, Zhang GN, et al: Synchronous and metachronous head and neck carcinomas. Cancer 1994;74:1933–1938.

75. Jones AS, Morar P, Phillips DE, et al: Second primary tumors in patients with head and neck squamous cell carcinoma. Cancer 1995;75:1343–1353.

76. Lippman SM, Spitz M, Trizna Z, et al: Epidemiology, biology, and chemoprevention of aerodigestive cancer. Cancer 1994;74:2719–2725.

77. Schwartz LH, Ozahin M, Zhang GN, et al: Synchronous and metachronous head and neck carcinomas. Cancer 1994;74:1933–1938.

78. Schantz SP, Spitz MR, Hsu TC: Mutagen sensitivity in patients with head and neck cancers: A biologic marker for risk of multiple primary malignancies. J Natl Cancer Inst 1990;82:1773–1775.

79. Gallo O, Bianchi S, Giovannucci ML, et al: p53 oncoprotein overexpression correlates with mutagen-induced chromosome fragility in head and neck cancer patients with multiple malignancies. Br J Cancer 1995;71:1008–1012.

Local and Distant Metastasis

80. Lindberg RD: Distribution of cervical lymph node metastasis of oral and oropharyngeal carcinomas. Cancer 1972;29:1446–1449.

81. Shah JP: Patterns of cervical lymph node metastasis from squamous carcinomas of the upper aerodigestive tract. Am J Surg 1990;160:405–409.

82. Shah JP, Cendon RA, Farr HW, et al: Carcinoma of the oral cavity. Factors affecting treatment failure at the primary site and neck. Am J Surg 1976;132:504–507.

83. Snow GB, Annyas AA, van Slooten EA, et al: Prognostic factors of neck node metastasis. Clin Otolaryngol 1982;7:185–192.

84. Stell PM, Morton RP, Singh SD: Cervical lymph-node metastasis. The significance of the level of the lymph node. Clin Oncol 1983;9:101–107.

85. Leemans CR, Tiwari RM, van der Waal I, et al: The efficacy of comprehensive neck dissection with or without postoperative radiotherapy in nodal metastases of squamous cell carcinoma of the upper respiratory and digestive tracts. Laryngoscope 1990;100:1194–1198.

86. Shah JP: Cervical lymph node metastasis-diagnostic, therapeutic, and prognostic implications. Oncology 1990;4:61–69.

87. Jones AS, Phillips DE, Helliwell TR, et al: Occult lymph node metastases in head and neck squamous carcinoma. Eur Arch Otorhinolaryngol 1993;250:446–449.

88. Johnson JT, Myers EN, Bedetti CD, et al: Cervical lymph node metastases incidence and implications of extracapsular carcinoma. Arch Otolaryngol 1985;111:534–537.

89. Carter RL, Bliss JM, Soo KC, et al: Radical neck dissections for squamous carcinomas: Pathological findings and their clinical implications with particular reference to transcapsular spread. Int J Radiat Oncol Biol Phys 1987;13:825–832.

90. Brasilino de Carvalho M: Quantitative analysis of the extent of extracapsular invasion and its prognostic significance: A prospective study

of 170 cases of carcinoma of the larynx and hypopharynx. Head Neck 1998;20:16–21.

91. Richard JM, Sancho-Garnier H, Micheau C, et al: Prognostic factors in cervical lymph node metastasis in upper respiratory and digestive tract carcinomas: Study of 1713 cases during a 15-year period. Laryngoscope 1987;97:97–101.

92. Olsen KD, Caruso M, Foote RL, et al: Primary head and neck cancers. Histopathologic predictors of recurrence after neck dissections in patients with lymph node involvement. Arch Otolaryngol Head Neck Surg 1994;120:1370–1374.

93. van den Brekel MWM, van der Waal I, Meijer CJLM, et al: The incidence of micrometastases in neck dissection specimens obtained from elective neck dissections. Laryngoscope 1996;106:987–991.

94. Vikram B, Strong EW, Shah JP, et al: Failure at distant sites following multimodality treatment for advanced head and neck cancer. Head Neck Surg 1984;6:730–733.

95. Leemans CR, Tiwari R, Nauta JJP, et al: Regional lymph node involvement and its significance in the development of distant metastases in head and neck carcinoma. Cancer 1993;71:452–456.

96. Calhoun KH, Fulmer P, Weiss R, et al: Distant metastases from head and neck squamous cell carcinomas. Laryngoscope 1994;104:1199–1205.

97. Crile GW: Carcinoma of the jaws, tongue, cheek and lips. Surg Gynecol Obstet 1923;36:159–184.

98. Braund RR, Martin HE: Distant metastasis in cancer of the upper respiratory and alimentary tracts. Surg Gynecol Obstet 1941;73:63–71.

99. Peltier LF, Thomas BL, Barclay THC, et al: The incidence of distant metastasis among patients dying with head and neck cancer. Surgery 1951;30:827–833.

100. Topazian DS: Distant metastasis of oral carcinoma. Oral Surg 1961;14:705–711.

101. Hoye RC, Herrold KMcD, Smith RR, et al: A clinicopathological study of epidermoid carcinoma of the head and neck. Cancer 1962;15:741–749.

102. Gowen GF, deSuto-Nagy G: The incidence and sites of distant metastasis in head and neck carcinoma. Surg Gynecol Obstet 1963;116:603–607.

103. Ju DMC: A study of the behaviour of cancer of the head and neck during its late and terminal phase. Am J Surg 1964;108:552–557.

104. O'Brien P, Carlson R, Steubner EA, et al: Distant metastases in epidermoid cell carcinoma of the head and neck. Cancer 1971;27:304–307.

105. Merino OR, Lindberg RD, Fletcher GH: An analysis of distant metastases from squamous cell carcinoma of the upper respiratory and digestive tracts. Cancer 1977;40:145–151.

106. Dennington ML, Carter DR, Meyers AD: Distant metastases in head and neck epidermoid carcinoma. Laryngoscope 1980;90:196–201.

107. Papac RJ: Distant metastases from head and neck cancer. Cancer 1984;53:342–345.

108. Bhatia R, Bahadur S: Distant metastasis in malignancies of the head and neck. J Laryngol Otol 1987;101:925–928.

109. Kotwall C, Sako K, Razack MS, et al: Metastatic patterns in squamous cell cancer of the head and neck. Am J Surg 1987;154:439–442.

110. Zbären P, Zehrmann W: Frequency and sites of distant metastases in head and neck squamous cell carcinoma. Arch Otolaryngol Head Neck Surg 1987;113:762–764.

111. Slootweg PJ, Hordijk GJ, Koole R: Autopsy findings in patients with head and neck squamous cell cancer and their therapeutic relevance. Eur J Cancer 1996;32b:413–415.

112. Nishijima W, Takooda S, Tokita N, et al: Analyses of distant metastases in squamous cell carcinoma of the head and neck and lesions above the clavicle at autopsy. Arch Otolaryngol Head Neck Surg 1993;119:65–68.

113. Grätz KW, Makek M: Fernmetastasen und Zweitkarzinome bei Mundhöhlenkarzinomen. Dtsch Z Mund Kiefer Gesichts Chir 1990;14:5–11.

114. Slootweg PJ, Rutgers DH, Wils IS: DNA ploidy analysis of squamous cell head and neck cancer to identify distant metastasis from second primary. Head Neck 1992;14:464–466.

115. Slootweg PJ, Giessen MCA, Rutgers DH, et al: DNA heterogeneity in metastasizing squamous cell head and neck cancer. J Craniomaxfac Surg 1993;21:348–350.

Histology and Prognosis

116. Shanmugaratnam K: Histological Typing of Tumours of the Upper Respiratory Tract and Ear, 2nd ed. Berlin: Springer, 1991:28–33.

117. Kershisnik M, Batsakis JG, Mackay B: Pathology consultation. Granular cell tumors. Ann Otol Rhinol Laryngol 1994;103:416–419.

118. Platz H, Fries R, Hudec M: Retrospective DÖSAK study on carcinomas of the oral cavity: Results and consequences. J Max Fac Surg 1985;13:147–153.

119. Broders AC: Carcinoma of the mouth: Types and degrees of malignancy. Am J Roentgenol Rad Ther Nucl Med 1927;17:90–93.

120. Arthur K, Farr HW: Prognostic significance of histologic grade in epidermoid carcinoma of the mouth and pharynx. Am J Surg 1972;124:489–492.

121. Zarbo RJ, Crissman JD: The surgical pathology of head and neck cancer. Semin Oncol 1988;15:10–19.

122. Kearsley JH, Thomas S: Prognostic markers in cancer of the head and neck region. Anticancer Drugs 1993;4:419–429.

123. Roland NJ, Caslin AW, Nash J, et al: Value of grading squamous cell carcinoma of the head and neck. Head Neck 1992;14:224–229.

124. Jakobsson PÅ, Eneroth CM, Killander D, et al: Histologic classification and grading of malignancy in carcinoma of the larynx. Acta Radiol Ther Phys Biol 1973;12:1–8.

125. Anneroth G, Batsakis J, Luna M: Review of the literature and a recommended system of malignancy grading in oral squamous cell carcinomas. Scand J Dent Res 1987;95:229–249.

126. Borges AM, Shrikhande SS, Ganesh B: Surgical pathology of squamous carcinoma of the oral cavity: Its impact on management. Semin Surg Oncol 1989;5:310–317.

127. Bryne M, Koppang HS, Lilleng R, et al: New malignancy grading is a better prognostic indicator than Broders' grading in oral squamous cell carcinomas. J Oral Pathol Med 1989;18:432–437.

128. Beltrami CA, Desinan L, Rubini C: Prognostic factors in squamous cell carcinoma of the oral cavity. Path Res Pract 1992;18:510–516.

129. Bryne M, Koppang HS, Lilleng R, et al: Malignancy grading of the deep invasive margins of oral squamous cell carcinomas has high prognostic value. J Pathol 1992;166:375–381.

130. Reichert T, Störkel S, Lippold R, et al: Vergleich histologischer Prognoseparameter beim Plattenepithelzelkarzinom der Mundhöhle. Dtsch Z Mund Kiefer Gesichts Chir 1992;16:89–92.

131. Odell EW, Jani P, Sheriff M, et al: The prognostic value of individual histologic grading parameters in small lingual squamous cell carcinomas. The importance of pattern of invasion. Cancer 1994;74:789–794.

132. Reichert T, Wagner W, Störkel S, et al: Pathohistologische Faktoren als Prognoseparameter des Plattenepithelzelkarzinoms. Dtsch Z Mund Kiefer Gesichts Chir 1994;18:31–35.

133. Bryne M, Jenssen N, Boysen M: Histological grading in the deep invasive front of T_1 and T_2 glottic squamous cell carcinomas has high prognostic value. Virchows Arch 1995;427:277–281.

134. Welkoborsky HJ, Hinni M, Dienes HP, et al: Predicting recurrence and survival in patients with laryngeal cancer by means of DNA cytometry, tumor front grading and proliferation markers. Ann Otol Rhinol Laryngol 1995;104:503–510.

135. McGavran MH, Bauer WC, Ogura JH: The incidence of cervical lymph node metastasis from epidermoid carcinoma of the larynx and their relationship to certain characteristics of the primary tumor: A study based on the clinical and pathological findings for 96 patients treated by primary en bloc laryngectomy and radical neck dissection. Cancer 1961;14:55–66.

136. Crissman JD, Liu WY, Gluckman JL, et al: Prognostic value of histopathologic parameters in squamous cell carcinoma of the oropharynx. Cancer 1984;54:2995–3001.

137. Yamamoto E, Miyakawa A, Kohama GI: Mode of invasion and lymph node metastasis in squamous cell carcinoma of the oral cavity. Head Neck Surg 1984;6:938–947.

138. Shingaki S, Suzuki I, Nakajima T, et al: Evaluation of histopathologic parameters in predicting cervical lymph node metastasis of oral and oropharyngeal carcinomas. Oral Surg Oral Med Oral Pathol 1988;66:683–688.

139. Sakr W, Hussan M, Zarbo RJ, et al: DNA quantitation and histologic characteristics of squamous cell carcinoma of the upper aerodigestive tract. Arch Pathol Lab Med 1989;113:1009–1014.

140. Wiernik G, Millard PR, Haybittle JL: The predictive value of histological classification into degrees of differentiation of squamous cell carcinoma of the larynx and hypopharynx compared with the survival of patients. Histopathology 1991;19:411–417.

141. Truelson JM, Fisher SG, Beals TE, et al: DNA content and histologic growth pattern correlate with prognosis in patients with advanced squamous cell carcinoma of the larynx. Cancer 1992;70:56–62.

142. Umeda M, Yokoo S, Take Y, et al: Lymph node metastasis in squamous cell carcinoma of the oral cavity: Correlation between histologic features and the prevalence of metastasis. Head Neck 1992;14:263–272.

143. Horiuchi K, Mishima K, Ohsawa M, et al: Prognostic factors for well-differentiated squamous cell carcinoma in the oral cavity with emphasis on immunohistochemical evaluation. J Surg Oncol 1993;53:92–96.

144. Ravasz LA, Hordijk GJ, Slootweg PJ, et al: Uni- and multivariate analysis of eight indications for post-operative radiotherapy and their significance for local-regional cure in advanced head and neck cancer. J Laryngol Otol 1993;107:437–440.

145. Kirita T, Okabe S, Izumo T, et al: Risk factors for the postoperative local recurrence of tongue carcinoma. J Oral Maxillofac Surg 1994;52:149–154.

146. Slootweg PJ, de Pagter M, de Weger RA, et al: Lymphocytes at tumor margins in patients with head and neck cancer. Relationship with tumor size, HLA molecules and metastasis. Int J Oral Maxillofac Surg 1994;23:286–289.

147. Resnick MJM, Uhlman D, Niehans GA, et al: Cervical lymph node status and survival in laryngeal carcinoma: Prognostic factors. Ann Otol Rhinol Laryngol 1995;104:685–694.

148. Rasgon BM, Cruz RM, Hilsinger RL, et al: Relation of lymph node metastasis to histopathologic appearance in oral cavity and oropharyngeal carcinoma: A case series and literature review. Laryngoscope 1989;99:1103–1110.

149. Hiratsuka H, Imamura M, Ishii Y, et al: Immunohistologic detection of lymphocyte subpopulations infiltrating in human oral cancer with special reference to its clinical significance. Cancer 1984;53:2456–2466.

150. Wolf GT, Hudson JL, Peterson KA, et al: Lymphocyte subpopulations infiltrating squamous carcinomas of the head and neck: Correlations with extent of tumor and prognosis. Otolaryngol Head Neck Surg 1986;95:142–151.

151. Guo M, Rabin BS, Johnson JT, et al: Lymphocyte phenotypes at tumor margins in patients with head and neck cancer. Head Neck Surg 1987;9:265–271.

152. Hirota J, Ueta E, Osaki T, et al: Immunohistologic study of mononuclear infiltrates in oral squamous carcinomas. Head Neck Surg 1990;12:118–125.

153. Lowe D, Fletcher CDM: Eosinophilia in squamous cell carcinoma of the oral cavity, external genitalia and anus—clinical correlations. Histopathology 1984;8:627–632

154. Goldsmith MM, Belchis DA, Cresson DH, et al: The importance of the eosinophil in head and neck cancer. Otolaryngol Head Neck Surg 1992;106:27–33

155. Thompson AC, Brailley PJ, Griffin NR: Tumor-associated tissue eosinophilia and long-term prognosis for carcinoma of the larynx. Am J Surg 1994;168:469–471.

156. Sassler AM, McClatchey KD, Wolf GT: Eosinophilic infiltration in advanced laryngeal squamous cell carcinoma. Laryngoscope 1995;105:413–416.

157. Crissman JD, Gluckman J, Whiteley J, et al: Squamous cell carcinoma of the floor of the mouth. Head Neck Surg 1980;3:2–7.

158. Spiro RH, Spiro JD, Strong EW: Surgical approach to squamous carcinoma confined to the tongue and the floor of the mouth. Head Neck Surg 1986;9:27–31.

159. Brown B, Barnes L, Mazariegos J, et al: Prognostic factors in mobile tongue and floor of mouth carcinoma. Cancer 1989;64:1195–1202

160. Mohit-Tabatabai MA, Sobel HJ, Rush BF, et al: Relation of thickness of floor of mouth stage I and II cancers to regional metastasis. Am J Surg 1986;152:351–353.

161. Moore C, Kuhns JG, Greenberg RA: Thickness as prognostic aid in upper aerodigestive tract cancer. Arch Surg 1986;121:1410–1414.

162. Spiro RH, Huvos AG, Wong GY, et al: Predictive value of tumor thickness in squamous carcinoma confined to the tongue and floor of the mouth. Am J Surg 1986;152:345–350.

163. Urist MM, O'Brien CJ, Soong SJ, et al: Squamous cell carcinoma of the buccal mucosa: Analysis of prognostic factors. Am J Surg 1987;154:411–414.

164. Maddox WA, Urist MM: Histopathological prognostic factors of certain primary oral cavity cancers. Oncology 1990;4:39–42.

165. Howaldt HP, Frenz M, Pitz H: Proposal for a modified T-classification for oral cancer. J Craniomaxfac Surg 1992;21:96–101.

166. Jones KR, Lodge-Rigal RD, Reddick RL, et al: Prognostic factors in the recurrence of stage I and II squamous cell cancer of the oral cavity. Arch Otolaryngol Head Neck Surg 1992;118:483–485.

167. Baredes S, Leeman DJ, Chen TS, et al: Significance of tumor thickness in soft palate carcinoma. Laryngoscope 1993;103:389–393.

168. Steinhart H, Kleinsasser O: Growth and spread of squamous cell carcinoma of the floor of the mouth. Eur Arch Otorhinolaryngol 1993;250:358–361.

169. Kligerman J, Lima RA, Soares JR, et al: Supraomohyoid neck dissection in the treatment of T1/T2 squamous cell carcinoma of oral cavity. Am J Surg 1994;168:391–394.

170. Karas DE, Baredes S, Chen TS, et al: Relationship of biopsy and final specimens in evaluation of tumor thickness in floor of mouth carcinoma. Laryngoscope 1995;105:491–493.

171. Woolgar JA, Scott J: Prediction of cervical lymph node metastasis in squamous cell carcinoma of the tongue/floor of mouth. Head Neck 1995;17:463–472.

172. Carter RL, Tanner NSB, Clifford P, et al: Perineural spread in squamous cell carcinomas of the head and neck. Clin Otolaryngol 1979;4:271–281.

173. Conte CC, Ergin MT, Ricci A, et al: Clinical and pathologic prognostic variables in oropharyngeal squamous cell carcinomas. Am J Surg 1989;157:582–584.

174. Lydiatt DD, Robbins KT, Byers RM, et al: Treatment of stage I and II oral tongue cancer. Head Neck 1993;15:308–312.

175. Morton RP, Ferguson CM, Lambie NK, et al: Tumor thickness in early tongue cancer. Arch Otolaryngol Head Neck Surg 1994;120:717–720.

176. Poleksic S, Kalwaic HJ: Prognostic value of vascular invasion in squamous cell carcinoma of the head and neck. Plast Reconstr Surg 1978;61:234–240.

177. Close LG, Brown PM, Vuitch MF, et al: Microvascular invasion and survival in cancer of the oral cavity and oropharynx. Arch Otolaryngol Head Neck Surg 1989;115:1304–1309.

178. Gasparini G, Weidner N, Maluta S, et al: Intratumor microvessel density and p53 protein: Correlation with metastasis in head and neck squamous cell carcinoma. Int J Cancer 1993;55:739–744.

179. Albo D, Granick MS, Jhala N, et al: The relationship of angiogenesis to biological activity in human squamous cell carcinomas of the head and neck. Ann Plast Surg 1994;32:588–594.

180. Leedy DA, Trune DR, Kronz JD, et al: Tumor angiogenesis, the p53 antigen and cervical metastasis in squamous cell carcinoma of the tongue. Otolaryngol Head Neck Surg 1994;111:417–422.

181. Williams JK, Carlson GW, Cohen C, et al: Tumor angiogenesis as a prognostic factor in oral cavity tumors. Am J Surg 1994;168:373–380.

182. Dray TG, Hardin NJ, Sofferman RA: Angiogenesis as a prognostic marker in early head and neck cancer. Ann Otol Rhinol Laryngol 1995;104:724–729.

183. Klijanienko J, El-Naggar AK, de Braud F, et al: Tumor vascularization, mitotic index, histopathologic grade, and DNA ploidy in the assessment of 114 head and neck squamous cell carcinomas. Cancer 1995;75:1649–1656.

184. Zätterström UK, Brun E, Willén R, et al: Tumor angiogenesis and prognosis in squamous cell carcinoma of the head and neck. Head Neck 1995;17:312–318.

185. Carrau RL, Barnes EL, Snyderman CH, et al: Tumor angiogenesis as a predictor of tumor aggressiveness and metastatic potential in squamous cell carcinoma of the head and neck. Invasion Metastasis 1995;15:197–202.

186. Penfold CN, Partridge M, Rojas R, et al: The role of angiogenesis in the spread of oral squamous cell carcinoma. Br J Oral Maxillofac Surg 1996;34:37–41.

187. Shpitzer T, Chaimoff M, Gal R, et al: Tumor angiogenesis as a prognostic factor in early oral tongue cancer. Arch Otolaryngol Head Neck Surg 1996;122:865–868.

188. Lutman GB: Epithelial nests in intraoral sensory nerve endings simulating perineural invasion in patients with oral carcinoma. Am J Clin Pathol 1974;61:275–286.

189. Danforth RA, Baughman RA: Chievitz's organ: A potential pitfall in oral cancer diagnosis. Oral Surg Oral Med Oral Pathol 1979;48:231–236.

190. Jensen JL, Wuerker RB, Correll RW, et al: Epithelial islands associated with mandibular nerves. Report of two cases in the walls of mandibular cysts. Oral Surg Oral Med Oral Pathol 1979;48:226–230.

191. Miko T, Molnár P: The juxtaoral organ. A pitfall for pathologists. J Pathol 1981;133:17–23.

192. Tschen JA, Fechner RE: The juxtaoral organ of Chievitz. Am J Surg Pathol 1979;3:147–150.

193. Wysocki GP, Wright BA: Intraneural and perineural epithelial structures. Head Neck Surg 1981;4:69–71.

194. Scholl P, Byers RM, Batsakis JG, et al: Microscopic cut-through of cancer in the surgical treatment of squamous carcinoma of the tongue. Prognostic and therapeutic implications. Am J Surg 1986;152:354–360.

195. Jones AS: Prognosis in mouth cancer: tumour factors. Eur J Cancer 1994;30b:8–15.

196. Wenig BL, Berry BW: Management of patients with positive surgical margins after vertical hemilaryngectomy. Arch Otolaryngol Head Neck Surg 1995;121:172–175.

197. Bradford CR, Wolf GT, Fisher SG, et al: Prognostic importance of surgical margins in advanced laryngeal squamous carcinoma. Head Neck 1996;18:11–16.

198. Bauer WC, Lesinski SG, Ogura JH: The significance of positive margins in hemilaryngectomy specimens. Laryngoscope 1975;85:1–13.

199. Looser KG, Shah JP, Strong EW: The significance of "positive" margins in surgically resected epidermoid carcinomas. Head Neck Surg 1978;1:107–111.

200. Chen TY, Emrich LJ, Driscoll DL: The clinical significance of pathological findings in surgically resected margins of the primary tumor in head and neck carcinoma. Int J Radiation Oncology Biol Phys 1987;13:833–837.

201. Loree TR, Strong EW: Significance of positive margins in oral cavity squamous carcinoma. Am J Surg 1990;160:410–414.

202. Brennan CT, Sessions DG, Spitznagel EL, et al: Surgical pathology of cancer of the oral cavity and oropharynx. Laryngoscope 1991;101:1175–1197.

203. Ravasz LA, Slootweg PJ, Hordijk GJ, et al: The status of the resection margin as a prognostic factor in the treatment of head and neck carcinoma. J Craniomaxfac Surg 1991;19:314–318.

204. van Es RJJ, Amerongen NV, Slootweg PJ, Egyedi P: Resection margin as a predictor of recurrence at the primary site for T1 and T2 cancers. Evaluation of histopathologic variables. Arch Otolaryngol Head Neck Surg 1996;122:521–525.

205. van den Brekel MWM, Snow GB: Assessment of lymph node metastases in the neck. Eur J Cancer 1994;30b:88–92.

206. Gnepp D, Barnes L, Crissman J, Zarbo R: Association of Directors of Anatomic and Surgical Pathology. Recommendations for the reporting of larynx specimens containing laryngeal neoplasms. Rev Virch Arch 1997;431:155–157.

207. Bryne M: Prognostic value of various molecular and cellular features in oral squamous cell carcinomas: A review. J Oral Pathol Med 1991;20:413–420.

208. Sano K, Takahashi H, Fujita S, et al: Prognostic implication of silver-binding nucleolar organizer regions (AgNORs) in oral squamous cell carcinoma. J Oral Pathol Med 1991;20:53–56.

209. Esser D, Theissig E, Willgeroth C: Nucleolar organizer regions in carcinomas of the oropharynx and hypopharynx. Eur Arch Otorhinolaryngol 1993;250:154–156.

210. Bourhis J, Bosq J, Wilson GD, et al: Correlation between p53 gene expression and tumor-cell proliferation in oropharyngeal cancer. Int J Cancer 1994;57:458–462.

211. Esser D, Meyer W, Willgeroth C, et al: Die Feststellung prognoserelevanter Faktoren bei Patienten mit einen Hypo- oder Oropharynxkarzinom. HNO 1994;42:413–417.

212. Michalides R, van Veelen N, Hart A, et al: Overexpression of cyclin D1 correlates with recurrence in a group of forty-seven operable squamous cell carcinomas of the head and neck. Cancer Res 1995;55:975–978.

213. Pich A, Chiusa L, Margaria E, et al: p53 overexpression correlates with proliferative activity and prognosis in carcinomas of the pyriform sinus. Int J Oncol 1995;6:1053–1058.

214. Ensley JF, Maciorowski Z: Clinical applications of DNA content parameters in patients with squamous cell carcinomas of the head and neck. Semin Oncol 1994;21:330–339.

215. Briggs RJS, Pienta KJ, Hruban RH, et al: Nuclear morphometry for prediction of metastatic potential in early squamous cell carcinoma of the floor of the mouth. Arch Otolaryngol Head Neck Surg 1992;118:531–533.

216. Bundgaard T, Sorensen FB, Gaihede M, et al: Stereologic, histopathologic, flowcytometric and clinical parameters in the prognostic evaluation of 74 patients with intraoral squamous cell carcinomas. Cancer 1992;70:1–13.

217. Bundgaard T, Bentzen SM, Wildt J: Histopathologic, stereologic, epidemiologic and clinical parameters in the prognostic evaluation of squamous cell carcinoma of the oral cavity. Head Neck 1996;18:142–152.

218. Slootweg PJ: Suppressor protein p53 and its occurrence in oral tumours. In Seifert G (ed): Current Topics in Pathology. Berlin: Springer, 1996:179–200.

219. Shin DM, Lee JS, Lippman SM, et al: p53 expression: Predicting recurrence and second primary tumors in head and neck squamous cell carcinoma. J Natl Cancer Inst 1996;88:519–529.

220. Brennan JA, Mao L, Hruban RH, et al: Molecular assessment of histopathological staging in squamous-cell carcinoma of the head and neck. N Engl J Med 1995;332:429–435.

Nasopharynx

221. Ali MY: Distribution and character of the squamous epithelium in the human nasopharynx. UICC Monograph Series, Vol 1. Copenhagen: Munksgaard, 1967; pp 138–141.
222. Loh LE, Chee TS, John AB: The anatomy of the fossa of Rosenmuller. Singapore Med J 1991;32:154–155.
223. Dickson RI: Nasopharyngeal carcinoma: An evaluation of 209 patients. Laryngoscope 1981;91:333–354.
224. Ho JHC: An epidemiologic and clinical study of nasopharyngeal carcinoma. Int J Radiat Oncol Biol Phys 1978;4:183–197.
225. McLaughlin MP, Mendenhall WM, Mancuso AA, et al: Retropharyngeal adenopathy as a predictor of outcome in squamous cell carcinoma of the head and neck. Head Neck 1995;17:190–198.
226. Fandi A, Cvitkovic E: Biology and treatment of nasopharyngeal cancer. Curr Opin Oncol 1995;7:255–263.
227. Bloom S: Cancer of the nasopharynx. Laryngoscope 1961;71:1207–1260.
228. Coffin CM, Rich SS, Dehner LP: Familial aggregation of nasopharyngeal carcinoma and other malignancies. A clinicopathologic description. Cancer 1991;68:1323–1328.
229. Kapadia SB, Janecka IP: Nasopharyngeal carcinoma. In Myers EN, Bluestone CD, Brackmann DE, Kranse CJ (eds): Advances in Otolaryngology-Head and Neck Surgery, Vol 9. St. Louis: Mosby, 1995:247–261.
230. Barnes L, Kapadia SB: The biology and pathology of selected skull base tumors. J Neuro Oncol 1994;20:213–240.
231. Ho HC: Nasopharyngeal carcinoma in Hong Kong. In Muir CS, Shanmugaratnam K (eds): Cancer of the nasopharynx, UICC Monograph Series, Vol 1. Copenhagen: Munksgaard, 1967:58–63.
232. Ho HC: Cancer of the nasopharynx. In Harris RJC (ed): Panel II, Ninth International Cancer Congress, UICC Monograph Series, Vol 10. Berlin: Springer, 1967:110–116.
233. Cvitkovic E, Bachouchi M, Armand JP: Nasopharyngeal carcinoma. Biology, natural history, and therapeutic implications. Hematol/Oncol Clin North Am 1991;5:821–838.
234. Vasef MA, Ferlito A, Weiss LM: Clinicopathological consultation. Nasopharyngeal carcinoma, with emphasis on its relationship to Epstein-Barr virus. Ann Otol Rhinol Laryngol 1997;106:348–356.
235. Hawkins EP, Krischer JP, Smith BE, et al: Nasopharyngeal carcinoma in children: A retrospective review and demonstration of Epstein-Barr viral genomes in tumor cell cytoplasm: A report of the Pediatric Oncology Group. Hum Pathol 1990;21:805–810.
236. Choi PHK, Suen MWM, Huang DP, et al: Nasopharyngeal carcinoma: Genetic changes, Epstein-Barr virus infection, or both. A clinical and molecular study of 36 patients. Cancer 1993;72:2873–2878.
237. Feinmesser R, Miyazakai I, Cheung R, et al: Diagnosis of nasopharyngeal carcinoma by DNA amplification of tissue obtained by fine-needle aspiration. N Engl J Med 1992;326:17–21.
238. Feinmesser R, Feinmesser M, Freeman JL, et al: Detection of occult nasopharyngeal primary tumours by means of *in situ* hybridization. J Laryngol Otol 1992;106:345–348.
239. Old L, Boyse EA, Oettgen, HF, de Harven E, et al: Precipitation of antibody in human sera to an antigen present in cultured Burkitt's lymphoma cells. Proc Nat Acad Sci (Washington), 1966;56:1699–1704.
240. Henle W, Henle G, Ho G, et al: Antibodies to Epstein-Barr virus in nasopharyngeal carcinoma, other head and neck neoplasms, and control groups. J Natl Cancer Inst 1970;44:225–231.
241. Easton J, Levine P, Connely R, Day N: Studies on nasopharyngeal carcinoma in the United States: A model for international comparisons. Comp Immunol Microbiol Infect Dis 1979;2:221–228.
242. Easton J, Levine P, Hyams V: Nasopharyngeal carcinoma in the United States. Arch Otolaryngol 1980;106:88–91.
243. Greene M, Fraumeni J, Hoover, R: Nasopharyngeal cancer among young people in the United States: Racial variation by cell type. J Natl Cancer Inst 1977;58:1267–1271.
244. Hidayatalla A, Malik MO, El Hadi AE, et al: Studies on nasopharyngeal carcinoma in the Sudan. I. Epidemiology and aetiology. Eur J Cancer Clin Oncol 1983;19:705–710.
245. Skinner DW, Van Haslett CA, Tsao SY: Nasopharyngeal carcinoma: Modes of presentation. Ann Otol Rhinol Laryngol 1991;100:549–551.
246. Su C-Y, Lui C-C: Perineural invasion of the trigeminal nerve in patients with nasopharyngeal carcinoma. Cancer 1996;78:2063–2069.

247. Werner-Wasik M, Winkler P, Uri A, Goldwein J: Nasopharyngeal carcinoma in children. Med Ped Oncol 1996;26:352–358.
248. Sham JT, Cheung YK, Choy D, Leong L: Cranial nerve involvement and base of the skull erosion in nasopharyngeal carcinoma. Cancer 1991;68:422–426.
249. Cvitkovic E, Bachouchi M, Boussen H, et al: Leukemoid reaction, bone marrow invasion, fever of unknown origin, and metastatic pattern in the natural history of advanced undifferentiated carcinoma of nasopharyngeal type: A review of 255 consecutive cases. J Clin Oncol 1993;11:2434–2442.
250. Tsai ST, Jin YT, Su IJ: Expression of EBER1 in primary and metastatic nasopharyngeal carcinoma tissues using in situ hybridization. A correlation with WHO histologic subtypes. Cancer 1996;77:231–236.
251. Derigs P: Lymphoepitheliales Carcinom de Rachens mit Metastasen. Virch Arch 1923;244:1–7.
252. Ahmad A, Stefani S: Distant metastases of nasopharyngeal carcinoma. A study of 256 male patients. J Surg Oncol 1986;33:194–197.
253. Vikram B, Mishra UB, Strong EW, et al: Patterns of failure in carcinomas of the nasopharynx: Failure at distant sites. Head Neck Surg 1986;8:276–279.
254. Teo PM, Leung SF, Yu P, et al: A comparison of the Ho's, International Union Against Cancer, and American Joint Committee stage classifications for nasopharyngeal carcinoma. Cancer 1991;67:434–439.
255. American Joint Committee Cancer Staging Manual, 5th ed. Philadelphia: J.B. Lippincott, 1997:31–39.
256. Sobin LH, Wittekind Ch (eds): TNM Classification of Malignant Tumours, International Union Against Cancer, 5th ed. New York: Wiley-Liss, 1997:25–32.
257. Teo PM, Tsao SY, Ho JH, et al: A proposed modification of the Ho stage-classification for nasopharyngeal carcinoma. Radiother Oncol 1991;21:11–23.
258. Svoboda D, Kirchner F, Shanmugaratnam K: Ultrastructure of nasopharyngeal carcinoma in American and Chinese patients. Exp Molecular Path 1965;4:189–204.
259. Shanmugaratnam K, Chan SH, de-The G, et al: Histopathology of nasopharyngeal carcinoma. Correlations with epidemiology, survival rates, and other biological characteristics. Cancer 1979;44:1029–1044.
260. Shanmugaratnam K: Histologic Typing of Upper Respiratory Tract Tumours. International Typing of Tumours, No. 19. Geneva: World Health Organization, 1978:32–33.
261. Zhu K, Levine RS, Brann EA, et al: A population-based case-control study of the relationship between cigarette smoking and nasopharyngeal cancer (United States). Cancer Causes Control 1995;6:507–512.
262. Shanmugaratnam K, Sobin LH: The World Health Organization Histological Classification of Tumours of the Upper Respiratory Tract and Ear. Cancer 1993;71:2689–2697.
263. McGuire LJ, Lee JCK: The histopathologic diagnosis of nasopharyngeal carcinoma. Ear Nose Throat J 1990;69:229–236.
264. Bailet JW, Mark RJ, Abemayor E, et al: Nasopharyngeal carcinoma: Treatment results with primary radiation therapy. Laryngoscope 1992;102:965–972.
265. Geara FB, Glisson BS, Sanguineti G, et al: Induction chemotherapy followed by radiotherapy versus radiotherapy alone in patients with advanced nasopharyngeal carcinoma. Cancer 1997;79:1279–1286.

Sinonasal Cavities

266. Robin PE, Powell DJ, Stansbie JM: Carcinoma of the nasal cavity and paranasal sinuses: Incidence and presentation of different histological types. Clin Otolaryngol 1979;4:432–456.
267. Roush GC: Epidemiology of cancer of the nose and paranasal sinuses: Current concepts. Head Neck Surg 1979;2:3–11.
268. Sisson GA Sr, Toriumi DM, Atiyah RA: Paranasal sinus malignancy: A comprehensive update. Laryngoscope 1989;99:143–150.
269. Mundy EA, Neiders ME, Sako K, et al: Maxillary sinus cancer: A study of 33 cases. J Oral Pathol 1985;14:27–36.
270. Rice DH: Benign and malignant tumors of the ethmoid sinus. Otolaryngol Clin North Am 1985;18:113–124.
271. Wang CC: Treatment of carcinoma of the nasal vestibule by irradiation. Cancer 1976;38:100–106.
272. Ohngren LS: Malignant tumors of the maxilloethmoidal region. Acta Otolaryngol Suppl 1938;19:1–476.
273. American Joint Committee Cancer Staging Manual, 5th ed. Philadelphia: JB Lippincott, 1997:47–52.
274. Sobin LH, Wittekind CH (eds): TNM Classification of Malignant Tumours, International Union Against Cancer, 5th ed. New York: Wiley-Liss, 1997:38–42.

275. Ringertz N: Pathology of malignant tumours arising in the nasal and paranasal cavities and maxilla. Acta Otolaryngol Suppl 1938;27:95–157.

276. Quick D, Cutler M: Radiation reaction of metastatic squamous cell carcinoma in cervical lymph nodes. AJR Am J Roentgenol 1925;14:529–540.

277. Geschikter CF: Tumors of the nasal and paranasal cavities. Am J Cancer 1935;2:637–660.

278. Osborn DA: Nature and behavior of transitional tumors in the upper respiratory tract. Cancer 1970;25:50–60.

279. Friedmann I, Osborn DA: Carcinoma of the surface epithelium (including ameloblastoma). In Friedmann I (ed): Pathology of Granulomas and Neoplasms of the Nose and Paranasal Sinuses. Edinburgh: Churchill-Livingstone, 1982:118–132.

280. Manivel C, Wick MR, Dehner LP: Transitional (cylindric) cell carcinoma with endodermal sinus tumor-like features of the nasopharynx and paranasal sinuses. Arch Pathol Lab Med 1986;110:198–202.

281. Michaels L: Malignant neoplasms of surface epithelium. In Michaels L (ed): Ear, Nose and Throat Histopathology. Berlin: Springer, 1981:71–67.

282. Hellquist HB: Tumours of the surface epithelium. In Pathology of the Nose and Paranasal Sinuses. London, Butterworth & Co, 1990:89–92.

283. Wenig BM: Neoplasms of the nasal cavity and paranasal sinuses. In Atlas of Head and Neck Pathology. Philadelphia: W.B. Saunders, 1993:57–58.

284. Hyams VJ, Batsakis JG, Michaels L: Tumors of the upper respiratory tract and ear. Atlas of Tumor Pathology, 2nd Series, no. 25. Washington: Armed Forces Institute of Pathology, 1988:58–66.

285. Rosai J: Respiratory track. In Rosai J (ed): Ackerman's Surgical Pathology, 8th ed. St Louis: Mosby–Year Book, 1996:294.

286. Michaels L, Young M: Histogenesis of papillomas of the nose and paranasal sinuses. Arch Pathol Lab Med 1995;119:821–826.

287. Patel P, Tiwari R, Karim ABM, et al: Squamous cell carcinoma of the nasal vestibule. J Laryngol Otol 1992;106:332–336.

288. Fradis M, Podoshin L, Gertner R, et al: Squamous cell carcinoma of the nasal septum mucosa. Ear Nose Throat J 1993;72:217–221.

289. Kraus DH, Sterman BM, Levine HL, et al: Factors influencing survival in ethmoid sinus cancer. Arch Otolaryngol Head Neck Surg 1992;118:367–372.

Larynx and Hypopharynx

290. Del Regato JAM, Spjut HJ, Cox JD (eds): Ackerman and Del Regato's Cancer. Diagnosis, Treatment, and Prognosis, 6th ed. St. Louis: Mosby, 1985:346.

291. Barnes L, Johnson JT: Pathologic and clinical considerations in the evaluation of major head and neck specimens resected for cancer. Path Annual 1986;21:173–250.

292. Michaels L: Squamous cell carcinoma of the hypopharynx. In Ear, Nose and Throat Histopathology. London: Springer Verlag, 1987:459–463.

293. Harrison DFN: Pathology of hypopharyngeal cancer in relation to surgical management. J Laryngol Otol 1970;84:349–367.

294. Spector JG, Sessions DG, Emami B, et al: Squamous cell carcinoma of the pyriform sinus: A nonrandomized comparison of therapeutic modalities and long-term results. Laryngoscope 1995;105:397–406.

295. Thabet HM, Sessions DG, Gado MH, et al: Comparison of clinical evaluation and computed tomographic diagnostic accuracy for tumors of the larynx and hypopharynx. Laryngoscope 1996;106:589–594.

296. Jones AS, Wilde A, McRae RD, et al: The treatment of early squamous cell carcinoma of the piriform fossa. Clin Otolaryngol 1994;19:485–490.

297. Jones AS, Roland NJ, Field JK, Phillips DE: The level of cervical lymph node metastases: Their prognostic relevance and relationship with head and neck squamous carcinoma primary sites. Clin Otolaryngol 1994;19:63–69.

298. Kirchner J, Owen J: Five hundred cancers of the larynx and pyriform sinus. Laryngoscope 1977;87:1288–1303.

299. Million R, Cassiss N: Management of head and neck cancer. A multidisciplinary approach. Philadelphia: JB Lippincott, 1994:431–497.

300. Myers EN, Alvi A: Management of carcinoma of the supraglottic larynx: Evolution, current concepts, and future trends. Laryngoscope 1996;106:559–567.

301. Pressman J, Simon M, Moncel C: Anatomical studies related to the dissemination of cancer of the larynx. Trans Am Acad Ophthalmol Otolaryngol 1960;64:628–638.

302. Fechner RE, Mills SE: In Sternberg S (ed): Histology for Pathologists. New York: Raven Press, 1992:443–455.

303. Olofsson J, van Nostrand AWP: Growth and spread of laryngeal and hypopharyngeal carcinoma with reflections on the effect of preoperative irradiation. 139 cases studied by whole organ sectioning. Acta Otolaryngol (Stockh) 1973;308(Suppl):1–84.

304. Beitler JJ, Mahadevia PS, Silver CE et al: New barriers to ventricular invasion in paraglottic laryngeal cancer. Cancer 1994;73:2648–2652.

305. Rosai J: In Rosai J (ed): Ackerman's Surgical Pathology, 8th ed. St Louis: Mosby–Year Book, 1996:321–328.

306. Wang CC: Head and neck neoplasms. In Mansfield CM (ed): Therapeutic Radiology: New Directions in Therapy. New Hyde Park, NY: Medical Examination Publishing Co, 1983:144–169.

307. Rucci L, Gammarota L, Gallo O: Carcinoma of the anterior commissure of the larynx. 2. Proposal of a new staging system. Ann Otol Rhinol Laryngol 1996;105:391–396.

308. Stell PM, Gregory I, Watt J: Morphology of the human larynx. II. The subglottis. Clin Otolaryngol 1980;5:389–395.

309. American Joint Committee on Cancer: Staging Manual, 5th ed. Philadelphia: JB Lippincott, 1997:41–46.

310. Kleinsasser O: Revision of classification of laryngeal cancer, is it long overdue? (Proposals for an improved TN-classification). J Laryngol Otol 1992;106:197–204.

311. Piccirillo JF, Wells CK, Sasaki CT, Feinstein AR: New clinical severity staging system for cancer of the larynx. Five-year survival rates. Ann Otol Rhinol Laryngol 1994;103:83–92.

312. Hirabayashi H, Koshii K, Uno K, et al: Extracapsular spread of squamous cell carcinoma in neck lymph nodes: Prognostic factor of laryngeal cancer. Laryngoscope 1991;101:502–506.

313. Yilmaz T, Hosal AS, Gedikoglu G, Turan E, Ayas A: Prognostic significance of depth of invasion in cancer of the larynx. Laryngoscope 1998;108:764–768.

314. Moe K, Wolf GT, Fisher SG, Hong WK. Regional metastases in patients with advanced laryngeal cancer. Arch Otolaryngol Head Neck Surg 1996;122:644–648.

315. Weidner N, Askin FB, Berthrong M, et al: Bizarre (pseudo malignant) granulation-tissue reactions following ionizing-radiation exposure. Cancer 1987;59:1509–1514.

316. Ferlito A, Carbone A, DeSanto LW, et al: Clinicopathological consultation. "Early" cancer of the larynx: The concept as defined by clinicians, pathologists, and biologists. Ann Otol Rhinol Laryngol 1996;105:245–246.

317. Ferlito A: The natural history of early vocal cord cancer. Acta Otolaryngol (Stockh) 1995;115:345–347.

318. Carbone A, Volpe R: Superficial extending carcinoma (SEC) of the larynx and hypopharynx. Path Res Pract 1992;188:729–735.

Trachea

319. McCarthy MJ, Rosado-de-Christensen ML: Tumors of the trachea. J Thorac Imag 1995;10:180–198.

320. Gilbert JG Jr, Mazzarella LA, Feit LA: Primary tracheal tumors in the infant and adult. Arch Otolaryngol 1953;58:1–9.

321. Houston HE, Payne WS, Harrison EG Jr, et al: Primary cancers of the trachea. Arch Surg 1969;99:132–140.

322. Manninen MP, Paakkala TA, Pukander JS, et al: Diagnosis of tracheal carcinoma at chest radiography. Acta Radiol 1992;33:546–547.

323. Morency G, Chalaoui J, Samson S, et al: Malignant neoplasms of the trachea. J Can Assoc Radiol 1989;40:198–200.

324. Theegarten D, Freitag L: Scar carcinoma of the trachea after tracheotomy. Case report and review of the literature. Respiration 1993;60:250–253.

325. Grillo HC, Mathiesen DJ: Primary tracheal tumors: Treatment and results. Ann Thorac Surg 1990;49:69–77.

326. Gelder CM, Hetzel MR: Primary tracheal tumours: A national survey. Thorax 1993;48:688–692.

327. Mornex F, Coquard R, Danhier S, Maingon P, El Husseini G, Van Houtte P: Role of radiation therapy in the treatment of primary tracheal carcinoma. Int J Radiat Oncol Biol Phys 1998;41:299–305.

Lip

328. Verbin RS, Bouquot JE, Guggenheimer J, et al: Cancer of the oral cavity and oropharynx. In Barnes L (ed): Surgical Pathology of the Head and Neck. New York: Marcel Dekker, 1985:333–401.

329. Schantz SP, Harrison LB, Hong WK: Cancer of the head and neck. In DeVita VT, Hellman S, Rosenberg SA (eds): Cancer: Principles and Practice of Oncology, 4th ed. Philadelphia: JB Lippincott, 1993:574–672.

330. Antoniades DZ, Styanidis K, Papanayotou P, et al: Squamous cell carcinoma of the lips in a northern Greek population. Evaluation of prognostic factors on 5-year survival rate-I. Eur J Cancer 1995;31b:340–345.

331. American Joint Committee on Cancer: Staging Manual, 5th ed. Philadelphia: JB Lippincott, 1997:24–30.

332. Frierson HF, Cooper PH: Prognostic factors in squamous cell carcinoma of the lower lip. Hum Pathol 1986;17:346–354.

333. Bagatin M, Orihovac Z, Mohammed AM: Perineural invasion by carcinoma of the lower lip. J Craniomaxfac Surg 1995;23:155–159.

Oral Cavity/Oropharynx

334. Daley TD, Lovas JGL, Peters E, et al: Salivary duct involvement in oral epithelial dysplasia and squamous cell carcinoma. Oral Surg Oral Med Oral Pathol 1996;81:186–192.

335. Slootweg PJ, Müller H: Mandibular invasion by oral squamous cell carcinoma. J Craniomaxfac Surg 1989;17:69–74.

336. Totsuka Y, Usui Y, Tei K, et al: Mandibular involvement by squamous cell carcinoma of the lower alveolus: Analysis and comparative study of histologic and radiologic features. Head Neck 1991;13:40–50.

337. Lukinmaa PL, Hietanen J, Söderholm AL, et al: The histologic pattern of bone invasion by squamous cell carcinoma of the mandibular region. Br J Oral Maxillofac Surg 1992;30:2–7.

338. Brown JS, Browne RM: Factors influencing the patterns of invasion of the mandible by oral squamous cell carcinoma. Int J Oral Maxillofac Surg 1995;24:417–426.

339. Huntley TA, Busmanis I, Desmond P: Mandibular invasion by squamous cell carcinoma: A computed tomographic and histological study. Br J Oral Maxillofac Surg 1996;34:69–74.

340. Eicker, SA, Overholt SM, El-Naggar AK: Lower gingival carcinoma. Clinical and pathologic determinants of regional metastases. Arch Otolaryngol Head Neck Surg 1996;122:634–638.

341. Barttelbort SW, Bahn SL, Ariyan S: Rim mandibulectomy for cancer of the oral cavity. Am J Surg 1987;154:423–428.

342. Müller H, Slootweg PJ: Mandibular invasion by oral squamous cell carcinoma. Clinical aspects. J Craniomaxfac Surg 1990;18:80–84.

343. Southam JC: The extension of squamous carcinoma along the inferior dental neuro vascular bundle. Br J Oral Surg 1970;7:137–145.

344. McGregor AD, MacDonald DG: Patterns of spread of squamous cell carcinoma within the mandible. Head Neck Surg 1989;11:457–461.

345. O'Brien CJ, Carter RL, Soo KC, et al: Invasion of the mandible by squamous carcinomas of the oral cavity and oropharynx. Head Neck Surg 1986;8:247–256.

346. McGregor AD, MacDonald DG: Routes of entry of squamous cell carcinoma to the mandible. Head Neck Surg 1988;10:294–301.

347. Cleary KR, Batsakis JG: Pathology consultation. Oral squamous cell carcinoma and the mandible. Ann Otol Rhinol Laryngol 1995;104:977–979.

348. Quigley LF, Cobb CM, Schoenfeld S, Hunt EE, Williams P: Reverse smoking and its oral consequences in Caribbean and South American peoples. J Am Dent Assoc 1964;69:427–442.

349. Reddy DG, Rao VK: Cancer of the palate in coastal Andhra due to smoking cigars with the burning end inside the mouth. Indian J Med Sci 1957;11:791–798.

350. Abrams AM, Melrose RJ, Howell FV: Necrotizing sialometaplasia. A disease simulating malignancy. Cancer 1973;32:130–135.

351. Micheau C, Cachin MY, Caillon B: Cystic metastases in the neck revealing occult carcinoma of the tonsil. A report of six cases. Cancer 1974;33:228–233.

352. Compagno J, Hyams VJ, Safavian M: Does branchiogenic carcinoma really exist? Arch Pathol Lab Med 1976;100:311–314.

353. Thompson LDR, Heffner DK: The clinical importance of cystic squamous cell carcinomas in the neck. A study of 136 cases. Cancer 1998;82:944–956.

Verrucous Carcinoma

354. Ackerman LV: Verrucous carcinoma of the oral cavity. Surgery 1948;23:670–678.

355. Goethals PL, Harrison EG, Devine KD: Verrucous squamous carcinoma of the oral cavity. Am J Surg 1963;106:845–851.

356. Kraus FT, Perez-Mesa C: Verrucous carcinoma. Clinical and pathologic study of 105 cases involving oral cavity, larynx and genitalia. Cancer 1966;19:26–38.

357. Fonts EA, Greenlaw RH, Rush BF, et al: Verrucous squamous cell carcinoma of the oral cavity. Cancer 1969;23:152–160.

358. Biller HF, Ogura JH, Bauer WC: Verrucous cancer of the larynx. Laryngoscope 1971;81:1323–1329.

359. Jacobson S, Shear M: Verrucous carcinoma of the mouth. J Oral Pathol 1972;1:66–75.

360. Elliott GB, McDougall JA, Elliott JDA: Problems of verrucose squamous carcinoma. Ann Surg 1973;177:21–29.

361. Burns HP, van Nostrand P, Bryce DP: Verrucous carcinoma of the larynx. Management by radiotherapy and surgery. Ann Otol 1976;85:538–543.

362. Ryan RE, De Santo LW, Devine KD, et al: Verrucous carcinoma of the larynx. Laryngoscope 1977;87:1989–1994.

363. Glanz H, Kleinsasser O: Verruköse Akanthose (verruköses Karzinom) des Larynx. Laryng Rhinol 1978;57:835–843.

364. Ferlito A, Recher G: Ackerman's tumor (verrucous carcinoma) of the larynx. A clinicopathologic study of 77 cases. Cancer 1980;46:1617–1630.

365. McCoy JM, Waldron CA: Verrucous carcinoma of the oral cavity. A review of forty-nine cases. Oral Surg Oral Med Oral Pathol 1981;52:623–629.

366. Batsakis JG, Hybels R, Crissman JD, et al: The pathology of head and neck tumors: Verrucous carcinoma. Head Neck Surg 1982;5:29–38.

367. McDonald JS, Crissman JD, Gluckman JL: Verrucous carcinoma of the oral cavity. Head Neck Surg 1982;5:22–28.

368. Medina JE, Dichtel MAJW, Luna MA: Verrucous squamous carcinomas of the oral cavity. Arch Otolaryngol 1984;110:437–440.

369. Ferlito A: Diagnosis and treatment of verrucous squamous cell carcinoma of the larynx. A critical review. Ann Otol Rhinol Laryngol 1985;94:575–579.

370. Lundgren JAV, van Nostrand P, Harwood AR, et al: Verrucous carcinoma (Ackerman's tumor) of the larynx: Diagnostic and therapeutic considerations. Head Neck Surg 1986;9:19–26.

371. Nair MK, Sankaranarayanan R, Padmanabhan TK, et al: Oral verrucous carcinoma. Treatment with radiotherapy. Cancer 1988;61:458–461.

372. Sllamniku B, Bauer W, Painter C, et al: Clinical and histopathological considerations for the diagnosis and treatment of verrucous carcinoma of the larynx. Arch Otorhinolaryngol 1989;246:126–132.

373. Vidyasagar MS, Fernandes DJ, Kasturi PD, et al: Radiotherapy and verrucous carcinoma of the oral cavity. A study of 107 cases. Acta Oncol 1992;31:43–47.

374. Abramson AL, Brandsma J, Steinberg B, et al: Verrucous carcinoma of the larynx. Possible human papillomavirus etiology. Arch Otolaryngol 1985;111:709–715.

375. Eisenberg E, Rosenberg B, Krutchkoff DJ: Verrucous carcinoma: A possible viral pathogenesis. Oral Surg Oral Med Oral Pathol 1985;59:52–57.

376. Brandsma JL, Steinberg BM, Abramson AL, et al: Presence of human papillomavirus type 16 related sequences in verrucous carcinoma of the larynx. Cancer Res 1986;46:2185–2188.

377. Adler-Storthz K, Newland JR, Tessin BA, et al: Human papillomavirus type 2 DNA in oral verrucous carcinoma. J Oral Pathol 1986;15:472–475.

378. Noble-Topham SE, Fliss DM, Hartwick WJ, et al: Detection and typing of human papillomavirus in verrucous carcinoma of the oral cavity using the polymerase chain reaction. Arch Otolaryngol Head Neck Surg 1993;119:1299–1304.

379. Shroyer KR, Greer RO, Fankhouser CA, et al: Detection of human papillomavirus DNA in oral verrucous carcinoma by polymerase chain reaction. Modern Pathol 1993;6:669–672.

380. Fliss DM, Noble-Topham SE, McLachlin CM, et al: Laryngeal verrucous carcinoma: A clinicopathologic study and detection of human papillomavirus using polymerase chain reaction. Laryngoscope 1994;104:146–152.

381. Johnson TL, Plieth DA, Crissman JD, et al: HPV detection by polymerase chain reaction (PCR) in verrucous lesions of the upper aerodigestive tract. Modern Pathol 1991;4:461–465.

382. Luna MA, Tortoledo ME: Verrucous carcinoma. In Gnepp DR (ed): Pathology of the Head and Neck. New York: Churchill-Livingstone, 1988:497–515.

383. Hyams VJ, Batsakis JG, Michaels L: Tumors of the upper respiratory tract and ear, 2nd series, Fascicle 25. Washington: Armed Forces Institute of Pathology, 1988:72–82.

384. Bouquot JE: Oral verrucous carcinoma: Incidence in two US populations. Oral Surg Oral Med Oral Pathol Oral Radiol Endod 1998;86:318–324.

385. Slootweg PJ, Müller H: Verrucous hyperplasia or verrucous carcinoma. An analysis of 27 patients. J Oral Maxillofac Surg 1983;11:13–19.

386. Ishiyama A, Eversole LR, Ross DA, et al: Papillary squamous neoplasms of the head and neck. Laryngoscope 1994;104:1446–1452.

387. Ferlito A, Antonutto G, Silvestri F: Histological appearances and nuclear DNA content of verrucous squamous carcinoma of the larynx. ORL J Otorhinolaryngol Relat Spec 1976;38:65–85.

388. Cooper JR, Hellquist HB, Michaels L: Image analysis in the discrimination of verrucous carcinoma and squamous papilloma. J Pathol 1992;166:383–387.

389. Shear M, Pindborg JJ: Verrucous hyperplasia of the oral mucosa. Cancer 1980;46:1855–1862.

390. Arendorf TM, Aldred MJ: Verrucous carcinoma and verrucous hyperplasia. J Dent Assoc South Africa 1982;37:529–532.

391. Murrah VA, Batsakis JG: Proliferative verrucous leukoplakia and verrucous hyperplasia. Ann Otol Rhinol Laryngol 1994;103:660–663.

392. Hansen LS, Olson JA, Silverman S: Proliferative verrucous leukoplakia. A long-term study of thirty patients. Oral Surg Oral Med Oral Pathol 1985;60:285–298.

393. Crissman JD, Gnepp DR, Goodman ML, et al: Preinvasive lesions of the upper aerodigestive tract: Histologic definitions and clinical implications (a symposium). Path Annual 1987;22:311–352.

394. Zakrewska JM, Lopes V, Speight P, Hopper C: Proliferative verrucous leukoplakia. A report of ten cases. Oral Surg Oral Med Oral Pathol Oral Radiol Endod 1996;82:396–401.

395. Hagen P, Lyons GD, Haindel C: Verrucous carcinoma of the larynx: Role of human papillomavirus, radiation, and surgery. Laryngoscope 1993;103:253–257.

396. Demian SDE, Bushkin FL, Echeverria RA: Perineural invasion and anaplastic transformation of verrucous carcinoma. Cancer 1973;32:395–401.

397. Ferlito A, Rinaldo A, Mannara GM: Review article. Is primary radiotherapy an appropriate option for the treatment of verrucous carcinoma of the head and neck? J Laryngol Otol 1998;112:132–139.

398. McCaffrey TV, Witte M, Ferguson MT: Verrucous carcinoma of the larynx. Ann Otol Rhinol Laryngol 1998;107:391–395.

399. Perez CA, Kraus FT, Evans JC, et al: Anaplastic transformation in verrucous carcinoma of the oral cavity after radiation therapy. Radiology 1966;86:108–115.

400. van Nostrand AWP, Olofsson J: Verrucous carcinoma of the larynx. A clinical and pathologic study of 10 cases. Cancer 1972;30:691–702.

401. Edström S, Johansson SL, Lindström J, et al: Verrucous squamous cell carcinoma of the larynx. Evidence for increased metastatic potential after irradiation. Otolaryngol Head Neck Surg 1987;97:381–384.

402. Tharp II ME, Shidnia H: Radiotherapy in the treatment of verrucous carcinoma of the head and neck. Laryngoscope 1995;105:391–396.

Spindle Cell Carcinoma

403. Batsakis JG: "Pseudosarcoma" of the mucous membranes in the head and neck. J Laryngol Otol 1981;95:311–316.

404. Brodsky G: Carcino (pseudo)sarcoma of the larynx: The controversy continues. Otolaryngol Clin North Am 1984;17:185–197.

405. Weidner N: Sarcomatoid carcinoma of the upper aerodigestive tract. Semin Diagn Pathol 1987;4:157–168.

406. Nappi O, Wick MR: Sarcomatoid neoplasms of the respiratory tract. Semin Diagn Pathol 1993;10:137–147.

407. Wick MR, Swanson PE: Carcinosarcomas: Current perspectives and an historical review of nosological concepts. Semin Diagn Pathol 1993;10:118–127.

408. Lane N: Pseudosarcoma (polypoid sarcoma-like masses) associated with squamous cell carcinoma of mouth, fauces and larynx. Cancer 1957;10:19–41.

409. Sherwin RP, Strong MS, Vaughn CW: Polypoid and junctional squamous cell carcinoma of the tongue and larynx with spindle-cell carcinoma ("pseudosarcoma"). Cancer 1963;16:51–60.

410. Goellner JR, Devine KD, Weiland LH: Pseudosarcoma of the larynx. Am J Clin Pathol 1973;59:312–326.

411. Appelman HD, Oberman HA: Squamous cell carcinoma of the larynx with sarcoma-like stroma. A clinicopathologic assessment of spindle cell carcinoma and "pseudosarcoma". Am J Clin Pathol 1965;44:135–145.

412. Himalstein MR, Humphrey TR: Pleomorphic carcinoma of the larynx. Arch Otolaryngol 1968;87:389–395.

413. Lichtiger B, MacKay B, Tessmer CF: Spindle-cell variant of squamous carcinoma. A light and electron microscopic study of 13 cases. Cancer 1970;26:195–200.

414. Leifer C, Miller AS, Putong PB, et al: Spindle cell carcinoma of the oral mucosa. A light and electron microscopic study of apparent sarcomatous metastasis to cervical lymph nodes. Cancer 1974;34:597–605.

415. Hyams VJ: Spindle cell carcinoma of the larynx. Can J Otolaryngol 1975;4:307–313.

416. Randall G, Alonso WA, Ogura JH: Spindle cell carcinoma (pseudosarcoma) of the larynx. Arch Otolaryngol 1975;101:63–66.

417. Someren A, Karcioglu Z, Clairmont AA: Polypoid spindle-cell carcinoma (pleomorphic carcinoma). Report of a case occurring on tongue and review of the literature. Oral Surg Oral Med Oral Pathol 1976;42:474–489.

418. Ellis GL, Corio RL: Spindle cell carcinoma of the oral cavity. A clinicopathologic assessment of fifty-nine cases. Oral Surg Oral Med Oral Pathol 1980;50:523–534.

419. Leventon GS, Evans HL: Sarcomatoid squamous cell carcinoma of the mucous membranes of the head and neck. A clinicopathologic study of 20 cases. Cancer 1981;48:994–1003.

420. Leonardi E, Dalri P, Pusiol T, et al: Spindle-cell squamous carcinoma of head and neck region. A clinicopathologic and immunohistochemical study of eight cases. ORL J Otorhinolaryngol Relat Spec 1986;48:275–281.

421. Zarbo RJ, Crissman JD, Venkat H, et al: Spindle-cell carcinoma of the upper aerodigestive tract mucosa. An immunologic and ultrastructural study of 18 biphasic tumors and comparison with seven monophasic spindle-cell tumors. Am J Surg Pathol 1986;10:741–743.

422. Slootweg PJ, Roholl PJM, Müller H, et al: Spindle-cell carcinoma of the oral cavity and larynx. Immunohistochemical aspects. J Craniomaxfac Surg 1989;17:234–236.

423. Takata T, Ito H, Ogawa J, et al: Spindle cell squamous carcinoma of the oral region. An immunohistochemical and ultrastructural study on the histogenesis and differential diagnoses with a clinicopathological analysis of six cases. Virchows Arch A Pathol Anat 1991;419:177–182.

424. Cassidy M, Maher M, Keogh P, et al: Pseudosarcoma of the larynx: The value of ploidy analysis. J Laryngol Otol 1994;108:525–528.

425. Minckler DS, Meligro CH, Norris HT: Carcinosarcoma of the larynx. Case report with metastases of epidermoid and sarcomatous elements. Cancer 1970;26:195–200.

426. Staley CJ, Ujiki GT, Yokoo H: "Pseudocarcinoma" of the larynx. Independent metastasis of carcinomatous and sarcomatous elements. Arch Otolaryngol 1971;94:458–465.

427. Srinivasan U, Talvalkar SV: True carcinosarcoma of the larynx: A case report. J Laryngol Otol 1979;93:1031–1035.

428. Sonobe H, Hayashi K, Takahashi K, et al: True carcinosarcoma of the maxillary sinus. Path Res Pract 1989;185:488–495.

429. Klijanienko J, Vielh P, Duvillard P, et al: True carcinosarcoma of the larynx. J Laryngol Otol 1992;106:58–60.

430. Hansen LT, Kristensen S, Moesner J: Polypoidal carcinosarcoma of the oropharynx: A clinicopathological and immunohistochemical study. J Laryngol Otol 1995;108:459–465.

431. Battifora H: Spindle cell carcinoma. Ultrastructural evidence of squamous origin and collagen production by the tumor cells. Cancer 1976;37:2275–2282.

432. Meijer JWR, Ramaekers FCS, Manni JJ, et al: Intermediate filament proteins in spindle cell carcinoma of the larynx and tongue. Acta Otolaryngol (Stockh) 1988;106:306–313.

433. Hellquist H, Olofsson J: Spindle cell carcinoma of the larynx. APMIS 1989;97:1103–1113.

434. Toda S, Yonemitsu N, Miyabara S, et al: Polypoid squamous cell carcinoma of the larynx. An immunohistochemical study for ras p21 and cytokeratin. Path Res Pract 1989;185:860–866.

435. Nakleh RE, Zarbo RJ, Ewing S, et al: Myogenic differentiation in spindle cell (sarcomatoid) carcinomas of the upper aerodigestive tract. Appl Immunohistochem 1993;1:58–68.

436. Ellis GL, Langloss JM, Heffner DK, et al: Spindle-cell carcinoma of the aerodigestive tract. An immunohistochemical analysis of 21 cases. Am J Surg Pathol 1987;11:335–342.

437. Goldman RL, Weidner N: Pure squamous cell carcinoma of the larynx with cervical nodal metastasis showing rhabdomyosarcomatous differentiation. Clinical, pathologic, and immunohistochemical study of a unique example of divergent differentiation. Am J Surg Pathol 1993;17:415–421.

438. Deshotels SJ, Sarma D, Fazio F, et al: Squamous cell carcinoma with sarcomatoid stroma. J Surg Oncol 1982;19:201–207.

439. Lambert PR, Ward PH, Berci G: Pseudosarcoma of the larynx. A comprehensive analysis. Arch Otolaryngol 1980;106:700–708.

440. Lasser KH, Naeim F, Higgins J, et al: "Pseudosarcoma" of the larynx. Am J Surg Pathol 1979;3:397–404.

441. Batsakis JG, Rice DH, Howard DR: The pathology of head and neck tumors: Spindle cell lesions (sarcomatoid carcinomas, nodular fasciitis and fibrosarcoma) of the aerodigestive tracts, part 14. Head Neck Surg 1982;4:499–513.

442. Ellis GL, Langloss JM, Enzinger FM: Coexpression of keratin and desmin in a carcinosarcoma involving the maxillary alveolar ridge. Oral Surg Oral Med Oral Pathol 1985;60:410–416.

443. Banerjee SS, Eyden BP, Wells S, et al: Pseudoangiosarcomatous carcinoma: A clinicopathological study of seven cases. Histopathology 1992;21:13–23.

444. Petri WH, Auclair PA, Branham GB, et al: Intraosseous tumor of the maxilla. J Oral Maxillofac Surg 1985;43:726–734.

445. Wenig BM, Devaney K, Bisceglia M: Inflammatory myofibroblastic tumor of the larynx. A clinicopathologic study of eight cases simulating a malignant spindle cell neoplasm. Cancer 1995;76:2217–2229.

446. Heffner DK, Hyams VJ: Teratocarcinosarcoma (malignant teratoma?) of the nasal cavity and paranasal sinuses. A clinicopathologic study of 20 cases. Cancer 1984;53:2140–2154.

447. Fernandez PL, Cardesa A, Alós L, Pinto J, Traserra J: Sinonasal teratocarcinosarcoma: An unusual neoplasm. Path Res Pract 1995;191:166–171.

448. Friedel W, Chambers RG, Atkins JP: Pseudosarcomas of the pharynx and larynx. Arch Otolaryngol 1976;102:286–290.

449. Berthelet E, Shenouda G, Black MJ, et al: Sarcomatoid carcinoma of the head and neck. Am J Surg 1994;168:455–458.

450. Ballo MT, Garden AS, El-Naggar AK, et al: Radiation therapy for early stage (T1-T2) sarcomatoid carcinoma of true vocal cords: Outcomes and patterns of failure. Laryngoscope 1998;108:760–763.

Basaloid Squamous Carcinoma

451. Wain SL, Kie R, Vollmer RT, et al: Basaloid—squamous carcinoma of the tongue, hypopharynx, and larynx: Report of 10 cases. Hum Pathol 1986;17:1158–1166.

452. Dougherty BG, Evans HL: Carcinoma of the anal canal: A study of 79 cases. J Clin Pathol 1985;83:159–164.

453. Ferry JA, Scully RE: "Adenoid cystic" carcinoma and adenoid basal carcinoma of the uterine cervix: A study of 38 cases. Am J Surg Pathol 1988;12:134–144.

454. Epstein JI, Sears DL, Tucker RS, et al: Carcinoma of the esophagus with adenoid cystic differentiation. Cancer 1984;53:1131–1136.

455. Tsang WYW, Chan JKC, Lee KC, et al: Basaloid-squamous carcinoma of the upper aerodigestive tract and so-called adenoid cystic carcinoma of the oesophagus: The same tumour type? Histopathology 1991;19:35–46.

456. Brambilla E, Moro D, Veale D, et al: Basal cell (basaloid) carcinoma of the lung: A new morphologic and phenotypic entity with separate prognostic significance. Hum Pathol 1992;23:993–1003.

457. Banks ER, Frierson HF, Mills SE, et al: Basaloid squamous cell carcinoma of the head and neck. Am J Surg Pathol 1992;16:939–946.

458. Cadier MA, Kelly SA, Parkhouse N, et al: Basaloid squamous carcinoma of the buccal cavity. Head Neck 1992;14:387–391.

459. Campman SC, Gandour-Edwards RF, Sykes JM: Basaloid squamous carcinoma of the head and neck. Arch Pathol Lab Med 1994;118:1229–1232.

460. Coppola D, Catalano E, Tang CK, et al: Basaloid squamous cell carcinoma of floor of mouth. Cancer 1993;72:2299–2305.

461. Gartlan MR, Goetz SP, Graham SM: Basaloid-squamous carcinoma (BSC) of the larynx. Arch Otolaryngol Head Neck Surg 1992;118:998–1001.

462. Ereño C, Lopez JI, Sanchez JM, et al: Basaloid-squamous cell carcinoma of the larynx and hypopharynx. A clinicopathologic study of 7 cases. Path Res Pract 1994;190:186–193.

463. Hellquist HB, Dahl F, Karlsson MG, et al: Basaloid squamous cell carcinoma of the palate. Histopathology 1994;25:178–180.

464. Klijanienko J, El-Naggar A, Ponzio-Prion A, et al: Basaloid squamous carcinoma of the head and neck. Immunohistochemical comparison with adenoid cystic carcinoma and squamous cell carcinoma. Arch Otolaryngol Head Neck Surg 1993;119:887–890.

465. Lovejoy HM, Matthews BL: Basaloid-squamous carcinoma of the palate. Otolaryngol Head Neck Surg 1992;106:159–162.

466. Luna MA, El Naggar A, Parichatikanond P, et al: Basaloid squamous carcinoma of the upper aerodigestive tract. Cancer 1990;66:537–542.

467. McKay MJ, Bilous AM: Basaloid-squamous carcinoma of the hypopharynx. Cancer 1989;63:2528–2531.

468. Muller S, Barnes L: Basaloid squamous cell carcinoma of the head and neck with a spindle cell component. Arch Pathol Lab Med 1995;119:181–182.

469. O'Malley BW Jr: Pathologic quiz case 2: Basaloid-squamous carcinoma of the right pyriform sinus. Arch Otolaryngol Head Neck Surg 1992;118:212–215.

470. Raslan WF, Barnes L, Krause JR, et al: Basaloid squamous cell carcinoma of the head and neck: A clinicopathologic and flow cytometric study of 10 new cases with review of the English literature. Am J Otolaryngol 1994;15:204–211.

471. Seidman JD, Berman JJ, Yost BA, et al: Basaloid squamous carcinoma of the hypopharynx and larynx associated with second primary tumors. Cancer 1991;68:1545–1549.

472. Shvili Y, Talmi YP, Gal R, et al: Basaloid-squamous carcinoma of larynx metastatic to the skin of the nasal tip. J Craniomaxfac Surg 1990;18:322–324.

473. Wan SK, Chan JKC, Tse KC: Basaloid-squamous carcinoma of the nasal cavity. J Laryngol Otol 1992;106:370–371.

474. Batsakis J, El-Naggar A: Basaloid-squamous carcinomas of the upper aerodigestive tracts. Ann Otol Rhinol Laryngol 1989;98:919–920.

475. Ferlito A, Rinaldo A, Altavilla G, Doglioni C: Basaloid squamous cell carcinoma of the larynx and hypopharynx. Ann Otol Rhinol Laryngol 1997;106:1024–1035.

476. Barnes L, Ferlito A, Altavilla G, et al: Clinicopathological consultation. Basaloid squamous cell carcinoma of the head and neck. Clinicopathological features and differential diagnosis. Ann Otol Rhinol Laryngol 1996;105:75–82.

477. Van der Wal JE, Snow GB, Karim ABMF, et al: Adenoid cystic carcinoma of the palate with squamous metaplasia or basaloid-squamous carcinoma? Report of a case. J Oral Pathol Med 1994;23:461–464.

478. Gnepp DR, Wick MR: Small cell carcinoma of the major salivary glands: An immunohistochemical study. Cancer 1990;66:185–192.

479. Gnepp DR: Small cell neuroendocrine carcinoma of the larynx. A critical review of the literature. ORL J Otorhinolaryngol Relat Spec 1991;53:210–219.

480. Morice WG, Ferreiro JA: Distinction of basaloid squamous cell carcinoma from adenoid cystic and small cell undifferentiated carcinoma by immunohistochemistry. Hum Pathol 1998;29:609–612.

481. Farmer ER, Helwig EB: Metastatic basal cell carcinoma: A clinicopathologic study of seventeen cases. Cancer 1980;46:748–757.

482. Tavin E, Persky MS, Jacobs J: Metastatic basal cell carcinoma of the head and neck. Laryngoscope 1995;105:814–817.

483. Snow SN, Sahl W, Lo JS: Metastatic basal cell carcinoma. Cancer 1994;73:328–335.

484. Larner JM, Malcolm RH, Mills SE, et al: Radiotherapy for basaloid squamous cell carcinoma of the head and neck. Head Neck 1993;15:249–252.

Adenoid Squamous Cell Carcinoma

485. Lever WF: Adenoacanthoma of sweat glands. Carcinoma of sweat glands with glandular and epidermal elements; report of four cases. Arch Dermatol Syphilol 1947;56:157–171.

486. Lever WF: Histopathology of the Skin. Philadelphia: J.B. Lippincott, 1954:480–481.

487. Muller SA, Wilhelmy CM Jr, Harrison EG Jr, et al: Adenoid squamous cell carcinoma (adenoacanthoma of Lever). Report of seven cases and review. Arch Dermatol 1964;89:589–597.

488. Johnson WC, Helwig EB: Adenoid squamous cell carcinoma (adenoacanthoma). A clinicopathologic study of 155 patients. Cancer 1966;19:1639–1650.

489. Wansker BA, Smith JG Jr, Okansky S: Adenoacanthoma-dyskeratotic squamous cell carcinoma with tubular and alveolar formations. Arch Dermatol 1957;75:96–104.

490. Lever WF: Histopathology of the Skin, 4th ed. Philadelphia: J.B. Lippincott, 1967:511–512.

491. Eusebi V, Lamovec J, Cattani MG, et al: Acantholytic variant of squamous cell carcinoma of the breast. Am J Surg Pathol 1986;10:855–861.

492. Nappi O, Pettinato G, Wick MR: Adenoid (acantholytic) squamous cell carcinoma of the skin. J Cutan Pathol 1989;16:114–121.

493. Jones AC, Freedman PD, Kerpel SM: Oral adenoid squamous cell carcinoma: A report of three cases and review of the literature. J Oral Maxillofac Surg 1993;51:676–681.

494. Jacoway JR, Nelson JF, Boyers RC: Adenoid squamous-cell carcinoma (adenoacanthoma) of the oral labial mucosa. A clinicopathologic study of fifteen cases. Oral Surg Oral Med Oral Pathol 1971;32:444–449.

495. Goldman RL, Klein HZ, Sung M: Adenoid squamous cell carcinoma of the oral cavity. Report of the first case arising in the tongue. Arch Otolaryngol 1977;103:496–498.

496. Takagi M, Sakota Y, Takayama S, et al: Adenoid squamous cell carcinoma of the oral mucosa. Cancer 1977;40:2250–2255.

497. Zaatari GS, Santoianni RA: Adenoid squamous cell carcinoma of the nasopharynx and neck region. Arch Pathol Lab Med 1986;110:542–546.

498. Hertenstein JC, Fechner RE: Acantholytic squamous cell carcinoma. Arch Otolaryngol Head Neck Surg 1986;112:780–782.

499. Batsakis JG, Huser J: Squamous carcinomas with gland like (adenoid) features. Ann Otol Rhinol Laryngol 1990;99:87–88.

500. Nappi O, Wick MR, Pettinato G, et al: Pseudo vascular adenoid squamous cell carcinoma of the skin. A neoplasm that may be mistaken for angiosarcoma. Am J Surg Pathol 1992;16:429–438.

501. Dodd LG: Fine-needle aspiration cytology of adenoid (acantholytic) squamous-cell carcinoma. Diag Cytopathol 1995;12:168–172.

502. Ferlito A, Devaney KO, Rinaldo A, et al: Clinicopathological consultation. Mucosal adenoid squamous cell carcinoma of the head and neck. Ann Otol Rhinol Laryngol 1996;105:409–413.

Adenosquamous Carcinoma

503. Gluckmann A, Cherry CP: Incidence, histology, and response to radiation of mixed carcinomas (adenoacanthomas) of the uterine cervix. Cancer 1956;9:971–979.

504. Cihak RW, Kawashima T, Steer A: Adenoacanthoma (adenosquamous carcinoma) of the pancreas. Cancer 1972;29:1133–1140.

505. Naunheim KS, Taylor JR, Skosey C, et al: Adenosquamous lung carcinoma, clinical characteristics, treatment and prognosis. Ann Thorac Surg 1987;44:462–466.

506. Gerughty RM, Hennigar GR, Brown FM: Adenosquamous carcinoma of the nasal, oral and laryngeal cavities. Cancer 1968;22:1140–1155.

507. Fujino K, Ito J, Kanaji M, et al: Adenosquamous carcinoma of the larynx. Am J Otolaryngol 1995;16:115–118.

508. Minic AJ, Stajcic Z: Adenosquamous carcinoma of the inferior turbinate: A case report. J Oral Maxillofac Surg 1994;52:764–767.

509. Ogawa T: A clinicopathological study of adenocarcinomas of the nasal cavity and paranasal sinuses. Nippon Jibiinkoka Gakkai Kaiho 1989;92:317–333.

510. Napier SS, Gormley JS, Newlands C, et al: Adenosquamous carcinoma. A rare neoplasm with an aggressive course. Oral Surg Oral Med Oral Pathol 1995;79:607–611.

511. Martinez-Madrigal F, Baden E, Casiraghi O, et al: Oral and pharyngeal adenosquamous carcinoma, a report of four cases with immunohistochemical studies. Eur Arch Otorhinolaryngol 1991;248:255–258.

512. Damiani JM, Damiani KK, Hauck K, et al: Mucoepidermoid-adenosquamous carcinoma of the larynx and hypopharynx: A report of 21 cases and a review of the literature. Otolaryngol Head Neck Surg 1981;89:235–243.

513. Aden KK, Adams GL, Niehans G, et al: Adenosquamous carcinoma of the larynx and hypopharynx with five new case presentations. Trans Am Laryngol Assoc 1988;109:216–221.

514. Zieske LA, Myers EN, Brown BM: Pulmonary lymphangitic carcinomatosis from hypopharyngeal adenosquamous carcinoma. Head Neck Surg 1988;10:195–198.

515. Sanderson RJ, Rivron RP, Wallace WA: Adenosquamous carcinoma of the hypopharynx. J Laryngol Otol 1991;105:678–680.

516. Siar CH, Ng KH: Adenosquamous carcinoma of the floor of the mouth and lower alveolus: A radiation-induced lesion? Oral Surg Oral Med Oral Pathol 1987;63:216–220.

517. Ellis GL, Auclair PL, Gnepp DR, Goode RKl: Other malignant epithelial neoplasms. In Ellis GL, Auclair PL, Gnepp DR (eds): Surgical Pathology of the Salivary Glands. Philadelphia: W.B. Saunders, 1991:455–459.

518. Hyams VJ, Batsakis JG, Michaels L: Tumors of the upper respiratory tract and ear. Atlas of Tumor Pathology, 2nd series, no. 25. Washington: Armed Forces Institute of Pathology, 1988:104–107.

519. Batsakis JG, Luna MA, El-Naggar AK: Pathology Consultation: Nonsquamous carcinomas of the larynx. Ann Otol Rhinol Laryngol 1992;101:1024–1026.

520. Fechner RE: Necrotizing sialometaplasia. A source of confusion with carcinoma of the palate. Am J Clin Pathol 1977;67:315–317.

521. Sanner JR: Combined adenosquamous carcinoma and ductal adenoma of the hard and soft palate: Report of a case. J Oral Surg 1979;37:331–334.

522. Ferlito A: A pathologic and clinical study of adenosquamous carcinoma of the larynx: Report of four cases and review of the literature. Acta Otorhinolaryngol Belg 1976;30:379–389.

523. El-Jabbour JN, Ferlito A, Friedmann I: Adenosquamous carcinoma. In Ferlito A (ed): Neoplasms of the Larynx. Edinburgh: Churchill-Livingstone, 1993:249–251.

524. Izumi K, Mnakajima T, Maeda T, Cheng J, Saku T: Adenosquamous carcinoma of the tongue. Report of a case with histochemical, immuno-histochemical, and ultra-structural study and review of the literature. Oral Surg Oral Med Oral Pathol Oral Radiol Endod 1998;85:178–184.

Papillary Squamous Cell Carcinoma

525. Crissman JD, Kessis T, Shah KV, et al: Squamous papillary neoplasia of the adult upper aerodigestive tract. Hum Pathol 1988;19:1387–1396.

526. Landman G, Taylor RM, Friedman KJ: Cutaneous papillary squamous cell carcinoma. A report of two cases. J Cut Pathol 1990;17:105–110.

527. Randall ME, Andersen WA, Mills SE: Papillary squamous cell carcinoma of uterine cervix: A clinicopathologic study of nine cases. Int J Gyn Pathol 1986;5:1–10.

528. Li WW, Pettit TH, Zakka KA: Intraocular invasion by papillary squamous cell carcinoma of the conjunctiva. Am J Ophthalmol 1980;90:697–701.

529. Leong AS, Brown JH: Malignant transformation in a thymic cyst. Am J Surg Pathol 1984;8:471–475.

530. Thompson LDR, Wenig, BM, Heffner DK, Gnepp DR: Exophytic and papillary squamous cell carcinomas of the larynx. A clinicopathologic series of 104 cases. Otolaryngol Head Neck Surg 1999;120:718—724.

531. McClatchey KD, Zarbo RJ: The jaws and oral cavity. In Sternberg SS (ed): Diagnostic Surgical Pathology, 2nd ed, Vol. II. New York: Raven Press, 1994:781–785.

532. Judd R, Zaki SR, Coffield LM, et al: Human papillomavirus 6 detected by the polymerase chain reaction in invasive sinonasal papillary squamous cell carcinoma. Arch Pathol Lab Med 1991;115:1150–1153.

533. Altmann F, Basek M, Stout AP: Papillomas of the larynx with intraepithelial anaplastic changes. Arch Otolaryngol 1986;11:423–429.

534. Lindeberg H, Oster S, Oxlund I, et al: Laryngeal papillomas: Classification and course. Clin Otolaryngol 1986;11:423–429.

535. Quick CA, Foucar E, Dehner LP: Frequency and significance of epithelial atypia in laryngeal papillomatosis. Laryngoscope 1979;89:550–560.

Lymphoepithelioma

536. Regaud C, Reverchon L: Sur un cas d'epithelioma epidermoide developpé dans le massif maxillaire superieure etendu aux ligaments de la face, aux cavites buccale, nasale et orbitaire ainsi que aux ganglions du cou gueri par la radiotherapie. Rev Laryngol Otol Rhinol (Bord) 1921;42:369–378.

537. Schmincke A: Ueber Lympho-epitheliale Geschwülste. Ziegler Beitr z Path Anat u.z. Allg Path 1921;68:161–170.

538. Frank DK, Cheron F, Cho H, et al: Nonnasopharyngeal lymphoepitheliomas (undifferentiated carcinomas) of the upper aerodigestive tract. Ann Otol Rhinol Laryngol 1995;104:305–310.

539. Iezzoni JC, Gaffey MJ, Weiss LM: The role of Epstein-Barr virus in lymphoepithelioma-like carcinomas. Am J Clin Pathol 1995;103:308–315.

540. MacMillan C, Kapadia SB, Finkelstein SD, et al: Lymphoepithelial carcinoma of the larynx and hypopharynx: Study of eight cases with relationship to Epstein-Barr virus and p53 gene alterations, and review of the literature. Hum Pathol 1996;27:1172–1179.

541. Weiss LM, Gaffey MJ, Shibata D: Lymphoepithelioma-like carcinoma and its relationship to Epstein-Barr virus. Am J Clin Pathol 1991;96:156–158.

542. Ferlito A, Weiss CM, Rinaldo A, et al: Clinicopathological consultation. Lymphoepithelial carcinoma of the larynx, hypopharynx and trachea. Ann Otol Rhinol Laryngol 1997;106:437–444.

543. Clifford P: On the epidemiology of nasopharyngeal carcinoma. Int J Cancer 1970;5:287–309.
544. De-The G: Epidemiological evidence implicating the Epstein-Barr virus in Burkitt's lymphoma and nasopharyngeal carcinoma etiology. IARC Sci Publ no. 20. Lyon, International Agency for Research on Cancer, 1978:285–299.
545. Lanier A, Bender T, Talbot M, et al: Nasopharyngeal carcinoma in Alaskan Eskimos, Indians and Aleuts. Cancer 1980;46:2100–2106.
546. Giffler RF, Gillespie JJ, Ayala AG, Newland JR: Lymphoepithelioma in cervical lymph nodes of children and young adults. Am J Surg Pathol 1977;1:293–301.
547. Zarate-Osorno A, Jaffe ES, Medeiros LJ: Metastatic nasopharyngeal carcinoma initially presenting as cervical lymphadenopathy. A report of two cases that resembled Hodgkin's disease. Arch Pathol Lab Med 1992;116:862–865.
548. Cappell DF: Lymphoepithelioma of the nasopharynx and tonsils. J Path Bact 1934;39:49–64.
549. Scofield HH: Epidermoid carcinoma of the nasal and pharyngeal regions: A statistical and morphological analysis of two hundred and fourteen cases. M.S. Thesis, Georgetown University, 1952.
550. Nomori H, Watanabe S, Nakajima T, et al: Histiocytes in nasopharyngeal carcinoma in relation to prognosis. Cancer 1986;57:100–105.
551. Looi LM: Tumour-associated tissue eosinophilia in nasopharyngeal carcinoma. A pathologic study of 422 primary and 138 metastatic tumors. Cancer 1987;59:466–470.
552. Carbone A, Micheau C: Pitfalls in microscopic diagnosis of undifferentiated carcinoma of nasopharyngeal type (lymphoepithelioma). Cancer 1982;50:1344–1351.
553. Sugimoto T, Hashimoto H, Enjoli M: Nasopharyngeal carcinoma and malignant lymphomas: An immunohistochemical analysis of 74 cases. Laryngoscope 1990;100:742–748.
554. Frierson HF, Bellafiore FJ, Gaffney MJ, et al: Cytokeratin in anaplastic cell large cell lymphoma. Mod Pathol 1994;7:317–321.
555. Shahab I, Osborne B, Butler J: Nasopharyngeal lymphoid tissue masses in patients with human immunodeficiency virus-1. Cancer 1994;74:3083–3088.
556. Melbye M, Cote TR, West D, et al: Nasopharyngeal carcinoma: An EBV-associated tumour not significantly influenced by HIV-induced immunosuppression. Br J Cancer 1996;73:995–997.

Unusual Features in Epidermoid Carcinoma

557. Norris CM, Mustoe TA, Ross JS, et al: Desmoplastic squamous cell carcinoma of the tongue simulating myositis or fasciitis. Head Neck Surg 1986;9:51–55.

Treatment

558. Terhaard CHJ, Snippe K, Ravasz LA, Hordijk GJ: Radiotherapy in T1 laryngeal cancer: Prognostic factors for locoregional control and survival. Int J Radiat Oncol Biol Phys 1991;21:1179–1186.
559. Wiggenraad RG, Terhaard CHJ, Hordijk GJ, Ravasz LA: The importance of vocal cord mobility in T2 laryngeal cancer. Radiother Oncol 1990;18:321–327.
560. Terhaard CHJ, Karim ABMF, Hoogenraad WJ, et al: Local control in T3 laryngeal cancer treated with radical radiotherapy: The concept of nominal standard dose and linear quadratic model. Int J Radiat Oncol Biol Phys 1991;20:1207–1214.
561. Terhaard CHJ, Hordijk GJ, Dolsma WV, et al: Morbidity associated with treatment for T3 laryngeal cancer. Laryngeal Cancer: Proceedings of the 2nd World Congress on Laryngeal Cancer, 1994:561–565.
562. Peters LJ, Ang KK: The role of altered fractionation in head and neck cancers. Sem Radiother Oncol 1992;2:180–194.
563. Horiot JC, Lefur R, N'Guyen T, et al: Hyperfractionation versus conventional fractionation in oropharyngeal cancer: Final analysis of a randomized trial of the EORTC cooperative group of radiotherapy. Radiother Oncol 1992;25:3231–3241.
564. Fowler JF, Tanner MA, Bataini JP, et al: Further analysis of the time factor in squamous cell carcinoma of the tonsillar region. Radiother Oncol 1990;19:237–244.
565. Whiters HR, Taylor JMG, Maciejewski B: The hazard of accelerated tumor clonogen repopulation during radiotherapy. Acta Oncol 1988;27:131–146.
566. Awwad HK, Khafagy Y, Barsoum M, et al: Accelerated versus conventional fractionation in the postoperative irradiation of locally advanced head and neck cancer: Influence of tumour proliferation. Radiother Oncol 1992;25:261–266.
567. Bataini JP, Bernier J, Asselain B, et al: Primary radiotherapy of squamous cell carcinoma of the oropharynx and pharyngolarynx: Tentative multivariate modelling system to predict the radiocurability of neck nodes. Int J Radiat Biol Phys 1988;14:653.
568. Stupp RS, Weichselbaum RR, Vokes EE: Combined modality therapy of head and neck cancer. Semin Oncol 1994;21:349–358.
569. Tannock IF, Browman G: Lack of evidence for a role of chemotherapy in the routine management of locally advanced head and neck cancer. J Clin Oncol 1986;4:1121–1126.
570. Merlano M, Benasso M, Corvo R, et al: Five-year update of a randomized trial of alternating radiotherapy and chemotherapy compared with radiotherapy alone in treatment of unresectable squamous cell carcinoma of the head and neck. J Natl Cancer Inst 1996;88:583–589.
571. Al-Sarraf M, Leblanc M, Giri PGS, et al: Superiority of chemoradiotherapy versus radiotherapy in patients with locally advanced nasopharyngeal cancer. Preliminary results of Intergroup randomized study. Proc Am Soc Clin Oncol 1996;15:313.
572. Adelstein DJ, Saxton JP, Lavertu P, et al: A phase III randomized trial comparing concurrent chemotherapy and radiotherapy with radiotherapy alone in resectable stage III and IV squamous cell head and neck cancer: Preliminary results. Head Neck 1997;19:567–575.
573. Munro AJ: An overview of randomised controlled trials of adjuvant chemotherapy in head and neck cancer. Br J Cancer 1995;71:83–91.
574. The Department of Veterans Affairs Laryngeal Cancer Study Group: Induction chemo therapy plus radiation compared with surgery plus irradiation in advanced laryngeal cancer. N Engl J Med 1991;324:1685–1690.
575. Lefebvre JL, Chevalier D, Luboinsky B et al: Larynx preservation in pyriform sinus cancer. Preliminary results of a European Organization for Research and Treatment of Cancer phase III trial. J Natl Cancer Inst 1996;88:890–899.
576. Browman GP, Cronin L: Standard chemotherapy in squamous cell head and neck cancer: What we have learned from randomized trials. Semin Oncol 1994;21:311–319.

3 : Nonsquamous Lesions of Nasal Cavity, Paranasal Sinuses, and Nasopharynx

Bayardo Perez-Ordóñez and Andrew G. Huvos

ANATOMY AND HISTOLOGY
Nasal Cavity

The nose is a complex organ formed by two components: the external and the internal nose. The external nose is triangular, with a wide base that contains two external openings, the nares or nostrils, separated by the columella. Inside the aperture of each nostril is a dilated area covered by skin known as the vestibule.

The internal nose is divided by the septum into right and left nasal cavities, or fossae. Posteriorly, it communicates with the nasopharynx through the choana. Each cavity is divided into four parts: superior (roof), inferior (floor), lateral, and medial walls. The superior wall is formed anteriorly by the cribriform plate of the ethmoid bone, which separates the nasal cavity from the anterior cranial fossa. The posterior portion of the roof is formed by the body of the sphenoid bone. The floor constitutes the largest portion of the nasal cavity and is formed by the palatine process of the maxillary bone and the horizontal plate of the palatine bone. The superior, middle, and inferior turbinates with their corresponding meatuses are located in the lateral wall, which is formed by the nasal portion of the maxillary bone, the perpendicular plate of the palatine bone, and the ethmoidal labyrinth, which separates the nasal cavity from the orbit.[1–3] The middle turbinate may occasionally be pneumatized.

Histologically, the nasal vestibule is covered by skin and is composed of keratinizing squamous epithelium and subcutaneous tissue with numerous hair follicles, sebaceous glands, and sweat glands. The squamous epithelium from the vestibule changes to ciliated pseudostratified (respiratory-type) epithelium, which covers the entire nasal cavity with the exception of a small portion of the posterior roof. The latter is lined by olfactory epithelium.[4] The submucosa contains seromucous glands and numerous thick vessels that resemble erectile tissue and are especially prominent in the turbinates. The olfactory epithelium consists of several types of cells: bipolar spindle cells with myelinated and non-myelinated axons traversing the cribriform plate, columnar sustentacular cells, round basal cells, and serous glands in the lamina propia.[1, 3, 4]

Paranasal Sinuses

The largest of the paranasal sinuses are the maxillary sinuses. These triangular cavities are located in the body of each maxilla. The base is formed by the lateral wall of the nasal cavity and the apex projects into the zygoma. Each sinus has a superior wall, or roof, an inferior wall, or floor, and posterior, medial, and anterolateral walls. The roof forms the floor of the orbit, whereas the floor is formed by the alveolar and palatine processes of the maxilla. The posterior wall relates to the infratemporal space and the pterygopalatine fossa. The anterior wall is the facial surface of the maxilla.

The ethmoid sinuses are formed by the frontal, maxillary, lacrimal, sphenoidal, and palatine bones. They are located in the ethmoidal labyrinth and consist of numerous air-filled cells divided into anterior, middle, and posterior groups according to their relation to the labyrinth. The frontal sinuses are located in the vertical portion of the frontal bone with only a thin plate of bone separating them

from the anterior cranial fossa and both orbits. The ostium of the frontal sinus opens into the anterior part of the medial meatus. The sphenoid sinuses are located within the sphenoid bone and are related to numerous vital structures in the cranial cavity; the internal carotid arteries are located laterally, whereas the optic chiasm and the hypophysis are located posteriorly.

All the paranasal sinuses are lined by ciliated pseudostratified respiratory-type epithelium similar to the nasal cavities. This epithelium is also known as schneiderian epithelium and is ectodermal in origin, unlike the endodermally derived mucosa of the nasopharynx. The mucous membrane in the sinuses is thinner and less vascular than that of the nasal cavity. The seromucous glands are also more sparse and are largely concentrated at the ostium of the maxillary sinus.

Nasopharynx

The pharynx is divided into three parts: nasopharynx, oropharynx, and hypopharynx. The nasopharynx is the portion of the pharynx that lies behind the nasal cavity and above the soft palate. It has anterior, posterior, and lateral walls. The anterior wall is continuous with the nasal cavity through the choana. The posterior wall is continuous with the roof of the nasal cavity and includes the roof of the nasopharynx anteriorly and a posterior portion located against the base of the skull and the body of the sphenoid. The posterior wall extends inferiorly to the free border of the soft palate where the oropharynx begins. The lateral walls contain the ostium of the eustachian tube, which is surrounded by a cartilaginous elevation called the *torus tubarius.* Posterior to this prominence there is a depression called the fossa of Rosenmüller.[5, 6]

Approximately 60% of the nasopharyngeal mucosa is lined by stratified squamous epithelium of endodermal origin. These areas include the lower half of the anterior and posterior walls and the anterior half of the lateral walls. Ciliated pseudostratified respiratory-type epithelium covers the areas around the nasal choanae and the roof of the posterior wall. The remainder of the nasopharynx contains irregular patches of squamous and ciliated epithelium. There are also areas with an intermediate or "transitional" type epithelium. The submucosa contains seromucinous glands, which can undergo oncocytic metaplasia especially in older individuals.[7] Bilateral oncocytic cysts and melanotic oncocytic metaplasia arising from these glands have been described.[8, 9] A prominent lymphoid component with germinal centers is also present beneath the mucosa. These lymphoid elements can be present within the mucosal epithelium, forming the so-called *lymphoepithelium.*[5, 6]

INFLAMMATORY DISORDERS
Rhinitis and Sinusitis

Rhinitis and sinusitis are the most common disorders of the sinonasal tract; however, tissue derived from these conditions is never, or rarely, seen by the surgical pathologist. Most cases are viral in origin, but they can be complicated by superimposed bacterial infections. Most examples are the result of adenoviruses, echoviruses, or rhinoviruses. Recently, cytomegalovirus has been reported as a cause of sinusitis in patients infected with human immunodeficiency virus (HIV).[10] Developmental anomalies that also may cause chronic sinusitis in children include hypoplasia of the maxillary sinuses, concha bullosa, a deviated uncinate process, and the so-called Haller's cells.[11] Complications of rhinosinusitis include secondary bacterial infection with extension into adjacent structures causing pharyngotonsillitis. In addition, chronic allergic rhinitis plays a significant role in the genesis of inflammatory pseudopolyps. The treatment of acute rhinitis and sinusitis is symptomatic. Chronic sinusitis may be medically managed with topical nasal steroids and antibiotics. Patients who have failed medical management may benefit from surgical intervention in the form of nasal lavage, the creation of a nasoantral window, or, more recently, functional endoscopic nasal surgery.[11] Chronic sinusitis is also a component of Kartagener's syndrome. This syndrome also includes bronchiectasis and situs inversus and is due to a defective ciliary cytoskeleton lacking dynein arms.[12–14] Occasionally, pathologists will be asked to perform ultrastructural assessment of nasal biopsies in cases suspicious of Kartagener's syndrome.

Mucous Impaction

Clinical Features. Mucous impaction is an uncommon inflammatory lesion that has also been called *inspissated mucus* or *snotoma*.[15] It is most commonly seen in children and young adults with a longstanding history of chronic rhinosinusitis of any etiology. It is a pseudoneoplastic process resulting from the impaction of a large amount of mucus within the maxillary antrum. This mucous mass produces opacification of the antrum, usually without sinus wall destruction or invasion. However, rare cases, similar to a mucocele, may present with pressure erosion and destruction of bone.

Pathologic Features. Grossly, the mass has a translucent appearance and a gray to pink color. Microscopically, it consists of mucin-positive acellular material containing numerous neutrophils, lymphocytes, and plasma cells admixed with desquamated respiratory-type epithelium.

Differential Diagnosis. The differential diagnosis of mucous impaction includes myxoma, well-differentiated mucinous adenocarcinoma, and embryonal rhabdomyosarcoma. The typical clinical history, the lack of destruction or invasion of the maxillary bone, the presence of degenerating inflammatory cells, and the absence of neoplastic cells should argue against the diagnosis of a neoplasm.

Treatment and Prognosis. This is a pseudoneoplastic condition with an excellent prognosis. The treatment of choice is removal of the impacted mucus with treatment of the underlying inflammatory process.

Sinonasal Inflammatory Polyps

Clinical Features. Sinonasal inflammatory polyps are nonneoplastic proliferations of the sinonasal mucosa composed of epithelial and stromal elements. The pathogenesis of these lesions is uncertain; however, mucosal edema and inflammation, cytokine secretion, and collagen synthesis stimulated by eosinophils have all been implicated.[16, 17] They have been divided into inflammatory nasal and antrochoanal polyps.

Inflammatory polyps are most often seen in adults with a longstanding history of chronic rhinitis accompanied by allergy, asthma, aspirin intolerance, or diabetes mellitus. They are multiple and often present as bilateral masses arising from the lateral nasal wall. Symptoms at presentation include nasal obstruction, rhinorrhea, and headaches. Radiologic studies usually reveal a soft tissue mass with air-fluid levels occupying the nasal cavity or paranasal sinuses. Large inflammatory polyps can destroy bone and extend into the nasopharynx, orbit, and cranial cavity.[18–20] Inflammatory nasal polyps develop in approximately 20% of children with cystic fibrosis, and, in some, they may be the initial clinical manifestation of the disease.

Unlike inflammatory polyps, polyps of the antrochoanal type are more frequently seen in children,[21, 22] although this finding has not been reproduced in other studies.[23] These lesions arise in the maxillary antrum and secondarily extend into the nasal cavity.[24] Approximately 90% are solitary. They are the least common nasal polyps.[23, 25]

Pathologic Features. Inflammatory polyps can measure up to several centimeters in diameter and have a myxoid or gelatinous appearance. Most have a broad stalk. Histologically, they are lined by respiratory epithelium with a variably thickened basement membrane.[26] The epithelium often exhibits some degree of squamous metaplasia. In some cases, this metaplastic epithelium shows a degree of atypia suggestive of dysplasia.[27] The stroma is abundant and highly edematous or myxoid and contains a mixed inflammatory infiltrate composed of eosinophils, lymphocytes, and plasma cells. In cases associated with infection, neutrophils may be present in large numbers. Epstein-Barr virus genome has been demonstrated in mucosal lymphocytes of Chinese patients with nasal polyposis.[28] The stroma contains a variable number of fibroblasts and blood vessels. Typically, inflammatory polyps do not contain seromucous glands. Secondary changes include surface ulceration, fibrosis, infarction, granulation tissue, deposition of a dense amyloid-like material, cartilaginous or osseous metaplasia, glandular hyperplasia, and granuloma formation. Polyps associated with cystic fibrosis lack basement thickening and submucosal hyalinization (Fig. 3–1, see p. 81).[29] The mucin present is acidic and stains blue or purple with alcian blue/periodic acid-Schiff stain, in contrast to inflammatory polyps of the usual type, which contain neutral mucin.

Antrochoanal polyps exhibit a long fibrous stalk. Histologically, they lack the thick basement membrane and the prominent inflammatory infiltrate of inflammatory polyps.[21, 22, 30] The stroma is variable but tends to be fibrotic and contains large vascular spaces with scant glandular elements.[23]

Differential Diagnosis. Many polyps contain spindle or polygonal stromal cells with slightly hyperchromatic nuclei. However, in some cases the number and the degree of atypia seen in these fibroblasts (Fig. 3–2, see p. 81) is sufficient to raise the possibility of a malignant tumor.[31, 32] In most cases, the differential diagnosis elicited is an embryonal rhabdomyosarcoma. The typical clinical history, the presence of a heavy inflammatory infiltrate, the lack of hypercellularity, and the absence of mitotic activity argue against this diagnosis. The atypical stromal cells are preferentially concentrated in the subepithelial region and in the vicinity of blood vessels. These atypical cells are immunoreactive to actin, suggesting a myofibroblastic derivation, and closely resemble "radiation fibroblasts."

Other lesions that should be separated from sinonasal polyps are nasopharyngeal angiofibroma, schneiderian papilloma, and squamous cell carcinoma. Nasopharyngeal angiofibroma contains stromal myofibroblasts with spindle or stellate shape admixed with thick abnormal vessels not seen in polyps. Nasal polyps also lack the thick fibrovascular papillary cores, the inverted growth pattern, the oncocytic epithelium, and the intraepithelial cysts of papillomas. The degree of atypia or invasion seen in squamous cell carcinoma is also absent.

Treatment and Prognosis. The treatment of sinonasal polyps is surgical resection. Identification and treatment of etiologic factors is necessary to prevent recurrences. Antrochoanal polyps may also recur if the stalk is incompletely resected.

Myospherulosis

Myospherulosis is a rare iatrogenic pseudomycotic lesion occurring in the nasal cavity, paranasal sinuses, middle ear, and soft tissues.[33–35] Typically, patients with myosperulosis have a history of surgery followed by packing of the nasal cavity with petrolatum-based ointment prior to the development of a nasal mass.[33, 35] His-

Text continued on page 89

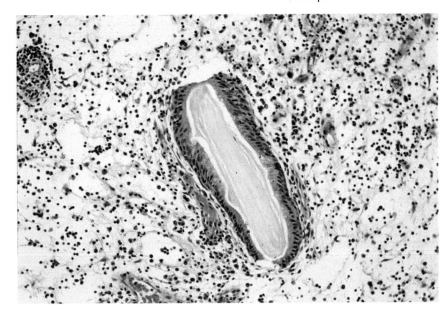

Figure 3–1. Inflammatory polyp in cystic fibrosis. Note the lack of thickening of the glandular basement membrane.

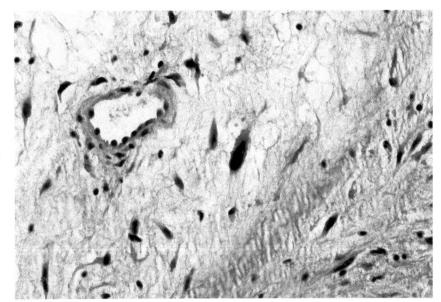

Figure 3–2. Atypical fibroblast in an inflammatory polyp. The nucleus is hyperchromatic but there is no associated hypercellularity or mitotic activity.

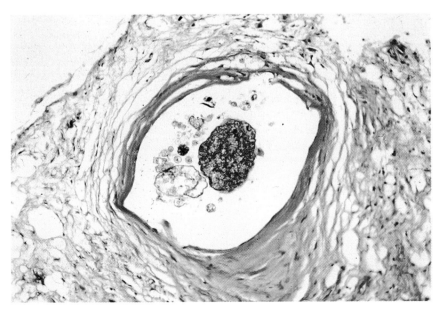

Figure 3–3. Myospherulosis of the sinonasal tract. Irregular cystic space containing larger "parent bodies," which are enveloping smaller spherules or "endobodies." (Courtesy of Dr. Bruce Wenig.)

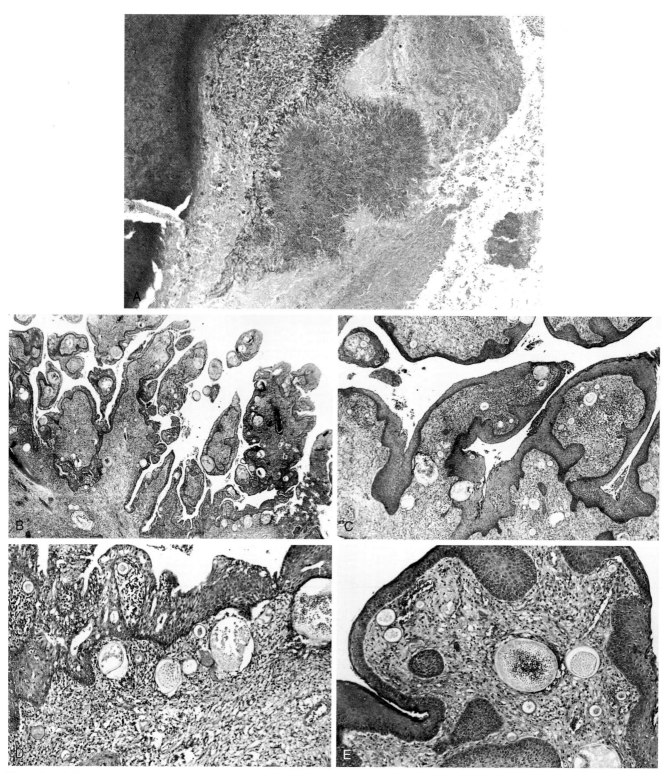

Figure 3–4. *A*, Chronic noninvasive fungal sinusitis. Typical mycetoma surrounded by mucus. *B* through *E*, Rhinosporidiosis is characterized by hyperplastic papillary epithelium with a prominent chronic submucosal infiltrate and sporangia containing numerous endospores.

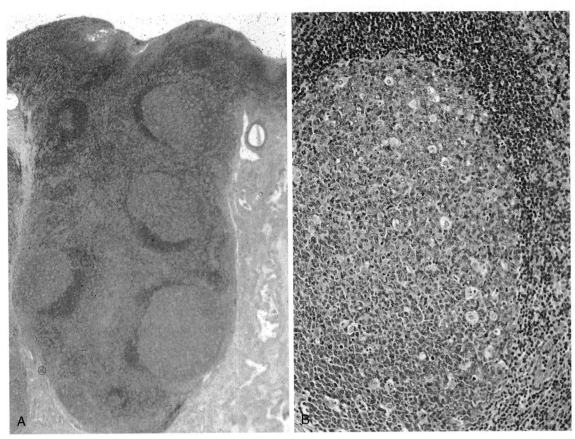

Figure 3–6. *A,* Lymphoid hyperplasia of the nasopharynx. There is formation of secondary germinal centers with prominent mantle zones. *B,* Reactive germinal center with numerous transformed follicular center cells, high mitotic rate, and numerous "tingible body" macrophages. Note the presence of "dark" and "pale" areas.

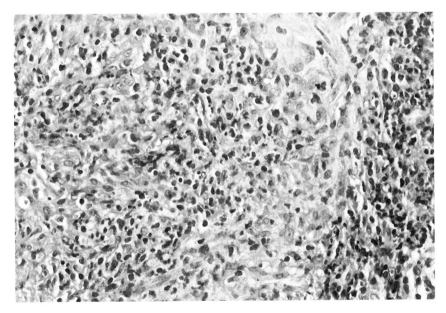

Figure 3–7. Wegener's granulomatosis. Invasion of blood vessels by a mixed inflammatory infiltrate composed of neutrophils, eosinophils, lymphocytes, and macrophages. A giant cell is also present.

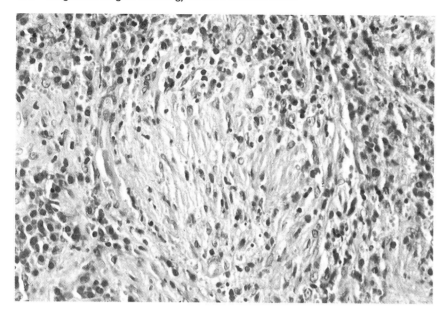

Figure 3–8. Wegener's granulomatosis. Poorly formed granuloma with numerous macrophages, small lymphocytes, and eosinophils.

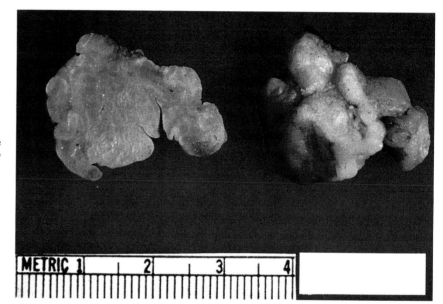

Figure 3–10. Nasal papilloma, inverted type. Note the lobulated appearance with formation of deep clefts.

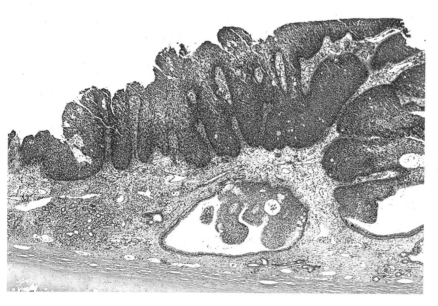

Figure 3–11. Inverted papilloma. Extension of neoplastic epithelium into seromucinous glands. This pattern of involvement is responsible for recurrences after a limited resection.

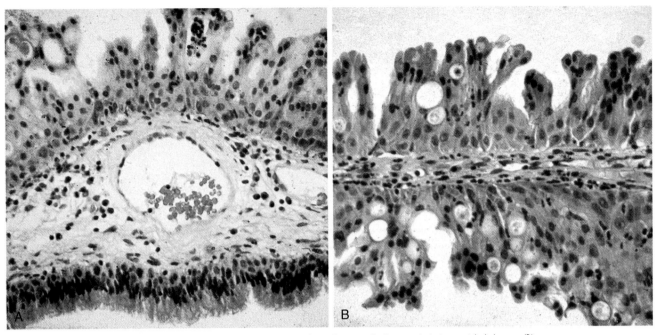

Figure 3–12. A, Cylindrical cell (oncocytic) papilloma with characteristic intraepithelial cysts (B).

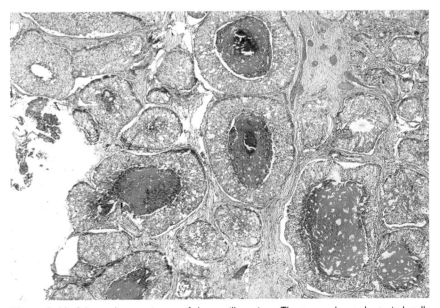

Figure 3–18. Salivary duct carcinoma of the maxillary sinus. The tumor shows the typical well-defined nests with central "comedonecrosis."

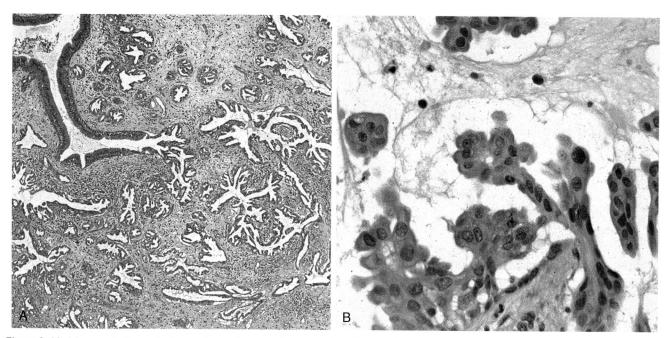

Figure 3–19. *A,* Low-grade sinonasal adenocarcinoma. The tumor is composed of infiltrative glands with a slit-like shape admixed with normal mucosa. *B,* Low-grade sinonasal adenocarcinoma. The papillary tufts are composed of cuboidal cells without significant pleomorphism.

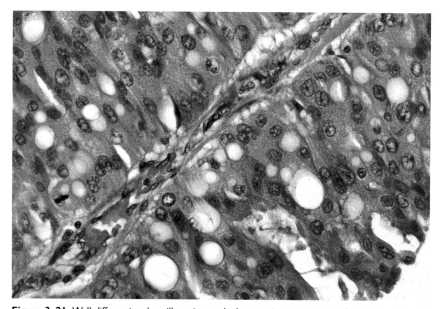

Figure 3–21. Well-differentiated papillary sinonasal adenocarcinoma containing basophilic cells with cytoplasmic vacuoles closely resembling those of acinic cell carcinoma.

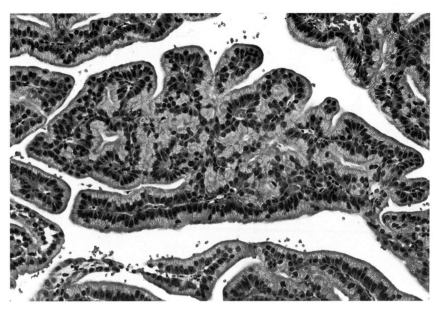

Figure 3–22. Well-differentiated intestinal-type adenocarcinoma of the sinonasal tract simulating small intestinal mucosa.

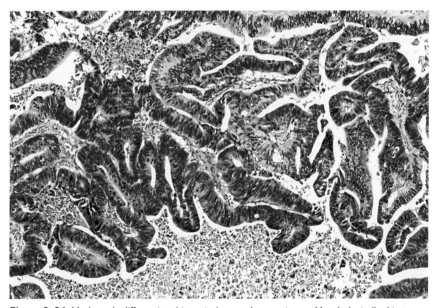

Figure 3–24. Moderately differentiated intestinal-type adenocarcinoma. Morphologically, this tumor is similar to a colorectal carcinoma of the usual type.

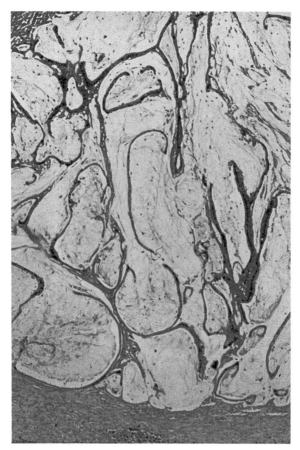

Figure 3–25. Well-differentiated mucinous adenocarcinoma.

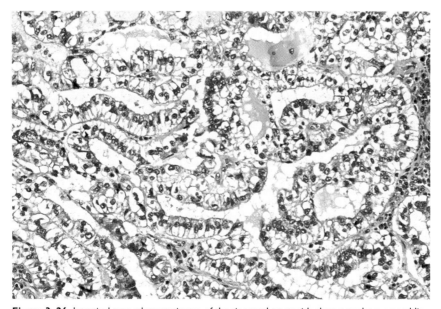

Figure 3–26. Intestinal-type adenocarcinoma of the sinonasal tract with clear cytoplasm resembling secretory-type endometrium.

tologically, there is a prominent fibrous and chronic inflammatory reaction with foreign-body type giant cells surrounding pseudocystic spaces. These spaces contain sac-like structures with a thick dark wall (Fig. 3–3, see p. 81) and are referred to as *parent bodies* with enclosed fungal-like "endobodies" or "spherules," which are simply degenerating erythrocytes. Fungal infections can be ruled out with a methenamine silver stain.[33]

Granulomatous Diseases

Tuberculosis

Tuberculosis in the upper respiratory mucosa is usually a manifestation of disseminated disease.[36, 37] The most common presentation is that of an ulcer or a polyp involving the septum and the inferior turbinate. In some cases, septal perforation can be seen. Microscopically, there are numerous poorly formed granulomas. Caseous necrosis is relatively infrequent and it is rare to find microorganisms in an acid-fast stain. The differential diagnosis of tuberculosis in the sinonasal tract includes other granulomatous diseases and Wegener's granulomatosis. The diagnosis is made by clinicopathologic correlation and cultures. The treatment consists of multiagent chemotherapy including a combination of isoniazid (INH), rifampicin, streptomycin, and ethambutol.

Sarcoidosis

Sarcoidosis is a multisystemic disorder that most often affects the lung and mediastinal lymph nodes. Rarely, it also involves the upper respiratory tract, including the nasal cavity and paranasal sinuses.[38–40] Grossly, the nasal mucosa is dry and crusty and is involved by yellow submucosal nodules. Histologically, the mucosa reveals numerous noncaseating epithelioid and giant cell granulomas. Stains for acid-fast bacilli are negative, and there is no vasculitis or necrosis.[39] The differential diagnosis includes other granulomatous diseases, especially cholesterol granulomas, tuberculosis, leprosy, and Wegener's granulomatosis. Virtually all patients with sinonasal sarcoidosis have pulmonary and hilar nodal involvement.[41] The treatment of sarcoidosis depends on the clinical manifestations of the disease and sites involved. Oral prednisone is usually the drug of choice. Chlorambucil may also be used when corticosteroids fail or are contraindicated.

Leprosy

Clinical Pathologic Features. Leprosy is a slowly progressive disease caused by *Mycobacterium leprae*. The infection affects the skin and peripheral nerves and results in disabling deformities. This infection has largely disappeared in the United States and most of Europe but still affects millions of people in underdeveloped countries. Leprosy is a disease with clinicopathologic manifestations determined by the host's cellular immune response. Two clinical forms of the disease occur, depending on whether the host is capable of mounting a T-cell–mediated immune response or is anergic. Those with an immune response develop tuberculoid leprosy. Anergy results in lepromatous leprosy.

M. leprae is transmitted from person to person via aerosols that originated from lesions in the upper respiratory tract. The vast majority of the lesions observed in the nasal cavity are of the lepromatous type and consist of large numbers of macrophages filled with massive quantities of acid-fast bacilli.[42, 43] Fibroblasts, neutrophils, eosinophils, and plasma cells can also be present. Occasionally, some of these cells are seen along nerves that show Schwann cells containing large numbers of bacilli. The bacilli may also be found within endothelial cells and fibroblasts, mucous glands and ducts, and vascular lumens. The bacilli are highlighted with the Fite-Faraco modification of the Ziehl-Neelsen stain.

Differential Diagnosis. The main differential diagnosis of tuberculous leprosy includes sarcoidosis, tuberculosis, certain fungal infections, and Wegener's granulomatosis. All of these latter entities have significantly different epidemiology, clinical manifestations, and serologic and microbiology tests that should allow their distinction from tuberculous leprosy. Rhinoscleroma may resemble lepromatous leprosy, but in leprosy the Fite-Faraco stain should demonstrate the presence of large numbers of acid-fast organisms.

Treatment and Prognosis. Dapsone, rifampin, clofazimine, and ethionamide are the main drugs used to treat leprosy. Adequate treatment requires the use of most of these drugs for several years. Supportive care is also important in reducing morbidity and injuries leading to blindness and mutilation. The prognosis depends on clinical stage of the disease, type of disease, availability of effective drugs, adherence to treatment, and supportive care measures.

Rhinoscleroma

Clinical Features. Rhinoscleroma is a chronic granulomatous disease that is endemic in parts of Central and South America, North and Central Africa, and certain areas of Eastern Europe.[44–47] It is uncommon in North America.[48] Rhinoscleroma is caused by the gram-negative rod *Klebsiella rhinoscleromatis* and affects primarily the nasal cavity and nasopharynx.[49, 50] Involvement of the lip, oropharynx, and palate is also common. In severe cases, the infection causes bone destruction and nasal obstruction with extension into the paranasal sinuses, orbit, middle ear, larynx, and tracheobronchial tree. Clinically, rhinoscleroma is characterized by three phases: rhinitic, florid, and fibrotic. The initial symptoms resemble a common cold, but in fully developed disease there is also dysphonia, aphonia, and anosmia. Clinically, anesthesia of the soft palate and hypertrophy of the uvula should suggest the diagnosis of rhinoscleroma. In advanced cases, the destruction of the nasal cartilage with the formation of nodules causes a severe deformity referred to as *Hebra nose*.[47] Recently, rhinoscleroma has been described as an opportunistic infection in HIV-affected individuals.[51]

Pathologic Features. Pathologically, rhinoscleroma is also characterized by three phases: rhinitis or catarrhal, florid or granulomatous, and fibrotic. In the catarrhal phase, the tissue changes are nonspecific and consist of abundant neutrophils, cellular debris, and granulation tissue. In the granulomatous phase, rhinoscleroma is characterized by pseudoepitheliomatous hyperplasia of the overlying mucosa, and a dense chronic inflammatory infiltrate composed of lymphocytes, plasma cells with numerous Russell bodies, and large macrophages with clear vacuolated cytoplasm. These macrophages are referred to as *Mikulicz's cells*. The microorganisms are present within the cytoplasm of these macrophages and can be demonstrated by a Warthin-Starry silver stain, a Giemsa stain, or a Gram stain. In inconclusive cases, the bacteria can be identified in 1 to 2 mm thick sections stained with toluidine blue. In the final fibrotic stage, there are variable degrees of fibrosis and the Mikulicz cells are absent or are difficult to identify.

Differential Diagnosis. The differential diagnosis of rhinoscleroma includes leprosy, sarcoidosis, tuberculosis, mycotic infections, and sinonasal sinus histiocytosis with massive lymphadenopathy (SHML; Rosai-Dorfman disease). Clinicopathologic features, special stains, and microbiologic cultures are helpful in excluding other granulomatous infections. In leprosy, the organisms are acid-fast and can be demonstrated by the Fite-Faraco stain. Rhinoscleroma lacks the large atypical cells with emperipolesis and S-100 protein immunostaining seen in SHML.

Treatment and Prognosis. The initial treatment of rhinoscleroma consists of prolonged antibiotic therapy using doxycycline, ciprofloxacin, ceforanide, rifampicin, or streptomycin. Antibiotic therapy is generally effective. Surgery and laser ablation can only be used until the patient has been proven clinically and histologically free of disease and cultures have been negative.

Fungal Diseases

Clinical Features. Sinonasal mycotic disease can be clinically classified as acute fulminant, chronic invasive, chronic noninvasive, and allergic.[52] Occasionally, the histologic distinction between invasive fungal disease and a "fungus ball," or mycetoma, is difficult or impossible and the distinction needs to be made on clinical and radiologic grounds. The histologic diagnosis of sinonasal mycotic infections often requires a heightened suspicion. In chronic noninvasive fungal infections, the mucosa shows a nonspecific inflammatory reaction, and often the use of Gomori's methenamine-silver and periodic acid-Schiff stains is required to identify the hyphae (Fig. 3–4, see p. 82). Chronic noninvasive infections have been associated with *Aspergillus* spp.,[53] *Pseudallescheria boydii*,[54] *Bipolaris* spp.,[55] *Sporothrix schenckii*,[56] *Schizophylum commune*,[57] and, rarely, mucor.[58]

Acute fulminant or angioinvasive fungal infections are common in immunocompromised hosts, particularly those with HIV infection and those with hematologic malignancies.[57, 59, 60] Acute fungal infections are characterized by acute inflammation, tissue necrosis, and numerous hyphae invading blood vessels. *Mucormycosis* (phycomycosis) is usually seen in association with poorly controlled diabetes mellitus, although it can also be seen in noncompromised hosts.[61] This is an aggressive infection that can quickly extend into soft tissues, orbit, and brain. Recognition is based on the identification of broad nonseptate hyphae. Other fungi capable of causing invasive fungal sinusitis include *Aspergillus*,[62–64] *Candida* spp.,[65] cryptococcosis,[66] *Curvularia lunata*,[67] *Pseudallescheria boydii*,[60] and *Alternaria* spp.[68]

Allergic fungal sinusitis is a noninvasive fungal pansinusitis that occurs in immunocompetent individuals with a longstanding history of atopy, elevated levels of total immunoglobulin-E and peripheral eosinophilia.[69] Initially, this condition was attributed to infection with *Aspergillus* spp. because of the presence of dichotomous fungal hyphae and the histologic similarities to allergic bronchopulmonary aspergillosis.[70] Subsequent studies, however, have demonstrated that nearly 80% of cases of allergic fungal sinusitis are due to members of the Dematiaceae family, with the most common genus being *Bipolaris* followed by *Curvularia, Exxerohilum, Alternaria,* and *Cladusporium*.[69, 71, 72]

Rhinosporidiosis is a chronic, superficial, mucocutaneous infection primarily involving the nasal cavities, nasopharynx, and oral cavity.[73] This infection, initially thought to be caused by *Rhinosporidium seeberi,* now appears to be caused by the waterborne organism cyanobacterium *Microcystis aeruginosa*.[74] It is endemic in India and Sri Lanka, where 90% of all infections occur. Rarely, cases are seen in the United States.[75] Clinically, the lesions are seen as friable polyps or papillomas.

Pathologic Features. Histologically, AFS consists of abundant pale eosinophilic or basophilic "allergic" mucin with a laminated appearance. The mucin contains numerous eosinophils, plasma cells, and lymphocytes admixed with cellular debris, sloughed respiratory epithelial cells, and edematous respiratory mucosa. Charcot-Leyden crystals with clusters of degenerated eosinophils are constant microscopic features. Fungal hyphae with dichotomous 45-degree branching and rare yeast forms are identified with Gomori's methenamine-silver or Fontana-Masson stain.[70, 72] No fungal balls or invasion of bone or mucosa is present. Because of morphologic similarities of the fungi causing AFS, cultures are mandatory for the exact identification of the organism responsible.

Microscopically, rhinosporidiosis is characterized by hyperplastic respiratory or squamous epithelium accompanied by a lymphoplasmacytic infiltrate. The subepithelial stroma contains numerous cysts or sporangia ranging in size from 100 to 300 μm with thick walls. The sporangia contain numerous endospores with a characteristic arrangement of immature and mature forms. The immature forms are small, whereas the mature forms are larger and contain eosinophilic cytoplasmic globules. The diagnosis rests on the identification of these structures in the surgical material or by smear preparations.[76]

Recently, Tadros et al.[77] described a case of fungal infection involving the right maxillary sinus in a 33-year-old woman with sickle cell disease caused by *Scedosporium apiospermum.* This is an additional case of hyalohyphomycosis, an emerging mycosis in immunodeficient individuals caused by nonpigmented septate hyphae that closely resemble *P. boydii.* Recognition of this infection is important, since scedosporial species are resistant to the most commonly used antimycotic agents, such as amphotericin B.

Differential Diagnosis. The differential diagnosis of fungal infections in the sinonasal tract includes a large number of non-neoplastic and neoplastic diseases. Sinonasal tuberculosis is generally accompanied by pulmonary disease and a positive skin test. Microscopically, there are large numbers of granulomas with caseous necrosis that are not seen in fungal infections. Gomori's methenamine-silver and acid-fast stains are helpful in revealing the responsible organism. Wegener's granulomatosis may be difficult to exclude based on morphologic grounds alone, since vasculitis may be a focal finding in nasal biopsies. However, most patients with Wegener's granulomatosis also have renal manifestations and serologic cytoplasmic antineutrophilic and myeloperoxidase antibodies. Sinonasal T cell or natural killer cell lymphomas may present with extensive tissue destruction with a polymorphous infiltrate involving the sinonasal tract. They also reveal the presence of an atypical lymphoid infiltrate not seen in sinonasal mycotic infections. Silver and periodic acid-Schiff stains may demonstrate the fungal organisms. Acute fulminant fungal infections may be present with similar clinical features to those of idiopathic midline destructive disease (IMDD), a controversial and extremely rare disorder of doubtful existence. The diagnosis of IMDD can be established only after other processes have been excluded by clinical manifestations, serologic studies, cultures, and biopsy with immunohistochemical and molecular pathology ancillary techniques.

Treatment and Prognosis. The treatment and prognosis of sinonasal fungal disease varies depending on the type of infection, causative organisms, and underlying medical conditions.[78, 79] The treatment of most noninvasive fungal disease usually consists of sinusotomy and curettage of all necrotic and diseased tissue. In some infections, such as blastomycosis, the role of surgery is more limited and is used only to establish a definitive diagnosis and to drain accumulations of pus that are not draining spontaneously. The invasive forms, especially opportunistic mycosis complicating the cases of patients with diabetes mellitus or immunosuppressed individuals, require radical surgical debridement and intravenous amphotericin B. In those affected by mucormycosis, surgery has an important role in removing devitalized tissues, since the vascular thrombosis present in necrotic tissues interferes with the delivery of amphotericin B. Surgery is also the mainstay in the treatment of chromoblastomycosis because the fungus shows little response to amphotericin B or flucytosine chemotherapy. Amphotericin B plays a major role in the treatment of invasive aspergillosis, mucormycosis, blastomycosis, candidiasis, coccidioidomycosis, histoplasmosis, paracoccidioidomycosis, and phaeohyphomycosis. Miconazole is the drug of choice in the treatment of *Pseudallescheria boydii*.[79] The management of hyalohyphomycosis is more difficult given the resistance that these organisms have demonstrated to amphotericin B, flucytosine, miconazole, ketoconazole, and, in some cases, itraconazole.[77] Surgical resection is the primary treatment of rhinosporidiosis. Surgery is also the treatment for recurrent lesions. Chemotherapy may play a role in the management of multiple recurrences.

The treatment of allergic fungal sinusitis varies according to clinical features and extent of disease.[78] The prognosis of noninvasive fungal infections in the sinonasal tract is excellent. The invasive forms have a guarded prognosis. In the case of mucormycosis, the most important determinant of survival is the underlying disorder. Patients with no underlying disease had a survival rate of approximately 75%, whereas those with leukemia or renal disease have a survival rate of 20%.[78] Adequate chemotherapy is also important in patient outcome; the addition of amphotericin B in the management of diabetic patients with mucormycosis has raised the survival rate from 37% to 79%.

▪ NON-NEOPLASTIC LESIONS INCLUDING CYSTS AND HAMARTOMAS

Necrotizing Sialometaplasia

Necrotizing sialometaplasia is rare in the sinonasal tract. This process is characterized by necrosis of the nasal seromucinous glands with secondary squamous metaplasia. It is usually seen following surgery or trauma in the sinonasal region.[80, 81] The metaplastic squamous cells may show focal nuclear atypia, but there is overall maintenance of the lobular acinar architecture and the individual acini maintain smooth contours.[82] The main significance of necrotizing sialometaplasia is its recognition and separation from squamous cell carcinoma and mucoepidermoid carcinoma. These tumors have a more infiltrative appearance, and, in the case of mucoepidermoid carcinoma, variable numbers of mucous and intermediate cells can also be identified. Rare cases may recur[83] or can obscure an underlying squamous cell carcinoma.[84]

Amyloidosis

Mufarrij et al.[85] reported a case of localized amyloidosis in the sinonasal tract. The patient had no evidence of systemic disease. The morphologic appearance and stains were typical of localized amyloidosis at other sites.

Paranasal Sinus Mucocele

Clinical Features. Paranasal mucoceles are chronic, nonneoplastic cystic lesions secondary to obstruction of the sinus outlet.[86, 87] They occur more frequently in the ethmoid sinuses and frontal sinus region (90%) and less commonly in the maxillary and sphenoid regions. In most instances, the blockage is secondary to an inflammatory or allergic process, although cystic fibrosis, trauma, or neoplastic processes have also been implicated.[88–90] The symptoms associated with these lesions vary depending on the location, size, and degree of extension into adjacent structures and include facial pain and swelling, proptosis, rhinorrhea, and nasal obstruction.[91] Radiologically, there is opacification of the affected sinus; in longstanding cases, erosion with destruction or sclerosis of the adjacent bone can also be present.[89, 92–94]

Pathologic Features. The gross appearance is characterized by a cyst filled with a mucoid or gelatinous secretion. Microscopically, the cysts are lined with flattened pseudostratified ciliated columnar epithelium accompanied by secondary changes such as fibrosis, granulation tissue, and recent and remote hemorrhage with cholesterol granulomas. In some instances, the epithelium exhibits a variable degree of squamous metaplasia. Sinus mucoceles have been divided into two groups: internal and external types. In the internal type, the cyst herniates into the submucosal tissues of the bony wall of the sinuses, whereas in the external type the cyst extends into the cranial cavity or subcutaneous tissues.

Differential Diagnosis. The clinical, radiologic, and pathologic features can closely simulate those of a neoplasm. The pathologic diagnosis of sinus mucocele should be closely correlated with the clinical history and radiologic and surgical findings. The characteristic clinical and radiologic findings and the absence of tumor cells in pathologic material should exclude the possibility of a neoplasm.

Treatment and Prognosis. The treatment of mucocele consists of surgical relief of the sinus obstruction and decompression of the mucocele. This may be accomplished by endoscopic surgery or by removal of the medial maxillary wall.

Respiratory Epithelial Adenomatoid Hamartoma

Clinical Features. Respiratory epithelial adenomatoid hamartoma is a rare lesion characterized by an adenomatoid proliferation of respiratory ciliated cells occurring in the nasal cavity, sinuses, and nasopharynx. This glandular process is derived from the schneiderian or surface nasopharyngeal epithelium, not from seromucous glands. Most patients are males in the fifth or sixth decade of life. In the study by Wenig and Heffner,[95] there were 27 males and 4 females with a median age of 58 years. The symptoms at presentation are nonspecific and include rhinosinusitis, allergies, nasal obstruction, stuffiness, septum deviation, and epistaxis. At physical examination, the lesion appears as a polypoid mass most commonly arising in the posterior septum. Involvement of the lateral wall, middle meatus, and inferior turbinate is less common.

Pathologic Features. Under low-power examination, these lesions have a polypoid appearance and are characterized by a benign proliferation of glands lined by ciliated respiratory epithelium (Fig. 3–5). The glands are round or oval and vary in size from small to large with a dilated appearance. The glandular lumina contains mucinous or amorphous material. Often the glandular lining is in direct contiguity with the surface epithelium, which occasionally reveals mucous metaplasia. The stroma is edematous and contains a mixed inflammatory infiltrate resembling the stroma of inflammatory polyps.[95]

Differential Diagnosis. The most important differential diagnosis is a well-differentiated adenocarcinoma. Respiratory adenomatoid hamartoma does not have the complex glandular growth with a back-to-back cribriform pattern and lacks the infiltrative growth and desmoplastic stroma of well-differentiated adenocarcinomas. Clinically, most sinonasal adenocarcinomas exhibit aggressive growth with invasion of bone and soft tissues, which is not seen in respiratory adenomatoid hamartoma. These lesions may also be misdiagnosed as schneiderian papilloma. However, respiratory hamartomas are not lined by squamous or cylindrical epithelium with intraepithelial mucous cysts, as is the case with papillomas.

Treatment and Prognosis. Respiratory adenomatous hamartoma is a benign condition with no risk of recurrence, persistence, or progression. The treatment should be conservative local excision or polypectomy.

Nasal Chondromesenchymal Hamartoma

Clinical Features. Nasal chondromesenchymal hamartoma is the suggested designation for a rare lesion of the nasal cavity preferentially affecting children under 3 months of age.[96] This lesion has morphologic similarities to the so-called chondromesenchymal hamartoma of the chest wall. The most common presentation is that of a nasal mass, often accompanied by respiratory difficulty. The mean size in the series by McDermott et al.[96] was 3.6 cm. Cystic changes, involvement of paranasal sinuses, and erosion of the cribriform plate with extension into the cranial cavity are frequent computed tomographic findings.

Pathologic Features. The tumors are composed of mesenchymal components. Irregular islands of mature cartilage give the tumors a lobular appearance. The cartilaginous nodules are surrounded by bland spindle cells with a myxoid background. Osteoclast-like multinucleated giant cells may be present at least focally. Uncommon findings are hemorrhagic spaces reminiscent of aneurysmal bone cyst, "chicken-wire" calcifications, perivascular hyalinization, and mitotic activity. Some of the cartilaginous nodules may be lined by respiratory epithelium.

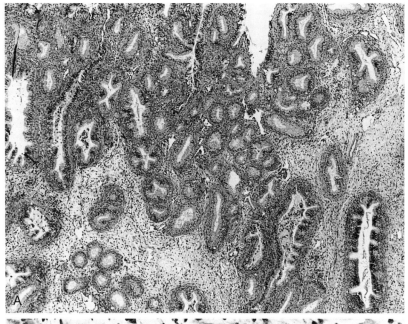

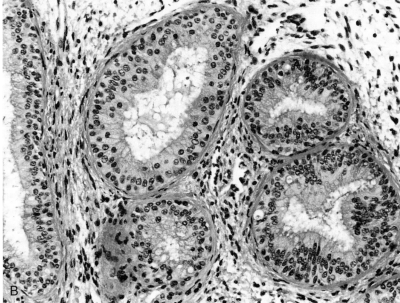

Figure 3–5. *A,* Respiratory epithelial adenomatoid hamartoma. The lesion consists of closely arranged glands lined by ciliated columnar epithelium. This benign lesion should not be confused with a well-differentiated adenocarcinoma. *B,* High-power detail demonstrating glandular pseudostratified ciliated epithelium with no cytologic atypia.

Differential Diagnosis. The main differential diagnosis of nasal chondromesenchymal hamartoma are cartilaginous neoplasms of the sinonasal tract. Awareness of this lesion, the patient's age, and the presence of noncartilaginous elements admixed with the cartilage nodules in their characteristic architecture should exclude a primary cartilaginous neoplasm.

Treatment and Prognosis. The treatment of nasal mesenchymal hamartomas is surgical resection. Complete resection is difficult and often necessitates a combined intranasal-neurosurgical approach. Five of the seven patients reported by McDermott et al.[96] had incomplete resection. Additional surgical resections are indicated in those patients with continued growth of the residual mass. No recurrences or deaths due to this lesion have reported.

Glial Heterotopia and Encephalocele

Clinical Features. Glial heterotopia represents a congenital displacement of neuroglial tissue and is considered a variant of encephalocele rather than a true neoplasm.[97, 98] Generally, it presents at birth or within the first few years of life. The most common loca-
tions are the subcutaneous tissues of the nose (60%), nasal cavity (30%), and, less frequently, the ethmoid sinus, palate, middle ear, tonsils, and pharyngeal area. Dumbell-shaped lesions with involvement of the subcutaneous tissues and subjacent nasal cavity may be seen. Radiologic studies are indicated to exclude communication with the cranial cavity.[97, 99, 100]

Encephalocele is a developmental anomaly closely related to glial heterotopia. When located in the nasal cavity, encephalocele is virtually indistinguishable from glial heterotopia.[97, 99] By definition, encephalocele maintains connection with the central nervous system via a defect in the cribriform plate. Meningitis can be a serious complication. Before any biopsy is attempted in children with a mass in the upper nasal cavity or the base of the external nose, communication with the central nervous system should be excluded.

Pathologic Features. Microscopically, glial heterotopia is composed of a mixture of mature astrocytes, gemistocytic astrocytes, glial fibers, and fibrovascular connective tissue. Neuronal elements are usually absent or scant, although in rare occasions they can be abundant.[101] In longstanding lesions, the degree of fibrosis may obscure the true nature of the lesion. Glial fibrillary acidic protein and S-100 protein immunohistochemical stains can be helpful in confirming the diagnosis.[102]

Microscopically, encephaloceles consist of a mixture of neural and glial tissues.[99, 100, 103]

Differential Diagnosis. The differential diagnosis of glial heterotopia includes typical encephalocele, nasal teratomas, and a true glioma. The absence of tissues other than glial elements should exclude the diagnosis of teratoma. True gliomas complicating glial heterotopia have been described.[104, 105]

The differential diagnosis of encephalocele includes glial heterotopia, nasal teratoma, and also a true glioma. The characteristic clinical and radiologic findings should distinguish this lesion from other developmental anomalies and cystic teratomas.

Treatment and Prognosis. The prognosis for children with encephalocele and nasal glial heterotopia is excellent after resection. In the case of glial heterotopia, simple excision is sufficient. In encephalocele, a craniotomy and repair of the craniofacial defect is required. Recurrences of glial heterotopia are due to incomplete resection.

Dermoid Cyst

Dermoid cyst is a non-neoplastic lesion that probably represents another developmental anomaly related to the midline closure of the face and juxtaposition of the central nervous system.[100] It is most frequently found as a mass in the midline of the bridge of the nose of infants. It may also be found in the nasopharynx, where the term *hairy polyps* has been used. Most cases show erosion of the underlying nasal bones. Microscopically, dermoid cysts are lined with keratinizing squamous epithelium and frequently contain hair follicles and sebaceous glands in the cyst wall. No neural elements are present. Bacterial contamination and cyst rupture may cause a prominent inflammatory reaction in the adjacent soft tissues. These lesions should be distinguished from cystic teratomas; the characteristic clinical and radiologic features of dermoid cyst and the absence of other tissues on microscopic examination are helpful in making this distinction. Treatment is complete resection, including excision of any discharging fistulous tract.[106]

Lymphoid Hyperplasia

Clinically significant lymphoid hyperplasia in the sinonasal region and nasopharynx is relatively uncommon.[107] Rimarenko et al.[108] described an example of this condition that simulated a nasal polyp. The histopathologic appearance of lymphoid hyperplasia in the sinonasal tract is similar to the one seen in lymph nodes (Fig. 3–6A, see p. 83). It is characterized by the presence of secondary germinal center formation composed of a mixture of tingible-body macrophages, small cleaved lymphocytes, large noncleaved cells, and large transformed lymphocytes admixed with plasma cells and numerous mitotic figures (Fig. 3–6B, see p. 83). The presence of a monomorphic cellular infiltrate and cytologic atypia should be viewed with suspicion by the surgical pathologist. Care should be taken to exclude a neoplasm with a prominent lymphoid infiltrate or a lymphoepithelioma-type carcinoma, particularly in the nasopharynx. Rarely, Castleman's disease or angiolymphoid hyperplasia can also present as a nasopharyngeal polypoid tumor.[109] Rare cases of plasma cell granuloma and inflammatory pseudotumors have also been reported in this location.[110–112]

Recently there have been reports of HIV-infected patients presenting with nasal obstruction, epistaxis, hearing loss, and sore throat due to enlarged nasopharyngeal and palatine tonsils.[113, 114] The nasopharyngeal biopsies and tonsillectomy specimens in this group of patients reveal moderate to marked follicular and interfollicular hyperplasia, with attenuated or partially lost mantle zones. Some cases have monocytoid B-cell hyperplasia and interfollicular zone expansion by aggregates of immunoblasts and plasma cells. Additional findings were infiltration of the germinal centers by small lymphocytes, resulting in fragmentation of the hyperplastic germinal

center, a phenomenon known as "follicle lysis," and follicular involution resulting in prominence of blood vessels accompanied by infiltration by sheets of plasma cells and immunoblasts.[113, 114] Wenig et al.[114] described the presence of multinucleated giant cells immunoreactive for CD68 and S-100 protein containing HIV p24 protein clustered adjacent to the surface squamous epithelium. The constellation of these morphologic findings was considered virtually diagnostic of HIV infection by these authors.[114]

Sinus Histiocytosis with Massive Lymphadenopathy (Rosai-Dorfman Disease)

Clinical Features. Sinus histiocytosis with massive lymphadenopathy (SHML) is a rare idiopathic disorder of histiocytes that presents primarily with massive enlargement of cervical lymph nodes[115, 116]; however, extranodal disease with involvement of the nasal cavity, orbit, and other head and neck sites is common.[117–119] The mean age at onset is approximately 20 years, and mild upper respiratory infection often precedes the development of cervical lymphadenopathy. Involvement of the sinonasal tract is often accompanied by nodal disease or extranodal lesions in other head and neck sites. In approximately 20% of cases of sinonasal SHML, the upper aerodigestive passages are the only site of disease. Laboratory manifestations include anemia, red cell autoantibodies, elevated erythrocyte sedimentation rate, and polyclonal hypergammaglobulinemia.[118, 119]

Pathologic Features. Sinonasal SHML presents as nasal polyps or nodules with partial obstruction of the nasal cavity and is histologically characterized by a diffuse polymorphic infiltrate composed of numerous plasma cells, often with abundant Russell's bodies, small lymphocytes, and histiocytes with large vesicular nuclei and abundant clear or eosinophilic cytoplasm. The cytoplasm of these histiocytes often contains numerous intact lymphocytes, many of them within vacuoles. This phenomenon has been referred to as *emperipolesis* or *lymphophagocytosis*. Plasma cells and erythrocytes can also be seen within these histiocytes. Fibrosis can be a prominent finding in extranodal disease and may hamper the recognition of the characteristic histiocytes of SHML. Lymphoid aggregates resembling a lymph node are also commonly seen in the nasal mucosa. S-100 protein, CD68, and Mac-387 antibodies are expressed by these cells.[117, 120, 121]

Differential Diagnosis. The differential diagnosis of SHML includes rhinoscleroma, leprosy, Langerhans cell granulomatosis, and malignant non-Hodgkin's lymphoma. Separation of SHML from these entities is based on recognition of its characteristic morphologic features and immunohistochemical profile.

Treatment and Prognosis. There is no systematic treatment study of SHML.[122] Most patients only require complete surgical resection of their masses. However, patients with systemic manifestations or respiratory obstruction may need chemotherapy or radiotherapy. In a literature review of all sites involved by SHML, Komp[122] states that a combination of vinca alkaloid, alkylating agents, and corticosteroids appear to be the most effective. Radiotherapy did not appear to be particularly effective. The responses with these agents appeared to be worse than with malignant lymphomas. Although in general SHML follows a benign clinical course,[118] in one study five of nine patients with sinonasal SHML experienced recurrences of their lesion and four had persistent disease when last seen.[117] In none of these cases was the diagnosis of SHML contemplated. Therefore it is imperative that the correct diagnosis be made so that complete removal of the mass is pursued.

Wegener's Granulomatosis

Clinical Features. Wegener's granulomatosis is a systemic vasculitis and necrotizing granulomatosis with involvement of the upper and lower respiratory tracts and kidneys.[123, 124] Wegener's granulomatosis was grouped in the past with lymphomatoid granulomatosis, polymorphic reticulosis, idiopathic midline destructive disease (IMDD) and a host of infectious processes under the vague clinical terms of *midfacial necrotizing lesion* and *lethal midline granuloma.*

Clinically, patients with involvement of the upper respiratory tract usually present with sinusitis, rhinorrhea, headache, nasal obstruction, anosmia, sinus pain, and, less often, otitis media and mastoiditis due to involvement of the eustachian tube.[125, 126] In most patients there are also pulmonary or renal manifestations.[125] "Classic" or cytoplasmic antineutrophilic cytoplasmic antibodies (cANCA) directed against neutrophilic proteinase 3 (PR3) are present in the serum of most patients; a minority have antibodies against myeloperoxidase (MPO) or (peri)nuclear ANCA (pANCA), whereas others lack these antibodies altogether.[127, 128] The presence of these antibodies and their titers appear to be related to levels of disease activity.

Pathologic Features. The diagnosis of Wegener's granulomatosis in biopsies of the head and neck is frequently difficult and inconclusive. The pathologic features to look for in these specimens are mucosal ulceration, acute and chronic inflammation, vasculitis, necrosis, and granulomatosis. The inflammation in Wegener's granulomatosis is generally mixed acute and chronic with neutrophils aggregating in small clusters and microabscesses (Fig. 3–7, see p. 83). Lymphocytes and plasma cells are usually abundant, and eosinophils are frequently seen. This inflammatory reaction may mask the underlying vasculitis, making it difficult to recognize it without the use of elastic stains. The necrotizing vasculitis involves arterioles and small arteries and veins. All stages of vasculitis may be present, ranging from acute to granulomatous to healed. The acute stage is characterized by patchy fibrinoid necrosis of the vessel wall accompanied by a prominent neutrophilic infiltrate. The inflammation and necrosis may involve part or the entire circumference of the affected vessel. Extravasated red blood cells, fibrin thrombi, and swollen endothelial cells are often seen. Multinucleated giant cells and histiocytes are present in granulomatous vasculitis. Healed vasculitis is characterized by concentric fibrosis surrounding an endothelial-lined vascular lumen. Frequently, recognition of involved blood vessels is difficult; in these instances, the use of elastic stains is helpful to identify the fragmented elastic remnants.

Coagulative necrosis is invariably present in Wegener's granulomatosis, but its detection in head and neck biopsies depends on tissue sampling and biopsy size. Usually it is patchy in distribution and may have a "geographic" appearance, with a prominent rim of palisaded epithelioid and spindle-shaped macrophages. Giant cells are also often present around the necrotic areas. A pathologic change not frequently recognized is the presence of microscopic foci of extravascular necrosis characterized by collagen with a clumped or granular appearance or fibrinoid degeneration.[126]

Giant cells unassociated with granulomas are typically present, but they tend to aggregate around areas of necrosis or are scattered in an edematous stroma. The granulomas in Wegener's granulomatosis are poorly formed and most often consist of loose aggregates of mononuclear and multinucleated macrophages (Fig. 3–8, see p. 84). The giant cells and granulomas can be found within the vessel wall, adjacent to the vessel, or distant from the affected vessels.

The utility of head and neck biopsies in establishing the diagnosis of Wegener's granulomatosis depends on a constellation of clinical and histopathologic findings. Devaney et al.[125] have proposed the following criteria for the diagnosis of Wegener's granulomatosis in head and neck biopsies: (1) The finding of necrosis, vasculitis, and granulomatous inflammation is diagnostic if the patient has involvement of lung, kidney, or both; (2) if two of the above-mentioned microscopic features are present, the biopsy is considered diagnostic only if both the kidney and the lung are involved; if only one site is involved, the biopsy is considered probable; (3) if only one of the three microscopic features is present, the biopsy is considered suggestive if both lung and kidney are affected and suspicious if only one site is involved; (4) if none of the microscopic features

tures is present, the biopsy is considered nonspecific even if there is clinical involvement of lung and kidney. In general, the diagnosis of Wegener's granulomatosis based on head and neck biopsies requires a careful correlation of clinical, serologic, microbiologic, and pathologic data. The less clinical support for Wegener's granulomatosis, the greater the number of pathologic findings needed to make a diagnosis.[123]

Differential Diagnosis. The differential diagnosis of Wegener's granulomatosis includes infectious processes, Churg-Strauss syndrome, sinonasal lymphoma, and IMDD. The diagnosis of aggressive sinonasal infections resides in close clinicopathologic correlation and the identification of an infectious agent in microbiologic cultures or biopsy material. Sinonasal infections generally do not have concurrent pulmonary and renal involvement and lack antineutrophilic cytoplasmic antibodies. Although the mucosa of the oral cavity, sinonasal tract, and nasopharynx can be inflamed and ulcerated, it is rare to find the extensive cartilage and bone destruction associated with sinonasal lymphoma and IMDD. Sinonasal lymphoma and IMDD should not have pulmonary or renal disease and also lack pANCA. In difficult cases, immunophenotyping and molecular pathology studies should be used to exclude the diagnosis of non-Hodgkin's lymphoma.

Treatment and Prognosis. The prognosis of patients with Wegener's granulomatosis largely depends on the extent of the disease and the treatment employed. Patients with the limited form of the disease may have only nasal and pulmonary involvement without glomerulonephritis or systemic involvement. A combined regimen of cyclophosphamide and prednisone is generally used for at least 1 year. Azathioprine has also been used as an alternative or adjunct to cyclophosphamide.

Idiopathic Midline Destructive Disease

Clinical Features. Idiopathic midline destructive disease (IMDD) is the term proposed by Tsokos et al.[129] for a locally destructive process involving the upper respiratory tract. The existence of this process as a distinctive clinicopathologic entity is controversial. The majority of the patients present with pansinusitis and destructive lesions involving the nasal septum, bone, and, less frequently, skin. The destructive process may extend into the orbit, nasopharynx, larynx, and trachea. None of the patients described by Tsokos et al. had systemic disease and there was no evidence of an infectious process by culture or special stains.[129] IMDD is extremely rare and is a diagnosis of exclusion. It requires ruling out an infectious process, Wegener's granulomatosis, carcinoma, and malignant lymphoma.[130]

Pathologic Features. Histologically, IMDD is characterized by the presence of mixed acute and chronic inflammation with a variable amount of karyorrhexis. Occasional giant cells and granulomas can be observed. Coagulative necrosis, atypical or frankly malignant cells, and fibrinoid necrosis are lacking and microorganisms are absent in cultures and special stains.

Differential Diagnosis. The diagnosis of IMDD resides in the exclusion of aggressive infections, vasculitis, or neoplastic processes, particularly non-Hodgkin's lymphomas (NHLs) in the sinonasal tract. Therefore, IMDD should be contemplated as a diagnostic possibility only after careful clinicopathologic correlation with serologic studies, microbiology cultures, and biopsies with adequate ancillary studies, including gene rearrangement, have failed to establish a diagnosis. Midline nasal destruction in cocaine abusers should also be separated from IMDD because of its better prognosis with more conservative treatment measures.[131] Because the histopathologic features of nasal destruction in cocaine abuse are not specific, the diagnosis rests heavily in a good clinical history and the identification of cocaine abuse.

Treatment and Prognosis. Tsokos et al.[129] reported a good response to local radiotherapy in their original series of patients.

Eight of their 11 patients had no evidence of disease after local radiotherapy. Two patients developed fatal radiation encephalomyelitis but had no disease at autopsy.

NEOPLASMS

Epithelial Tumors

Schneiderian Papillomas

Clinical Features. Sinonasal or schneiderian papillomas are benign neoplasms of the respiratory mucosa or schneiderian mucosa lining the nasal cavity and paranasal sinuses. Although there are no reliable data to estimate the incidence of schneiderian papillomas in the general population, they are relatively common. They accounted for 25% of nasal tumors seen in the Institute of Laryngology and Otology in London,[132] and Vrabec[133] and Suh et al.[134] reported large series of 101 and 57 cases of inverted papilloma, respectively, in 25- and 30-year study periods. These lesions have been designated by many names, reflecting dissimilar microscopic appearances; however, they are now classified in three histologic groups: fungiform (exophytic or everted) papillomas, inverted (squamous) papillomas, and cylindrical cell (oncocytic) papillomas.[135–137] Schneiderian papillomas have been regarded as variants of a single entity; however, Michaels recently contradicted this concept and regards these lesions as three separate entities.[136, 138] In a review of 191 cases, he did not find intermediate forms. He regards everted and cylindrical cell types as true papillomas, whereas inverted papilloma is seen as a mucosal polyp with extensive squamous metaplasia. No known etiologic or risk factors were associated with the development of schneiderian papillomas in the past; however, in recent years human papillomavirus DNA has been detected in the exophytic and inverted types using in situ hybridization and polymerase chain reaction.[139–141] Human papillomavirus 6/11 has been the most common type detected.[142] No association has been found between human papillomavirus and cylindrical cell papillomas.[142, 143]

Sinonasal papillomas occur in a wide age range, but most cases are seen in patients between 30 and 60 years of age.[135, 144, 145] They are uncommon in children. Males are affected at least twice as often as females.[133, 134, 146] Symptoms at presentation include unilateral nasal obstruction and stuffiness, and less commonly epistaxis, facial pain, and purulent discharge. Proptosis is generally seen in association with extensive bone erosion. Involvement of the middle ear and

mastoid has been rarely described.[147] In general, papillomas are unilateral[132, 144, 148]; however, they are often multifocal and, more rarely, bilateral.

Pathologic Features. All three types of schneiderian papillomas exhibit certain overlapping architectural and cytologic features, and several authors have described lesions with exophytic and endophytic components.[144, 148, 149] Exophytic papillomas constituted approximately 50% of the sinonasal tract papillomas reported by Hyams.[135] They are almost exclusively found in the nasal septum.[135, 150] Histologically, these lesions exhibit an exophytic pattern and are composed of papillary fronds with a thin central core of fibrovascular tissue (Fig. 3–9). The surface of the papilloma is lined with a thick nonkeratinizing squamous epithelium also referred to as *transitional epithelium*.[148] The lining may contain intraepithelial mucous cysts and, less frequently, ciliated respiratory epithelium with small numbers of goblet cells.[135] Unlike inverted papillomas, fungiform papillomas do not contain large glycogenated squamous cells. Surface keratinization with formation of a granular cell layer, a chronic inflammatory infiltrate, atypia, and mitotic activity are uncommon.[135]

In many authors' experience, inverted papilloma is the most common type of schneiderian papilloma.[134, 136, 144, 146, 148–150] Most tumors are confined to the lateral nasal wall and sinuses.[134, 135, 149] The maxillary sinus is most commonly affected, but involvement of ethmoid or sphenoid sinuses may also be seen. Under low-power examination, inverted papillomas have an endophytic growth pattern with invaginations of the surface epithelium into the underlying stroma (Fig. 3–10, see p. 84). This pattern gives the tumors a lobulated appearance. The neoplastic epithelium has a variable appearance and mostly consists of a markedly thickened layer of nonkeratinizing squamous epithelium overlying a thick basement membrane. The surface of the epithelial lining may be covered by a layer of ciliated respiratory epithelium, which often merges with a transitional-type epithelium (Fig. 3–11, see p. 84). The presence of numerous mucous cells with intraepithelial mucous cysts is also a common feature.[134, 145, 148, 150, 151] The squamous component may contain areas with large clear cells with abundant cytoplasmic glycogen and rarely may demonstrate a moderate degree of atypia.[135] Mitotic figures may be seen; however, they are usually few and are limited to the basal and parabasal layers.[135, 145, 149, 150] The stroma varies from fibrous to myxomatous. Chronic inflammation is more frequently seen in inverted papillomas than in exophytic papillomas and occasionally may closely resemble inflammatory polyps. Surface keratinization is uncommon; how-

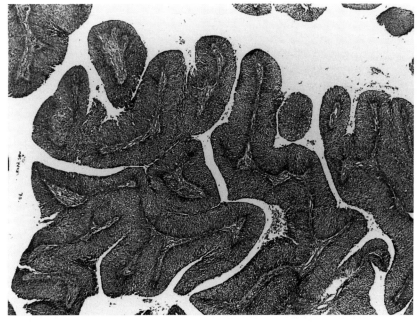

Figure 3–9. Exophytic or fungiform squamous papilloma. The lesion is characterized by thick squamous epithelium lining fibrovascular cores of variable size.

ever, when present, the possibility of a squamous cell carcinoma should be excluded.[134, 135, 144, 150]

The least common type of schneiderian papilloma is the cylindrical cell or so-called "oncocytic" schneiderian papilloma.[135, 136, 152, 153] The anatomic location and gross pathologic features of cylindrical cell papillomas are similar to those of inverted papillomas. Microscopically, they are lined with a multilayered epithelial proliferation of tall columnar cells with eosinophilic, granular cytoplasm (Fig. 3–12A, see p. 85). Scattered mucous cells with intraepithelial mucous cysts are also commonly seen (Fig. 3–12B). Architecturally, they also resemble inverted papillomas due to their endophytic growth pattern. The surface of these papillomas can also be lined by respiratory-type epithelium, and frequently they also have a nonkeratinizing "transitional" cell component.

Differential Diagnosis. Several lesions may be confused or need to be separated from schneiderian papillomas. Occasionally, inverted or cylindrical cell papillomas may be misdiagnosed as inflammatory polyps. Although inflammatory polyps may show squamous metaplasia, they do not have the thick nonkeratinizing squamous epithelium seen in inverted papillomas. Furthermore, they do not have an inverted growth pattern. Likewise, inflammatory polyps do not have the intraepithelial pseudocysts and oncocytic epithelium of cylindrical cell papillomas. Rhinosporidiosis may imitate the intraepithelial pseudocysts of cylindrical cell papillomas; however, papillomas do not have the degree of inflammation associated with rhinosporidiosis, the cysts are smaller and are intraepithelial rather than submucosal, and, more importantly, they do not contain microorganisms.

The differential diagnosis of cylindrical cell papilloma should also include low-grade sinonasal papillary adenocarcinoma. Low-grade adenocarcinomas are composed of infiltrative small acini and cribriform structures not seen in cylindrical cell papilloma. The surface epithelium in adenocarcinomas is generally normal, whereas in papillomas it is thickened by the neoplastic cells. Schneiderian papillomas should also be separated from nonkeratinizing squamous cell carcinoma. The degree of cytologic atypia seen in carcinomas is usually not seen in papillomas uncomplicated by a concurrent carcinoma. Attention to other features such as inverted pattern, invasive nests, and desmoplastic stroma is necessary to establish a definitive diagnosis.

Treatment and Prognosis. Most clinicians agree that the treatment of choice of schneiderian papillomas is surgical resection; however, there is no general agreement on the extent or type of surgery required. Most authors agree that recurrence of papillomas is a reflection of incomplete removal and recommend complete resection through a lateral rhinotomy incision with medial maxillectomy as adequate treatment.[133, 146, 154, 155] In selected patients with limited disease[156] or in those who refuse radical treatment, a more conservative approach using endoscopic removal may be recommended as an alternative. The recurrence rate with this approach has been as high as 17%.[133, 146] Patients with invasion of the skull base may require craniofacial resection.[146] Radiotherapy is primarily used as adjuvant therapy in tumors with associated carcinoma.[148]

The historic recurrence rate of all histologic types has ranged from 4% to 74%,[134, 135, 145, 148, 149, 154, 157] with many patients having a history of multiple recurrences. Today there is almost universal agreement that this high recurrence rate is probably due to incomplete resection, since papillomas have the tendency to widely spread along the respiratory mucosa through cylindrical cell or squamous metaplasia. A conservative resection such as polypectomy does not eliminate microscopic disease and has been associated with high recurrence rates.[134, 145, 149] The recurrence rate for inverted and cylindrical cell papillomas has been reduced to approximately 5% with lateral rhinotomy and medial maxillectomy.[133, 146, 154]

The prognosis of schneiderian papillomas of all histologic type without in situ or invasive carcinoma is excellent. As previously discussed, the local recurrence rate depends heavily on the initial surgical approach. No deaths directly caused by schneiderian papillomas have been described in several large studies.[133–135, 146, 149] In situ or invasive squamous cell carcinoma occurs in approximately 5% to 14% of patients with sinonasal papillomas (Fig. 3–13).[133–135, 148, 154, 155] This complication is almost exclusively seen in the inverted or cylindrical cell types. The carcinoma may be seen as part of a papilloma or it may present as a recurrence after resection of a benign lesion. Most of the carcinomas are of the squamous type; however, sarcomatoid carcinomas, clear cell carcinomas, high-grade mucoepidermoid carcinomas, and sinonasal undifferentiated carcinomas can also be seen.[144–146, 158, 159] Manivel et al.[160] described two cases with endodermal sinus tumor-like features. There are no histologic features that predict recurrences or malignant transformation.

Salivary Gland–Type Tumors

Clinical Features. Tumors of salivary gland–type reportedly constitute 4% to 8% of neoplasms of the sinonasal tract.[161–165] These tumors arise from the seromucous glands of the nasal cavity and paranasal sinuses and the overlying surface epithelium.[162, 166]

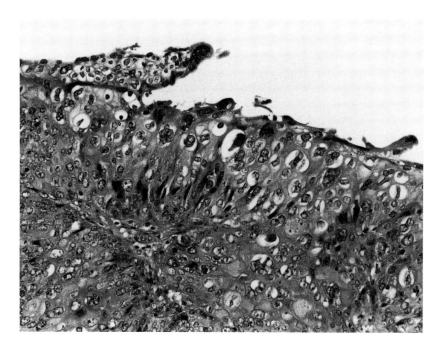

Figure 3–13. Carcinoma in situ arising in a squamous papilloma. There is significant cytologic atypia with nuclear pleomorphism and human papillomavirus effects in the dysplastic epithelium.

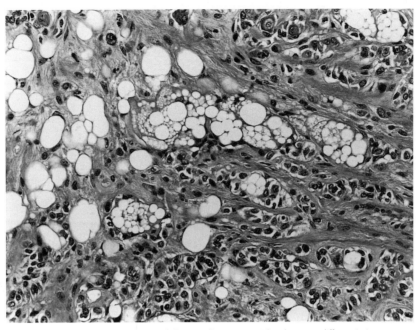

Figure 3–14. Mixed tumor of the maxillary sinus with sebaceous differentiation.

The clinical features of sinonasal salivary gland–type tumors are nonspecific, and most patients with malignant tumors present with clinical stages T3 and T4.[161, 163, 167, 168]

Pathologic Features. The pathologic features of these lesions are essentially similar to those of major and minor salivary glands with the notable exceptions of Warthin's tumor and pure sebaceous lesions that have not been reported in this location[164]; most other major histologic types of salivary gland–type neoplasms have been described in this region including benign (Fig. 3–14) and malignant mixed tumors (Fig. 3–15),[164, 169, 170] oncocytomas,[171, 172] myoepithelioma,[173–175] myoepithelial carcinoma,[176] adenoid cystic carcinoma (Fig. 3–16),[162, 163, 167, 177] mucoepidermoid carcinoma (Fig. 3–17),[165] acinic cell carcinoma,[178–180] basal cell adenocarcinoma,[181] polymorphous low-grade adenocarcinoma,[182–184] epithelial-myoepithelial carcinoma,[185] salivary duct carcinoma (Fig. 3–18, see p. 85), and clear cell carcinoma.[165] The most common histologic types are adenoid cystic carcinoma and mixed tumor.[161, 162, 165] An unusual case of a nasal pleomorphic adenoma with skeletal muscle differentiation has been described by Lam et al.[186]

Dehner et al.[187] described a peculiar lesion that they designated *salivary gland anlage tumor* or *congenital pleomorphic adenoma*. This lesion is characteristically located in the midline of the nasopharynx of newborns. The tumor is polypoid in appearance and, although benign, it may cause respiratory difficulties due to its location. Microscopically, the tumor is well circumscribed and is covered by an intact squamous mucosa, which appears to be in direct continuity with branching duct-like structures and cystic or solid epithelial nests within the substance of the lesion. These epithelial structures compartmentalize multiple solid nodules of ovoid and spindle cells with bland cytologic features. Immunohistochemical and ultrastructural studies have demonstrated a variable degree of myoepithelial differentiation within these nodules.[187]

Differential Diagnosis. The diagnosis of salivary gland tumors in the sinonasal tract rests in awareness of their occurrence in this location and recognition of their typical morphologic features. The main differential diagnoses of malignant salivary gland tumors are well-differentiated sinonasal adenocarcinoma and intestinal type adenocarcinoma.

Treatment and Prognosis. The treatment of salivary gland–type neoplasms in the sinonasal tract is complete surgical resection. The surgical approach employed and the extent of the surgery and, ultimately, prognosis depend on the location and structures involved by the tumor and its histologic type.[161] The reported 5-year survival

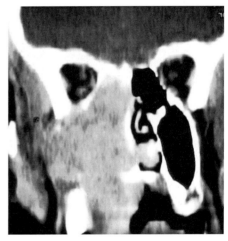

Figure 3–15. Recurrent malignant mixed tumor of the maxillary sinus. The tumor is destroying the lateral and medial walls and the floor of the maxilla.

rate for malignant salivary gland tumors in the sinonasal tract has varied from 40% to 63%,[161–163, 167] with adenoid cystic carcinoma being the most difficult to control owing to its advanced clinical stage at diagnosis and frequent involvement of surgical resection margins. Postoperative radiotherapy significantly increases the chances of local control.[161, 163, 167]

Low-Grade Adenocarcinoma

Clinical Features. Low-grade sinonasal adenocarcinomas are rare neoplasms with no sex predilection.[180, 188] Most cases arise in middle-aged adults with a median age of 54 years. The mean age for the cases reported as nasopharyngeal papillary adenocarcinoma was 37 years[188]. They also occur in children and the elderly (age range, 9–75 years). The nasal cavity is the most frequently involved site, followed by the ethmoid and maxillary sinuses. There is no known association with carcinogens. At presentation, most patients complain of nasal obstruction and epistaxis. Pain is uncommon. The most common site of involvement is the nasal cavity, followed by the ethmoid sinus.

Pathologic Features. Low-grade sinonasal adenocarcinomas

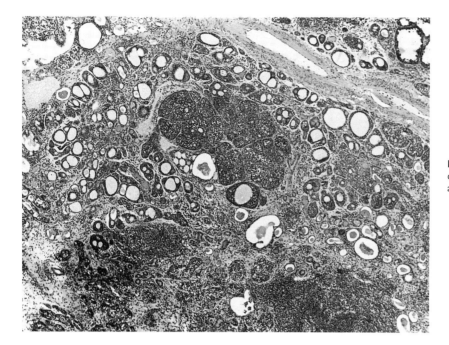

Figure 3–16. Adenoid cystic carcinoma of the nasal cavity. The tumor exhibits a mixture of dilated tubules and cribriform areas with a focal solid growth pattern.

are morphologically a heterogeneous group of tumors. In some, the architectural and cytologic uniformity frequently leads to a misdiagnosis of adenoma or papilloma. The majority of cases consist of small glands lined with a single layer of uniform cuboidal or columnar cells. The neoplastic glands have a back-to-back arrangement without intervening stroma. Some glands are cystically dilated or slit-like with epithelial tufts (Fig. 3–19, see p. 86), and others contain well-formed papillae (Fig. 3–20). Nuclear size varies from case to case but tends to be uniform within a given lesion. Mitotic figures are generally rare. Most tumors contain both intracellular and extracellular mucin. Origin from surface mucosa may be seen. Some neoplasms included in this group consist of cells with basophilic cytoplasm arranged in small, acinar-like nests.[180] These lesions closely resemble acinic cell carcinomas of salivary-gland type (Fig. 3–21, see p. 86) and probably should be regarded as such and be separated from the other nonsalivary tumors in this group.

Nasopharyngeal papillary adenocarcinoma shows papillary and glandular growth patterns. The papillae exhibit arborization and hyalinized fibrovascular cores. The glands have a crowded appearance with a cribriform pattern. The epithelial cells lining these structures are columnar or pseudostratified. They possess eosinophilic cytoplasm and round to oval nuclei with optically clear chromatin. Moderate nuclear pleomorphism is present but mitotic figures are uncommon. Psammoma bodies and focal necrosis are occasionally seen.

Differential Diagnosis. Low-grade sinonasal adenocarcinoma must be distinguished from intestinal-type adenocarcinoma described later because of the more aggressive clinical course of the latter. Distinction is usually straightforward, given the nuclear stratification and intestinal appearance of the latter neoplasms. In addition, intestinal-type tumors are cytologically more pleomorphic than low-grade adenocarcinomas, with the exception of rare nasal neoplasms resembling normal intestinal mucosa. Oncocytic schneiderian papillomas may be also confused with low-grade adenocarcinoma. Heffner et al.[180] listed the following differentiation features: (1) stratified epithelium in papillomas as opposed to single-layered cells in adenocarcinoma; (2) true glandular lumina in adenocarcinoma; and (3) more abundant, myxomatous stroma in papillomas.

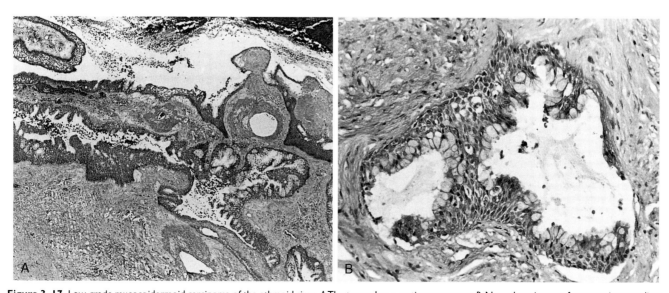

Figure 3–17. Low-grade mucoepidermoid carcinoma of the ethmoid sinus. A, The tumor has a cystic appearance. B, Note the mixture of mucous, intermediate, and squamous cells.

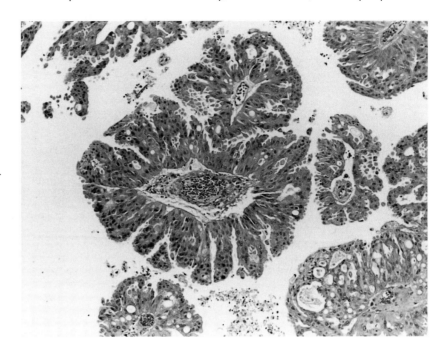

Figure 3–20. Well-differentiated papillary sinonasal adenocarcinoma.

The complex papillary pattern, vesicular nuclei, and focal psammoma bodies seen in some low-grade nasopharyngeal adenocarcinomas may mimic a metastatic papillary carcinoma of the thyroid gland[189]; however, nasopharyngeal carcinomas lack positivity with thyroglobulin antibodies.

Treatment and Prognosis. Patients with low-grade carcinoma have a good prognosis. Most patients have localized disease at presentation and do not require radical surgical procedures for complete resection of their tumors. The value of radiotherapy is unknown. Recurrences developed in up to 30% of the cases reported by Heffner et al.[180] but did not indicate intractable disease. After a median follow-up of 6 years, 78% of patients were disease-free.[180] Death from disease was seen in two cases and was due to local invasion rather than to metastases. None of the nine patients with low-grade nasopharyngeal adenocarcinoma reported by Wenig et al.[188] developed metastases, although one tumor recurred locally following radiation therapy.

Intestinal-Type Sinonasal Adenocarcinoma

Clinical Features. The second most common glandular neoplasm of the sinonasal region after adenoid cystic carcinoma is composed of cells mimicking normal, adenomatous, or carcinomatous intestinal mucosa.[159, 190–195] This lesion has been referred to as intestinal-type sinonasal adenocarcinoma (ITAC). The clinical features of these tumors are similar to those of other neoplasms in this region. Approximately 85% of patients affected are male; the age at presentation has ranged from 23 to 84 years, with a mean of 50 to 64 years. The ethmoid sinus is the most commonly involved site, followed by the nasal cavity and the maxillary antrum. Symptoms at presentation include nasal obstruction, epistaxis, facial pain, and the presence of a growing mass.

Intestinal-type sinonasal adenocarcinoma has a strong association with long-term exposure to fine hardwood dusts in the woodworking industry.[196] In such populations, the incidence approaches 1000 times that of the general public.[197–199] About 20% of ITAC cases occur in patients with industrial wood-dust exposure. Smoking and exposure to leather dust and nickel have also been incriminated.[191, 200] Although the morphologic features are similar, there seems to be clinical and prognostic differences between those cases arising in woodworkers and nonoccupational cases. Barnes[191] reported 17 cases of sporadic ITAC and compared them with published cases of ITAC arising in woodworkers and found that tumors related to industrial dust exposure occur predominantly in men (85–95%) and show a striking predilection for the ethmoid sinus. Tumors arising sporadically frequently occur in women and often arise in the maxillary antrum (20–50%).

Pathologic Features. These neoplasms recapitulate the entire range of appearances assumed by normal and neoplastic large and small intestinal mucosa. At the well-differentiated end of the spectrum are tumors that resemble normal intestinal mucosa (Fig. 3–22, see p. 87) replete with goblet, resorptive, Paneth's, and argentaffin cells, along with well-formed villi and a muscularis mucosae.[192] Although it is tempting to label such proliferations benign heterotopias, they are aggressive, invasive lesions. The papillary tumors consist of elongated fronds lined with stratified columnar goblet cells reminiscent of intestinal villous or tubular adenoma (Fig. 3–23). Papillary tumors may be invasive or intramucosal.

The most common form of sinonasal intestinal-type adenocarcinoma resembles conventional colonic adenocarcinoma (Fig. 3–24, see p. 87). In this variant, the neoplastic glands are lined with pleomorphic columnar cells arranged in a back-to-back pattern, vary in size, and widely invade the underlying stroma. Intracellular mucin is present focally, but goblet cells are not prominent. In less differentiated tumors, solid sheets of tumor cells may be present with only focal glandular lumina formation. Completing the analogy to intestinal neoplasms are the less frequent mucinous tumors. The predominant pattern in this variant consists of large glands distended with mucin or pools of extracellular mucin (Fig. 3–25, see p. 88) containing small clusters of neoplastic cells. Signet-ring cells form a minor component or, rarely, are predominant. The resemblance of intestinal-type adenocarcinoma to normal and neoplastic intestinal epithelium is not limited to the light microscopic appearance. Ultrastructural studies have confirmed the presence of resorptive, goblet, Paneth's, and argentaffin cells identical to their intestinal counterparts, and intestinal-type hormones have been documented immunocytochemically.[201] We have also seen rare examples of sinonasal adenocarcinomas with a clear cytoplasm and subnuclear vacuoles imitating an endometrioid carcinoma with a secretory pattern (Fig. 3–26, see p. 88).

Differential Diagnosis. The rare intestinal-type adenocarcinoma resembling normal intestinal mucosa and papillary carcinomas resembling villous adenoma can easily be recognized as primary nasal lesions because intestinal epithelium with this histology is not capable of metastasis. There are no morphologic features or immunocytochemical markers to distinguish nasal tumors resembling con-

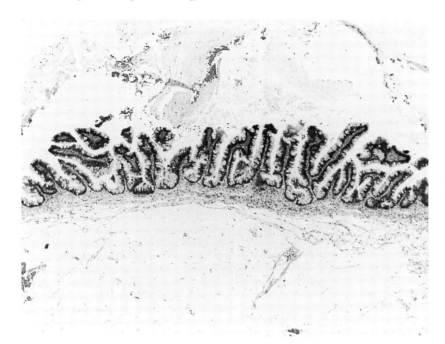

Figure 3–23. Well-differentiated intestinal-type adenocarcinoma of the sinonasal tract with the appearance of a colonic adenoma.

ventional or mucinous adenocarcinoma from a metastasis. In contrast to colonic carcinomas, molecular pathology studies have shown an absence of *K-ras* and *p*53 mutations in sinonasal carcinomas of the intestinal type.[202] In a review of 82 tumors metastatic to the nose and paranasal sinuses,[203, 204] 5 were primary in the gastrointestinal tract. In some patients, the sinonasal lesion was the initial clinical manifestation of disease. Barium radiographic studies should be performed in patients with sinonasal tumors resembling colorectal carcinomas.

Treatment and Prognosis. The treatment of ITAC is surgical resection with or without radiation, depending on the extent of disease.[197, 205] Lateral rhinotomy with partial maxillectomy or exenteration of the ethmoid sinus or nasal cavity are the approaches of choice, depending on the tumor location and extent. Patients with more advanced disease often require radical maxillectomy. External beam radiation alone has been employed as single-modality treatment, but a high incidence of local failure has been reported with this approach.[194, 195, 200] The role of adjuvant chemotherapy is unclear.

Intestinal-type sinonasal adenocarcinomas are aggressive neoplasms. In a review of 213 cases from the literature, Barnes[191] found that 53% of patients had developed local recurrences, 8% (range 0–22%) cervical lymph node metastases, 13% (range 0–29%) distant metastases, and 60% had died of their disease. Death usually results from uncontrollable local disease with intracranial extension or exsanguination. He also reported that tumors related to industrial wood dust exposure have a slightly better prognosis than tumors arising sporadically. He found a 50% survival rate at 5 years in the first group, whereas the latter had a 20% to 40% survival at 5 years.

Although all forms of intestinal-type neoplasia in the sinonasal region are at least locally aggressive, recent studies have suggested that grading these lesions provides additional prognostic information. Kleinsasser and Schroeder divided intestinal-type sinonasal adenocarcinomas into papillary-tubular cylindrical cell type, grades I to III; goblet cell type; signet-ring cell type; and mixed or transitional type.[190] Their study, and the subsequent study by Franquemont et al.[193] showed a better prognosis for the well-differentiated papillary-tubular neoplasms.

Small Cell Neuroendocrine Carcinoma

Clinical Features. Carcinomas with morphologic features indistinguishable from anaplastic small cell carcinoma of the lung occasionally arise in the nasal cavity and paranasal sinuses.[206–209] An origin from the minor salivary gland has been proposed for these neoplasms.[207] The age at presentation has ranged from 26 to 77 years with a mean age of approximately 51 years. The most common symptom at presentation is epistaxis followed by exophthalmos and nasal obstruction. Some of these tumors may have elevated hormonal levels; Kameya et al.[210] described increased levels of adrenocorticotropic hormone and calcitonin in two of their patients. Almost invariably the tumors are in advanced clinical stage with involvement of multiple sinuses (Fig. 3–27).

Pathologic Features. These are anaplastic small cell carcinomas with the typical features of pulmonary oat-cell carcinomas. Small cell neuroendocrine carcinomas (SNEC) are composed of sheets (Fig. 3–28, see p. 101) and nests of small to intermediate sized cells with high nucleoplasmic:cytoplasmic ratio, hyperchromatic nuclei with absent or occasional basophilic nucleoli, and high mitotic rate with frequent mitotic figures (Fig. 3–29, see p. 101). Nuclear molding and the DNA incrustation in vascular walls (Azzopardi phenomenon) can be seen. A peculiar "glomeruloid" vascular proliferation has also been described as a feature associated with neuroendocrine tumors in the sinonasal tract and other locations.[211]

Text continued on page 114

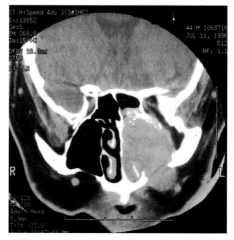

Figure 3–27. Sinonasal small cell carcinoma. This lesion is destroying the anterior wall of the maxilla and is involving the nasal cavity and the maxillary and ethmoid sinuses.

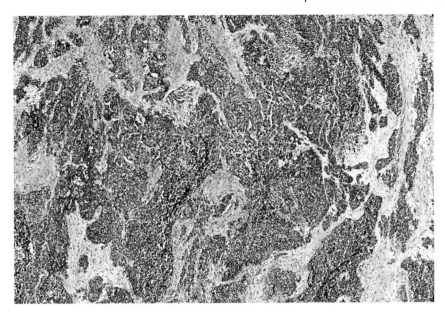

Figure 3–28. Sinonasal small cell carcinoma. The tumor cells are arranged in irregular sheets of variable size and lack the nested pattern seen in most olfactory neuroblastomas. Densely basophilic DNA material is also present.

Figure 3–29. Sinonasal small cell carcinoma. The tumor cells exhibit similar cytologic features to those of their pulmonary counterparts. The cells have a high nuclear:cytoplasmic ratio with oval nuclei containing stippled chromatin. Nucleoli are inconspicuous and the mitotic rate is high.

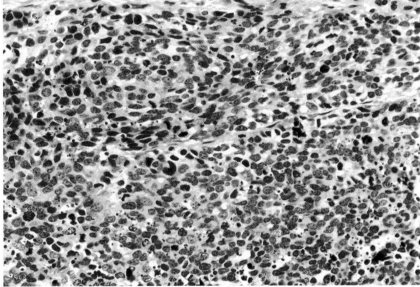

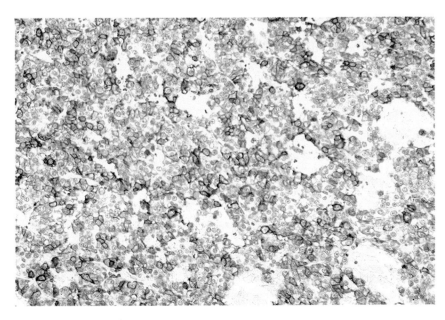

Figure 3–30. Keratin immunostaining in sinonasal small cell carcinoma. The tumor is diffusely positive for AE1 : AE3. This pattern differs from the focal or patchy expression seen in olfactory neuroblastoma.

Figure 3–31. Sinonasal undifferentiated carcinoma (SNUC). The cells are large and possess eosinophilic cytoplasm with a vesicular nucleus. Nucleoli are prominent.

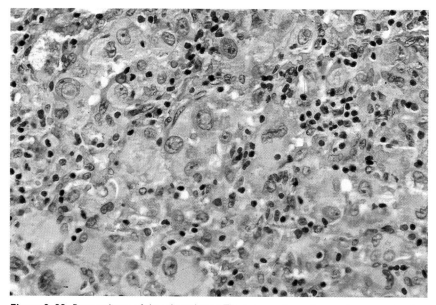

Figure 3–33. Paraganglioma of the ethmoid sinus. The tumor cells are large and possess abundant eosinophilic cytoplasm. Note the presence of intranuclear pseudoinclusions. The original diagnosis in this case was malignant melanoma due to the presence of S100-positive sustentacular cells.

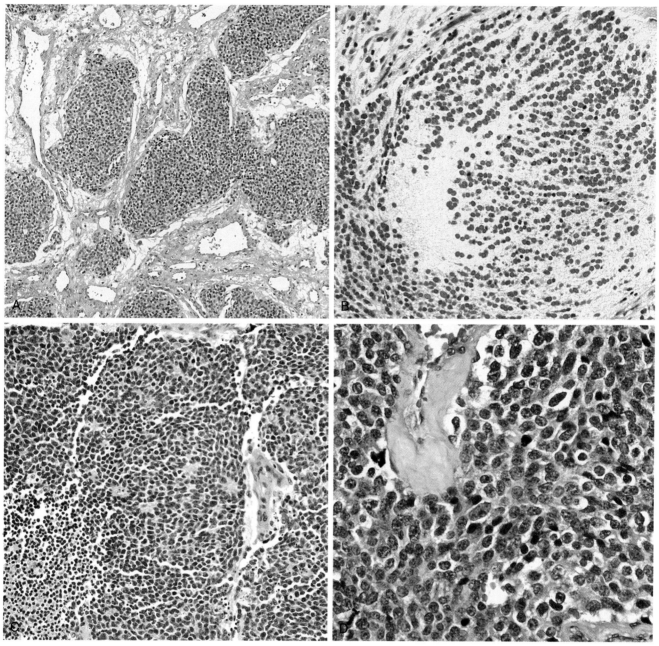

Figure 3–37. *A,* Typical low-power appearance of olfactory neuroblastoma. The tumor is composed of well-defined nests of round cells separated by fibrovascular septa. *B,* Olfactory neuroblastoma showing abundant neurofibrillary stroma with small cells containing round hyperchromatic nuclei. This morphologic appearance is closely reminiscent of a pediatric neuroblastoma. *C,* Olfactory neuroblastoma with extensive rosette formation. *D,* Moderate nuclear pleomorphism is found in this olfactory neuroblastoma.

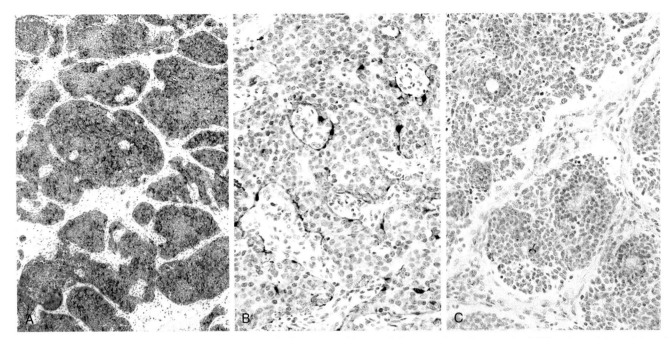

Figure 3–39. *A*, Diffuse expression of synaptophysin in a typical olfactory neuroblastoma. *B*, Sustentacular cells expressing S-100 at the periphery of the cell nests. *C*, Olfactory neuroblastoma with glandular differentiation immunoreactive for keratin.

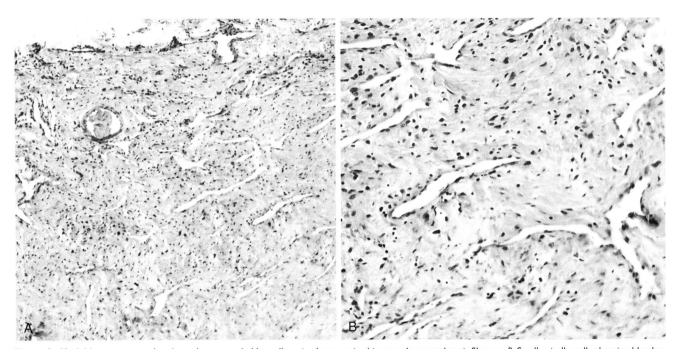

Figure 3–40. *A*, Numerous vascular channels surrounded by collagenized stroma in this nasopharyngeal angiofibroma. *B*, Small spindle cells showing bland cytologic features in stroma of angiofibroma.

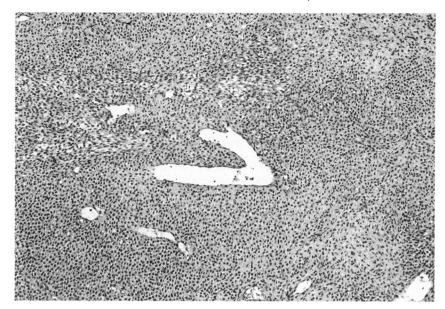

Figure 3–41. Sinonasal hemangiopericytoma. A "staghorn" shaped blood vessel is present in the center of the field. Note the uniform cellularity of the tumor.

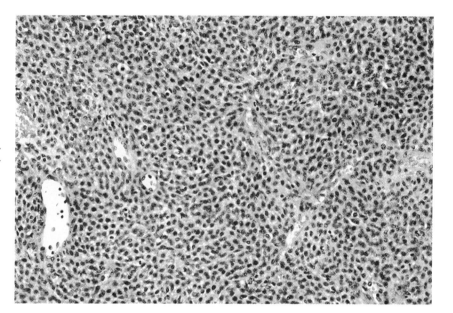

Figure 3–42. Sinonasal hemangiopericytoma. The tumor is quite cellular and uniform but no significant cytologic atypia is present.

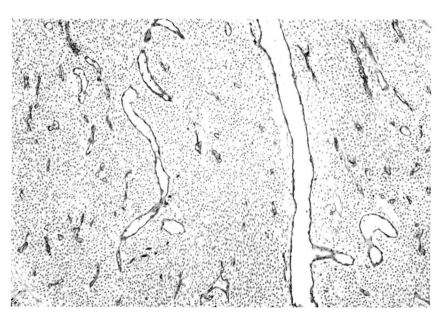

Figure 3–43. CD34 immunostaining in hemangiopericytoma. Only the endothelial cells are positive, whereas the other tumor cells are negative.

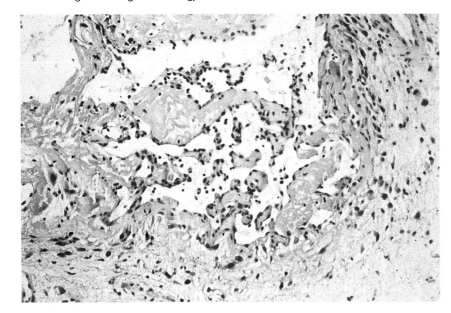

Figure 3–44. Papillary endothelial hyperplasia. Note the ectatic blood vessels with thin papillae containing hyalinized cores.

Figure 3–45. Well-differentiated angiosarcoma involving the nasal septum. The tumor is dissecting the normal collagen and is associated with a moderate lymphocytic infiltrate.

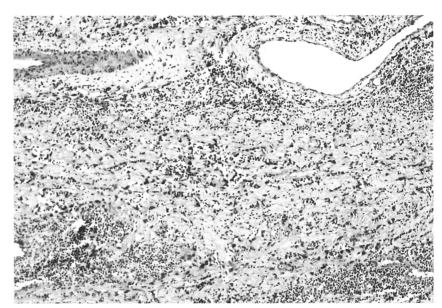

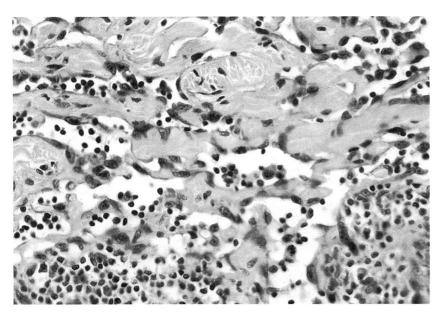

Figure 3–46. This angiosarcoma shows only mild to moderate cytologic atypia. The endothelium has a hobnail appearance.

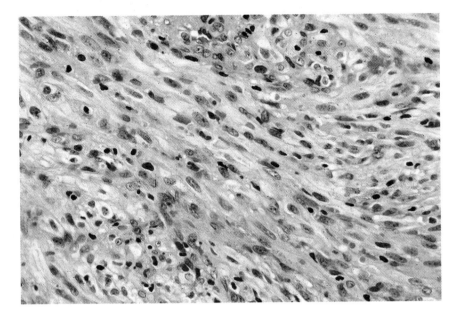

Figure 3–47. Kaposi's sarcoma of the nasal septum. The tumor is composed of spindle cells and contains numerous extravasated erythrocytes.

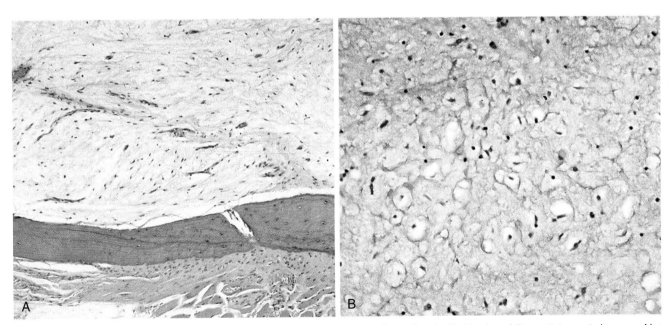

Figure 3–48. *A,* Craniofacial myxoma compressing and pushing cortical bone. *B,* Small stellate cells embedded in a basophilic matrix in a typical myxoma. Note the absence of blood vessels.

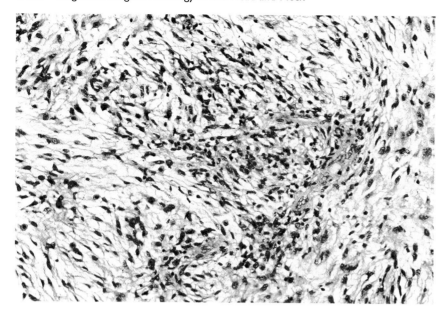

Figure 3–49. Hypercellular areas of a low-grade sarcoma composed of plump spindle cells surrounded by a myxoid matrix. This case could be classified as myxofibrosarcoma. The patient died 5 years after initial resection with uncontrollable local disease.

Figure 3–50. Post-radiation high-grade leiomyosarcoma. The tumor cells reveal an epithelioid appearance.

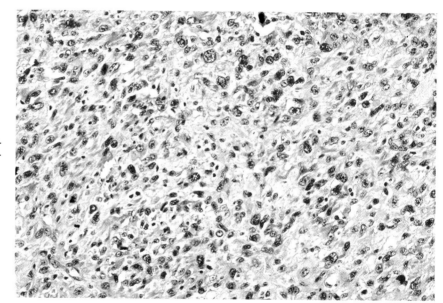

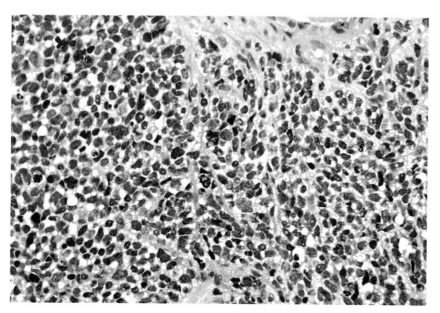

Figure 3–51. Solid variant of alveolar rhabdomyosarcoma involving the lateral nasal wall. The tumor cells are small and raise the traditional differential diagnosis of "small round blue cell tumors."

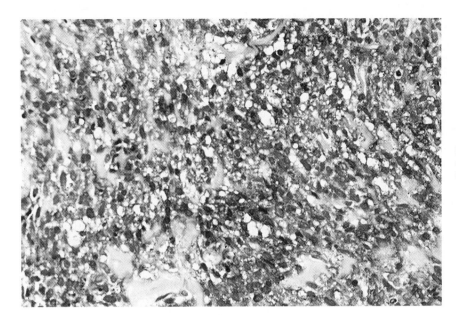

Figure 3–52. Periodic acid-Schiff stain demonstrating cytoplasmic glycogen in this sinonasal rhabdomyosarcoma.

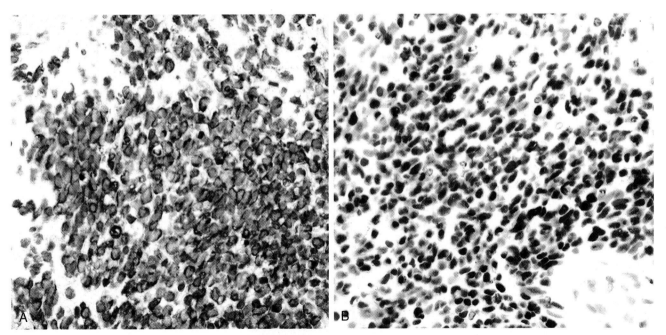

Figure 3–53. Desmin *(A)* and MyoD1 *(B)* are strongly positive in this alveolar rhabdomyosarcoma.

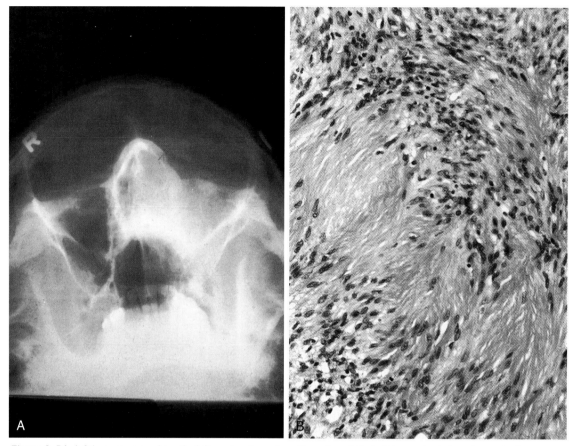

Figure 3–54. *A,* Schwannoma involving the left nasal cavity and maxillary sinus. *B,* Typical Verocay body in a sinonasal schwannoma.

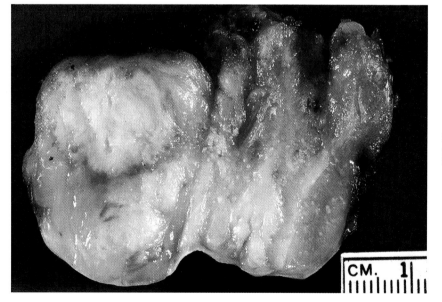

Figure 3–55. Large meningioma of the maxillary sinus. The tumor has a solid appearance and invades bone and antrum.

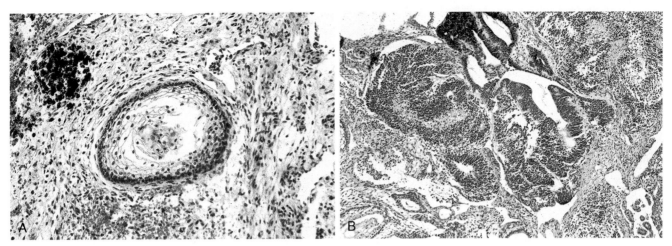

Figure 3–57. Teratocarcinosarcoma containing a well-defined nest of benign-looking squamous epithelium with clear cytoplasm *(A)* and primitive neuroepithelium with numerous rosettes and pigmentation *(B)*. (Courtesy of Dr. Bruce Wenig.)

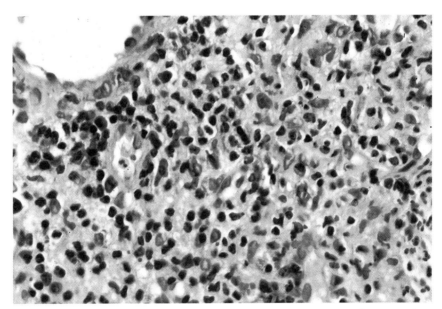

Figure 3–58. Angiocentric sinonasal T-cell lymphoma. The lymphoma cells are small to intermediate size with irregular hyperchromatic nuclei. Plasma cells are also present.

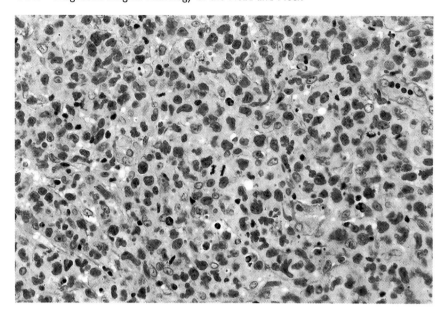

Figure 3–59. Malignant T-cell lymphoma of the sinonasal tract. The lymphoma cells exhibit moderate amounts of pale eosinophilic cytoplasm, markedly atypical nuclei, numerous mitotic figures, and frequent apoptotic cells.

Figure 3–60. Angiocentric sinonasal T-cell lymphoma. The neoplastic cells are invading and destroying the wall of an arteriole. There is extensive necrosis.

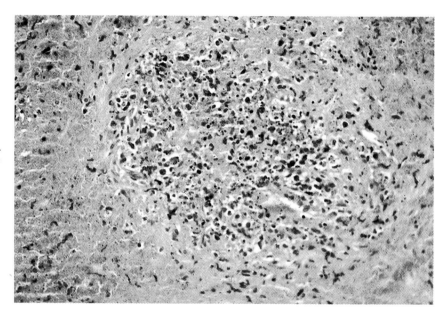

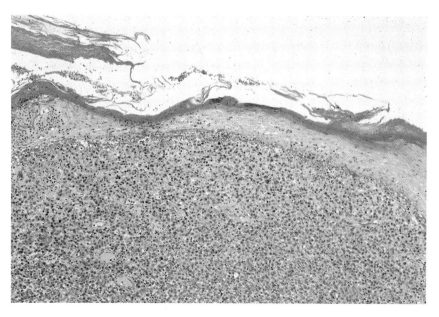

Figure 3–61. Well-differentiated plasmacytoma involving the nasal cavity. Sheets of plasma cells are seen beneath the squamous mucosa.

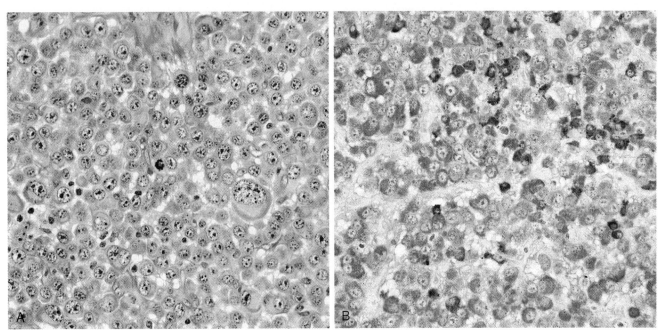

Figure 3–62. Plasmacytoma with a moderate degree of nuclear pleomorphism *(A)* and lambda light chain restriction *(B)*.

Immunohistochemical studies in a limited number of SNECs suggest that they are almost invariably positive for keratins (Fig. 3–30, see p. 101) with a variable expression of neuron-specific enolase, chromogranin, and synaptophysin.[206] No cells staining for S-100 protein or neurofilament are present. Unlike Merkel cell carcinomas, these tumors appear to be negative for cytokeratin 20.[212] Dense-core granules have been identified ultrastructurally in some cases.[209, 210, 213]

An unusual small-cell undifferentiated neoplasm with some features of small-cell undifferentiated carcinoma, but also showing divergent mesenchymal differentiation, has been described in the sinonasal region following radiation therapy for bilateral retinoblastoma.[214, 215]

Differential Diagnosis. The differential diagnosis of SNEC in the sinonasal tract includes olfactory neuroblastoma (ONB), sinonasal undifferentiated carcinoma (SNUC), poorly differentiated and basaloid squamous cell carcinomas, malignant lymphoma, and, rarely, Ewing's sarcoma or primitive neuroectodermal tumors (Table 3–1). This distinction may be difficult in some cases, but the combination of clinical, morphologic, immunohistochemical, and ultrastructural studies should allow a definitive diagnosis in most instances. Sinonasal SNEC should be distinguished from ONB because the latter has a better prognosis. The cells of ONBs are arranged in a lobular pattern and exhibit moderate amounts of cytoplasm, round nuclei, low nucleoplasmic:cytoplasmic ratio, and low mitotic activity. Necrosis is uncommon. In contrast, SNEC lacks lobular architecture, fibrovascular septa, and neurofibrillary stroma and does not contain neural or olfactory rosettes. The anaplastic cells of SNEC have scanty cytoplasm, high nucleoplasmic:cytoplasmic ratio, round or oval dense hyperchromatic nuclei, and numerous mitotic figures and apoptotic cells accompanied by extensive areas of necrosis. Immunohistochemically, sinonasal SNEC lacks the S-100 positive cells seen at the periphery of the cell nests of ONB and is negative for neurofilament. The expression of keratin in ONB is uncommon and when present is patchy or limited to areas with gland-like or olfactory differentiation, in contrast to the diffuse staining seen in SNEC.

Basaloid squamous cell carcinoma (BSCC) of the sinonasal tract[216] can be difficult to differentiate from SNEC.[217] Both neoplasms are composed of small pleomorphic cells with high nucleoplasmic:cytoplasmic ratio, inconspicuous nucleoli, high mitotic activity, and extensive areas of necrosis. However, SNEC does not have the well-defined tumor lobules with peripheral nuclear palisading, smooth contours, and hyaline basal lamina material seen in BSCC. No evidence of squamous differentiation has been reported in SNEC of the sinonasal tract, whereas in situ and invasive squamous cell carcinoma or tumor islands with abrupt keratinization are almost always found in BSCC. BSCC may express neuron-specific enolase,[218] but unlike SNEC, is negative for synaptophysin and chromogranin.

Treatment and Prognosis. SNECs are aggressive epithelial tumors with a high local and distant failure rate despite multimodal therapy. Given the poor prognosis associated with these tumors, there is need for a multidisciplinary treatment approach combining surgery or radiotherapy with chemotherapy. Surgery with adjuvant chemotherapy with a platinum-base regimen may be used in a curative attempt in patients with limited local disease. A platinum-based chemotherapeutic regimen similar to the one used for pulmonary small cell carcinomas may be used for control of systemic relapses.[132] Galanis et al.[132] reported a 72% response rate in 22 patients with extrapulmonary small cell carcinomas of all sites treated with a platinum-base regimen; however, the median duration of response was only 8.5 months. Owing to the poor long-term survival and the poor results obtained with surgery, radiotherapy may be an alternative for palliation in those patients with locally advanced disease.

Regardless of therapy employed, the long-term prognosis for sinonasal SNEC remains poor. Of 12 cases reported by several authors,[207–210, 219] 8 patients (67%) had died of disease and only 3 (25%) were alive with no evidence of disease. In a study of extrapulmonary small cell carcinomas from the Mayo Clinic,[220] the median survival of 14 patients with primary head and neck tumors was only 14.5 months. This group included seven cases involving the paranasal sinuses. It has been stated that the biologic behavior of these tumors differs from their pulmonary counterparts in that aggressive local disease, rather than systemic dissemination, appears to dominate the clinical picture[207–209, 219]; however, cervical lymph node and pulmonary metastases occur in a significant number of patients.[206, 220]

Carcinoid Tumor

Carcinoid tumors of the sinonasal tract are extremely uncommon, with only isolated case reports.[221, 222] Siwersson and Kindblom described a carcinoid tumor of the nasal cavity followed by a typical carcinoid tumor in the lung.[221] These lesions showed the trabecular and organoid architecture typical of carcinoid tumors in other organs; however, the tumor cells in both had an oncocytic cytoplasm closely resembling that of oncocytomas of minor salivary gland origin.[221, 222] One of these cases had low mitotic activity and at least focal areas of marked cytologic atypia.[221] The differential diagnosis of these uncommon lesions includes oncocytoma; in fact, it is recommended that any oncocytic lesion in this region be investigated for neuroendocrine differentiation.

McCluggage et al.[223] reported a widely invasive neoplasm with amphicrine differentiation. The tumor was composed of large cohesive cells with an organoid arrangement and small glandular spaces. There were areas composed of goblet cells with abundant intracellu-

Table 3–1. Ancillary Studies and Differential Diagnosis of Neuroendocrine and Small Cell Lesions of the Sinonasal Tract

Lesion	Keratin	Synaptophysin	Chromogranin	O-13	S100	Electron Microscopy	Molecular Pathology
ONB	−/+	+++	+++	−	+++/−	Neuronal processes Dense core granules Olfactory vesicles	
SCNec	+++	++/−	++/−	−	−−−	Absent or rare dense core granules	
SNUC	+++	−/?	−/?	−	−	Absent or rare dense core granules	
Lymphoma	−	−	−	−	−	No cell junctions Absent dense core granules	IgH or T-cell receptor rearrangements
ES/PNET	−	−/+	−/+	+++	−	Cytoplasmic glycogen Rare dense core granules	t(11;22)
RMS	−	−	−	−	−	Ribosome/myosin complex Thin and thick filaments	+2q, +8; t(2;13)

ES/PNET, Ewing sarcoma/peripheral neuroectodermal tumor; ONB, olfactory neuroblastoma; RMS, rhabdomyosarcoma; SCNec, small cell carcinoma; SNUC, sinonasal undifferentiated carcinoma.

lar mucin. Immunohistochemistry and electron microscopy demonstrated neuroendocrine differentiation. The overall appearance of the tumor was reminiscent of a goblet cell carcinoid of the appendix.

Sinonasal Undifferentiated Carcinoma

Clinical Features. Sinonasal undifferentiated carcinoma (SNUC) is an enigmatic lesion that has been recognized as a distinctive clinicopathologic entity only in recent years.[224–226] It appears to be an undifferentiated neoplasm with varying degrees of neuroendocrine differentiation.[224, 227] Some cases may have been reported simply as anaplastic carcinoma.[228] Epstein-Barr virus genome has been detected in several of these lesions[229, 230] and loss of the retinoblastoma tumor suppressor gene function has been implicated in their pathogenesis.[231]

The age range at presentation is broad, with both young adults and the elderly being affected. The median age in one study was 53 years.[226] There is a slight female predominance, and a strong association with smoking has been reported.[226, 232] Symptoms are related to a sinonasal mass. Physical examination usually demonstrates a large tumor obstructing the nasal cavity and invading surrounding structures.[233] Involvement of the nasal cavity, maxillary antrum, sphenoid sinus, frontal sinus, nasopharynx, orbit, and cranial cavity is frequent.[225, 228, 232, 233]

Pathologic Features. SNUCs consist of nests, trabeculae, ribbons, and sheets of medium-sized polygonal cells (Fig. 3–31, see p. 102), often with an "organoid" appearance. The nuclei are round to oval, slightly to moderately pleomorphic, and hyperchromatic. The chromatin varies from diffuse to coarsely granular and the nucleoli are typically large, but in some cases they may be inconspicuous. Most cells have small to moderate amounts of eosinophilic cytoplasm. Mitotic figures are numerous, and vascular invasion is extensive. Individual cell necrosis and central necrosis of cell nests are common. Homer Wright rosettes, intercellular fibrils, and argyrophil granules are absent, as are features of squamous or glandular differentiation. Occasional sinonasal undifferentiated carcinomas may be associated with severe dysplasia or carcinoma in situ of the surface mucosa. Immunocytochemical stains for cytokeratin and epithelial membrane antigen are positive for one or both markers in virtually all cases. About 50% of cases are positive for neuron-specific enolase, and electron-microscopic studies document rare dense-core granules occurring singly in individual cells.[224, 227] Interestingly, the expression of chromogranin and synaptophysin has not been studied in these tumors.

Differential Diagnosis. Differential diagnostic considerations for SNUC include olfactory neuroblastoma, nasopharyngeal carcinoma, small cell neuroendocrine carcinoma, large cell lymphoma, malignant melanoma, and embryonal rhabdomyosarcoma.[213, 234] The lack of junctional activity and melanin pigment and the absence of staining for S100 and HMB45 should help in the differential diagnosis between SNUC and melanoma. SNUC does not have the myxoid background or spindle cells seen in embryonal rhabdomyosarcoma and does not stain for muscle markers. The differentiation from large cell lymphoma on morphologic grounds alone is more difficult; however, lymphomas do not form cell nests or trabeculae, as seen in SNUC, and their immunophenotype is distinctly different. The use of a diagnostic panel that includes keratins, CD45, CD20 and other lymphoid markers, S-100 protein, HMB45, myoglobin, actins, and desmin should be used in difficult cases. Olfactory neuroblastoma consists of uniform to mildly pleomorphic cells with a diagnostic intercellular fibrillary background arranged in well-defined nests. Rosettes and ganglion cells are also diagnostic when present. These features are not seen in SNUC. S-100–positive sustentacular cells are scattered in neuroblastoma but are lacking in undifferentiated carcinoma. Both tumors, however, may stain for cytokeratin. Unlike SNUC, nasopharyngeal carcinoma grows as single cells or syncytial-like sheets often with a prominent inflammatory stroma in the undifferentiated type of nasopharyngeal carcinoma. Areas of spindling of tumor cells with maturation of tumor cords are

characteristic of the differentiated type of nonkeratinizing nasopharyngeal carcinoma and are not found in SNUC. Trabecular or organoid growth patterns are not seen. Small cell neuroendocrine carcinomas feature smaller cell size and denser hyperchromatic nuclei than SNUCs.

Treatment and Prognosis. Complete surgical resection usually cannot be achieved, and until recently radiation and chemotherapy had been of little value. Recent studies have shown an improved response to cisplatin-based chemotherapy and bone marrow transplantation.[227, 235] Despite this aggressive approach, the prognosis of SNUC is poor. Median survival in one study was only 4 months, with no disease-free patients.[226]

Neuroectodermal Tumors

Paraganglioma

Clinical Features. Paragangliomas have been reported as primary tumors in the nasopharynx, nasal cavity, and paranasal sinuses (Fig. 3–32)[236–239] or as secondary lesions extending from a carotid body or jugulotympanic or vagal paraganglioma.[238, 240] Most reported cases have occurred in females with a wide age range. Paragangliomas are most commonly seen as polypoid or exophytic masses in the middle or inferior turbinate. They have also been described in the posterior ethmoidal area, lateral and posterior pharyngeal walls, and posterior choana.

Pathologic Features and Differential Diagnosis. The recognition of paragangliomas in the sinonasal tract is mainly based on awareness of their occurrence in this region. The microscopic characteristics are similar to those of paragangliomas in other head and neck locations (Fig. 3–33, see p. 102). The differential diagnosis includes olfactory neuroblastoma, pituitary adenoma, malignant melanoma, and poorly differentiated carcinoma. The cell nests of paraganglioma and olfactory neuroblastoma are surrounded by S-100–positive sustentacular cells; however, the chief cells of paraganglioma have more abundant cytoplasm, and the nuclei are larger and often exhibit prominent nucleoli. Paragangliomas do not exhibit fibrillary background or rosettes, as seen in olfactory neuroblastomas. Pituitary adenomas may be distinguished from paragangliomas based on smaller tumor cell size and the immunohistochemical expression of specific pituitary hormones. Although the differential diagnosis of paraganglioma in the sinonasal tract includes malignant melanoma, the pathologic features of these neoplasms are different. Paragangliomas may show significant nuclear pleomorphism; however, they do not reveal significant mitotic activity. Furthermore, melanomas are diffusely positive for S100 and HMB45 and are negative for keratins, synaptophysin, and chromogranin. Electron

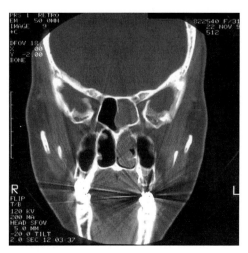

Figure 3–32. Paraganglioma of the ethmoid sinus.

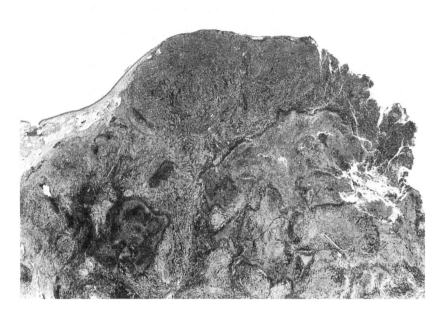

Figure 3–34. Nodular melanoma involving the maxillary sinus. The epithelium overlying the tumor is thin and focally ulcerated. No dysplastic epithelium or melanoma in situ is present, although melanoma in situ can occasionally be observed in these tumors.

microscopy in paragangliomas may demonstrate the presence of large numbers of dense core neuroendocrine granules, which should not be confused with melanosomes. Poorly differentiated carcinomas of the sinonasal tract usually reveal more nuclear pleomorphism, mitotic activity, and necrosis than paragangliomas and do not stain for neuroendocrine markers.

Treatment and Prognosis. Sinonasal paragangliomas generally behave in a benign fashion. However, rare cases of malignant paraganglioma of the nasal cavity have been described.[241, 242] These appear to be aggressive neoplasms characterized by the development of multiple local recurrences and brain metastases. The treatment of sinonasal paragangliomas is complete surgical resection if possible. In recurrent or malignant tumors, surgical debulking and radiotherapy may provide long-term local control.

Malignant Melanoma

Clinical Features. Primary malignant melanoma of the sinonasal tract constitutes approximately 1% of all melanomas.[243–247] In the material reviewed by Friedmann and Osborn at the Institute of Laryngology and Otology in London, melanomas represented 5% of all sinonasal tumors and were the second most common malignancy (23%) in that region.[248] The nasal cavity is more frequently affected than the paranasal sinuses. Within the nasal cavity, involvement of the anterior septum, inferior turbinate, and middle turbinate is most common. The maxillary antrum and the ethmoid sinuses are the most frequently involved paranasal sinuses.[249–251] Primary melanomas of the frontal and sphenoid sinuses and the nasopharynx are extremely rare. There is no sex predilection, and 80% of the patients are older than 50 years of age. Symptoms at presentation are nonspecific and are related to the location of the tumor; they include nasal obstruction, epistaxis, and facial pain.

Pathologic Features. Melanomas in the nasal cavity have a variable appearance. They appear as polypoid or sessile lesions with a brown or pink color. Mucosal ulceration is frequent (Fig. 3–34) and hemorrhage and necrosis are common in large lesions. Histologically, melanomas have a varied cytologic appearance.[252, 253] Most are composed of large epithelioid cells with abundant eosinophilic cytoplasm with round nuclei showing prominent eosinophilic nucleoli (Fig. 3–35A). Tumors composed of spindle cells (Fig.

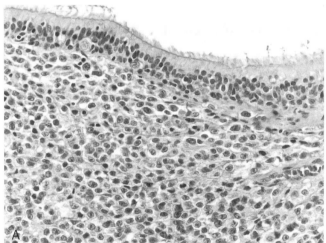
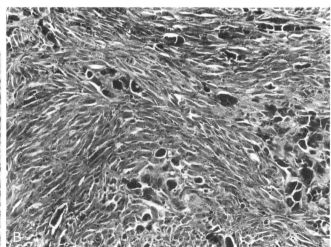

Figure 3–35. *A,* Amelanotic sinonasal malignant melanoma growing beneath an intact mucosa. The differential diagnosis of this lesion should include a large-cell non-Hodgkin's lymphoma. *B,* Spindle cell melanoma with abundant melanin content.

3–35*B*), mixed epithelioid and spindle cells, or small cells are not uncommon. In those tumors without mucosal ulceration, junctional or pagetoid changes and cellular nests or theques can be identified and strongly suggest the correct diagnosis. Approximately 30% of malignant melanomas in this region have cytoplasmic pigment. The neoplastic cells are arranged in an array of architectural patterns: solid, organoid, trabecular, alveolar, or any combination of these patterns. Cytologically, these are high-grade malignant lesions, similar to melanomas in other locations. They usually exhibit significant nuclear pleomorphism and numerous mitotic figures including atypical forms, hemorrhage, and necrosis. Not uncommonly, a myxoid background is also present. Melanomas are usually positive for vimentin, S-100, and HMB-45; therefore, the use of these stains as part of a diagnostic panel may be very helpful in establishing a definitive diagnosis.

Differential Diagnosis. The differential diagnosis of sinonasal malignant melanoma varies according to the predominant architectural and cytologic features present in the primary tumor. In lesions with epithelioid or spindle cell patterns, or both, the possibilities of a poorly differentiated carcinoma, sarcomatoid carcinoma, malignant fibrous histiocytoma, fibrosarcoma, and metastatic malignant melanoma should be excluded. Non-Hodgkin's lymphoma, rhabdomyosarcoma, Ewing sarcoma or peripheral neuroectodermal tumor, olfactory neuroblastoma, and small cell neuroendocrine carcinoma should be ruled out in those cases with a predominant small cell component. In these instances, the use of a panel of antibodies and electron microscopy are of great value in establishing a definitive diagnosis.

Treatment and Prognosis. Complete surgical resection is the treatment of choice. Radiotherapy and chemotherapy are of little value. In a study of 28 cases treated with radiotherapy alone, the reported local control rate was 79%; however, the 5-year survival rate was only 25%.[254] Malignant melanoma of the sinonasal tract is an aggressive disease with a 60% to 80% local recurrence rate and 10% 5-year survival rate.[248, 250, 255] Metastases to lung and brain are common.[249, 250, 256]

Olfactory Neuroblastoma

Clinical Features. Olfactory neuroblastoma (ONB) was first described by Berger in 1924.[257, 258] ONB has been described and referred to by numerous terms: esthesioneuroblastoma, esthesioneuroepithelioma, esthesioneurocytoma, and, of late, neuroendocrine carcinoma.[259–261] These tumors arise almost exclusively in the olfactory mucosa of the superior portion of the nasal cavity.[262] The putative cell of origin of ONB is a reserve cell that gives rise to both neuronal and epithelial (sustentacular) cells.[263] ONB affects men and women alike and is seen in a broad age range. Most cases present in the third and fourth decades,[264–267] with some studies reporting bimodal peaks at 15 and 50 years of age.[261, 268] The main presenting symptoms are nasal obstruction, epistaxis, and anosmia. Myers et al.[269] reported a case with invasion of the oral cavity and inappropriate antidiuretic hormone secretion. Physical examination usually demonstrates a large polypoid mass high in the nasal cavity, often extending into the paranasal sinuses.

Kadish et al.[270] proposed a staging system for these neoplasms: Stage A, disease confined to the nasal cavity; Stage B, disease confined to the nasal cavity and paranasal sinuses (Fig. 3–36); and Stage C, local or distant spread beyond the nasal cavity or paranasal sinuses. Stage B disease is the most common and occurs in approximately 40% to 50% of cases.

Pathologic Features. Under low-power magnification, most olfactory neuroblastomas consist of well-circumscribed cell nests and lobules separated by a fibrovascular stroma (Fig. 3–37*A*, see p. 103). The lobules may coalesce and interconnect, forming sheets of cells with a prominent capillary network. Approximately 60% to 70% of tumors have a variable amount of fibrillary stroma (Fig. 3–37*B*), although in some cases this may be only a focal finding (Fig. 3–38*A*). Rosettes are also a typical finding (Fig. 3–37*C*), but like the fibrillary stroma, they may also be found only in small foci.

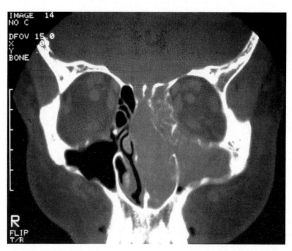

Figure 3–36. Olfactory neuroblastoma involving the nasal cavity and maxillary sinus.

The neoplastic cells are small or medium-sized and have pale eosinophilic cytoplasm with indistinct borders. The nuclei are round, somewhat vesicular, with fine chromatin and absent or small nucleoli. Most cases show only mild to moderate nuclear pleomorphism (Fig. 3–37*D*, see p. 103)[271] and a low mitotic rate. Necrosis is uncommon and is generally seen in cases with high mitotic counts.[271, 272] Rare cases have areas of glandular (Fig. 3–38*B*) or squamous differentiation.[263] A pigmented olfactory neuroblastoma was described by Curtis and Rubinstein.[273]

Immunohistochemical studies have shown that the cells of olfactory neuroblastomas are generally strongly positive for neuron-specific enolase, synaptophysin (Fig. 3–39*A*, see p. 104) and chromogranin. The periphery of the cell nests show numerous spindle or stellate cells positive for S-100 (Fig. 3–39*B*). Neurofilament protein and class III β-tubulin are seen within the cytoplasm and fibrillary matrix.[274] Keratin immunoreactivity is found in approximately 20% to 25% of olfactory neuroblastomas,[265, 274, 275] generally in areas with epithelial differentiation (Fig. 3–39*C*).

Most ONBs have a characteristic fibrillary background on hematoxylin-eosin stained sections. Ultrastructurally, these fibrils correspond to tangles of neuronal cell processes.[213, 272, 276, 277] Less common features are Flexner-Wintersteiner or Homer Wright rosettes. The former are gland-like structures indicative of olfactory differentiation.[272, 278] Ultrastructurally, true olfactory differentiation is characterized by cylindrical cells with thin apical microvilli and a bulbous tip or olfactory vesicle containing a few dense core granules.[272, 278] Homer Wright rosettes, also called *pseudorosettes,* are annular arrays of cells surrounding central zones of fibrils. They are most common in cases that contain a prominent fibrillary background. Maturation to ganglioneuroblastoma is rarely seen in ONB.[274]

The prognostic value of morphologic features in olfactory neuroblastoma is uncertain at best. Hyams et al.[271] introduced a four-tier grading system, which, in their series, was correlated with patient outcome. However, the clinical usefulness of this grading remains untested in other studies. Hirose et al.[274] found longer survival in those patients without metastases and in those with tumors with increased numbers of S-100–positive cells and a Ki-67 proliferation index less than 10%.

Recently, it has been postulated that olfactory neuroblastoma is a member of the Ewing sarcoma/peripheral neuroectodermal tumor family.[279] The chromosomal translocation t(11;22)(q24;q12) with fusion of the *EWS/FLI1* genes, typical of Ewing sarcoma or peripheral neuroectodermal tumor, was reported in two cell lines obtained from metastatic ONB and six primary olfactory neuroblastomas.[279, 280] However, immunohistochemical studies for the protein product of the *MIC-2* gene have not supported this hypothesis.[265, 281]

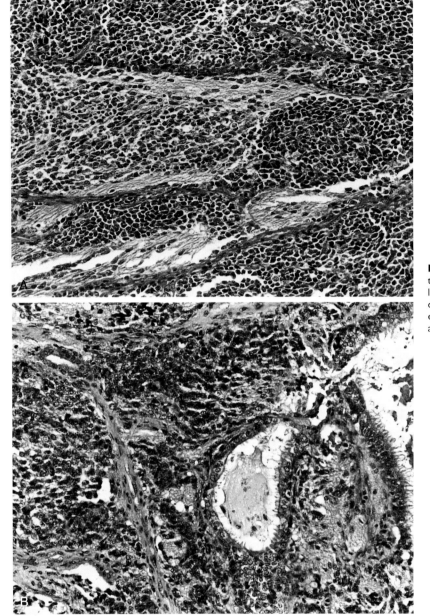

Figure 3–38. A, Poorly differentiated olfactory neuroblastoma with sheets of neoplastic cells and focal neurofibrillary stroma. B, Olfactory neuroblastoma with glandular differentiation. The glandular component is considered evidence of true olfactory differentiation by some authors and is usually immunoreactive for keratins.

We did not find *EWS/FLI* gene fusion messenger RNA in a series of well-characterized ONBs.[282] Wild-type *p53* hyperexpression appears to be a late event in the progression of olfactory neuroblastomas and tends to correlate with local aggressive behavior and development of metastasis.[283]

Differential Diagnosis. The differential diagnosis of ONB includes other neuroendocrine and small cell lesions of the sinonasal tract (see Table 3–1). Although olfactory neuroblastomas and sinonasal small cell neuroendocrine carcinomas share certain morphologic features in addition to expression of neuroendocrine and epithelial markers, they should be clearly separated because of significant prognostic differences. True sinonasal small cell neuroendocrine carcinomas resemble small cell carcinomas of the lung. The degree of mitotic activity and the extensive areas of necrosis present in small cell carcinomas are not seen in most olfactory neuroblastomas. Small cell carcinomas do not exhibit cell nests surrounded by S-100–positive cells. Keratin expression in olfactory neuroblastoma is usually limited to tumors with gland-like or olfactory differentiation, whereas small cell carcinomas are diffusely positive. Silva et

al.[261] and Ordóñez et al.[272] have proposed the separation of olfactory neuroblastomas into two groups: classic neuroblastoma and neuroendocrine carcinoma. However, the clinical and biologic value of this classification scheme remains unsettled.[260, 271, 274, 276, 284] We agree with Hyams et al.[271] and discourage the use of the term "neuroendocrine carcinoma" for lesions that fulfill the diagnostic criteria of ONB. The term, used in this context, fosters confusion with small cell neuroendocrine carcinomas and has not been proven to be of clinical value.[261, 274, 285]

Olfactory neuroblastomas should also be distinguished from rhabdomyosarcoma. The nests of alveolar rhabdomyosarcoma may be confused with the characteristic nests of ONB. The use of a panel of immunostains should be extremely helpful in establishing the correct diagnosis. Rhabdomyosarcomas are negative for neuroendocrine markers and do not possess S-100–positive cells at the periphery of the tumor nests. ONBs are negative for desmin and actin. Malignant melanoma predominantly composed of small cells is another lesion that may be confused with ONB. However, the degree of cytologic atypia and pleomorphism generally seen in melanoma is uncommon in ONB. Moreover, the immunophenotypes of these lesions are different. ONBs are diffusely positive for neuroendocrine markers, which are absent in melanomas. The characteristic location of the S-100–positive cells in ONB should also be helpful in making this distinction. The small undifferentiated cells of teratocarcinosarcoma may resemble the cells of ONB[286, 287]; however, the lack of nesting coupled with the presence of other epithelial and mesenchymal elements should point to the correct diagnosis. Sinonasal pituitary adenomas should also be considered in the differential diagnosis of ONBs, but the lack of fibrillary background and the expression of keratin and specific pituitary hormones in pituitary adenomas indicate the correct diagnosis.

Treatment and Prognosis. Complete surgical resection, if feasible, and adjuvant radiotherapy is the treatment of choice for olfactory neuroblastoma.[264, 266, 267, 274] Preliminary data concerning combined chemotherapy with cisplatin and etoposide and proton beam radiation in advanced or recurrent disease has shown promising early results.[260] The prognosis of olfactory neuroblastoma depends to a certain extent on the clinical stage; however, the clinical behavior is often unpredictable. The reported 5-year survival rate for stage A disease is 57% to 88%; for stage B, 58% to 60%; and for stage C, 0% to 50%.[262, 266] Recurrence or metastases may develop as late as 21 years after initial diagnosis; therefore, 5-year survival rates are meaningless. In a recent study, 38% of patients developed local recurrence, and 46% had nodal and distant metastases.[274]

▌ SOFT TISSUE TUMORS

Vascular Tumors

Lobular Capillary Hemangioma

Clinical Features. Lobular capillary hemangioma is a distinctive vascular lesion most commonly seen in the fourth and fifth decades of life. It frequently affects pregnant females or males under 16 years of age.[288, 289] The predominant sites of involvement are the anterior portion of the nasal septum (Little's area) and the tip of the turbinates. The most common clinical symptoms are epistaxis and nasal obstruction. Lesions arising in pregnant females often undergo spontaneous regression after delivery.

Pathologic Features. Grossly, lobular capillary hemangiomas are polypoid masses with smooth contours measuring up to 2.0 cm in diameter. Microscopically, they are composed of small, uniform vascular channels with a lobular architecture, often surrounding a larger central vessel. The individual capillaries vary from solid nests of plump endothelial cells without lumina to large vessels lined with prominent endothelial cells showing "tufting" and mitotic activity. The endothelium is surrounded by pericytes and stromal cells, which often exhibit a granulation tissue–like character and a variable infiltrate of neutrophils, lymphocytes, and plasma cells.[290] Secondary changes include mucosal ulceration with marked acute inflammation and intravascular papillary endothelial hyperplasia.

Differential Diagnosis. Perhaps the most clinically important lesions that need to be separated from lobular capillary hemangioma are nasopharyngeal angiofibroma, hemangiopericytoma, and angiosarcoma. The thick abnormal blood vessels and spindle or stellate fibroblasts of angiofibroma are significantly different from the small capillary-sized vessels with a lobular pattern seen in hemangiomas. The nuclear atypia and infiltrative pattern that characterizes angiosarcoma is also absent in hemangioma. Hemangiopericytomas are larger and more cellular lesions than hemangiomas. They have an attenuated endothelial lining surrounded by a somewhat uniform population of plump to spindled cells, in contrast to the more prominent endothelial cells and the array of capillary-sized blood vessels with a lobular architecture of hemangioma.

Treatment and Prognosis. Hemangiomas are benign lesions, are treated by simple surgical resection, and only rarely recur.

Nasopharyngeal Angiofibroma

Clinical Features. Angiofibromas are uncommon and constitute less than 1% of all head and neck tumors. They occur almost exclusively in males between 10 and 25 years of age. Well-documented examples of this tumor have been described in young children and middle-aged patients; however, its existence in females remains controversial. Hyams described no female patients among 150 cases reviewed at the Armed Forces Institute of Pathology.[291] An association with familial adenomatous polyposis has been reported.[292] Angiofibromas possess androgen, testosterone, and dihydrotestosterone receptors,[293, 294] and basic fibroblast growth factor.[295, 296] They lack estrogen or progesterone receptors.[294, 297] The most common presenting symptoms are unilateral nasal obstruction and epistaxis. Less commonly seen are facial swelling, diplopia, proptosis, headache, anosmia, and pain. Over one half of the patients have had symptoms for more than 1 year before diagnosis. The diagnosis of angiofibroma should be considered in any male under 30 years of age who presents with a nasopharyngeal mass.

It is believed that nasopharyngeal angiofibromas arise in the fibrovascular stroma normally present in the posterolateral wall of the roof of the nasal cavity where the sphenoidal process of the palatine bone meets the horizontal ala of the vomer and the pterygoid process. When the tumor becomes symptomatic, it is always found in the nasopharynx. On plain radiographs, the growing mass causes bowing of the posterior wall of the maxillary sinus. In the past, selective carotid arteriograms demonstrated a typical and highly diagnostic vascular pattern, which delimited the extension of the tumor; however, computed tomographic scans and magnetic resonance imaging have replaced this technique.

Pathologic Features. Grossly, angiofibromas are well circumscribed, lobulated, tan to purple-red masses measuring up to 6 cm in maximal dimension. The cut surface has a fibrous appearance. Often, blood vessels can be seen near the base of resection. Ulceration, necrosis, and cystic spaces are distinctly uncommon.

Histologically, these tumors are characterized by the presence of a collagenized vascular stroma containing numerous, irregularly shaped blood vessels (Fig. 3–40A, see p. 104).[289, 298, 299] The amount of collagen present in the stroma varies from fine to coarse strands embedded in a myxoid stroma, to a dense, acellular collagenous tissue. The stroma contains spindle (Fig. 3–40B) or stellate-shaped myofibroblasts with plump nuclei and numerous mast cells. Occasional multinucleated stromal cells and "ganglion-like" cells similar to those seen in proliferative myositis can be encountered. Mitotic figures can also be seen, but they are uncommon. The shape and distribution of the blood vessels and stroma is variable within angiofibromas. The periphery of the lesion contains numerous small, capillary-like vessels lined by a single layer of endothelial cells with little fibrous tissue, whereas larger vessels with thick muscular walls surrounded by dense collagenous tissue are found in the center of the tumor. These large vessels lack elastic fibers.[300] The stromal cells of nasopharyngeal angiofibroma appear to be of fibroblastic and myofibroblastic origin. They are immunoreactive for vimentin only with occasional expression of smooth muscle actin.[300, 301] Ultrastructurally, they contain actin filaments, dense bodies, and dilated rough endoplasmic reticulum.[301, 302]

Differential Diagnosis. The preoperative diagnosis of nasopharyngeal angiofibroma can be difficult. The diagnosis is based on clinical and radiologic findings. In fact, because of the characteristic radiologic appearance of angiofibroma, biopsy before definitive treatment is often unnecessary.[303] These tumors should be distinguished from lobular capillary hemangioma, a distinction that can be extremely difficult in superficial biopsy material; however, the distinctive location of angiofibroma, its larger size, and extension into adjacent structures makes this differentiation possible. The differential diagnosis of nasopharyngeal angiofibroma also includes other vascular lesions such as hemangiopericytoma, solitary fibrous tumor, and angiosarcoma, but the characteristic age, sex, and tumor location should strongly favor the diagnosis of angiofibroma. Furthermore, the thick blood vessels and the stellate stromal myofibroblasts seen in angiofibroma are not features of any of these neoplasms.

Treatment and Prognosis. Surgical removal is the treatment of choice for those lesions in which resection is possible. The preferred surgical approach depends on the surgeon's experience and extension of the tumor. For tumors limited to the nasopharynx, a transoral or lateral rhinotomy may be used. The recurrence rate for juvenile angiofibroma is approximately 20%.[303] This high recurrence rate is probably due to incomplete resection. With recent advances in imaging and interventional neuroradiology, this recurrence rate has declined considerably. Recurrent lesions may be managed with additional surgery. Disease with intracranial extension requires combined intracranial and extracranial procedures. Radiotherapy and chemotherapy may be necessary for unresectable or recurrent disease.[299, 304] Preoperative embolization has been recommended to reduce the risk of intraoperative hemorrhage and incomplete tumor removal. Spontaneous regression of a proven angiofibroma has been described.[305] Sarcomatous transformation has been reported in a few cases treated with radiotherapy,[306, 307] and a rare case with metastasizing lesions has been reported.[308] The prognosis for a patient with angiofibroma is excellent; the mortality rate varies from 0% to 9% and is related to uncontrollable hemorrhage and intracranial extension.

Hemangiopericytoma

Clinical Features. The nature of sinonasal hemangiopericytomas and their kinship to hemangiopericytomas of soft tissues remains controversial. Some authors regard these lesions as related but separate entities and have used the term *hemangiopericytoma-like* tumors to refer to the nasal tumors.[309–311] Others consider them as a hybrid between hemangiopericytoma and glomus tumor.[312] This uncommon soft tissue neoplasm can arise at any site in the head and neck region, but the nasal cavity and the paranasal sinuses are the most frequent sites of involvement. Most patients are middle-aged or elderly adults, and the most common clinical complaints are nasal obstruction and epistaxis. Physical and radiologic examination reveal the presence of a polypoid mass high in the nasal cavity or a mass involving the paranasal sinuses with secondary extension into the nasal cavity.[313, 314]

Pathologic Features. Hemangiopericytomas in the nasal cavity have histologic features similar to hemangiopericytomas in other locations.[315, 316] Under low-power magnification, these tumors are well circumscribed and have an uniform appearance. Blood vessels range from small capillaries to sinusoidal spaces with "staghorn" shape, often showing hyalinized walls (Fig. 3–41, see p. 105). Necrosis and hemorrhage are generally absent. The tumor cells are tightly packed with little intervening collagen. They have a monotonous appearance with round to oval shape and indistinct cytoplasm. The nuclei are regular and have a bland appearance, varying from small and dark to somewhat vesicular (Fig. 3–42, see p. 105). Nucleoli are inconspicuous. Mitotic activity is generally absent or is less than 1 per 10 high-power fields. Some tumors may have myxoid or lipomatous areas.[317] Reticulin stains show reticulin fibers encircling individual pericytes. Immunostains are helpful in excluding other lesions with a hemangiopericytoma-like pattern. Factor VIII-RA, *Ulex europaeus,* and CD34 highlight the endothelium but are negative in the tumor cells (Fig. 3–43, see p. 105). Vimentin is the only stain that is consistently positive. Rare tumors may show focal staining for actin.[318] Electron microscopy reveals basal lamina enveloping individual tumor cells.[318]

Differential Diagnosis. Solitary fibrous tumor is the most difficult lesion to distinguish from hemangiopericytoma. Fortunately, this distinction is mostly of academic interest, given the excellent prognosis associated with both lesions. Hemangiopericytomas have a homogeneous architecture, in contrast to the more varied appearance of solitary fibrous tumor, which exhibits hypercellular and hypocellular areas with abundant collagen. CD34 is reportedly expressed in a consistent fashion by solitary fibrous tumor, whereas

expression in hemangiopericytoma is more variable. The expression of CD99 and bcl-2 by solitary fibrous tumor may also help in the differential diagnosis of these entities.[319, 320] This distinction may be impossible in small specimens, and it is likely that many cases of hemangiopericytomas found in the literature in fact represent unrecognized solitary fibrous tumors.

Treatment and Prognosis. Most hemangiopericytomas of the nasal cavity have bland morphologic features and behave in an indolent fashion.[244, 309, 314, 318] They may recur locally, even decades later, but well-differentiated tumors do not appear to metastasize. Rare cases reported as malignant hemangiopericytomas do not have enough clinical follow-up to determine their true behavior,[321] although others appear to be similar to malignant tumors of soft tissues.[289, 309, 322] DNA content and S-phase fraction have not been useful in identifying aggressive clinical behavior.[244] The treatment of hemangiopericytomas in the sinonasal tract is total surgical resection whenever feasible. We consider these tumors to be well-differentiated hemangiopericytomas that owe their good prognosis to their relatively small size and early clinical presentation.

Other Vascular Tumors

Hemangiomas are relatively common lesions in the sinonasal tract.[289] Most are examples of capillary hemangiomas that involve the anterior nasal septum. Cavernous and venous hemangiomas are also found in this region. Cavernous hemangiomas are most often located in the lateral wall and can produce extensive bone destruction, thus simulating a malignant lesion.[323] The most uncommon is the venous type, which also appears to preferentially involve the anterior nasal septum. Histologically, these lesions are similar to hemangiomas arising in soft tissues. Cavernous hemangiomas do not have the cytologic atypia and anastomosing vessels seen in angiosarcoma, despite their occasional locally destructive growth. Hemangiomas are usually cured by simple excision; in some cases of the cavernous type, embolization can be of benefit to control bleeding and facilitate resection.[323]

Intravascular papillary endothelial hyperplasia is a reactive pseudoneoplastic proliferation of endothelial cells associated with thrombosis of benign vascular lesions that may simulate angiosarcoma.[324] Rare cases have been described in the nasal cavity and paranasal sinuses.[288, 325] Histologically, intravascular papillary endothelial hyperplasia is characterized by dilated vascular spaces containing endothelium-lined papillary fronds with a variable amount of stroma (Fig. 3–44, see p. 106). The stroma consists of a mixture of fibrin, red blood cells, and hypocellular hyaline material. The hyperplastic endothelial cells may have prominent but uniform nuclei with occasional mitotic activity. Thrombosis is usually present, and frank anaplasia or necrosis, unlike in angiosarcomas, is always absent. Rare cases of glomus tumor, angiomatosis, and hemangioendothelioma have been described in the sinonasal tract.[289, 326] Angiomatosis can be widespread and multifocal, but it is not a malignant lesion. The vascular channels of angiomatosis are lined by flat endothelium with no cytologic atypia.[289]

Angiosarcoma

Clinical Features. Primary angiosarcomas of the sinonasal tract are rare tumors[289, 327–331]; in contrast to angiosarcomas in other locations, primary lesions in this location appear to have a lower incidence of local recurrences and metastases. The age at presentation is broad but most reported cases are found in the sixth or seventh decade of life.[289, 328, 331] Symptoms at presentation are nonspecific and include unilateral nasal obstruction, epistaxis, purulent rhinorrhea, and proptosis in widely invasive tumors.

Pathologic Features. These tumors have a tendency to present as bleeding polypoid masses or less commonly as ill-defined nodules. Angiosarcomas of the sinonasal tract exhibit similar histologic features to angiosarcomas in other locations and are characterized by the presence of freely anastomosing "gaping" vascular channels dissecting the underlying stroma (Fig. 3–45, see p. 106). Solid areas, necrosis, and hemorrhage may be prominent features, particularly in high-grade tumors. The neoplastic vessels are lined with atypical endothelial cells with "hobnail" nuclei and epithelial tufts (Fig. 3–46, see p. 106). The individual tumor cells can be spindle, polygonal, or epithelioid in shape with plump cytoplasm, hyperchromatic nuclei, and increased mitotic activity. They can be classified as low-grade or high-grade based on their overall appearance. The diagnosis of angiosarcoma may be confirmed by the use of antibodies for CD31, CD34, factor VIII related antigen, and *Ulex europaeus.*

Differential Diagnosis. The differential diagnosis of angiosarcoma in this location includes hemangioma, hemangiopericytoma, solitary fibrous tumor, other soft tissue sarcomas, and sarcomatoid carcinoma. Benign lesions that should be kept in mind when considering a diagnosis of angiosarcoma are an antrochoanal polyp with a prominent vascular component and papillary endothelial hyperplasia.[325] Unlike hemangiomas and other benign vascular lesions, low-grade angiosarcomas reveal the presence of infiltrative interconnecting vascular channels lined with atypical endothelial cells. Angiosarcomas also lack the lobular architecture seen in hemangiomas. Hemangiopericytoma and solitary fibrous tumor do not have the infiltrative pattern or the cytologic atypia seen in angiosarcoma.

Treatment and Prognosis. Combined radical surgical resection followed by radiotherapy is the treatment of choice for sinonasal angiosarcomas,[328, 331] although small lesions can be treated by surgery alone.[289] The prognosis of angiosarcoma in the sinonasal tract is variable. The literature review by Bankaci et al.[328] revealed that 5 of 11 patients had no evidence of disease, 3 had local recurrences controlled by additional therapy, and 3 were alive with disease or had died with recurrences. One patient reported by Olsen et al.[331] and another reported by Kimura et al.[327] were alive with no evidence of disease.

Kaposi's Sarcoma and Bacillary Angiomatosis

Kaposi's sarcoma of the sinonasal tract is extremely rare and is usually a manifestation of advanced disease in HIV-infected patients, although it may rarely arise in patients without HIV infection.[332] The histologic appearance is similar to that of Kaposi's sarcoma in other locations (Fig. 3–47, see p. 107). Bacillary angiomatosis is a vasoproliferative lesion caused by *Rochalimaea henselae* infection in immunosuppressed individuals, particularly those with HIV infection.[333, 334] A case involving the nasal cavity has been described by Batsakis et al.[334] Histologically, bacillary angiomatosis resembles pyogenic granuloma; however, the endothelial cells are often larger and polygonal and may have some cytologic atypia. Numerous neutrophils are often present admixed with leukocytoclastic debris and a basophilic granular material. This material corresponds to large numbers of bacteria, easily demonstrable with Warthin-Starry or Steiner's silver stains.[333] The differential diagnosis of bacillary angiomatosis in the sinonasal tract includes pyogenic granuloma and Kaposi's sarcoma.

Fibrous and Fibrohistiocytic Tumors

Fibroma

Fibromas are uncommon benign lesions most frequently found in the nasal septum or vestibule.[335] The typical appearance is that of a small elevated nodule usually measuring less than 1 cm. Microscopically, they are composed of small spindle cells with bland cytologic features embedded in dense collagenous tissue. Fibromas are distinguished from aggressive fibrous lesions because of their small size and typical hypocellular appearance. They are treated by simple excision.

Benign Fibrous Histiocytoma

The nasal cavity and paranasal sinuses are, after the skin, the second most common location in the head and neck region for benign fibrous histiocytoma.[336] Symptoms at presentation are nonspecific. They are most often seen as tan to yellow nodules or polyps. Histologically, there are composed of a mixture of spindle-shaped fibroblastic and myofibroblastic cells admixed with histiocytes arranged in a typical fascicular and storiform pattern. Often, multinucleated giant cells, foamy and epithelioid histiocytes, hemosiderin-laden macrophages, lymphocytes, and plasma cells are present throughout the tumor. The stroma is variable and can be highly sclerotic with large amounts of collagen or focally myxoid. Benign fibrous histiocytoma should be distinguished from desmoid tumor (fibromatosis), malignant fibrous histiocytoma, and fibrosarcoma. These lesions differ from benign fibrous histiocytoma in their lack of histiocytes, multinucleated giant cells, and foam cells and in their infiltrative pattern, cellular atypia, and nuclear pleomorphism. The treatment is simple but complete surgical excision.

Fibromatosis (Desmoid Tumor)

Clinical Features. Fibromatoses or desmoid tumors are relatively common in the head and neck region, particularly in children. The soft tissue of the neck is the site most frequently affected; however, involvement of the nasal cavity and paranasal sinuses is seen rarely.[335, 337] Symptoms are not specific and are usually related to the presence of a mass, often accompanied by pain or tenderness. The maxillary sinus is the site most commonly affected, followed by the nasal cavity.

Pathologic Features. Histologically, fibromatosis is characterized by relatively uniform fibroblasts arranged in interlacing fascicles with a variable collagenous to myxoid background. These lesions exhibit little or no cellular pleomorphism, hypercellularity, or mitotic activity. Almost invariably, there is extensive infiltration of soft tissues and bone.

Differential Diagnosis. The differential diagnosis of fibromatosis in the sinonasal tract and nasopharynx includes other spindle cell lesions such as reactive fibrosis, fibrosarcoma, and solitary fibrous tumor. The distinction from reactive fibrosis may be difficult because both entities show overlapping features; however, the history of recurrent rhinosinusitis and an expansile rather than infiltrative lesion in radiologic studies favors reactive fibrosis. Furthermore, in reactive fibrosis there is little if any fascicular arrangement destruction and entrapment of normal tissues. Fibrosarcoma generally is more cellular and has a higher mitotic rate and more cellular pleomorphism than fibromatosis. Fibromatosis lacks the patternless arrangement, hemangiopericytoma-like blood vessels, and CD34 immunoreactivity of solitary fibrous tumor.

Treatment and Prognosis. Fibromatosis of the sinonasal tract has an excellent prognosis and seems to have a lower recurrence rate (21%) than lesions in other locations.[337] Complete surgical resection is the treatment of choice. Incompletely resected lesions may remain stable for many years.

Myxoma and Fibromyxoma

Clinical Features. Myxomas of the craniofacial bones are rare neoplasms with well-defined clinicopathologic characteristics.[338–340] Most cases affect children and young adults in the second and third decades of life, although they may also be seen in older individuals.[340–344] The most common presentation is that of a painless facial or nasal deformity. Other symptoms include nasal obstruction, exophthalmos, facial pain, and loose teeth. Radiologically, myxomas are seen as expansile unilocular or multilocular radiolucent masses involving the posterior or condylar regions of the mandible or the zygomatic process or alveolar bone of the maxilla. Extragnathic involvement is rare.

Pathologic Features. Grossly, myxomas are unencapsulated although they are well demarcated. The consistency is variable, depending on the amount of collagen within the tumor, and has been described as firm to gelatinous with a tan-yellow color. Myxomas are hypocellular tumors (Fig. 3–48A, see p. 107) composed of slender spindle or stellate cells with inconspicuous cytoplasm and benign-appearing nuclei (Fig. 3–48B). The chromatin is dense with no visible nucleoli. The tumor cells are embedded in an abundant myxoid or mucous background.[339, 340, 345, 346] A fibrous stroma may be found in some lesions and when this stroma is relatively abundant, many authors use the term *fibromyxoma*. Unlike other myxomatous neoplasms, myxomas exhibit a poorly developed vascular network with only occasional thin capillary-type vessels within their stroma. Myxomas may extensively invade bone and adjacent soft tissues. The invasive edges of myxomas are broad pushing rather than infiltrative (see Fig. 3–48A).

The immunophenotype of craniofacial myxomas has not been widely studied. The tumor cells express vimentin and laminin.[347, 348] Muscle specific actin, smooth muscle actin, desmin, CD31, CD34, collagen IV, and S100 have been shown to be negative. Electron microscopy of myxomas has shown features of embryonic mesenchyme fibroblasts. The tumor cells exhibit scanty cytoplasm with a paucity of organelles.

Differential Diagnosis. The differential diagnosis of myxomas in the sinonasal tract is limited and includes other odontogenic tumors, benign peripheral nerve tumors, myxoid liposarcoma, and rhabdomyosarcoma. Odontogenic tumors are basically excluded by the absence of odontogenic epithelium in adequately sampled lesions. Although peripheral nerve tumors may reveal hypocellular areas with myxoid background, the tumor cells are plumper than the spindle and stellate cells of myxomas. In addition, nuclear palisading and S-100 are absent in myxomas. Malignant myxoid neoplasms exhibit increased cellularity and marked cellular atypia that significantly differ from the characteristic hypocellular appearance and bland cytologic features of myxomas.

Treatment and Prognosis. Myxomas are benign tumors with an excellent long-term prognosis with no metastases and no tumor-related deaths. Nonetheless, myxomas have the capability of destroying bone and infiltrating soft tissues and the cranial cavity.[339, 340] The initial treatment should be aggressive, since limited resections increase the chances of local recurrences and are associated with a high local recurrence rate. Three of the six patients reported by Fu and Perzin[340] developed local recurrences. The treatment of craniofacial myxomas is surgical and should be complete resection with wide margins of normal tissue. Often, this requires subtotal or radical maxillectomy.[339, 340, 343, 344]

Recently, we saw a malignant myxoid neoplasm with hypercellularity and cytologic atypia closely resembling a so-called myxofibrosarcoma of soft tissues (Fig. 3–49, see p. 108).[347] The tumor developed multiple local recurrences with invasion of the cranial cavity, causing the patient's death 5 years after initial resection.

Solitary Fibrous Tumor

Clinical Features. Solitary fibrous tumor is an uncommon tumor in the head and neck[349–353]; however, the most common locations in this region are the nasal cavity and paranasal sinuses with isolated cases arising in the nasopharynx.[319, 349, 353] The age at presentation has ranged from 24 to 64 years and there is no sex predilection. Most patients present with chronic nasal obstruction.

Pathologic Features. Grossly, the tumors have been described as a polypoid white mass measuring up to 7 cm in maximal dimension. These lesions are morphologically and immunohistochemically analogous to those tumors arising in the pleura. The tumors are composed of a haphazard proliferation of spindle to oval cells with scant cytoplasm embedded in a tangle of collagen fibers with a keloid-like appearance. Typically the cellularity is variable from area to area with a mixture of hypocellular and hypercellular areas. The blood vessels usually exhibit a hyalinized wall and a hemangiopericytoma-

like pattern. The tumor cells do not have a significant degree of atypia or mitotic activity and there is no hemorrhage or necrosis. Immunohistochemically solitary fibrous tumors are usually positive for vimentin, CD34, CD99, and *bcl-2*.[319, 320]

Differential Diagnosis. The main differential diagnosis of solitary fibrous tumor in this location is sinonasal hemangiopericytoma, which usually does not possess a prominent collagenous background and, in addition, contains a more homogeneous cellularity and lacks staining for CD99 and *bcl-2*; in some cases, this distinction may be extremely difficult or impossible. A low-grade fibrosarcoma should be excluded. Given that low-grade fibrosarcomas may show no significant atypia, the use of an immunohistochemical panel that includes CD34, CD99, and *bcl-2* may be helpful in establishing a diagnosis of solitary fibrous tumor.

Treatment and Prognosis. The treatment of solitary fibrous tumor is complete surgical resection. These are benign neoplasms that do not require adjuvant therapy. Four of five patients reported by Witkin and Rosai were free of disease after a follow-up of 1 to 12 years.[349] The two patients reported by Zukenberg et al.[353] had no disease 6 and 12 months after surgery.[353] One patient had persistent but stable disease 4 years after surgery and tumor embolization.[349]

Fibrosarcoma

Clinical Features. Fibrosarcoma, like most soft tissue sarcomas, is uncommon in the sinonasal tract.[329, 354, 355] The symptoms at presentation are similar to those of other sarcomas in this region and include nasal obstruction and epistaxis.[329, 336, 356]

Pathologic Features. Histologically, fibrosarcomas are hypercellular lesions composed of thin elongated spindle cells arranged in long fascicles and bundles intersecting at different angles. Fascicles disposed at right angles, the so-called "herringbone" pattern, may be subtle or absent altogether.[356] Fibrosarcomas generally have a monotonous appearance and do not exhibit a marked degree of pleomorphism.[329, 336, 356] Heffner and Gnepp found that most fibrosarcomas in the sinonasal tract are low-grade malignancies with sparse mitotic activity.[356] Hemorrhage and necrosis are generally a focal finding. Although collagen is seen interwoven with the tumor cells, its presence is not as abundant as in fibromas or fibromatosis. Immunohistochemically, the cells are positive for vimentin, and by electron microscopy they reveal features typical of fibroblasts. Some cases may reveal S-100 staining and may be regarded as low-grade malignant peripheral nerve sheath tumors.[356] This distinction has no prognostic significance.

Differential Diagnosis. Due to the low-grade malignant features of fibrosarcomas in the sinonasal tract, many of these tumors are mistakenly interpreted as benign lesions. Heffner and Gnepp[356] recommended a high level of suspicion when dealing with fibrous lesions in this region. The main differential diagnosis includes fibroma, desmoid tumor (fibromatosis), solitary fibrous tumor, spindle cell squamous carcinoma, spindle cell melanoma, and malignant fibrous histiocytoma. Fibroma and desmoid tumors are not as cellular or mitotically active as fibrosarcomas and do not exhibit a herringbone pattern. Spindle cell carcinomas and malignant fibrous histiocytomas are usually high-grade neoplasms with numerous pleomorphic cells without a herringbone pattern; furthermore, spindle cell carcinoma usually contains areas of conventional carcinoma, and epithelial markers are generally demonstrated, at least focally, by immunohistochemistry. Solitary fibrous tumor is distinguished by its characteristic hypocellular dense collagen and hypercellular areas with hemangiopericytoma-like blood vessels and its characteristic staining for CD34 and CD99.

Treatment and Prognosis. Sinonasal fibrosarcomas exhibit a good long-term prognosis. The metastatic rate is low when compared with their counterparts in other locations[329, 354, 356]; however, local recurrences are common and represent the most common cause of death in these patients. The treatment of choice for these patients is aggressive complete surgical resection. However, the recognition of the malignant nature of these tumors is often difficult and it is possible that the high recurrence rate observed is due to incomplete removal. Fifteen of the 67 (22%) patients reported by Heffner and Gnepp[356] and only one of 13 cases (8%) reported by Fu and Perzin[336] died of disease. Male sex, mitotic rate higher than 4 mitotic figures per 50 high-power fields, high histologic grade, and local failure are poor prognostic indicators.[354, 356]

Malignant Fibrous Histiocytoma

Clinical Features. Malignant fibrous histiocytoma (MFH) is the most common soft tissue sarcoma in adults[357]; however, like other soft tissue sarcomas, its occurrence in the sinonasal tract is uncommon.[329, 336, 358] MFH shows no sex predilection and most patients are in the sixth or seventh decade of life at presentation. Most patients present with advanced disease with extensive bone destruction and involvement of more than one anatomic compartment.

Pathologic Features. These are high-grade sarcomas that exhibit significant cellular atypia with pleomorphic tumor cells, frequent mitotic figures, and extensive necrosis and hemorrhage. The neoplastic cells consist of a mixture of malignant spindle and multinucleated cells with abundant pale eosinophilic cytoplasm arranged in haphazard fascicles and areas with a storiform pattern. A non-neoplastic component composed of multinucleated cells, macrophages, xanthoma cells, and inflammatory cells is occasionally seen. Immunohistochemical studies show a variable phenotype in MFH. Most are only positive for vimentin. Staining is variable for CD68, trypsin, and α_1-chemotrypsin. Foci of cells positive for muscle actin or α-smooth muscle actin are often present, indicating myofibroblastic differentiation. Relatively few sinonasal MFHs have been studied immunohistochemically.[358]

Differential Diagnosis. MFH should be distinguished from other high-grade sarcomas, particularly osteosarcomas in which adjuvant chemotherapy is part of the primary line of treatment. This distinction may be difficult in small biopsies, but radiologic findings consistent with a primary bone lesion and the lack of neoplastic osteoid formation should be helpful in establishing a definitive diagnosis. It should be kept in mind that a large proportion of craniofacial osteosarcomas are the chondroblastic type; therefore, the identification of chondroid areas should suggest the diagnosis of osteosarcoma. Other tumors that need to be excluded are spindle cell carcinoma and high-grade leiomyosarcoma. Spindle cell carcinoma or sarcomatoid carcinoma should be excluded on the basis of malignant epithelium, expression of keratin, and the presence of epithelial differentiation by electron microscopy. High-grade leiomyosarcoma shows formation of longer fascicles than MFH; in addition, it shows a fibrillary cytoplasm with perinuclear vacuoles and cigar-shaped nuclei. Staining for muscle actin, smooth muscle actin, and desmin is more diffuse and stronger in leiomyosarcoma than in MFH.

Treatment and Prognosis. The treatment of MFH is radical resection with negative surgical margins. The extent and type of surgery depends on the location and extent of the tumor and includes partial or total maxillectomy or craniofacial resection. Postoperative adjuvant radiotherapy appears to be of value in the prevention of local recurrences. There are no data supporting the use of chemotherapy in the management of these tumors. The prognosis of sinonasal MFH is poor. Three of the four patients with sinonasal MFH reported by Barnes and Kanbour[358] died of disease 4, 19, and 24 months after treatment. Tanaka et al.[359] found in their review that 7 of 23 patients died of disease and 1 was alive with tumor. Most patients died as a result of local recurrences with intracranial extension within a year of diagnosis.

Muscle Tumors

Leiomyoma and Leiomyosarcoma

The sinonasal tract is a rare site for smooth muscle neoplasms. Leiomyomas,[360, 361] leiomyoblastomas,[362] and leiomyosarcomas

have been reported at this location.[361] Leiomyosarcomas in the sinonasal tract are clinically similar to other sarcomas in this region,[329, 361, 363, 364] and their morphologic features are also similar to their soft tissue counterparts (Fig. 3–50, see p. 108).[365] They should be distinguished from other malignant spindle cell proliferations seen in this region. Immunohistochemical stains for muscle markers, smooth muscle actin, muscle specific actin, and desmin may be necessary to establish a definitive diagnosis. Desmin can be negative in some of these tumors. The proposed origin of these tumors is the smooth muscle of vessel walls.[364] Leiomyosarcomas are aggressive neoplasms characterized by local recurrences and less commonly by distant metastases. However, tumors limited to the nasal cavity appear to have a better outcome.[361, 364] Seven patients reported by Kuruvilla et al.[364] with small lesions were alive without disease after follow-up periods ranging from 9 months to 9 years. In the review by Dropkin et al.,[363] 5 of 14 patients had developed metastases. The treatment of sinonasal leiomyosarcomas is complete resection. The role of radiotherapy is controversial.[361, 363]

Rhabdomyoma

Rhabdomyomas are rare benign neoplasms of striated muscle. These tumors have a predilection for the head and neck area but their occurrence in the nasopharynx is distinctly uncommon.[366, 367] They are classified into fetal and adult types according to their histologic appearance.[368] Adult-type rhabdomyomas are composed of large round or polygonal cells with abundant eosinophilic cytoplasm containing a variable amount of lipid and glycogen, which imparts to the cells a vacuolated, "spider cell," or clear appearance. Cross striations and intracytoplasmic rod-like inclusions are frequently identified. The fetal type resembles skeletal muscle of 7 to 10 weeks' gestation. Microscopically, this type is hypercellular, often with a myxoid background, and formed by immature slender muscle fibers and primitive spindle-shaped mesenchymal cells. Although this tumor may have infiltrative borders, there is no significant pleomorphism or mitotic activity as seen in embryonal rhabdomyosarcoma. These are benign neoplasms that may have local recurrences but should not be confused with rhabdomyosarcoma to avoid aggressive treatment.

Rhabdomyosarcoma

Clinical Features. Rhabdomyosarcoma is one of the most common sinonasal malignant tumors in children,[366, 369, 370] although occasional tumors are also encountered in adults.[329, 371, 372] The mean age in the study of sinonasal rhabdomyosarcomas by Fu and Perzin was 7 years.[366] The symptoms at presentation are nonspecific and include nasal obstruction, epistaxis, and recurrent nasal polyps. Most lesions are stage III or IV at presentation and frequently show extensive bone destruction.

Pathologic Features. The diverse morphologic appearance of rhabdomyosarcoma in the extremities is also present in those occurring in the nasal cavity and sinuses.[373] Most are of the embryonal type,[366, 369, 371] although alveolar, including the solid variant (Fig. 3–51, see p. 108), and mixed embryonal-alveolar types are also seen.[366, 372, 374] Chan et al.[375] described two alveolar rhabdomyosarcomas with clear cytoplasm; this appearance was due to the accumulation of cytoplasmic glycogen (Fig. 3–52, see p. 108). Rarely, cytologic differentiation can be seen in the embryonal type following chemotherapy.[376] The diagnosis of rhabdomyosarcoma in the sinonasal tract may be confirmed by an immunohistochemical panel that includes smooth muscle actin, muscle specific actin, sarcomeric actin, desmin (Fig. 3–53A, see p. 108), and myoD1 (Fig. 3–53B), among others.

Differential Diagnosis. The differential diagnosis of rhabdomyosarcoma in the sinonasal tract, as in other sites, is broad and includes other tumors with "small round blue cells" (see Table 3–1). Ewing's sarcoma, malignant melanoma, non-Hodgkin's lymphoma, olfactory neuroblastoma, small cell neuroendocrine carcinoma, and sinonasal undifferentiated carcinoma should be distinguished based on clinical findings and careful microscopic examination.

Nonetheless, the use of an appropriate panel of antibodies, which includes actins, desmin, and myoD1, is of the utmost importance, since ancillary studies are frequently needed to establish a definitive diagnosis. Uncommonly, a myxoma may also be misinterpreted as a rhabdomyosarcoma or vice versa. Myxomas generally are hypocellular lesions with low vascularity lacking staining for muscular markers.

Treatment and Prognosis. The optimal treatment of sinonasal rhabdomyosarcoma remains elusive and controversial; however, it appears that these tumors should be treated by combined radiotherapy and chemotherapy according to the Intergroup Rhabdomyosarcoma Study (IRS) protocol.[329] Drugs utilized in this regimen include vincristine, cyclophosphamide, Adriamycin, prednisone, and DTIC.[377] Because of the significant rate of central nervous system involvement seen in sinonasal rhabdomyosarcomas, the incorporation of central nervous system prophylaxis with cranial irradiation plus intrathecal chemotherapy has been recommended for high-risk patients.[74] Owing to high failure rates, poor overall prognosis, and high morbidity, surgery appears to be limited to biopsy in most cases.[329] These tumors are highly aggressive and most patients die with local and distant disease despite multimodal therapy.[329, 378] Most patients develop local recurrences with intracranial spread. Pulmonary, bone, and lymph node metastases are also frequently seen.[74] Rhabdomyosarcoma of the paranasal sinuses, nasal cavity, and nasopharynx are considered parameningeal tumors.[369] In 274 fatal lesions reported by the IRS-I and IRS-II, parameningeal tumors constituted 20% of cases in this group, although they only represented 15% of total cases enrolled in both studies. Eleven of 16 patients reported by Fu and Perzin[366] and only 4 of 14 reported by Sercarz et al.[329] were alive with no disease.

Peripheral Nerve Sheath Tumors

Clinical Features. Schwannomas, neurofibromas, plexiform neurofibromas, and malignant peripheral nerve sheath tumors can be encountered rarely in the nasal cavity and paranasal sinuses.[379–385] Sinonasal peripheral nerve sheath tumors affect males and females equally. The age at presentation ranges from 16 to 75 years. The median age in the series by Hasegawa et al.[386] was 52 years, whereas Robitaille et al.[387] reported a mean age of 28.8 years in their literature review. Most cases have not been associated with von Recklinghausen's disease, although some have been seen in this clinical setting.[387] The symptoms at presentation are variable and depend on tumor location. Patients with lesions primarily located in the nasal cavity usually complain of nasal obstruction and epistaxis, whereas those with tumors arising in the sinuses present with headaches and facial swelling. Radiologic studies show fullness of the involved sinus (Fig. 3–54A, see p. 110) and, not uncommonly, extensive bone destruction with extension into the skull base. It is important to remember that these radiologic features are not necessarily an indication of malignancy.[383, 386, 387]

Pathologic Features. The histologic features of schwannomas and neurofibromas in this location do not differ histologically or ultrastructurally from lesions arising in other locations. Schwannomas are composed of elongated monomorphic spindle cells with poorly defined eosinophilic cytoplasm with oval nuclei with tapering ends or a buckle configuration. Cellular Antoni A and myxoid Antoni B areas with palisading are variably seen (Fig. 3–54B), although Verocay bodies are uncommon. As in other locations, nuclear atypia may be present and is not an indication of aggressive behavior. Some tumors contain clusters of foamy macrophages, granular cell change, or hypercellular areas consistent with a diagnosis of *cellular schwannoma*. Neurofibromas are unencapsulated and infiltrative. They are composed of a mixture of Schwann cells, fibroblasts, and dendritic cells surrounded by thick collagen fibers and a myxoid matrix. As in schwannomas, atypical nuclei can also be found. The diagnosis of malignant peripheral nerve sheath tumor or malignant schwannoma

is more difficult to establish. Heffner and Gnepp found it difficult to establish that distinction based on morphologic features or S-100 immunoreactivity[356] and although some of these lesions have been seen in an otherwise typical neurofibroma,[379] it is not always possible to establish an origin from a nerve or a pre-existing benign peripheral nerve tumor. In general, most malignant peripheral nerve sheath tumors are poorly differentiated and hypercellular lesions and are composed of spindle cells with hyperchromatic nuclei with frequent mitotic figures and necrosis.[356, 379, 381] Some cases have shown rhabdomyoblastic differentiation and have been designated *"malignant triton tumors."*[356, 385] Fernandez et al.[382] reported a case of a malignant epithelioid schwannoma that elicited the differential diagnosis of malignant melanoma. The diagnosis of benign peripheral nerve sheath tumors in the sinonasal tract can be confirmed by their reactivity for S-100, CD34, neurofilament, and characteristic electron microscopic findings.[383, 388]

Differential Diagnosis. The differential diagnosis of peripheral nerve neoplasms in the sinonasal tract includes solitary fibrous tumor, fibromatosis, leiomyoma, benign fibrous histiocytoma, fibrosarcoma, and other malignant soft tissue neoplasms. Malignant epithelioid schwannoma needs to be separated from malignant melanoma. The differential expression of S-100 and HMB45 should allow differentiation between these two lesions. Although solitary fibrous tumor shares with peripheral nerve sheath tumors the expression of CD34, they also have hypocellular and hypercellular areas with a pattern-less appearance, storiform areas, and hemangiopericytoma-like vessels with *bcl-2* and CD99 immunoreactivity that is not seen in nerve sheath tumors. Furthermore, they are negative for S-100. The differential expression of S-100, desmin, and actins should allow differentiation between smooth muscle tumors and peripheral nerve sheath tumors. Occasionally, low-grade malignant schwannomas may be difficult to distinguish from fibrosarcomas; however, this distinction does not appear to be clinically significant.[356]

Treatment and Prognosis. The treatment of sinonasal peripheral nerve sheath tumors is complete surgical resection. If technically possible, an en bloc resection should be recommended; in some cases this requires a partial or total maxillectomy or a craniofacial resection, particularly in patients with neurofibroma or extensive bone involvement. Adjuvant radiotherapy appears to improve local control in cases of malignant tumors.[381, 384] Schwannomas and neurofibromas are benign lesions that only rarely show local recurrences and have an excellent prognosis.[379, 386, 387] Seven of eight benign tumors reported by Perzin et al.[379] showed no recurrences, and one recurrent lesion showed no radiologic evidence of progression. None of the four tumors with follow-up described by Hasegawa et al.[386] recurred after "piecemeal" resection only. The prognosis of malignant peripheral tumors in the sinonasal tract is more guarded and depends on the extent of disease, completeness of resection and use of adjuvant therapy, and grade of the tumor. In the combined experience of Perzin et al.,[379] Robitaille et al.,[387] and Fernandez et al.[382] of six patients with malignant tumors, three had died of disease, one was alive with recurrent tumor, one had no recurrences, and one was lost to follow-up. Four additional patients described in different reports[381, 384, 385, 389] were alive 3, 3, 11, and 3 years after treatment. Three of these patients received adjuvant radiotherapy. Most recurrences are seen within the first year after diagnosis.

Adipose Tissue Tumors

Although adipose tissue neoplasms represent one of the most common lesions of soft tissue, lipoma and liposarcoma are extremely uncommon in the sinonasal tract.[390] A myxoid liposarcoma arising in a 67-year-old woman was described by Fu and Perzin[390] in their review of nonepithelial neoplasms of the sinonasal tract. This lesion recurred locally, invaded the middle cranial fossa, and caused the patient's death.

∎ MISCELLANEOUS TUMORS

Meningioma

Clinical Features. Approximately 3% of all meningiomas secondarily involve the sinonasal tract[391]; however, there are rare primary nasal or paranasal tumors (Fig. 3–55, see p. 110).[392–395] As in other locations, there is a female predilection. Unlike primary intracranial lesions, a disproportionate number of tumors have been reported in younger patients. The mean age in the review by Ho[393] was 28 years. The most common symptoms are nasal obstruction, epistaxis, and exophthalmos. Some lesions may simulate a nasal polyp. The sphenoid sinus is the most common site of involvement.

Pathologic Features. Most meningiomas in the sinonasal tract are of the meningothelial or transitional type.[392, 396, 397] They consist of tumor cells with a syncytial appearance arranged in whorls, sheets, or broad bands with variable numbers of psammoma bodies. The cytoplasm is moderate to abundant with indistinct cell membranes (Fig. 3–56). The nuclei tend to be uniform with little pleomorphism and may exhibit nuclear pseudoinclusions. Bone invasion is frequent. Rare primary sinonasal fibroblastic meningiomas have also been described. Cases with mitotic activity and frank malignant histologic features have been described.[394, 395] Sadar et al.[395] reported a case of "angioblastic meningioma," which nowadays would have been classified as malignant hemangiopericytoma.

Differential Diagnosis. The differential diagnosis of meningioma in the sinonasal tract includes poorly differentiated carcinoma, malignant melanoma, and olfactory neuroblastoma. Identification of the typical cytologic features of meningioma, the absence of fibrillary stroma, the lack of significant cellular atypia and necrosis, and the lack of staining for keratins, S-100, HMB-45, and neuroendocrine markers are helpful in establishing a definitive diagnosis.

Treatment and Prognosis. Meningiomas are benign tumors, and complete local resection is curative. In the 19 cases reviewed by Ho,[393] no recurrences or deaths due to tumor were found. Nonetheless, they may exhibit recurrences and aggressive local behavior, and occasionally, owing to their location, complete resection may be difficult to achieve.[392] Two cases of frankly malignant sinonasal meningiomas causing patient death were described by Sadar et al.[395] Meningiomas do not seem to respond well to radiotherapy; however, postoperative radiation may be used as adjuvant therapy in incompletely resected tumors.

Sinonasal Ameloblastoma

Clinical Features. Primary sinonasal ameloblastomas are extremely rare with a dearth of case reports. The largest series reported consists of 24 cases seen at the Armed Forces Institute of Pathology during a period of 30 years.[398] Most patients are males and the mean age at diagnosis is 59.7 years. The most common symptom is that of a rapidly enlarging mass in the maxillary sinus or nasal cavity. Approximately one third of patients have sinusitis or epistaxis.

Pathologic Features. The histopathologic appearance of sinonasal ameloblastomas is similar to their gnathic counterparts. By far the most common is the plexiform type characterized by a network of anastomosing cords of odontogenic epithelium surrounded by a loose, myxomatous reticulum-like stroma. The tumor strands and cords are composed of columnar epithelium with hyperchromatic nuclei with reversed polarization and subnuclear cytoplasmic vacuolization. The acanthomatous pattern is less commonly seen and consists of epithelial islands showing squamous metaplasia and keratin pearl formation. Occasionally sinonasal ameloblastomas have a follicular pattern closely resembling enamel organ epithelium. Cytologic atypia is absent in sinonasal ameloblastomas.

Differential Diagnosis. The main differential diagnoses of sinonasal ameloblastoma is nasal extension of a gnathic tumor and a craniopharyngioma. Before establishing the diagnosis of a primary sinonasal ameloblastoma, the presence of a gnathic lesion should be excluded. Ameloblastomas lack the cyst formation, degenerative changes, calcifications, and cholesterol clefts of craniopharyngioma.

Treatment and Prognosis. Complete surgical resection is the treatment of choice. The type and extent of surgery is determined individually and dictated by tumor volume and structures involved. Some patients may require partial or radical maxillectomy. The prognosis of sinonasal ameloblastoma is excellent; however, local recurrences are seen in approximately 20% of patients, some of whom may have multiple recurrences. Most recurrences are seen within 24 months after the initial excision. No deaths due to tumor have been reported.

Ectopic Pituitary Adenoma

Clinical Features. The sphenoid sinus and bone is the most common location of ectopic pituitary adenomas.[399, 400] These lesions are generally considered to arise from the "pharyngeal pitu-

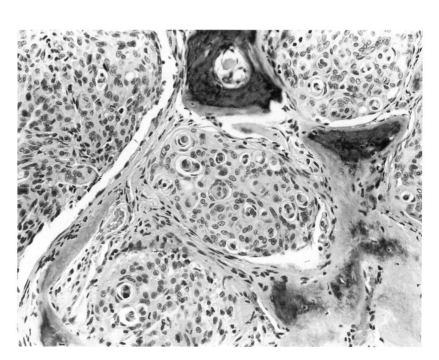

Figure 3–56. Invasive meningioma of the maxillary sinus. Note the characteristic whorls infiltrating bone.

itary gland." Remnants of embryonic adenohypophysis may be found along the path of the developing Rathke's cleft, and these remnants are known to contain all the hormone-producing cells found in the normal gland.[401] The so-called "pharyngeal pituitary gland" is found in the body of the sphenoid bone in over 90% of adults in autopsy studies.[402] Females are affected twice as often as males and more than 58% of patients have evidence of hormone hyperactivity. Patients with ectopic pituitary adenomas in the sinonasal tract may present with headaches, epistaxis, Cushing's disease, acromegaly, or hyperparathyroidism.[399, 401] Some lesions present as nasal polyps.[403]

Pathologic Features. Most of these lesions display a similar histologic appearance to those located in the sella turcica.[401] They have an endocrine architecture with nests, ribbons, trabeculae, papillae, and rosettes surrounded by a delicate vascular network. Most are of the chromophobe cell type.[399, 400, 402, 404] When studied by immunohistochemistry, the majority have been tumors that produce prolactin or growth hormone.

Differential Diagnosis. Sinonasal pituitary adenomas should be distinguished from pituitary adenomas extending from the sella turcica, neuroendocrine and sinonasal undifferentiated carcinoma, olfactory neuroblastoma, paraganglioma, and carcinoid tumor. Awareness of the existence of these lesions in ectopic locations and clinicopathologic correlation, particularly endocrine function and radiologic studies, are essential in arriving at a correct diagnosis. Immunohistochemical stains including hormonal markers are necessary to establish a definitive diagnosis. Although pituitary adenomas may show some significant nuclear atypia, they do not have the degree of cellular pleomorphism, mitotic activity, and necrosis that characterize small cell neuroendocrine carcinoma and sinonasal undifferentiated carcinoma. They can be distinguished from olfactory neuroblastoma by the absence of fibrillary stroma and their consistent expression of keratin and specific pituitary hormones.

Treatment and Prognosis. Complete surgical removal is the treatment for ectopic pituitary adenoma. In large, invasive lesions this goal may not be achieved. For incompletely resected tumors, postoperative radiation is indicated.[399, 403] Dopamine-agonist drugs such as bromocriptine are effective in reducing the size of pituitary adenomas, especially prolactinomas. The prognosis of patients with these lesions is good. Lloyd et al.[400] reported that 4 of 11 patients were cured by surgery alone or surgery followed by radiotherapy. Four patients died less than 1 year after surgery of unrelated causes or due to hormonal insufficiency.[404] All three patients reported by Luk et al.[403] were alive after surgery alone or surgery followed by radiotherapy.

Craniopharyngioma

Craniopharyngiomas are complex benign epithelial neoplasms most commonly seen in the sellar and third ventricle regions. Their proposed origin is the obliterated craniopharyngeal duct of Rathke's pouch, although origin from misplaced odontogenic epithelium has also been proposed.[405] Rarely, craniopharyngiomas arise in the nasopharynx and extend to the nasal cavity and sphenoid sinuses.[406, 407] The microscopic appearance of nasopharyngeal tumors has been similar to that of sellar adamantinomatous craniopharyngiomas with their epithelial lobules, peripheral palisading, and internally loose epithelial cells reminiscent of "stellate reticulum." Most lesions also have squamous metaplasia and cysts filled with keratin. These lesions are extremely uncommon in this location and should not be confused with a well-differentiated squamous cell carcinoma. A high index of suspicion is necessary to make the diagnosis if one is ever faced with this lesion.

Teratomas and Other Germ Cell Tumors

Rarely, the sinonasal tract and the nasopharynx are the setting for teratomas and other germ cell tumors.[408, 409] Most of the reported cases have occurred in children and are often congenital,[408–412] but they have also been described in older adults.[413] Most patients have nasal obstruction and a mass at presentation.

Teratomas in the sinonasal tract and nasopharynx are composed of a mixture of mature and immature ectodermal, mesodermal, and endodermal elements as seen in gonadal lesions.[414] Given the intrinsic difficulty of distinguishing immature cell elements in a teratoma from malignancy, we believe that it is advisable to approach these uncommon lesions in a similar manner to gonadal lesions and to classify them into mature and immature groups.[415] Most cases reported in children have been mature teratomas.[410, 411] Petrovich et al.[413] reported a case of a left nasal "malignant" teratoma in a 63-year-old male that seems to represent an immature teratoma with papillary areas reminiscent of a yolk sac tumor.

Examples of yolk sac tumor involving the nasopharynx have also been reported.[409, 410] These are aggressive neoplasms characterized by the presence of Schiller-Duval bodies admixed with papillae, tubules, microcysts and macrocysts, and sheets of primitive cells with a myxomatous background and deposits of eosinophilic basement material as well as periodic acid-Schiff–positive hyaline droplets. Immunohistochemically, the tumor cells are positive for alfa-fetoprotein.[409, 410] In the case reported by Byard et al.,[410] the tumor arose 3 years after excision of a congenital mature teratoma.

The differential diagnosis of germ cell tumors in the sinonasal region and nasopharynx is complex and depends on the tissues seen in the surgical material. Mature teratoma should be distinguished from nasal "glioma" or a meningocele. The latter entities probably represent developmental defects of the craniofacial skeleton and do not contain elements other than glia. Olfactory neuroblastoma and rhabdomyosarcoma may resemble the neuroepithelium or the mesenchyme of immature teratoma but lack other neoplastic elements. Yolk sac tumor should be separated from poorly differentiated adenocarcinoma. Extensive sampling and identification of tissues arising from all three germinal layers are the keys for a diagnosis of teratoma. Yolk sac tumor can be distinguished by the array of architectural patterns present in the tumor and the characteristic Schiller-Duval bodies in addition to positive staining for alpha-fetoprotein. The morphologic differentiation of malignant teratomas from teratocarcinosarcomas and nasal blastomas is difficult and subjective, and it is likely that most of the reported cases of malignant or immature teratomas in adults represent examples of teratocarcinosarcomas.[415] The treatment of sinonasal germ cell neoplasms is complete surgical resection. The prognosis of teratomas in children is extremely favorable and they generally do not require adjuvant chemotherapy or radiotherapy. It is important to recognize areas of yolk sac, since these tumors are aggressive and require adjuvant cisplatin chemotherapy for adequate management.

Teratocarcinosarcoma

Clinical Features. This unique neoplasm is extremely uncommon. It shows a male predominance and affects adults with an age range of 18 to 79 and mean age of 60 years.[416–419] The most common symptoms at presentation are nasal obstruction and epistaxis. Only a few patients complain of pain or proptosis. Radiologic studies generally show a nasal mass with bone destruction and extension into ethmoidal or maxillary sinuses.

Pathologic Features. Grossly, the tumors may have a polypoid appearance and are friable and hemorrhagic.[416, 418] Histologically, they are characterized by a heterogeneous combination of epithelial and mesenchymal elements. The epithelial components are composed of a mixture of clear cell nonkeratinizing epithelium (Fig. 3–57A, see p. 111), squamous epithelium without clear cell elements, squamous cell carcinoma, and benign, atypical, or clearly malignant glandular elements. Immature neuroepithelial tissue (Fig. 3–57B) resembling olfactory neuroblastoma with rosette formation and ganglion and glial differentiation is also present.[420] The mesenchymal tissues also have a variable appearance with areas of nonspecific myxomatous tissue, cellular areas of benign and malignant-appearing fibroblasts, and smooth muscle admixed with foci of rhabdomyosarcoma, chondrosarcoma, or fetal cartilage.[416–418] Unlike gonadal or extragonadal germ cell tumors, there are no areas of seminoma, yolk sac tumor, or choriocarcinoma.[419]

The immunohistochemical findings are dependent on the areas studied.[417, 420] The primitive neuroepithelial tissue may be positive for CD99 (O13/MIC2), neuron specific enolase, synaptophysin, and chromogranin. Keratin and rarely alpha-fetoprotein may also be seen in the neuroepithelial component. S-100 and glial fibrillary acidic protein are expressed by those areas with glial differentiation. Epithelial membrane antigen and keratin are seen in the epithelial elements. Desmin and myoglobulin are positive in the sarcomatous area with rhabdomyoblastic differentiation.

Differential Diagnosis. The distinction of teratocarcinosarcomas from nasal blastomas and malignant teratomas is tenuous and controversial. These tumors are regarded by some authors as similar, if not related, entities.[416, 417] The differential diagnosis of these uncommon lesions is broad and includes squamous cell carcinoma, sarcomatoid carcinoma, adenocarcinoma, olfactory neuroblastoma, craniopharyngioma, and other sarcomas. The histologic complexity of teratocarcinosarcomas and the presence of mixed epithelial and mesenchymal elements should suggest the diagnosis. A definitive diagnosis may not be possible in small biopsies.

Treatment and Prognosis. The average survival is less than 2 years. Approximately 67% of patients with adequate follow-up developed uncontrollable local recurrences and 35% developed metastases to cervical nodes. Some patients have prolonged survival periods.[416, 418]

Nasal Blastoma

Nasal blastomas rare malignant neoplasms with controversial morphology and histogenesis. The relationship of nasal blastoma with and its differentiation from teratocarcinosarcomas and carcinosarcomas of the sinonasal tact are still controversial; they probably represent the same pathologic entities. There have been only isolated reports of these lesions.[421–423] Microscopically, nasal blastomas are composed of a mixture of primitive epithelial and mesenchymal elements resembling fetal lung. The epithelial component consists of poorly developed glands and squamous epithelium. The stroma is formed by a variable mixture of malignant myxoid, chondromyxoid, fibrous, and muscular tissues.[421, 422] Distinction of blastoma from immature teratoma is difficult and often impossible. Clinically, they are distinguished from teratoma by the older age at first occurrence and morphologically by the absence of ectodermal and endodermal components. Nasal blastoma may be regarded as a type of carcinosarcoma. The treatment and prognosis are similar to those of teratocarcinosarcoma.

Alveolar Soft Part Sarcoma

A case of alveolar soft part sarcoma involving the left nasal cavity and maxillary sinus was reported in a 21-year-old female by Chatter et al.[424] The mass decreased in size after radiotherapy, but the patient had persistent disease at last follow-up. The tumor had initially been diagnosed as clear cell carcinoma.

Post-radiation Malignant Tumors

Therapeutic irradiation of primary lesions of the head and neck can rarely be complicated by the development of secondary sarcomas[425–427] in the sinonasal tract. Clinically, most patients present with nasal obstruction, epistaxis, and facial pain. The interval from radiation treatment to the development of the secondary malignancies has ranged from 3.5 to 30 years,[427] with a median latency period of 10 years.[425, 426]

▍ LYMPHOPLASMACYTIC TUMORS

Primary sinonasal and nasopharyngeal non-Hodgkin's lymphomas (NHLs) are uncommon in North America. NHLs of the sinonasal region have been the subject of numerous studies; however, a clear understanding of their morphologic spectrum and behavior has been complicated by their rarity and by the use of outdated terminology and various classification systems. In recent years, evolving concepts in cell differentiation of lymphoid neoplasms and the development of sophisticated techniques in immunohistochemistry and molecular biology are rapidly changing our understanding of these neoplasms and are facilitating their diagnosis and classification. For practical reasons and recognizing the existence of overlapping clinical and pathologic features in both groups, we have divided this section in those cases that can be readily classified using the terminology of the International Working Formulation[428] and those cases that have been reported in the past few years as sinonasal T cell natural killer cell lymphomas.[429]

Malignant Non-Hodgkin's Lymphoma

Clinical Features. The clinical symptoms at presentation are nonspecific and consist of nasal obstruction, epistaxis, rhinorrhea, and the presence of a mass.[430–433] The mean age at presentation has ranged from 59 to 70 years, with the vast majority of patients in their sixth or seventh decades of life. Most tumors are locally advanced at presentation, with frequent bone destruction and extension into adjacent sinuses, nasopharynx, or palate.

Pathologic Features. The most common histologic types are diffuse large cell and diffuse large cell immunoblastic type.[430–434] Diffuse small noncleaved, Burkitt's and non-Burkitt's types are frequent in the nasopharynx of children.[434–436] Small lymphocytic, small cleaved cell, and monocytoid B-cell type have been described in this location, although they are distinctly uncommon.[431, 432, 434] The majority of sinonasal lymphomas included in this group are B cell type.

Differential Diagnosis. The diagnosis and classification of lymphomas in the sinonasal region should be based on the same parameters used in other locations. An adequate biopsy with good cell preservation is of utmost importance. The differential diagnosis of NHL includes sinonasal undifferentiated carcinoma, small cell carcinoma, olfactory neuroblastoma, rhabdomyosarcoma, malignant melanoma, and nasopharyngeal carcinoma. Close attention to architectural and cytologic details and the use of an immunohistochemical panel that includes epithelial, lymphoid, muscular, and melanocytic markers is necessary to establish a definitive diagnosis.

Treatment and Prognosis. The treatment of choice for sinonasal NHL is radiotherapy for control of local disease with or without chemotherapy, depending on the histologic type of lymphoma and the stage of the disease. The survival rate in general is poor and has ranged from 55% to 17% at 5 years, depending on the stage of the disease and histologic type.[430, 432, 433] Most patients who died of disease developed systemic relapses.[430, 433, 434] The median survival for patients with diffuse large cell lymphoma is less than 1 year.[430, 431]

Sinonasal T Cell and Natural Killer Cell Lymphoma (Angiocentric Lymphoma, Polymorphic Reticulosis)

Clinical Features. The nature of this group of neoplasms remains controversial[429]; however, large advances have been made in the understanding of their behavior, morphologic appearance, and molecular biology. Numerous terms have been used to describe the clinical and pathologic features of these lesions; among those are *lethal midline granuloma*,[437, 438] *midline malignant reticulosis*,[439] *lymphomatoid granulomatosis, angiocentric peripheral T-cell lymphoma,*[440, 441] and *angiocentric lymphoproliferative lesion.*[442] Recent studies indicate that these tumors represent a distinctive group of malignant lymphomas with a T-cell/natural killer cell (T/NK-cell) phenotype.[429, 437, 443–446] We believe that the term *polymorphic reticulosis* should be avoided as a diagnostic term and that an effort should be made to establish a precise pathologic diagnosis with the help of immunohistochemical and molecular pathology studies.

This tumor is most commonly seen in Asia and an increased incidence has also been described in Latin American countries such as Mexico, Guatemala, and Peru.[447–449] T/NK-cell sinonasal lymphoma has a strong association with Epstein-Barr virus (EBV) infection and the presence of EBER-1, EBER-2, and, less commonly, LMP-1 has been identified in the neoplastic lymphoid cells.[437, 450–453] Mutations of the *EBV-LMP-1* gene have been found in 26% of T/NK sinonasal lymphomas in Mexico City; however, this study also found a similar proportion of mutations in reactive tonsils of healthy control subjects.[454] Sinonasal T/NK lymphoma in this study was most commonly associated with EBV strain A.[454]

Sinonasal T/NK-cell lymphomas are most frequently seen in males, with a male:female ratio of 2:1 to 3:1. The age of presentation ranges from 13 to 80 years, with a mean age of approximately 45 years in most series.[251, 441, 444, 449, 455, 456] Common symptoms are nasal obstruction, epistaxis, rhinorrhea, and the presence of an ulcerated nasal mass, frequently with extension to paranasal sinuses and palate. Bone destruction may also be present. Approximately 50% to 60% of patients have localized disease at presentation and 25% may have involvement of cervical lymph nodes, skin, bone marrow, spleen or liver, or other extranodal sites.[441, 455, 456]

Pathologic Features. Nasal or nasopharyngeal T/NK-cell lymphomas exhibit a broad morphologic spectrum, the hallmark being the presence of a polymorphic cellular infiltrate composed of atypical lymphoid cells admixed with a variable number of plasma cells, small lymphocytes, histiocytes, eosinophils, and neutrophils. The atypical cells vary in number, cell size, and cytologic atypia. In some cases, the neoplastic lymphoid cells are small to intermediate in size and possess dark, twisted hyperchromatic nuclei with irregular contours (Fig. 3–58, see p. 111). In other cases, the cells are large with abundant pale to clear cytoplasm and exhibit large nuclei with prominent nucleoli (Fig. 3–59, see p. 112). Giemsa-stained cytologic preparations from involved lymph nodes or peripheral blood have revealed azurophilic cytoplasmic granules.[457] The distribution of the neoplastic cells in the tissue is irregular and may vary from field to field, and in some instances they may be obscured by the reactive inflammatory cells. Most cases show prominent angiocentricity with infiltration and destruction of the vessel wall (Fig. 3–60, see p. 112). Although this feature is characteristic of T/NK-cell lymphomas, its presence is not required for the diagnosis. Necrosis is almost invariably present in all cases of sinonasal T/NK-cell lymphoma, and recently it was proposed that the extensive apoptosis seen in these neoplasms is due to the cytolytic effects of cytolytic granular proteins perforin, TIA-1, and granzymes.[454, 458, 459] Often, it has a zonal distribution and is accompanied by extensive mucosal ulceration and destruction of cartilage or bone. The presence of granulomas and multinucleated giant cells is not a feature of these tumors.

The immunophenotype of T/NK-cell lymphomas is characteristic. The tumor cells are positive for the NK-cell marker CD56 (neural cell adhesion molecule, N-CAM) but are generally negative for other NK-cell markers such as CD57 and CD16.[460, 461] They are also positive for CD2, CD45RO, and CD43. CD3 is negative in frozen tissue sections but it may be seen in the tumor cell cytoplasm in paraffin-embedded tissues.[440, 456, 462, 463] CD4, CD5, CD7, CD8, βF1, and TRCδ are generally negative, although occasional tumors may show expression of some of these T-cell markers.[437, 440, 443, 444, 456, 460] As expected, all B-cell markers are negative. Staining for granzyme B, an antibody-detecting cytoplasmic cytotoxic granule, and the expression of perforin and *TIA*-1 appear to be specific for these tumors.[454, 456] Most gene rearrangement studies have shown a germline configuration for the *TCR*-α, -β, -γ, and

-δ genes,[461] although some cases have demonstrated rearrangement of some of these genes.[443, 452, 460, 462]

Differential Diagnosis. The differential diagnosis of nasal T/NK-cell lymphomas includes sinonasal infections, especially fungal infections, Wegener's granulomatosis, other NHLs, and idiopathic midline destructive disease. The diagnosis of these neoplasms requires a high index of suspicion and rests on a combination of clinicopathologic findings, microbiologic cultures, characteristic immunophenotype, and, when necessary, molecular pathology analysis. The presence of a polymorphic lymphoid infiltrate with variable degrees of cytologic atypia, angioinvasion, and necrosis should strongly suggest a diagnosis of sinonasal T/NK-cell lymphoma, especially in patients with no serum antineutrophilic cytoplasmic antibodies (ANCA) and no evidence of pulmonary or renal abnormalities.

Treatment and Prognosis. Traditionally, the prognosis of sinonasal T/NK-cell lymphomas has been poor, with many patients dying of disease within 2 years of diagnosis.[439, 464–466] Recent studies suggest, however, that patients with localized disease may respond well to aggressive radiotherapy or combined chemotherapy, or both. In the study by Liang et al.,[455] 78% of patients with stage I-II disease had a 78% response, although their disease-free survival rate at 5 years was only 60%. The 5-year survival rate for patients with stage III-IV disease was 17%. The 5-year and 15-year survival rates reported by Strickler et al.[446] were 63% and 50%, whereas Ho et al.[441] reported a 5-year survival rate of 64% in patients with *polymorphic reticulosis.* Most studies indicate that radiotherapy with or without chemotherapy is superior to chemotherapy alone as the initial treatment for sinonasal T/NK-cell lymphomas.[446, 455, 456] The combination of cyclophosphamide, doxorubicin, vincristine, and prednisone (CHOP) has been the most commonly used chemotherapy regimen. Patients with recurrent disease may be treated with combined therapy or chemotherapy alone. Involvement of central nervous system, skin, or lung or systemic involvement is common in patients who fail therapy. A hemophagocytic syndrome is a common complication that adversely affects survival.

Plasmacytoma

Clinical Features. Extramedullary plasmacytomas are uncommon, representing 5.7% of all plasmacytomas.[467] Approximately 90% of them occur in the head and neck, the sinonasal tract being involved in approximately 75% of these cases. Sinonasal plasmacytomas most commonly affect males in their sixth and seventh decades of life.[467–469] The symptoms at presentation are nonspecific and include unilateral nasal obstruction, rhinorrhea, epistaxis, and facial pain. The finding of Bence-Jones protein in urine is distinctly uncommon in the absence of disseminated disease.

Pathologic Features. Extramedullary plasmacytomas are composed of plasma cells with a diffuse pattern of infiltration and variable degrees of differentiation (Fig. 3–61, see p. 112). In well-differentiated tumors, the neoplastic cells closely resemble mature plasma cells, although occasional mitotic figures can be seen. In moderately or poorly differentiated neoplasms, the cells are more pleomorphic and show a significant degree of atypia with frequent mitotic figures, large vesicular nuclei with coarse chromatin, and often prominent nucleoli (Fig. 3–62A, see p. 113). Binucleated atypical plasma cells are common in poorly differentiated lesions. The high-grade tumors may closely resemble immunoblastic large cell lymphomas. Most lesions show a monotypic pattern of staining, usually for κ light chain (Fig. 3–62B).

Differential Diagnosis. The differential diagnosis of sinonasal plasmacytoma varies according to the degree of differentiation of the neoplasm. Well-differentiated tumors need to be distinguished from plasma cell granuloma, reactive plasmacytosis, and small lymphocytic lymphoma, plasmacytic, or plasmacytoid types. Plasma cell granuloma can be excluded by the absence of other inflammatory cell types and Russell's bodies. Reactive plasmacytosis is characterized by a polytypic immunoglobulin expression and numerous Russell's bodies. Unlike plasmacytomas, NHLs with plasmacytoid or plasmacytic differentiation express CD20, CD45RB, and other lymphoid markers. Plasma cells express epithelial membrane antigen and CD38.

Poorly differentiated lesions should be differentiated from immunoblastic large cell lymphoma, granulocytic sarcoma, malignant melanoma, and poorly differentiated carcinomas. The systematic use of an antibody panel including keratins, epithelial membrane antigen, lymphoid markers and immunoglobulins, S-100, and HMB-45 should be useful in establishing a definite diagnosis.

Treatment and Prognosis. The treatment of solitary plasmacytomas of the sinonasal tract is radiotherapy with doses of 30 Gy. Large lesions may require surgical debulking. Extramedullary plasmacytomas may follow one of several clinical courses. Most patients have localized disease and are cured by surgery and radiotherapy. In a second group, the disease may recur locally after initial therapy but can be controlled with good long-term prognosis. A third group will succumb to local tumor recurrences or to disseminated disease. Classic multiple myeloma develops in 30% to 50% of patients sometimes decades after the initial diagnosis. The 5-year survival rate has ranged from 30% to 70%.[467, 469]

METASTATIC TUMORS

Clinical Features. Metastatic involvement of the sinonasal tract is rare.[470, 471] The most common malignancies that secondarily involve the sinonasal tract are kidney, lung, and breast.[470] Other tumors that may occasionally metastasize to the nasal cavity and sinuses are malignant melanoma and carcinomas of thyroid, pancreas, prostate, stomach, colon and rectum, testis, and adrenal gland. In most instances, metastases to the sinonasal tract are a manifestation of disseminated disease; however, a sinonasal metastasis has been the initial presentation of carcinomas from the gastrointestinal tract, lung, liver, kidney, and thyroid.[189, 203, 472-474] Clinically, most patients will present with facial pain and swelling of variable duration. Other symptoms include nasal obstruction, epistaxis, and enlarged cervical lymph nodes.

Pathologic Features. Renal cell carcinoma in the sinonasal tract maintains its characteristic morphology of medium-sized or large clear cells arranged in nests or sheets surrounded by thin-walled blood vessels. Unlike the clear cells of carcinomas of other sites, the cytoplasm in renal cell carcinomas does not have a vacuolated, granular, or pale eosinophilic appearance; instead, it is truly clear and often appears "empty" under light microscopy. The main differential diagnoses of renal cell carcinoma in the sinonasal tract are mucoepidermoid carcinoma and acinic cell carcinoma. In most instances, adequate sampling will solve this quandary, since these neoplasms are only rarely entirely composed of clear cells.[475] Renal cell carcinoma does not contain the typical epidermoid or intermediate cells of mucoepidermoid carcinoma. The presence of mucous cells is also helpful in establishing the correct diagnosis. In those rare cases in which no diagnostic cells are present, electron microscopy may be helpful, since renal cell carcinoma contains fat, which should be absent in mucoepidermoid carcinoma. Clear cells are seen in only 6% of acinic cell carcinomas.[475] The presence of other cell types, particularly acinar cells with their characteristic periodic acid Schiff–diastase resistant granules should exclude the diagnosis of metastatic renal cell carcinoma.

There are no reliable morphologic features that allow distinction between metastatic colorectal carcinomas and moderately differentiated sinonasal intestinal type adenocarcinomas. In this situation, correlation with medical history and clinical findings, including colonoscopy, is necessary to establish the correct diagnosis. Well-differentiated, intestinal-type adenocarcinomas are, in most cases, primary sinonasal tumors, since these lesions resemble normal intestinal mucosa or villous adenomas. Intestinal lesions with this mor-

phology do not have metastatic potential. Nonetheless, close attention to morphologic findings and correlation with clinical findings is still necessary to exclude a metastatic neoplasm.

The main differential diagnosis of other metastatic adenocarcinomas such as lung, breast, thyroid, pancreas, prostate, and stomach is mainly a poorly differentiated sinonasal intestinal-type adenocarcinoma. In this setting, the use of antibodies for thyroglobulin and prostatic specific antigen may be useful to exclude a metastasis from those sites. The differential expression of keratins such as CK7 and CK20 in sinonasal adenocarcinomas and secondary carcinomas has not been investigated.

Treatment and Prognosis. Metastatic involvement of the sinonasal tract is in most cases evidence of advanced disease and is associated with a dismal prognosis.[470] Two thirds of patients generally die within 1 year of diagnosis and less than 10% survive 5 years. Given the bleak prognosis of these patients and the disseminated nature of their disease, no radical treatment appears warranted. However, palliative treatment with radiotherapy with or without surgery may help control local disease and pain. Radiotherapy with or without surgery has also been reported to prolong life in some cases. According to Harrison and Lund,[470] craniofacial resection offers excellent palliation without significant morbidity.

REFERENCES

Anatomy and Histology

1. Barnes L, Johnson JT: Pathologic and clinical considerations in the evaluation of major head and neck specimens resected for cancer. *Pathol Annu* 1986;21:175–250.
2. Walike JW: Anatomy of the nasal cavities. *Otolaryngol Clin North Am* 1973;6:609–621.
3. Wenig BM: Nasal cavity and paranasal sinuses. In Wenig BM: *Atlas of Head and Neck Pathology.* Philadelphia: W.B. Saunders, 1993:3–95.
4. Nakashima T, Kimmelman CP, Snow GB: Structure of the human fetal and adult olfactory neuroepithelium. *Arch Otolaryngol* 1984;110:641–646.
5. Wenig BM: Anatomy and histology of the oral cavity, nasopharynx, and neck. In: *Atlas of Head and Neck Pathology.* Philadelphia: W.B. Saunders, 1993:101–102.
6. Fechner RE, Mills SE: Larynx and pharynx. In Sternberg SS (ed): *Histology for Pathologists.* New York: Raven Press, 1992:443–455.
7. Erlandson RA: Oncocytes in the nasopharynx. *Arch Otolaryngol* 1977;103:175–178.
8. Benke TT, Zitsch RP, Nashelsky MB: Bilateral oncocytic cysts of the nasopharynx. *Otolaryngol Head Neck Surg* 1995;112:321–324.
9. Shek TWH, Lu ISC, Nichols JM, et al.: Melanotic oncocytic metaplasia of the nasopharynx. *Histopathology* 1996;26:273–275.

Rhinitis and Sinusitis

10. Marks SC, Upadhyay S, Crane L: Cytomegalovirus sinusitis: A new manifestation of AIDS. *Arch Otolaryngol Head Neck Surg* 1996;122:789–791.
11. Milczuk HA, Dalley RW, Wessbacher FW, et al.: Nasal and paranasal sinus abnormalities in children with chronic sinusitis. *Laryngoscope* 1993;103:247–252.
12. Zamboni L: Clinical relevance of evaluation of sperm and ova. In Kraus FT, Damjanov I (eds): *Pathology of Reproductive Failure.* Baltimore: Williams & Wilkins, 1991:10–31.
13. Robson AM, Smallman LA, Gregory J, et al.: Ciliary ultrastructure in nasal brushings. *Cytopathology* 1993;4:149–159.
14. Armengot M, Juan G, Barona R, et al.: Immotile cilia syndrome: Nasal mucociliary function and nasal ciliary abnormalities. *Rhinology* 1994;32:109–111.

Mucous Impaction

15. Hyams VJ: Unusual tumors and lesions. In Gnepp DR (ed): *Pathology of the Head and Neck: Contemporary Issues in Surgical Pathology.* New York: Churchill Livingstone, 1988;459–495.

Sinonasal Inflammatory Polyps

16. Jankowski R: Eosinophils in the pathophysiology of nasal polyps. *Acta Otolaryngol (Stockh)* 1996;116:160–163.
17. Petruson B, Hansson HA, Petruson K: Insulin-like growth factor I is a possible pathogenic mechanism in nasal polyps. *Acta Otolaryngol (Stockh)* 1988;106:156–160.
18. Hao SP, Chang C-N, Chen H-C: Transtubal nasal polyposis masquerading as a skull base malignancy. *Otolaryngol Head Neck Surg* 1996;115:556–559.
19. Winestock DP, Bartlett PC, Sondheimer FK: Benign nasal polyps causing bone destruction in the nasal cavity and paranasal sinuses. *Laryngoscope* 1978;88:675–679.
20. Yazbak PA, Phillips JM, Ball PA, et al.: Benign nasal polyposis presenting as an intracranial mass: Case report. *Surg Neurol* 1991;36:380–383.
21. Heck WE, Hallberg OE, Williams HL: Antrochoanal polyp. *Arch Otolaryngol* 1950;52:538–548.
22. Ryan RE, Neel HB: Antrochoanal polyps. *J Otolaryngol* 1979;8:344–346.
23. Cook PR, Davis WE, McDonald R, et al.: Antrochoanal polyposis: A review of 33 cases. *Ear Nose Throat J* 1993;72:401–410.
24. Berg O, Carenfelt C, Silversward C: Origin of the choanal polyp. *Arch Otolaryngol Head Neck Surg* 1988;114:1270–1271.
25. Chen JM, Scholoss MD, Azouz ME: Antrochoanal polyp: A 10-year retrospective study in the pediatric population with a review of the literature. *J Otolaryngol* 1989;18:160–172.
26. Tos M, Morgensen C: Mucous glands in nasal polyps. *Arch Otolaryngol* 1977;103:407–413.
27. Baird AR, Hilmi O, White PS, et al.: Epithelial atypia and squamous metaplasia in nasal polyps. *J Laryngol Otol* 1998;112:755–757.
28. Tao Q, Srivastava G, Dickens P, et al.: Detection of Epstein-Barr virus–infected mucosal lymphocytes in nasal polyps. *Am J Pathol* 1996;143:1111–1118.
29. Oppenheimer EH, Rosenstein BJ: Differential diagnosis of nasal polyps in cystic fibrosis and atopy. *Lab Invest* 1979;40:445–449.
30. Batsakis JG, Sneige N: Choanal and angiomatous polyps of the sinonasal tract. *Ann Otol Rhinol Laryngol* 1992;101:623–625.
31. Batsakis JG: Stromal cell atypia in sinonasal polyposis. *Ann Otol Rhinol Laryngol* 1986;95:321–322.
32. Compagno J, Hyams VJ, Lepore ML: Nasal polyposis with stromal atypia: Review of follow-up study of 14 cases. *Arch Pathol Lab Med* 1976;100:224–226.

Myospherulosis

33. Rosai J: The nature of myospherulosis of the upper respiratory tract. *Am J Clin Pathol* 1978;69:475–481.
34. Shimada K, Kobayashi S, Yamadori I, et al.: Myospherulosis in Japan: A report of two cases and an immunohistochemical investigation. *Am J Surg Pathol* 1988;12:427–432.
35. Kyriakos M: Myospherulosis of the paranasal sinuses, nose, and middle ear: A possible iatrogenic disease. *Am J Clin Pathol* 1977;67:118–130.

Granulomatous Diseases

36. Lecointre F, Marandas P, Micheau C, et al.: Tuberculosis of the mucosa of the naso-pharynx: A clinical study of 37 cases seen at the Gustave-Roussy institute between 1961 and 1978. *Ann Otolaryngol Chir Cervicofac* 1980;97:423–433.
37. Waldman SR, Levine HL, Sebek BA, et al.: Nasal tuberculosis: A forgotten entity. *Laryngoscope* 1981;91:11–16.
38. McCaffrey TV, McDonald TJ: Sarcoidosis of the nose and paranasal sinuses. *Laryngoscope* 1983;93:1281–1284.
39. Coup AJ, Hopper IP: Granulomatous lesions in nasal biopsies. *Histopathology* 1980;4:293–308.
40. Krespi YP, Kuriloff DB, Aner M: Sarcoidosis of the sinonasal tract: A new staging system. *Otolaryngol Head Neck Surg* 1995;112:221–227.
41. Postma D, Fry TL, Malenbaum BT: The nose, minor salivary glands and sarcoidosis. *Arch Otolaryngol* 1984;110:28–30.
42. McDougall AC, Rees RJL, Weddell AGM, et al.: The histopathology of lepromatous leprosy in the nose. *J Pathol* 1975;115:215–226.
43. Pollack JD, Pincus RL, Lucente FE: Leprosy of the head and neck. *Otolaryngol Head Neck Surg* 1987;97:93–96.

44. Wabinga HR, Wamukota W, Mugerwa JW: Scleroma in Uganda: A review of 85 cases. *East Afr Med J* 1993;70:186–188.
45. Sherif M, Eissa S, Bakry MW: Scleroma (rhinoscleroma): An immunologic and histopathologic study. *J Egypt Soc Parasitol* 1986;16:293–301.
46. Sedano HO, Roman CB, Koutlas IG: Respiratory scleroma: A clinicopathologic and ultrastructural study. *Oral Surg Oral Med Oral Pathol Oral Radiol Endod* 1996;81:665–671.
47. Schwartz DA, Geyer SJ: Klebsiella and rhinoscleroma. In Connor DH, Chandler FW, Schwartz DA, et al (eds): *Pathology of Infectious Diseases.* Stamford: Appleton & Lange, 1997;589–595.
48. Andraca R, Edson RS, Kern EB: Rhinoscleroma: A growing concern in the United States? Mayo Clinic experience. *Mayo Clin Proc* 1993;68:1151–1157.
49. Batsakis JG, El-Naggar AK: Rhinoscleroma and rhinosporidiosis. *Ann Otol Rhinol Laryngol* 1992;101:879–882.
50. Berger SA, Pollock AA, Richmond AS: Isolation of *Klebsiella rhinoscleroma* in a general hospital. *Am J Clin Pathol* 1977;67:499–502.
51. Paul C, Pialoux G, Dupont B, et al.: Infection due to *Klebsiella rhinoscleromatis* in two patients infected with human immunodeficiency virus. *Clin Infect Dis* 1993;16:441–442.

Fungal Diseases

52. Brandwein M: Histopathology of sinonasal fungal disease. *Otolaryngol Clin North Am* 1993;26:949–981.
53. Stammberger HR, Jakes R, Beaufort F: Aspergillosis of the paranasal sinuses. X-ray diagnosis, histopathology and clinical aspects. *Ann Otol Rhinol Laryngol* 1984;93:251.
54. Watters GW, Milford CA: Isolated sphenoid sinusitis due to *Pseudallescheria boydii. J Laryngol Otol* 1993;107:344–346.
55. Rao A, Forgan-Smith R, Miller S, et al.: Phaeohyphomycosis of the nasal sinuses caused by bipolaris species. *Pathology* 1989;21:280–281.
56. Zieske LA, Kopke RD, Hamill R: Dematiaceous fungal sinusitis. *Otolaryngol Head Neck Surg* 1991;105:567–577.
57. Rosenthal J, Katz R, Du Bois DB, et al.: Chronic maxillary sinusitis associated with the mushroom schizophyllum commune in a patient with aids. *Clin Infect Dis* 1992;14:46–48.
58. Henderson LT, Robbins KT, Weitzner S, et al.: Benign mucor colonization (fungus ball) associated with chronic sinusitis. *South Med J* 1988;81:846–850.
59. Grigg AP, Phillips P, Durham S, et al.: Recurrent *Pseudallescheria boydii* sinusitis in acute leukemia. *Scand J Infect Dis* 1993;25:263–267.
60. Meyer RD, Gaultier CR, Yamashita JT, et al.: Fungal sinusitis in patients with AIDS: Report of 4 cases and review of the literature. *Medicine (Baltimore)* 1994;73:69–78.
61. Del Valle Zapico A, Rubio Suarez A, Mellado Encinas P, et al.: Mucormycosis of the sphenoid sinus in an otherwise healthy patient: Case report and literature review. *J Laryngol Otol* 1996;110:471–473.
62. Lansford BK, Bower CM, Seibert RW: Invasive fungal sinusitis in the immunocompromised pediatric patient. *Ear Nose Throat J* 1995;74:566–573.
63. Drakos PE, Nagler A, Or R, et al.: Invasive fungal sinusitis in patients undergoing bone marrow transplantation. *Bone Marrow Transplant* 1993;12:203–208.
64. McGill TJ, Simpson G, Healy GB: Fulminant aspergillosis of the nose and paranasal sinuses: A new clinical entity. *Laryngoscope* 1980;90:748–754.
65. Kriesel JD, Adderson EE, Gooch WM, et al.: Invasive sinonasal disease due to scopulariopsis candida: Case report and review of scopulariopsosis. *Clin Infect Dis* 1994;19:317–319.
66. Choi SS, Lawson W, Bottone E, et al.: Cryptococcal sinusitis: A case report and review of literature. *Otolaryngol Head Neck Surg* 1988;99:414–418.
67. Ismail Y, Johnson RH, Wells MV, et al.: Invasive sinusitis with intracranial extension caused by curvularia lunata. *Arch Intern Med* 1993;153:1604–1606.
68. Valenstein P, Schell WA: Primary intranasal *fusarium* infection: Potential for confusion with rhinocerebral zygomycosis. *Arch Pathol Lab Med* 1986;110:751–754.
69. Torres C, Ro JY, El-Naggar AK, et al.: Allergic fungal sinusitis: A clinicopathologic study of 16 cases. *Hum Pathol* 1996;27:793–799.
70. Katzenstein AL, Sale SR, Greenberger PA: Pathologic findings in allergic aspergillus sinusitis: A newly recognized form of sinusitis. *Am J Surg Pathol* 1983;7:439–443.

71. Corey JP, Delsuphe KG, Ferguson BJ: Allergic fungal sinusitis: Allergic, infectious, or both? *Otolaryngol Head Neck Surg* 1995;113:110–119.

72. Friedman GC, Hartwick RW, Ro JY, et al.: Allergic fungal sinusitis: Report of three cases associated with dematiaceous fungi. *Am J Clin Pathol* 1991;96:368–372.

73. Watts JC, Chandler FW: Rhinosporidiosis. In Connor DH, Chandler FW, Schwartz DA, et al. (eds): *Pathology of Infectious Diseases.* Stamford: Appleton & Lange, 1997;1085–1088.

74. Ahluwalia KB, Maheshwari N, Deka RC: Rhinosporidiosis: A study that resolves etiologic controversies. *Am J Rhinology* 1997, 11:479–483

75. Gaines JJ, Clay JR, Chandler FW, et al.: Rhinosporidiosis: Three domestic cases. *South Med J* 1996;89:65–67.

76. Kamal MM, Luley AS, Mundhada SG, et al.: Rhinosporidiosis: Diagnosis by scrape cytology. *Acta Cytol* 1995;39:931–935.

77. Tadros TS, Workowski KA, Siegel RJ, et al.: Pathology of hyalohyphomycosis by *Scedosporium apiospermum (Pseudallescheria boydii):* An emerging mycosis. *Hum Pathol* 1998;29:1266–1272.

78. Blitzer A, Lawson W: Fungal infections of the nose and paranasal sinuses: Part I. *Otolaryngol Clin North Am* 1993;26:1007–1035.

79. Lawson W, Blitzer A: Fungal infections of the nose and paranasal sinuses: II. *Otolaryngol Clin North Am* 1998;26:1037–1068.

Necrotizing Sialometaplasia

80. Brannon RB, Fowler CB, Hartman KS: Necrotizing sialometaplasia: A clinicopathologic study of sixty-nine cases and review of the literature. *Oral Surg Oral Med Oral Pathol* 1991;72:317–325.

81. Johnston WH: Necrotizing sialometaplasia involving the mucous glands of the nasal cavity. *Hum Pathol* 1977;8:589–592.

82. Wenig BM, Devaney K, Wenig BL: Pseudoneoplastic lesions of the oropharynx and larynx simulating cancer. *Pathol Annu* 1995;30:143–187.

83. Close LG, Cowan DF: Recurrent necrotizing sialometaplasia of the nasal cavity. *Otolaryngol Head Neck Surg* 1985;93:422–425.

84. Franchi A, Gallo O, Santucci M: Pathologic quiz case 1. Necrotizing sialometaplasia obscuring recurrent well-differentiated squamous cell carcinoma of the maxillary sinus. *Arch Otolaryngol Head Neck Surg* 1995;121:584–586.

Amyloidosis

85. Mufarrij AA, Busaba NY, Zaytoun GM, et al.: Primary localized amyloidosis of the nose and paranasal sinuses: A case report with immunohistochemical observations and a review of the literature. *Am J Surg Pathol* 1990;14:379–383.

Paranasal Sinus Mucocele

86. Natvig K, Larssen TE: Mucocele of the paranasal sinuses: A retrospective and histological study. *J Laryngol Otol* 1978;92:1075–1082.

87. Feldman M, Lowry LD, Rao VM, et al.: Mucoceles of the paranasal sinuses. *Trans Pa Acad Ophthalmol Otolaryngol* 1987;39:614–617.

88. Schaeffer BT, Som PM, Sacher M, et al.: Coexistence of a nasal mucoepidermoid carcinoma and sphenoid mucoceles: CT diagnosis and treatment implications. *J Comput Assist Tomogr* 1985;9:803–805.

89. Crain MR, Dolan KD, Maves MD: Maxillary sinus mucocele. *Ann Otol Rhinol Laryngol* 1990;99:321–322.

90. Tunkel DE, Naclerio RM, Baroody FM, et al.: Bilateral maxillary sinus mucocele in an infant with cystic fibrosis. *Otolaryngol Head Neck Surg* 1994;111:116–120.

91. Delfini R, Missori P, Iannetti G, et al.: Mucoceles of the paranasal sinuses with intracranial and intraorbital extension: Report of 28 cases. *Neurosurgery* 1993;32:901–906.

92. Hashim H, Asakura T, Awa H, et al.: Giant mucocele of paranasal sinuses. *Surg Neurol* 1985;23:69–74.

93. Hesselink JR, Weber AL, New PF, et al.: Evaluation of mucoceles of the paranasal sinuses with computed tomography. *Radiology* 1979;133:397–400.

94. Weissman JL, Curtin HD, Eibling DE: Double mucocele of the paranasal sinuses. *AJNR Am J Neuroradiol* 1994;15:1263–1264.

Respiratory Epithelial Adenomatoid Hamartoma

95. Wenig BM, Heffner DK: Respiratory epithelial adenomatoid hamartomas of the sinonasal tract and nasopharynx: A clinicopathologic study of 31 cases. *Ann Otol Rhinol Laryngol* 1995;104:639–645.

Nasal Chondromesenchymal Hamartoma

96. McDermott MB, Ponder TB, Dehner LP: Nasal chondromesenchymal hamartoma. An upper respiratory tract analogue of the chest wall mesenchymal hamartoma. *Am J Surg Pathol* 1998;22:425–433.

Glial Heterotopia, Encephalocele, and Dermoid Cyst

97. Yeoh GP, Bale PM, de Silva M: Nasal cerebral heterotopia: The so-called nasal glioma or sequestered encephalocele and its variants. *Pediatr Pathol* 1989;9:531–549.

98. Karma P, Rasanen O, Karja J: Nasal gliomas: A review and report of two cases. *Laryngoscope* 1977;87:1169–1179.

99. Zinreich SJ, Borders JC, Eisele DW, et al.: The utility of magnetic resonance imaging in the diagnosis of intranasal meningoencephaloceles. *Arch Otolaryngol Head Neck Surg* 1992;118:1253–1256.

100. Stoll W, Nieschalk M: Kongenitale Fehlbildungen des pranasalen Raumes: Gliome, Fisteln, Epidermoidzysten. *Laryngo-Rhino-Otol* 1996;75:739–744.

101. Mirra SS, Pearl GS, Hoffman JC, et al.: Nasal "glioma" with prominent neuronal component: Report of a case. *Arch Pathol Lab Med* 1981;105:540–541.

102. Theaker JM, Fletcher CD: Heterotopic glial nodules: A light microscopic and immunohistochemical study. *Histopathology* 1991;18:255–260.

103. Kane AM, Lore J Jr: Meningoencephalocele of the paranasal sinuses. *Laryngoscope* 1975;85:2087–2091

104. Chan JK, Lau WH: Nasal astrocytoma or nasal glial heterotopia? *Arch Pathol Lab Med* 1989;113:943–945.

105. Bossen EH, Hudson WR: Oligodendroglioma arising in heterotopic brain tissue of the soft palate and nasopharynx. *Am J Surg Pathol* 1987;11:571–574.

106. Gnepp DR: Teratoid neoplasms of the head and neck. In Barnes L (ed): *Surgical Pathology of the Head and Neck.* New York: Marcel Dekker, 1985:1411–1433.

Lymphoid Hyperplasia

107. Mabry RL: Lymphoid pseudotumor of the nasopharynx and larynx. *J Laryngol Otol* 1967;81:441–443.

108. Rimarenko S, Schwartz IS: Polypoid nasal pseudolymphoma. *Am J Clin Pathol* 1985;83:507–509.

109. Chen TC, Kuo T: Castleman's disease presenting as a pedunculated nasopharyngeal tumour simulating angiofibroma. *Histopathology* 1993;23:485–488.

110. Seider MJ, Cleary KR, van Tassel P, et al.: Plasma cell granuloma of the nasal cavity treated by radiation therapy. *Cancer* 1991;67:929–932.

111. Muzaffar M, Hussain SI, Chughtai A: Plasma cell granuloma: Maxillary sinuses. *J Laryngol Otol* 1994;108:357–358.

112. Som PM, Brandwein MS, Maldjian C, et al.: Inflammatory pseudotumor of the maxillary sinus: CT and MRI findings in six cases. *AJR* 1994;163:689–692.

113. Shahab I, Osborne BM, Butler JJ: Nasopharyngeal lymphoid tissue masses in patients with human immunodeficiency virus-1: Histologic findings and clinical correlation. *Cancer* 1995;74:3083–3088.

114. Wenig BM, Thompson LDR, Frankel SS, et al.: Lymphoid changes of the nasopharyngeal and palatine tonsils that are indicative of human immunodeficiency virus infection: A clinicopathologic study of 12 cases. *Am J Surg Pathol* 1996;20:572–587.

Sinus Histiocytosis with Massive Lymphadenopathy (Rosai-Dorfman Disease)

115. Rosai J, Dorfman RF: Sinus histiocytosis with massive lymphadenopathy: A newly recognized benign clinicopathologic entity. *Arch Pathol* 1969;87:63–70.

116. Rosai J, Dorfman RF: Sinus histiocytosis with massive lymphadenopathy: A pseudolymphomatous benign disorder: Analysis of 34 cases. *Cancer* 1972;30:1174–1188.

117. Wenig BM, Abbondanzo SL, Childers EL, et al.: Extranodal sinus histiocytosis with massive lymphadenopathy (Rosai-Dorfman disease) of the head and neck. *Hum Pathol* 1993;24:483–492.

118. Foucar E, Rosai J, Dorfman R: Sinus histiocytosis with massive lymphadenopathy (Rosai-Dorfman disease): Review of the entity. *Semin Diagn Pathol* 1990;7:19–73.
119. Foucar E, Rosai J, Dorfman RF: Sinus histiocytosis with massive lymphadenopathy: Ear, nose, and throat manifestations. *Arch Otolaryngol* 1978;104:687–693.
120. Eisen RN, Buckley PJ, Rosai J: Immunophenotypic characterization of sinus histiocytosis with massive lymphadenopathy (Rosai-Dorfman disease). *Semin Diagn Pathol* 1990;7:74–82.
121. Paulli M, Rosso R, Kindl S, et al.: Immunophenotypic characterization of the cell infiltrate in five cases of sinus histiocytosis with massive lymphadenopathy (Rosai-Dorfman disease). *Hum Pathol* 1992;23:647–654.
122. Komp DM: The treatment of sinus histiocytosis with massive lymphadenopathy (Rosai-Dorfman disease). *Semin Diagn Pathol* 1990;7:83–86.

Wegener's Granulomatosis

123. Colby TV, Tazelaar HD, Specks U, et al.: Nasal biopsy in Wegener's granulomatosis. *Hum Pathol* 1991;22:101–104.
124. Gaudin PB, Askin FB, Falk RJ, et al.: The pathologic spectrum of pulmonary lesions in patients with anti-neutrophil cytoplasmic autoantibodies specific for anti-proteinase 3 and anti-myeloperoxidase. *Am J Clin Pathol* 1995;104:7–16.
125. Devaney KO, Travis WD, Hoffman G, et al.: Interpretation of head and neck biopsies in Wegener's granulomatosis: A pathologic study of 126 biopsies in 70 patients. *Am J Surg Pathol* 1990;14:555–564.
126. Del Buono EA, Flint A: Diagnostic usefulness of nasal biopsy in Wegener's granulomatosis. *Hum Pathol* 1991;22:107–110.
127. Fienberg R, Mark EJ, Goodman M, et al.: Correlation of antineutrophil cytoplasmic antibodies with the extrarenal histopathology of Wegener's (pathergic) granulomatosis and related forms of vasculitis. *Hum Pathol* 1993;24:160–168.
128. Batsakis JG, El-Naggar AK: Wegener's granulomatosis and antineutrophil cytoplasmic autoantibodies. *Ann Otol Rhinol Laryngol* 1993;102:906–908.

Idiopathic Midline Destructive Disease (IMDD)

129. Tsokos M, Fauci AS, Costa J: Idiopathic midline destructive disease (IMDD). A subgroup of patients with the "midline granuloma" syndrome. *Am J Clin Pathol* 1982;77:162–168.
130. Costa J, Delacretaz F: The midline granuloma syndrome. *Pathol Annu* 1986;21:159–171.
131. Sercarz JA, Strasnick B, Newman A, et al.: Midline nasal destruction in cocaine abusers. *Otolaryngol Head Neck Surg* 1991;105:701.

Schneiderian Papillomas

132. Friedmann I, Osborn DA: Papillomas of the nose and sinuses. In: *Pathology of Granulomas and Neoplasms of the Nose and Paranasal Sinuses*. Edinburgh: Churchill Livingstone, 1982:104–116.
133. Vrabec DP: The inverted schneiderian papilloma: A 25-year study. *Laryngoscope* 1994;104:582–605.
134. Suh KW, Facer GW, Devine KD, et al.: Inverting papilloma of the nose and paranasal sinuses. *Laryngoscope* 1977;87:35–46.
135. Hyams VJ: Papillomas of the nasal cavity and paranasal sinuses: A clinicopathological study of 315 cases. *Ann Otol Rhinol Laryngol* 1971;80:192–206.
136. Michaels L, Young M: Histogenesis of papillomas of the nose and paranasal sinuses. *Arch Pathol Lab Med* 1995;119:821–826.
137. Shanmugaratnam K, Sobin LH: Histological typing of tumors of the upper respiratory tract and ear. In: World Health Organization. *International Histological Classification of Tumours,* 2nd ed. Berlin: Springer-Verlag, 1991.
138. Michaels L: Benign mucosal tumors of the nose and paranasal sinuses. *Semin Diagn Pathol* 1996;13:113–117.
139. Judd R, Zaki SR, Coffield LM, et al.: Sinonasal papillomas and human papillomavirus: Human papillomavirus 11 detected in fungiform schneiderian papillomas by in situ hybridization and the polymerase chain reaction. *Hum Pathol* 1991;22:550–556.
140. Brandwein M, Steinberg B, Thung S, et al.: Human papillomavirus 6/11 and 16/18 in schneiderian inverted papillomas: In situ hybridization with human papillomavirus RNA probes. *Cancer* 1989;63:1708–1713.

141. McLachlin CM, Kandel RA, Colgan TJ, et al.: Prevalence of human papillomavirus in sinonasal papillomas: A study using polymerase chain reaction and in situ hybridization. *Mod Pathol* 1992;5:406–409.
142. Gaffey MJ, Frierson HF Jr, Weiss LM, et al.: Human papillomavirus and Epstein-Barr virus in sinonasal schneiderian papillomas. An in situ hybridization and polymerase chain reaction study. *Am J Clin Pathol* 1996;106:475–482.
143. Sarkar FH, Visscher DW, Kintanar EB, et al.: Sinonasal schneiderian papillomas: Human papillomavirus typing by polymerase chain reaction. *Mod Pathol* 1992;5:329–332.
144. Lasser A, Rothfeld PR, Shapiro RS: Epithelial papilloma and squamous cell carcinoma of the nasal cavity and paranasal sinuses: A clinicopathological study. *Cancer* 1976;38:2503–2510.
145. Vrabec DP: The inverted schneiderian papilloma: A clinical and pathological study. *Laryngoscope* 1975;85:186–220.
146. Lawson W, Ho BT, Shaari CM, et al.: Inverted papilloma: A report of 112 cases. *Laryngoscope* 1995;105:282–288.
147. Seshul MJ, Eby TL, Crowe DR, et al.: Nasal inverted papilloma with involvement of middle ear and mastoid. *Arch Otolaryngol Head Neck Surg* 1995;121:1045–1048.
148. Snyder RN, Perzin KH1: Papillomatosis of nasal cavity and paranasal sinuses (inverted papilloma, squamous papilloma): A clinicopathologic study. *Cancer* 1972;30:668–690.
149. Ridolfi RL, Lieberman PH, Erlandson RA, et al.: Schneiderian papillomas: A clinicopathologic study of 30 cases. *Am J Surg Pathol* 1977;1:43–53.
150. Nielsen PL, Buchwald C, Nielsen LH, et al.: Inverted papilloma of the nasal cavity: Pathological aspects in a follow-up study. *Laryngoscope* 1991;101:1094–1101.
151. Katenkamp D, Stiller D, Kuttner K: Inverted papillomas of nasal cavity and paranasal sinuses: Ultrastructural investigations on epithelial-stromal interface. *Virchows Arch [Pathol Anat]* 1982;397:215–226.
152. Barnes L, Bedetti C: Oncocytic schneiderian papilloma: A reappraisal of cylindrical cell papilloma of the sinonasal tract. *Hum Pathol* 1984;15:344–351.
153. Bawa R, Allen GC, Ramadan HH: Cylindrical cell papilloma of the nasal cavity. *Ear Nose Throat J* 1995;74:179–181.
154. Calcaterra TC, Thompson JW, Paglia DE: Inverting papillomas of the nose and paranasal sinuses. *Laryngoscope* 1980;90:53–60.
155. Myers EN, Schramm VL Jr, Barnes EL Jr: Management of inverted papilloma of the nose and paranasal sinuses. *Laryngoscope* 1981;91:2071–2084.
156. Sham CL, Woo JKS, van Hasselt CA: Endoscopic resection of inverted papilloma of the nose and paranasal sinuses. *J Laryngol Otol* 1998;112:758–764.
157. Harrison D, Lund VJ: Papillomas of the nasal cavity and paranasal sinuses. In: *Tumours of the Upper Jaw.* Edinburgh: Churchill-Livingstone, 1993:73–80.
158. Kapadia SB, Barnes L, Pelzman K, et al.: Carcinoma ex oncocytic schneiderian (cylindrical cell) papilloma. *Am J Otolaryngol* 1993;14:332–338.
159. Walter P, Stebler S, Schaffer P, et al.: Cylindrical epithelioma of nasal cavities and accessory sinuses. Anatomoclinical study of 26 cases. *Ann Anat Pathol (Paris)* 1976;21:463–476.
160. Manivel C, Wick MR, Dehner LP: Transitional (cylindric) cell carcinoma with endodermal sinus tumor-like features of the nasopharynx and paranasal sinuses: Clinicopathologic and immunohistochemical study of two cases. *Arch Pathol Lab Med* 1986;110:198–202.

Salivary Gland-Type Tumors

161. Miller RH, Calcaterra TC: Adenoid cystic carcinoma of the nose, paranasal sinuses and palate. *Arch Otolaryngol* 1980;106:424–426.
162. Manning JT, Batsakis JG: Salivary-type neoplasms of the sinonasal tract. *Ann Otol Rhinol Laryngol* 199;100:691–694.
163. Goepfert H, Luna MA, Lindberg RD, et al.: Malignant salivary gland tumors of the paranasal sinuses and nasal cavity. *Arch Otolaryngol* 1983;109:662–668.
164. Batsakis JG, Rice DH, Solomon AR: The pathology of head and neck tumors: Squamous and mucous-gland carcinomas of the nasal cavity, paranasal sinuses, and larynx, part 6. *Head Neck Surg* 1980;2:497–508.
165. Heffner DK: Sinonasal and laryngeal salivary gland lesions. In Ellis GL, Auclair PL, Gnepp DR (eds): *Surgical Pathology of the Salivary Glands.* Philadelphia: W.B. Saunders, 1991:544–559.
166. Gnepp DR, Heffner DK: Mucosal origin of sinonasal tract adenomatous neoplasms. *Mod Pathol* 1989;2:365–371.

167. Tran L, Sidrys J, Horton D, et al.: Malignant salivary gland tumors of the paranasal sinuses and nasal cavity. A UCLA experience. *Am J Clin Oncol* 1989;12:387–392.

168. Spiro RH, Koss LG, Hajdu SI, et al.: Tumors of minor salivary origin: A clinicopathologic study of 492 cases. *Cancer* 1973;31:117–129.

169. Cho KJ, El-Naggar AK, Mahanupab P, et al.: Carcinoma ex-pleomorphic adenoma of the nasal cavity: A report of two cases. *J Laryngol Otol* 1995;109:677–679.

170. Compagno J, Wong RT: Intranasal mixed tumors (pleomorphic adenomas): A clinicopathologic study of 40 cases. *Am J Clin Pathol* 1977;68:213–218.

171. DiMaio SJ, DiMaio JVJM, DiMaio T-M, et al.: Oncocytic carcinoma of the nasal cavity. *South Med J* 1980;73:803–806.

172. Chui RT, Liao SY, Bosworth H: Recurrent oncocytoma of the ethmoid sinus with orbital invasion. *Otolaryngol Head Neck Surg* 1985;93:267–270.

173. Begin LR, Rochon L, Frenkiel S: Spindle cell myoepithelioma of the nasal cavity. *Am J Surg Pathol* 1991;15:184–190.

174. Begin LR, Black MJ: Salivary-type myxoid myoepithelioma of the sinonasal tract: A potential diagnostic pitfall. *Histopathology* 1993;23:283–285.

175. Alos L, Cardesa A, Bombi JA, et al.: Myoepithelial tumors of salivary glands: A clinicopathologic, immunohistochemical, ultrastructural, and flow-cytometric study. *Semin Diagn Pathol* 1996;13:138–147.

176. Graadt Van Roggen JF, Baatenburg-De Jong RJ, Verschuur HP, et al.: Myoepithelial carcinoma (malignant myoepithelioma): First report of an occurrence in the maxillary sinus. *Histopathology* 1998;32:239–241.

177. Ralfa S: Mucous gland tumors of paranasal sinuses. *Cancer* 1969;24:683–691.

178. Ordonez NG, Batsakis JG: Acinic cell carcinoma of the nasal cavity: Electron-optic and immunohistochemical observations. *J Laryngol Otol* 1986;100:345–349.

179. Perzin KH, Cantor JO, Johannessen JV: Acinic cell carcinoma arising in nasal cavity: Report of a case with ultrastructural observations. *Cancer* 1981;47:1818–1822.

180. Heffner DK, Hyams VJ, Hauck KW, et al.: Low-grade adenocarcinoma of the nasal cavity and paranasal sinuses. *Cancer* 1982;50:312–322.

181. Fonseca I, Soares J: Basal cell adenocarcinoma of minor salivary and seromucous glands of the head and neck region. *Semin Diagn Pathol* 1996;13:128–137.

182. Dardick I, van Nostrand P: Polymorphous low-grade adenocarcinoma: A case report with ultrastructural findings. *Oral Surg Oral Med Oral Pathol* 1988;66:459–465.

183. Lloreta J, Serrano S, Corominas JM, et al.: Polymorphous low-grade adenocarcinoma arising in the nasal cavities with an associated undifferentiated carcinoma. *Ultrastructural Pathology* 1995;19:365–370.

184. Kleinsasser O: Terminal tubulus adenocarcinoma of the nasal seromucous glands: A specific entity. *Arch Otorhinolaryngol* 1985;241:183–193.

185. Michal M, Sklalova A, Simpson RHW, et al.: Clear cell myoepithelioma of the salivary gland. *Histopathology* 1996;28:309–315.

186. Lam PWY, Chan JKC, Sin VC: Nasal pleomorphic adenoma with skeletal muscle differentiation: Potential misdiagnosis as rhabdomyosarcoma. *Hum Pathol* 1997;28:1299–1302.

187. Dehner LP, Valbuena L, Perez-Atayde A, et al.: Salivary gland anlage tumor ("congenital pleomorphic adenoma"). A clinicopathologic, immunohistochemical and ultrastructural study of nine cases. *Am J Surg Pathol* 1994;18:25–36.

Low-Grade Adenocarcinoma

188. Wenig BM, Hyams VJ, Heffner DK: Nasopharyngeal papillary adenocarcinoma: A clinicopathologic study of a low-grade carcinoma. *Am J Surg Pathol* 1988;12:946–953.

189. Cinberg JZ, Solomon MP, Ozbardacki G: Thyroid carcinoma and secondary malignancy of the sinonasal tract. *Arch Otolaryngol* 1980;106:239–241.

Intestinal-Type Sinonasal Adenocarcinoma

190. Kleinsasser O, Schroeder H-G: Adenocarcinomas of the inner nose after exposure to wood dust. Morphological findings and relationships between histopathology and clinical behavior in 79 cases. *Arch Otolaryngol* 1988;245:1–15.

191. Barnes L: Intestinal-type adenocarcinoma of the nasal cavity and paranasal sinuses. *Am J Surg Pathol* 1986;10:192–202.

192. Mills SE, Fechner RE, Cantrell RW: Aggressive sinonasal lesion resembling normal intestinal mucosa. *Am J Surg Pathol* 1982;6:803–809.

193. Franquemont DW, Fechner RE, Mills SE: Histologic classification of sinonasal intestinal-type adenocarcinoma. *Am J Surg Pathol* 1991;15:368–375.

194. Sanchez-Casis G, Devine KD, Welland LH: Nasal adenocarcinomas that closely simulate colonic carcinomas. *Cancer* 1971;28:714–720.

195. Gamez-Araujo JJ, Ayala AG, Guillamondegui O: Mucinous adenocarcinoma of nose and paranasal sinuses. *Cancer* 1975;36:1100–1105.

196. Elwood JM: Wood exposure and smoking: Association with cancer of the nasal cavity and paranasal sinuses in British Columbia. *Can Med Assoc J* 1981;124:1573–1577.

197. Klintenberg C, Olofsson J, Hellquist H, et al.: Adenocarcinoma of the ethmoid sinuses: A review of 28 cases with special reference to wood dust exposure. *Cancer* 1984;54:482–488.

198. Ironside P, Matthews J: Adenocarcinoma of the nose and paranasal sinuses in woodworkers in the state of Victoria, Australia. *Cancer* 1975;36:1115–1121.

199. Moran CA, Wenig BM, Mullick FG: Primary adenocarcinoma of the nasal cavity and paranasal sinuses. *Ear Nose Throat J* 1995;70:821–828.

200. Urso C, Ninu MB, Franchi A, et al.: Intestinal-type adenocarcinoma of the sinonasal tract: A clinicopathologic study of 18 cases. Tumori 1993;79:205–210.

201. McKinney CD, Mills SE, Franquemont DW: Sinonasal intestinal-type adenocarcinoma: Immunohistochemical profile and comparison with colonic adenocarcinoma. *Mod Pathol* 1995;8:421–425.

202. Wu TT, Barnes L, Bakker A, et al.: *K-ras-2* and *p53* genotyping of intestinal-type adenocarcinoma of the nasal cavity and paranasal sinuses. *Mod Pathol* 1996;9:199–204.

203. Bernstein JM, Montgomery WW, Balogh K: Metastatic tumors to the maxilla, nose, and paranasal sinuses. *Laryngoscope* 1966;76:621–650.

204. Gillmore JR, Gillespie CA, Hudson WR: Adenocarcinoma of the nose and paranasal sinuses. *Ear Nose Throat J* 1987;66:120–123.

205. Alessi DM, Trapp TK, Fu YS, et al.: Nonsalivary sinonasal adenocarcinoma. *Arch Otolaryngol Head Neck Surg* 1988;114:996–999.

Small Cell Neuroendocrine Carcinoma

206. Perez-Ordonez B, Caruana SM, Huvos AG, et al.: Small cell neuroendocrine carcinoma of the nasal cavity and paranasal sinuses. *Hum Pathol* 1998;29:826–832.

207. Koss LG, Spiro RH, Hajdu S: Small cell (oat cell) carcinoma of minor salivary gland origin. *Cancer* 1972;30:737–741.

208. Rejowski JE, Campanella RS, Block LJ: Small cell carcinoma of the nose and paranasal sinuses. *Otolaryngol Head Neck Surg* 1982;90:516–517.

209. Weiss MD, deFries HO, Taxy JB, et al.: Primary small cell carcinoma of the paranasal sinuses. *Arch Otolaryngol* 1983;109:341–343.

210. Kameya T, Shimosato Y, Adachi I, et al.: Neuroendocrine carcinoma of the paranasal sinus: A morphological and endocrinological study. *Cancer* 1980;45:330–339.

211. Gaudin PB, Rosai J: Florid vascular proliferation associated with neural and neuroendocrine neoplasms: A diagnostic clue and potential pitfall. *Am J Surg Pathol* 1995;19:642–652.

212. Chan JKC, Suster S, Wenig BM, et al.: Cytokeratin 20 immunoreactivity distinguishes Merkel cell (primary cutaneous) neuroendocrine carcinomas and salivary gland small cell carcinomas from small cell carcinomas of various sites. *Am J Surg Pathol* 1997;21:226–234.

213. Kyung-Whan M: Usefulness of electron microscopy in the diagnosis of "small round cell tumors of the sinonasal region. *Ultrastructural Pathology* 1995;19:347–363.

214. Saw D, Chan JK, Jagirdar J, et al.: Sinonasal small cell neoplasm developing after radiation therapy for retinoblastoma: An immunohistologic, ultrastructural, and cytogenetic study. *Hum Pathol* 1992;23:896–899.

215. Frierson HF, Ross GW, Stewart FM, et al.: Unusual sinonasal small-cell neoplasms following radiotherapy for bilateral retinoblastomas. *Am J Surg Pathol* 1989;13:947–954.

216. Wan SK, Chan JK, Tse KC: Basaloid-squamous carcinoma of the nasal cavity. *J Laryngol Otol* 1992;106:370–371.

217. Mills SE: Neuroendocrine tumors of the head and neck: A selected review with emphasis on terminology. *Endocr Pathol* 1996;7:329–343.

218. Banks ER, Frierson HF, Mills SE, et al.: Basaloid squamous cell carcinoma of the head and neck: A clinicopathologic and immunohistochemical study of 40 cases. *Am J Surg Pathol* 1992;16:939–946.

219. Raychowdhuri RN: Oat-cell carcinoma and paranasal sinuses. *J Laryngol Otol* 1965;79:253–255.
220. Galanis E, Frytak S, Lloyd RV: Extrapulmonary small cell carcinoma. *Cancer* 1997;79:1729–1736.

Carcinoid Tumor

221. Siwersson U, Kindblom LG: Oncocytic carcinoid of the nasal cavity and carcinoid of the lung in a child. *Pathol Res Pract* 1984;178:562–569.
222. Perdigou JB, Pages M, Le Bodic MF, et al.: Tumeur oncocytarie avec granulations neuro-secretoires de la muqueuse nasale. *Arch Anat Cytol Path* 1981;29:75–78.
223. McCluggage WG, Napier SS, Primrose WJ, et al.: Sinonasal neuroendocrine carcinoma exhibiting amphicrine differentiation. *Histopathology* 1995;27:79–82.

Sinonasal Undifferentiated Carcinoma

224. Frierson HF, Mills SE, Fechner RE, et al.: Sinonasal undifferentiated carcinoma. *Am J Surg Pathol* 1986;10:771–779.
225. Pitman KT, Lassen LF1: Pathologic quiz case 2. Sinonasal undifferentiated carcinoma (SNUC). *Arch Otolaryngol Head Neck Surg* 1995;121:1201–1203.
226. Frierson HF Jr, Mills SE, Fechner RE, et al.: Sinonasal undifferentiated carcinoma: An aggressive neoplasm derived from schneiderian epithelium and distinct from olfactory neuroblastoma. *Am J Surg Pathol* 1986;10:771–779.
227. Deutsch B, Levine PA, Stewart M, et al.: Sinonasal undifferentiated carcinoma: A ray of hope. *Otolaryngol Head Neck Surg* 1993;108:697–700.
228. Helliwell TR, Yeoh LH, Stell PM: Anaplastic carcinoma of the nose and paranasal sinuses: A light microscopy, immunohistochemistry and clinical correlation. *Cancer* 1986;58:2038–2045.
229. Gallo O, Di Lollo S, Graziani P, et al.: Detection of Epstein-Barr virus genome in sinonasal undifferentiated carcinoma by use of in situ hybridization. *Otolaryngol Head Neck Surg* 1995;112:659–664.
230. Lopategui JR, Gaffey MJ, Frierson HF, Jr, et al.: Detection of Epstein-Barr viral RNA in sinonasal undifferentiated carcinoma from Western and Asian patients. *Am J Surg Pathol* 1994;18:391–8.
231. Greger V, Schirmacher P, Bohl J, et al.: Possible involvement of the retinoblastoma gene in undifferentiated sinonasal carcinoma. *Cancer* 1990;66:1954–1959.
232. Gallo O, Graziani P, Fini-Storchi O: Undifferentiated carcinoma of the nose and paranasal sinuses. *Otolaryngol Head Neck Surg* 1995;72:588–595.
233. Ascaso FJ, Adiego MI, Garcia J, et al.: Sinonasal undifferentiated carcinoma invading the orbit. *Eur J Ophthalmol* 1994;4:234–236.
234. Mills SE, Fechner RE: "Undifferentiated" neoplasms of the sinonasal region: Differential diagnosis based on clinical, light microscopic, immunohistochemical, and ultrastructural features. *Semin Diagn Pathol* 1989;6:316–328.
235. Hewan-Lowe K, Dardick I: Ultrastructural distinction of basaloid-squamous carcinoma and adenoid cystic carcinoma. *Ultrastructural Pathology* 1995;19:371–381.

Paraganglioma

236. Ueda N, Yoshida A, Fukunishi R, et al.: Nonchromaffin paraganglioma in the nose and paranasal sinuses. *Acta Pathol Jpn* 1985;35:489–495.
237. Himelfarb MZ, Ostrzega NL, Samuel J, et al.: Paraganglioma of the nasal cavity. *Laryngoscope* 1983;93:350–352.
238. Lack EE, Cubilla AL, Woodruff JM: Paragangliomas of the head and neck region: A pathologic study of tumors from 71 patients. *Hum Pathol* 1979;10:191–218.
239. Parisier SC, Sinclair GM: Glomus tumor of the nasal cavity. *Laryngoscope* 1968;78:2013–2024.
240. Lack EE, Cubilla AL, Woodruff JM, et al.: Paragangliomas of the head and neck region: A clinicopathologic study of 69 patients. *Cancer* 1977;39:397–409.
241. Nguyen QA, Gibbs PM, Rice DH: Malignant nasal paraganglioma: A case report and review of the literature. *Otolaryngol Head Neck Surg* 1995;113:157–161.
242. Branham GH, Gnepp DR, O'McMenomey S, et al.: Malignant paraganglioma: A case report and literature review. *Otolaryngol Head Neck Surg* 1989;101:99–103.

Malignant Melanoma

243. Franquemont DW, Mills SE: Sinonasal malignant melanoma: A clinicopathologic and immunohistochemical study of 14 cases. *Am J Clin Pathol* 1991;96:689–697.
244. El-Naggar AK, Batsakis JG, Garcia GM, et al.: Sinonasal hemangiopericytomas: A clinicopathologic and DNA content study. *Arch Otolaryngol Head Neck Surg* 1992;118:134–137.
245. Guzzo M, Grandi C, Licitra L, et al.: Mucosal malignant melanoma of head and neck: Forty-eight cases treated at Istituto Nazionale Tumori of Milan. *Eur J Surg Oncol* 1993;19:316–319.
246. Shah JP, Huvos AG, Strong EW: Mucosal melanomas of the head and neck. *Am J Surg* 1977;134:531–535.
247. Barton RT: Mucosal melanomas of the head and neck. *Laryngoscope* 1975;85:93–99.
248. Friedmann I, Osborn DA: Melanotic tumours of the nose and sinuses. In: *Pathology of Granulomas and Neoplasms of the Nose and Paranasal Sinuses.* Edinburgh: Churchill Livingstone, 1982:162–172.
249. Kingdom TT, Kaplan MJ: Mucosal melanoma of the nasal cavity and paranasal sinuses. *Head Neck* 1995;17:184–189.
250. Lund VL: Malignant melanoma of the nasal cavity and paranasal sinuses. *J Laryngol Otol* 1982;96:347–355.
251. Lund VL: Malignant melanoma of the nasal cavity and paranasal sinuses. *Ear Nose Throat J* 1993;72:285–290.
252. Nakhleh RE, Wick MR, Rocamora A, et al.: Morphologic diversity in malignant melanomas. *Am J Clin Pathol* 1990;93:731–740.
253. Freedman HM, De Santo LW, Devine KD, et al.: Malignant melanoma of the nasal cavity and paranasal sinuses. *Arch Otolaryngol* 1973;97:322–325.
254. Raben A, Pfister D, Harrison LB: Radiation therapy and chemotherapy in the management of cancers of the nasal cavity and paranasal sinuses. In Kraus DH, Levine HL (eds): *Nasal Neoplasia.* New York: Thieme, 1997;183–212.
255. Thompson AC, Morgan DA, Bradley PJ: Malignant melanoma of the nasal cavity and paranasal sinuses. *Clin Otolaryngol* 1993;18:34–36.
256. Robertson DM, Hungerford JL, McCartney A: Malignant melanomas of the conjunctiva, nasal cavity, and paranasal sinuses. *Am J Ophthalmol* 1989;108:440–442.

Olfactory Neuroblastoma

257. Berger L, Luc G, Richard D: L'esthésioneuroépithéliome olfactif. *Bull Cancer* 1924;13:410–421.
258. Berger L, Coutard H: L'esthésioneurocytome olfactif. *Bull Assoc Etude Cancer* 1924;13:404–414.
259. Mendeloff J: The olfactory neuroepithelial tumors: A review of the literature and report of six additional cases. *Cancer* 1957;10:944–956.
260. Bhattacharyya N, Thornton AF, Joseph MP, et al.: Successful treatment of esthesioneuroblastoma and neuroendocrine carcinoma with combined chemotherapy and proton radiation. *Arch Otolaryngol Head Neck Surg* 1997;123:34–40.
261. Silva EG, Butler JJ, Mackay B, et al.: Neuroblastomas and neuroendocrine carcinomas of the nasal cavity: A proposed new classification. *Cancer* 1982;50:2388–2405.
262. Appelblatt NH, McClatchey KD: Olfactory neuroblastoma: A retrospective clinicopathologic study. *Head Neck Surg* 1982;5:108–113.
263. Miller DC, Goodman ML, Pilch BZ, et al.: Mixed olfactory neuroblastoma and carcinoma: A report of two cases. *Cancer* 1984;54:2019–2028.
264. Hutter RVP, Lewis JS, Foote FWJ, et al.: Esthesioneuroblastoma: A clinical and pathologic study. *Am J Surg* 1963;106:748–753.
265. Perez-Ordonez B, Huvos AG: Olfactory neuroblastoma and sinonasal small cell neuroendocrine carcinoma: Immunohistochemical features and differential diagnosis. *Mod Pathol* 1997;10:116A
266. Dulguerov P, Calcaterra TC: Esthesioneuroblastoma: The UCLA experience 1970–1990. *Laryngoscope* 1992;102:843–849.
267. Mills SE, Frierson HF: Olfactory neuroblastoma: A clinicopathologic study of 21 cases. *Am J Surg Pathol* 1985;9:317–327.
268. Shah JP, Feghali J: Esthesioneuroblastoma. *Am J Surg* 1981;142:456–458.
269. Myers SL, Hardy DA, Weibe CB, et al.: Olfactory neuroblastoma invading the oral cavity in a patient with inappropriate antidiuretic hormone secretion. *Oral Surg Oral Med Oral Pathol* 1994;77:645–650.
270. Kadish S, Goodman M, Wang CC: Olfactory neuroblastoma: A clinical analysis of 17 cases. *Cancer* 1976;37:1571–1576.
271. Hyams VJ, Batsakis JG, Michaels L: Tumors of the upper respiratory tract and ear: Neuroectodermal lesions. In: *Atlas of Tumor Pathology,*

2nd series. Washington, D.C.: Armed Forces Institute of Pathology, 1988:226–257.

272. Ordóñez NG, Mackay B: Neuroendocrine tumors of the nasal cavity. *Pathol Annu* 1993;28:77–111.

273. Curtis JL, Rubinstein LJ: Pigmented example of melanotic neuroepithelial neoplasm. *Cancer* 1982;49:2136–2143.

274. Hirose T, Scheithauer BW, Lopes MBS, et al.: Olfactory neuroblastoma: An immunohistochemical, ultrastructural, and flow cytometric study. *Cancer* 1995;76:4–19.

275. Frierson HF, Ross GW, Mills SE, et al.: Olfactory neuroblastoma. *Am J Clin Pathol* 1990;94:547–553.

276. Taxy JB, Bharani NK, Mills SE, et al.: The spectrum of olfactory neural tumors: A light-microscopic immunohistochemical and ultrastructural analysis. *Am J Surg Pathol* 1986;10:687–695.

277. Kahn LB: Esthesioneuroblastoma: A light and electron microscopic study. *Hum Pathol* 1974;5:364–371.

278. Griego JE, Mackay B, Ordóñez NG, et al.: Olfactory neuroblastoma: A case report. *Ultrastruct Pathol* 1996;20:399–406.

279. Sorensen PHB, Wu JK, Berean KW, et al.: Olfactory neuroblastoma is a peripheral primitive neuroectodermal tumor related to Ewing sarcoma. *Proc Natl Acad Sci U S A* 1996;93:1038–1043.

280. Whang-Peng J, Freter CE, Knutsen T, et al.: Translocation t(11;22) in ONB. *Cancer Genet Cytogenet* 1987;29:155–157.

281. Nelson RS, Perlman EJ, Askin FB: Is esthesioneuroblastoma a peripheral neuroectodermal tumor? *Hum Pathol* 1995;26:639–641.

282. Argani P, Perez-Ordóñez B, Xiao H, et al.: Olfactory neuroblastoma is not related to the Ewing family of tumors: Absence of EWS/FLI1 gene fusion and MIC2 expression. *Am J Surg Pathol* 1998;22:391–398.

283. Papadaki H, Kounelis S, Kapadia SB, et al.: Relationship of p53 gene alterations with tumor progression and recurrence in olfactory neuroblastoma. *Am J Surg Pathol* 1996;20:715–721.

284. Chaudhry MR, Akhtar S, Kim DS: Neuroendocrine carcinoma of the ethmoid sinus. *Eur Arch Otorhinolaryngol* 1994;251:461–463.

285. Eden BV, Debo RF, Larner JM, et al.: Esthesioneuroblastoma: Long-term outcome and patterns of failure. The University of Virginia experience. *Cancer* 1994;73:2556–2562.

286. Chang KC, Jin YT, Chen RMY, et al.: Mixed olfactory neuroblastoma and craniopharyngioma: An unusual pathologic finding. *Histopathology* 1997;30:378–382.

287. Naresh KN, Pai SA: Foci resembling olfactory neuroblastoma and craniopharyngioma are seen in sinonasal teratocarcinosarcomas. *Histopathology* 1998;32:84.

Lobular Capillary Hemangioma

288. Heffner DK: Problems in pediatric otorhinolaryngic pathology: II. Vascular tumors and lesions of the sinonasal tract and nasopharynx. *Int J Pediatr Otorhinolaryngol* 1983;5:125–138.

289. Fu YS, Perzin KH1: Non-epithelial tumors of the nasal cavity, paranasal sinuses, and nasopharynx: A clinicopathologic study: I. General features and vascular tumors. *Cancer* 1974;33:1275–1288.

290. Mills SE, Cooper PH, Fechner RE: Lobular capillary hemangioma: The underlying lesion of pyogenic granuloma. A study of 73 cases from the oral and nasal mucous membranes. *Am J Surg Pathol* 1980;4:470–479.

Nasopharyngeal Angiofibroma

291. Hyams VJ: Tumors of the upper respiratory tract: Vascular tumors. In Hyams VJ, Batsakis JG, Michaels L (eds): *Atlas of Tumor Pathology*, 2nd series. Washington, D.C.: Armed Forces Institute of Pathology 1986:130–145.

292. Giardiello FM, Hamilton SR, Krush AJ, et al.: Nasopharyngeal angiofibroma in patients with familial adenomatous polyposis. *Gastroenterology* 1993;105:1550–1552.

293. Hwang HC, Mills SE, Patterson K, et al.: Expression of androgen receptors in nasopharyngeal angiofibroma: An immunohistochemical study of 24 cases. *Mod Pathol* 1998;11:1122–1126.

294. Lee DA, Rao BR, Meyer JS, et al.: Hormonal receptor determination in juvenile nasopharyngeal angiofibromas. *Cancer* 1980;46:547–551.

295. Schiff M, Gonzalez AM, Ong M, et al.: Juvenile nasopharyngeal angiofibroma contain an angiogenic growth factor: Basic FGF. *Laryngoscope* 1992;102:940–945.

296. Nagai MA, Butugan O, Logullo A, et al.: Expression of growth factors, proto-oncogenes, and *p53* in nasopharyngeal angiofibromas. *Laryngoscope* 1996;106:190–195.

297. Johns ME, MacLeod RM, Cantrell RW: Estrogen receptors in nasopharyngeal angiofibromas. *Laryngoscope* 1980;90:628–634.

298. Sternberg SS: Pathology of juvenile nasopharyngeal angiofibroma: A lesion of adolescent males. *Cancer* 1954;7:15–28.

299. Neel HB, Whicker JH, Devine KD, et al.: Juvenile angiofibroma. Review of 120 cases. *Am J Surg* 1973;126:547–556.

300. Beham A, Fletcher CDM, Kainz J, et al.: Nasopharyngeal angiofibroma: An immunohistochemical study of 32 cases. *Virchows Arch A Pathol Anat Histopathol* 1993;423:281–285.

301. Beham A, Kainz J, Stammberger HR, et al.: Immunohistochemical and electron microscopical characterization of stromal cells in nasopharyngeal angiofibromas. *Eur Arch Otorhinolaryngol* 1997;254:199.

302. Taxy JB: Juvenile nasopharyngeal angiofibroma. An ultrastructural study. *Cancer* 1977;39:1044–1054.

303. Wanamaker JR, Lavertu P, Levine HL: Juvenile angiofibroma. In Kraus DH, Levine HL (eds): *Nasal Neoplasia*. New York: Thieme, 1997:61–84.

304. Goepfert H, Cangi A, Lee Y-Y: Chemotherapy for aggressive juvenile nasopharyngeal angiofibroma. *Arch Otolaryngol* 1985;111:285–289.

305. Dohar JE, Duvall AJ 3d: Spontaneous regression of juvenile nasopharyngeal angiofibroma. *Ann Otol Rhinol Laryngol* 1992;101:469–471.

306. Spagnolo DV, Papadimitriou JM, Archer M: Postirradiation malignant fibrous histiocytoma arising in juvenile nasopharyngeal angiofibroma and producing alpha-1-antitrypsin. *Histopathology* 1984;8:339–352.

307. Chen KTK, Bauer FW: Sarcomatous transformation of nasopharyngeal angiofibroma. *Cancer* 1982;49:369–371.

308. Hormia M, Koskinen O: Metastasizing nasopharyngeal angiofibroma: A case report. *Arch Otolaryngol* 1969;89:107–110.

Hemangiopericytoma

309. Compagno J, Hyams VJ: Hemangiopericytoma-like intranasal tumors: A clinicopathologic study of 23 cases. *Am J Clin Pathol* 1976;66:672–683.

310. Compagno J: Hemangiopericytoma-like tumors of the nasal cavity: A comparison with hemangiopericytoma of soft tissues. *Laryngoscope* 1978;88:460–469.

311. Sugimoto T, Masuda T, Uemura T, et al.: Hemangiopericytoma-like intranasal tumor: A case report with an immunohistochemical study. *Otolaryngol Head Neck Surg* 1995;113:323–327.

312. Rosai J: Respiratory tract. In: *Ackerman's Surgical Pathology*, 7th ed. St. Louis: Mosby-Year Book, 1996:289–434.

313. Abdel-Fattah HM, Adams GL, Wick MR: Hemangiopericytoma of the maxillary sinus and skull base. *Head Neck* 1990;12:77–83.

314. Chawla OP, Oswal VH: Haemangiopericytoma of the nose and paranasal sinuses. *J Laryngol Otol* 1987;101:729–737.

315. Purdy Stout A, Murray MR: Hemangiopericytoma: A vascular tumor featuring Zimmermann's pericytes. *Ann Surg* 1942;116:26–33.

316. Enzinger FM, Smith BH: Hemangiopericytoma. *Hum Pathol* 1976;7:61–82.

317. Nielsen GP, Dickersin GR, Provenzal JM, et al.: Lipomatous hemangiopericytoma: A histologic, ultrastructural and immunohistochemical study of a unique variant of hemangiopericytoma. *Am J Surg Pathol* 1995;19:748–756.

318. Eichhorn JH, Dickersin GR, Bhan AK, et al.: Sinonasal hemangiopericytoma: A reassessment with electron microscopy, immunohistochemistry, and long-term follow-up. *Am J Surg Pathol* 1990;14:856–866.

319. Mentzel T, Bainbridge TC, Katenkamp D: Solitary fibrous tumour: Clinicopathological, immunohistochemical, and ultrastructural analysis of 12 cases arising in soft tissues, nasal cavity and nasopharynx, urinary bladder and prostate. *Virchows Arch* 1997;430:445–453.

320. Chilosi M, Facchetti F, Dei Tos AP, et al.: *Bcl-2* expression in pleural and extrapleural solitary fibrous tumours. *J Pathol* 1997;181:362–367.

321. de Campora E, Calabrese V, Bianchi PM, et al.: Malignant hemangiopericytoma of the nasal cavity: Report of a case and review of the literature. *J Laryngol Otol* 1983;97:963–968.

322. Gorenstein A, Facer GW, Weiland LH: Hemangiopericytoma of the nasal cavity. *ORL J Otorhinolaryngol Relat Spec* 1978;86:405–415.

Other Vascular Tumors

323. Kim HJ, Kim JH, Hwang EG: Bone erosion caused by sinonasal cavernous hemangioma: CT findings in two patients. *AJNR Am J Neuroradiol* 1995;16:1176–1178.

324. Kuo TT, Sayers CP, Rosai J: Masson's "vegetans intravascular heman-

gioendothelioma": A lesion often mistaken for angiosarcoma. Study of seventeen cases located in the skin and soft tissues. *Cancer* 1976;38:1227–1236.

325. Stern Y, Braslavsky D, Segal K, et al.: Intravascular papillary endothelial hyperplasia in the maxillary sinus: A benign lesion that may be mistaken for angiosarcoma. *Arch Otolaryngol Head Neck Surg* 1991;117:1182–1184.

326. Dass AA, Saleem Y: Hemangioendothelioma of the maxillary sinus. *Otolaryngol Head Neck Surg* 1995;112:735–737.

Angiosarcoma

327. Kimura Y, Tanaka S, Furukawa M: Angiosarcoma of the nasal cavity. *J Laryngol Otol* 1992;106:368–369.

328. Bankaci M, Myers EN, Barnes L, et al.: Angiosarcoma of the maxillary sinus: Literature review and case report. *Head Neck Surg* 1979;1:274–280.

329. Sercarz JA, Mark RJ, Tran L, et al.: Sarcomas of the nasal cavity and paranasal sinuses. *Ann Otol Rhinol Laryngol* 1994;103:699–704.

330. Degos R, Labayle J, Belaich S, et al.: Nasal angiosarcoma. *Ann Dermatol Syphiligr (Paris)* 1971;98:406–407.

331. Aust MR, Olsen KD, Meland NB, et al.: Angiosarcomas of the head and neck: Clinical and pathologic characteristics. *Ann Otol Rhinol Laryngol* 1997;106:943–951.

Kaposi's Sarcoma and Bacillary Angiomatosis

332. Gnepp DR, Chandler W, Hyams VJ: Primary Kaposi's sarcoma of the head and neck. *Ann Intern Med* 1984;100:107–114.

333. Le Boit PE, Berger TG, Egbert BM, et al.: Bacillary angiomatosis: The histopathology and differential diagnosis of a pseudoneoplastic infection in patients with human immunodeficiency virus disease. *Am J Surg Pathol* 1989;13:909–920.

334. Batsakis JG, Ro JY: Bacillary angiomatosis. *Ann Otol Rhinol Laryngol* 1995;104:668–672.

Fibroma

335. Fu YS, Perzin KH: Nonepithelial tumors of the nasal cavity, paranasal sinuses, and nasopharynx. a clinicopathologic study: VI. fibrous tissue tumors (fibroma, fibromatosis, fibrosarcoma). *Cancer* 1976;37:2912–2928.

Benign Fibrous Histiocytoma

336. Perzin KH, Fu YS: Non-epithelial tumors of the nasal cavity, paranasal sinuses and nasopharynx: A clinico-pathologic study XI. fibrous histiocytomas. *Cancer* 1980;45:2616–2626.

Fibromatosis (Desmoid Tumor)

337. Gnepp DR, Henley J, Weiss SW, et al.: Desmoid fibromatosis of the sinonasal tract and nasopharynx: A clinicopathologic study of 25 cases. *Cancer* 1996;78:2572–2579.

Myxoma and Fibromyxoma

338. Ghosh BC, Huvos AG, Gerold FP, et al.: Myxoma of the jaw bones. *Cancer* 1973;31:237–240.

339. Fu Y-S, Perzin KH: Non-epithelial tumors of the nasal cavity, paranasal sinuses and nasopharynx: A clinico-pathologic study. *Cancer* 1977;39:195–203.

340. Heffner DK: Problems in pediatric otorhinolaryngic pathology. I. Sinonasal and nasopharyngeal tumors and masses with myxoid features. *Int J Pediatr Otorhinolaryngol* 1983;5:77–91.

341. Hayes DK, Madsen JM, Simpson R, et al.: Myxomas of the maxilla in infants and children. *Otolaryngol Head Neck Surg* 1991;105:464–468.

342. Canalis RF, Smith GA, Konrad HR: Myxomas of the head and neck. *Arch Otolaryngol Head Neck Surg* 1976;102:300–305.

343. Gregor RT, Loftus-Coll B: Myxoma of the paranasal sinuses. *J Laryngol Otol* 1994;108:679–681.

344. Stout AP: Myxoma, the tumor of primitive mesenchyme. *Ann Surg* 1948;127:706–719.

345. Oliver DS, DiNardo LJ, Monahan M, et al.: Pathologic Quiz Case 2.

Odontogenic fibromyxoma. *Arch Otolaryngol Head Neck Surg* 1995;121:805–807.

346. Harrison D, Lund VJ: Mesenchymal malignancy. In: *Tumours of the Upper Jaw.* Edinburgh: Churchill-Livingstone, 1993;135–156.

347. Perez-Ordóñez B, Shah JP, Huvos AG: Myxomas and fibromyxosarcoma of craniofacial bones. A study of 5 cases [abstract]. *Proceedings of the 4th International Conference on Head and Neck Cancer.* Toronto, Canada, 1996:235.

348. Moshiri S, Oda D, Worthington P, et al.: Odontogenic myxoma: Histochemical and ultrastructural study. *J Oral Pathol Med* 1992;21:401–403.

Solitary Fibrous Tumor

349. Witkin GB, Rosai J: Solitary fibrous tumor of the upper respiratory tract: A report of six cases. *Am J Surg Pathol* 1991;15:842–848.

350. Ferreiro JA, Nascimento AG: Solitary fibrous tumor of the major salivary glands. *Histopathology* 1996;28:261–264.

351. Lucas DR, Campbell RJ, Fletcher CDM, et al.: Solitary fibrous tumor of the orbit. *Int J Surg Pathol* 1995;2:193–198.

352. Batsakis JG, Hybels RD, El-Naggar AK: Solitary fibrous tumor. *Ann Otol Rhinol Laryngol* 1993;102:74–76.

353. Zukerberg LR, Rosenberg AE, Randolph G, et al.: Solitary fibrous tumor of the nasal cavity and paranasal sinuses. *Am J Surg Pathol* 1991;15:126–130.

Fibrosarcoma

354. Koka V, Vericel R, Lartigau E, et al.: Sarcomas of nasal cavity and paranasal sinuses: Chondrosarcoma, osteosarcoma and fibrosarcoma. *J Laryngol Otol* 1994;108:947–953.

355. Frankenthaler R, Ayala AG, Hartwick RW, et al.: Fibrosarcoma of the head and neck. *Laryngoscope* 1990;100:799–802.

356. Heffner DK, Gnepp DR: Sinonasal fibrosarcomas, malignant schwannomas, and "triton" tumors: A clinicopathologic study of 67 cases. *Cancer* 1992;70:1089–1101.

Malignant Fibrous Histiocytoma

357. Enzinger FM: Malignant fibrous histiocytoma 20 years after Stout. *Am J Surg Pathol* 1986;10(Suppl 1):43–53.

358. Barnes L, Kanbour A: Malignant fibrous histiocytoma of the head and neck. a report of 12 cases. *Arch Otolaryngol Head Neck Surg* 1988;114:1149–1156.

359. Tanaka T, Saito R, Kajiwara M, et al.: Fibrous histiocytoma of the nasal cavity and maxillary sinus. *Acta Pathol Jpn* 1982;32:657–669.

Leiomyoma and Leiomyosarcoma

360. Harcourt JP, Gallimore AP: Leiomyoma of the paranasal sinuses. *J Laryngol Otol* 1993;107:740–741.

361. Fu YS, Perzin KH: Nonepithelial tumors of the nasal cavity, paranasal sinuses, and nasopharynx: A clinicopathologic study. IV. smooth muscle tumors (leiomyoma, leiomyosarcoma). *Cancer* 1975;35:1300–1308.

362. Papavasiliou A, Michaels L: Unusual leiomyoma of the nose (leiomyoblastoma). Report of a case. *J Laryngol Otol* 1981;95:1281–1286.

363. Dropkin LR, Tang CK, Williams JR: Leiomyosarcoma of the nasal cavity and paranasal sinuses. *Ann Otol Rhinol Laryngol* 1976;85:(3 Pt 1):399–403

364. Kuruvilla A, Wenig BM, Humphrey DM, et al.: Leiomyosarcoma of the sinonasal tract: A clinicopathologic study of nine cases. *Arch Otolaryngol Head Neck Surg* 1990;116:1278–1286.

365. Enzinger FM, Weiss SW: Leiomyosarcoma. In: *Soft Tissue Tumors,* 3rd ed. St. Louis: Mosby-Year Book, 1995;491–510.

Rhabdomyoma

366. Fu YS, Perzin KH: Nonepithelial tumors of the nasal cavity paranasal sinuses, and nasopharynx: A clinicopathologic study. V. skeletal muscle tumors (rhabdomyoma and rhabdomyosarcoma). *Cancer* 1976;37:364–376.

367. Kapadia SB, Meis JM, Frisman DM, et al.: Adult rhabdomyoma of the head and neck: A clinicopathologic and immunophenotypic study. *Hum Pathol* 1993;24:608–617.

368. Weiss SW, Enzinger FM: Rhabdomyoma. In: *Soft Tissue Tumors,* 3rd ed. St. Louis: Mosby-Year Book, 1995:523–537.

Rhabdomyosarcoma

369. Newton WA Jr, Soule EH, Hamoudi AB, et al.: Histopathology of childhood sarcomas. Intergroup Rhabdomyosarcoma studies I and II: Clinicopathologic correlation. *J Clin Oncol* 1988;6:67–75.
370. Horn RC, Enterline HT: Rhabdomyosarcoma: A clinicopathological study and classification of 39 cases. *Cancer* 1958;11:181–199.
371. Suzuki M, Kobayashi Y, Harada Y, et al.: Rhabdomyosarcoma of the maxillary sinus: A case report. *J Laryngol Otol* 1984;98:405–415.
372. El-Naggar AK, Batsakis JG, Ordonez NG, et al.: Rhabdomyosarcoma of the adult head and neck: A clinicopathological and DNA ploidy study. *J Laryngol Otol* 1993;107:716–720.
373. Enzinger FM, Weiss SW: Rhabdomyosarcoma. In: *Soft Tissue Tumors,* 3rd ed. St. Louis: Mosby-Year Book, 1995:523–577.
374. Enterline HT, Horn RC: Alveolar rhabdomyosarcoma. *Am J Clin Pathol* 1958;29:356–366.
375. Chan JK, Ng HK, Wan KY, et al.: Clear cell rhabdomyosarcoma of the nasal cavity and paranasal sinuses. *Histopathology* 1989;14:391–399.
376. Molenaar WM, Oosterhuis JW, Kamps WA: Cytologic "differentiation" in childhood rhabdomyosarcomas following polychemotherapy. *Hum Pathol* 1984;15:973–979.
377. Maurer HM, Beltangady M, Gehan EA, et al.: The Intergroup Rhabdomyosarcoma Study: I. A final report. *Cancer* 1988;61:209–220.
378. Shimada H, Newton WA, Soule EH, et al.: Pathology of fatal rhabdomyosarcoma. Report from Intergroup Rhabdomyosarcoma Study (IRS-I and IRS-II). *Cancer* 1987;59:459–465.

Peripheral Nerve Sheath Tumors

379. Perzin KH, Panyu H, Wechter S: Nonepithelial tumors of the nasal cavity, paranasal sinuses and nasopharynx: A clinicopathologic study. XII: Schwann cell tumors (neurilemoma, neurofibroma, malignant schwannoma). *Cancer* 1982;50:2193–2202.
380. Franquemont DW, Fechner RE, Mills SE: Histologic classification of sinonasal intestinal-type adenocarcinoma. *Am J Surg Pathol* 1991;15:368–375.
381. Nagayama I, Nishimura T, Furukawa M: Malignant schwannoma arising in a paranasal sinus. *J Laryngol Otol* 1993;107:146–148.
382. Fernandez PL, Cardesa A, Bombi JA, et al.: Malignant sinonasal epithelioid schwannoma. *Virchows Arch A Pathol Anat Histopathol* 1993;423:401–405.
383. Hillstrom RP, Zarbo RJ, Jacobs JR: Nerve sheath tumors of the paranasal sinuses: Electron microscopy and histopathologic diagnosis. *Otolaryngol Head Neck Surg* 1990;102:257–263.
384. Younis RT, Gross CW, Lazar RH: Schwannomas of the paranasal sinuses: Case report and clinicopathologic analysis. *Arch Otolaryngol Head Neck Surg* 1991;117:677–680.
385. Shajrawi I, Podoshin L, Fradis M, et al.: Malignant triton tumor of the nose and paranasal sinuses: A case study. *Hum Pathol* 1989;20:811–814.
386. Hasegawa SL, Mentzel T, Fletcher CDM: Schwannomas of the sinonasal tract and nasopharynx. *Mod Pathol* 1997;10:777–784.
387. Robitaille Y, Seemayer TA, El Deiry A: Peripheral nerve tumors involving paranasal sinuses: A case report and review of the literature. *Cancer* 1975;35:1254–1258.
388. Dickersin GR: The electron microscopic spectrum of nerve sheath tumors. *Ultrastruct Pathol* 1987;11:103–146.
389. Hoffman DF, Everts EC, Smith JD, et al.: Malignant nerve sheath tumors of the head and neck. *Otolaryngol Head Neck Surg* 1988;99:309–314.

Adipose Tissue Tumors

390. Fu YS, Perzin KH: Non-epithelial tumors of the nasal cavity, paranasal sinuses and nasopharynx: A clinicopathologic study: VIII. Adipose tissue tumors (lipoma and liposarcoma). *Cancer* 1977;40:1314–1317.

Meningioma

391. Farr HW, Gray GF, Vrana M, et al.: Extracranial meningioma. *J Surg Oncol* 1973;4:411–420.
392. Perzin KH, Pushparaj N: Nonepithelial tumors of the nasal cavity, para-

nasal sinuses, and nasopharynx: A clinicopathologic study. XIII: Meningiomas. *Cancer* 1984;54:1860–1869.
393. Ho KL: Primary meningioma of the nasal cavity and paranasal sinuses. *Cancer* 1980;46:1442–1447.
394. Taxy JB: Meningioma of the paranasal sinuses: A report of two cases. *Am J Surg Pathol* 1990;14:82–86.
395. Sadar ES, Conomy JP, Benjamin SP, et al.: Meningiomas of the paranasal sinuses, benign and malignant. *Neurosurgery* 1979;4:227–232.
396. Kershisnik M, Callender DL, Batsakis JG: Extracranial, extraspinal meningiomas of the head and neck. *Ann Otol Rhinol Laryngol* 1993;102:967–970.
397. Leyva WH, Gnepp DR: Pathologic quiz case 2. Meningioma. *Arch Otolaryngol Head Neck Surg* 1987;113:206–209.

Sinonasal Ameloblastoma

398. Schafer DR, Thompson LDR, Smith BC, et al.: Primary ameloblastoma of the sinonasal tract: A clinicopathologic study of 24 cases. *Cancer* 1998;82:667–674.

Ectopic Pituitary Adenoma

399. Langford L, Batsakis JG: Pituitary gland involvement of the sinonasal tract. *Ann Otol Rhinol Laryngol* 1995;104:167–169.
400. Lloyd RV, Chandler WF, Kovacs K, et al.: Ectopic pituitary adenomas with normal anterior pituitary glands. *Am J Surg Pathol* 1986;10:546–552.
401. Asa SL: Tumors of the pituitary gland: Pituitary adenomas. In: *Atlas of Tumor Pathology,* 3rd series. Washington, DC: Armed Forces Institute of Pathology, 1998:47–147.
402. Lloyd RV: Ectopic pituitary adenomas. In Lloyd RV: *Major Problems in Pathology: Surgical Pathology of the Pituitary Gland* (Major Problems in Pathology, Vol 27). Philadelphia: W.B. Saunders, 1993:116–120.
403. Luk SC, Chan JKC, Chow SM, et al.: Pituitary adenoma presenting as sinonasal tumor: Pitfalls in diagnosis. *Hum Pathol* 1996;27:605–609.
404. Matsushita H, Matsuya S, Endo Y, et al.: A prolactin producing tumor originated in the sphenoid sinus. *Acta Pathol Jpn* 1984;34:103–109.

Craniopharyngioma

405. Burger PC, Scheithauer BW: Tumors of the central nervous system: Craniopharyngiomas. In: *Atlas of Tumor Pathology,* 3rd series. Washington, DC: Armed Forces Institute of Pathology, 1994:349–354.
406. Byrne MN, Sessions DG: Nasopharyngeal craniopharyngioma: Case report and literature review. *Ann Otol Rhinol Laryngol* 1990;99:633–639.
407. Akimura T, Kameda H, Abiko S, et al.: Infrasellar craniopharyngioma. *Neuroradiology* 1989;31:180–183.

Teratomas, Teratocarcinosarcoma, and Nasal Blastoma

408. Gonzalez-Crussi F: Extragonadal teratomas: Teratomas of the head (extracranial). In: *Atlas of Tumor Pathology,* 2nd series. Washington, DC: Armed Forces Institute of Pathology, 1982:109–117.
409. Byard RW, Smith CR, Chan HSL: Endodermal sinus tumor of the nasopharynx and previous mature congenital teratoma. *Pediatr Pathol* 1991;11:297–302.
410. Lack EE: Extragonadal germ cell tumors of the head and neck region. Review of 16 cases. *Hum Pathol* 1985;16:56–64.
411. Byard RW, Jimenez CL, Carpenter BF, et al.: Congenital teratomas of the neck and nasopharynx: A clinicopathologic study of 18 cases. *J Pediatr Child Health* 1990;26:12–16.
412. Guarisco JL, Butcher RB: Congenital cystic teratoma of the maxillary sinus. *Otolaryngol Head Neck Surg* 1990;103:1035–1038.
413. Petrovich Z, Wollman J, Acquarelli M, et al.: Malignant teratoma of the nasal cavity. *J Surg Oncol* 1977;9:21–28.
414. Ulbright TM: Neoplasms of the testis. In Bostwick DG, Eble JN (eds): *Urologic Surgical Pathology.* St. Louis: Mosby-Year Book, 1997:566–645.
415. Batsakis JG, El-Naggar AK, Luna MA: Teratomas of the head and neck with emphasis on malignancy. *Ann Otol Rhinol Laryngol* 1995;104:496–500.
416. Heffner DK, Hyams VJ: Teratocarcinosarcoma (malignant teratoma?)

of the nasal cavity and paranasal sinuses. A clinicopathologic study of 20 cases. *Cancer* 1984;53:2140–2154.

417. Fernandez PL, Cardesa A, Alos L, et al.: Sinonasal teratocarcinosarcoma: An unusual neoplasm. *Pathol Res Pract* 1995;191:166–171.

418. Shanmugaratnam K, Kunaratnam N, Chia KB, et al.: Teratoid carcinosarcoma of the paranasal sinuses. *Pathology* 1983;15:413–419.

419. Luna MA: Critical commentary to "sinonasal teratocarcinoma." *Pathol Res Pract* 1995;191:172.

420. Pai SA, Naresh KN, Masih K, et al.: Teratocarcinosarcoma of the paranasal sinuses: A clinicopathologic and immunohistochemical study. *Hum Pathol* 1998;29:718–722.

421. Patterson SD, Ballard RW: Nasal blastoma: A light and electron microscopic study. *Ultrastruct Pathol* 1980;1:487–494.

422. Meinecke R, Bauer F, Skouras J, et al.: Blastomatous tumors of the respiratory tract. *Cancer* 1976;38:818–823.

423. Shindo ML, Stanley RB Jr, Kiyabu MT: Carcinosarcoma of the nasal cavity and paranasal sinuses. *Head Neck* 1990;12:516–519.

Alveolar Soft Part Sarcoma

424. Chatterji P, Purohit GN, Ramdev IN, et al.: Alveolar soft part sarcoma of the nasal cavity and paranasal sinuses. *J Laryngol Otol* 1977;91:1003–1008.

Postirradiation Malignant Tumors

425. Coia LR, Fazekas JT, Kramer S: Postirradiation sarcoma of the head and neck: A report of three late sarcomas following therapeutic irradiation for primary malignancies of the paranasal sinus, nasal cavity, and larynx. *Cancer* 1980;46:1982–1985.

426. Maisel RH, Manivel JC, Porto DP, et al.: Postirradiation sarcomas of the head and neck. *Ear Nose Throat J* 1989;68:684–701.

427. Huvos AG, Woodard HQ, Cahan WG, et al.: Postirradiation osteogenic sarcoma of bone and soft tissues: A clinicopathologic study of 66 patients. *Cancer* 1985;55:1244–1255.

Malignant Non-Hodgkin's Lymphoma

428. National Cancer Institute: National Cancer Institute sponsored study of classification of non-Hodgkin's lymphomas. Summary and description of a Working Formulation for Clinical Usage. The non-Hodgkin's Lymphoma Pathologic Classification Project. *Cancer* 1982;49:2112–2135.

429. Jaffe ES, Chan JKC, Su I-J, et al.: Report of the Workshop on Nasal and Related Extranodal Angiocentric T/Natural Killer Cell Lymphomas: Definitions, differential diagnosis, and epidemiology. *Am J Surg Pathol* 1996;20:102–111.

430. Tran LM, Mark R, Fu YS, et al.: Primary non-Hodgkin's lymphomas of the paranasal sinuses and nasal cavity: A report of 18 cases with stage IE disease. *Am J Clin Oncol* 1992;15:222–225.

431. Kapadia SB, Barnes L, Deutsch M: Non-Hodgkin's lymphoma of the nose and paranasal sinuses: A study of 17 cases. *Head Neck Surg* 1981;3:490–439.

432. Abbondanzo SL, Wenig BM: Non-Hodgkin's lymphoma of the sinonasal tract: A clinicopathologic and immunophenotypic study of 120 cases. *Cancer* 1995;75:1281–1291.

433. Frierson HF Jr, Mills SE, Innes DJ Jr: Non-Hodgkin's lymphomas of the sinonasal region: Histologic subtypes and their clinicopathologic features. *Am J Clin Pathol* 1984;81:721–727.

434. Fu YS, Perzin KH: Nonepithelial tumors of the nasal cavity, paranasal sinuses and nasopharynx: A clinicopathologic study. X. Malignant lymphomas. *Cancer* 1979;43:611–621.

435. Kristensen S: Immunoblastic sarcoma of the nasal cavity. *Arch Otorhinolaryngol* 1984;240:227–230.

436. Harrinson D, Lund VJ: Lymphoreticular tissue neoplasia and destructive lesions. In: *Tumours of the Upper Jaw.* Edinburgh: Churchill-Livingstone, 1993:265–281.

Sinonasal T/NK Cell Lymphoma (Angiocentric Lymphoma, Polymorphic Reticulosis)

437. Lippman SM, Grogan TM, Spier CM, et al.: Lethal midline granuloma with a novel T-cell phenotype as found in peripheral T-cell lymphoma. *Cancer* 1987;59:936–939.

438. Gaulard P, Henni T, Marolleau J-P, et al.: Lethal midline granuloma (polymorphic reticulosis) and lymphomatoid granulomatosis. Evidence

for a monoclonal T-cell lymphoproliferative disorder. *Cancer* 1988;62:705–710.

439. Kassel SH, Echevarria RA, Guzzo FP: Midline malignant reticulosis (so-called lethal midline granuloma). *Cancer* 1969;23:920–935.

440. Ferry JA, Sklar J, Zukerberg LR, et al.: Nasal lymphoma: A clinicopathologic study with immunophenotypic and genotypic analysis. *Am J Surg Pathol* 1991;15:268–279.

441. Ho FC, Choy D, Loke SL, et al.: Polymorphic reticulosis and conventional lymphomas of the nose and upper aerodigestive tract: A clinicopathologic study of 70 cases, and immunophenotypic studies of 16 cases. *Hum Pathol* 1990;21:1041–1050.

442. Medeiros LJ, Jaffe ES, Chen YY, et al.: Localization of Epstein-Barr viral genomes in angiocentric immunoproliferative lesions. *Am J Surg Pathol* 1992;16:439–447.

443. Suzumiya J, Takeshita M, Kimura N, et al.: Expression of adult and fetal natural killer cell markers in sinonasal lymphomas. *Blood* 1994;83:2255–2260.

444. Chan JK, Ng CS, Lau WH, et al.: Most nasal/nasopharyngeal lymphomas are peripheral T-cell neoplasms. *Am J Surg Pathol* 1987;11:418–429.

445. Tsang WYW, Chan JKC, Ng CS, et al.: Utility of a paraffin section-reactive CD56 antibody (123C3) for characterization and diagnosis of lymphomas. *Am J Surg Pathol* 1996;20:202–210.

446. Strickler JG, Meneses MF, Habermann TM, et al.: Polymorphic reticulosis: A reappraisal. *Hum Pathol* 1994;25:659–665.

447. Arber DA, Weiss LM, Albujar PF, et al.: Nasal lymphomas in Peru. High incidence of T-cell immunophenotype and Epstein-Barr virus infection. *Am J Surg Pathol* 1993;17:392–399.

448. Aviles A, Rodriguez L, Guzman R, et al.: Angiocentric T-cell lymphoma of the nose, paranasal sinuses and hard palate. *Hematol Oncol* 1992;10:141–147.

449. van de Rijn M, Bhargava V, Molina-Kirsch H, et al.: Extranodal head and neck lymphomas in Guatemala: High frequency of Epstein-Barr virus-associated sinonasal lymphomas. *Hum Pathol* 1997;28:834–839.

450. Chan JK, Yip TT, Tsang WY, et al.: Detection of Epstein-Barr viral RNA in malignant lymphomas of the upper aerodigestive tract. *Am J Surg Pathol* 1994;18:938–946.

451. Kanavaros P, Briere J, Lescs MC, et al.: Epstein-Barr virus in non-Hodgkin's lymphomas of the upper respiratory tract: Association with sinonasal localization and expression of NK and/or T-cell antigens by tumor cells. *J Pathol* 1996;178:297–302.

452. Luzi P, Leoncini L, Funto I, et al.: Epstein-Barr virus infection in sinonasal non-Hodgkin's lymphomas. *Virchows Arch [Pathol Anat]* 1995;425:121–125.

453. Ott G, Kalla J, Ott M, et al.: The Epstein-Barr virus in malignant non-Hodgkin's lymphoma of the upper aerodigestive tract. *Diagn Mol Pathol* 1997;6:134–139.

454. Elenitoba-Johnson KSJ, Zarate-Osorno A, Meneses A, et al.: Cytotoxic granular expression, Epstein-Barr virus strain type, and latent membrane protein-1 oncogene deletions in nasal T-cell lymphocyte/natural killer cell lymphomas from Mexico. *Mod Pathol* 1998;11:754–761.

455. Liang R, Tood D, Chan TK, et al.: Nasal lymphoma: A retrospective analysis of 60 cases. *Cancer* 1990;66:2205–2209.

456. Van Gorp J, de Bruin PC, Sie-Go DMDS, et al.: Nasal T-cell lymphoma: A clinicopathological and immunophenotypic analysis of 13 cases. *Histopathology* 1995;27:139–148.

457. Aozasa K, Ohsawa M, Tomita Y, et al.: Polymorphic reticulosis is a neoplasm of large granular lymphocytes with CD3+ phenotype. *Cancer* 1995;75:894–901.

458. Ng CS, Lo STH, Chan JKC, et al.: CD56+ putative natural killer cell lymphomas: Production of cytolytic effectors and related proteins mediating tumor cell apoptosis. *Hum Pathol* 1997;28:1276–1282.

459. Oshima K, Suzumiya J, Shimazaki K, et al.: Nasal T/NK cell lymphomas commonly express perforin and Fas ligand: Important mediators of tissue damage. *Histopathology* 1997;31:444–450.

460. Harabuchi Y, Imai S, Wakashima J, et al.: Nasal T-cell lymphoma casually associated with Epstein-Barr virus. Clinicopathologic, phenotypic, and genotypic studies. *Cancer* 1996;77:2137–2149.

461. Petrella T, Delfau-Larue M-H, Caillot D, et al.: Nasopharyngeal lymphomas: Further evidence for a natural killer cell origin. *Hum Pathol* 1996;27:827–833.

462. Chiang AKS, Srivastava G, Lau PWF, et al.: Differences in T-cell-receptor gene rearrangement and transcription in nasal lymphomas of natural killer and T-cell Types: Implications on cellular origin. *Hum Pathol* 1996;27:701–707.

463. Chott A, Rappersberger K, Scholossarek W, et al.: Peripheral T cell lymphoma presenting primarily as lethal midline granuloma. *Hum Pathol* 1988;19:1093–1101.

464. Crissman JD, Weiss MA, Gluckman J: Midline granuloma syndrome: A clinicopathologic study of 13 patients. *Am J Surg Pathol* 1982;6:335–346.

465. Wong KF, Chan JKC, Ng CS, et al.: CD56 (NKH1)-positive hematolymphoid malignancies: An aggressive neoplasm featuring frequent cutaneous/mucosal involvement, cytoplasmic azurophilic granules, and angiocentricity. *Hum Pathol* 1992;23:798–804.

466. Ratech H, Burke JS, Blayney DW, et al.: A clinicopathologic study of malignant lymphomas of the nose, paranasal sinuses, and hard palate, including cases of lethal midline granuloma. *Cancer* 1989;64:2525–2531.

Plasmacytoma

467. Castro EB, Lewis JS, Strong EW: Plasmacytoma of paranasal sinuses and nasal cavity. *Arch Otolaryngol* 1973;97:326–329.

468. Fu YS, Perzin KH: Nonepithelial tumors of the nasal cavity, paranasal sinuses and nasopharynx. a clinicopathologic study. IX. plasmacytomas. *Cancer* 1978;42:2399–406.

469. Kapadia SB, Desai U, Cheng VS: Extramedullary plasmacytoma of the head and neck: A clinicopathologic study of 20 cases. *Medicine* 1982;61:317–329.

Metastatic Tumors

470. Harrinson D, Lund VJ: Tumours of the upper jaw. Edinburgh: Churchill-Livingstone, 1993:124–134.

471. Friedmann I, Osborn DA: Metastatic tumours of the nose and sinuses. In: *Pathology of Granulomas and Neoplasms of the Nose and Paranasal Sinuses.* Edinburgh: Churchill-Livingstone, 1982:300–303.

472. Frigy AF: Pathologic quiz case 2: Metastatic hepatocellular carcinoma of the nasal cavity. *Arch Otolaryngol* 1984;110:624–627.

473. Yamasoba T, Kikuchi S, Sugasawa M, et al.: Occult follicular carcinoma metastasizing to the sinonasal tract. *ORL J Otorhinolaryngol Relat Spec* 1994;56:239–243.

474. Cinberg JZ, Terrife D: Follicular adenocarcinoma of the thyroid in the maxillary sinus. *Otolaryngol Head Neck Surg* 1980;88:157–158.

475. Ellis GL: Clear cell neoplasms in salivary glands: Clearly a diagnostic challenge. *Ann Diagn Pathol* 1998;2:61–78.

4 Lesions of the Oral Cavity

Jerry E. Bouquot and Hiromasa Nikai

FIBROUS, FIBROHISTIOCYTIC, AND FIBROVASCULAR LESIONS

The great majority of soft tissue masses of the mouth are hyperplastic inflammatory responses to local, usually chronic, trauma or infection.[1–11] These benign reactive lesions result from the proliferation of one or more components of the normal connective tissue stroma and are sometimes unique to the mouth because of their origin from periodontal or odontogenic tissues. Reactive lesions are much more common in the mouth than in other parts of the body, presumably because of the close proximity of mucosa to hard, often sharp, teeth and prosthetic appliances. Found in the mouths of 3% of adults, these lesions collectively represent more than 80% of biopsied oral masses.[1–3, 7]

Also included in this first section are benign neoplastic lesions with fibrous proliferation as a major characteristic. Look-alike "fibrous" tumors of peripheral nerves and smooth muscle are discussed separately in this chapter under the sections relating to benign nerve tumors and benign muscle tumors. Altogether, neoplastic fibrous lesions are much less common than inflammatory hyperplasias of the mouth, they are more likely to represent a localized manifestation of a systemic process or syndrome.

Irritation Fibroma and Localized Fibrous Hyperplasia

Irritation fibroma, or *traumatic fibroma,* is a common submucosal response to trauma from teeth or dental prostheses and was first reported in 1846 as *fibrous polyp* and *polypus.*[12] It is universally understood that the use of the term "fibroma" is not intended in this case to convey neoplastic origin, as is the usual intent of its use for fibrous tumors in other anatomic sites. Found in 1.2% of adults (Table 4–1), this inflammatory hyperplasia is the most common oral mucosal mass submitted for biopsy and is usually composed of types I and III collagen.[1–3, 7] Gingival lesions are also common, although at that location they probably result from chronic infection rather than trauma.[13] A number of variations on the theme of inflammatory fibrous hyperplasia are mentioned in the following discussion.

Clinical Features. The irritation fibroma has a 66% female predilection and can occur at any age, but is usually biopsied in the fourth through sixth decades of life. It is extremely rare during the first decade of life. Patients with multiple fibromas may represent cases of *familial fibromatosis,* fibrotic *papillary hyperplasia of the palate, tuberous sclerosis,* or *multiple hamartoma syndrome (Cowden syndrome).*[5, 7] Those with a generalized fibrous overgrowth of the gingival tissues are said to have *fibrous gingival hyperplasia* or *gingival fibromatosis,* which is discussed elsewhere in this chapter.

Within the mouth, buccal, labial, and lateral tongue sites account for 71% of all fibromas.[2] The mass may be sessile or pedunculated and usually reaches its maximum size within a few months (Fig. 4–1A). Seldom does it exceed 1.5 cm in size, and once fully formed it remains indefinitely.[7, 14] It is an asymptomatic, moderately firm, immovable mass with a surface coloration that is most often normal but may show pallor from decreased vascularity, whiteness from thickened surface keratin, or ulceration from recurring trauma.

A fibroma beneath a denture has no room to expand uniformly in all directions and so develops as a flat, pancake-shaped mass with small surface papules along the outer edges. This *leaf-shaped fibroma* may be associated with an underlying cupped-out area of bony erosion (Fig. 4–1B).

Another unique variant of denture-related fibroma, *epulis fissuratum* (epulis means "mass on the gingiva"), is an irregular, linear, fibrous hyperplasia occurring in the mucosal vestibule or sulcus adjacent to the alveolar ridge, where the edge of a loose-fitting denture chronically pounds into the tissue.[7, 9, 15–17] The mass runs parallel to the edge of the denture (Fig. 4–2A). Eventually, three or more "waves" of fibrous *redundant tissue* may be seen, with deep grooves between them. The superior edges of these masses may have a line of papules or secondary growths, perhaps explaining why the lesion was first reported in 1858 as "mamillated epulis."[18] The lesion accounts for approximately 3% of submitted oral biopsies and is usually found in persons 40 to 50 years of age.[15]

Yet another rather unique fibrous hyperplasia is the *giant cell fibroma.*[7, 19–21] Usually a small mucosal mass less than 0.5 cm in size (Fig. 4–3A), this lesion differs from routine fibrous hyperplasia in that it is typically lobulated, has a greater tendency to recur, and has unique fibroblasts. It represents approximately 5% of all oral and pharyngeal fibromas and is similar to the *fibrous papule of the face,* which is now thought to represent a variant of *angiofibroma.*[8] The most common sites of occurrence, in descending order of frequency, are gingiva, tongue, palate, and buccal mucosa. This occurs at a younger age than routine irritation fibromas, with almost 70% of lesions reported in persons less than 30 years of age.

The *retrocuspid papilla (retrocuspid papule)* is a final fibrous oral mass, one which appears to be a unique variation of normal anatomy. It occurs as a small, asymptomatic, firm papule of the lingual aspect of the mandibular cuspid, either on the gingiva or the adjacent oral floor mucosa. The mass is usually sessile but may be pedunculated and is typically bilateral.[9, 22] It is found in the majority of children but in less than 20% of older adults. Biopsied cases are often red and edematous.

Pathologic Features and Differential Diagnosis. The irritation fibroma is composed of a dense and minimally cellular stroma of collagen fibers arranged randomly or organized into interlacing fascicles (Fig. 4–1C&D). The stromal cells are bipolar fibroblasts with plump nuclei and fibrocytes with thin, elongated nuclei and minimal cytoplasm. As with *keloids* of the skin, the mucosal fibroma may be remarkably avascular, but areas of necrosis are not seen unless associated with overlying mucosal ulceration. Keloids do not, moreover, occur in the mouth.

Usually scattered, mature capillaries are found; often a few of these are dilated. In cases resulting from the slow fibrosis of granulation tissue or *pyogenic granuloma,* focal areas of edema and neovascularity may be seen in the midportion or lower third of the mass. Occasional lesions may still contain residual granulation tissue, prompting some pathologists to prefer the term *fibrotic pyogenic granuloma.* Such lesions may be indistinguishable from the *angiofibroma* of *tuberous sclerosis.*

Table 4–1. Prevalence Rates for Selected Oral Mucosal Masses and Surface Alterations in U.S. Adults

Diagnosis	Number of Lesions per 1000 Population*		
	Males	*Females*	*Total*
Torus	22.8	30.0	27.1
Irritation fibroma	13.0	11.4	12.0
Fordyce granules	17.7	5.2	9.7
Hemangioma	8.4	4.1	5.5
Papilloma	5.3	4.2	4.6
Epulis fissuratum	3.4	4.4	4.1
Lingual varicosities	3.5	3.4	3.5
Papillary hyperplasia	1.7	3.8	3.0
Mucocele	1.9	2.6	2.5
Enlarged lingual tonsil	2.4	1.2	1.6
Lichen planus	1.2	1.1	1.1
Buccal exostosis	0.9	0.9	0.9
Median rhomboid glossitis	0.8	0.5	0.6
Epidermoid cyst	0.7	0.4	0.5
Oral melanotic macule	0.5	0.3	0.4
Oral tonsils (except lingual)	0.5	0.3	0.4
Lipoma	0.2	0.1	0.2
Ranula	0.2	0.1	0.2
Buccinator node, hyperplastic	0.1	0.07	0.08
Pyogenic granuloma	0.0	0.07	0.04
Nasoalveolar cyst	0.0	0.07	0.04
Neurofibroma	0.0	0.07	0.04

*Total examined population = 23,616 adults; total number of masses = 1453. Data from Bouquot,[1] Bouquot and Gundlach,[2] and Gnepp.[3]

The lesional fibrosis typically extends to the overlying stratified squamous epithelium but may be separated from it by a thin layer of normal fibrovascular connective tissue. Although usually nonencapsulated, some lesions show a pseudoencapsulation and may, therefore, be mistaken for *neurofibroma* or *palisaded encapsulated neuroma.* Scattered chronic inflammatory cells are seen in small numbers, usually beneath the epithelium or around blood vessels. Occasional fibromas demonstrate extreme elongation of rete processes and are called *fibroepithelial polyps* by some authorities, presumably because of their similarity to the dermal lesion of that name.[8] These polyps are seen on the tongue in patients with *Gorlin syndrome (nevoid basal cell carcinoma syndrome).*[5]

The surface epithelium is usually atrophic but may show signs of continued trauma, such as excess keratin, intracellular edema of the superficial layers, or traumatic ulceration. The hyperkeratinized epithelium is not dysplastic or precancerous and is essentially a *frictional keratosis.* Rarely, melanin deposition is seen in the basal layer. This has no diagnostic significance, but its presence has led some to refer to such a lesion as *pigmented fibroma.*

Epulis fissuratum is microscopically similar to routine irritation fibroma (Fig. 4–2B) except that the chronic inflammatory cells are more numerous and the surface epithelium is much more likely to be ulcerated, especially in the base of the clefts between the redundant folds of tissue. The intact surface epithelium is often quite acanthotic, with occasional lesions showing enough elongation of rete processes to justify a secondary diagnosis of *pseudoepitheliomatous hyperplasia* (Fig. 4–2C). The pathologist must be very cautious about misinterpreting this epithelial hyperplasia as well-differentiated *squamous cell carcinoma* or *verrucous carcinoma,* especially with samples showing elongated rete processes cut tangentially or at right angles, appearing as separate islands of epithelium deep in the stroma. It is important, in this regard, to understand that carcinoma in association with epulis fissuratum is extremely rare.

Giant cell fibroma differs from routine irritation fibroma in that it contains moderate numbers of large, stellate fibroblasts with large, angular, pale-staining nuclei (Fig. 4–3B). Some lesional fibroblasts contain two or more nuclei. These cells are most often seen imme-

diately beneath the epithelium and are seldom numerous. They may impart a "glial" appearance to the fibrous stroma and their similarity to giant nevus cells may be remarkable. Giant cells in the dermal counterpart, *fibrous papule of the face,* express factor XIIIa but not S-100 protein, indicating an origin from fibroblasts rather than melanocytic nevus cells.[8, 21] The *angiofibroma* of *tuberous sclerosis* may also demonstrate similar glial-like stroma.

The *retrocuspid papule* consists of dense collagenic tissue with large, stellate fibroblasts, sometimes with multiple nuclei.[22] The stroma often has a whorled pattern and the surface epithelium may demonstrate considerable rete peg hyperplasia; rests of odontogenic epithelium are occasionally noted. Without the latter features, the histopathologic distinction between this lesion and the giant cell fibroma is slight indeed.

Many soft tissue nodules of the mouth have a moderately dense fibrous stroma but contain various nonfibrous components. These components are used to classify the nodule as a distinctly different entity.[7, 9] Scattered islands of benign and innocuous-looking squamous epithelium, for example, are seen in the *peripheral squamous odontogenic tumor* and the *peripheral Pindborg tumor.* Islands of benign odontogenic or basaloid epithelium are found in the *peripheral odontogenic fibroma, odontogenic gingival epithelial hamartoma,* the *peripheral ameloblastoma,* the *peripheral adenomatoid odontogenic tumor,* and the *peripheral Gorlin cyst.*

Nodules with metaplastic or osteoblastic bone production are usually termed *peripheral ossifying fibroma,* whereas dark globular cementoid inclusions are seen in the *peripheral cementifying fibroma.* Cementoid inclusions or dystrophic calcification may be admixed with epithelial islands in the *peripheral Pindborg tumor,* the *peripheral Gorlin cyst,* or the *peripheral adenomatoid odontogenic tumor.* Cartilage in the center of a fibrous nodule is seen in the *Cutright tumor.*

Entrapped minor salivary glands may also be seen in the lower portion of any focal fibrous hyperplasia; this incidental finding must not be confused with *adenomatoid hyperplasia* or salivary neoplasia. In a similar fashion, *herniated buccal fat pad* can present as a mass with deep fatty tissue and overlying fibrosis.

Treatment and Prognosis. Irritation fibroma and other localized fibrous hyperplasias are easily removed by conservative surgical excision, with no need to remove a margin of surrounding normal mucosa.[7] Recurrence is unlikely unless the inciting trauma continues or is repeated. The bony concavity associated with some leaf-shaped fibromas under dentures will recontour to normal after removal of the offending mass. For epulis fissuratum, the treatment includes both surgical removal and reline or remake of the offending denture. Giant cell fibroma is also treated by conservative surgical excision, but it is more likely to recur than routine irritation fibroma.

Fibromatosis

The upper aerodigestive tract is home to several rather generalized fibrous and myofibromatous proliferative disorders. Broadly called *fibromatosis* or *desmoplastic fibroma,* such proliferations typically behave in a benign manner but sometimes are locally aggressive and may have an alarming, infiltrative histopathologic appearance.[7, 23–30] The more aggressive lesions are frequently called *juvenile aggressive fibromatoses* or *extra-abdominal desmoids.* *Myofibromatosis* is an admixture of smooth muscle cells and fibroblasts within a fibrous stroma; it is discussed elsewhere in this chapter, as are *generalized fibromatosis of gingival tissues* and *gingival fibrous hyperplasia,* special forms of fibrous proliferation.

Clinical Features. Soft tissue *fibromatosis* of the oral region is rare but is, after the vascular developmental lesions, the most common of the congenital masses of the oral soft tissues.[25, 26] It occurs primarily in children and young adults but may be seen in middle-aged individuals as well.[30] There is no gender predilection.

This lesion presents as a broad-based, firm, sometimes lobulated, painless, slowly enlarging mass with normal coloration. The

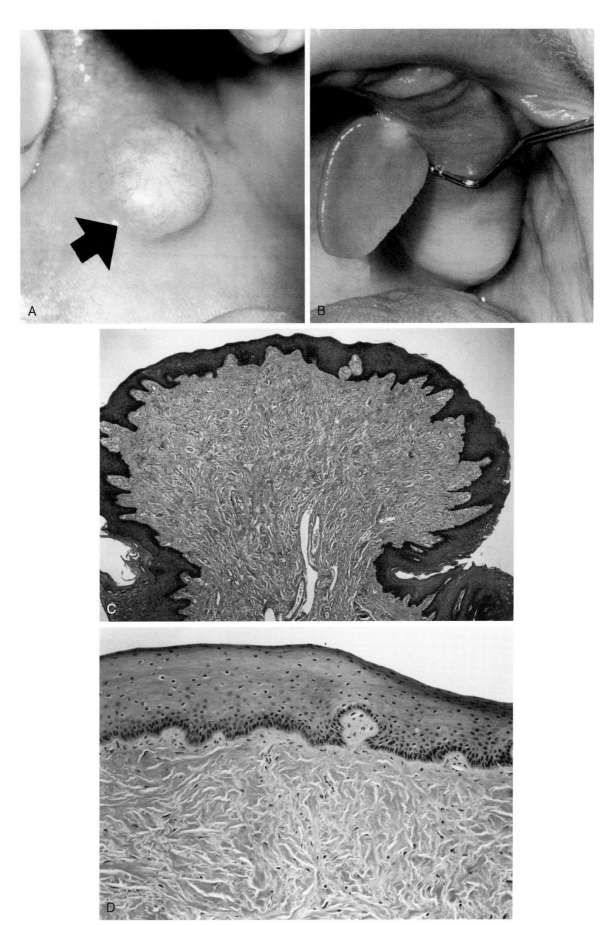

Figure 4–1. *A,* Slightly pedunculated irritation fibroma of the right buccal mucosa; *B,* leaf-shaped fibroma of the hard palate has been forced by an overlying denture to enlarge laterally and remain flat; *C,* the irritation fibroma is usually pedunculated, is covered by a somewhat hyperplastic epithelium, and is composed of dense collagenic tissue, sometimes with a few dilated veins; *D,* thick collagen bundles are irregularly arranged, with few visible blood vessels.

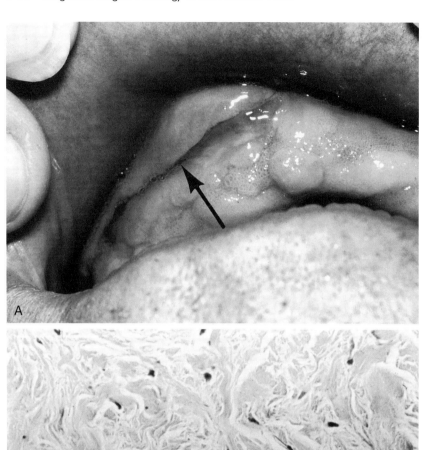

Figure 4–2. *A,* An epulis fissuratum of the right maxillary vestibule presents as a redundant fold of tissue (*arrow* points to groove where denture usually seats). *B,* The epulis is composed predominantly of dense collagenic tissue, as seen here, but may show areas of edema and chronic inflammatory cell infiltration.

speed of enlargement is variable and should not be used as a reliable predictor of aggressive future behavior.[25] Fibromatosis usually develops adjacent to the mandible, where underlying bone may be eroded or destroyed by "invasion."[23] Lesions average 3 to 4 cm in size at diagnosis, but lesions as large as 9 cm have been reported, as have multiple lesions in the same patient.[25] Larger lesions may develop secondary surface lobulation.

Pathologic Features. Fibromatosis is characterized by a proliferation of spindle-shaped, somewhat primitive mesenchymal cells arranged in streaming fascicles. Reticulin stains and Masson trichrome stain will confirm the collagenic nature of the stroma. Thin-walled vascular spaces are invariably present but not in large numbers. The lesional periphery is poorly demarcated from surrounding tissues, appearing often to be infiltrating those tissues. Erosion of underlying bone or actual destruction of bone may be seen. The degree of cellularity is variable, with some cases demonstrating moderate numbers of lesional cells in a background stroma of abundant mature collagen, and others showing minimal stroma with large numbers of active mesenchymal cells. In both types, cellularity is most evident at the periphery of the tumor. Hyperchromatic and pleomorphic nuclei are seldom seen. Occasional normal-appearing mitotic figures may be found, but should not exceed 4 mitoses per high-power field. The presence of dysplastic mesenchymal cells should make the pathologist suspicious for *fibrosarcoma, malignant fibrous histiocytoma,* or *fibroblastic osteosarcoma* (if attached to bone).

Occasional fibromatoses infiltrating striated muscle will induce atrophy, degeneration, and regeneration of muscle cells, resulting in the presence of osteoclast-like multinucleated giant cells and imparting a *giant cell lesion* appearance.

Treatment and Prognosis. Oral fibromatosis is treated by wide excision, including a thin margin of adjacent normal tissues. It has a locally aggressive behavior with a recurrence rate of more than 20%.[25, 26] This rate is similar to the rate for lesions of the sinonasal area but is far below the rate for lesions of the neck or other extraabdominal locations (40–70%).[29] Recurrences are treated by reexcision. Severe, multicentric lesions with visceral involvement are much more serious and may lead to respiratory distress or diarrhea. The oral lesions are, however, usually of minimal consequence in such cases.

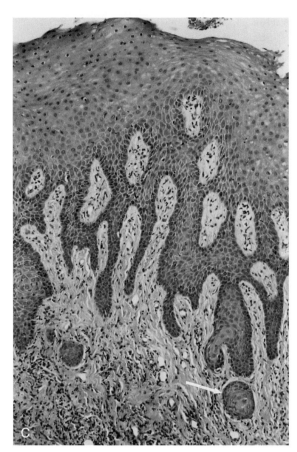

Figure 4–2. *Continued. C,* Repeated trauma from the denture edge may result in severe elongation of rete pegs, or pseudoepitheliomatous hyperplasia, with some pegs appearing like independent islands of "invading" squamous epithelium when cut tangentially *(arrow).*

Gingival Fibromatosis and Drug-Induced Fibrous Hyperplasia

By far, the most common of the oral fibromatoses involves the gingiva, usually affecting all gingival surfaces of both arches.[7, 9, 31] The term *fibrous gingival hyperplasia* is often used for this phenomenon when it is induced by one of a variety of drugs (Table 4–2),[32–34] whereas *gingival fibromatosis* is used for those cases that have an hereditary pattern,[31, 35–40] are part of a more extensive syndrome (Table 4–3),[5, 7–9] or are idiopathic.[7, 31] *Hereditary gingival fibromatosis* and *idiopathic gingival fibromatosis* first present in childhood, whereas *drug-induced gingival hyperplasia* first becomes noticeable 3 or more months after the onset of drug use. Some cases occur years after drug use is initiated.

As the fibrous hyperplasia is significantly enhanced by poor oral hygiene, gingivitis and periodontitis may be associated with the fibrosis. This entity was first reported in 1856 by Goddard and

Table 4–2. Drugs Associated with Fibrous Gingival Hyperplasia

Amlodipine	Nifedipine
Bepridil	Nimodipine
Bleomycin	Nisoldipine
Cyclosporine	Nitrendipine
Diltiazem	Oxidipine
Felodipine	Phenytoin
Isradipine	Sodium valproate
Nicardipine	Verapamil

Data from Neville et al.[7] and Thompson et al.[24]

Table 4–3. Syndromes Associated with Gingival Fibromatosis

With Generalized Gingival Fibromatosis
    Byars-Jurkiewicz syndrome (gingival fibromatosis, hypertrichosis, giant fibroadenomas of the breast, and kyphosis)
    Cross syndrome (gingival fibromatosis, microphthalmia, mental retardation, athetosis, and hypopigmentation)
    Gingival fibromatosis and growth hormone deficiency
    Gingival fibromatosis, hypertrichosis, epilepsy, and mental retardation syndrome
    Jones-Hartsfield syndrome (gingival fibromatosis and sensorineural hearing loss)
    Laband syndrome (gingival fibromatosis; ear, nose, bone, and nail defects; and hepatosplenomegaly)
    Murray syndrome (gingival fibromatosis with juvenile hyaline fibromatosis)
    Prune-belly syndrome (hypoplastic abdominal muscle, cryptorchidism, obstructive nephropathy, and gingival fibromatosis)
    Ramon syndrome (gingival fibromatosis, hypertrichosis, cherubism, mental and somatic retardation, and epilepsy)
    Rutherford syndrome (gingival fibromatosis and corneal dystrophy)
With Papular Gingival Fibromatosis (Papulosis)
    Acanthosis nigricans
    Cowden syndrome (multiple hamartoma syndrome)
    Tuberous sclerosis

Gross[41] under the rather descriptive term, *fungus excrescence of the gingiva.*

Occasional adults develop a large, smooth, fleshy hyperplasia of the soft tissues overlying the bone of the maxillary tuberosity. This *symmetrical fibromatosis of the tuberosity* is a localized variant of gingival fibromatosis and appears to be a developmental type of phenomenon, although its true etiology is unknown.[7] This form of hyperplasia may actually be more common than generalized gingival fibromatosis.

Clinical Features. Gingival fibromatosis presents as a generalized but often irregular enlargement of the facial and lingual aspects of the attached and marginal gingiva (Fig. 4–4A). A portion of one quadrant may be involved, or all four quadrants of the gingival tissues may be involved. Enlargement is painless, slowly progressive, and dependent to a great extent on the oral hygiene of the individual.[31] Although the hyperplastic tissues are usually firm to palpation, inflammation and edema may make some surface areas (facing the teeth) spongy, erythematous, and easily bleeding. It is not unusual for the fibromatosis to completely cover the teeth.

Symmetrical fibromatosis of the tuberosity is typically bilateral and presents as a generalized, soft, smooth-surfaced, painless enlargement of the tissues overlying the posterior maxillary alveolus.[7] Slow growth may eventuate in lesions so large as to actually touch one another across the arch of the hard palate, or to become traumatized by contact with mandibular teeth. Most cases, however, remain much smaller.

Pathologic Features. Gingival fibromatosis and drug-induced fibrous hyperplasia are composed of dense or moderately dense, rather avascular, bland collagenic connective tissue with scattered chronic inflammatory cells, especially beneath the surface epithelium (Fig. 4–4B). The attached gingival epithelium may have extreme elongation of rete processes. The crevicular epithelium facing the tooth surfaces usually shows considerable degeneration, subepithelial edema, and more extensive inflammatory cell infiltration because of the gingivitis or periodontitis that is so often present.

When evaluating the inflammatory cell infiltrate, the pathologist must be careful to differentiate the polyclonal, mixed infiltrate from a diffuse submucosal infiltration of atypical leukocytes in *leukemia* or *diffuse lymphoma (MALT [mucosal associated lymphoid tissue] lymphoma).* Both chronic and acute leukemic patients may develop a generalized gingival hyperplasia secondary to massive infiltration of neoplastic leukocytes, presumably because these cells retain a certain amount of normal chemotactic ability and are drawn to an area of inflammation, such as gingivitis. The clinical presentation is often called *leukemic gingivitis* or *leukemic gingival hyperplasia.*[7] The criteria used for the determination of leukemia or lymphoid malignancy are the same as those used for leukemic or extranodal (MALT) lymphoma infiltrations anywhere in the body.

Some cases of generalized gingival hyperplasia show focal collections of histiocytes intermixed with lymphocytes and foreign-body type multinucleated giant cells. This *granulomatous gingivitis* may be a foreign body reaction to toothpaste or may be indicative of a more systemic chronic granulomatous disease, such as *sarcoidosis, Crohn's disease,* or *Wegener's granulomatosis.*[7, 42] Other gingival hyperplasias have large numbers of plasma cells scattered throughout the subepithelial stroma. This *plasma cell gingivitis* is presumed to be an unusual allergic reaction.[7, 43]

Juvenile hyaline fibromatosis, a hereditary condition that may involve the gingiva, can be distinguished from gingival fibromatosis by its prominent periodic acid-Schiff (PAS)-positive background matrix of chondroitin sulfate.[8] Amyloid infiltration of the gingival tissues is not uncommon in primary or secondary *amyloidosis.* It can be identified via Congo red stain under polarized light, thioflavine T stain under fluorescent light, or immunoreactivity with antibodies for immunoglobulin light chains.[8]

Symmetrical fibromatosis of the tuberosity is composed of a moderately dense fibrous stroma with a more myxoid appearance than is found in generalized gingival fibromatosis. Focal areas may demonstrate edema or dense fibrosis, and inflammatory cells are quite sparse. Stromal cells are inactive bipolar and stellate mesenchymal cells lacking in mitotic activity or variation in size. The surface epithelium is usually atrophic but may be acanthotic with narrow, elongated rete ridges.

Treatment and Prognosis. Gingival fibromatosis is removed by gingivectomy, with recurrences being treated in the same fashion or by more conservative removal of local areas of hyperplasia. Improved oral hygiene will greatly diminish the risk of recurrence.[7, 31] Drug-induced gingival hyperplasia may also be treated by gingivectomy and plaque control. Discontinuation of drug use often results in cessation and even regression of the gingival enlargement.

Symmetrical fibromatosis of the tuberosity usually requires no treatment.[8] Large lesions or those that interfere with function or denture placement may be removed with conservative surgical excision. Recurrence has not been reported. Granulomatous gingivitis and plasma cell gingivitis are treated by addressing the underlying etiologies.[42, 43]

Oral Submucous Fibrosis

On the Indian subcontinent, the use of smokeless tobacco in various forms is very popular. This habit, which usually involves the chewing of a betel quid (combined areca nut, betel leaf, tobacco, and slack lime), has led to the development, in a large proportion of users, of a unique generalized fibrosis of the oral soft tissues called *oral submucous fibrosis.*[7, 44–51] Though not producing soft tissue

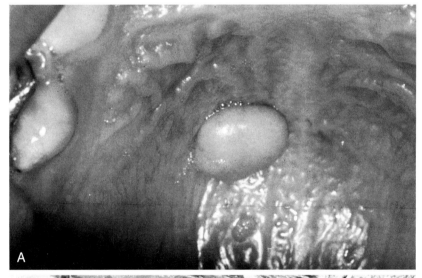

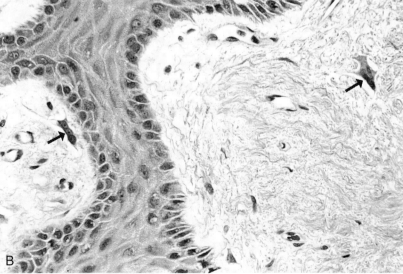

Figure 4–3. *A,* The giant cell fibroma, here on the hard palate, is usually pedunculated and slightly lobulated; *B,* the key diagnostic feature is a scattering of enlarged, stellate, sometimes multinucleated, pale-staining fibroblasts *(arrows),* seen most frequently in the subepithelial stroma.

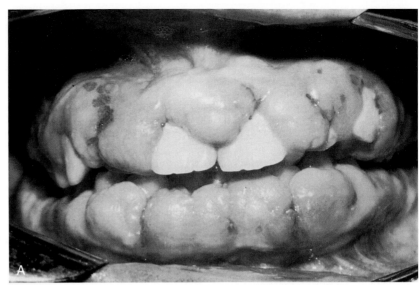

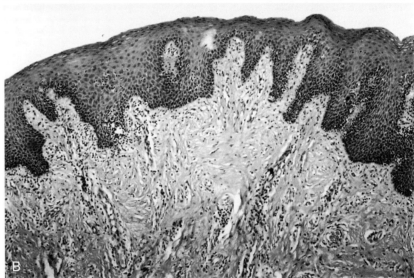

Figure 4–4. *A,* Generalized fibrous enlargement of a patient's entire gingiva is the classic presentation of gingival fibromatosis. *B,* Dense and rather avascular collagen makes up almost all of the hyperplasia in this disease, usually with scattered subepithelial and perivascular lymphocytes, while the overlying epithelium is often hyperplastic, may appear degenerated, and may contain lymphocytes.

masses in the usual sense, the fibrosis may be confused with generalized fibromatosis and, hence, is included in this section of this chapter.

The condition is found in 4 of 1000 adults in rural India and is caused by the areca nut in the quid. Additionally, it is estimated that as many as 5 million young Indians are suffering from this precancerous condition as a result of the increased popularity of the habit of chewing pan masala. It results in a marked rigidity with progressive inability to open the mouth.[44, 45] There is a fibroelastic transformation of the juxta-epithelial connective tissues and an increased risk of oral carcinoma from the tobacco of the quid.[38, 49, 51]

Clinical Features. Submucous fibrosis typically affects the buccal mucosa, lips, retromolar areas, and soft palate. Occasional involvement of the pharynx and esophagus is seen. Early lesions present as a blanching of the mucosa, imparting a mottled, marble-like appearance. Later lesions demonstrate palpable fibrous bands running vertically in the buccal mucosa and in a circular fashion around the mouth opening or lips.[45] As the disease progresses, the mucosa becomes stiff, causing difficulty in eating and considerably restricting the patient's ability to open the mouth (trismus). If the tongue is involved, it becomes stiff and has a diminished size.

Mucosal petechiae are seen in more than 10% of cases and most patients complain of a burning sensation, often aggravated by spicy foods.[45] Salivary flow is diminished and blotchy melanotic mucosal pigmentation is often seen. More than one fourth of affected persons develop precancerous leukoplakia of one or more oral

surfaces. Once present, oral submucous fibrosis does not regress, either spontaneously or with cessation of betel quid chewing.[45]

Pathologic Features and Differential Diagnosis. The early cases of oral submucous fibrosis present as chronic inflammatory cell infiltration of subepithelial connective tissues. This otherwise nonspecific infiltrate usually contains a number of eosinophils, cells seldom found in oral inflammation. Older lesions demonstrate a reduced vascularity, reduced numbers of inflammatory cells, and dense bundles and sheets of collagen immediately beneath the epithelium. The eventual thick band of hyalinized subepithelial collagen shows varying extension into submucosal tissues, typically replacing the fatty or fibrovascular tissues normal to the site.

Minor salivary glands in the area of habitual quid placement often demonstrate a chronic inflammatory infiltrate and replacement of acinar structures by the hyalinized fibrosis. The hyalinized stroma can be distinguished from the amyloid infiltration of *amyloidosis* through the use of Congo red staining and thioflavin-T staining under polarized and immunofluorescent light.

The epithelium is atrophic, with or without excess surface keratin, and demonstrates intracellular edema. One fourth of the biopsied cases will demonstrate *epithelial dysplasia* at the time of biopsy. When *squamous cell carcinoma* is seen, it has the same features of carcinoma as those seen in persons without the betel quid chewing habit.

Treatment and Prognosis. There is no effective treatment for oral submucous fibrosis and the condition is irreversible once formed.[45, 46] Plastic surgery may be required to allow for improved opening of the mouth. Surface leukoplakias are handled by close follow-up and repeated biopsies of areas of severe involvement. All dysplasias and carcinomas are treated in the routine manner for those entities. Epidemiologic studies have shown that as many as 10% of oral submucous fibrosis patients develop an oral carcinoma. Since the tobacco is the component of the quid most associated with cancer development, cessation of the quid chewing habit or eliminating the tobacco from the quid will reduce the risk of oral cancer. Likewise, a certain proportion of precancerous keratoses will diminish or disappear with habit cessation.[49]

Fibrosarcoma

Malignancies of fibroblasts are decidedly rare in the oral and oropharyngeal region, but *fibrosarcoma* is, nevertheless, the most common mesenchymal cancer of the region, representing more than half of all sarcomas.[7, 9, 28, 52–56] Twenty-three percent of head and neck fibrosarcomas occur within the oral cavity.[56] Radiotherapy to the local site is known to increase the risk of fibrosarcoma development but there are no other known etiologic factors.[53] On the perioral skin, occasional cases develop at the site of thermal damage or of a pre-existing scar.

Clinical Features. Persons affected by oral/pharyngeal fibrosarcoma are usually 30 to 50 years of age, but there is a wide age range and many patients are less than 20 years of age.[52] Fibrosarcoma has been diagnosed in the oral region of infants.[53] There is no apparent gender predilection and any submucosal site may be involved, although the buccal mucosa and tongue account for three fourths of oral lesions.[53]

Fibrosarcoma most often presents as a clinically innocuous, lobulated, sessile, painless, and nonhemorrhagic submucosal mass of normal coloration. It may, however, be a rapidly enlarging, hemorrhagic mass similar in clinical appearance to an ulcerated *pyogenic granuloma, peripheral giant cell granuloma,* or *peripheral ossifying fibroma.* Even lesions that do not demonstrate surface ulceration or rapid growth may show destruction of underlying muscle and bone.[56]

Pathologic Features and Differential Diagnosis. Fibrosarcoma is a lesion with a varied microscopic appearance. The low-grade or well-differentiated variant is usually somewhat circumscribed and composed of such mature spindle cells that differentiation from benign fibrous hyperplasia and proliferation may be quite difficult. The presence of focal anaplasia and increased mitotic activity becomes paramount in such cases, and aggressive clinical

behavior must be taken into account when making a histopathologic diagnosis. Fibrosarcoma of infancy and early childhood demonstrates smaller, more numerous, and more primitive cells than the adult lesion.

Lesional cells are spindle-shaped with pale eosinophilic cytoplasm and spindled nuclei with tapered ends (Fig. 4–5). Cells flow in interweaving fascicles or bundles, often producing a herringbone pattern in focal areas. The lesion is typically quite cellular, but moderate amounts of mature collagen may be produced, perhaps with areas of hyalinization. Scattered, histologically normal mitotic figures are seen in small numbers, but cells and nuclei are not pleomorphic.

Less well-differentiated fibrosarcoma shows minimal collagen production and marked cellularity. Lesional cells exhibit larger, more hyperchromatic, more pleomorphic, and more rounded nuclei, although the pleomorphism is seldom pronounced. Multinucleated giant cells are rarely seen. There seems to be an association between patient age at diagnosis and lesional differentiation, with less differentiated neoplasms occurring in the younger patients.

Focal areas of tumor necrosis may be seen in the poorly differentiated fibrosarcoma, and myxoid areas, as well as occasional chronic inflammatory cells, may be seen in infantile fibrosarcoma. Stromal hemorrhage is not seen.

Fibrosarcoma of the oral region must be differentiated from a variety of other malignant and benign spindle cell proliferations. The most problematic malignancies in this regard include the *malignant fibrous histiocytoma, malignant peripheral nerve sheath tumor (malignant schwannoma), dermatofibrosarcoma protuberans, leiomyosarcoma,* and certain carcinomas such as *desmoplastic (sarcomatoid) melanoma, spindle cell (sarcomatoid) carcinoma,* and *myoepithelial carcinoma.* The carcinomas are distinguished by focal transition areas with epithelioid or pigmented cells, perhaps requiring immunoperoxidase confirmation of their epithelial nature via positive reactivity for cytokeratins (using MNF116 and CAM 5.2) and S-100 protein (Table 4–4).[57–60] It is important to remember that fibrosarcoma, especially in adults, is extremely rare in the mouth and that the diagnosis is many times one of exclusion in a lesion that is negative to appropriate immunohistochemical markers.

Malignant fibrous histiocytoma can usually be differentiated from fibrosarcoma by the more pronounced pleomorphism of its cells and nuclei, and by the presence of a storiform or whorling stromal pattern rather than a herringbone pattern, and by immunoreactivity for factor XIIIa or α-1-antichymotrypsin antibodies (see Table 4–4).

Leiomyosarcoma has the fascicular pattern and uniform cellularity of a low-grade fibrosarcoma, but nuclei have more blunted

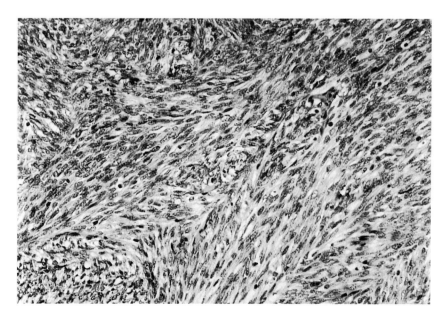

Figure 4–5. Well-differentiated fibrosarcoma is composed of mature spindled cells with pointed ends, arranged in interweaving fascicles forming a herring-bone pattern.

Table 4–4. Immunohistochemical Features of Various Malignancies of the Oral and Pharyngeal Region

Diagnosis	Vimentin	S100 Protein	Smooth Muscle Actin	Desmin	BCL2	CD34	SMA/MSA	Pankeratin	Cytokeratin	EMA	Ulex europaeus I Lectin	Alpha-1-antichymotrypsin
Fibrosarcoma	+	–	–	–	–	–	+/–		–	–	–	–
Malignant fibrous histiocytoma	+	–	–	–					–	–	–	+
Leiomyosarcoma	+	+	+	+	–	+/–	+		+/–	+/–	–	–
Synovial sarcoma	+	–	–	–					+	+	+/–	+/–
Spindle cell carcinoma	–	–	–	–				+	+			
Desmoplastic melanoma		+										
Malignant schwannoma	+	+/–	–	–	+/–	+/–	–		+/–	+/–	–	+/–
Angiosarcoma									+/–			
Kaposi's sarcoma	+	–	+/–	–		+			–	–	+/–	+/–

ends ("cigar-shaped") and fuchsinophilic fibers can be demonstrated by the Masson trichrome stain. Lesional cells are immunoreactive for a variety of antibodies, including vimentin, desmin, alpha-smooth muscle actin, muscle-specific actin, and S-100 protein (see Table 4–4).

Malignant peripheral nerve sheath tumors can usually be differentiated by their greater degree of pleomorphism and by the presence of wavy or comma-shaped bipolar nuclei with pointed ends or with one pointed and one blunted end (arrowhead nucleus). The stroma often demonstrates large whorls or nodules with a neural or myxoid appearance, and many tumors show alternating patterns of hypercellular, and perhaps herringboned fascicles with hypocellular myxoid zones. This tumor often contains cells that are immunoreactive for S-100 protein, NSE, cytokeratin (CK), BCL2, and CD34, but negative cases do not eliminate it as a viable diagnosis so long as lesional cells are not reactive for vimentin, smooth muscle actin, desmin, or HMB45 (see Table 4–4).

Another sarcoma that may mimic fibrosarcoma is the *synovial sarcoma,* especially the monophasic type. The examination of multiple microscopic sections may be needed to identify an area with the classic biphasic pattern. Lacking this, it should be understood that the spindle cell phase of synovial sarcoma typically has significantly more collagen, has areas of myxoid stroma, and has an extremely uniform cellular pattern. Electron microscopy may be necessary to demonstrate the epithelioid cells of synovial sarcoma, and immunohistochemistry may be helpful (see Table 4–4). The recently described *sclerosing epithelioid fibrosarcoma* may also present with numerous polygonal epithelioid cells, but these grow in distinct nests and chords.[57]

Spindle cell carcinoma is discussed elsewhere in this text (Chapter 2), but it can be said here that it differs from fibrosarcoma in that it has a "separated bundle" growth pattern and the nuclei are large and open with a retained nucleolus, that is, they remain similar to the nuclei of routine squamous cell carcinoma. There are no perinuclear vacuoles and some cells should appear epithelioid. Immunohistochemical markers of epithelial differentiation may be negative in spindle cell carcinoma, and the most likely markers to elicit positive reactivity include EMA, CK (AE1/3, CAM52), vimentin and muscle-specific actin (scattered cells only).[10, 58, 59] Spindle cells in *myoepithelial carcinoma* frequently co-express S-100 protein, smooth muscle actin, calponin, vimentin, and CK of low molecular weight.

Fibromatosis may be histologically and clinically indistinguishable from well-differentiated fibrosarcoma. The spindle cells may be numerous but are uniformly bland. Stroma contains abundant mature collagen and there is a lack of herringbone change. Areas of fibromatosis may show increased cellularity and mitotic activity, but this is not seen uniformly throughout lesional tissues. Some authorities insist on the presence of areas with more than 5 mitotic figures per high-power field for a diagnosis of fibrosarcoma.[60]

Nodular fasciitis can be distinguished from well-differentiated fibrosarcoma by its rapid growth, superficial location, and mixture of fibroblasts, myofibroblasts, and chronic inflammatory cells, including occasional histiocyte-like cells demonstrating pleomorphism. The stroma is often myxoid with focal areas of mucoid change; the latter is a feature not seen in fibrosarcoma.

Treatment and Prognosis. Well-differentiated fibrosarcoma is treated by wide local excision, whereas more poorly differentiated tumors require radical surgery, including removal of potentially invaded muscle and bone.[56] Fibrosarcoma seldom metastasizes except late in its clinical course, but when this does occur the metastatic deposits are usually blood-borne and carried to distant sites, especially the lungs, liver, and bones. Radiotherapy may be used as salvage for recurrences. The 5-year survival rate for this disease in poor, ranging from 20% to 35%.[7, 9, 56]

Fibrous Histiocytoma

Fibrous histiocytoma represents a benign but diverse group of neoplasms that exhibit both fibroblastic and histiocytic differentiation.[6–9, 61–66] The cell of origin is believed to be the histiocyte, but the varied microscope appearances of the lesion has led to the use of numerous alternative diagnostic terms, including *dermatofibroma, sclerosing hemangioma, xanthogranuloma, fibroxanthoma,* and *nodular subepidermal fibrosis.* A malignant variant of this neoplasm is discussed in the following section.

Clinical Features. The most common location of fibrous histiocytoma occurrence is the skin of the extremities, where it usually presents as a small, firm nodule.[8, 62] Oral and perioral lesions are uncommon, but when seen they occur predominantly on the buccal mucosa and vestibule.[7, 65, 66] The oral lesion is typically found in middle-aged and older adults, where it presents as a painless submucosal nodule that can vary in size from a few millimeters to several centimeters. Deeper tumors tend to be larger and most lesions cannot be easily moved about beneath the epithelium.

Pathologic Features and Differential Diagnosis. Fibrous histiocytoma is characterized by a submucosal, cellular aggregation of spindle-shaped, fibroblast-like cells with relatively pale, oval nuclei; scattered rounded histiocytic cells are also present. Foamy histiocytes and Touton-type multinucleated giant cells, with nuclei pushed to the periphery, may be seen to contain phagocytosed lipid or he-

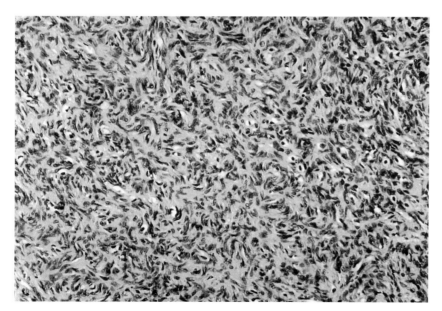

Figure 4–6. The classic fibrous histiocytoma shows a swirling or storiform pattern at low power examination, with lesional cells resembling fibroblasts but with more plump and open nuclei. The amount of background fibrous stroma is variable.

mosiderin; these cells sometimes are so numerous that they form xanthomatous aggregates. A background stroma of variably dense collagenic tissue and vascularity is seen. The spindled cells may be arranged randomly, but usually there are large areas with tumor cells streaming in interlacing fascicles from a central nidus and intersecting with cells from adjacent aggregates, imparting a storiform or criss-cross pattern on low-power magnification (Fig. 4–6).

The fibrous histiocytoma is poorly demarcated from surrounding tissues and is separated from the overlying mucosa by a zone of fibrovascular connective tissue (grenz zone). The overlying epithelium often demonstrates considerable acanthosis, with regular elongation of rete processes. Chronic inflammatory cells, especially lymphocytes, are usually scattered throughout the tumor in small numbers. The lesional stroma is occasionally very densely fibrotic or hyalinized, leading some in the past to use the diagnostic misnomer *sclerosing hemangioma*. Deeper lesions may contain focal areas of dystrophic calcification or metaplastic osteoid.

Acid phosphatase, nonspecific esterase, and succinate dehydrogenase enzymes are consistently present in lesional cells, especially those resembling rounded histiocytes.[6, 66] A significant proportion of cases will be immunoreactive for α_1-antitrypsin and factor XIIIa antigen. CD68, a macrophage antigen, usually does not mark the tumor cells. Electron microscopy has shown a spectrum of cell types from spindled fibroblastic cells to rounded histiocyte-like cells; endothelial lesional cells are not seen.

When the lesion is composed predominantly of proliferating sheets of histiocytes with few Touton giant cells and foamy cytoplasm, the terms *xanthogranuloma* or *juvenile xanthogranuloma* have traditionally been applied. These are typically better circumscribed and less fibrosed than the more routine fibrous histiocytoma. This lesion is usually diagnosed during the first two decades of life and must be differentiated from soft tissue lesions of *Langerhans cell disease (histiocytosis X)* and from routine *xanthoma,* or reactive histiocyte proliferations as seen after trauma, or in persons with *hyperlipidemia* or *hypercholesterolemia*. The histiocytic cells of a xanthoma typically express S-100 protein, while the lesional cells of the fibrous histiocytoma do not. Cholesterol clefts, moreover, are commonly seen in the xanthoma. The multinucleated giant cells of Langerhans disease do not typically have their nuclei pushed to the cell periphery.

Benign fibrous histiocytoma is often confused with other benign fibrous lesions and must be differentiated from *nodular fasciitis, myofibroma, palisading encapsulated neuroma, neurofibroma, leiomyoma,* and the spindle cell type of *myoepithelioma*. It is important, moreover, to separate this tumor from aggressive forms of fibrous and fibrohistiocytic neoplasms such as *dermatofibrosarcoma protuberans, malignant fibrous histiocytoma,* and *fibrosarcoma*.

Treatment and Prognosis. Benign fibrous histiocytoma is treated by wide surgical excision, with 5% to 10% of cases recurring locally.[6, 64–66] Deeper and larger lesions have a higher rate of recurrence. More aggressive examples usually show the microscopic features of dysplasia, such as marked cellularity, mitotic activity, focal necrosis, even atypical giant cells. It is sometimes, however, very difficult to predict biologic behavior on the basis of cellular features, as illustrated by the occasional case that metastasizes despite its bland histopathologic appearance. For this reason, extended follow-up is recommended after surgical removal.

Malignant Fibrous Histiocytoma

Malignant fibrous histiocytoma (MFH) was first described in 1964 under the name *malignant fibrous xanthoma*.[67] Since that time, several major variants have been identified and it has become the most commonly diagnosed of all the sarcomas of adults.[68–72] Oral and maxillofacial sites are seldom involved, however, and the tumor occurs primarily in the soft tissues of the extremities and retroperitoneum.[6]

Clinical Features. The MFH occurs primarily in adults, especially those 50 to 70 years of age, but rare cases have been described in children.[6, 68–73] Regardless of the histopathologic subtype, men are affected almost twice as frequently as women.

Within the maxillofacial region, the most common complaint is a moderately firm submucosal mass expanding slowly or moderately fast, with or without pain and surface ulceration.[7, 68, 69, 71] The irregular nodular lesion is typically unencapsulated and attached to surrounding tissues and adjacent structures. It is usually less than 4 cm in greatest diameter at the time of biopsy. The myxoid variant often has quite a soft consistency and the angiomatoid variant is often found in a location more superficial than that of the other variants.

Pathologic Features and Differential Diagnosis. MFH has a wide spectrum of cellular and tissue alterations. The cellular differentiation and density vary markedly, even within the same tumor. The classic histopathologic features, however, include at least mild cellular and nuclear pleomorphism, an admixture of fibroblastic and histiocytic elements, and focal areas with a storiform or cartwheel pattern of streaming spindle cells. This classic pattern is the one most frequently encountered in head and neck sites and is often referred to as the *storiform-pleomorphic MFH*.[71]

Most lesional cells are spindled fibroblast-like cells that tend to be arranged in short woven fascicles or bundles with scattered areas showing a storiform pattern where fascicles intertwine. The spindle cells may be long and thin with minimal atypia, but there are usually areas with plump spindle cells containing enlarged, hyperchromatic, and irregular nuclei. Varying numbers of rounded, polygonal, and irregularly shaped histiocyte-like cells may dominate some areas of the lesion, often with very pleomorphic, multinucleated giant cells interspersed. The histiocytic cells have either abundant eosinophilic cytoplasm or pale foamy cytoplasm, and cell membranes are not easily visualized. Areas with histiocytic predominance usually have a haphazard structural appearance.

Chronic inflammatory cells are often scattered sparsely throughout the tumor, including foamy histiocytes, lymphocytes, and plasma cells. Multinucleated Touton giant cells are occasionally seen. Mitotic activity varies widely and is directly related to the degree of cellular pleomorphism.

The fibrous stroma of MFH varies in density, being less pronounced in areas of lesser cellular differentiation. Myxoid stroma may be found and, rarely, foci of osteoid or cartilage metaplasia are present. Although blood vessels are usually inconspicuous, some lesions present with numerous dilated, branching vessels. Depending on the dominant morphology, MFH is currently subclassified as one of several major variants: *pleomorphic-storiform, myxoid, angiomatoid (aneurysmal),* and *giant cell MFH*.[6, 70–75]

The myxoid variant is defined as a MFH with more than half of its stroma represented by myxoid change with spindle cells and scattered pleomorphic epithelioid cells. The vasculature is quite prominent and vessel walls appear thickened. To differentiate this tumor from myxoid liposarcoma, staining for hyaluronidase-sensitive mucopolysaccharides may be necessary. The liposarcoma, moreover, has a meshwork of thin-walled capillaries and tends to have a more uniform cellular histology with less spindling of lesional cells. The rare *extraskeletal myxoid chondrosarcoma* can be easily differentiated by its lack of stromal vascularity and structure, whereas the *myxoid leiomyosarcoma* almost always contains areas suggestive of smooth muscle differentiation.

The angiomatoid MFH has a prominent network of capillaries and arching veins with somewhat thickened walls and with plump endothelial nuclei. The vessels may be dilated to the point of appearing cystic, and stromal hemorrhage may be found. Myxoid stroma is seen in focal areas. Angiomatoid areas are interspersed with diffuse sheets of histiocytoid oval or spindled cells with minimal pleomorphism. Such cells are often concentrated around vascular channels and there may be occasional to moderate numbers of peripherally located lymphocytes. Lymphocytes also may be seen within the fibrous pseudoencapsulation of some lesions, sometimes associated with germinal centers. Multinucleated giant cells may demonstrate marked nuclear atypia.

The giant cell variant of MFH *(giant cell tumor of soft tissue)* is characterized by large numbers of osteoclast-like multinucleated giant cells scattered throughout a cellular stroma of histiocytoid and fibroblastic cells arranged in storiform nodules separated by fibrous septa. Stromal cells usually demonstrate moderate nuclear pleomorphism with occasional bizarre, hyperchromatic nuclei. A large proportion of cases show osteoid, even calcified bone, at the periphery.

The MFH often mimics the histopathologic appearance of other sarcomas, especially *fibrosarcoma, pleomorphic liposarcoma, pleomorphic rhabdomyosarcoma,* and *hemangiopericytoma.* Some lesions may, moreover, mimic *benign fibrous histiocytoma* or *nodular fasciitis.* The former is typically smaller, is more superficially located, and has much less cellular atypia, although mitotic activity might be abundant.[70, 73] The latter also has less cellular atypia and lacks evidence of peripheral invasion.

Fibrosarcoma may contain areas with a storiform pattern but it typically lacks significant pleomorphism and has no histiocytic or bizarre multinucleated giant cells. Pleomorphic liposarcoma may contain large numbers of pleomorphic giant cells, and fat stains may not help to distinguish between it and MFH because the histiocytic cells of the latter may contain lipids and the pleomorphic cells of the former may not contain lipids. The diagnosis of liposarcoma is aided considerably by the finding of signet-ring lipoblasts, especially when differentiating myxoid liposarcoma from myxoid MFH.

Pleomorphic rhabdomyosarcoma can be separated from MFH by the presence of cross-striations or longitudinal myofibrils in lesional cells. In the absence of these, it may not be possible to differentiate these two malignancies without positive immunoreactivity with myogenic markers or the demonstration of rhabdomyoblasts by electron microscopy.

Hemangiopericytoma typically has a more uniform cell population than does the angiomatoid variant of MFH.[72, 75] There is usually much less cellular and nuclear pleomorphism and there is a pericellular network of reticulin fibers demonstrated by silver reticulin stains.

Treatment and Prognosis. MFH of the oral region is usually treated by radical surgical resection, but at least 40% of lesions recur locally and a similar proportion metastasize within 2 years.[68, 71] The 5-year survival rate is poor, no more than 30%, although it is somewhat better for the myxoid variant.

Myofibromatosis

Myofibromatosis is an admixture of myofibroblasts and fibroblasts within a fibrous stroma.[6, 8, 76–84] It is usually less aggressive than pure fibromatosis of the oral region, but it may be part of a *congenital generalized fibromatosis* or *generalized hamartomatosis.*[82–84] Multiple lesions tend to fall into two categories: superficial myofibromatosis, with nodules confined to subcutaneous and submucosal stroma, with occasional involvement of skeletal muscle or bone[8]; and generalized myofibromatosis, with visceral lesions and a mortality rate approaching 80%.[78, 83, 84] Some authorities prefer to use the term *myofibroma* for single lesions, especially those with adult onset, and myofibromatosis for multifocal involvement.[8]

This is considered to be a developmental anomaly, but some lesions occur in adults.[77] Many cases have a close clinical and microscopic similarity to fibromatosis, hence its inclusion in this section of this chapter. Myofibromatosis presents in the paraoral region as a single or as multiple submucosal nodules, usually in neonates and infants.[79, 81]

Pathologic Features. Myofibromatosis or myofibroma presents with a microscopic appearance similar to that of *fibromatosis* but the peripheral cells demonstrate eosinophilic cytoplasm reminiscent of smooth muscle.[76] There is usually a biphasic pattern of lightly staining fibrous areas separated by regions of pericyte-like vascular cell or smooth muscle-like spindle cell proliferations. The lesion is most vascular centrally, where it may mimic a *hemangiopericytoma* or *glomus tumor,* with lesional cells proliferating around blood vessels. Collagen is present but seldom abundant. The more fibrotic lesions, of course, must be differentiated from *fibromatosis, irritation fibroma, neurofibroma, angiofibroma,* and fibrotic *pyo-*

genic granuloma, according to criteria described for those lesions elsewhere in this chapter.

Lesional cells show features of both myofibroblastic and fibroblastic cells, with fuchsinophilic and phosphotungstic acid hematoxylin (PTAH)-positive intracellular fibrils. These cells are immunoreactive for vimentin and actin, but not for desmin or S-100 protein.[76] These stains help demonstrate the smooth muscle nature of the lesion and separate myofibromatosis from *neurofibroma* and *fibrous histiocytoma,* although they are less helpful for *nodular fasciitis,* which also contains myofibroblasts.

Treatment and Prognosis. Myofibromatosis is much more innocuous than fibromatosis and spontaneous regression may occur, although multifocal involvement may produce serious extragnathic difficulties for the patient. The typical treatment for oral lesions is conservative surgical removal, with minimal recurrence expected.

Nodular Fasciitis

Nodular (pseudosarcomatous) fasciitis is a presumably reactive vascular and fibroproliferative response to injury.[6–8, 85–91] The lesion is benign but has a rapid rate of growth and a histopathologic appearance that can be quite alarming. Although relatively common, it was not recognized as a separate histopathologic entity until 1955.[8] Approximately 17% of all cases occur in the head and neck region, usually the neck and face.[7, 86, 87]

Clinical Features. In the mouth, nodular fasciitis is usually a discrete submucosal nodule that is slightly tender and is not freely movable beneath the mucosa.[7] It seldom achieves more than 2 cm in size and is usually more superficially located than *fibromatosis* of the oral region. While occurring at all ages, this entity is most often diagnosed in persons 30 to 40 years of age, with no gender predilection.

Pathologic Features and Differential Diagnosis. Nodular fasciitis presents as haphazardly arranged bundles of fibroblasts in a myxoid or mucoid background. An important diagnostic feature is a fine capillary network arranged in a radial pattern around a larger central vessel or vessels. The fibroblasts are typically large and plump, similar to those of granulation tissue. Pleomorphic fibroblasts may be present, and mitoses are common but not plentiful or abnormal. A variable amount of collagen and acid mucopolysaccharide are seen in the intercellular matrix, although the latter may not be readily visible without special staining with alcian blue or colloidal iron. Scattered chronic inflammatory cells are typically present in small to moderate numbers, and long-standing lesions may demonstrate foamy histiocytes and osteoclast-like multinucleated giant cells with 2 to 6 nuclei. When striated muscle is involved *(intramuscular fasciitis),* it is completely replaced by the fibrovascular proliferation, unlike *proliferative myositis,* which infiltrates between muscle fibers.[90]

The spindle-shaped fibroblasts in this lesion tend to be arranged in long fascicles that are slightly curved, whorled, or S-shaped. They seem especially prone to extension along the fibrous septa of submucosal fatty tissues. Small slit-like spaces often separate the fibroblasts, and extravasation of erythrocytes is commonly seen, although it is seldom extensive. Occasional microcysts are seen in older lesions, perhaps coalesced into larger cystic spaces. The lesion is not often encapsulated but is usually well demarcated from surrounding tissues.

Ultrastructural studies have confirmed the presence of myofibroblasts in nodular fasciitis, with a basic fibroblast appearance but with peripherally located bundles of myofilaments with dense patches similar to those of smooth muscle cells. Lesional cells are immunoreactive to vimentin, smooth muscle actin, and muscle-specific actin, but not for desmin.

The differential diagnosis of this lesion includes *fibrosarcoma, fibrous histiocytoma,* and *liposarcoma,* few of which demonstrate the vascular component of nodular fasciitis. The scattered inflammatory cells also help differentiate the lesion. Occasional lesions will demonstrate very small foci of metaplastic bone or cartilage *(ossifying fasciitis, fasciitis ossificans, parosteal fasciitis),* tempting the pathologist to diagnose the case as *osteosarcoma.* Nodular fasciitis can also arise within blood vessels *(intravascular fasciitis)* and in deep fascia *(fascial fasciitis).*[6, 8, 91]

Treatment and Prognosis. Despite its often aggressive microscopic appearance, nodular fasciitis is a self-limiting lesion that is readily treated by simple local excision. Deeper lesions tend to be somewhat larger and less well demarcated, and hence require a wider local excision. Recurrence rates vary from 1% to 6% with this treatment and some lesions have been reported to regress and disappear without treatment.[86, 87]

The major prognostic factor here is an accurate diagnosis, and recurrences should, therefore, be evaluated very carefully. Earlier studies have shown that as many as one fourth of all cases were erroneously interpreted as malignant and, conversely, numerous cases of well-differentiated fibrosarcoma have been misdiagnosed as nodular fasciitis.

Proliferative Myositis

Another pseudosarcomatous lesion is *proliferative myositis,* a reactive fibroproliferative lesion of injured striated muscle.[6–8, 92–94] Some authorities consider it to be an early stage of *heterotopic ossification* or *myositis ossificans,* whereas others consider it to be a separate clinical and histopathologic entity. As with *nodular fasciitis,* accurate microscopic diagnosis is extremely important. In some investigations, more than 40% of proliferative myositis cases have been erroneously diagnosed as *sarcoma,* especially *rhabdomyosarcoma.*[92] This reactive lesion is usually seen in the flat muscles of the shoulder girdle, but occasionally presents in the head and neck region, particularly in the sternocleidomastoid muscle.[94] It was first described by Kern[92] in 1960.

Clinical Features. Proliferative myositis of the oral region is a rapidly enlarging, immovable, perhaps tender submucosal mass. Children are rarely affected and the typical patient is 45 to 65 years of age at tumor onset.[94] There is a slight female predilection. The lesion is usually 1.5 to 5.0 cm. in greatest dimension at the time of diagnosis and involves the muscle in a diffuse, infiltrative fashion.

Pathologic Features. This lesion appears almost scar-like on gross examination, with a poorly circumscribed periphery and a grayish-white cut surface. Microscopically, plump fibroblast-like cells are the predominant cell type, but giant ganglion-like cells with

deeply staining basophilic cytoplasm and prominent nucleoli are the hallmark of proliferative myositis. These cells are also myofibroblasts but are often so bizarre as to impart a strong similarity to rhabdomyosarcoma or other sarcoma. Likewise, atrophic or degenerated muscle cells may contribute to the overall impression of striated muscle malignancy.

Fibrosis is seen to involve the endomysium, perimysium, and epimysium. Lesional cells are immunoreactive for vimentin, actin, smooth-muscle actin, factor XIIIa, and fibronectin and are usually not reactive for desmin or myosin.[6] Occasionally, however, they will also react for desmin and myosin. Ultrastructurally, they appear to be myofibroblasts.[8, 93] Focal ossification or dystrophic calcification may be observed in some cases, but never is it as pronounced as in *heterotopic ossification.*

Treatment and Prognosis. Spontaneous regression and disappearance have been rarely reported. Treatment of this self-limiting lesion is conservative surgical excision, and recurrence should not be expected.[6, 8] The major prognostic difficulty is arriving at a correct diagnostic interpretation of the tissue, hence, recurrent lesions should be carefully evaluated for an alternative diagnosis.

Oral Focal Mucinosis

Oral focal mucinosis is the microscopic counterpart of the *cutaneous focal mucinosis* or *cutaneous myxoid cyst.*[7, 9, 95–101] It is not common and its cause is uncertain, but the lesion appears to represent overproduction of hyaluronic acid by local fibroblasts.

Clinical Features. This lesion has a strong female predilection (2 : 1) and occurs primarily in young adults.[95, 97, 98] Most maxillofacial cases are seen on bone-bound mucosa. Three fourths of all cases occur on the gingiva, and the hard palate is the site for most of the rest. The lesion presents as a sessile, soft, painless nodule with normal surface coloration. Some cases are lobulated, but surface ulceration is very rare. Lesions are typically less than 2 cm in greatest dimension.

Pathologic Features and Differential Diagnosis. Oral focal mucinosis consists of a submucosal, well-localized but nonencapsulated nidus of very loose, myxomatous, or "mucinous" connective tissue (Fig. 4–7). More superficial lesions may produce atrophy and loss of rete ridges of the overlying squamous epithelium. Fibroblasts are seen in minimal to moderate numbers within the mucinous area, often demonstrating delicate, fibrillar processes. The mucinous zone is much less vascular than surrounding connective tissues, and inflammatory cells are not associated with the lesion except as a

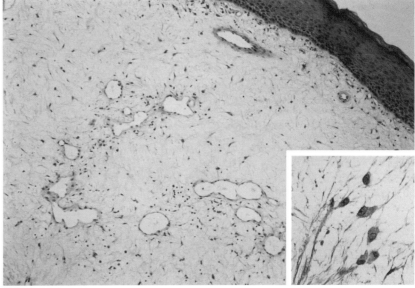

Figure 4–7. Focal mucinosis is characterized by a loose myxoid stroma admixed with scattered bipolar and stellate fibroblasts, here with stroma extending to the surface epithelium. Lesional cells may be somewhat alarming *(inset),* but mitotic figures are not seen.

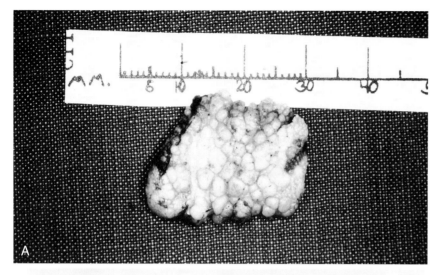

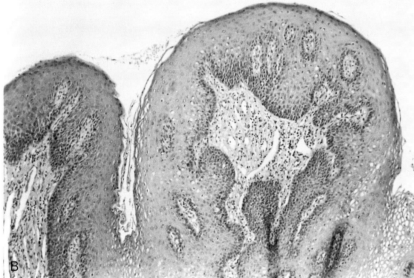

Figure 4–8. Papillary hyperplasia. *A,* Gross specimen from the hard palate shows clustered nodules on the mucosal surface; *B,* connective tissue papillae are greatly enlarged to produce the individual nodules and papules, often with areas of edema and with scattered chronic inflammatory cells.

perivascular infiltrate of lymphocytic T-cells at the periphery. The hyaluronic acid of the lesion will stain positive with alcian-blue (pH 2.5) in frozen sections, but this is not always the case with paraffin-embedded sections.[8]

Special staining may be necessary to differentiate this lesion from other disorders with perivascular infiltrates, such as *lupus erythematosus.* There are microscopic similarities between oral focal mucinosis and *cutaneous mucinosis of infancy,* which may represent a localized form of *papular mucinosis* or *lichen myxedematosus.*[99–101]

Differentiation from another look-alike lesion, the oral *mucocele,* is usually not difficult. The mucocele is more strongly demarcated from surrounding fibrovascular tissues by a peripheral "encapsulation" of granulation tissue, and it has bloated inflammatory cells floating within the extravasated mucus. Mucicarmine staining, of course, will demonstrate mucus in the mucocele.

A slight similarity is also seen between mucinosis and the *nerve sheath myxoma (neurothekeoma, bizarre neurofibroma, pacinian neurofibroma),* a variant of *neurofibroma* that rarely affects mucosa of the upper aerodigestive tract.[6] The nerve sheath myxoma, however, is more circumscribed, has fibrous septa between multiple myxoid nodules, and has more plump stromal cells.

Treatment and Prognosis. Oral focal mucinosis is treated by conservative surgical removal. It does not recur with this treatment.[97, 98]

Inflammatory Papillary Hyperplasia

Inflammatory papillary hyperplasia, also known as *papillary hyperplasia of the palate* and erroneously as *palatal papillomatosis,* is almost always restricted to the mucosa under a denture base.[7, 9, 102–105] First reported by Berry[106] in 1851, it results from selective but severe edema and eventual inflammatory fibrosis of the connective tissue papillae between the rete processes of the palatal epithelium. It is found in 3 of every 1000 adults.[1–3]

The great majority of cases are seen beneath ill-fitting dentures of long use and in persons who do not take their dentures out overnight. The lesion seems to result from a combination of chronic, mild trauma and low-grade infection by bacteria or candida yeast. It is occasionally seen in patients without dentures but with high palatal vaults or with the habit of breathing through the mouth.

Clinical Features. Papillary hyperplasia is seen in middle-aged and older persons and there is a strong female predilection (2:1).[103] The disease occurs on the bone-bound oral mucosa of the hard palate and alveolar ridges. It presents as a cluster of individual papules or nodules that may be erythematous, somewhat translucent, or normal in surface coloration (Fig. 4–8*A*). Often the entire vault of the hard palate is involved, with alveolar mucosa being largely spared. White cottage cheese–like colonies of candida may be seen in clefts between papules.[105] There is seldom pain, but a burning sensation may be produced by the yeast infection. Early papules are more edematous, whereas older ones are more fibrotic and firm, being individually indistinguishable from *irritation fibroma.*

Pathologic Features and Differential Diagnosis. Connective tissue papillae are greatly enlarged by edematous connective tissue, granulation tissue, densely fibrotic tissue, or a combination thereof, depending on the duration of the lesion (Fig. 4–8B). Small to moderate numbers of chronic inflammatory cells are present, perhaps admixed with occasional polymorphonuclear leukocytes. Each enlarged papilla produces a surface nodule that may be pedunculated or sessile, with deep clefts between nodules.

Covering epithelium is often atrophic but may be acanthotic, especially near the base of the internodal troughs. Occasional lesions demonstrate extensive *pseudoepitheliomatous hyperplasia.* Basal cell hyperchromatism and basal layer hyperplasia often impart a false appearance of mild *epithelial dysplasia.* Surface ulceration is surprisingly rare, and deeper tissues show few alterations beyond a mild chronic inflammatory cell infiltration.

Although individual nodules may appear identical to pyogenic granuloma and irritation fibroma, the palatal location and the multinodularity of the lesion makes the diagnosis of papillary hyperplasia an easy one. Some of the more edematous papules may mimic the mucus extravasation of *mucocele,* but will be negative for mucus with the mucicarmine stain. A silver or PAS stain will frequently identify candida spores and hyphae in the superficial portions of the epithelium, especially in cases with severe acanthosis or pseudoepitheliomatous hyperplasia.

Treatment and Prognosis. The old concern that papillary hyperplasia of the palate held increased risk for cancer is no longer accepted. Even extensive lesions will continue indefinitely, waxing and waning in the early years but remaining more constant as nodules become more and more fibrotic. Occasional proliferations are so exuberant that clefts between nodules may be more than a centimeter deep.

Early lesions may completely disappear with cessation of denture use for 2 to 4 weeks, perhaps aided by topical antibiotic or antifungal therapies.[105] Persistent lesions must be surgically removed or laser ablated if a proper base is to be prepared for a new and better-fitting denture.

Pericoronitis

The mandibular retromolar pad or operculum is often hyperplastic, pushing against or even overlapping the last molar in the arch. Food debris and bacteria may become entrapped between this pad and the tooth, resulting in acute infection and extreme pain. This *pericoronitis* was first reported by Gunnel[107] in 1844 as "painful affection."

Clinical Features. Pericoronitis typically occurs in teenagers and young adults, presenting shortly after the eruption of the second or third mandibular molars. It presents as an erythematous, tender, sessile swelling of the retromolar pad, sometimes with surface ulceration from continuous trauma from the opposing maxillary molars.[7, 9, 108] Pus may be expressed from the tissue-tooth interface, and a foul taste may be present. Pain may be mild but is usually quite intense and may radiate to the external neck, the throat, the ear, or the oral floor. The patient often cannot close the jaw because of tenderness, and extreme pain may, conversely, result in the inability to open the jaws more than a few millimeters (trismus or "lock jaw"). Cervical lymphadenopathy, fever, leukocytosis, and malaise are common signs and symptoms, and the malady may be associated with an ipsilateral tonsillitis or upper respiratory infection.[109–111]

Pathologic Features. Pericoronitis is usually surgically removed after a course of antibiotic therapy to prevent future painful episodes, so active pus production is seldom seen in biopsy samples. The retromolar mass is composed of an admixture of moderately dense collagenic tissue and edematous granulation tissue, with moderate to large numbers of mixed chronic inflammatory cells throughout. The superior mucosa may be ulcerated, with an ulcer bed of fibrinoid necrotic debris. The epithelium immediately adjacent to the offending tooth typically presents with a combination of rete process hyperplasia, degeneration, and necrosis, perhaps with associated neutrophils. Bacterial colonies, dental plaque, and necrotic food debris may be attached to the epithelium. The pathologist should distinguish this lesion from *pyogenic granuloma* and routine *gingivitis,* and this often requires correlation with clinical features.

Treatment and Prognosis. Acute pericoronitis is treated by local antiseptic lavage and gentle curettage under the flap, with or without systemic antibiotics.[108] Once the acute phase is controlled, the offending molar is extracted or a wedge of hyperplastic pad tissue is removed surgically. Recurrence is unlikely with either of these treatments.

Pyogenic Granuloma

Pyogenic granuloma of the oral and oropharyngeal region is similar to its counterparts in other parts of the body, although it may occur under rather unique circumstances.[7–9, 112–116] During pregnancy, for example, hormonal excesses combine with poor oral hygiene to produce a generalized inflammatory enlargement of the gingiva, occasionally with one or more interdental papillae increasing to more than 2.0 cm in size.[117–119] This *pregnancy tumor (granuloma or epulis gravidarum)* usually regresses after the birth of the child, possibly to reappear with the next pregnancy. Hullihen's description in 1844 was most likely the first pyogenic granuloma reported in the English literature.[120]

Another special pyogenic granuloma is the *epulis granulomatosa (epulis haemangiomatosa),* a hemorrhagic gingival mass of granulation tissue protruding from the poorly healing bony socket of a recently extracted tooth. A third unique presentation is a draining granulation tissue mass, or *parulis,* surrounding and often hiding the end of a fistulous tract from an underlying intraosseous dental infection.

The term pyogenic granuloma is not well chosen, as there is seldom pus production and there is never granuloma formation. It has, nevertheless, become entrenched in our vocabulary and is widely used today.

Clinical Features. In addition to these special events, pyogenic granuloma can occur at any mucosal location of acute or chronic trauma, or infection.[7–9, 112–114] In the mouth, the vast majority of these very common lesions occur on the gingiva (Fig. 4–9A), where they may develop as dumb-bell–shaped masses on the facial and lingual surfaces of the dental arch, connected by a thin isthmus between adjacent teeth. Other sites of common involvement include the tongue, the lip mucosa and vermilion, and the buccal mucosa.

All ages and both genders are susceptible to this exuberant inflammatory response.[112] The lesion is usually a pedunculated, bright red mass with or without white areas of surface ulceration; some lesions have a normal coloration. Rarely does pyogenic granuloma exceed 2.5 cm in size and it usually reaches its full size within weeks or months, remaining indefinitely thereafter.[7]

A newly identified and rather unique form of granulation tissue proliferation is the *traumatic eosinophilic ulcer (traumatic eosinophilic granuloma).*[7, 121] This lesion of young adults and middle-aged individuals appears to be trauma-induced and routinely demonstrates surface ulceration. It differs from the typical oral or pharyngeal *traumatic ulcer* in that it is larger (1.5–3.0 cm), has often alarming proliferation of the granulation tissue of the ulcer bed (similar to pyogenic granuloma, but with a central indentation or crater), and has a much greater rate of recurrence.

Pathologic Features and Differential Diagnosis. Pyogenic granuloma is characterized by a rich profusion of anastomosing vascular channels, usually with plump endothelial cell nuclei, that is, neovascularity (Fig. 4–9B&C). The background stroma is typically edematous, but fibroplasia is often active and older lesions may have undergone considerable fibrosis (*fibrotic pyogenic granuloma*). The fibroblasts are typically plumb and mitotic activity may be noted in the stromal cells. Older lesions demonstrate fewer and more mature cells, that is, fibrocytes.

The blood vessels often show a clustered or medullary pattern separated by less vascular fibrotic septa, leading some authorities to consider the pyogenic granuloma to be a polypoid form of *capillary hemangioma* or nothing more than an inflamed *lobular hemangioma* occurring on the skin or mucosal surfaces; others prefer to use the term *granulation tissue-type hemangioma* (Fig. 4–9D).[6, 116] A mixed chronic and acute inflammatory cell infiltrate is scattered throughout the stroma, with early lesions containing more neutrophils than older lesions. Occasional lesions demonstrate an extreme predominance of plasma cells, prompting some pathologists to call them *plasma cell granuloma* (see Fig. 4–9C), a term that is best avoided because of the potential confusion with mucosal *solitary plasmacytoma* or *multiple myeloma*. Rare examples of *intravenous pyogenic granuloma* have been reported.[6]

The overlying stratified squamous epithelium may be atrophic or hyperplastic, and it is usually degenerated or ulcerated in large areas. When ulcerated, the ulcer bed is composed of fibrinoid necrotic debris, and regenerating epithelium at the ulcer edge may have a primitive or dysplastic appearance. The more aggressive variant, traumatic eosinophilic ulcer, shows considerable proliferation of granulation tissue, pushing the ulcer bed as much as a centimeter

above the normal mucosal surface. The required diagnostic feature is a scattering of eosinophils, usually in deeper areas associated with chronic rather than acute inflammatory cells. The inflammatory changes in this lesion have a greater tendency to extend deeply into underlying tissues, including muscle, than do those of a more typical pyogenic granuloma.

The histopathologic differentiation of pyogenic granuloma from *hyperplastic gingival inflammation* is sometimes impossible, and the pathologist must depend on the surgeon's description of a distinct clinical mass to make the granuloma diagnosis. Usually, however, routine *gingivitis* has edema confined to the subepithelial regions of crevicular mucosa (facing the teeth) with more exposed epithelium demonstrating a normal or hyperplastic appearance without ulceration. Quite often, the differentiation of pyogenic granuloma from inflamed capillary hemangioma is also impossible.

The reader is reminded that granulation tissue may be associated with many other oral soft tissue lesions, including *peripheral ossifying fibroma, peripheral giant cell granuloma,* and *mucocele.* The older and more fibrotic pyogenic granuloma can be distinguished from *irritation fibroma* by the presence of plump endothelial cell nuclei in the stromal blood vessels, but this is probably an

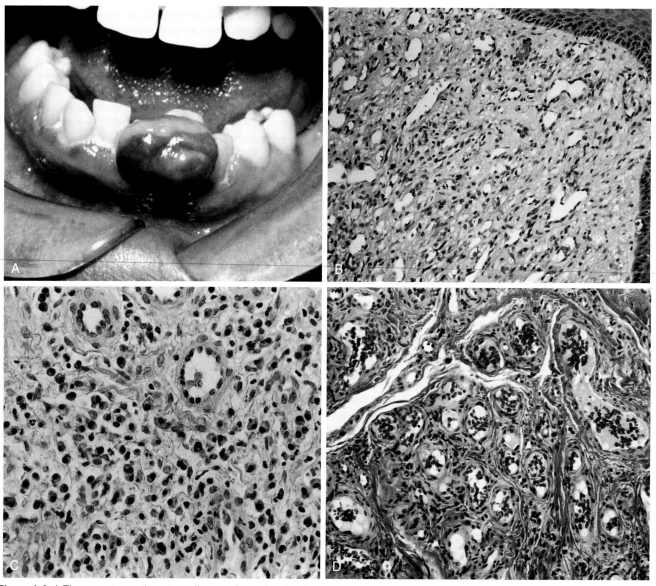

Figure 4–9. *A,* The pyogenic granuloma is usually somewhat pedunculated and lobulated, with an ulcerated surface; *B,* active vessels are admixed with inflammatory cells in an edematous background stroma; *C,* plasma cells may dominate the inflammatory cell infiltrate; *D,* occasional lesions will show a lobular pattern identical to the lobular capillary hemangioma.

unnecessary distinction as we presume that at least some irritation fibromas begin life as pyogenic granulomas.

Kaposi's sarcoma, bacillary angiomatosis, and *epithelioid hemangioma* must also be distinguished from pyogenic granuloma. Kaposi's sarcoma of acquired immunodeficiency syndrome (AIDS) shows proliferation of dysplastic spindle cells, vascular clefts, extravasated erythrocytes, and intracellular hyaline globules, none of which are features of pyogenic granuloma. Bacillary angiomatosis, also AIDS-related, shows dense, extracellular deposits of pale hematoxyphilic granular material representing masses of bacilli that stain positive with the Warthin-Starry stain. Epithelioid hemangioma has more plump, histiocytoid, endothelial cell proliferation without an acute inflammatory cell infiltrate.[6, 8]

Treatment and Prognosis. *Pyogenic granuloma* is treated by conservative surgical excision with removal of potential traumatic or infective etiologic factors.[6, 9] Recurrence occurs in approximately 15% of lesions thus removed, with gingival cases showing a much higher recurrence rate than lesions from other oral mucosal sites.[113] Therefore, pyogenic granuloma of the gingiva, such as epulis granulomatosa, should not only be excised, but the surgical wound bed should be curetted and adjacent teeth should be scaled and root-planed. If at all possible, removal in a pregnant woman should be postponed until after the birth. Lesional shrinkage at that time may make surgery unnecessary.

GRANULOMA-LIKE MUCOSAL LESIONS WITH GIANT CELLS

The oral soft tissues are associated with a variety of lesions containing multinucleated giant cells. With a few of these, as discussed in this section, the giant cells become the most significant part of the diagnosis.

Peripheral Giant Cell Granuloma

Peripheral giant cell granuloma is, for all practical purposes, a site-specific variant of pyogenic granuloma embedded with osteoclast-like multinucleated giant cells and arising exclusively from the periodontal ligament enclosing the root of a tooth.[7, 9, 122–126] This unique origin, of course, means that such a lesion can only be found within or upon the gingiva or alveolar ridge; no other site is acceptable. Called variously *giant cell reparative granuloma, osteoclastoma, giant cell epulis,* and *myeloid epulis,* this lesion was first reported as *fungus flesh* in 1848.[127] Almost half of all cases have lesional cells containing surface receptors for estrogen and this has led to speculation that some peripheral giant cell granulomas are responsive to hormonal influences.[125]

Clinical Features. The usual age at diagnosis is the fourth through sixth decades, but there is no marked age predilection. More than 60% of cases occur in females and this female predilection is more pronounced in the older age groups.[7, 124] Individual lesions are nodular and pedunculated, frequently with an ulcerated surface, and frequently with a red, brown, or bluish hue (Fig. 4–10A). Generally larger than pyogenic granuloma, the lesion may exceed 4 cm in size, but most lesions remain less than 2 cm in diameter.[126] Any alveolar region may be affected, and radiographs may show either a saucerization of underlying bone, periodontitis of underlying tissues, or an isthmus of soft tissue connecting to an intraosseous *central giant cell granuloma.*

Pathologic Features and Differential Diagnosis. The peripheral giant cell granuloma is composed of an unencapsulated aggregation of rather primitive but uniform mesenchymal cells with oval, pale nuclei and with a moderate amount of eosinophilic cytoplasm. Mitotic activity is not unusual in the lesion and may even be pronounced in lesions developing in children and adolescents. Mitotic activity within the giant cells is, however, not seen and if present should be considered to be a sign of sarcomatous change.

Stromal cells may be spindled with a background of collagenic fibers or may be rounded with a less fibrotic background. There may be occasional chronic inflammatory cells admixed with the mesenchymal cells or within surrounding fibrovascular tissues. A thin band of routine fibrovascular tissue separates the lesion from the overlying epithelium, often with dilated veins and capillaries. When surface ulceration is present, the ulcer bed consists of routine fibrinoid necrotic debris over granulation tissue.

Admixed throughout the stroma are numerous osteoclast-like multinucleated giant cells containing varying numbers of pale vesicular nuclei similar to those within the surrounding stromal cells (Fig. 4–10B). These cells have eosinophilic cytoplasm, which electron microscopy has shown to contain large numbers of mitochondria.[123] Immunohistochemistry has shown the giant cells to be only slightly different from true osteoclasts. The origin of the multinucleated cells is still unknown, but they are assumed to arise from syncytial fusion of mononuclear preosteoclasts of bone marrow origin.

Blood vessels within the lesional stroma show plump endothelial cell nuclei and scattered extravasation of erythrocytes is commonly seen. Hemosiderin deposition may be seen in areas of old hemorrhage. Metaplastic or osteoblastic new bone formation may be seen, usually in the lower third of the lesion. Dystrophic calcification may be present as well.

Occasional lesions show an admixture of tissue types compatible with peripheral giant cell granuloma, *peripheral ossifying fibroma,* and *pyogenic granuloma,* presumably because of the common pathoetiology of these lesions. Such lesions are traditionally diagnosed according to the dominant tissue type.

Peripheral giant cell granuloma can be differentiated from *osteoblastic osteosarcoma* by the uniformity of the stromal cells and by the lack of dysplasia in these cells. In young persons, however, numerous mitotic figures and active proliferation of stromal cells may make this distinction difficult. Peripheral giant cell granuloma may be indistinguishable from the rare extraosseous *brown tumor* of *hyperparathyroidism.*[128]

Treatment and Prognosis. Peripheral giant cell granuloma is treated by conservative surgical excision followed by curettage of any underlying bony defect and careful scaling and root-planing of associated teeth.[7, 124] A recurrence rate of 10% or more has been reported, so re-excision may be necessary. Very large or recurring lesions may represent brown tumors of hyperparathyroidism and will require treatment of the underlying endocrine dysfunction prior to surgical removal.[128]

Orofacial Granulomatosis and Granulomatous Mucositis

Granulomatous inflammation of the oral and oropharyngeal submucosal tissues is not common, but when found it presents a definite diagnostic dilemma because of the wide variety of possible etiologic diseases and the rather generic appearance of the individual lesions. The matter is made more confusing by the common use of the term "granuloma" to describe maxillofacial diseases with little or no resemblance to true granulomas, such as *pyogenic granuloma, periapical granuloma, peripheral giant cell granuloma, pulse granuloma, traumatic eosinophilic granuloma,* and *epulis granulomatosa.* The group of true granulomatous diseases is collectively called *orofacial granulomatoses.*[7, 129–147]

Until the latter two-thirds of the 20th century, the most common of the oral granulomatous lesions were those produced by *tuberculosis* and *tertiary syphilis.*[130] Today they are more likely to represent oral manifestations of autoimmune disorders, such as Crohn's disease and sarcoidosis, or localized allergic reactions, or deep fungal infections.[131–133, 136–139, 142, 144, 147] The name of the associated systemic disease is traditionally applied to oral lesions, whenever possible, but a certain number of cases remain idiopathic and are diagnosed simply as *granulomatous mucositis* or *orofacial granulomatosis.*[7, 129, 137] Before such generic terminology can be applied,

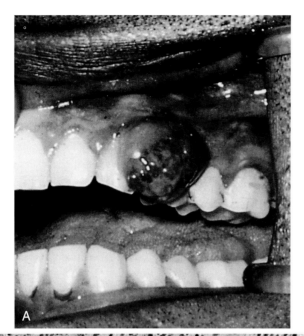

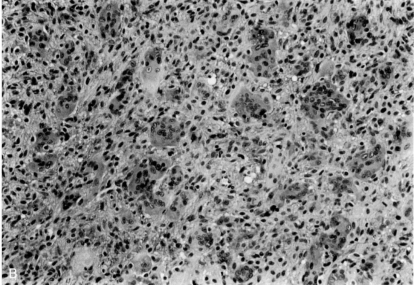

Figure 4–10. *A,* The peripheral giant cell granuloma must be located on alveolar bone and often shows surface ulceration. *B,* Osteoclast-like cells are scattered throughout a primitive mesenchymal stroma with few visible blood vessels but with extravasated erythrocytes.

however, the pathologist must make every effort to rule out histologically distinctive granulomatous diseases and specific granulomatous infectious processes (Table 4–5). Cases associated with systemic disease may present with or without involvement of extraoral regions at the time of diagnosis.

Clinical Features. Granulomatous lesions of the oral and oropharyngeal mucosa usually present as sessile, lobulated, moderately firm and relatively nontender nodules and papules with normal coloration and with little or no surrounding inflammatory mucosal erythema. With time, some of the granulomas may ulcerate centrally and present as a deep, painless ulcer with a nonerythematous rolled border, reminiscent of *squamous cell carcinoma.* The granulomas of tertiary syphilis, tuberculosis, and deep mycotic infections may reach a size of more than 2 cm, but those related to autoimmune phenomena, especially sarcoidosis, cheilitis granulomatosa, and Crohn's disease, typically remain small and often present as multiple nodules and papules, sometimes clustered together to impart a cobblestone appearance to the mucosa.

Several granulomatous diseases have unique clinical features. The granulomas of deep fungal infections, *Langerhans cell disease (eosinophilic granuloma), sarcoidosis,* and *Wegener's granulomatosis* may destroy underlying bone when located on gingival or alveolar mucosa. This is also true for palatal lesions of tertiary syphilis and tuberculosis, which have a special affinity for perforating the hard palate. Granulomatous gingivitis is the only granulomatous lesion typically associated with pain and, of course, by definition must occur on gingival mucosa.[136, 147] Extensive involvement of submucosal areas may produce a generalized enlargement of the affected site, especially noticeable on the lips and tongue, as in cheilitis granulomatosa, *Melkersson-Rosenthal syndrome,* and syphilitic glossitis.

Pathologic Features and Differential Diagnosis. Most granulomatous lesions of the oral region present as small, noncaseating granulomas with peripheral lymphocytes, central epithelioid histiocytes and, usually, multinucleated giant cells (Fig. 4–11). Foreign bodies within the giant cells and histiocytes may polarize (Fig. 4–11, inset) and microorganisms may be identified by appropriate bacterial and fungal stains (see Table 4–5). Wegener's granulomatosis may have no granulomas visible but will show a pattern of mixed inflammatory infiltrates around blood vessels, with focal areas of necrosis and areas with heavy neutrophilic infiltration and nuclear dust. The oral epithelium in this disease may demonstrate severe acanthosis or pseudoepitheliomatous hyperplasia, as may granulomatous infection by *blastomycosis,* and it is the granulomatous disease most likely to be associated with extravasated erythrocytes.

Table 4–5. Granulomatous Lesions Affecting the Oral and Oropharyngeal Submucosa (Collectively Called Orofacial Granulomatosis)

Diagnosis	Distinguishing Diagnostic Features
Tuberculosis	Bacillus demonstrated by acid-fast stain; areas of caseous necrosis
Tertiary syphilis (gumma)	Spirochetes demonstrated by immunostain for *Treponema pallidum*
Sarcoidosis	No microorganisms identified
Crohn's disease	Gastrointestinal involvement, no microorganisms identified
Wegener's granulomatosis	Destruction of underlying bone, vasculitis, no microorganisms identified
Granulomatous gingivitis	Gingival location only
Eosinophilic granuloma	Combination of eosinophils, multinucleated giant cells, histiocytes
Mycotic granulomatous infection	Fungus identified by silver stains
Foreign body reaction	Identification of associated foreign material
Cholesterol granuloma	Identification of associated submucosal inclusion cyst and cholesterol clefts
Cheilitis granulomatosa	Association with Melkersson-Rosenthal syndrome; involvement of lips alone is called cheilitis granulomatosa of Miescher
Idiopathic orofacial granulomatosis	No etiologic factor can be identified
Hairy cell leukemia	In addition to multinucleated and histiocytic cells, dysplastic lymphocytes are seen
Salmonella infection	Bacteria identified by Gram stain

Many of the granulomatous diseases listed in Table 4–5 require physical examination and laboratory evaluation for an appropriate diagnosis. These are beyond the scope of this chapter and will not be discussed further.

Treatment and Prognosis. The treatment of orofacial granulomatosis and the various forms of granulomatous mucositis will depend on the underlying or systemic cause. Localized lesions without systemic connection can be treated by conservative surgical removal and plastic surgical reconstruction. Prior to surgery, a host of medications may be used with variable results: intralesional and systemic corticosteroids, low-dose radiotherapy, methotrexate, dapsone, salazosulfapyridine (sulfasalazine), and hydroxychloroquine sulfate, among others. No therapy has proven to be universally effective in orofacial granulomatosis without systemic involvement.

Many lesions eventually resolve spontaneously with or without therapy, but others continue to progress despite rather aggressive therapy. For those oral lesions that are manifestations of systemic disease, the prognosis of oral lesions will depend on the patient's response to therapies for the systemic disease.

▋ SOFT TISSUE LESIONS WITH BONE OR CARTILAGE

The oral soft tissues are the site of a variety of developmental and reactive proliferations composed of tissue types not normal to the site, such as bone or cartilage, or of an admixture of multiple tissue types in an unusual fashion, such as teratoma. These are often small and innocuous malformations that are not biopsied or formally diagnosed.

Those formally diagnosed seldom require more than a clinical diagnosis. Some cases, however, in particular the reactive masses, have a nonspecific clinical appearance or are located in sites that interfere with proper function or proper oral hygiene and, hence, are biopsied for microscopic interpretation. Although many of the developmental anomalies are present in early life, they are often not noticed until adult life and are usually excised to rule out recent neoplastic growth. The reader is reminded, furthermore, that focal deposits of bone and cartilage may be present in a variety of other benign and malignant lesions discussed in other sections of this chapter: *peripheral giant cell granuloma, malignant peripheral nerve sheath tumor, liposarcoma,* and *malignant fibrous histiocytoma.*

Torus and Bony Exostosis

While not technically soft tissue masses, the *torus palatinus, torus mandibularis* and *bony exostosis (buccal exostosis)* are all lesions that present as surface masses and are removed with minimal disturbance of deeper cancellous bones.[7, 148–151] As such, they are submitted to the pathologist as palatal or alveolar masses and might be confused with *peripheral ossifying fibroma* or other bone-producing soft tissue masses of the oral mucosa. For this reason, these lesions are included in the present section.

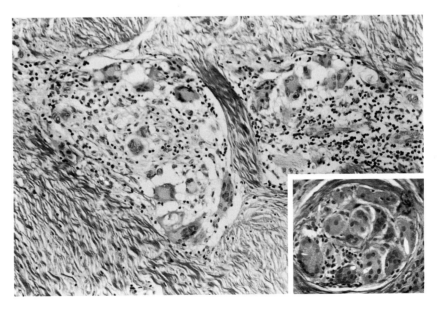

Figure 4–11. Submucosal granulomas are seen in a variety of oral conditions; here, the Touton-type cells represent sarcoidosis of the gingival tissues. With polarized light *(inset),* birefringent foreign fibers or particles may be seen within giant cells of a foreign body reaction.

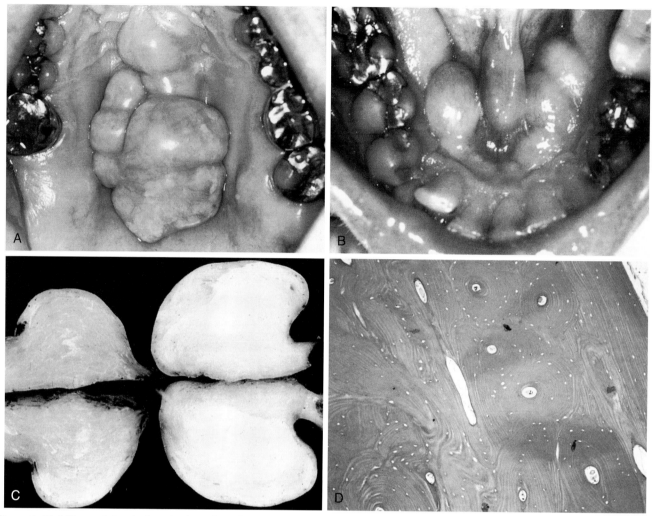

Figure 4–12. *A,* Torus palatinus is always in the midline of the hard palate and is often multilobulated; *B,* torus mandibularis is always on the lingual aspect of the mandibular alveolus and is frequently bilateral; *C,* cut surfaces usually demonstrate dense, lamellated cortical bone; *D,* there are few marrow spaces in the bone of the typical torus and many lesions show considerable loss of osteocytes, indicative of ischemic damage.

The torus is considered to be a developmental anomaly, although it does not present until adult life and often will continue to grow slowly throughout life.[150] It may be the outcome of mild, chronic periosteal ischemia secondary to mild nasal septum pressures (palatal torus) or the torquing action of the arch of the mandible (mandibular torus) or lateral pressures from the roots of the underlying teeth (buccal exostosis), but this is largely speculation. The most similar bony growth outside the jaws is the *bunion* of the lateral foot, and the earliest dental journal report of a torus palatinus was probably in an 1857 essay by Parmentier[152] relating to tumors of the palate.

Clinical Features. These entities are all very site-specific. The palatal torus is found only in the midline of the hard palate (Fig. 4–12*A*).[7, 150] The mandibular torus is found only on the lingual surface of the mandible, near the bicuspid teeth (Fig. 4–12*B*).[7, 151] The buccal exostosis is found only on the facial surface of the alveolar bone, usually the maxillary alveolus.[7] Bony surface proliferations found in another site are typically given the generic diagnosis of bony exostosis or osteoma; that is, they are considered to be trauma-induced inflammatory periosteal reactions or true neoplasms. Unless such a bony prominence is specifically located, is pedunculated, or is associated with an osteoma-producing syndrome such as the *Gardner syndrome,* there may be no means by which to differentiate an exostosis from an osteoma, even under the microscope.

As previously stated, these lesions are not present until the late

teen and early adult years, and many, if not most, continue to slowly enlarge over time. Fewer than 3% occur in children. Taken as a group, these lesions are found in at least 3% of adults and are more common in females than in males.[1, 2] The torus may be bosselated or multilobulated, but the exostosis is typically a single, broad-based, smooth-surfaced mass, perhaps with a central sharp, pointed projection of bone producing tenderness immediately beneath the surface mucosa. Lesions may become 3 to 4 cm in greatest diameter, but are usually less than 1.5 cm at biopsy. A definite hereditary basis, usually autosomal dominant, has been established for some cases of tori, and Asians, especially Koreans, have a much higher prevalence rate than do other ethnic groups.[149, 151]

Pathologic Features. On cut surface, the torus and exostosis show dense bone with a lamellar or laminated pattern (Fig. 4–12*C*). They are usually composed of dense, mature, lamellar bone with scattered osteocytes and small marrow spaces filled with fatty marrow or a loose fibrovascular stroma. Some lesions have a thin rim of cortical bone overlying inactive cancellous bone with considerable fatty or hematopoietic marrow present. Minimal osteoblastic activity is usually seen, but occasional lesions will show abundant periosteal activity. Large areas of bone may show enlarged lacunae with missing or pyknotic osteocytes (Fig. 4–12*D*), indicative of ischemic damage to the bone. Ischemic changes such as marrow fibrosis and dilated veins may also be found in the marrow, with rare examples showing actual infarction of fatty marrow.[153]

Treatment and Prognosis. Neither the torus nor the bony exostosis requires treatment unless it becomes so large that it interferes with function, interferes with denture placement, or suffers from recurring traumatic surface ulceration (usually from sharp foods, such as potato chips or fish bones).[7, 9, 150] When treatment is elected, the lesions may be chiseled off of the cortex or removed via bone burr cutting through the base of the lesion.

Slowly enlarging, recurrent lesions occasionally are seen, but there is no malignant transformation potential. The patient should be evaluated for Gardner syndrome should he or she have multiple bony growths or lesions not in the classic torus or buccal exostosis locations. Intestinal polyposis and cutaneous cysts or fibromas are other common features of this autosomal dominant syndrome.[7]

Peripheral Ossifying/Cementifying Fibroma

In addition to the *peripheral giant cell granuloma,* mesenchymal cells of the periodontal ligament are capable of producing another unique inflammatory hyperplasia, the *peripheral ossifying fibroma,* also referred to as the *peripheral cementifying fibroma,* depending on whether or not bone or cementum is seen microscopically.[7, 9, 154–157] The pluripotential cells of the ligament have the apparent ability to transform or metaplastically alter into osteoblasts, cementoblasts, or fibroblasts. The reader is reminded that this is a reactive lesion, not the peripheral counterpart of the intraosseous neoplasm called *central cemento-ossifying fibroma.* Odontogenic lesions of the gingiva, moreover, may produce various calcified materials and are discussed elsewhere in this text (Chapter 9).

By definition, the peripheral ossifying fibroma must be associated with gingival tissues, and the diagnosis cannot be used for lesions of other oral sites. The presence of teeth is not, however, required for the diagnosis, as periodontal ligament fibers remain within and above alveolar bone long after their associated teeth have been extracted. Shepherd[158] first reported this entity as *alveolar exostosis* in 1844.

Clinical Features. Peripheral ossifying fibroma presents as a painless, hemorrhagic, and often lobulated mass of the gingiva or alveolar mucosa (Fig. 4–13*A*), perhaps with large areas of surface ulceration.[7, 9, 155] Early lesions are quite irregular and red, but older lesions may have a smooth salmon pink surface and may be indistinguishable clinically from the more common *irritation fibroma.*[156] Most lesions are 1 to 2 cm in size, but some may slowly enlarge to more than 4 cm.[157] Early growth is often alarmingly rapid.

A lesion may vary somewhat in size over time, depending on the amount of superficial inflammation and edema. Although this tumor is typically diagnosed in teenagers and young adults, it may occur at any age, especially in individuals with poor oral hygiene. Radiographs may show irregular, scattered radiopacities in the lesion.

Pathologic Features and Differential Diagnosis. An aggregated submucosal proliferation of primitive oval and bipolar mesenchymal cells is the hallmark of peripheral ossifying fibroma.[154] The lesion may be very cellular or may be somewhat fibrotic, but scattered throughout are islands and trabeculae of woven or lamellar bone, usually with abundant osteoblastic rimming (Fig. 4–13*B*). Metaplastic bone may also be seen. The calcified tissues may have the dark-staining, acellular, rounded appearance of cementum, in which case the term peripheral cementifying fibroma has traditionally been used (Fig. 4–13*C*). Many examples show an admixture of bone and cementum, that is, *peripheral ossifying/cementifying fibroma,* and early lesions may contain only small ovoid areas of dystrophic calcification. Although the lesional stroma is similar to that of *peripheral giant cell granuloma,* the erythrocyte extravasation of the latter lesion is not a feature of peripheral ossifying fibroma and osteoclast-like cells are quite rare.

The lesional nidus is not encapsulated but is rather well demarcated from the surrounding fibrovascular stroma. Surrounding tissues are often edematous, with neovascularity and variable numbers of chronic and acute inflammatory cells. By way of

differential diagnosis, the *exuberant callus* so common to the long bones is almost never found at the surface of jawbones and so is not a serious diagnostic distinction from peripheral ossifying fibroma. Some gingival masses, however, contain large areas of classic *pyogenic granuloma, irritation fibroma,* or peripheral giant cell granuloma as well as peripheral ossifying fibroma. In such cases, the pathologist usually chooses for the appropriate diagnosis the lesional type that predominates. Also, individual cells must be carefully examined for dysplastic changes to rule out *osteoblastic* or *juxtacortical osteosarcoma,* but frequent mitotic figures of normal configuration are acceptable for the benign diagnosis, especially in lesions found in children.

Treatment and Prognosis. Conservative surgical excision must be followed by diligent curettage of the wound and root-planing of adjacent teeth if recurrence is to be avoided. With simple removal, the recurrence rate is greater than 20%.[7, 10] Malignant transformation has not been reported for this lesion.

Heterotopic Ossification

Heterotopic ossification, widely known as *myositis ossificans,* is a reactive bone-producing soft tissue proliferation of muscle or other connective tissues.[6–8, 159–163] When occurring in subcutaneous or submucosal fat, it is often referred to as *panniculitis ossificans* or *fasciitis ossificans.* A more serious and extensive form, *myositis ossificans progressiva* or *fibrodysplasia ossificans progressiva,* involves skeletal muscle, tendons, fascia, aponeuroses, and ligaments.[164, 165] The progressive form is also associated with assorted congenital anomalies, especially of the toes and thumbs, with ankylosis of the digits and a history of joint pain and swelling. Multiple and sometimes massive heterotopic ossification and calcification may develop. Several other conditions, such as *fibro-osseous pseudotumor, florid reactive periostitis,* and *bizarre parosteal osteochondromatous proliferation,* are probably variations of heterotopic ossification.[6, 163]

Heterotopic ossification may occur after acute or chronic trauma to a muscle. The musculature of the head and neck region is an uncommon site for this phenomenon, but occasional cases have occurred in the masseter and other facial muscles.[162] Most authorities presume this lesion to originate from an intramuscular hematoma with metaplastic transformation of pleuripotential stromal cells, but traumatic implantation of periosteum is another logical explanation for selected cases.

Clinical Features. Heterotopic ossification of the head and neck region typically occurs in the masseter muscle of a young person after a single severe injury.[159, 162] There is no gender predilection. Shortly after the injury, a painful mass begins enlarging to 2 to 4 cm in greatest dimension. The tumor usually reaches its maximum size within 1 to 2 weeks. It is minimally movable beneath the skin or mucous membrane and may be rather firm to palpation. Radiographs of early lesions will reveal feathery opacities caused by ossifications along muscle fibers. Older lesions show more solid opaque masses that may coalesce to appear as one large, irregularly opaque mass, often with a central or acentric zone of radiolucency. The mass is not attached to adjacent bone.

Computed tomograms show the lesion to be well circumscribed, usually with a shell of ossification surrounding a less mineralized core. Conversely, the lesion may appear to be poorly defined and infiltrative on magnetic resonance images.[163]

Myositis ossificans progressiva is rare, slowly progressive, inherited, and associated with a microdactyly or adactyly of the thumbs and great toes, and with the eventual onset of fibroblastic proliferations and calcification during the first decade of life.[164, 165] Sporadic examples have been reported and there is no gender predilection. Diffuse or multinodular, doughy, soft tissue involvement is seen most commonly on the back, shoulders, and upper arms. Facial and lip involvement have been reported, with masseter muscle involvement sometimes severe enough to interfere with jaw opening.[164] Muscles become progressively stiffened and contraction deformities may occur. Joint ankylosis is a frequent problem, as are *exostoses* and *osteoporosis*.

Pathologic Features and Differential Diagnosis. Active, poorly organized fibroblastic proliferation is seen throughout the lesion. The stromal cells are plump and bipolar and may demonstrate considerable mitotic activity, but they never demonstrate cytologic atypia or true dysplasia. The background consists of loosely arranged collagen and reticulin fibers with neovascularity becoming more pronounced toward the lesional periphery. The fibroblasts also form into fascicles toward the periphery, with an admixture of osteoblasts and reactive new bone.

The bone is woven or immature in early lesions but in older lesions it is mature lamellar bone, perhaps with fatty or hematopoietic marrow. Large amounts of cartilage may also be seen, tempting the pathologist to call the tumor *soft tissue chondroma* or *soft tissue chondrosarcoma*. Those ossifications with very active stromal cells might, likewise, tempt the pathologist to consider a *soft tissue osteosarcoma*. Some lesions contain cystic spaces centrally, where the tissues can take on the appearance of *aneurysmal bone cyst,* a bone lesion with rare examples in soft tissues.

Treatment and Prognosis. Treatment is usually not necessary, as most tumors of heterotopic ossification regress spontaneously.[159, 162] The lesion for which treatment is elected, however, can be removed by conservative surgical excision. Occasional recurrences do occur, often with rapid onset after surgery and with rapid growth after onset. There have been a few reported cases of malignant transformation of heterotopic ossification into extraskeletal osteosarcoma, but there is some concern that these may actually have been misdiagnosed at the outset.[8] Patients with myositis ossificans progressiva or fibrodysplasia ossificans progressiva will, of course, have more serious, perhaps life-threatening sequelae, such as *anorexia* from difficult mouth opening and *pneumonia* or respiratory failure in early life.[164]

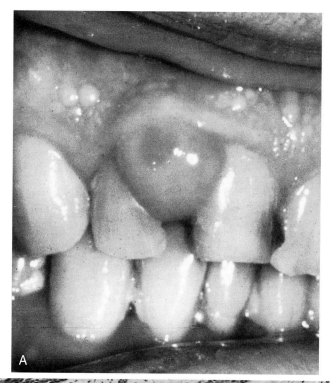

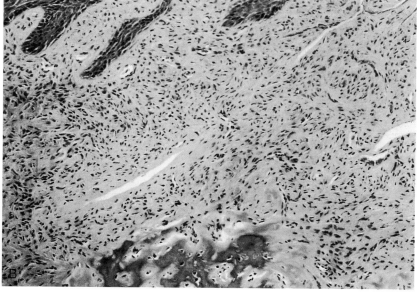

Figure 4–13. *A,* Peripheral ossifying fibroma must be located on the alveolar mucosa or gingiva and is typically located between teeth in the area of the gingival papilla. *B,* Metaplastic bone (lower portion of photo) often shows irregular osteoblastic rimming in some areas.

Soft Tissue Osseous/Cartilaginous Choristoma

Extraskeletal proliferation of bone and cartilage in oral and maxillofacial soft tissues probably reflects the multipotential nature of primitive mesenchymal cells throughout the region. Usually developmental in origin, some of these proliferations seem to occur as a result of local trauma.[166, 167] Several terms are used for them.

Choristoma (aberrant rest, heterotopic tissue) is defined as a histologically normal tissue proliferation or nodule of a tissue type not normally found in the anatomic site of proliferation.[7, 8, 168–175] *Hamartoma* is defined as a benign tumor-like nodule composed of an overgrowth of mature cells and tissues that are normally found in the affected part, but with disorganization and often with one element predominating. The occurrence of multiple hamartomas in the same patient is called *hamartomatosis*. It is possible that some or many examples of *osseous choristoma* are nothing more than old cases of *heterotopic ossification,* but the two lesions have traditionally been classified as separate and distinct entities. Likewise, the presence of ectopic tissue elements from more than one germ cell layer has traditionally been called *teratoma* (see elsewhere in this section), and it is not unusual for an oral or cervicofacial teratoma to contain bone or cartilage.

Clinical Features. *Osseous/cartilaginous choristoma* is characteristically seen as a painless, firm nodule in young adults, especially in females, and has most frequently been reported on the tongue, although no submucosal site is immune.[169–175] It seldom reaches a size greater than 1.5 cm, although even small lesions may produce local dysfunction if located on the lateral border of the tongue. A similar lesion, *osteoma cutis,* is found beneath the skin of the face and other areas, but is usually considered to be a different entity.

A unique cartilage-producing form of this tissue-level disorder is found on the edentulous alveolar ridge of a denture wearer, especially in the anterior maxilla. Presumably trauma-induced, this self-limiting *Cutright tumor (chondroid choristoma, traumatic osseous and chondromatous metaplasia)* may produce pressure atrophy of underlying bone, may become tender, and may contain bone in addition to cartilage.[166, 167] Another chondroid choristoma, mistakenly termed *chondroid hamartoma* is frequently found in the anterior tongue of individuals with the *orofaciodigital (OFD) syndrome, type I.*[5]

When multiple *primary cutaneous ossification* is encountered, it may be part of *Albright's hereditary osteodystrophy,* which is associated with congenital or early subcutaneous ossifications of the extremities, trunk, and scalp. Oral mucosal involvement is very rare. The bony spicules in this disease may produce surface ulceration or may extrude from the surface. *Pseudohypoparathyroidism* and *pseudopseudohypoparathyroidism* are frequently observed in this condition, which is inherited as an X-linked or autosomal dominant trait.

Pathologic Features and Differential Diagnosis. The osseous/cartilaginous choristoma is composed of a submucosal proliferation of benign and normal (perhaps immature) bone or cartilage. These "abnormal" tissues are embedded within a background stroma of fibrovascular connective tissue, usually without true encapsulation but often with a pseudoencapsulation. Cartilage may be active and mimic *synovial chondromatosis (joint mice)* or *soft tissue chondroma* (Fig. 4–14*A&B*) Bone maturation often results in lamellar bone, perhaps with hematopoietic or fatty marrow (Fig. 4–14*C*). Choristomas and hamartomas given other specific diagnostic names, such as *Fordyce granules (ectopic sebaceous glands)* and *oral tonsils (benign lymphoid aggregates),* are discussed under those names in this text.

Osseous choristoma may be confused with *heterotopic ossification (myositis ossificans),* but the latter is typically located in muscle and has more osteoblastic activity than the choristoma. Differentiation of osseous choristoma from *peripheral ossifying fibroma* is not usually difficult because the latter has a unique cellular stroma of oval, primitive mesenchymal cells and is found exclusively on alveolar bone surfaces. Neither cartilage nor marrow is produced by the peripheral ossifying fibroma and, by tradition, a cartilaginous choristoma of the crest of the alveolar ridge in a denture wearer is called a Cutright tumor.

Osseous choristoma should not be confused with the dystrophic calcification so frequently found in old thrombi, hematomas and keratin-filled soft tissue cysts. This darkly staining aggregation of precipitated salts does not have a bone-like organization.

Treatment and Prognosis. The choristoma is best treated by conservative surgical excision. No recurrences have been reported with this therapy.[7, 174]

Juxtacortical (Periosteal/Parosteal) Osteosarcoma

Several variants of *osteosarcoma* or *osteogenic sarcoma* arise on the surface of bone rather than within the medullary spaces. These initially grow outward but eventually will perforate through the underlying cortex and proliferate within cancellous bone. This *juxtacortical osteosarcoma* occurs most frequently on the surfaces of long bones, but rare reported examples have involved the jaws.[7, 176–178] The disease is included here to help differentiate from the *peripheral ossifying fibroma,* which is completely benign but may show high mitotic activity and somewhat alarming stromal cells.

This malignancy was first reported as a benign *parosteal osteoma* by Geschickter and Copeland[179] in 1951, but is today considered to be a low-grade malignancy and is usually subdivided into two types: *parosteal osteosarcoma* and *periosteal osteosarcoma.* Juxtacortical osteosarcoma is different from the *soft tissue osteosarcoma,* which arises completely within connective tissues some distance from the cortex and is not physically associated with a bone. Soft tissue osteosarcoma is not further discussed in this chapter.

Clinical Features. Juxtacortical osteosarcoma presents as an irregular, lobulated or fungating, nonmovable submucosal mass of the attached gingiva or alveolar mucosa covering the mandible or maxilla. It is seldom painful but may present with a dull ache. The malignancy occurs more frequently on the surface of the mandible than the maxilla, and there seems to be a strong predilection for males.[177, 178] The typical patient is 35 years of age at diagnosis, but lesions have been present for 1 to 5 years prior to diagnosis and the age range is quite broad: 17 to 63 years.[176] Irregular radiopacities are seen on 75% to 90% of routine radiographs of the lesion.

Pathologic Features and Differential Diagnosis. *Parosteal osteosarcoma* is characterized by a high degree of tissue differentiation and the bland histology may lead the pathologist to a benign diagnosis such as *osteoblastoma, peripheral ossifying fibroma,* or *heterotopic ossification.* The criteria, however, for intramedullary malignancy are also used for the peripheral lesions, namely, dysplasia or anaplasia of the mesenchymal stroma and the production of bone by that neoplastic stroma. *Periosteal osteosarcoma* is more poorly differentiated and often has a prominent chondroid component.

The classic juxtacortical osteosarcoma demonstrates scattered trabeculae of immature or woven bone, which may run parallel one to the other. The bone shows only mild osteoblastic rimming and only occasional lesional cells become incorporated into the new bone. Small foci of osteoid and chondroid metaplasia may also be seen. The fibrous stroma is usually hypocellular and the cellular dysplasia required for a malignant diagnosis may be rather sparse in the parosteal osteosarcoma, but periosteal osteosarcoma typically has numerous lesional cells that are moderately or poorly differentiated. The latter may have so much cartilage production that there is a strong similarity to *chondroblastic intramedullary osteosarcoma.*

The differentiation of juxtacortical osteosarcoma from peripheral ossifying fibroma, reactive cortical *exostosis, heterotopic ossification, osseous choristoma,* and *peripheral giant cell granuloma* with reactive bone is based predominantly on the identification of pleomorphic or otherwise dysplastic stromal cells producing bone in the osteosarcoma. The other lesions, all of which are discussed elsewhere in this chapter, may show many plump, active stromal cells

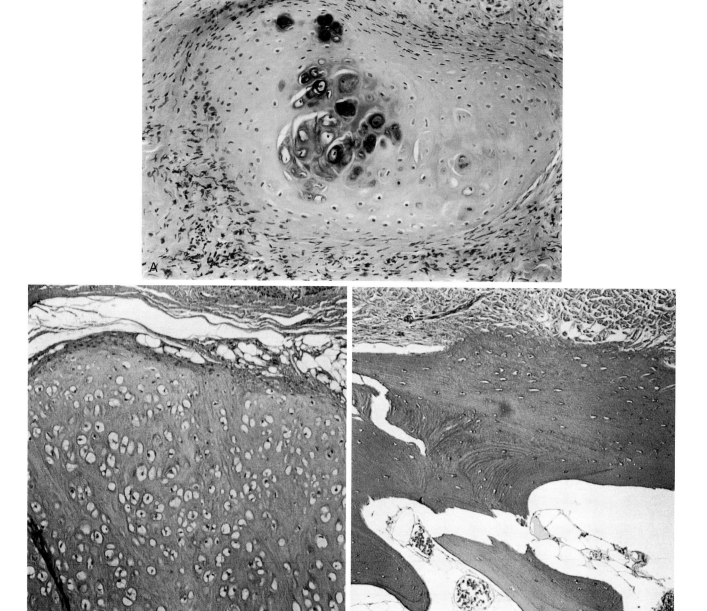

Figure 4–14. *A,* The Cutright tumor is a cartilaginous choristoma with very mature and localized submucosal cartilage. *B,* Cartilaginous choristoma may show enough lack of maturity that a distinction between it and a soft tissue chondroma or low-grade chondrosarcoma may be problematic. *C,* Osseous choristomas of the oral region may show so much maturity that bone marrow is present.

with moderate mitotic activity, but true dysplasia is lacking. Moreover, heterotopic ossification has its most active stromal proliferation centrally located, while the juxtacortical osteosarcoma has the most active regions toward its periphery. Finally, although some lesions may mimic *osteochondroma,* that benign lesion has not yet been reported to arise from the surface of the jawbones.

Once malignancy has been established, radiographic and clinical information may be required to ensure that the lesion is not an intramedullary osteosarcoma that has perforated through to the periosteal surface. This task is sometimes made impossible by the converse invasion of a juxtacortical lesion into cancellous bone.

Treatment and Prognosis. Lesions are treated by extensive surgical removal.[177] Well-differentiated lesions may be handled more conservatively than poorly differentiated ones, but it is important to remember that different sites within the same tumor may show different tissue grades. Juxtacortical osteosarcoma has a considerably better prognosis than its intraosseous counterpart, although the few jawbone cases reported do not allow for specific commentary to be made for that anatomic site.

Well differentiated lesions of long bones have an approximate 80% 5-year survival rate, whereas the survival rate of those with poorly differentiated lesions is less than half that. However, no deaths have been reported from the few cases of juxtacortical osteosarcoma of the jaws.[177]

NONCALCIFIED SOFT TISSUE TUMORS WITH MIXED OR ECTOPIC TISSUES

Glial Choristoma

Rare cases of lingual choristoma have been reported with glial tissue as the predominant or only tissue type present. This *glial choristoma* presents as a soft, painless, submucosal or deep nodule that is 1 to 2 cm in diameter and is only slightly movable.[3, 180, 181] It has been reported in teenagers and young adults and may be an example of *teratoma* with glial predominance rather than true heterotopic brain tissue. The tumor is not associated with central nervous system pathosis or syndromes; in the head and neck region, the most common sites of presentation are the cribriform area of the nasal sinus *(nasal glioma)* and the bridge of the nose *(extranasal glioma).*[180]

Pathologic Features. Glial choristoma is composed of an unencapsulated but fairly well demarcated submucosal aggregation of loose glial fibers intermixed with a variable number of mononuclear and multinucleated oval and stellate astrocytes with moderate eosinophilic cytoplasm (Fig. 4–15). Ganglion cells may be numerous. Bands of fibrous tissue may be intermingled with the lesional cells or may surround clusters of cells. There is no evidence of cellular dysplasia or tissue necrosis.

Glial tissues with astrocytic differentiation are immunoreactive for glial fibrillary acidic protein (GFAP), S-100 protein, and sometimes for vimentin. In general, the number of GFAP-positive cells is proportional to the degree of differentiation, and with glial choristoma there is enough cellular maturity to provide strong and diffuse reactivity. This diffuse reactivity will help to differentiate the lesion from *neurilemoma,* which lacks glial filaments, and from lingual metastasis of an anaplastic brain neoplasm.

Treatment and Prognosis. Glial choristoma should be removed by conservative surgical excision.[180, 181] No recurrence has been reported, nor has malignant transformation been reported.

Teratoma

A *teratoma* (pleural, *teratomata*) is a germ cell tumor derived from pluripotential cells and made up of elements of different types of tissue from all three germ cell layers.[7, 182–187] Most often found in the ovary or testis, the rare teratoma of the head and neck region arises primarily from Rathke's pouch remnants of the sphenoid bone region, from the lateral neck, and from the tongue. Rathke's pouch teratomas may extend into the mouth through a cleft palate. Although typically congenital, the teratoma is a true neoplasm of multiple tissue types foreign to the site from which it arises. Tissues derived from different embryonic germ layers are the rule rather than the exception.

This tumor varies considerably in the differentiation and maturation of its involved tissues, with some lesions containing fingers, teeth, jawbone, or diminutive skeletons, whereas others demonstrate no more than an admixture of various tissue types with no attempt at maturation or structural development. Most paraoral cases are cystic and relatively undifferentiated. Oral lesions have, however, been known to contain tissues from all parts of the body, including brain, bone, cartilage, skin, lung, and the gastrointestinal tract.[7, 8, 183, 184]

Pathologic Features. The various tissue types found in a teratoma for the most part are mature, although full differentiation is often lacking. The tissues are randomly admixed one with another, showing little or no correlation with their normal anatomic relationships. The lesion is typically encapsulated and well demarcated from the surrounding normal tissues. There may or may not be a fibrovascular background stroma separating the different tissue types.

The keratin-filled *dermoid cyst* of the oral floor midline has abortive sebaceous glands, perhaps even hair follicles, in its walls. Many authorities consider this to be a teratoma, going so far as to call such a lesion a *teratoid cyst* and equating it with the *ovarian dermoid cyst.* It is best, however, to refer to such a lesion as a dermoid cyst since it contains elements from only two germ cell layers.

Malignant teratomas do occur, usually with only a single component demonstrating dysplastic changes. When a rhabdomyoblastic component is seen, a variety of heterologous or mixed tumors must be ruled out, and when multiple components appear malignant, terms such as *malignant mesenchymoma* and *malignant ectomesenchymoma* may be applied.[6]

Treatment and Prognosis. Treatment of a teratoma consists of conservative surgical removal, a procedure that often requires finesse and delicacy because of the close proximity to important anatomic structures of the head and neck region.[183, 187] With conservative removal, occasional recurrence is to be expected, especially when portions of the teratoma must be left in place to preserve normal anatomic structures. Careful and long-term follow-up is recommended. Malignant teratoma is treated according to its most prominent malignant component, usually by radical surgery, with or without radiotherapy. Rarely, a benign teratoma has been reported to transform into malignancy, especially carcinoma.[188]

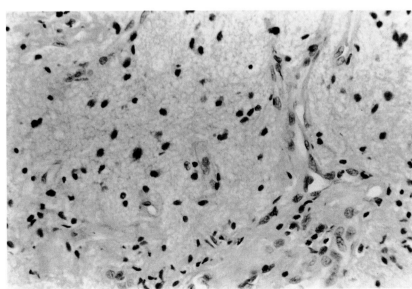

Figure 4–15. Oval and stellate astrocytes in the glial choristoma are scattered throughout a stroma of glial fibers. (Courtesy of Dr. Sidney Schochet, West Virginia University, Morgantown, West Virginia.)

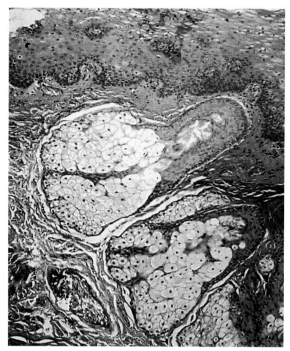

Figure 4–16. Fordyce granules are submucosal sebaceous glands with rudimentary excretory ducts or no visible ducts.

Fordyce Granules

Sebaceous glands are normal adnexal structures of the dermis but may also be found within the mouth, where they are referred to as *Fordyce granules* or *ectopic sebaceous glands.*[7, 9, 189–191] This variation of normal anatomy is seen in the majority of adults, perhaps as much as 80% of them, but seldom are granules found in large numbers. When seen as a streak of individual glands along the interface between the skin of the lip and the vermilion border, the terms *Fox-Fordyce disease* and *Fordyce's condition* have been used. Fordyce[192] first described this condition in 1896.

Clinical Features. Fordyce granules appear as rice-like, white or yellow-white, asymptomatic papules of 1 to 3 mm in greatest dimension.[190] There is no surrounding mucosal change and the granules remain constant throughout life. The most common sites of occurrence are the buccal mucosa (often bilateral), the upper lip vermilion, and the mandibular retromolar pad and tonsillar areas, but any oral surface may be involved. Some patients will have hundreds of granules while most have only one or two.

Occasionally, several adjacent glands will coalesce into a larger cauliflower-like cluster similar to *sebaceous hyperplasia* of the skin. In such an instance, it may be difficult to determine whether to diagnose the lesion as sebaceous hyperplasia or *sebaceous adenoma.*[193, 194] The distinction may be moot because both entities have the same treatment, although the adenoma has a greater growth potential. It should be mentioned that *sebaceous carcinoma* of the oral cavity has been reported, presumably arising from Fordyce granules or hyperplastic foci of sebaceous glands.[194, 195]

Pathologic Features and Differential Diagnosis. Fordyce granules are usually not biopsied because they are readily diagnosed clinically, but they are often seen as incidental findings of mucosal biopsies of the buccal, labial, and retromolar mucosa.[7, 9] The granules are similar to normal sebaceous glands of the skin but lack hair follicles and almost always lack a ductal communication with the surface (Fig. 4–16). The glands are located just beneath the overlying epithelium and often produce a local elevation of the epithelium. Individual sebaceous cells are large, with central dark nuclei and abundant foamy cytoplasm. The surrounding stroma may contain occasional chronic inflammatory cells because of trauma with adjacent teeth.

Large numbers of lobules coalescing into a definitely elevated mass may be called benign sebaceous hyperplasia, and occasional small keratin-filled *pseudocysts* may be seen and must be differentiated from *epidermoid cyst* or *dermoid cyst* with sebaceous adnexa. The pathologist must be careful to differentiate such lesions from salivary neoplasms with sebaceous cells, such as *sebaceous lymphadenoma* and *sebaceous adenoma,* and their malignant counterparts *sebaceous lymphadenocarcinoma* and *sebaceous carcinoma.*[193–195]

Treatment and Prognosis. No treatment is required for Fordyce granules, except for cosmetic removal of labial lesions.[191] Inflamed glands can be treated topically with clindamycin.[196] When surgically excised, there is no recurrence. Neoplastic transformation is very rare but has been reported.[197]

Juxtaoral Organ of Chievitz

The juxtaoral organ was first described by Chievitz[198] in 1885 and is considered to be a vestigial organ, perhaps of the developing parotid gland, or to be epithelium entrapped during the embryonic development of the interface between the maxillary and mandibular processes.[197–201] A neuroendocrine receptor function has been suggested. It is present in almost all individuals and is located bilaterally in buccotemporal fascia on the medial surface of the mandible, near the angle. Until recently, it was thought that the organ produces no visible or palpable mass; it was an occasional incidental finding in biopsied tissue samples from the region. A proliferative mass of the lingual aspect of the posterior mandible has, however, now been reported as the first example of a tumor of the juxtaoral organ.[197] A similar structure has been found within the anterior maxillary bone, but no embryonic explanation has been offered for its presence in that location.[201]

Pathologic Features. The juxtaoral organ is a multilobulated nest or aggregation of 2 to 10 discrete islands of moderately large, oval or angular cells with a distinct squamoid appearance but with no keratin formation and with few, if any, intercellular bridges (Fig. 4–17). Most islands also have smaller, darkly staining basaloid cells, usually aligned at the periphery, and a few show central epithelioid cells with clear cytoplasm. There is a definite glandular or organoid pattern. The background stroma is moderately dense fibrous tissue with no inflammatory infiltrate, no obvious encapsulation, and perhaps with extracellular melanin deposits.

Characteristically, there is a prominent PAS-positive basement membrane around the epithelial islands and there are numerous small, myelinated, often degenerated nerves admixed with the epithelial islands. Occasional epithelial islands will demonstrate focal areas of dystrophic calcification.

A word of caution is warranted. Because the organ of Chievitz is located so deep in the soft tissues, it may be mistakenly interpreted by the pathologist as well-differentiated *squamous cell carcinoma, mucoepidermoid carcinoma,* or metastatic deposits from a visceral organ.[201]

Treatment and Prognosis. Although the function of this structure is completely unknown, it is a very innocuous variation of normal anatomy and requires no treatment.[199] The single reported case of tumorous growth of the organ had no recurrence 8 months after conservative surgical removal.[197]

Benign Lymphoid Aggregate

Nodules of tonsillar tissue, usually called *benign lymphoid aggregates, lingual tonsils* (posterior lateral tongue), *oral tonsils,* or *oral tonsil tags,* are found in several oral and pharyngeal regions besides the tonsillar beds of the lateral pharynx.[7, 202, 203] This tissue, which corresponds to the adenoidal tissue of the nasopharynx, responds to infection and antigenic challenges, undergoing proliferation and appearing to become more numerous as very small, clinically invisible aggregates enlarge to a visible size.[204] *Lymphoid hyperplasia* is the state in which many of these variants of normal anatomy are biopsied. The prevalence of hyperplastic oral tonsils is 1 to 2 per 1000 adults.[1, 205]

It should be mentioned that 1 in 10 individuals have a small buccinator lymph node of the anterior buccal region below the occlusal plane. Some of these are located immediately beneath the mucosal epithelium and may enlarge to a size of 1 to 2 cm as a result of local trauma, dental infection, or upper respiratory infection. Histopathologic inflammatory changes are consistent with those found in cervical and other lymph nodes.

Clinical Features. Intraoral and pharyngeal lymphoid aggregates are more prominent in younger individuals, reaching their peak size during the adolescent and teenage years.[7, 9] Although they may become especially large in young people, the hyperplastic state may be seen in persons of any age.

Sites of occurrence, in decreasing order of frequency, are the posterior pharyngeal wall, the lateral posterior tongue, the soft palate, and the oral floor.[7, 203] During and for several days after an upper respiratory or other acute infection, benign lymphoid aggregates become enlarged, erythematous, and perhaps somewhat tender, but they do not reach a size greater than 0.8 cm except on the posterior lateral tongue, where reported cases have been 1.5 cm or greater in diameter. Without hyperplasia, the aggregates are 0.1 to 0.4 cm. in size and have a pale yellow, semitransparent appearance (Fig. 4–18A, see p. 169).[7]

Pathologic Features. The benign lymphoid aggregate is composed predominantly of well differentiated lymphocytes collected into a single aggregation, usually with one or more germinal centers containing reactive lymphoblasts, predominantly B-cell types (Fig. 4–18B, see p. 169). Mitotic figures are seen in the germinal centers, as are macrophages containing phagocytized "tingible bodies" of nuclear debris from the surrounding proliferating lymphocytes. Linear streaking, or "Indian filing," of lymphocytes may be seen at the periphery of the aggregate, and scattered lymphocytes are occasionally present in the surrounding fibrovascular stroma. There is no nodal encapsulation and vascular channels are minimally present, perhaps invisible without special staining.

The surface epithelium is often atrophic but occasional nodules of lymphoid aggregation show deep "tonsillar" clefts from the surface, perhaps filled with sloughed keratin. These clefts may crimp off at the surface, resulting in a keratin-filled *lymphoepithelial cyst,* or they may be considerably widened by the keratin build-up. In the latter case, the keratin may mushroom above the surface and become clinically visible as a tonsillar *keratin plug.*

The lymphoid cells of a lymphoid aggregate must be carefully evaluated to differentiate it from extranodal *lymphoma* and to determine whether the aggregate is hyperplastic. Microscopic criteria for hyperplasia and lymphoma are the same as those used for other lymphoid tissues of the body. Differentiation from a simple chronic inflammatory cell infiltrate is usually not difficult because the inflammatory infiltrate is much less abruptly demarcated from surrounding stroma, has many more lymphocytes in the surrounding stroma, has a greater admixture of inflammatory cell types, and lacks germinal centers.

It should be mentioned that certain very chronic inflammatory or immune-related conditions, such as *lichen planus* or *lupus erythematosus,* may demonstrate small lymphoid aggregates deep in the submucosal tissues. These never produce surface nodules.

Treatment and Prognosis. The benign lymphoid aggregate requires no treatment but may have to be excisionally biopsied to provide an appropriate diagnosis and to rule out lymphoid or other malignancy.[7, 206, 207]

Lingual Thyroid

Late in the first month of life, the anlage of the thyroid gland descends from the posterior dorsal midline of the tongue (actually the floor of the pharyngeal gut) to its final position in the lower neck. The initial site of descent eventually becomes the foramen caecum, located in the midline at the junction of the anterior (oral) tongue and the tongue base. If the embryonic gland does not descend normally, ectopic or residual thyroid tissue (technically either a *choristoma* or *hamartoma*) may be found between the foramen caecum and the epiglottis.

Of all ectopic thyroids, 90% are found on the lingual dorsum, where they are called *lingual thyroid* or *ectopic lingual thyroid.*[7, 9, 208–210] Rarely, parathyroid glands are associated with the ectopic thyroid tissue. Other sites of ectopic thyroid deposition include the cervical lymph nodes, submandibular glands, and the trachea. Approximately two thirds of patients with lingual thyroid lack thyroid tissue in the neck.[208]

Clinical Features. The lingual thyroid is four times more common in females than in males. It presents as an asymptomatic nodular mass of the posterior lingual midline, usually less than a centimeter in size but sometimes reaching more than 4 cm (Fig. 4–19A, see p. 170).[208] Larger lesions can interfere with swallowing and breathing, but most patients are unaware of the mass at the time of diagnosis, which is usually in the teenage or young adult years.

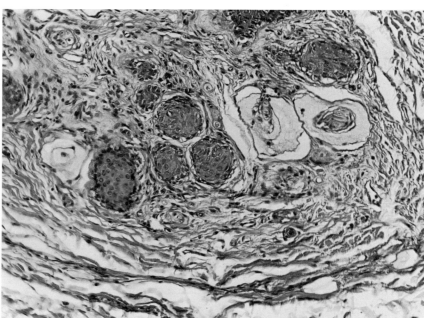

Figure 4–17. The juxtaoral organ of Chievitz consists of multilobulated nests of squamoid cells with mild polarization of peripheral basaloid cells. (From Danforth RA, Baughman RA: Chievitz's organ: A potential pitfall in oral cancer diagnosis. Oral Surg Oral Med Oral Pathol 1979;48:231.)

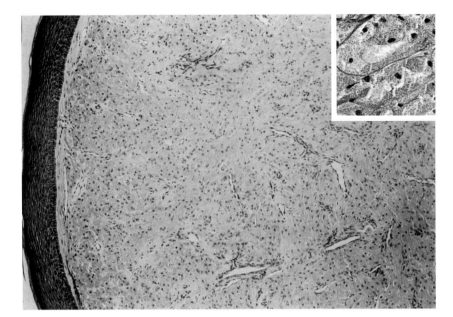

Figure 4–20. The congenital epulis is composed almost entirely of histiocyte-like granular cells; the overlying epithelium is always atrophic, with a general loss of rete ridges. High power view of the lesional cells (*inset*) shows granular cytoplasm and acentrically located, small, dark nuclei.

Up to 70% of patients with lingual thyroid have *hypothyroidism* and 10% suffer from *cretinism*.[7, 209]

Pathologic Features. The lingual thyroid consists of a nonencapsulated collection of embryonic or mature thyroid follicles which may extend between muscle bundles, raising suspicions of malignant invasion. The follicular cells, however, are normal or atrophic in appearance (Fig. 4–19B, see p. 170). All diseases capable of affecting the normal thyroid gland can, of course, affect the glandular tissue entrapped in the tongue. *Thyroid adenoma, goiter, hyperplasia, inflammation,* and *carcinoma* occur in lingual thyroids and must, therefore, be evaluated in the same fashion as would any biopsied thyroid gland.[211] Parathyroid tissue may be seen but has not been neoplastic in reported cases.

Treatment and Prognosis. Surgical excision or radioiodine therapy are effective treatments for lingual thyroid, but no treatment should be attempted until an iodine-131 radioisotope scan has determined that there is adequate thyroid tissue in the neck.[209, 210] In those patients lacking thyroid tissue in the neck, the lingual thyroid can be excised and autotransplanted to the muscles of the neck. Most cases require no treatment and biopsy should be considered with caution because of the potential for hemorrhage, infection, or release of large amounts of hormone into the vascular system (thyroid storm). Occasional patients with parathyroid tissue associated with their lingual thyroid have developed tetany after the inadvertent removal of this tissue.

Rare examples of *thyroid carcinoma* arising in the mass have been reported, almost always in males, but an enlarged lingual thyroid is more likely to reflect a normal compensatory response to thyroid hypofunction.[211] Endocrine evaluation for *hypothyroidism* should, therefore, be done in such cases. In this light, it is important to know that three of every four patients with *infantile hypothyroidism* have ectopic thyroid tissue.

Congenital (Granular Cell) Epulis

The *congenital epulis (congenital granular cell myoblastoma, granular cell epulis of infancy, granular cell fibroblastoma)* is a unique and rare congenital tumor of the alveolar mucosa of the jaws.[6–9, 212–217] The exact nature of this entity is not clear. Once thought to be a form of odontogenic dysgenesis, it is now thought to originate from primitive mesenchymal cells of neural crest origin, although the evidence for this is less than conclusive.[214–216] This gingival growth was first described by Neumann[218] in 1871.

Clinical Features. The congenital epulis is almost exclusively found on the anterior alveolar ridges of newborns, although a few cases have reportedly developed shortly after birth.[212, 213, 219] Approximately 90% of cases occur in girls and 10% present with multiple lesions.[212] It presents as a 0.5 to 2.0 cm soft, pedunculated, and perhaps lobulated nodule of the alveolar mucosa, especially the mucosa of the maxilla. A few lesions have been as much as 9 cm in size at birth and several cases have had involvement of both jaws. The earliest reported case was identified by ultrasonography in a 31-week fetus.[219] There is no tenderness or surface change and the lesion does not increase in size after birth. In fact, many of the smaller examples will spontaneously regress after birth.

Pathologic Features and Differential Diagnosis. The mucosal mass is composed almost entirely of large, rounded and polyhedral, histiocyte-like cells with small, dark oval nuclei and abundant eosinophilic granular cytoplasm (Fig. 4–20). Lesional cells are usually rounded but may be somewhat spindled. There are vascular channels between granular cells, but fibrous stroma is minimally present and often appears to be completely lacking. The tumor cells extend to the overlying epithelium, which is atrophic and never demonstrates the *pseudoepitheliomatous hyperplasia* so commonly seen in the *granular cell tumor* of adults.

Lesional cells do not immunoreact for laminin or S-100 protein, as do the granular cells of the granular cell tumor.[217] They are also negative for Leu7, NSE, and other neural markers, and reactive only toward vimentin.[10] These cells also are strongly positive for acid phosphatase. There is no other congenital alveolar mucosal lesion that is similar to the congenital epulis, but oral involvement by *Langerhans cell disease* might have enough tissue histiocytes to somewhat mimic the epulis. Occasional odontogenic tumors contain abundant granular cells, but these are almost never congenital and seldom located outside the bone. Conversely, 30% to 50% of cases show odontogenic epithelial rests among the granular cells.

The granular cell tumor (myoblastoma) has cells that are histopathologically identical to those of the granular cell epulis, but the early onset, unique location, and pedunculated appearance make the epulis easily differentiated from the tumor. The tumor, moreover, is not encapsulated and infiltrates into underlying tissues, and many of the lesional cells have a spindled appearance, especially at the deep margin of the tumor. Similar granular cells are found in the connective tissue papillae of *verruciform xanthoma,* but the association of this lesion with overlying papillomatosis and the older age at onset make it easily distinguished from granular cell epulis.

Text continued on page 181

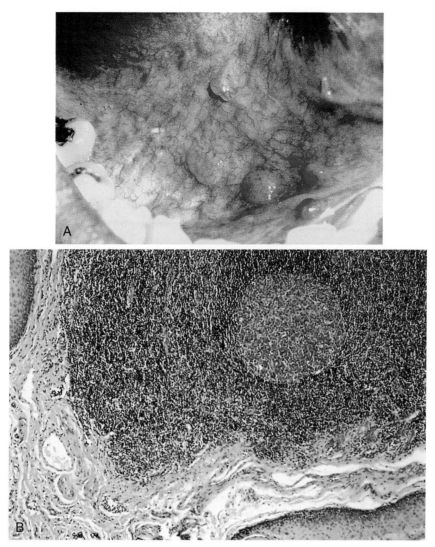

Figure 4–18. *A,* "Oral tonsils" or benign lymphoid aggregates are often multiple and present as slightly yellowish almost translucent nodules here of the oral floor. *B,* The deep margin of one nodule shows tightly aggregated, mature lymphoid cells with one germinal center.

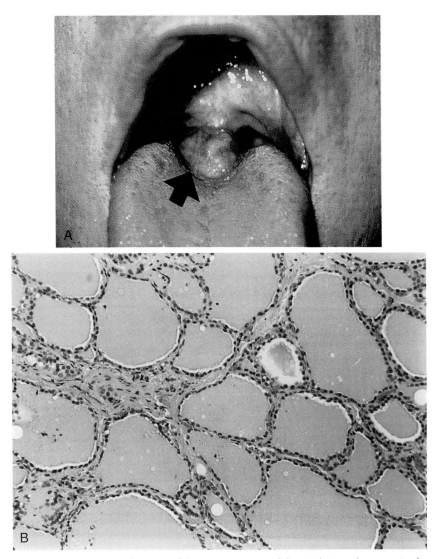

Figure 4–19. *A*, The lingual thyroid presents as a midline mass of the posterior tongue; *B*, biopsied tissue shows routine features of the thyroid gland.

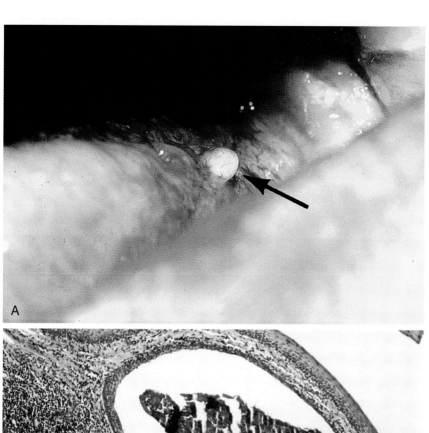

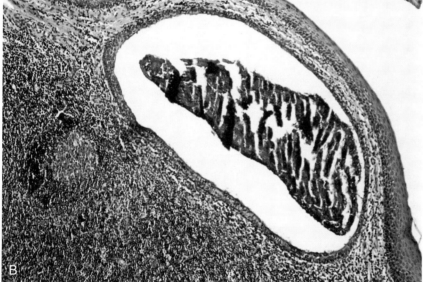

Figure 4–22. *A,* Oral lymphoepithelial cyst usually presents as a small, sessile, yellow-white, submucosal mass; *B,* the submucosal cyst is filled with sloughed keratin, has a thin epithelial lining, and is adjacent to or surrounded by a benign lymphoid aggregate.

Figure 4–23. The traumatic angiomatous lesion presents as a focal dilation of a vein, often with a partially organized thrombus.

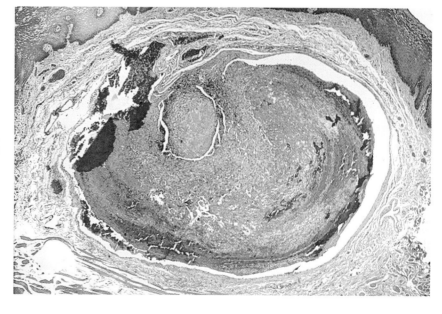

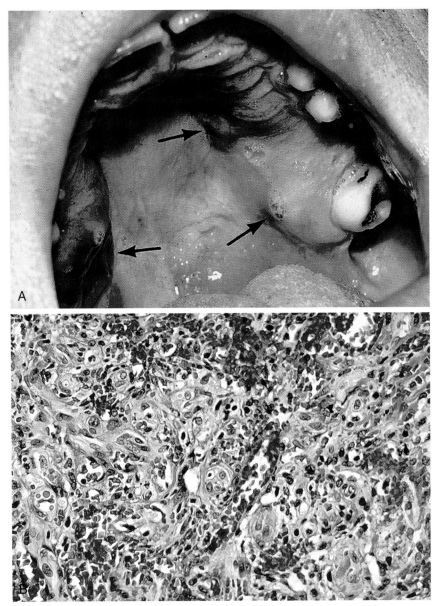

Figure 4–26. *A*, Oral Kaposi's sarcoma may present as either flattened or sessile nodules, usually with a red or purplish discoloration. *B*, Vascular channels are lined by atypical endothelial cells and the background stroma shows erythrocyte extravasation with pleomorphic spindled and rounded lesional cells.

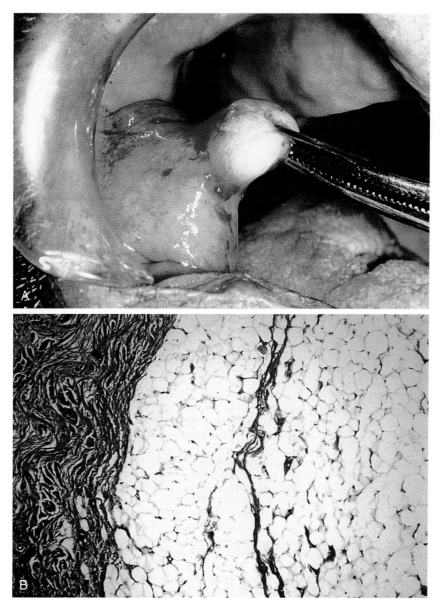

Figure 4–28. *A,* The lipoma presents as a smooth-surfaced sessile mass with yellow/white discoloration; *B,* mature adipocytes are admixed with fibrous streaks, and oral lesions also may show scattered chronic inflammatory cells from recurring trauma to the lesion.

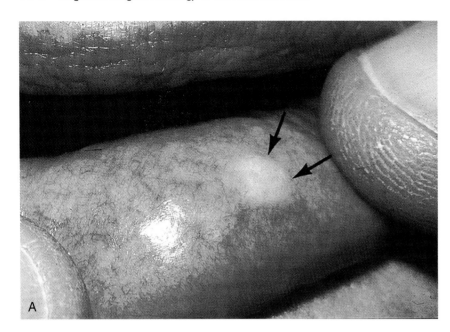

Figure 4–31. *A,* The granular cell tumor typically presents as a slightly elevated, smooth-surfaced area of pallor.

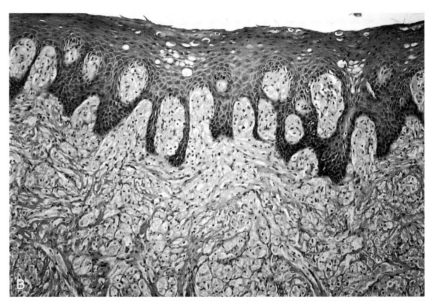

Figure 4–31 *Continued. B,* histiocyte-like lesional cells with small, acentrically located nuclei are diffusely infiltrated between fibrous stroma and muscle fibers, extending to the surface epithelium; *C,* higher power view of lesional cells shows obvious granular cytoplasm.

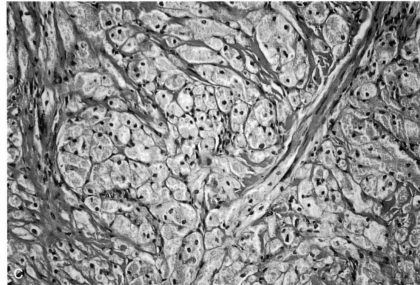

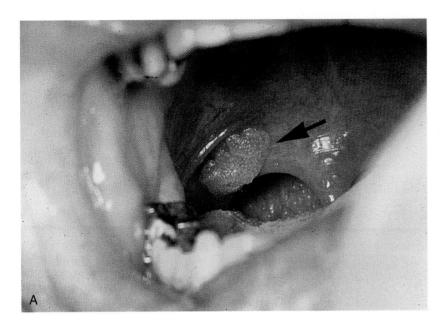

Figure 4–34. *A,* Unlike the papilloma, the condyloma is broad-based with blunted surface projections and minimal surface keratinization.

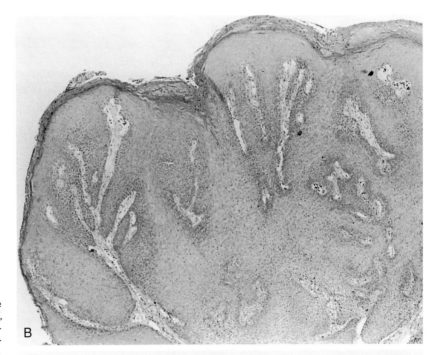

Figure 4–34 *Continued. B,* low-power view shows the more blunted surface configuration of the condyloma; *C,* higher power view shows broad, short surface projections with acanthotic rete pegs and occasional koilocytes with pyknotic nuclei surrounded by clear spaces.

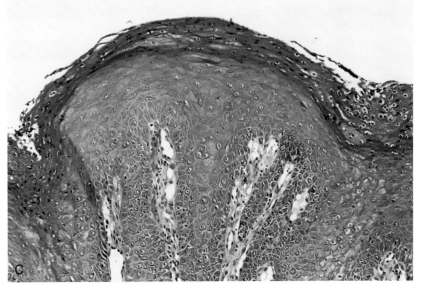

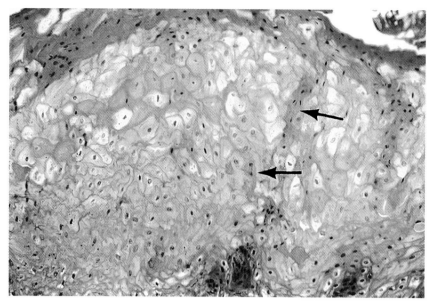

Figure 4–43. Vertical keratin streaks *(arrows)* and individually keratinized cells deep in the epithelium are features that distinguish hereditary benign intraepithelial dyskeratosis from other acanthotic mucosal entities with hyperkeratosis and abundant intracellular edema of the spindle cell layer.

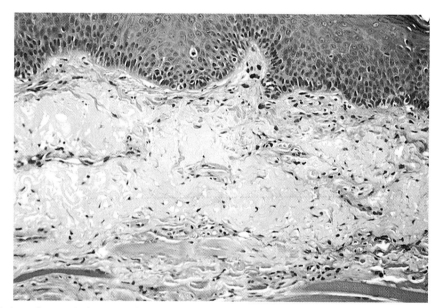

Figure 4–44. *A,* The epithelium of actinic cheilosis is usually atrophic, with scattered chronic inflammatory cells associated with the subepithelial streaking of solar elastosis, which here extends as deep as the underlying muscle of the lip.

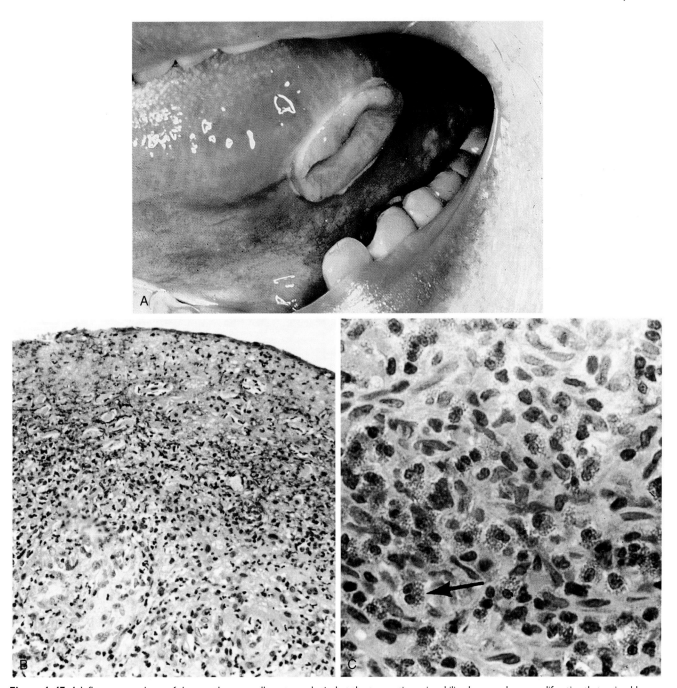

Figure 4–47. *A,* Inflammatory ulcers of the mouth are usually not exophytic, but the traumatic eosinophilic ulcer may be so proliferative that a sizeable mass is formed, usually with a central cupped-out area, as seen here. *B,* The ulcer bed is fibrinoid necrotic debris overlying granulation tissue with scattered inflammatory cells. *C,* Eosinophils within the granulation tissue of the ulcer bed are the key to diagnosis of traumatic eosinophilic ulcer.

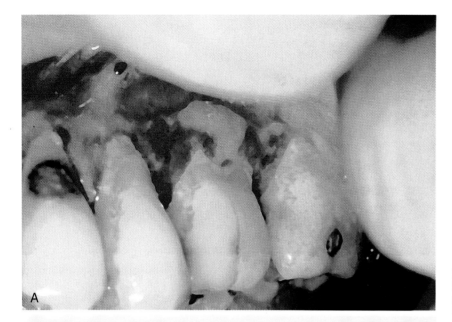

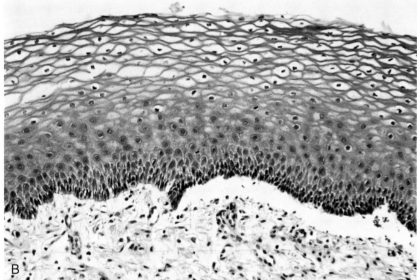

Figure 4–49. *A,* The bullae of benign mucous membrane pemphigoid are usually broken at the time of examination; they may remain confined to the alveolar mucosa. *B,* The blister forms by the pulling away of the entire epithelium from the basement membrane, with very few inflammatory cells in underlying stroma, as would be seen in bullous lichen planus.

Figure 4–50. The heavy metals of an amalgam tattoo present as small brown-black particles scattered throughout this subepithelial stroma, often coating reticulin fibers and blood vessels.

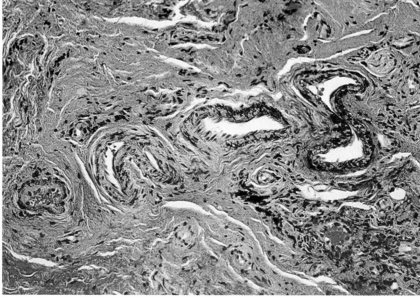

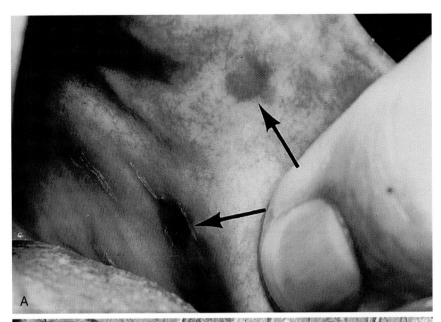

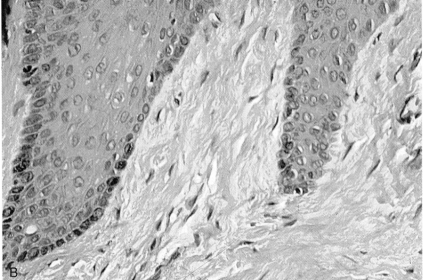

Figure 4–51. A, Oral melanotic macules *(arrows)* are flat, brownish, well-demarcated discolorations of the mucosa. B, Melanin in the oral melanotic macule is present primarily in the basal cell layer but it is not unusual for pigment incontinence to occur in the macule, with extracellular melanin and melanophages seen within subjacent stroma.

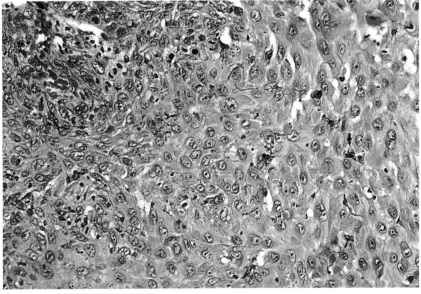

Figure 4–52. The epithelium of the melanoacanthoma is very bland but shows brown dendritic streaks between keratinocytes throughout all layers.

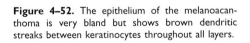

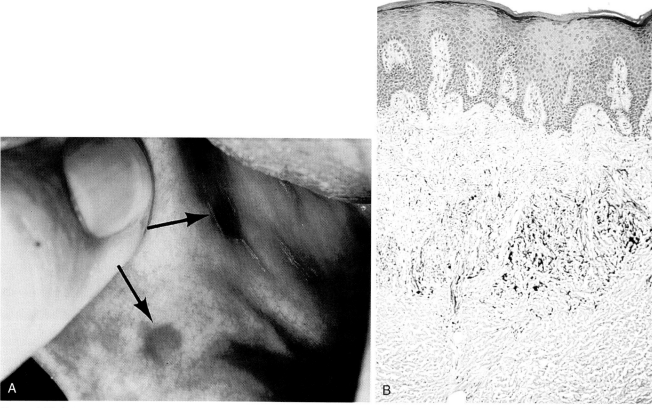

Figure 4–53. *A,* A blue nevus of the hard palate demonstrates the characteristically well-demarcated blue discoloration. (Courtesy of Dr. Sadru Kabani, Boston University, Boston, Massachusetts.) *B,* Thin, spindling, branching melanocytes of the blue nevus are located deep in the submucosal stroma.

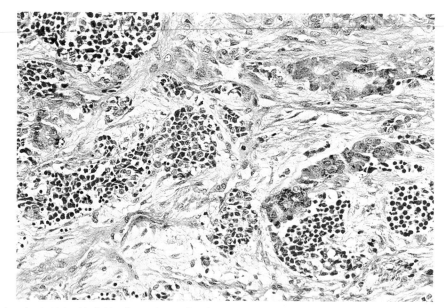

Figure 4–54. Pigment-ladened cuboidal epithelioid cells are clustered in the neuroectodermal tumor of infancy, while a second type of lesional cell consists of a small, dark, round cell with a hyperchromatic nucleus and minimal cytoplasm.

Treatment and Prognosis. Prior to birth, the congenital epulis enlarges at a rate similar to that of the growing fetus, but after birth the mass tends to spontaneously regress and disappear over the first 8 months of life.[7, 9, 212] Residual remnants do not interfere with tooth eruption. There is, therefore, no need to treat a small congenital lesion. A larger lesion may interfere with eating or drinking, requiring conservative excision as soon as the child is large enough to safely undergo surgery. There is no tendency for recurrence and malignant transformation has not been reported.

Median Rhomboid Glossitis

The embryonic tongue is formed by two lateral processes (lingual tubercles) meeting in the midline and fusing above a central structure from the first and second branchial arches, the tuberculum impar. The posterior dorsal point of fusion is occasionally defective, leaving a rhomboid-shaped, smooth erythematous mucosa lacking in papillae or taste buds. This *median rhomboid glossitis (central papillary atrophy, posterior lingual papillary atrophy)* is a focal area of susceptibility to recurring or chronic atrophic candidiasis, prompting a recent movement toward the use of *posterior midline atrophic candidiasis* as a more appropriate diagnostic term.[7, 9, 220–222]

The latter term has certain difficulties, however, because not all cases improve with antifungal therapy or show initial evidence of fungal infection. The erythematous clinical appearance, moreover, is due primarily to the absence of filiform papillae, rather than to local inflammatory changes, as first suggested in 1914 by Brocq and Pautrier.[223] The lesion is found in 1 of every 300 to 2000 adults, depending on the rigor of the clinical examinations.[1–3, 224] It is seldom biopsied unless the red discoloration is confused with precancerous *erythroplakia* or its surface shows pronounced nodularity.

Clinical Features. Median rhomboid glossitis presents in the posterior midline of the dorsum of the tongue, just anterior to the V-shaped grouping of the circumvallate papillae.[7, 220] The long axis of the rhomboid or oval area of red depapillation is in the anterior-posterior direction. Most cases are not diagnosed until the middle age of the affected patient, but the entity is, of course, present in childhood. There appears to be a 3 : 1 male predilection.[224]

Those lesions with *atrophic candidiasis* are usually more erythematous but some respond with excess keratin production and, therefore, show a white surface change. Infected cases may also demonstrate midline soft palate erythema in the area of routine contact with the underlying tongue involvement; this is euphemistically referred to as a *kissing lesion.*[222]

Lesions are typically less than 2 cm in greatest dimension and most demonstrate a smooth, flat surface, although it is not unusual for the surface to be lobulated. Occasional lesions have surface mamillations raised more than 5 mm above the tongue surface, and occasional lesions are located somewhat anterior to the usual location. None have been reported posterior to the circumvallate papillae.

Prior to biopsy, the clinician should be certain that the midline lesion does not represent a *lingual thyroid,* as it may be the only thyroid tissue present in the patient's body. Additional clinical look-alike lesions include the gumma of tertiary *syphilis,* the granuloma of *tuberculosis, deep fungal infections,* and *granular cell tumor.*

Pathologic Features. Median rhomboid glossitis shows a smooth or nodular surface covered by atrophic stratified squamous epithelium overlying a moderately fibrosed stroma with somewhat dilated capillaries. Fungiform and filiform papillae are not seen, although surface nodules may mimic or perhaps represent anlage of these structures. A mild to moderately intense chronic inflammatory cell infiltrate may be seen within subepithelial and deeper fibrovascular tissues.

Chronic candida infection may result in excess surface keratin or extreme elongation of rete processes and premature keratin production within individual cells or as epithelial pearls (dyskeratosis) deep in the processes.[7, 221] Silver staining for fungus will often reveal candida hyphae and spores in the superficial layers of

the epithelium. This *pseudoepitheliomatous hyperplasia* may be quite pronounced, and the tangential cutting of such a specimen may result in the artifactual appearance of cut rete processes as unconnected islands of squamous epithelium, leading to a mistaken diagnosis of well differentiated *squamous cell carcinoma.* Because of this difficulty, it is recommended that the patient be treated with topical antifungals prior to biopsy of a suspected median rhomboid glossitis.

Treatment and Prognosis. No treatment is necessary for median rhomboid glossitis, but nodular cases are often removed for microscopic evaluation.[7, 9, 220] Recurrence after removal is not expected, although those cases with pseudoepitheliomatous hyperplasia should be followed closely for at least a year after biopsy to be certain of the benign diagnosis. Antifungal therapy (topical troches or systemic medication) will reduce clinical erythema and inflammation due to candida infection. This therapy, as stated earlier, should ideally be given prior to the biopsy, to reduce the candida-induced pseudoepitheliomatous hyperplasia features. Some lesions will disappear entirely with antifungal therapy.[221]

▌ SOFT TISSUE CYSTS

Epithelium-lined cystic spaces are occasionally found beneath the oral and pharyngeal mucosa. These may have their origins in the embryonic development of teeth *(odontogenic cysts),* in epithelial remnants left over from maxillofacial embryogenesis and development *(nonodontogenic cysts, fissural cysts, ductal cysts),* or in viable epithelial fragments traumatically embedded beneath the oral mucosa *(inclusion cysts, entrapment cysts).* Such cysts usually have a very limited growth potential, with slow enlargement presumably generated by the slightly elevated hydrostatic pressures within the cystic lumina. Taken as a group, oral soft tissue cysts are found in at least 1 of every 2000 adults.[1–3]

Several soft tissue cysts are discussed elsewhere in this text. The *true salivary retention cyst,* for example, is an epithelium-lined cyst arising from a plugged salivary gland duct; it is discussed with salivary diseases. The *eruption cyst,* discussed with odontogenic lesions, occurs on the crest of the alveolar process and is actually a *dentigerous cyst* associated with an underlying erupting tooth. In this instance the cortical bone separating the dentigerous cyst from the surface mucosa has been resorbed and only a thin layer of fibrovascular stroma separates the cyst epithelium from the surface epithelium. Also, a small proportion of *nasopalatine duct cysts* arise at the oral orifice of the incisive canal, presenting as soft tissue cysts. When this occurs, the cyst is traditionally referred to as a *cyst of the incisive papilla;* it is discussed with other bone cysts elsewhere in this text.

There are also *pseudocysts* of the oral and pharyngeal soft tissues. By traditional definition, these lack an epithelial lining. The *mucocele* is one such lesion, consisting of a submucosal pool of extravasated mucus from a ruptured minor salivary gland. This entity is much more common than true soft tissue cysts of the mouth and throat, with 1 case diagnosed in every 200 to 300 adults.[1] The mucocele and its sublingual gland counterpart, the *ranula,* are discussed with other salivary diseases elsewhere in this text. A second type of pseudocyst is an artifact, produced by tangential cutting of a deep surface indentation during laboratory processing. It is mentioned throughout the text when appropriate.

Epidermoid and Dermoid Cyst

The *epidermoid cyst,* often mistakenly called a *sebaceous cyst* or *wen,* is a very common skin lesion that arises from traumatic entrapment of surface epithelium *(epidermal inclusion cyst)* or, more often, from aberrant healing of the infundibular epithelium during an episode of follicular inflammation or *folliculitis.*[8] Oral and pharyngeal epidermoid cysts of the inclusion cyst variety also occur, but are rare in adults and are frequently so small that they are not biopsied.[7, 9, 225] Syndromes associated with multiple cutaneous epidermoid cysts, such as *Gardner syndrome, Gorlin syndrome,* and *pachyonychia congenita,* do not demonstrate cysts of the oral mucosa, but facial cysts may occur.[5]

The epidermoid cyst of the oral floor midline has a much greater growth potential than epidermoid cysts occurring at other oral/pharyngeal sites. These large cysts are often given the label *dermoid cyst* by authorities who believe it to be a *forme fruste* of benign, *cystic teratoma.*[7, 225–231] Since its first description in 1852 as a *sublingual cyst* or *wen,*[232] the distinction between the oral floor epidermoid and dermoid cyst has been rather confused. As it is likely that most examples represent cystic degeneration of embryonically entrapped epidermis, and as the microscopic features of this cyst are almost always identical to those of the epidermoid cyst of the skin or other oral locations, we suggest that the use of the term *dermoid cyst* be reserved only for those cysts with epidermal adnexa beneath the lining epithelium. *Congenital teratoid cyst* contains elements derived from all three germ layers, ectoderm, mesoderm, and entoderm.[229–231]

Clinical Features. The epidermoid cyst of the oral and pharyngeal mucosa is usually located on the attached gingiva, where it has traditionally been called *gingival cyst of adult.*[7, 233–235] At this site, the lesion is presumably secondary to cystic degeneration of odontogenic embryonic rests or traumatic inclusions of surface epithelium. Other common locations are the lateral tongue, oral floor, lateral pharyngeal wall, and soft palate. Most cases are diagnosed during the teen or young adult years.

The epidermoid cyst typically remains less than 1 cm in diameter and may be somewhat movable beneath the surface, except on bone-bound mucosa.[7, 234] The cyst is almost always superficial, producing a sessile nodule with a white or yellow-white discoloration (Fig. 4–21*A*); the occasional deeper lesions may show a normal color. The larger "dermoid cyst" is usually found in the oral floor midline above the mylohyoid muscle, although the occasional dumbbell-shaped cyst will penetrate through a hiatus in the muscle and extend into the submental area, possibly imparting a double chin appearance.[229–234] In this location, the cyst may reach 6 to 7 cm in greatest diameter, may become infected, and may interfere with swallowing or the proper function of the tongue.

Pathologic Features. The epidermoid cyst is lined by a thin stratified squamous epithelium with few rete processes (Fig. 4–21*B*). Quite often, there is no granular cell layer and keratin from the surface of the epithelium can be seen to be sloughing into the cystic lumen, which is usually filled with degenerated and necrotic keratinaceous detritus. Areas of epithelial degeneration or ulceration may be seen, usually associated with a mild to moderately intense chronic inflammatory cell reaction. Inflammation may extend deeply into subepithelial fibrovascular stroma. Occasional cysts have contained fungi, bacteria, or necrotic food debris in their lumina, and darkly hematoxylophilic precipitated salts (dystrophic calcification) may be seen within the necrosed keratin.

When keratin degenerates within an ulcer bed of the cyst wall, cholesterol crystals form elongated, sharp-ended clefts (cholesterol clefts), which are clear spaces in stained tissue sections because of the dissolution of the associated fats by laboratory processing. Foreign-body multinucleated giant cells are frequently seen adjacent to or surrounding such clefts. This *cholesterol granuloma* will occasionally proliferate into the lumen of the cyst from an area of ulceration.

The dermoid cyst differs from epidermoid cyst only in the presence within its walls of normal or dysmorphic adnexal appendages, usually sebaceous glands or abortive hair follicles (Fig. 4–21*C*). If the cyst wall contains other elements, such as muscle (other than pilar arrector smooth muscle) or bone, the term *teratoid cyst* is preferred.

Treatment and Prognosis. Treatment consists of conservative surgical removal, trying not to rupture the cyst, as the luminal contents may act as irritants to fibrovascular tissues, producing postoperative inflammation.[7, 9, 230] Recurrence is unlikely after treatment. Malignant transformation of oral cysts has not been reported.

Palatal and Gingival Cysts of the Newborn

A special form of odontogenic cyst is found in as many as 80% of newborn infants.[7, 9, 236] Although this *gingival cyst of the newborn* has the microscopic appearance of an *epidermoid cyst,* it arises from epithelial remnants of the deeply budding dental lamina during tooth development, after the fourth month in utero, and is, therefore, discussed with the odontogenic lesions in this text (Chapter 9).[237] A similar *palatal cyst of the newborn* is commonly found in the posterior midline of the hard palate, where it arises from epithelial remnants remaining in the stroma after fusion of the palatal processes, which meet medially to form the palate.[7, 238–240] As originally described, the cysts along the median raphe of the palate were called *Epstein's pearls* and the term *Bohn's nodules* was used for cysts that originated from palatal gland structures and were scattered more widely over the hard and soft palates.[238] Today these two terms are used interchangeably for both palatal and gingival cysts of newborns.

Clinical Features. Palatal cysts of the newborn typically present as multiple (usually less than six) 1 to 4 mm yellow-white, sessile mucosal papules of the posterior hard palate, and occasionally of the anterior soft palate.[238–240] Occasional cysts are located some distance from the midline. The cysts are usually somewhat larger and less numerous than the gingival cysts of the alveolar processes in newborns, but the two entities are otherwise clinically identical. Both types of cyst are so superficial that several may be ruptured at the time of examination.

Pathologic Features. Both gingival and palatal cysts of the newborn show a thin stratified squamous epithelium cyst lining with a routine fibrovascular connective tissue stroma, usually without an inflammatory cell infiltrate. The cystic lumen is filled with degenerated keratin, usually formed into concentric layers or "onion rings," and the epithelium lacks rete processes. Occasional cysts will demonstrate a communication with the surface.

Treatment and Prognosis. No treatment is required for gingival or palatal cysts of the newborn.[7, 239] The cysts are very superficial and within weeks will rupture to harmlessly spill their contents into the oral or pharyngeal environment. The cyst lining then fuses with the overlying mucosa and becomes part of it. Occasionally, a larger cyst or a cyst situated more deeply in the submucosal stroma will remain for 6 to 8 months before rupturing.[7]

Nasolabial Cyst

The *nasolabial cyst (nasoalveolar cyst, Klestadt's cyst)* is now considered to originate from remnants of the embryonic nasolacrimal duct or the lower anterior portion of the mature duct, although a popular past theory presumed it to arise from epithelial rests remaining from the "fusion" of the globular process with the lateral nasal process and the maxillary process.[7, 241–243] Zuckerkandl[244] may have been the first to describe this cyst, and at least 200 examples have thus far been reported, including one family with a father and daughter having similar involvement.

Clinical Features. The nasolabial cyst has a strong female predilection (75% occur in women) and appears to occur more frequently in blacks than in whites.[241–243] It is found near the base of the nostril, just above the periosteum, or in the superior aspect of the upper lip, and is bilateral in approximately 10% of all cases. The cyst usually obliterates the nasolabial fold and may elevate the ala of the nose on the affected side. It also obliterates the maxillary vestibule and frequently extends into the floor of the nasal vestibule, occasionally causing nasal obstruction or pressure erosion of the bone of the nasal floor. When located in the lip, there almost always is a fibrous or epithelial attachment to the nasal mucosa.

Most examples are less than 1.5 cm in greatest diameter, but some have reached much larger sizes.[243, 245] Injection of a radiopaque dye into the lumen will help define the cyst outline, which may be somewhat irregular, even bilobed. It is not unusual for this cyst to be secondarily inflamed and somewhat tender to palpation. Occasional cysts rupture or drain into the oral cavity or nose.

Pathologic Features. The nasolabial cyst is lined by respiratory epithelium, stratified squamous epithelium, pseudostratified columnar epithelium or a combination of these. Mucus-filled goblet cells may be scattered within the epithelium and chronic inflammatory cells may be seen in the surrounding fibrovascular stroma.

Treatment and Prognosis. This cyst is treated by conservative surgical excision, usually using access from the anterior maxillary vestibule.[241–243] The surgical procedure may have to be extended

deeply into the nasal sinus and it is sometimes necessary to remove part of the nasal mucosa to remove the entire cyst.

Lymphoepithelial Cyst

The *oral lymphoepithelial cyst* develops within a *benign lymphoid aggregate* or *accessory tonsil* of the oral or pharyngeal mucosa.[7, 9, 246, 247] The surface of such aggregates may be indented with tonsillar crypts, as are the much larger pharyngeal tonsils of the lat-

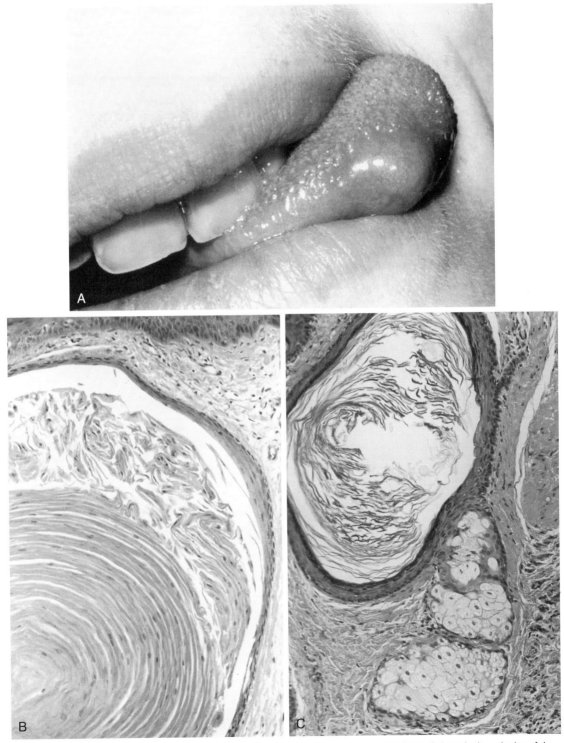

Figure 4–21. *A,* Epidermoid cyst presents as a sessile, yellowish, smooth-surfaced, submucosal mass, here located along the lateral edge of the tongue. *B,* The cyst is filled with sloughed keratin and is lined by a thin stratified squamous epithelium with few rete ridges. *C,* Adnexa in the cyst wall alters the diagnosis to dermoid cyst.

eral pharyngeal walls. The crypts may become obstructed by keratin or other debris, or the surface opening may become constricted during episodes of inflammatory hyperplastic responses. Certain cases develop a complete disunion of the crypt epithelium from the surface epithelium, resulting in a subepithelial cyst lined by the old crypt epithelium. This cyst was first reported by Parmentier[232] in 1857 as *hydatid cyst.* Outside of the head and neck region, lymphoepithelial cyst is found most frequently in the pancreas and testis.[248]

A similar but much larger *cervical lymphoepithelial cyst (branchial cleft cyst)* most probably develops from entrapped salivary duct epithelium in the lymph nodes of the lateral neck, rather than from the branchial cleft.[7, 249, 250] These are discussed in a separate chapter of this text (Chapter 10). Another similar cyst, the *parotid cyst,* is found in major salivary glands, especially in AIDS patients, although it often lacks a surrounding lymphoid aggregate.[251, 252] This cyst is also discussed elsewhere in this text (Chapter 6).

Clinical Features. Oral lymphoepithelial cyst presents as a movable, painless submucosal nodule with a yellow or yellow-white discoloration (Fig. 4–22*A,* see p. 171). Occasional cysts are transparent. Almost all cases are less than 0.6 cm in diameter at the time of diagnosis, which is usually during the teen years or the third decade of life.[7, 246, 247] Approximately half of all intraoral examples are found on the oral floor, but the lateral and ventral tongue are not uncommon sites of occurrence, nor is the soft palate, especially the mucosa above the pharyngeal tonsil. Of course, this cyst may also occur within the pharyngeal tonsils themselves. Occasional superficial cysts rupture to release a foul-tasting, cheesy, keratinaceous material.

This cyst has a clinical appearance similar to that of an *epidermoid cyst* or a *dermoid cyst* of the oral and pharyngeal mucosa, but its growth potential is much less than that of the other cysts. The lymphoepithelial cyst never occurs on the alveolar mucosa, so it can easily be distinguished from a *gingival cyst of adults* or from an unruptured *parulis* or "pus pocket" at the terminus of a fistula (extending from the apical or lateral region of an abscessed tooth).

Pathologic Features and Differential Diagnosis. The lymphoepithelial cyst is lined by atrophic and often degenerated stratified squamous epithelium, usually lacking in rete processes and usually demonstrating a minimal granular cell layer (Fig. 4–22*B,* see p. 171). Orthokeratin is seen to be sloughing from the epithelial surface into the cystic lumen, often completely filling the lumen and sometimes showing dystrophic calcification. Rarely, mucus-filled goblet cells may be seen within the superficial layers of the epithelium, and occasional cysts will demonstrate an epithelium-lined communication with the overlying mucosal surface. The cyst is entrapped within a well-demarcated aggregate of mature lymphocytes. The aggregate or "tonsil" will have a variable number of germinal centers, sometimes none at all. The lymphoid aggregate may be hyperplastic.

This combination of epithelium-lined cyst with lymphoid aggregates is unique enough to make the diagnosis an easy one, but the pathologist must differentiate this lesion from the *Warthin tumor (papillary cystadenoma lymphomatosum).*[253] The latter lesion is lined not by squamous epithelium but by a bilayered cuboidal, columnar, or oncocytic ductal epithelium. It is almost always found in the parotid gland, but rare oral examples have been reported.

Occasional cysts have very small lumina with degenerated epithelial linings and may mimic metastatic deposits of well-differentiated *squamous cell carcinoma.* Deeper sections will reveal the true nature of the benign lesion.

Treatment and Prognosis. No treatment is usually necessary for the oral lymphoepithelial cyst unless its location is such that it is constantly being traumatized.[7, 246, 247] Most lesions are, however, removed by conservative surgical excision to arrive at a definitive diagnosis. There is no malignant potential to this lesion but the lymphoid stroma, as with all lymphoid tissues, can become involved with an extranodal *lymphoma.*[7]

Thyroglossal Duct Cyst

The anlage of the median lobe of the thyroid gland arises in the foramen caecum area of the posterior dorsal tongue, at the junction between the anterior one third and the posterior two thirds tongue. During its descent to the lower neck, it retains an attachment with its point of origin, the thyroglossal duct or tract. Normally this duct is obliterated by the sixth week of life, but remnants can remain and undergo cystic degeneration to form a *thyroglossal duct cyst* or *thyroglossal duct fistula* later in life.[7, 9, 253–255] Autosomal dominant inheritance has been reported in some cases.[256, 257]

Clinical Features. The thyroglossal duct cyst may occur anywhere along the thyroglossal duct itself, with 70% arising in the anterior midline of the neck, below the level of the hyoid bone.[253–255] Oral examples are usually found deep in the muscle of the tongue. There is no gender predilection. Normally diagnosed during the first two decades of life, more than a third of cases are not diagnosed until middle age. The typical case is less than 3 cm in diameter at diagnosis, but examples 10 cm in size have been recorded. If the cyst maintains an attachment to the hyoid bone or tongue it will move vertically during swallowing or protrusion of the tongue.

The thyroglossal duct cyst, which is visible in the mouth, is seen as a sessile, movable, often tender nodule of the posterior dorsum of the tongue. It is usually in a midline location, but 20% are found at a somewhat lateral location. Other possible masses occurring at this site include *median rhomboid glossitis, lingual thyroid,* granulomatous infection, and *granular cell tumor.* It is important to remember that the lingual dorsum is an extremely rare site of *carcinoma* development outside of specific systemic diseases, such as tertiary *syphilis (syphilitic glossitis)* and chronic, severe *iron deficiency anemia (Plummer-Vinson syndrome).*

Deep cysts have normal color, but more superficial ones appear semi-translucent, filled with a watery or serous fluid. Dorsal surface lesions may produce dysphagia, hoarseness, difficulty in phonation, or mild choking attacks. Those that occur in the posterior oral floor or deep tongue tissues may elevate the tongue to the point of causing protrusion of the tongue or difficulty with swallowing. As many as a third of these cysts have a fistulous connection to the oral or dermal surface, allowing repeated infections, and occasional cysts have developed a *parathyroid adenoma* from parathyroid tissue within their stroma.[255]

Pathologic Features. The thyroglossal duct cyst is lined by stratified squamous epithelium, ciliated columnar epithelium, nonciliated columnar epithelium, an intermediate epithelium, or a combination thereof. There may be an epithelium-lined fistula to the surface. Mucous glands may be seen in the subepithelial fibrovascular stroma and mucus may be seen in the lumen of the cyst. Aberrant thyroid tissue may also be seen in the stroma, and these must be carefully evaluated for *thyroid carcinoma,* especially *papillary carcinoma,* which occasionally occurs in these cysts.[7, 171–173a] Chronic inflammatory cells are typically scattered throughout the cyst stroma.

Treatment and Prognosis. Thyroglossal duct cyst is treated by wide surgical excision to remove all aberrant thyroid tissue.[7, 253, 255] This may necessitate a rather major surgical procedure (the Sistrunk procedure) in which the lesion is approached through the hyoid bone or the anterior neck. In this procedure, the entire thyroglossal tract is removed from the neck to the base of the tongue. Rare cases of thyroid carcinoma have been reported to arise from untreated thyroglossal duct cysts.[258, 259]

Heterotopic Oral Gastrointestinal Cyst

Ectopic or heterotopic gastric mucosa has been found all up and down the gastrointestinal tract, including the esophagus, small intestines, pancreas, gallbladder, and Meckel's diverticulum. Moreover, there have been several reported cases of *heterotopic gastric cyst* or *heterotopic intestinal cyst* of the tongue or oral floor.[7, 260–262] These cystic choristomas are either embedded deeply in the tongue or present as superficial, movable nodules of the lingual dorsum or oral floor. Some have communication with the surface.

Pathologic Features. The cyst wall is usually composed of routine gastric mucosa of the type seen in the body and fundus of the stomach.[260, 262] Ciliated columnar epithelium and stratified squamous epithelium may be admixed with the gastric mucosa, and a muscularis mucosae may be present. Both parietal and chief cells may be found, and pancreatic tissue was noted in one cyst.[262]

Treatment and Prognosis. The heterotopic gastrointestinal cyst of the mouth is treated by conservative excision.[7, 260, 262] Recurrence has not been reported, nor has malignant transformation. This cyst is not associated with any known syndrome.

VASCULAR LESIONS

Vascular tumors of the oral and pharyngeal soft tissues constitute a group of lesions that often have poorly understood pathoetiologies, frustrating treatment options, and unpredictable biologic behaviors. For the pathologists, nomenclature is an additional problem. It is not unusual, furthermore, for vasoformative abnormalities to be multiple or diffuse, or to be simply one component of a syndrome with serious manifestations outside the head and neck region (Table 4–6).[5]

Some of the vascular lesions are, moreover, clinically obvious but do not present as elevated or submucosal masses. These may not be very demonstrable in a biopsy sample and are better diagnosed using clinical criteria. *Lingual varicosities* and *telangiectasias* are examples that are seldom biopsied because experience has taught us that the clinical diagnosis is much more reliable than the histologic identification of collapsed venous channels beneath the oral mucosa.

Some vascular lesions may be the result of a more generalized or systemic phenomenon. *Spider nevi* or submucosal telangiectasias may, for example, result from liver *cirrhosis,* from *pregnancy,* or from association with a syndrome (see Table 4–6).[6–8]

Table 4–6. Syndromes Associated with Oral and Paraoral Vascular Malformations

With Hemangiomas
Bannayan-Riley-Ruvalcaba syndrome
Beckwith-Wiedemann syndrome
Disseminated hemangiomatosis
Epidermal nevus syndrome
Klippel-Trenaunay-Weber syndrome
Maffucci's syndrome (enchondromatosis and hemangiomatosis)
Multiple angiomas with thrombocytopenia
Proteus syndrome
Pseudoxanthoma elasticum
Sotos' syndrome (cerebral gigantism)
Sturge-Weber angiomatosis (Sturge-Weber syndrome)
Tuberous sclerosis
von Recklinghausen neurofibromatosis
With Telangiectasias or Varicosities
Acrolabial telangiectasia
Bean syndrome (blue rubber bleb nevus syndrome)
Coats' disease (telangiectatic retinal detachment)
CREST syndrome (calcinosis, Raynaud's phenomenon, esophageal dysfunction, sclerodactyly, telangiectasia syndrome)
Cutis marmorata telangiectatica congenita
Fabry syndrome (angiokeratoma corporis diffusum universale)
Hereditary hemorrhagic telangiectasia (Osler-Rendu-Parkes Weber syndrome)
Kasabach-Merritt syndrome
Scleroderma

Data from Gorlin et al.,[5] Enzinger and Weiss,[6] Neville et al.,[7] and Elder et al.[8]

Traumatic Angiomatous Lesion

The *traumatic angiomatous lesion (venous pool, venous lake, venous aneurysm)* is a small, focal area of venous aneurysm or dilation (telangiectasia?), which occurs after trauma and remains indefinitely thereafter.[7, 9] It presents as a bluish, sessile, soft, discrete, painless nodule that is somewhat movable beneath the epithelium. It is usually seen after 40 years of age, with no gender predilection, and almost all head and neck cases are located on the lower lip mucosa or vermilion, or on the buccal mucosa.[7, 263, 264] Pressure on the feeder vessel will produce blanching, and the lesion is almost never larger than 6 mm in greatest diameter. It differs from *varicose veins* in location (varicosities are usually on the ventral tongue), in the lack of multiple vessel involvement, and in the nodular rather than serpiginous appearance.[265, 266] It differs from the telangiectasias of *hereditary hemorrhagic telangiectasia* and similar developmental disorders by the pattern and increased numbers of vascular lesions associated with the latter.[267]

Pathologic Features. The traumatic angiomatous lesion is seen as a single, perhaps tortuous, dilated vein located superficially beneath the surface epithelium, above the striated muscle.[267] The endothelial nuclei are quite inactive and flattened and the vessel lumen is filled with erythrocytes. There may be a slight encirclement by fibrous tissues and there often is an organizing thrombus in the lumen (Fig. 4–23, see p. 171). Lesions that are continuously traumatized by the teeth will have chronic inflammatory cells in the background stroma. There is no way to distinguish this lesion from varicose veins on the basis of histopathology; both lesions may present with intravascular thrombi.[263, 265]

Treatment and Prognosis. No treatment is necessary for this entity, because it remains small indefinitely.[7, 264] Occasional lesions may be conservatively excised, however, for esthetic reasons or for reasons of tenderness from recurring trauma.

Caliber-Persistent Labial Artery

Miko et al.[268] first described, in 1980, a developmental anomaly referred to by them as *persistent caliber artery* of the lower lip. Also called *retained caliber labial artery* and *caliber-persistent labial artery,* the lesion is exactly what the name implies. The inferior alveolar artery retains its large size and thickened walls even after it leaves the bone through the mental foramen and travels through the orbicularis oris muscle to supply the mucosal aspects of the lower lip. The artery becomes superficial toward the midline of the lower lip, and the persistent size makes it palpable, usually a few millimeters inferior to the vermilion border.[268–270] This is also a phenomenon of the lower gastrointestinal tract, specifically of the gastric and jejunal mucosa, where it has produced lethal hemorrhage.[268, 271]

Clinical Features. Of the few examples of oral persistent caliber artery reported to date, more than 80% have been on the lower lip and a few have been on the upper lip and hard palate.[268–270] Patients have been 40 to 88 years of age at diagnosis, but lesions are present for months and years prior to diagnosis. The artery typically presents as a sessile, elongated nodule that may be pulsatile.[269] It may be tender or ulcerated as a result of recurrent trauma or irritation from the anterior teeth, and this has led some to confuse the lesions clinically with ulcerative lip *carcinoma.*[268, 271] Multiple lesions have been reported.[271]

Pathologic Features and Differential Diagnosis. A large artery with thick smooth muscle walls (Fig. 4–24) is separated from the overlying stratified squamous epithelium by a variable amount of routine fibrovascular connective tissue in this lesion. The "retained caliber" of this artery is obvious and the vessel is typically somewhat parallel to the surface. Excess keratin on the surface and scattered chronic inflammatory cells in the stroma are evidence of chronic trauma.

This lesion is easily distinguished from its venous counterpart, the *traumatic angiomatous lesion (venous pool, venous lake, venous*

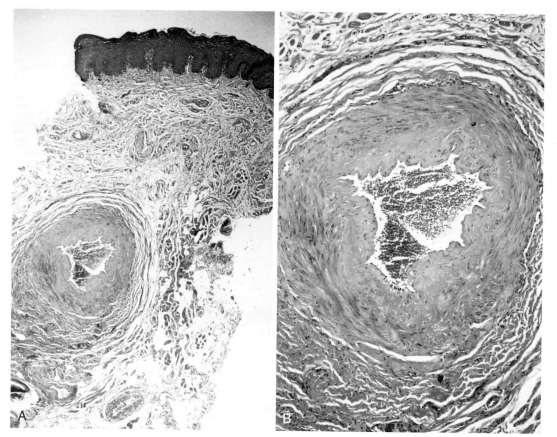

Figure 4–24. *A,* The thick-walled, caliber-persistent artery is normal in every way except that it is too large a vessel to be found so close to the mucosal surface in the anterior midline of the body; *B,* higher power view of the thickened arterial wall.

aneurysm) by the thickness of its muscled walls. It may, at times, be difficult to differentiate caliber-persistent artery from *arteriovenous malformation (A-V shunt),* but typically the latter entity involves multiple intertwining arterioles rather than a single large artery. The A-V shunt also has a greater admixture of arteriole and venous vessels. There is no encapsulation of either lesion.

Treatment and Prognosis. No treatment is necessary for caliber-persistent labial artery unless it becomes tender or excessively enlarged from recurring trauma.[269, 270] Simple surgical removal of the offending vessel will provide cure, although excessive hemorrhage may be a surgical problem. The suggestion by Miko et al[271] that chronic ulceration of such a lesion may lead to malignant transformation has not been substantiated by others.

Hemangioma

The most likely vasoformative tumor to be submitted for biopsy from the oral/pharyngeal region is the *hemangioma.* Hemangioma of the head and neck region is relatively common, representing at least one third of all hemangiomas in humans.[7, 272–275] Oral hemangioma represents 14% of all human hemangiomas and is found in 5.5 of every 1000 U.S. adults.[1–3, 6] It was first reported in 1841 as *bluish excrescence* and *erectile tissue.*[276]

Composed of a proliferation or excess of vascular channels, it is usually present at birth but may arise in young adults or older individuals. Most lesions appear to be developmental anomalies or hamartomas, seen in 2% of newborns (all anatomic sites). Some result from abnormal vessel proliferation after trauma, and a few appear to be true benign neoplasms. In this light, it should be mentioned that some authorities reserve the term *hemangioma* exclusively for the neoplastic variant.[6]

Many maxillofacial entities of a nonvascular nature have vascular subtypes, such as *angioleiomyoma* and *angiolipoma.* Likewise, a paraoral hemangioma may rarely be associated with an overlying reactive hyperkeratosis and papillomatosis *(verrucous hemangioma).* The *cherry angioma (senile angioma, De Morgan's spots)* so common to the skin of older adults is not seen on the mucosa of the mouth and throat.

Clinical Features. The oral or pharyngeal hemangioma has an older age at diagnosis than lesions from other sites. In adults, the mucosal hemangioma most often arises from the frequently traumatized mucosal sites: the lip mucosa (63% of oral cases), the buccal mucosa (14% of cases) and the lateral borders of the tongue (14% of cases), but it may occur at any oral or pharyngeal location.[7, 273] In population studies, there is a strong (2 : 1) male predilection, although there is minimal gender predilection in hospital-based studies.[2] Congenital and neonatal lesions do occur, especially in the lips and parotid glands.[7, 277]

The mucosal hemangioma is typically a soft, moderately well circumscribed, painless mass that is red or blue in coloration (Fig. 4–25A). The more superficial ones are often lobulated and will blanch under finger pressure. Deeper lesions tend to be dome-shaped with normal or blue surface coloration; they seldom blanch. A lesion with a thrill or bruit, or with an obviously warmer surface, is most likely a special vascular malformation, called *arteriovenous hemangioma (arteriovenous aneurysm, A-V shunt, arteriovenous malformation),* with direct flow of blood from the venous to the arterial system, bypassing the capillary beds.

The lesion is usually less than 2 cm in greatest dimension, but may be so extensive as to encompass much of the oral and pharyngeal tissues. Congenital lesions tend to keep pace with body growth, whereas adult-onset lesions tend to slowly enlarge over a period of months or years. Extension into underlying muscle or pressure atrophy of underlying bone may occur and, of course, the hemangioma may be part of a syndrome (see Table 4–6).[5]

Pathologic Features. The hemangioma is characterized by an excess of blood vessels, usually veins and capillaries, in a focal area of submucosal connective tissue. It is almost never encapsulated. Lesions are subdivided into several categories. *Capillary hemangioma* is the most common type and is composed of numerous intertwining capillary-sized vessels lined by endothelium with relatively flat or plump nuclei, depending on the duration of the lesion (Fig. 4–25B). Those with plump endothelial nuclei are younger and often demonstrate mitotic activity, a feature not present in older lesions.

While lacking a capsule, the capillary hemangioma is often well circumscribed and there is typically a central feeder vessel with radiating, lobular extensions or vascular proliferations, leading some to prefer the diagnosis of *lobular hemangioma* (Fig. 4–25C). Lobular vascular architecture is used to confirm the benign nature of such lesions and is characteristic of several vascular subtypes, such as *cellular hemangioma of infancy (strawberry nevus, benign hemangioendothelioma of infancy, juvenile hemangioma)* and *epithelioid hemangioma*. The relationship between the lobular capillary hemangioma and the *pyogenic granuloma* is somewhat unclear at this time.

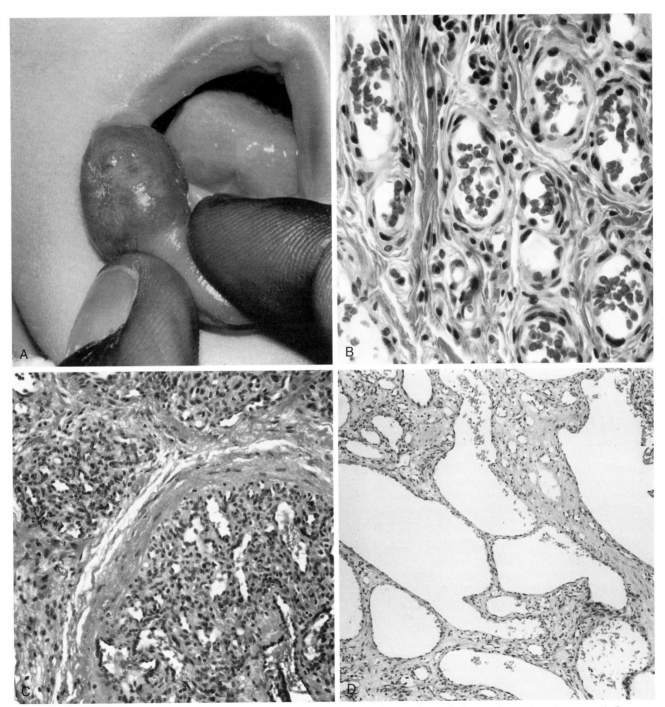

Figure 4–25. *A*, The hemangioma typically presents as discoloration of a soft, sessile, submucosal mass. *B*, Capillary hemangioma is composed of numerous capillary-sized endothelium-lined vessels with plump endothelial nuclei projecting into the lumina. *C*, Vessels of the lobular hemangioma are arranged in clusters or lobules. *D*, Large, dilated vessels lined by endothelial cells with relatively flat nuclei represent features of the cavernous hemangioma.

The lumina in capillary hemangioma are typically small, perhaps to the point of masking the vascular nature of the lesion. Reticulin stains will more easily demonstrate the vessels and factor XIII-positive interstitial cells are consistently seen in this lesion.

Endothelial proliferation that takes place completely or almost completely within a venous lumen, typically with tufts and papillary projections, may also be seen. This is usually termed papillary *endothelial hyperplasia (intravascular hemangioendothelioma, intravascular angiomatosis)* and is presumed to arise from abnormal organization of a thrombus.[278, 279]

The *epithelioid hemangioma* deserves special mention.[4, 280–282] Often called *angiolymphoid hyperplasia with eosinophilia, histiocytoid hemangioma,* or, mistakenly, *Kimura's disease,* this superficial, often multifocal lesion has a strong predilection for the head and neck region and may be associated with an unidentified infectious agent. The vessels in this lesion are lined by epithelioid or histiocytoid endothelial cells that extend considerably into the lumen, imparting a "tombstone" effect to the vessel walls. The lesional cells have rounded nuclei and abundant eosinophilic cytoplasm with occasional vacuoles. Electron microscopy will reveal excess mitochondria, endoplasmic reticulum, and cytofilaments in the cytoplasm. Another epithelioid change is seen: there are gaps between endothelial cells, with desmosome-like attachments between them.

A mixed chronic inflammatory cell infiltrate, including eosinophils and occasional germinal centers, is seen to surround the lesional vessels of epithelioid hemangioma. It should be mentioned that Kimura's disease is a chronic inflammatory condition endemic to Asian populations and presents with lesions bearing superficial resemblance to epithelioid hemangioma. This disease presents with peripheral eosinophilia, increased serum IgE, proteinuria, and nephrotic syndrome, and has a strong predilection for males. Submucosal or subcutaneous lesions are characterized by abundant, aggregated lymphoid tissue with prominent germinal centers, but the associated vessels are thin walled and the number of eosinophils is often much more marked ("eosinophilic abscess") than in epithelioid hemangioma.

Intramuscular hemangioma shows capillaries in a loose fibrous stroma interspersed between striated muscle bundles in a pseudoinfiltrative fashion that may mimic malignancy.[275] Vessel lumina are usually well developed in this tumor, but occasional cases have a more solid cellular appearance. Mitotic activity is usually not pronounced and intraluminal tufts of endothelial cells may be seen to project into vessel lumina. Capillaries may occasionally proliferate within perineural sheaths.

When lesional vascular channels are considerably enlarged, the term *cavernous hemangioma* has traditionally been applied (Fig. 4–25D). This differs from capillary hemangioma in that it is less well circumscribed, is larger, and is usually deeper in submucosal tissues. Sluggish blood flow may result in organized or dystrophically calcified thrombi within dilated vessels. The vessels may be arranged in a haphazard or a somewhat lobular pattern and there may be areas with fibrosis of the background stroma. Occasional vascular lesions, in fact, are dominated so much by a dense fibrous stroma that they are called *sclerosing hemangioma.* Chronic inflammatory cells may be scattered in multiple foci.

Some examples of hemangioma have minimal stroma and demonstrate excess anastomosis of adjacent cavernous channels, often with a papillary infolding of the endothelium at points of contact between vessels. The term *sinusoidal hemangioma* has been used for such lesions. The *arteriovenous hemangioma,* on the other hand, presents as a nonencapsulated aggregation of intertwining, tortuous medium-sized or larger arteries and veins in the submucosal tissues. This may show excessive or dilated lymphatic channels in addition to the blood vessels.

Treatment and Prognosis. The hemangioma is usually treated by conservative surgical excision, but it is known to respond well to the following:[7, 272–275]

- intralesional injections of sclerosing chemicals, such as sodium morrhuate

- implanted or external irradiation
- cryosurgery
- laser ablation
- strangulation of the feeder vessel
- intralesional injections of corticosteroid

The lack of encapsulation and the infiltrating nature of the lesional border, especially in intramuscular hemangioma, often forces the surgeon to perform a simple debulking procedure, with remnants of tumor deliberately left behind to preserve the maximum amount of surrounding normal tissues. Recurrence is not unusual unless the tumor is completely excised. Epithelioid hemangioma responds to low-dosage radiotherapy, but not to cryotherapy or intralesional steroids.

Most congenital capillary hemangiomas will spontaneously regress or disappear by the fifth or sixth years of life, but cavernous types tend less to do this, as do those associated with *Sturge-Weber syndrome.*[283, 284] When hemangioma admixes with lymphatic proliferations, such as *hemangiolymphangioma,* the lesion tends to behave more like a *lymphangioma* than a hemangioma.

Hemangioendothelioma

A varied group of proliferative and neoplastic vascular lesions, called collectively *hemangioendothelioma,* seems to have a biologic behavior that falls somewhere between the benign *hemangioma* and malignant *angiosarcoma.*[4, 6–9] Most cases present as red or blue nodules that may be multiple and are usually quite superficial.[285–289] Diagnosis is typically made during the second and third decades of life and there is no gender predilection. Approximately 10% of cases are associated with other developmental anomalies or syndromes, including early-onset *varicose veins, lymphedema, Klippel-Trenaunay-Weber syndrome,* and *Maffucci's syndrome.*[7, 285]

Pathologic Features and Differential Diagnosis. The hemangioendothelioma is a poorly circumscribed, usually biphasic proliferation of venous or capillary vessels. There are dilated and congested veins with inactive endothelial cell nuclei and with occasional thrombi or pheboliths. These vessels are intermixed with solid sheets of epithelioid *(epithelioid hemangioendothelioma)* or spindle-shaped *(spindle cell hemangioendothelioma)* mesenchymal cells with minimal dysplasia, few mitotic figures, and minimal differentiation toward a vascular lumen or channel.[285, 287, 288]

Slit-like vascular channels, similar to those of *Kaposi's sarcoma,* are often seen, perhaps with mild extravasation of erythrocytes and hemosiderin deposition within or outside of macrophages. It should be mentioned that the *kaposiform hemangioendothelioma,* with its histopathologic admixture of tissues similar to both *capillary hemangioma* and Kaposi's sarcoma, has not yet been reported from an oral or pharyngeal location.[290, 291]

The clustering or grouping of the endothelial cells of hemangioendothelioma is more readily apparent with the use of reticulin staining, which shows fibers surrounding solid clusters with or without a small central vascular lumen ("microlumen"). Thick-walled vascular channels may be seen at the lesional periphery, and the tumor frequently demonstrates areas of necrosis or dense fibrosis.

The epithelioid cells have abundant eosinophilic cytoplasm, may contain vacuoles (primitive lumina), and may be admixed with smooth muscle bundles. These cells stain positively with *Ulex europaeus* and many will show cytoplasmic factor VIII-associated antigen reactivity with immunohistochemistry. Tumor cells also stain for endothelial markers such as CD31 and CD34 in approximately one fifth of cases.[289] Some epithelioid hemangioendotheliomas have a myxoid or hyaline stroma, and aldehyde fuchsin (pH 1.0) staining may reveal sulfated acid mucopolysaccharides in this stroma.[286]

The lesional cells of the spindle cell hemangioendothelioma are rather bland, bipolar mesenchymal fibroblast-like cells that may contain vacuoles, presumed to be abortive or primitive vascular lumina. Epithelioid cells are usually seen in small numbers in scattered areas and the associated dilated venous channels are more prone to contain thrombi and phleboliths than are those of the epithelioid hemangioendothelioma. Factor VIII-associated antigen is often found within the endothelium of the venous channels, but the spindle cells are typically negative.[286]

The pathologist must be careful to rule out *metastatic carcinoma* or *melanoma,* which typically display much more dysplasia than hemangioendothelioma. The various epithelioid *sarcomas* must also be ruled out, especially *epithelioid angiosarcoma.* These are discussed elsewhere in the present chapter.

Treatment and Prognosis. Hemangioendothelioma is treated with wide surgical excision, with more than half of all cases recurring at the operative site or several centimeters distant.[284–288] Those tumors with significant cellular atypia and mitotic activity are associated with more aggressive clinical behavior, but not all tumors that metastasize have these changes at initial biopsy.

Almost a third of epithelioid hemangioendotheliomas develop metastases in regional lymph nodes (at least 50% or more of all metastatic cases) or in the lungs, liver, or bones.[288] Patients who develop metastases have a 50% 5-year survival rate. The spindle cell hemangioendothelioma is rarely associated with metastasis but has a higher rate of local recurrence than does the epithelioid variant of this tumor (60% vs. 13%, respectively).[288]

Hemangiopericytoma

Stout and Murray[292] in 1942 were the first to suggest *hemangiopericytoma* as a distinctly different vascular neoplasm. Stout[293] also was the first to report an oral hemangiopericytoma, just a few years after its initial delineation. It is a neoplasm that is usually benign but has a definite malignant counterpart. Head and neck lesions represent 16% to 25% of all reported hemangiopericytomas, and the tumor represents 2% to 3% of all soft tissue sarcomas in humans.[4, 6, 7, 294–298] Chromosomal translocations t(12;19) and t(13;22) have been observed in lesional cells.[6]

Clinical Features. The oral hemangiopericytoma is typically a rapidly enlarging red or bluish mass that arises in all age groups but is rare prior to the second decade or after the seventh decade.[7, 294, 296] There is no gender predilection. It is soft or rubbery, is usually painless, and is relatively well demarcated from the surrounding mucosa. The lesion may be sessile or somewhat pedunculated, and may demonstrate a surface lobularity or telangiectasis. Intraosseous examples have been reported.[299]

The oral/pharyngeal mucosa is, additionally, one of the most common locations for the rarely reported *infantile hemangiopericytoma.*[300, 301] This lesion is usually multiple and congenital and often demonstrates an alarmingly rapid rate of enlargement after birth. Although this entity tends to recur after surgical excision, there is no potential for metastasis.

Pathologic Features and Differential Diagnosis. Hemangiopericytoma consists of numerous vascular channels with plump endothelial nuclei and a surrounding, tightly packed proliferation of oval and spindled cells with dark nuclei and a moderate amount of cytoplasm. Areas with more spindled pericytes may show an interlacing pattern of cells, but usually there is a medullary tissue pattern, sometimes with palisading of cells, reminiscent of a neural tumor. Older, less aggressive lesions tend to have less cellularity and may have a largely mucoid interstitial appearance, which can be mistaken for *myxoid lipoma* or *myxoid liposarcoma.* Focal cartilage production may rarely be seen and such lesions must be differentiated from *mesenchymal chondrosarcoma.*

The number of mitotic figures is variable and of prognostic significance, with lesions showing fewer than 2 to 3 mitotic figures per high-power field having a slower growth, lesser recurrence rate, and fewer metastases than lesions with 4 or more mitotic figures per high-power field. Lesions with pleomorphic cells and areas of necrosis or hemorrhage usually have a more aggressive behavior than those without these features.

Reticulin staining will demonstrate lesional vessels lined by a single layer of endothelial cells, with the pericytes lying outside the basal lamina, although they are often individually surrounded by reticulin and collagen fibers. Lesional cells are immunoreactive for vimentin (variable intensity), factor XIIIa antigen, HLA-DR antigen, and QBEND10 (CD34).[6, 8] They do not stain for or react with factor VIII-related antigen, *Ulex europaeus I* lectin, alpha-smooth muscle actin, desmin, myoglobin, low molecular weight cytokeratin, high molecular weight cytokeratin, or epithelial membrane antigen.

The differential diagnosis of this lesion includes, in addition to the tumors just named, *fibrous histiocytoma, MFH, synovial sarcoma,* other stromal *sarcomas, juxtaglomerular tumor, vascular leiomyoma,* and *juvenile hemangioma.*

Treatment and Prognosis. The treatment of hemangiopericytoma is dependent on the amount of cellular dysplasia and mitotic activity. The more bland lesions with minimal mitotic activity are treated by wide local excision, but the more active and dysplastic lesions are treated by radical surgical excision, with or without adjunctive radiotherapy.[294–298] Surgical removal is usually preceded by ligation of the feeder vessels or by embolization to reduce the size of the tumor and the risk of operative hemorrhage.

The rate of metastasis for this tumor during the first 5-year postoperative period varies from 17% to 56%, and metastasis occasionally occurs up to 10 years after surgery.[7, 294–298] Metastases are usually to the lungs and bones; lymph node metastasis is uncommon. Most recurrent tumors will eventually demonstrate metastasis. The overall 5-year survival rate for the microscopically dysplastic hemangiopericytoma is somewhat less than 50%.[298]

Angiosarcoma

The term *angiosarcoma* is still used to designate the vascular neoplasm with a definitively aggressive, malignant clinical course and a histopathologic appearance that is more atypical than the low-grade lesion called *hemangioendothelioma.*[302–307] It is a decidedly rare entity, representing less than 1% of all sarcomas in humans, and there is often so little microscopic evidence for the vessels of origin, that is, blood or lymphatic vessels, that it seems best to use the rather generic term, angiosarcoma, rather than *hemangiosarcoma* or *lymphangiosarcoma.*[6] More than half of all cases are found in the head and neck region, and in this area the scalp and facial skin are the most commonly affected sites; about 8% of head and neck lesions arise from oral cavity sites.[6, 302, 304, 305] Trauma, long-standing lymphedema, and irradiation of benign vascular lesions appear to be contributory factors in the onset of some cases, but most cases present with no obvious etiology.

Clinical Features. Angiosarcoma of the oral region is a disease of older individuals, averaging more than 65 years of age.[302, 304] There is no gender predilection and the tumor is typically a solitary or multifocal submucosal nodule that may be bosselated, may be ulcerated, and may bleed spontaneously. The clinical appearance may be indistinguishable from that of oral pyogenic granuloma.[303, 307]

The lesion is rather painless and is fixed to surrounding soft tissues and adjacent bony structures; margins are difficult to define. Some tumors grow rapidly whereas others take many months to reach a size of 4 to 5 cm. Occasional lesions will be deceptively small at clinical examination, only to reveal deep and widespread submucosal extension at surgery.

Pathologic Features and Differential Diagnosis. The histopathologic appearance of this neoplasm varies greatly, depending on the degree of cellular differentiation. The well-differentiated lesions may be quite similar to hemangioendothelioma, with distinct, endothelium-lined vascular channels with relatively flattened endothelial nuclei. There is, however, a tendency for the channels in angiosarcoma to anastomose with one another and to produced dilated sinusoids. The sarcoma, moreover, has a more infiltrative, dissecting pattern at its interface with the normal surrounding tissues.

Occasional proliferation of lesional cells will produce islands and sheets of tumor endothelial cells with large, hyperchromatic nuclei. These proliferations often protrude into the vascular lumina to form papulations similar to those found in *intravascular papillary endothelial hyperplasia.*[308] Chronic inflammatory cells may be seen in small numbers at the periphery of the lesion.

The less-differentiated angiosarcoma may have scattered areas of well-differentiated lesional tissues, but it is usually composed of pleomorphic and hyperchromatic epithelioid cells with abundant mitotic activity. It may resemble a *carcinoma* or poorly differentiated *fibrosarcoma,* in which case a reticulin stain will often demonstrate the vascular channels with tumor cells lying on the luminal side of the vessel. *Ulex europaeus* staining for endothelial cells is also helpful, although it must be remembered that it is also positive in some examples of *synovial sarcoma* and *epithelioid sarcoma.*

Less than one in four angiosarcomas will be immunoreactive for factor VIII-associated antigen. Antibodies to thrombomodulin are reactive in most cases, but have also been reactive in trophoblastic tumors and occasional carcinomas.[6] CD34 is also expressed by most angiosarcomas but may be seen in the occasional epithelioid sarcoma. Perhaps the most specific immunohistochemistry is reactivity to the CD31 antibody, the platelet-endothelial cell adhesion molecule.[6] To date, nonvascular soft tissue tumors have been completely nonreactive to this antibody.

Treatment and Prognosis. Angiosarcoma of the oral region is treated by wide local excision, although radiotherapy is sometimes used for multifocal lesions.[305] It is not unusual for tumor cells to be found more than a centimeter beyond the grossly evident lesional periphery. Positive necks are treated by radical neck dissection. The prognosis is very much dependent on two features: the degree of cellular differentiation and the clinical size of the tumor. The overall survival is poor, approximately 10% to 15% after 5 years, with most recurrences and metastases occurring within 2 years of treatment. In some series, no patients survived who had lesions with diameters greater than 5 cm.[305]

Kaposi's Sarcoma

Kaposi's sarcoma is a multicentric proliferation of vascular and spindle cell components, which was first described in 1872.[309] Now considered to be a viral-induced or viral-associated tumor, it is unclear whether the lesion is a true neoplasm or a simple hyperplasia.[6, 10, 310–315] Today it is strongly affiliated with AIDS and its course is greatly influenced by the immune status of the affected individual. Although found predominantly in persons infected with human immunodeficiency virus (HIV), HIV does not seem to be the direct cause of the tumorous proliferation and HIV amino acid sequences have not been identified within lesional cells.[314, 315] These cells produce several cytokines capable of stimulating their own growth, and HIV-infected lymphocytes are also capable of producing their own set of similar cytokines.

Clinical Features. Kaposi's sarcoma has four major clinical presentations: *classic (chronic), endemic (lymphadenopathic; African), immunosuppression-associated (transplant),* and *AIDS-related.*[6, 10, 311] The classic variant affects older males of Italian, Slavic, or Jewish ancestry and is rare in the United States. It is often associated with altered immune states as well as lymphoreticular and other malignancies. It has no association with HIV infection. Cutaneous multifocal blue-red nodules develop on the lower extremities and slowly increase in size and numbers, with some lesions regressing while new ones are forming on adjacent or distant skin. Oral involvement in this form of the disease is quite unusual, but when it occurs it does so as soft, bluish nodules of the palatal mucosa or gingiva.

Lymphadenopathic Kaposi's sarcoma is endemic to young African children and presents as a localized or generalized enlargement of lymph node chains, including the cervical nodes. The disease follows a fulminating course with visceral involvement and minimal skin or mucous membrane involvement. In the head and neck region, salivary glands may be affected. This variant does not appear to be HIV related.

Transplantation-associated Kaposi's sarcoma is seen in 1% to 4% of renal transplant patients, usually becoming manifest 1 to 2 years after transplantation.[6, 311] The extent and progression of the disease correlate directly with the loss of cellular immunity of the host. Sarcomatous involvement occurs on the skin as well as internal organs, but oral mucosal lesions are decidedly rare.

In the United States, AIDS-related Kaposi's sarcoma is found primarily in male homosexuals, but in Africa, heterosexual transmission and needle-stick contamination seem to be much more strongly associated. Approximately 40% of homosexual AIDS patients will develop Kaposi's sarcoma, often as an early sign of the disease.[6] Affected patients are usually young adults or early middle-aged males, with the average age at sarcomatous diagnosis being 39 years in the United States. Individual lesions occur in many cutaneous locations, especially along lines of cleavage and on the tip of the nose. Oral lesions can also occur on any mucosal surface but have a strong predilection for palatal and gingival mucosa.[310, 312]

Early oral mucosal sarcomas are flat and slightly blue, red, or purple. With time, lesions become more deeply discolored and surface papules and soft nodules develop, usually remaining less than 2 cm in size (Fig. 4–26A, see p. 172).[7, 310, 313] Individual lesions may coalesce and occasional patients never develop the nodular variant. Cervical lymph nodes and salivary gland enlargement may also be seen. The patient may have oral candidiasis and AIDS-related gingivitis as well.

Pathologic Features and Differential Diagnosis. Kaposi's sarcoma has a similar histopathologic appearance in all of its clinical subtypes.[6, 8, 10] The early lesion (patch stage) is characterized by a proliferation of small veins and capillaries around one or more dilated vessels. A pronounced mononuclear inflammatory cell infiltrate, including mast cells, is often noted, as are scattered erythrocytes and hemosiderin deposits. There may be an inconspicuous perivascular proliferation of spindle cells, but cellular atypia is minimal.

More advanced lesions are nodular and show increased numbers of small capillaries or dilated vascular channels interspersed with proliferating sheets of sarcomatous or atypical spindle cells, often with large numbers of extravasated erythrocytes and abundant hemosiderin deposition (Fig. 4–26B, see p. 172). Slit-like vascular channels without a visible endothelial lining are typically interspersed with the spindle cells. Lesional cells have somewhat enlarged, hyperchromatic nuclei with mild to moderate pleomorphism. Mitotic activity is quite variable but is usually minimal. Infiltration by chronic inflammatory cells is also variable. Occasional lesions show such exuberance of the spindled component that the vascular features become minimally visible. Rarely, the vascular component dominates with anastomosing channels lined by anaplastic endothelial cells, similar in appearance to *angiosarcoma.*

Intracellular and extracellular hyaline globules occur with some frequency in the earlier stages of this tumor. They occur in clusters of faintly eosinophilic spheres smaller than erythrocytes. These are PAS positive and diastase resistant and probably represent partially digested or degenerated erythrocytes (ghost erythrocytes). Immunoreactivity is somewhat variable, but the spindle cells are consistently reactive for CD34 and the delicate, flattened endothelial cells lining the vascular clefts are reactive for both CD31 and CD34.[8, 313] The vascular channels are often reactive for *Ulex europaeus* agglutinin, but nonreactive for factor XIIIa.

As a proliferative vascular and spindled lesion, Kaposi's sarcoma may mimic a variety of other soft tissue lesions, especially *pyogenic granuloma, hemangioma, lymphangioma, hemangioendothelioma, hemangiopericytoma,* and *bacillary angiomatosis.* The vascular channels of pyogenic granuloma and hemangioma are more widely spaced, seldom appear slit-like, and have much more prominent endothelial cells. The hemangioma lacks the inflammatory cell infiltrate of Kaposi's sarcoma, but the pyogenic granuloma abounds with these.

Hemangioendothelioma, especially when the spindle cell component is prominent, differs from Kaposi's sarcoma by showing dilated vascular spaces admixed with collections of epithelioid cells with and without early lumina. The angiosarcoma typically shows more endothelial cell atypia and enlargement, even intraluminal shedding, than is found in Kaposi's sarcoma. The reader is referred to descriptions of these lesions elsewhere in this chapter.

Treatment and Prognosis. Various treatments have been used with oral Kaposi's sarcoma with variable success. Small or localized lesions can be surgically excised with a small surrounding margin of clinically normal tissue, but more recent therapies have concentrated on low-dose irradiation and intralesional chemotherapy and sclerosing solutions.[6–9, 313, 316] For larger and multifocal lesions, systemic chemotherapy is often effective.[6–8]

Lymphangioma

The *lymphangioma* is a benign hamartomatous hyperplasia of lymphatic vessels, with three-fourths of all cases occurring in the head and neck region.[6–9, 317–321] Although occasional adult-onset cases occur, this tumor is thought to be a developmental malformation of vessels that have poor communication with the normal lymph system. Very large cystic spaces may be seen in lesions proliferating in loose connective tissues and fascial spaces.[320, 321] Diagnosed cases are typically superficial but may extend deeply into underlying connective tissues. Rarely, multiple lesions are seen in infancy and childhood in *lymphangiomatosis,* the lymphatic counterpart to *angiomatosis* of blood vessels and a potentially life-threatening disease when visceral involvement occurs.[322]

Clinical Features. Oral mucosal lymphangioma almost always becomes apparent prior to the third year of life; half of all cases are congenital.[7, 318–320] There is no gender predilection. Oral lesions are most frequently found on the tongue, where they may produce considerable macroglossia and dysfunction.[318] Any oral or pharyngeal site may, however, be affected and the most common head and neck location is the lateral neck, where this lesion typically contains large cystic spaces and is commonly called *cystic lymphangioma* or *cystic hygroma,* discussed elsewhere in this text.[320, 321]

The cervical lymphangioma occurs most frequently in the posterior triangle, but lesions of the anterior triangle tend to be more problematic, interfering with the patient's ability to breath or swallow and extending upward into the oral cavity, or downward into the mediastinum.[320] Torticollis or wry neck may develop from cervical involvement and cervical lesions tend to be much larger than oral or pharyngeal lesions, sometimes larger than the patient's head at birth.

Superficial oral mucosal lymphangiomas often demonstrate a pebbled or botryoid appearance, once referred to as chronic "clustered blisters" because of the translucent appearance of the lymphatic channels, which may have only sparse fibrovascular tissue separating their endothelial walls from the surface epithelium (Fig. 4–27*A*.)[323] Secondary hemorrhage into the lymphatic vessels may cause some of the surface "vesicles" to appear red or blue. Satellite lesions several millimeters from the main lesional mass may be seen.

Occasional lesions show only widely scattered clear "vesicles" interspersed with blood-filled papules or blebs. Such lesions are, presumably, a combination of lymphangioma and hemangioma and are termed *hemangiolymphangioma.* They behave more like lymphatic than vascular tumors.

A unique *congenital alveolar lymphangioma* is seen on the alveolar mucosa of African-American neonates.[317, 319] This lesion is seldom greater than a centimeter in size and is often bilateral on the alveolar ridge. The mandible is more often affected than the maxilla and the lesion typically disappears during the months after birth.

Deeper lymphangiomas present with an irregular surface nodularity and are quite soft and painless. They may feel like a "ball of worms" on palpation, but are usually rather nonspecific and ill-defined.

Pathologic Features and Differential Diagnosis. The lymphangioma consists of multiple, intertwining lymph vessels in a loose fibrovascular stroma, sometimes with scattered aggregates of lymphoid tissue. The lymphatic vessels of a lymphangioma are lined by a single layer of endothelial cells with flattened, occasionally plump, nuclei (Fig. 4–27*B&C*).

The vessels may be capillary in size, with a very attenuated lumen or may be so dilated that the cystic areas can be visualized at surgery. Oral examples are more likely to contain the dilated vessels. The vessels are filled with an uniform, eosinophilic, proteinaceous fluid with occasional erythrocytes and leukocytes. Those vessels just beneath the surface epithelium tend to fill or replace the connective tissue papillae, perhaps producing a papillary surface change. It is not unusual for a superficial lesion to have little or no fibrous stroma separating it from the overlying epithelium.

There is no encapsulation of lymphatic vessels, even with the tumors that appear well circumscribed clinically. Deeper lesions show vessels interspersed between adipocytes and striated muscle bundles. Deeper lesions also tend toward greater vessel dilation.

Some authorities prefer to subclassify lymphangioma into four categories[6]:

- *lymphangioma simplex (capillary lymphangioma, lymphangioma circumscriptum)*—composed of small, thin-walled lymphatics
- *cavernous lymphangioma*—composed of dilated lymphatic vessels with surrounding adventitia
- *cystic lymphangioma (cystic hygroma)*—consisting of huge, macroscopic lymphatic spaces with surrounding fibrovascular tissues and smooth muscle
- *benign lymphangioendothelioma (acquired progressive lymphangioma)*— lymphatic channels appear to be dissecting through dense collagenic bundles

These categories are somewhat artificial and many lesions are combinations of categories. Microscopic features of cystic hygroma are discussed elsewhere in this text (Chapters 8, 10). Occasional lesions demonstrate proliferation of lymphatic channels with another connective tissue component, primarily smooth muscle cells *(lymphangiomyoma).*

The lymphatic endothelial cells in these or more routine lymphangiomas can be identified via positive immunoreactivity with factor VIII-associated antigen and CD31, as well as positive staining with *Ulex europaeus.*[6] Immunohistochemistry is not a particularly reliable means of distinguishing lymphangioma from *hemangioma,* but this is not usually a problem because of the large number of erythrocytes in the vessels of the latter.

In addition to distinguishing lymphangioma from hemangioma, the pathologist must also delineate it from well-differentiated *angiosarcoma* and patch-stage *Kaposi's sarcoma.* Recently, a lymphangioma-like variant of Kaposi's sarcoma has been reported.[324]

Treatment and Prognosis. Because of the nonencapsulated and "infiltrating" nature of the lymphangioma, complete removal is often inadvisable and may be impossible without excessive removal of surrounding normal structures.[7, 318, 321] Surgical debulking of the tumor is, therefore, the typical treatment provided, with the understanding that additional debulking procedures will most likely be required as the affected child grows. Most patients will need two to four procedures before full growth and development have been achieved. Recurrence is possible but unlikely for those lesions able to be removed completely via excisional surgery. Radiotherapy and chemical cauteries are much less effective with the lymphangioma than they are with the hemangioma.

▌ TUMORS OF FATTY TISSUE

Tumors of fatty tissue are seldom encountered in biopsied oral and pharyngeal soft tissues. When this does occur, the lesion is almost always benign and will represent a traumatic herniation of submuco-

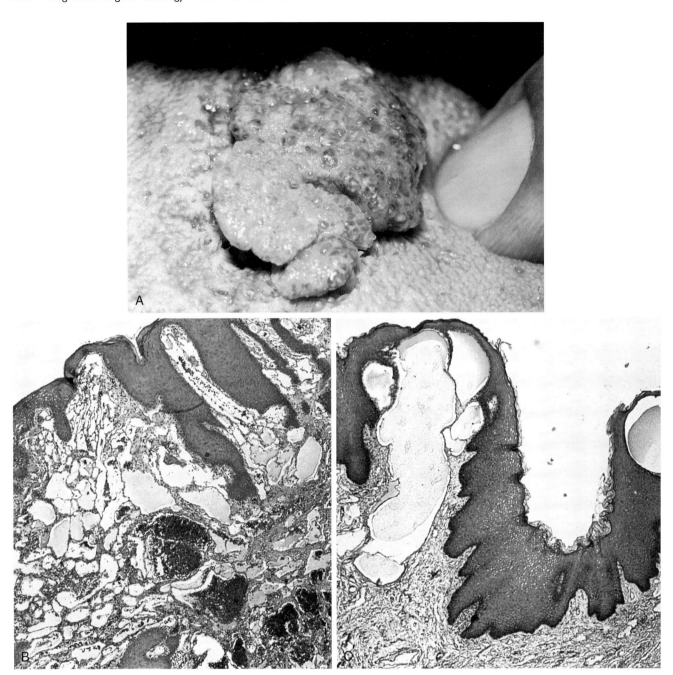

Figure 4–27. *A*, Oral lymphangioma frequently appears as a cluster of bubbles or blisters; *B*, lymph vessels are scattered throughout submucosal connective tissues with occasional vessels filled with blood; *C*, lesional vessels may show minimal separation from overlying epithelium.

sal adipose tissue, a developmental anomaly, or a true neoplasm. The frequency of these lesions in the adult or childhood populations is unknown.

Herniated Buccal Fat Pad

Many adults have a rather thick, diffuse layer of fatty tissue, the buccal fat pad (buccal sucking pad), between the submucosal fibrovascular stroma and the underlying masseter muscle of the buccal region, or between the masseter and buccinator muscles. This bilateral condition is common in infants and is occasionally seen in adults, especially in obese persons and persons with rounded faces. Acute trauma from biting the buccal tissues may rupture this fatty tissue, allowing a portion of it to herniate as a sessile or pedunculated submucosal mass that may be several centimeters across. Once

this occurs, the *herniated buccal fat pad* does not further increase in size but seems not to revert to normal.[7, 325–328] It must usually be surgically excised to prevent further injury of the resultant exophytic mass. The histopathology is that of normal, mature adipose tissue interspersed with a variable number of fibrous bands or trabeculae.[328]

Lipoma

The *lipoma* is a very common benign tumor of adipose tissue, but its presence in the oral and oropharyngeal region is relatively uncommon.[6–9, 329, 330] The first description of an oral lesion was provided in 1848 by Roux[331] in a review of alveolar masses; he referred to it as a "yellow epulis." Although most lesions are developmental anomalies, those that occur in the maxillofacial region usually arise late in life and are presumed to be neoplasms of adipocytes, occasionally associated with trauma. As with all fatty tissue, a lipoma will float on the surface of formalin rather than sink to the bottom of a biopsy specimen jar.

Clinical Features. The lipoma is a slowly enlarging, soft, smooth-surfaced mass of the submucosal tissues (Fig. 4–28A, see p. 173).[7, 329, 330] When superficial, there is a yellow surface discoloration. When well-encapsulated, tumors are freely movable beneath the mucosa, but less well-demarcated lesions are not movable. The lesion may be pedunculated or sessile and occasional cases show surface bosselation. The tumor has a less dense and more uniform appearance than surrounding fibrovascular tissues when it is transilluminated. Magnetic resonance imaging scans are very useful in the clinical diagnosis; computed tomography scans and ultrasonography are less reliable.

Few oral or pharyngeal lesions occur before the third decade of life and there is no gender predilection.[7, 330] Once present, a mucosal oral lipoma may increase to 5 to 6 cm over a period of years, but most cases are less than 3 cm in greatest dimension at diagnosis. Rarely, a lipoma will occur within maxillary bones or sinuses, but usually this entity is found in the buccal, lingual, or oral floor regions. Multiple head and neck lipomas have been observed in *neurofibromatosis, Gardner syndrome, encephalocraniocutaneous lipomatosis, multiple familial lipomatosis,* and *Proteus syndrome.*[7, 9] Generalized lipomatosis has been reported to contribute to unilateral facial enlargement in *hemifacial hypertrophy.*[332, 333]

Pathologic Features and Differential Diagnosis. The lipoma is composed predominantly of mature adipocytes, possibly admixed with collagenic streaks, and is often well demarcated from the surrounding connective tissues (Fig. 4–28B, see p. 173). A thin fibrous capsule may be seen and a distinct lobular pattern may be present. Quite often, however, lesional fat cells are seen to "infiltrate" into surrounding tissues, perhaps producing long, thin extensions of fatty tissue radiating from the central tumor mass. When located within striated muscle, this infiltrating variant is called *intramuscular lipoma (infiltrating lipoma),* but extensive involvement of a wide area of fibrovascular or stromal tissues might best be termed *lipomatosis.*

Occasional lesions exhibit excessive fibrosis between the fat cells *(fibrolipoma),* excess numbers of small vascular channels *(angiolipoma),* a myxoid background stroma *(myxoid lipoma, myxolipoma),* or areas with uniform spindle-shaped cells interspersed between normal adipocytes *(spindle cell lipoma).*[334–336] When spindle cells appear somewhat dysplastic or mixed with pleomorphic giant cells with or without hyperchromatic, enlarged nuclei, the term *pleomorphic lipoma* is applied.[337] When the spindled cells are of smooth muscle origin, the term *myolipoma* may be used, or *angiomyolipoma* when the smooth muscle appears to be derived from the walls of arterioles.

Rarely, chondroid or osseous metaplasia may be seen in a lipoma *(osteolipoma, ossifying lipoma, chondroid lipoma, ossifying chondromyxoid lipoma).*[338] When bone marrow is present, the term *myelolipoma* is used. Also on rare occasions, isolated ductal or tubular adnexal structures are scattered throughout fat lobules, in which case the term *adenolipoma* is applied. *Perineural lipoma* has also been reported.

On occasion, lipoma of the buccal mucosa cannot be distinguished from a *herniated buccal fat pad,* except by the lack of a history of sudden onset after trauma. Otherwise, lipoma of the oral and pharyngeal region is not difficult to differentiate from other lesions, although spindle cell and pleomorphic types must be distinguished from *liposarcoma.* When metaplastic calcified tissue is present, the lesion may be confused with *soft tissue chondroma* or *soft tissue osteoma.*

The benign neoplasm of brown fat, *hibernoma,* has been reported in the oral/pharyngeal region only rarely.[339] This childhood tumor is composed of lobules of highly vascular stroma admixed with three types of adipocytes: a large, univacuolated fat cell with a peripheral nucleus; a moderate-sized multivacuolated fat cell with

scanty granular, eosinophilic cytoplasm and a centrally located rounded nucleus; and a smaller cell with the same cytoplasm but with only small circular spaces representing fat microvacuoles.

A fat tumor composed of a central core of mature adipocytes and a peripheral envelope of cells containing variably sized fat vacuoles is called *lipoblastoma.*[340] Affected cells are smaller than normal, with one to four vacuoles, perhaps with a light, wispy cytoplasm between vacuoles. Some cells have nuclei centrally located, as seen in the moderately sized cells of hibernoma, whereas others show the nucleus to be pushed toward the cytoplasmic membrane (signet-ring cell). Mitotic activity is extremely rare and fibrous septa separate fat lobules in this tumor. An abnormality of the long arm of chromosome 8q11-13 is a rather consistent finding in the lesional cells.[341]

Treatment and Prognosis. Conservative surgical removal is the treatment of choice for oral lipoma, with occasional recurrences expected.[7, 329, 330] An infiltrating lipoma often must be simply debulked, a portion of the infiltrating fat being deliberately allowed to remain to preserve as much normal tissue as possible.

Liposarcoma

Liposarcoma, the malignancy of adipocytes, constitutes approximately 17% of all sarcomas, and 3% of all liposarcomas occur in the head and neck region, usually in the neck and cheek areas.[6, 342–349] Oral involvement is decidedly rare.[349] No well-established causative factor has been identified, although trauma has been implicated. Development from a pre-existing benign lipoma is very rare and most cases arise de novo.

Clinical Features. Oral liposarcoma can develop at any age but most cases occur in middle-aged individuals, with an average age of 45 years.[343, 346, 348] This is approximately a decade earlier than liposarcoma development in other anatomic sites. The tumor has a slight male predilection, but the number of reported cases is small and this may reflect a case-selection bias. The typical example is a slowly enlarging, painless, deep, moderately soft mass without surface ulceration or hemorrhage. Occasional cases grow with alarming rapidity, however, and these tend to metastasize very early as well. Any oral site may be affected, but the most commonly involved sites are the cheek, floor of mouth, lips, and soft palate.[343]

Transillumination may show an area of decreased density, but magnetic resonance imaging is the best imaging method for identifying and outlining the lesion. The fatty tissue of liposarcoma gives a bright signal on T1-weighted MRI scans, with progressively decreasing signal on T2-weighted images.[6, 349] Fat-suppression images show signal dropout within the neoplastic mass.

Pathologic Features and Differential Diagnosis. The liposarcoma demonstrates considerable microscopic variability. *Well-differentiated liposarcoma* represents 5% to 15% of all liposarcomas and is often so mature in appearance and so innocuous in its clinical behavior that some authorities advocate using the term *atypical lipoma* for those located in superficial dermal or mucosal regions.[6] The lesion is composed of broad sheets and streaks of adipocytes admixed with occasional lipoblasts, separated by fibrous septa containing spindle cells with hyperchromatic and mildly pleomorphic nuclei. Signet-ring cells are usually present and are important to the diagnosis; multivacuolar lipoblasts may be seen as well.

The size of available fat cells is variable and some lesions are infiltrated by a small to moderate number of chronic inflammatory cells *(well differentiated inflammatory liposarcoma).* Some tumors show lesional cells within a matrix of loose or moderately dense collagenic fibers *(well-differentiated sclerosing liposarcoma).* In the absence of inflammatory and sclerosing features, the term *well-differentiated "lipoma-like" liposarcoma* has been applied.

The less well-differentiated lesions are typically subclassified into one of four categories: myxoid, round cell, pleomorphic, or dedifferentiated liposarcoma.[6–8] The *myxoid liposarcoma* represents half of all liposarcomas and is composed of variably mature multivacuolar and univacuolar lipoblasts, often with numerous signet-ring types scattered throughout a myxomucinous stroma with a sparse or sometimes abundant fibrillar network. A delicate network of inter-twining small capillaries is also seen. The stroma is rich in nonsul-fated glycosaminoglycans and there is a lobular pattern to the tis-sue.[6] Lesional cells may be rounded or spindled, and in the less differentiated tumors the spindle forms may proliferate so exten-sively that the appearance of the tissue closely resembles the primi-tive mesenchymal proliferation of the *malignant mesenchymoma.* Most cases, however, are relatively well differentiated and the usual diagnostic dilemma is among *well-differentiated liposarcoma, myx-oid liposarcoma,* and *myxoid lipoma.* Multinucleated lipoblasts may be present in small numbers, as may mitotic figures. Focal chondroid and osseous metaplasia may be seen.

Round cell liposarcoma, also known as *poorly differentiated myxoid liposarcoma* represents 10% to 20% of all liposarcomas. This very aggressive variant is probably a poorly differentiated myx-oid liposarcoma, with many more cells, with a loss of the vascular network and lobular pattern, and with very little lipid within lesional cells. Transition toward myxoid liposarcoma and the occasional sig-net ring cell may be the key identifying feature. The round cells have a small to moderate amount of finely vacuolated or granular cyto-plasm and may appear epithelioid or pericytoid.

Pleomorphic liposarcoma represents 25% to 35% of all lipo-sarcomas and is characterized by a disorderly growth pattern, ex-treme cellularity, and extreme cellular pleomorphism, including bi-zarre giant cells.[6] Lesional cells are polygonal or stellate with pale eosinophilic cytoplasm and poorly demarcated cell boundaries. These are interspersed with giant lipoblasts containing greatly en-larged, very hyperchromatic, angular, or globular nuclei. The latter cells are reminiscent of the giant cells of *pleomorphic rhabdomyo-sarcoma* and *malignant fibrous histiocytoma.* Uncoalesced lipid droplets may be seen in the giant cells, but this is not common.

Dedifferentiated liposarcoma is characterized by an admixture of well-differentiated and poorly differentiated lipoblastic compo-nents. This is extremely rare in the oral region and is more common in the retroperitoneum and the extremities. The undifferentiated component can resemble a round cell or pleomorphic liposarcoma, and two thirds of cases bear a strong resemblance to *malignant fi-brous histiocytoma.*[6]

Stains for lipids are often useful in the diagnosis of liposar-coma, but this material may be scarce and is sometimes produced by unrelated mesenchymal and epithelial neoplasms. The mucinous matrix, when present, will stain with alcian blue and is metachro-matic with toluidine blue and cresyl violet stains; it is weakly posi-tive with Meyer's mucicarmine stain. Intracellular glycogen (diastase-sensitive, PAS positive) may be seen in some lesional cells. Adipocytes and lipoblasts react positively for vimentin and S-100 protein immunostains, but these vary in intensity and may not be ex-pressed in poorly differentiated lesions.[6–8] Smooth muscle actin may also be immunoreactive in some lesional cells and is present in all liposarcomas showing smooth muscle differentiation.

Treatment and Prognosis. Liposarcoma of the oral region is typically treated by wide local excision.[6–9, 344, 348] Radiotherapy may be used to control local recurrence and lessen the risk of metas-tasis. Five-year survival rates are similar to those of other anatomic sites and are very much dependent on lesional size and the histopathologic grade or subtype. Patients with well differentiated lesions have an 85% to 100% 5-year survival, whereas those with myxoid liposarcoma have a somewhat lesser survival rate (75–95%) and those with round cell and pleomorphic liposarcoma show an even worse survival rate (20–50%).[6, 348] Those with dedifferentiated liposarcoma have a 30% 5-year survival rate.

▮ NEURAL TUMORS

A variety of reactive proliferations and benign neoplasms of periph-eral nerves may be seen within the oral and pharyngeal soft tissues.

Except for the *traumatic neuroma,* these neural tumors are paradoxi-cally painless and nontender and seldom present serious clinical problems. Many of the head and neck examples, however, are asso-ciated with syndromes having very serious consequences, such as *neurofibromatosis* and *multiple mucosal neuroma syndrome.* Two as-sociated lesions, the *glial choristoma* and *juxtoral organ of Chievitz,* are discussed separately in this chapter's section on developmental anomalies.

Traumatic Neuroma

The *traumatic neuroma (amputation neuroma)* is a reactive prolif-eration of nerve fibers that occurs as a result of poor healing after damage to the peripheral nerve.[6–9, 350–352] The proximal portion of a severed nerve regenerates and attempts to re-establish its normal dis-tribution by sending axons toward the distal segment. When granu-lation or scar tissue interferes with this process, the regenerating fi-bers turn back on themselves and proliferate randomly to produce a mass somewhat akin to a "ball of worms." A similar phenomenon in an area of simple myelin destruction may produce a very small *nerve tuft* along the side of an axon.

Because many of the new nerve fibers lack myelin sheathing, aphactic or abnormal pain signals may be generated when mild physical pressure on the neuroma forces several adjacent nerve fi-bers into contact *(cross-talk).* Other abnormal sensations can be pro-duced, such that a patient may feel the presence of an amputated limb *(phantom limb)* or spontaneous pain *(phantom pain).* Within the bone, a traumatic neuroma may produce a toothache-like pain *(phantom toothache),* even after extraction of all teeth in the area.

Clinical Features. The traumatic neuroma of mucosal sur-faces tends to be a smooth-surfaced submucosal nodule of the men-tal foramen area, the lateral tongue, and the lower lip.[350] The lesion can occur at any age but is most common in middle-aged adults and is slightly more common in females than in males. It can occur within the jawbones after tooth extraction or other surgery, or it can occur within the oral submucosal tissues.[351] Intraosseous examples present as well-demarcated radiolucencies if they are visible at all.

At least two thirds of traumatic neuromas of the mouth and pharynx are nonpainful, but when pain is present, it may occur as a mild tenderness, a constant or intermittent aching, a burning sensa-tion, or a severe radiating pain.[7, 350] The neuroma of the mental fo-ramen area may be chronically painful because of constant irritation from overlying dentures.

Pathologic Features. The traumatic neuroma consists of a moderately loose fibrovascular stroma admixed with numerous in-tertwining or haphazardly arranged nerve fibers. The nerves them-selves are normal except for their tortuous and exuberant prolifera-tion and the frequent appearance of immaturity or "regeneration." Luxol fast blue stain will show some fibers to be myelinated while others are not. There is seldom an attempt toward encapsulation of this tumor, and tumor growth is rather asymmetrical. With matura-tion, perineuria form around the proliferated axons and the back-ground stroma may become quite densely fibrotic. Early lesions may demonstrate wallerian degeneration of recently severed nerve stumps incorporated into the proliferative mass.

Treatment and Prognosis. Traumatic neuroma is best treated by conservative surgical removal, but lesions associated with larger nerves may require selective microsurgical removal of the irregular neural mass.[7, 350] Occasional lesions recur.

Mucosal Neuroma

The *multiple endocrine neoplasia (MEN) syndromes* are character-ized by tumors of neuroendocrine origin.[4–8] The third of these to be reported, *MEN III syndrome,* also called *MEN IIB syndrome* or *mul-tiple mucosal neuroma syndrome,* was initially described by Wagen-mann[353] in 1922.

The disease is associated with adrenal *pheochromocytoma, medullary thyroid carcinoma,* diffuse alimentary tract *ganglioneuromatosis,* and multiple small submucosal neuroma nodules of the upper aerodigestive tract.[5, 354–359] The disease is inherited as an autosomal dominant trait, although many cases appear to be spontaneous mutations.

The affected individual has a tall, lanky, marfanoid body type, with a narrow face and perhaps with muscle wasting. The adrenal and thyroid tumors typically do not present until after puberty, whereas the oral mucosal neuromas usually develop during the first decade of life. *Mucosal neuromas* are extremely rare, perhaps unheard of, outside of the MEN III syndrome.[5, 359]

Clinical Features. The oral mucosal neuroma of this disease presents as a 2 to 7 mm yellowish-white, sessile, painless nodule of the lips, anterior tongue, and buccal commissures.[5, 357] Usually there are two to eight (or more) neuromas, with deeper lesions having normal coloration. There may be enough neuromas in the body of the lips to produce enlargement and a "blubbery lip" appearance. Similar nodules may be seen on the eyelids, sometimes producing eversion of the lid, and on the sclera. Facial skin, especially around the nose, may also be involved.

Abnormal laboratory values are part of this syndrome.[5, 359] When a medullary thyroid carcinoma is present, serum and urinary calcitonin levels are elevated. When a pheochromocytoma is present, there often is an increase in the serum levels of vanillylmandelic acid and altered epinephrine/norepinephrine ratios.

Pathologic Features and Differential Diagnosis. The mucosal neuroma is composed of a partially encapsulated aggregation or proliferation of nerves, often with thickened perineurium, intertwined with one another in a plexiform pattern (Fig. 4–29). This tortuous pattern of nerves is seen within a background of loose endoneurium-like fibrous stroma. Individual nerves flow in fascicles of two to three fibers and are histologically normal except for occasional hyperplasias and bulbous expansions.

Luxol fast blue staining will identify myelin sheathing of some fibers, and lesional cells react immunohistochemically for S-100 protein, collagen type IV, vimentin, neuron-specific enolase, and neural filaments.[5, 6] More mature lesions will react also for EMA, indicating a certain amount of perineurial differentiation. Early lesions have a stroma rich in acid mucopolysaccharides, and so will stain positively with alcian blue.

Inflammatory cells are not seen in the stroma and dysplasia is not present in the neural tissues. There may be close microscopic similarity with *traumatic neuroma,* but the streaming fascicles of mucosal neuroma are usually more uniform and the intertwining nerves of the traumatic neuroma lack the thick perineurium of the mucosal neuroma.

Treatment and Prognosis. The mucosal neuromas of this syndrome are asymptomatic and self limiting, and present no problem requiring treatment.[5, 357] They may, however, be surgically removed for esthetic purposes or if they are being constantly traumatized. The patient should be followed by an internist, endocrinologist, or other appropriate clinician relative to his or her potential adrenal or thyroid cancer. Because of the serious nature of the latter conditions, it is strongly suggested that other family members be evaluated for MEN III.

Palisaded Encapsulated Neuroma

A benign neural neoplasm, the *palisaded encapsulated neuroma (PEN, solitary circumscribed neuroma)* was first reported as a distinct entity in 1972.[6–8, 360–365] It is now recognized as one of the more common of the superficial nerve tumors of the head and neck region, although neural tumors in general are rather rare events in that anatomic site. The etiology of this lesion is unknown, but trauma is considered by some to induce or trigger its development. Nine of every 10 examples of PEN have been reported as facial lesions, usually from the region of the nose and midface.[8] Oral and pharyngeal lesions are not uncommon but are often misdiagnosed as *neurofibroma* or *neurilemoma.* The lesion is not associated with *MEN* syndromes.

Clinical Features. Oral examples of PEN are seen most frequently on the hard palate, although any oral or pharyngeal mucosal surface may be affected.[7, 362, 365] The diagnosis is typically made during the fifth through seventh decades of life, but many lesions have been present for years prior to biopsy and formal diagnosis. There is no gender predilection. The lesion usually presents as a sessile, smooth-surfaced nodule of less than 1 cm diameter; it may have a rubbery feel on palpation.

Pathologic Features. The PEN consists of interlacing bundles or fascicles of spindle cells (Schwann cells) with thin, wavy, pointed nuclei and with no dysplasia or mitotic activity. The cellular fascicles are typically four to six cells thick and are arranged in parallel streams in some areas, and nuclear palisading is seldom pronounced, as it is in *neurilemoma.* Nuclear pleomorphism and mitotic activity are not seen. Silver stains for axons and luxol fast blue stain for myelin will confirm the presence of neural tissue within the tumor, and the fascicles are immunoreactive for neural filaments.[365]

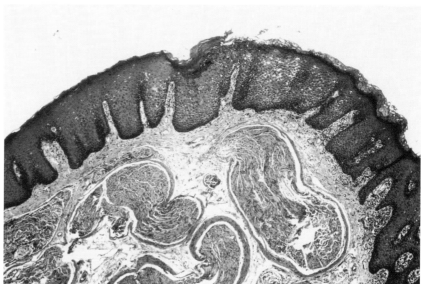

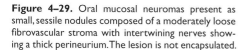

Figure 4–29. Oral mucosal neuromas present as small, sessile nodules composed of a moderately loose fibrovascular stroma with intertwining nerves showing a thick perineurium. The lesion is not encapsulated.

The neural tissue of this lesion is well circumscribed and usually encapsulated, but large areas of the periphery may lack a capsule, especially along the superficial aspects. Pseudoepitheliomatous hyperplasia of the overlying epithelium has been reported. Occasional lesions demonstrate areas reminiscent of the palisading Verocay bodies of Antoni A tissue in neurilemoma, but true Verocay bodies are not seen. This lesion should be differentiated from *neurilemoma* and *neurofibroma,* as described subsequently.

Treatment and Prognosis. The treatment for this self-limiting lesion is conservative excision, with few recurrences reported.[7, 362] Unlike neurofibroma and neurilemoma, the PEN is not a feature of *von Recklinghausen neurofibromatosis* or of *multiple mucosal neuroma syndrome (MEN IIB, MEN III).*

Neurilemoma

Neurilemoma (schwannoma) is a benign neoplasm of the Schwann cells of the neural sheath.[6–9, 366–371] At least a fourth, and perhaps as much as half of all cases of neurilemoma and *neurofibroma* occur in the head and neck region.[370] In some series, one fourth of the head and neck cases were found in patients with *von Recklinghausen neurofibromatosis (neurofibromatosis I).*

Clinical Features. The neurilemoma of the oral region is a slowly enlarging, painless submucosal nodule that is somewhat movable beneath the surface and rarely becomes larger than 2 cm in greatest diameter.[7, 366, 367, 370] It is most frequently diagnosed in the 25 to 55 year age group, but can occur at any age; there is no gender predilection. The tongue is the most frequent site of occurrence, perhaps resulting in macroglossia, but any oral site is susceptible. Almost all lesions are sessile with a normal surface coloration, but larger ones may be lobulated and dorsal tongue lesions may show a loss of papillae of the overlying epithelium.

Pathologic Features. The neurilemoma is characterized by two basic tissue types. Antoni type A tissue shows fascicles of spindle-shaped Schwann cells streaming around numerous acellular, eosinophilic areas surrounded by paralleled or palisaded spindled cells with blunt, elongated nuclei. The cells of these Verocay bodies all orient their long axes toward the acellular area, and the areas themselves are oval, linear, or serpiginous in shape. A low-power microscopic view of this tissue is reminiscent of an aerial view of soldiers aligned against each other across multiple battlefields.

The second tissue type, Antoni type B, lacks the organoid, homogeneous Verocay bodies and consists entirely of less cellular and more randomly arranged spindle cells in a loose, myxomatous stroma. Neurites usually cannot be demonstrated in either tissue type.

The tumor is typically encapsulated and the associated peripheral nerve may be seen in the microscopic section. Occasional older lesions show degenerative changes consisting of hemorrhage, hemosiderin deposition, mild chronic inflammatory cell infiltration, dense fibrosis, and nuclear pleomorphism. This *ancient neurilemoma* is benign but must be differentiated from *neurofibrosarcoma* and *malignant neurilemoma.*[372]

Treatment and Prognosis. The neurilemoma is treated by conservative surgical excision, with minimal risk of recurrence.[366, 370] Malignant transformation in untreated lesions has been reported but is uncommon. Patients with multiple neural tumors should be evaluated for von Recklinghausen neurofibromatosis or *MEN III.*

Neurofibroma

The most common of the peripheral nerve tumors is the benign *neurofibroma,* derived from an admixture of Schwann cells and perineural fibroblast proliferations.[4–9, 373–376] Multiple lesions are seen in persons with *von Recklinghausen neurofibromatosis (neurofibromatosis type I)* and certain melanotic macules are considered by some to be a variant of neurofibroma.[5, 377–379]

Clinical Features. The oral or pharyngeal neurofibroma is usually diagnosed in teenagers and young adults, although all ages are susceptible.[7, 373–376] There is no gender predilection and most examples arise from the tongue, buccal, or labial mucosa. The lesion presents as a slowly enlarging, painless, soft nodule that is readily movable if situated immediately beneath the mucosa but is less so when located in deeper tissues. Many lesions feel like a "bag of worms" on palpation.

Typically less than 2 cm in largest diameter at the time of diagnosis, some lesions have reached more than 8 cm in size, and even larger oral lesions have been reported in patients with von Recklinghausen neurofibromatosis.[375] Larger lesions may be lobulated or may produce a generalized local enlargement, such as macroglossia. Neurofibromas have been reported as well-demarcated radiolucencies within the jawbones, usually within the mandible, in patients with neurofibromatosis.

Von Recklinghausen neurofibromatosis is a hereditary condition that occurs in one of every 2000 to 3000 adults and is associated with multiple neurofibromas of the skin, mucous membranes, and visceral tissues.[5, 377, 378] Surface lesions may number in the hundreds and will vary from small, firm papules to huge, baggy, pendulous masses (elephantiasis neuromatosa); two thirds of affected individuals have only mild involvement.

Oral involvement in neurofibromatosis is seen in approximately 70% of cases, usually represented by a generalized enlargement of fungiform papillae of the tongue (50% of cases) and by one to three relatively small submucosal nodules of neurofibroma (25% of cases).[5, 377, 378] Pendulous examples of neurofibroma have not been reported for oral or pharyngeal sites.

Another feature of this syndrome is the presence of melanotic macules of the skin, called *café au lait* ("coffee with milk") spots. These macules are smooth, dark brown or tan, and measure from a few millimeters to several centimeters across. They are usually congenital but may develop during the first years of life; they do not occur on oral or pharyngeal mucosa. The macule is characterized by an increase in melanin pigment in the basal cell layer of the epidermis, but some authorities consider it to be a variant of neurofibroma.[379] Lisch nodules, translucent brown macules of the iris, are seen in almost all persons affected by neurofibromatosis. Various other anomalies affect the central nervous system and the skeleton, producing sometimes severe bony deformities, CNS tumors, macrocephaly, seizures, and mental deficiency.

Pathologic Features and Differential Diagnosis. The neurofibroma consists of a cellular proliferation of randomly arranged spindle-shaped cells with elongated, wavy nuclei and few, if any, of the Verocay bodies so characteristic of the *neurilemoma* (Fig. 4–30A&B). The neural cells are associated with a variable amount of background stroma, usually a loose fibrosis with areas of myxoid matrix. Occasional areas show lesional cells in a whorled pattern reminiscent of pacinian bodies or the storiform pattern of *fibrous histiocytoma.* Mast cells are often abundant and can be helpful in the diagnosis; these can be more readily demonstrated with the Giemsa or toluidine blue stains, or can be detected immunohistochemically using antibody to the serine proteinase, chymase.[380]

Sparsely distributed and usually small axons are frequently seen to traverse the tumor, especially with the use of silver stains. Tumorous proliferation may occur outside the perineurium, in which case there is poor demarcation from the surrounding fibrovascular tissues, or it may occur within the perineurium, resulting in a fibrous capsule or pseudoencapsulation of the neural mass.

Distinguishing the neurofibroma from benign fibrous proliferations is usually not difficult because the latter lack the unique wavy appearance of lesional cell nuclei. Those entities with myxoid stroma, especially the *myxoid lipoma, nodular fasciitis,* and *focal mucinosis,* are more problematic, but again lack the thin, wavy nuclei of the neurofibroma. *Palisaded encapsulated neuroma* usually has parallel cellular streams or fascicles, a feature uncommon in neurofibroma. Nuclear pleomorphism and mitotic activity is more-

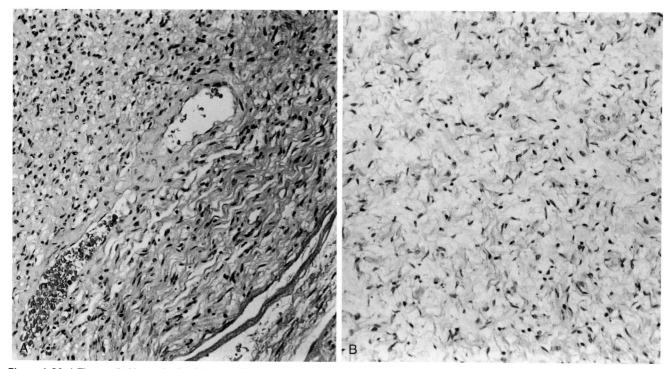

Figure 4–30. *A,* The spindled lesional cells of the neurofibroma often show thin wavy nuclei that are rounded when cut tangentially and are randomly oriented with a hint of streaming and whorling patterns. *B,* The background stroma may be quite myxoid, with spindled cells rather sparsely scattered.

over, quite unusual in the neurofibroma, thereby aiding in its differentiation from *malignant peripheral nerve sheath tumor.*

Treatment and Prognosis. Solitary neurofibroma not associated with a syndrome is surgically excised with minimal risk of recurrence. The malignant transformation potential of this tumor when not associated with a syndrome is minimal to nonexistent, but as many as 12% of persons affected by neurofibromatosis will develop cancer, usually *neurofibrosarcoma* or *malignant neurilemoma (malignant schwannoma)* transforming from a long-term neurofibroma of the skin of the trunk or extremities.[5, 381] Oral lesions in neurofibromatosis very seldom transform into sarcoma but may become large enough to interfere with proper function. Genetic counseling and evaluation of other family members should be performed for those suspected to be affected by a syndrome.

Malignant Peripheral Nerve Sheath Tumor

Malignant peripheral nerve sheath tumor (MPNST, malignant schwannoma, malignant neurilemoma) is now the preferred name for the spindle cell malignancy of peripheral nerve Schwann cells.[6, 8, 382–389] It represents approximately 10% of all soft tissue sarcomas and its diagnosis has been called "one of the most difficult and elusive diagnoses in soft tissue diseases."[6] It is found in at least 4% of patients with neurofibromatosis I, where its development is thought to be a multi-step, multi-gene process.[6, 381] Conversely, up to half of all cases of MPNST are diagnosed in persons with neurofibromatosis I. About one in ten cases are associated with irradiation. The tumor is usually found in the lower extremities, but one-ninth of all lesions occur in the head and neck region, usually associated with the large cranial nerves, especially the trigeminal nerve.[383] Intraosseous examples have been reported.[389]

Clinical Features. MPNST occurs usually in persons 20 to 50 years of age, but children and elderly persons may also be affected.[382–387] Lesions that develop in persons with neurofibromatosis I typically occur a decade or more earlier than those in non-syndrome patients.[381] The most common head and neck area of involvement is the neck, but when this tumor occurs in the mouth, it usually arises from the tongue or soft palate. There is a slight predilection toward males in sporadic cases, but within the subgroup of patients with neurofibromatosis I, 80% of lesions are found in males.

The oral lesion appears as a bosselated, usually sessile, circumscribed submucosal mass that may be associated with pain or paresthesia, or with muscle weakness and atrophy.[382, 383] Two thirds of lesions are larger than 5 cm at the time of diagnosis, but the tumor is considered to be a slow-growing one. At surgery, attachment to a major nerve trunk is not unusual and the surgeon may notice cystic degeneration or hemorrhage within the lesional stroma.

Pathologic Features and Differential Diagnosis. The MPNST resembles routine *fibrosarcoma* in its overall organization, but the spindled lesional cells demonstrate the wavy or comma-shaped outline and nuclear contour of Schwann cells. Cellular and nuclear pleomorphism may be quite pronounced and mitotic activity is usually high. The cytoplasm of lesional cells is usually indistinct and slightly eosinophilic. The spindle cells form into tightly packed bundles or fascicles, although these typically show greater variation than the fascicles of fibrosarcoma. Densely cellular areas are typically interspersed with hypocellular and myxoid regions in which the spindle cells are much less organized but may be focally arranged into nondescript whorled patterns, similar to the pacinian body-like areas found in the *neurofibroma.* An anaplastic MPNST does occur but is rare.

Nuclear palisading may be a striking feature but is not seen in approximately half of all cases, and when present is found only in scattered, focal areas. Other distinctive but uncommon histopathologic features include hyalinized cords surrounded by rounded lesional cells (in cross-section these resemble rosettes), perineural and intraneural spread of tumor, and lesional proliferation or herniation into the lumina of small vessels. Heterotopic islands of bone, cartilage, skeletal muscle, or mucous glands are seen in more than 10% of MPNST lesions.

The MPNST may be classified into three major categories with *epithelioid, mesenchymal,* or *glandular* characteristics. The epithelioid variant demonstrates plump, rounded or ovoid epithelioid cells scattered throughout the spindled lesional cells, usually in rather small numbers and in well-defined clusters. These cells may have vesicular or hyperchromatic nuclei and may bear slight resemblance to the cells of the *amelanotic melanoma.*

Some MPNST lesions show rhabdomyoblastic differentiation leading to the common use of the diagnostic term *Triton tumor.* The spindle cells are interspersed with large, plump, rounded, or strap cells with eosinophilic, fibrillar cytoplasm and with cross-striations in the cytoplasm. These cells may be clustered and must be distinguished from simple entrapment of striated muscles fibers.

The glandular MPNST contains areas with usually well-differentiated ductal structures lined by simple, stratified, cuboidal or columnar epithelial cells with occasional goblet cells. The lumina may contain PAS-positive, diastase-resistant mucus.

Rare MPNST cases contain multiple sarcomatous tissue types, especially *osteosarcoma, chondrosarcoma,* and *angiosarcoma.* These have sometimes been indistinguishable from the *malignant mesenchymoma* of soft tissue.

The following antigens can be used to identify nerve sheath differentiation: S-100 protein, Leu-7, myelin basic protein.[6, 388] S-100 immunoreactivity is focal and scattered in 50% to 90% of MPNSTs; diffuse reactivity suggests a benign neural tumor. The other two antigens show immunoreactivity in approximately half of the tumors. With electron microscopic examination, the spindled lesional cells are seen to have non-tapering, branching cytoplasmic processes extending for great distances from the cell body; these contain microtubules and neurofilaments. In well-differentiated lesions, the processes are covered with basal laminae.

As previously stated, most MPNSTs resemble fibrosarcoma and may require immunohistochemistry and electron microscopic evaluation to discern useful diagnostic differences. The other sarcomas most closely resembling this tumor are *leiomyosarcoma* and *monophasic synovial sarcoma.* In the oral cavity, the synovial sarcoma is so rare as to be excluded from the differential diagnosis, whereas the spindle cell of the leiomyosarcoma has a more distinct eosinophilic cytoplasm and a quite blunted nucleus. The cytoplasm of the latter cell is, moreover, fuchsinophilic, contains a moderate amount of PAS-positive glycogen, and demonstrates longitudinal striations with Masson trichrome staining.

Distinguishing the MPNST from a benign nerve sheath tumor is usually not difficult, but some neurofibromas may be quite cellular and may contain occasional pleomorphic cells. In such cases, the presence or absence of mitotic activity is usually the determining feature.

Treatment and Prognosis. The MPNST of the oral region is treated by wide surgical excision, but local recurrence is a common occurrence and hematogenous metastasis occurs in at least half of treated cases.[7, 382, 389] The tumor is resistant to radiotherapy and chemotherapy, and those occurring in neurofibromatosis I behave in a more aggressive fashion than those not associated with the syndrome. Overall, the 5-year survival rate for MPNST is 40% to 75%.[6, 381]

Granular Cell Tumor and Malignant Granular Cell Tumor

It is not clear whether *granular cell tumor (granular cell myoblastoma, granular cell schwannoma)* is a true neoplasm, a developmental anomaly, or a trauma-induced proliferation.[6–8, 390–397] The basic cell of origin is now thought to be neural, although past reports frequently indicated an origin from striated muscle, or less frequently an origin from histiocytes, fibroblasts, or pericytes.[4–9, 394, 397] The tumor is widely distributed throughout the body, but more than half of all cases occur in the oral cavity.[392] The other head and neck site likely to be involved is the larynx.

Malignant variants represent approximately 1% of all cases, with some representing neoplasia in *Cowden syndrome (multiple hamartoma syndrome).*[5, 395] However, other authors consider these malignancies to be simply variants of the distinctive and rare *alveo-*

lar soft part sarcoma (ASPS), a look-alike malignancy composed largely of granular epithelioid cells organized in alveolar-like nests.[5, 7, 398–401] Once considered an organoid variant of malignant granular cell tumor or a *malignant nonchromaffin paraganglioma,* ASPS also has immunohistochemical features of skeletal muscle. Its true histogenesis, however, remains debatable and it is included here only for purposes of convenience. Approximately one in four lesions occur in the head and neck region, usually the oral cavity, pharynx, and orbit.[398, 401] The most common location, however, is the thigh.[6]

Clinical Features. More than a third of all granular cell tumors occur on the lingual dorsum, usually as a sessile, painless, somewhat firm, immovable nodule less than 1.5 cm in greatest diameter.[390, 392, 393] Lesions often demonstrate a pallor or a yellowish discoloration and typically have a smooth surface (Fig. 4–31A, see p. 174). When it occurs on the lingual dorsum, the surface papillae are separated one from another but do not usually disappear.

Other oral and pharyngeal sites of involvement include the soft palate, uvula, labial mucosa, oral floor, and gingiva. There is no gender predilection for oral cases, but overall almost twice as many cases are diagnosed in women as in men. The lesion is typically diagnosed between the ages of 30 and 60, but it can arise at any age.[394] As many as 15% of patients will have granular cell tumors of multiple anatomic sites, with as many as 50 individual lesions in one patient.[391, 395]

Oral malignant granular cell tumor is rare but has been reported to grow rapidly, to become ulcerated and bosselated, and to achieve a size greater than 4 to 5 cm by the time of diagnosis. It usually occurs in young adults.

Alveolar soft part sarcoma of the head and neck region accounts for 25% of all such sarcomas and has a decided predilection for children and young adults, especially females.[398, 399, 401] More peripheral lesions tend to occur in older individuals. Oral lesions are usually found in the tongue and the typical case is a slowly enlarging, asymptomatic, submucosal mass.[401]

Pathologic Features. The granular cell of diagnostic necessity is a large polygonal, oval, or bipolar cell with abundant, fine, or coarsely granular eosinophilic cytoplasm, and a small, pale-staining or vesicular nucleus acentrically located in the cell (Fig. 4–31B&C, see p. 174). The cell membrane is moderately distinct, and some cells may contain large clumps of the granular cytoplasmic material, perhaps with clear haloes surrounding the clumps. Ultrastructural studies have described the cytoplasmic granules as autophagic vacuoles containing cellular debris, including mitochondria and fragmented endoplasmic reticulum, as well as myelin.[6, 394]

Granular cells often occur in ribbons separated by fibrous septa, giving the appearance of infiltrating or "invading" into underlying tissues, especially muscle, with the bipolar shape being more frequently noted at the leading edge. The cells may also appear to be streaming off from or metaplastically arising from underlying muscle fibers. Older lesions tend to become desmoplastic with a few scattered nests of granular cells in a densely fibrotic background.[390] Granular cells demonstrating nuclear enlargement, hyperchromatism and pleomorphism, or with mitotic activity or increased cellularity, are elements of the malignant variant of this tumor.

The more oval granular cells near the surface tend to occur in broad sheets with minimal background stroma. They have a remarkable resemblance to macrophages and are S-100 protein positive with immunostaining.[388, 391] Immunohistochemistry will also be reactive for NSE, laminin, and various myelin proteins. Staining is negative for neurofilament proteins and GFAP. The interstitial cells stain for myelin protein.

The granular cells of oral and pharyngeal lesions typically extend to the surface epithelium, where they often induce a remarkable *pseudoepitheliomatous hyperplasia.* The pathologist must be very cautious about misdiagnosing this as well-differentiated *squamous cell carcinoma* and, almost by definition, a carcinoma-like surface lesion with underlying granular cells should be considered to be a benign, reactive change. No granular cell tumor of the mouth has yet been associated with a true squamous cancer, and the lingual dorsum is one of the oral sites least likely to develop such a cancer. The inductive mechanism responsible for the pseudoepitheliomatous hyperplasia is poorly understood, but it is seen in several other head and neck lesions, most notably *histoplasmosis* and other deep fungal infections, *median rhomboid glossitis (posterior atrophic candidiasis),* and *keratoacanthoma.*

The malignant granular cell tumor has two distinct variations or subtypes. The first variant has a benign histopathology, not different from a typical granular cell tumor except for increased mitotic activity and mild nuclear pleomorphism. The clinical features of large size, rapid growth, and surface ulceration must, therefore, be used to arrive at a malignant diagnosis, and the pathologist should carefully evaluate the lesional periphery for signs of true invasion. The second variant shows transition from typical benign granular cells to pleomorphic granular cells to pleomorphic nongranular spindle cells and giant cells with numerous mitotic figures. Malignant granular cell tumors are often negative for immunoreactivity for S-100 protein, NSE, and vimentin.

The histopathology of ASPS is remarkably uniform from one tumor to the next, being characterized by organoid or nest-like clusters of epithelioid cells with a central loss of cellular cohesion resulting in a pseudoalveolar pattern.[398–401] Cell nests are separated by thin-walled, sinusoidal vascular spaces. Although the clusters vary somewhat in size, they do not demonstrate the irregular alveolar pattern of *alveolar rhabdomyosarcoma.* The lesional cell is large and polygonal with a distinct cell border, a vesicular nucleus, and dense, abundant granular, eosinophilic, or vacuolated cytoplasm. There is minimal variation in size and shape between cells and mitotic activity is sparse. Vascular invasion is a frequent finding. Reticulin stains will enhance the organoid arrangement of the tumor cells and the cells typically contain PAS-positive, diastase-resistant, rod-shaped crystals.[400]

Treatment and Prognosis. Conservative excision is the treatment of choice for granular cell tumor. Recurrence is seen in fewer than 7% of cases thus treated, even if granular cells extend beyond the surgical margins of the biopsy sample.[7, 390, 394] A few reported metastasizing granular cell tumors have appeared to be histologically benign, and for this reason, tumors that recur, grow rapidly, or reach a size greater than 5 cm should be viewed with grave suspicion.[397]

The malignant granular cell tumor and the ASPS are treated by wide surgical excision, but lung, brain, and skeletal metastases tend to occur early and frequently in the former lesion, while occurring much later in the ASPS. Oral lesions carry a better prognosis than those elsewhere, and the overall 5-year survival rate is approximately 65%.[10, 399, 401]

MUSCLE TUMORS

Leiomyoma

The benign neoplasm of smooth muscle, the *leiomyoma,* is rare in the upper aerodigestive tract, being far more common in the genitalia, skin (*leiomyoma cutis,* arising from pilar arrector muscles), and gastrointestinal tract.[4–8, 402–409] Leiomyomas of the head and neck region probably arise from vascular smooth muscle and almost all cases fall into one of two general types, *solid leiomyoma* (sometimes referred to as the *leiomyoma of deep soft tissue*) and *vascular leiomyoma (angiomyoma, angioleiomyoma).*[405, 406] The latter accounts for almost three fourths of all oral cases, and rare examples of a third type, *epithelioid leiomyoma (leiomyoblastoma)* have been reported.[409]

Clinical Features. Leiomyoma of the head and neck region occurs at all ages and has no gender predilection.[403, 404, 409] It typically presents as a slowly enlarging, asymptomatic, firm submucosal mass or nodule, although occasional lesions are tender or painful, especially the vascular leiomyoma.[406] The lesion may continue to slowly enlarge for several years and may reach several centimeters in diameter, although most lesions are quite small at biopsy. The solid leiomyoma routinely appears normal in color, but the vascular lesion often exhibits a blue or red discoloration. Tumors usually occur as single lesions of the tongue, lips, palate, and buccal mucosa, but 20% occur on other mucosal sites.[404] Rare examples of *intravenous* and *disseminated leiomyomatosis* have been reported, but not from the head and neck regions.

Pathologic Features and Differential Diagnosis. All forms of leiomyoma are well encapsulated and show little cellular pleomorphism or mitotic activity. The solid tumor is composed of interlacing bundles of spindle-shaped smooth muscle cells with elongated, blunt-ended, pale-staining nuclei (Fig. 4–32). Nuclei may be palisaded and must then be differentiated from *neurilemoma,* a task usually made easy by the lack of Verocay bodies and wavy, thin, spindled nuclei. Lesions are rather cellular, but collagenic strands often separate the streaming bundles of tumor cells, and occasional leiomyomas have a prominent fibroblastic or myxoid component.

Older and larger solid tumors may show degenerative changes, even dystrophic calcifications similar to psammoma bodies. The angiomyoma demonstrates numerous tortuous blood vessels with hyperplastic smooth muscle walls and with intertwining bundles of smooth muscle cells between the vessels. The smooth muscle cells often appear to swirl away from the vessel and may demonstrate perinuclear vacuolization. Adipose cells may be intermixed with tumor

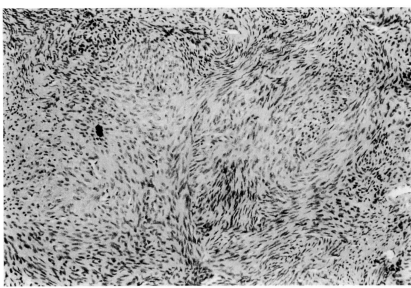

Figure 4–32. The leiomyoma shows interlacing bundles of spindle-shaped smooth muscle cells with cigar-shaped nuclei.

cells and the lesional vessels typically lack internal and external elastic laminae. These lesions have a remarkable lack of morphologic variation between cases.

The tumor cells of the rare *palisaded myofibroblastoma,* of course, are derived from myofibroblasts, modified smooth muscle cells, usually those within a lymph node.[408] The cells are typically palisaded and the tumor almost always demonstrates rather unique eosinophilic bands and islands of acellular collagen (amianthoid fibers).

Diagnosis is rarely difficult, but the leiomyoma must be differentiated from *nodular fasciitis, myxoma, neurilemoma, fibrous histiocytoma (dermatofibroma),* and hamartomatous aggregates of smooth muscle tissues. The smooth muscle nature of the spindle cells can be confirmed by Masson's trichrome stain as well as positive immunohistochemical staining for smooth muscle or muscle specific actin and desmin. Myofibrils can be demonstrated by Mallory's phosphotungstic acid (PTAH) stain.

Treatment and Prognosis. Conservative surgical excision is the definitive treatment for leiomyoma.[404, 409] Very few recurrences have been reported.

Leiomyosarcoma

Leiomyosarcoma is a rare malignancy of the oral and pharyngeal region.[410–415] It arises from smooth muscle cells, especially those found in blood vessel walls, and from undifferentiated mesenchymal cells.[6] Often, the tumor completely obliterates its origin in blood vessel walls. The epithelioid variant, called *malignant leiomyoblastoma* or *epithelioid leiomyosarcoma,* is most prevalent in the gastrointestinal and genitourinary tracts and has rarely been reported in oral or pharyngeal locations.[414]

Clinical Features. Oral leiomyosarcoma typically presents as a painless, lobulated, fixed mass of the submucosal tissues in a middle-aged or older individual.[7, 412, 414] It is exceedingly rare in children and often has a rubbery or semi-firm consistency to palpation. Lesions are usually less than 2 cm in diameter at diagnosis and are slow-growing, but secondary ulceration of the mucosal surface has been reported.

Pathologic Features. Leiomyosarcoma is composed of fascicles of interlacing spindle-shaped cells with abundant eosinophilic cytoplasm and moderately large, blunt-ended nuclei, often with mild atypia. Cellularity and cellular differentiation can vary considerably between tumors and between different areas of the same tumor. The well-differentiated lesion shows the spindled cells streaming or interweaving in fascicles in a fashion similar to that seen in *leiomyoma.* Nuclear palisading may be seen in several areas of the tumor, as may ischemic areas of stromal fibrosis and hyalinization.

Eosinophilic myofibrils are occasionally noted but are much more readily discerned with the Masson trichrome stain (bright pink) or the PTAH stain (deep blue-purple). Increased mitotic activity is commonly seen, as are hyperchromatic nuclei. The presence of mitoses is valuable for separating benign from malignant smooth muscle neoplasms, and numbers as low as 2 per 10 high-power fields have been associated with metastasis.

Lesional cells in poorly differentiated leiomyosarcoma are less elongated, more fusiform or rounded, enlarged, and more pleomorphic. Hyperchromatism of nuclei is often pronounced and numerous normal and abnormal mitotic figures are scattered throughout the lesion. Focal areas may contain giant cells with multiple, pleomorphic, even bizarre nuclei. The stroma is typically sparse, but cellular streaming is usually far less regular than in the low-grade lesions, although the fascicles may be as uniform as those of well-differentiated tumors. There occasionally are perinuclear vacuoles, presumably from dissolving glycogen. Hemorrhage, focal necrosis, increased vascularity, and focal myxoid change are not uncommon features of poorly differentiated lesions.

Epithelioid leiomyosarcoma demonstrates numerous rounded epithelioid cells with either eosinophilic or clear cytoplasm. These cells seldom display obvious myoblastic differentiation and are easily demonstrated with the PAS-diastase reaction; electron microscopy will usually show the classic features of leiomyoblasts.[413] Pleomorphism may be minimal or extreme, and mitotic activity is often the key to determining whether a smooth muscle tumor is malignant: lesions with 5 or more mitotic figures per 10 high-power fields should definitely be considered malignant, but those with a lesser number are also probable sarcomas.

As with other leiomyosarcomas, the epithelioid variant has glycogen granules demonstrated with PAS staining, and the cells appear bright-red with the Masson's trichrome staining of intracellular myofibrils. Longitudinal striations of myofibrils may be seen within lesional cells with the PTAH stain and reticulin staining of well-differentiated lesions will demonstrate a delicate meshwork of reticulin fibers surrounding individual tumor cells (or clusters of tumor cells, in the case of epithelioid lesions). Well-differentiated lesions are likely to be immunoreactive for desmin, alpha smooth muscle actin, and muscle-specific actin (see Table 4–4).

Treatment and Prognosis. Radical surgery is the treatment of choice for leiomyosarcoma, with adjunctive chemotherapy or radiotherapy used occasionally. The prognosis is poor, with numerous recurrences and distant metastases.[412, 414] The exact location of the tumor, especially relating to the surgeon's ability to adequately remove it, appears to be almost as important in determining the prognosis as tumor size at diagnosis. Overall 5-year survival is approximately 35% to 50%.[6, 414]

Rhabdomyoma

Adult rhabdomyoma, the benign neoplasm of striated muscle, is more common in the head and neck region than in any other anatomic site, but it is still a rare neoplasm of the maxillofacial region.[4–8, 416–421] The *fetal rhabdomyoma* was first reported on the tongue in 1897 and is considered to be a developmental lesion, not a neoplasm.[6, 419] It has been reported in persons affected by the *basal cell nevus (Gorlin) syndrome.*[422] The term *rhabdomyoma* is also used to describe a hamartomatous cardiac mass associated with *tuberous sclerosis.*[6]

Clinical Features. The adult form of rhabdomyoma occurs primarily in middle-aged and older individuals, usually (70% of cases) in males.[6, 418] The most frequent head and neck sites of involvement are the pharynx and the oral cavity, although laryngeal lesions have also been reported.[417, 421] Within the mouth, the oral floor is most often affected; pharyngeal lesions occur most frequently in the base of the tongue and the soft palate.

Fetal rhabdomyoma usually occurs in newborns and young children, but the lesion has been reported in patients as old as 50 years of age.[419] This type also has a strong male predilection, but cases are usually found within the muscles of the face and the preauricular region, not in the mouth.

Both tumor types present as a nodule or submucosal mass that can become several centimeters in size. Multinodular tumors have been described, with two or more discrete nodules closely adjacent to one another.[420] Rarely, separate tumors may be found at different anatomic sites.

Pathologic Features. The adult rhabdomyoma is composed of an encapsulated mass of large, uniform, polygonal cells with granular eosinophilic cytoplasm. Vacuoles beneath the cell membrane often give the cytoplasm a stellate or "spider web" appearance. With careful observation, cells with cross-striations can be found in almost all cases. A fibrous stroma is present and mitotic activity is extremely low. Many cases demonstrate occasional degeneration vacuoles or clear spaces between the tumor cells.

The fetal rhabdomyoma is composed of less mature, somewhat pleomorphic, polygonal muscle cells admixed with spindle-shaped cells. This type is typically more cellular than the adult type and often has a myxoid stroma. Mitotic activity is minimal, but the more pleomorphic examples can be mistaken for *rhabdomyosarcoma.*

Cross-striations and crystalline structures are more readily identified with the PTAH stain, and oil red O staining will often reveal intracellular lipid. Lesional cells are immunoreactive with myoglobin, desmin, and alpha-smooth muscle actin.

Treatment and Prognosis. Both variants of rhabdomyoma are treated by conservative surgical excision.[6, 416–420] Recurrence has been reported but is uncommon. Malignant transformation has not been reported.

Rhabdomyosarcoma

The first published example of *rhabdomyosarcoma,* the malignancy of striated muscle, was probably a tongue lesion reported in 1854.[423] The head and neck region is a likely site for this neoplasm to originate, and tumors from this site generally occur at a younger age than do rhabdomyosarcomas of other sites. Although an uncommon lesion, this tumor is among the most common head and neck cancers in young persons.[423–430] Congenital cases have been reported.[424, 428]

Clinical Features. Oral and pharyngeal rhabdomyosarcoma is typically a rapidly enlarging, painless submucosal mass in children and young adults (mean age at diagnosis: 20 years).[10, 423–429] It is rare after 45 years of age. There is a slight male predilection (1.5:1.0 male:female ratio). The tumor surface may be smooth or lobulated, sometimes botryoid or grape-cluster in appearance, and the tumor becomes fixed to surrounding tissues at an early stage. Very few patients have waited beyond 6 months for a diagnosis; most present for evaluation within 1 to 2 months of tumor onset.[10, 429]

Pathologic Features and Differential Diagnosis. Rhabdomyosarcoma is subdivided into three general types, often with combined features, and there is little variation in biologic behavior between the types. The majority of head and neck lesions are *embryonal rhabdomyosarcoma,* with small, round or oval tumor cells resembling embryonal or developing voluntary muscle cells.[7] These cells have a finely granular eosinophilic cytoplasm with infrequent cells demonstrating fasciculation or cross-striations. There often is a fibrillar material imparting a clear zone around the nucleus and the nucleus itself is typically enlarged. The more well-differentiated tumors demonstrate elongated, strap-shaped or tadpole-shaped rhabdomyoblasts. Occasional giant cells with enlarged or multiple nuclei can be seen, as can muscle-like cells with rather bizarre nuclear and cellular shapes. Mitotic figures are often seen and may be abnormal, but are not necessary to the diagnosis. The background stroma consists of moderately loose to dense fibrous tissue and may be quite scant. A background of poorly differentiated ovoid mesenchymal cells is frequently noted and myxoid zones are commonly seen in the stroma.

Alveolar rhabdomyosarcoma is comprised of relatively small, poorly differentiated round and oval cells aggregated into irregular clusters or nests separated by fibrous septa. Degenerated cells in the center of the clusters show a decided lack of cohesiveness, whereas the peripheral cells adhere in a single layer to the septal walls. Multinucleated giant cells may be seen and mitotic figures are common and sometimes bizarre. It is differentiated from the *alveolar soft part sarcoma* by its less regular tissue pattern and more pleomorphic cells. An occasional variant, referred to as the *botryoid type,* demonstrates a diffuse myxoid or mucoid matrix with sparsely scattered primitive mesenchymal cells. The characteristic feature of this type is a peripheral zone of increased cellularity, sometimes known as the "cambium layer."

Pleomorphic rhabdomyosarcoma shows randomly arranged eosinophilic cells with considerable variation in cell size and shape, as well as variation in nuclear size and shape. The pleomorphic cells are often admixed with small, primitive mesenchymal cells. This tumor is often so undifferentiated that the identification of the cell of origin is difficult or impossible. Positive immunostains for desmin and myoglobin are very helpful in such cases.

Regardless of the histologic subtype, special stains are often quite useful for differentiating rhabdomyosarcoma from other neoplasms. The trichrome stain is especially useful because it colors rhabdomyoblasts bright red while myofilaments and cross-striations have fuchsinophilic properties, also highlighted by PTAH (deep purple color). Myxoid stroma may be positive for hyaluronidase with acid mucopolysaccharide staining, although many other tumors also have positive stroma with these stains.

The most useful immunoreactions are toward myoglobin and anti-skeletal muscle actin.[431, 432] Antibodies to desmin and myosin will also be reactive, but cannot differentiate rhabdomyosarcoma from *leiomyosarcoma* (see Table 4–4). Desmin is more reactive than myoglobin in poorly differentiated rhabdomyosarcoma.

The most problematic tumors to differentiate from alveolar rhabdomyosarcoma are neuroblastoma, lymphoma, soft tissue Ewing's sarcoma, and undifferentiated small cell carcinoma. The *neuroblastoma* has a much more uniform and diffuse distribution of lesional cells and often contains rosettes with neurofilament cores. It also is nonreactive for desmin, myoglobin, and skeletal muscle actin, as are the *lymphomas, Ewing's sarcoma,* and the carcinoma. The latter is an especially important distinction because *oat cell carcinoma* can present with a rather distinctive pseudoalveolar pattern.

Pleomorphic rhabdomyosarcoma must be differentiated from other pleomorphic sarcomas such as *pleomorphic liposarcoma* and *pleomorphic MFH,* and the pathologist must also be careful not to confuse degenerated or metaplastic rhabdomyoblasts in other sarcomas, especially the *Triton tumor (malignant peripheral nerve sheath tumor),* the *malignant mesenchymoma* and *carcinosarcoma.* The latter malignancies must demonstrate an obvious component, somewhere in the specimen, of their classic histopathologic appearance.

Treatment and Prognosis. Rhabdomyosarcoma is treated by radical surgical excision followed by multi-agent chemotherapy, usually a combination of vincristine, dactinomycin, and cyclophosphamide.[7, 426, 431] Postoperative radiotherapy is used for those cases that cannot be completely resected. Five-year survival rates have improved dramatically from less than 10% prior to the 1960s to 65% today.[6] Stage I lesions have an even better prognosis (80%). Metastasis, when it occurs, is via either blood or lymphatic vessels, usually to cervical lymph nodes, lungs, bones, or brain.

▌ BENIGN EPITHELIAL PROLIFERATIONS

Many of the biopsied lesions of the oral mucosa represent generic or unique proliferations of the stratified squamous epithelium, with or without inductive changes of the underlying stroma. Most of these entities are innocuous enough in clinical appearance but are removed for microscopic evaluation to rule out early malignancy. These proliferations fall into three natural subtypes: papillary masses, broad verruciform excesses of surface keratin, and flat hyperplasias of the keratin or the spindous cell layer. Many lesions have overlapping features both clinically and microscopically. Therefore, close communication between the surgeon and the pathologists is necessary to establish the most appropriate diagnosis. With all such lesions, however, the primary objective is to evaluate the epithelium for dysplasia or signs of invasion.

Papillary and Verruciform Masses

Papillary and verruciform epithelial proliferations are quite common in the oral and paraoral region, representing at least 3% of biopsied oral lesions.[1–3] Many are thought to be induced by viral infection of the epithelium, especially from human papillomavirus (HPV). HPV encompasses a group of double-stranded DNA viruses of the papovavirus subgroup A capable of integration with host DNA. At the present time there are more than 68 known HPV subtypes, many which are associated with lesions of the head and neck. These viruses often can be identified by in situ hybridization, immunohistochemistry, and polymerase chain reaction techniques, but are seldom visible with routine histopathologic staining.

Additional focal epithelial proliferations are either neoplastic or of unknown origin. Some are malignancies, discussed elsewhere in this text (see Chapters 2 and 6), while others mimic malignant epithelial changes. The pathologist must be ever alert for these distinctions, which are often very subtle ones.

Squamous Papilloma

Of the several types of papillomas, the one occurring in the mouth and oropharynx is almost always the squamous papilloma.[7, 434–438] It is the fourth most common oral mucosal mass and is found in 4 of every 1000 U.S. adults (see Table 4–1).[2] Accounting for 3% to 4% of all biopsied oral soft tissue lesions, this entity was first reported as a gingival "wart" by Tomes[127] in 1848 and is a localized, benign HPV-induced epithelial hyperplasia.[426–431] The virus subtypes most often isolated from oral papillomas, HPV-6 and HPV-11, are not among those associated with malignancy or precancer.[438] Moreover, although all HPV lesions are infective, the squamous papilloma appears to have an extremely low virulence and infectivity rate; it does not seem to be contagious.[7]

It is important to recognize that the squamous papilloma of the mouth behaves differently from those of the nasal, paranasal, and laryngeal regions. Although the others are clinically and microscopically identical to their oral counterparts, they have a much higher recurrence rate, are almost always multiple, and will often proliferate continuously over time.[7] Laryngeal papillomas may, in fact, be so relentlessly proliferative that they cause life-threatening asphyxiation, and some worry about malignant transformation in long-standing cases.[9, 10, 439]

That said, it is also important to remember that, in rare circumstances, an innocuous oral squamous papilloma may herald the serious precancer *proliferative verrucous leukoplakia.*[440] Papillomas of the head and neck region with special histopathologic features, such as *schneiderian papillomas,* have their own biologic behaviors, but are not discussed in this section because they do not occur in the mouth.

Verruca vulgaris, condyloma acuminatum, verruciform xanthoma, and some of the oral masses of *Heck's disease* and *multiple hamartoma syndrome* may be clinically indistinguishable from squamous papilloma, as may multilobulated soft tissue lesions with a mulberry appearance, such as *giant cell fibroma, pyogenic granuloma* without surface ulceration, and *papillary hyperplasia.* In addition, extensive coalescing papillary lesions *(papillomatosis)* of the oral mucosa may be seen in several dermatologic disorders, including *nevus unius lateris (ichthyosis hystrix), acanthosis nigricans, tuberous sclerosis,* and *focal dermal hypoplasia (Goltz-Gorlin) syndrome.*[5, 7]

Because the squamous papilloma may be clinically and microscopically indistinguishable from *verruca vulgaris,* the virus-induced focal papillary hyperplasia of the epidermis, it is briefly discussed in this section. The associated viruses in verruca are the subtypes HPV-2, HPV-4, and HPV-40.[8, 441–445] Verruca vulgaris is contagious and capable of spread to other parts of an affected person's skin or membranes by way of autoinoculation. It is uncommon on oral mucous membranes but extremely common on the skin.[42]

Clinical Features. Epidemiologic studies have demonstrated that the squamous papilloma of the mouth and oropharynx occurs at all ages of life but is usually diagnosed in persons 30 to 50 years of age.[1–3] There is no gender predilection and any oral surface may be affected, although lesions are usually found on lingual, labial, or buccal mucosa.[2]

The typical lesion is a soft, pedunculated mass with numerous finger-like surface projections (papilla means "nipple-shaped projection") (Fig. 4–33A&B). Projections may be pointed and the surface may be covered with a considerable amount of keratin, producing a white surface change. The heavily keratinized lesion with short rounded projections is cauliflower-like, while a similar but less ke-

ratinized lesion resembles a raspberry or mulberry with a pink or red coloration.

Verruca vulgaris of the oral mucosa is typically a childhood problem, but occasional lesions may arise even into middle age.[7, 8, 442] The skin of the hands is the site of predilection, but when oral mucosa is involved, the lesion is usually found on the vermilion border, labial mucosa, or anterior tongue. The typical lesion may be identical to a squamous papilloma, but it tends to have pointed or verruciform surface projections, to have a very narrow stalk, to be white from considerable surface keratin, and to present as multiple or clustered individual lesions. As with the papilloma, the verruca vulgaris enlarges rapidly to its maximum size, seldom achieving more than 5 mm in greatest diameter.

Pathologic Features and Differential Diagnosis. The squamous papilloma typically has a narrow stalk below a mass with numerous blunted and pointed surface projects, often characterized as finger-like (Fig. 4–33C&D). Submucosal fibrovascular connective tissues are contiguous with the stroma of the stalk, the body of the mass, and the surface projections. Scattered chronic inflammatory cells in small numbers are common in the stroma, presumably from chronic low-grade trauma to the lesion. The surface keratin is often quite thickened, usually with parakeratin. The covering squamous epithelium shows a normal maturation pattern, although occasional papillomas demonstrate pronounced basilar hyperplasia and mild mitotic activity that could be mistaken for *mild epithelial dysplasia.* Koilocytes (HPV-altered epithelial cells with perinuclear clear spaces and nuclear pyknosis) may or may not be found in the superficial layers of the epithelium, and occasional lesions have focal areas covered by mixed bacterial colonies, perhaps with mild, irregular destruction of the otherwise smooth surface of the keratin beneath the colonies.

The verruca vulgaris is also characterized by a proliferation of hyperkeratotic stratified squamous epithelium arranged into finger-like or pointed projections, each with its connective tissue core. It differs from papilloma in that elongated rete ridges tend to converge toward the center of the lesion, producing a "cupping" effect. Also, a prominent granular cell layer (hypergranulosis) exhibiting coarse, clumped keratohyaline granules is typically found and abundant koilocytes are often seen in the superficial spinous layer. Eosinophilic intranuclear viral inclusions are sometimes noted within the cells of the granular layer, a feature never found in the squamous papilloma.

The pathologist must be mindful of the occasional similarity between a sessile papilloma and the other oral verruciform lesions, most of which are described in this section. The squamous papilloma differs from the oral *condyloma acuminatum* in that its surface projections are typically more elongated and more often pointed. It will usually have considerably more keratin on its surface and is much less likely to contain koilocytes in large numbers. The condyloma, moreover, is seldom pedunculated with a stalk, as is typical of the papilloma. Both lesions may show active basal layer cells, but true epithelial dysplasia is only found in the condyloma.

The subepithelial connective tissue, in particular, must be evaluated for the presence of foamy histiocytes or granular cells, which may be the only distinguishing feature between a papilloma and a *verruciform xanthoma* or a focal *pseudoepitheliomatous hyperplasia* above a *granular cell tumor.* Relative to the latter change, an additional difference is that the rete ridges of the papilloma do not extend below the level of the ridges of adjacent epithelium, while the ridges in pseudoepitheliomatous hyperplasia typically extend deeply into underlying stroma.

Treatment and Prognosis. Conservative surgical excision including the base of the lesion is adequate treatment for squamous papilloma, and recurrence is unlikely.[7, 425, 428] Frequently, lesions have been left untreated for years with no reported transformation into malignancy, continuous enlargement, or dissemination to other parts of the oral cavity. It should be emphasized that squamous papillomas of the larynx behave differently from their oral counterparts. Laryngeal lesions tend to recur more often after therapy and have a greater tendency to be multiple and continuously proliferative.

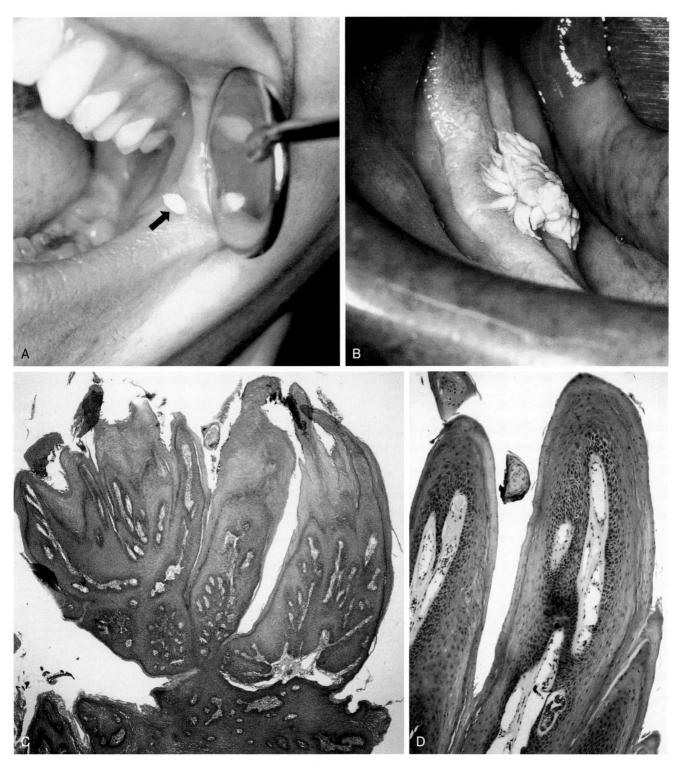

Figure 4–33. *A,* The squamous papilloma with its clustered, pointed projections is often so heavily keratinized that it is pure white. *B,* Large lesions may appear somewhat alarming. (Courtesy of Dr. William Young, University of Queensland, St. Lucia, Queensland, Australia.) *C,* Low-power view shows the pedunculated nature of the lesion, as well as pointed, heavily keratinized surface projections. *D,* Higher power view shows the connective tissue core in each surface projection, with a thick keratin surface layer and, in this example, no visible koilocytes.

Skin and intraoral verruca vulgaris is also treated effectively by conservative surgical excision or curettage, but liquid nitrogen cryotherapy and topical application of keratinolytic agents (usually containing salicylic acid and lactic acid) are also effective.[8, 435] All destructive or surgical treatments should extend to include the base of the lesion. Recurrence is seen in a small proportion of treated cases. Lesions do not transform into malignancy, and two thirds will disappear spontaneously within 2 years, especially those in children.

Condyloma Acuminatum

Yet another papilloma look-alike lesion is the HPV-induced *condyloma acuminatum* (condyloma means "knuckle" or "knob"), an epithelial proliferation considered to be a sexually transmitted disease.[445–450] The condyloma develops at a site of sexual contact or trauma and is, therefore, much more common in the anogenital region, where it represents approximately 20% of all sexually transmitted diseases.[8, 448] Not surprisingly, the virus involved with oral condyloma acuminatum is HPV, especially subtypes HPV-6, HPV-11, HPV-16, and HPV-18.[7, 446] The latter two subtypes are among those associated with carcinoma and epithelial dysplasia of genital mucosa, perhaps explaining why the condyloma is considered a premalignant lesion by many.[8] For reasons unknown, this precancerous character does not seem to be a part of condylomas arising from oral and oropharyngeal mucosa.[7]

It is not unusual for a patient with a condyloma to have multiple sexually transmitted diseases and so caution is advised relative to infection control procedures in the dental office. This multi-disease feature is so strong, in fact, that the genital condyloma was once thought to be a characteristic feature of syphilis rather than a separate entity. The condyloma is very contagious and may spread by autoinoculation to other sites of trauma.

Clinical Features. Condyloma usually is diagnosed in teenagers and young adults, but all ages are susceptible.[448] Oral lesions occur most frequently on the lip mucosa, the lingual frenum, and the soft palate, all points of potential trauma during cunnilingus and fellatio.[446, 450] The lesion presents as a broad-based, pink mass with the surface covered by short, blunted projections, giving it a raspberry or mulberry appearance (Fig. 4–34A, see p. 175). Many lesions have a mild semitransparency to the surface nodules. Condylomata tend to be larger than papillomas and are characteristically multiple and clustered. The average lesional size is 1.0 to 1.5 cm, but lesions as large as 3 cm have been reported.[446] Even large oral condylomata are seldom elevated more than a few millimeters above the surface.

Pathologic Features and Differential Diagnosis. Condyloma acuminatum presents as a benign proliferation of acanthotic stratified squamous epithelium with mildly keratotic papular or nodular surface projections. Thin connective tissue cores support the papillary epithelial projections, which are more blunted and broad than those of squamous papilloma and verruca vulgaris (Fig. 4–34B&C, see p. 175). The appearance of keratin-filled crypts between prominences of the latter disease are seldom found in the condyloma.

The covering epithelium is mature and differentiated, but superficial keratinocytes commonly contain pyknotic nuclei surrounded by clear zones (koilocytes), a classic microscopic feature of HPV infections. Ultrastructural examination will reveal virions within the cytoplasm or nuclei of koilocytes or both, and the virus also can be demonstrated by immunohistochemistry, in situ hybridization, and polymerase chain reaction techniques. The diagnosis, however, seldom requires the use of special methods. The reader is referred to the pathology section of the preceding discussion of the squamous papilloma for a review of the differential diagnosis of oral papillary lesions with similarities to condyloma.

Treatment and Prognosis. Condyloma is treated by conservative surgical excision, topical application of podophyllin, or laser ablation.[7–9, 446] The latter treatment has raised some question as to the airborne spread of HPV through the aerosolized microdroplets created by the vaporization of lesional tissue. Regardless of the method used, a condyloma should be removed because it is contagious and capable of spreading to other oral surfaces as well as to other persons through direct, usually sexual, contact.

In the anogenital area, this lesion may demonstrate a premalignant character, especially when infected with HPV subtypes 16 and 18, but this has not been demonstrated in oral lesions. It should be remembered that condyloma may be an oral manifestation of a greater problem, such as child sexual abuse or HIV infection.[445, 446, 450]

Focal Epithelial Hyperplasia

One of the most contagious of the oral papillary lesions is *focal epithelial hyperplasia* or *Heck's disease,* another HPV-induced epithelial proliferation first described in 1965 in Native Americans.[451–457] The level of contagion is exemplified by the fact that in some isolated populations up to 40% of children have been affected.[7, 453] Today it is known to exist in numerous populations and ethnic groups and to be produced by one of the subtypes of the human papillomavirus, HPV-13, and possibly HPV-32.[7, 455] Where the infection is endemic among children, adults seem to have minimal evidence of residual oral lesions and so the lesions are presumed to eventually disappear on their own.[454]

Focal epithelial hyperplasia is somewhat different from other HPV infections in that it is able to produce extreme acanthosis or hyperplasia of the prickle cell layer of the epithelium with minimal production of surface projections or induction of connective tissue proliferation. The mucosa may be 8 to 10 times thicker than normal.

Clinical Features. Heck's disease primarily occurs in children, but lesions may occur in young and middle-aged adults.[452, 456] There is no gender predilection. Sites of greatest involvement include the labial, buccal, and lingual mucosa, but gingival and tonsillar lesions have also been reported.[456]

Individual lesions are broad-based or so slightly elevated as to present as well demarcated plaques. Lesions are frequently papillary in nature, but relatively smooth-surfaced, flat-topped lesions are more commonly seen. Papules and plaques are usually the color of normal mucosa but may be pale or, rarely, white. Hyperplastic lesions are small (0.3–1.0 cm), discrete, and well-demarcated, but they frequently cluster so closely together that the entire mucosal area takes on a cobblestone or fissured appearance.

Pathologic Features and Differential Diagnosis. Epithelial hyperplasia in this disease presents microscopically as an abrupt and sometimes considerable focal acanthosis of the oral epithelium. The thickened mucosa extends upward, not down into underlying connective tissues; hence, the lesional rete ridges are at the same depth as the adjacent normal rete ridges. The ridges themselves are widened, often confluent, and sometimes club-shaped; they are not long and thin as in *psoriasis* and other diseases. Some superficial keratinocytes show a koilocytic change similar to that seen in other HPV infections, while occasionally others demonstrate a collapsed nucleus that resembles a mitotic figure (mitosoid cell). These presumably result from viral alteration of the cells. Virus-like particles have been noted ultrastructurally within both cytoplasm and nuclei of cells within the spinous layer, and this layer is positive for HPV antigen with in situ hybridization.

The lesion is usually easily differentiated from *squamous papilloma, verruca vulgaris,* and *condyloma* by its lack of pronounced surface projections; the presence of mitosoid cells; and the lack of connective tissue cores in the surface projections, when present. The sessile nature of focal epithelial hyperplasia also serves to separate it from the former two lesions, although this is not a guaranteed distinction.

Focal epithelial hyperplasia also tends to lack the pronounced elongation of thin rete ridges seen in *keratoacanthoma* and *pseudoepitheliomatous hyperplasia,* and it lacks the central keratin-filled core of the keratoacanthoma. It also lacks the subepithelial foamy or granular histiocyte-like cells required for the diagnosis of *verruciform xanthoma.*

Treatment and Prognosis. Conservative excisional biopsy may be required to establish the proper diagnosis, but additional treatment is unnecessary, except perhaps for esthetic reasons relating to visible labial lesions.[7–9, 454, 457] Spontaneous regression has been reported after months or years, and the disease is rather rare in adults.[454] No case of focal epithelial hyperplasia has been reported to transform into carcinoma. It should be remembered that focal epithelial hyperplasia may be an oral manifestation of AIDS.[457]

Verruciform Xanthoma

The *verruciform xanthoma* is a papilloma look-alike lesion that seems not to be associated with HPV but is perhaps a response to local trauma.[7, 458–461] The lesion contains abundant lipid-laden histiocyte-like cells and is histopathologically similar to dermal xanthomas, although there appears to be no association with *diabetes mellitus, Langerhans cell disease (histiocytosis X), hyperlipidemia,* or any other metabolic disorder. Some authors have suggested that the lesion may represent an unusual reaction to localized epithelial trauma or damage. This hypothesis is supported by cases of verruciform xanthoma that have developed in association with disturbed epithelium *(melanocytic nevus, epidermolysis bullosa, epithelial dysplasia, pemphigus vulgaris,* and so on).[459] First reported as an oral lesion in 1971, it has subsequently been reported on the skin and vulvar mucosa, although it remains a predominantly oral lesion.[458, 461] There is evidence for an association with immune suppression in some cases.[460]

Clinical Features. This unique lesion occurs in middle-aged and older individuals, usually 40 to 70 years of age.[458, 459, 461] There is a strong female predilection (1:2 male:female ratio) and the usual intraoral locations are the gingiva and alveolar mucosa, but any oral mucosal site may be involved.

Verruciform xanthoma appears as a well-demarcated, soft, painless, sessile, slightly elevated mass with a white, yellow/white, or red color and a papillary or roughened surface (*verruciform* means "with pointed projections, warty"). It is usually less than 2 cm in diameter and no oral lesion larger than 4 cm has been reported. Multiple lesions have occasionally been described.[461] Aggregated xanthoma cells may be so numerous as to be visible

clinically as a cluster of small yellow surface nodules resembling fish eggs.

Verruciform xanthoma may be very similar in clinical appearance to *squamous papilloma, condyloma acuminatum,* or early *carcinoma,* and biopsy may be the only means by which to distinguish one from the other.

Pathologic Features and Differential Diagnosis. There is an obvious verruciform or papillary surface change, often with clefts or crypts between the epithelial projections, sometimes filled with parakeratin (Fig. 4–35A). The surface layer of parakeratin is typically thickened, and on routine hematoxylin and eosin staining exhibits a distinctive orange coloration. The rete ridges are elongated to a uniform depth.

The required histopathologic feature of verruciform xanthoma is found within the connective tissue papillae, which contain foamy histiocytes or xanthoma cells (*xanthos* means "yellow"). These cells are not seen beneath the level of the adjacent rete ridges and may completely fill the papilla (Fig. 4–35B). They contain lipid as well as PAS-positive, diastase-resistant granules. There has been no plausible explanation for the strong localization of lesional cells in the papillae.

The pathologist must be careful not to confuse xanthoma cells with lingual dorsum taste buds in the connective tissue papillae, but

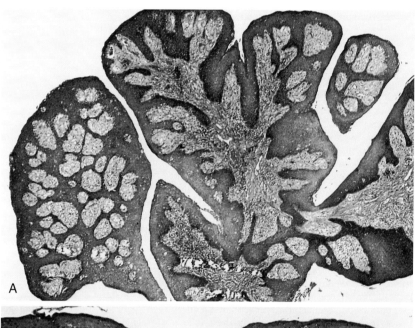

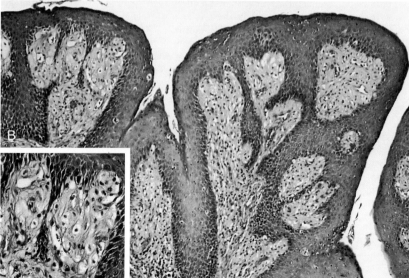

Figure 4–35. *A,* The verruciform xanthoma has a papillary configuration. *B,* Surface epithelium shows elongated rete pegs with foamy histiocyte-like cells seen in the connective tissue papillae; high-power view *(inset)* shows the lesional foamy histiocytes.

differentiation from other maxillofacial lesions with foamy or granular histiocyte-like cells is not difficult because verruciform xanthoma is the only lesion to have these cells confined to the papillae. *Granular cell epulis, granular cell tumor,* and *fibrous histiocytoma* all present with extensive foamy or granular histiocyte-like cells throughout the lesional stroma and, in fact, typically present with a subepithelial zone free of such cells.

Treatment and Prognosis. Verruciform xanthoma is treated by conservative surgical excision and recurrence is rare with this treatment.[7, 458, 461] Although no malignant transformation has been reported, a few cases of verruciform xanthoma have been reported in association with carcinoma in situ or squamous cell carcinoma. This might imply that it is a potentially premalignant lesion, but is probably best explained as representing degenerative changes in response to dysplastic epithelium.[7, 458]

Keratoacanthoma and Pseudoepitheliomatous Hyperplasia

Occasionally a localized epithelial hyperplasia will strongly mimic the microscopic appearance of well-differentiated *squamous cell carcinoma* or *verrucous carcinoma.* Primarily a cutaneous lesion referred to as *keratoacanthoma ("self-healing" carcinoma; pseudocarcinoma),* this entity is a benign, self-limiting proliferation of the epithelial component of the follicular infundibulum.[8, 462–468] The average annual incidence rates in white males and females, respectively, are 144 in 100,000 and 73 in 100,000 population.[8, 463]

The etiology of this lesion is unknown. Sun damage is suggested by the fact that the vast majority of solitary lesions are found on sun-exposed skin, predominantly in elderly persons. Human papillomaviruses, usually the HPV-26 or HPV-37 subtypes, have been found in some lesions.[466] Cutaneous keratoacanthoma-like lesions have been produced in animals by the application of known carcinogens.[8] The lesions occur with increased frequency in immunosuppressed patients and in the *Muir-Torre syndrome* (sebaceous neoplasms, keratoacanthomas, and gastrointestinal carcinomas), and multiple lesions tend to be hereditary in nature.[8, 467, 468]

Keratoacanthoma of the oral epithelium is almost always a lesion of the lower lip vermilion. Intraoral examples have been reported but are decidedly rare and obviously require a different theory to explain their origin.[464–466] The characteristically exuberant, downgrowing proliferation of rete pegs, however, does occur in the mouth, but not with the same distinctive clinical or microscopic features as keratoacanthoma. For this reason, the more generic term, *pseudoepitheliomatous hyperplasia,* is usually applied to oral lesions.[469]

Pseudoepitheliomatous hyperplasia has a different biologic behavior than keratoacanthoma and is most often associated with chronic denture irritation and *papillary hyperplasia of the palate* or *epulis fissuratum.*[469] It is also associated with cases of *chronic candidiasis,* especially the form called *median posterior atrophic candidiasis (median rhomboid glossitis),* with the deep fungi *blastomycosis* and *histoplasmosis,* and with the *granular cell tumor.*

Clinical Features. Keratoacanthoma occurs almost always in patients older than 45 years of age and shows a male predilection.[8, 462, 466] Solitary lesions arise on sun-exposed skin in all but 5% of cases, and 8% of all cases are found on the outer edge of the vermilion border, affecting the upper and lower lips with equal frequency.[464, 466]

The skin or vermilion lesion appears as a firm, nontender, well-demarcated, dome-shaped nodule with a central plug of keratin, often resembling a volcano. Except for the yellow, brown, or black keratin plug, the nodule has normal texture and color but may be erythematous. The central core has an irregular, crusted, often verruciform surface. Intraoral keratoacanthoma usually lacks this volcano-like appearance because it has minimal crater formation. It presents as a solitary nodule with a somewhat granular surface change.

Rapid enlargement is typical, with the lesion attaining a diameter of 1 to 2 cm within 6 weeks. This critical feature helps distinguish keratoacanthoma from the much more slowly enlarging *squamous cell carcinoma.* When a large number of keratoacanthomas is seen early in life, it most likely represents the *Ferguson Smith type,* which is hereditary, and lesions are not likely to spontaneously involute.[8] The *eruptive Grzybowski type* manifests as hundreds of small papules of the skin and upper digestive tract and has been associated with internal malignancy.[468]

The typical intraoral example of pseudoepitheliomatous hyperplasia is a broad-based, well-demarcated plaque with a granular or verruciform surface alteration. It may be white or pink, depending on the amount of surface keratin and by definition there is no central keratin-filled crater or surface indentation. The lesion is painless and nonhemorrhagic and seldom reaches a size larger than 1 cm in greatest diameter. Of course, for those cases stimulated by an underlying stromal change, such as a granular cell tumor or deep fungal infection, the hyperplasia may be found on the surface of a sessile or somewhat pedunculated mass. Most affected patients are middle-aged.

Pathologic Features and Differential Diagnosis. The overall pattern of the keratoacanthoma is diagnostically more important than the appearance of individual cells, so excisional or large incisional biopsy with inclusion of adjacent clinically normal epithelium is suggested for proper histopathologic interpretation. The cells are mature and the epithelium shows good differentiation from the basal layer to the surface keratin but dyskeratosis (abnormal or premature keratin production) is often seen as individually keratinizing lesional cells and keratin pearls identical to those of well-differentiated squamous cell carcinoma.

At the lip of the central crater, an acute angle is formed between the overlying epithelium and the periphery of the lesion. The central crater is filled with keratin and the base of the crater shows broad, proliferating rete ridges that seldom extend below the level of the sweat glands in skin lesions or to the underlying muscle in oral lesions. A pronounced chronic inflammatory cell response may be found within adjacent stroma. Late-stage lesions have considerably more keratinization of cells deep in the tumor than do early lesions.

Differentiation of keratoacanthoma from well-differentiated squamous cell carcinoma may be problematic. The malignancy, however, lacks the characteristic acute angle between normal and lesional epithelial margins of the keratoacanthoma, and the rete pegs of the keratoacanthoma show a "pushing" extension into underlying stroma, rather than the invading islands and individual dysplastic cells of the carcinoma.

The keratoacanthoma can easily be distinguished from crater-producing or volcano-like *molluscum contagiosum* of labial, buccal, or other oral mucosa by the presence in the latter of large, basophilic viral inclusions (molluscum bodies) within keratinocytes at the base of the central "volcanic" core. These cells are commonly seen to be sloughing into the central cratered area.[471]

Pseudoepitheliomatous hyperplasia of the intraoral mucosa is characterized by extreme elongation or downgrowth of rete pegs along a broad expanse of hyperkeratinized surface epithelium, without the nodule formation or the central crater of the keratoacanthoma (Fig. 4–36*A*). Individual cells are very mature and only occasional dyskeratosis is present, usually as a keratin pearl rather than individually keratinized cells. Long, intertwining rete pegs and rete ridges, when cut tangentially, can give a rather strong impression of invading squamous cell carcinoma (Fig. 4–36*B*). The pathologist should look carefully for granular cells of a granular cell tumor or deep fungi (with silver staining) in the subepithelial stroma, to avoid mistakenly diagnosing this as a malignancy. Sarda et al[470] have proposed the use of AgNOR evaluation to help distinguish pseudoepitheliomatous hyperplasia from squamous cell carcinoma.

Treatment and Prognosis. Keratoacanthoma tends to involute of its own accord, but surgical excision is often performed to confirm a benign diagnosis.[464, 465] Large lesions of the vermilion or labial skin should be removed for esthetic reasons because significant

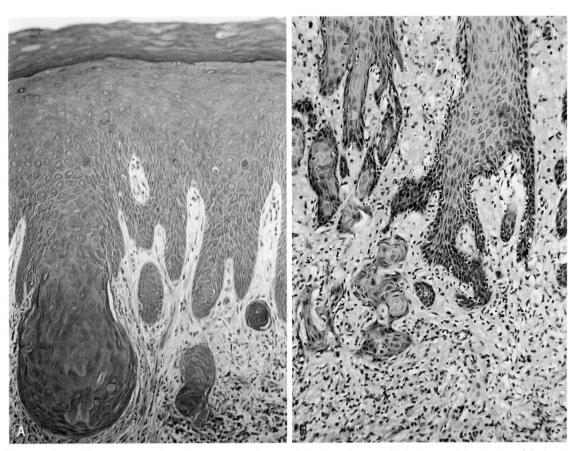

Figure 4–36. *A,* Pseudoepitheliomatous hyperplasia shows excess surface keratin but lacks the central indentation and keratin plug of the keratoacanthoma; its proliferating rete ridges extend deeply into underlying stroma, often appearing as independent islands of well-differentiated squamous epithelium. *B,* Dyskeratotic proliferating rete pegs, as seen here, can mimic superficially invading squamous carcinoma.

scarring may result from involution. Recurrence occurs after excision in approximately 2% of skin cases.[8] Aggressive behavior and malignant transformation into carcinoma have been reported in a few keratoacanthomas, but the similarity between this lesion and squamous cell carcinoma tends to raise doubts as to the appropriateness of the initial diagnosis in such cases.[8]

Pseudoepitheliomatous hyperplasia of intraoral mucosa is treated by conservative surgical removal or laser ablation, with minimal chance of recurrence.[469] The greatest danger lies not in the lesion itself but in the risk of its being misdiagnosed as a well-differentiated squamous cell carcinoma.

Hairy Leukoplakia

A well-demarcated, painless, verruciform hyperkeratotic lesion of the lateral tongue in HIV-infected male homosexuals was first reported in 1981 as *hairy leukoplakia.*[472–475] It appears to represent an Epstein-Barr virus–induced proliferation in an area of chronic trauma and is found in approximately 80% of AIDS patients.[475] It is eventually also found in one of every four HIV-infected individuals. Its presence usually heralds progression into AIDS and is positively correlated with the depletion of peripheral CD4 cells. Occasional patients with other immunosuppression diseases, or without evidence of immunosuppression, will present with hairy leukoplakia.[474]

Clinical Features. Hairy leukoplakia varies in its clinical appearance from a flat, white plaque to one with small or long white projections with pointed or blunted ends. Almost all AIDS-related cases have been on the lateral lingual margin, but occasional cases creep onto the ventral or dorsal surfaces or are found at another oral site, especially the buccal commissure. The lesion is asymptomatic, although a secondary infection by *Candida albicans* may produce

tenderness or a burning sensation. It is important to remember that, despite its name, this is not a true leukoplakia and does not exhibit precancerous behavior.

Pathologic Features and Differential Diagnosis. A hyperkeratotic surface is seen, usually with verruciform projections, sometimes with keratin-filled clefts between them (Fig. 4–37*A*). Immediately beneath the parakeratosis is the characteristic feature of this lesion: a koilocytic appearance of large keratinocytes with intracellular "edema" and basophilic nuclear viral inclusions with peripheral displacement of chromatin (Fig. 4–37*B*). The latter changes often impart a smudged appearance to the nucleus. Ballooning degeneration and perinuclear clearing may also be seen in occasional deeper cells and silver stains will often reveal candidal hyphae within the superficial layers of the epithelium. There is usually only a mild chronic inflammatory cell response within underlying connective tissues. Immunohistochemistry or electron microscopy will demonstrate intranuclear Epstein-Barr virions.

This lesion must be differentiated from the previously mentioned verruciform lesions (see discussion in the pathology section relating to the papilloma), and must likewise be differentiated from *verrucous carcinoma* and *hairy tongue.* The carcinoma lacks the abrupt onset, early age at diagnosis, and keratinocytes with viral inclusions. It also demonstrates a blunt, pushing invasion of the underlying stroma, which is not seen in hairy leukoplakia. Hairy tongue is poorly demarcated clinically and produces a generalized keratotic change of the entire dorsum of the tongue.[476, 477] It may show occasional koilocytes but lacks the large virally affected keratinocytes of hairy leukoplakia. Occasional cases of *hyperplastic lichen planus* will show verruciform surface changes, but the ballooning degeneration of that disease is confined to the basal layer and there are no viral inclusions in affected cells. Lichen planus also demonstrates a subepithelial band of chronic inflammatory cells, a feature not found in hairy leukoplakia.

Treatment and Prognosis. Hairy leukoplakia is a self-limiting lesion with no known potential for malignant transformation.[475] Larger lesions may require conservative surgical removal because of constant trauma with adjacent teeth and interference with chewing, but most lesions can be left alone. The lesion may disappear spontaneously or with antiviral medications or with systemic AIDS therapies, but it often recurs.[7, 475] An incisional biopsy is almost always performed to confirm the diagnosis because of the close association with HIV infection and the high probability of an infected individual with hairy leukoplakia progressing to AIDS within 1 to 2 years of the leukoplakia diagnosis.

Nonpapillary Keratotic Mucosal Hyperplasias

Keratotic oral mucosal changes with few surface projections are found in 3% of adults and represent a diverse group of lesions.[1, 478] Several of these are premalignant entities and are discussed elsewhere in this text (Chapter 1), but others have no malignant transformation potential or have a potential so low that it is not considered significant. All of these present as white clinical macules and several have such similar histopathology that corroborating clinical information may be necessary for an appropriate final diagnosis.

Frictional, Chemical, and Thermal Keratosis

Frictional keratosis is the oral counterpart of a *callus* on the skin. It is a common alteration, especially in areas of recurring, mild mechanical trauma or irritation from malposed teeth, dental prosthetics, or patient habit, such as smokeless tobacco use *(smokeless tobacco keratosis),* exuberant toothbrushing with an overly firm brush *(toothbrush keratosis),* constant rubbing of the tongue against the teeth *(tongue thrust keratosis),* or the frequent clenching of the facial muscles, thereby pushing cheek and lips firmly against the dentition *(chronic cheek bite keratosis, chronic lip bite keratosis).*[7, 478, 479] In most cases the cause is obvious, but without a known etiology the clinician is forced to presume the keratotic plaque to be *leukoplakia* and to manage it as a premalignancy.

Chemical keratosis may also occur as the result of the compounds in smokeless tobacco, certain toothpastes, acid medication used inappropriately (aspirin placed on the gingiva to alleviate

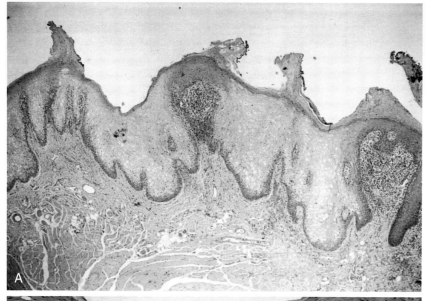

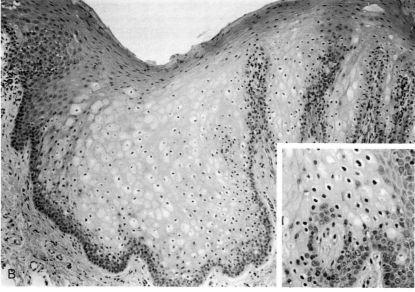

Figure 4–37. *A,* Hairy leukoplakia presents as acanthotic epithelium with excessively keratinized, pointed surface projections separated by mucosal "valleys." *B,* Intracellular edema of spindle cell keratinocytes is typically pronounced, and scattered chronic inflammatory cells are usually seen in underlying stroma; *inset* shows higher power view of the intracellular edema and nuclear pyknosis.

toothache pain), and certain spices in candies or chewing gum, especially cinnamon and peppermint.

A special form of thermally or chemically induced keratosis is seen as a generalized whiteness of the hard palate in persons who smoke cigars and pipes. Once a common mucosal change, this *nicotine stomatitis (nicotine palatinus, smoker's palate)* has become less common as cigar and pipe smoking have lost popularity. Although this lesion is a white keratotic change obviously associated with tobacco smoking, it does not appear to have a premalignant nature, perhaps because it develops in response to the heat rather than the chemicals of tobacco smoke.[481–483] It can also be produced by the long-term use of extremely hot beverages.[481] In some South American and Southeast Asian cultures, hand-rolled cigarettes and cigars are smoked with the lit end held within the mouth. This "reverse smoking" habit produces a similar but more pronounced palatal keratosis, called *reverse smoker's palate,* which is definitely a premalignant lesion.[7, 9]

Clinical Features. Frictional keratosis is usually found in teenagers and young adults of both genders. Many individuals have a thin, slightly raised white keratotic line along the occlusal plane of the buccal mucosa, often bilateral. This *linea alba* is considered to be a variation of normal anatomy but is called frictional keratosis, chronic cheek bite keratosis, or *morsicatio buccarum* when it becomes pronounced (Fig. 4–38A). There is usually a clenching or bruxing habit and the most severe lesions are found in persons with the habit of constantly pushing the cheeks between the teeth with a finger while gently biting on the buccal tissues. The surface of a frictional keratosis may be quite rough and irregular, and on the buccal mucosa may show a scalloped effect as the tissues take on the contours of adjacent teeth. Focal oval areas of pink mucosa may be seen, representing areas in which the patient has peeled off the thick surface keratin with his or her teeth. The resulting combination of red and white mucosa may be mistaken for the precancerous *granular leukoplakia* or *erythroleukoplakia.*

A similar linear line of excess keratin may be found along the lateral edges of the tongue, often with crenations from chronically pushing the tongue against the teeth. Rounded or irregularly shaped white plaques may be seen on the anterior dorsal surface of the tongue from a chronic tongue thrust habit and may be seen in the retromolar region because of trauma from the maxillary dentition.

Nicotine stomatitis is found in males older than 45 years of age with long-term tobacco use. The palatal mucosa becomes diffusely gray and then white, with scattered white papules with punctate red centers, representing inflamed salivary glands and ducts. In severe cases, the palate becomes fissured and takes on the appearance of a dried lake bed.

Smokeless tobacco keratosis is a white, nonelevated plaque with a poorly demarcated periphery and usually with regular and intertwining fissures running through it. It occurs in the area of habitual tobacco placement and is a completely painless lesion.

Pathologic Features. Acanthosis and hyperkeratosis, usually orthokeratosis, are the hallmarks of frictional keratosis. The keratin may become ragged and delaminated by the patient's habit and it is not unusual to find bacterial colonies lodged in surface irregularities. The granular cell layer is often quite prominent, a feature lacking in most other oral hyperkeratoses. The cells of the spinous layer often demonstrate intraepithelial edema and occasional vacuolated cells with pyknotic nuclei resemble koilocytes (Fig. 4–38B&C). Dysplasia is not seen in the epithelium and there is no increase in mitotic activity. There is a mild scattered chronic inflammatory cell infiltrate within underlying fibrovascular stroma (Fig. 4–38D).

Frictional keratosis with prominent intracellular edema and koilocyte-like cells may be difficult to distinguish from *leukoedema, white-sponge nevus, smokeless tobacco keratosis, chemical keratosis,* and *hairy leukoplakia.* The differential diagnosis of these lesions is discussed elsewhere in this text.

Nicotine stomatitis shows hyperkeratosis and acanthosis of palatal epithelium with scattered chronic inflammatory cells within subepithelial stroma and mucous glands (Fig. 4–39). Squamous

metaplasia and hyperplasia of excretory ducts are often seen and neutrophils may fill some ducts. The degree of epithelial hyperplasia and hyperkeratosis correlates positively with the duration and the amount of smoking. Epithelial dysplasia is rare.

Smokeless tobacco keratosis is predominantly a chemical burn; hence, the major changes are seen in the more superficial epithelium, where hyperparakeratosis may be pronounced and where the cells often show considerable intraepithelial edema (Fig. 4–40). As the mucosa is habitually stretched during smokeless tobacco use but is not in the biopsy specimen, surface verruciform change is commonly seen as a "shrinkage" artifact. Underlying stroma usually contains small numbers of chronic inflammatory cells, and minor salivary glands may show a hyalinized stroma.

Treatment and Prognosis. No treatment is required for frictional keratosis and there is no potential for malignant transformation. The patient's habit, however, may produce aching facial or tongue muscles or dysfunction of the temporomandibular joint. This may be reason to stop the habit. The white keratotic plaques will completely disappear within a few days or weeks of the elimination of the chronic trauma. Any keratosis remaining after 4 weeks should be considered to be true leukoplakia or another diagnosis, and biopsy would be in order to evaluate for dysplastic epithelial cells.

Within a month or two of smoking cessation, the palate affected by nicotine palatinus will usually return to normal, even when the keratosis has been present for many decades.[469–481] Although this is not a precancerous lesion and requires no treatment, the patient nevertheless should be encouraged to stop smoking, and other high-risk areas should be examined closely. Any white lesion of the palatal mucosa that persists after 2 months of habit cessation should be considered a true leukoplakia and managed accordingly.

The smokeless tobacco keratosis will almost always disappear within a few weeks or months of cessation of the tobacco habit. Any residual white keratosis after two months should be considered a leukoplakia and viewed with suspicion.

Leukoedema

Leukoedema is a common developmental alteration of the oral mucosa that appears to be a simple variation of normal anatomy.[484–487] When the most mild cases are included, it is seen in almost 90% of adult blacks and half of adult whites, although it presents as a much less pronounced alteration in whites.[487] Tobacco smoking and chewing has been shown to enhance the whiteness and size of the lesion, but most cases are so subtle that they are not formally diagnosed. Similar mucosal changes have been reported on vaginal and laryngeal mucosa.[7, 8]

Clinical Features. Leukoedema presents most typically as an asymptomatic, bilateral, whitish gray, semitransparent macule of the buccal mucosa. Occasional patients show fine grooves or folds crisscrossing the macule in a delicate lace-like pattern. This mucosal change may begin as early as 3 to 5 years of age, but is not usually noticeable until adolescence.[7, 485, 487] By the end of the teenage years, 50% of black children demonstrate the altered mucosa.[487]

The opalescent macule is usually poorly demarcated from surrounding mucosa and is occasionally seen on the soft palate and oral floor. When the cheeks are stretched outward, the leukoedema typically disappears.

Pathologic Features and Differential Diagnosis. Leukoedema is characterized by a variable intracellular edema of the superficial half of the epithelium (Fig. 4–41). The vacuolated cells are large and often have pyknotic nuclei. They may extend to the basal layer and may cluster into inverted wedge-shaped regions separated by normal spinous epithelial cells. The epithelium is hyperplastic and rete ridges are often broad and elongated. Parakeratosis is commonly seen but is not pronounced unless there has been chronic trauma.

Intracellular edema is characteristic of several other oral lesions, many of which may be found on the buccal mucosa: *smokeless tobacco keratosis, frictional keratosis (chronic cheek bite kera-*

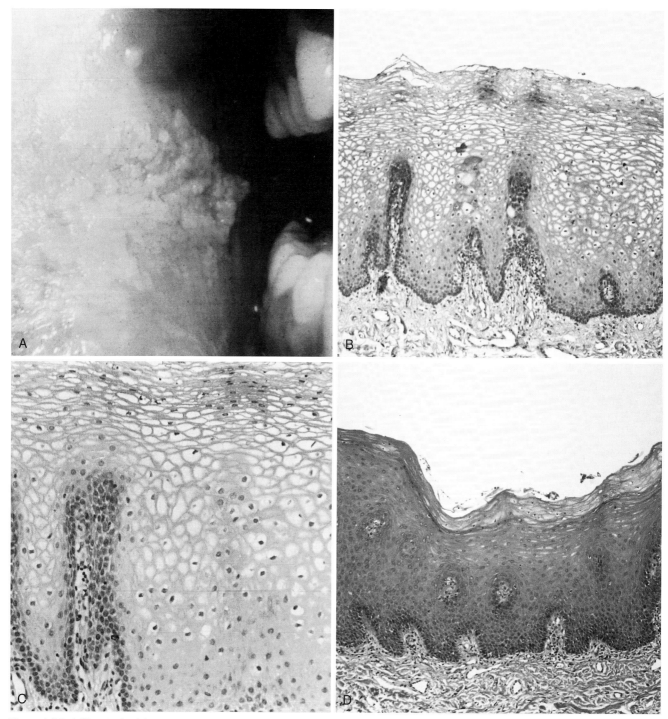

Figure 4–38. *A*, Chronic cheek bite presents as an irregular white keratosis of the buccal mucosa along the biting plane of the teeth; *B*, severe cheek biting may result in considerable acanthosis from intracellular edema of the spindle cell layer; *C*, higher power view of intracellular edema with koilocyte-like change; *D*, more typically, the epithelium shows excess surface parakeratin with less pronounced intracellular edema.

tosis), white sponge nevus, and *Witkop's disease.* The identification of etiologic habits will greatly ease the difficulty of establishing a final diagnosis for smokeless tobacco keratosis and frictional keratosis. Microscopically, these typically present with a more pronounced surface keratosis and have scattered chronic inflammatory cells within underlying stroma.

Since leukoedema and white sponge nevus both have innocuous onsets in the childhood and teenage years, it may be impossible to distinguish between them except by the clinical "stretch test." The nevus will remain visible when the affected mucosa is stretched, whereas leukoedema will disappear. *Hereditary benign intraepithe-*

lial dyskeratosis (Witkop's disease) also shows pronounced intracellular edema but can be distinguished from the others by the scattered presence in the spinous layer of individually keratinized cells. The reader is referred to the following section pertaining to white sponge nevus for a more thorough discussion of the differential diagnosis of these lesions.

Treatment and Prognosis. No treatment is necessary for leukoedema. It has no malignant potential and does not change significantly after 25 to 30 years of patient age.[7, 487] Should the affected individual stop using tobacco products, the lesion will likely become less pronounced.

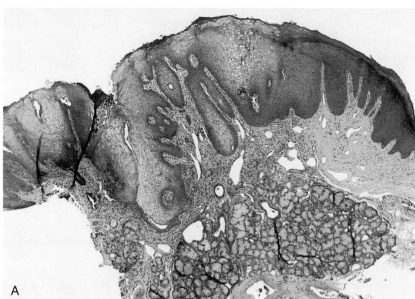

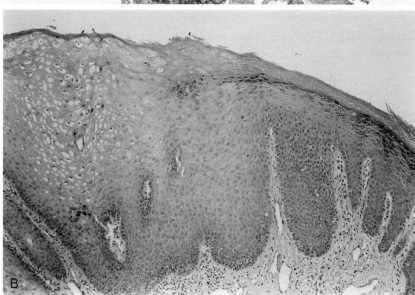

Figure 4–39. *A,* Focal acanthosis, excess surface keratin, squamous metaplasia of the salivary duct lining, and chronic inflammatory cells in underlying stroma characterize the papules overlying the inflamed salivary glands of nicotine palatinus. *B,* Higher power view shows acanthosis with a prominent granular layer toward the right and koilocyte-like cells toward the left.

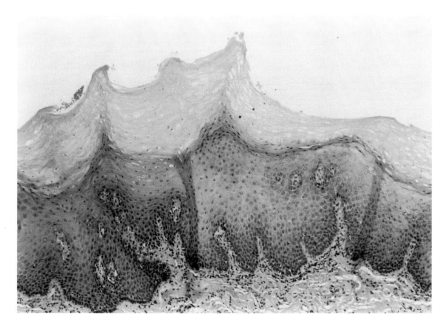

Figure 4–40. The excess parakeratin of smokeless tobacco keratosis may be pronounced and show considerable intracellular edema of superficial cells, often with intermittent verruciform projections of the surface, as seen here. Scattered lymphocytes are beneath the epithelium.

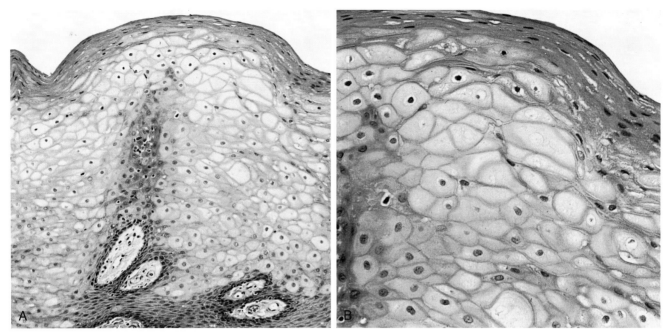

Figure 4–41. *A,* Leukoedema has a thin layer of surface parakeratin and is characterized by intracellular edema of the superficial epithelial layers, although this may be difficult to differentiate from chronic chemical or mechanical trauma; *B,* higher power view of the vacuolated cells shows some with pyknotic nuclei.

White Sponge Nevus

Initially described by Cannon[488] in 1935, *white sponge nevus* is a rare developmental anomaly inherited as an autosomal dominant trait with variable expressivity and a high degree of penetrance.[489–493] Sometimes called the *nevus of Cannon,* this keratotic mucosal alteration may be seen on vaginal and rectal mucosa but the great majority of cases involve oral mucosa.[7–9] The underlying pathophysiology responsible for the altered epithelial cells is unclear, but a mutation in the mucosal keratin K4 has been identified.[492]

Oral changes in *hereditary benign intraepithelial dyskeratosis* or *Witkop's disease* are identical to those of white sponge nevus, but the former disease shows unique microscopic cells and clinically evident ocular changes.[494, 495] Clinically similar white macules or plaques may also be seen in the mouths of persons with *pachyonychia congenita* and *dyskeratosis congenita.*[7, 496, 497]

Clinical Features. White sponge nevus almost always presents during childhood and there is no gender predilection.[489–491] Typically, bilateral white keratotic macules and plaques are found on the buccal mucosae, but labial, lingual, and other sites may be involved. Individual lesions are seen as a relatively thick, white, often corrugated plaque that may cover most of the buccal mucosa (Fig. 4–42A). Usually asymptomatic, rare examples of mild discomfort has been reported from secondary infection.[491]

Occasional lesions are less thickened and reveal a "watery" or semitransparent appearance. Lesions are usually well demarcated from the surrounding normal mucosa, as opposed to the poor demarcation of *leukoedema* and *smokeless tobacco keratosis.* The plaques do not change significantly when the cheeks are stretched, and, rarely, the plaques are small, multiple, and scattered about the affected mucosa rather than being a single more diffuse keratosis.

Pathologic Features and Differential Diagnosis. The hallmark microscopic feature of this disease is an extensive and often marked intracellular edema of the superficial epithelial cells, predominantly within the spinous layer (Fig. 4–42B). The nuclei are typically pyknotic, and the cells may mimic the koilocytes of viral infections. Edematous cells may be organized into inverted triangles with broad bases along the surface, and there may be a thickened parakeratin layer. Deep indentations or grooves may be seen to extend from the surface almost to the basal layer, but the lower portions of the epithelium are otherwise not involved. There are few

mitotic figures and there is never evidence of dysplasia. In cytologic smears, occasional cells will have condensed eosinophilic cytoplasm immediately surrounding the nucleus.

Intracellular edema is not pathognomonic for white sponge nevus. Leukoedema is another developmental phenomenon with childhood onset and abundant superficial epithelial cells with edema. It typically lacks the parakeratosis and vertical grooves of white sponge nevus, but there are times when the only viable means of distinguishing between the two is to stretch the affected mucosa; leukoedema tends to diminish or disappear when this is done, while no change is seen in white sponge nevus or other look-alike lesions.

Frictional keratosis, especially *chronic cheek bite keratosis,* may also present with intracellular edema of superficial epithelial cells, but there is usually extensive surface keratosis, vertical infolding is absent, and only occasional nuclei are pyknotic. Scattered chronic inflammatory cells are usually found within the subepithelial stroma.

Smokeless tobacco keratosis may demonstrate pronounced intracellular edema of superficial cells, sometimes extending to the parabasal region. It is also characterized by surface parakeratosis and occasional grooves or corrugations. This keratotic lesion may, therefore, exactly mimic the histopathology of white sponge nevus and may require clinical correlation for proper diagnosis. The smokeless tobacco lesion is white and corrugated, but its onset is associated with the smokeless tobacco habit and it is typically found in the mandibular vestibule, where the tobacco is habitually placed. Such lesions are, moreover, very seldom bilateral and they will usually disappear after cessation of the tobacco habit. It is important to differentiate these two entities because smokeless tobacco keratosis is a low-grade precancer and requires follow-up examinations.

Another oral precancer, *leukoplakia,* is easily distinguished from white sponge nevus by its adult onset and its usual lack of intracellular edema. Leukoplakia is essentially a phenomenon of excess keratosis of the surface with acanthosis of the spinous layer and with occasional dysplasia of basal cells (see Chapter 1).

The final disease that may mimic the oral white macules of white sponge nevus is *Witkop's disease* or *hereditary benign intraepithelial dyskeratosis (HBID).* The histopathology is identical to white sponge nevus except that scattered spinous cells demonstrate premature keratinization and loss or pyknosis of nuclei (Fig. 4–43, see p. 176). This change is often seen as streaks of dyskeratotic cells. It is important for the pathologist to recognize this unique feature because persons affected by the autosomal dominant Witkop's disease may develop gelatinous plaques of the bulbar conjunctiva, which may eventuate in blindness.

Treatment and Prognosis. White sponge nevus remains essentially unchanged after the first few months of onset.[490, 491] The occasional mildly symptomatic case may respond to topical applications of tetracycline.[493] There is no malignant potential and it does not interfere with normal masticatory functions, and so no treatment is required except for the rare example of a plaque that extends onto the lip vermilion and is surgically removed for esthetic reasons.

Actinic Cheilosis

Actinic cheilosis (actinic cheilitis) is a diffuse, degenerative, irreversible alteration of the vermilion border of the lips that results from excessive exposure to ultraviolet light.[498–502] It primarily affects persons with light complexions, especially those with a tendency to sunburn easily.

Clinical Features. Actinic cheilosis is a disease of persons older than 50 years of age, and its frequency increases with advancing age thereafter. The male to female ratio is as high as 10:1 in some studies.[7, 500, 502] Almost all cases occur on the lower lip vermilion, probably because of the more direct sunlight exposure of that site.

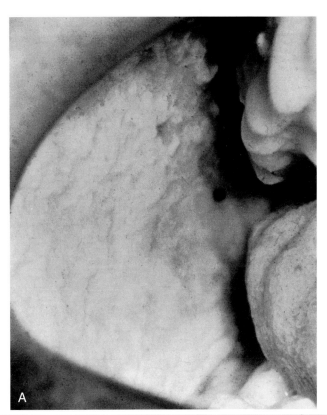

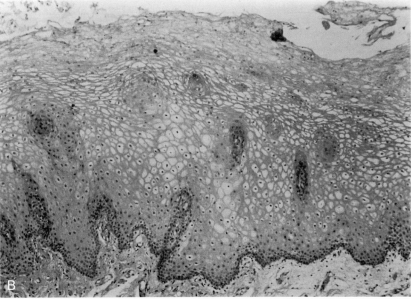

Figure 4–42. *A,* White sponge nevus presents as a corrugated white plaque of the buccal mucosa. (Courtesy of Dr. Robert Gorlin, University of Minnesota, Minneapolis, Minnesota.) *B,* The intracellular edema of superficial cells may be indistinguishable from those of leukoedema or severe chronic cheek bite.

The labial changes develop so slowly that the patient is frequently unaware of a change, beginning with mild puffiness and vermilion atrophy with admixed blotchy areas of pallor and erythema, perhaps with a bluish background hue. The normal demarcation between the vermilion zone and the skin of the lip becomes blurred or disappears. As the lesion progresses, rough, scaly areas develop on the drier portions of the vermilion, appearing in some cases as *leukoplakia*. Painless ulceration may develop in one or more sites, especially in areas of mild trauma. Ulcers may last for months, even years, and may be difficult to differentiate from ulcerated *squamous cell carcinoma*, although the latter is typically more indurated. Ulcers more than 2 months old should be biopsied to evaluate for malignancy.

Pathologic Features. Atrophic stratified squamous epithelium is seen, often with marked parakeratin production and possibly with epithelial dysplasia of the basal and parabasal layers. Rete ridges may be lost. The subepithelial stroma invariably demonstrates an amorphous, acellular, lightly basophilic change (solar elastosis, actinic elastosis) from the ultraviolet light–induced breakdown of collagen fibers (Fig. 4–44, see p. 176). Fibrovascular tissues above and below the elastosis are often scattered with lymphocytes. The lower margin of the elastosis is relatively uniform throughout the lip, but areas of involvement may be separated laterally by less damaged stroma.

Treatment and Prognosis. Actinic cheilosis is an irreversible change, and squamous cell carcinoma, almost always well-differentiated, develops in 6% to 10% of cases.[7, 500] Malignant transformation seldom occurs prior to 60 years of age and the resulting carcinoma typically enlarges so slowly and metastasizes so late that one population study found no deaths and minimal morbidity from the carcinomas.[3]

Follow-up is recommended and patients should use lip balm with sunscreens to prevent further degeneration.[499–501] Occurrence of induration, thickening, ulceration, or leukoplakia should lead to biopsy for histopathologic evaluation. In severe cases without malignancy, a lip shave procedure (vermilionectomy) can remove the vermilion mucosa and replace it with a portion of the intraoral labial mucosa.

Benign Migratory Glossitis

Benign migratory glossitis is a psoriasiform mucositis of the dorsum of the tongue.[503–505] Its dominant characteristic is a constantly changing pattern of serpiginous white lines surrounding areas of smooth, depapillated mucosa. The changing appearance has led some to call this the *wandering rash of the tongue,* whereas the depapillated areas have reminded others of continental outlines on a globe, hence the use of the popular term *geographic tongue.* As with psoriasis, the etiology of benign migratory glossitis is unknown, but it does seem to become more prominent during conditions of psychologic stress and it is found with increased frequency (10%) in persons with psoriasis of the skin.[7, 506] The great majority of those with oral involvement, however, lack psoriatic skin involvement. Approximately 1% to 2% of the population are affected, although most cases are so mild that they are never formally diagnosed.[1, 224]

Clinical Features. Geographic tongue affects all ages and both genders, with no particular age group more affected than others.[503–505] The entire lingual dorsum is often involved with serpiginous, irregular, slightly raised and separated white lines that generally surround variably sized areas of smooth, red or pink mucosa without papillae (Fig. 4–45A). Occasionally there will be a shallow, nonhemorrhagic cleft between the line and the smooth mucosal patch, and more than one fifth of all examples are associated with a generalized fissuring of the tongue. Some smooth patches lack the white rimming.

The white lines advance outward from the smooth patches, with healing occurring in some areas while extension is occurring in others. Individual smooth macules often coalesce and the overall appearance usually changes on a daily or weekly basis. Most examples are asymptomatic, but some patients complain of intermittent tingling, mild tenderness, or pain with spicy foods. Lesions with secondary *candidiasis* may present with a burning sensation of the lingual dorsum, especially toward the tip of the tongue.

Rarely, patients will present with an unchanging pattern, referred to as *stationary geographic tongue* or *nonmigratory glossitis,* or with extension onto the nonpapillated ventral surfaces of the tongue, or even with involvement of the buccal, labial, or soft palate mucosa. The latter cases are called *benign migratory stomatitis* or *erythema migrans* and may present with either white or red serpiginous lines.[506–508]

Erythematous patches without such lines but with psoriasiform histopathology are referred to simply as *psoriasis* and are decidedly rare.[509, 510] *Reiter's syndrome,* a combination of *conjunctivitis, urethritis,* and *arthritis* demonstrates oral psoriasiform, erythematous macules in 1 of every 10 cases.[7] The macules occur in young adults after a variety of infections and may have the serpiginous white outlines of erythema migrans, called *circinate balanitis,* on penile skin. Deep, painful oral ulcers in Reiter's syndrome are common but not universal; they help distinguish oral lesions from simple geographic tongue or mouth.

Pathologic Features and Differential Diagnosis. All of the microscopic features of psoriasis are present in benign migratory glossitis and migratory stomatitis, but these will not be obvious unless the biopsy is taken from a prominent serpiginous line at the periphery of a depapillated patch. A thickened layer of keratin is infiltrated with neutrophils, as are lower portions of the epithelium to a lesser extent (Fig. 4–45B). These inflammatory cells often produce small microabscesses, called Monro's abscesses, in the keratin and spinous layers. Rete ridges are typically thin and considerably elongated, with only a thin layer of epithelium overlying connective tissue papillae. When rete ridges are not elongated, the pathologist should consider Reiter's syndrome as a diagnostic possibility. Chronic inflammatory cells can be seen in variable numbers within the stroma and silver or PAS staining will often demonstrate candidal hyphae or spores in the superficial layers of the epithelium. There is no liquefactive degeneration of basal cells, as seen in lichenoid lesions, and there is no ulceration except in cases of Reiter's syndrome.

Few other pustular diseases affect the oral mucosa. True psoriasis of the oral mucosa would present, of course, an identical appearance under the microscope. Other pustular diseases include *pyostomatitis vegetans, stomatitis herpetiformis,* and the hyperplastic inflammatory response *(parulis)* at the orifice of a fistula extending to the surface from a dental or periodontal abscess. These lesions all present with microabscess or neutrophilic infiltration of the lower portions of the epithelium or of the underlying connective tissue papillae. None are present with abscesses of the keratin or superficial layers. Also, occasional examples of *subcorneal pustular dermatitis* are encountered in the mouth as *subcorneal pustular mucositis,* but the separation of the keratin layer from the spinous layer makes it rather easy to differentiate from migratory stomatitis.

Treatment and Prognosis. No treatment is usually necessary for benign migratory glossitis and stomatitis. Symptomatic lesions can be treated with topical prednisolone and a topical or systemic antifungal medication can be tried if a secondary candidiasis is suspected. Occasional symptomatic cases respond well to topical tetracycline or systemic, broad-spectrum antibiotics, but this should not be expected.

Lichen Planus

Lichen planus is a lichenoid autoimmune mucositis with a clinically different but microscopically similar dermal counterpart.[511–517] On the skin, the disease is usually of shorter duration, approximately 3 years, and does not have the ulcerating and blistering effects seen frequently in oral lesions. In the mouth, lichen planus has several clinical variants with considerable cross-over between variants, and with occasional shifting from one variant to another.

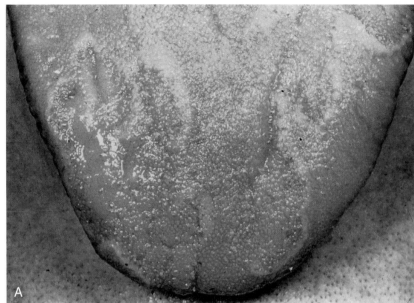

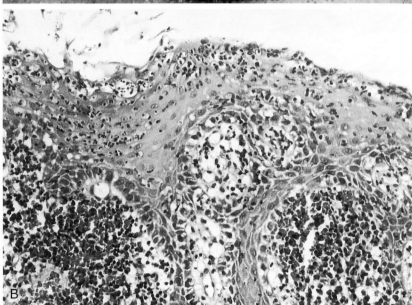

Figure 4–45. *A,* Benign migratory glossitis typically presents with serpiginous white lines admixed with grooves and areas of denuded papillae on the dorsum of the tongue. *B,* Neutrophils diffusely infiltrate the keratin layer, often producing Monro's abscesses.

Some of these variants are thought to represent an elevated cancer risk but there is ongoing debate as to the validity of this hypothesis.[7, 514–518] Some authors, including us, believe that the cancers do, in fact, arise from the long-standing lichenoid lesions, but others presume that the occurrence is simply the fortuitous simultaneous development of two independent entities.[7, 517, 518] The controversy, unfortunately, is fueled more by opinion than substantial facts. Numerous case reports have not resolved this issue, but several follow-up studies have found an increased frequency of cancer, and the cancers that develop are usually in areas of the lichenoid change. No definitive epidemiologic study, however, has been performed.

Malignant "degeneration" or transformation, if it does ensue, is most likely to occur in lesions subclassified as atrophic or erosive lichen planus, with a broad erythematous background. Most bullous and ulcerative lichen planus lesions also have this red surrounding mucosa; therefore, these also are thought to be susceptible to malignant change.

Some cases of lichenoid oral mucosal change have obvious etiologic associations, usually a systemic medication or mucosal contact with dental materials or certain spices, but the etiology in most cases remains unknown. There is no strong association between oral and dermal lesions, and most persons with oral involvement never have skin involvement. Oral lichen planus is found in 1 in 1000 adults.[1]

Clinical Features. Population studies have shown a similar prevalence rate for men and women, but clinical investigations have always found a relatively strong female predilection, usually with a 1 : 2 male : female ratio.[1, 11, 514, 517] All ages are affected, but the disease is rare in children and is most likely to be first seen in young and middle-aged adults. The great majority of cases present as irregular bilateral plaques of the buccal mucosa, but any oral surface can be affected and occasional patients present with extensive involvement throughout the mouth. Lichen planus of the keratinized oral mucosa, such as gingiva, lingual dorsum, and hard palate, may be so excessively keratinized that lesions are clinically indistinguishable from *leukoplakia* or *frictional keratosis.*

The most common oral presentation is a reticular or "spider web" pattern of slightly raised, white keratotic streaks, mistakenly termed Wickham's striae after the fine checkerboard pattern found on the dermal plaques of lichen planus (Fig. 4–46*A*). The intersecting white lines characteristically show numerous very fine perpendicular white lines along their length, and areas of intersection often have punctate nodules of keratin hyperplasia. Some individuals will show only these punctate nodules, whereas others will show serpiginous or circinate white lines, with or without a background of reticulated lines.

In addition to the keratotic changes, half of affected mucosa shows a diffuse background of mild to intense erythema, which may extend some distance from the white lines. This red macule is poorly demarcated from the surrounding normal mucosa and apparently represents epithelial atrophy, allowing underlying vascular flow to become more visible. Occasional lesions are primarily erythematous, with very few white streaks, and these must be distinguished by biopsy from *erythroplakia* and *erythroleukoplakia,* as well as from oral *psoriasis.* Occasional lesions also will present with intermittent, sometimes severe, ulceration or blistering of the mucosa.

Most cases of lichen planus are asymptomatic, but atrophic and ulcerative cases may be somewhat tender and sensitive to abrasive

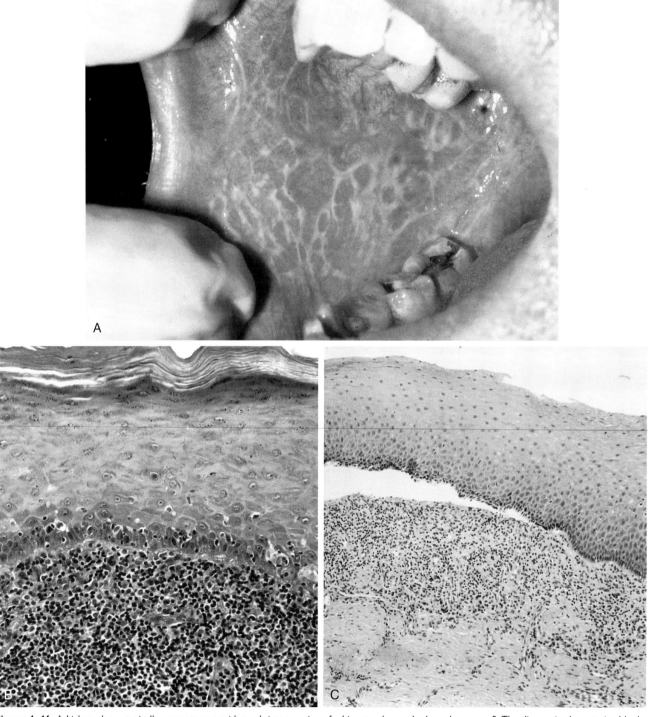

Figure 4–46. *A,* Lichen planus typically presents as a spider-web interweaving of white streaks on the buccal mucosa. *B,* The disease is characterized by hyperkeratosis with ballooning degeneration of basal cells and with a subepithelial band of chronic inflammatory or immune cells. *C,* Blister formation in lichen planus occurs at the level of the basement membrane, with ballooning degeneration of the basal cells often noted in areas where the epithelium pulls away from the connective tissue.

contacts or acidic foods. The pruritus so common to the dermal lesions is not present in the oral lesions. The clinician must be diligent in the attempt to relate the oral lesion to adjacent dental materials or a patient habit, such as chewing gum with cinnamon or peppermint flavoring. When a specific contact hypersensitivity is suspected, the diagnostic term *lichenoid reaction* is preferred. The clinician must also be diligent in his or her search for induration, ulceration, and other clinical signs of malignancy.

Pathologic Features and Differential Diagnosis. Oral lichen planus, like its dermal counterpart, is characterized by a subepithelial band of chronic inflammatory cells, predominantly lymphocytes, which has a lower border well demarcated from deeper connective tissues. When plasma cells or Langerhans cells are numerous, lichenoid reaction rather that autoimmune lichen planus should be suspected. If the biopsy is performed during an episode of quiescent activity, this band of infiltrate might be quite sparse, and if a stria is cut cross-wise, the band will appear as a subepithelial lymphoid aggregate.

Liquefactive or ballooning degeneration of cells of the basal and suprabasal layers is also characteristic of lichen planus (Fig. 4–46B), although it may be patchy and minimally present. Degenerated apoptotic cells may be seen in the epithelium, and occasional cases will show eosinophilic colloid or Civatte bodies between the spinous cells. Patchy areas often demonstrate squamoid change of basal cells, and rete ridges may show one of two patterns: complete loss of the ridges with flattening of the inferior surface of the epithelium, or a morphologic shift into an inverted triangle or "sawtoothed" ridge, as is more frequently seen in the skin counterpart. Many cases will show a thickened or hyalinized basement membrane, perhaps with scattered clear microvesicles, and in dark-skinned individuals melanin pigmentation may be seen within and beneath the basal cell layer (pigment incontinence).

Bullous lichen planus is represented by blister formation at the level of the basement membrane (Fig. 4–46C), and ulcerative lichen planus will show typical inflammatory degeneration and necrosis of epithelium adjacent to the ulcer. In the latter, no epithelium remains along the ulcer bed itself, and in the former, small epithelial tags may be seen to lift away from the basement membrane at the ulcer edge. When lesions are ulcerated, the lichenoid band of inflammatory cells may be replaced by the more randomly distributed chronic and acute inflammatory cells of granulation tissue. The band is still present beneath bullous lesions for several hours after the blister has ruptured.

The surface is excessively keratinized by parakeratin, orthokeratin, or a combination thereof, except in the most atrophic cases. On mucosal surfaces that are normally heavily keratinized, this keratin hyperplasia may represent more than half of the entire epithelial thickness and may show short, pointed surface projections similar to those seen in *verruciform leukoplakia.* The granular cell layer may become pronounced, but only in lesions with secondary frictional trauma of long duration.

The pathologist must always be careful to evaluate the basal epithelium for evidence of dysplasia, especially in atrophic and ulcerated cases. When dysplasia is found, it is graded as it would be without the surrounding lichenoid changes, but the diagnosis is often changed to *lichenoid dysplasia.* It is not yet known whether such cases represent transformation of a true lichen planus or an unusual T-cell response to altered basal cells.

The differential diagnosis of intraoral lichen planus includes the aforementioned lichenoid dysplasia and *contact stomatitis* or lichenoid reaction. Distinguishing features of lichenoid drug reaction include infiltration of lymphocytes high into the epithelium, quite pronounced liquefactive degeneration of basal cells, and loss of the sharp demarcation of the lower margin of the infiltrated band.

Cases with very thick subepithelial immunologic infiltrates, especially those with lymphoid aggregates deep in subepithelial connective tissues, are more likely associated with hypersensitivity reactions, as are lesions with numerous plasma and Langerhans cells.[517, 519, 520] Deep aggregates may, moreover, be perivascular,

may contain germinal centers, and may be indicative of a secondary *candidiasis* or a systemic lichenoid disease such as *lupus erythematosus.*[521] Because of the latter associations, fungal stains should be used, especially if there are neutrophils in the keratin layers, and signs of vasculitis should be sought, although a negative result in either examination does not necessarily rule out yeast or systemic autoimmunity.

Another lichenoid mucositis to be considered in the differential diagnosis is *graft versus host disease,* which likely has a common pathoetiology in T-cell damage to the epithelium.[7, 522, 523] The lymphocytic band in graft versus host disease is usually more sparse and less well-defined than that of idiopathic lichen planus, and marked fibrosis of subepithelial stroma is common in long-standing cases. Subepithelial blistering is rare except during acute stage disease, in which case skin involvement is quite likely and greatly aids in the diagnosis. It is important to remember that almost all individuals with graft versus host disease demonstrate some form of oral involvement, slight though it may be.

Direct immunofluorescence is of some value in the differential diagnosis of lichen planus, but it is seldom used because other features are adequate to the task. In more than three quarters of all cases there is a slightly irregular linear deposition of fibrinogen along the basement membrane. This rather nonspecific change is not diagnostic in and of itself but can be quite helpful, when combined with the clinical features and with the absence of immunoglobulin or complement reactivity, to rule out other autoimmune disorders such as *pemphigoid* and lupus erythematosus. The pathologist must be cautious, however, as occasional patchy complement-associated immunofluorescence may be seen in the basement membrane adjacent to an ulcerative or atrophic area of lichen planus.

Discoid and systemic lupus erythematosus may present with oral keratotic and ulcerative lesions that are clinically identical to lichen planus and show a strong histopathologic similarity as well. Elongated, thin rete ridges are more likely to be associated with lupus, as is deep extension of the subepithelial lymphocytic band, especially with lymphoid aggregates present. Rete hyperplasia in lupus may, in fact, be so extensive that dyskeratosis occurs and the epithelium takes on the localized appearance of *pseudoepitheliomatous hyperplasia.* Thickened or degenerated endothelium with perivascular infiltrates is, of course, very helpful for the identification of lupus vasculitis, but these changes are often missing in oral examples. Cutaneous lupus lesions usually show a positive IgG and IgA reactivity along the basement membrane, and a patchy band of complement reactivity may be seen on immunofluorescence. Circulating antinuclear antibodies may also be present in cases of systemic disease, but an extensive discussion of the extraoral characteristics of lupus is beyond the scope of this chapter.

Lichen sclerosus et atrophicus is the final lesion to differentiate from oral lichen planus. Extremely rare in the mouth, this typically genital mucositis may be clinically indistinguishable from oral lichen planus. The epithelium is uniformly atrophic, often extremely so, and only a thin layer of surface keratin is seen. There is typically extensive subepithelial fibrosis or hyalinization and a lesser inflammatory infiltrate is noticed; the infiltrate is often separated from the epithelium by a hyalinized band. Subepithelial hyalinization is also a feature of *systemic sclerosis* or *scleroderma, amyloidosis,* and *oral submucous fibrosis.* Congo red birefringence and thioflavin T fluorescence can help to rule out amyloidosis, but differences in clinical features may be needed to rule out the other disorders.

Treatment and Prognosis. There is no cure for this disease, and therapy is only palliative.[515, 517, 524] Fortunately, oral lichen planus lesions wax and wane and are typically asymptomatic. For those patients suffering from tenderness and sensitivity to acidic foods, topical or systemic prednisolone is usually effective but should be used sparingly because of the potential systemic side effects. Persons affected with oral lesions seldom develop skin lesions, although the clinician should be on the lookout for evidence of lupus erythematosus during follow-up examinations, especially in patients with arthritic joint pains.

Table 4–7. Inflammatory Ulcers of the Oral Mucosa

Diagnosis	Special Features
Flat, shallow ulceration (bullous ulcers)	
Benign mucous membrane pemphigoid	Subepithelial blister may be evident in epithelium at ulcer edge
Pemphigus vulgaris	Intraepithelial blister may be evident in epithelium at ulcer edge
Bullous lichen planus	Subepithelial blister at ulcer edge; other signs of lichen planus
Epidermolysis bullosa	Subepithelial blister may be evident in epithelium at ulcer edge
Linear IgA disease	Subepithelial blister may be evident in epithelium at ulcer edge
Coalesced viral vesicles	Intraepithelial vesicle, often with neutrophils in vesicle fluids; may show syncytial epithelial cells with multiple nuclei
Aphthous-like (saucerized) ulcers	
Aphthous stomatitis	Ulcer bed of fibrinoid necrotic debris over granulation tissue
Traumatic ulcer	Same ulcer as aphthous; may be factitial
Traumatic eosinophilic ulceration	Scattered eosinophils in granulation tissue of the ulcer bed
Squamous cell carcinoma, early	Dysplastic squamous epithelium
Necrotizing sialometaplasia	Squamoid metaplastic salivary cells; infarction and necrosis of fat and gland
Ulcerative colitis/Crohn's disease	May be granulomatous or consist of granulation tissue
Fungating ulceration	
Tuberculosis	Caseating granulomatous inflammation
Tertiary syphilis (gumma)	Noncaseating granulomatous inflammation
Deep fungal infections	Noncaseating granulomatous inflammation, special stains show fungus
Squamous cell carcinoma	Dysplastic epithelial cells
Necrotizing sialometaplasia	Squamoid metaplastic salivary cells; infarction and necrosis of fat and gland
Traumatic eosinophilic ulcer	Scattered eosinophils in granulation tissue of the ulcer bed
Eosinophilic granuloma (Langerhans' cell disease)	Eosinophils, histiocytes, and lymphocytes, perhaps with multinucleated giant cells
Keratoacanthoma	Well-differentiated down-growing squamous epithelium; ulcer bed is actually cleft filled with keratin plug
Ulcerative colitis/Crohn's disease	May be granulomatous or consist of granulation tissue

For patients with atrophic or ulcerative or bullous forms of the disease, an examination for early oral cancer should be performed every 4 to 6 months. This follow-up may entail repeat biopsies of areas of nonhealing ulceration, induration, or deep erythema. The estimated risk of malignant transformation, if real, is less than 2% over a 10-year period.[7, 517] Lichen sclerosus et atrophicus of the mouth carries no malignant potential, as it does in the genital region.

ULCERATIVE AND BLISTERING MUCOSAL LESIONS

The oral epithelium is prone to traumatic, autoimmune hypersensitivity and inflammatory damage resulting in surface ulceration and blisters of varying sizes. Mucocutaneous viral infections, such as those from the herpes simplex, varicella zoster, and coxsackie viruses, produce small, clear vesicles within the spinous and other layers of the epithelium, often attracting chronic and acute inflammatory cells into the epithelium. Autoimmune damage is usually antibody mediated and may be demonstrated by a breakdown of intercellular attachments in the spinous layer, as in *pemphigus* or *Darier's disease,* or by a loss of attachment to the basement membrane or subepithelial stroma, as in *benign mucous membrane pemphigoid, bullous lichen planus,* and *linear IgA disease.* Occasional allergic reactions will also produce intraepithelial or subepithelial bullae and vesicles, especially in *contact mucositis* and *erythema multiforme.* Rarely, a developmental disorder such as *hereditary epidermolysis bullosa* will result in subepithelial blisters.

The major role of the histopathologist in oral vesiculobullous disease is to confirm the working clinical diagnosis prior to the use of systemic or topical therapies. The first task is to determine the size of the biopsied lesion (vesicles are less than 3 mm in diameter; bullae are larger) and the vertical location of the blister within the epithelium.

The role of the pathologist in noncancerous oral ulcerative disease is often more difficult because microscopic changes can be rather subtle or nonspecific. Many inflammatory ulcers have a similar clinical appearance and the histopathology becomes especially important in these cases. The discussion following begins with generic changes and discusses the wide variety of potential diagnoses as differential diagnosis rather than devoting separate sections to each ulcerative disorder.

Inflammatory Mucosal Ulceration

Inflammatory ulceration of the oral mucosa is quite common (Table 4–7). As many as 20% of adults suffer from *aphthous stomatitis* or *canker sores,* and certainly more than that experience occasional traumatic ulceration from teeth and dental prostheses. At any one time, however, only 1 of 800 adults has such an ulcer active in the mouth.[1, 7] Only those ulcers that do not heal quickly, clinically mimic oral malignancy, or exist as part of a larger scheme of mucosal changes are biopsied. The correct histopathologic interpretation of such lesions may be confusing and often requires close communication between pathologist and submitting surgeon. Because of this, they are discussed here as a common group.

Clinical Features. The two most important features of oral ulcerations not associated with keratosis are the inflammatory response of surrounding mucosa and the depth of the ulcer bed; the presence or absence of pain is of secondary importance. Mucosal ulcers are typically surrounded by an erythematous halo, indicating a normal and healthy inflammatory response. Often there will be a very thin line of coagulation necrosis separating the halo from the ulcer bed. Without the inflammatory halo, a nonhealing ulcer may represent a local manifestation of immunoincompetence, especially *diabetes mellitus, AIDS,* or *leukemia,* or it may represent the end-stage healing of an innocuous ulcer.

Oral ulcers resulting from blistering disorders present with a flat, shallow ulcer bed, sometimes with small epithelial tags at the margin. Only rarely is an intact blister seen in the mouth. A deep or moderately deep ulcer has a cupped-out, saucerized appearance and is described as aphthous-like because of a clinical similarity to the recurring *aphthous ulcer* of *aphthous stomatitis.*[525–528] Such ulcers are usually quite painful, but very deep examples representing malignancy or granulomatous inflammation are often entirely without pain. The only ulcer that becomes painful before the appearance of the ulcer itself (prodromal pain) is the aphthous ulcer. The *traumatic ulcer* is, of course, linked to an obvious episode of local trauma.

Multiple saucerized ulcers associated with moderately severe pain may represent, in addition to aphthous stomatitis, *Behçet's disease, ulcerative colitis, chronic ulcerative stomatitis,* or nonhealing traumatic ulceration in immunoincompetence or *neutropenia.*[529–531] A dirty brownish-yellow ulcer bed is indicative of necrosis of underlying fat or of hemorrhage into the ulcer bed. These are seen primarily in *necrotizing sialometaplasia* and in *purpura, leukemia,* and *aplastic anemia.*

Ulcerating oral *squamous cell carcinoma* is usually deeply ulcerated and has an indurated, rolled border surrounding it, usually without an inflammatory halo and usually without tenderness or pain until the late stages of growth. Malignancy and granulomatous inflammation may also present as fungating growths prior to central ulceration and destruction. A special form of traumatic ulcer, the *traumatic eosinophilic ulcer,* may show so much exophytic growth that it can easily be mistaken for *pyogenic granuloma* or ulcerated carcinoma (Fig. 4–47A, see p. 177).[532]

A unique and quite site-specific ulceration of the gingival papillae between the teeth, *acute necrotizing ulcerative gingivitis (ANUG, trench mouth)* is exquisitely painful even though the necrotic ulcers remain small and localized.[533] Although normally self-limiting, ANUG in immunocompromised individuals may extend to adjacent oral soft tissues to produce a life-threatening destruction of the maxillofacial region, called variously *necrotizing ulcerative stomatitis, gangrenous stomatitis, cancrum oris,* or *noma.*[7, 533]

Destruction of bone beneath a mucosal ulcer is a serious event, most likely indicative of malignancy, *Wegener's granulomatosis, lethal midline granuloma, granulomatous osteomyelitis (tuberculosis,* tertiary *syphilis),* or *noma.*[7, 534–537]

Pathologic Features and Differential Diagnosis. Saucerized or aphthous-like ulcer beds consist of fibrinoid necrotic debris of the surface with abundant neutrophil dust and other cell remnants (Fig. 4–47B, see p. 177). This typically overlies granulation tissue with variable numbers of chronic and acute inflammatory cells, neovascularity, and edema. Erythrocyte extravasation is seldom seen and if present should make one suspicious of *Wegener's vasculitis, angiosarcoma,* or *Kaposi's sarcoma.* The inflammatory infiltrate should be carefully evaluated for dysplastic cells to rule out leukemic infiltration or *MALT lymphoma,* and an overwhelming predominance of plasma cells may be indicative of *plasmacytoma* or *multiple myeloma.* Filamentous bacterial colonies coated by neutrophils may be seen as a feature of oral *actinomycosis,* and mucosal ulceration in such cases may be associated with the orifice of a fistulous tract extending deeply into underlying soft or hard tissues.[538–540]

Scattered or numerous eosinophils in the granulation tissue are consistent with either traumatic eosinophilic ulcer (Fig. 4–47C, see p. 177) or *Langerhans' cell disease.* Eosinophils are decidedly rare in oral inflammatory lesions and are associated with more aggressive biologic behavior than the typical saucerized ulcer; they rarely may be associated with a protozoan infection. There may be so much proliferation of granulation tissue in these types of ulcerations that the resultant fungating appearance may mimic pyogenic granuloma.

The presence of multinucleated giant cells beneath an ulcer bed is also significant and may indicate serious systemic disease or more aggressive local disease. These are discussed elsewhere in this chapter under the topic of granulomatous inflammations.

Fat necrosis is rarely a feature of oral inflammatory ulceration, but when present it is most likely indicative of necrotizing sialometaplasia. This localized infarction of soft tissues may have a strong chronic inflammatory cell response and is characterized by squamous metaplasia of salivary duct epithelium, fibrous replacement of acinar tissues, ductal ectasia, and edema of surrounding stroma. The pathologist must be very cautious in evaluating the islands of squamous epithelium; many of the early cases of necrotizing sialometaplasia were mistakenly diagnosed as well-

differentiated *squamous cell carcinoma* or *mucoepidermoid carcinoma* and treated accordingly.

Treatment and Prognosis. The treatment of an oral ulceration is very much dependent on the final histopathologic diagnosis. Traumatic ulcers, of course, will heal without therapy in 4 to 10 days unless there is an underlying immunoincompetence. Granulomatous ulcers require conservative surgical removal and attention to the underlying systemic problem or local foreign material. Traumatic eosinophilic ulcer is excised conservatively the first time, with recurrences removed with a larger margin of normal tissue and with the removal of tipped teeth or other local causes of trauma.

Pemphigus Vulgaris and Other Intraepithelial Blisters

The most serious of the bullous diseases affecting the oral mucosa is *pemphigus vulgaris,* a life-threatening autoimmune disorder of skin and mucous membranes. It is relatively rare but shows an increased frequency in Ashkenazi Jews.[8, 541–544] The mouth is the only site of involvement in half of all cases of pemphigus and is the initial site of presentation in almost three of four cases.[7, 11, 544] An association between pemphigus vulgaris, *myasthenia gravis,* and *thymoma* has been reported, and a variety of drugs have been implicated in its induction, especially penicillamine, phenylbutazone, rifampin, and captopril, although most cases are idiopathic.[8] It is also known to occur in association with a variety of internal malignancies *(paraneoplastic pemphigus).*[11, 545, 546]

Patients with pemphigus vulgaris produce IgG autoantibodies to desmoglein 3 (the "PV antigen"), a transmembrane glycoprotein that mediates cell adhesion.[8, 11, 541] Although the exact mechanism is unclear, autoantibodies theoretically produce an allosteric change in the desmoglein, impairing its adhesive abilities, and increase active plasmin in the area, producing cell degradation and acantholysis. Complement may be actively involved in this process.[8]

Clinical Features. Pemphigus vulgaris is a disease of older individuals, usually 50 years or older, but rare examples in children and adolescents have been reported.[7, 11, 544] There is no gender predilection. The oral lesion is a fragile bulla, almost always ruptured by the time of diagnosis. There is little or no erythematous inflammatory halo and a fresh lesion may retain epithelial tags at its periphery. In contradistinction to *traumatic* and *aphthous ulcers,* the base of a pemphigus ulcer is not concave or saucerized and there is considerably less associated pain. The bullae tend not to become secondarily infected but may reach more than 4 cm in diameter and may be so numerous as to represent most of the oral mucosa. Blisters can be created by pressure or friction upon a normal-appearing area of mucosa *(Nikolsky sign).*

Bullae may present on any oral or oropharyngeal surface, but typically arise in the buccal, palatal, and gingival regions. Occasional patients have lesions restricted completely to the gingiva.[11, 544] Skin lesions are similar except that the more heavily keratinized epidermis allows blisters to remain intact much longer. Most patients have circulating autoantibodies, which can be detected by indirect immunofluorescence using serum from other affected individuals. Titers are directly proportionate to the severity of the disease.[11]

A special subset of patients demonstrates internal malignancy in addition to mucosal and skin erosions and bullae. Called paraneoplastic pemphigus, its oral manifestations may resemble *erythema multiforme* or *bullous lichen planus* and may be extremely severe and resistant to treatment.[546] The associated autoantibodies are different from those of routine pemphigus vulgaris, and can be demonstrated by indirect immunofluorescence using rat bladder transitional epithelium as the substrate.[8, 11] Pemphigus vulgaris shows positive indirect immunofluorescence only on stratified squamous epithelium, such as monkey esophagus. Neoplasms most often associated with this form of pemphigus include *lymphoma, leukemia, sarcoma,* and *thymus tumors. Waldenstrom's macroglobulinemia* and *Castleman's disease* have also been reported as associated.

Rare variants of pemphigus may affect the oral mucosa. *Pemphigus vegetans* presents with much smaller blisters than pemphigus vulgaris. The blisters are often filled with pus and coalesce to impart an appearance of vegetative growth. The vermilion border of the lips is especially prone to involvement. The oral disease most likely to clinically mimic this form of pemphigus is *pyostomatitis vegetans,* a rare oral manifestation of *inflammatory bowel disease,* particularly *ulcerative colitis* and *Crohn's disease.*[7, 547] Oral lesions in this disease are characterized by yellow, partially ulcerated pustules arranged in serpentine strands or "snail tracks" on an erythematous background. Minimal discomfort is felt, and the oral lesions may precede intestinal involvement.

Pemphigus foliaceus may affect perioral and other facial skin. The least severe form of pemphigus, *pemphigus erythematosus,* presents on the face and scalp with scaly dermal erythema reminiscent of *seborrheic dermatitis.* There may be a "butterfly" erythema of the nose and midface, mimicking *lupus erythematosus.* Oral and pharyngeal lesions in these subtypes are extremely rare.

Pathologic Features and Differential Diagnosis. The blistering or cleavage in this disease occurs above the basal layer of the epithelium, typically leaving a layer of basal cells with rounded tops, reminiscent of tombstones (Fig. 4–48*A*). The intact bulla is filled with serum and occasional sloughed, rounded keratinocytes resembling fried eggs, with large, hyperchromatic nuclei and a rim of eosinophilic cytoplasm. The latter acantholytic cells, called *Tzanck cells,* are best seen in the smear sample of a fresh blister *(Tzanck test).* They are strongly suggestive of pemphigus vulgaris but may also be encountered in *Darier's disease* and in regenerating thermally or chemically damaged epithelium.[8, 548] The suprabasal bulla frequently contains chronic and acute inflammatory cells, including eosinophils. The presence of eosinophils in oral vesiculo-ulcerative lesions is somewhat specific, but they may also occur in *pemphigoid, epidermolysis bullosa acquisita, eosinophilic granuloma,* parasitic infection, and *traumatic eosinophilic ulcer.*

When the bulla has ruptured, the associated ulcer bed slowly becomes covered with fibrinoid necrotic debris, with neovascularity and mixed inflammatory cells in the underlying stroma. The epithelium at the edge of a fresh ulcer will show intraepithelial cleavage.

Direct immunofluorescence of perilesional mucosa shows a lacy or chicken-wire pattern of deposits around individual spinous cells of the epithelium (Fig. 4–48*B*). IgG is almost always the deposited immunoglobulin, but IgM and IgA are seen in almost half of all cases.[9, 11, 543] Some authorities have suggested direct immunofluorescence of cytologic smears as a reliable and noninvasive method of diagnostic confirmation.[11, 541] Direct immunofluorescence of paraneoplastic pemphigus mucosa demonstrates both intercellular and basement membrane IgG and complement deposits.[8, 546]

Differentiation from other oral and pharyngeal bullous diseases is easily made, because most of them produce subepithelial blisters (pemphigoid, epidermolysis bullosa, bullous lichen planus, *linear IgA disease*), but small lesions may be mistaken for intraepithelial viral vesicles and any lesion may be confused with the oral keratinized blisters of Darier's disease.[7, 548, 549] Clinical history or the presence of syncytial multinucleated epithelial cells will usually lead to a diagnosis of infection by a dermatotrophic virus capable of damaging oral mucosa, such as herpes simplex, herpes zoster, and coxsackie viruses, whereas the presence of excessive surface keratinization and corps ronds (round bodies) within intact bullae will help differentiate Darier's disease.

Finally, it is important to remember that mucosal lesions of erythema multiforme may demonstrate either intraepithelial or subepithelial blistering, or both.[550, 551] This unique allergic response, however, typically occurs in much younger patients, has a much more abrupt onset, and has a limited duration, making it relatively easy to distinguish it from pemphigus.

Treatment and Prognosis. Systemic corticosteroid therapy is effective in reducing or eliminating the clinical manifestations of pemphigus vulgaris, although doses of prednisone may have to be as high as 400 mg daily for patients with severe involvement.[11, 544] Topical corticosteroids can be used as an adjunct therapy if the bullae are confined to oral mucosa. Oral or intravenous administration of cyclophosphamide, azathioprine, cyclosporine, and methotrexate may have enough beneficial effect to allow reduced dosages of corticosteroids.[8, 11] Even with immunosuppressive therapy, however, almost 10% of patients will die from their disease, from electrolyte loss, wound infection, or treatment complications.[8, 11] Patients with paraneoplastic pemphigus may have to forgo treatment of their vesiculobullous disease until the underlying neoplasm is controlled, although supportive therapy can be instituted.[546]

Benign Mucous Membrane Pemphigoid and Other Subepithelial Blisters

Benign mucous membrane pemphigoid (BMMP, cicatricial pemphigoid) is an autoimmune disorder of mucous membranes that is produced by an antibody attack against the basement membrane, specifically against at least two hemidesmosome antigens, BPAG1 and BPAG2 (collectively called the *bullous pemphigoid antigen*), which bind the basal cell layer of the epithelium to the basement membrane.[552–560] The effect may be quite localized, as circulating autoantibodies are not present in a large proportion of affected individuals, or are present only at low titers using indirect immunofluorescence techniques.[11, 555] The disease results in separation of the epithelium from the underlying stroma at the level of the lamina lucida, the electron lucent zone found between the basal cell membrane and lamina densa.

Compared to pemphigus vulgaris, the disease runs a rather benign, protracted course, with at least one third of patients eventually developing skin involvement of the head and neck region, legs, or genitalia. Additionally, half of all patients will develop bullae of other membranes of the upper aerodigestive tract, the anus, or genitalia. There is an increased frequency of certain HLA tissue types, especially HLA-B12 and HLA-DR4 and Dqw7, and some drug-induced cases have also been associated with different HLA types.[11, 555, 560]

Clinical Features. This disease is characterized by bullous lesions of mucous membranes, especially oral and conjunctival membranes. Eye involvement results in scar formation or fibrous synechiae of palpebral and bulbar conjunctivae, with entropion and blindness occurring in almost one third of untreated cases.[7, 552, 555] Disease onset is usually between 40 and 60 years of patient age, and oral lesions are the first manifestation of disease in two thirds of cases.[11, 552, 553] There is no racial or ethnic predilection, but the disease is much more common in women than in men (male : female ratio, 1 : 2).[7, 555]

Individual lesions develop slowly and are usually smaller and less frequent during the early months or years of the disease (Fig. 4–49*A*, see p. 178). Bullae may, however, become more than 3 cm in diameter and may remain intact long enough for the clinician to see them as clear or slightly bluish blisters. Although there is seldom a surrounding inflammatory halo, the mucosa in the affected region may be quite diffusely erythematous and at least 10% of patients will have a positive Nikolsky test (creation of a blister by pressure or friction).[553] A ruptured blister leaves a shallow, mildly tender ulcer bed that heals in 7 to 10 days. Large or secondarily infected lesions may result in scar formation, but this phenomenon is much less severe than it is with conjunctival involvement.

Oral sites most often involved include the gingiva (90% of oral cases), palate, and buccal mucosa.[7, 552, 554] Although individual blisters do not necessarily recur at the same exact site, new lesions do seem to remain contained within a limited anatomic region. When only the gingiva or alveolar mucosa are involved, the disease has a special tendency to remain localized, and this has led some authorities to prefer the more generic term, *desquamative gingivitis.*[557–560]

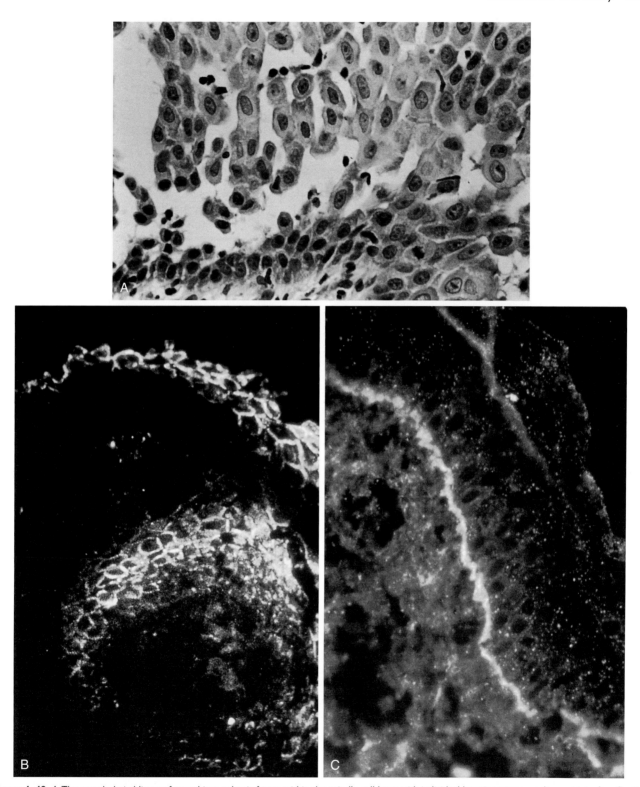

Figure 4–48. *A,* The acantholytic blister of pemphigus vulgaris forms within the spindle cell layer with individual keratinocytes rounding out into free-floating Tzanck cells within the blister; notice the tombstone effect of the basal cells, which remain attached to the basement membrane. *B,* Immunoglobulin is deposited around individual epithelial cells in pemphigus, imparting a chicken-wire pattern. *C,* Immunoglobulins are deposited along the basement membrane in benign mucous membrane pemphigoid.

Desquamative gingivitis is, however, a term also used to describe gingival manifestations of *pemphigus* and *bullous lichen planus.*

Pathologic Features and Differential Diagnosis. Oral bullae demonstrate separation of the epithelium from the basement membrane (Fig. 4–49*B,* see p. 178), often with small numbers of chronic and acute inflammatory cells, including eosinophils, in the extracellular serous fluid of the blister. Only rarely will chronic inflammatory cells be seen within the subepithelial stroma of a fresh, unruptured lesion. Most lesions, however, are ruptured at the time of biopsy, so the subepithelial separation may only be found at the edge of an otherwise nonspecific inflammatory ulceration. Direct immunofluorescence will demonstrate in almost all cases a continuous linear band of IgG and C3 immunoreactants along the basement membrane (see Fig. 4–48C). More than half of all patients will also have circulating autoantibodies identifiable in the serum through indirect immunofluorescence.

Pemphigoid is distinguished from pemphigus by the location of the blister: the latter produces acantholysis with cleavage of the spinous cell layer, whereas the former produces cleavage of the basement membrane region. Other entities can create subepithelial cleavage or blistering, including *linear IgA disease, bullous lichen planus, epidermolysis bullosa* (hereditary and acquired forms), *bullosa hemorrhagica, erythema multiforme, bullous pemphigoid,* and *dermatitis herpetiformis.*[11, 552, 553, 560–564]

The ruptured blisters of adult-onset linear IgA are very similar except that there is typically a neutrophilic infiltrate along the basement membrane and surrounding the blood vessels of the subepithelial stroma.[561] Neutrophilic microabscesses may be present within the connective tissue papillae, and on direct immunofluorescence linear deposits of IgA are seen along the basement membrane. Eruptions identical in every way to linear IgA have occurred with the use of lithium, vancomycin, diclofenac, and glibenclamide.[11, 561]

Dermatitis herpetiformis has an histopathologic appearance similar to linear IgA disease, except that the basement membrane deposits of IgA have a more irregular or granular appearance. It also presents typically with small, viral-like vesicles rather than the larger bullae of pemphigoid or linear IgA.

Bullous lichen planus has a distinct band of chronic inflammatory or immunologic cells immediately beneath the epithelium, which usually makes it easy to distinguish it from pemphigoid. A loss of rete ridges or the formation of saw-toothed ridges is also characteristically found, as is liquefactive (hydropic, ballooning) degeneration of the basal cells and a thickened surface layer of parakeratin. There are, however, occasional cases with lichenoid light microscopic changes and characteristic pemphigoid immunofluorescence.[556]

Routine histopathologic examination will often not distinguish between *epidermolysis bullosa acquisita (EBA)* and pemphigoid, and at least half of EBA patients have involvement of the oral mucosa.[562] Immunofluorescence will, however, show IgG isoantibody deposition on the floor of the EBA bulla, whereas antibodies coat the roof of the blister in pemphigoid.[11] In EBA, the blisters arise beneath the basal lamina, where the anchoring fibrils (type VII collagen) are destroyed. EBA may, moreover, be associated with *Crohn's disease* and other *inflammatory bowel diseases, rheumatoid arthritis, systemic lupus erythematosus, idiopathic pulmonary fibrosis,* and *chronic thyroiditis.* Hereditary epidermolysis bullosa is more easily distinguished by its childhood onset and its classic acral distribution.[563, 564]

Erythema multiforme bullosa can present with subepithelial or intraepithelial cleavage, or both together, but it typically also has subepithelial edema and infiltration by mixed inflammatory cells, including eosinophils. Subepithelial vesiculation is seen in association with necrotic basal keratinocytes, whereas pemphigoid basal cells remain intact. Many cases cannot, however, be distinguished from pemphigoid using histopathologic and immunoreactive features, and the diagnosis is often based on the clinical presentation and exclusion of other vesiculobullous disorders. Erythema multiforme not only occurs at a younger age than pemphigoid, but it typically has a duration limited to weeks or months, whereas pemphigoid remains an incurable disease.

Treatment and Prognosis. Oral pemphigoid can often be controlled by topical or systemic corticosteroids or other immunosuppressive agents, particularly cyclophosphamide, but there is no cure for this disease. Lesions occur intermittently and may affect different parts of the oral mucosa at different times. Seldom do blisters occur elsewhere in the upper aerodigestive tract, but patients with laryngeal or esophageal involvement will develop dysphagia or esophageal webs. Ocular involvement eventually becomes manifested in 50% to 85% of cases and skin involvement is eventually

seen in up to 30% of cases.[11, 553] The patient should be followed carefully by an ophthalmologist whether or not conjunctival involvement is seen at the time of oral lesion diagnosis.

PIGMENTED MUCOSAL LESIONS

Focal mucosal discoloration is not uncommon in the mouth, although it usually represents an underlying vascular change, as discussed previously in this chapter. Nonvascular mucosal pigmentations are found in approximately 1 of every 500 adults, although they are not commonly biopsied.[1] Submucosal foreign material will often become embedded within small injuries created inadvertently during dental restorative procedures or in association with a wound occurring while holding a pencil or some other object in the mouth. These produce permanent brown, black, or gray mucosal discolorations or *tattoos,* which may require biopsy to rule out *malignant melanoma* or *lentigo maligna.* Occasional systemic poisoning by certain metals may show visible deposits within the oral mucosa, especially the gingival tissues. These metals include mercury *(acrodynia),* lead *(gingival "lead line"),* cadmium or bismuth *("bismuth line"),* and silver *(argyria),* among others. Although the skin pigmentation in *hemochromatosis (bronze diabetes)* is largely caused by increased amounts of melanin in the basal cell layer of the epidermis, iron from hemosiderin may also be deposited in the dermis of many patients, producing a brown-black discoloration.

Melanin-containing oral lesions also, of course, occur in the mouth in the absence of systemic disease, usually as *racial pigmentation* or innocuous *melanotic macules,* but their similarity to early melanoma often requires a biopsy evaluation. It should be remembered that melanin deposition might not just be a local change but may represent systemic diseases, such as *Addison's disease, Albright's disease,* or *Peutz-Jeghers syndrome,* or induction from a systemic medication, such as chloroquine or another of the quinine derivatives.

Amalgam Tattoo

The implantation of dental materials into mildly injured or periodontally inflamed mucosal tissues during the restoration of carious teeth is not an unusual event. The material most likely to present as a mucosal discoloration is amalgam from the "silver fillings," hence, the lesion is usually called an *amalgam tattoo,* but other metals may produce the same effect.[7, 565–568] Most of the time these "biocompatible" materials do not illicit a local inflammatory response, but occasional cases are associated with chronic inflammatory changes compatible with a foreign body reaction. Amalgam is a combination of mercury, silver, tin, copper, and, sometimes, zinc. The mercury usually constitutes half of the mixture and rarely produces obvious tissue necrosis despite its rather high level of toxicity in other settings. Overall, amalgam tattoo is found in approximately 1 per 1000 adults.[1]

Occasional deposits of amalgam are found intraosseously, usually as a result of the material being inadvertently scraped from an adjacent restoration during tooth extraction or other surgical procedure, including the deliberate placement of amalgam into the apical canal of a root during endodontic surgery.

Clinical Features. The amalgam tattoo presents as a soft, painless, nonulcerated, blue-gray-black macule with no surrounding erythematous reaction.[7, 9, 565] It is most frequently found on the gingival or alveolar mucosa, but many cases are seen on the buccal mucosa and no anatomic site is immune from this change. The tattoo is found more frequently in females than in males, perhaps because women more frequently seek dental care. It is also seen more frequently with advancing patient age, presumably because of increased exposure to dental procedures over time.

The tattoo is only moderately demarcated from the surrounding mucosa and is usually less than 0.5 cm in greatest diameter, although rare examples have been more than 3.0 cm in size. Lesions with larger particles will be visible on routine dental radiographs.

Pathologic Features. The amalgam tattoo is characterized by an unencapsulated area of submucosal stroma with clusters of small black-brown rounded particles, often seen to coat blood vessels and reticulin fibers (Fig. 4–50, see p. 178). Occasional larger, angular particles are seen, but seldom is there a noticeable inflammatory cell response. When present, this response is usually represented by chronic inflammatory cells aggregated in the areas of foreign material. Histiocytes and foreign body multinucleated giant cells may be associated with the amalgam particles, in which case the lesion is said to be a *foreign body reaction.* Neutrophils and eosinophils are not part of this reaction.

Treatment and Prognosis. Once present, the amalgam tattoo remains indefinitely, and occasional lesions slowly enlarge over time, presumably as amalgam-ladened histiocytes try to move the material out of the local site. No treatment is necessary, but excisional biopsy is often performed to rule out melanoma or another pigmented lesion. Lesions visible on radiographs are usually not biopsied and those occurring on the visible vermilion border of the lips are usually removed for esthetic reasons. There is no malignant potential for this lesion.

Oral Melanotic Macule

The oral mucosa is usually not pigmented despite the fact that it has the same density of melanocytes as the skin. Occasional patients, however, will show a focal area of melanin deposition, either as a response to local chronic conditions (mechanical trauma, tobacco smoking, chronic autoimmune mucositis), racial background (the darker a person's skin color the more likely he or she is to have oral pigmentation), or systemic medications, especially chloroquine (Table 4–8). Moreover, certain syndromes and systemic diseases have oral pigmentation as part of their spectrum (Table 4–8), as mentioned previously in this section.

Most focal melanin deposits of the oral mucosa that are not associated with race or an appropriate syndrome are innocuous surface discolorations called *oral melanotic macule (focal melano-*

Table 4–8. Associations with Melanin Pigmentation of Oral Mucosa

Physiologic or Syndromic Associations
  Addison's disease
  Bloom syndrome
  Cronkhite-Canada syndrome
  Dunnigan syndrome
  Dyskeratosis congenita
  Endocrine candidosis
  Incontinentia pigmenti
  LEOPARD syndrome (lentiginosis profusa; no intraoral melanosis)
  McCune-Albright syndrome
  Neurofibromatosis
  Oculocerebrocutaneous syndrome
  Peutz-Jeghers syndrome
  Racial or physiologic pigmentation
  Rothmund-Thomson syndrome
  Trisomy 14 mosaicism
  Unusual facies, vitiligo, spastic paraplegia syndrome
  Xeroderma pigmentosum
Chronic Trauma or Irritation
  Chronic autoimmune disease (e.g., erosive lichen planus, pemphigoid)
  Chronic mucosal trauma/irritation (e.g., chronic cheek bite)
  Smoker's melanosis
Systemic Medications
  Chloroquine and other quinine derivatives
  Estrogen
  Medications for acquired immunodeficiency syndrome
  Phenolphthalein

sis).[7, 569–571] This entity represents not only a focal increase in melanin deposition but a concomitant increase in the number of melanocytes. Unlike the cutaneous *ephelis (freckle),* the oral melanotic macule is not dependent on sun exposure, nor does it show the elongated rete ridges of *actinic lentigo.* Some authorities have questioned the purported lack of an association with actinic irradiation for melanotic macule located on the vermilion border, preferring to consider the lesion at this site to be a distinct entity called *labial melanotic macule.*[572] Melanotic macules are found in the mouths of 1 of every 1000 adults.[1]

Clinical Features. The oral melanotic macule has a 2:1 female predilection with an average age of 43 years at the time of diagnosis, although it can develop at any age.[7, 571] One third of lesions occur on the vermilion border of the lower lip, but the buccal mucosa, gingiva, and palate are other sites of common occurrence.[1] Almost one fifth of the lesions are multiple.

The typical macule is a well-demarcated, uniformly tan to dark brown, asymptomatic, round or oval discoloration less than 7 mm in diameter (Fig. 4–51A, see p. 179). The lesion is not thickened and has the same consistency as surrounding mucosa. It tends to have an abrupt onset and seldom enlarges after diagnosis.

A special case of oral melanosis, called *smoker's melanosis,* is found on the gingival or buccal mucosa in heavy smokers.[7, 9, 573, 574] It has an adult onset and is often associated with a concomitant superficial white-gray keratosis. The keratosis may become thick enough to mimic *leukoplakia,* although it is not known whether it is a true precancer. Both the pigmentation and the keratosis diminish or disappear once the tobacco habit is stopped.[574]

Although the melanotic macule is an innocuous lesion, it must be remembered that focal oral and oropharyngeal pigmentation might represent an internal malignancy (usually lung), an oral manifestation of a systemic disease, or one facet of a genetic syndrome (see Table 4–8).[7, 575, 576]

Pathologic Features. The oral melanotic macule is characterized by an otherwise normal stratified squamous epithelium with abundant melanin deposits within the keratinocytes of the basal and parabasal layers (Fig. 4–51B, see p. 179). Deposits may also be seen within subepithelial stroma (melanin incontinence), perhaps within macrophages or melanophages. There is no underlying inflammatory response. The melanin can be distinguished from iron deposits with melanin stains or by the loss of brown color after bleaching. Brown formalin deposits can be differentiated by their association with erythrocytes rather than with basal layer epithelial cells.

Treatment and Prognosis. No treatment is required for oral melanotic macule except for esthetic considerations.[577] The intraoral melanotic macule has no malignant transformation potential, but an early melanoma could have a similar clinical appearance. For this reason, pigmented macular lesions of recent onset, large size, irregular pigmentation, unknown duration, or with a history of recent enlargement should be excised and examined histopathologically.

Melanoacanthoma

Oral *melanoacanthoma (melanoacanthosis)* is a benign, focal melanosis of the oral mucosa characterized by dendritic melanocytes dispersed throughout the epithelium.[578–583] It is a reactive lesion that appears to be unrelated to the melanoacanthoma of skin.[8]

Clinical Features. The lesion occurs almost exclusively in blacks and has a female predilection.[578, 582] It is seen most frequently on the buccal mucosa in 20- to 40-year-old persons but can occur at any oral site and at any age. Usually presenting as a single smooth, flat or slightly raised, dark brown to black macule, the lesion often demonstrates an alarmingly rapid increase in size and occasionally will reach a diameter of several centimeters within a period of a few weeks. It is asymptomatic and not indurated, and bilateral examples have been reported.[581]

Pathologic Features. The pathognomonic feature of oral melanoacanthoma, sometimes the only obvious feature, is the occurrence of numerous brown dendritic melanocytes scattered throughout all layers of the epithelium, instead of being confined to the basal cell layer, as is the normal case (Fig. 4–52, see p. 179). Basal layer melanocytes also are increased in numbers. Spongiosis and mild acanthosis are usually seen, as are occasional eosinophils and scattered subepithelial chronic inflammatory cells. The epithelial cells demonstrate no dysplasia.

Treatment and Prognosis. Incisional biopsy is recommended because of the rapid rate of enlargement. Once the diagnosis has been established and it is shown that there is no evidence of *melanoma,* no further treatment is necessary.[580, 582] Occasionally the melanoacanthoma will undergo spontaneous resolution following incisional biopsy; none have transformed into malignancy.

Mucosal Melanocytic Nevus

The oral mucosa is a rare location for the presentation of the *melanocytic nevus (pigmented nevus, nevocellular nevus, mole),* the benign proliferation of nevus cells within subepithelial stroma.[7–9, 584–589] All cutaneous subtypes have been reported on the oral mucosa, including *congenital nevus, blue nevus, Spitz nevus,* and *halo nevus,* but the great majority of identified cases are the *intradermal nevus,* usually referred to as *intramucosal nevus.* As with skin lesions, the oral nevus is considered to be a developmental anomaly or hamartoma of nevus cells (nevocytes) rather than a true neoplasm. Although rare in the mouth, the cutaneous melanocytic nevus is probably the most common of all human tumors, with white adults averaging 10 to 40 nevi each.[8]

Clinical Features. The cutaneous melanocytic nevus is first seen during childhood and most lesions are present before 35 years of age; most oral examples are biopsied during the young adult or middle-age years. Although there is no gender bias for cutaneous lesions, two thirds of oral nevi are found in females.[8, 585]

The intraoral nevus is usually an intramucosal (or submucosal?) nevus. It has an appearance similar to its cutaneous counterpart but usually lacks the papillary surface change and has a greater tendency to be nonpigmented.[590] The lesion is usually 4 to 6 mm in greatest diameter and the most common sites of oral involvement are the hard palate, buccal mucosa, and gingiva.

Both types of blue nevus *(dermal melanocytoma, Jadassohn-Tieche nevus)* are found in the mouth. The *common blue nevus* is the second most common benign melanocytic proliferation encountered in the mouth, usually seen in females in the fourth decade of life (Fig. 4–53A, see p. 180).[587, 588] Typically found on the hard or soft palate, it presents as a macular or dome-shaped, blue or blue-black lesion less than 1 cm in diameter. The *cellular blue nevus* is very rarely found on the oral mucosa but appears as a slow-growing blue-black papule or nodule that is typically less than 8 mm in diameter and is seldom larger than 2 cm. This lesion is usually diagnosed in females between 10 and 30 years of age, but congenital examples have been reported.[588]

The oral halo nevus appears as a central pigmented papule or macule with a surrounding zone of pallor that may be as much as 1.5 cm in diameter.[7] The oral Spitz nevus *(benign juvenile melanoma, spindle and/or epithelioid cell nevus)* occurs as a dome-shaped, pink to reddish-brown papule less than 6 mm in diameter. It presents as a solitary mass and usually develops during childhood. The small lesional size and young age at diagnosis are useful in clinically distinguishing the Spitz nevus from a true *melanoma.*

Pathologic Features. The oral intramucosal nevus presents as an unencapsulated proliferation of nevus cells within the subepithelial stroma. Lesional cells are often clustered together and are usually ovoid and uniform in size, but their appearance may vary in different parts of the nodule. More superficial cells are usually epithelioid and frequently contain intracellular melanin, whereas nevus cells of the mid-portion of the nodule have less cytoplasm, are

seldom pigmented, and appear much like lymphocytes. Deeper nevus cells appear elongated and spindle-shaped, much like Schwann cells or fibroblasts. Some authorities classify these variations as type A (epithelioid), type B (lymphocyte-like), and type C (spindle-shaped) nevus cells.[8] There may be a complete lack of melanin production within submucosal nevus cells, and multinucleated giant nevus cells may be found with or without intracellular melanin deposits. A grenz zone of uninvolved connective tissue separates lesional cells from the overlying epithelium.

The *junctional nevus* is extremely rare on oral mucosa, but when present it demonstrates sharply demarcated nests or thèques of type A nevus cells at the interface (junction) of the subepithelial stroma and the mucosal epithelium. Supposedly, nests of type A and type B nevus cells appear within subepithelial stroma with age, at which time the diagnostic term *compound nevus* is applied.[7, 8, 585] Over time, the intraepithelial nests disappear, leaving nevus cells only in the subepithelial connective tissues, producing the intramucosal nevus described earlier.

The oral example of the common blue nevus presents as a submucosal aggregation of elongated, slender melanocytes with intracellular melanin deposition and branching dendritic extensions (Fig. 4–53B, see p. 180). These cells usually align themselves parallel to the surface epithelium and may be quite deep within the subepithelial stroma. The cellular blue nevus appears as a well-circumscribed, highly cellular aggregation of plump, melanin-producing spindle cells within the lamina propria or submucosa. Pigmented dendritic spindle cells are seen at the periphery of the lesion. A blue nevus may be found in conjunction with an overlying melanocytic nevus, in which case the term *combined nevus* is used.

The oral Spitz nevus has the same histopathology as its cutaneous counterpart, with the general appearance of a compound nevus with zonal differentiation from the superficial to deep portions of the nodule. Lesional cells are spindle-shaped or epithelioid, with the two types often intermixed. The epithelioid cells may be multinucleated, may appear somewhat bizarre, and may lack cellular cohesiveness. Mitotic figures with a normal appearance may be seen in superficial areas of the lesion. Ectatic superficial blood vessels, which probably impart much of the reddish color of some lesions, are frequently seen.

Treatment and Prognosis. No treatment is required for any of the histologic subtypes of the oral mucosal nevus. However, most adult-onset pigmented lesions are removed by excisional biopsy when encountered, to rule out melanoma. The oral nevus is, therefore, routinely removed by default.[7, 585] Recurrence has not been reported, nor has spontaneous regression or malignant transformation into an oral mucosal melanoma.

Oral Melanotic Neuroectodermal Tumor of Infancy

The rare *oral melanotic neuroectodermal tumor of infancy (pigmented epulis of infancy)* is a congenital neoplasm of unclear histogenesis that was first described by Krompecher[591] in 1918. Referred to additionally as *retinal anlage tumor, melanotic progonoma, pigmented ameloblastoma, melanotic adamantinoma,* and *congenital melanocarcinoma,* it is considered to arise from neural crest cells, the cells that are embryologically responsible for much of the development of the maxillofacial region.[6–9, 591–599] Extraoral examples have been reported from the mediastinum, brain, anterior fontanelle, epididymis, and soft tissues of the arm.[6] Malignant variants represent approximately 5% of reported cases.[6]

Clinical Features. More than 90% of cases of neuroectodermal tumor of infancy present during the first year of life, and four of five occur in or on the anterior maxillary alveolus.[593, 595] Occasional cases are congenital, and males and females are equally affected. The lesion appears as a sessile or slightly pedunculated, lobulated, firm mass that typically has a deep blue or black surface discoloration. The tumor is usually 2 to 4 cm in diameter at diagnosis and radiographs often reveal a destructive, poorly demarcated radiolucency of the underlying bone, perhaps with a faint "sunburst" appearance from mild calcification along vessels radiating from the center of the tumor. The surface mucosa is not ulcerated and the lesion is asymptomatic. High levels of urinary vanillylmandelic acid are usually found, as they are in the presentation of a number of other neural crest tumors, such as *pheochromocytoma, ganglioneuroblastoma, neuroblastoma,* and *retinoblastoma.*[595]

Pathologic Features. The tumor in gross cross-section has a whitish, gray, or blue-black appearance, depending on the amount of melanin present. There is a biphasic microscopic pattern with one cell population consisting of cuboidal epithelioid cells with open, vesicular nuclei clustered in alveolar or tubular patterns (Fig. 4–54, see p. 180). These cells typically have abundant brown intracellular melanin granules. Ultrastructural studies have shown the lesional cells to have features of epithelial and melanocytic cells, bounded by basal laminae and interdigitating with adjacent cells, with desmosomal attachments. Melanosomes are present in the cytoplasm and the cells are immunoreactive for cytokeratin and melanoma-associated antigen (HMB-45). Some lesional cells react for neuron-specific enolase, synaptophysin, and Leu-7 as well.[6, 7]

The second lesional cell is a small dark round cell with a hyperchromatic nucleus and minimal cytoplasm; it has the appearance of a neuroblast. The cells aggregate in loose nests or islands within the background fibrovascular stroma (see Fig. 4–54). The neuroblastic cells are often surrounded by the larger pigmented cells and may be associated with neurofibrillar material resembling glial tissue. This second cell type contains few organelles but demonstrates intracytoplasmic neurofilamentous material, elongated cell processes, and dense core vesicles under electron microscopic examination. Mitoses are rarely seen, and the tumor cells extend to the overlying mucosa.

Many of the tumors show pseudoencapsulation, perhaps with reactive bone formation at the lesional periphery. Developing tooth buds are typically included in the specimen, tempting the pathologist to presume an odontogenic origin or diagnosis for the lesion.

There appear to be no microscopic parameters able to distinguish the benign from the malignant neuroectodermal tumors of infancy, unless lesional cells are obviously dysplastic or demonstrate abundant or abnormal mitoses.

Treatment and Prognosis. Because of its locally aggressive behavior, the melanotic neuroectodermal tumor of infancy is treated by wide surgical excision.[591, 593, 595] When bone is involved, a 0.5 cm margin of radiographically normal bone should also be removed. Elevated vanillylmandelic acid levels usually return to normal once the tumor is resected. Recurrence occurs in 15% of treated cases and in 50% of cases treated without wide resection, so careful follow-up is important. Malignant variants of this tumor must, of course, be treated more radically, usually by excisional surgery with a wider margin of normal surrounding tissue.[592]

Melanoma

Melanoma is a malignant neoplasm of melanocytes and their precursor cells.[8, 600–610] It accounts for 5% of cutaneous cancers, with an annual incidence rate of approximately 9 per 100,000 persons in the United States.[7, 8, 609] Almost 30% of cutaneous melanomas arise in the head and neck region, but involvement of the oral and pharyngeal mucosa is decidedly rare, representing less than 1% of all melanomas in hospital-based studies and showing an annual incidence rate of only 1 per 2,000,000 persons.[7, 9, 609] An alarming increase has been noted for skin melanoma in white populations and some authors have suggested, from clinical experience, that the frequency of oral melanoma may be increasing as well.[605]

Actinic damage is a strong etiologic factor for the skin lesions, but no etiology has thus far been determined for the mucosal lesions

of the mouth and throat. The first reported example of an oral melanoma appears to be a mandibular gingival lesion in a young man, discussed by the British physician Heinter in 1787.[609]

Clinical Features. Four of every five oral melanomas occur on the palate and maxillary alveolar mucosa, but any site can be affected. There is no gender predilection for oral or pharyngeal melanoma. It occurs most commonly in the 50 to 65 year age group, but age at diagnosis is rather uniformly distributed throughout the 30 to 80 year age bracket.[7, 600–602, 607, 608] Cases have been reported in teenagers and adolescents.

The most common forms of oral melanoma are the *mucosal (acral) lentiginous melanoma* and the *superficial spreading melanoma.*[7–10, 608] These begin with an irregularly pigmented brown macule and enlarge laterally for a period of time prior to the development of a vertical growth phase with exophytic surface growth and invasion of underlying stroma. Lesions have irregular outlines, and satellite lesions may be seen a few millimeters from the primary site. Occasional lesions, called *nodular melanomas,* begin in the vertical growth phase as soft, dark brown or black, lobulated masses that may eventually show surface ulceration and hemorrhage.[7, 8] Rarely, a nodular melanoma will be composed of lesional cells so poorly differentiated that no melanin pigment is produced and no mucosal discoloration is clinically evident *(amelanotic melanoma).* Regardless of the tumor type, lesions are typically painless and quite soft to palpation. Oral melanoma almost always arises de novo from the mucous membrane; it rarely develops within benign melanocytic lesions.

The least common form of oral melanoma is the *lentigo maligna melanoma,* which develops from a precursor *lentigo maligna* or *Hutchinson's freckle.*[9–10, 603, 605] Lentigo maligna usually occurs as a sun-damage lesion of the midface skin and probably represents melanoma in situ or melanoma in a slowly expanding, purely radial growth phase.[8, 603] On the skin, the average duration prior to development of a vertical growth phase is 15 years, but duration is unknown for the oral examples. The appearance of nodularity within a lentigo maligna signals the onset of the invasive phase and the transition to lentigo maligna melanoma.

Pathologic Features. The histopathologic features of oral melanoma are identical to those of cutaneous melanoma. Atypical melanocytes initially are seen at the epithelial-connective tissue junction and proliferate toward the surface and laterally along the basal cell layer. Dysplastic melanocytes demonstrate increased cellular and nuclear size, pleomorphism, hyperchromatism, and scattered intracellular melanin deposits. Pleomorphism and enlargement may be extreme, and some lesions contain variable numbers of cells with clear cytoplasm. Intraepithelial lesional melanocytes often have prominent dendritic processes, especially in the mucosal lentiginous melanoma.

Lesional cells in the early stages are scattered singly among the basal epithelial cells or clustered as nests within the basal cell layer. The superficial spreading melanoma often shows so many nests that it is said to have a "pagetoid spread" because of its resemblance to the cutaneous *intraepithelial adenocarcinoma of Paget's disease.* Spread is lateral or radial in this stage, with dysplastic cells sometimes found above the basal and parabasal layers, perhaps all the way to the surface layers.

With the onset of the vertical growth phase, atypical melanocytes are observed invading subepithelial connective tissues as individual cells, clusters, or cords of cells. In nodular melanoma, this vertical growth phase occurs early in the course of tumor development and, by definition, no radial growth of cells can be observed in the overlying epithelium beyond the edge of the invasive tumor. Invading cells usually appear either spindle-shaped or epithelioid, but the tumor is notorious for its ability to mimic a wide variety of other malignancies. This is especially true for amelanotic melanoma. Immunohistochemical evaluation for S-100 and HMB-45 reactivity is beneficial in distinguishing melanoma from other malignancies.[7, 8, 607] A detailed discussion of histologic look-alike lesions and descriptions of the numerous specific melanoma subtypes is beyond the scope of this chapter; the reader is referred to Chapter 13 and the excellent text by Elder et al. [8] for additional information.

It is important to assess the depth of invasion of a cutaneous melanoma, but this assessment is much more difficult for oral melanomas and it is not known whether it has the same prognostic significance. Nevertheless, it should be attempted. The Clark system of measurement for cutaneous lesions assigns a "level" of invasion to the lesion, depending on the deepest anatomic form of stroma invaded.[8] Oral submucosal connective tissues are more varied and less layered than the cutaneous stromal tissues, so the more recent Breslow classification appears more appropriate for evaluation of oral lesions. On the skin, the Breslow categories appear to most accurately correlate with prognosis, but this correlation has not been adequately assessed for the rare oral lesions. The Breslow system is based on the actual measurement of the distance from the top of the granular cell layer to the deepest identifiable point of tumor invasion. As much of the oral mucosa lacks an identifiable granular cell layer, the surface keratin layer is alternatively used for oral melanoma.[607]

Treatment and Prognosis. Radical surgical excision of oral melanoma is the only curative treatment, and that is only effective with early detection of the lesion.[7, 9, 609] The older literature suggests a surgical margin of 3 to 5 cm around the clinically visible cutaneous tumor, but more recent studies indicate that a 1 cm margin is adequate for small, early lesions.[8] For larger, more invasive tumors, wide surgical excision is still recommended. The oral melanoma, even when small, is still treated with radical surgical excision, with more than a 1 cm margin of clinically normal mucosa surrounding it. Underlying bone must be removed as well, usually requiring a hemimaxillectomy for palatal lesions.

Surgical removal of regional lymph nodes is recommended for lesions with a histopathologic depth of invasion exceeding 1.24 mm.[7, 8] Radiation therapy, chemotherapy, and immunotherapy have shown no significant impact on survival. Overall, the prognosis for oral melanoma is extremely poor. Only 4% to 20% of affected patients survive for 5 years or more.[7, 9, 608–610] At all times, it must be remembered that many melanomas of the oral region are, in fact, metastases from the trunk or from a cutaneous head and neck site.[606]

Metastasis to Oral Soft Tissues

The metastasis of malignant neoplasms to the region of the oral cavity is not a common event.[7, 9, 611–618] When present, metastatic deposits are usually found within the mandible or the nodes of the parotid glands.[7, 615–617] In population studies, metastases to the head and neck region, excluding deposits in the cervical lymph nodes, account for almost 4% of all malignancies of this anatomic area.[614] Almost half of these lesions present as the first evidence of malignancy, and approximately two thirds metastasize from below the clavicles.[614] Fewer than one tenth of such metastases, however, are to the oral soft tissues.

The mechanism by which tumors spread to the oral region are poorly understood, but certainly those from cancers located below the clavicles must be blood-borne. Lesional cells are apparently not adequately filtered by the lungs, although it has also been suggested that Batson's plexus, a valveless vertebral venous plexus, might allow retrograde spread of tumor cells, bypassing filtration through the lungs.[7]

Clinical Features. Oral soft tissue metastases are more common in males and are seen most frequently in middle-aged and older adults. The most common site for deposition of metastatic tumor cells from other sites is the gingiva (50% of all cases), primarily from the growth of an intraosseous lesion with perforation through the overlying cortex or extension up the periodontal ligament space.[7, 9] The tongue is the second most likely site of involvement, followed by the oral floor.[7, 614]

The typical lesion is a rapidly enlarging, irregular nodule, often resembling a *pyogenic granuloma* or other reactive hyperplastic

growth. Surface ulceration and hemorrhage are not uncommon, and for gingival lesions, adjacent teeth may be loosened. Radiographic examination of underlying bone may show considerable destruction, but the damage might also be quite subtle. Pain is a common feature, often leading to a working diagnosis of traumatic ulceration or toothache (gingival lesions only), which can considerably delay biopsy and the establishment of a correct diagnosis.

Malignancies from all body sites have been reported to have metastasized to the oral region. The most frequent examples depend in large part on the most common tumors found in any given population. Within the U.S. population, the most common cancers to metastasize to the mouth include those from the lungs (one third of oral metastases), kidneys, breasts (one fourth of oral examples in females), skin (predominantly melanoma), and prostate (rarely to soft tissue). The primary tumor is discovered shortly after the time of diagnosis for the oral metastasis, but is usually not known to the patient prior to the development of the oral lesion.[614]

Pathologic Features. The microscopic appearance of the metastatic deposit will resemble that of the primary tumor. Most cases are carcinomas, but metastatic sarcomas to the oral region do occur.[616]

Treatment and Prognosis. Management of the oral lesion is usually palliative and should be coordinated with the patient's overall treatment.[7, 9, 612, 617] The overall prognosis is poor because metastatic deposits are frequently present in other anatomic sites.

▋ REFERENCES

General Topics

1. Bouquot JE: Common oral lesions found in a large mass screening. J Am Dent Assoc 1986;112:50–57.
2. Bouquot JE, Gundlach KKH: Oral exophytic lesions in 23,616 white Americans over 35 years of age. Oral Surg Oral Med Oral Pathol 1986;62:284–291.
3. Gnepp DR (ed): Pathology of the Head and Neck. Philadelphia: Churchill-Livingstone, 1988:263–314.
4. Wenig BM: Atlas of Head and Neck Pathology. Philadelphia: W.B. Saunders, 1993.
5. Gorlin RJ, Cohen MM, Levine S: Syndromes of the Head and Neck, 4th ed. Oxford: Oxford University Press, 1994.
6. Enzinger FM, Weiss SW: Soft tissue tumors, 3rd ed. St. Louis: Mosby, 1995.
7. Neville BW, Damm DD, Allen CM, Bouquot JE: Oral and Maxillofacial Pathology. Philadelphia: W.B. Saunders, 1995.
8. Elder D, Elenitsas R, Jaworsky C, Johnson B Jr: Lever's Histopathology of the Skin, 8th ed. Philadelphia: Lippincott-Raven, 1997.
9. Sapp JP, Eversole LR, Wysocki GP: Contemporary Oral and Maxillofacial Pathology. St. Louis: Mosby, 1997.
10. Odell EW, Morgan PR: Biopsy Pathology of the Oral Tissues. London: Chapman & Hall Medical, 1998.
11. Reich RF, Kerpel SM, Freedman PD: Differential diagnosis and treatment of ulcerative, erosive, and vesiculobullous lesions of the oral mucosa. Oral Maxillofac Surg Clin North Am 1998;10:95–129.

Irritation Fibroma and Localized Fibrous Hyperplasias

12. Tomes J: A course of lectures on dental physiology and surgery (lectures I–XV). Am J Dent Sc 1846–1848; 7:1–68,121–134; 8:33–54,120–147,313–350.
13. Bouquot JE, Crout RJ: Odd gums: The prevalence of common gingival and alveolar lesions in 23,616 white Americans over 35 years of age. Quint Internat 1988;19:747–753.
14. Barker DS, Lucas RB: Localized fibrous overgrowth of the oral mucosa. Br J Oral Surg 1967;5:86–92.
15. Cutright DE: The histopathologic findings in 583 cases of epulis fissuratum. Oral Surg Oral Med Oral Pathol 1974;37:401–411.
16. Budtz-Jorgensen E: Oral mucosal lesions associated with the wearing of removable dentures. J Oral Pathol 1981;10:65–80.
17. Buchner A, Begleiter A, Hansen LS: The predominance of epulis fissuratum in females. Quintessence Int 1984;15:699–702.

18. Saurel L: Memoirs upon the tumors of the gums, known under the name epulis. Am J Dent Sc 1858; 8(new series):33–43, 212–231.

19. Weathers DR, Callihan MD: Giant cell fibroma. Oral Surg Oral Med Oral Pathol 1974;37:374–384.

20. Houston GD: The giant cell fibroma: Review of 464 cases. Oral Surg Oral Med Oral Pathol 1982;53:582–587.

21. Magnusson BC, Rasmusson LG: The giant cell fibroma: A review of 103 cases with immunohistochemical findings. Acta Odontol Scand 1995;53:293–296.

22. Buchner A, Merrell PW, Hansen LS, et al: The retrocuspid papilla of the mandibular lingual gingiva. J Periodontol 1990;61:585–589.

Fibromatosis

23. Larsson A, Bjorlin G: Aggressive fibrous lesions of the oral cavity. J Oral Pathol 1976;5:241–251.

24. Thompson DH, Khan A, Gonzales C, Auclair P: Juvenile aggressive fibromatosis: Report of three cases and review of the literature. Ear Nose Throat J 1991;70:462–468.

25. Fowler CB, Hartman KS, Brannon RB: Fibromatosis of the oral and paraoral region. Oral Surg Oral Med Oral Pathol 1994;77:373–386.

26. Vally IM, Altini M: Fibromatoses of the oral and paraoral soft tissues and jaws. Review of the literature and report of 12 new cases. Oral Surg Oral Med Oral Pathol 1990;69:191–198.

27. Plaited BEC, Balm TJM, Loftus BM, et al: Fibromatosis of the head and neck. Clin Otolaryngol 1995;20:103–108.

28. Fisher C: Fibromatosis and fibrosarcoma in infancy and childhood. Eur J Cancer 1996;32A:2094–2100.

29. Gnepp DR, Henley J, Weiss S, Heffner D: Desmoid fibromatosis of the sinonasal tract and nasopharynx: A clinicopathological study of 25 cases. Cancer 1996;78:2572–2579.

30. Coffin CM, Dehner LP: Fibroblastic-myofibroblastic tumors in children and adolescents: A clinicopathologic study of 108 examples in 103 patients. Ped Pathol 1991;11:559–588.

Gingival Fibromatosis

31. Carranza FA: Glickman's Clinical Periodontology, 7th ed. Philadelphia: W.B. Saunders, 1990.

32. Butler RT, Kalkwarf KL, Kaldahl WB: Drug-induced gingival hyperplasia: Phenytoin, cyclosporine, and nifedipine. J Am Dent Assoc 1987;114:56–60.

33. Miller CS, Damm DD: Incidence of verapamil-induced gingival hyperplasia in a dental population. J Periodontol 1990;63:453–456.

34. Dongari A, McDonnell HT, Langlais RP: Drug-induced gingival overgrowth. Oral Surg Oral Med Oral Pathol 1993;76:543–548.

35. Jorgenson RJ, Cocker ME: Variation in the inheritance and expression of gingival fibromatosis. J Periodontol 1974;45:472–477.

36. Oikarinen K, Salo T, Kaar ML, et al: Hereditary gingival fibromatosis associated with growth hormone deficiency. Br J Oral Maxillofac Surg 1990;28:335–339.

37. Takagi M, Yamamoto H, Mega H, et al: Heterogeneity in the gingival fibromatoses. Cancer 1991;2202.

38. Ramer M, Marrone J, Stahl B, Burakoff B: Hereditary gingival fibromatosis: Identification, treatment, control. J Am Dent Assoc 1996; 127:493–495.

39. Piattelli A, Scarano A, Dibellucci A, Matarasso S: Juvenile hyaline fibromatosis of gingiva: A case report. J Periodont 1996;67:451–453.

40. Wynne SE, Aldred MJ, Bartold PM: Hereditary gingival fibromatosis associated with hearing loss and supernumerary teeth: A new syndrome. J Periodontol 1995;66:75–79.

41. Goddard WH, Gross L: Case of hypertrophy of the gums. Dent Regist West 1856;9:276–282.

42. Daley TD, Wysocki GP: Foreign body gingivitis: An iatrogenic disease? Oral Surg Oral Med Oral Pathol 1990;69:708–712.

43. Sollecito TP, Greenberg MS: Plasma cell gingivitis: Report of two cases. Oral Surg Oral Med Oral Pathol 1992;73:690–693.

Oral Submucous Fibrosis

44. Pindborg JJ, Mehta FS, Gupta PC, Daftary DK: Prevalence of oral submucous fibrosis among 50,915 Indian villagers. Br J Cancer 1968;22:646–654.

45. Murti PR, Gupta PC, Bhonsle RB, et al: Smokeless tobacco use in India: Effects on oral mucosa. In: Stotts RC, Schroeder KL, Burns DM

(eds): Smokeless Tobacco or Health, an International Perspective. NIH Publ 93-3461. Bethesda, MD: US Department of Health and Human Services, National Institutes of Health, 1992: 51–65.

46. Borle RM, Borle SR: Management of oral submucous fibrosis: A conservative approach. J Oral Maxillofacial Surg 1991;49:788–791.

47. Jayanthi V, Probert CSJ, Sher KS, Mayberry JF: Oral submucous fibrosis: A preventable disease. Gut 1992;33:4–6.

48. Pindborg JJ: Oral precancer. In: Barnes L (ed): Surgical Pathology of the Head and Neck. New York: Marcel Dekker Co, 1985: 279–331.

49. Murti PR, Bhonsle RB, Pindborg JJ, et al: Malignant transformation rate in oral submucous fibrosis over a 17-year period. Community Dent Oral Epidemiol 1985;13:340–341.

50. Sinor PN, Gupta PC, Bhonsle RB, et al: A case-control study of oral submucous fibrosis with special reference to the etiologic role of areca nut. J Oral Pathol Med 1990;19:94–98.

51. Bouquot JE, Glover ED, Schroeder KL: Leukoplakia and smokeless tobacco keratosis are two separate precancers. In: Varma AD (ed): Oral Oncology, vol 2. Delhi: MacMillan India, Ltd, 1991 :67–69.

Fibrosarcoma

52. Batsakis JG, Rice DH, Howard DR: The pathology of head and neck tumors: Spindle cell lesions (sarcomatoid carcinomas, nodular fasciitis, and fibrosarcoma) of the aerodigestive tracts, part 14. Head Neck Surg 1982;4:499–513.

53. Barnes L: Tumors and tumorlike lesions of the soft tissues. In: Barnes L (ed): Surgical Pathology of the Head and Neck. New York: Marcel Dekker, 1985: 725–780.

54. Fletcher CD, McKee PH: Sarcomas: A clinicopathologic guide with particular reference to cutaneous manifestations. III: Angiosarcoma, malignant hemangiopericytoma, fibrosarcoma and synovial sarcoma. Clin Exp Dermatol 1985;10:332–349.

55. Oppenheimer RW, Friedman M: Fibrosarcoma of the maxillary sinus. Ear Nose Throat J 1988;67:193–198.

56. Mark RJ, Sercarz JA, Tran L, et al: Fibrosarcoma of the head and neck. The UCLA experience. Arch Otolaryngol Head Neck Surg 1991;117:396–401.

57. Meis-Kindblom JM, Kindblom LG, Enzinger FM: Sclerosing epithelioid fibrosarcoma: A variant of fibrosarcoma simulating carcinoma. Am J Surg Pathol 1995;19:979–993.

58. Ellis GL, Corio RL: Spindle cell carcinoma of the oral cavity: A clinicopathologic assessment of fifty-nine cases. Oral Surg Oral Med Oral Pathol 1980;50:523–533.

59. Slootweg PJ, Roholl PJ, Muller H, et al: Spindle-cell carcinoma of the oral cavity and larynx. Immunohistochemical aspects. J Craniomaxillofac Surg 1989;17:234–236.

60. Brooks JSJ: Soft tissue lesions of the oral and maxillofacial region. Proceedings of the Annual Meeting of the American Academy of Oral and Maxillofacial Pathology, Dallas, Texas; May, 1998.

Fibrous Histiocytoma

61. Hoffman S, Martinez MG Jr: Fibrous histiocytomas of the oral mucosa. Oral Surg Oral Med Oral Pathol 1981;52:277–283.

62. Gonzalez S, Duarte I: Benign fibrous histiocytoma of the skin: A morphologic study of 290 cases. Pathol Res Pract 1982;174:379–391.

63. Thompson SH, Shear M: Fibrous histiocytomas of the oral and maxillofacial regions. J Oral Pathol 1984;13:282–294.

64. Fletcher CD: Benign fibrous histiocytoma of subcutaneous and deep soft tissue: A clinicopathologic analysis of 21 cases. Am J Surg Pathol 1990;14:801–809.

65. Gray PB, Miller AS, Loftus MJ: Benign fibrous histiocytoma of the oral/perioral regions: Report of a case and review of 17 additional cases. J Oral Maxillofac Surg 1992;50:1239–1242.

66. Bielamowicz S, Dauer MS, Chang B, Zimmerman MC: Noncutaneous benign fibrous histiocytoma of the head and neck. Otolaryngol Head Neck Surg 1995;113:140–146.

Malignant Fibrous Histiocytoma

67. Stout AP: Pathological aspects of soft part sarcomas. Ann NY Acad Sci 1964;114:1041–1046.

68. Bras J, Batsakis JG, Luna MA: Malignant fibrous histiocytoma of the oral soft tissues. Oral Surg Oral Med Oral Pathol 1987;64:57–67.

69. Nuamah IK, Browne RM: Malignant fibrous histiocytoma presenting as perioral abscess. Int J Oral Maxillofac Surg 1995;24:158–159.
70. Oshiro Y, Fukuda T, Tsuneyoshi M: Atypical fibroxanthoma versus benign and malignant fibrous histiocytoma. Cancer 1995;75:1128–1134.
71. Poli P, Floretti G, Tessitori G: Malignant fibrous histiocytoma of the floor of the mouth: Case report. J Laryngol Otol 1995;109:680–682.
72. Meister P: Malignant fibrous histiocytoma: Histomorphological pattern or tumor type. Pathol Res Pract 1996;192:877–881.
73. Lazova R, Mynes R, May D, Scott G: Ln-2 (CD74): A marker to distinguish atypical fibroxanthoma from malignant fibrous histiocytoma. Cancer 1997;79:2115–2124.
74. Grossman LD, White RR, Arber DA: Angiomatoid fibrous histiocytoma. Ann Plast Surg 1996;36:649–651.
75. Zelger BW, Zelger BG, Steiner H, Ofner D: Aneurysmal and hemangiopericytoma-like fibrous histiocytoma. J Clin Pathol 1996;49:313–318.

Myofibromatosis

76. Fletcher CDM, Ach P, Van Noorden S, McKee PH: Infantile myofibromatosis: A light microscopic, histochemical and immunohistochemical study suggesting true smooth muscle differentiation. Histopathology 1987;11:245–258.
77. Daimaru Y, Hashimoto H, Enjoji M: Myofibromatosis in adults: Adult counterpart of infantile myofibromatosis. Am J Surg Pathol 1989;13:859–865.
78. Smith KJ, Skelton HG, Barrett TL, et al: Cutaneous myofibroma. Mod Pathol 1989;2:603.
79. Speight PM, Dayan D, Fletcher CDM: Adult and infantile myofibromatosis: A report of three cases affecting the oral cavity. J Oral Pathol Med 1991;20:380–384.
80. Sugatani T, Inui M, Tagawa T, et al: Myofibroma of the mandible: Clinicopathological study and review of the literature. Oral Surg Oral Med Oral Pathol Oral Radiol Endodont 1995;80:303–309.
81. Magid MS, Campbell WG, Ngadiman S, et al: Infantile myofibromatosis with hemangiopericytoma-like features of the tongue: A case-study including ultrastructure. Pediat Pathol Lab Med 1997;17:303–313.
82. Spraker MK, Stack C, Esterly NB: Congenital generalized fibromatosis. J Am Acad Dermatol 1984;10:365.
83. Venencie PV, Bigtel P, Desguelles C, et al: Infantile myofibromatosis. Br J Dermatol 1987;117:255.
84. Coffin CM, Neilson KA, Ingels S, et al: Congenital generalized myofibromatosis: A disseminated angiocentric myofibromatosis. Ped Pathol Lab Med 1995;15:571–587.

Nodular Fasciitis

85. Price EP Jr, Siliphant WM, Shuman R: Nodular fasciitis: A clinicopathologic analysis of 65 cases. Am J Clin Pathol 1961;35:122.
85a. Soule EH: Proliferative (nodular) fasciitis. Arch Pathol 1962;73:437.
86. Werning JT: Nodular fasciitis of the orofacial region. Oral Surg Oral Med Oral Pathol 1979;48:441–446.
87. DiNardo LJ, Wetmore RF, Potsic WP: Nodular fasciitis of the head and neck in children. A deceptive lesion. Arch Otolaryngol Head Neck Surg 1991;117:1001–1002.
88. Lai FM-M, Lam WY: Nodular fasciitis of the dermis. J Cutan Pathol 1993;20:66–69.
89. Diaz-Flores L, Martin Herrera AI, Garcia Montelongo R, Gutierrez Garcia R: Proliferative fasciitis: Ultrastructure and histogenesis. J Cutan Pathol 1989;16:85–92.
90. Montgomery EA, Meis JM: Nodular fasciitis. Its morphologic spectrum and immunohistochemical profile. Am J Surg Pathol 1991;15:942–945.
91. Price S, Kahn LB, Saxe N: Dermal and intravascular fasciitis: Unusual variants of nodular fasciitis. Am J Dermatopathol 1993;15:539–543.

Proliferative Myositis

92. Ushigome S, Takakuwa T, Takagi M, et al: Proliferative myositis and fasciitis. Report of five cases with an ultrastructural and immunohistochemical study. Acta Pathol Jpn 1986;36:963.
93. Dent CD, DeBoom GW, Hamlin ML: Proliferative myositis of the head and neck. Report of a case and review of the literature. Oral Surg Oral Med Oral Pathol 1994;78:354–358.
94. Turner R, Robson A, Motley R: Proliferative myositis: An unusual

cause of multiple subcutaneous nodules. Clin Exper Dermatol 1997;22:101–103.

Oral Focal Mucinosis

95. Tomich CE: Oral focal mucinosis: A clinicopathologic and histochemical study of eight cases. Oral Surg Oral Med Oral Pathol 1974;38:714–724.
96. Lum D: Cutaneous mucinosis of infancy. Arch Dermatol 1980;116:198–200.
97. Buchner A, Merrell PW, Leider AS, Hansen LS: Oral focal mucinosis. Int J Oral Maxillofac Surg 1990;19:337–340.
98. Gnepp DR, Vogler C, Sotelo-Avita C, Kielmovitch IH: Focal mucinosis of the upper aerodigestive tract in children. Human Pathol 1990;21:856–858.
99. Stephens CJM, McKee PH, Black MM: The dermal mucinoses: Advances in dermatology 1993;21:293.
100. Caputo R, Grimalt R, Gelmetti C: Self-healing juvenile cutaneous mucinosis. Arch Dermatol 1995;131:459–461.
101. Clark BJ, Mowat A, Fallowfield ME, Lee FD: Papular mucinosis: is the inflammatory cell infiltrate neoplastic? The presence of a monotypic plasma cell population demonstrated by in-situ hybridization. Br J Dermatol 1996;135:467–470.

Inflammatory Papillary Hyperplasia

102. Bhaskar SN, Beasley JD III, Cutright DE: Inflammatory papillary hyperplasia of the oral mucosa: Report of 341 cases. J Am Dent Assoc 1970;81:949–952.
103. Priddy RW: Inflammatory hyperplasias of the oral mucosa. J Can Dent Assoc 1992;58:311–315,319–321.
104. Bouquot JE, Wrobleski GJ: Papillary (pebbled) masses of the oral mucosa, so much more than simple papillomas. Pract Periodontics Aesthet Dent 1996;8:533–543.
105. Salonen MAM, Raustia AM, Oikarinen KS: Effect of treatment of palatal inflammatory papillary hyperplasia with local and systemic antifungal agents accompanied by renewal of complete dentures. Acta Odont Scand 1996;54:87–91.
106. Berry A: A partial set of teeth sustained by air chambers instead of clasps. Dent Reg West 1851; 9:114–116.

Pericoronitis

107. Gennell JS: A remedy for the painful affection produced when cutting the lower dens salientia or wisdom tooth, etc. Am J Dent Sc 1844;4:43–44.
108. Blakey GH, White RP, Offenbacher S, et al: Clinical/biological outcomes of treatment for pericoronitis. J Oral Maxillofac Surg 1996;54:1150–1160.
109. Neissen LC: Pericoronitis as a cause of tonsillitis. Lancet 1996;348:1602–1603.
110. Rajasuo A, Jousimiessomer H, Savolainen S, et al: Bacteriological findings in tonsillitis and pericoronitis. Clin Infect Dis 1996;23:51–60.
111. Meurman JH, Rajasuo A, Murtomaa H, Savolainen S: Respiratory tract infections and concomitant pericoronitis of the wisdom teeth. Br Med J 1995;310:834–836.

Pyogenic Granuloma

112. Bhaskar SN, Jacoway JR: Pyogenic granuloma: Clinical features, incidence, histology, and result of treatment. Report of 242 cases. J Oral Surg 1966;24:391–398.
113. Vilmann A, Vilmann P, Vilmann H: Pyogenic granuloma: Evaluation of oral conditions. Br J Oral Maxillofac Surg 1986;24:376–382.
114. Mooney MA, Janniger CK: Pyogenic granuloma. Cutis 1995;55:133–136.
115. Patrice SJ, Wiss K, Mulliken JB: Pyogenic granuloma (lobular capillary hemangioma): A clinicopathologic study of 178 cases. Pediatr Dermatol 1991;8:267–276.
116. Mills SE, Cooper PH, Fechner RE: Lobular capillary hemangioma: The underlying lesion of pyogenic granuloma—a study of 73 cases from the oral and nasal mucous membranes. Am J Surg Pathol 1980;4:471–479.
117. Daley TD, Nartey NO, Wysocki GP: Pregnancy tumor: An analysis. Oral Surg Oral Med Oral Pathol 1991;72:196–199.

118. Silverstein LH, Burton CH, Singh BB: Oral pyogenic granuloma in pregnancy. Int J Gynecol Obstet 1995;49:331–332.
119. Sills ES, Zegarelli DJ, Hoschander MM, Strider WE: Clinical diagnosis and management of hormonally responsive oral pregnancy tumor (pyogenic granuloma). J Reproduct Med 1996;41:467–470.
120. Hullihen SP: Case of aneurism by anastomosis of the superior maxillae. Am J Dent Sc 1844; 4:160–162.
121. Gerber ME, Myer CM: Eosinophilic ulcer of the tongue. Otolaryngol Head Neck Surg 1997;117:715–716.

Peripheral Giant Cell Granuloma

122. Giansanti JS, Waldron CA: Peripheral giant cell granuloma: Review of 720 cases. J Oral Surg 1969;17:787–791.
123. Sapp JP: Ultrastructure and histogenesis of peripheral giant cell reparative granuloma of the jaws. Cancer 1972;30:119–129.
124. Katsikeris N, Kakarantza-Angelopoulou E, Angelopoulos AP: Peripheral giant cell granuloma: Clinicopathologic study of 224 new cases and review of 959 reported cases. Int J Oral Maxillofac Surg 1988;17:94–99.
125. Whitaker SB, Bouquot JE: Identification and semi-quantification of estrogen and progesterone receptors in peripheral giant cell lesions of the jaws. J Periodontol 1994;65:280–283.
126. Bodner L, Peist M, Gatot A, Fliss DM: Growth potential of peripheral giant cell granuloma. Oral Surg Oral Med Oral Pathol Oral Radiol Endodont 1997;83:548–551.
127. Tomes J: A course of lectures on dental physiology and surgery (lectures I-XV). Am J Dent Sc 1846-48; 7:1–68, 121–134; 8:33–54, 120–147, 313–350.
128. Smith BR, Fowler CB, Svane TJ: Primary hyperparathyroidism presenting as a "peripheral" giant cell granuloma. J Oral Maxillofac Surg 1988;46:65–69.

Orofacial Granulomatosis and Granulomatous Mucositis

129. Wysocki G, Brooke R: Oral manifestations of chronic granulomatous disease. Oral Surg Oral Med Oral Pathol 1978;46:815–819.
130. Michaud M, Blanchette G, Tomich C: Chronic ulceration of the hard palate: First clinical sign of undiagnosed pulmonary tuberculosis. Oral Surg Oral Med Oral Pathol 1984;57:63–67.
131. Coenen C, Borsch G, Muller K, Fabry H: Oral inflammatory changes as an initial manifestation of Crohn's disease antedating abdominal diagnosis. Dis Colon Rectum 1988;31:548–552.
132. Melson RD, et al: Sarcoidosis in a patient presenting with clinical and histologic features of primary Sjögren's syndrome. Ann Rheum Dis 1988;47:166–168.
133. Allen CM, et al: Cheilitis granulomatosa: Report of six cases and review of the literature. J Am Acad Dermatol 1990;23:444–450.
134. Devaney K, Travis W, Hoffman G, et al: Interpretation of head and neck biopsies in Wegener's granulomatosis. Am J Surg Pathol 1990;14:555–564.
135. Allen CM, Camisa C, Salewski C, Weiland JE: Wegener's granulomatosis: Report of three cases with oral lesions. J Oral Maxillofac Surg 1991;49:294–298.
136. Daley TD, Wysocki GP: Foreign body gingivitis: an iatrogenic disease? Oral Surg Oral Med Oral Pathol 1991;71:451–453.
137. Ghandour K, Issa M: Oral Crohn's disease with late intestinal disease. Oral Surg Oral Med Oral Pathol 1991;72:565–567.
138. Oliver AJ, Rich Am, Reade PC, et al: Monosodium glutamate-related orofacial granulomatosis: Review and case report. Oral Surg Oral Med Oral Pathol 1991;71:560–564.
139. Sharma OP: Histoplasmosis: a masquerader of sarcoidosis. Sarcoidosis 1991;8:10–13.
140. Hoffman G, Kerr G, Leavitt R, et al: Wegener's granulomatosis: An analysis of 158 patients. Ann Intern Med 1992;116:488–498.
141. Kuno Y, Sakakihara S, Mizumo N: Actinic cheilitis granulomatosa. J Dermatol 1992;19:556–562
142. Mendelsohn SS, Field EA, Woolgar J: Sarcoidosis of the tongue. Clin Exp Dermatol 1992;17:47–48.
143. Lilly J, Juhlin T, Lew D, Vincent S, et al: Wegener's granulomatosis presenting as oral lesions. A case report. Oral Surg Oral Med Oral Pathol Oral Radiol Endod 1998;85:153–157.
144. Samaranayake LP: Oral mycoses in HIV infection. Oral Surg Oral Med Oral Pathol 1992;73:171–180.

145. Winnie R, DeLuke DM: Melkersson-Rosenthal syndrome: Review of the literature and case report. Int J Oral Maxillofac Surg 1992;21:115–117.
146. Zimmer WM, Rogers RS 3d, Reeve CM, Sheridan PJ: Orofacial manifestations of Melkersson-Rosenthal syndrome: A study of 42 patients and review of 220 cases from the literature. Oral Surg Oral Med Oral Pathol 1992;74:610–619.
147. Gordon SC, Daley TD: Foreign body gingivitis: Clinical and microscopic features of 61 cases. Oral Surg Oral Med Oral Pathol Oral Radiol Endod 1997;83:562–570.

Torus and Bony Exostosis

148. Miller SC, Roth H: Torus palatinus: A statistical study. J Am Dent Assoc 1940;27:1950–1957.
149. Johnson CC, Gorlin RJ, Anderson VE: Torus mandibularis: A genetic study. Am J Hum Genet 1965;17:433–422.
150. Rezai RF, Jackson JT, Salamat K: Torus palatinus, an exostosis of unknown etiology: Review of the literature. Compend Contin Educ Dent 1985;6:149–152.
151. Indignities DZ, Bailees M, Papanayiotou P: Concurrence of torus palatinus with palatal and buccal exostoses: Case report and review of the literature. Oral Surg Oral Med Oral Pathol Oral Radiol Endod 1998;85:552–557.
152. Parmentier: Essay on tumors in the palatine region. Am J Dent Sc 1857; 7 (new series): 324–339, 456–465, 545–561.
153. Bouquot JE: Ischemic change and necrosis in maxillofacial tori and exostoses. Proceeding of the 53rd Annual Meeting of the American Academy of Oral and Maxillofacial Pathology; Hawaii, June, 1999.

Peripheral Ossifying Fibroma

154. Buchner A, Hansen LS: The histomorphologic spectrum of peripheral ossifying fibroma. Oral Surg Oral Med Oral Pathol 1987; 63:452–461.
155. Kenney JN, Kaugers GE, Abbey LM: Comparison between the peripheral ossifying fibroma and peripheral odontogenic fibroma. J Oral Maxillofac Surg 1989;47:378–382.
156. Zain RB, Fei YJ: Fibrous lesions of the gingiva: A histopathologic analysis of 204 cases. Oral Surg Oral Med Oral Pathol 1990;70:466–470.
157. Poon CK, Kwan PC, Chao SY: Giant peripheral ossifying fibroma of the maxilla: Report of a case. J Oral Maxillofac Surg 1995;53:695–698.
158. Shepherd SM: Alveolar exostosis. Am J Dent Sc 1844;4:43–44.

Heterotopic Ossification

159. Clapton WK, James CL, Morris LL, et al: Myositis ossificans in childhood. Pathology 1992;24:311–314.
160. El-Labban NG, Hopper C, Barber P: Ultrastructural finding of vascular degeneration in myositis ossificans circumscripta (fibrodysplasia ossificans). J Oral Pathol Med 1993;22:428–431.
161. Merchan EC, Sanchez-Herrera S, Valdazo DA, Gonzalez JM: Circumscribed myositis ossificans: Report of nine cases without history of injury. Acta Orthop Belg 1993;59:273–277.
162. Adderson EE, Bohnsack JF: Traumatic myositis ossificans simulating soft tissue infection. Ped Infect Dis J 1996;15:551–553.
163. Unni KK: Dahlin's Bone Tumors: General Aspects and Data on 11,087 cases, 5th ed. Philadelphia: Lippincott-Raven, 1996.
164. Cohen RB, Hahn GV, Tabas JA, et al: The natural history of heterotopic ossification in patients who have fibrodysplasia ossificans progressiva: A study of forty-four patients. J Bone Joint Surg 1993;75A:215–219.
165. Kaplan FS, Tabas JA, Gannon FH, et al: The histopathology of fibrodysplasia ossificans progressiva: An enchondral process. J Bone Joint Surg 1993;75:220–230.

Osseous/Cartilaginous Choristoma

166. Cutright DE: Osseous and chondromatous metaplasia caused by dentures. Oral Surg Oral Med Oral Pathol 1972;34:625–633.
167. Cutilli BJ, Quinn PD: Traumatically induced peripheral osteoma: Report of a case. Oral Surg Oral Med Oral Pathol 1992;73:667–669.
168. Gardner DG, Paterson JC: Chondroma or metaplastic chondrosis of soft palate. Oral Surg Oral Med Oral Pathol 1968;26:601.

169. Cabbabe EB, Sotelo-Avila C, Moloney ST, Makhlouf MV: Osseous choristoma of the tongue. Ann Plast Surg 1986;16:150–152.

170. Hodder SC, MacDonald DG: Osseous choristoma of buccal mucosa: Report of a case. Br J Oral Maxillofac Surg 1988;26:78–80.

171. Tohill MJ, Green JG, Cohen DM: Intraoral osseous and cartilaginous choristomas: Report of three cases and review of the literature. Oral Surg Oral Med Oral Pathol 1987;63:506–510.

172. Chou L, Hansen SI, Daniels E: Choristomas of the oral cavity: A review. Oral Surg Oral Med Oral Pathol 1991;72:584–593.

173. Long DE, Koutnik W: Recurrent intraoral osseous choristoma: Report of a case. Oral Surg Oral Med Oral Pathol 1991;72:337–339.

174. Ishikawa M, Mizukoshi T, Notani K, et al: Osseous choristoma of the tongue: Report of two cases. Oral Surg Oral Med Oral Pathol 1993;76:561–563.

175. Psimopoulou M, Indignities K: Submental osseous choristoma: A case report. J Oral Maxillofac Surg 1998;666–667.

Peripheral (Juxtacortical) Osteosarcoma

176. Brass JM, Donner R, van der Kwast WAM: Juxtacortical osteogenic sarcoma. Oral Surg Oral Med Oral Pathol 1980;50:535–544.

177. Zarbo RJ, Regezi JA, Baker SR: Periosteal osteogenic sarcoma of the mandible. Oral Surg Oral Med Oral Pathol 1984;57:643–647.

178. Slootweg PJ, Muller H: Osteosarcoma of the jawbones. J Maxillofac Surg 1985;13:158–166.

179. Geschickter CF, Copeland MM: Parosteal osteoma of bone: A new entity? Ann Surg 1951;133:790–807.

Glial Choristoma

180. Strome SE, McClatchey K, Kileny PR, Koopman CF: Neonatal choristoma of the tongue containing glial tissue: Diagnosis and surgical considerations. Int J Pediatr Otorhinolaryngol 1995;33:265–273.

181. Ide F, Shimoyama T, Horie N: Glial choristoma in the oral cavity: Histopathologic and immunohistochemical features. J Oral Pathol Med 1997;26:147–150.

Teratoma

182. Batsakis JG, Littler ER, Oberman HA: Teratomas of the neck: A clinicopathological appraisal. Arch Otolaryngol 1964;79:619–625.

183. Gorlin RJ: Developmental anomalies of the face and oral structures. In: Gorlin RJ, Goldman HM: Thoma's Oral Pathology, vol. 1, 6th ed. St. Louis: C.V. Mosby, 1970: 21–95.

184. Kountakis SE, Minotti AM, Maillard A, Steinberg CM: Teratomas of the head and neck. Am J Otolaryngol Head Neck Surg 1994;15:292–296.

185. McKiernan DC, Koay B, Vinayak B, et al: A case of submandibular teratoma. J Laryngol Otol 1995;109:992–994.

186. Biglioli F, Gianni AB, Difrancesco A: Congenital teratoma of the cheek: Report of a case. Int J Oral Maxillofac Surg 1996;25:208–209.

187. McMahon MJ, Chescheir NC, Kuller JA, et al: Perinatal management of a lingual teratoma. Obstet Gynecol 1996;87:848–851.

188. Kuhn JJ, Schoem SR, Warnock GR: Squamous cell carcinoma arising in a benign teratoma of the maxilla. Otolaryngol Head Neck Surg 1996;114:447–452.

Fordyce Granules

189. Miles AEW: Sebaceous glands in the lip and cheek mucosa of man. Br Dent J 1958;105:235–239.

190. Gorsky M, Buchner A, Fundoianu-Dayan D, Cohen C: Fordyce's granules in the oral mucosa of adult Israeli Jews. Community Dent Oral Epidemiol 1986;14:231–232.

191. Rhodus NL: An actively secreting Fordyce granule: A case report. Clin Prev Dent 1986;8:24–26.

192. Fordyce J: A peculiar affection of the mucous membrane of the lip and oral cavity. J Cutan Genito-Urin Dis 1896;14:413–419.

193. Miller AS, McCrea MW: Sebaceous gland adenoma of the buccal mucosa. J Oral Surg 1968;26:593–595.

194. Ellis GL, Auclair PL, Gnepp DR: Surgical Pathology of the Salivary Glands. Philadelphia: W.B. Saunders, 1991.

195. Abuzeid M, Gangopadhyay K, Rayappa CS, Antonios JI: Intraoral sebaceous carcinoma. J Laryngol Otol 1996;110:500–502.

196. Miller ML, Harford RR, Yeager JK: Fox Fordyce disease treated with topical clindamycin solution. Arch Dermatol 1995;131:1112–1113.

Juxtaoral Organ of Chievitz

197. Vadmal MS, Rossi MB, Teichberg S, Hajdu SI: Intraoral tumor of Chievitz in a child. Pediatr Dev Pathol 1998;1:230–233.

198. Chievitz JH: Beitrage zur Entwicklungsgeschichte der Speicheldrusen. Arch Anat Physiol 1885;9:401–436.

199. Danforth RA, Baughman RA: Chievitz's organ: A potential pitfall in oral cancer diagnosis. Oral Surg Oral Med Oral Pathol 1979;48:231–236.

200. Miko T, Molnar P: The juxtaoral organ: A pitfall for pathologists. J Pathol 1981;133:17–23.

201. Eversole LR, Leider AS: Maxillary intraosseous neuroepithelial structures resembling those seen in the organ of Chievitz. Oral Surg Oral Med Oral Pathol 1978;46:555–558.

Benign Lymphoid Aggregates

202. Simpson HE: Lymphocyte hyperplasia in foliate papillitis. J Oral Surg 1964;22:209–214.

203. Bhargava D, Raman R, Alabri RK, Bushnurmath B: Heterotopia of the tonsil. J Laryngol Otol 1996;110:611–612.

204. Endo LH, Altemani A, Chone C, et al: Histopathological comparison between tonsil and adenoid responses to allergy. Acta Oto-Laryngol 1996;S523:17–19.

205. Bouquot JE, Gundlach KKH: Odd tongues: The prevalence of common tongue lesions in 23,616 white Americans over 35 years of age. Quintessence Int 1986;17:719–730.

206. Joseph M, Ricardon E, Goodman H: Lingual tonsillectomy: A treatment for inflammatory lesions of the lingual tonsil. Laryngoscope 1984;94:179–183.

207. Napier SS, Newlands C: Benign lymphoid hyperplasia of the palate: Report of two cases and immunohistochemical profile. J Oral Pathol Med 1990;19:221–225.

Lingual Thyroid

208. Baughman RA: Lingual thyroid and lingual thyroglossal tract remnants. A clinical and histopathologic study with review of the literature. Oral Surg Oral Med Oral Pathol 1972;34:781–799.

209. Kansal P, Sakati N, Rifai A, Woodhouse N: Lingual thyroid: A diagnosis and treatment. Arch Intern Med 1987;147:2046–2048.

210. Williams JD, Sclafani AP, Slupchinskij O, Douge C: Evaluation and management of the lingual thyroid gland. Ann Otol Rhinol Laryngol 1996;105:312–216.

211. Diaz-Arias AA, Bickel JT, Loy TS, et al: Follicular carcinoma with clear cell change arising in lingual thyroid. Oral Surg Oral Med Oral Pathol 1992;74:206–211.

Congenital (Granular Cell) Epulis

212. O'Brien FV, Pielou WD: Congenital epulis: Its natural history. Arch Dis Child 1971;46:559–560.

213. Lack EE, Worsham GF, Callihan MD, et al: Gingival granular cell tumors of the newborn (congenital "epulis"): A clinical and pathologic study of 21 patients. Am J Surg Pathol 1981;5:37–46.

214. Slootweg P, de Wilde P, Vooijs P, et al: Oral granular cell lesions: An immunohistochemical study with emphasis on intermediate-sized filament proteins. Virchows Arch (Pathol Anat Histopathol) 1983;402:35–45.

215. Tucker MC, Rusnock EJ, Axumi N, et al: Gingival granular cell tumors of the newborn: An ultrastructural and immunohistochemical study. Arch Pathol Lab Med 1990;114:895–898.

216. Damm DD, Cibull ML, Giessler RH, et al: Investigation into the histogenesis of congenital epulis of the newborn. Oral Surg Oral Med Oral Pathol 1993;76:205–212.

217. Kaiseling E, Ruck P, Xiao JC: Congenital epulis and granular cell tumor: A histologic and immunohistochemical study. Oral Surg Oral Med Oral Pathol Oral Radiol Endodont 1995;80:687–697.

218. Neumann E: Ein Fall von congenitaler Epulis. Arch Heilk 1871;12:189–194.

219. Kusukawa J, Kulara S, Koga C, Inoue T: Congenital granular cell tu-

mor (congenital epulis) in the fetus: A case report. J Oral Maxillofac Surg 1997;55:1356–1359.

Median Rhomboid Glossitis (Posterior Lingual Papillary Atrophy)

220. Baughman RA: Median rhomboid glossitis: A developmental anomaly? Oral Surg Oral Med Oral Pathol 1971;31:56–65.
221. Allen CM: Animal models of oral candidiasis: A review. Oral Surg Oral Med Oral Pathol 1994;78:216–221.
222. Brown RS, Krakow AM: Median rhomboid glossitis and a kissing lesion of the palate. Oral Surg Oral Med Oral Pathol Oral Radiol Endodont 1996;82:472–473.
223. Brocq L, Pautrier LM: Glossite losangue mediane de la face dorsale de la langue. Ann Derm Syph (Paris) 1914;5:1–18.
224. Bouquot JE, Gundlach KKH: Odd tongues: The prevalence of common tongue lesions in 23,616 white Americans over 35 years of age. Quint Internat 1986;17:719–730.

Epidermoid and Dermoid Cysts

225. Gold BD, Sheinkipf DE, Levy B: Dermoid, epidermoid and teratomatous cysts of the tongue and floor of the mouth. J Oral Surg 1974;32:107–111.
226. Howell CJT: The sublingual dermoid. Oral Surg Oral Med Oral Pathol 1985;59:578.
227. Flom GS, Donavan TJ, Landgraf JR: Congenital dermoid cyst of the anterior tongue. Otolaryngol Head Neck Surg 1989;101:388–391.
228. Shaari CM, Ho BT, Shah K, Biller HF: Lingual dermoid cyst. Otolaryngol Head Neck Surg 1995;112:476–478.
229. Harada H, Kusukawa J, Kameyama T: Congenital teratoid cyst of the floor of the mouth: A case report. Int J Oral Maxillofac Surg 1995;24:361–362.
230. Bonilla JA, Szeremeta W, Yellon RF, Nazif MM: Teratoid cyst of the floor of the mouth. Int J Ped Otorhinolaryngol 1996;38:1:71–75.
231. Kitagawa Y, Hashimoto K, Tanaka N, Ishii Y: Congenital teratoid cyst with a median fistula in the submental region: Case report and ultrastructural findings. J Oral Maxillofac Surg 1998;56:254–262.
232. Bouquot JE, Lense E: The birth of oral pathology: Part I, first dental journal reports of benign oral tumors and cysts, 1839–1859. Oral Surg Oral Med Oral Pathol 1992;74:599.
233. Buchner A, Hansen LS: The histomorphologic spectrum of the gingival cyst in the adult. Oral Surg Oral Med Oral Pathol 1979;48:532–539.
234. Nxumalo TN, Shear M: Gingival cyst in adults. J Oral Pathol Med 1992;21:309–313.
235. Breault LG, Billman MA, Lewis DM: Report of a gingival surgical cyst developing secondarily to a subepithelial connective-tissue graft. J Periodontol 1997;68:392–395.

Palatal and Gingival Cysts of the Newborn

236. Nichamin SJ, Kaufman M: Gingival microcysts in infancy. Pediatrics 1963;31:412–415.
237. Moskow BS, Bloom A: Embryogenesis of the gingival cyst. J Clin Periodontol 1983;10:119–130.
238. Fromm A: Epstein's pearls, Bohn's nodules and inclusion-cysts of the oral cavity. J Dent Child 1967;34:275–287.
239. Cataldo E, Berkman MD: Cyst of the oral mucosa in newborns. Am J Dis Child 1968;116:44–48.
240. Jorgenson RJ, Shaprio SD, Salinas CF, Levin LS: Intraoral findings and anomalies in neonates. Pediatrics 1982;69:577–582.

Nasolabial Cyst

241. Wesley RK, Scannell T, Nathan LE: Nasolabial cyst: Presentation of a case with a review of the literature. J Oral Maxillofac Surg 1984;42:188–192.
242. Adams A, Lovelock DJ: Nasolabial cyst. Oral Surg Oral Med Oral Pathol 1985;60Z:118–119.
243. David VC, O'Connell JE: Nasolabial cyst. Clin Otolaryngol 1986;11:5–8.
244. Zuckerkandl E: Normale und pathologische Anatomie der Nasenhohle. Vienna: W. Braunmuller, 1882.

245. Cohen MA, Hertzanu Y: Huge growth potential of the nasolabial cyst. Oral Surg Oral Med Oral Pathol 1985;59:441–445.

Lymphoepithelial Cyst

246. Buchner A, Hansen LS: Lymphoepithelial cysts of the oral mucosa. Oral Surg Oral Med Oral Pathol 1980;50:441–449.
247. Chaudhry AP: A clinicopathologic study of intraoral lymphoepithial cysts. J Oral Med 1984;39:79–84.
248. Schinkenickl DA, Muller MF: Lymphoepithelial cyst of the pancreas. Br J Radiol 1996;69:876–878.
249. Skouteris CA, Patterson GT, Sotereanos GC: Benign cervical lymphoepithelial cyst: report of cases. J Oral Maxillofac Surg 1989;47:1106–1112.
250. Janicke S, Kettner R, Kuffner HD: A possible inflammatory reaction in a lateral neck cyst (branchial cyst) because of odontogenic infection. Int J Oral Maxillofac Surg 1994;23:369–371.
251. Gnepp DR, Sporck FT: Benign lymphoepithelial parotid cyst with sebaceous differentiation: Cystic sebaceous lymphadenoma. Am J Clin Pathol 1980;74:683–687.
252. Smith FB: Benign lymphoepithelial lesion and lymphoepithelial cyst of the parotid gland in HIV infection. Prog AIDS Pathol 1990;2:61–72.

Thyroglossal Duct Cyst

253. Wampler HW, Krolls SO, Johnson RP: Thyroglossal tract cyst. Oral Surg Oral Med Oral Pathol 1978;45:32–38.
254. Brereton RJ, Symonds E: Thyroglossal cysts in children. Br J Surg 1978;65:507–508.
255. Katz AD, Hachigian M: Thyroglossal duct cysts: A thirty-year experience with emphasis on occurrence in older patients. Am J Surg 1988;155:741–744.
256. Klin B, Seroor F, Fried K, et al: Familial thyroglossal duct cyst. Clin Genet 1993;43:101–103.
257. Castillo-Taucher S, Castillo P: Autosomal dominant inheritance of thyroglossal duct cyst. Clin Genet 1994;45:111–112.
258. Yanagisawa K, Eisen RN, Sasaki CT: Squamous cell carcinoma arising in a thyroglossal duct cyst. Arch Otolaryngol Head Neck Surg 1992;118:538–541.
259. Wigley TL, Chonkich GD, Wat BY: Papillary carcinoma arising in the thyroglossal duct cyst. Otolaryngol Head Neck Surg 1997;116:386–388.

Heterotopic Oral Gastrointestinal Cyst

260. Daley TD, Wysocki GP, Lovas JL, Smouth MS: Heterotopic gastric cyst of the oral cavity. Head Neck Surg 1984;7:168–171.
261. Lipsett J, Sparnon AL, Byard RW: Embryogenesis of enterocystomas: Enteric duplication cysts of the tongue. Oral Surg Oral Med Oral Pathol 1993;75:626–630.
262. Ohbayashi Y, Miyake M, Nagahata S: Gastrointestinal cyst of the tongue: A possible duplication cyst of foregut origin. J Oral Maxillofac Surg 1997;55:626–628.

Traumatic Angiomatous Lesion (Venous Lake)

263. Alcalay J, Sandbank M: The ultrastructure of cutaneous venous lakes. Int J Dermatol 1987;26:645–646.
264. Mirowski GW, Rozycki TW: Common skin lesions. In: Regezi JA, Sciubba JJ (eds): Oral Pathology: Clinical Pathologic Correlations, 3rd ed. Philadelphia: W.B. Saunders, 1999: 479–518.
265. Weathers DR, Fine RM: Thrombosed varix of oral cavity. Arch Dermatol 1971;104:427–430.
266. Southam JC, Ettinger RL: A histologic study of sublingual varices. Oral Surg Oral Med Oral Pathol 1974;38:879–886.
267. Guttmacher AE, Marchuk DA, White RI: Hereditary hemorrhagic telangiectasia. N Engl J Med 1995;333:918–924.

Caliber-Persistent Labial Artery

268. Miko TL, Adler P, Endes P: Simulated cancer of the lower lip attributed to a "caliber persistent" artery. J Oral Pathol 1980;9:137–144.
269. Lovas JGL, Rodu B, Hammond HL, Allen CM, et al: Caliber-persistent

labial artery: A common vascular anomaly. Oral Surg Oral Med Oral Pathol Oral Radiol Endod 1998;86:308–312.

270. Manganaro AM: Caliber-persistent artery of the lip: Case report. J Oral Maxillofac Surg 1998;56:895–897.

271. Miko TL, Molnar P, Verseckei L: Interrelationship of caliber persistent artery, chronic ulcer and squamous cancer of the lower lip. Histopathology 1983;7:595–599.

Hemangioma

272. Woods WR, Tulumello TN: Management of oral hemangioma. Review of the literature and report of a case. Oral Surg Oral Med Oral Pathol 1977;44:39.

273. Batsakis JG: Tumors of the Head and Neck: Clinical and Pathological Considerations, 2nd ed. Baltimore: Williams & Wilkins, 1979.

274. Hart B, Schwartz HC: Cavernous hemangioma of the masseter muscle: Report of a case. J Oral Maxillofac Surg 1995;53:467–469.

275. Rossiter JL, Hendrix RA, Tom LW, Potsic WP: Intramuscular hemangioma of the head and neck. Otolaryngol Head Neck Surg 1993; 108:18–26.

276. Harris CA: A physiological and pathological inquiry concerning the physical characteristics of the human teeth and gums, the salivary calculus, the lips and the tongue, and the fluids of the mouth. Am J Dent Sc 1842;3:20–132,153–189.

277. Wawro NM, Fredrickson RW, Tennant RW: Hemangioma of the parotid gland in the newborn and in infancy. Cancer 1955;8:595–599.

278. Clearkin KP, Enzinger FM: Intravascular papillary endothelial hyperplasia. Arch Pathol Lab Med 1976;100:441–444.

279. Pesce C, Valente S, Gandolfo AM, Lenti E: Intravascular lobular capillary hemangioma of the lip. Histopathology 1996;29:382–384.

280. Chan JKC, Hui PK, Ng CS, et al: Epithelioid hemangioma (angiolymphoid hyperplasia with eosinophilia) and Kimura's disease in Chinese. Histopathology 1989;15:557–574.

281. Fetsch JF, Weiss SW: Observations concerning the pathogenesis of epithelioid hemangioma (angiolymphoid hyperplasia). Mod Pathol 1991;4:449–455.

282. Toeg A, Kermish M, Grishkan A, Temkin D: Histiocytoid hemangioma of the oral cavity: A report of two cases. J Oral Maxillofac Surg 1993;51:812–814.

283. Marti-Bonmati L, Menor F, Mulas F: The Sturge-Weber syndrome: Correlation between the clinical status and radiological CT and MRI findings. Childs Nerv Syst 1993;9:107–109.

284. Oakes WJ: The natural history of patients with the Sturge-Weber syndrome. Pediatr Neurosurg 1992;18:287–290.

Hemangioendothelioma

285. Ellis GL, Kratochvil FJ: Epithelioid hemangioendothelioma of the head and neck: A clinicopathologic report of twelve cases. Oral Surg Oral Med Oral Pathol 1986;61:61–68.

286. Weiss SW, Ishak KG, Dail DH, et al: Epithelioid hemangioendothelioma and related lesions. Semin Diagn Pathol 1986;3:259–287.

287. Scott GA, Rosai J: Spindle cell hemangioendothelioma: Report of seven additional cases of a recently described entity vascular neoplasm. Am J Derrmatopathol 1988;10:281–288.

288. Lai FM, Allen PW, Yuen PM, et al: Locally metastasizing vascular tumor: Spindle cell, epithelioid, or unclassified hemangioendothelioma. Am J Clin Pathol 1991;96:660–663.

289. Polk P, Webb JM: Isolated cutaneous epithelioid hemangioendothelioma. J Am Acad Dermatol 1997;36:1026–1028.

290. Zukerberg LR, Nickoloff BJ, Weiss SW: Kaposiform hemangioendothelioma of infancy and childhood: An aggressive neoplasm associated with Kasabach-Merritt syndrome and lymphangiomatosis. Am J Surg Pathol 1993;17:321–328.

291. Fukunaga M, Ushigome S, Ishikawa E: Kaposiform hemangioendothelioma associated with Kasabach-Merritt syndrome. Histopathology 1996;28:281–284.

Hemangiopericytoma

292. Stout AP, Murray MR: Hemangiopericytoma: Vascular tumor featuring Zimmermann's pericytes. Ann Surg 1942;116:26.

293. Stout AP: Hemangiopericytoma: A study of twenty-five new cases. Cancer 1949;3:1027–1037.

294. Walike JW, Bailey BJ: Head and neck hemangiopericytoma. Arch Otolaryngol 1971;93:345–353.

295. Daniels RL, Haller JR, Harnsberger HR: Hemangiopericytoma of the masticator space. Ann Otol Rhinol Laryngol 1996;105:162–165.

296. Delgaudio JM, Garetz SL, Bradford CR, Stenson KM: Hemangiopericytoma of the oral cavity. Otolaryngol Head Neck Surg 1996;114:339–340.

297. Kothari PS, Murphy M, Howells GL, Williams DM: Hemangiopericytoma: A report of 2 cases arising on the lip. Br J Oral Maxillofac Surg 1996;34:454–456.

298. Lin JC, Hsu CY, Jan JS, Chen JT: Malignant hemangiopericytoma of the floor of the mouth: Report of a case and review of the literature. J Oral Maxillofac Surg 1996;54:1020–1023.

299. Abdel-Fattah HM, Adams GL, Wick MR: Hemangiopericytoma of the maxillary sinus and skull base. Head Neck 1990;12:77–83.

300. Seibert JJ: Multiple congenital hemangiopericytomas of the head and neck. Laryngoscope 1978;88:1006–1012.

301. Alpers CE, Rosenau W, Finkbeiner WE, et al: Congenital (infantile) hemangiopericytoma of the tongue and the sublingual region. Am J Clin Pathol 1984;81:377–382.

Angiosarcoma

302. Bardwil JM, Mocega EE, Butler JJ, et al: Angiosarcomas of the head and neck region. Am J Surg 1968;116:548–553.

303. Wesley RK, Mintz SM, Wertheimer FW: Primary malignant hemangioendothelioma of the gingiva: Report of a case and review of the literature. Oral Surg Oral Med Oral Pathol 1975;39:103–112.

304. Cochran JH Jr, Fee WE Jr: Angiosarcoma of the head and neck. Otolaryngol Head Neck Surg 1979;87:409–416.

305. Oliver AJ, Gibbons SD, Radden BG, et al: Primary angiosarcoma of the oral cavity. Br J Oral Maxillofac Surg 1991;29:38–41.

306. Fletcher CD, Beham A, Bekir S, et al: Epithelioid angiosarcoma of deep soft tissue: A distinctive tumor readily mistaken for an epithelial neoplasm. Am J Surg Pathol 1991;15:915–924.

307. Munoz M, Monje F, Alonzo del Hoyo JR, Martin-Granizo R: Oral angiosarcoma misdiagnosed as a pyogenic granuloma. J Oral Maxillofac Surg 1998;56:488–491.

308. Tosios K, Hkoutlas IG, Papanicolaou SI: Intravascular papillary endothelial hyperplasia of the oral soft tissues: Report of 18 cases and review of the literature. J Oral Maxillofac Surg 1994;52:1263–1268.

Kaposi's Sarcoma

309. Kaposi M: Idiopathisches multiples Pigmentsarkom der Haut. Arch Dermatol Syph 1872;4:265–276.

310. Ficarra G, Berson A, Silverman S Jr, et al: Kaposi's sarcoma of the oral cavity: A study of 134 patients with a review of the pathogenesis, epidemiology, clinical aspects, and treatment. Oral Surg Oral Med Oral Pathol 1988;66:543–550.

311. Friedman-Kien AE, Saltzman BR: Clinical manifestations of classical, endemic African, and epidemic AIDS-associated Kaposi's sarcoma. J Am Acad Dermatol 1990;22:1237–1250.

312. Searles GE, Markman S, Yazdi HM: Primary oral Kaposi's sarcoma of the hard palate. J Am Acad Dermatol 1990;23:518–519.

313. Regezi JA, MacPhail LA, Daniels TE, Greenspan JS, et al: Oral Kaposi's sarcoma: A 10-year retrospective histopathologic study. J Oral Pathol Med 1993;22:292–297.

314. Ensoli B, Gendelman R, Markham P, et al: Synergy between basic fibroblast growth factor and HIV-1 tat protein in induction of Kaposi's sarcoma. Nature 1994;371:674–680.

315. Miles SA: Pathogenesis of AIDS-related Kaposi's sarcoma. Evidence of a viral etiology. Hematol Oncol Clin North Am 1996; 10:1011–1021.

316. Lucatorto FM, Sapp JP: Treatment of oral Kaposi's sarcoma with a sclerosing agent in AIDS patients. Oral Surg Oral Med Oral Pathol 1993;75:192–198.

Lymphangioma

317. Levin LS, Jorgenson RJ, Jarvey BA: Lymphangiomas of the alveolar ridges in neonates. Pediatrics 1976;58:881–884.

318. Goldberg MH, Nemarich AN, Danielson P: Lymphangioma of the tongue: Medical and surgical therapy. J Oral Maxillofac Surg 1977; 35:841–844.

319. Wilson S, Gould AR, Wolff C: Multiple lymphangiomas of the alveolar ridge in a neonate: Case study. Pediatr Dent 1986;8:231–234.

320. Kennedy TL: Cystic hygroma-lymphangioma: A rare and still unclear entity. Laryngoscope 1989;99:1–10.

321. Ricciardelli EJ, Richardson MA: Cervicofacial cystic hygroma: Patterns of recurrence and management of the difficult case. Arch Otolaryngol Head Neck Surg 1991;117:546–553.

322. Ramani P, Shah A: Lymphangiomatosis: Histologic and immunohistochemical analysis of four cases. Am J Surg Pathol 1993;17:329–335.

323. Herron GS, Rouse RV, Kosek JC, et al: Benign lymphangioendothelioma. J Am Acad Dermatol 1994;31:362–368.

324. Cossu S, Satta R, Cottoni F, Massarelli G: Lymphangioma-like variant of Kaposi's sarcoma: Clinicopathological study of 7 cases with review of the literature. Am J Dermatopathol 1997;19:16–22.

Herniated Buccal Fat Pad

325. Clawson JR, Kline KK, Armbrecht EC: Trauma-induced avulsion of the buccal fat pad into the mouth: Report of a case. J Oral Surg 1968;26:546–547.

326. Brooke RI, MacGregor AJ: Traumatic pseudolipoma of the buccal mucosa. Oral Surg Oral Med Oral Pathol 1969;28:223–225.

327. Browne WG: Herniation of buccal fat pad. Oral Surg Oral Med Oral Pathol 1970;29:181–183.

328. Berk CW, Gibson WS Jr: Pathologic quiz case 1: Traumatic herniated gangrenous buccal fat pad (traumatic pseudolipoma). Arch Otolaryngol Head Neck Surg 1994;120:340–342.

Lipoma

329. de Visscher JGAM: Lipomas and fibrolipomas of the oral cavity. J Maxillofac Surg 1982;10:177–181.

330. Rapidis AD: Lipoma of the oral cavity. Int J Oral Surg 1982;11:263–275.

331. Roux M: On exostoses: Their character. Am J Dent Sc 1848; 9:133–134.

332. Macmillan ARG, Oliver AJ, Reade PC, et al: Regional macrodontia and regional bony enlargement associated with congenital infiltrating lipomatosis of the face presenting as unilateral facial hyperplasia. Int J Oral Maxillofac Surg 1990;19:283–286.

333. Kang N, Ross D, Harrison D: Unilateral hypertrophy of the face associated with infiltrating lipomatosis. J Oral Maxillofac Surg 1998;56:885–887.

334. Chen SY, Fantasia JE, Miller AS: Myxoid lipoma of oral soft tissue: A clinical and ultrastructural study. Oral Surg Oral Med Oral Pathol 1984;57:300–307.

335. McDaniel RK, Newland JR, Chiles DG: Intraoral spindle cell lipoma: Case report with correlated light and electron microscopy. Oral Surg Oral Med Oral Pathol 1984;57:52–57.

336. Zelger BWH, Zelger BG, Plorer A, et al: Dermal spindle cell lipoma: Plexiform and nodular variants. Histopathology 1995;27:533–540.

337. Guillou L, Dehon A, Charlin B, et al: Pleomorphic lipoma of the tongue: Case report and literature review. J Otolaryngol 1986;15:313–316.

338. Fujimura N, Enomoto S: Lipoma of the tongue with cartilaginous change: A case report and review of the literature. J Oral Maxillofac Surg 1992;50:1015–1017.

339. Rigor VU, Goldstone SE, Jones J, et al: Hibernoma: A case report and discussion of a rare tumor. Cancer 1986;57:2207–2211.

340. Shear M: Lipoblastomatosis of the cheek. Br J Oral Surg 1967;5:173–179.

341. Tallini G, Dalcin P, Rhoden KJ, et al: Expression of Hmgi-C and Hmgi(Y) in ordinary lipoma and atypical lipomatous tumors: Immunohistochemical reactivity correlates with karyotypic alterations. Am J Pathol 1997;151:37–43.

Liposarcoma

342. Sauk JJ Jr: Liposarcoma of the head and neck. J Oral Surg 1971;29:38–40.

343. Sadeghi EM, Sauk JJ: Liposarcoma of the oral cavity: Clinical, tissue culture, and ultrastructure study of a case. J Oral Pathol 1982;11:263–275.

344. Eidinger G, Katsikeris N, Gullane PI: Liposarcoma: Report of a case and review of the literature. J Oral Maxillofac Surg 1990;48:984–988.

345. Guest PG: Liposarcoma of the tongue: A case report and review of the literature. Br J Oral Maxillofac Surg 1992;30:268–269.

346. McCulloch TM, Makielski KH, McNutt MA: Head and neck liposarcoma: A histopathologic reevaluation of reported cases. Arch Otolaryngol Head Neck Surg 1992;118:1045–1049.

347. Stewart M, Schwartz M, Alford B: Atypical and malignant lipomatous lesions of the head and neck. Arch Otolaryngol Head Neck Surg 1994;120:1151–1155.

348. Zheng J, Wang Y: Liposarcoma in the oral and maxillofacial region: An analysis of 10 consecutive patients. J Oral Maxillofac Surg 1994;52:595–598.

349. Kamikaidou N, Kirita T, Kenji M, Masahito S: Liposarcoma of the cheek: Report of a case. J Oral Maxillofac Surg 1998;662–665.

Traumatic Neuroma

350. Sist TC Jr, Greene GW: Traumatic neuroma of the oral cavity: Report of thirty-one new cases and review of the literature. Oral Surg Oral Med Oral Pathol 1981;51:394–402.

351. Peszkowski MJ, Larsson A: Extraosseous and intraosseous oral traumatic neuromas and their association with tooth extraction. J Oral Maxillofac Surg 1990;48:963–967.

352. Haring JI: Case #4: Traumatic neuroma. RDH 1994;14:11.

Mucosal Neuroma

353. Wagenmann A: Multiple neurome des Auges und der Zunge. Ber Dtsch Opthalmol Ges 1922;43:282–285.

354. Gorlin RJ, Sedano HO, Vickers RA, Cervenka J: Multiple mucosal neuromas, pheochromocytoma and medullary carcinoma of the thyroid: A syndrome. Cancer 1968;22:293–299.

355. Miller RL, Burzynski NJ, Giammara BL: The ultrastructure of oral neuromas in multiple mucosal neuromas, pheochromocytoma, medullary thyroid carcinoma syndrome. J Oral Pathol 1977;6:253–263.

356. Dyck PJ, Carney JA, Sizemore GW, et al: Multiple endocrine neoplasia, type 2b: Phenotype recognition; neurological features and their pathological basis. Ann Neurol 1979;6:302–314.

357. Schenberg ME, Zajac JD, Lim-Tio S, et al: Multiple endocrine neoplasia syndrome, type 2b: Case report and review. Int J Oral Maxillofac Surg 1992;21:110–114.

358. Morrison PJ, Nevin NC: Multiple endocrine neoplasia type 2B (mucosal neuroma syndrome, Wagenmann-Froboese syndrome). J Med Genet 1996;33:779–782.

359. Pujol RM, Matias-Guiu X, Miralles J, et al: Multiple idiopathic mucosal neuromas: A minor form of multiple endocrine neoplasia type 2B or a new entity? J Am Acad Dermatol 1997;37:349–352.

Palisaded Encapsulated Neuroma

360. Reed RJ, Fine RM, Meltzer HD: Palisaded encapsulated neuromas of the skin. Arch Dermatol 1972;106:865–870.

361. Fletcher CDM: Solitary circumscribed neuroma of the skin (so-called palisaded, encapsulated neuroma): A clinicopathologic and immunohistochemical study. Am J Surg Pathol 1989;13:574–580.

362. Chauvin PJ, Wysocki GP, Daley TD, Pringle GA: Palisaded encapsulated neuroma of oral mucosa. Oral Surg Oral Med Oral Pathol 1992;73:71–74.

363. Dakin MC, Leppard B, Theaker JM: The palisaded, encapsulated neuroma (solitary circumscribed neuroma). Histopathology 1992;20:405–410.

364. Megahed M: Palisaded encapsulated neuroma (solitary circumscribed neuroma): A clinicopathologic and immunohistochemical study. Am J Dermatopathol 1994;16:120–125.

365. Magnusson B: Palisaded encapsulated neuroma (solitary circumscribed neuroma) of the oral mucosa. Oral Surg Oral Med Oral Pathol Oral Radiol Endodont 1996;82:302–304.

Neurilemoma (Schwannoma)

366. Hatziotis JC, Asprides H: Neurilemoma (schwannoma) of the oral cavity. Oral Surg Oral Med Oral Pathol 1967;24:510–526.

367. Wright BA, Jackson D: Neural tumors of the oral cavity. Oral Surg Oral Med Oral Pathol 1980;49:509–522.

368. Sharma S, Sarkar C, Mathur M, et al: Benign nerve sheath tumors: A

light microscopic, electron microscopic and immunohistochemical study of 102 cases. Pathology 1990;22;191–195.

369. White W, Shui MH, Rosenblum MK, et al: Cellular schwannoma: A clinicopathologic study of 57 patients and 58 tumors. Cancer 1990; 66:1266–1275.

370. Williams HK, Cannell H, Silvester K, Williams DM: Neurilemmoma of the head and neck. Br J Oral Maxillofac Surg 1993;31:32–35.

371. Woodruff JM: The pathology and treatment of peripheral nerve tumors and tumor-like conditions. CA Cancer J Clin 1993;43:290–308.

372. Colmenero C, Rivers T, Patron M, et al: Maxillofacial malignant peripheral nerve sheath tumours. J Craniomaxillofac Surg 1991;19:40–46.

Neurofibroma

373. Alatil C, Oner B, Unur M, Erseven G: Solitary plexiform neurofibroma of the oral cavity: A case report. Int J Oral Maxillofac Surg 1996;25:379–380.

374. Tsutsumi T, Oku T, Komatsuzaki A: Solitary plexiform neurofibroma of the submandibular salivary gland. J Laryngol Otol 1996;110:1173–1175.

375. Sahota JS, Viswanatha A, Nayak DR, Hazarika P: Giant neurofibroma of the tongue. Int J Ped Otorhinolaryngol 1996;34:153–157.

376. Devarebeke SJ, Deschepper A, Hauben E, et al: Subcutaneous diffuse neurofibroma of the neck: A case report. J Laryngol Otol 1996; 110:182–184.

377. Shapiro SD, Abramovitch K, Van Dis ML, et al: Neurofibromatosis: Oral and radiographic manifestations. Oral Surg Oral Med Oral Pathol 1984;58:493–498.

378. D'Ambrosio JA, Langlais RP, Young RS: Jaw and skull changes in neurofibromatosis. Oral Surg Oral Med Oral Pathol 1988;66:391–396.

379. Pique E, Olivarese M, Farina MC, et al: Pseudoatrophic macules: A variant of neurofibroma. Cutis 1996;57:100–102.

380. Johnson MD, Kamso-Pratt J, Federspiel CF, Whetsell WO: Mast cell and lymphoreticular infiltrates in neurofibromas. Arch Pathol Lab Med 1989;113:1263–1270.

381. Neville BW, Hann J, Narang R, Garen P: Oral neurofibrosarcoma associated with neurofibromatosis type I. Oral Surg Oral Med Oral Pathol 1991;72:546–561.

Malignant Peripheral Nerve Sheath Tumor

382. DeVore DT, Waldron CA: Malignant peripheral nerve tumors of the oral cavity: Review of the literature and report of a case. Oral Surg Oral Med Oral Pathol 1961;14:56–68.

383. Hutcherson RW, Jenkins HA, Canalis RF, Handler SD, Eichel BS: Neurogenic sarcoma of the head and neck. Arch Otolaryngol 1979; 105:267–270.

384. Tsuneyoshi M, Enjoji M: Primary malignant peripheral nerve tumors (malignant schwannomas). A clinicopathologic and electron microscopic study. Acta Pathol Jpn 1979;29:363–375.

385. Ducatman BS, Scheithauer BW: Malignant peripheral nerve sheath tumor with divergent differentiation. Cancer 1984;54:1049–1057.

386. Johnson MD, Glick AD, Davis BW: Immunohistochemical evaluation of Leu-7, myelin basic protein, S-100 protein, glial fibrillary acidic protein, and LN3 immunoreactivity in nerve sheath tumors and sarcomas. Arch Pathol Lab Med 1988;112:155–160.

387. Meis JM, Enzinger FM, Martz KL, et al: Malignant peripheral nerve sheath tumors (malignant schwannoma) in children. Am J Surg Pathol 1992;16:694–707.

388. Daimaru Y, Hashimoto H, Enjoji M: Malignant peripheral nerve-sheath tumor (malignant schwannoma). An immunohistochemical study of 29 cases. Am J Surg Pathol 1985;9:434–444.

389. Hamakawa H, Kayabara H, Sumida T, Tanioka H: Mandibular malignant schwannoma with multiple spinal metastases: A case report and a review of the literature. J Oral Maxillofac Surg 1998;56:1191–1195.

Granular Cell Tumor and Malignant Granular Cell Tumor

390. Regezi JA, Batsakis JG, Courtney RM: Granular cell tumors of the head and neck. J Oral Surg 1979;37:402–406.

391. Lamey PJ, Rennie JS, James J: Multiple granular cell tumors of the palate. Int J Oral Maxillofac Surg 1987;16:236–238.

392. Stewart CM, Watson RE, Eversole SR, et al: Oral granular cell tumors:

A clinicopathologic and immunocytochemical study. Oral Surg Oral Med Oral Pathol 1988;65:427–435.

393. Fliss DM, Puterman M, Zirkin H, Leiberman A: Granular cell lesions in head and neck: A clinicopathological study. J Surg Oncol 1989;42:154–160.

394. Mirchandani R, Scuibba JJ, Mir R: Granular cell lesions of the jaws and oral cavity: A clinicopathologic, immunohistochemical, and ultrastructural study. J Oral Maxillofac Surg 1989;47:1248–1255.

395. Goodstein ML, Eisele DW, Hyams VJ, et al: Multiple synchronous granular cell tumors of the upper aerodigestive tract. Otolaryngol-Head Neck Surg 1990;103:664–668.

396. Garlick JA, Dayan D, Buchner A: A desmoplastic granular cell tumour of the oral cavity: Report of a case. Br J Oral Maxillofac Surg 1992: 30:119–121.

397. Junquera LM, de Vicente JC, Losa JL, et al: Granular-cell tumours: An immunohistochemical study. Br J Oral Maxillofac Surg 1997;35:180–184.

398. Donald PJ: Alveolar soft part sarcoma of the tongue. Head Neck Surg 1987;9:172–178.

399. Cetik F, Ozsahinoglu C, Kivanc F, et al: Alveolar soft part sarcoma of the tongue. J Laryngol Otol 1989;103:952–954.

400. Ordonez JG, Ro JY, Mackay B: Alveolar soft part sarcoma: An ultrastructural and immunocytochemical investigation of its histogenesis. Cancer 1989;63:1721–1736.

401. Takita MA, Morishita M, Iriki-In M, et al: Alveolar soft-part sarcoma of the tongue: Report of a case. Int J Oral Maxillofac Surg 1990; 19:110–112

Leiomyoma

402. Stout AP: Leiomyoma of the oral cavity. Am J Cancer 1938;34:31.

403. Galili D, Shteyer A: Leiomyoma of the oral cavity. J Oral Med 1974;3:69–71

404. Damm DD, Neville BW: Oral leiomyomas. Oral Surg Oral Med Oral Pathol 1979;47:343–348.

405. Hachisuga T, Hashimoto H, Enjoji M: Angioleiomyoma: A clinicopathologic reappraisal of 562 cases. Cancer 1984;54:126–130.

406. Epivatianos A, Trigonidis G, Papanayotou P: Vascular leiomyoma of the oral cavity. J Oral Maxillofac Surg 1985;43:377–382.

407. Leung K-W, Wong DY-K, Li W-Y: Oral leiomyoma: Case report. J Oral Maxillofac Surg 1990;48:735–738.

408. Alguacil-Garcia A: Intranodal myofibroblastoma in a submandibular lymph node: A case report. Am J Clin Pathol 1992;97:69–72.

409. Koutlas IG, Manivel JC: Epithelioid leiomyoma of the oral mucosa. Oral Surg Oral Med Oral Pathol Oral Radiol Endodont 1996;82:670–673.

Leiomyosarcoma

410. Brandjord RM, Reaume CE, Wesley RK: Leiomyosarcoma of the floor of the mouth: Review of the literature and report of a case. J Oral Surg 1977;35:590–594.

411. Poon CK, Kwan PC, Yin NT, et al: Leiomyosarcoma of the gingiva: Report of a case and review of the literature. J Oral Maxillofac Surg 1987;45:888–892.

412. Freedman PD, Jones AC, Kerpel SM: Epithelioid leiomyosarcoma of the oral cavity. J Oral Maxillofac Surg 1993;51:928–932.

413. Schenberg ME, Slootweg PJ, Koole R: Leiomyosarcoma of the oral cavity: Report of four cases and review of the literature. J Craniomaxillofac Surg 1993;21:342–347.

414. Mesquita RA, Migliari DA, de Sousa SO, Alves MR: Leiomyosarcoma of the buccal mucosa: A case report. J Oral Maxillofac Surg 1998;56:504–507.

415. Savastano G, Palombini L, Muscariello V, Erra S: Leiomyosarcoma of the maxilla: A case report. J Oral Maxillofac Surg 1998;56:1101–1103.

Rhabdomyoma

416. Corio RL, Lewis DM: Intraoral rhabdomyomas. Oral Surg Oral Med Oral Pathol 1979;48:525–531.

417. Kapadia SB, Meis JM, Frisman DM, et al: Adult rhabdomyoma of the head and neck: A clinicopathologic and immunophenotypic study. Hum Pathol 1993;24:608–617.

418. Box JC, Newman CL, Anastasiades KD, et al: Adult rhabdomyoma:

Presentation as a cervicomediastinal mass (case-report and review of the literature). Am Surg 1995;61:271–276.

419. Kapadia SB, Meis JM, Frisman DM, Ellis GL, et al: Fetal rhabdomyoma of the head and neck: A clinicopathologic and immunophenotypic study. Hum Pathol 1993;24:754–765.

420. Neville BW, McConnel FMS: Multifocal adult rhabdomyoma: Report of a case and review of the literature. Arch Otolaryngol 1981;107:175–178.

421. Helmberger RC, Stringer SP, Mancuso AA: Rhabdomyoma of the pharyngeal musculature extending into the prestyloid parapharyngeal space. Am J Neuroradiol 1996;17:1115–1118.

422. Hardisson D, Jimenezheffernan JA, Nistal M, et al: Neural variant of fetal rhabdomyoma and nevoid basal cell carcinoma syndrome. Histopathology 1996;29:247–252.

Rhabdomyosarcoma

423. Masson JK, Soule EH: Embryonal rhabdomyosarcoma of the head and neck. Report on eighty-eight cases. Am J Surg 1965;110:585–591.

424. Wharam MD, Beltangady MS, Heyn RM, Lawrence W, et al: Pediatric orofacial and laryngopharyngeal rhabdomyosarcoma. An Intergroup Rhabdomyosarcoma Study report. Arch Otolaryngol Head Neck Surg 1987;113:1225–1227.

425. Peters E, Cohen M, Altini M, Murray J: Rhabdomyosarcoma of the oral and paraoral region. Cancer 1989;63:963–966.

426. Nayar RC, Prudhomme F, Parise O Jr, Gandia D, et al: Rhabdomyosarcoma of the head and neck in adults: A study of 26 patients. Laryngoscope 1993;103:1362–1366.

427. Don DM, Newman AN, Fu YS: Spindle cell variant of embryonal rhabdomyosarcoma. Otolaryngol Head Neck Surg 1997;116:529–532.

428. Kraus DH, Saenz NC, Gollamudi S, Heller G, et al: Pediatric rhabdomyosarcoma of the head and neck. Am J Surg 1997;174:754–765.

429. Pavithran K, Doval DC, Mukherjee G, Kannan V, et al: Rhabdomyosarcoma of the oral cavity: Report of eight cases. Acta Oncol 1997;36:819–821.

430. Barr FG: Molecular genetics and pathogenesis of rhabdomyosarcoma. J Pediatr Hematol Oncol 1997;19:483–491.

431. Coffin CM, Rulon J, Smith L, Bruggers C, et al: Pathologic features of rhabdomyosarcoma before and after treatment: A clinicopathologic and immunohistochemical analysis. Mod Pathol 1997;10:1175–1187.

432. Lai R, Tian Y, An J, Zhou MW, Sou G, et al: A comparative study on morphology and immunohistochemistry of rhabdomyosarcoma and embryonal skeletal muscles. Chin Med J Engl 1997;110:392–396.

433. Rubin BP, Hasserjian RP, Singer S, Janecka I, et al: Spindle cell rhabdomyosarcoma (so-called) in adults: Report of two cases with emphasis on differential diagnosis. Am J Surg Pathol 1998;22:459–464.

Squamous Papilloma

434. Abbey LM, Page DG, Sawyer DR: The clinical and histopathologic features of a series of 464 oral squamous cell papillomas. Oral Surg Oral Med Oral Pathol 1980;49:419–424.

435. Batsakis JG, Raymond AK, Rice DH: The pathology of head and neck tumors: Papillomas of the upper aerodigestive tract, part 18. Head Neck Surg 1983;5:332–344.

436. Bouquot JE, Wrobleski GJ: Papillary (pebbled) masses of the oral mucosa, so much more than simple papillomas. Pract Perio Aesth Dent 1996;8:533–543.

437. Miller CS, White DK, Royse DD: In situ hybridization analysis of human papillomavirus in orofacial lesions using a consensus biotinylated probe. Am J Dermatopath 1993;15:256–259.

438. Ward KA, Napier SS, Winter PC, et al: Detection of human papillomavirus DNA-sequences in oral squamous-cell papillomas by the polymerase chain-reaction. Oral Surg Oral Med Oral Pathol 1995;80:63–66.

439. Sakakura A, Yamamoto Y, Takasaki T, et al: Recurrent laryngeal papillomatosis developing into laryngeal carcinoma with human papilloma-virus (HPV) Type-18. A case report. J Laryngol Otol 1996;110:75–77.

440. Zakrzewska JM, Lopes V, Speight P, Hopper C: Proliferative verrucous leukoplakia. Oral Surg Oral Med Oral Pathol 1996;82:396–401.

441. Adler-Storthz K, Newland JR, Tessin BA, et al: Identification of human papillomavirus types in oral verruca vulgaris. J Oral Pathol 1986;15:230–233.

442. Green TL, Eversole LR, Leider AS: Oral and labial verruca vulgaris:

Clinical, histological, and immunohistochemical evaluation. Oral Surg Oral Med Oral Pathol 1986;62:410–416.

443. Eversole LR, Laipis PJ, Green TL: Human papillomavirus type 2 DNA in oral and labial verruca vulgaris. J Cutan Pathol 1987;14:319–325.

444. Premoli-de-Percoco G, et al: Detection of human papillomavirus-related oral verruca vulgaris among Venezuelans. J Oral Pathol Med 1993;22:113–116.

Condyloma Acuminatum

445. Silverman S Jr, Migliorata CA, Lazada-Nur F, et al: Oral findings in people with or at high-risk for AIDS: A study of 375 homosexual males. J Am Dent Assoc 1986;112:187–192.

446. Zunt S, Tomich CE: Oral condyloma acuminatum. J Dermatol Surg Oncol 1989;15:591–594.

447. Barone R, Ficarra G, Gaglioti D, et al: Prevalence of oral lesions among HIV-infected intravenous drug abusers and other risk groups. Oral Surg Oral Med Oral Pathol 1990;69: 169–173.

448. Sykes NL: Condyloma acuminatum. Int J Dermatol 1995;34:297–302.

449. Suskind DL, Mirza N, Rosin D, et al: Condyloma acuminatum presenting as a base-of-tongue mass. Otolaryngol Head Neck Surg 1996;114:487–490.

450. Simon PA: Oral condyloma acuminatum as an indicator of sexual abuse: Dentistry's role. Quintessence Int 1998;29:455–458.

Focal Epithelial Hyperplasia

451. Archard HO, Heck JW, Stanley HR: Focal epithelial hyperplasia: An unusual and mucosal lesion found in Indian children. Oral Surg Oral Med Oral Pathol 1965;20:201–212.

452. Witkop CJ Jr, Niswander JD: Focal epithelial hyperplasia in Central and South American Indians and Latinos. Oral Surg Oral Med Oral Pathol 1965;20:213–217.

453. Starink TM, Woerdeman MJ: Focal epithelial hyperplasia of the oral mucosa. Report of two cases from the Netherlands and review of the literature. Br J Dermatol 1977;96:375–380.

454. Harris AM, van Wyk CW: Heck's disease (focal epithelial hyperplasia): A longitudinal study. Community Dent Oral Epidemiol 1993;21:82–85.

455. Padayachee A, van Wyk CW: Human papillomavirus (HPV) DNA in focal epithelial hyperplasia by in situ hybridization. J Oral Pathol Med 1991;20:210–214.

456. Carlos R, Sedano HO: Multifocal papilloma virus epithelial hyperplasia. Oral Surg Oral Med Oral Pathol 1994;77:631–635.

457. Viraben R, et al: Focal epithelial hyperplasia (Heck disease) associated with AIDS. Dermatology 1996;193:261–262.

Verruciform Xanthoma

458. Neville B: The verruciform xanthoma. A review and report of eight new cases. Am J Dermatopathol 1986;8:247–253.

459. Nowparast B, Howell FV, Rick GM: Verruciform xanthoma: A clinicopathologic review and report of 54 cases. Oral Surg Oral Med Oral Pathol 1981;51:619–625.

460. Allen CM, Kapoor N: Verruciform xanthoma in a bone marrow transplant recipient. Oral Surg Oral Med Oral Pathol 1993;75:591–594.

461. Huang JS, Tseng CC, Jin YT, et al: Verruciform xanthoma: Case report and literature review. J Periodontol 1996;67:162–165.

Keratoacanthoma and Pseudoepitheliomatous Hyperplasia

462. Rook A, Whimster I: Keratoacanthoma: A 30-year retrospective. J Am Acad Dermatol 1986;14:226–234.

463. Chuang TY, Reizner GT, Elpern DJ, et al: Keratoacanthoma in Kauai, Hawaii, first documented incidence in a defined population. Arch Dermatol 1993;129:317–319.

464. Eversole LR, Leider AS, Alexander G: Intraoral and labial keratoacanthoma. Oral Surg Oral Med Oral Pathol 1982;54:663–667.

465. de Visscher JG, van der Wal JE, Starink TM: Giant keratoacanthoma of the lower lip: Report of a case of spontaneous regression. Oral Surg Oral Med Oral Pathol Oral Radiol Endod 1996;81:193–196.

466. Janette A, Pecaro B, Lonergan M, Lingen MW: Solitary intraoral keratoacanthoma: Report of a case. J Oral Maxillofac Surg 1996;54:1026–1030.

467. Fahmy A, Burgdorf WH, Schosser WH, et al: Torre-Muir syndrome: Report of a case and re-evaluation of the dermatopathological features. Cancer 1982;49:1898–1903.
468. Jaber PW, Cooper PH, Greer KE: Generalized eruptive keratoacanthoma of Grzybowski. J Am Acad Dermatol 1993;29:299–304.
469. Elzay RP, O'Keefe EM: Unusual gingival epithelial proliferation: Primary pseudoepitheliomatous hyperplasia. Oral Surg Oral Med Oral Pathol 1979;47:436–440.
470. Sarda R, Sankaran V, Ratnaker C, Veliath AJ, et al: Application of the AgNOR method to distinguish pseudoepitheliomatous hyperplasia from squamous cell carcinoma. Indian J Cancer 1995;32:169–174.
471. Whitaker SB, Wiegand SE, Budnick SD: Intraoral molluscum contagiosum. Oral Surg Oral Med Oral Pathol 1991;72:334–336.

Hairy Leukoplakia

472. Green TL, Greenspan JL, Greenspan D, DeSouza YG: Oral lesions mimicking hairy leukoplakia: A diagnostic dilemma. Oral Surg Oral Med Oral Pathol 1989;67:422–426.
473. Sciubba JJ, Brandsma J, Schwartz M: Hairy leukoplakia: An AIDS-associated opportunistic infection. Oral Surg Oral Med Oral Pathol 1989;67:404–410.
474. Lozada-Nur F, Robinson J, Regezi JA: Oral hairy leukoplakia in immunosuppressed patients. Oral Surg Oral Med Oral Pathol 1994;78:599–602.
475. Greenspan JS, Greenspan D, Palefsky JM: Oral hairy leukoplakia after a decade. Epstein-Barr Virus Report 1995;2:123–128.
476. Farman AG: Hairy tongue (lingua villosa). J Oral Med 1977;32:85–91.
477. Sarti GM, Haddy RI, Schaffer D, Kehm J: Black hairy tongue. Am Fam Physician 1990;41:1751–1755.

Frictional, Chemical and Thermal Keratosis

478. Bouquot JE, Gorlin RJ: Leukoplakia, lichen planus and other oral keratoses in 23,616 white Americans over 35 years of age. Oral Surg Oral Med Oral Pathol 1986;61:373–381.
479. Salons L, Axell T, Hellden L: Occurrence of oral mucosal lesions, the influence of tobacco habits and an estimate of treatment time in an adult Swedish population. J Oral Pathol Med 1990;19:170–176.
480. Díaz-Guzmán L, Castellanos JL: Lesiones de la mucosa bucal; estudio epidemiologico en 7,297 pacientes. Revista adm 1991;48:75–80.
481. Saunders WH: Nicotine stomatitis of the palate. Ann Otol Rhinol Laryngol 1958;67:618–627.
482. Schwartz DL: Stomatitis nicotina of the palate: Report of two cases. Oral Surg Oral Med Oral Pathol 1965;20:306–315.
483. Rossi KM, Guggenheimer J: Thermally induced "nicotine" stomatitis: A case report. Oral Surg Oral Med Oral Pathol 1990;70:597–599.

Leukoedema

484. Archard HO, Carlson KP, Stanley HR: Leukoedema of the human oral mucosa. Oral Surg Oral Med Oral Pathol 1968;25:717–728.
485. Martin JL: Leukoedema: A review of the literature. J Natl Med Assoc 1992;84:938–940.
486. Hernandez-Martin A, Fernandez-Lopez E, de Unamuno P, Armijo M: Diffuse whitening of the oral mucosa in a child. Pediatr Dermatol 1997;14:316–320.
487. Martin JL: Leukoedema: An epidemiological study in white and African Americans. J Tenn Dent Assoc 1997;77:18–21.

White Sponge Nevus

488. Cannon AB: White nevus of the mucosa (naevus spongiosus albus mucosae). Arch Dermatol Syph 1935;31:365–373.
489. Jorgenson RJ, Levin LS: White sponge nevus. Arch Dermatol 1981;117:73–76.
490. Nichols GE, Cooper PH, Underwood PB Jr, Greer KE: White sponge nevus. Obstet Gynecol 1990;76:545–548.
491. Marcushamer M, King DL, McGuff S: White sponge nevus: case report. Pediatr Dent 1995;17:458–459.
492. Rugg EL, McLean WH, Allison WE, et al: A mutation in the mucosal keratin K4 is associated with oral white sponge nevus. Nat Genet 1995;11:450–452.
493. Lim J, Ng S: Oral tetracycline rinse improves symptoms of white sponge nevus. J Am Acad Dermatol 1992;26:1003–1005.

494. Reed JW, Cashwell LF, Klinworth GK: Corneal manifestations of hereditary benign intraepithelial dyskeratosis. Arch Ophthalmol 1979;97:297–300.
495. Sadeghi EM, Witkop CJ: The presence of Candida albicans in hereditary benign intraepithelial dyskeratosis: An ultrastructural observation. Oral Surg Oral Med Oral Pathol 1979;48:342–346.
496. Feinstein A, Friedman J, Schewach-Miller M: Pachyonychia congenita. J Am Acad Dermatol 1988;19:705–711.
497. Yavazyilmaz E, Yamalik N, Yetgin S, Kansu O: Oral-dental findings in dyskeratosis congenita. J Oral Pathol Med 1992;21:280–284.

Actinic Cheilosis

498. Schmitt C, Folsom T: Histologic evaluation of degenerative changes of the lower lip. J Oral Surg 1968;26:51–56.
498a. Cataldo E, Doku HC: Solar cheilitis. J Dermatol Surg Oncol 1981;7:989–993.
499. Piscascia DD, Robinson JK: Actinic cheilitis: A review of the etiology, differential diagnosis, and treatment. J Am Acad Dermatol 1987;17:255–264.
500. Manganaro AM, Will MJ, Poulous E: Actinic cheilitis: A premalignant condition. Gen Dent 1997;5:492–494.
501. Dufresne RG Jr, Curlin MU: Actinic cheilitis. A treatment review. Dermatol Surg 1997;23:15–21.
502. Wright K, Dufresne R: Actinic cheilitis. Dermatol Surg 1998;24:490–491.

Migratory Glossitis and Erythema Migrans

503. Marks R, Radden BG: Geographic tongue: A clinico-pathological review. Austral J Dermatol 1981;22:75–79.
504. Waltimo J: Geographic tongue during a year of oral contraceptive cycles. Br Dent J 1991;171:94–96.
505. Sigal MJ, Mock D: Symptomatic benign migratory glossitis: Report of two cases and literature review. Pediatr Dent 1992;14:392–396.
506. Littner M, Dayan D, Gorsky M, et al: Migratory stomatitis. Oral Surg Oral Med Oral Pathol 1987;63:555–559.
507. Zunt SL, Tomich CE: Erythema migrans: A psoriasiform lesion of the oral mucosa. J Dermatol Surg Oncol 1989;15:1067–1070.
508. Espelid M, Bang G, Johannessen AC, et al: Geographic stomatitis: Report of 6 cases. J Oral Pathol Med 1991;20:425–428.
509. Morris LF, Phillips CM, Binnie WH, et al: Oral lesions in patients with psoriasis: A controlled study. Cutis 1992;49:339–344.
510. Sklavounou A, Laskaris G: Oral psoriasis: Report of a case and review of the literature. Dermatologica 1990;180:157–159.

Lichen Planus

511. Batsakis JG, Cleary KR, Cho KJ: Lichen planus and lichenoid lesions of the oral cavity. Ann Otol Rhinol Laryngol 1994;103:495–497.
512. Vincent SD, Fotos PG, Baker KA, Williams TP: Oral lichen planus: The clinical, historical and therapeutic features of 100 cases. Oral Surg Oral Med Oral Pathol 1990;70:165–171.
513. Silverman S Jr: Lichen planus. Curr Opin Dent 1991;1:769–772.
514. Bricker SL: Oral lichen planus: A review. Semin Dermatol 1994;13:87–90.
515. Sanchis-Bielsa JM, Bagan-Sebastian JV, Jorda-Cuevas E, et al: Oral lichen planus: An evolutive clinical and histological study of 45 patients followed up on for five years. Bull Group Int Rech Sci Stomatol Odontol 1994;37:45–49.
516. Porter SR, Kirby A, Olsen I, Barrett W: Immunologic aspects of dermal and oral lichen planus. Oral Surg Oral Med Oral Pathol 1997;83:358–366.
517. Scully C, Beyli M, Feirrero M, Ficarra G, et al: Update on oral lichen planus: Aetiopathogenesis and management. Crit Rev Oral Bio Med 1998;9:86–122.
518. Eisenberg E: Lichen planus and oral cancer: Is there a connection between the two? J Am Dent Assoc 1992;12:104–108.
519. Torres V, Mano-Azul AC, Correia T, Soares AP: Allergic contact cheilitis and stomatitis from hydroquinone in an acrylic dental prosthesis. Contact Dermatitis 1993;29:102–103.
520. Veien NK, Borchorst E, Hattel T, Laurberg G: Stomatitis or systemically-induced contact dermatitis from metal wire in orthodontic materials. Contact Dermatitis 1994;30:210–213.

521. Rhodus NL, Johnson DK: The prevalence of oral manifestations of systemic lupus erythematosus. Quintessence Int 1990;21:461–465.

522. Schubert MM, Sullivan KM, Morton TH, et al: Oral manifestations of chronic graft vs host disease. Arch Intern Med 1984;133:1591–1595.

523. Nakamura S, Hiroki A, Shinohara M, et al: Oral involvement in chronic graft-versus host disease after allogenic bone marrow transplantation. Oral Surg Oral Med Oral Pathol 1996;82:556–563.

524. Zegarelli DJ: The treatment of oral lichen planus. Ann Dent 1993; 52:3–8.

Inflammatory Mucosal Ulceration

525. Bagan JV, Sanchis JM, Milian MA, Penarrocha M, et al: Recurrent aphthous stomatitis: A study of the clinical characteristics of lesions in 93 cases. J Oral Pathol Med 1991;20:395–397.

526. Field EA, Brookes V, Tyldesley WR: Recurrent aphthous ulceration in children: A review. Int J Paediatr Dent 1992;2:1–10.

527. Pedersen A, Hougen HP, Kenrad B: T-lymphocyte subsets in oral mucosa of patients with recurrent aphthous ulcerations. J Oral Pathol Med 1992;21:176–180.

528. Porter SR, Kingsmill V, Scully C: Audit of diagnosis and investigations in patients with recurrent aphthous stomatitis. Oral Surg Oral Med Oral Pathol 1993;76:449–452.

529. Jaremko WM, Beutner EH, Kumar V, Kipping H, et al: Chronic ulcerative stomatitis associated with a specific immunologic marker. J Am Acad Dermatol 1990;22:215–220.

530. Church LF Jr, Schosser RH: Chronic ulcerative stomatitis associated with stratified epithelial specific antinuclear antibodies: A case report of a newly described disease entity. Oral Surg Oral Med Oral Pathol 1992;73:579–582.

531. Worle B, Wollenberg A, Schaller M, Kunzelmann KH, et al: Chronic ulcerative stomatitis. Br J Dermatol 1997;137:262–265.

532. Chung HS, Kim NS, Kim YB, Kang WH: Eosinophilic ulcer of oral mucosa. Int J Dermatol 1998;37:432.

533. Horning GM, Cohen ME: Necrotizing ulcerative gingivitis, periodontitis, and stomatitis: Clinical staging and predisposing factors. J Periodontol 1995;66:990–998.

534. Aozasa K, Ohsawa M, Tajima K, et al: Nation-wide study of lethal midline granuloma in Japan: Frequencies of Wegener's granulomatosis, polymorphic reticulosis, malignant lymphoma and other related conditions. Int J Cancer 1989;44:63–66.

535. Grange C, Cabane J, Dubois A, et al: Centrofacial malignant granulomas: Clinicopathologic study of 40 cases and review of the literature. Medicine 1992;71:179–196.

536. Strickler JG, Meneses MF, Habermann TM, et al: Polymorphic reticulosis: A reappraisal. Human Pathol 1994;25:659–665.

537. Sobrevilla-Calvo P, Meneses A, Alfaro P, et al: Radiotherapy compared to chemotherapy as initial treatment of angiocentric centrofacial lymphoma (polymorphic reticulosis). Acta Oncol 1993;32:69–72.

538. Miller M, Haddad AJ: Cervicofacial actinomycosis. Oral Surg Oral Med Oral Pathol Oral Rad Endod 1998;85:496–508.

539. Ficarra G, Di Lollo S, Pierleoni F, Panzoni E: Actinomyces of the tongue: A diagnostic challenge. Head Neck 1993;15:53–55.

540. Herman WW, Whitaker SB, Williams MF, Sangueza OP: Acute actinomycosis presenting as an ulcerated palatal mass. J Oral Maxillofac Surg 1998;56:1098–1101.

Pemphigus Vulgaris and Other Intraepithelial Blisters

541. Williams DM: Vesiculobullous mucocutaneous disease: Pemphigus vulgaris. J Oral Pathol Med 1989;18:544–553.

542. Lamey PJ, Rees TD, Binnie WH, et al: Oral presentation of pemphigus vulgaris and its response to systemic steroid treatment. Oral Surg Oral Med Oral Pathol 1992;74:54–57.

543. Mignogna MD, Lo Muzio L, Gallors G, et al: Oral pemphigus: Clinical significance of esophageal involvement. Report of eight cases. Oral Surg Oral Med Oral Pathol Oral Radiol Endod 1997;84:179–184.

544. Robinson JC, Lozada-Nur F, Frieden I: Oral pemphigus vulgaris: A review of the literature and a report on the management of 12 cases. Oral Surg Oral Med Oral Pathol Oral Radiol Endod 1997;84:349–355.

545. Anhalt GJ, Kim S-C, Stanley JR, et al: Paraneoplastic pemphigus: An autoimmune mucocutaneous disease associated with neoplasia. N Engl J Med 1990;323:1729–1735.

546. Helm TN, Camisa C, Valenzuela R, Allen CM: Paraneoplastic pemphigus: A distinct autoimmune vesiculobullous disorder associated with neoplasia. Oral Surg Oral Med Oral Pathol 1993;75:209–213.

547. Thornhill MH, Zakrzewska JM, Gilkes JJH: Pyostomatitis vegetans: Report of three cases and review of the literature. J Oral Pathol Med 1992;21:128–133.

548. Burge SM, Fenton DA, Dawber RP, Leigh IM: Darier's disease: A focal abnormality of cell adhesion. J Cutan Pathol 1990;17:160–169.

549. Miller CS, Redding SW: Diagnosis and management of orofacial herpes simplex virus infections. Dent Clin North Am 1992;36:879–895.

550. Stampien TM, Schwartz RA: Erythema multiforme. Am Fam Physician 1992;46:1171–1176.

551. Roujeau JC: The spectrum of Stevens-Johnson syndrome and toxic epidermal necrolysis: A clinical classification. J Invest Dermatol 1994;102:28S–30S.

Benign Mucous Membrane Pemphigoid and Other Subepithelial Blisters

552. Williams DM: Vesiculobullous mucocutaneous disease: Benign mucous membrane and bullous pemphigoid. J Oral Pathol Med 1990;19:16–23.

553. Boh EE, Millikan LE: Vesiculobullous disease with prominent immunologic features. JAMA 1992;268:2893–2898.

554. Lamey P-J, Rees TD, Binnie WH, et al: Mucous membrane pemphigoid: Treatment experience at two institutions. Oral Surg Oral Med Oral Pathol 1992;74:50–53.

555. Weinberg MA, Insler MS, Campen RB: Mucocutaneous features of autoimmune blistering diseases. Oral Surg Oral Med Oral Pathol Oral Radiol Endod 1997;84:517–534.

556. Allen CM, Camisa C, Grimwood R: Lichen planus pemphigoides: Report of a case with oral lesions. Oral Surg Oral Med Oral Pathol 1987;63:184–188.

557. Markopoulos AK, Antoniades D, Papanayotou P, Tregonidis G: Desquamative gingivitis: A clinical, histopathologic, and immunologic study. Quintessence Int 1996;27:763–767.

558. Scully C, Porter SR: The clinical spectrum of desquamative gingivitis. Semin Cutan Med Surg 1997;16:308–313.

559. Bozkurt FY, Celenligil H, Sungur A, Ruacan S: Gingival involvement in mucous membrane pemphigoid. Quintessence Int 1998;29:438–441.

560. Yih WY, Maier T, Kratochvil FJ, Zieper MB: Analysis of desquamative gingivitis using direct immunofluorescence in conjunction with histology. J Periodontol 1998;69:678–785.

561. Cowan CG, Lamey PJ, Walsh M, Irwin ST, et al: Linear IgA disease (DAD): Immunoglobulin deposition in oral and colonic lesions. J Oral Pathol Med 1995;24:374–378.

562. Matsumura Y, Hamanaka H, Horiguchi Y, et al: Epidermolysis bullosa acquisitive (EBA) with nonclassical distribution of eruptions. J Dermatol 1993;20:159–163.

563. Sedano HO, Gorlin RJ: Epidermolysis bullosa. Oral Surg Oral Med Oral Pathol 1989;67:555–565.

564. Wright JT, Fine J-D, Johnson LB: Hereditary epidermolysis bullosa: Oral manifestations and dental management. Pediatr Dent 1993; 15:242–248.

Amalgam Tattoo

565. Buchner A, Hansen LS: Amalgam pigmentation (amalgam tattoo) of oral mucosa: A clinicopathologic study of 268 cases. Oral Surg Oral Med Oral Pathol 1980;49:139–147.

566. Harman LC, Natiella JR, Meenaghan MA: The use of elemental microanalysis in verification of the composition of presumptive amalgam tattoo. J Oral Maxillofac Surg 1986;44:628–633.

567. Shiloah J, Covington JS, Schuman NJ: Reconstructive mucogingival surgery: The management of amalgam tattoo. Quintessence Int 1988;19:489–492.

568. Slabbert H, Ackermann GL, Altini M: Amalgam tattoo as a means for person identification. J Forensic Odontostomatol 1991;9:17–23.

Oral Melanotic Macule

569. Buchner A, Hansen LS: Melanotic macule of the oral mucosa: A clinicopathologic study of 105 cases. Oral Surg Oral Med Oral Pathol 1979;48:244–249.

570. Watkins KV, Chaudhry AP, Yamane GM, et al: Benign focal melanotic lesions of the oral mucosa. J Oral Med 1984;39:91–96.

571. Kaugars GE, Heise AP, Riley WT, et al: Oral melanotic macules: A review of 353 cases. Oral Surg Oral Med Oral Pathol 1993;76:59–61.
572. Ho KK, Dervan P, O'Loughlin S, Powell FC: Labial melanotic macule: A clinical, histopathologic, and ultrastructural study. J Am Acad Dermatol 1993;28:33–39.
573. Brown FH, Houston GD: Smoker's melanosis: A case report. J Periodontol 1991;62:524–527.
574. Hedin CA, Pindorf JJ, Axell T: Disappearance of smoker's melanosis after reducing smoking. J Oral Pathol Med 1993;22:228–230.
575. Merchant HW, Haynes LE, Ellison LT: Soft-palate pigmentation in lung disease, including cancer. Oral Surg Oral Med Oral Pathol 1976;41:726–733.
576. Barrett AW, Porter SR, Scully C, et al: Oral melanotic macules that develop after radiation therapy. Oral Surg Oral Med Oral Pathol 1994;77:431–434.
577. Trelles MA, Verkruysse W, Segui JM, Udaeta A: Treatment of melanotic spots in the gingiva by argon laser. J Oral Maxillofac Surg 1993;51:759–761.

Oral Melanoacanthoma

578. Goode RK, Crawford BE, Callihan MD, Neville BW: Oral melanoacanthoma. Oral Surg Oral Med Oral Pathol 1983;56:622–628.
579. Wright JM: Intraoral melanoacanthoma: Reactive melanocytic hyperplasia. Case report. J Periodontol 1988;59:53–55.
580. Tomich CE, Zunt SL: Melanoacanthosis (melanoacanthoma) of the oral mucosa. J Dermatol Surg Oncol 1990;16:231–236.
581. Heine BT, Drummond JF, Damm DD, Heine RD 2nd: Bilateral oral melanoacanthoma. Gen Dent 1996;44:451–452.
582. Chandler K, Chaudhry Z, Kumar N, et al: Melanoacanthoma: A rare cause of oral hyperpigmentation. Oral Surg Oral Med Oral Pathol Oral Radiol Endod 1997;84:492–494.
583. Seoane Leston JM, Vazquez Garcia J, Aguado Santos A, et al: Dark oral lesions: Differential diagnosis with oral melanoma. Cutis 1998;61:279–282.

Mucosal Melanocytic Nevus

584. Buchner A, Hansen LS: Pigmented nevi of the oral mucosa: A clinicopathologic study of 36 new cases and review of 155 cases from the literature. Parts I & II. Oral Surg Oral Med Oral Pathol 1987;63:566–572, 676–682.
585. Buchner A, Leider AS, Merrell PW, et al: Melanocytic nevi of oral mucosa: A clinicopathologic study of 130 cases from northern California. J Oral Pathol Med 1990;19:197–201.
586. Allen CM, Oellegrini A: Probable congenital melanocytic nevus of the oral mucosa: Case report. Pediatr Dermatol 1995;12:145–148.
587. Barker GR, Sloan P: An intraoral combined blue naevus. Br J Oral Maxillofac Surg 1988;26:165–168.
588. Percinoto C, Cunho RF, Delbem AC, et al: The oral blue nevus in children: A case report. Quintessence Int 1993;24:567–569.
589. Nikai H, Miyauchi M, Ogawa I, et al: Spitz nevus of the palate. Oral Surg Oral Med Oral Pathol 1990;69:603–608.
590. Laskaris G, Kittas C, Triantafyllou A, et al: Unpigmented intramucosal nevus of palate. An unusual clinical presentation. Int J Oral Maxillofac Surg 1994;23:39–40.

Melanotic Neuroectodermal Tumor of Infancy

591. Krompecher E: Zur Histogenese und Morphologie der Adamantinome und sonstiger Kiefergeschwuelste. Beitr Pathol Anat 1918;64:169–197.
592. Borello ED, Gorlin RJ: Melanotic neuroectodermal tumor of infancy: A neoplasm of neural crest origin. Cancer 1966;19:196–203.
593. Nikai H, Ijuhin N, Yamasaki A, et al: Ultrastructural evidence for neural crest origin of the melanotic neuroectodermal tumor of infancy. J Oral Pathol 1977;6:221–232.
594. Dehner LP, Sibley RK, Sauk JJ, et al: Malignant melanotic neuroectodermal tumor of infancy: A clinical, pathologic, ultrastructural, and tissue culture study. Cancer 1979;43:1389–1410.
595. Kapadia SB, Frisman DM, Hitchcock CL, et al: Melanotic neuroectodermal tumor of infancy: Clinicopathological, immunohistochemical, and flow cytometric study. Am J Surg Pathol 1993;17:566–573.
596. Nelson ZL, Newman L, Loukota RA, Williams DM: Melanotic neuroectodermal tumor of infancy: An immunohistochemical and ultrastructural study. Br J Oral Maxillofac Surg 1995;33:375–380.
597. Kim YG, Oh JH, Lee SC, Ryu DM: Melanotic neuroectodermal tumor of infancy. J Oral Maxillofac Surg 1996;54:517–520.
598. Bouckaert MMR, Raubenheimer EJ: Gigantiform melanotic neuroectodermal tumor of infancy. Oral Surg Oral Med Oral Pathol Oral Radiol Endod 1998;86:569–572.
599. Batsakis JG, Mackay B, El Naggar AK: Ewing sarcoma and peripheral primitive neuroectodermal tumor: An interim report. Ann Otol Rhinol Laryngol 1996;105:838–843.

Melanoma

600. Rapini RP, Golitz LE, Greer RO Jr, et al: Primary malignant melanoma of the oral cavity: A review of 177 cases. Cancer 1985;55:1543–1551.
601. Berthelsen A, Andersen AP, Jensen TS, Hansen HS: Melanomas of the mucosa in the oral cavity and the upper respiratory passages. Cancer 1984;54:907–912.
602. Stern SJ, Guillamondegui OM: Mucosal melanoma of the head and neck. Head Neck 1991;13:22–27.
603. Langford FP, Fisher SR, Molter DW, Seigler HF: Lentigo maligna melanoma of the head and neck. Laryngoscope 1993;103:520–524.
604. Medina JE: Malignant melanoma of the head and neck. Otolaryngol Clin North Am 1993;26:73–85.
605. Smyth AG, Ward-Booth RP, Avery BS, To EW: Malignant melanoma of the oral cavity: An increasing clinical diagnosis? Br J Oral Maxillofac Surg 1993;31:230–235.
606. Patton LL, Brahim JS, Baker AR: Metastatic malignant melanoma of the oral cavity: A retrospective study. Oral Surg Oral Med Oral Pathol 1994;78:51–60.
607. Umeda M, Shimada K: Primary malignant melanoma of the oral cavity: Its histological classification and treatment. Br J Oral Maxillofac Surg 1994;32:39–47.
608. Rapini RP: Oral melanoma: Diagnosis and treatment. Semin Cutan Med Surg 1997;16:320–322.
609. Clarkeson EI: Current management of oral melanoma. Oral Maxillofac Surg Clin North Am 1998;10:131–140.
610. Pandey M, Abraham EK, Mathew A, Ahamen IM: Primary malignant melanoma of the upper aero-digestive tract. Int J Oral Maxillofac Surg 1999;28:45–49.

Metastasis to the Oral Soft Tissues

611. Oikarinen VJ, Calonius PEB, Sainio P: Metastatic tumours to the oral region. I: Analysis of cases in the literature. Proc Finn Dent Soc 1975;71:58–65.
612. Luna MA: The occult primary and metastatic tumors to and from the head and neck. In: Barnes L (ed): Surgical Pathology of the Head and Neck. New York: Marcel Dekker, 1985: 1211–1232.
613. Sokalosky MS, Bouquot JE, Graves RW: Metastatic esophageal carcinoma to the oral cavity. J Oral Maxillofac Surg 1986;44:825–827.
614. Bouquot JE, Weiland LH, Kurland LT: Metastases to and from the upper aerodigestive tract in the population of Rochester, Minnesota, 1935–1984. Head Neck 1989;11:212–218.
615. Zachariades N: Neoplasms metastatic to the mouth, jaws and surrounding tissues. J Craniomaxillofac Surg 1989;17:283–290.
616. Allen CM, Neville B, Damm DD, Marsh W: Leiomyosarcoma metastatic to the oral region: Report of three cases. Oral Surg Oral Med Oral Pathol 1993;76:752–756.
617. Hirshberg A, Leibovich P, Buchner A: Metastases to the oral mucosa: Analysis of 157 cases. J Oral Pathol Med 1993;22:385–390.
618. Tomita T, Inouye T, Shinden S, Mukai M: Palliative radiotherapy for lingual metastasis of renal cell carcinoma. Auris Nasus Larynx 1998;25:209–214.

5 Nonsquamous Pathology of the Larynx, Hypopharynx, and Trachea

■ Margaret S. Brandwein, Silloo B. Kapadia, and Douglas R. Gnepp

▪ LARYNGEAL/HYPOPHARYNGEAL ANATOMIC BARRIERS AND PATHWAYS FOR TUMOR SPREAD

The hypopharynx is in continuity with the oropharynx, from the level of the hyoid bone to the opening of the esophagus; it is composed of the inferior aspect of the middle constrictor and the inferior pharyngeal constrictor. The hypopharynx sits behind the larynx, and its lateral-most walls—the piriform sinuses—are nestled medial to the thyroid lamina and lateral to the endolarynx. Immediately posterior to the hypopharynx is the potential retropharyngeal space, and posterior to that is the prevertebral fascia. Patients with tumors of the hypopharynx present with progressive difficulty and pain with swallowing, first to solids then to liquids; they often complain of referred otalgia.

The larynx can be anatomically divided into three compartments: supraglottic, glottic, and infraglottic (Fig. 5–1). The supraglottis is composed of the epiglottis, aryepiglottic folds, vestibular folds (false cords), ventricle, and saccule. The ventricle is the "pocket" between the vocal fold (true cord) and the vestibular fold. The lateral superior extension, or "cul-de-sac," of the ventricle is variably sized and referred to as the saccule. The glottis refers to the vocal folds from the edge of the ventricle to the free edge of the vocal fold. The boundary, which divides the glottic from infraglottic compartments, is defined as the tissue of the free edge of the vocal fold to the level of the inferior cricoid margin. From a compartmental viewpoint, the supraglottis is distinct and separate from the glottis and infraglottis, which are contiguous. American Joint Committee on Cancer (AJCC) and the International Union Against Cancer (IUAC) classifications will stage tumors on the undersurface of the vocal fold as glottic tumors.

The exact laryngeal site for a tumor may determine or influence (1) the type of presenting symptoms, (2) stage at presentation, (3) surgical options (conservative, voice-sparing versus radical), and (4) patient prognosis. Although the vast majority of malignancies of the supraglottis and glottis are squamous cell carcinomas, nonsquamous malignancies (e.g., salivary tumors, neuroendocrine carcinoma) are more likely encountered in the supraglottis than the glottis (Fig. 5–2). Glottic tumors present with changes in voice quality,

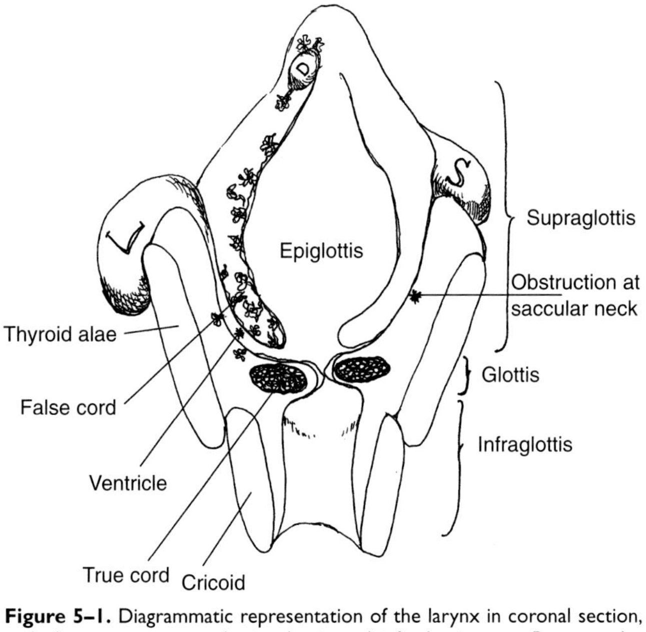

Figure 5–1. Diagrammatic representation of the larynx in coronal section, with divisions into supraglottic, glottic, and infraglottic areas. Between the false (ventricular) fold and the true cords is the laryngeal ventricle, which ends in a saccule. An air-filled expansion of the saccule forms a laryngocele (L), which retains its patency with the endolarynx. A saccular cyst (S) is a mucin-filled expansion of the saccule, akin to a mucocele. A ductal cyst (D) is the result of blockage of a minor salivary duct.

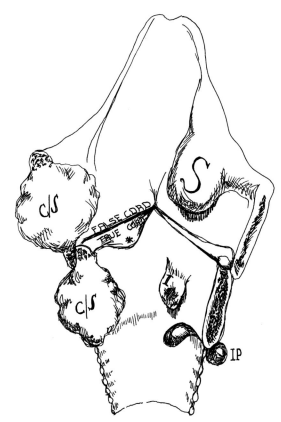

Figure 5–2. Diagrammatic representation of likely nonsquamous tumor presentations: Expansile tumors of the cricoid and thyroid alae are most likely chondrosarcomas (C/S), whereas the most common malignancies of the supraglottis (S) and infraglottis (I) are squamous carcinomas. Other diagnostic possibilities for polypoid tumors of these sites include basaloid squamous carcinoma, neuroendocrine carcinoma, and salivary neoplasia. Additionally, the differential diagnosis of supraglottic polypoid masses should also include paraganglioma and oncocytic cystadenoma. Inferior paragangliomata (IP) may have a unique dumbbell shape.

such as hoarseness; patients tend to seek medical care when these tumors are relatively small (1–2 cm). Large glottic tumors or bilateral glottic tumors may present with worsening upper airway obstruction and stridor. Supraglottic tumors may reach a larger size before becoming symptomatic. Epiglottic tumors may cause a change in vocal quality (a muffled, or "hot potato," voice). Tumors at the base of the epiglottis may be asymptomatic and escape visualization at indirect laryngoscopy (Winkelkarzinom, or "cancer in the corner"). Primary tumors of the ventricle are rare,[1] and the majority of carcinomas encountered here are the result of direct spread from glottic primary sites. Primary ventricular carcinomas are noteworthy in that they remain hidden from the observer on laryngeal examination, merely forming a bulge under the intact vestibular fold mucosa.

The piriform sinuses are extralaryngeal gutters that flank the thyroid lamina. The lateral wall of the piriform is the thyroid lamina; the medial wall is the cricoid ring. On swallowing, the larynx is raised upward, the epiglottis moves inferiorly, partially covering the endolarynx, and the vocal folds close. Fluids are deflected laterally and inferiorly down the piriform sinuses and are led into the opened cricopharyngeus—the opening to the esophagus. Tumors of the piriform sinus, as they are not in the endolarynx, do not present with vocal or respiratory symptoms. They are usually large ulcerating tumors and produce symptoms when they reach considerable size; patients may complain of pain on swallowing, which may radiate to the ear.

Most tumors that appear infraglottic actually arise from the undersurface of the vocal fold and so are still considered glottic tumors. Tumors at or below the cricoid may be considered infraglottic tumors, for example cricoid chondrosarcomas (see Fig. 5–2). These tumors have a more insidious course of onset, with patients complaining of increasing exertional dyspnea. Primary tracheal malignancies are extremely rare: It is more likely to encounter a primary carcinoma of the esophagus eroding into the trachea than a primary neoplasm.

The supraglottis is derived, embryologically, from the buccopharyngeal anlage (branchial arches 3 and 4), whereas the glottic compartment is derived from the laryngotracheal anlage (arches 5 and 6). The fascial compartmentalization, as well as the lymphatic drainage, is distinct for the supraglottic and glottic compartments. This anatomic fact is the basis for the oncologic soundness of the supraglottic horizontal laryngectomy. Dye injected in the supraglottic space remains confined and does not travel to the ventricular or glottic tissues. Likewise, glottic dye injections do not pass superiorly to the ventricle or inferiorly to the mucosa overlying the cricoid.[2] In fact, the mucosa overlying the lamina propria of this space (Reinke's space, or the laryngeal bursa) may burst from fluid distention rather than to allow injected dye to extend into the ventricle or cross the

anterior commissure. These studies also confirm that the larynx is divided into right and left compartments.

Two membranes serve as barriers and result in tissue compartmentalization: the quadrangular membrane and the conus elasticus (Fig. 5–3). The quadrangular membrane is present in the supraglottis; the conus elasticus in the glottis and infraglottis meet and fuse in the area of the perichondrium. These membranes act as a curtain containing tumor medially. The quadrangular membrane originates from the lateral aspects of the epiglottis and extends to the vestibular folds and arytenoid cartilages. Deeper, it fuses with the perichondrium of the thyroid lamina. It continues inferiorly to connect the thyroid cartilage with the cricoid ring (cricothyroid ligament). The conus elasticus (cricovocal membrane) is the continuation of the cricothyroid ligament; it ensheathes the vocalis muscle, separating it from Reinke's space. The conus elasticus merges with the vocalis ligament (vocal tendon). This vocalis ligament serves to initially limit the spread of carcinoma from the vocal fold. A subepithelial periventricular membrane (central membrane) has been identified that spans the paraglottic region and, in effect, connects the conus elasticus and quadrangular membranes centrally (see Fig. 5–3).[3]

The vocalis muscles originate from the vocal ligaments, which have their attachment at the anterior commissure and insert upon the arytenoid processes. The attachment of the vocal ligaments also limits the spread of carcinoma from one lateral side to the other. The vocal folds have a relative paucity of lymphatics, as compared with the supraglottis and the pre-epiglottic space. This paucity of lymphatic vessels is most marked in the anterior vocal folds and accounts for the rarity of cervical metastases of T1 glottic carcinomas. The lymphatic channels of the vocal fold become denser posteriorly in the region of the arytenoids.[4] Glottic carcinomas may spread by undermining the tissue around the ventricles (paraglottic region), escaping the endolarynx, and spreading laterally by invading the cricothyroid ligament and the inferior aspect of the thyroid lamina. Ossified thyroid lamina is more prone to tumor invasion, as compared with the relatively avascular nonossified cartilage. Carcinoma may also spread superiorly into the vestibular fold by undermining paraglottic ventricular tissue.

The epiglottis is composed of fenestrated cartilage, which allows for early tumor spread from the laryngeal surface to the lingual surface and into the pre-epiglottic space. The latter contains abundant lymphatics; tumor spread into this space increases the risk for cervical metastasis and worsens prognosis. The pre-epiglottic space is bound anteriorly by the thyrohyoid membrane. Tumor that breeches this space invades into the base of the tongue. The superior boundary of the pre-epiglottic space is the hyoepiglottic ligament, which connects the hyoid bone to the epiglottis. Epiglottic carcinomas that are inferior to the hyoepiglottic ligament (infrahyoid tu-

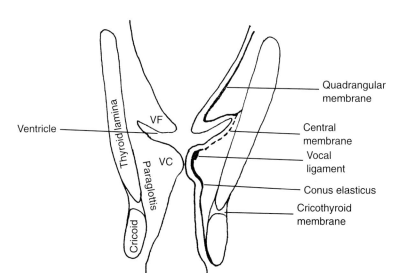

Figure 5–3. Diagrammatic representation of laryngeal barriers: The quadrangular membrane originates from the lateral aspects of the epiglottis and extends to the vestibular folds and arytenoid cartilages, fusing with the perichondrium of the thyroid lamina. The conus elasticus is the continuation of the cricothyroid ligament; it merges superiorly with the vocalis ligament; the central membrane spans the paraglottic region.

mors) are more commonly encountered than those superior to the hyoepiglottic ligament (suprahyoid tumors). The hyoepiglottic ligament provides a barrier blocking the inferior passage of the infrequent suprahyoid carcinomas into the pre-epiglottic space.[5]

A complete laryngeal resection pathology report should contain vital prognostic information, as well as record the extent of surgical intervention. The type of laryngectomy specimen (e.g., total, hemi-, extended hemi-, anterior vertical partial, or supraglottic laryngectomy) should be noted. The exact tumor site should be recorded (e.g., supraglottic, glottic, transglottic), along with whether the tumor crosses the midline. Involvement of the paraglottic space, pre-epiglottic space, and soft tissue of the anterior neck should be described. Reporting of the neoplasm should include (1) histologic subtyping, (2) tumor grade, (3) greatest dimension in centimeters, (4) maximum tumor thickness in centimeters, (5) presence of perineural spread, (6) presence of vascular invasion, (7) invasion of cartilage or ossified cartilage, (8) multicentric invasive carcinoma, and (9) diffuse/multicentric carcinoma in situ. Status of the inked resection margins should include a measurement of the closest margins in millimeters, if possible, and should note the presence of high-grade dysplasia at the margin when pertinent. The neck dissection should not only include a count of the involved number of nodes and the level at which they are present (I-V) but also include the diameter of the largest positive lymph node and the presence or absence of extracapsular spread.

NON-NEOPLASTIC DISEASE
Mycobacterial and Bacterial Infections

Laryngeal Tuberculosis

Clinical Features. Laryngeal tuberculosis (laryngeal phthisis; *phthisis* means to dry up) was one of the most common causes of laryngeal pathology prior to the advent of antibiotics.[6] An autopsy study in the pre-antibiotic era revealed that almost 40% of patients dying from tuberculosis had laryngeal infection.[7] The majority of these patients also had gastrointestinal tuberculosis, presumably a result of swallowed infectious sputum.[7] Laryngeal tuberculosis was usually accompanied by the stigmata of cavitary pulmonary disease, highly infectious sputum, progression to end-stage miliary infection, and a poor prognosis.

Currently, laryngotracheal tuberculosis is quite uncommon. Initial symptoms include hoarseness, cough, hemoptysis, and dysphagia. The mode of spread to the larynx and trachea is still mostly through expectorated sputum. Although the association of laryngeal tuberculosis with advanced cavitary pulmonary disease is uncommon, most patients with laryngeal tuberculosis also have bacilli in their sputum,[8, 9] a finding that favors direct pulmonary spread rather than hematogenous seeding. Laryngeal lesions may be nodular and ulcerated, clinically mimicking carcinoma.[10] Seventy percent of these lesions affect the anterior two thirds of the vocal cords, similar to the distribution of most vocal cord carcinomas (Fig. 5–4A, see p. 243).[8, 11] This is in contrast to the previously held belief that tuberculosis mainly affected the posterior interarytenoid area.[12] This posterior commissure predisposition for infection documented in the older literature most likely related to the clinical practice of encouraging patients to lie supine for most of their illness.[9]

Pathologic Features. The usual histology of late infection is that of necrotizing granulomas, epithelioid histiocytes, giant cells, and lymphoplasmacytic infiltrates (Fig. 5–4B to D, see p. 243). Early infection may be histologically nonspecific, with an acute inflammatory infiltrate and a lack of well-formed granulomas. The diagnosis of tuberculosis requires a Ziehl-Neelsen stain and patience, as one might have to examine many step sections to find a solitary "red snapper." The acid-fast bacilli (AFB) do not stain with hematoxylin-eosin stain or Gram stain.

Special Studies. If laryngeal tuberculosis is suspected (based on the presence of a pulmonary lesion and/or positive sputum or a strongly positive skin reaction), and the biopsy fails to reveal AFB, another diagnostic possibility would be to submit additional fresh or formalin fixed paraffin–embedded tissue for polymerase chain reaction (PCR) analysis.[13]

Differential Diagnosis. Normal laryngeal mucosa rarely harbors significant inflammation; therefore, any moderate to severe acute or chronic inflammation should be viewed as pathologic, and the possibility of infection should be considered. Granulomatous and dense chronic inflammation can also be seen in other, albeit rare, laryngeal pathogens such as *Coccidioidomycosis, Cryptococcus,* and *Blastomycosis.* The granulomatous infiltrate of sarcoid is characteristically non-necrotizing, although, rarely, necrosis may be present. Positive special studies (cultures, special stains, or PCR) are necessary to establish the diagnosis of tuberculosis. Tuberculoid leprosy can be distinguished from tuberculosis because (1) tuberculoid leprosy may involve nerves, which is uncommon for tuberculosis, and (2) *Mycobacterium leprae* will not stain with a Ziehl-Neelsen stain, but will stain with a Fite-Faraco stain. Foreign body granulomas may mimic infectious granulomas; they may be seen after Teflon injection or with laryngeal amyloidosis.

Treatment. Empirical therapy (isoniazid, rifampin, pyrazinamide, and streptomycin or ethambutol) is recommended for 8 weeks followed by isoniazid and rifampin for 16 weeks for susceptible strains. Multi-drug–resistant *Mycobacterium tuberculosis* requires the above four drugs, plus any three of the following: ethionamide, capreomycin, ciprofloxacin, or cycloserine. The course of therapy may need to be lengthened if the patient's sputum remains positive after 3 months.

Laryngeal Leprosy

Mycobacterium leprae is the causative agent of leprosy, which is seen mostly in tropical climates. Leprosy is endemic to rural areas of Latin America, South and Southeast Asia, Saharan Africa, the Mediterranean basin, and Northern Europe.[14] In the United States, endemic states include Florida, Louisiana, Texas, California, and Hawaii. The rate of indigenous United States cases of leprosy has remained stable over the last two decades, but the rate of imported cases reported in the United States has dramatically increased, starting in the late 1970s, because of the influx of Vietnamese, Cambodian, Laotian, and Philippine immigrants. Of interest, this increase did not lead to increased transmission within the United States.[14] The rate of household transmission for lepromatous leprosy patients (see subsequent discussion) is much higher than for tuberculoid leprosy patients, indicating the importance of exposure dose, which is greater in lepromatous leprosy.[15]

Clinical Features. Leprosy has a predisposition to affect cooler peripheral areas such as digits, ears, and nose. It presents as cutaneous hypopigmented or hyperpigmented, hypoesthetic isolated macular lesions. Early lesions may also be tender, erythematous, and indurated (erythema nodosum leprosum) and can ulcerate. Neural involvement is common to all types of leprosy and results in severe pain and muscular atrophy. Sensory loss ultimately leads to repeat mechanical trauma and secondary infections.

Lepromatous leprosy presents with a widespread symmetrical facial distribution of lesions, leading to coarsening of features (leonine facies). The earlobes and nose are especially enlarged and infiltrated. Intranasal and paranasal sinus involvement is common and occurs after cutaneous nasal involvement. Sinus involvement may present with mucopurulent rhinitis, producing copious mucus rife with mycobacteria. Early mucosal lesions are plaque-like, whereas late sinonasal lesions are nodular or ulcerative, or both, and may ultimately lead to nasal collapse.

The larynx usually becomes infected retrograde to the nasal disease. In a study of 973 untreated leprous patients, laryngeal involvement was related to mycobacterial load: it was seen in 65% of patients with lepromatous leprosy, with the greatest association seen with the most advanced cases.[16] The epiglottis was most often involved, appearing thickened and irregular, probably mirroring *M.*

leprae's predisposition for cooler sites. Vocal cord paralysis, secondary to recurrent laryngeal nerve involvement, was present in 9% of patients.

Pathologic Features. Tuberculoid leprosy reveals epithelioid granulomas and relatively few organisms. The organisms are seen only on Fite-Faraco or modified Fite stains. Nerves are surrounded by cuffs of lymphocytes or by granulomas, or may contain free acid-fast bacilli. Lepromatous leprosy, the opposite clinical and immunologic pole, reveals diffuse infiltration of tissues by histiocytic cells, which are incapable of undergoing "epithelioid" transformation and unable to form granulomas. These foamy histiocytes (lepra cells, Virchow cells) may be "stuffed" with abundant mycobacilli (globi), which remain uncleared by the host. Free bacilli may also be abundant within nerves. Between these two extremes, there are borderline cases (i.e., borderline tuberculoid and borderline lepromatous)[17] with variable immunologic response (e.g., mixture of ill-formed granulomas and foamy histiocytes). The histoid form of leprosy is seen in late leprosy and is characterized by spindle-shaped histiocytes forming dermatofibroma-like tumors.[18]

The diagnosis of leprosy is more difficult to determine early in the disease course when mycobacilli may be sparse and granulomas not fully developed. Mycobacteria may be sparsely present or absent in tuberculoid leprosy. In a biopsy study of 30 cases of lepromatous leprosy, only seven revealed histologic evidence of bacilli—most often, as expected, in those cases with foamy histiocytes.[19]

Differential Diagnosis. The differential diagnosis for tuberculoid leprosy includes *Mycobacterium tuberculosis* infection; however, the clinical history should be helpful in ruling out *M. tuberculosis* and atypical mycobacteria and in establishing the diagnosis of leprosy. Perineural involvement by lymphocytes, granulomas, or free organisms is an important diagnostic feature of leprosy and is not seen with *M. tuberculosis* infections. An acute suppurative reaction is lacking in leprosy (except for erythema nodosum leprosum) and is present in cutaneous manifestations of *M. tuberculosis.* The Fite-Faraco stain is specific for *M. leprae* and is not known to stain other mycobacteria.

Polymerase chain reaction has been applied to the detection of DNA sequences from *M. leprae* extracted from formalin-fixed paraffin-embedded tissue,[20, 21] with excellent sensitivity and specificity over other related mycobacterial species. This method would have the greatest usefulness in tuberculoid and borderline tuberculoid leprosy, in which the mycobacterial counts are lowest.

Treatment. Tuberculoid leprosy may be treated with dapsone and rifampin. Lepromatous leprosy requires the addition of a third agent, such as clofazimine.

Laryngeal Syphilis

Clinical Features. Syphilis is a venereal illness transmitted by *Treponema pallidum* (pale turning thread). Primary syphilis results in a localized chancre at the mucosal site of infection 1 week to 3 months after initial exposure. In additional to genitourinary sites, chancres can develop in the oral cavity after oral-genital contact and may incidentally infect the unwary, ungloved examiner. Affected oral sites include lips, palate, gingiva, tongue, and tonsil. Biopsies from these areas may come to the pathologist from a patient with a nonspecific history of "ulcer." Typically, cutaneous chancres are painless, hard, raised lesions that develop shallow ulcerations with sharp, raised borders. On mucosal surfaces, primary chancres may appear as silvery gray erosions, granulation tissue, or nonspecific ulcers, or may even mimic carcinoma. Chancres are self-healing with minimal scarring.

Secondary syphilis occurs weeks to months after the primary chancre and is the result of systemic spread of the infection. The disease usually manifests in patients with fever, pharyngitis, and a generalized macular/papular rash; the latter may affect the hair follicles of the scalp, eyebrows and beard, causing a patchy "moth-eaten" alopecia (alopecia syphilitica). The diffuse maculopapular rash can be seen intraorally and often is associated with laryngeal hyperemia.

The macular/papular lesions coalesce in warm moist areas, like the anogenital and intertriginous areas, to form hyperplastic lesions—condyloma latum, or flat condylomas. As condylomata lata arise from a systemic spread of *T. pallidum,* they are not dependent on the initial site of inoculation, but are also infectious. "Mucous patches" are infectious, raised, and flattened macerated lesions with a thin grayish membranous covering; they are seen intraorally and may also be seen on the epiglottis.[22, 23] Condyloma latum, the hyperplastic lesion of secondary syphilis, may occur in the larynx, ears, and nasolabial folds. Generalized lymphadenopathy occurs during the secondary stage, with a predisposition for periarticular lymph nodes, such as in epitrochlear and inguinal areas. Secondary syphilis will lapse into a latent state, but patients may frequently experience recurrent mucocutaneous symptoms of secondary syphilis.

Tertiary syphilis is the long-term chronic systemic parenchymal result of untreated infection, which may become manifest years to decades after primary infection. Tertiary syphilis has a predisposition to affect the central and peripheral nervous system and the cardiovascular system. Gummas, the destructive lesions of late, tertiary syphilis, have a proclivity for membranous bones, commonly affecting the palate. Laryngeal framework, nasal, and temporal bones and ossicles may also develop gummas. Gummas are painless raised ulcerative masses, which may rapidly progress to necrotic destructive masses. Chondritis/perichondritis may involve the epiglottis and cricoarytenoid joint.[22] Infraglottic tracheal stenosis is a possible sequel to tertiary syphilis.

Pathologic Features. Nonspecific lymphoplasmacytic infiltrates may be seen in all stages of syphilis and are most dense in the primary chancre. The overlying epidermis is thinned and eventually ulcerates. Lymphoplasmacytic vasculitis in a coat sleeve–like arrangement and endothelial proliferation are seen. The Steiner modification of Warthin-Starry or Dieterle stains will reveal the spirochetes, especially around vessels, but they may be localized in the squamous mucosa or submucosa (Fig. 5–5, see p. 244). Interpretation of these silver stains is made difficult by the presence of melanocytes and reticulin fibers, as well as spirochetes other than *T. pallidum.*

In secondary syphilis, one also sees a dense lymphoplasmacytic infiltrate. Granulomas with multinucleated giant cells and epithelioid histiocytes may be a late finding. Plasma cells may be sparse or absent in these lesions. Spirochetes may be seen in the secondary lesions, again predominantly around vessels. Vascular endothelial proliferation is not a constant finding in secondary lesions and is more likely seen in older lesions. Condyloma latum is composed of epithelial hyperplasia (rather than the attenuated epithelium of chancres), with elongated rete pegs and dense lymphoplasmacytic infiltrates with perivascular cuffing of plasma cells. Lymph nodes contain noncaseating granulomas, perivascular cuffing of plasmacytes, and capsular fibrosis. The gummas of late secondary and tertiary syphilis reveal necrotizing granulomas with multinucleated Langerhans-type giant cells and obliterative endarteritis. Spirochetes are sparse and are only rarely observed in gummas by special stains. Recurrent laryngeal nerve paralysis may be seen in neurosyphilis as a manifestation of central nervous system disease, along with other cranial nerve deficits, or as an isolated nerve palsy.

Special Studies. The classic "dark field" examination is made by examining transudate from a chancre suspended in saline for the motile spirochetes and is not feasible for usual formalin-fixed paraffin-embedded laryngeal biopsies. A more specific form of this examination is the dark field direct immunofluorescent antibody test for *T. pallidum* (DFA-TP), which can be performed on dried, fixed tissue smears.[24] Immunohistochemical staining with commercially available polyclonal antibody may be helpful in cases that clinically and histologically suggest primary or secondary syphilis but fail to reveal spirochetes by silver staining.[25]

Differential Diagnosis. Lymphoplasmacytic infiltrates may be seen in nonspecific laryngitis and in the early stages of scleroma (see later discussion). *Blastomyces* infection is classically known for inducing a hyperplastic hyperkeratotic mucosal reaction, similar to condyloma latum. Special stains and cultures should help rule this

Text continued on page 255

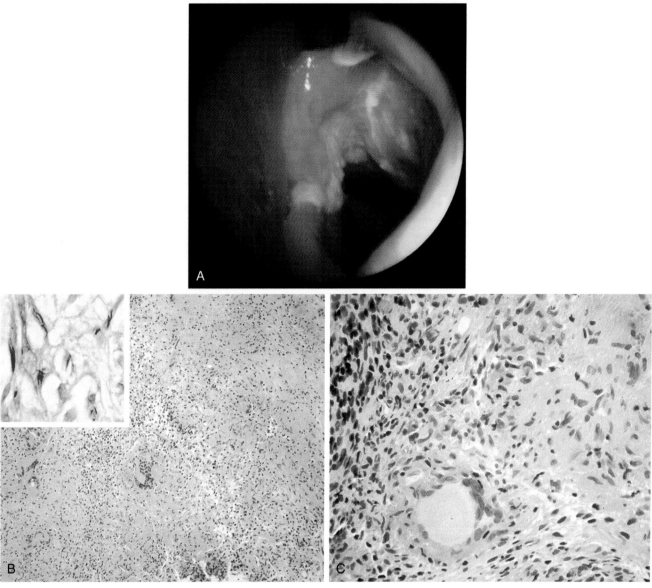

Figure 5–4. Tuberculosis laryngitis. A, Endoscopic view of supraglottic mass with an irregular surface. (Courtesy of Dr. Peak Woo.) B, C, Histology of laryngeal tuberculosis. Note diffuse inflammatory granulomatous infiltrate *(B)* with high-power detail demonstrating epithelioid granulomata *(C)* with a Langhans'-type multinucleated giant cell. The peripheral location of the nuclei is characteristic for these giant cells and distinguishes them from foreign body giant cells, which have centrally located nuclei. *Inset:* Acid fast stain reveals characteristic bacilli. (Courtesy of Dr. Jodi-Sasoon.)

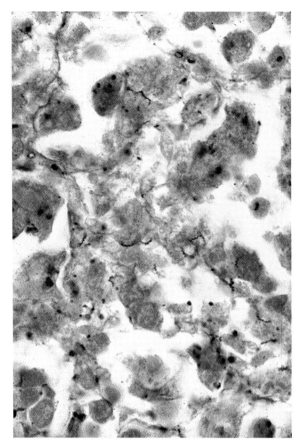

Figure 5–5. *Treponema pallidum.* A Dieterle stain reveals a "cork-screw" configuration of spirochetes.

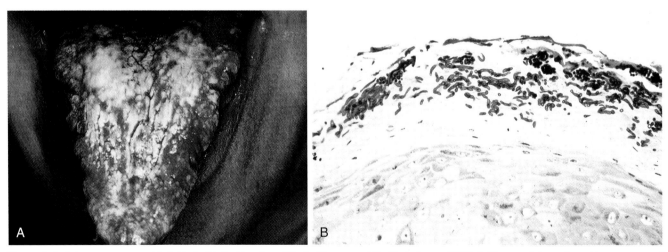

Figure 5–6. *A,* Immunosuppressed individual with florid oral candidiasis. (Courtesy of Dr. Marie Ramer, DDS.) *B,* Characteristic nonbranching, nonseptated "pseudo"-hyphae and rounded yeast forms of *Candida* in superficial keratin layer of surface epithelium. (Gomori's methenamine silver stain.)

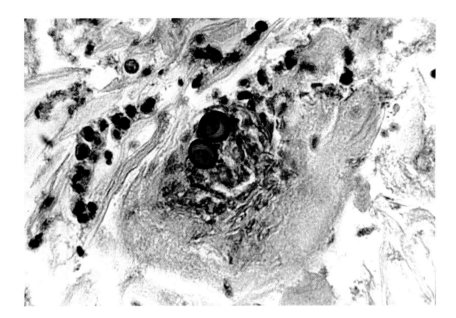

Figure 5–8. Blastomycoses. These yeasts have a thick outer wall, which will also stain with periodic acid-Schiff. Blastomyces stain weakly or not at all with a mucin stain. Note the characteristic space between the thick wall and the protoplasm in the yeast marked; this is not seen in *Cryptococcus*, the main differential diagnosis.

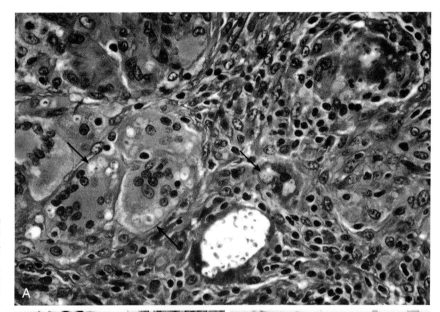

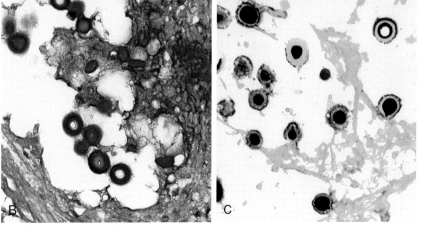

Figure 5–9. Case of primary laryngeal *cryptococcosis* in a nonimmunosuppressed woman. *A,* Laryngeal biopsy revealing microabscess formation in the lamina propria with multinucleated giant cells containing small yeast forms *(arrows)*. (Courtesy of Dr. Leslie Smallman.) *B,* Mucicarmine stain accentuates the inner and outer limits of the polysaccharide capsule. *C,* Gomori's methenamine silver stain, which densely stains the entire organism, leaving a negative impression of the capsule.

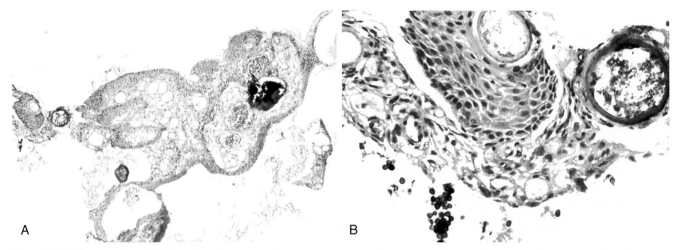

Figure 5–11. Rhinosporidiosis. *A,* Papillary hyperplasia, seen at low power, may mimic other entities such as papillomata or adenocarcinoma. Note large cysts within the lamina propria. *B,* Note: Mature spherules, approximately 240 μm in diameter, with thick walls approximately 6 to 9 μm in the submucosa.

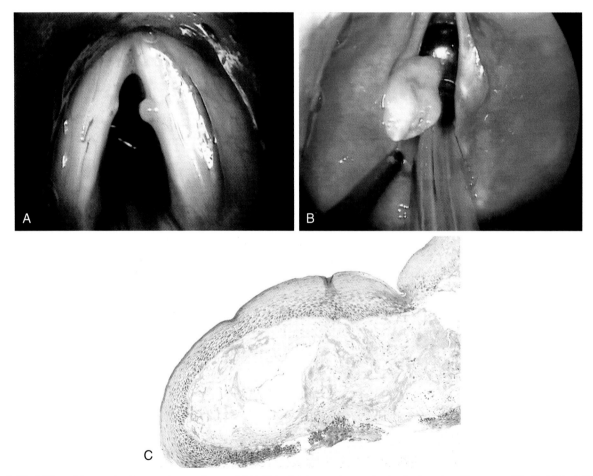

Figure 5–13. *A,* Bilateral laryngeal polyps on the anterior vocal folds. This clinician was known for her husky voice. (Courtesy of Dr. Peak Woo.) *B,* Contact granuloma. Polypoid lesion with saucer-like traumatic ulceration projecting from the arytenoid process as a result of vocal abuse. (Courtesy of Dr. Peak Woo.) *C,* Laryngeal polyps. Histologically, one sees dilated venous channels and extravasated fibrin within the lamina propia.

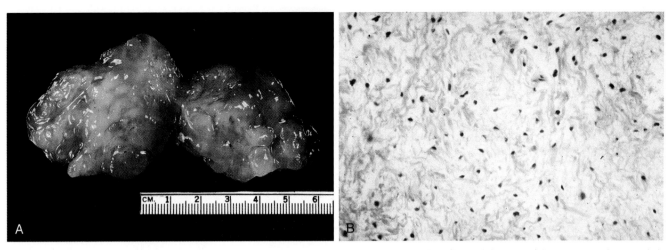

Figure 5–14. Supraglottic myxoma—a rarity. *A*, Cut surface reveals a lobulated pale myxoid tumor. The differential diagnosis of this tumor grossly may include a lipomatous tumor with myxoid change, and pleomorphic adenoma with prominent myxoid change. *B*, Histologically, one sees small bland spindle cells in a loose myxoid stroma. The uniform pattern and relatively low vascularity aid in distinguishing myxomas from other tumors.

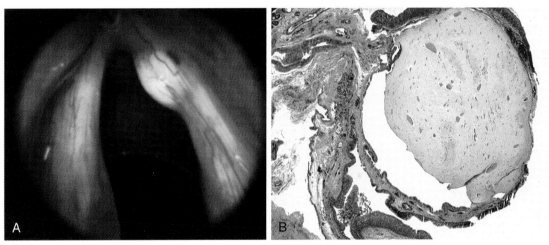

Figure 5–17. Ductal cyst. *A*, Endoscopic view of cyst of right anterior vocal fold. (Courtesy of Dr. Peak Woo.) *B*, Cystically dilated duct composed of oncocytic columnar epithelium.

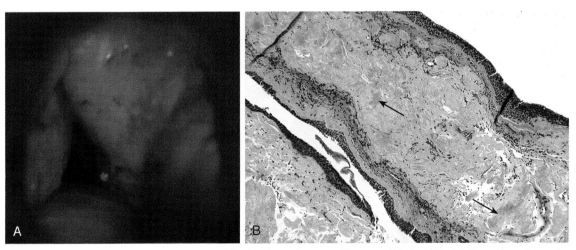

Figure 5–18. Laryngeal amyloid. *A*, Endoscopic view revealing diffusely indurated mucosa. (Courtesy of Dr. Peak Woo.) *B*, Deposition of amorphous material of varying eosinophilia. The more dense areas *(arrows)* result in a "waxy" appearance akin to pink crayons.

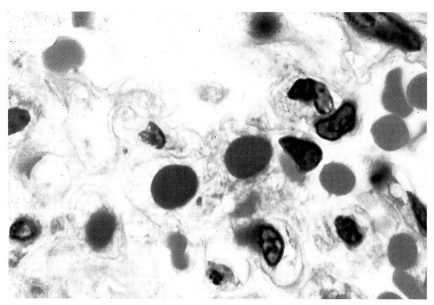

Figure 5–22. Lupus erythematosis cells: Mononuclear cells with engulfed hematoxylin bodies. Note the homogenized remains of nuclei exposed to antinuclear antibodies, which appear as large amphophilic cytoplasmic inclusions.

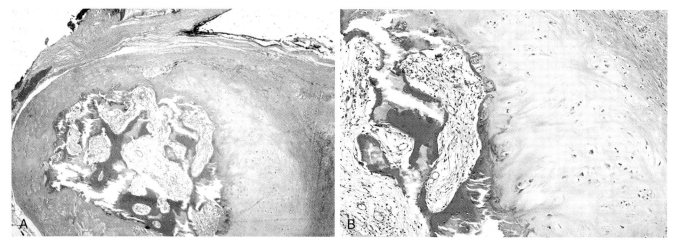

Figure 5–24. *A&B,* Chondrometaplasia. This lesion was seen as a polypoid mass arising from the mid-vocal fold. Mature chondroid matrix is seen, which "blends" into the surrounding fibroconnective tissue. Central ossification is also noted, an unusual feature of this case.

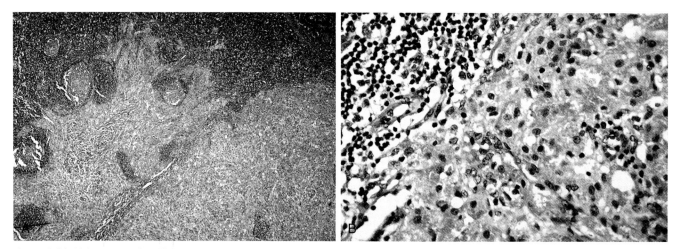

Figure 5–30. Malignant granular cell tumor presenting as a large (4.7 cm) hypopharyngeal/laryngeal tumor in a 29-year-old woman with locoregional metastasis. *A&B,* Metastatic tumor to the lymph node. Only a mild degree of nuclear pleomorphism is seen with prominent nucleoli.

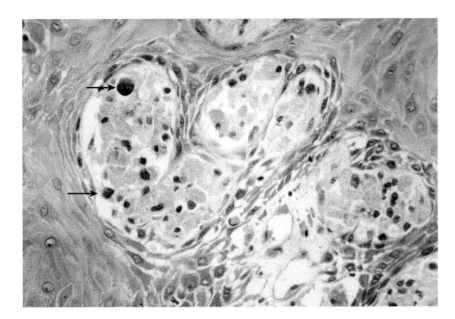

Figure 5–31. Atypical granular cell tumor presenting as a recurrent, nonmetastasizing tumor. Pleomorphic granular cells are seen at the mucosal basement membrane *(arrows);* elsewhere they could be seen coursing through the mucosa. Spindling and pleomorphism were also present.

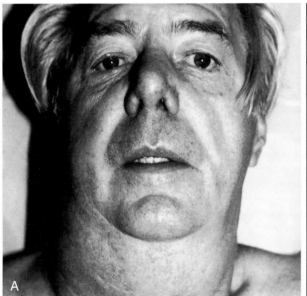

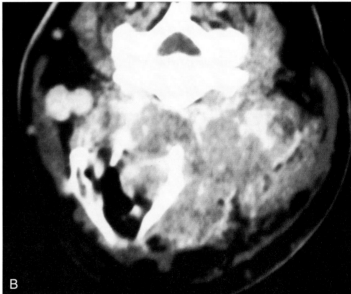

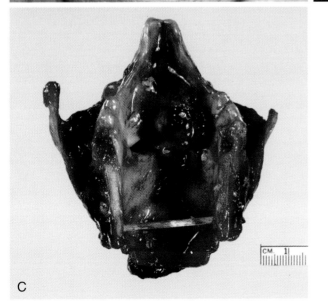

Figure 5–34. *A&B,* Laryngeal neuroendocrine carcinoma, presenting as a neck mass. (Courtesy of Dr. Hugh Biller.) *C,* Neuroendocrine carcinoma presenting as an epiglottic tan polypoid tumor.

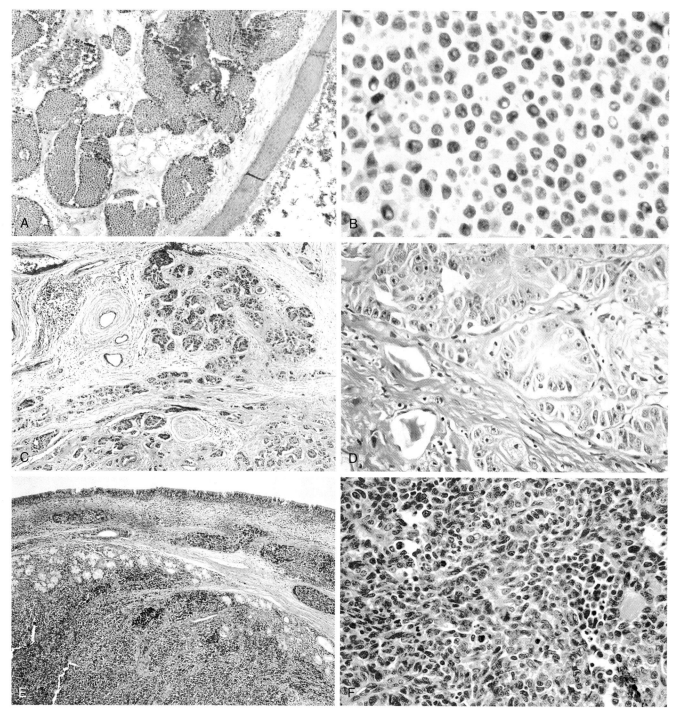

Figure 5–35. *A,* Well-differentiated neuroendocrine carcinoma (WDNEC) with an organoid pattern. *B,* Detail of WDNEC. Note round, relatively non-pleomorphic nuclei with stippled chromatin and prominent intranuclear holes. *C,* Moderately differentiated neuroendocrine carcinoma (MDNEC) with an infiltrating glandular pattern. *D,* Note: increased nuclear pleomorphism of this MDNEC with finely stippled chromatin. *E,* Poorly differentiated neuroendocrine carcinoma (PDNEC) (small cell carcinoma). Note diffuse submucosal infiltrate with several vessels filled with tumor. *F,* Detail of PDNEC. Note plump to elongated nuclei with fine chromatin pattern and inconspicuous nucleoli and minimal cytoplasm.

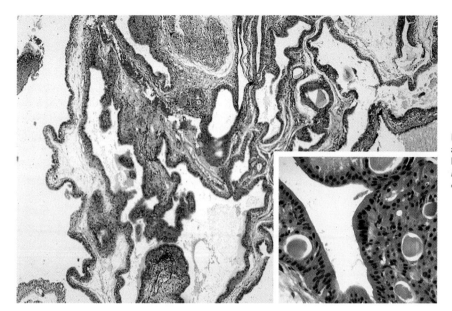

Figure 5–36. Oncocytic cystadenoma. *A,* Multicystic and papillocystic lesion composed of cuboidal and co-lumnar oncocytes forming cystic cribriform spaces. *Inset,* The cytoplasm of tumor cells is typically abundant, granular, and intensely eosinophilic.

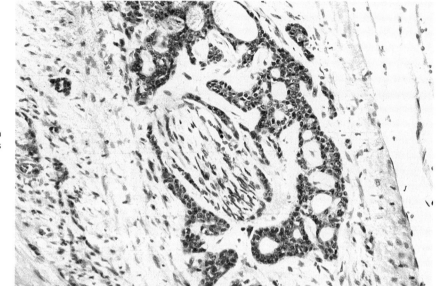

Figure 5–38. Adenoid cystic carcinoma. A cribriform (sieve-like) pattern can be seen as the tumor infiltrates a laryngeal nerve.

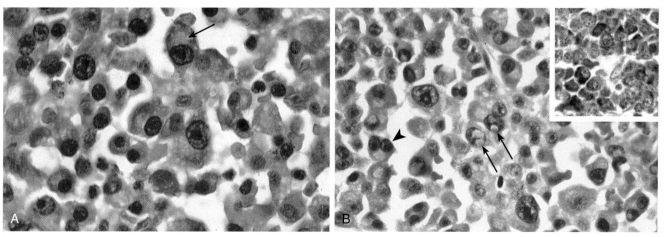

Figure 5–40. Plasmacytoma. *A,* Infiltrate of mature and immature plasma cells. The perinuclear hof is still prominent in the larger, more pleomorphic cells *(arrow). B,* Pleomorphic plasmacytoma. The plasmacytic nature can be recognized by finding binucleated cells *(arrowhead)* and intranuclear Dutcher bodies *(straight arrows). Inset,* Cytoplasmic light chain restriction.

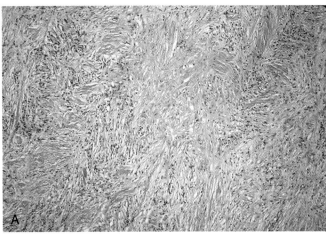

Figure 5–41. Inflammatory myofibroblastic tumor. *A*, At low power, a storiform pattern is seen with scattered lymphocytes. *B*, The fibroblasts are reactive in appearance. Necrosis and hemorrhage are not seen. *C*, The inflammatory component is predominantly lymphoplasmacytic. This degree of inflammation would not be expected in a desmoid tumor.

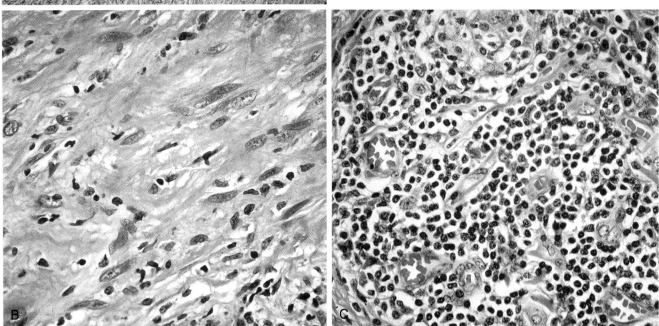

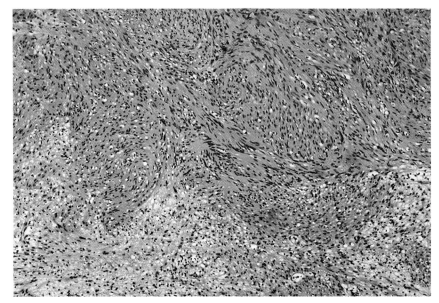

Figure 5–45. Schwannoma (neurilemmoma). An alternating pattern of relative cellularity and collagenized matrix (top of photomicrograph) and somewhat less cellularity and myxoid background (bottom). The spindle cells palisade, forming a tiger-striped pattern with Verocay bodies (center).

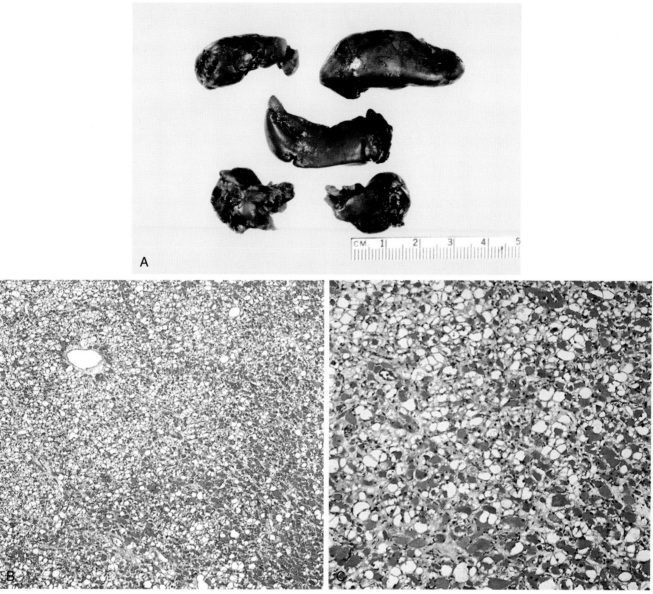

Figure 5–49. Pharyngeal adult rhabdomyoma. *A,* Grossly, this tumor is polypoid and brown, mimicking an oncocytic tumor. *B&C,* Microscopically, one sees closely packed, uniform, large polygonal cells with abundant eosinophilic, granular or vacuolated cytoplasm ("spider" cells) and one or more small, round, centrally or peripherally located, vesicular nuclei. Haphazard cytoplasmic cross-striations can be seen more easily on phosphotungstic acid-hematoxylin stain (not illustrated).

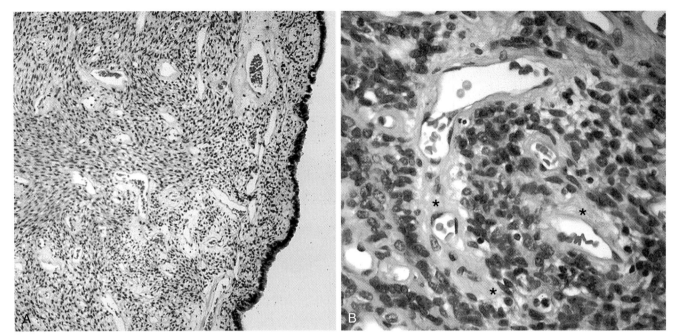

Figure 5–55. Hemangiopericytoma. *A,* Note the submucosal tumor composed of a uniform population of bland short spindle cells in fibrillary background around thin-walled blood vessels. *B,* Perivascular hyalinization is a more sensitive finding than "staghorn" type vessels (*). Factor XIIIa expression (not shown) is characteristic for hemangiopericytoma and aids in establishing the diagnosis.

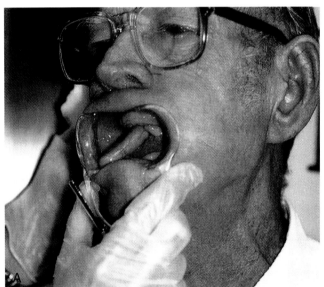

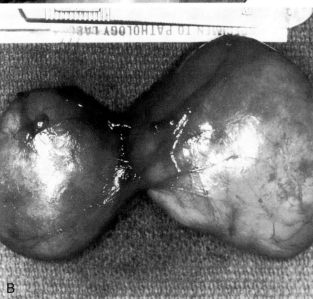

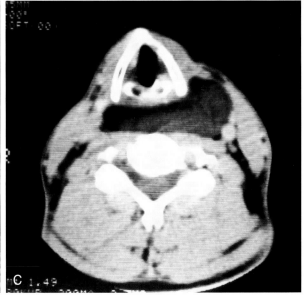

Figure 5–56. *A,* Hypopharyngeal lipomatous tumors. Within hollow organs, these polypoid tumors may reach enormous proportions. This patient is regurgitating his tumor. Note the sausage-like grey-pink intraoral mass. (Courtesy of Dr. J. Mark Reed.) *B,* Retropharyngeal lipoma. This encapsulated dumbbell-shaped tumor was composed entirely of mature adipose tissue. (Courtesy of Dr. Hugh Biller.) *C,* On radiograph, the lipoma can be seen as a well-demarcated, low-density retropharyngeal mass.

out. The hyperplasia of condyloma latum may also be confused with laryngeal malignancy. Careful histologic sampling will usually allow separation of these two entities. The differential diagnosis of the granulomatous inflammation of tertiary syphilis includes mycobacterial and fungal infections. These latter infections can be separated on the basis of culture and special stains. Laryngeal inflammatory pseudotumor (inflammatory myofibroblastic tumor) may also be characterized by a dense lymphoplasmacytic infiltrate but will have a more prominent reactive myofibroblastic component.

Treatment. Penicillin G is the drug of choice for syphilis. Penicillin-allergic patients may be treated with erythromycin, tetracycline, or ceftriaxone.

Laryngeal "Scleroma" (Rhinoscleroma)

The term *rhinoscleroma* was minted by Ferdinand von Hebra and Moritz Kohn (aka Kaposi) to describe the condition of patients presenting with hard *(sclero)* noses *(rhino)*,[26] which they originally concluded must be secondary to indolent malignancy. Mikulicz substantiated that this entity was actually inflammatory and von Frisch identified bacillary organisms in 1882.[27] Interestingly, aniline dye workers in San Salvador were noted in the late 19th century to have an increased prevalence of rhinoscleroma. The dye, indigo, was derived from *Indigofera tinctoria,* a legume. Alvarez discovered a bacillus in the legume, which he called *Bacillus indigogenous,* and concluded that it was identical to von Frisch's bacillus.[28]

Klebsiella rhinoscleromatis is endemic to tropical and subtropical areas (Central America, Chili, Central Africa, India, Indonesia, Egypt, Algeria, Morocco) as well as temperate latitudes (Eastern and Central Europe and the Russian republics).[29, 30] It is an uncommon pathogen in the United States but may be seen in immigrant populations. It is an organism of low infectivity and not a normal commensal organism. Human-to-human transmission of *K. rhinoscleromatis* has been assumed to be the only mode of contact (legume-to-human transmission notwithstanding), and infection will result only after prolonged exposure.[28] Increased incidence among family members and contacts has been noted by some reports, but this remains controversial.[28–30] Rhinoscleroma has been referred to as the "disease of the great unwashed."[28] Social conditions may vary, but it has been stressed that poor hygiene and crowded environments are common features. In one mountainous endemic site in Indonesia, many families sleep together in large, poorly ventilated houses, huddled together with their dogs and domestic fowl for warmth.[29, 30]

Clinical Features. Usually, scleroma initially presents within the second and third decades of life and more frequently affects women than men.[31] The nasal cavity and sinuses are most frequently involved, although it can involve the entire upper respiratory tract, including the larynx, so much so that the general name *scleroma* has been advocated rather than the term *rhinoscleroma.* The natural course evolves through three stages. The early stage is the atrophic catarrhal stage: the mucosa is reddened and atrophic, with foul purulent discharge and crusting. The clinical differential diagnosis in this early stage includes infection with *Klebsiella pneumoniae ozaenae.* The granulomatous stage occurs months to years later, with waxy, ulcerating inflammatory masses that distend and deform the mucosal surfaces. The inflammatory masses extend through the external nares in severe cases and may distort the soft tissues of the midface, resulting in a "rhinoceros-like" appearance.[32] The clinical differential diagnosis includes leprosy and syphilis. The final sclerotic stage is characterized by fibrosis along with the inflammation, culminating in stenosis. Common clinical symptoms of laryngeal involvement include cough and hoarseness. The infraglottis is the most frequently involved laryngeal site[31] and may culminate in infraglottic stenosis.

Pathologic Features. Histologically, one sees a dense chronic inflammatory infiltrate with collections of foamy macrophages (Mikulicz's cells). The catarrhal stage is dominated by nonspecific lymphoplasmacytic infiltrate; the Mikulicz cells are sparse. They are most abundant in the nodular granulomatous stage. True granulomas

with epithelioid histiocytes are not seen in this infection. Plasma cell infiltrates and Russell's bodies are prominent in early infection. The final sclerotic stage reveals dense fibroconnective tissue with a relative paucity of inflammatory cells.

Special Studies. *K. rhinoscleromatis* (Frisch's bacillus) is a gram-negative bacillus. Special stains such as periodic acid–Schiff, with and without diastase, HotchKiss-McManus, and Warthin-Starry will reveal the bacterial rods within these histiocytes; the latter stain is the most sensitive for revealing the bacilli.[33] Immunohistochemistry on formalin-fixed paraffin-embedded tissues against type III *Klebsiella* antigen is also sensitive and specific. Routine cultures for *K. rhinoscleromatis* (MacConkey's medium) may be positive in only 50% of cases and are more likely to be positive in the nodular stage.

Differential Diagnosis. The differential diagnosis includes atypical mycobacterial infection, which also appears as a histiocytic infiltrate rather than a granulomatous reaction. A Ziehl-Neelsen stain can rule this out. Lepromatous leprosy also appears as a diffuse histiocytic infiltrate (Virchow cells) and should be ruled out by a Fite-Faraco stain. When a lymphoplasmacytic infiltrate dominates the histology, the diagnosis of syphilis should also be considered.

Treatment and Prognosis. Parenteral antibiotic therapy, such as with tetracycline, streptomycin, or chloramphenicol, may be effective in arresting disease progression. Surgery for early acute disease may increase disease dissemination. Reconstruction may be indicated in the sclerotic stage. Fatal sclerotic airway obstruction may occur. Squamous carcinoma has purportedly been associated with scleroma, but adequate documentation is lacking.[34]

Laryngeal Actinomycoses

Harz studied actinomycosis in the bovine form of the illness lumpyjaw in 1877. The causative agent was named *Actinomyces bovis* (*Actinomyces:* "Strahlenpilz" or "ray-fungus"). It was originally thought to be associated with the habit, by both human and cow, of chewing straw.[35] However, the *Actinomyces* are now known to be commensal organisms of human and bovine hosts; unlike most true fungi, they have not been identified as environmental saprophobes. The human pathogen, *Actinomyces israelii,* is normally present around teeth, especially carious teeth, in saliva, and in tonsillar crypts. It is classified as a filamentous bacterium rather than a fungus because (1) it reproduces by fission rather than sporulation (as perfect fungi do) or filamentous budding (as imperfect fungi do) and (2) it contains muramic acid in cell walls and has an absence of mitochondria, both features of bacteria.[36]

Actinomyces is thought to have limited potential as a pathogen in normal hosts and may contribute to gingivitis and caries.[37] Antecedent trauma or other precursors are necessary predisposing factors for invasive infection. Three sites for *Actinomyces* infections are cervicofacial, thoracic, and abdominal; cervicofacial infection is the most common form. Soft tissue abscesses and draining cervical fistulas develop as a result of secondary actinomyces infection of periapical abscesses. These sinuses may occasionally have long tracts communicating with the soft tissues of the back and chest. Actinomycosis can also present as a neck mass without the characteristic sinuses. As an anaerobe, *Actinomyces* would not be expected to cause a primary endolaryngeal infection, but rather cause laryngeal, infraglottic, and hypopharyngeal infection via secondary extension of extralaryngeal cervical abscesses.[37–41]

Pathologic Features. The pale yellow "sulfur granules" or grains, observed clinically, are microcolonies of bacilli. On hematoxylin-eosin stain, one sees only blue amorphous masses: the slender filamentous nature of these bacilli becomes more apparent on Brown and Brenn (gram-positive) or Gomori's methenamine-silver stains. The filaments have a club-shaped, or beaded, end. The filaments may mimic fungi in their tendency to branch. However, their very narrow width (approximately 0.5 μm) is less than the range of fungal hyphal diameters. In disseminated disease, the organism is less likely to form the "sulfur granule" clumps, and also there is a tendency for it to be mixed with other bacteria.

Differential Diagnosis. The main differential diagnosis is between *Actinomyces* and *Nocardia. Actinomyces* are not acid fast and do not stain with Ziehl-Neelsen, although occasionally they may be weakly acid fast. This point can help distinguish *Actinomyces* from *Nocardia* on tissue sections. The latter filamentous bacteria do not stain well with hematoxylin-eosin but do stain well with a modified Ziehl-Neelsen. The distinction between these two filamentous bacteria is important because their sensitivities to antibiotics differ: penicillin is the drug of choice for *Actinomyces,* whereas *Nocardia* is unresponsive to penicillin and can be treated with sulfa drugs. The diagnosis of actinomycosis is confirmed by anaerobic culture. A significant number of reported cases lack confirmatory cultures, owing to lack of anaerobic conditions or overgrowth of other bacteria plus the failure to recognize *Actinomyces* as a pathogen and perform appropriate subcultures.

Treatment. Surgical drainage of an abscess cavity is indicated. Penicillin G is the antibiotic of choice; allergic patients may be treated with tetracycline, clindamycin, or erythromycin.

Fungal Infections

Laryngeal Candidiasis

Clinical Features. Laryngeal candidiasis would not occur in immunocompetent hosts but may be seen in diabetic patients and patients immunosuppressed by steroid therapy, chemotherapy, or severe chronic illness (Fig. 5–6, see p. 244).[42] Patients present with hoarseness, dysphagia, and odynophagia. The mucosa reveals suppurative laryngitis with ulceration and pseudomembrane formation with a white creamy or milky curd-like exudate, which is left raw and bleeding after biopsy.

Pathologic Features. The pseudohyphae of *Candida* are thin, regular, and "pinched" at the point of pseudoseptation without true branching. Small, oval, globose yeast cells result in a "spaghetti and meatballs" appearance (see Fig. 5–6). The inflammatory infiltrate may be acute and nonspecific or granulomatous.

Differential Diagnosis. The differential diagnosis includes other thin, hypha-forming fungi, but the hypopharynx and larynx are not usually involved with infections by hyphal fungi. There have been only rare well-documented cases of laryngeal aspergillosis, reported in the setting of neutropenia or acquired immunodeficiency syndrome (AIDS).[43–47]

Treatment. Parenteral antibiotic therapy would include fluconazole or ketoconazole. If disseminated disease is present, then systemic antifungal therapy (amphotericin B, or flucytosine) is indicated.

Laryngeal Coccidioidomycosis

Clinical Features. *Coccidioides immitis* is endemic to southern Texas, New Mexico, Arizona, California, Northern Mexico, Guatemala, Honduras, Venezuela, and Argentina.[48] Coccidioidomycosis (also referred to as San Joaquin Valley fever, desert rheumatism, and the bumps) is an infection of the immunocompetent, and in endemic areas may be as common as chickenpox.[49] Approximately 20% of yearly reported cases are diagnosed outside the endemic areas.[50]

Coccidioides endospores germinate to form hyphae and barrel-shaped arthrospores; the latter are infectious. Airborne arthrospores come to rest in soil and germinate in cool, moist conditions. Exposure to aerosolized soil in endemic areas places one at risk for coccidioidomycosis: point source epidemics have been the result of archeologic digs. There is an especially high rate of symptomatic pulmonary infection and an erythema multiforme hypersensitivity rash among individuals visiting from nonendemic areas.[51, 52] *Coccidioides* is extraordinarily infectious—10 arthroconidia will cause infection in animals.[53] Handling Petri dishes of laboratory cultures has caused disease, as have handling and washing glassware. Coc-

cidioidomycosis is not the result of direct human-to-human transmission as only the germinating arthrospores, not the endospores, are infectious. However, several hospital staff have developed coccidioidomycosis after removing a plaster cast from a patient with *Coccidioides* osteomyelitis, caused by germination within the cast.[54]

Pulmonary infection occurs through inhalation of arthrospores and commonly causes self-limiting pulmonary and mediastinal disease. Laryngotracheal coccidioidomycosis is rare and may be seen with or without concurrent pulmonary disease.[55, 56] Patients with upper airway involvement present with hoarseness and stridor, and endoscopically have edematous, erythematous polypoid laryngotracheal mucosa.

Pathologic Features. *Coccidioides* evokes a granulomatous foreign body–type reaction with a dense chronic inflammatory infiltrate. The fungal spherules are large (30 to 80 μm), and the capsule is thick, with internal and external limits giving it a double-walled appearance. The endospores are small (2 to 5 μm) and numerous. The overlying squamous mucosa may be hyperplastic and hyperkeratotic. Serum acute antibodies and a newly converted skin reaction to coccidioidin antigen may be helpful clinical diagnostic adjuncts; these tests may be falsely negative early in the course of infection.

Differential Diagnosis. The differential diagnosis of the spherules includes *Rhinosporidium seeberi*, which are much larger (350 μm) than *Coccidioides. Rhinosporidium seeberi* also has a thicker, obviously bilaminated capsule. The *Rhinosporidium* capsule stains with the mucicarmine stain; the *Coccidioides* capsule does not. Free endospores may be confused with other yeast within their size range: *Blastomyces, Cryptococcus, Paracoccidioides, Sporothrix, Pneumocystis*, and *Torulopsis*, but only the first four have been reported to infect the larynx.[57–63] Morphologic features should allow for proper classification.

Treatment. Transient acute pulmonary infection usually goes untreated. If the patient has laryngeal infection as part of a cavitating pulmonary process, surgical débridement may be necessary in addition to antifungal therapy (either ketoconazole, amphotericin B, fluconazole, or itraconazole).

Laryngeal Paracoccidioidomycosis

Clinical Features. Paracoccidioidomycosis (South American *Blastomycosis* infection) is endemic to South America, especially Brazil, Colombia, Venezuela, Uruguay, and Argentina. A wide clinical range may be seen, from subclinical to clinically apparent infections, in both immunocompetent and immunosuppressed populations. Infection is acquired by aspiration, and pulmonary involvement is common. It has also been suggested that the act of teeth cleaning with wooden sticks may cause oral infections by the fungus.[64] Paracoccidioidomycosis has a predilection for facial skin and upper airway mucosal surfaces, especially the oral mucosa.[65] Lesions are painful and reddened, granular, mulberry-like (framboesiform), or ulcerative.[66, 67] Laryngeal involvement secondary to pulmonary infection is possible and should be considered in the differential diagnosis of laryngeal infections from South American patients.

Pathologic Features. Paracoccidioidomycosis causes an ulcerative, densely inflamed granulomatous response. Multinucleated giant cells containing ingested yeast fragments can be seen. The yeast are round, 4 to 20 μm in diameter. The characteristic feature is multiple budding daughter yeasts that may virtually rim the mother yeast capsule, giving the appearance of spokes on a mariner's wheel. This is best-observed on Gomori's methenamine-silver and periodic acid-Schiff stains (Fig. 5–7A,B). *Paracoccidioides* may be birefringent and polarize with a Maltese cross appearance, although this finding may also be seen with other yeast forms.

Differential Diagnosis. The small, newly released daughter spores may be confused with other smaller yeast (e.g., *Histoplasma*). Single budding yeast also may resemble *Blastomyces,* which is the main differential diagnosis (hence the synonym South American *Blastomyces*) (Fig. 5–7C,D). The diagnosis can be secured

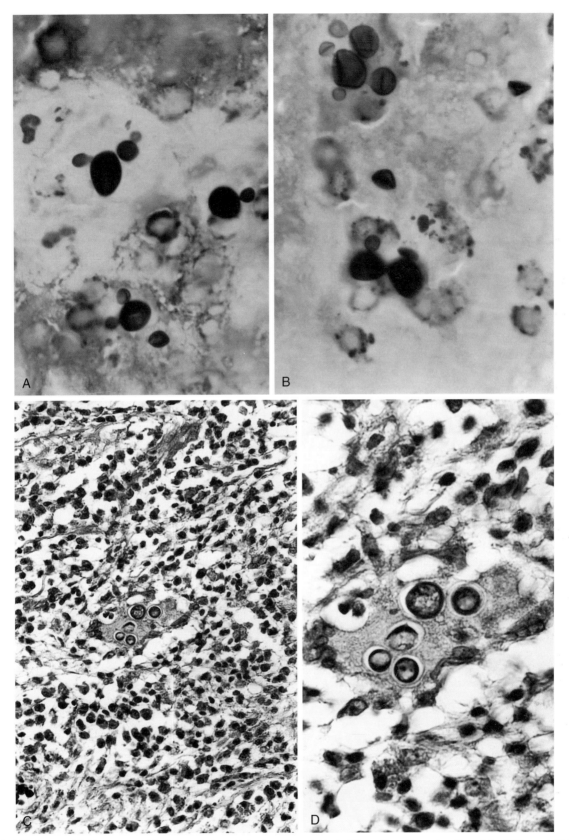

Figure 5–7. *A&B,* Paracoccidioidomycoses with characteristic multiple circumferential buds. (Gomori's methenamine-silver stain. 400× mag.) *C&D,* The size of paracoccidioidomycoses overlaps with blastomyces; the latter, which is illustrated, lacks circumferential budding.

by observing the multiple spoke-wheel budding on Gomori's methenamine-silver stain. The budding of *Blastomyces* is invariably singular and has a wider neck than that of *Paracoccidioides*. *Blastomyces* also has retraction artifact between the yeast form and the capsule (Fig. 5–7C,D).

Treatment. Antifungal therapy is indicated (ketoconazole, amphotericin B, or itraconazole).

Laryngeal Blastomycosis

Clinical Features. *Blastomyces dermatitidis* (North American blastomycosis, Gilchrist's disease, Chicago disease) is endemic in the Ohio and Mississippi River basins and in the Great Lakes area. Small epidemics have been reported in North Carolina, Minnesota, Illinois, Wisconsin, Kentucky, and Virginia.[62, 68, 69] Despite the name, it is not confined to North America and has been detected in South America and Africa. Avid bird hunters, for reasons stated subsequently, have a noted risk.[69] Canine blastomycosis follows the same geographic distribution as human disease in the United States, and hunting dogs have been especially noted to develop blastomycosis.[71]

Blastomyces has been occasionally isolated from soil specimens, especially near water. As with other fungi, only the arthrospores are infectious, not the yeast forms. Point sources are usually associated with woodsy and watery environments, such as one traced to beaver ponds or lakeside construction sites.[72] Proximity to arthrospores affects the rate of infection: individuals picking up objects off the ground to examine them are more vulnerable to infection than those examining from a distance. This would also explain the association of blastomycosis with bird hunters, as they "lie in wait" for their prey by crouching or lying on the ground, and also with their hunting dogs, which sniff at the ground.

Blastomyces may cause disease through inhalation or traumatic inoculation into skin. It may present with acute onset of fever, productive cough, and myalgias or with insidious onset of weight loss, malaise, anorexia, and a chronic cough, mimicking tuberculosis. Patients suffering direct inoculation into soft tissues or the upper airway present with local symptoms such as an ulcerating mass but no systemic symptoms.

In a recent report of 102 patients with blastomycosis seen at the Mayo clinic, five patients had laryngeal lesions.[73] Laryngeal blastomycosis appears as an erythematous or white mass with irregular borders that may immobilize the vocal cords—an appearance that mimics carcinoma. Deep laryngeal fissures or laryngocutaneous fistulas may form. Quite a number of unfortunate "laryngeal carcinomas" have been reported for which re-review of the biopsies or laryngectomy specimens revealed not cancer but blastomycosis.[74, 75]

Pathologic Features. *Blastomyces* is distinctive in its ability to induce a hyperplastic, hyperkeratotic verrucous response mimicking squamous carcinoma or verrucous carcinoma. Acute and chronic granulomatous reaction with necrosis is seen, reminiscent of tuberculosis. The organism is round, 6 to 15 μm wide, with very distinctive, thick "double" cell walls and characteristic broad-based single buds. Another characteristic feature for *Blastomyces* is the retraction artifact between the cell wall and the protoplasm seen on hematoxylin-eosin stain (Fig. 5–8, see p. 245).

Differential Diagnosis. The differential diagnosis includes infection with *Paracoccidioides, Cryptococcus,* and *Sporothrix schenckii.* The broad budding dumbbell- or lollipop-shaped appearance of *Blastomyces* aids in distinguishing it from the similarly sized *Cryptococcus* and *Sporothrix schenckii.* However, *Blastomyces* budding is not always observed. Both *Blastomyces* and *Cryptococcus* have cell walls that stain strongly with periodic acid-Schiff and Gomori's methenamine-silver. The cell wall of *Blastomyces* will stain weakly or not at all with the mucicarmine stain, whereas *Cryptococcus* will react strongly with the mucicarmine stain.

Treatment. Antifungal therapy is indicated (ketoconazole, amphotericin B, or itraconazole), and surgical reconstruction may be necessary.

Laryngeal Cryptococcosis

Clinical Features. *Cryptococcus neoformans* is a ubiquitous yeast-like organism of worldwide distribution. Emmons first reported its association with pigeon nesting sites and excreta in the 1950s.[76] *C. neoformans* is a dimorphic fungus, seen in vivo as the yeast form. The hyphal sexual form is *Filobasidiella neoformans.* Cryptococcal laryngitis has been seen in patients with AIDS either with previous or concurrent pneumonia or as isolated laryngeal lesions. It may also occur in immunocompetent hosts, with or without intercurrent pulmonary disease.[57–59, 77] Clinically, cryptococcal laryngitis typically has an exudative or a warty appearance because of the epithelial hyperplasia, but may rarely present as a smooth-surfaced mass.[78]

Pathologic Features. The yeast-like organisms are not readily stained by hematoxylin-eosin, although it may accentuate their nuclei. Gomori's methenamine-silver will stain the organism, whereas mucicarmine and digested periodic acid–Schiff stain will accentuate the polysaccharide capsule (Fig. 5–9, see p. 245). Uncollapsed round yeast-like organisms are the size of erythrocytes (6–7 μm) but may be as large as 20 μm. Collapsed deformed yeast take on a boat-like or sickle-type shape, similar to *Pneumocystis.* Single budding yeast with narrow necks may be seen. Capsule-deficient *Cryptococcus,* seen in AIDS, may confound the diagnosis.[79]

Differential Diagnosis. The differential diagnosis includes yeast forms such as *S. schenckii, Pneumocystis carinii, Torulopsis glabrata, B. dermatitidis,* and *Histoplasma capsulatum.* The latter yeast is much smaller than *Cryptococcus* and the others listed. *B. dermatitidis* and *Cryptococcus* are the only two yeast forms with a polysaccharide cell wall that stains with digested periodic acid–Schiff. *Blastomyces* can be distinguished from *Cryptococcus* by its wider budding isthmus, its protoplasmic retraction artifact, and its lack of strong reaction with the mucicarmine stain. The other organisms can be distinguished from *Cryptococcus* based on their size and shape. *H. capsulatum* is smaller and intracellular; *S. schenckii* has football-shaped yeast in addition to the rounded forms; *P. carinii* is approximately the same size as *Cryptococcus* but lacks the variation in size, the mucinophilic capsule, and the budding forms of *Cryptococcus.*

Treatment. Amphotericin B, possibly in conjunction with flucytosine, is indicated for extrapulmonary cryptococcal infection; however, localized disease may be amenable to excisional surgical biopsy.[78]

Laryngeal Histoplasmosis

Histoplasmosis (Darling's disease) was elucidated early in the 20th century by Samuel Darling, a pathologist working in Panama.[80] The intracellular organisms he found were within histiocytes, so he coined the name *Histoplasma. Capsulatum* was derived from the "refractile rim" observed around the organisms. Histoplasmosis is ubiquitous worldwide; it is endemic in the Midwest and Central United States (Ohio and Mississippi River Valley), and in the Southeast United States, Mexico, Central and South America (Guatemala, Venezuela, Peru) as well as Europe, Russia, and the Far East. A dimorphic fungus, its infectious hyphal form, *Emmonsiella capsulatum* can be isolated from starling roosts, bat caves, pigeon excrement, and chicken coops.[81, 82] Epidemics have been associated with construction and renovation sites, either through turning contaminated soil, or by working on sites where birds had been roosting.[83]

Clinical Features. The most common manifestation of histoplasmosis is a subclinical pulmonary infection, usually because of small exposure source and normal patient immunity. Massive inhalation can lead to acute pneumonia. Serious sequelae include chronic cavitating and fibrosing pulmonary infection, sclerosing mediastinitis, and disseminated infection with bone marrow and adrenal involvement. Prior to the AIDS epidemic, disseminated histoplasmosis was rarely seen, and then usually in elderly patients or those immunosuppressed by chemotherapy or hematologic malignancy. Disseminated disease is thought to be due to reinfection or, less frequently, reactivation of latent disease.[84] Cervical adenopathy, pharyngitis, tonsillitis, and ulcerating oral lesions may occur in disseminated AIDS cases.[85] Laryngeal histoplasmosis usually occurs in association with active pulmonary histoplasmosis, although it may also be seen in the absence of detectable lung infection.[86] Oropharyngeal histoplasmosis, on occasion, may precede disseminated infection. Oral histoplasmosis presents as extremely painful, indurated, ulcerating, or verrucous lesions that may erode underlying bone. Nodular masses may be seen in the oral cavity and larynx and exophytic lesions may clinically mimic carcinoma. Ulcerating facial lesions occur around the nose, mouth, and other sites.[87]

Pathologic Features. *Histoplasma* are 2 to 4 μm oval to spherical "intracellular and extracellular petite hematoxylinophilic bodies, each surrounded by a small halo."[88] The halo is due to cytoplasmic retraction from the capsule. Careful observation will reveal intracellular nuclei. A granulomatous reaction may be present. The overlying mucosa can be hyperplastic. Hematoxylin-eosin is the best stain to observe these organisms as it (1) emphasizes the intracellular site and (2) emphasizes the "halo" effect around each organism, allowing observation of the nuclei (Fig. 5–10). The organism does stain with Gomori's methenamine-silver, but the high background of this stain makes it unsuitable for evaluation. Periodic acid-Schiff will stain the organisms and their capsule with less background. The "halo" is not evident with either Gomori's methenamine-silver or periodic acid-Schiff stains. Solitary and multiple thin-necked budding may be seen. A touch preparation from a mucosal lesion is superior in revealing the fine morphology of *Histoplasma* and, if possible, should be an adjunct to tissue biopsy.

Differential Diagnosis. The histologic differential diagnosis includes other small intracellular organisms such as *Leishmania tropica* and *Leishmania mexicana* complex, *Trypanosoma cruzi,* poorly encapsulated *Cryptococcus,* and small tissue forms of *Blastomyces dermatitidis,* which may also cause mucocutaneous lesions. Laryngeal leishmaniasis (originally diagnosed as histoplasmosis) has been reported as a sequel of a cutaneous infection (Oriental sore).[89, 90]

Leishmania and *Trypanosoma* are within the same size range as *Histoplasma* but lack the prominent clear halo. *Leishmania* and *Trypanosoma* can be seen by hematoxylin-eosin and reticulin stains. *Histoplasma* is a round to oval organism; *Leishmania* and *Trypanosoma cruzi* have a diaper-pin shape. *Histoplasma* will stain with Gomori's methenamine-silver and periodic acid-Schiff stains, *Trypanosoma* and *Leishmania* will not. Also, both *Trypanosoma* and *Leishmania* have intracellular kinetoplasts, which are not visualized on hematoxylin-eosin sections but may be seen on Giemsa-stained

touch preparations. Poorly encapsulated *Cryptococcus* usually retains some mucinophilia and so may be distinguished from *Histoplasma. B. dermatitidis* may be distinguished from *Histoplasma* by its broad-based pattern of budding.

Treatment. The distinction between *Histoplasma* and *Leishmania* is particularly important in cases of disseminated infection, as the treatments are very different (antifungal agents versus antiprotozoal agents). Histoplasmosis can be treated with itraconazole, ketoconazole, or amphotericin B.

Laryngeal Rhinosporidiosis

Clinical Features. *Rhinosporidium seeberi* has a worldwide distribution but is endemic in India, Sri Lanka, Malaysia, Brazil, and Argentina. In the United States, cases have been reported from the rural South and West.[91–94] Preceding mucosal trauma (e.g., by digital contamination, dust storms) is considered necessary in establishing infection. Stagnant pools of water (e.g., bathing in the Ganges, humans and animals bathing together in ponds in the Durg district, Madhya Pradesh) have been associated with many cases. *Rhinosporidium* most commonly infects the nasal cavity, causing friable lobulated red or pink polyps that may become massive and extend posteriorly to fill and obstruct the nasopharynx, oropharynx, and hypopharynx. Conjunctival infection may also occur, usually after local injury. Endolaryngeal involvement by *Rhinosporidium* is secondary to nasopharyngeal involvement and can be seen as "satellite polyps."[95, 96]

Rhinosporidiosis will not grow on synthetic culture media; therefore, the diagnosis is dependent on tissue examination. The nature of *Rhinosporidium* is as yet unsettled. *Rhinosporidium* has only occasionally been successfully cultured in liquid media: only sporangia were formed.[97–99] One report claimed positive cultures in 24 of 25 patients with rhinosporidiosis, with the dimorphic growth of hyphal forms, consistent with the view that *Rhinosporidium* is a fungus.[100] Until these findings have been confirmed by others, it appears more likely that this report represents a consistent contaminant. Asworth noted that the thick cyst wall appears identical to that of cellulose, and its reaction with iodine and weak sulfuric acid is likewise identical.[99] He regarded the presence of a cyst pore and the cellulose-like nature of the wall to be consistent with a fungal classification. As rhinosporidiosis has been associated with stagnant pools of water, it was suggested that *Rhinosporidium* is an algae-like organism. The supporting data for this are rather weak. Spherules of an unknown nature had been identified ultrastructurally; one pos-

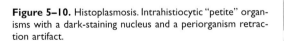

Figure 5–10. Histoplasmosis. Intrahistiocytic "petite" organisms with a dark-staining nucleus and a periorganism retraction artifact.

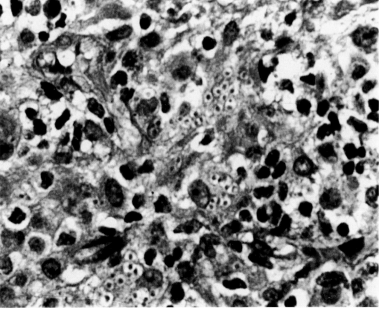

sible suggestion is that they may be chlorophyll precursors; however, important plant and algae components (protoplastids, plastids) were not identified.[101] Recent evidence suggests that *Rhinosporidium* may be related to the freshwater *Cyanobacterium* (blue green algae) *microcystis;* however, further study is warranted.[102]

Pathologic Features. In hematoxylin-eosin stained tissue, an intense acute and lymphoplasmacytic infiltrate is present. Submucosal cysts (also referred to as spherules or sporangia) are numerous, round, large (100–350 μm), and thick-walled (Fig. 5–11, see p. 246). This thick cyst wall stains with hematoxylin-eosin, Gomori's methenamine-silver, digested periodic acid-Schiff, and mucicarmine and is birefringent. The most mature, largest cysts are closest to the mucosal surface. Hundreds to thousands of small (2 to 9 μm) spores are seen within mature cysts. (see Fig. 5–11) The spores are initially uninuclear and range in size from 10 to 100 μm in diameter, but upon maturation are multinucleated, forming clusters of 12 to 16 "naked nuclei." Mitotic figures within these spores are infrequently observed. Upon maturation, the cysts extrude the "spore morulas" into the surrounding tissue from a pore. In cases of disseminated rhinosporidiosis, it is possible to find single spores in body fluids such as urine.

Differential Diagnosis. The differential diagnosis of *Rhinosporidium* is mainly with mucosal *Coccidioides immitis.* In fact, Seeber initially believed that *Rhinosporidium* was related to *C. immitis;* but its spherules are not as large (60 μm), its walls are not as thick, birefringent, or mucinophilic, and its endospores are not as numerous. If one sees only the extruded mature spores, which range from 2 to 9 μm in diameter, one might consider all other yeast forms within that range.

Oncocytic schneiderian papilloma (OSP, or cylindrical cell papilloma) may also be confused histologically with rhinosporidiosis; however, the cysts are intramucosal for OSP and contain mucin and polymorphonuclear cells, versus the spore-filled submucosal cysts of the rhinosporidiosis.

Treatment. Surgical débridement is indicated for these polypoid lesions. There is no known medical agent to which *Rhinosporidium* is responsive.

Viral Infections

Laryngeal Cytomegalovirus Infection

Clinical Features. Cytomegalovirus, a double-stranded DNA herpesvirus of high worldwide prevalence, is trophic for endothelial cells, B and T lymphocytes, mononuclear cells, and salivary gland epithelium. Cytomegalovirus infection may be subclinical in healthy, nonimmunocompromised patients. In utero or neonatal infections, or infections in the AIDS population, can cause serious multiorgan infection involving lung, kidney, gastrointestinal tract, and retina. The larynx and trachea may be sites for ulcerative cytomegalovirus infections, in the absence of cytomegalovirus pneumonitis.[103–107] The clinical differential diagnosis of ulcerative laryngeal lesions in AIDS patients would also include candidal and herpetic infection, and may be resolved by tissue biopsy, touch preparation, or smear, plus cultures.

Vocal cord paralysis (without mucosal ulceration) has been seen due to laryngeal neuritis: cytomegalovirus inclusions have been demonstrated at autopsy within the recurrent laryngeal nerve.[108] Concomitant supraglottic diffuse large-cell lymphoma and cytomegalovirus epiglottitis have been reported.[109] Although cytomegalovirus is not firmly established as having oncogenic potential, it may reactivate latent Epstein-Barr virus infection, which is associated with lymphogenesis.

Pathologic Features. Cytomegalovirus cells can be seen in the endothelial cells adjacent to foci with ulceration. The "classic" cytomegalovirus-infected cell has a large pink intranuclear inclusion, surrounded by a clear halo and, less commonly, an amphophilic cytoplasmic inclusion (Fig. 5–12). The combination of intranuclear and intracytoplasmic inclusions is seen only once the viral infection undergoes a replicative phase, which occurs in a minority of infected cells.

Special Studies. Prior to replication, infected cells produce great quantities of immediate early antigens (IEA) and early antigens (EA), which may be detected immunohistochemically as intranuclear inclusions. This accentuates the importance of special studies in the absence of "classic" cytomegalovirus inclusions. This also explains the enhanced sensitivity to immunohistochemistry for EA as compared to in situ hybridization for cytomegalovirus genome in early infections lacking classic histology.

Differential Diagnosis. The characteristic appearance of productively infected cytomegalic cells, with their intranuclear and intracytoplasmic inclusions, leaves little room for other possibilities. However, in early infections, enlarged "funny-looking" cells are seen, which may raise the possibility of other infections such as herpes simplex virus (HSV) infection. Slowly resolving mucocutaneous herpetic ulcers and disseminated infection can occur in AIDS patients, and possibly extend to the hypopharynx and larynx. HSV-infected cell nuclei become enlarged and reveal peripheral chromatin beading and homogeneous ground-glass inclusions, which may be basophilic or "cleared out." Multinucleated HSV syncytial cells also contain intranuclear inclusions and cytoplasmic inclusions. The nuclei of these multinucleated cells may mold with each other, rather

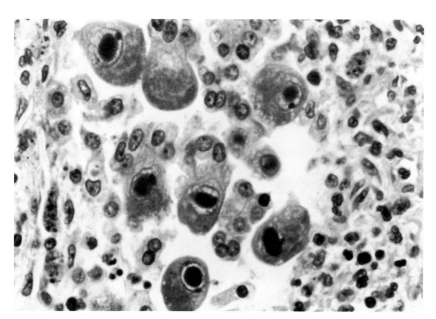

Figure 5–12. Cytomegalic cell with classic large intranuclear inclusion with a peri-inclusion halo, abundant cytoplasm with fine inclusions indicative of late, productive infection. Cells that have early, preproductive infection are not as large and lack the pronounced intranuclear and cytoplasmic inclusions.

than overlap. Immunohistochemistry on formalin-fixed paraffin-embedded biopsies for HSV 1 and HSV 2 and cytomegalovirus antigens can be helpful in making the distinction between HSV and cytomegalovirus infections.

Treatment. Gancyclovir or foscarnet may be used to treat cytomegalovirus laryngitis.

Protozoal Infections

Trichinella

Clinical Features. *Trichinella*, a nematode commonly found in temperate zones, is transmitted by ingestion of smoked, preserved, or inadequately cooked or frozen infected meat. Heating meat to at least 60°C for 30 minutes per pound, or deep-freezing it for at least 3 weeks at −15°C will kill the parasites. Owing to current meat regulations in the United States, most current cases of trichinosis can be traced to noncommercial, home-slaughtered meats. Cases are usually due to pork ingestion, but other meats such as bear, horse, wallaby, and kangaroo have caused trichinosis.[110]

Most cases of trichinosis are self-limited; severity generally depends on inoculum size. A patient with trichinosis initially presents with fever, nausea, vomiting, headache, fatigue, and diarrhea. After migration from the host's small intestine, the initial site of infestation, *Trichinella* becomes encysted in skeletal muscle. *Trichinella* especially favors muscles with a rich blood supply, such as the extraocular muscles, intrinsic laryngeal muscles, diaphragm, and deltoid and gastrocnemius muscles. After the first week, the symptoms correspond to peripheral migration of the larvae into muscle: they include periorbital or facial edema, myositis, blurry vision, and peripheral eosinophilia. Eye movement and swallowing may be painful and there is profound diffuse muscle weakness. Parasite invasion into the lungs, heart, and central nervous system is infrequent and fatalities are rare. The parasite alters the myocyte intracellular environment so that both can remain viable for years. Accordingly, *Trichinella* may be an incidental finding, many years after infection in the sternocleidomastoid muscle of radical neck dissections, or in laryngectomy specimens.[111, 112]

Pathologic Features. The larvae appear as a tightly coiled worm within an intramuscular double-walled capsule. If the larvae are missed on muscle biopsy because of sampling error, nonspecific myositis may be seen. Calcified cysts denote remote infection.

Treatment. If *Trichinella* is an incidental finding in a laryngectomy specimen, no treatment is indicated. Steroids may be used for relief of the acute migratory symptoms, plus mebendazole.

Schistosoma

Schistosoma is a parasitic blood fluke. *Schistosoma mansoni* is endemic to Africa, South America, the West Indies, and Puerto Rico; *Schistosoma japonicum* is endemic to China, Japan, and the Philippines; *Schistosoma haematobium* is endemic to the Nile Valley and India; *Schistosoma mekongi* is endemic to the Mekong River basin in Cambodia; and *Schistosoma intercalatum* is endemic to Western and Central Africa. *Schistosoma* derives its name ("split body") from the fact that the male parasite's body curves in ventrally to form an enclosed gynecophoral canal, in which the female fluke "reposes."[113] *Schistosoma* enters the host in the aqueous larval stage (cercaria) by penetrating the skin, which causes intense pruritus. They migrate to the vasculature and are carried to the nutritious hepatic portal system, where they mature and produce eggs. The eggs, as well as dead flukes, evoke severe chronic granulomatous inflammation and fibrosis in the liver and intestines *(S. mansoni, S. japonicum)*, and rectum, bladder, and pelvis *(S. haematobium)*. Occasional cases of laryngeal involvement by *Schistosoma* have been reported.[114–116]

Pathologic Features. The ova of *Schistosoma* may be calcified and are usually within a granulomatous reaction or in receding inflammation. *S. mansoni* and *S. haematobium* ova are elongate and oval. *S. mansoni* has a prominent, pointed lateral spine, *S. haematobium* a prominent terminal spine. *S. japonicum* ova are rounder and "plumper" than *S. mansoni* and *S. haematobium* ova, with a small lateral spine.

Leishmania

Leishmaniasis is a protozoan infection transmitted to humans and animals through the bites of *Phlebotomus* sandflies. In tropical and subtropical areas, the animal population maintains the disease reservoir. There are three forms of infection: cutaneous, mucocutaneous, and visceral leishmaniasis. Cutaneous leishmaniasis (Oriental sore, tropical sore) is endemic to Central and Eastern Asia, the Middle East, India, Central Africa, and Central and South America. Mucocutaneous leishmaniasis *(Leishmania braziliensis)* is endemic to Central and South America. It usually follows late in the course of cutaneous leishmaniasis. Visceral leishmaniasis (Kala-Azar) *(Leishmania donovani)* is endemic in Italy, Sicily, Greece, Turkey, China, India, South America, and Africa. Infection with *L. donovani* results in intrahistiocytic infection affecting liver, spleen, bone marrow, lymph nodes, heart, and kidneys and causing weight loss, hepatosplenomegaly, anemia, and thrombocytopenia.

Pathologic Features. Isolated ulcerating lesions may develop in the oropharyngeal nasal and laryngeal mucosa, as well as in the anogenital mucosa. Mucocutaneous leishmaniasis is characterized by surface ulceration, dense lymphoplasmacytic infiltrates with necrosis, and granulation tissue. The leishmanial amastigotes are seen within histiocytes under oil immersion. The number of amastigotes varies with host immunity status: tissues from patients with isolated lesions and adequate immunity will reveal epithelioid histiocytes and sparse organisms, whereas those from anergic patients with diffuse involvement will reveal foamy macrophages with abundant amastigotes.

Vocal Cord Nodules/Polyps/Contact Ulcers

Clinical Features. Vocal cord nodules (also called laryngeal nodules, or singer's, preacher's, or screamer's nodes) are nonneoplastic stromal reactions occurring in Reinke's space, an area normally devoid of vessels.[117–124] They are usually related to trauma due to misuse or excess vocal abuse (hence screamer's nodules or singer's nodules), although other factors, such as smoking, may also play some role.[121] Polyps have a male predominance and are usually unilateral; by contrast, vocal nodules are usually bilateral and symmetrical, with a female predominance. Vocal cord polypoid degeneration, or Reinke's edema, causes bilateral diffuse vocal polyps in the middle-aged to elderly population; it is unrelated to vocal abuse but associated with smoking. From a histopathologic standpoint, these entities have a similar appearance and so are discussed together.

These lesions may be seen in any age group, but most patients are 20 to 60 years of age. The most frequent symptom is hoarseness or voice change. The involved site is the vibratory surface of the true vocal cord, usually the junction of the anterior and middle third, which is the point of maximum vibratory impact (Fig. 5–13A, see p. 246). Occasionally, polyps may originate from adjacent ventricular fold or cavity, and rarely they may be associated with hypothyroidism. They may appear gray or white, translucent, sessile, or polypoid, and usually measure a few millimeters in diameter.

Contact ulcers (contact granulomas) are distinguished from vocal cord nodules/polyps in that they occur on the vocal process of the arytenoids, as a result of forceful apposition during vocalization. They may be unilateral or bilateral (Fig. 5–13B, see p. 246). They occur with a male predominance, characteristically in lawyers, salesmen, managers, and preachers (hence, preacher's nodules) who must affect a deep, low-frequency, forceful voice.

Pathologic Features. Microscopically, vocal cord nodules and polyps are characterized by the finding of a sparsely cellular stromal change, either myxoid or edematous, fibrous, vascular, and fibrinous or hyaline, underlying the stratified squamous epithelium (Fig.

5–13C). Dilated vascular spaces or foci of hemorrhage may be present. Inflammatory cell infiltrates are infrequent, and glandular elements are absent. The squamous epithelium may be normal, atrophic, or keratotic[117–121] or at times dysplastic. Ulceration is infrequent. The presence of atypical stromal cells has been sporadically observed in vocal cord polyps.[125]

Gray et al.[120] found two patterns of injury in these laryngeal lesions as indicated by deposition of fibronectin and type IV collagen on immunohistochemical study. One pattern showed prominent fibronectin deposition in the superficial lamina propria with thick collagen type IV bands, indicating basement membrane injury. The other pattern showed rare injury to the basement membrane zone and little fibronectin deposition.

Differential Diagnosis. When prominent, the myxoid stromal change may be mistaken for a myxoma, and the hyaline variant for laryngeal amyloid. Myxomas are extremely rare in the larynx (Fig. 5–14, see p. 247).[126] Amyloid deposits tend to be more nodular and may even be associated with the presence of a granulomatous reaction with multinucleated giant cells. The usual stains for amyloid, namely Congo red, crystal violet, or thioflavine T, are negative in vocal cord nodules (polyps), and, therefore, the possibility of amyloid can be easily excluded when suspected. Systemic diseases such as hypothyroidism and mucopolysaccharidosis may cause diffuse, edematous laryngeal thickening with deposition in the lamina propria.[127]

Treatment and Prognosis. Treatment for vocal nodules is voice therapy to eliminate the source of voice abuse. Vocal polyps are excised. These lesions have a benign clinical course but may persist if the etiologic factors remain.

Cysts: Laryngoceles/Saccular Cysts/Dermoid Cysts

Laryngeal cysts can be divided into three categories: (1) they can be mucin-filled, arising from minor salivary ducts (ductal cysts: squamous, oncocytic, or "tonsillar"); (2) they may result from obstruction of the saccule (saccular cysts); or (3) they may be air-filled pulsion diverticulum of the saccule (laryngocele). In a review of two decades of laryngeal cysts (190 cases) from the Mayo Clinic, ductal cysts were most commonly encountered (75%), usually in the vocal cords and lingual epiglottis.[128]

Laryngocele

The laryngeal ventricle (sinus of Morgagni) is the space, or "pocket," between the vocal fold (true cord) and the ventricular fold (false cord). The bilateral upward extension, or "cul-de-sac," of the ventricle is the laryngeal saccule. A laryngocele is the symptomatic dilation of the laryngeal saccule by entrapped air, that is, a pulsion diverticulum, which still communicates with the laryngeal lumen. A laryngocele may remain confined to the endolarynx (internal laryngocele) as a supraglottic submucosal bulge. It may also undermine the paraglottic space superiorly, protrude over the superior rim of the thyroid lamina, and herniate through the foramen of the superior laryngeal neurovascular bundle in the thyrohyoid membrane. This type of laryngocele (mixed external/internal, or foramina cyst) presents as an anterior neck mass (Fig. 5–15). It stands to reason that external laryngoceles must have some internal component and so may be termed "mixed" laryngoceles. Patients with internal and mixed laryngoceles complain of hoarseness, dyspnea, and chronic cough. Newborn infants with laryngoceles present with a feeble cry, difficulty in feeding, cough, and a neck mass.[129, 130] The air-filled nature of laryngoceles is easily confirmed on radiographic examination (see Fig. 5–15). Sometimes, laryngoceles undergo intermittent obstruction, and secretions will result in a mucus-filled sac. Coughing may clear the obstruction, dispelling the secretions. As long as a communication exists between the sac and the laryngeal lumen, this can still be classified as a laryngocele. A laryngopyocele is an ob-

structed laryngocele, or a saccular cyst, that has become secondarily infected.

Laryngoceles are usually unilateral, less often bilateral (see Fig. 5–15), and may be seen over a wide age range, from neonates to incidental autopsy findings in the middle-aged and elderly.[131] Only a small subset of patients with laryngoceles are engaged in activities involving increased intralaryngeal pressure (glass blowers, trumpet blowers). It is thought that asymptotically enlarged saccules may be prevalent in the general population and render persons more vulnerable to laryngocele formation. These enlarged saccules may be a phylogenous laryngeal remnant akin to primate lateral laryngeal air sacs.[132] MacFie[132] radiographically demonstrated a high incidence of asymptomatic laryngoceles (56%) occurring in 93 musicians (wind instrumentalists). These laryngoceles could be demonstrated upon forceful expiration with an open glottis (see Fig. 5–15) (a maneuver similar to playing a wind instrument), yet could not be demonstrated on forced exhalation with a closed glottis (Valsalva's maneuver).

Treatment. Laryngoceles are cured by simple excision. Histologically, they are lined by respiratory mucosa. Lymphoid tissue, as the inferior extension of Waldeyer's ring, may also be present. No other neck cyst would present as an air-filled cyst; therefore, this history is pathognomonic.

Saccular Cyst

A saccular cyst is a mucin-filled dilatation of the laryngeal saccule secondary to obstruction, either acquired or congenital in origin, analogous to a sinonasal mucocele. "Mucus under pressure points" and saccular cysts are no exception; they may point either medially or laterally. Medial saccular cysts obscure the anterior vocal fold but are limited in size and extension by the anterior commissure. Lateral saccular cysts point superior-laterally and, like external laryngoceles, may herniate through the thyrohyoid membrane and reach massive proportions if neglected (Fig. 5–16).[133]

Pathologic Features. Histologically, saccular cysts are lined by saccular mucosa—usually respiratory type, but occasionally squamous or oncocytic mucosa—and filled with mucinous material. This latter point distinguishes saccular cysts from laryngoceles. Saccular cysts may be indistinguishable from thyroglossal duct cysts, as remnant thyroid tissue may be absent from thyroglossal duct cysts. The majority of thyroglossal duct cysts are present in the anterior midline, inferior to the hyoid bone. However, rare thyroglossal duct cysts may push on the thyrohyoid membrane to encroach on the pre-epiglottic space.[134] In this case, one relies on the anatomic location to make the distinction between the two: the stalk or tract of a thyroglossal duct cyst is midline and should lead to the hyoid bone, whereas the stalk of a large saccular cyst is lateral and herniates through the thyrohyoid membrane. The differential diagnosis of saccular cysts may also include a branchial cleft cyst. The anatomic location of the duct or tract will also aid in the distinction. The tract of a branchial cleft cyst will not lead through the thyrohyoid membrane but will continue superiorly along the anterior border of the sternocleidomastoid muscle and may end at the angle of the mandible or in the tonsillar bed. Squamous cell carcinomas may also cause saccular obstruction resulting in a secondary mucocele, or laryngocele.[135]

Treatment. Saccular cysts and symptomatic mixed laryngoceles may be cured by surgical excision.

Ductal Cysts (Squamous, "Tonsillar," and Oncocytic)

Laryngeal cysts may also result from the blockage of a minor salivary gland duct. In this case, the cyst lining is actually the dilated ductal epithelium (Fig. 5–17, see p. 247). It may be squamous, oncocytic (see subsequent discussion on salivary lesions), or squamous with surrounding lymphoid stroma—referred to as "tonsillar" cysts.[136] Squamous cysts and oncocytic cysts have a predisposition for the

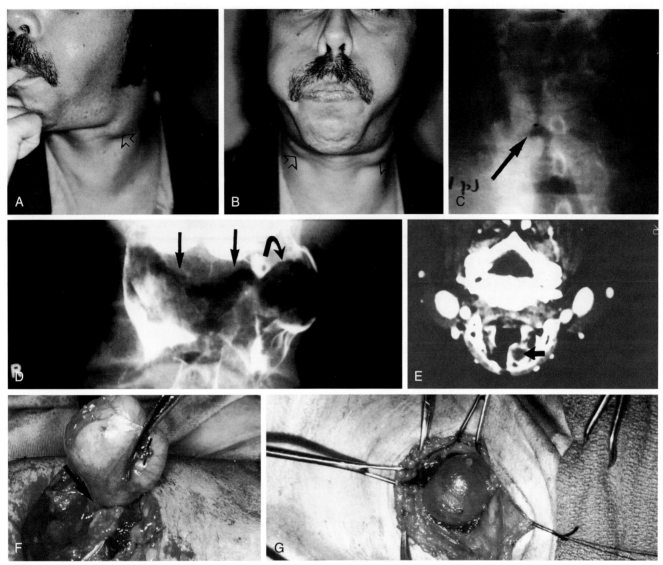

Figure 5–15. Laryngoceles: *A&B*, Bilateral upper neck masses *(arrows)* are seen on forceful expiration with an opened glottis. *C&D*, Plain radiographs demonstrate the internal and external air-filled components of these bilateral laryngoceles. Straight arrows indicate the internal component, the curved arrow indicates the external component. *E*, This air-filled cyst is confined to the endolarynx and therefore may be classified as an internal laryngocele. *F&G*, Delivery of two laryngoceles from an external cervical approach. The neck of the cyst may be seen in part *F (arrow)*. (Courtesy of Dr. Hugh Biller.)

Figure 5–16. *A&B*, Mucus-filled cyst of the anterior neck consistent with saccular cyst. The distinction with a thyroglossal duct cyst is made at the time of surgery by the location of the tract: the thyroglossal duct cyst tracks back to the hyoid bone, whereas the saccular cyst herniates through the thyrohyoid membrane.

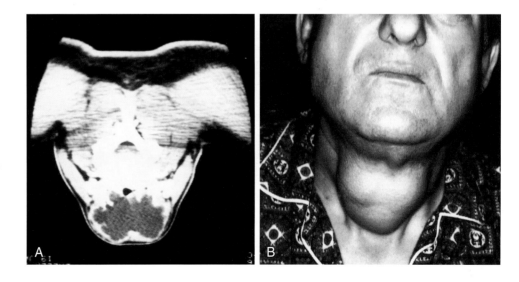

ventricular bands, ventricle, aryepiglottic folds and epiglottis.[137] Tonsillar cysts have a predisposition for the valecula—an area with tonsillar remnants.[136] Simple conservative excision is curative.

Other Laryngeal Cysts and Sinuses

Cysts such as epidermal inclusion cysts, dermoid cysts, and branchial cleft cysts may occur in the endolarynx. An epidermoid cyst, a keratin-filled cyst lined by stratified squamous mucosa, may be the result of a traumatic mucosal inclusion, or a congenital rest. More rare still are dermoid cysts, which contain skin adnexal structures and are purely mature benign growths of presumed congenital rests.[136] Branchial cleft anomalies primarily involving the supraglottis are extremely rare. The supraglottis is derived, embryologically, from branchial arches 3 and 4, whereas the glottic compartment is derived from arches 5 and 6. Fourth branchial pouch sinuses manifest as sinus tracts leading from the piriform to skin, or may follow the course of the left recurrent laryngeal nerve, into the mediastinum, and back to the cricothyroid joint ending in the piriform sinus. Retrograde excision, beginning at the piriform apex, ensures complete removal of the tract.[138, 139] Histologically, branchial cleft cysts can be lined by columnar epithelium, stratified squamous mucosa, or a combination of the two. Foamy histiocytes, cholesterol crystals, and inflammatory cells may be present within the cyst; a prominent lymphoid stroma usually accompanies the cyst lining.

Laryngeal Amyloidosis

Amyloidosis is the term applied to a diverse group of disorders that have in common the deposition of an amorphous, extracellular material in various tissues.[140, 141] The amyloid protein in these conditions is morphologically, histochemically, and ultrastructurally similar. By x-ray diffraction, amyloid fibers in general have a crossed beta-pleated sheet configuration that is responsible for the fibers specific staining properties. Previous classifications included primary or secondary systemic, myeloma-associated, localized, and hereditary-familial forms. However, because of the significant overlap in organ distribution and protein composition in these diverse disorders, the current classification of amyloidosis is based on the biochemical composition of its subunit protein. It is now recognized that the amyloid in primary systemic, myeloma-associated, and, more recently, upper aerodigestive localized amyloidosis is composed of immunoglobulin light chains (AL amyloid). The protein in secondary amyloidosis is composed of amyloid protein A (apolipoprotein, AA amyloid).

Amyloid localized to the upper aerodigestive tract is rare and most commonly affects the larynx or tongue.[142–147] In contrast to lingual amyloid, which is invariably part of a primary systemic or myeloma-associated amyloidosis, laryngeal amyloid is most often a localized form, and only rarely is it a component of systemic amyloidosis.

Clinical Features. Amyloid localized to the larynx presents as either a nodule or a diffusely infiltrating process (Fig. 5–18, see p. 247). Hoarseness is the most common symptom. The false cord is the single most common site of laryngeal amyloid, followed by the true vocal cord and the ventricle. Primary amyloid deposits can occur at any location within the larynx, however, and multiple sites of involvement are not unusual. In a recent study, Lewis et al.[144] found that the mean age of 22 patients with laryngeal amyloid was 56 years. The common sites were the false vocal cords (12 cases), ventricle (8 cases), infraglottis (8 cases), true vocal cords (6 cases), arytenoids and aryepiglottic folds (5 cases), and anterior commissure (3 cases). In 6 cases there was concomitant involvement of the trachea, usually when the infraglottis was involved. The diagnosis of laryngeal amyloidosis is established by biopsy.

Pathologic Features. Laryngeal amyloid usually presents as a firm polypoid lesion covered by an intact mucosa. Microscopically, amyloid is seen as a discrete nodular mass or a diffuse subepithelial deposit of amorphous eosinophilic material in the stroma, blood ves-

sel walls, or basement membranes of mucoserous glands resulting in atrophy (see Fig. 5–18). Amyloid may also be seen as hyaline "rings" around adipose tissue cells and may be associated with a granulomatous reaction surrounding nodular deposits. An associated infiltrate of plasma cells, lymphocytes, or histiocytes may be present. Histochemically, amyloid of any type can be confirmed by demonstrating the typical apple-green birefringence on polarized microscopy after staining with Congo red. Metachromasia on staining with crystal violet or thioflavine T immunofluorescence may also be used.

Special Studies. In a recent study of 20 cases, laryngeal amyloid was confirmed as a form of localized amyloid immunohistochemically characterized by monoclonal or light chains deposition (AL amyloid)[144] in 12 cases, with light chains in 5 and absence of light chains in 3. Most were positive for amyloid P component. Plasma cells in the interstitium showed polyclonal staining. Laryngeal amyloid was negative for amyloid A protein, prealbumin, and β_2-microglobulin. Ultrastructurally, amyloid is composed of linear, nonbranching fibers, 10 to 15 nm in width.

Differential Diagnosis. Laryngeal amyloid may be confused on routine sections for vocal cord nodules with hyalinized stroma; however, the diagnosis is easily made on Congo red stain because vocal cord nodules lack the apple-green birefringence. Localized amyloid should be distinguished from plasmacytoma that may be associated with amyloid.[145]

Treatment and Prognosis. Most patients with localized amyloid can be successfully treated by simple excision via direct laryngoscopy. In one study, recurrence or persistence of the laryngeal amyloid occurred in 60% of patients, usually within 5 years after initial therapy, although some had multiple recurrences more than 10 years later.[144] Recurrence is related to difficulty in removal of extensive, multifocal submucosal disease. In these cases, death may result from progressive tracheobronchial involvement; however, association with systemic amyloidosis is rare. The latter possibility can be excluded by Congo red stain of fine needle aspirates of abdominal fat, a simple, safe technique.[148]

Endotracheal Intubation

Clinical Features. Prolonged endotracheal intubation results in endolaryngeal pressure necrosis and ulceration. Vocal cord ulceration is a common complication of prolonged intubation; it was observed in 76% of 79 men intubated 3 to 58 days (mean 9 days), and it resolved in a mean of 4 weeks.[149] Granulation tissue (clinically referred to as granulomas) and scar formation may follow, impairing cord mobility. This directly correlates with duration of intubation and the use of a larger endotracheal tube.[149] Other possible intubation sequelae include arytenoid dislocation, synechia (dense scar), and transient unilateral or bilateral vocal cord paralysis (the latter resulting in post-extubation airway obstruction) as a result of pressure neuropraxis.[150] Focal infraglottic mucinosis has been described as a post-intubation sequela.[151]

Pathologic Features. Donnelly[152] described the sequelae of intubation in a series of 99 autopsy cases. The majority of damage is in the posterior larynx and the infraglottic region. The earliest changes, seen after 1 to 3 hours, were loss of epithelium of the posterior cricoid and vocal processes. Loss of basement membrane was seen after 4 to 6 hours. Between 12 and 48 hours, mucosal ulceration could be seen in the vocal processes and the infraglottis, with inflammation of the perichondrium. After 96 of hours intubation, the perichondrium of the vocal process and cricoid lamina were invariably exposed with cartilaginous "excavation." These changes can all be attributed to the constant pressure and abrasion of the tube, which moves with each respiration, against the relatively stationary larynx. Further, the endotracheal cuff, which is inflated against the trachea to prevent backflow of expressed air from the ventilator, will result in infraglottic erosion. Infraglottic stenosis and collapse are possible sequelae of this damage.

Persistent post-extubation hoarseness should lead to laryngoscopy. Biopsy will reveal hyperplastic mucosa, acute and chronic inflammation, and exuberant granulation tissue. A giant cell reaction or storiform fibroblastic proliferation may be seen. Dilated vessels may have a ramifying and staghorn appearance. Wenig and Heffner[153] have noted that these biopsies often may lead to diagnostic confusion with neoplastic processes, including hemangioma, hemangiopericytoma, angiosarcoma, inflammatory pseudotumor, squamous cell carcinoma, and verrucous carcinoma.

Focal mucinosis is rare and probably related to previous trauma. It appears as relatively avascular basophilic myxoid matrix within the lamina propria, with small spindled or stellate cells. Focal mucinosis lacks infiltrating borders and extensive reticulin and collagen fiber network, all features present in myxomas.[151]

Differential Diagnosis. Vocal cord ulcerations and changes due to vocal abuse or chronic gastroesophageal reflux may have similar histologies. Distinguishing contact ulcers from benign or malignant vascular tumors should not be difficult in light of a history of recent intubation. The proliferative squamous component with pseudoepitheliomatous hyperplasia may mimic squamous carcinoma and verrucous carcinoma. A pronounced inflammatory and granulation tissue component, as well as pertinent clinical history, should lead one to reconsider a malignant diagnosis in this situation.

Foreign Body Granulomas

In the early 1960s, the technique of injecting foreign material into the vocal fold for the treatment of vocal cord paralysis was introduced. Material such as Teflon was injected into the lateral thyroarytenoid muscle tissue of the paralyzed vocal fold, to bring it toward the midline. Medializing a paralyzed vocal fold results in a more complete glottic closure on cord adduction and may fortify a "breathy" voice and improve vocal quality. However, misplaced injections or over-injections can cause symptomatic foreign body granulomas. The clinician may recognize these masses as being secondary to Teflon, or may assume the presence of malignancy. Teflon migration into the neck may also simulate malignancy.

Pathologic Features. One sees foreign body giant cell reaction with typical multinucleated giant cells. Asteroid-type bodies may be seen.[154] The intracellular and extracellular Teflon is abundant, colorless, glass-like, refractile, and amorphous material that polarizes (Fig. 5–19). Dense fibroconnective tissue accumulates over time, apparently peaking and remaining unchanged after 6 months.[154] Teflon may also migrate from the endolarynx and be detected in cervical lymph nodes. The nature of this material can be confirmed by dispersive x-ray analysis, which shows peaks for carbon and fluorine, or infrared absorption spectrophotometry, which reveals fluorocarbon bonds. The differential diagnosis includes other foreign materials that may, historically, have been injected for symptomatic relief of unilateral vocal cord paralysis. This may include paraffin, cartilage, bone, silicon, Gelfoam, glycerin, tantalum oxide, and tantallym powder.[154–156] Injection of these materials has been abandoned, however.

Treatment. Conservative excision of the foreign body–induced granulation tissue is indicated for relief of upper airway symptoms. To date, no case of foreign body–induced malignancy after Teflon injection has been reported.

Sarcoidosis

Clinical Features. Sarcoidosis is most often diagnosed between the second and fourth decade of life and is more common in women. The highest incidences are seen in Sweden, Norway, the Netherlands, and England. In the United States, it is tenfold more common among African-Americans than whites and is most prevalent in the Southeast. There is an increased incidence in people who have migrated from the South. Generally, there is an inverse relationship between susceptibility to *Mycobacteria tuberculosis* and sarcoid: sarcoid is virtually nonexistent among populations with a high susceptibility to *Mycobacteria tuberculosis* (Eskimos, Indians, and Chinese).[157, 158]

Patients may present with lymphadenopathy, hepatosplenomegaly, pulmonary, arthritic, and ocular symptoms or nonspecific symptomatology such as fever, malaise, weight loss, and erythema nodosum. Yet others are totally asymptomatic and the diagnosis will be picked up on an incidental chest radiograph, which reveals enlarged hilar lymph nodes and a diffuse pulmonary reticular pattern. Among those clinically symptomatic individuals, the majority of patients follow a self-limiting course, the disease "burns out," usually within 2 years. Fewer individuals will progress to severe pulmonary fibrosis and renal involvement.

The anterior or posterior cervical lymph nodes are most commonly involved in the head and neck. Extranodal head and neck involvement can be seen in 38% of sarcoid patients—usually ophthalmic manifestations. Less commonly, the parotid gland, lacrimal gland, and upper respiratory tract submucosa may be involved. Laryngeal involvement, which occurs in up to 5% of patients with sarcoidosis, results in upper airway symptoms such as progressive dyspnea or upper airway obstruction.[159] The lamina propria of the supraglottis appears preferentially involved. The mucosa may be edematous and "boggy" or reveal granular coalescent fleshy nodules in the epiglottis, arytenoids, or aryepiglottic folds.[160, 161] At later stages, the mucosa appears fibrotic. There is no tendency toward ulceration. The vocal folds seem to be spared, which may relate to the relative paucity of lymphatics in the vocal cords. Vocal cord paralysis may occur, usually in the setting of polyneuritis, although recurrent laryngeal nerve compression by mediastinal adenopathy has been proposed as another mechanism.[159, 162]

The exact etiologic agent of sarcoidosis is uncertain, but the current evidence points to sarcoidosis being the result of infection by an L-form atypical mycobacterium of limited pathogenicity in a susceptible population. Moscovic[163] studied the Hamazaki-Wesenberg inclusions in great detail by histochemistry and electron microscopy; he concluded that these pleomorphic, spindled, almond-shaped and round bodies with electron-dense cores (nucleoids) were consistent with mycobacterial L-forms resulting from bacteriophage infection.

Mycobacterium avium complex, *Mycobacterium paratuberculosis* sequences, and *M. paratuberculosis*–related antigen (36K antigen) have been detected in specimens and isolated by culture from sarcoid patients, further implicating mycobacteria as causative agents for susceptible populations.[164]

Pathologic Features. Sarcoid granulomas are characteristically small, nonconfluent, non-necrotic, and densely hyalinized. Rarely, however, they may be associated with necrosis. The pathologist must then rule out *M. tuberculosis* or fungal infection through multiple cultures and histologic studies. Pathognomonic features of sarcoid include asteroid bodies, Schaumann bodies, and Hamazaki-Wesenberg inclusions. Asteroid bodies are star-like crystalline inclusions seen within multinucleated giant cells. Schaumann described calcified laminated concretions within multinucleated giant cells of patients with sarcoid.[165] Akin to Michaelis-Gutmann bodies, Schaumann bodies may be the result of degenerating organisms. Hamazaki-Wesenberg inclusions are seen within histiocytes, unrelated to granulomas, and are round (coccoid), oval, or rod-shaped golden-brown inclusions, 3 to 15 μm in greatest dimension, which autoflouresce with ultraviolet light and may also stain with Ziehl-Neelsen and the intensified Kinyoun stains.

Differential Diagnosis. Sarcoid granulomas are not entirely specific: in addition to tuberculosis and fungal infections, they may be observed with rheumatoid arthritis,[166] and also can be seen in lymph nodes adjacent to malignancy. Despite the characteristic appearance, the diagnosis of sarcoidosis should remain an exclusionary one, to be rendered only after ancillary studies rule out infection.

Treatment and Prognosis. The majority of patients with sarcoidosis do not require therapy, and they undergo spontaneous remission. Parenteral steroid therapy is indicated for airway compro-

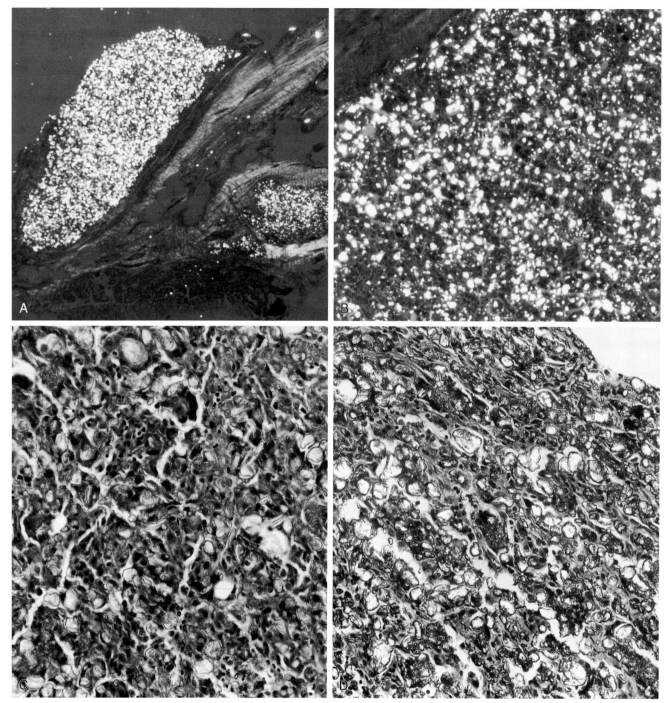

Figure 5–19. Teflon granuloma as viewed with polarized microscopy *(A,B,&C)* and by conventional light microscopy *(D)*. Note prominent polarization of teflon intermixed with numerous histiocytes and chronic inflammatory cells.

mise. Intralaryngeal steroid injection may be attempted for chronically inflamed mucosa.

Gout

Gout is the metabolic disorder resulting from hyperuricemia. Uric acid is the end product of the metabolism of purines—part of the nucleic acid backbone. Primary gout may be due to increased uric acid production (e.g., increased dietary uric acid from purine-rich food such as meat, sweetbread, anchovies or in the face of an inherent biochemical defect). Secondary gout may be caused by decreased urinary uric acid excretion (lead poisoning,[167] lead ne-

phropathy [saturnine gout], thiazide diuretics) or purine overproduction due to increased cell turnover (myeloproliferative diseases). There is a pronounced male predisposition.

Clinical Features. Acute arthritic gout is episodic, monoarticular, and self-limiting. Acute episodes may be provoked by alcohol ingestion or medication (diuretics, insulin, and penicillin). Sodium urate crystal deposition in a synovial space results in an acutely inflamed and exquisitely tender joint. The large toe is most commonly involved (podagra); other joints (fingers, wrists, and elbows) may be involved. Symptomatic urate crystal deposition leads to acute or chronic arthritis. Chronic gout results from the long-term deposition of sodium urate crystals, usually in distal, cooler sites, resulting in pathognomonic tophi.

In the head and neck, gouty tophi present as asymptomatic depositions seen on the outer helix of the pinna; other head and neck sites, like the larynx, are less frequent. Guttenplan et al.[168] collected eight cases, plus one observed by him, of laryngeal gout, although it is suspected that more cases go unreported, and even more unrecognized. The cricoarytenoid joint,[169] vocal folds,[170] ventricles, and infraglottis may be involved sites. Involvement of the cricoarytenoid joint may result in hoarseness, pain, dysphagia, and cord fixation. Clinically, the deposits may appear as an exophytic papillary lesion, with a fixed vocal cord, mimicking carcinoma,[171] and a discrete spur on the vocal fold,[172] or as grains or specks on the mucosal surface.[167]

Pathologic Features. On gross examination, gouty tophi are filled with cheesy, curd-like material. Microscopically, tophi appear as large deposits of amorphous, amphophilic material with surrounding foreign body reaction, foamy histiocytes, and lymphoplasmacytic infiltrates (Fig. 5–20). The urate crystals may be seen as closely packed birefringent, needle-like structures. They are best observed in ethanol-fixed tissue, as the urate crystals dissolve out in aqueous fixatives such as formalin. The massive urate deposition in the cricoarytenoid joint results in destruction of the articular cartilage and fibroinflammatory joint fixation.[169]

Differential Diagnosis. Other deposits such as amyloid or Teflon may be considered in the differential diagnosis. Amyloid is more eosinophilic, rather than amphophilic, with areas of varying density. Although a scattering of lymphoplasmacytic cells might be present, the intense histiocytic and foreign body giant cell infiltrate of a tophus is not seen. Injected foreign material (Teflon, paraffin) will not pick up stain, and appears as refractile noncrystalline material or as empty space in the tissue.

Treatment. Acute episodes of gout may be treated with colchicine and nonsteroidal anti-inflammatory drugs. Chronic hyperuricemia is managed by avoiding provocative agents such as alcohol, purine-rich foods, aspirin, and diuretics. Allopurinol, a xanthine oxidase inhibitor, or probenecid, a uricosuric agent, can be used to manage, and prevent, the sequelae of chronic hyperuricemia.

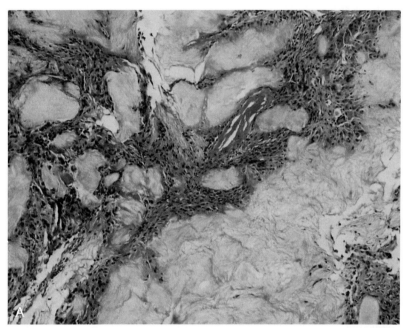

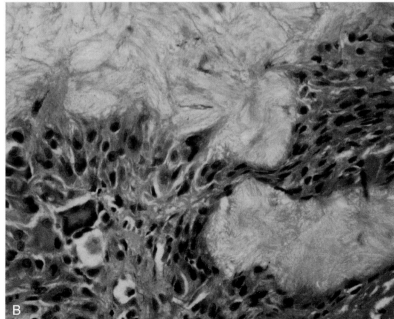

Figure 5–20. Gouty tophus. *A,* Low power view of large deposits of amorphous material with intense foreign body reaction. *B,* High power view. The urate deposition has a fibrillary appearance, unlike amyloid, which is more amorphous (see Fig. 5–18). The inflammatory reaction is greater in gouty tophus than in amyloid.

Autoimmune Diseases and Diseases of Uncertain Mechanisms

Rheumatoid Arthritis

Rheumatoid arthritis (RA) is an autoimmune-mediated polyarticular arthritis with a female predominance. The majority of patients with RA are serum-positive for rheumatoid factor (RF), which represents autoantibodies against the Fc fragment of IgG (anti-idiotype antibodies). RF is not specific for RA, as it may also be elevated in other autoimmune illnesses such lupus erythematosus, pernicious anemia, Hashimoto's thyroiditis, and nonautoimmune chronic illnesses. The synovium is the primary target of RA, which becomes hyperplastic, papillary, and villiform (pannus) in the face of a chronic lymphoplasmacytic infiltrate. The pannus acts to erode the articular surfaces of the joint space. Rheumatoid nodules are necrotizing inflammatory nodules that may form in soft tissues adjacent to joints, skin and tendons, extensor surfaces, and bony prominences and within visceral organs such as heart, lungs, and gastrointestinal tract. Like RF, rheumatoid nodules may be seen in other autoimmune diseases.

Clinical Features. Upper airway laryngeal symptoms are common in patients with RA. Laryngeal symptoms have been noted in 26% of patients with generalized RA.[173] A female predominance is seen. Cricoarytenoid involvement can cause joint fixation, resulting in hoarseness, exertional dyspnea, and stridor. Patients may complain of a sensation of a foreign body in their throat. Speaking, coughing, or swallowing may elicit pain, as does anterior pressure on the larynx. On examination, the arytenoid mound is erythematous and edematous.[174] The cords may be fixed and immobile to manipulation. Arytenoid fixation and edema may cause acute upper airway obstruction.[175] Rheumatoid nodules in the vocal cord soft tissues have also been reported in RA.[176]

Pathologic Features. The cricoarytenoid joint may reveal pannus (cloak-like) formation of the synovium with synovial papillary hyperplasia and dense lymphoplasmacytic infiltrates, often with germinal center formation. Uniarticular or bilateral joint involvement may be seen. The articular surface may be destroyed and reveal an irregular widened joint space filled with fibrous adhesions.[173] Rheumatoid nodules may be present in the soft tissue adjacent to the joint or in the vocal fold. They are characterized by areas of fibrinoid necrosis rimmed by pallisading macrophages and other chronic inflammatory cells.

Differential Diagnosis. Cricoarytenoid fixation, mucosal swelling, and rheumatoid nodules are not specific findings for RA; they may be seen in other autoimmune illnesses such as lupus erythematosus. Discovering a rheumatoid nodule will at least categorize the disease process as autoimmune. If necrosis were seen in vocal cord biopsy, it would still be wise to rule out acid-fast bacilli and fungal organisms.

Treatment. There is a step-wise progression for the therapy of RA, based on disease severity. Salicylates and nonsteroidal anti-inflammatory drugs can be used as a first-line regimen to reduce joint symptoms. Hydrochloroquine has been moderately effective for early RA. Unrelenting disease can be treated with gold injections, penicillamine, and immunosuppressive drugs such as methotrexate and azathioprine, all of which have significant toxicities. Corticosteroids may be used, episodically, in conjunction with the above drugs. RA of the cricoarytenoid joint may be treated with laser arytenoidectomy, or by fixation of the arytenoid in abduction using a wire, thereby increasing the glottic airway space and improving symptoms.

Lupus Erythematosus

Lupus erythematosus (LE) is an autoimmune disease characterized by autoantibodies to double-stranded DNA and nuclear histones. The circulating immune complexes deposit within vessel walls and along skin and mucosal basement membranes and elicit an inflammatory cascade. LE primarily affects the skin, joints, kidneys, nervous system, and mucous membranes—usually intraorally. LE tends to affect younger individuals, in the third and fourth decades of life, with a pronounced female predominance. Patients complain of polyarthralgias, malar rash, photosensitivity, fever, and malaise. Pulmonary involvement may take the form of pleural effusions, pleuritis, capillaritis, vasculitis, and pulmonary hypertension. Pericarditis, myocarditis, coronary vasculitis, and valvular dysfunction may occur. Glomerulonephritis may progress to renal insufficiency. The neurologic manifestations of LE include seizure disorder, transverse myelitis, and emotional disturbances.

Clinical Features. Laryngeal involvement in LE is thought to be underappreciated, but may occur in as many as one third of patients with LE.[177] The laryngeal findings may be similar to those of RA—hoarseness, decreased cricoarytenoid mobility, and rheumatoid nodules. Acute symptoms include hypopharyngeal and laryngotracheal edema; oral, hypopharyngeal, and supraglottic ulceration, or an inflammatory mass obstructing the upper airway. The mucosal edema, especially of the epiglottis, may necessitate intubation.[177] Sequelae include laryngitis sicca, laryngeal scarring, vocal cord paralysis, and infraglottic stenosis.[178] Superimposed infectious laryngitis, unresponsive solely to corticosteroids, may also occur in LE; therefore, bacterial and fungal cultures are important at the time of laryngoscopy. Although laryngeal symptoms usually occur during active, generalized lupus, occasionally vocal cord rheumatoid nodules or infraglottic stenosis may be the initial presentation for LE (Fig. 5–21).[178, 179]

Vocal cord paralysis in LE may be due to either cricoarytenoid arthritis or joint fixation, or to neurogenic causes. The distinction between neurogenic origin versus joint fixation may be made by the clinician at the time of laryngoscopy: if the arytenoid is freely mobile upon spatula palpation, then the joint obviously is not fixed, and the vocal cord paralysis has a neurogenic etiology. This paralysis may be due to compression of the left recurrent laryngeal nerve (RLN) as a result of dilated pulmonary arteries secondary to lupus-associated pulmonary hypertension. The left RLN may be compressed between the engorged left pulmonary artery and the aortic arch, as it wraps around it to return to the neck.[180] As additional indirect proof, (1) six of the seven patients with unilateral paralysis in Teitel et al.'s review had left-sided vocal cord paralysis, (2) pulmonary hypertension was present in three of these patients, and (3) the paralysis did not respond to steroids in four of these cases.[177] Recurrent laryngeal nerve palsy in systemic LE may also be the result of other mechanisms, such as vasculitis.[181] However, there has been no documented case of vasculitis of the vasa vasorum of the vagus nerve or RLN.

Serologically, patients may have positive rheumatoid factor and antinuclear antibodies such as anti-double stranded DNA, and anti-Smith antibodies, which are specific for LE. Drug-induced systemic LE may occur secondary to a number of drugs (procainamide, hydralazine, isoniazid, methyl-dopa, quinidine, chlorpromazine) usually in patients who are slow drug acetylators, have received large daily doses of the drug, or, in the case of hydralazine-induced lupus, have the HLA-DR4 genotype. Laryngeal lupus secondary to drug-induced LE (hydralazine hoarseness) has been described.[182] The mechanism of hydralazine-induced LE is uncertain, but hydrazine metabolites have been shown to induce and stabilize conformational DNA changes (Z-DNA conformation), which may then elicit formation of anti-DNA antibodies.[183]

Pathologic Features. The rheumatoid nodules seen in LE are identical to those of RA. Hematoxylin bodies or LE cells, when seen, are fairly specific for LE (Fig. 5–22, see p. 248). Hematoxylin bodies are enlarged, amphophilic "naked" nuclei. The nuclear chromatin, which has been exposed to antinuclear antibodies, appears homogeneous, without morphology. LE cells are mononuclear cells that have engulfed these hematoxylin bodies and now appear as large amphophilic cytoplasmic inclusions. Both hematoxylin bodies and LE cells stain strongly with the Feulgen stain.

Fibrinoid vasculitis is another histologic hallmark of LE. The vasculitis affects small and medium-sized arteries, and one sees varying degrees of vessel wall replacement by amorphous fibrinous

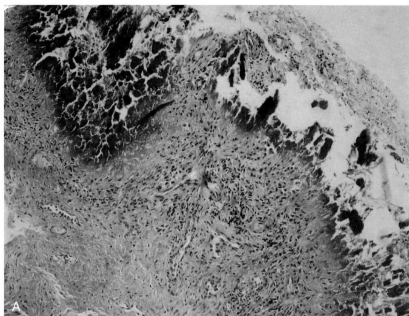

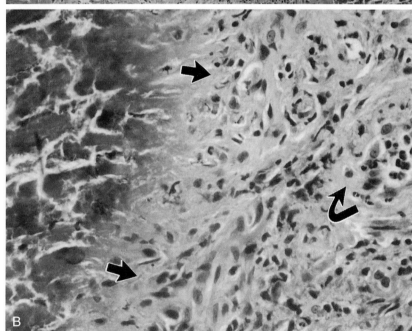

Figure 5–21. Laryngeal rheumatoid nodule as a presenting finding in lupus erythematosis. *A*, Zones of fibrinoid necrosis. *B*, Fibrinoid necrosis (left) with rimming of histiocytes *(small arrows)* and leukocytoclastic vasculitis *(curved arrow)*.

material. Perivascular edema and acute and chronic inflammatory infiltrates are seen. Teitel et al.[177] searched the literature for cases of LE with laryngeal involvement and found definitive evidence of necrotizing vasculitis in only 2 of 24 cases.

Differential Diagnosis. In the absence of hematoxylin bodies or LE cells, the histology may be indistinguishable from RA. Vasculitis is not specific for LE and may also be seen in relapsing polychondritis, Wegener's granulomatosis, polyarteritis nodosum, and RA. Superimposed infectious laryngitis may also be present and should be considered when evaluating biopsies. *Nocardia* laryngitis has been reported in LE patients.[184] *Nocardia* are filamentous bacteria that do not stain well with hematoxylin-eosin stain but are best seen with a modified Ziehl-Neelsen stain. Chronic mucosal inflammation may be reminiscent of the early stages of scleroma.

Cricoarytenoid fixation may be seen in rheumatoid arthritis, gout, Reiter's syndrome, costochondritis (Tietze's syndrome), traumatic arytenoid subluxation, and infections such as gonorrhea, syphilis, and mumps. Infraglottic stenosis may also be a sequel

of relapsing polychondritis, Wegener's granulomatosis, previous trauma, prolonged endotracheal intubation, tracheopathica-chondro-osteoplastica, perichondritis of syphilis, and severe pulmonary/tracheal infections such as tuberculosis, scleroma, and histoplasmosis.

Treatment and Prognosis. Corticosteroids are the mainstay of controlling active disease. Most cases of lupus laryngitis will resolve with corticosteroid immunosuppression. Epinephrine inhalation may also be necessary for acute laryngeal edema, and patients may require emergency tracheostomy for airway management. Superimposed infection should be considered for cases nonresponsive to immunosuppression. Laryngotracheal stenosis may be corrected with surgical reconstruction during quiescent periods.

Wegener's Granulomatosis

Clinical Features. Wegener's granulomatosis (WG) is a systemic necrotizing vasculitis that affects the upper and lower respiratory tract and also causes renal glomerulonephritis. Although the etiology currently remains unknown, circulating antineutrophil antibodies are present in the vast majority of patients during active disease and can be helpful in establishing diagnosis. WG has a male predominance, and the disease usually presents at the fifth decade of life onward. Involvement of the head and neck is common, either in the classic, multisystem form of WG or in the less intense form limited to the upper airway. Upper respiratory symptoms include severe chronic sinusitis. Nasal septal collapse leads to a saddle nose deformity. Otologic manifestations include serous otitis media, otitis externa, and sensorineural loss. Oropharyngeal ulcerative inflammation and hyperplastic gingivitis may occur. Laryngotracheal disease may be seen in up to one quarter of patients with WG, and rarely may be a presenting symptom of WG.[185] Endoscopically, the infraglottis appears erythematous and indurated. Laryngotracheal involvement can lead to intractable infraglottic stenosis requiring tracheostomy for airway maintenance. Patients with juvenile-onset WG were found to be five times more likely to develop infraglottic stenosis than adult-onset WG patients.[186]

Pulmonary involvement commonly leads to cavitating necrotic lesions that radiologically may mimic carcinoma. Other pulmonary manifestations include interstitial fibrosis, alveolar hemorrhage, bronchopneumonia, and bronchiolitis. Renal involvement occurs in 20% of patients, resulting in a crescentic glomerulonephritis. Patients may complain of rashes, migratory arthritis, and ocular, genitourinary, and gastrointestinal symptoms, all related to ischemic vasculitis. Cranial nerve deficits and posterior pituitary intracranial manifestations (diabetes insipidus) may also be seen.

Pathologic Features. The classic histologic triad of WG includes (1) granulomatous inflammation, (2) vasculitis, and (3) parenchymal necrosis. The inflammatory infiltrate can be mixed acute and chronic granulomatous, with scattered giant cells and pallisading histiocytes. The vasculitis may affect medium-sized and small arteries, veins, and capillaries, with fibrinoid necrosis, granulomatous inflammation, and chronic healing scars. The necrosis mirrors the vasculitic process; large, confluent geographic zones of necrosis are seen with medium arterial involvement, small microabscesses occur with small vessel and capillary involvement (Fig. 5–23). In the study by Devaney et al.,[187] two of the three histologic findings deemed suggestive for WG were found in 44% of patients. The classic triad was found in only 16%. Usually, the diagnosis is established on finding two histologic features, elevated antineutrophil cytoplasmic antibodies, plus involvement of at least one of the three organ systems (upper airway, lungs, kidneys).

Differential Diagnosis. The differential diagnosis of laryngotracheal granulomatous inflammation with necrosis includes a long list of infections: tuberculosis, syphilis, histoplasmosis, cryptococcosis, blastomycosis, paracoccidioidomycosis, coccidioidomycosis, and candidiasis. Infraglottic stenosis may also be a sequel of relapsing polychondritis, LE, and previous trauma including prolonged endotracheal intubation; it may also be of idiopathic origin. Vasculitis, when present, brings to mind other disease processes such as LE or polyarteritis nodosa (PAN).

Special Studies. Antineutrophil cytoplasmic antibodies are measured by indirect immunofluorescence using normal neutrophils fixed in ethanol, and patient sera. Two patterns may be observed: coarse, diffuse, cytoplasmic staining (C-ANCA) and perinuclear cytoplasmic staining (P-ANCA). C-ANCA is highly specific for WG and corresponds to antibodies directed against serine protease 3. It is positive in more than 90% of patients with active disease and 65% of those with active limited disease. Occasionally, C-ANCA may also be present in PAN and Churg-Strauss vasculitis. P-ANCA is a nonspecific pattern of staining, which disappears when the test is repeated on formalin-fixed neutrophils. P-ANCA may also be present in other diseases such as PAN, Churg-Strauss vasculitis, LE, Goodpasture's syndrome, Crohn's disease, and Sjögren's syndrome.[188]

Treatment. Trimethoprim/sulfamethoxazole therapy can be initiated for patients with disease limited to the paranasal sinuses and upper and lower airways, without systemic vasculitis and renal

involvement. Prednisone and long-term cyclophosphamide are used to manage patients with severe pulmonary and renal involvement. Tracheostomy may be necessary for airway control. Surgical laryngeal reconstruction may be necessary during the quiescent stage.

Mucosal Bullous Diseases: Benign Mucosal Pemphigoid and Pemphigus Vulgaris

Pemphigoid

Clinical Features. Cicatricial pemphigoid (benign mucosal pemphigoid [BMP], bullous pemphigoid) is a chronic, progressive autoimmune disease with a female:male ratio of 2:1. Bullous pemphigoid is a more intense variant of cicatricial pemphigoid, with a predilection for the skin rather than mucous membranes. The incidence of cicatricial pemphigoid increases with advancing age. In a series of 142 patients (93 women and 49 men) with BMP from the Mayo Clinic, 94% of patients were older than 50, and the peak age of onset was in the eighth decade of life.[189] The mucous membranes are primarily affected, usually oral (88%) and ocular (60%) mucosa; additionally, 18% of patients have mild skin lesions usually of the limb flexor surfaces. The larynx and oropharynx/hypopharynx are involved in 10% and 8% of patients, respectively, and usually in the setting of disseminated disease. Laryngeal involvement is an unusual primary manifestation of mucosal pemphigoid.[190] Patients complain of hoarseness, odynophagia, or increasing dyspnea. Laryngeal erosive bullae tend to form on the epiglottis and aryepiglottic folds. The lesions of BMP are erythematous and usually noncrusting. The Nikolsky sign is indicative of the general mucosal fragility: a small amount of pressure applied to the "normal" mucosa (finger, pencil eraser, air blast) will result in mucosal shearing and ulceration. This test is nonspecific and may also be positive in other mucocutaneous diseases such as pemphigus vulgaris, erythema multiforme, and bullous lichen planus. The lesions characteristically heal by intense scarring, hence the appellation *cicatricial*. Mucous membrane scarring leads to stenosis, whereas ocular involvement and scarring lead to conjunctival symblepharon, corneal ulceration, and opacification. Laryngeal scarring can result in vocal cord fixation and airway compromise.[191]

Pathologic Features. Pemphigoid is the result of autoantibodies formed against type IV basement membrane collagen, which is reflected in the histology and immunopathology. Characteristically, the diagnosis is made on seeing separation or clefting of the mucosa from the lamina propria at the level of the basement membrane. The lamina propria has a chronic inflammatory infiltrate and increased vascularity. Acantholysis (Tzanck cells, tombstone cells) is a feature of pemphigus, but not of pemphigoid.

Special Studies. Direct immunofluorescence on the biopsy reveals a linear deposition of IgG or IgM, or both, and complement directed against the basement membrane. Indirect immunofluorescence is performed utilizing patient serum and control tissue and reveals the same pattern of deposition.

Differential Diagnosis. The differential diagnosis includes artifactual submucosal clefting, pemphigus vulgaris, erosive lichen planus, herpetic vesicles, and epidermolysis bullosa acquisita. Artifactual clefting may be difficult to distinguish from pemphigoid by light microscopy, especially if the lamina propria is inflamed. Clinical history and immunofluorescence can distinguish between pemphigoid and artifact. The distinction between pemphigus and pemphigoid is made on the basis of the location of the mucosal clefting (intraepithelial with acantholysis for pemphigus vulgaris, subepithelial for pemphigoid). Re-epithelization of the floor of the blister in pemphigoid may be confused with intramucosal clefting.

Pemphigus

Clinical Features. Pemphigus is a progressive mucocutaneous autoimmune vesiculobullous disease. It occurs most commonly in the fourth and fifth decades of life, and there appears to be a predis-

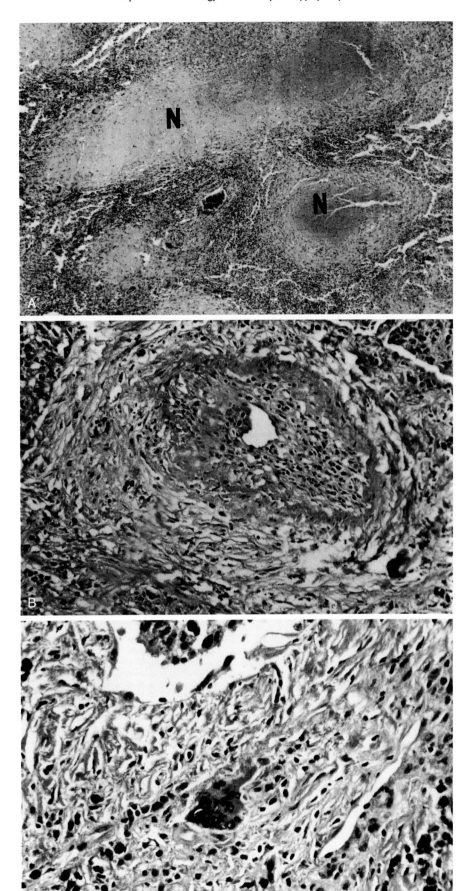

Figure 5–23. A, Geographic zones of necrosis (N) seen in this case of pulmonary Wegener's granulomatosis. B, Tangential section through vessel with chronic intramural vasculitis. C, Multinucleated giant cells are seen within the vasculitis.

position for Jewish and Mediterranean individuals. Pemphigus may be subclassified as pemphigus foliaceous, pemphigus erythematosus, pemphigus vegetans, and pemphigus vulgaris. Pemphigus foliaceous is characterized by an extensive dermal exfoliative component with little or no mucosal involvement. Pemphigus erythematosus (Senear-Usher syndrome) mimics LE in its malar distribution of the erythematous scaling crusting lesions; there is also little or no mucosal involvement. The lesions of pemphigus vegetans and pemphigus vulgaris initially appear on the mucous membranes, with subsequent dermal involvement. The actual oral vesicles are often not clinically observed because the acantholysis is suprabasilar (intra-epithelial), resulting in early rupture of the flaccid vesicles. Such ulcers are usually not serosanguineous, and they crust readily. Oral pemphigus involves the oral mucosa more diffusely than pemphigoid. The eroded bullae of pemphigus vegetans develop hypertrophic granulation tissue, producing hyperplastic lesions in the skin and vermilion border of the lips. Upper airway involvement by pemphigus vulgaris occurs in about 10% of patients and results in supraglottic laryngeal edema, which can lead to airway obstruction. Laryngotracheal (16%) and pharyngeal (49%) involvement usually occurs in the setting of clinically disseminated disease (oral and skin involvement).[192, 193] Laryngeal/pharyngeal bullae have been reported, at times, as initial indicators of disease.[192, 194, 195] Patients can complain of sore throat, a burning sensation, and hoarseness. The hypopharynx, epiglottis, and aryepiglottic folds may reveal edema, ulceration, and inflamed mucosa.[196]

Patients with pemphigus have circulating IgG autoantibodies against desmosome tonofilament complexes. A group of polypeptides (85 kD, 130 kD, and 210 kD), termed the *vulgaris complex,* located on the keratinocyte surface may be the specific antigenic targets. Pemphigus may also be drug-induced, usually by thiol-containing drugs such as penicillin, and laryngeal involvement has been reported in drug-induced pemphigus.[197] We have observed pemphigus as a paraneoplastic syndrome associated with a hematologic malignancy.

Pathologic Features. Epithelial cell separation or acantholysis and intraepithelial clefting are diagnostic features of pemphigus due to loss of intercellular bridges. The basal cell layer is uninvolved, remaining intact with the underlying lamina propria. The cells below the intra-epithelial cleft have a tombstone-like effect: they are irregular, with decreased cytoplasm and almost naked, rounded nuclei that protrude into the clefts, resembling tombstones on a hill. Individual spherical acantholytic cells—Tzanck cells—are seen floating within the intra-epithelial clefts; they are rounded, enlarged, and have large hyperchromatic nuclei.

Special Studies. Immunofluorescence reveals intercellular deposition of IgG and complement throughout the mucosal thickness, especially concentrated in the "prickle layer," corresponding to deposition of autoantibodies against desmosome tonofilament complexes.

Treatment. Systemic corticosteroids and immunosuppressant agents such as methotrexate, azathioprine, and cyclophosphamide are indicated for mucocutaneous vesicular bullous disease. Tracheostomy may be necessary for airway management in acute disease. The major clinical problem, once disease control is achieved, is compliance and long-term effects of corticosteroid therapy.

Crohn's Disease

Clinical Features. Crohn's disease, or regional enteritis, is a chronic, severe, debilitating inflammatory process of unknown etiology. The intestine is primarily involved, and the inflammatory process may progress to fistula formation and bowel obstruction. The entire gastrointestinal tract, including the oral cavity, may be involved. Extraintestinal manifestations of Crohn's disease include inflammation of the joints, eyes, liver, skin, and marrow cavity.

Upper airway involvement by Crohn's disease is extremely rare. Croft and Wilkenson[198] reviewed 332 patients with Crohn's disease and found that 6.1% had some form of oral ulceration. They document one patient with severe Crohn's disease who developed

severe edema and ulceration of the oral cavity, pharynx, and larynx post-ileocolectomy. Gianoli and Miller[199] identified five cases of laryngeal involvement, plus one case of their own—a 44-year-old woman with ulcerations of the palate, nasal cavity, and vocal cords, and genital ulcers and evidence of small intestinal disease. In general, a female predominance is noted, with a peak incidence in the third decade of life. Supraglottic edema and cricoarytenoid edema can be seen. Limited cricoarytenoid motility may occur, possibly as a result of joint arthritis. Five of the six patients had evidence of generalized systemic involvement at the time of laryngeal symptoms. Upper airway involvement may be diffuse, with ulceration involving the entire oral and laryngotracheobronchial tract.[200, 201]

Pathologic Features. In the small intestine, transmural chronic inflammatory infiltrates with interposed "skip areas" of relatively uninflamed mucosa are characteristic for Crohn's disease. Noncaseating granulomas and giant cells may be seen in Crohn's disease and aid in distinguishing it from ulcerative colitis. However, these granulomas are not common and have been observed in only 28% of cases.[202] Crohn's disease involvement of the upper airway may be histologically nonspecific, revealing only nongranulomatous chronic inflammation.[198] Occasionally, non-necrotic microgranulomas may be seen in laryngeal biopsies, reminiscent of the intestinal findings.[200, 201, 203]

Differential Diagnosis. In the absence of granulomas, the histology is entirely nonspecific, and correlation with the clinical picture is necessary to establish an association. If granulomas are seen, mycobacterial and fungal infection or sarcoidosis are included in the differential diagnosis.

Treatment. Acute upper airway ulcerative lesions can be managed with corticosteroid therapy.

Necrotizing Sialometaplasia

Clinical Features. Necrotizing sialometaplasia (NSM) is a benign, self-healing, necrotizing, ulcerative, inflammatory condition that arises in the minor salivary glands. The oral cavity, typically the palate, is the most common site; less commonly, the major salivary glands, the trachea, and the larynx may be involved.[204–207] Abrams et al.[204] initially described the clinicopathologic entity in 1973 as a benign lesion that may clinically and pathologically mimic mucoepidermoid or epidermoid carcinoma.[205] In the larynx, NSM only rarely produces a visible lesion.[206] It is not uncommonly encountered as an incidental post-biopsy finding within seromucinous glands.[208] In this setting, NSM may cause difficulty during evaluation of laryngectomy surgical margins, particularly during intraoperative frozen sections evaluation.

Pathologic Features and Differential Diagnosis. Histologically, NSM is characterized by lobular necrosis and sialadenitis intermixed with squamous metaplasia of excretory ducts and acini. In the larynx it is usually easy to separate NSM from tumor extension into excretory ducts by looking for smooth-edged squamous nests arranged in a lobular fashion with residual ductal lumina. Occasionally, however, severe regenerative atypia may accompany NSM, making it difficult to distinguish, with complete certainty, from "cancerization" of seromucinous glands.[208] Deeper histologic sections will usually clarify this dilemma by demonstrating extension of the atypical epithelial population from the overlying mucosa in the latter situation. Rarely, an additional adjacent piece of tissue during the frozen section procedure should be requested from the surgeon to further evaluate the surgical margin. This will usually resolve the problem.

Treatment and Prognosis. No treatment is necessary for NSM, as it will heal spontaneously without intervention.

Chondrometaplasia

Clinical Features. Laryngeal chondrometaplasia refers to an expansile formation of benign, metaplastic cartilaginous tissue of limited growth potential.[209, 210] These lesions have also been referred to as chondromas. They are invariably small (1 cm or less), polypoid tumors on the middle or posterior vocal fold, or arytenoid. They have been incidental findings in less than 2% of autopsy larynges and are thought to be a degenerative consequence following vocal nodule formation.[211] As the clinical course of these lesions is distinct from that of laryngeal chondrosarcomas, the term *chondrometaplasia* or *chondroma* is justifiable. Hyams and Rabuzzi[209] identified nine cases in the vocal fold. The lesions varied in size from 0.3 to 1.0 cm in maximum dimension and patients typically presented with hoarseness.

Pathologic Features. Chondrometaplasia is composed of bland cartilage with no direct attachment to underlying cartilaginous structures; it typically "blends" into the adjacent soft tissues. Hyams does point out that some "cordal lesions . . . seemed to infiltrate along seromucinous glands." Elastic stain will reveal a high content of elastic fibers within the chondrometaplasia.

Differential Diagnosis. Polypoid laryngeal mucosa and submucosa can be present in and divert one's attention from the chondrometaplastic nature of the lesion. One might mistakenly assume that the cartilage present is part of normal anatomy rather than a pathologic process. Correlation with clinical impression and confirmation of site of biopsy will be helpful in establishing the diagnosis. On the other hand, one may question whether the cartilage is metaplastic or neoplastic. Neoplastic cartilage has a lobular growth pattern with tumor islands being sharply demarcated from the surrounding tissue, whereas chondrometaplasia "blends" into the surrounding soft tissue.

Treatment and Prognosis. Conservative endoscopic excision is usually curative. Hyams and Rabuzzi[209] reported no recurrence of vocal cord chondrometaplasia. Anecdotally, we have seen one case of polypoid chondrometaplasia of the vocal cord, distinct from the arytenoid, which recurred after 6 years (Fig. 5–24, see p. 248).

Relapsing Polychondritis

Clinical Features. *Relapsing polychondritis* (RPC) is the term coined by Pearson et al.[212] for a multisystem, autoimmune disease resulting from an array of antibodies to cartilaginous components. RPC can occur over a wide age range, without gender preponderance. The majority of affected sites are in the head and neck and in the chest. The external ears are commonly involved, and one third of cases present with chondritis of the pinna resulting in a soft and flabby ear. Recurrent episodes of pinna chondritis result in a scarred, deformed ear (cauliflower ear). Seventy-five percent of patients develop nasal involvement, which commences as a painful erythematous nose and progresses to septal collapse and saddle nose deformity. At least half of patients develop upper airway symptoms, most commonly chronic progressive bronchitis and stridor, due to laryngotracheal chondritis.[213, 214] The thyroid cartilage is tender to palpation. Laryngotracheal edema may lead to early upper airway obstruction. Stenosis may be infraglottic and localized, or diffuse. Late complications include chronic obstructive pneumonia and fatal tracheal stenosis. Patients complain of arthralgias as a result of involvement of articular cartilages (78%). Other manifestations include costochondritis (47%), episcleritis (60%), iritis (27%), and cataracts (33%).[213] Temporal bone manifestations include cranial nerve VIII deafness, tinnitus, vertigo, otitis media, and mastoiditis. Cardiovascular involvement may lead to aortic ring insufficiency and aortic aneurysm. The audiovestibular symptoms and cardiovascular complications may be the result of a vasculitic component that can be present in RPC.[214] One third of patients with RPC will also have other autoimmune disorders such as rheumatoid arthritis, Sjögren's syndrome, lupus erythematosus, and polyarteritis nodosum.[215] Patients are usually anemic and have elevated erythrocyte sedimentation rates and positive rheumatoid factor. During active disease, the chondrolysis results in elevated urinary acid mucopolysaccharides.

Pathologic Features. The diagnosis is usually made clinically. It would be uncommon for pathologists to receive biopsies for diagnostic purposes; rather, the pathologist may see involved tissue after reconstructive surgery during disease quiescence. During acute periods, acute and chronic inflammatory cells infiltrate cartilage, and chondrocyte "drop-out" is present. The cartilaginous matrix lacks the normal basophilic hue and becomes fragmented, "leached out," and disintegrated (chondrolysis). The laryngotracheal mucosa is edematous and inflamed. Eventually, granulation tissue and fibrosis replace the cartilaginous structures and metaplastic ossification may be seen.[214] A vasculitic component may also be present in RPC.

Differential Diagnosis. Clinically, the erythema and painful nodules of the helix may mimic chondrodermatitis nodularis chronica helica (CNCH). The entire pinna is not swollen and erythematous in CNCH, and the remaining aerodigestive tract and audiovestibular system are unaffected. Saddle nose deformity may be seen in other entities, such as Wegener's granulomatosis, tertiary or congenital syphilis, and cocaine abuse. The otic symptoms may also be seen in Wegener's granulomatosis, polyarteritis nodosum, and Cogan's (oculovestibulo-auditory) syndrome. The latter is characterized by abrupt onset of tinnitus and vertigo, with progression to sensorineural deafness, often occurring in conjunction with other autoimmune diseases.

Treatment and Prognosis. Corticosteroid suppression or dapsone, or both, is indicated for active disease. Many patients will require tracheostomy for airway management. Most fatalities are the result of airway collapse or chronic pneumonia and sepsis.

Tracheopathia Chondro-osteoplastica

Clinical Features. Tracheopathia chondro-osteoplastica (TCO) is a disease of unknown etiology, limited to the trachea, which causes progressive ossification and increasing tracheal rigidity. Symptoms appear in the third and fourth decades of life but have occurred as early as 12 years of age.[216] Patients usually have a long history of chronic cough and "asthma," which may progress to chronic hemoptysis, inspiratory stridor, and laryngotracheobronchitis. Associated atrophic rhinitis is common. There is a wide spectrum for the degree of tracheal involvement; accordingly, the exact incidence of TCO is unknown. Rare familial involvement has been reported.[217] An association between TCO and amyloidosis has been described, and it has been suggested that TCO represents an end stage of primary localized tracheal amyloidosis or a variant of primary pulmonary amyloidosis[218]; an autopsy series failed to confirm an association between the two.[219] Chronic infection has been cited as another possible etiologic factor. Virchow[220] suggested in 1863 that TCO might be a localized form of ecchondroses, a theory that still is currently in vogue.

Laryngoscopy and bronchoscopy reveal gritty small submucosal nodularities (less than 0.5 cm) giving a beaded or "rock garden" appearance. The projections arise from the lateral and anterior tracheal walls, and the membranous posterior trachea is usually, but not exclusively, spared. Serum calcium and phosphorus levels are generally normal.[216] The trachea may be severely narrowed as the tracheal walls become more rigid and thickened. The vocal cords are only occasionally involved. Rarely, TCO exclusively affects the larynx.[219, 221]

Pathologic Features. Heterotopic calcification and ossification with mature bone formation resembling osteomas are seen in the lamina propria.[222] Marrow spaces can be seen within the ossification. Some of the ossifications are distinct from, and unconnected to, the tracheal rings, whereas others are contiguous with the tracheal rings. Osseous metaplasia of the tracheal rings may also be seen. Areas of atypical disorganized cartilaginous tissue resembling ecchondrosis may be seen (Fig. 5–25). Young et al.[223] maintain that serial sectioning always reveals a connection between the ossified projection and the internal perichondrium of the tracheal rings, favoring Virchow's theory. Amyloid deposits can be seen in some cases.[224] Coincidental bronchial mucoepidermoid carcinoma and TCO have been reported.[225]

Differential Diagnosis. If disorganized cartilaginous tissue is present on a tracheal biopsy, the differential diagnosis includes a low-grade cricoid chondrosarcoma. Clinical and radiographic correlation can aid in this distinction. Mature ossification, on biopsy, may be difficult to distinguish from metaplastic ossification seen as part of the aging process. The latter can be ruled out if the ossification is seen in the lamina propria, separate from the tracheal ring.

Heterotopic bone formation (myositis ossificans) has been rarely reported in the larynx[226] and would enter the differential diagnosis of TCO, which, as mentioned, rarely exclusively affects the larynx.[219, 221] Histologically, TCO involves ossification of metaplastic cartilage, whereas myositis ossificans typically has a zonation effect of a central immature, proliferative, fibroblastic component with osteoid formation, and an outer shell of varying thickness composed of maturing bone. Importantly, endochondral ossification is not a usual component of myositis ossificans, as it is of TCO. The clinical distinction between localized TCO and laryngeal myositis ossificans is not important, as laryngeal function may be restored in both with conservative excision.

Treatment and Prognosis. Severely symptomatic patients may be treated with laser bronchoscopy in an attempt to increase the tracheal lumen size. Occasional patient deaths have been attributed to complications of TCO, while other cases are incidental autopsy findings.

Post-radiation Changes

Clinical Features. Radiation is a treatment option for patients with T1 laryngeal squamous carcinoma, with the option for surgical salvage if recurrence develops. The surgical pathologist should be familiar with the appearance of radiation effects, and not overdiagnose these changes as recurrent carcinoma. It appears, from personal experience, that the tendency is to overdiagnose recurrent carcinoma in these situations, rather than to miss recurrence. In addition to radiation failure tumor recurrence and radiation-induced malignancy, other sequelae to laryngeal irradiation include laryngeal edema and ulceration, fibrosis, perichondritis, cartilaginous necrosis, osteomyelitis, and osteonecrosis, which may clinically mimic tumor recurrence. Post-biopsy chondritis and osteonecrosis rarely occur as com-

plications of postirradiation biopsies.[227, 228] Secondary infection and fistula formation may follow chondronecrosis.[229]

Pathologic Features. Radiation increases the size of mucosal cells; the nuclei are especially large and cells may be multinucleated. Nucleoli may be prominent. However, in "pure" radiation change, the chromatin is "washed out," smudged, blurry, and homogeneous, not coarse and dysplastic-appearing.[230] The nuclear:cytoplasmic ratio is preserved, not increased. Nuclear and cytoplasmic vacuolization are present; the latter results in pseudoglandular spaces seen in post-radiation squamous cell carcinoma (Fig. 5–26). Radiation-induced changes are chronic and may persist lifelong.

Dysplasia may be superimposed on radiation changes; the resultant effect is that the degree of dysplasia may be overestimated, or the dysplasia may mimic invasive carcinoma. These cases should be read out carefully and prudently, with awareness of the histologic pall cast by radiation. Tangentially sectioned superimposed epithelial hyperplasia, either from the surface mucosa (Fig. 5–27) or within salivary ducts is especially prone to be overdiagnosed as invasive carcinoma. Although it may be distorted, recognizing the basic structure of a duct, such as smooth contours, basement membrane, and the suggestion of a lumen, may be helpful. Invasive carcinoma usually has jaggedly contoured tumor nests. Other changes that bespeak prior irradiation include acinar atrophy of minor salivary glands, perivascular hyalinization, multinucleated myocytes, endothelial hyperplasia (see Fig. 5–27C,D), stromal atypia, and squamous metaplasia of ducts. Dense fibrosis is a typical post-radiation change and may lead to glottic stenosis.

Osteomyelitis with microabscess formation and osteonecrosis of the laryngeal structures may also be seen. A case of extensive reactive bone formation with osteomyelitis was illustrated among a series of 265 post-radiation larynges.[228] Keene et al.[228] noted that chondronecrosis and osteonecrosis were equally likely to occur in nonirradiated as well as irradiated larynges with high stage (T3/T4) tumors (24% versus 27%, respectively), usually within the first 12 months, but was a very unlikely occurrence with T1/T2 tumors. They did see a marked propensity for arytenoid necrosis in irradiated patients. Brandenburg et al.[231] also evaluated post-radiation surgical salvage laryngectomy specimens, and compared them to nonirradiated resections. Irradiated larynges were more likely to have cartilage invasion and extension into infraglottic and extralaryngeal soft tissues. Not surprisingly, recurrent carcinoma in radiation failure is seen as smaller and more widely dispersed tumor islands ("leaner and meaner tumor"), which may be entirely subepithelial, thus accounting for the difficulties clinicians have in evaluating the postirradiated larynx.

▪ BENIGN AND MALIGNANT LARYNGEAL NEOPLASIA

Laryngeal Papillomatosis: Juvenile-Onset and Adult-Onset Papillomas, and Aggressive Papillomatosis

Clinical Features. Laryngeal papillomas (fungiform papillomas, exophytic papillomas) are histologically benign human papillomavirus (HPV)–induced lesions. Juvenile-onset laryngeal papillomatosis (JOLP) usually follows an exuberant course distinct from that of adult-onset laryngeal papilloma (AOLP). JOLP often presents before the age of 5 years, without gender predominance. The papillomas are multiple and may carpet the endolarynx and infraglottis, resulting in extreme hoarseness and upper airway obstruction (Fig. 5–28). The clinical course of JOLP is often one of innumerable recurrences. Airway patency is maintained by multiple laser excisions. Most cases resolve by puberty, but some cases of JOLP may persist into young adulthood. By contrast, AOLP occurs after the second decade of life, with a strong male predominance. These lesions are usually singular and amenable to endoscopic excision. Oc-

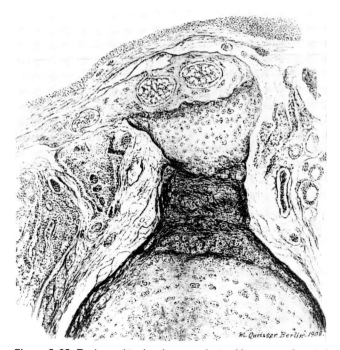

Figure 5–25. Tracheopathia chondro-osteoplastica. Note areas of atypical disorganized cartilaginous tissue that here is connected with underlying tracheal cartilage. (From Muckleston HS: On so-called "multiple osteomata" of the tracheal mucous membrane. Laryngoscope 1909;19:881-893.)

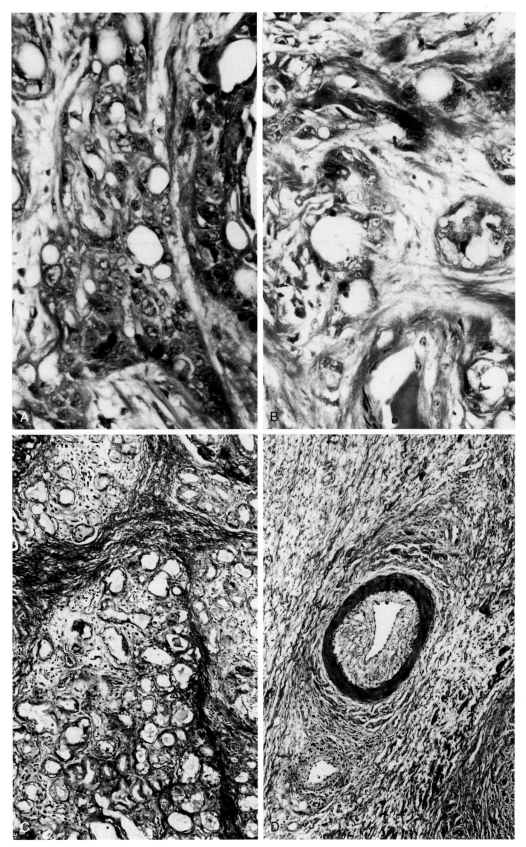

Figure 5–26. Radiation changes. *A&B,* Vacuolization within an irradiated squamous cell carcinoma results in a pseudoglandular pattern that may mimic adeno-carcinoma. *C,* Acinar atrophy and periglandular fibrosis of minor salivary glands. *D,* Endothelial hyperplasia and perivascular fibrosis.

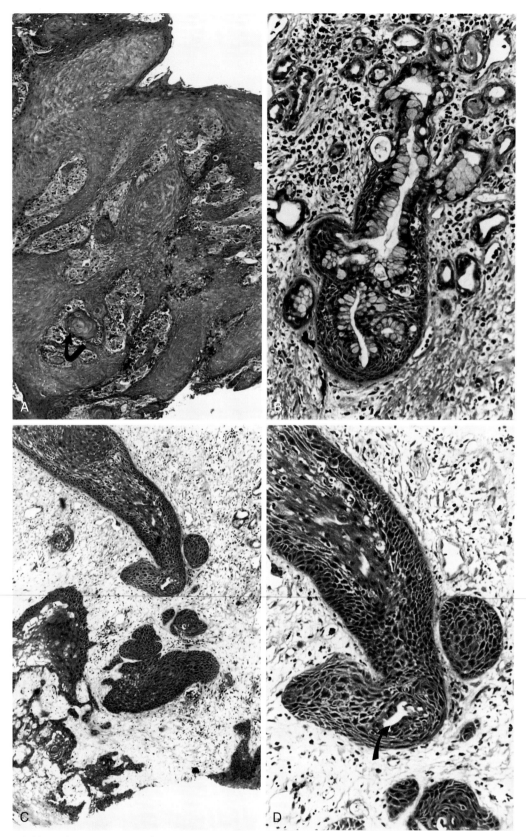

Figure 5–27. Epithelial hyperplasia in the setting of previous irradiation for carcinoma. *A,* The elongated rete pegs with deep pearl formation *(curved arrow)* tempts the diagnosis of infiltrating squamous cell carcinoma (SCC), which need not be accompanied by surface carcinoma in situ. The smooth borders of the islands speak against carcinoma. *B,* Recognizing squamous metaplasia and acinar atrophy in adjacent ducts sets the context for radiation change. *C&D,* It is helpful to look for ductal lumina (arrow) within deep epithelial nests. Overall, pathologists should shy away from diagnosing infiltrating SCC in the setting of generalized pseudoepitheliomatous hyperplasia.

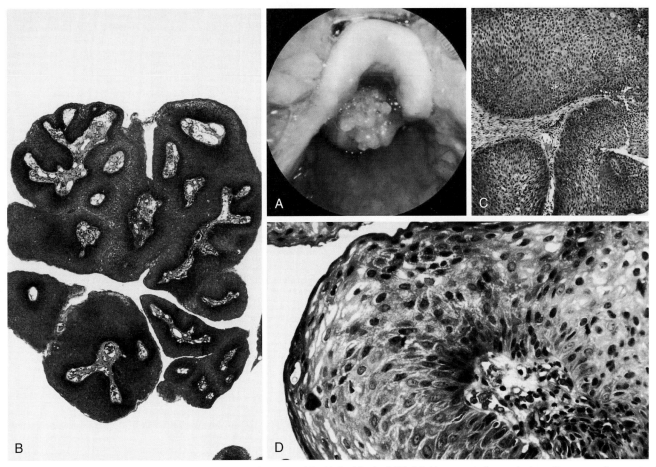

Figure 5–28. *A,* Endoscopic view of juvenile papillomatosis. (Courtesy of Dr. Michael Rothschild.) *B-D,* Microscopically, exophytic papillomas are characterized by maturing hyperplastic squamous mucosa on fibrovascular cores. Keratinization may be seen. Normally, atypia and mitotic figures are minimal.

casionally, AOLP may present with multiple lesions that recur after excision.

Ullman, in 1923,[232] suspected an infectious etiology for laryngeal papillomas; he successfully produced papilloma-like growths on his arm and on the arm of his assistant after injection of cell free tissue extracts derived from a laryngeal papilloma from a child. The association of HPV with JOLP and AOLP has been clearly established; HPV 6 and 11 are most commonly detected.[233–235] HPV is present in normal tissue surrounding the papillomatous lesions and becomes reactivated, resulting in recurrences.[236]

The upper airway may be first exposed to HPV during vaginal delivery. Thirty-one patients with laryngeal papillomas were surveyed, and 67% of their mothers had a positive clinical history for condylomas. The exposure rate for neonates of HPV-positive mothers is significant: HPV DNA was isolated from the nasopharyngeal secretions of 47% of vaginally delivered neonates whose mothers had been demonstrated to have HPV-positive cervical cells. The infection rate, however, appears to be low, in keeping with the relative rarity of laryngeal papillomas despite the high incidence of genitourinary condylomas. Transplacental hematogenous transmission is also possible.[237, 238]

Pathologic Features. Exophytic papillomas are histologically defined by stratified squamous epithelium over fibrovascular cores. The fibrovascular cores result in their characteristic fungiform architecture and distinguish these lesions from condylomas, which are more sessile and broad-based. The squamous mucosa of exophytic papillomas is usually immature without significant hyperkeratosis (see Fig. 5–28); mild to moderate dysplasia may be present. However, dense keratinization, intramucosal keratinization, diffuse dysplasia of any degree, or full-thickness dysplasia should make one

consider squamous carcinoma-ex-fungiform papilloma or a papillary/exophytic squamous carcinoma. Increased atypia has been correlated with clinical recurrence,[239] although opinions as to the predictive value of dysplasia in laryngeal papillomas differ.[240]

Differential Diagnosis. The main distinction, especially in adults, is with that of papillary carcinoma in situ and exophytic squamous carcinoma (also referred to as papillary squamous carcinoma). Papillary carcinoma in situ produces finger-like growths with fibrovascular cores and a dysplastic epithelial lining. Adjacent surface dysplasia frequently extends into seromucinous ducts. Exophytic squamous carcinoma has a cauliflower-like appearance and is composed of an exophytic papillary tumor composed of ribbons of stratified squamous cells aligned atop a basement membrane, thus bearing superficial resemblance to a papilloma. This tumor has a more complicated and crowded exophytic papillary arrangement than does squamous papilloma. The presence of dysplasia and greater degree of keratinization, especially intraepithelial keratin pearls, may distinguish it from papillomas. Intraepithelial keratin pearls are not routinely seen in papillomas and should raise the suspicion of either dysplastic progression or exophytic squamous cell carcinoma. Papillary squamous cell carcinoma may be in situ or have an infiltrating component. True verruca vulgaris is uncommon in the larynx and has been associated, as with papillomas, with HPV 6/11.[241] Verruca vulgaris lacks the fibrovascular cores of exophytic papillomas, has a thick "coating" of hyperkeratosis and parakeratosis, and usually contains areas with prominent keratohyaline granules.

Treatment and Prognosis. As mentioned, patients with JOLP may require innumerable endoscopic laser procedures to maintain airway patency. Interferon therapy may increase the interval between relapses. AOLP may be treated by conservative endoscopic excision. Those patients with dysplastic papillomas require close clinical follow-up. In one series of 63 cases of laryngeal papillomas, 12 patients (19%) initially presented as JOLP with disease persistence into adulthood.[242] No case underwent malignant change. Twenty patients (32%) had solitary lesions, cured by endoscopic excision, 30 patients (47%) had multiple lesions—60% of them required multiple (five or fewer) excisions. Seven patients (8%) developed florid papillomatosis. Aggressive papillomatosis or florid aggressive papillomatosis refers to diffuse laryngotracheal squamous metaplasia and papillomatosis, which carpets the endolarynx and may extend into the tracheobronchial tree and the pulmonary parenchyma. Generally, florid papillomatosis may occur in up to 25% of patients with either JOLP or AOLP.[243–245] These patients require tracheostomy for airway control and may require laryngectomy for disease control.

Malignant change is known to occur in laryngeal and laryngotracheopulmonary papillomatosis. This change may occur in concert with external promoters such as irradiation and cigarette smoking, or may happen de novo.[246–249] While malignant transformation of JOLP and AOLP has been the subject of sporadic reports, retrospective series place the rate of malignant transformation for all laryngeal papillomas between 2% and 17%.[248–252] Transformation may occur in localized as well as diffuse cases. Malignant transformation can occur in both JOLP and AOLP and is usually related to long disease duration. A large series of 102 patients with JOLP (52%) and AOLP (48%) revealed that eight patients (7.8%, three with JOLP, five with AOLP) developed malignant transformation; seven developed laryngeal carcinoma and one patient with laryngotracheal papillomatosis developed bronchial carcinoma.[249] The time between onset of papilloma and transformation was 4 to 55 years (mean 24 years). The ratio of observed to expected cases of laryngeal carcinoma was 88. Cofactors promoting carcinogenesis (irradiation, smoking, bleomycin) were present in at least six of these patients including two of the three JOLP patients. Factors that suggested malignant transformation included decreased vocal fold mobility, the presence of cervical lymph nodes, exuberant and rapid growth requiring very frequent excisions, and laryngeal edema. Interestingly, carcinomas arising in squamous papillomas contain "low risk" HPV types (types 6/11) not associated with malignant transformation.[234, 246] An associated carcinoma was found to contain episomal HPV-6a genomes with duplications of the upstream regulatory region, the late region, and a portion of the early region. These duplications were absent from the associated benign laryngeal papilloma, suggesting that viral mutation may be necessary for "low risk" HPV types to induce carcinogenesis.[253]

Granular Cell Tumor

Clinical Features. Granular cell tumors (GCTs) are benign, slow-growing tumors of schwannian or pre-schwannian origin. This tumor occurs, with a female preponderance, in a greater than expected proportion of African-Americans. A wide age range is seen, with an incidence peak in the third to fifth decades of life. GCTs are the most common, benign, nonepithelial neoplasm listed in the Armed Forces Institute of Pathology (AFIP) Otolaryngic Tumor Registry.[255] About half of all cases involve the head and neck, most commonly the anterior tongue and subcutaneous tissues of the head and neck.[256, 257] The larynx and trachea are less commonly involved, representing 1.6% to 3.7% of involved sites.[257, 258] Other common sites for GCT include the breast, anogenital region, and subcutaneous tissue of the trunk. GCTs rarely are larger than 3 cm in greatest dimension. Multiple synchronous or metachronous tumors at various sites occur in approximately 5% of patients.[257]

Laryngeal GCTs are smooth, white, polypoid tumors arising from the posterior true vocal folds or, less often, from the anterior commissure, false cords, infraglottis, and trachea.[258] Eighteen cases of pediatric laryngeal granular cell tumors have been reported in the literature, which, unlike their adult counterparts, have a predisposi-

tion for the anterior infraglottis.[259–262] Tracheal GCTs represented 4% (6 of 145) of referred cases of GCT to the AFIP; a recent literature review identified 30 tracheal tumors in total.[256] Eighty-four percent of cases occurred in women; 63% of them were African-American. Twenty percent of tracheal GCTs were multiple. Patients with laryngeal GCT usually complain of hoarseness, those with tracheal tumors invariably have a long history of "intractable asthma." The white mucosal surface is caused by squamous mucosal hyperplasia that accompanies about half of these cases.

Pathologic Features. GCTs typically have an infiltrative growth pattern and a histiocytoid-type cytologic appearance. The tumor cells grow in small nests and cords; their nuclei are small and generally eccentric, their cytoplasm abundant, granular, or stippled (Fig. 5–29). They have indistinct cytoplasmic boundaries, and the granules are periodic acid-Schiff–positive and resistant to digestion. Nuclear pleomorphism and mitotic figures are not usually seen in GCT.[257]

Pseudoepitheliomatous hyperplasia may be present in up to 50% of cases; on occasion, it may even mimic infiltrating squamous carcinoma. Rare cases can have a moderate degree of epithelial atypia. The pseudoepitheliomatous hyperplasia can be a clue, on superficial biopsies, that one may be dealing with a granular cell tumor. It should lead the pathologist to look for granular cells in the subepithelial layer or to order deeper sections. Marked desmoplasia may be seen in older or larger tumors; here, the typical granular cells are seen in the periphery of the tumor.

True malignant GCTs are only rarely encountered. Malignant GCTs may be either histologically benign, yet large (usually over 9 cm) or metastasizing, or they may be histologically malignant.[263] Histologically malignant cases reveal nuclear pleomorphism, increased mitoses, and necrosis. Rare cases are particularly disturbing in that they appear, histologically, perfectly benign, yet manage to metastasize (Fig. 5–30, see p. 248). Histologically benign metastases need to be distinguished from benign multifocal tumor.

Special Studies. Ultrastructural examination of GCT confirms a relationship to Schwann cells. The cytoplasmic granules are actually lysosomal structures that contain infoldings of cell membranes similar to schwannian extensions.[264] Typically, both GCTs and Schwann cells express S-100 protein strongly, and both may also express markers of histiocytic differentiation (antibody KP-1, which detects CD 68).[265]

Differential Diagnosis. The overall benign appearance of GCT limits the differential diagnosis to rhabdomyoma, paraganglioma, and histiocytic infiltrates, either reactive or inflammatory. The cells of rhabdomyoma are much larger than granular cells and contain cross-striations. Paraganglioma characteristically has a nesting pattern and will stain with neuroendocrine markers. GCT can be distinguished from histiocytic infiltrates by the lack of inflammatory cells. Histiocytes assembled as a reaction to foreign body or infection will appear in diffuse sheets, or in clumps, without the infiltrating, nesting, and ribboning pattern seen in granular cell tumors.

Treatment and Prognosis. Conservative endoscopic removal will be curative for most cases. GCTs have a very low rate of recurrence (8%), even after incomplete excision.[252] Recurrent tumors or frankly malignant tumors require resection with free margins. Twelve of 20 patients reported in the literature with metastatic malignant GCT ultimately died of the disease.[265, 266] One case of malignant laryngeal GCT reported in 1958 in the German literature ultimately resulted in the patient's demise after 24 months.[266] We have seen a large (4.7 cm) hypopharyngeal GCT in a 29-year-old woman that was ultimately fatal after locoregional metastasis (see Fig. 5–30). She died after 2 years of disseminated disease. Malignant GCTs appear insensitive to chemotherapy. We have also seen a recurrent, non-metastasizing laryngeal GCT with atypical features (nuclear pleomorphism, spindling of cells, pagetoid spread into overlying mucosa) that could be classified as an atypical GCT (Fig. 5–31, see p. 249).[267] This patient with an atypical, recurrent laryngeal granular cell tumor remains recurrence-free after partial laryngectomy.

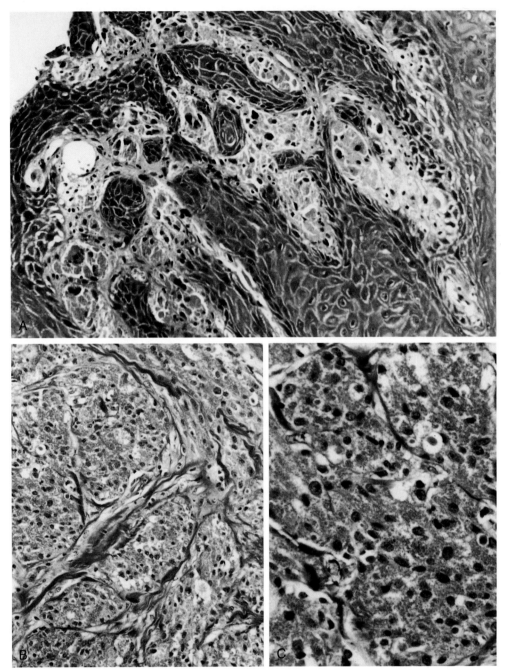

Figure 5–29. Laryngeal granular cell tumor. *A,* Marked pseudoepitheliomatous hyperplasia is present. *B&C,* Note syncytial cells with abundant pink granular cytoplasm and small eccentric nuclei typical for granular cell tumor.

Laryngeal Paraganglioma

Clinical Features. Paraganglia are organs of neural crest origin, situated adjacent to sympathetic or parasympathetic nerves, with capacity for production of an array of neuroendocrine products. In the head and neck, paraganglia are normally present in the middle ear, along the glossopharyngeal and vagus nerves, at the common carotid bifurcation, and along the superior and inferior laryngeal nerves (Fig. 5–32). Head and neck paraganglia are usually parasympathetic, with the exception of those derived from the superior sympathetic cervical ganglia. Neoplasms of the head and neck paraganglia (paragangliomas) most commonly arise from the carotid bodies (carotid body tumor, chemodectoma), vagus nerve, or the middle ear paraganglia (glomus tumor).

The ratio of superior laryngeal paraganglioma to inferior laryngeal paraganglioma is approximately 6:1.[268] Superior laryngeal paragangliomas are polypoid, submucosal, intralaryngeal tumors. Inferior laryngeal paraganglioma are usually dumbbell-shaped, with intralaryngeal and extralaryngeal extension (see Fig. 5–32).[269–272] Their hypervascularity imparts a red to blue hue and may result in hemoptysis. When situated deep to the thyroid fascia, they may be clinically confused with thyroid tumors. Clinically, supraglottic paragangliomas usually present with hoarseness and dyspnea. Infraglottic tumors may present with dyspnea and hoarseness due to nerve palsy of the recurrent laryngeal nerve. Severe pain has been occasionally noted, presumably due to neuroendocrine activity of the neoplasm.[273] Bleeding may be profuse during biopsy. Of further interest, Barnes[268] noted the female:male ratio of these tumors to be

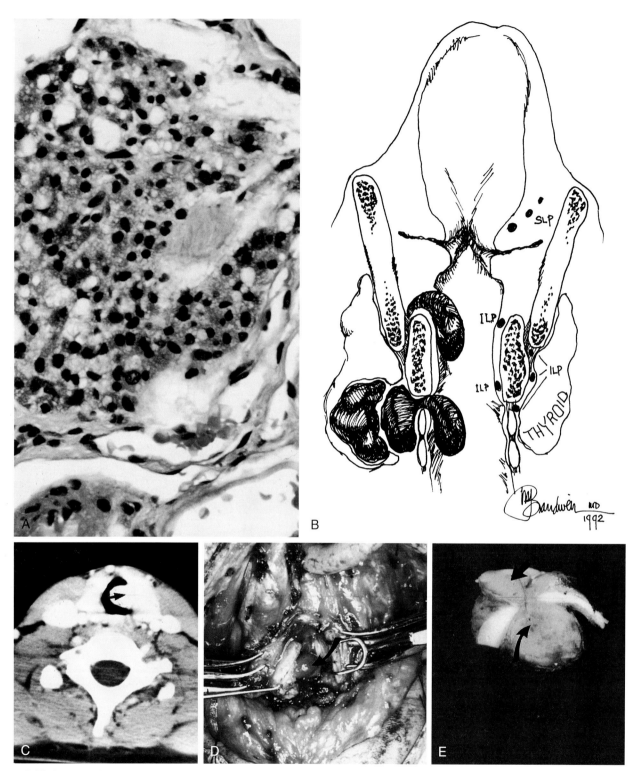

Figure 5–32. *A*, Laryngeal paraganglion. Note cells with small nuclei and vacuolated cytoplasm sometimes forming gland-like spaces. *B*, The right side of the larynx demonstrates sites where the superior laryngeal paraganglia (SLP) and inferior laryngeal paraganglia (ILP) are located. The left side of the larynx demonstrates the configuration of reported inferior laryngeal paragangliomas. *C*, The radiograph reveals the intratracheal component of an inferior laryngeal paraganglioma *(arrow)*. *D*, Intraoperative view. The cricoid has been cut and retracted. The intratracheal tumor component is seen as a vascular polypoid tumor *(arrow)*. *E*, The resection specimen revealed a dumbbell-shaped subcricoid mass *(arrows)* protruding between the inferior cricoid and the first tracheal ring.

3:1. He noted a right-sided laryngeal predisposition, with a right:left ratio of 2.3:1. Laryngeal paragangliomas may be associated with paragangliomas elsewhere,[274] or with a family history of paragangliomas.[271] Apparent hormonal sensitivity with increased growth during pregnancy has been reported.[275] Rare tumors may be clinically functional.[276]

Pathologic Features. Paragangliomas are vascular, epithelioid neoplasms. Toward the center of the tumor, "balls of cells" (Zellballen) are formed: the cells are separated into ball-like organoid compartments by fibrovascular tissue. This pattern is highlighted by reticulin stain (Fig. 5–33). Cells have abundant granular cytoplasm and round nuclei with salt-and-pepper stippling of chromatin. Cellular pleomorphism can be present in paragangliomas and occasionally may be marked, but the Zellballen pattern is maintained, at least focally. The pleomorphism is of no independent prognostic value.

Special Studies. Paragangliomas are usually positive for neuroendocrine immunohistochemical markers such as neuron-specific enolase, synaptophysin, and chromogranin. The S-100 stain highlights the Schwann-like sustentacular cells that unsheathe the Zellballen. Paragangliomas are usually negative for epithelial markers such as cytokeratin, carcinoembryonic antigen, and epithelial membrane antigen and also calcitonin.[277] Ultrastructurally, these tumors contain abundant membrane-bound dense core granules typical of neuroendocrine neoplasia.

Differential Diagnosis. The main differential diagnosis is with typical carcinoid tumor (well-differentiated neuroendocrine carcinoma [NEC]) and atypical carcinoid tumor (moderately differentiated NEC).[278] The latter two may also have finely stippled chromatin and focally have a Zellballen pattern. Moderately differentiated NEC has a higher nuclear:cytoplasmic ratio than paraganglioma. Infiltration, necrosis, or mitotic figures may be appreciated. Calcitonin expression, and expression of epithelial markers (cytokeratin, carcinoembryonic antigen, and epithelial membrane antigen) may be useful in distinguishing carcinoids/NEC from paragangliomas (Table 5–1).

Treatment and Prognosis. Laryngeal paragangliomas are curable by conservative surgery. Paragangliomas are sensitive to radiotherapy; unresectable skull base paragangliomas may be palliated with radiotherapy. Many of the reported "malignant paragangliomas" of the larynx can be better classified as moderately differentiated NEC. True malignant laryngeal paragangliomas, that is, histologically confirmed paragangliomas that develop metastatic disease, are extremely rare.[277]

Neuroendocrine Carcinomas

Neuroendocrine tumors of the larynx are divided into two broad categories based on their tissue of origin: epithelial and paraganglionic. The epithelial-derived tumors known as NEC are uncommon neoplasms accounting for 0.06% of laryngeal malignancies.[279] Owing to differences in biologic behavior and histologic growth patterns, this group of neoplasms is further subclassified into three distinct subtypes: carcinoid tumor (well-differentiated neuroendocrine carcinoma [WDNEC]), atypical carcinoid tumor (moderately differentiated neuroendocrine carcinoma [MDNEC]), and small cell carcinoma including both the intermediate and oat cell variants (poorly differentiated neuroendocrine carcinoma [PDNEC]). Patients with WDNEC survive longer with less morbidity than those with

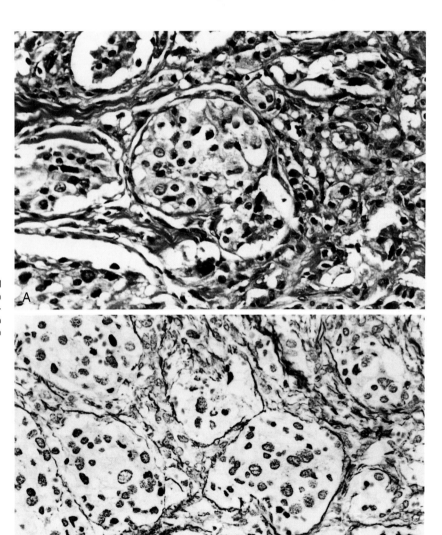

Figure 5–33. Paraganglioma. *A,* The tumor is composed of nests of cells with finely stippled nuclear chromatin and abundant cytoplasm that form a prominent, well-vascularized nesting pattern. Nuclear pleomorphism may be pronounced, as is seen here. *B,* Reticulin stain highlighting the "Zellballen" effect.

Table 5–1. Comparison of Laryngeal Neuroendocrine Tumors

	Paraganglioma	Carcinoid (WDNEC)	Atypical Carcinoid (MDNEC)	Small Cell Carcinoma (PDNEC)
Clinical Aspects				
Age (decades)	Fifth	Seventh to eighth	Sixth to seventh	
Sex ratio (M:F)	1:3	12:1	3:1	
Location	Supraglottic and submucosal			
Symptoms	Hoarseness			
Behavior	Benign	Usually benign	Malignant	
Metastasis	None	Rare	Often (lymph nodes, lung, bone, liver, brain, skin)	
Paraneoplastic syndromes	None	Rarely associated		
Treatment	Surgery			Radiation and chemotherapy
Adjuvant chemotherapy/radiation	Not indicated		Questionable benefit	Indicated
Prognosis	Excellent	92% survival	48% 5-year survival 30% 10-year survival	16% 2-year survival 5% 5-year survival
Histologic, Ultrastructural, and Immunohistochemical Aspects				
Surface involvement	Absent		Generally absent	Absent
Ulceration	Absent		Common	
Growth pattern	Organoid	Trabecular, glandular	Cribriform, ribbons, solid sheets	
Squamoid differentiation	None	May be present		
Crush artifact	Absent			Prominent
Necrosis	Absent		Uncommon	Prominent
Mitoses	Rare/absent		Usually few	Prominent
Nuclear pleomorphism	May be marked	Absent	Mild to marked	Prominent
Nuclear shape	Round/oval, ± hyperchromasia	Round/oval, vesicular, central	Round/oval, hyperchromatic	Oval/spindle ± eccentric
Nucleoli	Occasional	Absent	Variable	Absent
Cytoplasm	Eosinophilic to clear	Eosinophilic, oncocytic	Variable	Minimal
Nuclear:cytoplasmic ratio	Variable	Low	Variable	High
Epithelial mucin	Absent	Common	Variable	
Argyrophilia	+++	++		Rarely positive
Argent-affinity	Absent		Rarely present	
Neurosecretory granules	100–250 nm	90–230 nm, abundant	70–420 nm, common	50–200 nm, rare
Junctional complexes	Infrequent	Present		Scanty
Lumina	Absent	Present		Usually absent
Expression of epithelial markers (cytokeratin, EMA, CEA)	Absent	Present		
Expression of neuroendocrine markers (NSE, chromogranin, S-100)	Present			
Expression of neuroendocrine polypeptides (calcitonin, bombesin)	Absent	Present		

CEA, carcinoembryonic antigen; EMA, epithelial membrane antigen; MDNEC, moderately differentiated neuroendocrine carcinoma; NSE, neuron-specific enolase; PDNEC, poorly differentiated neuroendocrine carcinoma; WDNEC, well-differentiated neuroendocrine carcinoma; ±, with or without.

PDNEC, while MDNEC has a biologic behavior intermediate between the other two.[280–288]

Clinical Features. MDNEC is the most frequently encountered type of NEC, followed by PDNEC. True, typical, carcinoid WDNECs are the least common subtype and are extremely rare. A recent review from the AFIP indicated a ratio of 54:14:2 for MDNEC, PDNEC, and WDNEC, respectively, out of 8469 malignant laryngeal neoplasms.[285] Most of the tumors reported as carcinoid tumors are better categorized as atypical carcinoid or MDNEC, from both their histologic appearance and biologic potential. Data contrasting the clinical and pathologic aspects of these tumors are summarized in Table 5–1. Patients most often present in the sixth to eighth decade of life. There is a strong male predisposition, with the most frequent presenting symptom being hoarseness. In addition, patients with PDNECs often present with a neck mass (Fig. 5–34A,B, see p. 249). There is a strong association of MDNEC and PDNEC with a history of smoking. Tumors most commonly arise in the supraglottis, and only occasionally from other laryngeal areas.

Pathologic Features. Patients present with submucosal or polypoid masses, usually ranging in size from a few millimeters up to 4 cm in greatest dimension (Fig. 5–34C, see p. 249). WDNECs are characterized by nests of uniform cells separated by a fibrovascular or hyalinized connective tissue stroma (Fig. 5–35, see p. 250). Nuclei are round to oval with stippled or vesicular chromatin and eosinophilic cytoplasm. A glandular component is common. Cellular pleomorphism, mitotic activity, and necrosis are usually absent in WDNEC. MDNEC is characterized by infiltrative growth and a varied histologic pattern that may include glandular, organoid, acinar, trabecular, solid, and nesting architectures (see Fig. 5–35). The tumor cells are polyhedral to round, are at least twice the size of the small cell variant of PDNEC, and contain varying amounts of eosinophilic cytoplasm. Occasionally, oncocytic differentiation may be observed.[289] Nuclei are round to oval with a stippled chromatin, are often eccentrically located, and display mild to severe pleomorphism. Mitotic figures are rare or absent. PDNECs are characterized by sheets and, rarely, interconnecting ribbons of undifferentiated small cells with minimal cytoplasm (oat cell variant), or slightly larger cells with minimal to moderate cytoplasm (intermediate variant) and hyperchromatic, pleomorphic, oval, round, or spindle-shaped nuclei with delicate chromatin and absent or inconspicuous nucleoli. Individual cell necrosis, vascular and perineural invasion, and prominent mitotic activity are common. Glandular or squamous differentiation and rosette formation may occasionally be observed.

Ultrastructural studies demonstrate neurosecretory granules in all three types in varying numbers and sizes (see Table 5–1); desmosomes and tonofilaments are frequent in WDNEC and MDNEC but are less common in PDNEC, whereas lumina (true and intracellular) are frequent in WDNEC and MDNEC and are usually absent in PDNEC. Argyrophil silver stains are frequently positive in WDNEC and MDNEC and are usually negative or focally positive in PDNEC. Classic neuroendocrine markers (e.g., chromogranin, neuron-specific enolase [NSE], synaptophysin, Leu-7) will usually be positive. Calcitonin is also positive in all three types of neuroendocrine carcinoma.[277]

Differential Diagnosis. Frequent considerations include melanoma, paraganglioma, medullary thyroid carcinoma, and squamous carcinoma. S100, a common marker for melanoma, may be positive in laryngeal NEC; therefore, HMB-45,[290] a melanin-specific antibody, should be added to the immunohistochemical profile. Ultrastructural studies may be helpful to evaluate for melanosomes or premelanosomes. Calcitonin positivity or ultrastructural evidence of glandular lumina with microvilli can distinguish NEC from paraganglioma. Medullary thyroid carcinoma shares many histologic and immunohistochemical features of MDNEC. Both contain intracellular calcitonin and may contain extracellular amyloid.[291, 292] Clinicopathologic correlation should establish the proper diagnosis. Additionally, although both may secrete calcitonin, an elevated serum calcitonin is much more frequently associated with medullary thyroid carcinoma; however, we have observed symptomatic serum calcitonin elevation in one patient with a primary laryngeal NEC.[280, 291] Poorly differentiated squamous carcinoma may occasionally have ribbons or cords of tumor cells and can grow in sheets somewhat similar to moderately or poorly differentiated NEC; however, immunohistochemical and ultrastructural studies for neuroendocrine markers (NSE ubiquity notwithstanding) are negative in the squamous carcinomas.

Treatment and Prognosis. Surgery is the primary therapy for WDNEC and MDNEC, and a lymph node dissection is indicated for MDNEC because of the high rate of cervical nodal metastases. PDNEC should be treated with a combination of radiation and chemotherapy similar to the protocols used for pulmonary oat cell carcinoma of the lung due to early hematogenous spread.[285–288]

WDNEC is associated with a very good prognosis. In a recent review, 8 of 12 patients were disease-free 1.5 to 8 years after treatment. One patient died of unrelated causes at 2.25 years; one patient was disease free 8 years after one recurrence; and one patient was alive with metastatic disease and the carcinoid syndrome at 4 years.[287] Only one patient died of disease, 5 years after surgical treatment.

The MDNECs are more aggressive neoplasms, with 5- and 10-year cumulative survival rates of 48% and 30%, respectively.[282] Tumors larger than 1 cm appear to be more aggressive, and patients developing skin or subcutaneous involvement have a worse prognosis.[282] In a recent review of 119 MDNECs with follow-up information, 74% of the 66 patients treated with neck dissections during their disease course had metastatic disease.[282]

The most aggressive type of laryngeal NEC is PDNEC. In a recent series, 73% of patients with PDNEC died with an average survival of only 9.8 months (range 1 to 26 months).[281] Two- and 5-year survivals were 16% and 5%, respectively. Additionally, these tumors may be associated with paraneoplastic syndromes, including Cushing,[293] Eaton-Lambert,[294] and Schwartz-Bartter syndromes.[295]

Salivary-Type Lesions

Salivary gland–type neoplasms are rare tumors in the larynx, accounting for less than 0.7% of laryngeal carcinomas.[296] They account for 56% of laryngeal glandular tumors; malignancies outnumber benign tumors by a ratio of 2.6:1.[297] The most common benign tumors are oncocytic lesions; benign mixed tumors are a distant second, unlike their frequent occurrence in the salivary glands (Table 5–2).[297] The four most common malignant salivary tumors are adenosquamous carcinoma (discussed in Chapter 2), followed with equal incidence by adenoid cystic and mucoepidermoid carcinoma,[297–299] and lastly malignant mixed tumors. Other salivary tumors that arise, albeit rarely, in the larynx include myoepithelioma (benign and malignant), acinic cell carcinoma, epithelial myoepithelial carcinoma, clear cell carcinoma, and salivary duct carcinoma.[296–300]

Oncocytic Cysts and Cystadenomas

Clinical Features. Laryngeal oncocytic cysts and their proliferative counterparts, oncocytic cystadenomas, are uncommonly encountered lesions and have been found in 0.1% to 1% of laryngeal biopsies.[301, 302] The majority occur in the false cords or ventricles, where seromucinous glands are most dense; a compilation of 142 cases revealed the distribution of supraglottic, glottic, and infraglottic cases to be 74%, 22%, and 4%, respectively.[304] A female predominance has been noted, with a female:male ratio of 2:1.[305] Most patients are in their seventh and eighth decades of life. Bilateral and diffuse distribution has been noted, which accounts for symptomatic recurrence after biopsy.[302–308] The majority of cases are under 1 cm in greatest dimension. The largest of 19 cases from the AFIP was 2.8 cm in greatest dimension.[304] Rarely, obstructing "extensive" or "bulky" tumors are reported.[308]

Pathologic Features. These lesions have acinar, mucinous, or ductal epithelial cells that have undergone oncocytic metaplasia and some degree of hyperplasia. Oncocytic cystadenomas range from predominantly simple cystic lesions (oncocytic cysts) to more complex multicystic and papillocystic lesions (oncocytic cystadenoma). Lymphocytic infiltrates may be prominent and reminiscent of Warthin's tumors. Simple cysts without papillations should be classified as oncocytic cysts, whereas more complex multicystic lesions with a papillary component should be classified as cystadenoma (Fig. 5–36, see p. 251). Atypia is usually absent.

Differential Diagnosis. Cystic, papillary oncocytic cystadenomas are histologically benign and should pose no diagnostic problem for the pathologist. The differential diagnosis of non-squamous papillary laryngeal tumors is limited to papillary thyroid carcinoma and salivary duct carcinoma. The latter is rarely seen in the larynx[300] but may be papillary. We have recently seen a case of papillary oncocytic cystadenoma diagnosed as low-grade papillary adenocarcinoma. Reversal of this diagnosis obviously saved the patient needless surgery (see subsequent discussion). Careful attention to cytology should allow for recognition of cuboidal oncocytes. Small nests of oncocytes may be closely packed together, but the ductal/

Table 5–2. Laryngeal Glandular Tumors

Tumor Type	Number of Cases
Adenosquamous carcinoma	19
Oncocytic tumors	12
Adenoid cystic carcinoma	11
Mucoepidermoid carcinoma	11
Mixed tumor	3
Cystadenoma	1
Malignant mixed tumor	1
Total salivary gland tumors	58
Adenocarcinomas (mostly neuroendocrine)	45
TOTAL FOR ALL TUMORS	103

Adapted from Heffner DK: Sinonasal and laryngeal salivary gland lesions. In: Ellis GL, Auclair PL, Gnepp DR, eds. *Surgical Pathology of the Salivary Glands.* Philadelphia: WB Saunders, 1991:544–559.

cystic nature of oncocytic cystadenomas should be obvious. Predominantly solid, diffuse, noncystic true oncocytic tumors of the larynx are not known to occur in humans (although they have been seen in dogs[309, 310]). Thus, a laryngeal biopsy of a predominantly noncystic, diffuse, seemingly "oncocytic" tumor should raise suspicions of other diagnoses. For instance, neuroendocrine carcinoma of the larynx may masquerade as an "oncocytic" tumor.[311, 312] Mucoepidermoid carcinoma and squamous cell carcinoma may be extremely eosinophilic and appear "oncocytic." Nuclear pleomorphism can be seen in all the tumors mentioned and would not be seen in oncocytic cystadenoma. Electron microscopic investigation or immunohistochemical staining may be necessary for unusual cases that are difficult to classify.

Treatment. Simple conservative endoscopic excision is curative for most cases. Occasionally, laryngeal oncocytic cystadenomas may recur, more likely as a manifestation of diffuse or multifocal oncocytic metaplasia, rather than oncologic aggressiveness.

Benign Mixed Tumor

Clinical Features. Benign mixed tumors (BMT) commonly present in the third to sixth decades; rarely, they may arise in the pediatric age range.[313, 314] To date, less than 20 cases have been reported (Fig. 5–37).[297, 313–319] The majority of tumors involve the supraglottis, usually epiglottis, and may reach up to 4 cm in greatest dimension.

Pathologic Features and Differential Diagnosis. The histologic appearance of laryngeal BMT is similar to that of BMT arising in the salivary glands (see Fig. 5–37). (See salivary gland chapter for histologic description.) Because of its rarity, a diagnosis of laryngeal BMT should be approached with caution, with every possible effort made to exclude other more common neoplasms, such as mucoepidermoid, mucinous, or adenoid cystic carcinoma and chondrosarcoma.[296, 297] The presence of chondroid or myxoid stroma eliminates mucoepidermoid and mucinous adenocarcinoma from consideration. Adenoid cystic carcinoma does not exhibit the varied growth patterns typical of BMT and is infiltrative; chondroid or myxoid stroma and plasmacytic myoepithelial cells favor the latter. BMT can be distinguished from chondrosarcoma by the presence of both epithelial and myoepithelial components.

Treatment and Prognosis. Complete surgical excision is the treatment of choice; BMTs are benign and should be cured if completely removed.

Adenoid Cystic Carcinoma

Clinical Features. Adenoid cystic carcinoma (ACC) of the larynx accounts for 0.07% to 0.25% of laryngeal carcinomas.[320–322] To date, approximately 125 cases have been reported.[296, 322–324] There is a broad age range of occurrence, with a slightly increased incidence in the fourth to sixth decades of life.[297] Approximately 60% involve the infraglottis, 33% the supraglottis, and 6% the vocal fold.[296] Voice change or hoarseness, pain radiating to the ear, and dysphagia are the most common presenting symptoms for supraglottic tumors; infraglottic tumors may be associated with "asthma," pain, hoarseness, or dyspnea on exertion.[296, 297] Extralaryngeal invasion may result in initial presentation as a thyroid mass.

Pathologic Features. The majority of tumors diffusely invade the submucosa and adjacent soft tissues without protruding into the laryngeal lumen. ACCs of the larynx are morphologically similar to those arising in the salivary glands and are composed of a somewhat uniform population of basaloid tumor cells. (See salivary chapter for description.) They are widely infiltrative and may grow in a dense scar-like fashion. Perineural invasion is common (Fig. 5–38, see p. 251). Intraoperative frozen section examination is extremely useful to map out disease extent and type of resection required.[297]

Differential Diagnosis. The differential diagnosis consists of BMT, basaloid squamous cell carcinoma, and neuroendocrine carcinoma and, for infraglottic tumors, thyroid carcinoma. BMTs are usually well circumscribed, contain myxoid or chondroid stroma, often with plasmacytic myoepithelial cells, usually have more varied growth patterns, and do not exhibit perineural invasion. Basaloid squamous cell carcinoma (BSCC) commonly has an adenoid growth pattern similar to that seen in ACC (Fig. 5–39); however, ACC lacks the malignant squamous component typical of BSCC and there is much less cytologic atypia, mitotic activity, and necrosis in ACC than is found in BSCC. Neuroendocrine carcinoma does not exhibit a cribriform growth pattern and ACC does not contain rosettes; however, with small biopsies this differential diagnosis may be problematic. Immunohistochemistry may be necessary to establish the specific nature of the tumor. Neuroendocrine carcinoma, ACC, and BSCC may all express low molecular weight cytokeratin, S-100, and NSE to varying degrees. Strong synaptophysin and chromogranin expression is consistent with neuroendocrine carcinoma, whereas expression of high molecular weight cytokeratin would favor BSCC. Thyroid tumors usually have a distinctive histologic pattern different from ACC; however, if difficulties do arise, immuno-

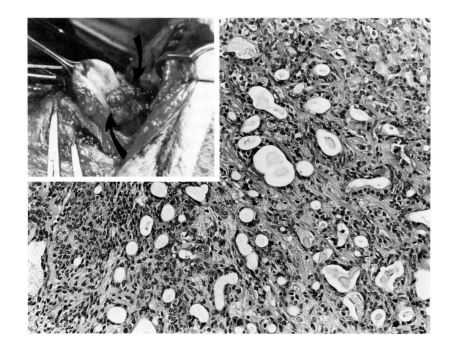

Figure 5–37. Epiglottic benign mixed tumor. *Inset,* Lobulated exophytic mass *(arrows).* (Courtesy of Dr. Hugh Biller.) Note: epithelial and myoepithelial cells forming ductal structures, within a myxoid background.

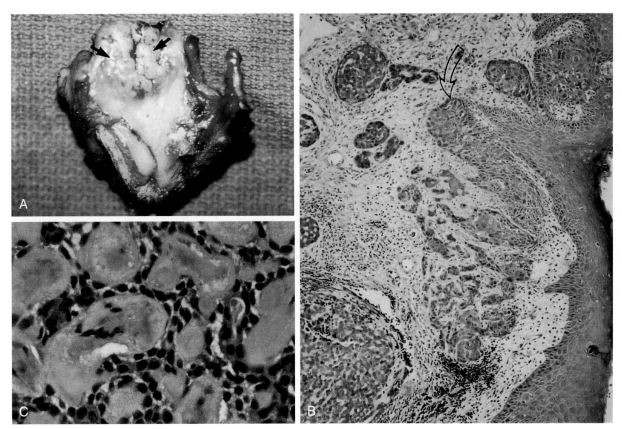

Figure 5–39. Laryngeal basaloid squamous carcinoma. A, Gross specimen with submucosal epiglottic tumor *(arrows)*. B&C, Cord formation and hyaline deposition are reminiscent of adenoid cystic carcinoma, which in fact was the initial diagnosis for this case. Right focal keratinization and attachment to the rete pegs can be seen focally *(arrow)*.

histochemical staining for thyroglobulin and calcitonin should resolve the problem.

Treatment and Prognosis. Complete surgical excision consisting of partial or complete laryngectomy is the treatment of choice. Recurrence rates have historically been in the range of 50%[297]; therefore, adjuvant radiation therapy is indicated. Cervical lymph node dissection is not usually recommended[296] unless there is palpable lymphadenopathy. Isolated pulmonary metastasis, if present, should be treated aggressively and not alter treatment of the primary tumor.[296] ACC has a slow relentless clinical course marked by high local recurrence rates and late distant metastases. Patients with infraglottic tumors have an average survival of 8 years, with occasional patients surviving for 15 years.[296] Tumors with perineural invasion appear to have a higher risk of local recurrence.[325] Occasional patients may have rapid progression of disease or transition from a slow to a more rapid clinical course.[296] Similar to ACC of other upper aerodigestive sites, most patients will eventually die from their tumor.

Mucoepidermoid Carcinoma

Clinical Features. Laryngeal mucoepidermoid carcinomas (MEC) have a similar incidence to ACC.[297] To date, less than 100 cases have been described in the literature.[296, 297, 325–331] In a series of 85 cases of MEC reviewed at our institution, 6% occurred in the larynx. These tumors usually occur between the ages of 45 and 75 years and rarely may arise in children.[326] They most frequently arise in the supraglottic area.[327] Presenting symptoms are similar to those of squamous carcinoma, with patients frequently complaining of hoarseness and rarely presenting with a neck mass.[327]

Pathologic Features. Tumors usually originate in the submucosa and range up to 5 cm in greatest dimension. They have an appearance similar to their salivary gland counterpart, composed of mucin-secreting intermediate and squamous cells in varying proportions arranged in solid or cystic nests. For a detailed histologic description, refer to the salivary gland chapter. Occasional tumors may arise from surface mucosa; a clear cell variant has also been reported.[330, 332]

Differential Diagnosis. The differential diagnosis includes a hamartomatous proliferation of mucinous glands, necrotizing sialometaplasia (NSM), and adenosquamous carcinoma. Benign hamartomatous mucinous gland proliferations will occasionally arise in the larynx and may have dilated ductal structures similar to MEC. The mucinous glands are usually better formed than those in MEC and squamous and intermediate cells are lacking in the hamartomas. NSM retains a lobular pattern and is noninvasive. The most problematic differential diagnosis is between high-grade MEC and adenosquamous carcinoma (ADSC), the latter is more frequent than MEC.[327] ADSC always involves the surface mucosa with two distinct components. The most superficial portion of the tumor is usually a squamous carcinoma with easily recognizable intracellular junctions and keratin production; deeper portions of the tumor frequently differentiate toward a poorly differentiated adenocarcinoma. The presence of an in situ component or of a superficial squamous carcinoma strongly supports the diagnosis of ADSC. Additionally, ADSC does not usually contain goblet cells as MEC does and, unlike MEC, frequently contains distinct separate areas of squamous and adenocarcinoma.

Treatment and Prognosis. Total laryngectomy has been the most commonly employed treatment; however, small or limited tumors may be treated by partial laryngectomy. A neck dissection should be performed for palpable lymphadenopathy; however, the decision to perform an elective neck dissection relates to histologic grade on the preoperative biopsy. Elective neck dissection and/or cervical radiation therapy is indicated for high-grade MEC. If the preoperative diagnosis is an intermediate-grade MEC, it is unclear whether elective neck dissection is also indicated, as (1) the tumor grading on the biopsy may not be representative of the overall tumor grade and (2) metastatic disease may also occur with truly intermediate-grade MEC. What is clear is the rarity with which low-grade MEC metastasize.

Mucoepidermoid carcinomas should be graded after thorough sampling. (See salivary gland chapter for more specific information on grading.) Low-grade tumors have a good prognosis with an actuarial survival of 100% at 3, 5, and 10 years and a recurrence rate of 50% in one series.[327] A literature review has revealed a 5-year survival rate for low-grade MEC of 91%, whereas high-grade tumors (many of which most likely are adenosquamous carcinomas, as previously discussed) have survival rates on the order of 50% at 3 years.[327]

Melanoma

Clinical Features. Mucosal melanoma constitutes less than 2% of all melanomas in Western populations. For the Japanese, by comparison, melanomas of the mucosal surfaces constitute one quarter to one third of all melanoma cases.[333–335] The vast majority of upper aerodigestive tract mucosal melanomas occur in the sinonasal tract and oral cavity. Laryngeal and hypopharyngeal melanomas are much more rare—representing only 3.8% to 8% of upper aerodigestive mucosal melanomas.[333–342] Eneroth and Lundberg[343] did not find any laryngeal melanomas among their 41 cases of upper aerodigestive tract melanoma. Nine cases had been coded as laryngeal melanomas at the Otolaryngic Tumor Registry at the AFIP over a 77-year period (0.09% of 10,270 primary laryngeal neoplasms).[342] Only four of those cases were immunohistochemically confirmed as melanomas; the others proved to be neuroendocrine carcinoma (3), lymphoma (1), or metastatic melanoma (1). To date, fewer than 50 cases have been reported, with the majority of these tumors arising in elderly Caucasian males. Mucosal melanomas generally appear as brown, tan, or bluish polypoid tumors, most frequently involving the supraglottic region. Patients present with hoarseness, hemoptysis, sore throat, neck pain, and foreign body sensation.

Pathologic Features. Melanoma has earned the histologic reputation as the great masquerader: sarcoma-like, epithelioid, or pleomorphic patterns may be seen. Melanoma can have a plasmacytic, spindle cell, or epithelioid cytology. With the plasmacytic appearance, the nuclei are eccentric, and the cytoplasm is bright pink to "dirty" brown and granular. Intranuclear vacuolations (intranuclear holes) or pink nucleoli are helpful "giveaways" to the true diagnosis. Spindle cell morphology can mimic a sarcoma and the nuclei often have a variable morphology. Melanin deposition may still be observable in the cytoplasm. The epithelioid form of melanoma forms sheets of large plump cells that have a nesting tendency. Intranuclear vacuolations are seen, and again, melanin may be seen in the cytoplasm.

Junctional activity may be observed in primary mucosal melanomas and is not seen in metastatic tumors, but its absence does not preclude the diagnosis of primary mucosal melanoma. Intramucosal spread of melanocytes in the adjacent epithelium histologically favors a primary tumor. The question may arise, when a laryngeal or pharyngeal melanoma is diagnosed, as to whether it represents a primary or a metastatic tumor. Certainly, this is a significant question as metastatic cutaneous melanoma is one of the most common secondary malignancies (along with renal cell carcinoma) to occur in the larynx. It is unlikely, in the absence of a history of dermal melanoma, that a screening examination will uncover an occult primary tumor. If the patient has a history of a prior dermal melanoma, the laryngeal/pharyngeal tumor should be considered a metastasis, and probably forebears disseminated disease.

Benign mucosal melanosis has been observed in the larynx, albeit rarely, and is more likely observed in smokers.[344]

Differential Diagnosis. The differential diagnosis of melanoma varies with its particular appearance. As a "small blue round cell tumor," the differential diagnosis includes poorly differentiated neuroendocrine carcinoma, lymphoma, and plasmacytoma. As a pleomorphic tumor, the differential diagnosis includes undifferentiated carcinoma and rhabdomyosarcoma. As a spindle cell tumor, the differential diagnosis includes spindle cell carcinoma and sarcomas such as leiomyosarcoma and malignant fibrous histiocytoma. The immunohistochemical profile of staining with anti-S100, HMB-45, and anti-vimentin can secure the diagnosis. Cytokeratin and epithelial membrane antigen are generally not expressed, but occasional expression of both has been noted[345] that may result in confusion in a biopsy. Additionally, the following patterns of antigen expression are not seen in a melanoma: lymphoma will express leukocyte common antigen (CD45) and B cell antigen (CD20) in paraffin sections; plasmacytomas may or may not express CD45 and CD20; they will also express epithelial membrane antigen. A muscle tumor expresses muscle specific actin and desmin; myoglobin is expressed in a rhabdomyosarcoma.

Treatment and Prognosis. Complete resection with negative margins will probably prolong the disease-free interval at the primary site. A careful clinical and radiographic evaluation of the neck should be performed. If positive nodes are found, a neck dissection should also be performed. Radiation and chemotherapy have never been shown to have efficacy. Generally, the prognosis of mucosal melanoma is poorer as compared with cutaneous melanoma, probably related to overall tumor load at the time of initial diagnosis. Average survival rates for mucosal malignant melanoma, including laryngeal melanoma, is less than 3.5 years; the 5-year survival is less than 21%.[336–339] Patients with laryngeal melanoma usually progress to widespread disseminated disease. In contrast to mucosal melanomas of other sites, laryngeal melanomas appear to have a somewhat better local recurrence rate (32%).[341] This may relate to overall resectability of laryngeal tumors as compared with other sites. Unlike melanomas of the skin, Clark's levels and Breslow thickness have no relationship to clinical outcome.

Lymphoid Neoplasia

A wide variety of primary or secondary hematologic neoplasms may involve the larynx.[346] Of these, extramedullary plasmacytomas (EMP)[346–354] and non-Hodgkin's lymphomas (NHL) are the most common. However, even these are quite rare and constitute far less than 1% of all laryngeal tumors.[346] Waldeyer's ring and the sinonasal tract are much more frequent sites of EMP and extranodal NHL. Hodgkin's disease is even less common at these extranodal sites. Rarely, leukemic infiltrates may also involve the larynx.

Extramedullary Plasmacytoma

Extramedullary plasmacytoma is a soft tissue malignant neoplasm composed of a monoclonal proliferation of plasma cells.[347] The neoplastic cells display monotypic cytoplasmic immunoglobulin expression and an absence of immature B cell antigens. EMP may be primary or secondary to underlying multiple myeloma.

Clinical Features. Most EMPs (80%) occur in the head and neck. About 80% of head and neck EMPs are primary tumors and 20% are secondary to myeloma.[347] The mean age of patients is 59 years (range 34–78 years), with a male predominance of 4:1.[347] About 80% occur in the sinonasal tract and Waldeyer's ring. The larynx is involved in 5% and the pharynx in 5%. Most EMPs are solitary (2 to 5 cm); 10% are multiple at presentation. On examination, mucosal EMPs appear polypoid and smooth without ulceration. Laryngeal EMPs generally involve the supraglottis, most often the epiglottis, followed by the false cord, ventricle, arytenoid, and infraglottis. Cervical lymph nodes are enlarged in 10% of patients. The extent of primary tumor is best determined on radiographic imaging. The diagnosis usually requires biopsy of the mass.

Gorenstein et al.[352] described six males with solitary EMP of the larynx, ranging in age from 32 to 63 years (mean 53 years). The first symptom was usually hoarseness. The vocal cord was the site in four, and the infraglottis in two cases. In three cases there was also involvement of adjacent ventricle, trachea, or base of tongue. Most were well differentiated EMP.

Pathologic Features. On gross examination, the tumor is often red-brown, lobulated, smooth, or nodular and has a fleshy or rubbery consistency. Histologically, EMP is composed of sheets of plasma cells that vary in maturation from well to moderately or poorly differentiated and has a diffuse pattern of proliferation with a scant stroma.[347, 348] The neoplastic cells infiltrate the subepithelial layer of the mucosa and are similar to those seen in multiple myeloma (Fig. 5–40, see p. 251). Amyloid may be seen in 5% of EMP.[347]

Special Studies. Immunohistochemistry or, less frequently, electron microscopy may be essential for diagnosis. The diagnosis of EMP is easily confirmed in most cases by demonstrating cytoplasmic light chain restriction using immunostains for κ and λ light chains or in situ hybridization for κ and λ mRNA.[347–353] Ig heavy chain gene rearrangement can be found using molecular techniques. Ultrastructurally, plasma cells are rich in rough endoplasmic reticulum and have a prominent Golgi apparatus.

Differential Diagnosis. The differential diagnosis of well differentiated EMP includes reactive plasmacytosis of the mucous membranes, plasma cell granuloma, granulomatous infections, rhinoscleroma, and extranodal Rosai-Dorfman disease. Rosai-Dorfman disease usually presents with enlarged cervical lymph nodes. It has been reported as a rare cause of infraglottic narrowing due to paratracheal nodal and tracheal involvement.[355] Unlike EMP, however, immunoperoxidase staining of reactive plasma cells in these conditions will demonstrate a polyclonal pattern (both κ and λ light chains). Moderately or poorly differentiated EMP may be confused with other small cell malignancies, mainly immunoblastic lymphoma, melanoma, carcinoma, neuroendocrine carcinoma, and rhabdomyosarcoma. EMP is negative for S-100 protein, HMB45, cytokeratin, and muscle markers. The diagnosis of EMP is confirmed by demonstrating cytoplasmic light chain restriction. However, B cell NHL may also demonstrate this finding, and immunohistochemical studies for other B-cell lineage markers may be useful.[356] A plasmacytic lymphocyte infiltrate secondary to Waldenström's macroglobulinemia has been reported in the larynx and thus may also enter the differential diagnosis.[357]

Treatment and Prognosis. The treatment of primary EMP is radiation therapy, which has a good local response in most patients. Since the prognosis of secondary EMP is markedly different, it is essential to first exclude the presence of systemic disease.[347] Primary EMP may produce a small monoclonal component, but excessive production is suspicious for myeloma.[347]

Extramedullary plasmacytoma of the larynx appears to have a good prognosis. In the group reported by Gorenstein et al.,[352] patients were treated by excision or radiation therapy or both. Only one tumor recurred after radiation therapy. None of the six patients died of their disease, with follow-up ranging from 3 to 25 years (median 5 years).

The median survival in patients with primary EMP is 114 months for those with locoregional disease versus 16 months for those with myeloma.[358] The extent of primary tumor, differentiation of plasma cells, and dissemination are important prognostic factors. The presence of regional lymphadenopathy, amounts or type of paraprotein, local bone destruction, and persistence of primary tumor after irradiation do not necessarily indicate a poor prognosis.[347] Despite good local response, about 30% of primary EMP will progress to myeloma, often within 2 years but at times after decades.[347] However, it is difficult to predict from the clinicopathologic features, which of the cases will progress to myeloma.

Malignant Lymphomas

Clinical Features. Malignant lymphomas usually present primarily as a lymph nodal mass. However, in about 25% of cases, extranodal sites of the head and neck or gastrointestinal tract may be the primary sites. Lymphomas of the larynx are rare; a group of investigators culled and reviewed 65 reported cases.[346, 349–365] Most patients are older (mean age 58 years) and there is a male predominance (1.5:1). The most frequent presenting symptoms are hoarseness and dysphagia. Most tumors are localized to the larynx and may involve regional cervical lymph nodes (Stage IE or IIE). The supraglottic larynx, especially the epiglottis and aryepiglottic folds, is the most common site, followed by the ventricle and infraglottis.[346] The tumors are generally polypoid and smooth, without ulceration of the overlying mucosa.

Pathologic Features. Lymphomas presenting in extranodal sites of the head and neck are mainly NHL of low or high grade. Depending on the extranodal site, these may be predominantly of B cell (Waldeyer's ring) or T cell type (nasopharynx and sinonasal). NHL presenting with extranodal laryngeal involvement may be primary[359–365] or part of multicentric or systemic involvement.[346, 366] These are of varied histologic types, although most are B cell lymphomas. T cell lymphomas are less common but have been reported in the larynx.[365] Using the NHL working formulation, extranodal NHL may be classified as low, intermediate, or high grade.[367] They may have a diffuse or follicular pattern of proliferation. Low-grade lymphoplasmacytic lymphomas and those having features of low-grade B cell lymphomas of mucosal-associated lymphoid tissue (MALT) type have been observed at this site.[346, 360, 361] (For a more detailed description, see Chapter 12.)

Differential Diagnosis. Small lymphocytic lymphomas need to be distinguished from inflammatory pseudotumor and atypical or reactive lymphoid infiltrates such as infectious mononucleosis. Immunophenotypic study in these lesions shows a mixture of B and T cells in reactive lesions with a polyclonal pattern of staining for immunoglobulin light chains. When there is a suspicion of low-grade NHL, molecular genetic studies for Ig heavy chain gene rearrangement may be helpful in the diagnosis. If fresh tissue is unavailable for the demonstration of B cell antigens (CD19, 20, 22) on frozen tissue, immunohistochemistry may be performed on formalin-fixed, paraffin-embedded sections using CD20 (L26) or the expression of monotypic Ig κ or λ light chains. T cell markers helpful in evaluating these lesions include CD3, CD45, and CD43. Polymerase chain reaction (PCR) may now be performed on both fresh tissue and paraffin-embedded sections to demonstrate Ig heavy chain gene rearrangements, consistent with a diagnosis of NHL.

Treatment and Prognosis. Extranodal laryngeal lymphomas limited to the primary site or with regional lymphadenopathy may be managed by biopsy followed by radiation therapy. Systemic chemotherapy is indicated for recurrent or disseminated NHL. Most laryngeal lymphomas have a good initial response to radiation therapy and the prognosis is generally favorable.[346]

Inflammatory Myofibroblastic Tumor (Inflammatory Pseudotumor, Plasma Cell Granuloma)

Clinical Features. Inflammatory myofibroblastic tumor (IMT) is a fibroinflammatory space-occupying lesion or, most likely, a *number* of entities with overlapping histologic features, the true nature of which is only beginning to be elucidated. The lung, liver, and gastrointestinal tract (omentum and mesentery) are the most common sites for IMT. In the head and neck, IMTs have been reported in the epiglottis, endolarynx, parapharyngeal space, maxillary sinus, submandibular region, and oral cavity.[368–380] In a series of 84 patients with IMT from all extrapulmonary sites, no pronounced gender predominance was seen (female:male 1.3:1),[371] and a predisposition for the first two decades of life was noted. Wenig et al.[369] reported on a series of eight patients with laryngeal IMT. These lesions caused hoarseness and foreign body sensation, usually over a period of months. Only one of these patients had a history of previous trauma—a difficult endotracheal intubation. The lesions appeared as nodular, pedunculated polypoid fleshy tumors.

Pathologic Features. It is quite common for patients with IMT to undergo multiple biopsy procedures to establish a diagnosis. On biopsy evaluation, IMT appears to be a diagnosis of exclusion. Excised tumors have been described as fleshy, whorled, and firm or myxoid. Coffin et al.[371] described 19% of tumors to be multinodular. The polymorphous appearance of IMT may reflect its variable etiology or its shifting histology during disease course. Lymphocytes, plasma cells, histiocytes, fibroblasts, and myofibroblasts are the basic components of IMT, with mutable proportions. Four basic histologic patterns emerge: (1) a dominant lymphoplasmacytic infiltrate, (2) a dominant lymphohistiocytic infiltrate, (3) a predominantly "young and active" myofibroblastic process, (4) a predominantly collagenized process with lymphoplasmacytic infiltrate (Fig. 5–41, see p. 252). The lymphoplasmacytic IMT consists of a mature lymphoid infiltrate with germinal centers, and a rich plasma cell infiltrate, hence the name plasma cell granuloma. Lymphohistiocytic IMT most resembles an infectious process, as foamy histiocytes are prominent. The "young and active" IMT has a densely cellular fascicular and storiform pattern, resembling fibrous histiocytoma except for the inflammatory infiltrate or nodular fasciitis. Overlapping histologic features between IMT, nodular fasciitis, and fibrous histiocytoma corroborate the place of these entities in the pathologic spectrum between reactive and neoplastic processes. Collagenized IMT is paucicellular and resembles a desmoid tumor but with a prominent inflammatory infiltrate. A zonation/maturation effect may be observed. Progression of patterns may also be seen in some long-standing cases necessitating multiple procedures.

Special Studies. Immunohistochemical study on these cases reveals that the majority of fibroblastic spindle cells express markers of smooth muscle differentiation (muscle-specific actin, smooth muscle actin, and desmin). Coffin et al.[371] noted that one third of the cases also focally expressed cytokeratin, which may also speak for myofibroblastic differentiation. Ultrastructural examination has confirmed a myofibroblastic population—fibroblast-like spindle cells with intracytoplasmic microfilament bundles and pinocytotic vesicles.

Differential Diagnosis. The differential diagnosis depends on the predominant histologic pattern and includes plasmacytoma, nodular fasciitis, fibromatosis, fibrous histiocytoma, inflammatory fibrosarcoma, inflammatory malignant fibrous histiocytoma, and spindle cell carcinoma. Mitotic figures and plump spindle cells are present in IMT, but nuclear pleomorphism and apoptosis are not usually seen in IMT; their presence should lead one to consider an inflammatory sarcomatous process or spindle cell carcinoma. IMT may overlap, in terms of biologic potential and histology, with the entity described as a "low-grade inflammatory fibrosarcoma."[381] The diagnoses of nodular fasciitis, fibrous histiocytoma, and fibromatosis can come to mind when examining IMT. Perhaps IMT is also related to these processes, but the constellation of histologic features of IMT (storiform pattern, lack of necrosis, pronounced chronic inflammatory component) is inconsistent with these processes. The plasmacytic and histiocytic component to IMT may raise the possibility of infections such as syphilis and atypical mycobacterium. In such cases, special stains (acid-fast bacillus, silver stains) are warranted. Autoimmune diseases (lupus erythematosus, rheumatoid arthritis) can cause intense laryngeal inflammation and hence appear as an inflammatory pseudotumor.

The distinction between laryngeal IMT and spindle cell carcinoma may be difficult on biopsy. IMT lacks the extreme nuclear pleomorphism usually seen in carcinoma, which is the basis for distinguishing the two. Spindle cell carcinoma lacks the myxoid "feathery" reactive appearance of IMT. Spindle cell carcinoma may be recognized as such by the presence of carcinoma in situ, superficially infiltrating islands of keratinizing carcinoma, or origin from dysplastic basilar surface epithelium. However, the absence of these features does not rule out this diagnosis. Keratin positivity and expression of smooth muscle markers in spindle cells may be seen in both IMT and spindle cell carcinoma, hence immunohistochemistry may not be helpful with this differential diagnosis.

The distinction between IMT and spindle cell carcinoma, inflammatory fibrosarcoma, and malignant fibrous histiocytoma (MFH) is obviously crucial, not only from a prognostic viewpoint but also for the initial therapeutic approach (see subsequent discussion).

Treatment and Prognosis. In the head and neck, many IMT may resolve or regress with conservative excisional biopsy or steroid therapy, or both. However, some cases may persist and worsen. Single or multiple recurrences developed in 25% of patients with IMT from all body sites after excision, two of which developed histologic evidence of sarcomatous transformation. Recurrence or transformation was more likely to occur in patients with mesenteric or retroperitoneal multinodular tumors; these cases still tended to remain localized.[371]

It may be important, from initial therapeutic and prognostic viewpoints, to subclassify laryngeal IMT into primarily lymphoplasmacytic/lymphohistiocytic versus active myofibroblastic/collagenized myofibroblastic. The eight patients with laryngeal IMT reported by Wenig et al.[369] were all initially treated by conservative laryngoscopic excision. All of these tumors were of proliferative, active myofibroblastic histology; none were purely lymphoplasmacytic (plasma cell granuloma). One of these patients experienced two recurrences within 2 years, and was treated with radiotherapy and finally total laryngectomy. He died of other causes, but with evidence of persistent tracheal disease. Anecdotally, laryngeal lymphoplasma cell–rich IMTs (laryngeal plasma cell granuloma) have responded to initial corticosteroid/antibiotic therapy.[379, 380]

Langerhans Cell Granulomatosis

Langerhans cell granulomatosis (LCG, or histiocytosis X) is the term applied to a group of childhood disorders, including eosinophilic granuloma, Hand-Schüller Christian disease, and Letterer-Siwe disease.[382–385] Eosinophilic granuloma is a localized form of LCG, usually manifesting as a solitary bone lesion, whereas the latter two syndromes have multifocal or disseminated disease, with involvement of lymph nodes, skin, liver, spleen, lung, head and neck, or gastrointestinal tract. The etiology is unknown, although a recent report suggests that all forms of LCG are clonal.[386] Other investigators, however, believe LCG to be a benign, possibly reactive process.[385]

Clinical Features. Although the head and neck area is frequently involved in LCG,[387–391] involvement of the larynx is extremely rare, and only individual cases have been reported in the literature.[392, 393] In a recent study, 23 of 28 patients (82%) with LCG had head and neck disease, causing the presenting symptom in 40% of patients.[389] Facial rash and cervical adenopathy are common. The skull is the most frequently involved flat bone; the mandible and temporal bone are also common sites. Otitis media or destructive lesions of the temporal bone, or both, may be the initial presentation in up to 60% of cases. Radiographic evaluation including magnetic resonance imaging scans is important in the evaluation of patients with LCG.[394]

Pathologic Features. The histology of LCG is distinctive but it is important to use other methods (electron microscopy, CD1a stains) to confirm the diagnosis whenever possible.[382, 385] LCG is characterized by a polymorphous cellular infiltrate of mononuclear or multinucleated histiocytes (Langerhans cells) having reniform to oval, lobulated or grooved (cleft) nuclei, mixed with varying numbers of eosinophils, granulocytes, and lymphocytes.[382, 385] These cells (10–12 μm in diameter) have an eosinophilic cytoplasm on hematoxylin-eosin stain. Immunohistochemically, they are typically positive for S-100 protein and, more specifically, CD1a.[395, 396] Intracytoplasmic "Birbeck" granules are diagnostic of LCG cells on ultrastructural analysis.[395]

Differential Diagnosis. The mixed infiltrate of histiocytes and eosinophils, and the presence of phagocytosis, in LCG may be mistaken for reactive histiocytosis, Hodgkin's disease, and sinus histiocytosis with massive lymphadenopathy (SHML, or Rosai-Dorfman disease). SHML has been described as causing infraglottic narrowing as a result of extrinsic compression from a lymph node, and intrinsic tracheal involvement.[355] LCG cells are S-100 protein and CD1a positive, whereas SHML cells are S-100 positive and CD1a negative.[396] The characteristic feature of SHML is prominent lymphophagocytosis (emperipolesis). SHML cells lack the typical nuclear features of LCG cells and, furthermore, lack the characteristic intracytoplasmic "Birbeck" granules seen on ultrastructural analysis.[385, 395]

Treatment and Prognosis. Treatment of LCG is based on the degree of disease involvement.[385] Biopsy or curettage of osseous lesions, and, at times, low-dose radiation therapies are the mainstays of treatment for localized LCG; chemotherapy is reserved for aggressive and refractory disease. The variable histologic features bear little correlation with prognosis of LCG. Rather, classification schemes based on the extent of organ involvement are more significant for treatment and prognosis. Alessi et al.[389] subclassified 28 children with LCG as either type I (monostotic disease, 7 children), type II (multiple sites without visceral involvement, 15 children) and type III (presentation with disseminated disease including visceral involvement, 6 children). Generally, the greater the degree of organ involvement, the worse the prognosis. Patients with type I disease had an excellent prognosis after local curettage, whereas patients with type III disease all succumbed to disease despite treatment with chemotherapy.

Fibroblastic Tumors

Desmoid (Fibromatosis)

The desmoid or aggressive fibromatoses are a group of nonmetastasizing fibrous proliferations with an infiltrative growth pattern and a tendency to locally recur.[397–399] Nine to 23% of extraabdominal desmoid fibromatoses involve the head and neck region: this frequency increases to over one third in children.[398–408] Within the head and neck area, desmoid fibromatosis most frequently involves the neck; this has been seen in 40% to 85% of patients in several large series.[399, 401, 407, 409] The second most frequent site of involvement is the face, followed by oral cavity, scalp, paranasal sinuses, and orbital areas.[407, 409] The larynx and thyroid gland are the least frequent sites involved by desmoids.[409–413] To date, only scattered cases of fibromatosis involving the larynx have been reported.[410–413] They appear as submucosal masses with a predisposition for the anterior glottis and infraglottis (Fig. 5–42).[413]

Pathologic Features. On gross examination, desmoid fibromatoses are firm and rubbery with a grayish-white cut surface. They usually are poorly circumscribed and characteristically infiltrate into adjacent soft tissues. Microscopically, they are composed of interlacing fascicles of elongated, relatively uniform, spindle-shaped fibroblasts, often in a collagenous to myxoid background (see Fig. 5–42). The collagenous background may be emphasized by trichrome stain. Pleomorphism is minimal; cellularity ranges from 1+ to 2+ on a scale of 1 to 4. Mitoses and necrosis are only rarely observed. Scattered mild acute and chronic inflammatory infiltrates may be found focally within the fibromatoses, often associated with mucosal surfaces. The differential diagnosis includes other spindle cell tumors such as leiomyoma, low-grade fibrosarcoma, nerve sheath tumors, low-grade liposarcoma, and solitary fibrous tumor.[413]

Treatment and Prognosis. Owing to the limited number of cases of desmoids involving the larynx, their biologic behavior is difficult to predict. However, it would be safe to assume, as with desmoids of other anatomic sites, that there is a tendency for local recurrence but no metastatic potential (in the absence of radiation therapy). Treatment should consist of complete surgical excision of the neoplastic tissue with conservation of vocal function. Total laryngectomy should be reserved for advanced disease in which a conservative laryngectomy has failed or is technically inappropriate and

other more conservative methods such as anti-estrogen treatment and nonsteroidal anti-inflammatory drugs were not efficacious.[399]

Fibrosarcoma

Fibrosarcomas of the head and neck regions are uncommon, and their true incidence is uncertain because of the lack of immunohistochemical and ultrastructural confirmatory studies in the older literature.[415] True laryngeal fibrosarcomas are extremely rare[410, 414, 416, 417] and few generalizations can be made as to clinicopathologic features and prognosis.

Pathologic Features. Fibrosarcomas appear as densely cellular spindle cell malignancies producing a collagenous matrix. The fascicles of tumor cells grow in a variable intersecting pattern, which can be seen on cross section as "herringbone" areas: intersecting tumor bundles forming deep Vs. The spindle cells are tapered and may be wavy. Nuclear pleomorphism, a significant mitotic rate, and necrosis are generally found. Transition from low-grade fibrosarcoma to high-grade areas may be seen.[410] Trichrome stain will accentuate the collagen background. On ultrastructural examination, abundant rough endoplasmic reticulum and Golgi's apparatus characterize fibroblastic cells. Features suggestive of nonfibroblastic origin (e.g., pinocytotic vesicles, dense bodies, desmosomes, cellular processes, and basement membrane) are lacking. Immunohistochemistry can exclude other specific diagnoses (they are negative for cytokeratin, S-100, HMB-45, smooth muscle actin, myoglobulin, and FXIIIa). The differential diagnosis includes other laryngeal spindle cell malignancies such as spindle cell carcinoma, leiomyosarcoma, rhabdomyosarcoma, and so on.

Treatment and Prognosis. Surgical resection with negative resection margins is the treatment of choice. Unfortunately, prognostic information is not available, given the paucity of well-documented reports on laryngeal fibrosarcoma with clinical follow-up. Shin and Abramson[416] documented a patient with a high-grade laryngeal fibrosarcoma who refused laryngectomy. He died of disease 10 months after treatment with radiotherapy. It is reasonable to assume that, as with other sarcomas, the overall prognosis depends on tumor size at presentation, nature (invasive versus polypoid), and tumor grade. As with fibrosarcomas at other sites, the potential for regional and distant metastases exists.

Nerve Sheath Tumors

Peripheral nerve sheath neoplasms may be divided into benign and malignant types.[418–421] Nerve sheath tumors of the larynx are rare. The benign nerve sheath tumors include neurofibroma, plexiform neurofibroma, and neurilemmoma (schwannoma); the malignant neoplasms are referred to as malignant peripheral nerve sheath tumors (malignant schwannoma or neurogenic sarcoma).

Benign Nerve Sheath Tumors

Neurofibromas

Neurofibromas are benign, expansile swellings contained within epineurium. Most patients with neurofibromas are young; there is no gender predilection. Most tumors are sporadic and not associated with the syndrome of von Recklinghausen's disease (neurofibromatosis type 1 [NF-1]). Although the head and neck region is a common location for benign nerve sheath tumors, neurofibromas of the larynx are rare, accounting for approximately 0.1% of benign laryngeal tumors.[422, 423] However, they should be included in the differential diagnosis of a submucosal supraglottic mass.[422–435] Occasionally, they may also arise from the vocal cord or infraglottis.[430, 432] Laryngeal neurofibromas may be solitary, a harbinger of neurofibromatosis type 2, or an uncommon component of NF-1.[425, 427, 437] Unlike neurilemmomas, neurofibromas have the potential to undergo malignant change.[418–420] Submucosal neurofibroma-like lesions

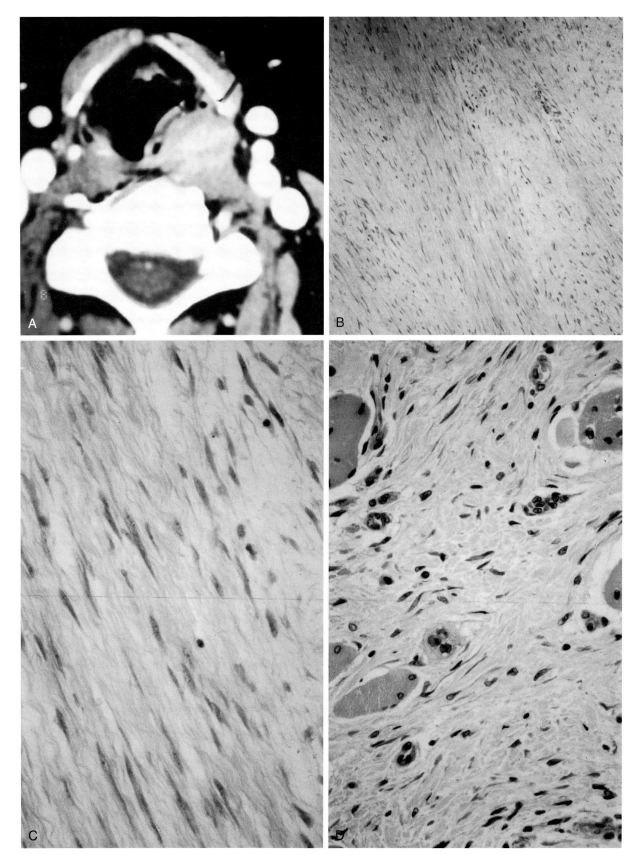

Figure 5–42. *A*, Computed tomographic scan demonstrating a desmoid tumor presenting as a posterior hypopharyngeal/piriform sinus mass. *B&C*, Histologically, one sees interlacing fascicles of elongated, relatively uniform, spindle-shaped fibroblasts in a collagenous background. Pleomorphism is minimal and there is no necrosis. *D*, The fibroblasts may be seen dissecting through adjacent skeletal muscle.

(submucosal neuromas) are seen in multiple endocrine neoplasia syndrome (MEN IIb or III). This syndrome is also associated with thyroid neoplasia (medullary carcinoma), adrenal pheochromocytomas, parathyroid adenomas, gastrointestinal ganglioneuromatosis, and marfanoid habitus. The submucosal neuromas may diffusely involve the lips, tongue, oral mucosa, and larynx.

Pathologic Features. Neurofibromas are composed of spindled cells having an irregular, wavy nucleus, with varying cellularity.[418-420] The overall cellular distribution is fairly uniform from field to field. Comma-shaped cells may be seen (Fig. 5–43). The cells may be arranged in fascicles in a fibrous or myxoid stroma rich in mucopolysaccharides. Mast cells can be scattered throughout. Histologically, plexiform neurofibromas reveal a tortuous collection of diffusely hyperplastic hypercellular nerve fascicles, arising in a background of diffuse neurofibroma—spindled, wavy cells in a fibrocollagenous and myxoid background. Focal atypia or rare mitoses are common in all variants of neurofibroma. However, when seen to a marked degree, malignant transformation should be considered. The nerve sheath origin of neurofibromas can be confirmed by the demonstration of S-100 protein immunopositivity or on ultrastructural examination.[418-421]

Differential Diagnosis. The differential diagnosis includes traumatic neuromas, the proliferative result of nerve repair after injury. These are painful lesions that histologically appear as nerve trunks, embedded in dense collagenous scar. Small proliferating nerve twigs can be seen sprouting from the damaged trunk. The presence of dense scar and the absence of proliferating spindled neural supporting cells distinguish a traumatic neuroma from a neurofibroma. Schwannomas may be distinguished from neurofibromas by the variation in cellular/collagen density from field to field (Antoni A and B areas) and the presence of prominent cellular pallisading (Verocay bodies).

Treatment. When possible, complete excision is the treatment of choice; however, aggressive debilitating surgery should be avoided.[425, 433, 434]

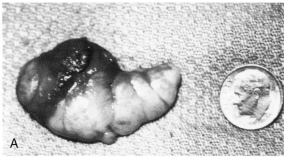

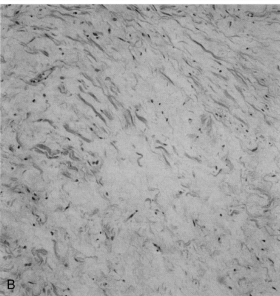

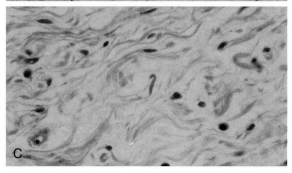

Figure 5–43. *A,* Endolaryngeal pedunculated plexiform neurofibroma from a patient with von Recklinghausen's disease. (Courtesy of Dr. Hugh Biller.) *B,* Low power reveals uniform distribution of small spindled cells, some quite wavy, in a myxoid matrix. *C,* Bland, comma-shaped cells in a myxoid matrix can be seen.

Neurilemmoma

Neurilemmomas or schwannomas are benign nerve sheath tumors that present in young individuals, although any age group may be involved. Most are solitary and arise in soft tissues, including the head and neck, and sites such as the cranial or spinal nerve roots and cervical nerves.[420] Acoustic neuromas are neurilemmomas of cranial nerve VIII. Vagal neurilemmomas of the parapharyngeal space bulge medially and can present as peritonsillar or superior palatal masses. Neurilemmomas of the larynx are extremely uncommon (Fig. 5–44).[435-440] The exact incidence of these neoplasms is difficult to ascertain, as many reports do not separate schwannomas from neurofibromas. Our review of the literature supports the rare occurrence of these neoplasms, which appear to have an estimated incidence similar to neurofibromas: 0.1% of benign neoplasms of the larynx. They present as a discrete submucosal nodule.

Pathologic Features. On gross examination, neurilemmomas present as eccentric, discrete, globular, expansile masses, which are confined to the nerve of origin by an epineurial capsule.[418, 420] Neurilemmomas are distinctively composed of mixed architectural patterns: fusiform cells with wavy nuclei, moderate amounts of cytoplasm and indistinct borders, and loosely arranged fascicles having a whorled or pallisading arrangement (Verocay body) with stromal hyalinization; this pattern is referred to as Antoni A (Fig. 5–45, see p. 252). In the Antoni B pattern, the tumor cells are found in a loose matrix with microcyst formation.[418-420] The S-100 positivity and ultrastructural characteristics of tumor cells confirm their nerve sheath origin.

Treatment. Conservative dissection of a schwannoma represents adequate therapy. As schwannomas are derived from the tissues investing nerve trunks, surgeons are usually able to dissect the lesion away from the trunk without sacrificing the nerve. Endoscopic surgical removal may be performed under direct laryngoscopy. This is unlike the situation of neurofibromas, which must be resected together with the nerve trunk from whence they arose.

Malignant Peripheral Nerve Sheath Tumors

Malignant peripheral nerve sheath tumors (malignant schwannoma, neurogenic sarcoma) are aggressive tumors of neural origin. Malignant schwannomas of the head and neck region and larynx are rare.[441-443] They may arise de novo, from a pre-existing benign neurofibroma or plexiform neurofibroma, especially in patients with NF-1, or as a complication of prior radiation therapy.

On gross examination, these tumors may be partly surrounded by epineurium and may be necrotic or hemorrhagic. More advanced tumors invade adjacent soft tissue. Histologically, these neoplasms are usually high grade, quite cellular, and composed of fascicles of spindle cells with a wavy appearance in a myxoid stroma. Nuclear

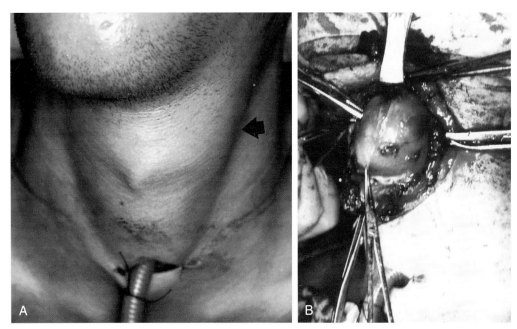

Figure 5–44. *A,* Hypopharyngeal schwannoma presenting with an anterior neck mass *(arrow) B,* The tumor is well circumscribed.

atypia and mitoses can be prominent. The differential diagnosis includes other sarcomas, such as fibrosarcoma and malignant fibrous histiocytoma, and at times neurotrophic or spindle cell melanoma. Association of the tumor with a nerve or the clinical association with von Recklinghausen's disease aid in establishing a sarcoma as being neurogenic. In difficult cases, immunoperoxidase stains (50–75% are S-100 positive) and electron microscopy (reduplicated basement membrane, abundant collagen, cell processes) may be essential to confirm their nerve sheath origin.[418–421]

Wide excision is the treatment of choice. Prognosis is poor and depends on tumor size, association with NF-1, and adequacy of surgical excision. Patients with malignant schwannoma and NF-1 have a poorer prognosis (21% 5-year survival), compared to those without NF-1 (56% 5-year survival). Large tumors (>5 cm) are associated with a worse prognosis.[420]

Cartilaginous Tumors

Clinical Features. Laryngeal cartilaginous neoplasms have a decidedly male predominance. In all likelihood this relates to the fact that the larynx is a sexually dimorphic organ sensitive to the effects of androgen. Laryngeal chondrosarcomas occur mostly in hyaline cartilage structures: the ratio of cricoid to thyroid lamina tumors is approximately 3 : 1.[444–447] Cricoid tumors often occur in the posterior aspect of the ring. Clinically, patients present with slowly evolving dyspnea. Thyroid lamina tumors grow anterolaterally and tend to present earlier as palpable neck masses (Fig. 5–46), which may be clinically confused with thyroid tumors. Chondrosarcomas occur infrequently in the epiglottis, which is composed of elastic cartilage and remains nonossified throughout life, or in the arytenoid cartilages,[448–453] the latter composed essentially of hyaline cartilage with elastic cartilage at the vocalis insertion, which undergoes ossification inconsistently. The hyoid bone ossifies early in life and chondrosarcomas in this site are extremely uncommon,[454, 455] although hyoid bone chondrosarcoma has been reported as part of the spectrum of Gardner's syndrome.[455]

Laryngeal ossification commences at puberty and may be seen radiographically from the third decade onward.[456, 457] The peak incidence of laryngeal chondrosarcomas occurs when cartilage ossification is more likely to be present: fifth to eighth decades.[458–461] The first sites of laryngeal ossification usually follow muscle insertions,

i.e., the posterior cricoid ring and the oblique line of the posterior thyroid lamina.[456, 457, 462] The site preference for chondrosarcomas (posterior and posterior-lateral cricoid, and inferior-lateral thyroid lamina) corresponds to areas of laryngeal muscle insertion. Perhaps ossification brings with it pluripotential mesenchymal cells or cartilaginous rests not normally present in cartilage, which can be the source for these tumors.

There appears to be a small association with previous radiation with only a few reported cases.[463, 464] Interestingly, one case revealed the tumor to have a circumferential pattern not typical of most laryngeal chondrosarcomas.[463]

The diagnosis may be established by preoperative radiographic studies that can reveal an expansile tumor of the cricoid or thyroid alae with calcifications; however, some tumors may fail to reveal calcifications.

Pathologic Features. The gross appearance of laryngeal chondrosarcomas is characteristic; they appear as expansile tumors with a glassy firm white/gray cut surface (see Fig. 5–46C,D). Tumoral calcification lends a gritty feel to the tumor. Laryngeal chondrosarcomas follow the diagnostic criteria of chondrosarcomas of the axial skeleton. Grade I tumors grow in a lobulated fashion with abundant cartilage tissue (Fig. 5–47). Crowding of chondrocytes and double nuclei within single lacunae are seen. Cytologically, grade I tumors have minimal atypia, but nucleoli—not normally seen in chondrocytes—are present. Mitotic figures are usually not seen. Grade II tumors have greater cellularity and more nuclear crowding than grade I tumors. Obvious cytologic pleomorphism and hyperchromatism and mitotic activity can be appreciated. Grade III tumors begin to lose their chondroblastic differentiation: elaboration of chondroid material is sparser and solid areas of malignant cells are present (Fig. 5–48); there is brisk mitotic activity.

Uncommonly, chondrosarcomas can progress to develop a histologically high-grade "dedifferentiated" component, referred to as *additional malignant mesenchymal component;* this can occur in up to 10% of pelvic chondrosarcomas.[465, 466] A few cases of "dedifferentiated" laryngeal chondrosarcomas have been reported.[445, 467–470] Grossly, the dedifferentiated component loses its glassy cartilaginous appearance and has a softer tan-gray component that may "spring forth from the tumor" (see Fig. 5–46D). The significance of an additional malignant mesenchymal component is that the dedifferentiated component generally augurs poor patient survival. Tumors with additional mesenchymal component histologically appear as a spindle cell sarcoma, which was sharply demarcated from the grade I-II chondrosarcoma. The spindle component differs from a grade III chondrosarcoma in that there is no tendency toward histologic cartilage differentiation (see Fig. 5–48). The dedifferentiated component may take the form of an osteosarcoma, fibrosarcoma, rhabdomyosarcoma, malignant fibrous histiocytoma, or leiomyosarcoma, or it may be unclassifiable.

Myxoid chondrosarcoma (extraskeletal myxoid chondrosarcoma) represents a histologically distinct subset of chondrosarcoma. It is characterized by strands and trabeculae of relatively small chondrocytes with a plasmacytic rim of eosinophilic cytoplasm. The background is predominantly basophilic and myxoid, rather than a mixture of myxoid and eosinophilic hyaline chondroid matrix. Myxoid chondrosarcomas are thought to represent a less differentiated form of chondrosarcoma; they have rarely been described in the larynx.[448, 452]

Differential Diagnosis. Given the "firm" nature of this tumor, attempts at preoperative tissue biopsy diagnosis are commonly difficult. Preoperative differential diagnostic issues may be (1) cartilaginous tumor versus normal cartilaginous structure, chondrometaplasia, tracheopathica chondroplastica, or fracture callus; and (2) "chondroma" versus a chondrosarcoma. Aggressive biopsies from the supraglottis might show foci of epiglottic cartilage, which

may raise the first issue. Cartilaginous neoplasms have a lobulated growth pattern and are quite sharply demarcated from the surrounding soft tissue. Chondrometaplasia will "blend" into the surrounding soft tissue (see Fig. 5–47B). Normal cartilage will be rimmed by perichondrium which also "blends" into the surrounding tissue. When in doubt, correlation with clinical radiographic appearance will be helpful. Ossified laryngeal cartilage or the hyoid bone might be traumatically fractured; it is conceivable that fracture callus may result in a mass mimicking a cartilaginous neoplasm. Osteoblastic activity may be seen in both entities, and might not aid in the differential diagnosis. Certainly the clinically history of trauma would be evident. Secondly, the cartilaginous tissue produced in the fracture callus would not be discretely lobulated, pushing, and sharply demarcated, but have a more "blending" quality with the surrounding tissue. Previous hemorrhage (hemosiderin deposition, hemosiderin-laden macrophages) would be seen with fracture callus but is not seen in a previously unbiopsied, untreated cartilaginous neoplasm.

The second issue, sampling problems of a cartilaginous neoplasm, is a well-known problem as tumor grade on biopsy may not be representative of the entire tumor. For laryngeal lesions, the distinction between "chondroma" and chondrosarcoma is a moot one, even though many articles, especially those authored by surgeons,

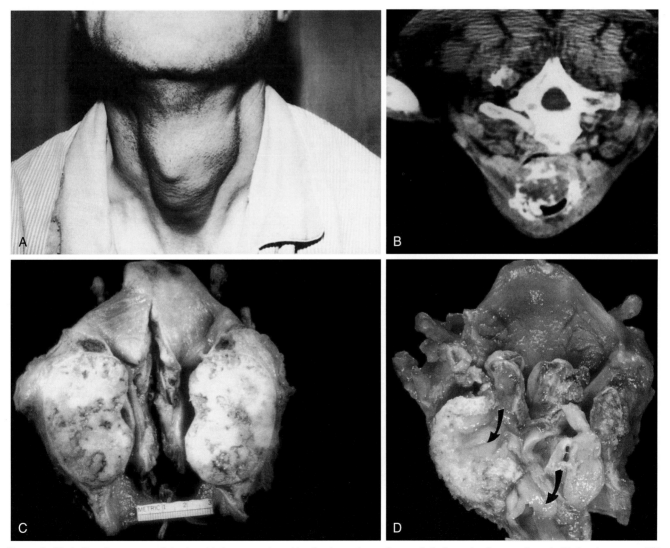

Figure 5–46. *A,* Chondrosarcoma of the thyroid alae presenting with a hard anterior neck mass. *B,* Radiograph of a posterior cricoid chondrosarcoma. This expansile tumor contains a variable degree of calcification; the absence of calcifications on radiographs does not rule out the possibility of a chondrosarcoma. *C,* Cut section reveals a firm glistening tumor with lobulated glassy areas typical of a chondrosarcoma. *D,* An unusual case of "dedifferentiated" laryngeal chondrosarcoma. A soft tan polypoid "dedifferentiated" tumor component can be seen arising from the center of the cartilaginous component *(arrows).*

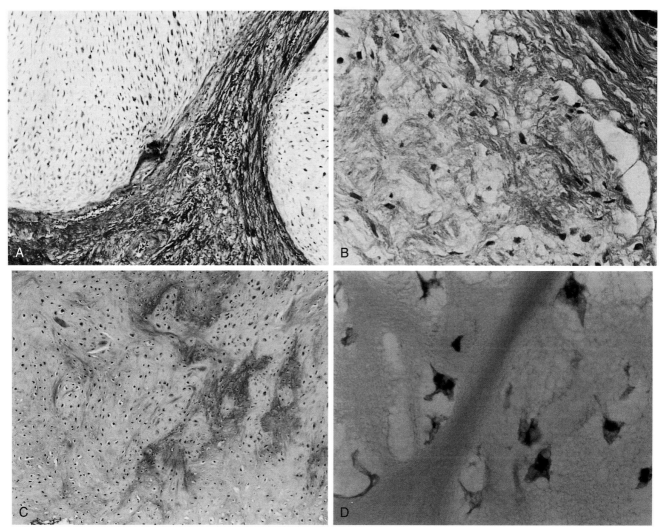

Figure 5–47. *A,* Note lobulations of chondrosarcoma that are well demarcated from the surrounding tissue. Compare with part *B,* chondrometaplasia, which is photographed here at the periphery, "blending" into the surrounding tissue. *C&D,* Grade I chondrosarcoma. Note degree of cellularity and chondrocyte nuclear atypia.

present the concept of chondroma as if it was rigidly delineated from grade I chondrosarcoma. In the axial skeleton, the distinction between chondromas (enchondromas) and chondrosarcomas, one that dictates the initial surgical approach, is based on clinical, radiographic and histologic grounds. Radiographically, skeletal enchondromas may expand the medullary space but have well-defined margins and lack evidence of cortical destruction. The medullary space of the larynx is small, and so (by analogy to axial skeletal tumors [enchondromas] all cartilaginous tumors of the bony framework (both benign and malignant) will result in cortical destruction and remodeling. Given the potential for tumor grade variation due to sampling, the potential for radiologically "benign" axial skeletal enchondromas to contain pleomorphism, and given the known capacity of chondromas to progress to chondrosarcomas, there is little justification for the persistence of distinguishing laryngeal "chondromas" from grade I chondrosarcomas.

Immunohistochemistry is generally not necessary for the diagnosis of laryngeal chondrosarcomas. In the rare case of "dedifferentiated" chondrosarcoma, immunohistochemical studies can reveal that the spindle cell component will have a profile that generally differs from that of the cartilaginous component, which expresses S-100 protein strongly. Spindle cell carcinoma may have areas of cartilaginous differentiation. Immunohistochemistry will reveal keratin expression in approximately 50% of tumors, confirming its nature.

Treatment and Prognosis. The clinicopathologic experience at Mount Sinai Hospital with laryngeal chondrosarcoma confirms its generally indolent nature.[467] The majority of these tumors are either grade I or II. In the larynx, experience dictates that it is wiser to treat all cartilaginous tumors as potential chondrosarcomas in that they require complete resection with negative margins. Recurrence is very rare if the tumor is completely resected. "Shelling out" even a small "chondroma" will guarantee eventual recurrence. This usually occurs after a few years, but may take up to a decade or longer. Recurrence might "convert" an initial potentially curative plan of partial laryngectomy to a salvage total laryngectomy after recurrence. The literature supports the idea that recurrent laryngeal chondrosarcomas do not generally result in a compromised patient outcome: A metastatic rate of 8.5% has been estimated from reported cases,[468] and metastatic potential appears to correlate with histologic grade.[461]

Della Palma et al.[454] culled a handful of hyoid bone chondrosarcomas from the European literature and noted a high tendency for recurrence. It may be that the marrow space of the hyoid is quite prone to harbor satellite foci of tumor. Anecdotally, the only patient with hyoid bone chondrosarcoma seen in our institution developed a local recurrence after 3 years, requiring re-excision. It would appear reasonable to recommend removing the entire hyoid bone, rather than partial hyoid resection.

"Dedifferentiated" laryngeal chondrosarcomas appear to live up to their ominous reputation, although they have rarely been re-

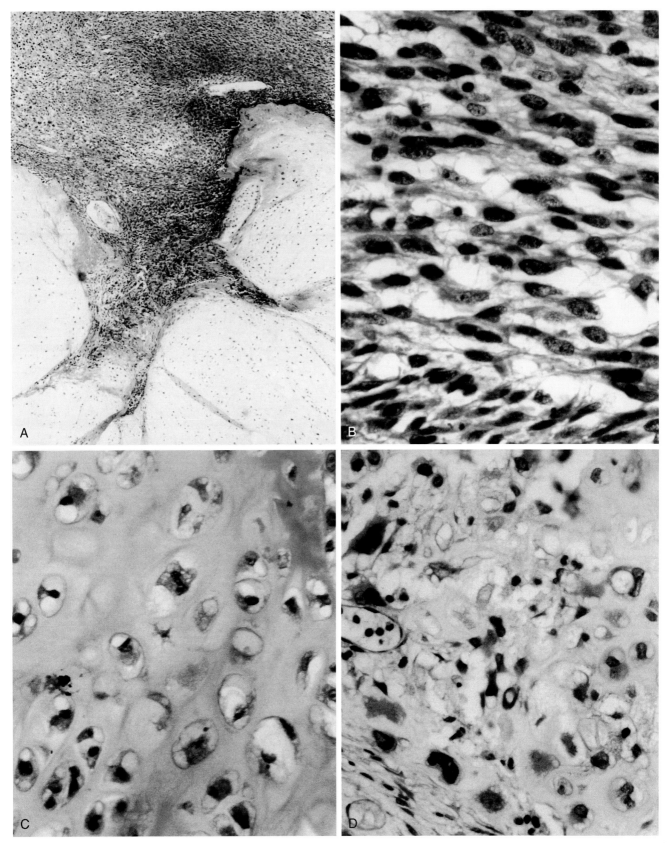

Figure 5–48. *A&B,* Dedifferentiated chondrosarcoma. *A,* Note abrupt transition from low grade chondrosarcoma to high grade undifferentiated spindle cells. *B,* Undifferentiated spindle cells, higher power. *C&D,* Grade III chondrosarcoma. Despite extreme cellular pleomorphism, lacunae formation and chondroid elaboration are retained.

ported, and cases with clinical follow-up are even rarer.[445, 467–470] Of the patients with follow-up, we reported a patient with laryngeal "dedifferentiated" chondrosarcoma who died of disease 17 years after first onset of chondrosarcoma, 3 years after the onset of the "dedifferentiated" component.[467] Ferlito et al.'s patient died 30 months after total laryngectomy.[445] Nakayama et al.[470] described two patients: one was convincingly reported and illustrated as having a progression from a grade I to a higher grade "dedifferentiated" chondrosarcoma—this patient was alive with persistent local and metastatic disease. Only one patient reported with clinical follow-up appears to have had a positive outcome.[469] One reported case of laryngeal myxoid chondrosarcoma has been associated with aggressive metastatic disease consistent with the concept that these tumors are less differentiated and more aggressive than typical chondrosarcomas.[452] The patient with epiglottic myxoid chondrosarcoma reported by Wilkenson et al.[448] was disease-free at 30 months. Greater experience will determine whether laryngeal myxoid chondrosarcoma is associated with a distinctly poor prognosis.

Osteogenic Sarcoma

Clinical Features. Laryngeal osteosarcoma (LOS) is a more rarely encountered entity than laryngeal chondrosarcoma (LCS). Although over 300 cases of the latter have been reported in the literature, and many more cases have gone unreported, few cases of LOS have been identified.[471–477] Unlike LCS, which expands out from the cricoid ring or thyroid lamina, LOS usually presents as a polypoid soft tissue tumor of the endolarynx. However, some cases do primarily involve the bony/cartilaginous framework.[476–478] While LCS is usually associated with an indolent history of progressive dyspnea, patients with LOS manifest rapid onset of symptoms matching the tumor's rapid growth. Pinsolle et al.[471] tabulated seven cases of LOS, six of which were pathologically documented. These six cases occurred in males in the seventh and eight decades of life. One case was found to occur after radiation.[472]

Pathologic Features. Grossly, these tumors can grow as fleshy submucosal polyps, mimicking other sarcomas. Calcification may be noted grossly. The laryngeal cartilaginous/bony framework is usually intact but can be involved. One case was accompanied by invasion of the anterior laryngeal cartilage, which was probably related to previous thyrotomy.[473] Microscopically, the reported cases of LOS are high-grade neoplasms with either a fibrosarcomatous or an osteoblastic osteosarcoma appearance. Malignant stellate or spindled sarcoma cells are seen with a variable component of osteoid. The latter can form a delicate eosinophilic latticework pattern, or a denser, well-formed osteoid matrix. Chondroid areas can be seen but are not predominant. Osteoclastic multinucleated giant cells are frequently found in LOS; they are usually not observed in LCS.

Differential Diagnosis. The differential diagnosis includes chondrosarcoma with osteoid formation, spindle cell carcinoma, and, lastly, metastatic osteosarcoma. As a general rule, when a chondroblastic malignancy also contains malignant osteoid, it is referred to as a chondroblastic osteogenic sarcoma rather than an osteoblastic chondrosarcoma. On preoperative biopsy, LCS can be distinguished from LOS generally by the preponderance of grade I to grade II malignant chondroid areas. Spindled sarcoma cells may be seen in a grade III LCS, a "dedifferentiated" LCS, spindle cell carcinoma, other sarcomas, and LOS.

Spindle cell carcinoma also enters the differential diagnosis, since it may contain benign and rarely malignant osteoid. The overlying mucosa of a spindle cell carcinoma, when intact, often reveals carcinoma in situ or severe dysplasia and the spindle cell component often will appear to arise directly from the epithelial rete pegs. Evidence of squamous differentiation is best seen near the mucosal component; immunohistochemical confirmation (positive keratin stains) may still be required to confirm the diagnosis. Metastatic osteogenic sarcoma to the larynx has also been reported.[479] This unlikely event can be ruled out with clinical correlation.

Treatment and Prognosis. Complete surgical resection with adequate margins is indicated for LOS. Given its general high morbidity, conservative surgery with plans for reconstruction is probably not warranted. Five of the six reported patients died from metastatic disease 3 months to 2 years after diagnosis (mean 1 year); one patient was alive after 40 months.[471] The distinction between LCO and LOS has important prognostic implications, as LCS is generally associated with a low mortality due to low tumor grade.

Aneurysmal Bone Cyst

Aneurysmal bone cyst (ABC) is a benign expansile cyst-like process of bone that usually involves long tubular bones of the extremities, the vertebrae, or the sacrum.[480] About one quarter of cases can occur in the head and neck, usually the craniofacial bones or cervical vertebrae.[481] ABC of the ossified laryngeal cartilages is extremely rare. They have been reported in the anterior thyroid lamina,[482] cricoid ring,[483] and hyoid bone.[484] As with axial skeletal ABC, a history of prior trauma may be associated with these lesions and is thought to contribute to their formation.

Pathologic Features. These lesions are composed of large, variably sized, blood-filled cystic and sinusoidal nonendothelial lined spaces traversed by fibroblastic cells. New bone formation is evident; osteoid formation, osteoclast giant cells, and plump background spindle cells are seen. Hemorrhage and hemosiderin depositions are present and suggest the possibility of an ABC.

Differential Diagnosis. Osteogenic sarcoma and giant cell tumor, both quite rare, must also be considered in the differential diagnosis. Laryngeal osteogenic sarcoma presents as a destructive soft tissue polypoid tumor, rather than an expansile tumor situated within the laryngeal framework. Laryngeal osteogenic sarcomas are uniformly high-grade, pleomorphic tumors. Biopsies of ABC may reveal reactive bony matrix, but not frank pleomorphism. Traumatic fracture callus may also enter the differential diagnosis, but this would usually lack the dilated blood-filled spaces delineated by fibrous septae that define ABC. The spindle cell background of ABC may mislead the pathologist into thinking about an intermediate-grade or low-grade sarcoma, on biopsy or at the time of frozen section, which may lead to unnecessarily aggressive surgery. It would be useful to remember that most primary sarcomas of the larynx, including osteogenic sarcoma, are soft tissue–based and would involve the cartilaginous framework secondarily, whereas the clinical differential diagnosis of expansile tumors arising in the cartilaginous framework is limited to cartilaginous tumors, ABC, and giant cell tumor (see subsequent discussion). Also, rare metastatic tumors may present as isolated lesions of the ossified thyroid cartilage.

Treatment and Prognosis. Conservative resection or curettage is indicated once the diagnosis is established.

Giant Cell Tumor

Giant cell tumors are histologically benign, yet expansile and possibly locally aggressive tumors formed by osteoclastic giant cells. Giant cell tumors of the laryngeal cartilages are extremely rare; eight cases were found within the AFIP consultation files[485] and Kleinsasser[486] compiled another 10 cases from the literature. Most tumors arise from the thyroid lamina.

Pathologic Features. Giant cell tumors are characterized by a diffuse population of osteoclastic giant cells spread across a background of short spindled cells with nuclei identical to those within the giant cells. Hemorrhage and hemosiderin deposition are not prominent features of giant cell tumors. There may be dozens to hundreds of nuclei within the osteoclastic giant cells. Reactive bone may be seen in the periphery of the tumor as the ossified cartilage may undergo some remodeling.

Differential Diagnosis. The differential diagnosis in the larynx is limited to aneurysmal bone cyst, brown tumor, and fracture callus. Osteoclastic giant cells with numerous nuclei may be seen in all three entities. But osteoclastic giant cells with "hundreds" of nuclei would only be expected in giant cell tumors, and dilated vascular spaces typical for ABC are usually not found in a giant cell tumor. In general, giant cell tumors are histologically indistinguishable from brown tumors of hyperparathyroidism. The latter possibility can be ruled out with the appropriate clinical pathologic correlation.

Treatment and Prognosis. In the axial skeleton, curettage would be indicated for a giant cell tumor. Therefore, due to the anatomy and function of the laryngeal cartilages, it would seem appropriate to recommend conservative yet complete resection. Hyams et al.[485] reported that none of their eight cases were known to have metastasized. Kleinsasser[486] noted that two cases did metastasize to the lungs—an occurrence that occasionally is seen in axial skeletal giant cell tumors. It is questionable, however, as to whether these cases truly represent giant cell tumor versus malignant fibrous histiocytoma or another osteoclast-rich neoplasm.[487, 488]

Skeletal Muscle Tumors

Rhabdomyomas

Rhabdomyomas are benign mesenchymal tumors that show skeletal myogenic differentiation and may be cardiac or extracardiac in origin.[489–492] The latter have a tendency to occur in the head and neck (90%) and, in contrast to cardiac rhabdomyomas, are not associated with tuberous sclerosis. They are classified into adult type, which exhibit mature skeletal myogenic differentiation, and fetal type, which exhibit immature skeletal muscle differentiation.[489–492] It is unclear whether they are hamartomas or true neoplasms, but one study[493] found cytogenetic abnormalities in a recurrent adult rhabdomyoma, lending support to the suggestion that they may be neoplasms rather than hamartomas.

Adult Rhabdomyoma

Clinical Features. Kapadia et al.[489] have described the largest series (27 cases) of adult rhabdomyoma of the head and neck reported to date. The median age was 60 years (range, 33 to 80 years) with a male predominance (3:1). The lesions presented as a mucosal mass in the upper aerodigestive passage with airway obstruction or as a soft tissue mass. Occasionally, large tumors involved contiguous sites. The larynx was the third most common mucosal site, after the oral cavity and pharynx, and the neck was the most common soft tissue site, with a rare case involving the face.[489] The median duration of symptoms was 2 years (range, 2 weeks to 3 years); occasionally an asymptomatic mass was found on routine physical examination or at autopsy.[489] Adult rhabdomyoma is usually solitary but may be multinodular (25% of cases) in the same anatomic location; only rarely does adult rhabdomyoma involve separate sites, such as the larynx and the neck.[489]

Pathologic Features. On gross examination, adult rhabdomyoma appears as tan to red-brown, circumscribed, lobulated, soft or fleshy nodules (Fig. 5–49, see p. 253). Median tumor size is 3 cm (range, 1.5 to 7.5 cm). Tumors are composed of well-demarcated, unencapsulated lobules of closely packed, uniform, large polygonal cells having abundant eosinophilic, granular, or vacuolated cytoplasm ("spider" cells) that is glycogen-rich. One or more small, round, centrally or peripherally located, vesicular nuclei are present (see Fig. 5–49). Haphazardly arranged, rod-like cytoplasmic cross striations are seen focally, which may be visualized more easily on phosphotungstic acid–hematoxylin stain or immunostains.

Special Studies. Immunohistochemistry confirms the skeletal myogenic differentiation of adult rhabdomyoma. Kapadia et al.[489] found cytoplasmic immunoreactivity for muscle-specific actin and myoglobin in 21 of 21 cases, and for desmin in 16 of 21 cases. Variable rare or weak positivity may be present for vimentin, smooth muscle actin (SMA), and S-100 protein.[489] There is no immunoreac-

tivity for glial fibrillary acidic protein, cytokeratin, epithelial membrane antigen or CD68. Focal expression of SMA in adult rhabdomyoma may represent divergent differentiation or aberrant expression of SMA in tumor cells. Ultrastructurally, glycogen granules, myofilaments, and modified Z-bands consisting of densely packed intermediate filaments are seen.[494–497]

Differential Diagnosis. Immunopositivity for S-100 protein is potentially a source of confusion in distinguishing adult rhabdomyoma from granular cell tumor; therefore, skeletal muscle markers are also important. Adult rhabdomyoma cells stain weakly for S-100 protein, whereas granular cell tumor is strongly positive; the converse is true for muscle markers with adult rhabdomyoma staining strongly and granular cell tumor staining weakly or not at all.[498]

Granular cell tumor, a tumor of Schwann cell origin, is composed of closely packed polyhedral cells having small nuclei and an acidophilic, granular cytoplasm with indistinct cell borders and a syncytial growth pattern. In contrast to adult rhabdomyoma, the cytoplasmic granules are periodic acid-Schiff–positive and diastase-resistant. Pseudoepitheliomatous hyperplasia of the squamous epithelium is a distinctive feature (65%). Ultrastructurally, the cytoplasmic granules represent abundant phagolysosomes.

Other lesions that may be confused with adult rhabdomyoma include oncocytoma and paraganglioma. Most oncocytomas occur in the parotid or submandibular gland. Grossly, they are tan-brown and nodular, not unlike adult rhabdomyoma. However, they are composed histologically of polyhedral cells seen in acinar, trabecular, or solid patterns.[499] Tumor cells have abundant granular, eosinophilic cytoplasm, which may be periodic acid-Schiff–positive (glycogen) but diastase-negative. Cells are immunoreactive for cytokeratin but not for muscle markers. On ultrastructural examination, the cytoplasm is rich in mitochondria.

Paragangliomas are neuroendocrine neoplasms that rarely arise in the larynx. Paragangliomas are composed of polyhedral cells (chief cells) arranged in characteristic organoid nests (Zellballen) surrounded by inconspicuous sustentacular cells. Ultrastructural demonstration of membrane-bound dense-core granules and reactivity of tumor cells confirm their neuroendocrine nature for NSE, synaptophysin or chromogranin. Only the sustentacular cells stain for S-100 protein or glial fibrillary acidic protein.

Treatment and Prognosis. Complete surgical excision is the treatment of choice. Kapadia et al.[489] reported local recurrences after excision in 8 of 20 adult rhabdomyoma cases (40%), from 2 to 11 years after diagnosis, often after incomplete excision. However, rhabdomyomas lack local aggressiveness or malignant potential.

Fetal Rhabdomyoma

Clinical Features. Patients with fetal rhabdomyoma have a median age of 4 years (range, 3 days to 58 years) with a male predominance of 2:1.[500–503] In a recent large series (24 cases), Kapadia et al. found 42% of patients were less than 1 year old, 25% of cases were congenital, and 50% of cases occurred in patients older than 15 years of age.[501] Median tumor size was 3.0 cm (range 1–12.5 cm). Symptoms included a solitary mass (duration 3 days–19 years; median 8 months) involving soft tissue or mucosa.[501] Classic fetal rhabdomyoma tends to occur in the posterior auricular soft tissues of infants, but it may arise in the larynx.[500, 501]

Pathologic Features. On gross examination, fetal rhabdomyoma has a circumscribed, soft, gray-white to tan-pink, glistening appearance. Histologically, a spectrum of changes is seen, from "classic" immature fetal rhabdomyoma, to cases with a wider spectrum of differentiation (referred to as "intermediate" or "juvenile" or "cellular" fetal rhabdomyoma). Classic fetal rhabdomyoma shows bland, primitive spindled cells associated with delicate fetal myotubules haphazardly arranged in a myxoid stroma. Intermediate fetal rhabdomyoma has a variety of patterns, including ganglion cell-like rhabdomyoblasts, interlacing large strap-like cells with striated cytoplasm, and fascicles of spindled leiomyoma-like rhabdomyoblasts.[501]

Special Studies. Electron microscopy demonstrates cytoplasmic thick and thin myofilaments with Z-bands and glycogen. Kapadia et al. have shown a skeletal muscle immunophenotype of fetal rhabdomyoma in all cases (muscle-specific actin, myoglobin, and desmin positive).[501] Focal reactivity may be seen for smooth muscle actin, S-100 protein, glial fibrillary acidic protein, or vimentin.

Differential Diagnosis. Fetal rhabdomyoma may be mistaken for rhabdomyosarcoma, since they occur in childhood and have overlapping clinical and histologic features. In contrast to rhabdomyosarcoma, however, fetal rhabdomyoma is well circumscribed and superficially located and does not invade adjacent tissue. It also lacks the "cambium" layer and degree of hypercellularity seen in rhabdomyosarcoma. Necrosis and mitoses are very rare in fetal rhabdomyoma; however, the absence of prominent nuclear atypia is the single most important criterion in distinguishing fetal rhabdomyoma from rhabdomyosarcoma.[501]

Treatment and Prognosis. Excision is the treatment of choice. Kapadia et al.[489] reported local recurrence in only 1 of 15 cases with available follow-up (median follow-up 48 months, range 2 months to 52 years). None of the cases metastasized. Fetal rhabdomyoma does not have a tendency for local aggressive behavior or malignant transformation.

Rhabdomyosarcoma

Clinical Features. Rhabdomyosarcoma is a malignant mesenchymal tumor characterized by skeletal myogenic differentiation.[504–506] It accounts for 20% of all soft tissue sarcomas and is the most common soft tissue sarcoma in children (75%). In childhood, about 50% of all rhabdomyosarcomas occur in the head and neck. There is no sex predilection. About 80% of patients with head and neck rhabdomyosarcoma are younger than 12 years old. The orbit is the most frequent site, followed by the nasopharynx, middle ear, and sinonasal tract[504–506]; in 25% of patients, nonorbital, nonparameningeal sites are involved,[507, 508] including the larynx (Fig. 5–50).[509–513]

Pathologic Features. Histologically, rhabdomyosarcomas are divided into embryonal, botryoid (a variant of embryonal rhabdomyosarcoma), alveolar, and pleomorphic types based on the growth pattern, differentiation, and shape of tumor cells. Approximately 85% of head and neck rhabdomyosarcomas belong to the embryonal type or its botryoid variant, and 15% are alveolar. Pleomorphic rhabdomyosarcoma is not seen in children often enough to warrant a specific subtype.

Embryonal rhabdomyosarcoma has a varying cellularity with hypercellular areas and less cellular myxoid areas. Round cells with darkly staining hyperchromatic nuclei and scant cytoplasm and short spindled cells are seen with a central elongated nucleus, tapered ends, and eosinophilic or amphophilic cytoplasm in a fibromyxoid stroma. Mitoses are present. Botryoid embryonic rhabdomyosarcoma (5% of cases), the subtype with the most favorable survival, typically presents in the upper aerodigestive tract in children aged 2 to 5 years. It has a characteristic polypoid, "bunch of grapes" appearance. Histologically, it displays a prominent myxoid stroma in which hypocellular and more cellular areas are seen with a subepithelial condensation of tumor cells, the cambium layer. Small, round, spindled or strap-like tumor cells show marked nuclear atypia and rhabdomyoblastic differentiation.

Alveolar rhabdomyosarcoma occurs mainly in patients aged 10 to 25 years and has an anatomic distribution similar to that of embryonic rhabdomyosarcoma. Microscopically, it is composed of noncohesive cells, 10 to 15 μm in diameter, arranged in an alveolar pattern with tumor cells peripherally attached to the fibrous septa. The nuclei are hyperchromatic and round or spindled with inconspicuous nucleoli. The acidophilic or amphophilic cytoplasm is more abundant than that of a lymphocyte. The alveolar pattern may be focal.

Special Studies. The diagnosis of rhabdomyosarcoma can be confirmed by the demonstration of rhabdomyoblastic differentiation,

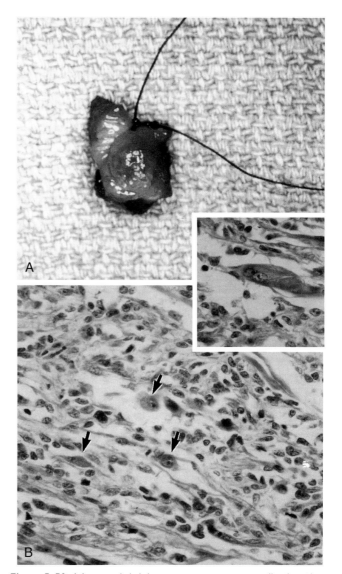

Figure 5–50. *A,* Laryngeal rhabdomyosarcoma seen as a small polypoid endolaryngeal neoplasm. (Courtesy of Dr. Hugh Biller.) *B,* Embryonal rhabdomyosarcoma with prominent "strap cells" *(arrows* and *inset).*

either on immunohistochemistry or electron microscopy. Immunoreactivity of tumor cells for desmin, muscle-specific actin, and MyoD1 protein is found in 75% to 90% of cases and for myoglobin in only 20% to 50% of cases.[514] Myoglobin, although specific for striated muscle, is the least sensitive marker. Rarely, rhabdomyosarcoma may unexpectedly express cytokeratin or SMA. Ultrastructural features include cytoplasmic thick and thin filaments with Z-band material forming sarcomeres, amorphous masses of Z-band material with thin, intermediate or thick filaments radiating from them, and thick filaments lined by ribosomes.

Differential Diagnosis. In the larynx, embryonic rhabdomyosarcoma should be distinguished from fetal rhabdomyoma, which is well circumscribed and not invasive, as compared with embryonic rhabdomyosarcoma, which is poorly circumscribed and invasive, as well as lymphoma, carcinoma, plasmacytoma, and malignant melanoma. In difficult cases, rhabdomyosarcoma can be diagnosed by the ultrastructural or immunohistochemical demonstration of features supporting myogenous differentiation.

Treatment and Prognosis. Advancements in the management of rhabdomyosarcoma, with multimodality treatment regimens, have markedly improved survival. Regional lymph node sampling is appropriate; however, prophylactic lymph node dissection is not necessary. Resection followed by chemotherapy is the mainstay of therapy. Radiation therapy is not necessary in the management of totally resected nonalveolar rhabdomyosarcoma. Survival depends on site (orbit better than parameningeal), histologic type (botryoid and embryonal better than alveolar), and stage. Tumors of nonorbital and nonparameningeal sites such as the larynx also have a favorable prognosis. The Intergroup Rhabdomyosarcoma-1 study has shown that localized tumors completely resected (group I) have a 5-year survival rate of 83%, compared to 70% for group II, 52% for group III, and 20% for group IV rhabdomyosarcoma.[504, 505]

Smooth Muscle Tumors

Leiomyoma

Clinical Features. Leiomyomas are benign tumors of smooth muscle origin most commonly found in smooth muscle–lined hollow organs; approximately 95% of all leiomyomas arise in the uterus, 3% occur subcutaneously, and 0.8% arise from the gastrointestinal tract.[515] Farman[515] observed only one laryngeal leiomyoma (0.001%) in his series of 7748 cases. Lindholm et al.[516] collected 33 cases of laryngeal leiomyomas from the literature; they found a male:female ratio of 2:1 with a mean age at diagnosis in the fifth decade; four of these cases occurred in children. Laryngeal leiomyomas are submucosal pedunculated or sessile tumors; the majority occur in the supraglottis (ventricle, false cord, and aryepiglottic fold) and are 3.0 cm in size or smaller.[516–522] Leiomyomas may be simple, epithelioid, or with a prominent vascular component (vascular leiomyoma). Soft tissue vascular leiomyomas are characteristically associated with extreme tenderness, presumably because of vascular contraction and ischemia. Laryngeal vascular leiomyomas have accordingly been associated with a sense of laryngeal stricture,[523] in addition to the nonspecific complaints of dyspnea, hoarseness, and dysphagia.[524]

Pathologic Features. Simple leiomyoma is composed of benign spindle cells with blunt-ended, cigar-shaped nuclei and abundant pink cytoplasm. The spindle cells form bundles and swirled fascicles. Background hyalinization and perivascular hyalinization may be seen. Epithelioid leiomyoma (leiomyoblastoma) is composed of nests and sheets of cells with relatively abundant cytoplasm, which may be clear or have perinuclear clearing. Cell membranes may be especially prominent. The nuclei are round or ovoid, bean-shaped, and centrally placed. Epithelioid areas are usually intermixed with more usual spindle cell areas. It has been noted that one quarter of reported laryngeal leiomyomas could be classified as vascular leiomyomas.[516] Vascular leiomyomas contain abundant capillary, cavernous, or venous-type vessels. Capillary angioleiomyomas are composed of bundles of leiomyocytes with interspersed capillary clusters. Tumors of the cavernous type have dilated, cystic-appearing vascular spaces separated by leiomyocytes. Venous angioleiomyomas contain numerous thick-walled blood vessels with intervening bundles of leiomyocytes, which may merge with these vessel walls.[525]

Leiomyocytes express muscle cell actin, desmin, and vimentin, are usually S-100 negative, and ultrastructurally are characterized by elongated, cleft nuclei, thin myofilaments with dense bodies, pinocytotic vesicles, and basal lamina.

Differential Diagnosis. The differential diagnosis includes other benign and uncommon spindle cell neoplasias such as peripheral nerve sheath tumors and desmoid tumors. Leiomyomas may be differentiated from the above-mentioned tumors by expression of smooth-muscle actin and desmin. Leiomyomas are distinguished from leiomyosarcoma primarily by the lack of mitotic figures. Necrosis and pleomorphism are also lacking in a leiomyoma; however, any benign tumor that has been embolized preoperatively may contain areas of necrosis that can confound the resection histology. The term *leiomyoblastoma* is especially unfortunate, as it has been associated with benign as well as malignant tumors; therefore, the terms

epithelioid leiomyoma and *epithelioid leiomyosarcoma* are preferred. The differential diagnosis of epithelioid leiomyoma includes other epithelial tumors such as granular cell tumor and well-differentiated squamous carcinoma. In terms of likelihood, well-differentiated squamous cell carcinoma is most likely to be encountered on biopsy. A well-differentiated squamous cell carcinoma is cytologically relatively bland, but is quickly distinguished from epithelioid leiomyoma by its abundant keratinization. Laryngeal granular cell tumor is more commonly encountered than epithelioid leiomyoma; it is distinguished from the latter by its "histiocytic" appearance, with indistinct cell boundaries and strong S-100 positivity. Granular cell tumors have a multinodular, infiltrating pattern with small clusters of granular cells; in distinction, leiomyomas are well-circumscribed and demarcated from the surrounding tissue. Clear cell change within leiomyoma may bring up a differential diagnosis of other clear cell tumors (metastatic tumors such as renal cell carcinoma, melanoma, and adenocarcinoma), especially on limited biopsy. These neoplasms are pleomorphic, unlike epithelioid leiomyoma, and the latter also lacks evidence of lipid, mucin, or melanin. Clear cell tumors of salivary origin (clear cell carcinoma, acinic cell carcinoma, oncocytoma) would be exceptionally rare in the larynx.

Treatment and Prognosis. These benign tumors are cured by conservative excision. Incomplete tumor resection may result in persistence and clinical recurrence.[526, 527] Endoscopic excision may allow for adequate excision of small tumors. It has been recommended that vascular leiomyomas, even when small, be excised by an external approach, as they bleed profusely.[523]

Leiomyosarcoma

Clinical Features. Leiomyosarcomas are malignant tumors with smooth muscle differentiation. They constitute about 5% to 6% of all soft tissue sarcomas. Three to 10% of all leiomyosarcomas occur in the head and neck, most commonly arising from the sinonasal tract, skin, cervical esophagus, and larynx.[528] Based on 12 published reports of confirmed laryngeal leiomyosarcomas,[526] a male predominance is noted with a mean age in the fifth decade (range 8–70 years). Six cases were supraglottic, four were transglottic, one arose from the infraglottis, and one was confined to the true cords (Fig. 5–51).[521, 529–534]

Pathologic Features. Leiomyosarcomas are composed of elongated spindle cells forming interlacing bundles with long, blunt-ended nuclei (see Fig. 5–51). Nuclear pleomorphism with coarse chromatin is seen. Usually, the mitotic count is 5 or more mitoses per 10 high power fields. Necrosis is also usually present. Leiomyocytes express muscle cell actin, desmin, and vimentin; are usually S-100 negative; and ultrastructurally are characterized by elongated, cleft nuclei, thin myofilaments with dense bodies, pinocytotic vesicles, and basal lamina.

Differential Diagnosis. The differential diagnosis of leiomyosarcoma includes spindle cell carcinoma (SpCC) and other sarcomas such as fibrosarcoma and malignant fibrous histiocytoma (MFH). The spindle cells of SpCC may be keratin-positive[535]; however, focal cytokeratin positivity may be seen in a large proportion of leiomyosarcomas, thus the distinction between these two tumors might be difficult on limited biopsy. Prominent keratin positivity, origin from the overlying mucosa, and severe dysplasia or carcinoma in situ of overlying mucosa support a diagnosis of SpCC. MFH does not usually stain with muscle markers. However, as leiomyosarcomas, as well as other sarcomas and SpCC, are initially approached by surgery, this preoperative distinction may not be crucial.

Treatment and Prognosis. Complete resection is the primary treatment choice for laryngeal leiomyosarcoma. The clinical follow-up on the 12 cases described averaged 29 months (range 2–168 months). Locoregional metastasis developed in three patients; one of them developed fatal widespread metastatic disease.[533, 534] As with other laryngeal sarcomas, the prognosis is likely to be dependent on tumor grade and resectability.

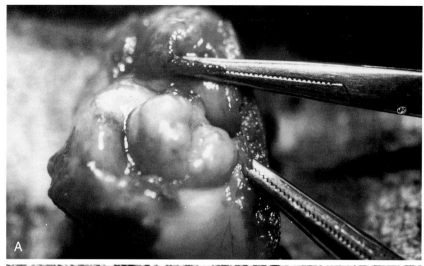

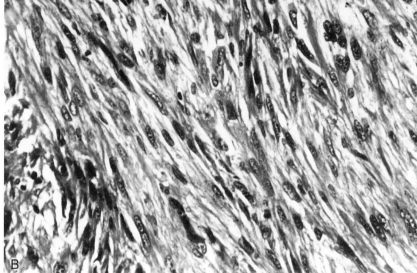

Figure 5–51. *A,* Laryngeal leiomyosarcoma seen as a polypoid and ulcerated endolaryngeal neoplasm. (Courtesy of Dr. Hugh Biller.) *B,* Fascicles of closely packed spindle cells with elongated, blunt-ended nuclei characterize leiomyosarcoma.

Vascular Tumors

Hemangioma and Lymphangioma

Clinical Features. Hemangiomas are benign tumors of blood vessels occurring most commonly as cutaneous lesions on the face or extremities. Mucosal hemangiomas are most often seen in the oral cavity. Laryngeal hemangiomas are uncommon and can be seen as two distinct clinicopathologic entities: neonatal and adult forms. A female:male ratio of 1.5:1 has been noted for neonatal laryngeal hemangiomas.[536, 537] Neonatal hemangiomas present within the first 6 months of life, resulting in progressive stridor that may wax and wane. Intermittent laryngoscopies may be noted as normal.[536, 538] The intermittent symptomatology presumably is due to variable engorgement of vessels, aggravated by upper respiratory infection, inflammation, and edema. Neonatal laryngeal hemangiomas are primarily infraglottic tumors that appear as circumferential or asymmetric infraglottic swellings, or sessile growths that may appear pink, red, or blue.[536, 537, 539] They are not well delineated and often have indistinct submucosal borders. Infraglottic hemangiomas may also be situated in the deep lamina propria and hence be virtually undetectable at laryngoscopy. Occasionally, they may be seen in the neonatal supraglottis.[540] Half of babies with infraglottic hemangiomas also have cutaneous lesions and involvement of other upper aerodigestive mucosal sites (Fig. 5–52*A,B*). Infraglottic hemangiomas are rarely biopsied for fear of bleeding; the diagnosis is made on infraglottic endoscopic examination.[541]

Adult laryngeal hemangiomas may arise from the true vocal fold or supraglottic structures. They form discrete polypoid submucosal tumors that cause hoarseness and sensation of an upper airway foreign body. A marked male predominance has been noted.[542] Hemangiomas are sensitive to the effects of steroidal hormones and can increase in size during pregnancy (Fig. 5–52*C*).[543]

The larynx is only rarely involved by lymphangiomas. In the pediatric population, they are almost always deep extensions of hypopharyngeal cystic hygromas of the neck and tongue base.[544] In children and young adults, isolated laryngeal lymphangiomas have been reported as rare entities and have been observed in the supraglottis.[545–549]

Pathologic Features. Hemangiomas can be classified as capillary, cavernous (venous), or arteriolovenous hemangiomas. Capillary hemangiomas are histologically cellular lesions forming small, often compressed, indistinct vascular spaces containing erythrocytes. The endothelial cells, the predominant component, are large, plump, and immature, with cleared nuclei and fine chromatin. Inflammatory cells may be prominent. Pyogenic granuloma (lobular hemangioma), a variant of the capillary hemangiomas, is neither "pyogenic" nor granulomatous. It grows as a polypoid lesion with a "collarette" of mucosa and is often superficially ulcerated, and the capillary proliferations are separated into distinct lobulations. Cavernous hemangiomas (venous hemangiomas) are composed of large, dilated, thin-walled vascular spaces, separated by a variable amount of fibroconnective tissue. Arteriolar (arteriovenous) hemangiomas contain thick-walled arterial vessels in addition to thin-walled vessels. Neonatal infraglottic hemangiomas can be seen on the undersurface of the vocal folds, at the superior cricoid where they may encircle the infraglottis or project into the lumen. They may also be subtle to detect, as they can be situated quite deep to the submucosal minor salivary glands.[538] The possibility exists that symptomatic and fatal neonatal infraglottic hemangiomas, once collapsed, may escape notice at postmortem gross examination.[536]

Lymphangiomas are composed of dilated, very thin walled vascular spaces lined by flattened endothelium and filled with eosinophilic proteinaceous material. Thin strands of fibroconnective tissue separate the spaces. Erythrocytes may also be present at times, usually focally within these spaces and usually as a result of surgical trauma.

Special Studies. Immunohistochemistry is rarely necessary for benign vascular and lymphatic neoplasia. Endothelial markers (FVIII, CD 31, CD 34, and Ulex) can be expressed by endothelial cells in both hemangiomas and lymphangiomas.

Differential Diagnosis. The differential diagnosis of benign laryngeal vascular lesions is with reactive processes, vocal cord nodules, and traumatic granulation tissue. The neovascularity of reactive processes is more inflamed and less compact than hemangiomas. Fibrin- and hemosiderin-laden macrophages suggest a reactive process. Pediatric infraglottic hemangiomas may be extremely cellular.

A case from the older literature of "infraglottic hemangiopericytoma"[550] in all likelihood represents a hemangioma. Again, strong expression of endothelial markers can be helpful in supporting this diagnosis. When hemangiopericytomas do express endothelial markers, they do so weakly and focally.

Traumatized lymphangiomas may resemble cavernous hemangiomas, and, conversely, hemangiomas devoid of erythrocytes may resemble lymphangiomas. Further, the two processes can co-exist. There are no *independent* therapeutic/prognostic implications in distinguishing between lymphangiomas and hemangiomas. Clinically, the extent of the lesion is the most significant prognosticator.

Treatment and Prognosis. The prognosis of hemangiomas and lymphangiomas is largely dependent on the clinicopathologic situation. Neonatal infraglottic hemangiomas may regress within the first year of life; therefore, these babies may be treated supportively. Hemangiomas and lymphangiomas may cause symptomatic recurrence after excision, as these tumors have an insidiously noncircumscribed, dissecting growth pattern that does not allow for complete resection. The regression of cutaneous hemangiomas, when present, may parallel regression of the infraglottic hemangioma. The expectation of regression must be balanced with the need for airway adequacy and the necessity of avoiding aggressive excision that may lead to infraglottic stenosis. Systemic steroid therapy may be admin-

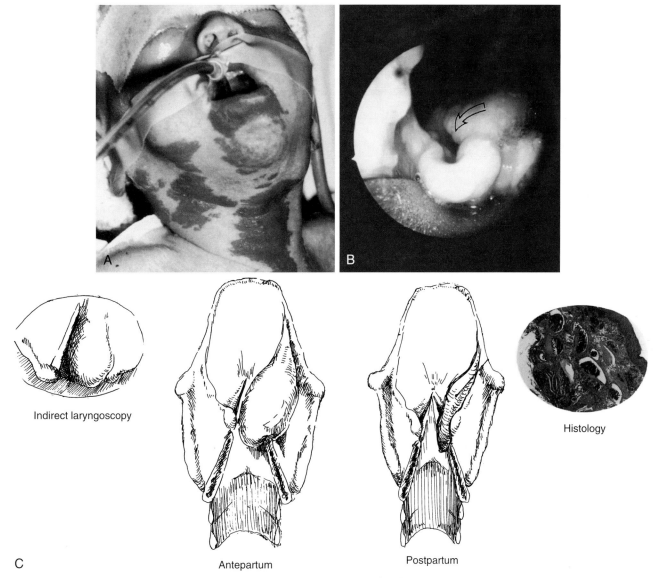

Figure 5–52. *A,* Infantile infraglottic hemangioma associated with cutaneous hemangiomata. *B,* Endoscopic view. A submucosal erythematous compressible mass is seen *(arrow).* (Courtesy of Dr. Michael Rothschild.) *C,* A case of a supraglottic hemangioma: the patient's symptoms waxed and waned with each pregnancy.

Indirect laryngoscopy

Histology

C   Antepartum   Postpartum

istered, and tumor size may be decreased with CO_2 laser excision. Tracheostomy may be necessary for large tumors.[537] Localized adult polypoid hemangiomas or lymphangiomas may be effectively excised endoscopically with laser electrocautery, or from an external approach.

Hemangiomatosis or lymphangiomatosis—the diffuse, aggressive involvement of contiguous structures by dissecting vascular/lymphangitic tissue—may result in enormous patient morbidity. Angiomatosis results in deformity, hemorrhage, and infection. Its noncircumscribed nature defies attempts at complete resection. Cervicofacial cystic hygroma (lymphangiomatosis) may cause upper airway obstruction as well as deformity. Supportive treatment (tracheostomy) may be necessary.

Angiosarcoma

Clinical Features. Angiosarcomas (malignant hemangioendothelioma) are malignant neoplasms forming vascular-type tissue. They most commonly occur as a subcutaneous or deep soft tissue neoplasm affecting the head and neck, lower extremities, or the trunk. In a compilation of 168 cases of all head and neck angiosarcomas,[528] 72% occurred in cutaneous, subcutaneous, and deep soft tissue sites, affecting the scalp and cheeks most frequently. Twenty-three percent of these angiosarcomas directly involved the upper aerodigestive tract, usually the nasal cavity and oral cavity. Laryngeal angiosarcomas are extremely rare. They have been reported as supraglottic tumors of the epiglottis and aryepiglottic folds. They may appear as red or bluish polypoid or friable tumors. A laryngeal angiosarcoma has been reported following irradiation for squamous cell carcinoma.[436] McRae et al.[550] report a fatal case of laryngeal angiosarcoma, which, they claim, is the first documented transformation from a benign, nonirradiated infraglottic hemangioma. However, as the primary lesion was only biopsied, it is more likely that this was a heterogeneous vascular malignancy, which increased in tumor grade with time.

Pathologic Features. The histologic appearance of angiosarcoma varies dramatically with tumor grade. Well-differentiated angiosarcoma (malignant hemangioendothelioma) produces obvious blood-filled vascular spaces. There is a combination of "closed" lumina, which are finite and delineated, and serpiginous "open" lumina, which are insidiously infiltrating interanastomosing spaces (Fig. 5–53). Cytologically, one sees "tombstone" types of cells protruding into lumina with increased nuclear:cytoplasmic ratios and nuclear anaplasia. Low-grade angiosarcomas produce abundant "open" vascular lumina and have a minimal solid component and a low-grade cytology. High-grade angiosarcomas are densely cellular, infiltrative

sarcomas. The amount of malignant vascular lumen formation varies and may be focal. Cytologically, these tumors are frankly malignant, with nuclear pleomorphism and atypical mitotic figures.

Special Studies. Immunohistochemistry may be necessary to distinguish high-grade tumors from other sarcomas. In these cases, factor VIII is invariably disappointing, as it is usually associated with a high background. Ulex, CD31, and CD34 staining may be associated with less background, and hence higher specificity. As with all neoplasia, the less differentiated a tumor, the less likely its expression of specific markers. Ultrastructural examination may aid in distinguishing true vascular spaces (with luminal pinocytotic vesicles, abluminal basal lamina, and tight junctions) from "pseudovascular" spaces, which lack the above ultrastructural features. Weibel-Palade bodies—the tubular structures associated with benign endothelial cells—are sparse if present at all in angiosarcomas.

Differential Diagnosis. The differential diagnosis of high-grade angiosarcoma includes other high-grade sarcomas and pseudoangiosarcomatous squamous cell carcinoma.[551] As squamous cell carcinoma is by far the most common malignant laryngeal diagnosis, it should still be considered in the differential diagnosis in spite of the apparent "vascular" formation. The dissecting pseudoangiomatous spaces ("acantholytic" squamous cell carcinoma) may be the result of tumor hyaluronic acid secretion (Fig. 5–54).[551] These tumors still express cytokeratins and would be negative for endothelial markers (FVIII, CD31, CD34). However, 25% of cases express the lectin Ulex, which is commonly expressed in endothelium as well as epithelial tumors, and may be a potential source of confusion. Epithelioid angiosarcoma may also express cytokeratin, but in conjunction with endothelial markers.[552]

Endolaryngeal Kaposi's sarcoma may also enter the differential diagnosis, which has important prognostic and therapeutic implications, as endolaryngeal Kaposi's sarcoma in unlikely to occur in the absence of acquired immunodeficiency syndrome (AIDS).[553] Further, the diagnosis of Kaposi's sarcoma may open other therapeutic options such as interferon-α.[554] Kaposi's sarcoma is composed of slit-like spaces without an endothelial lining, which differs from the incomplete, anastomosing channels with malignant endothelial cells seen in high-grade angiosarcomas. Intracellular eosinophilic globules, or "red bodies," usually smaller than erythrocytes, are often seen and have a high sensitivity and specificity for Kaposi's sarcoma.

Treatment and Prognosis. Generally, angiosarcomas are associated with a dismal prognosis. To date, there have been only a few reported, well-documented laryngeal cases with follow-up. Most of these patients had rapidly progressive malignant courses with hematogenous distant spread.[436, 555, 556] However, the patient reported by Ferlito et al.[557] died of other causes, tumor-free, after 6 years.

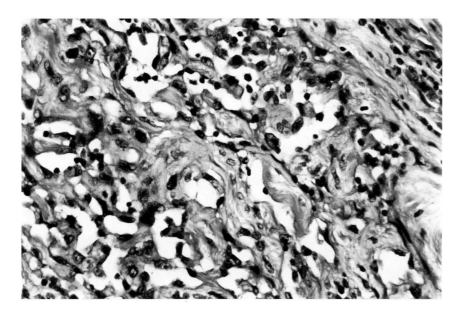

Figure 5–53. Angiosarcoma. Dissecting ramifying vascular spaces. The atypical nuclei are somewhat prominent, protruding into the lumen.

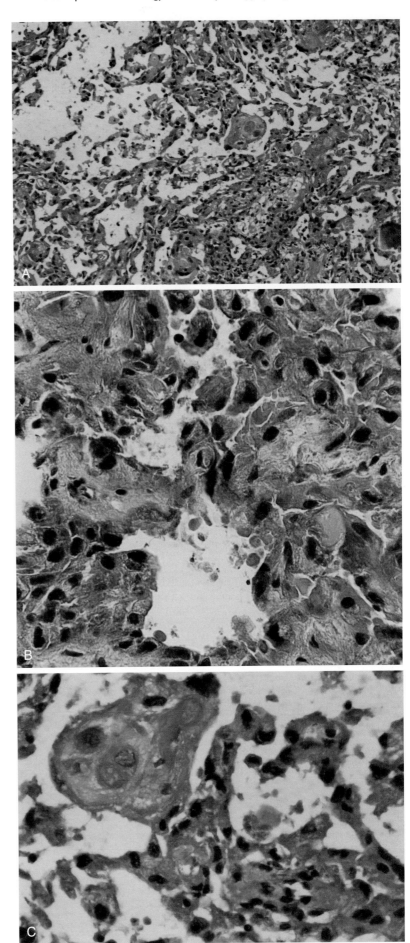

Figure 5–54. Acantholytic squamous cell carcinoma forming a pseudovascular pattern (A&B). Keratin pearls (C) give this away as epithelial in origin.

Kaposi's Sarcoma

Clinical Features. Kaposi's sarcoma is a vascular soft-tissue neoplasm with two distinct clinical presentations: (1) AIDS-related Kaposi's sarcoma, which is a widespread invasive sarcoma affecting viscera, mucosa, and skin; and (2) "classic" Kaposi's sarcoma, which forms indolent skin tumors of the extremities occurring in middle-aged to elderly individuals of Mediterranean descent. Gnepp et al.[553] compiled a total of 83 cases of "classic" Kaposi's sarcoma affecting the head and neck from the literature and the files of the Armed Forces Institute of Pathology (AFIP). Eight percent of all classic Kaposi's sarcoma affected the skin of the head and neck, and only 2% primarily affected the mucosa. Mucosal sites included conjunctiva, palate, tongue, gingiva, and tonsil; skin sites included eyelids, nose, ears, and face. By comparison, Kaposi's sarcoma cases in AIDS commonly affect skin of the head and neck (32%) and upper airway mucosal surfaces (19%). Common sites for AIDS Kaposi's sarcoma cases in the head and neck include palate, gingiva, buccal mucosa, tongue, larynx, trachea, and sinuses.[558–560] Patients with classic Kaposi's sarcoma are usually over the age of 50 at the time of tumor diagnosis although 3% to 4% of cases of the classic form are diagnosed in patients less than 15 years old. Patients with AIDS diagnosed with head and neck Kaposi's sarcoma tend to be decades younger than patients with classic cases (mean age 38 years), with occasional tumors arising in older persons.[553] Early lesions present clinically as flat bluish plaques; older lesions form nodular and ulcerating vascular tumors.

Pathologic Features. Early Kaposi's sarcoma appears as flat pigmented macules. In early lesions, or in sites adjacent to tumor-stage lesions, one sees a proliferation of thin-walled irregularly shaped vascular spaces, often lined by plump endothelial cells and surrounded by an inflammatory infiltrate.

The nodular (tumoral or late) stage of Kaposi's sarcoma appears as a variably cellular infiltrate of long, plump, pleomorphic spindle-shaped nuclei. Mitotic figures are easily recognized. Architecturally, the degree of "vascular space" formation correlates with tumor differentiation. Well-differentiated tumors produce dilated ectatic spaces, angiosarcomatous anastomotic spaces—likened to blood-filled mazes—and "glomeruloid" formations—loose "skein-like" clusters of capillaries resembling glomeruli.[561] Poorly differentiated Kaposi's sarcoma contains packed spindle cells with or without slit-like or cleft-like spaces. Intracellular eosinophilic globules, or red bodies, are seen, usually smaller than erythrocytes, that have been mistaken for Russell's bodies and even fungal conidia. These eosinophilic bodies have a high sensitivity and specificity for Kaposi's sarcoma. They stain with phosphotungstic acid–hematoxylin, periodic acid-Schiff, and trichrome stains.[562] Erythrocytes are usually abundant within the slit-like spaces, and hemosiderin deposition is also present. However, areas of Kaposi's sarcoma may be depleted of erythrocytes, focally mimicking other soft tissue sarcomas.

The tumor will react with antibodies against lectin Ulex, an endothelial and epithelial marker, and variably with anti-factor VIII, which is specific for endothelium. It is the better-differentiated vascular areas (glomeruloid, ectatic vascular spaces) that tend to express these markers; the spindled cells express them inconsistently. The spindled cells reliably express vimentin, CD31, and CD34; the latter two are markers of vascular endothelium and hematopoietic cells.

Differential Diagnosis. The differential diagnosis includes other spindle cell laryngeal sarcomas (e.g., neurogenic, myogenic). The diagnosis of Kaposi's sarcoma may be especially difficult with limited material, which may have compressed vascular slits and be devoid of erythrocytes. The eosinophilic bodies can be helpful in establishing the diagnosis. Vascular markers (factor VII, CD31, and CD34) will be helpful, but the absence of their expression cannot rule out Kaposi's sarcoma. The differential diagnosis also includes high-grade angiosarcoma. This tumor forms incomplete, anastomosing channels, with protrusion of the malignant nuclei into the lumina, in contrast to the slit-like spaces of Kaposi's sarcoma. Kaposi's sarcoma spindle cells are larger and more hyperchromatic that those seen in hemangiopericytoma.

Treatment. Laryngeal Kaposi's sarcoma requires some form of immediate therapy, as it may rapidly progress to cause airway obstruction. Radiotherapy, interferon-α therapy, or laser debulking may provide regression or palliation.[554, 563]

Hemangiopericytoma

Clinical Features. In 1923, Zimmerman[564] first described the features of a smooth muscle-like cell surrounding small vessels and coined the name *pericyte*. The cellular processes of pericytes are perpendicular to its long axis and surround the vessel's exterior; they are thought to have contractile ability. Zimmerman likened these cells to a "hand with slightly spread fingers gripping the other arm," the fingers being the cellular processes. Stout and Murray[565] described vascular tumors composed of short spindle cells and suggested that they originate from these pericytes, hence the designation *hemangiopericytoma*. Hemangiopericytomas are extremely rare, accounting for a small minority of all vascular tumors. The lower extremities and the retroperitoneum/pelvis are the most common sites for hemangiopericytoma.[566] The head and neck are the third most common site, occurring in the soft tissues of the neck, mouth, and, lastly, sinonasal tract. Rarer sites for head and neck hemangiopericytoma include the orbit, parotid gland, skull base, temporal bone, and sphenoid sinus.[567–572] Documented primary cases of laryngeal hemangiopericytoma are rare.[542, 573–575] An unusual multifocal fatal case of hemangiopericytoma has been described involving the lips, tongue, soft palate, and epiglottis. This woman had been treated with high-dose steroids for oral and cutaneous pemphigus vulgaris.[574] Rarely, a thyroid hemangiopericytoma may secondarily obstruct the larynx.[576]

Pathologic Features. The diagnosis of hemangiopericytoma is based on identifying uniform, fusiform, and spindled cells, which are condensed around large and medium-sized vessels (Fig. 5–55, see p. 254). The tumor background has bountiful small vascular spaces and medium-sized vessels containing elastica and abundant hyaline material within their ill-defined walls. This hyaline provides a Grenze zone, or border between tumor cells and vessels. The vascular spaces are rounded or serpiginous; the classic "staghorn" type vessels are seen rarely, if at all. Reticulin stain might be helpful as it reveals the characteristic meshwork of reticulin fibers surrounding each of the spindle cells. The spindle cells generally are bland, short to medium length, tapered, without much cytoplasm, distinguishing them from higher-grade sarcomas such as leiomyosarcomas and fibrosarcomas. Cellular processes may be seen extending from the spindle cells. Nucleoli are usually single and not prominent, nuclear chromatin is finely dispersed. The pattern of hemangiopericytoma is one of short fascicles, small whorls, and perpendicular orientation around vessels.

Special Studies. Immunohistochemistry may help differentiate hemangiopericytoma from other spindle-cell tumors. Vimentin and CD34 have been touted as the only antigens consistently and strongly detected in all tumor cells. Other antigens such as actin and S-100 are detected in only a small number of cases. Factor XIIIa is a clotting cascade factor that has been found to be expressed by tissue macrophages and perivascular (presumably pericytic) cells; it shows promise as being yet another antigen expressed by hemangiopericytoma.[577, 578] Nine cases of soft tissue hemangiopericytoma were studied and compared against 16 other neoplasms, 12 of which were spindle cell sarcomas. All of the hemangiopericytoma expressed factor XIIIa. Malignant fibrous histiocytoma was the only other soft tissue sarcoma to express factor XIIIa. In a study on sinonasal hemangiopericytoma, 67% of cases expressed factor XIIIa, confirming that the profile of vimentin and factor XIIIa positivity can be helpful in establishing the diagnosis of hemangiopericytoma.[579] Factor XIIIa might also accentuate cellular processes when present.

Differential Diagnosis. The differential diagnosis of laryngeal hemangiopericytoma includes other spindle cell sarcomas, spindle cell carcinoma (SpCC), and solid adenoid cystic carcinoma. The characteristic "staghorn" vessels described are neither specific nor entirely sensitive findings for hemangiopericytoma. "Staghorn" vessels may be seen in many other soft tissue spindle cell neoplasms, such as malignant peripheral nerve sheath tumor, leiomyosarcoma, fibrosarcoma, and synovial sarcoma. Hemangiopericytoma lacks long sweeping fascicles, herringbone or storiform pattern, and nuclear pleomorphism, seen in sarcomas such as fibrosarcoma, leiomyosarcoma, monophasic synovial sarcoma, and malignant fibrous histiocytoma.

Treatment and Prognosis. Surgical excision with adequate margins is the primary treatment for hemangiopericytoma. There is inadequate reporting on clinical follow-up of patients with laryngeal hemangiopericytoma; therefore, conclusions cannot be drawn regarding prognosis. The patient reported by Walike and Bailey[574] died with multifocal upper airway disease, but apparently no distant metastases. The woman reported by Schwartz and Donovan[575] was disease-free 3.5 years after resection. One of the laryngeal tumors reported by Ferlito[580] revealed histologic evidence of malignancy—necrosis, cellular pleomorphism, and local infiltration. However, at autopsy, no evidence of metastatic disease was found. In a review of the literature and report of seven patients with sinonasal hemangiopericytoma, an overall low rate of locoregional metastatic disease (3 patients [2.5%]) and patient mortality (4 patients [3.3%]) was found.[579] This confirms the general low-grade malignant potential of this neoplasm. Tumor recurrence was not necessarily a harbinger of poor outcome, as it is for axial-skeletal hemangiopericytoma. However, tumor recurrence can occur after the first 5 years, and patients with hemangiopericytoma require long-term follow-up.

Adipose Tumors

Lipomas

Clinical Features. Lipomas are among the most common benign tumors encountered, usually involving subcutaneous and deep soft tissues. Benign fatty tumors are rare in the endolarynx and hypopharynx, accounting for about 0.6% of benign lipomas.[581] A male predominance is noted.[582] Lipomas may be subdivided into those affecting the hypopharynx and those of the intrinsic larynx; the former are more common.[581] Hypopharyngeal/parapharyngeal lipomatous tumors may be clinically silent and can reach large proportions before coming to diagnosis. As parapharyngeal space tumors, they may distort and compress the neurovascular structures of the carotid sheath and bulge into the tonsillar fossae. They have a predisposition for the supraglottis: aryepiglottic folds, false cords—sites with more adipose tissue than the glottis. Epiglottic lipomas and infraglottic lipomas are more unusual.[582–587] The infraglottis is the least common site for upper airway lipomas.[582] A case of laryngeal lipomatosis with progressive airway obstruction has been reported as part of a generalized syndrome of multifocal symmetrical lipomas (Madelung's disease or Launois-Bensaude adenolipomatosis).[588]

Pathologic Features. Grossly, these tumors are soft and yellow and may be encapsulated (Fig. 5–56A, see p. 254). In the hypopharynx, they may form long, pedunculated, sausage-like tumors causing progressive dysphagia with solid foods (Fig. 5–56B,C). These polypoid masses can prolapse into the endolarynx, causing airway obstruction, or into the oral cavity, resulting in gagging.[589, 590] The tumor reported by Holt in 1854 is the longest to date—9 inches long![591] Lipomas are well circumscribed, noninfiltrative tumors composed of mature adipose tissue and fine fibrous septate. True lipoblasts (see subsequent discussion) and atypia are not present. The adipose tissue may be admixed with other mature, benign mesenchymal tissue, necessitating diagnostic subclassification; that is, tumors with somewhat thicker collagenous septae and bland fibroblasts in addition to the mature adipose tissue are fibrolipomas. Laryngeal spindle cell lipomas have denser infiltrates of bland fibroblastic-like spindle cells in addition to collagen bundles.[592] Intramuscular lipomas show interspersed bundles of ma-

ture skeletal muscle, enveloped and surrounded by mature adipose tissue.[593] Myxolipomas have a prominent myxoid background. Hibernomas are benign tumors composed of brown fat with adipocytes having prominent eosinophilic granular cytoplasm. The granularity represents increased mitochondrial population within these cells.[594] Hibernomas are usually reported in the cervical area, which contains remnants of mitochondria-rich "brown fat," although a case has been seen in the pre-epiglottic fat.[587]

Generally, immunohistochemistry and ultrastructural studies are diagnostically unnecessary for benign lipomatous tumors—generous tissue sampling is more germane.

Differential Diagnosis. The distinction between lipoma and well-differentiated liposarcoma may be made with difficulty on limited biopsy of a fatty tumor. It is always possible that features of well-differentiated liposarcoma lurk beyond the preoperative slide. Likewise, older literature reports of laryngeal lipomas may in fact represent well-differentiated liposarcomas, so that the actual incidence of true laryngeal lipomas is still difficult to establish. Unfortunately, since true laryngeal lipomas may be small (2 cm in diameter), and liposarcomas may be enormous, clinical correlation may be of no use. Shades of gray can always be expected in real life, as is reflected by the case reported by Dinsdale et al.[595]: this pediatric lipomatous laryngeal tumor contained lipoblasts, myxoid areas, and a plexiform vascular network suggestive of myxoid liposarcoma; yet by analogy to pediatric lipoblastoma, an overall benign yet cautious diagnosis was rendered.

Treatment and Prognosis. Lipomas are usually cured by conservative excision. Some reported benign lipomas have been treated by "decompressive" subtotal excision, which would appear a risky approach in the event that tumor histology reveals more than a lipoma.[596] Eagle[586] reported two metachronous hypopharyngeal and epiglottic tumors, occurring 14 years apart. It is questionable as to whether a laryngeal/hypopharyngeal lipoma may degenerate into a liposarcoma. It is probably best to view such cases as unrecognized well-differentiated liposarcomas ab initio.

Liposarcoma

Clinical Features. Liposarcoma is one of the most common soft tissue sarcomas of adulthood, usually occurring in the lower extremities, and in the retroperitoneum. The head and neck are involved in (5.6%) of liposarcomas.[418] The soft tissues of the neck, scalp, and face are the most common sites for liposarcomas above the clavicles, comprising 54% of head and neck cases.[598] Hypopharyngeal and laryngeal sites occurred in 38% of 76 cases of head and neck liposarcomas reviewed from the Royal Marsden Hospital over a 50-year period.[598] A pronounced male predominance is noted: only two reported cases occurred in females.[599, 600] Liposarcomas have been reported with a wide age range, from the third decade[598–605] of life onward. A supraglottic predisposition is seen. Tumors may extensively involve the hypopharynx, piriform sinuses, supraglottic, and glottic compartments, causing progressively increasing airway obstruction and vocal changes. Liposarcomas appear as submucosal polypoid pedunculated tumors that are soft and yellow/tan/gray upon sectioning. They may be as small as 2 cm in greatest dimension[600] or be massive and transglottic.[602] Submucosal tumors may present endoscopically as small bulges, with overlying edematous yet benign mucosa, rendering superficial biopsies nondiagnostic.[603] As with liposarcomas at other sites, occasional laryngeal tumors may be part of a multicentric clinical picture: an obese man with a previous myxoid liposarcoma of the thigh developed a higher-grade supraglottic liposarcoma.[604]

Pathologic Features. Hypopharyngeal/laryngeal liposarcomas of the larynx reflect the spectrum of histology seen in the skeletal soft tissues. Tumors may be low-grade (lipoblastic liposarcoma or lipoma-like, sclerosing liposarcoma or atypical lipoma) or intermediate- to high-grade (myxoid liposarcoma, pleomorphic liposarcoma, round cell liposarcoma, dedifferentiated liposarcoma). Wenig et al.[600] noted that the sclerosing pattern was the most common one encountered for hypopharyngeal/laryngeal tumors.

Low-grade tumors are characterized by an abundance of mature, histologically benign adipose tissue, coursed by collagenous fibrous tissue. Lipoblasts may be focal; they have characteristic "chicken claw"-shaped nuclei that are indented by cytoplasmic fat globules. Their chromatin is usually dense and pyknotic, but enlarged nucleoli may be found. Atypical lipoblasts, which have large, irregular nuclei and smudged chromatin, and florette cells, with multiple nuclei in a wreath-like pattern, can be seen (Fig. 5–57).[606] An abundant collagenous, bland fibroblastic background may dominate the picture—hence the tumor may be classified as sclerosing liposarcoma; the same histologic picture in the subcutis may be diagnosed as an atypical lipoma.[607]

Myxoid liposarcoma is a common histologic pattern generally seen in soft tissue liposarcoma. The stromal background is loose and myxoid, perforated by a fine chicken-wire–like meshwork of arborizing vessels. The lipoblasts appear as univacuolated signet ring cells and multivacuolated cells. The lipoblasts may be scarce, congregated at the periphery of the expanding tumor lobules. The poorly, differentiated forms of liposarcoma may appear as pleomorphic, round cell, or dedifferentiated forms. Pleomorphic liposarcomas are characterized by densely packed malignant spindle cells and bizarre, highly pleomorphic forms; the lipoblastic component (lipoblasts and signet ring cells) may be minimal. Focal cartilaginous differentiation may be seen in high-grade liposarcomas, a tribute to the multipotentiality of mesenchymal cells. Round cell liposarcoma is the small-cell version of this sarcoma, composed of closely packed signet ring–type lipoblasts with little intervening myxoid or adipose stroma. The term dedifferentiated liposarcoma describes a well-differentiated liposarcoma which, after single or multiple recurrences, gives rise to a dominant undifferentiated clone. An alternative meaning to this term, not yet described for laryngeal liposarcomas, is a sarcoma that, upon initial presentation, reveals a dominant undifferentiated clone adjacent to well-differentiated liposarcoma.[608]

Special Studies. Special studies may be necessary for high-grade liposarcoma. The immunohistochemical profile of liposarcomas is nonspecific; strong staining with vimentin and S-100 can be expected. Formalin-fixed paraffin-embedded tissue is suboptimal for identification of fat droplets by fat stains. If fresh tissue for oil-red O stains is unavailable, and the diagnosis of either pleomorphic or round cell liposarcoma is suspected, it can be confirmed by ultrastructural identification of cytoplasmic non-membrane–bound lipid droplets.

Differential Diagnosis. Low-grade liposarcomas may not be recognized as such on biopsy and may be diagnosed as "fibroadipose polyps," lipomas, fibromas, and so on. Lipoblasts are a focal finding and may not be present on biopsy. Higher grade tumors may not be recognized as adipose in nature on limited biopsy. Intramuscular lipomas may recur as they have a nonencapsulated burrowing manner of growth, but a recurrent "fibrolipoma" should be viewed with suspicion and, in its place, a low-grade liposarcoma should be suspected.[609] Chondroid metaplasia[600] may be present, thereby mimicking a laryngeal cartilaginous tumor. Pleomorphic liposarcomas may be confused with other pleomorphic sarcomas such as malignant fibrous histiocytoma, which may have lipid droplets as a degenerative change; extensive sectioning of the resection specimen will aid in confirming the adipose nature of a tumor.

Treatment and Prognosis. These tumors are properly treated by resection with adequate margins. Wenig et al. argue that while tumors of similar low-grade histology may be called "atypical lipomatous tumors" of the subcutaneous or intramuscular tissues, this might encourage inadequate removal in the upper aerodigestive tract. Conservative, function-sparing yet curative, partial laryngectomy is preferable to salvage total laryngectomy in the face of an inadequately treated, recurrent tumor. The majority of reported tumors developed single or multiple recurrences, after initial polypectomy or subtotal resection, and if high tumor grade.[599, 600, 610, 611] Occasional tumors may develop higher grade clones as they recur.[612] Radical neck dissection is not usually warranted for low-grade tumors. High-grade tumors may develop locoregional metastases.[612]

Adjuvant radiotherapy may be indicated for high-grade tumors. The 5-year survival for laryngeal liposarcomas (89%) is significantly better than for some other head and neck sites such as soft tissue of neck (60%), pharynx (59%), and oral cavity (50%). This relates to the inherent resectability of laryngeal tumors, as well as a predisposition for laryngeal liposarcomas to be low grade (ratio of low:high grade is 2:3) as compared to other head and neck sites (ratio of low:high grade is 1:2 for neck and pharynx).[598]

Synovial Sarcoma

Clinical Features. Synovial sarcoma (SS) is a soft tissue sarcoma that typically occurs in para-articular soft tissue sites. It has a wide age range (all decades of life), with a pronounced peak incidence in the second and third decades and a male predominance. Enzinger and Weiss[613] note it to be the fourth most common soft tissue sarcoma at the AFIP after malignant fibrous histiocytoma, liposarcoma, and rhabdomyosarcoma. The most commonly affected body sites are the thigh and knee, then the distal extremities. Nine percent (31 cases) of the 345 AFIP cases occurred in head and neck sites, including soft tissue of the neck (12 cases), pharynx (7 cases), and larynx (7 cases). To date, less than 20 synovial sarcomas primarily involving the larynx have been reported.[614] They may present as expansile nodular, pedunculated, and pedicled tumors of the endolarynx[615] and hypopharynx, causing dyspnea and hoarseness.[616–618]

Pathologic Features. SS may be either a biphasic or monophasic phenotype. Biphasic SS is a tumor of malignant spindle cells with interposed epithelial elements; the latter may appear as large or small solid islands, glandular or papilloglandular elements. Smaller interposed epithelial elements may be apparent only after immunohistochemical studies (see subsequent discussion). The epithelial elements may have a characteristic cleft-like glandular pattern, mimicking, or rather parodying, papillary synovial proliferation. The spindled elements form whorls and fascicles of closely packed, somewhat uniform-appearing tumor cells. Hemangiopericytoma-like areas of increased vascularity with perivascular hyalinization and "staghorn"-type vessels may be seen. Palisading peripheral nerve sheath-like areas may be found. Monophasic synovial sarcoma lacks the obvious epithelial elements by light microscopy—although cytokeratin may accentuate interposed epithelial cells.

Special Studies. The glandular elements often produce mucinophilic material that stains with Alcian blue and is hyaluronidase resistant. The epithelial elements, as well as the spindle cells, may express low and high molecular weight cytokeratin and epithelial membrane antigen. Many monophasic SSs also express cytokeratin. The spindle cells, but not the epithelial cells, express vimentin. Electron microscopic studies reveal the epithelial elements to produce basal lamina, hemidesmosomes, microvilli, and interdigitating processes. The spindled cells are simpler, less differentiated, without any specific attachments, and are surrounded by collagenous material.

Differential Diagnosis. Monophasic synovial sarcoma is a challenging diagnosis. The differential diagnosis includes other sarcomas such as fibrosarcoma, malignant schwannoma, hemangiopericytoma, solitary fibrous tumor, and, in the periparotid region, a spindle cell myoepithelioma. Extensive histologic sampling of the tumor together with immunohistochemistry and electron microscopy will usually allow proper classification. Epithelioid sarcoma is yet another sarcoma expressing both vimentin and keratin. Epithelioid sarcoma usually affects the superficial tissues of the distal extremities; supraclavicular involvement is usually limited to the scalp. Histologically, epithelioid sarcoma does not have the distinct biphasic spindled and epithelial populations of SS but is, as the name implies, entirely epithelial. Malignant mesothelioma can be considered in the differential diagnosis of biphasic SS, but clinical correlation (absence of pleural pathology) can easily rule out this possibility.

Treatment and Prognosis. Surgical resection with negative soft tissue margins is the recommended therapy. Adjuvant radiotherapy is usually offered for incompletely resected cases. Locore-

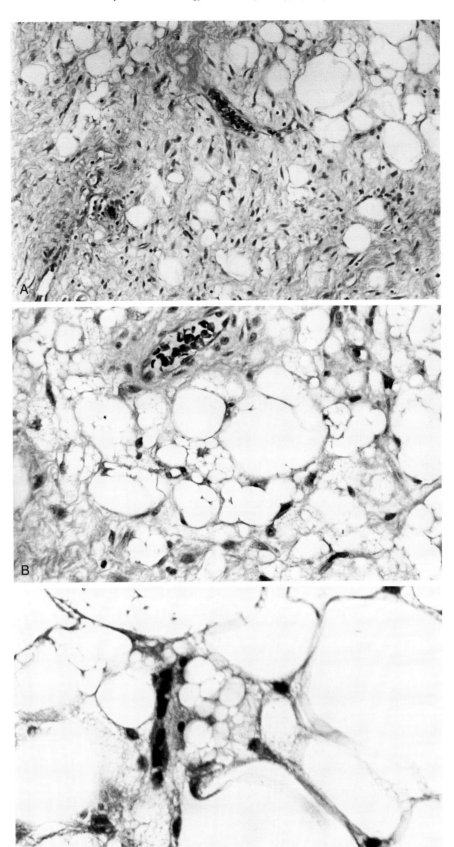

Figure 5–57. *A,* A collagenized and fibroblastic background within a lipomatous tumor should hint at the diagnosis of low-grade liposarcoma. *B,* Numerous lipoblasts may be seen. Note the nuclear indentation from the lipid vesicles. *C,* Lipoblasts, high power detail.

gional recurrence may develop within the first few years, but late recurrences (more than 5 years after diagnosis) are also possible. Polypoid exophytic tumors are anecdotally noted to be associated with long disease-free survival rates,[620] which probably relates to

degree of infiltration and resectability. Metastatic disease usually augurs fatal disease. As with most sarcomas, metastases are usually hematogenous, involving the lungs. Metastases to cervical lymph nodes are an uncommon occurrence.[617]

Malignant Fibrous Histiocytoma

Clinical Features. Malignant fibrous histiocytoma (MFH) is one of the most common soft tissue sarcomas below the clavicles. The dual composition of fascicles of malignant fibroblastic cells and multinucleated histiocytic cells historically raised questions as to whether MFH was derived from malignant fibroblasts undergoing facultative histiocytic change, or the converse, histiocytic tumors undergoing facultative fibroblastic change. Although it has been recognized that MFH has become a "waste-basket" category for some sarcomas, there remains a group of sarcomas that truly reveal both fibroblastic and histiocytic phenotype. In the head and neck, such sarcomas are rare and few have been documented to occur in the larynx.[486, 622–629] Ferlito[627] reported seven patients and collected nine more from the literature. There is a pronounced male predominance and a wide age range, from the first decade of life onward. These tumors appear as polypoid exophytic soft tumors that cause nonspecific vocal and airway symptoms.

Pathologic Features. A number of histologies, either uniform or a mixture of patterns, may be seen in MFH. Most MFHs have a storiform/pleomorphic pattern. Whorls and fascicles of malignant fibroblastic spindle cells forming a "rush-mat" or radiating "star-like" (storiform) pattern characterize MFH. The putative "histiocytic" component is composed of plump epithelioid cells and larger multinucleated giant cells that have bizarre nuclei. If a prominent myxoid background is present, these sarcomas can be classified as myxoid MFH. As with other sarcomas, focal metaplastic mesenchymal elements such as cartilaginous or osseous differentiation may be seen in MFH. A marked inflammatory infiltrate may be present, thus warranting the designation of inflammatory MFH.

Special Studies. Immunohistochemistry can be helpful in ruling out non-sarcomas, as epithelioid areas within an MFH may bring to mind diagnoses such as pleomorphic carcinoma, anaplastic thyroid carcinoma, and melanoma. Diffuse and strong S-100 expression is inconsistent with an MFH, and suggests the diagnosis of a neural neoplasm or melanoma. Likewise, diffuse keratin expression would be inconsistent with the diagnosis of MFH, although focal keratin reactivity has been described.[630] MFH expresses vimentin diffusely, and other markers such as desmin may be seen focally. The immunohistochemical pattern for MFH is also fraught with nonspecific markers: antibodies to lysozyme, α_1-antitrypsin, and acid phosphatase mark some MFH. Expressions of these markers have been argued as evidence of histiocytic derivation/differentiation. Unfortunately, nonspecific tumor imbibement of these serum enzymes will result in non-specific antibody uptake. Nemes et al.[577, 578] have shown that factor XIIIa, a marker of histiocytes and pericytes, can be expressed in MFH and hemangiopericytomas. Therefore, strong diffuse expression of factor XIIIa in the right circumstances may be supportive of the diagnosis of MFH.

Differential Diagnosis. The differential diagnosis on biopsy includes inflammatory myofibroblastic tumors (inflammatory pseudotumor). This is obviously an important distinction, as the latter entity is treated more conservatively. Superficial biopsy of an inflammatory MFH may reveal a pronounced inflammatory component and a relatively bland fibroblastic component. The emergence of atypical mitotic figures, cell necrosis, or nuclear atypia among the spindle cells should steer one away from the diagnosis of inflammatory myofibroblastic tumor. Spindle cell carcinoma should be considered in the differential diagnosis of laryngeal MFH.[631] Evidence of focal keratinizing squamous cell carcinoma, or keratin positivity within the spindle cells leads to the diagnosis of spindle cell carcinoma. The differential diagnosis of MFH includes other laryngeal soft tissue sarcomas (pleomorphic liposarcoma, osteogenic sarcoma, leiomyosarcoma, etc.). However, this preoperative distinction is less crucial, as the surgical approach to laryngeal sarcomas is not dictated by particular histologic subtype. An exception to this would be pediatric laryngeal rhabdomyosarcoma which might require neoadjuvant chemotherapy.

What of the clinicopathologic benign counterpart in the larynx: fibrous histiocytoma or fibrous xanthoma? Some cases reported as such, in fact, are malignant.[632] Truly benign laryngeal fibrous histiocytomas have been illustrated[417] but they surely must be rare. Histologically fibrous histiocytomas are composed of whorls of benign fibroblastic cells with a radiating, storiform pattern, admixed with multinucleated giant cells. They can be distinguished from MFH, as they are less cellular and lack nuclear pleomorphism, abnormal mitotic figures, and necrosis. A variable degree of chronic inflammation may be present, thus sometimes blurring the distinction between fibrous histiocytoma and inflammatory myofibroblastic tumor.

Treatment and Prognosis. Hematogenous metastatic disease, usually to the lungs, has been reported; survival is short after the development of metastatic disease.[626] On the other hand, many of the 11 patients collected by Ferlito were recurrence free after surgery (with or without adjuvant radiotherapy) after a mean of 50 months.[623] Although an inflammatory component has been associated with a somewhat improved prognosis for soft tissue MFH, laryngeal factors such as tumor stage, degree of infiltration into the larynx, initial resectability, as well as tumor grade, are probably more important prognosticators.

Spindle Cell Carcinomas

Clinical Features. Squamous cell carcinomas may be associated with a prominent malignant spindle cell component with a wide spectrum of appearances; the general term *spindle cell carcinoma* (SpCC) has been advocated for these tumors, which may cause diagnostic problems on preoperative biopsies. SpCCs are uncommon; they account for 0.6% (12 of 2052) of laryngeal malignancies seen by Ferlito.[320] Yet, for all upper aerodigestive tract SpCCs, the larynx/hypopharynx are common sites; 65% of these cases occurred in the larynx, epiglottis, vocal cords, pyriform sinuses, and hypopharynx.[633–635] There is a pronounced male predisposition and most patients are between the fifth and ninth decades of life. The tumors may be polypoid and exophytic, or ulcerating and infiltrating, but the tendency for laryngeal tumors is to retain an exophytic polypoid growth pattern.

The histology and differential diagnosis of SpCC is covered in Chapter 2.

Treatment and Prognosis. Wide resection is indicated; the role of adjuvant chemotherapy and radiotherapy is uncertain. Generally, polypoid exophytic tumors have an improved prognosis over invasive and ulcerating tumors as a function of presenting stage.[636–640] Of the 20 patients reported by Hyams, 5 died of aggressive tumor behavior (no time period was given).[635] Three additional patients suffered fatal upper airway obstruction due to tumor; however, these deaths cannot be attributed to the oncologic aggressiveness of SpCC.[635] Hellquist and Olofsson[636] reported 13 cases, with only 1 tumor-related death (at 2 years); 12 patients were disease free, 5 of them for 5 years or longer. Olsen et al. reported a number of interesting findings from their series of 34 patients with laryngeal (25) and hypopharyngeal (9) SpCC. The 3-year survival rate with laryngeal SpCC was improved (76.2%) as compared with that of hypopharyngeal SpCC (56.8%), which probably relates to the inherent resectability of laryngeal tumors.[638] Another interesting finding was the correlation of immunohistochemistry with survival; keratin expression was significantly related to decreased survival. The authors concluded that this may relate to the metastatic potential of the tumor element with carcinomatous differentiation.[638]

Teratoma

Clinical Features. Teratoma (Greek: monstrous tumor) is a tumor of variable maturity and organization; its elements represent differentiation from all three embryonic germ layers. Teratomas represent true neoplasms rather than hamartomatous malformations. The term teratoma is also loosely applied to dermoid cysts or tumors, even though they show only bivergent differentiation into ectodermal and mesodermal tissue. The presentation of teratomas may be as broad as their histologic appearances.[639] Teratomas involve midline structures (skull base, sinonasal cavity, neck, mediastinum, and sacrococcygeus) and gonads. They can present as congenital tumors, or occur throughout all decades of life. They vary greatly in maturity and oncogenic potential: teratomas may be mature and benign (e.g., the common dermoid cyst of ovary, the rare pediatric "hairy polyp" of nasopharynx) or they may be immature and oncologically benign (e.g., neonatal nasopharyngeal teratomas) or malignant (e.g., adult cervical teratomas). A generalization that usually holds true for head and neck sites is that neonatal/congenital teratomas tend to be histologically immature but oncologically benign, with few instances of metastases and fewer instances still of tumor-related deaths. Adult head and neck teratomas, on the other hand, also tend to be immature but histologically and oncologically are malignant; a greater percentage of these tumors will metastasize and be the direct cause of patient death.

Primary laryngeal teratomas are extremely rare, with only four primary laryngeal cases having been identified, one in a child and three in adults.[614, 640–643] They ranged in size from a 3-mm tumor of the true cord to a "quite large" tumor of the cord.

Pathologic Features. Teratomas have a mixture of immature and maturing elements of ectodermal, mesodermal, and endodermal origin. Concerning the four laryngeal cases, three tumors (including the pediatric case)[640–642] were composed of mature tissues, whereas the last case[643] was predominantly composed of immature and fetal tissue including cartilage, epithelial, neuronal, and retinal tissue. Central nervous system tissue and primitive neuroectodermal type tissue may generally predominate in some head and neck cases, yet be sparse in others. The ectodermal structures include "fetal-type" squamous cysts with clear cell change and sebaceous elements. The mesodermal elements may be sparse and include immature yet bland loose myxoid stroma, maturing cartilage (although the latter may often be absent), and occasional muscle differentiation. The endodermal elements include cysts lined by ciliated cells or gastrointestinal type epithelium with goblet cells. Disorganized but maturing nerve-like structures, pigmented retinal type epithelium, neurofibrillary-rich central nervous system–like tissue, and immature neuroepithelium-like areas with rosette formation may all be seen.

Metastatic elements in adult teratomas can arise from either immature elements or histologically malignant elements. The latter appear in areas with necrosis, a significant mitotic rate, and sufficient nuclear atypia. Evidence of germ cell tumors (yolk-sac tumors, germinomas, embryonal carcinoma, or choriocarcinoma) is usually not seen in head and neck teratomas.

Differential Diagnosis. A broad differential diagnosis exists with these tumors when initially evaluated on small biopsies, for example, neuroendocrine carcinoma, undifferentiated carcinoma, and spindle cell carcinoma. Attention to the nondescript "mesenchymal" background and heterogeneity of elements encountered provides clues for this rare diagnosis. Mature teratomas may suggest the diagnosis of hamartoma. However, the ectodermal elements of mature teratomas (squamous cysts) have a decidedly fetal, "cleared out" appearance, and the sebaceous elements, if present, are nonindigenous and therefore inconsistent with the diagnosis of hamartoma.

Treatment and Prognosis. Clinical follow-up is available for three of the four reported cases. Two of these tumors were mature[640, 642] and one had a primitive, immature, yet histologically benign tissue (lacking necrosis and mitotic figures).[643] All three patients were disease-free after primary excision (two patients were known to have 15 months and 5 years follow-up time).

Blastoma

Clinical Features. A blastoma (embryoma) is a malignant neoplasm of mixed mesenchymal, epithelial, and nondifferentiated blastomatous elements that mimics embryonic development of the particular organ. They can occur both in pediatric and adult populations: pulmonary blastomas occur with a male predominance, usually in adults; hepatoblastomas and pancreatoblastomas occur mostly in children. Eble et al.[644] reported an exophytic tumor of the piriform sinus that developed in a 65-year-old man, an employee of a glass factory and smoker, which microscopically was analogous to a pulmonary blastoma.

Pathologic Features. The three elements—mesenchymal, epithelial, and blastomous—exist in varying proportions; transformation can be seen from one element to another. The mesenchymal element forms primitive-appearing spindle cells, chondroid, and myxoid elements. The epithelial elements form strands of primitive-appearing cells, glandular elements, and squamous elements. The blastomous elements are small, nondifferentiated primitive-appearing cells which may be poorly cohesive, and lack definite epithelial or mesenchymal characteristics.

Differential Diagnosis. The differential diagnosis includes spindle cell carcinoma (SpCC) and malignant teratoma. SpCC is the most common of these three tumors. The spindle cell elements dominate SpCC, with little in the way of epithelial components that are usually squamous, not glandular. The blastomous element is lacking in SpCC. Malignant teratoma contains nonindigenous elements (e.g., central nervous tissue, retinal tissue). In children, the diagnosis of metastatic Wilms' tumor should be considered.

Treatment and Prognosis. Blastomas of other sites (lungs, liver, and pancreas) are malignant tumors with the potential to metastasize. Surgical resection is the primary treatment. The patient reported by Eble et al.[644] was disease free 13 months after total laryngectomy.

Hamartoma

Clinical Features. A hamartoma is a benign tumor-like growth composed of mature tissue indigenous to the region. In the larynx, the majority of hamartomas have been reported in infants and children, in association with posterior cleft larynx. Over 60 cases of cleft larynges have been reported.[614, 645–652] The cricoid cartilage, rather than forming a complete ring, is U-shaped and discontinuous posteriorly. Endoscopically, this may be a subtle finding, with abundant soft mucosa in the posterior commissure. Cleft larynx is also associated with cleft palate, tracheoesophageal fistula, esophageal atresia, hypospadia, and imperforate anus.[645] Only rare cases of cleft larynges are also associated with hamartoma.[645–647] Occasional laryngeal hamartomas have also been reported in adults, not associated with posterior cleft defect,[648, 649] which may reach large proportions up to 3.5 cm in greatest dimension.[647] The term *mesenchymoma* has also been applied to tumors of benign indigenous mesenchymal histology, however the designation hamartoma conveys unquestionable benignity. Despite oncologic benignity, these masses, with or without associated laryngeal malformations, may be the cause of severe upper airway obstruction.

Pathologic Features. The hamartoma may form a "septum-like" mass originating from the posterior larynx, covered with epithelium, and composed of mature but disorganized skeletal muscle, mature cartilage, minor salivary tissue, and adipose tissue.[645, 651] In other cases, the "hamartoma" may appear as redundant mucosa forming a polypoid lesion.[646] The cartilaginous component has been noted to "blend" or "merge" into the surrounding stroma.[648]

Differential Diagnosis. The diagnosis of pediatric lesions should be straightforward, especially in the presence of laryngeal malformation. In adults, the differential diagnosis may include chondrometaplasia, pleomorphic adenoma, low grade cartilaginous neoplasms, teratoma, and adult rhabdomyoma. Chondrometaplasia is an expansile formation of benign, metaplastic cartilaginous tissue of limited growth potential, usually of the vocal fold. It appears as bland cartilage that typically "blends" into the surrounding soft tissue rather than pushes against it. The cartilaginous tissue of the polyp has no direct attachment to underlying cartilaginous structures and is not associated with other tissue types (e.g., muscle, glands). Pleomorphic adenoma can be distinguished from the other lesions by the presence of myoepithelial cells within the chondroid stroma and surrounding glandular/ductular tumor cells. The overall tissue maturity and lack of nonindigenous tissue types will distinguish a hamartoma from a cervical teratoma, which is usually a mixture of immature and maturing tissue of ectodermal, mesodermal, and endodermal origin. A hamartoma may be distinguished from an adult-type rhabdomyoma by the presence of other mature endogenous tissues such as adipose tissue and fibrous bands.

Treatment and Prognosis. The lesions require excision to improve the airway and voice. Multiple debulking procedures may be necessary as these tumors may enlarge and infiltrate.[652] However, overall oncologic aggression has not been reported.

Secondary Tumors (Intratracheal Thyroid Ectopia, Metastatic Tumors)

It is not uncommon for malignancies to invade the larynx by contiguous extension. This is a familiar scenario for large squamous carcinomas of the tongue base, which may insinuate into the soft tissues of the pre-epiglottic space, destroy the epiglottis and invade supraglottic soft tissue. Piriform sinus carcinomas invariably involve soft tissues lateral to the thyroid lamina, and may extend over and around it to involve the supraglottis. Unlike the fenestrated elastic cartilage of the epiglottis, nonossified hyaline cartilage is relatively resistant to tumor invasion.

Thyroid carcinomas, either papillary or anaplastic, may directly invade the trachea via intratracheal ring spaces. Follicular thyroid carcinomas and Hürthle cell carcinomas tend to spread through vascular invasion. Locoregional vascular invasion into the trachea has been reported with Hürthle cell carcinomas.[653] Importantly, not all intratracheal thyroid tissue represents extension of malignant disease: tracheal rests may be found in the infraglottis and present as symptomatic masses.[654–661] Intratracheal thyroid rests represent the rarest form of thyroid ectopia. Intratracheal thyroid ectopia may be histologically benign and enlarged, may give rise to malignancy[655] (usually papillary carcinoma), or may be an incidental finding in the setting of thyroid carcinoma (Fig. 5–58). The last situation may lead to some confusion with regard to tumor staging as a papillary thyroid carcinoma, confined to the gland, may be clinically staged inappropriately as a T4 tumor due to incidental intratracheal rests. Infra-

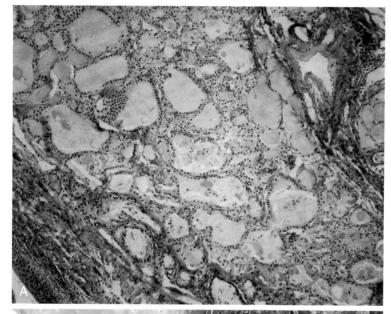

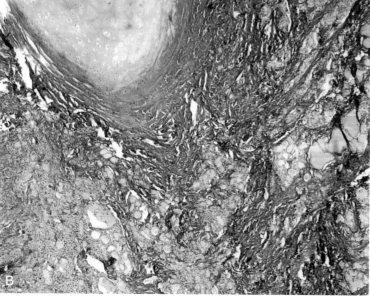

Figure 5–58. A, Ectopic thyroid beneath tracheal mucosa. B, The thyroid tissue is seen traversing thyrohyoid membrane.

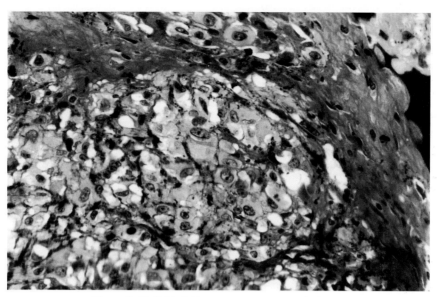

Figure 5–59. Epithelioid sarcoma, metastatic to the larynx.

glottic, submucosal thyroid rests have been identified in 2 of 250 laryngectomy specimens.[655] A 4 : 1 preponderance for left-sided thyroid ectopia has been noted.[661]

Metastatic tumors to the larynx are rarer phenomena. In a series of 900 laryngeal malignancies over a three-decade period, one case was seen.[662] In a recent review, El Naggar[663] identified 142 cases of metastatic tumors to the larynx. The majority (59.2%) occurred in the supraglottis, 28.5% occurred in the infraglottis, 8.2% in the glottic region, and 4.1% in the paraglottic piriform region. Metastatic cutaneous melanomas and renal cell carcinomas were the two leading metastatic diagnoses.[663, 664] Cutaneous melanoma metastatic to the upper aerodigestive tract had been found in 53 (0.6% of almost 9000) patients with cutaneous melanoma.[665] The distribution of these 53 cases was as follows: tonsil, 24%; tongue base, 10%; anterior tongue, 6%; lip, 10%; gingiva, 6%; palate, 3%; nasal cavity, 4%; nasopharynx, 13%; pharyngeal wall, 7%; piriform sinus, 4%; and larynx, 12%.[666] Owing to the rarity of primary laryngeal melanomas, metastatic laryngeal melanomas are a more likely occurrence. Any intralaryngeal site might potentially be involved by metastatic melanoma.[667] Characteristic of melanoma, laryngeal metastasis may occur after more than a decade of disease quiescence. No cases of secondary laryngeal melanoma have been noted in which an occult skin primary tumor was discovered after the laryngeal tumor. Thus, despite its rarity, a laryngeal melanotic malignancy diagnosed in the absence of a previous skin malignancy is more likely to be primary to the larynx. However, the clinician should be urged to investigate all previous "skin biopsies."

In the case of renal cell carcinoma, the laryngeal metastasis will usually occur with a known primary site. Only occasionally, the laryngeal or tracheal metastasis may be the primary harbinger of renal cell carcinoma.[667–670] Given the known capricious natural history of renal cell carcinoma, patients with isolated laryngeal metastasis may go on to have a reasonable disease free survival, thus justifying an aggressive surgical approach for certain cases. It is in these circumstances that the pathologist's recognition of a metastatic renal cell carcinoma may be lifesaving.[670]

Breast carcinoma is another potential source of metastatic disease, found in 10% of secondary laryngeal tumors,[663] usually in the setting of a known breast primary. However laryngeal metastasis may occasionally herald the onset of disseminated disease.[671] Laryngeal metastasis from prostate carcinoma,[672] lung adenocarcinoma,[662] seminoma,[673] embryonal carcinoma,[674] colonic adenocarcinoma,[675] gastric adenocarcinoma,[676] and angiosarcoma[677] has been reported.

Metastatic squamous cell carcinoma can occur from sites such as lung.[678] The preoperative question in such a case would be, does this squamous carcinoma represent a new primary tumor or a metastatic focus? Depending on the patient's overall health status, this may influence therapy decision-making. The presence of in situ disease, when seen, is consistent with a primary site, whereas its absence on preoperative biopsy does not rule out that possibility. On the other hand, if the overall squamous cell carcinoma grade on the laryngeal biopsy is better differentiated than that of the previous carcinoma, this is more consistent with a laryngeal primary.

Other Tumors

Immunohistochemistry may be helpful in establishing the nature of the laryngeal tumor. Surfactant apoprotein was demonstrated in a lung papillary adenocarcinoma and its laryngeal metastasis, confirming the metastatic nature of the laryngeal tumor.[662] We have seen a case of epithelioid sarcoma metastatic to the larynx (Fig. 5–59). In this case, had the pathologist not been supplied with a clinical history, and had the immunohistochemical profile been limited to the keratins, an erroneous diagnosis of poorly differentiated carcinoma might have been made.

ACKNOWLEDGMENTS

I (MSB) would like to thank Drs. Hugh Biller, Mike Rothschild, Ira Sanders, and Peak Woo for sharing their endoscopic and surgical clinical photographs and Drs. Biller and Woo for their constructive comments. The strength and ability of a pathologist is inherently linked to the breadth of diagnostic opportunities afforded to that individual; in this way I consider myself quite lucky to be associated with the Mount Sinai Medical Center Department of Otolaryngology.

We would also like to thank Dr. Carol Adair from the Otolaryngic branch of the Armed Forces Institute of Pathology for loaning the material to photograph for Figure 5–19 (Teflon granuloma).

REFERENCES

Anatomic Considerations

1. Kirchner JA, Carter D: Intralaryngeal barriers to the spread of cancer. *Acta Otolaryngol* 1987;103:503–513.
2. Pressman J, Dowdy A, Libby R, et al: Further studies upon the submucosal compartments and lymphatics of the larynx by the injection of dyes and radioisotopes. *Ann Otol Rhinol Laryngol* 1956;65:766–980.

3. Beitler JJ Mahadevia PS, Silver CE, et al: New barriers to ventricular invasion in paraglottic laryngeal cancer. *Cancer* 1994;73:2648–2652.

4. Werner JA, Schunke M, Rudert H, Tillmann B: Description and clinical importance of the lymphatics of the vocal fold. *Otolaryngol Head Neck Surg* 1990;102:13–19.

5. Zeitels SM, Vaughan CW: Preepiglottic space invasion in "early" epiglottic cancer. *Ann Otol Laryngol* 1991;100:789–792.

Infectious Disease: Mycobacterial and Bacterial

6. Thompson, SC: *Tuberculosis of the Larynx: Ten Years Experience in a Sanitarium.* 1924, London: HMSO.

7. Auerbach O: Laryngeal tuberculosis. *Arch Otolaryngol* 1946;44:191–201.

8. Bailey CM, Windle-Taylor PC: Tuberculosis laryngitis: A series of 37 patients. *Laryngoscope* 1981;91:93–100.

9. Soda A, Rubio H, Salazar M, et al: Tuberculosis of the larynx: Clinical aspects in 19 patients. *Laryngoscope* 1989;99:1147–1150.

10. Thaller SR, Gross JF, Pilch BZ, et al: Laryngeal tuberculosis as manifested in the decades 1963–1983. *Laryngoscope* 1987;97:848–850.

11. Rupa V, Bhanu TS: Laryngeal tuberculosis in the eighties: An Indian experience. *J Laryngol Otol* 1989;103:864–868.

12. Dworetsky JP, Risch OC: Laryngeal tuberculosis: A study of 500 cases of pulmonary tuberculosis with a resume based on 28 years of experience. *Ann Otol Rhinol Laryngol* 1941;50:745–757.

13. Pao CC, Lin SS, Wu SY, et al: The detection of mycobacterial DNA sequences in uncultured clinical specimens with cloned *Mycobacterium tuberculosis* DNA as probes. *Tubercle* 1988;69:27–36.

14. Mastro TD, Redd SC, Breiman RF: Imported leprosy in the United States, 1978 through 1988: An epidemic without secondary transmission. *Am J Pub Health* 1992;82:1127–1130.

15. Fine PM: Leprosy: The epidemiology of a slow bacterium. *Epidemiol Rev* 1982;4:162–188.

16. Yoshie Y: Clinical and histopathological studies on leprosy of the larynx. *Int J Leprosy* 1955;24:352–353.

17. Ridley DS, Jopling WH: Classification of leprosy according to immunity: A five group system. *Int J Leprosy* 1965;34:255–273.

18. Wade HW: The histoid variety of lepromatous leprosy. *Int J Leprosy* 1963;31:129–141.

19. Gupta JC, Gandagule VN, Nigam JP, et al: A clinicopathological study of laryngeal lesions in 30 cases of leprosy. *Leprosy in India* 1980;52:557–565.

20. Nishimura M, Kwon KS, Shibuta K, et al: An improved method for DNA diagnosis of leprosy using formaldehyde-fixed paraffin-embedded skin biopsies. *Mod Pathol* 1994;7:253–256.

21. Williams DL, Gillis TP, Booth RJ, et al: The use of a specific DNA probe and PCR for the detection of *Mycobacterium leprae. J Infect Dis* 1990;162:193–200.

22. McNulty JS, Fassett RL: Syphilis: An otolaryngological perspective. *Laryngoscope* 1981;91:889–905.

23. Meyer I, Shklar G: The oral manifestations of acquired syphilis. *Oral Surg Oral Med Oral Pathol* 1967;23:45–57.

24. Larsen S: Syphilis. *Clin Lab Med* 1989;9:545–557.

25. Knispel J, Saruk M, Ceraianu G, Phelps RG: The use of a novel immunoperoxidase technique to detect spirochetes in tissue sections. *Lab Invest* 1993;6:35a.

26. von Hebra F, Kohn M: Ueber ein eigentümliches Neugebilde an der Nase. *Wien Med Wochenschr* 1876;20:1–5.

27. von Frisch A: Zur Aetiologie des Rhinscleroms. *Wien Med Wochenschr* 1882;32:96–97.

28. Quevedo J: Scleroma in Guatemala with a study of the disease based on the experience of 108 cases. *Ann Otol Rhinol Laryngol* 1945;58:613–645.

29. Muzyka MM, Gubina KM: Problems of the epidemiology of scleroma. I. Geographical distribution of scleroma. *J Hyg Epidemiol Microbiol Immunol* 1971;15:233–242.

30. Muzyka MM, Gubina KM: Problems of the epidemiology of scleroma. II. Some aspects of the problem of endemic focus formation. *J Hyg Epidemiol Microbiol Immunol* 1972;16:8–18.

31. Friedmann I, Ferlito A: Specific granulomas. In: *Granulomas and Neoplasms of the Larynx.* New York: Churchill Livingstone, 1988:39–48.

32. Reyes E: Rhinoscleroma. *Arch Dermatol Syphilol* 1946;54:532–537.

33. Meyer PR, Shum TK, Becker TS, Taylor CR: Scleroma (rhinoscleroma). A histologic immunohistochemical study with bacterial correlates. *Arch Pathol Lab Med* 1983;107:377–383.

34. Attia OM: Two cases of rhinoscleroma associated with carcinoma. *J Laryngol Otol* 1958; 72:412–415.

35. Peabody JW, Seabury JH: Actinomycosis and nocardiosis. *J Chron Dis* 1957;5:374–400.

36. Rippon JW: *Medical Mycology. The Pathogenic Fungi and the Pathogenic Actinomyces,* 3rd ed. Philadelphia: WB Saunders, 1988:15.

37. Bennhoff DF: Actinomycosis: Diagnostic and therapeutic considerations and a review of 32 cases. *Laryngoscope* 1984;94:1198–1217.

38. Brandenburg JH, Finch WW, Kirkham WR: Actinomycosis of the larynx and pharynx. *Ann Otol Rhinol Laryngol* 1993;86:739–742.

39. Tsuji DH, Fukada H, Kawasaki Y: Actinomycosis of the larynx. *Auris Nasus Larynx* 1991;18:79–85

40. Hughes RA, Paonessa DF, Conway WF: Actinomycosis of the larynx. *Ann Otol Rhinol Laryngol* 1984;93:520–524.

41. Friedmann I, Ferlito A: Mycotic diseases. In: *Granulomas and Neoplasms of the Larynx.* New York: Churchill Livingstone, 1988:49–59.

Infectious Disease: Fungal

42. Fisher EW, Richards A, Anderson G, et al: Laryngeal candidiasis: A cause of airway obstruction in the immunocompromised child. *J Laryngol Otol* 1992;106:168–170.

43. Kingdom TT, Lee KC: Invasive aspergillosis of the larynx in AIDS. *Otolaryngol Head Neck Surg* 1996;115:135–140.

44. Friedmann I, Ferlito A: Mycotic diseases. *Granulomas and Neoplasms of the Larynx.* New York: Churchill Livingstone, 1988:49–59.

45. Smith AG, Schultz RB: Observations on the disposition of *Aspergillus fumigatus* in the respiratory tract. *J Clin Path* 1965;44:271–279.

46. Bodey GP, Bolivar R, Gomez LG, Luna M, Hopfer R: Aspergillus epiglottitis. *Cancer* 1983;51:367–370.

47. Moss JA, Kheir SM, Flint A: Primary aspergillosis of the larynx simulating carcinoma. *Hum Pathol* 1983;14:184–186.

48. Ajello L: Coccidioidomycosis and histoplasmosis: A review of their epidemiology and geographical distribution. *Mycopath Mycolog Appl* 1971;45:221–230.

49. Drutz DJ, Catanzaro A: State of the art: Coccidioidomycosis. Part I. *Am Rev Respir Dis* 1978;117:559–585.

50. Dudley JE: Coccidioidomycosis and neck mass "single lesion" disseminated disease. *Arch Otolaryngol Head Neck Surg* 1987; 113:553–555.

51. Werner SB, Pappagianis D, Heindl I, et al: An epidemic of coccidioidomycosis among archeology students in northern California. *N Engl J Med* 1972;286:507–512.

52. Werner SB, Pappagianis D: Coccidioidomycosis in northern California. *Calif Med* 1973;119:16–20.

53. Pappagianis D: Epidemiology of coccidioidomycosis. *Curr Top Med Mycol* 1988;2:199–238.

54. Eckmann BH, Schaeffer GL, Huppert M: Bedside interhuman transmission of coccidioidomycosis via growth on fomites. An epidemic involving six persons. *Am Rev Respir Dis* 1964;89:175–185.

55. Boyle JO, Coulthard SW, Mandel RM: Laryngeal involvement in disseminated coccidioidomycosis. *Arch Otolaryngol Head Neck Surg* 1991;117:433–438.

56. Hajare S, Rakmusan TA, Kalia A, et al: Laryngeal coccidioidomycosis causing airway obstruction. *Ped Infect Dis J* 1989;8:54–56.

57. Smallman LA, Stores OPR, Watson MG, et al: Cryptococcus of the larynx. *J Laryngol Otol* 1989;103:214–215.

58. Reese MC, Colclasure JB: Cryptococcus of the larynx. *Arch Otolaryngol* 1975;101:698–701.

59. Browning DG, Schwartz DA, Jurado RL: Cryptococcosis of the larynx in a patient with AIDS: An unusual cause of fungal laryngitis. *South Med J* 1992;85:762–764.

60. Lyons GD: Mycotic disease of the larynx. *Ann Otol Rhinol Laryngol* 1966;75:162–175.

61. Suen JY, Wetmore SJ, Wetzel WG, et al: Blastomycosis of the larynx. *Ann Otol Rhinol Laryngol* 1980;89:563–566.

62. Ferguson GB: North American blastomycosis. A review of the literature and a report of two cases primary in the larynx. *Laryngoscope* 1951;9:851–873.

63. Dumich PS, Neel HB: Blastomycosis of the larynx. *Laryngoscope* 1983;93:1266–1270.

64. Furtaldo T: Infection versus disease in South American blastomycosis. *Int J Dermatol* 1975;14:117–125.

65. Lazow SK, Seldin RD, Solomon MP: South American blastomycosis of the maxilla: Report of a case. *J Oral Maxillofac Surg* 1990;48:68–71.

66. Sposto MR, Scully C, Almeida OP, et al: Oral paracoccidioidomycosis.

A study of 36 South American patients. *Oral Surg Oral Med Oral Pathol* 1993;75:461–465.

67. Almeida OP, Jorge J, Scully C, et al: Oral manifestations of paracoccidioidomycosis (South American *Blastomycosis*). *Oral Surg Oral Med Oral Pathol* 1991;72:430–435.

68. Kitchen MS, Reiber CD, Eastin GB: An urban epidemic of North American *Blastomycosis*. *Am Rev Respir Dis* 1977;115:1063–1066.

69. Klein BS, Vergeront JM, Weeks RJ, et al: Isolation of *Blastomyces dermatitidis* in soil associated with a large outbreak of blastomycosis in Wisconsin. *N Engl J Med* 1986;314:529–534.

70. Sarosi GA, Davies SF: Blastomycosis. *Am Rev Respir Dis* 1979;120:911–938.

71. Armstrong CW, Jenkins SR, Kaufman L, et al: Common-source outbreak of blastomycosis in hunters and their dogs. *J Infect Dis* 1987;155:568–570.

72. Tosh FE, Hammerman KJ, Weeks RJ, et al: A common source epidemic of North American blastomycosis. *Am Rev Respir Dis* 1974;109:525–529.

73. Reder PA, Neel HB: Blastomycosis in otolaryngology: Review of a large series. *Laryngoscope* 1993;103:53–58.

74. Payne J, Koopman C: Laryngeal carcinoma: Or is it laryngeal blastomycosis? *Laryngoscope* 1984;94:608–611.

75. Pirozzi DJ, Schwartzmann SW, Lewis AD: An unusual case of North American blastomycosis. *Arch Dermatol* 1978;114:1370–1371.

76. Emmons CW: Saprophytic sources of *Cryptococcus neoformans* associated with the pigeon (Columba livia). *Am J Hyg* 1955;62:227–232.

77. Isaacson, JE, Frable MAS. Cryptococcosis of the larynx. *Otolaryngol Head Neck Surg* 1996;114:106–109.

78. Gnepp DR, Frisch M: Primary cryptococcal infection of the larynx: Report of a case. *Otolaryngol Head Neck Surg* 1995;113:477–480.

79. Bottone EJ, Wormser GP: Capsule-deficient *Cryptococci* in AIDS [letter]. *Lancet* 1985;2:553.

80. Darling ST: A protozoon general infection producing pseudotubercles in the lungs and focal necrosis in the liver, spleen and lymph nodes. *JAMA* 1906;46:1283–1285.

81. Furcolow ML, Tosh FE, Larsh HW, et al: The emerging pattern of urban histoplasmosis. Studies on an epidemic in Mexico, Missouri. *N Engl J Med* 1961;264:1226–1230.

82. Tosh FE, Weeks RJ Pfeiffer FR, et al: The use of formalin to kill *Histoplasma capsulatum* at an epidemic site. *Am J Epidemiol* 1967;85:259–265.

83. Parrott T, Taylor G, Poston M, et al: An epidemic of histoplasmosis in Warrenton, North Carolina. *South Med J* 1955;48:1147–1150.

84. Wheat LJ, Conolly-Stringfield PA, Baker RL, et al: Disseminated histoplasmosis in acquired immune deficiency disease: Clinical findings, diagnosis and treatment and review of the literature. *Medicine* 1990;69:361–374.

85. Oda D, McDougal L, Fitsche T, et al: Oral histoplasmosis as a presenting disease in AIDS. *Oral Surg Oral Med Oral Pathol* 1990;70:631–636.

86. Bennett DE: Histoplasmosis of the oral cavity and larynx. *Arch Intern Med* 1967;120:417–427.

87. Young LL, Dolan T, Sheridan PJ, et al: Oral manifestations of histoplasmosis. *Oral Surg* 1972;33:191–204.

88. Cobb CM, Shultz RE, Brewer JH, et al: Chronic pulmonary histoplasmosis with an oral lesion. *Oral Surg Oral Med Oral Pathol* 1989;67:73–76.

89. Zinneman HH, Hall WH: Chronic pharyngeal and laryngeal histoplasmosis successfully treated with ethyl vanuillate. *Minnesota Med* 1953;36:249–252.

90. Zinneman HH, Hall WH, Wallace FG: Leishmania of larynx. *Am J Med* 1961;31:654–658.

91. Wright J: A nasal sporozoon (*Rhinosporidium kinealyi*). *NY Med J* 1907;86:1149–1153.

92. Norman WG: Rhinosporidiosis in Texas. *Arch Otolaryngol* 1960;72:361–362.

93. Lasser A, Smith HW: Rhinosporidiosis. *Arch Otolaryngol* 1976;102:308–310.

94. Jimenez JF, Young DE, Hough AJ: Rhinosporidiosis. A report of two cases from Arkansas. *Am J Clin Pathol* 1984;82:611–615.

95. Naik RS, Siddiqui RS, Naik V: Urethronasal rhinosporidiosis. *J Ind Med Assoc* 1979;72:238–239.

96. Pillai OSR: Rhinosporidiosis of the larynx. *J Laryngol Otol* 1974;88:277–280.

97. Grover S: *Rhinosporidium seeberi:* A preliminary study of the morphology and life cycle. *Sabouraudia* 1970;7:249–251.

98. Thianprait M, Thagerngpol K: Rhinosporidiosis. *Curr Top Med Mycol* 1989;3:64–85.

99. Ashworth JH: On *Rhinosporidium seeberi* (Wernicke 1903) with special reference to its sporulation and affinities. *Trans Royal Soc Edin* 1923;53:301–342.

100. Krishnamoorthy S, Sreedharan VP, Koshy P, et al: Culture of *Rhinosporidium seeberi:* Preliminary report. *J Laryngol Otol* 1989;103:178–180.

101. Vanbreseghem R: Ultrastructure of *Rhinosporidium seeberi. Int J Dermatol* 1973;12:20–28.

102. Ahluwala KB: Rhinosporidiosis: A study that resolves etiologic controversies. *Am J Rhinol* 1997;11:1–5.

Viral Infection

103. Lalwani AK, Snyderman NL: Pharyngeal ulceration in AIDS patients secondary to CMV infections. *Ann Otol Rhinol Laryngol* 1991;100:484–487.

104. Kanas R, Jensen JL, Abrams AM, et al: Oral mucosal CMV as a manifestation of AIDS. *Oral Surg Oral Med Oral Pathol* 1987;64:183–189.

105. Imoto EM, Stein RM, Shellito JE, et al: Central airway obstruction due to CMV-induced necrotizing tracheitis in a patient with AIDS. *Am Rev Respir Dis* 1990;142:884–886.

106. Marelli RA, Biddinger PW, Gluckman JL: CMV infection of the larynx in AIDS. *Otolaryngol Head Neck Surg* 1992;106:296–301.

107. Langford A, Kunze R, Timm H, et al: CMV associated oral ulcerations in HIV-infected patients. *J Oral Pathol Med* 1989;19:71–76.

108. Small PM, McPhaul LW, Sooy CD, et al: CMV infection of the laryngeal nerve presenting as hoarseness in AIDS patients. *Am J Med* 1989;86:108–110.

109. Siegel RJ, Browning D, Schwartz DA, et al: CMV laryngitis and probable malignant lymphoma of the larynx in a patient with AIDS. *Arch Pathol Lab Med* 1992;116:539–541.

Protozoal Infections

110. Feldmeier H, Bienzle U, Jansen-Rossek R, et al: Sequelae after infection with *Trichinella spiralis:* A prospective cohort study. *Wien Klin Wochenschr* 1991;103:111–116.

111. Kean H: Cancer and trichinosis of the larynx. *Laryngoscope* 1966;76:1766–1768.

112. Lewy RB: Carcinoma of the larynx and trichinosis. *Arch Otolaryngol* 1964;80:320–321.

113. Voge M, Markell EK, John DT: The trematodes. In: Markell EK, Voge M, John DT: *Medical Parasitology.* Philadelphia: WB Saunders, 1986:149–184.

114. Shaheen HB: Bilharziasis of the larynx. *Arch Otolaryngol* 1942;35:286–287.

115. Toppozada HH: Laryngeal bilharzia. *J Laryngol Otolaryngol* 1985;99:1039–1041.

116. Manni HJ Lema PN, van Raalte JA, Westerbeek GF: Schistosomiasis in otolaryngology: Review of the literature and case report. *J Laryngol Otol* 1983;97:1177–1181.

Vocal Polyps

117. Ash JE, Schwartz L: The laryngeal (vocal cord) node. *Trans Am Acad Ophthalmol Otolaryngol* 1944;48:323–332.

118. Barnes L, Gnepp DR: Diseases of the larynx, hypopharynx, and esophagus. In: Barnes L, ed. *Surgical Pathology of the Head and Neck.* New York: Marcel Dekker, 1985:141–226.

119. Epstein SS, Winston P, Friedmann I, Ormerod FC: The vocal cord polyp. *J Laryngol Otol* 1957;71:673–688.

120. Gray SD, Hammond E, Hanson DF: Benign pathologic responses of the larynx. *Ann Otol Rhinol Laryngol* 1995;104:13–18.

121. Kambic V, Radsel Z, Zargi M, et al: Vocal cord polyps: Incidence histology, and pathogenesis. *J Laryngol Otol* 1981;95:609–618.

122. Kleinsasser O: Pathogenesis of vocal cord polyps. *Ann Otol Rhinol Laryngol* 1982;91:378–381.

123. Steinberg BM, Abramson AL, Kahn LB, et al: Vocal cord polyps: Biochemical and histologic evaluation. *Laryngoscope* 1985;95:1327–1331

124. Strong MS, Vaughn CW: Vocal cord nodules and polyps: The role of surgical treatment. *Laryngoscope* 1971;81:911–923.

125. Ferlito A: Vocal cord polyp with stromal atypia. A pseudosarcomatous lesion. *Acta OtoRhinoLaryngol Belg* 1985;39:955–960.
126. Sena T, Brady S, Huvos AG, et al: Laryngeal myxoma. *Arch Otolaryngol Head Neck Surg* 1991;117:430–432.
127. Friedmann I, Ferlito A: Laryngeal manifestations in systemic nonneoplastic diseases. In: *Granulomas and Neoplasms of the Larynx*. New York: Churchill Livingstone, 1988:349–357.

Cysts

128. DeSanto LW, Devine KD, Weiland LH: Cysts of the larynx: Classification. *Laryngoscope* 1970;80:145–176.
129. Civantos FJ, Holinger LD: Laryngoceles and saccular cysts in infants and children. *Arch Otolaryngol Head Neck Surg* 1992;118:296–300.
130. Zelman WH, Burke LI: External laryngocele: An unusual cause of respiratory distress in a newborn. *ENT Journal* 1994;73:19–22.
131. Stell PM, Maran AGD: Laryngocele. *J Laryngol* 1975;89:915–925.
132. MacFie DD: Asymptomatic laryngoceles in wind-instrument bandsmen. *Arch Otolaryngol* 1966;83:270–275.
133. Raveh E, Inbar E, Shvero J, Feinmesser R: Huge saccular cyst of the larynx: A case report. *J Laryngol Otol* 1995;109:653–656.
134. Shaari CM, Ho BT, Som PM, Urken ML: Large thyroglossal duct cyst with laryngeal extension. *Head Neck* 1994;16:586–588.
135. Micheau C: Relationship between laryngoceles and laryngeal carcinomas. *Laryngoscope* 1978;88:680–689.
136. Newman BH, Taxy JB, Laker HI: Laryngeal cysts in adults: A clinicopathologic study of 20 cases. *Am J Clin Pathol* 1984;81:715–720.
137. Dada MA: Laryngeal cyst and sudden death. *Med Sci Law* 1995;35:72–74.
138. Chatzimanolis E, Dokianakis G, Gavalas G: Congenital fistula of the 4th pharyngeal pouch and cleft. *HNO* 1990;38:217–219.
139. Rosenfeld RM, Biller HF: Fourth branchial pouch sinus: Diagnosis and treatment. *Otolaryngol Head Neck Surg* 1991;105:44–50.

Amyloidosis

140. Glenner GG: Amyloid deposits and amyloidosis. The B-fibrillosis. *N Engl J Med* 1980;302:1283–1292.
141. Kyle RA, Greipp PR: Amyloidosis (AL). Clinical and laboratory features in 229 cases. *Mayo Clin Proc* 1983;58:665–683.
142. Barnes EL, Zafar T: Laryngeal amyloidosis. Clinicopathologic study of seven cases. *Ann Otol Rhinol Laryngol* 1977;86:856–863
143. Chen KTK: Amyloidosis presenting in the respiratory tract. *Pathol Annu* 1989;24:253–273.
144. Lewis JE, Olsen KD, Kurtin PJ, et al: Laryngeal amyloidosis: A clinicopathologic and immunohistochemical review. *Otolaryngol Head Neck Surg* 1992;106:372–377.
145. Michaels L, Hyams VJ: Amyloid in localized deposits and plasmacytomas of the respiratory tract. *J Pathol* 1979;128:29–38.
146. Mitrani M, Biller HF: Laryngeal amyloidosis. *Laryngoscope* 1985;95:1346–1347.
147. Talbot AR: Laryngeal amyloidosis. *J Laryngol Otol* 1990;104:147–149.
148. Libbey CA, Skinner M, Cohen AS: Use of abdominal fat tissue aspirate in the diagnosis of systemic amyloidosis. *Arch Int Med* 1983;143:1549–1552.

Intubation Effects

149. Santos PM, Afrassiabi A, Weymuller EA: Risk factors associated with prolonged intubation and laryngeal injury. *Otolaryngol Head Neck Surg* 1994;111:453–459
150. Brandwein M, Abramson AL, Shikowitz MJ; Bilateral vocal cord paralysis following endotracheal intubation. *Arch Otolaryngol* 1986;112:877–882.
151. Gnepp DR, Vogler C, Sotelo-Avila C, Keilmovitch IH: Focal mucinosis of the upper aerodigestive tract in children. *Human Pathol* 1990;21:856–858.
152. Donnelly WH: Histopathology of endotracheal intubation. An autopsy study of 99 cases. *Arch Pathol* 1969;88:511–520.
153. Wenig BM, Heffner DK: Contact ulcers of the larynx. A reacquaintance with the pathology of an often underdiagnosed entity. *Arch Pathol Lab Med* 1990;114:825–828.

Teflon Granulomas

154. Dedo HH, Carlsoo B: Histologic evaluation of Teflon granulomas of human vocal cords. *Acta Otolaryngol* 1982;93:475–484.
155. Valvares MA, Montgomery WW, Hillman RE: Teflon granuloma of the larynx: Etiology, pathophysiology and management. *Ann Otol Laryngol* 1995;104:511–515.
156. Wenig BM, Heffner DK, Oertel YC, Johnson FB: Teflonomas of the larynx and neck. *Hum Pathol* 1990;21:617–623.

Sarcoidosis

157. Siltzbach LE: Editorial: Current thoughts on the epidemiology and etiology of sarcoidosis. *Am J Med* 1965;39:361–368.
158. Siltzbach LE: Sarcoidosis: Clinical features and management. *Med Clin North Am* 1967;51:483–502.
159. Devine KD: Sarcoidosis and sarcoidosis of the larynx. *Laryngoscope* 1965;75:533–569.
160. Rybak LP, Falconer R: Pediatric laryngeal sarcoidosis. *Ann Otol Rhinol Laryngol* 1987;96:670–673.
161. Mochizuki H, Morikawa A, Tokuyama K, et al: Laryngeal sarcoidosis in a young child. *Clin Pediatr* 1987;26:486–488.
162. Lerner DM, Deeb Z: Acute upper airway obstruction resulting from systemic diseases. *South Med J* 1993;86:623–627.
163. Moscovic EA: Sarcoidosis and mycobacterial L-forms. A critical reappraisal of pleomorphic chromogenic bodies (Hamazaki corpuscles) in lymph nodes. *Pathol Annu* 1978;2:69–164.
164. El Zaatari FA, Naser SA, Markesich DC, et al: Identification of *Mycobacterium avium* complex in sarcoidosis. *J Clin Microbiol* 1996;34:2240–2245.
165. Schaumann J, Hallberg VL: Koch's bacilli manifested in the tissue of lymphogranulomatosis benigna (Schaumann) by using Hallberg's staining method. *Acta Med Scand* 1941;152:499–501.
166. McCluggage WG, Bharucha H: Lymph node hyalinization in rheumatoid arthritis and systemic sclerosis. *J Clin Pathol* 1994;47:138–142.

Gout

167. Moore N: Specimens from a case of gout viz. right knee-joint, left patella, metacarpo-phalangeal joint of right index finger, larynx, the pons varolii, part of the pia mater and the kidneys. *Transact Path Soc London* 1882;33:271–279.
168. Gutterplan MD, Townsend MJ Hendrix RA, Balsara G: Laryngeal manifestations of gout. *Ann Otol Laryngol* 1991;100:899–902.
169. Goodman M, Montgomery W, Minette L: Pathologic findings in gouty cricoarytenoid arthritis. *Arch Otolaryngol* 1976;102:27–29.
170. Marrion RB, Alperin JE, Maloney WH: Gouty tophus of the true vocal cord. *Arch Otolaryngol* 1972;96:161–162.
171. Jackson C, Jackson CL: *Diseases and Injuries of the Larynx*. New York: Macmillan, 1942:plate IX.
172. Lefkovitz AM: Gouty involvement of the larynx. Report of a case and review of the literature. *Arthritis Rheumatism* 1965;8:1019–1025.

Autoimmune Diseases: Rheumatoid Arthritis

173. Bienenstock H, Ehrlich GE, Freyberg RH: Rheumatoid arthritis of the cricoarytenoid joint: A clinicopathologic study. *Arthritis Rheumatism* 1963;6:48–63.
174. Curley JWA, Byron MA, Bates GJ: Cricoarytenoid joint involvement in acute systemic lupus erythematosus. *J Laryngol Otol* 1986;100:727–732.
175. Guerra LG, Lau KY, Marwah R: Upper airway obstruction as the sole manifestation of rheumatoid arthritis. *J Rheumatol* 1992;19:974–976.
176. Woo P, Mendelshohn JU, Humphrey D: Rheumatoid nodules of the larynx. *Otolaryngol Head Neck Cancer* 1995;133:147–150.

Autoimmune Disease: Lupus Erythematosus

177. Teitel AD, MacKenzie R, Stern R, Paget SA: Laryngeal involvement in systemic lupus erythematosus. *Semin Arthritis Rheumatism* 1992;22:203–214.
178. Martin L, Edworthy SM, Ryan P, Fritzler MJ: Upper airway disease in systemic lupus erythematosus: A report of 4 cases and a review of the literature. *J Rheumatol* 1992;19:1186–1190.

179. Schwartz IS, Grishman E: Rheumatoid nodules of the vocal cords as the initial manifestation of systemic lupus erythematosus. *JAMA* 1980;244:2751–2752.
180. Aszkenasy OM, Clarke TJ Hickling P, Marshall AJ: Systemic lupus erythematosus, pulmonary hypertension, and left recurrent laryngeal nerve palsy. *Ann Rheumatic Dis* 1987;46:246–247.
181. Saluja S, Singh RR, Misra A, et al: Bilateral recurrent laryngeal nerve palsy in systemic lupus erythematosus. *Clin Exp Rheumatol* 1989;7:81–83.
182. Weiser GA, Fourouhar FA, White WB: Hydralazine hoarseness. A new appearance of drug-induced systemic lupus erythematosus. *Arch Intern Med* 1984;144:2271–2272.
183. Thomas TJ, Seibold JR, Adams LE, Hess EV: Triplex–DNA stabilization by hydralazine and the presence of anti-(triplex DNA) antibodies in patients treated with hydralazine. *Biochem J* 1993;294:419–425.
184. Petri M, Katzenstein P, Hellman D: Laryngeal infection in lupus: Report of nocardiosis and review of laryngeal involvement in lupus. *J Rheumatol* 1988;15:1014–1015.

Autoimmune Disease: Wegener's Granulomatosis

185. Leavitt RY, Fauci AS: Less common manifestations and presentations of Wegener's granulomatosis. *Curr Opin Rheumatol* 1992;4:16–22.
186. Lebovics RS, Hoffman GS, Leavitt RY, et al: The management of infraglottic stenosis in patients with Wegener's granulomatosis. *Laryngoscope* 1992;102:1341–1345.
187. Devaney KO, Travis WD, Hoffman G, et al: Interpretation of head and neck biopsies in Wegener's granulomatosis. *Am J Surg Pathol* 1990;14:555–564.
188. Hoffman GS: Advances in Wegener's granulomatosis. *Hosp Pract* 1995;30:33-40.

Autoimmune Disease: Mucosal Bullous Disease

189. Hanson RD, Olsen KD, Rogers RS: Upper aerodigestive tract manifestations of cicatricial pemphigoid. *Ann Otol Rhinol Laryngol* 1988;97:493–499.
190. Fischer I, Dahl MV, Christiansen TA: Cicatricial pemphigoid confined to the larynx. *Cutis* 1980;25:371–373.
191. Wilhelm T: Vernarbendes Schleimhautpemphigoid mit laryngealer Beteiligung. Fallbericht und Literaturübersicht. *HNO* 1992;40:495–499.
192. Rosenberg F, Sanders S, Nelson C: Pemphigus: A 20 year review of 107 patients treated with corticosteroids. *Arch Dermatol* 1976;112:962–970.
193. Sculley R, Mark EJ, McNeely WF, McNeely BU: Case records of the Massachusetts General Hospital. *N Engl J Med* 1992;326:1276–1284.
194. Obregon G: Pemphigus of the larynx. *Ann Otol Rhinol Laryngol* 1957;66:575–586.
195. Saunders MS, Gentile RD, Lobritz RW: Primary laryngeal and nasal septal lesions in pemphigus vulgaris. *J Am Osteopath Asso* 1992;92:933–937.
196. Samy LL, Girgis IH, Wasef SA: Pharyngeal and laryngeal pemphigus. *J Laryngol Otol* 1968;82:111–121.
197. Fragoggiannis NG, Gangopadhyay S, Cate T: Pemphigus of the larynx and esophagus. *Ann Intern Med* 1995;122:803–804.

Autoimmune Disease: Crohn's Disease

198. Croft CB, Wilkenson AR: Ulceration of the mouth, pharynx and larynx in Crohn's disease of the intestine. *Br J Surg* 1972;59:249–252.
199. Gianoli GJ, Miller RH: Crohn's disease of the larynx. *J Laryngol Otol* 1994;108:596–598.
200. Lemann M, Messing B, D'Agay F, Modigliani R: Crohn's disease with respiratory tract involvement. *Gut* 1987;28:1669–1672.
201. Ramsdell WM, Shulman RJ, Lifschift CH: Unusual appearance of Crohn's disease. *Am J Dis Child* 1984;138:500–501.
202. Petras RE: Non-neoplastic intestinal diseases. In: Sternberg S, ed. *Diagnostic Surgical Pathology.* New York: Raven Press, 1989:982.
203. Kelly JH, Montgomery WW, Goodman ML, Mulvaney TJ: Upper airway obstruction associated with regional enteritis. *Ann Otol* 1979;88:95–99.

Necrotizing Sialometaplasia

204. Abrams AM, Melrose RJ, Howell FV: Necrotizing sialometaplasia: A disease simulating malignancy. *Cancer* 1973;32:130–135.
205. Jensen JL: Idiopathic diseases. In: Ellis GL, Auclair PL, Gnepp DR, eds. *Surgical Pathology of the Salivary Glands.* Philadelphia: WB Saunders, 1991:60–82.
206. Walker GK, Fechner RE, Johns ME: Necrotizing sialometaplasia of the larynx secondary to atheromatous embolization. *Am J Clin Pathol* 1982;77:221–223.
207. Ben-Izhak O, Ben-Arieh Y: Necrotizing squamous metaplasia in herpetic tracheitis following prolonged intubation: A lesion similar to necrotizing sialometaplasia. *Histopathol* 1993;22:265–269.
208. Gnepp DR: Frozen sections. In: *Pathology of the Head and Neck.* New York: Churchill Livingstone, 1988:1–24.

Chondrometaplasia

209. Hyams VJ, Rabuzzi DD: Cartilaginous tumors of the larynx. *Laryngoscope* 1970;80:755–767.
210. Ferlito A, Recher G: Chondrometaplasia of the larynx. *ORL J Otorhinolaryngol Relat Spec* 1985;47:174–177.
211. Hill MJ, Taylor CL, Scott GBD: Chondromatous metaplasia in the human larynx. *Histopathology* 1980;4:205–214.

Polychondritis

212. Pearson CM, Kline HM, Newcomer VD: Relapsing polychondritis. *N Engl J Med* 1960;263:51–58.
213. Dolan DL, Lemmon GB, Teitelbaum SL: Relapsing polychondritis. Analytical literature review and studies on pathogenesis. *Am J Med* 1966;41:285–299.
214. McAdam LP, O'Hanlan MA, Bluestone R, Pearson CM: Relapsing polychondritis: Prospective study of 23 patients and a review of the literature. *Medicine* 1976;55:193–215.
215. Eng J, Sabanathan S: Airway complications in relapsing polychondritis. *Ann Thorac Surg* 1991;51:686–692.

Tracheopathia Chondro-osteoplastica

216. Härmä RA, Suurkari S: Tracheopathia chondro-osteoplastica. A clinical study of 30 cases. *Acta Otolaryngol* 1977;84:118–123.
217. Prakash UBS, McCullough AE, Edell ES, Nienhuis DM: Tracheopathia osteoplastica: Familial occurrence. *Mayo Clin Proc* 1989;64:1091–1096.
218. Alroy GG, Lichtig C, Kaftori JK: Tracheobronchopathia osteoplastica: End stage of primary lung amyloidosis. *Chest* 1972;61:465–468.
219. Way SPB: Tracheopathia osteoplastica. *J Clin Pathol* 1967;20:814–820.
220. Pounder DJ, Pieterse AS: Tracheopathia osteopiastica: A study of the minimal lesion. *J Pathol* 1982;138:235–239.
221. Nienhuis DM, Prakash UBS, Edell ES: Tracheobronchopathia osteochondroplastica. *Ann Otol Rhinol Laryngol* 1990;99:689–694.
222. Muckleston HS: On so-called "multiple osteomata" of the tracheal mucous membrane. *Laryngoscope* 1909;19:881–893.
223. Young RH, Sandstrom RE, Mark RE: Tracheopathia osteoplastica. *J Thorac Cardiovasc Surg* 1980;79:537–541.
224. Sakula A: Tracheopathia osteoplastica. Its relationship to primary tracheobronchial amyloidosis. *Thorax* 1968;23:105–110.
225. Roggenbuck C, Hau T, de Wall N, Buss H: Gleichzeitiges auftreten von Tracheobroncopathia Osteochondroplastica und Mucoepidermoidcarcinom. *Der Chirug* 1995;66:231–234.
226. Pappas DG, Johnson LA: Laryngeal myositis ossificans. *Arch Otolaryngol* 1965;81:227–231.

Radiation Changes

227. Ackerman LV: The pathology of radiation effect on normal and neoplastic tissue. *Am J Roentgenol* 1972;114:447–459.
228. Keene M, Harwood AR, Bryce DP, Van Nostrand AWP: Histopathological study of radionecrosis in laryngeal carcinoma. *Laryngoscope* 1982;92:173–180.
229. Berger G, Freeman JL, Briant DR, et al: Late post radiation necrosis and fibrosis of the larynx. *J Otolaryngol* 1984;13:160–164.
230. Seaman WB, Ackerman LV: The effect of radiation on the esophagus.

A clinical and histologic study of the effects produced by the betatron. *Radiology* (Syracuse) 1957;86:534–541.

231. Brandenburg JH, Condon KG, Frank TW: Coronal sections of larynges from radiation-therapy failures: A clinical-pathologic study. *Otolaryngol Head Neck Surg* 1986;95:213–218.

Papillomas

232. Ullman EV: On the aetiology of laryngeal papillomas. *Acta Otolaryngol* 1928;5:317–338.

233. Mounts P, Shah K, Kashima HL: Viral etiology of juvenile and adult onset squamous papilloma of the larynx. *Proc Natl Acad Sci U S A* 1982;79:5425–5429.

234. Lindeberg H, Syrjänen S, Karja J, et al: HPV 11 DNA in squamous cell carcinomas and pre-existing multiple laryngeal papillomas. *Acta Otolaryngol* 1989;107:141–149.

235. Tsutsumi K, Nakajima T, Gotoh M, et al: In situ hybridization and immunohistochemical study of HPV in adult laryngeal papillomas. *Laryngoscope* 1989;99:80–85.

236. Steinberg BS, Topp WC, Schneider PS, et al: Laryngeal papillomavirus infection during clinical remission. *N Engl J Med* 1983;308:1261–1264.

237. Quick CA, Krzyzek RA, Watts SL, et al: Relationship between condylomata and laryngeal papillomata. Clinical and molecular virological evidence. *Ann Otol* 1980;89:467–471.

238. Smith EM, Johnson SR, Cripe TP, et al: Perinatal vertical transmission of HPV and subsequent development of respiratory tract papillomatosis. *Ann Otol Rhinol Laryngol* 1991;100:479–482.

239. Quick CA, Foucar E, Dehner LP: Frequency and significance of epithelial atypia in laryngeal papillomatosis. *Laryngoscope* 1979;89:550–560.

240. Michaels L: Squamous cell papillomas. In: Michaels L, ed. *Pathology of the Larynx.* New York: Springer-Verlag, 1984:159–173.

241. Barnes L, Yunis EJ, Krebbs FJ, et al: Verruca vulgaris of the larynx. *Arch Pathol Lab Med* 1991;115:895–899.

242. Capper JWR, Bailey CM, Michaels L: Squamous papillomas of the larynx in adults. A review of 63 cases. *Clin Otolaryngol* 1983;8:109–119.

243. Byrne JC, Tsao MS, Fraser RS, et al: HPV–11 DNA in a patient with chronic laryngotracheobronchial papillomatosis and metastatic squamous cell carcinoma of the lung. *N Engl J Med* 1987;317:873–878.

244. Guillou L, Sahli R, Chaubert P, et al: Squamous cell carcinoma of the lung in a nonsmoking nonirradiated patient with juvenile laryngotracheal papillomatosis. *Am J Surg Pathol* 1991;15:891–898.

245. Weiss MD, Kashima HK: Tracheal involvement in laryngeal papillomatosis. *Laryngoscope* 1983;93:45–48.

246. Michaels L: Papilloma. In: Ferlito A, ed. *Surgical Pathology of Laryngeal Neoplasms.* New York: Chapman and Hall, 1996:93–105.

247. Zarod AP, Rutherford JD, Corbitt G: Malignant progression of laryngeal papilloma associated with HPV 6 DNA. *J Clin Pathol* 1988;41:280–283.

248. Hasan Dutt SN, Kini U, et al: Laryngeal carcinoma ex-papilloma in a non-irradiated no-smoking patient: A clinical record and review of the literature. *J Laryngol Otol* 1995;109:762–766.

249. Lie ES, Engh V, Boysen-M, et al: Squamous cell carcinoma of the respiratory tract following laryngeal papillomatosis. *Acta Otolaryngol* (Stockh) 1994;114:209–214.

250. Pou AM, Rimeel FL, Jordan JA, et al: Adult respiratory papillomatosis: HPV type and viral coinfections as predictors of prognosis. *Ann Otol Rhinol Laryngol* 1995;104:758–762.

251. Mahnke, CG, Frohlich O, Lippert BM, et al: Recurrent laryngeal papillomatosis. Retrospective analysis of 95 patients and review of the literature [editorial]. *Otolaryngol Pol* 1996;50:567–578.

252. Ramsaroop R, Singh B: Clinical features of malignant transformation in benign laryngeal papillomata. *J Laryngol Otol* 1994;108:642–648.

253. Cohen SR, Geller KA, Seltzer S, Thimpson JW: Papilloma of the larynx and tracheobronchial tree in children. A retrospective study. *Ann Otol* 1980;89:497–503.

254. Steinberg BM, DiLorenzo TP, Tamsen A, Abramson AL: Human papillomavirus type 6a DNA in the lung carcinoma of a patient with recurrent laryngeal papillomatosis is characterized by a partial duplication. *J Gen Virol* 1992;73:423–428.

Granular Cell Tumor

255. Hyams V, Heffner D: Laryngeal pathology. In: Tucker H, ed. *The Larynx.* New York: Thieme, 1987:33–78.

256. Burton DM, Heffner DK, Patow CA: Granular cell tumors of the trachea. *Laryngoscope* 1992;102:807–813.

257. Lack EE, Worja GF, Callihan LD, et al: Granular cell tumor: A clinicopathologic study of 110 patients. *J Surg Oncol* 1980;13:301–306.

258. Compagno J, Hyams VJ, Ste-Marie P: Benign granular cell tumors of the larynx: A review of 36 cases with clinicopathologic data. *Ann Otol Rhinol Laryngol* 1975;84:504–507.

259. Conley SF, Milbrath MM, Beste DJ: Pediatric laryngeal granular cell tumor. *J Otolaryngol* 1992;21:450–453.

260. Shapiro AM, Rimell FL, Kenna MA: Pathologic quiz case 1. *Arch Otolaryngol Head Neck Surg* 1995;121:1058–1061.

261. Hamid AM, Alshaikhly A: Granular cell tumor of the larynx in an eight year old girl. *J Laryngol Otol* 1993;107:940–941.

262. Lazar RH, Younis RT, Kluka EA, et al: Granular cell tumor of the larynx: Report of two pediatric cases. *ENT J* 1992;71:440–443.

263. Gamboa LG: Malignant granular cell myoblastoma. *Arch Pathol* 1955;60:663–668.

264. Mittal KR, True LD: Origin of granules in granular cell tumor. Intracellular myelin formation with autodigestion. *Arch Pathol Lab Med* 1988;112:302–303.

265. Bonin DMSO, Kurtin PJ: Immunohistochemical demonstration of the lysozomal associated glycoprotein CD68 (KP-1) in granular cell tumors and schwannomas. *Hum Pathol* 1994;25:1172–1181.

266. Robertson AJ, McIntosh W, Lamont P, et al: Malignant granular cell tumor (myoblastoma) of the vulva: Report of a case and review of the literature. *Histopathology* 1981;5:69–79.

267. Brandwein M, LeBenger J, Strauchen J, Biller H: Atypical granular cell tumor of the larynx: An unusually aggressive tumor clinically and microscopically. *Head Neck* 1990;12:154–159.

Paraganglioma and Neuroendocrine Carcinoma

268. Barnes L: Paraganglioma of the larynx. A critical review of the literature. *ORL Otorhinolaryngol Relat Spec* 1991;53:220–234.

269. Martinson FD: Chemodectoma of the glomus laryngicum inferior. *Arch Otolaryngol* 1967;85:70–73.

270. Olofsson J, Grontoft O, Sokjer H, Risberg B: Paraganglioma involving the larynx. *ORL Otorhinolaryngol Relat Spec* 1984;46:57–65.

271. Brandwein M, Levy G, Som P, Urken M: Paraganglioma of the inferior laryngeal paraganglion. *Arch Otolaryngol Head Neck Surg* 1992;118:994–996.

272. Peterson KL, Fu YS, Calcaterra T: Subglottic paraganglioma. *Head Neck J Sci Spec Head Neck* 1997;19:54–56.

273. Stanley RJ, Weiland LH, Neel HB III: Pain-inducing laryngeal paraganglioma. Report of the ninth case and review of the literature. *Otolaryngol Head Neck Surg* 1986;95:107–112.

274. Hartmann E: Chemodectoma laryngis. *Acta Otolaryngol* (Stockh) 1960;51:528–532.

275. Werner JA, Hansmann ML, Lippert BM, Rudert H: Laryngeal paraganglioma and pregnancy. *ORL Otorhinolaryngol Relat Spec* 1992;54:163–167.

276. Laudadio P: Chemodectoma (paraganglioma non chromaffin) del glomo laringeo superiore. *Otorinolaringol Ital* 1971;39:19–31.

277. Ferlito A, Barnes L, Wenig BM: Identification, classification, treatment and prognosis of laryngeal paraganglioma. Review of the literature and eight new cases. *Ann Otol Rhinol Laryngol* 1994;103:525–536.

278. Ferlito A, Milroy C, Wenig BM, et al: Laryngeal paraganglioma versus atypical carcinoid tumor. *Ann Otol Rhinol Laryngol* 1995;104:78–83.

279. Meyer-Breitling E, Burkhardt A: *Tumours of the Larynx.* Berlin: Springer-Verlag, 1988:79.

280. Wenig BM, Gnepp DR: The spectrum of neuroendocrine carcinomas of the larynx. *Semin Diagn Pathol* 1989;6:329–350.

281. Gnepp DR, Ferlito A, Hyams V: Primary anaplastic small cell (oat cell) carcinoma of the larynx. *Cancer* 1983;51:1731–1745.

282. Woodruff JM, Senie RT: Atypical carcinoid tumor of the larynx. A critical review of the literature. *ORL Otorhinolaryngol Relat Spec* 1991;53:194–209.

283. El-Naggar AK, Batsakis JG: Carcinoid tumor of the larynx. A critical review of the literature. *ORL Otorhinolaryngol Relat Spec* 1991;53:188–193.

284. Ferlito A, Barnes L, Rinaldo A, Gnepp DR, Milroy CM: A review of neuroendocrine neoplasms of the larynx: Update on diagnosis and treatment. *J Laryngol Otol* 1998;112:827–834.

285. Wenig BM, Hyams VJ, Heffner DK: Moderately differentiated neuroendocrine carcinoma of the larynx. A clinicopathologic study of 54 cases. *Cancer* 1988;62:2658–2676.

286. Ferlito A, Friedmann I: Review of neuroendocrine carcinomas of the larynx. *Ann Oto Rhinol Laryngol* 1989;98:780–790.

287. Batsakis JG, El-Naggar AK, Luna MA: Neuroendocrine tumors of the larynx. *Ann Oto Rhinol Laryngol* 1992;101:710–714.

288. Watters GWR, Molyneux AJ: Pathology in focus: Atypical carcinoid tumour of the larynx. *J Laryngol Otol* 1995;109:455–458.

289. Stanley RJ, Desanto LW, Weiland LH: Oncocytic and oncocytoid carcinoid tumors (well-differentiated neuroendocrine carcinoma) of the larynx. *Arch Otolaryngol Head Neck Surg* 1986;112:529–536.

290. Gown AM, Vogel AM, Hoak D, et al: Monoclonal antibodies specific for melanocytic tumors distinguish subpopulations of melanocytes. *Am J Pathol* 1986;123:195–203.

291. Batsakis JG, El-Naggar AK, Luna MA: Pathology consultation: Neuroendocrine tumors of larynx. *Ann Otol Rhinol Laryngol* 1992;101:710–714.

292. El-Naggar AK, Batsakis J, Vassilopoulou-Sellin R, et al: Medullary (thyroid) carcinoma-like carcinoids of the larynx. *J Laryngol Otol* 1991;105:683–686.

293. Bishop J, Osamura RY, Tsutsumi Y: Multiple hormone production in an oat cell carcinoma of the larynx. *Acta Pathol Jpn* 1985;35:915–923.

294. Medina JE, Moran M, Goepfert H: Oat cell carcinoma of the larynx and Eaton-Lampert syndrome. *Arch Otolaryngol* 1984;110:123–126.

295. Trotoux J, Glickmanas M, Sterkers O, et al: Syndrome de Schwartz-Bartter: Revelateur d'un cancer larynge sous-glottique a petites cellules. *Ann Oto Laryngol (Paris)* 1979;96:349–358.

Salivary Tumors

296. Luna MA: Salivary gland neoplasms. In: Ferlito A, ed. *Surgical Pathology of Laryngeal Neoplasms.* London: Chapman and Hall Medical, 1996:257–294.

297. Heffner DK: Sinonasal and laryngeal salivary gland lesions. In: Ellis GL, Auclair PL, Gnepp DR, eds. *Surgical Pathology of the Salivary Glands.* Philadelphia: WB Saunders, 1991:544–559.

298. Hamlyn, PJ, O'Brien CJ, Shaw HJ: Uncommon malignant tumours of the larynx: A 25 year review. *J Laryngol Otol* 1986;100:163–168.

299. El-Jabbour JN, Ferlito A, Friedmann I: Salivary gland neoplasms. In: Ferlito A, ed. *Neoplasms of the Larynx.* London: Churchill Livingstone, 1993:231–264.

300. Ferlito A, Gale N, Hvala H: Laryngeal salivary duct carcinoma. *J Laryngol Otol* 1981;95:731–738.

301. Steiner W, Pesch HJ: Endoskopisch-histomorphologische differentiale Diagnose seltener gutartiger Proliferationen des Endolarynx. *Laryngol Rhinol* 1976;55:111–118.

302. Busuttil A: Oncocytic lesions of the upper respiratory tract. *J Laryngol* 1976;90:277–288.

303. Brandwein MS, Huvos AG: Laryngeal oncocytic cystadenomas. A report of eight cases and a literature review. *Arch Otolaryngol Head Neck Surg* 1995;121:1302–1305.

304. Gallagher JC, Puzon BQ: Oncocytic lesions of the larynx. *Ann Otol Rhinol Laryngol* 1969;78:307–318.

305. Yamase HT, Putnam HC: Oncocytic papillary cystadenomatosis of the larynx. A clinicopathologic entity. *Cancer* 1979;44:2306–2311.

306. Le Jeune FE, Putnam HC, Yamase HT: Multiple oncocytic papillary cystadenomas of the larynx: A case report. *Laryngoscope* 1980;90:501–504.

307. Robinson AC, Kaberos A, Cox PM, Stearns MP: Oncocytoma of the larynx. *J Laryngol Otol* 1990;104:346–349.

308. Som ML, Peimer R: Oncocytic cystadenoma of the larynx. *Ann Otol* 1949;58:234–242.

309. Mays MBC: Laryngeal oncocytoma in two dogs. *J Am Vet Med Assoc* 1984;185:677–679.

310. Pass DA, Huxtable CR, Cooper BJ, et al: Canine laryngeal oncocytomas. *Vet Pathol* 1980;17:672–677.

311. Johns ME, Regezi JA, Batsakis JG: Oncocytic neoplasm of salivary glands: An ultrastructural study. *Laryngoscope* 1977;87:862–871.

312. Johns ME, Batsakis JG, Short CD: Oncocytic and oncocytoid tumors of the salivary glands. *Laryngoscope* 1973;83:1940–1952.

313. MacMillan RH, Fechner RE: Pleomorphic adenoma of the larynx. *Arch Pathol* 1986;110:245–247.

314. Zakzouk MS: Pleomorphic adenoma of the larynx. *J Laryngol Otol* 1985;99:611–616.

315. Gierek T, Namysowski G, Kamienski J: Pleomorphic adenoma of atypical localization. *Otolaryngol Pol* 1990;44:249–251.

316. Suttner HJ, Stoss H, Iro H: Pleomorphes Adenom der Epiglottis: Kasuistik und Literaturübersicht. *HNO* 1992;40:453–455.

317. Baptista PM, Garcia-Tapia R, Vazquez JJ: Pleomorphic adenoma of the epiglottis. *J Otolaryngol* 1992;21:355–357.

318. Bizal JC, Righi PF, Kesler KA: Pleomorphic adenoma of the trachea. *Otolaryngol Head Neck Surg* 1997;116:139–140.

319. Sawatsubashi M, Tuda K, Tokunaga O, Shin T: Pleomorphic adenoma of the larynx: A case and review of the literature in Japan. *Otolaryngol Head Neck Surg* 1997;117:415–417.

320. Ferlito A: Histologic classification of larynx and hypopharynx cancers and their clinical implications. Pathologic aspects of 2052 malignant neoplasms diagnosed at the ORL Department of Padua University from 1966 to 1976. *Acta Otolaryngol Suppl* (Stockh) 1976;342:1–88.

321. Avanzini F, Ferri T, Ferrari G, et al: Unusual laryngeal cancers: a clinical statistical study. In: Sacristan T, Alvarez-Vincent JJ, Bartual K, Antoli-Candeta F, eds. Proceedings of the XIV World Congress of Otorhinolaryngology, September 10–11, 1989. Madrid: Kugler and Ghedini Publications, Amsterdam Head and Neck Surgery, 1991.

322. Stillwagon GB, Smith RRL, Highstein C, Lee DJ: Adenoid cystic carcinoma of the supraglottic larynx: Report of a case and review of the literature. *Am J Otolaryngol* 1985;6:309–314.

323. Olofsson J, van Nostrand AWP: Adenoid cystic carcinoma of the larynx: A report of four cases and a review of the literature. *Cancer* 1977;40:1307–1313.

324. Bignardi L, Aimoni C, Franceschetti E, et al: Adenoid cystic carcinoma of the larynx: Review of the literature. *Acta Otorrinolaringol Esp* 1993;44:141–145.

325. Cohen J, Guillamondegui OM, Batsakis JG, et al: Cancer of the minor salivary glands of the larynx. *Am J Surg* 1985;150:513–518.

326. Mitchel DB, Humphreys S, Kearns DB: Mucoepidermoid carcinoma of the larynx in a child. *Int J Pediatr Otorhinolaryngol* 1988;15:211–215.

327. Damiani JM, Damiani KA, Hauck K, Hyams VJ: Mucoepidermoid-adenosquamous carcinoma of the larynx and hypopharynx: A report of 21 cases and a review of the literature. *Otolaryngol Head Neck Surg* 1981;89:235–243.

328. Ferlito A, Recher G, Bottin R: Mucoepidermoid carcinoma of the larynx. A clinicopathologic study of 11 cases with review of the literature. *ORL J Otorhinolaryngol Relat Spec* 1981;43:280–299.

329. Cumberworth VL, Marula A, MacLennan KA, et al: Mucoepidermoid carcinoma of the larynx. *J Laryngol Otol* 1989;103:420–423.

330. Gomes V, Costarelli L, Cimino G, et al: Mucoepidermoid carcinoma of the larynx. *Eur Arch Otorhinolaryngol* 1990;248:31–34.

331. Snow RT, Fox AR: Mucoepidermoid carcinoma of the larynx. *J Am Osteopath Assoc* 1991;91:182–184.

332. Seo IS, Warfel KA, Tomich CE, et al: Clear cell carcinoma of the larynx. A variant of mucoepidermoid carcinoma. *Ann Otol Rhinol Laryngol* 1980;89:168–172.

Melanoma

333. Mori W: A geo-pathological study on malignant melanoma. *Pathol Microbiol* 1971;37:169–180.

334. Uehara T, Matsubara O, Kasuga T: Melanocytes in the nasal cavity and paranasal sinus. Incidence and distribution in Japan. *Acta Pathol Jpn* 1987;37:1105–1114.

335. Seiji M, Ohsumi T: Statistical study on malignant melanoma in Japan (1961–1970). *Tohoku J Exp Med* 1972;107:115–125.

336. Guzzo M, Grandi C, Licitra L, et al: Mucosal malignant melanoma of head and neck: Forty-eight cases treated at Instituto Nazionale Tumori of Milan. *Eur J Surg Oncol* 1993;19:316–319.

337. Panje WR, Moran WJ: Melanoma of the upper aerodigestive tract: A review of 21 cases. *Head Neck Surg* 1986;8:309–321.

338. Conley J Pack GT: Melanoma of the mucous membranes of the head and neck. *Arch Otolaryngol* 1974;99:315–319.

339. Shah JP, Huvos AG, Strong EW: Mucosal melanomas of the head and neck. *Am J Surg* 1977;134:531–535.

340. Kim H, Park CI: Primary malignant laryngeal melanoma: Report of a case with review of literature. *Yonsei Med J* 1982;23:118–122.

341. Reuter VE, Woodruff JM: Melanoma of the larynx. *Laryngoscope* 1986;96:389–393.

342. Wenig BM: Laryngeal mucosal malignant melanoma. A clinicopathologic, immunohistochemical and ultrastructural study of four patients and a review of the literature. *Cancer* 1995;75:1568–1577.

343. Eneroth CM, Lundberg C: Mucosal malignant melanomas of the head and neck. *Acta Otolaryngol* 1975;80:452–458.

344. Gonzalez-Vela MC, Fernandez FA, Mayorga M, et al: Laryngeal melanosis: Report of four cases and literature review. *Otolaryngol Head Neck Surg* 1997;117:708–712.

345. Franquemont DW, Mills SE: Sinonasal malignant melanoma. A clini-

copathologic and immunohistochemical study of 14 cases. *Am J Clin Pathol* 1991;96:689–697.

Hematopoietic Neoplasms

346. Horny HP: Hematopoietic neoplasms. In: Ferlito A, ed. *Surgical Pathology of Laryngeal Neoplasms*. London: Chapman & Hall Medical, 1996:425-439.
347. Kapadia SB, Desai U, Cheng VS: Extramedullary plasmacytoma of the head and neck. A clinicopathologic study of 20 cases. *Medicine* 1982;61:317–329.
348. Weissman JL, Myers JN, Kapadia SB: Extramedullary plasmacytoma of the larynx. *Am J Otolaryngol* 1993;14:128–131.
349. Aquilera NS, Kapadia SB, Nalesnik MA, et al: Extramedullary plasmacytoma of the head and neck: Use of paraffin sections to assess clonality with *in situ* hybridization, growth fraction, and the presence of Epstein-Barr virus. *Mod Pathol* 1995;8:503–508.
350. Bjelkenkrantz K, Lundgren J, Olofsson J: Extramedullary plasmacytoma of the larynx. *J Otolaryngol* 1981;10:28–34.
351. Maniglia AJ, Xue JW: Plasmacytoma of the larynx. *Laryngoscope* 1983;93:741–744.
352. Gorenstein A, Neel HB III, Devine KD, et al: Solitary plasmacytoma of the larynx. *Arch Otol* 1977;103:159–161.
353. Aguilera NS; Kapadia SB; Nalesnik MA; Swerdlow SH: Extramedullary plasmacytoma of the head and neck: Use of paraffin sections to assess clonality with in-situ hybridization, growth fraction, and the presence of EBV. *Mod Pathol* 1995; 8: 503–508.
354. Ferreiro JA, Egorshin EV, Olsen KD, et al: Mucous membrane plasmacytosis of the upper aerodigestive tract. A clinicopathologic study. *Am J Surg Pathol* 1994;18:1048–1053.
355. Courtney-Harris RG, Goddard MJ: Sinus histiocytosis with massive lymphadenopathy (Rosai-Dorfman disease): A rare case of infraglottic narrowing. *J Laryngol Otol* 1992;106:61–62.
356. Strickler JG, Audeh W, Copenhauer CM, et al: Immunophenotypic difference between plasmacytoma/multiple myeloma and immunoblastic lymphoma. *Cancer* 1988;61:1782–1786.
357. Spanio M, Varini A, Silvestri F, Bussani R: Laryngeal involvement in Waldenström's macroglobulinemia: A case report. *Otolaryngol Head Neck Surg* 1996;114:642–644.
358. Soesan M, Paccagnella A, Chiarion-Sileni, et al: Extramedullary plasmacytoma: Clinical behavior and response to treatment. *Ann Oncol* 1992;3:51–57.
359. Swerdlow JB, Merl SA, Davey FR, et al: Non-Hodgkin's lymphoma limited to the larynx. *Cancer* 1984;53:2546–2549.
360. Diebold J, Audouin J, Viry B, et al: Primary lymphoplasmacytic lymphoma of the larynx. A rare localization of MALT-type lymphoma. *Ann Otol Rhinol Laryngol* 1990;99:577–580.
361. Chen KT: Localized laryngeal lymphoma. *J Surg Oncol* 1984;26:208–209.
362. Bickerton RC, Brockbank MJ: Lymphoplasmacytic lymphoma of the larynx, soft palate and nasal cavity. *J Laryngol Otol* 1988;102:468–470.
363. Hisashi K, Komune S, Inoue H: Coexistence of MALT-type lymphoma and squamous cell carcinoma of the larynx. *J Laryngol Otol* 1994;108:995–997.
364. Morgan K, MacLennan KA, Narula A: Non-Hodgkin's lymphoma of the larynx (stage IE). *Cancer* 1989;64:1123–1127.
365. Nakashima T, Inamitsu M, Uemura T, et al: Immunopathology of polymorphic reticulosis of the larynx. *J Laryngol Otol* 1989;103:955–960.
366. Wells P, Wotherspoon A, Burnet NG, et al: Cutaneous B-cell lymphoma with subsequent laryngeal involvement. *Clin Oncol* 1995;7:62–64.
367. The Non-Hodgkin's Lymphoma Pathologic Classification Project: National Cancer Institute sponsored study of classification of non-Hodgkin's lymphomas: Summary and description of a working formulation for clinical usage. *Cancer* 1982;49:2112– 2135.

Inflammatory Myofibroblastic Tumor

368. Batsakis JG, El-Naggar AK, Luna MA, Goepfert H: Pathology consultation—"Inflammatory pseudotumor": What is it? How does it behave? *Ann Otol Rhinol Laryngol* 1995;104:329–331.
369. Wenig BM, Devaney K, Bisceglia M: Inflammatory myofibroblastic tumor of the larynx. *Cancer* 1995;76:2217–2229.
370. Scalafani AP, Kimmelman CP, McCormick SA: Inflammatory pseudotumor of the larynx: Comparison with orbital inflammatory pseudotu-

mor with clinical implications. *Otolaryngol Head Neck Surg* 1993;109:548–551.
371. Coffin CM, Watterson J, Priest JR, Dehner LP: Extrapulmonary inflammatory myofibroblastic tumor (inflammatory pseudotumor): A clinicopathologic and immunohistochemical study of 84 cases. *Am J Surg Pathol* 1995;19:859–872.
372. Hytiroglu P, Brandwein MS, Strauchen JA, et al: Inflammatory pseudotumor of the parapharyngeal space: Case report and review of the literature. *Head Neck* 1992;14:230–234.
373. Som PM, Brandwein MS, Maldjian C, et al: Inflammatory pseudotumor of the maxillary sinus: CT and MR findings in six cases. *AJR* 1994;163:689–692.
374. Chan YF, Ma LT, Young CK, Lam KH: Parapharyngeal inflammatory pseudotumor presenting as a fever of unknown origin in a 3 year old girl. *Ped Pathol* 1988;8:195–203.
375. Keen M, Cho HT, Savetsky L: Pseudotumor of the larynx: An unusual cause of airway obstruction. *Otolaryngol Head Neck Surg* 1986;94:243–246.
376. Keen M, Conley J, McBride T, et al: Pseudotumor of the pterygomaxillary space presenting as anesthesia of the mandibular nerve. *Laryngoscope* 1986;96:560–563.
377. Takimoto T, Kathoh T, Ohmura T, et al: Inflammatory pseudotumor of the maxillary sinus mimicking malignancy. *Rhinol* 1990;28:123–127.
378. Olsen KD, DeSanto LW, Wold LE, Weiland LH: Tumefactive fibroinflammatory lesions of the head and neck. *Laryngoscope* 1986;96:940–944.
379. Albizzati C, Ramesar CRB, Davis BC: Plasma cell granuloma of the larynx (Case report and review of the literature). *J Laryngol Otol* 1988;102:187–189.
380. Fradis M, Rosenman D, Podoshin L, et al: Steroid therapy for plasma cell granuloma of the larynx. *Ear Nose Throat J* 1988;67:558–564.
381. Meis JM, Enzinger FM: Inflammatory fibrosarcoma of the mesentery and retroperitoneum. A tumor closely simulating inflammatory pseudotumor. *Am J Surg Pathol* 1991; 15:1146–1156.

Langerhans' Cell Histiocytosis

382. Jaffe HL, Lichtenstein L: Eosinophilic granuloma of bone: Condition affecting one, several or many bones, but apparently limited to skeleton, and representing mildest clinical expression of peculiar inflammatory histiocytosis also underlying Siwe disease and Schüller-Christian disease. *Arch Pathol* 1944;37:99–118.
383. Lichtenstein L: Histiocytosis X: Integration of eosinophilic granuloma of bone Letterer Siwe's disease and Schüller-Christian disease as related manifestations of a single nosologic entity. *Arch Pathol* 1953;55:84–102.
384. Lieberman PH, Jones CR, Dargeon HWK, Begg CFA: A reappraisal of eosinophilic granuloma of bone Hand-Schüller-Christian syndrome and Letterer-Siwe syndrome. *Medicine* 1969;48:375–398.
385. Lieberman PH, Jones CR, Steinman RM, et al: Langerhans' cell (eosinophilic) granulomatosis. A clinicopathologic study encompassing 50 years. *Am J Surg Pathol* 1996;20:519–552.
386. Willman CL, Busque L, Griffith B, et al: Langerhans'-cell histiocytosis (histiocytosis X) a clonal proliferative disease. *N Engl J Med* 1994;331:154–160.
387. Kapadia SB: Histiocytosis X. In: Barnes L, ed. *Surgical Pathology of the Head and Neck*. New York: Marcel Dekker, 1985:1149–1152.
388. DiNardo LJ, Wetmore RF: Head and neck manifestations of histiocytosis-X in children. *Laryngoscope* 1989;99:721–724.
389. Alessi DM, Maceri D: Histiocytosis X in the head and neck in a pediatric population. *Arch Otolaryngol Head Neck Surg* 1992;118:945–948.
390. Jones RO, Pillsbury HC: Histiocytosis X of the head and neck. *Laryngoscope* 1984;94:1031–1035.
391. Smoler J, Rivera-Camacho R, Vivar-Mejia G, Levy-Pinto S: Otolaryngologic manifestations of histiocytosis X. *Laryngoscope* 1971;81:1903–1911.
392. Friedmann I, Ferlito A: Primary eosinophilic granuloma of the larynx. *J Laryngol Otol* 1981;95:1249–1254.
393. Lhoták J, Dvoracková I: Histiocytosis X of the larynx. *J Laryngol Otol* 1975;89:771–777.
394. De Schepper AM, Ramon F, Van Marck E: MR imaging of eosinophilic granuloma: Report of 11 cases. *Skeletal Radiology* 1993;22:163–166.
395. Ide F, Iwase T, Saito I, et al: Immunohistochemical and ultrastructural analysis of the proliferating cells in histiocytosis X. *Cancer* 1984;53:917–921.
396. Emile J-F, Wechsler J, Brousse N, et al: Langerhans' cell histiocytosis.

Definitive diagnosis with the use of monoclonal antibody 010 on routinely paraffin-embedded samples. *Am J Surg Pathol* 1995;19:636–641.

Fibroblastic Tumors

397. Lattes R: Tumors of the soft tissues. *Atlas of Tumor Pathology.* Vol. 1 Fascicle, second series. Washington, DC: Armed Forces Institute of Pathology, 1982.
398. Allen PW: The fibromatoses: A clinicopathologic classification based on 140 cases. Part I. *Am J Surg Pathol* 1977;1:255–270.
399. Enzinger FM, Weiss SW. *Soft Tissue Tumors,* 3rd ed. St. Louis: C.V. Mosby, 1995:210–220.
400. Gnepp DR, Henley J, Weiss S, Heffner D: Desmoid fibromatosis of the sinonasal tract and nasopharynx: A clinicopathologic study of 25 cases. *Cancer* 1996;78:2572–2579.
401. Masson JK, Soule EH: Desmoid tumors of the head and neck. *Am J Surg* 1966;112:615–622.
402. Das Gupta TK, Brasfield RD, O'Hara J: Extra-abdominal desmoids: Pathologic study. *Ann Surg* 1969;170:109–121.
403. Dehner LP, Askin FB: Tumors of fibrous tissue origin in childhood. A clinicopathologic study of cutaneous and soft tissue neoplasms in 66 children. *Cancer* 1976;38:888–900.
404. Stout AP: Juvenile fibromatoses. *Cancer* 1954;7:953–978.
405. Rao BN, Horowitz ME, Parham DM, et al: Challenges in the treatment of childhood fibromatosis. *Arch Surg* 1987;122:1296–1298.
406. Ayala AG, Ro JY, Goepfert H, et al: Desmoid fibromatosis: A clinicopathologic study of 25 children. *Semin Diagnost Pathol* 1986;3:138–150.
407. Conley J, Healey W, Stout P: Fibromatosis of the head and neck. *Am J Surg* 1966;112:609–614.
408. Allen PW: The fibromatoses: A clinicopathologic classification based on 140 cases. Part 2. *Am J Surg Pathol* 1977;1:305–321.
409. Fasching MC, Saleh J Woods JE: Desmoid tumors of the head and neck. *Am J Surg* 1988;156:327–330.
410. McIntosh WA, Kassner GW, Murray JF: Fibromatosis and fibrosarcoma of the larynx and pharynx in an infant. *Arch Otolaryngol* 1985;111:478–480.
411. Rosenberg HS, Vogler C, Close LG, Warshaw HE: Laryngeal fibromatosis in the neonate. *Arch Otolaryngol* 1981;107:513–517.
412. Jamal MN, Dajani SS, Tarawneh MS: Idiopathic subcutaneous and laryngeal fibromatosis. *J Laryngol Otol* 1986;100:851–855.
413. Safneck JR, Alguacil-Garcia A, Dort JC, et al: Solitary fibrous tumor: report of 2 new locations in the upper respiratory tract. *J Laryngol* 1993;107:252–256.
414. Rohn GN, Close LG, Vuitch F, Merkel MA: Fibrous neoplasms of the adult larynx. *Head Neck* 1994;16:227–231.
415. Ferlito A, Nicolai P, Barion U: Critical comments in laryngeal fibrosarcoma. *Acta OtoRhinoLaryngol Belg* 1983;37:918–925.
416. Shin WY, Abramson AL: The value of electron microscopy in the diagnosis of fibrosarcoma of the larynx. *Trans Am Acad Ophthal Otolaryngol* 1976;82:582–587.
417. Devaney KO: Fibrous and histiocytic tissue neoplasms. In: Ferlito A, ed. *Surgical Pathology of Laryngeal Neoplasms.* New York: Chapman & Hall, 1996:295–320.

Peripheral Nerve Sheath Tumors

418. Enzinger FM, Weiss SW: *Soft Tissue Tumors,* 3rd ed. St. Louis: CV Mosby, 1995.
419. Hajdu SI: Peripheral nerve sheath tumors: histogenesis, classification, and prognosis [editorial]. *Cancer* 1993;72:3549–3552.
420. Swanson PE, Scheithauer BW, Wick MR: Peripheral nerve sheath neoplasms. Clinicopathologic and immunochemical observations. *Pathol Ann* 1995;30:1–82.
421. Erlandson RA, Woodruff JM: Peripheral nerve sheath tumors: An electron microscopic study of 43 cases. *Cancer* 1982;49:273–287.
422. New GB, Erich JB: Benign tumors of the larynx: A study of seven hundred and twenty two cases. *Arch Otolaryngol* 1938;28:841–910.
423. Hollinger PH, Johnston KC: Benign tumors of the larynx. *Ann Otol Rhinol Laryngol* 1951;60:496–509.
424. Stanley RJ, Scheithauer BW, Weiland LH, et al: Neural and neuroendocrine tumors of the larynx. *Ann Otol Rhinol Laryngol* 1987;96:630–638.
425. Martin DS, Smith J, Awwad EE, et al: MR in neurofibromatosis of the larynx. *Am J Neuroradiol* 1995;16:503–506.
426. Czinger J, Fekete-Szabo G: Neurofibroma of the supraglottic larynx in childhood. *J Laryngol Otol* 1994;108:156–158.
427. Willcox TO Jr, Rosenberg SI, Handler SD: Laryngeal involvement in neurofibromatosis. *Ear Nose Throat J* 1993;72:811–815.
428. Maceri DR, Saxon KG: Neurofibromatosis of the head and neck. *Head Neck Surg* 1984;6:842–850.
429. Supance JS, Quenelle DJ, Crissman J: Endolaryngeal neurofibromas. *Otolaryngol Head Neck Surg* 1980;88:74–78.
430. Fukuda I, Ogasawara H, Kumoi T, et al: Subglottic neurofibroma in a child. *Int J Pediatr Otorhinolaryngol* 1987;14:161–170.
431. Pearlman SJ, Friedman EA, Appel M: Neurofibroma of the larynx. *Arch Otolaryngol* 1950;52:8–14.
432. Mevio E, Galioto P, Scelsi M, et al: Neurofibroma of vocal cord: Case report. *Acta Otorhinolaryngol Belg* 1990;44:447–450.
433. Hisa Y, Tatemoto K, DeJima K, et al: Laser vestibulectomy for endolaryngeal neurofibroma. *Otolaryngol Head Neck Surg* 1995;113:459–461.
434. Sidman J, Wood RE, Poole M, et al: Management of plexiform neurofibroma of the larynx. *Ann Otol Rhinol Laryngol* 1987;96:53–55.
435. Smith BC, Wenig BM: Neurogenic neoplasms including melanoma. In: Ferlito A, ed. *Surgical Pathology of Laryngeal Neoplasms.* New York: Chapman & Hall, 1996.
436. Thomas RL: Nonepithelial tumors of the larynx. *J Laryngol Otol* 1979;93:1131–1141.
437. Jamal MN: Schwannoma of the larynx: case report and review of the literature. *J Laryngol Otol* 1994;108:788–790.
438. Dekker PJ, Haidar A: Neurilemmoma of the larynx. *Br J Clin Prac* 1994;48:159–160.
439. Newman D, Youngs R: Neurilemmoma of the larynx. *J Otolaryngol* 1992;21:72–73.
440. Takumida M, Taira T, Suzuki M, et al: Neurilemmoma of the larynx (a case report). *J Laryngol Otol* 1986;100:847–850.
441. DeLozier HL: Intrinsic malignant schwannoma of the larynx. A case report. *Ann Otol Rhinol Laryngol* 1982;91:336–338.
442. Greager JA, Reichard KW, Campana JP, et al: Malignant schwannoma of the head and neck. *Am J Surg* 1992;163:440–442.
443. Hujala K, Martikainen P, Minn H, et al: Malignant nerve sheath tumors of the head and neck. *Eur Arch Oto Rhino Laryngol* 1993;250:379–382.

Cartilaginous Tumors

444. Neel HB, Unni KK: Cartilaginous tumors of the larynx: A series of 33 patients. *Otolaryngol Head and Neck Surg* 1982;90:201–207.
445. Ferlito A, Nicholai P, Montaguti A, et al: Chondrosarcoma of the larynx: Review of the literature and report of 3 cases. *Am J Otolaryngol* 1984;5:350–359.
446. Moore I: Cartilaginous tumors of the larynx: A study of all recorded cases. *J Laryngol Otol* 1925;40:145–164.
447. Cocke EW: Benign cartilaginous tumors of the larynx. *Laryngoscope* 1962;72:727–730.
448. Wilkenson AH, Beckford NS, Babin RW, et al: Extraskeletal myxoid chondrosarcoma: Case report and review of the literature. *Otolaryngol Head Neck Surg* 1991;104:257–260.
449. Jacobs RD, Stayboldt C, Harris JP: Chondrosarcoma of the epiglottis with regional and distant metastasis. *Laryngoscope* 1989;99:861–864.
450. Kasanew M, John DG, Newman P, et al: Chondrosarcoma of the epiglottis. *J Laryngol Otol* 1988;102:374–377.
451. Rao ABN: A case of chondroma of the epiglottis. *J Laryngol* 1964;78:315–319.
452. Moran CA, Suster S, Carter D: Laryngeal chondrosarcoma. *Arch Pathol Lab Med* 1993;117:914–917.
453. Finn DG, Goepfert H, Batsakis JG: Chondrosarcoma of the head and neck. *Laryngoscope* 1984;94:1539–1544.
454. Della Palma PD, Piazza P: Peripheral chondrosarcoma of the hyoid bone. Report of a case. *Appl Pathol* 1983;1:333–338.
455. Greer JA, Devine KD, Dahlin DC: Gardiner's syndrome and chondrosarcoma of the hyoid bone. *Arch Otolaryngol* 1977;103:425–427.
456. Keen JA, Wainwright J: Ossification of the thyroid cricoid and arytenoid cartilages. *S Afr J Lab Clin Med* 1958;4:83–108.
457. Hately W, Evison G, Samuel E: The pattern of ossification in the laryngeal cartilages: A radiological study. *Br J Radiol* 1965;38:585–591.
458. Batsakis JG, Raymond AK: Cartilage tumors of the larynx. *So Med J* 1988;81:481–484.
459. Hellquist H, Olofsson J, Grontoft O: Chondrosarcoma of the larynx. *J Laryngol Otol* 1979;93:1037–1047.

460. Devaney KO, Ferlito A, Silver CE: Cartilaginous tumors of the larynx. *Ann Otol Rhinol Laryngol* 1995;104:251–255.
461. Huizenga C, Balogh K: Cartilaginous tumors of the larynx. A clinicopathologic study of 10 new cases and a review of the literature. *Cancer* 1970;26:201–210.
462. Harrison DFN, Denny S: Ossification within the primate larynx. *Acta Otolaryngol* 1983;95:440–446.
463. Glaubiger DL, Casler JD, Garrett WL, et al: Chondrosarcoma of the larynx after radiation treatment for vocal cord cancer. *Cancer* 1991;68:1828–1831.
464. Ghalib SH, Warner ED, DeGowin EL: Laryngeal chondrosarcoma after thyroid irradiation. *JAMA* 1969;210:1762–1763.
465. Johnson S, Tetu B, Ayala AG, Chawla SP: Chondrosarcoma with additional mesenchymal component (dedifferentiated chondrosarcoma) I. A clinicopathologic study of 26 cases. *Cancer* 1986;58:278–286.
466. Dahlin DC, Beabout JW: Dedifferentiation of low-grade chondrosarcomas. *Cancer* 1971;28:461–466.
467. Brandwein M, Moore S, Som P, Biller H: Laryngeal chondrosarcomas: A clinicopathologic study of 11 cases including two chondrosarcomas with additional malignant mesenchymal component. *Laryngoscope* 1992;8:858–867.
468. Nicholai P, Sasaki CT, Ferlito A, Kirshner JA: Laryngeal chondrosarcoma: Incidence, pathology, biological behavior and treatment. *Ann Otol Rhinol Laryngol* 1990;99:515–523.
469. Bleiweiss IJ, Kaneko M: Chondrosarcoma of the larynx with additional malignant mesenchymal component (dedifferentiated chondrosarcoma). *Am J Surg Pathol* 1988;12:314–320.
470. Nakayama M, Brandenberg JH, Hafez GR: Dedifferentiated chondrosarcoma of the larynx with regional and distant metastases. *Ann Otol Rhinol Laryngol* 1993;102:785–791.

Osteogenic Tumors

471. Pinsolle J, Demeaux H, Laur P, et al: Osteosarcoma of the soft tissue of the larynx: Report of a case with electron microscopic studies. *Otolaryngol Head Neck Surg* 1990;102:276–280.
472. Sheen TS, Wu CT, Hsieh T, Hsu MM: Postirradiation laryngeal osteosarcoma. Case report and literature review. *Head Neck* 1997;19:57–62.
473. Sprinkle PM, Allen MS, Brookshire PFL: Osteosarcoma of the larynx. A true primary sarcoma of the larynx. *Laryngoscope* 1966;76:325–333.
474. Suchatlampong V, Sriumpai S, Khawcharoenporn V: Osteosarcoma of the larynx. The first case report in Thailand with ultrastructural study. *J Med Assoc Thailand* 1981;64:307–310.
475. Remagen W, Lohr J, Westernhagen BV: Osteosarkom des Kehlkopfes. *HNO* 1983;31:366–368.
476. Berge JK, Kapadia SB, Myers EN: Osteosarcoma of the larynx. *Arch Otolaryngol* 1998;124:207–210.
477. Haar JG, Chaudhry AP, Karanjia MD, Milley PS: Chondroblastic osteosarcoma of the larynx. *Arch Otolaryngol* 1978;104:477–481.
478. van Laer CG, Helliwell TR, Atkinson MW, Stell PM: Osteosarcoma of the larynx. *Ann Otol Rhinol Laryngol* 1989;98:971–974.
479. Shimizu KT, Selch MT, Fu YS, et al: Osteosarcoma metastatic to the larynx. *Ann Otol Rhinol Laryngol* 1994;103:160–163.
480. Lichtenstein L: Aneurysmal bone cyst. *J Bone Joint Surg* 1957;39:873–882.
481. Huvos A: Simple bone cyst and aneurysmal bone cyst. In: *Bone Tumors: Diagnosis, Treatment and Prognosis,* 2nd ed. Philadelphia: WB Saunders, 1991:728.
482. Schilling HE, Neal D, Nathan M, Aufdemorte TB: Aneurysmal bone cyst of the larynx. *Am J Otolaryngol* 1986;7:370–374.
483. Sercarz JA, Robert M, Alessi D, et al: Aneurysmal bone cyst of the cricoid cartilage: An unusual cause of infraglottic stenosis. *Head Neck* 1991;13:457–460.
484. Shadaba A, Zaidi S: Aneurysmal bone cyst of the hyoid. *J Laryngol Otol* 1992;106:71–72.

Giant Cell Tumors

485. Hyams VJ, Batsakis JG, Michaels L: Tumors of the upper respiratory tract and ear. *Atlas of Tumor Pathology,* 2nd ed, fascicle 25. Washington, DC: Armed Forces Institute of Pathology, 1982.
486. Kleinsasser O: *Tumors of the Larynx and Hypopharynx: Tumors of the Laryngeal Skeleton.* New York: George Thieme Verlag, 1988:335.
487. Coyas AO, Anastassiades OT, Kyriakos I: Malignant giant cell tumor of the larynx. *J Laryngol* 1974;88:799–803.
488. Kotarba E, Niezabitoski A: Giant cell tumor of laryngeal soft tissue. *Otolaryngol Pol* 1974;28:331–335.

Skeletal Muscle Tumors

489. Kapadia SB, Meis JM, Frisman DM, et al: Adult rhabdomyoma of the head and neck. Clinicopathologic and immunophenotypic study. *Hum Pathol* 1993;24:608–617.
490. Willis J, Abdul-Karim FW, di Sant'Agnese PA: Extracardiac rhabdomyomas. *Semin Diagn Pathol* 1994;11:15–25.
491. Di Sant'Agnese PA, Knowles DM: Extracardiac rhabdomyoma: A clinicopathologic study and review of the literature. *Cancer* 1980;46:780–789.
492. Eusebi V, Ceccarelli C, Daniele E, et al: Extracardiac rhabdomyoma: An immunocytochemical study and review of the literature. *Appl Pathol* 1988;6:197–207.
493. Gibas Z, Miettinen M: Recurrent parapharyngeal rhabdomyoma. Evidence of neoplastic nature of the tumor from cytogenetic study. *Am J Surg Pathol* 1992;16:721–728.
494. Cleveland DB, Chen S-Y, Allen CM, et al: Adult rhabdomyoma. A light microscopic, ultrastructural virologic, and immunologic analysis. *Oral Surg Oral Med Oral Pathol* 1994;77:147–153.
495. Battifora HA, Eisenstein R, Schild JA: Rhabdomyoma of larynx. Ultrastructural study and comparison with granular cell tumors (myoblastomas). *Cancer* 1969;23:183–190.
496. Helliwell TR, Sisson MCJ, Stoney PJ, et al: Immunohistochemistry and electron microscopy of head and neck rhabdomyoma. *J Clin Pathol* 1988;41:1058–1063.
497. Rosenman D, Gertner R, Fradis M, et al: Rhabdomyoma of the larynx. *J Laryngol Otol* 1986;100:607–610.
498. Regezi JA, Zarbo RJ, Courtney RM, Crissman JD: Immunoreactivity of granular cell lesions of skin, mucosa and jaw. *Cancer* 1989;64:1455–1460.
499. Brandwein M, Huvos AG: Oncocytic tumors of major salivary glands. A study of 68 cases with follow-up on 44 patients. *Am J Surg Pathol* 1991;15:514–528.
500. Dehner LP, Enzinger FM, Font RL: Fetal rhabdomyoma: An analysis of nine cases. *Cancer* 1972;30:160–166.
501. Kapadia SB, Meis JM, Frisman D, et al: Fetal rhabdomyoma of the head and neck. Clinicopathologic and immunophenotypic study. *Hum Pathol* 1993;24:754–765.
502. Crotty PL, Nakhleh RE, Dehner LP: Juvenile rhabdomyoma. An intermediate form of skeletal muscle tumor in children. *Arch Pathol Lab Med* 1993;117:43–47.
503. Konrad EA, Meister P, Huber G: Extracardiac rhabdomyoma. Report of different types with light microscopic and ultrastructural studies. *Cancer* 1982;49:898–907.
504. Maurer HM, Beltangady M, Gehan EA, et al: The Intergroup Rhabdomyosarcoma Study-I: a final report. *Cancer* 1988;61:209–220.
505. Maurer HM, Gehan EA, Beltangady M, et al: The Intergroup Rhabdomyosarcoma Study-II. *Cancer* 1993;71:1904–1922.
506. Tsokos M: The diagnosis and classification of childhood rhabdomyosarcoma. *Semin Diag Pathol* 1994;11:26–38.
507. Wharam MD Jr, Foulkes MA, Lawrence W Jr, et al: Soft tissue sarcoma of the head and neck in childhood: Nonorbital and nonparameningeal sites. A report of the Intergroup Rhabdomyosarcoma Study (IRS-1). *Cancer* 1984;53:1016–1019.
508. Wharam MD, Beltangady MS, Heyn RM, et al: Pediatric orofacial and laryngopharyngeal rhabdomyosarcoma. An Intergroup Rhabdomyosarcoma Study Report. *Arch Otolaryngol Head Neck Surg* 1987;113:1225–1227.
509. Balazs M, Egerszegi P: Laryngeal botryoid rhabdomyosarcoma in an adult. Report of a case with electron microscopic study. *Pathol Res Pract* 1989;184:643–649.
510. Batsakis JG, Fox JE: Rhabdomyosarcoma of the larynx. *Arch Otolaryngol* 1970;91:136–140.
511. Dodd OJM, Wieneke KF, Rosman P: Laryngeal rhabdomyosarcoma. Case report and literature review. *Cancer* 1987;59:1012–1018.
512. Fernandes P, Tandon DA, Tickoo SK, Rath GK: Embryonal rhabdomyosarcoma of the larynx in a child: Report of a case and review of literature. *Indian J Cancer* 1988;25:89–93.
513. Gross M, Gutjahr P: Therapy of rhabdomyosarcoma of the larynx. *Int J Pediatr Otorhinolaryngol* 1988;15:93–97.
514. Parham DM, Webber B, Holt H, et al: Immunohistochemical study of childhood rhabdomyosarcoma and related neoplasms. Results of an In-

tergroup Rhabdomyosarcoma Study Project. *Cancer* 1991;67:3072–3080.

Smooth Muscle Tumors

515. Farman AG: Benign smooth muscle tumors. *S Afr Med J* 1975;49:1333–1340.
516. Lindholm CE, Hellquist HB, Hellquist H, Vejlens L: Epithelioid leiomyoma of the larynx. *Histopathology* 1994;24:155–159.
517. Mori H, Kumoi T, Hashimoto M, et al: Leiomyoblastoma of the larynx: Report of a case. *Head Neck* 1992;14:148–152.
518. Mochizuki T, Kamata T, Ogawa Y, et al: A case of vascular leiomyoma in the larynx. *Nippon Jibiinkoka Gakkai Kaiho* 1995;98:1119–1124.
519. Fujii M, Hirakawa K, Harada Y, et al: A case of vascular leiomyoma of the larynx. *J Laryngol Otol* 1994;108:593–595.
520. Bulun E, Cenik Z, Uyar Y, et al: An unusual laryngeal hamartoma: Ipofibroleiomyoma. *J Otolaryngol* 1993;22:136–137.
521. Watters GW, McKiernan DC: Smooth muscle tumours of the larynx. *J Laryngol Otol* 1995;109:77–79.
522. Uematsu K, Mori H, Kumoi T, Hashimoto M: Leiomyoblastoma of the larynx: Report of a case. *Head Neck* 1992;14:148–152.
523. Shibata K, Komune S: Laryngeal angiomyoma (vascular leiomyoma) clinicopathologic findings. *Laryngoscope* 1980;90:1880–1886.
524. Nuutinen J, Syrjanen K: Angioleiomyoma of the larynx. Report of a case and review of the literature. *Laryngoscope* 1983;93:941–943.
525. Hachisuga T, Hashimoto H, Enjoji M: Angioleiomyoma. A clinicopathologic reappraisal of 564 cases. *Cancer* 1984;54:126–130.
526. Kapadia SB, Barnes L: Muscle tissue neoplasms. In: Ferlito A, ed. *Surgical Pathology of the Larynx.* New York: Chapman & Hall Medical, 1996:321–340.
527. Kaya S, Saydam L, Ruacan S: Laryngeal leiomyoma. *Int J Ped Otorhinolaryngol* 1990;19:285–288.
528. Barnes L: Tumors and tumor-like lesions of the soft tissues, In: Barnes L, ed. *Surgical Pathology of the Head and Neck.* New York: Marcel Dekker, 1985.
529. Ratcliffe NA, Rowe-Jones JM, Solomons NB: Leiomyosarcoma of the larynx. *J Laryngol Otol* 1994;108:359–362.
530. Boudard P, Carles D, Devars F, et al: Leiomyosarcoma of the larynx: presentation of a case. *Rev Laryngol Otol Rhinol Bord* 1992;113:115–117.
531. Bertheau P, Deboise A, De Roquancourt A, et al: Leiomyosarcoma du larynx. Etude histologique immunohistochemique et ultrastructurale d'une observation avec revue de la litterature. *Ann Pathol* 1991;11:122–127.
532. Tewary AK, Pahor AL: Leiomyosarcoma of the larynx: Emergency laryngectomy. *J Laryngol Otol* 1991;105:134–136.
533. Kleinsasser O, Glanz H: Myogenic tumors of the larynx. *Arch Otolaryngol* 1979;225:107–119.
534. Gryczynski M: Laryngeal leiomyosarcoma. *Otolaryngol Pol* 1971;25:545–548.
535. Mientinen M: Immunoreactivity for cytokeratin and epithelial membrane antigen in leiomyosarcoma. *Arch Pathol Lab Med* 1988;112:637–640.

Vascular Neoplasia

536. Campbell JS, Wigglesworth FW, Latarrocca R, Wilde H: Congenital infraglottic hemangiomas of the larynx and trachea in infants. *Pediatrics* 1958;22:727–737.
537. Seikaly H, Cuyler JP: Infantile infraglottic hemangioma. *J Otolaryngol* 1994;23:135–136.
538. Cameron AH, Cant WHP, MacGregor ME, Prior AP: Angioma of the larynx in laryngeal stridor of infancy. *J Laryngol* 1960;74:846–857.
539. Doermann P, Lunseth J, Segnitz RH: Obstructing infraglottic hemangioma of the larynx in infancy. *N Engl J Med* 1958;258:68–71.
540. Abdul-Wahab BRJ, Olusegun OA: Haemangioma of the vallecula causing acute upper airway obstruction in a 6 1/2 week old Nigerian infant with strawberry naevus. *Trop Geograph Med* 1993;45:33–35.
541. Feurstein SS: Subglottic hemangioma in infants. *Laryngoscope* 1973;83:466–475.
542. Devaney KO: Vascular neoplasms. In: Ferlito A, ed. *Surgical Pathology of Laryngeal Neoplasms.* New York: Chapman & Hall, 1996:341–374.
543. Brandwein M, Abramson A, Shikowitz M: Supraglottic hemangioma during pregnancy. *Obstet Gynecol* 1987;69:450–453.
544. Myer CM, Bratcher GO: Laryngeal cystic hygroma. *Head Neck Surg* 1983;6:706–709.
545. Kleinsasser O: Tumors of the vascular system. In: *Tumors of the Larynx and Hypopharynx.* Stuttgart: George Thieme Verlag, 1988.
546. El-Serafy S: Rare benign tumors of the larynx. *J Laryngol Otol* 1971;85:837–851.
547. Claros P, Viscasillas S, Claros A, Claros A: Lymphangioma of the larynx as a cause of progressive dyspnea. *Int J Ped Otorhinolaryngol* 1985;9:263–268.
548. Jaffe BF: Unusual laryngeal problems in children. *Ann Otol* 1973;82:637–642.
549. Ruben RJ, Kucinski SA, Greenstein N: Cystic lymphangioma of the vallecula. *Can J Otolaryngol* 1975;4:180–184.
550. McRae RDR, Gatland DJ, Jones FRM, Khan S: Malignant transformation in a laryngeal hemangioma. *Ann Otol Rhinol Laryngol* 1990;99:562–565.
551. Banerjee SS, Eyden BP, Well S, et al: Pseudoangiosarcomatous carcinoma: A clinicopathological study of seven cases. *Histopathol* 1992;21:13–23.
552. Gray MH, Rosenberg AE, Dickersin GR, Bhan AK: Cytokeratin expression in epithelioid vascular neoplasm. *Hum Pathol* 1990;21:212–217.
553. Gnepp DR, Chandler W, Hyams V: Primary Kaposi's sarcoma of the head and neck. *Ann Intern Med* 1984;100:107–114.
554. Gridell C, Palmieri G, Airoma G, et al: Complete regression of laryngeal involvement by classic Kaposi's sarcoma with low dose alpha 2b interferon. *Tumori* 1990;76:292–293.
555. Pratt J, Loring W, Goodof II: Hemangioendotheliosarcoma of the larynx. *Arch Otolaryngol* 1968;87:484–489.
556. Sciott R, Delaere P, Van Damme B, Desmet V: Angiosarcoma of the larynx. *Histopathol* 1995;26:177–180.
557. Ferlito A, Nicolai P, Caruso G: Angiosarcoma of the larynx. Case report. *Ann Òtol Rhinol Laryngol* 1985;94:93–95.
558. Greenberg JE, Fischl MA, Berger JR: Upper airway obstruction secondary to AIDS-related Kaposi's sarcoma. *Chest* 1985;88:638–640.
559. Levy FE, Tansek KM: AIDS-associated Kaposi's sarcoma of the larynx. *Ear Nose Throat J* 1990;69:177–183.
560. Fliss DM, Parikh J, Freeman JL: AIDS-related Kaposi's sarcoma of the sphenoid sinus. *J Otolaryngol* 1992;21:235–237.
561. Ioachim HL, Adsay V, Giancotti FR, et al: Kaposi's sarcoma of internal organs. *Cancer* 1995;75:1376–1385.
562. Green TL, Beckstead JH, Lozada-Nur F, et al: Histopathologic spectrum of oral Kaposi's sarcoma. *Oral Surg* 1984;58:306–314.
563. Coyas A, Eliadellis E, Anastassiades O: Kaposi's sarcoma of the larynx. *J Larygol Otol* 1983;97:647–649.
564. Zimmerman KW: Der feinere Bau der Blutcapillaren. *Z Anat Entwicklungsgesch* 1923;68:29–109.
565. Stout AP, Murray MR: Hemangiopericytoma: Vascular tumor featuring Zimmermann's pericytes. *Ann Surg* 1942;116:26–33.
566. Enzinger FM, Smith BH: Hemangiopericytoma: An analysis of 106 cases. *Hum Pathol* 1976;7:61–82.
567. Kimmelman CP: Hemangiopericytoma of the sphenoid sinus. *Otolaryngol Head Neck Surg* 1981;89:713–716.
568. Whittam DE, Hellier W: Haemangiopericytoma of the parotid salivary gland: Report of a case with literature review. *J Laryngol Otol* 1993;10:1159–1162.
569. Carrillo R, Rodriquez-Peralto JL, Batsakis JG, El-Naggar AK: View from beneath—Pathology in focus. Primary haemangiopericytomas of the parotid gland. *J Laryngol Otol* 1992;106:659–661.
570. Chin LS, Rabb CH, Hinton DR, et al: Hemangiopericytoma of the temporal bone presenting as a retroauricular mass. *Neurosurg* 1993;33:728–732.
571. Croxatto JO, Font RL: Hemangiopericytoma of the orbit: A clinicopathologic study of 30 cases. *Hum Pathol* 1982;13:210–218.
572. Philippou S, Gellrich NC: Hemangiopericytoma of the head and neck region. A clinical and morphological study of three cases. *Int J Oral Maxillofac Surg* 1992;21:99–103.
573. Pesavento G, Ferlito A: Haemangiopericytoma of the larynx. *J Laryngol Otol* 1982;96:1065–1073.
574. Walike JW, Bailey BJ: Head and neck hemangiopericytoma. *Arch Otolaryngol* 1971;93:345–353.
575. Schwartz MR, Donovan DT: Hemangiopericytoma of the larynx: A case report and review of the literature. *Head Neck Surg* 1987;96:369–372.
576. Dictor M, Elner A, Andersson T, Ferno M: Myofibromatosis-like hemangiopericytoma metastasizing as a differentiated vascular smooth muscle and myosarcoma. *Am J Surg Pathol* 1992;16:1239–1247.

577. Nemes Z, Thomazy V, Adany R, Muszbek L: Identification of histiocytic reticulum cells by immunohistochemical demonstration of Factor XIII (F-XIIIa) in human lymph nodes. *J Pathol* 1986;149:121–132.

578. Nemes Z: Differentiation markers in hemangiopericytoma. *Cancer* 1992;69:133–140.

579. Catalano PJ, Brandwein MS, Shah DK, et al: Sinonasal hemangiopericytomas: A clinicopathological and immunohistochemical study of seven cases. *Head Neck Surg* 1996;18:42–53.

580. Ferlito A: Primary malignant haemangiopericytoma of the larynx (A case report with autopsy). *J Laryngol Otol* 1978;92:511–519.

Adipose Tumors

581. Batsakis JG, Fox JE: Supporting tissue neoplasms of the larynx. *Surg Gynecol Obstet* 1970;131:989–997.

582. Zakrzewski A: Subglottic lipoma of the larynx. Case report and literature review. *J Laryngol Otol* 1965;79:1039–1048.

583. Birkett HS: Lipoma of the larynx: Intrinsic in origin. *J Laryngol Otol* 1934;49:733–740.

584. Grant JH: Lipoma of the larynx. *J Laryngol* 1961;75:765–767.

585. Kennedy KS, Wotoxic PJ, St John JN: Parapharyngeal fibrolipoma. *Head Neck* 1990;12:84–87.

586. Eagle WW: Lipoma of the epiglottis and lipoma of the hypopharynx in the same patient. *Ann Otol Rhinol* 1965;74:851–862.

587. Franceschini SS, Segnini G, Berrettini S, et al: Hibernoma of the larynx. Review of the literature and a new case. *Acta OtoRhinoLaryngolog Belg* 1993;47:51–53.

588. Moretti JA, Miller D: Laryngeal involvement in benign symmetric lipomatosis. *Arch Otolaryngol* 1973;97:495–496.

589. Som ML, Wolff L: Lipoma of the hypopharynx producing menacing symptoms. *Arch Otolaryngol* 1952;56:524–531.

590. Månsson LJ, Wilske LG, Kindblom LG: Lipoma of the hypopharynx. *J Laryngol* 1978;92:1037–1043.

591. Holt H: Fatty pendulous tumor of the pharynx and larynx. *Trans Path Soc* 1854;5:123–125.

592. Nonaka S, Enomoto K, Kawabori S, et al: Spindle cell lipoma within the larynx: A case report with correlated light and electron microscopy. *ORL Otorhinolaryngol Relat Spec* 1993;55:147–149.

593. Chen KTK, Weinberg RA: Intramuscular lipoma of the larynx. *Am J Otolaryngol* 1984;5:71–72.

594. Gaffney EF, Hargreaves HK, Semple E, Vellios F: Hibernoma: Distinctive light and electron microscopic features and relationship to brown adipose tissue. *Hum Pathol* 1983;14:677–687.

595. Dinsdale RC, Manning SC, Brooks DJ, Vuitch F: Myxoid laryngeal lipoma in a juvenile. *Otolaryngol Head Neck Surg* 1990;103:653–657.

596. Reid AP, Hussain SSM, Pahor AL: Lipoma of the larynx. *J Laryngol Otol* 1987;101:1308–1311.

597. Kapur TR: Recurrent lipomata of the larynx and the pharynx with late malignant change. *J Laryngol Otol* 1968;82:761–768.

598. Golledge J, Fisher C, Rhys-Evans PH: Head and neck liposarcoma. *Cancer* 1995;76:1051–1058.

599. Jesberg N: Fibrolipoma of the piriform sinuses: Thirty–seven year follow-up. *Laryngoscope* 1982;92:1157–1159.

600. Wenig BM, Weiss SW, Gnepp DR: Laryngeal and hypopharyngeal liposarcoma. A clinicopathologic study of 10 cases with a comparison to soft-tissue counterparts. *Am J Surg Pathol* 1990;14:134–141.

601. Shah MC, Lowry LD: Primary liposarcoma of the larynx. *Trans Pa Acad Ophthalmol Otolaryngol* 1984;37:49–52.

602. Velek VP: Liposarcoma of the larynx. *Trans Am Acad Ophthalmol Otolaryngol* 1976;87:569–570.

603. Miller D, Goodman M, Weber A, Goldstein A: Primary liposarcoma of the larynx. *Trans Am Acad Ophthalmol Otolaryngol* 1975;80:444–447.

604. Krausen AS, Gall AM, Garza R, et al: Liposarcoma of the larynx: A multicentric or metastatic malignancy. *Laryngoscope* 1977;87:1116–1124.

605. Meis JM, Mackay B, Goepfert H: Liposarcoma of the larynx. Case report and literature review. *Arch Otolaryngol* 1986;112:1289–1292.

606. Evans HL: Liposarcoma and atypical lipomatous tumors: A study of 66 cases followed for a minimum of 10 years. *Am J Surg Pathol* 1988;1:41–54.

607. Evans HL: Liposarcoma: a study of 55 cases with a reassessment of its classification. *Am J Surg Pathol* 1979;3:507–523.

608. Coindre JM, de Loynes B, Bui NB, et al: Dedifferentiated liposarcoma: A clinicopathologic study of 6 cases. *Ann Pathol* 1992;12:20–28.

609. Reibel JF, Green WM: Liposarcoma arising in the pharynx nine years after fibrolipoma excision. *Otolaryngol Head Neck Surg* 1995;112:599–602.

610. Allsbrook WC, Harmon JD, Chongchitnant N, Erwin S: Liposarcoma of the larynx. *Arch Pathol Lab Med* 1985;109:294–296.

611. Ferlito A: Primary pleomorphic liposarcoma of the larynx. *J Otolaryngol* 1978;7:161–162.

612. Narula A, Jefferis AF: Squamous cell carcinoma and liposarcoma of the larynx occurring metachronously. *J Laryngol Otol* 1985;99:509–511.

Synovial Sarcoma

613. Pack GT, Ariel IM: Synovial sarcoma (malignant synovioma). A report of 60 cases. *Surgery* 1950;28:1047–1084.

614. Fischer C: Miscellaneous neoplasms. In: Felito A, ed. *Surgical Pathology of the Larynx*. New York: Chapman & Hall Medical, 1996.

615. Miller LH, Latimer LS, Miller T: Synovial sarcoma of the larynx. *Trans Am Acad Ophthal Otol* 1975;80:448–451.

616. Jernstrom P: Synovial sarcoma of the pharynx. Report of a case. *Am J Clin Pathol* 1954;24:957–961.

617. Roth JA, Enzinger FM, Tannenbaum M: Synovial sarcoma of the neck: A follow-up study of 24 cases. *Cancer* 1975;35:1243–1253.

618. Mitcherling JJ, Collins EM, Tomich CE, et al: Synovial sarcoma of the neck: Report of case. *J Oral Surg* 1976;34:64–69.

619. Moore DM, Berke GS: Synovial sarcoma of the head and neck. *Arch Otolaryngol Head Neck Surg* 1987;113:311–313.

620. Shmookler BM, Enzinger FM, Brannon RB: Orofacial synovial sarcoma. A clinicopathologic study of 11 new cases and review of the literature. *Cancer* 1982;50:269–276.

621. Miscler NE, Chuprevich T, Tormey DC, et al: Synovial sarcoma of the neck associated with previous head and neck radiation therapy. *Arch Otolaryngol* 1978;104:482–483.

622. Barnes L, Kanbour A: Malignant fibrous histiocytoma of the head and neck. A report of 12 cases. *Arch Otolaryngol Head Neck Surg* 1988;114:1149–1156.

623. Ferlito A, Nikolai P, Recher G, et al: Primary laryngeal malignant fibrous histiocytoma: Review of the literature and report of seven cases. *Laryngoscope* 1983;93:1351–1358.

624. Ferlito A, Recher G, Polidoro F, Rossi M: Malignant pleomorphic fibrous histiocytoma of the larynx. *J Laryngol Otol* 1979;93:1021–1029.

625. Johnson JT, Poushter DL: Fibrous histiocytoma of the infraglottic larynx. *Ann Otol* 1977;86:243–246.

626. Canalis RF, Green M, Konard HR, et al: Malignant fibrous xanthoma (xanthofibrosarcoma) of the larynx. *Arch Otolaryngol* 1975;101:135–137.

627. Ferlito A: Histiocytic tumors of the larynx. A clinicopathological study with review of the literature. *Cancer* 1978;42:611–622.

628. Ribári O, Elemér G, Bálint A: Laryngeal giant cell tumor. *J Laryngol Otol* 1975;89:857–861.

629. Hall-Jones J: Giant cell tumour of the larynx. *J Laryngol Otol* 1972;86:371–381.

630. Weiss SW, Bratthauer GL, Morris PA: Postirradiation malignant fibrous histiocytoma expressing cytokeratin. Implications for the immunodiagnosis of sarcomas. *Am J Surg Pathol* 1988;12:554–558.

631. Alguacil-Garcia A, Alonso A, Pettigrew NM: Sarcomatoid carcinoma (so-called pseudosarcoma) of the larynx simulating malignant giant cell tumor of soft parts. A case report. *Am J Clin Pathol* 1984;82:340–343.

632. Rolander T, Kim OJ Shumrick DA: Fibrous xanthoma of the larynx. *Arch Otolaryngol* 1972;96:168–170.

Spindle Cell Carcinoma

633. Slootweg PJ, Roholl PJM, Muller H, Lubsen H: Spindle-cell carcinoma of the oral cavity and larynx. Immunohistochemical aspects. *J Craniomaxillofac Surg* 1989;17:234–236.

634. Nakleh RE, Zarbo RJ, Ewing S, et al: Myogenic differentiation in spindle cell (Sarcomatoid) carcinomas of the upper aerodigestive tract. *Appl Immunohistochemistry* 1993;1:58–68.

635. Hyams VJ: Spindle cell carcinoma of the larynx. *Can J Otolaryngol* 1975;4:307–313

636. Hellquist H, Olofsson J: Spindle cell carcinoma of the larynx. *APMIS* 1989;97:1103–1113.

637. Zarbo RJ, Crissman JD, Venkat H, Weiss MA: Spindle cell carcinoma of the upper aerodigestive tract mucosa. An immunohistologic and ultrastructural study of 18 biphasic tumors and comparison with seven monophasic spindle cell tumors. *Am J Surg Pathol* 1986;10:741–753.

638. Olsen KD, Lewis JE, Suman VJ: Spindle cell carcinoma of the larynx and hypopharynx. *Otolaryngol Head Neck Surg* 1997;116:47–52.

Teratomas

639. Gonzalez-Crussi F: Extragonadal teratomas, vol. 18. *Atlas of Tumor Pathology*, 2nd ed. Washington DC: Armed Forces Institute of Pathology, 1982.

640. Chumakov FI, Voinova VG: Unusual case of teratoma of the larynx. *Vestn Otorinolarungol* 1973;73:92–94.

641. Johnson LF, Strong MS: Teratoma of the larynx. *Arch Otolaryngol* 1953;58:435–441.

642. Fleischer K: Drei seltene Kehlkopftumoren. Speicheldrusenmischtumo Granuloblastom. *Laryngorhino-otologie* 1956;35:346–354.

643. Cannon CR, Johns ME, Rechner RE: Immature teratoma of the larynx. *Otolaryngol Head Neck Surg* 1987;96:366–368.

Blastoma

644. Eble JN, Hull MT, Bojrab D: Laryngeal blastoma. A light and electron microscopic study of a novel entity analogous to pulmonary blastoma. *Am J Clin Pathol* 1985;84:378–385.

Hamartoma

645. Holinger LD, Tansek KM, Tucker GF: Cleft larynx with airway obstruction. *Ann Otol Rhinol Laryngol* 1985;94:622–626.

646. Cohen SR: Posterior cleft larynx associated with hamartoma. *Ann Otol Rhinol Laryngol* 1984;93:443–446.

647. Lyons TJ, Variend S: Posterior cleft larynx associated with hamartoma. A case report and literature review. *J Laryngol Otol* 1988;102:471–472.

648. Weinberger J, Kassim O, Birt BD: Hamartoma of the larynx. *J Otolaryngol* 1985;14:305–308.

649. Patterson HC, Dickerson GR, Pilch BZ, Bentkover SH: Hamartoma of the hypopharynx. *Arch Otolaryngol* 1981;107:767–772.

650. Binns PM: Mesenchymoma of larynx and neck. *Otolaryngol Head Neck Surg* 1979;87:590–593.

651. Fine ED, Dahms B, Arnold JE, Laryngeal hamartoma: A rare congenital abnormality. *Ann Otol Rhinol Laryngol* 1995;104:87–89.

652. Archer SM, Crockett DM, McGill TJI: Hamartoma of the larynx: Report of two cases and review of the literature. *Int J Ped Otorhinolaryngol* 1988;16:237–243.

Thyroid Ectopia, Secondary Tumors

653. White SA, Goddard MJ: Metastatic Hürthle cell tumor causing central airway obstruction. *J Laryngol Otol* 1993;107:957–959.

654. Ogden CW, Goldstraw P: Intratracheal thyroid tissue presenting as stridor. *Eur J Cardiothorac Surg* 1991;5:108–109.

655. Rotenberg D, Lawson VG, van Nostrand P:Thyroid carcinoma presenting as a tracheal tumor. *J Otolaryngol* 1979;8:401–410.

656. Donegan, JO, Wood MD: Intratracheal thyroid—Familial occurrence. *Laryngoscope* 1985;95:6–8.

657. Bone R, Biller HF, Irwin TM: Intralaryngotracheal thyroid. *Ann Otol Rhinol Laryngol* 1972;81:424–428.

658. Chanin LR, Greenberg LM: Pediatric upper airway obstruction due to ectopic thyroid: Classification and case reports. *Laryngoscope* 1986;98:422–427.

659. Brandwein M, Som PM, Urken M: Benign intratracheal thyroid: A possible cause for preoperative overstaging. *Arch Otolaryngol Head Neck Surg* 1998;124:1266–1269.

660. Myers E, Pantangco IP: Intratracheal thyroid. *Laryngoscope* 1975;85:1833–1840.

661. Falk P: Anatomische Studien ueber Bezichurgen von Schildreussengewebe zum Kehlopfund Luftroehre bein Neugeboren. *Arch Ohren Nasen Kohlkpfs* 1937;143:304.

662. Ogata H, Ebihara S, Mukai K, et al: Laryngeal metastasis from a pulmonary papillary adenocarcinoma: A case report. *Jpn Clin Oncol* 1993;23:199–203.

663. El-Naggar AK: Secondary neoplasms. In: Ferlito A, ed. *Surgical Pathology of Laryngeal Neoplasms.* New York: Chapman & Hall Medical, 1996:465–474.

664. Batsakis JG, Luna MA, Byers RM: Metastasis to the larynx. *Head Neck Surg* 1985;7:458–460.

665. Henderson LT, Robbins KT, Weizner S: Upper aerodigestive tract metastasis in disseminated malignant melanoma. *Arch Otolaryngol* 1986;112:659–663.

666. Patel JK, Didolkar M, Pickren JW, Moore RH: Metastatic pattern of malignant melanoma: A study of 216 autopsy cases. *Am J Surg* 1978;135:807–810.

667. Ferlito A, Caruso G: Secondary malignant melanoma of the larynx. Report of 2 cases and review of 79 laryngeal secondary cancers. *ORL Otorhinolaryngol Relat Spec* 1984;46:117–133.

668. Mochimatsu I, Tsukuda M, Furukawa S, Sawaki S: Tumor metastasizing to the head and neck: A report of seven cases. *J Laryngol Otol* 1993;107:1171–1173.

669. Marlowe SD, Swartz JD, Koenigsberg R, et al: Metastatic hypernephroma to the larynx: An unusual presentation. *Neuroradiology* 1993;35:242–243.

670. Greenberg RE, Richter RM, Cooper J, et al: Hoarseness: A unique clinical presentation for renal cell carcinoma. *Urology* 1992;40:159–161.

671. Wanamaker JR, Kraus DH, Eliachar I, Lavertu P: Manifestations of metastatic breast carcinoma to the head and neck. *Head Neck* 1993;15:257–262.

672. Park YW, Park MH: Vocal cord paralysis from the prostatic carcinoma metastasizing to the larynx. *Head Neck* 1993;15:455–458.

673. Bolgnesi C, Caliceti G: Seminoma metastatico della laringe. *Otorinolar Ital* 1960;29:15–25.

674. Glanz H, Kleinsasser O: Metastasen in Kehlkopf. *HNO* 1978;26:163–167.

675. Levine HL, Appelbaum EL: Metastatic adenocarcinoma to the larynx: Report of a case. *Trans Am Acad Ophthalmol Otolaryngol* 1976;82:536–541.

676. Refoyo JLP, Vicente P, Fonseca E: Metastasis de adenocarcinoma gastrico en laringe. *Anales ORL Iber Amer* 1991;23:281–287.

677. Maddox JC, Evans HL: Angiosarcoma of skin and soft tissue: A study of 44 cases. *Cancer* 1981;48:1907–1921.

678. Bernáldez R, Toledano A, Alvarez J: Pulmonary carcinoma metastatic to the larynx. *J Laryngol Otol* 1994;108:898–901.

6 ∷ Salivary and Lacrimal Glands

Douglas R. Gnepp, Margaret S. Brandwein, and John D. Henley

DEVELOPMENT AND ANATOMY

Embryology

The oropharyngeal membrane divides the primitive oral cavity from the primitive pharynx. The oral cavity structures originating external to the oropharyngeal membrane are of ectodermal derivation; those arising internal to the oropharyngeal membrane are of endodermal origin. In the adult, the boundary of this remote membrane is less than certain. It is generally accepted that the parotid gland is of ectodermal origin. Both ectodermal and endodermal origins have been described for the sublingual and submandibular glands, although the consensus rests with the former for both glands. Regardless of their origin, each gland develops from a primitive bud of epithelium growing into the underlying mesenchyme. Development proceeds via dynamic epithelial-mesenchymal cell interactions and relies, in part, on an intact basement membrane[1] and matrix-degrading enzymes.[2]

The primordial parotid, submandibular, and sublingual glands become apparent during the sixth to eighth week of development. The first to develop are the parotid glands, then the submandibular glands, then the sublingual glands, and last the minor salivary glands, which are initiated by the 10th week. Three stages in the development of salivary glands are distinguished.[3] In the first stage, dichotomous branching ducts develop from the salivary anlage. In the second stage, canalization of the ducts and the production of gland lobules continues through the seventh embryonal month. The third stage begins in the fifth embryonal month with differentiation of acini and further maturation of the gland, with considerable reduction of the initially abundant connective tissue. Complete maturation of the salivary glands does not occur until after birth.[4]

Cervical lymph nodes develop simultaneously and in close proximity with the parotid gland. Although the parotid is the first of the major glands to develop, it is the last to become encapsulated. After the submandibular and sublingual glands become encapsulated and before the parotid glands develop their capsules, the lymphatic system in the area of the major salivary glands develops from mesoderm.[5] This intimacy and late encapsulation explains the frequent presence of intraparotid lymph nodes and of epithelial salivary gland inclusions within periparotid and intraparotid lymph nodes.

Anatomy

The salivary glands are responsible for the production, modification, and secretion of saliva, which aids mastication, deglutition, digestion, and protection of teeth and soft tissues. They are exocrine glands that are structurally organized into three major bilaterally paired glands and the minor salivary glands. The *parotid, submandibular,* and *sublingual* glands constitute the major glands, and the *minor* salivary glands are collectively represented by mucosa-based seromucinous glands located throughout the oral and oropharyngeal mucosa.

The fundamental structure of all salivary glands is the acinar-ductal unit. The terminal acinus empties into a duct system that, in the major glands, is divided into *intercalated, striated,* and *excretory* segments. Acini are variably composed of serous or mucous cells or both. These acini are arranged in small, pear-shaped groups surrounded by a distinct basement membrane; they have an inconspicuous central lumen.[6] Serous cells are pyramidal-shaped with cytoplasm filled with highly refractile zymogen granules. They have basally oriented nuclei and abundant rough endoplasmic reticulum; their cytoplasm characteristically stains basophilic. Mucinous cells have a round basal nucleus and are distended by vacuoles containing acidic and neutral, optically clear mucin. The acini produce saliva, which flows into the intercalated duct system. The intercalated ducts, connecting the acini to the striated ducts, are relatively short, lined by cuboidal cells, and generally inconspicuous at a light microscopic level. Striated ducts are much larger than intercalated ducts and are approximately three to six times the diameter of an acinus.[7] They modify saliva, succeed the intercalated duct system, and are lined with tall columnar cells rich in mitochondria and show numerous basal cytoplasmic invaginations arranged in a parallel fashion. The striated ducts are followed by the excretory (interlobular) ducts that are lined by multiple layers of duct epithelium. The lining ranges from pseudostratified columnar epithelium with occasional goblet cells to stratified columnar to squamous type epithelium as the duct approaches the oral epithelium.

Myoepithelial cells are present at the periphery of the acini, along the outside of the intercalated ducts, and infrequently along the striated ducts. These contractile cells, which contain cytoplasmic actin, myosin, and intermediate filaments, are enclosed within the basement membrane and the basilar surface of acini and duct cells; they have a stellate shape with numerous dendritic processes that cradle the acini; hence, these cells have been referred to as "basket cells."[8]

The *parotid gland* is the largest of the three major glands and weighs on average between 14 and 30 g.[9] It is enclosed within a delicate fibrous capsule. The gland is located in the retromandibular fossa and is anatomically divided into superficial and deep lobes by the facial nerve. Although this latter terminology is commonly utilized, it is not completely correct on an anatomic basis. Therefore, a more anatomically correct terminology has become popular: the superficial portion of the gland is that region that overlies the ramus of the mandible and masseter muscle; the retromandibular portion refers to the smaller region behind and deep to the mandibular ramus.[9] The parotid gland is composed almost entirely of serous cells; however, in the area of the parotid tail adjacent to the submandibular gland, one may occasionally find mucinous acini. Frequently intermixed with the serous acini one finds abundant adipose tissue, which becomes more conspicuous with age. This can be appreciated on gross inspection: the gland is lobulated with a yellow-tan hue. Microscopically the abundant adipose tissue helps to histologically separate parotid tissue from submandibular gland. Sebaceous glands may be observed in 10% to 42% of normal parotid glands (Fig. 6–1); with serial sectioning, virtually all glands will contain sebaceous glands.[6, 10] Parotid melanocytes have been described recently in one patient.[11] The parotid glands contain 3 to 32 (average 20) intraglandular lymph nodes that are interconnected by a plexus of lymph vessels, which drain the skin from the side of the head above the parotid gland and the orbital region, as well as the nose, upper lip, external

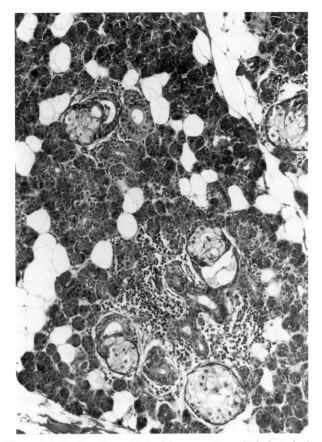

Figure 6–1. Portion of parotid gland demonstrating multiple foci of sebaceous differentiation. Sebaceous foci are commonly associated with the intercalated ducts.

auditory canal, eustachian tube, and tympanic membrane.[12, 13] These lymph nodes frequently contain entrapped or ectopic salivary gland acini and ducts.

An accessory parotid gland is present in up to 56% of individuals.[14] Accessory parotids are discrete masses of serous salivary gland that connect to the main excretory duct of the parotid; they are most frequently found on the anterior surface of the main gland or anterior to the parotid along the masseter in the area of the excretory duct.[6] These accessory glands are subject to all the pathologies afflicting the main gland. The main excretory duct, Stensen's duct, opens to the oral cavity opposite the second maxillary molar.

The *submandibular gland* is the second largest salivary gland weighing about 7 to 8 g.[6] It is also enclosed by a delicate fibrous capsule. This gland is located in the submandibular triangle behind and below the free border of the mylohyoid muscle. The main excretory duct, Wharton's duct, opens at the side of the lingual frenulum on the floor of the mouth. This gland is mixed, with both serous and mucous cells; serous units predominate, accounting for approximately 90% of the acinar cells.[7, 9] Serous cells are typically arranged as crescent-shaped caps or demilunes at the periphery of mucinous acinar cells.[7] Unlike the parotid gland, the submandibular gland proper does not contain any intraparenchymal lymph nodes. Sebaceous glands may also be found in the submandibular gland in 5% to 6% of submandibular glands.[6, 10] For any given age, the amount of intraglandular adipose tissue is less than that found in the parotid gland.[7]

The *sublingual gland* is poorly encapsulated and lies between the floor of the mouth and the mylohyoid muscle, lying against the anterior lingual surface of the mandible. It is the smallest major salivary gland, weighing about 2 to 3 g.[6, 9] Unlike the other major glands, the sublingual gland has multiple excretory ducts. The main duct, Bartholin's duct, is accompanied by several surrounding ducts (Rivinus' ducts) that open into the mouth in the plica sublingualis or

join the submandibular duct.[6] This gland contains both serous and mucous cells; however, mucous cells heavily outnumber serous cells, which are frequently arranged as demilunes at the periphery of mucinous acinar cells.[7] Intraparenchymal lymph nodes are not found, and sebaceous glands are only occasionally seen (4%).[10]

Minor salivary glands are unencapsulated seromucinous glands located immediately beneath the mucosa throughout the oral cavity except for the anterior hard palate and gingiva, which are generally devoid of glands.[7] Several groups of secretory units open via short ducts directly into the mouth. These glands are in close contact with surrounding soft tissues, especially the muscle of the tongue and lips. This anatomic arrangement should be carefully considered when evaluating for the presence or absence of invasive growth of a minor salivary gland tumor.[7] Mucous-only glands are limited to the palate, retromolar pad, and anterior ventral tongue (glands of Blandin and Nuhn); in the region of the posterior tongue lateral and posterior to the circumvallate papillae there are serous glands (von Ebner's glands).[7] Other anatomic sites have mixed acini with a prominent mucinous component. Takeda studied minor salivary glands in 445 patients and found melanocytes in 8 (1.8%) glands distributed in fibrous tissue around the interlobular and intralobular ducts and acini.[14a]

DEVELOPMENTAL DISORDERS

Aside from heterotopic salivary glands, developmental disorders of these glands are rare oddities for the pathologist. Reported congenital anomalies include aplasia or absence of one or more of the major glands[15, 16]; gland duplication[17]; and congenitally atretic, imperforate, ectatic, and duplicated ducts.[18, 19] Diffuse structural abnormalities may be seen in syndromes affecting branchial arch development, such as the lacrimo-auriculo-dento-digital syndrome (LADD).[16, 20]

Tumor-like presentations of maldevelopment include rare hamartomas of the hard palate[21] and unusual cystic choristomas of the submandibular gland.[22] These latter lesions appear to be a mixture of epithelium of both ectodermal and endodermal derivation. The congenital salivary gland anlage tumor or "congenital pleomorphic adenoma" is thought to represent a hamartoma of minor salivary gland origin.[23] This lesion characteristically involves the sinonasal area. An additional rare developmental anomaly important to consider, as it can simulate a neoplasm, is polycystic (dysgenetic) disease.

Salivary Gland Heterotopia

Heterotopic salivary gland is most commonly encountered as an incidental finding in periparotid and intraparotid lymph nodes. Less frequently, ectopic glands are seen in soft tissues of the anterior neck, usually along the anterior border of the sternocleidomastoid muscle, particularly in the area of the sternoclavicular joint,[24] and in cervical lymph nodes. Other reported sites of involvement include the middle ear,[25–28] posterior triangle of the neck,[29] mandible and maxilla,[30, 31] gingiva,[32, 33] tonsils, sella turcica,[34] thyroid,[28, 35] mediastinum,[28, 36] rectum,[37] vulva,[38] prostate,[39] larynx, lacrimal gland, cerebellopontine angle, and stomach. In addition, we have recently seen a case of ectopic salivary gland tissue associated with an anterior neck thyroglossal duct cyst. This finding has also been noted by other observers.[28]

Clinical Features. Typically, heterotopic or choristomatous salivary gland is an incidental finding. However, potential clinical presentations include a mass or draining sinus of the anterior neck, which is often associated with a branchial cleft anomaly.[40–42] Heterotopic salivary gland tissue may also be associated with the branchio-otorenal syndrome.[43]

An unusual clinical occurrence is the neoplastic transformation of heterotopic salivary gland. A variety of benign and malignant neoplasms have been described to arise in this manner, including various adenomas,[44–48] mucoepidermoid carcinoma,[45] acinic cell carcinoma,[49, 50] and adenoid cystic carcinoma.[51] This phenomenon presumably accounts for intramandibular primary salivary gland tumors, the majority of which are mucoepidermoid carcinomas.[31]

Pathologic Features. Heterotopic salivary gland recapitulates normal salivary gland with the exception of excretory ducts. The glands are serous or seromucinous in type. Neoplasms arising from heterotopia are indistinguishable from those arising from the major and minor glands.

Treatment and Prognosis. Non-neoplastic choristomatous masses are amenable to simple excision. Neoplasms, however, should be treated as their respective histology warrants.

When a malignant tumor is presumed to arise from heterotopia, an occult primary tumor must be excluded. This entails appropriate imaging studies, which include the deep parotid lobe and possibly a superficial or total parotidectomy.

Polycystic (Dysgenetic) Disease

Clinical Features. *Polycystic (dysgenetic) disease* is a very rare developmental abnormality involving the salivary gland duct system that has histologic similarity to polycystic disease of the kidney. It has an incidence in three large salivary gland registries ranging from 1 in 3500 to 1 in 6875 tumors.[28, 52] It was first described by Seifert and colleagues in 1981[53] and represents 0.2% of benign salivary gland cysts.[54] To date there are 17 cases reported; 16 involved the parotid gland and only 1 the submandibular gland.[28, 52, 53, 55–58] One of the patients in the original series of Seifert and colleagues had an affected father, suggesting that some cases have an autosomal dominant mode of transmission.[16, 53] Almost all cases have occurred in females ranging in age from 6 to 65 years.[56] The majority presented in childhood, but some are also reported in adults. Most patients have bilateral involvement; however, occasionally a single gland will be involved. Patients typically present with recurrent, painless swelling of the affected gland with no abnormality of salivary flow. Sialography exhibits multicystic change.

Pathologic Features. Microscopically, although the lobular architecture of the gland is preserved, the parenchyma is replaced by varying degrees of honeycombed cystic change (Fig. 6–2, see p. 337). Cysts vary in size but are usually not more than several millimeters in diameter. They are lined with a flat, cuboidal, or columnar epithelium; apocrine-like snouting, cytoplasmic vacuolation or eosinophilia, and degenerative changes are common. The cysts are often interconnected and irregular with incomplete fibrous septa. In addition, they may be filled to varying degrees by inspissated proteinaceous secretions and contain eosinophilic bodies with concentric radial patterns similar to spheroliths and microliths.

The stroma is fibrous, and entrapped acini and ducts are present between the cysts. Inflammation is absent and squamous metaplasia is unusual. Although these lesions may be mistaken for adenocarcinoma, the diffuse nature of polycystic disease with persistence of the lobular architecture should allow separation from neoplasia. This cystic process may affect ectopic salivary gland tissue in cervical lymph nodes.[57] Therefore, involvement of cervical nodes should not be construed as evidence of a malignancy.

The differential diagnosis consists predominantly of a cystadenoma and cystadenocarcinoma, both of which are localized masses and, unlike polycystic disease, do not involve the entire gland.

Treatment and Prognosis. Polycystic disease is a completely benign process. It may be necessary to surgically remove the involved glands for cosmetic reasons or to establish the diagnosis.

Congenital Sialectasis and Merkel's Cysts

Congenital sialectasis is a rare cystic condition arising in children and adults, accounting for 1.4% of non-neoplastic salivary gland cysts.[59] It usually affects one or both of the parotid glands. Scattered ducts are dilated, often contain secretory material, and are always connected directly to an intact ductal system. The ectatic ducts are lined by a single-layered or multilayered, somewhat flattened to cuboidal epithelium and, if secondarily infected, with an associated inflammatory infiltrate. The lack of an inflammatory infiltrate helps separate this condition from a secondarily acquired duct ectasia in infants and young children. However, since stagnation of secretions aids in the development of recurrent sialadenitis, it is difficult to separate a secondarily infected congenital sialectasis from acquired duct ectasia.

Merkel's cysts of the submandibular gland are somewhat similar and may also be developmental in origin.[59] These cysts are lined by flattened epithelium and are caused by distortion and segmentation of the submandibular duct.

Adenomatoid Hyperplasia of Minor Salivary Glands

Giansanti et al.[60] described this unusual lesion of oral mucous glands in 1971. Despite nomenclature, the nature (hyperplastic versus hamartomatous) of *adenomatoid hyperplasia of the mucous glands* is unclear. The etiology of this lesion has remained idiopathic, although it has been suggested that chronic, local trauma may be an important factor in its development.[61]

Clinical Features. To date, 58 cases have been documented in the literature.[62] Adenomatoid hyperplasia presents as a painless, firm mass or an elevated nodule covered by intact oral mucosa. The mucosa may appear normal or slightly bluish. Greater than 80% of lesions occur on the hard or soft palate; other sites (e.g., retromolar trigone) are less commonly affected. Typically, men and women in the fourth to sixth decades of life are affected. The male to female ratio is approximately 3 : 2.[62] Histologic examination is essential in establishing the diagnosis, since these lesions cannot be clinically discriminated from neoplasia.

Pathologic Features. Grossly, these lesions may measure up to 3 cm in greatest dimension.[63] Microscopically, coalescing lobules of normal-appearing mucinous acini appear in excess within the lamina propria and submucosa (Fig. 6–3). In a few cases, the acinar tissue has been described as hyperplastic, but this has not been confirmed, to date, by morphometry.[62] Although well-circumscribed, the lesions are unencapsulated. The overlying epithelium may exhibit pseudoepitheliomatous hyperplasia.[64] Ducts appear normal and inflammation is inconspicuous. Connective tissue surrounding acini may appear dense and prominent. Low-grade mucoepidermoid carcinoma is a differential diagnostic consideration in any case sampled via fine needle aspiration biopsy.[65]

Treatment and Prognosis. The biology of these lesions is benign. Treatment is simple excision; recurrence has not been reported.

SIALADENITIS, SIALOLITHIASIS, AND SIALADENOSIS

Infectious Sialadenitis

Infections of the salivary glands are caused by a variety of microbial agents including bacteria, mycobacteria, viruses, fungi, parasites, and protozoa.

Acute Suppurative Sialadenitis

Clinical Features. Acute suppurative sialadenitis occurs in children and adults in a variety of clinical settings. Reduced or absent salivation is an important factor in its genesis, and infection typically accompanies states of dehydration. The pathogenesis is attributable to ascending infection of the canalicular system. Preterm infants are at risk for developing neonatal sialadenitis when dehydration is a predisposing factor. *Staphylococcus aureus*[66] and

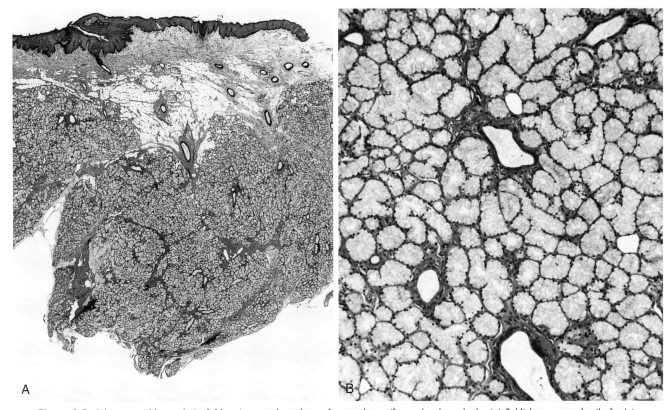

Figure 6–3. Adenomatoid hyperplasia. A, Note increased numbers of somewhat uniform, closely packed acini. B, Higher power detail of acini.

Pseudomonas aeruginosa[67] are described pathogens in such cases. Recurrent juvenile parotitis, principally affecting 3- to 6-year-olds,[68] is characterized by recurrent episodes of parotid gland swelling accompanied by purulent secretion from Stensen's duct. This condition is typically associated with sialectasis on sialography, thus aiding the distinction from other inflammatory conditions. Duct abnormalities,[68] heredity, and allergy are among the implicated causes. *Streptococcus pneumoniae* and *Haemophilus influenzae* were recovered frequently in a series of patients.[69] Nosocomial infections are attributable to gram-negative and anaerobic organisms. *Staphylococcus aureus* is common in chronic infections. In adults, the elderly and malnourished are at highest risk for suppurative sialadenitis. Postoperative sialadenitis, a particularly morbid form of sialadenitis, has become a less frequent complication of major surgery. Obstructive sialadenitis secondary to lithiasis is most common in the submandibular glands of elderly patients.

The presenting symptom of acute suppurative parotitis is tenderness associated with diffuse or localized swelling that may be fluctuant. A fistula draining purulent material may form.[70]

Pathologic Features. Microscopically there is edema, hyperemia, and acute inflammation. A periductal and intraductal accumulation of neutrophils is associated with destruction of the ductal epithelium. Acini are lost and parenchymal microabscesses form as the inflammatory process progresses.

Treatment. Therapy involves appropriate antibiotic treatment. Surgical drainage is desirable in the event of abscess formation.

Tuberculosis

Clinical Features. Mycobacterial lymphadenitis of the parotid gland is the most common form of mycobacterial infection to affect the salivary glands. Both tuberculous and atypical infections occur.[71] Parenchymal infection is rare.[72] Intraparotid and periparotid lymph nodes become infected as the result of lymphatic drainage of the glandular duct system, from an infection originating in the mouth and pharynx, or as a result of dissemination of pulmonary disease.[73]

Tuberculous lymphadenitis may go unrecognized for an extended period, since constitutional symptoms typically are not present. Signs and symptoms may precede diagnosis for weeks to years. The disease usually manifests as a painless, discrete, solid nodule and is commonly mistaken for a neoplasm.[70, 74] There may be multiple masses. The overlying skin is usually smooth and lacks erythema. However, scrofula (suppurative, draining cervical mycobacterial lymphadenitis) may occur. The submandibular and sublingual salivary glands are much less frequently involved.

Pathologic Features. Necrotizing granulomatous inflammation is present microscopically. Epithelioid macrophages, foreign-body and Langhans' giant cells, and lymphocytes surround the caseous centers. Acid-fast bacilli are extremely difficult to demonstrate in tissue sections. Bacterial cultures are usually required, and they too may fail to demonstrate the pathogen. Polymerase chain reaction may be used to establish the diagnosis.[75]

Treatment. The diagnosis is commonly established in surgically excised affected tissues. Treatment is antimycobacterial drug therapy.

Viral Sialadenitis

Several viruses have been causally associated with sialadenitis, including paramyxovirus (mumps), coxsackievirus, lymphocytic-choriomeningitis virus, herpes virus, influenza A, parainfluenza, cytomegalovirus, and adenovirus.[76–78] Of these, paramyxovirus (mumps) is the best known of the sialoadenotropic viruses.

Mumps

Clinical Features. Mumps is a self-limiting disease that predominantly affects children. It is caused by droplet infection of the upper respiratory tract. Viremia develops during an incubation period lasting 16 to 18 days, after which one or both of the parotid glands become painful and swollen. Stimulation of salivation intensifies the pain. Diagnosis is usually made on clinical grounds and is supported by the serologic findings.

Pathologic Features. The glands are very rarely examined microscopically. When reported,[70] dense interstitial lymphoplasmacytic infiltrates, acinar cell vacuolization, and ductal dilatation are the microscopic features. The changes are reversible.

Treatment and Prognosis. Orchitis, meningoencephalitis, pancreatitis, and arthritis are extremely rare complications that usually affect adults and lead to serious consequences such as sterility and deafness. Treatment is predominantly symptomatic.

Human Immunodeficiency Virus

Clinical Features. Patients with human immunodeficiency virus (HIV) infection are at risk for the development of infectious sialadenitis. Potential opportunistic pathogens include cytomegalovirus (CMV),[78] *Pneumocystis carinii,*[78] adenovirus,[77] and *Histoplasma.*[79] Clinical presentations are variable and either infection or neoplasm may be suspected. Pronounced CMV salivary gland disease is rare, even though many patients with acquired immunodeficiency syndrome (AIDS) excrete CMV in their saliva.[80] The chronic parotid swelling observed in some infants with AIDS is believed to be due to acute CMV parotitis.

Pathologic Features. The diagnosis is based on histologic recognition of the offending organisms or characteristic viral cytopathic changes. Dual infections may occur. CMV-infected cells are large, with characteristic amphophilic nuclear and cytoplasmic inclusions.

Treatment. Treatment is appropriate antimicrobial drug therapy.

Chronic Sialadenitis and Related Conditions

The potential etiologies of chronic sialadenitis are manifold and include mechanical, physical, microbial, and immunologic factors. Chronic inflammation with or without gland destruction is a common incidental finding in oral minor salivary glands. The etiology is often unclear, although, occasionally, inspissated intraductal secretion or a sialolith may be demonstrable. Inflammation of the major glands generally accompanies mechanical obstruction of the excretory ducts. In one study of surgically excised glands, calculi were associated with chronic sialadenitis of the parotid and submandibular glands in 24% and 73% of cases, respectively.[81] Moreover, decreased salivary flow, increased salivary viscosity, and ascending infection all play a potential role in chronic sialadenitis.[81] While sialoliths are the most common cause of ductal obstruction, duct stricture or severance or extrinsic duct compression may compromise salivary flow. Ascending infection is a potential complication of ductal obstruction. Long-standing obstruction leads to chronic sialadenitis with acinar atrophy and fibrosis. The so-called "Kuttner tumor" is the end-stage fibrotic result of chronic sclerosing sialoadenitis of the submandibular gland. Affected glands are stony hard and clinically simulate tumors.

Sialadenitis is a common complication of radiotherapy, including high-dose radioiodine therapy,[82] used in the treatment of head and neck cancers. The serous acini of the parotid glands are particular sensitive to radiation injury.[83] Chronic (juvenile) recurrent parotiditis is a disorder primarily affecting children and has exhibited autosomal dominant inheritance in some cases.[84] After mumps, it is the most common inflammatory salivary gland disease in children.[85] Congenital duct malformations, ascending infection, allergy, and dehydration have been implicated in the development of this disorder.[83, 84] Patients with cystic fibrosis are predisposed to developing chronic sialadenitis, particularly involving the sublingual and minor (mucus-rich) salivary glands.

Granulomatous sialadenitis is a form of chronic sialadenitis with many potential causes. Duct obstruction secondary to stones or tumor is the most commonly identified cause.[86] Many cases, however, remain idiopathic. Infectious agents responsible for granulomatous inflammation include mycobacteria, fungi, and the agent of cat-scratch disease (see infectious sialadenitis). Up to 6% of patients with sarcoidosis will have parotid involvement.[83] Moreover, the lesions of Wegener's granulomatosis may involve the parotid gland, so that the disorder presents as a parotid swelling or mass lesion.[87]

Clinical Features. The symptoms of chronic obstructive sialadenitis are similar to those of sialolithiasis. In the absence of lithiasis, patients may be asymptomatic. Others may present with swelling with or without tenderness or pain. Xerostomia is generally uncommon and disease is unilateral. Acute radiation injury becomes clinically evident within 24 hours after exposure, producing swelling and tenderness.[83] Chronic (juvenile) recurrent parotiditis is a long-standing disorder characterized by bilateral fluctuating parotid enlargement, as frequent as every 3 to 4 months.[85] Sialectasis is characteristic on sialography, thus aiding its distinction from other inflammatory conditions. *Streptococcus pneumoniae* and *Haemophilus influenzae* were frequently recovered in a series of patients.[88] Boys are affected more commonly than girls, and the disease commonly becomes asymptomatic at puberty,[84] although it may extend into adulthood.[85] Sialadenitis may also be associated with sarcoidosis. These patients frequently have co-existent pulmonary symptoms. Typically, parotid involvement causes painless, diffuse swelling. Salivary gland sarcoidosis may simulate Sjögren's syndrome presenting with sicca complex. Mycobacterial disease is likely to simulate tumor and may be unexpected prior to surgical excision of a suspected neoplasm.

Pathologic Features. Chronic obstructive sialadenitis is associated with lymphoplasmacytic inflammation, fibrosis, and acinar atrophy to varying degrees. Mild neutrophilic inflammation may be present. Inflammation tends to aggregate periductally. Lymphoid aggregates with germinal centers are common. Acinar atrophy may be marked so that acini are completely lacking. Ducts and acini often appear ectatic. The ductal epithelium is prone to metaplastic changes, including squamous cell, mucous cell, and ciliary cell metaplasia. Oncocytic change is common in inflamed minor salivary glands.[89] A granulomatous inflammatory response may be seen, with extravasation of saliva secondary to duct rupture.[90] The Kuttner tumor is characterized by periductal lymphoplasmacytic inflammation with incorporation of the interlobular and intralobular ducts in thick fibrous trabeculae.[90]

Acute radiation injury of the parotid manifests with swelling, vacuolation, and potential necrosis of the serous cells.[83] With a significant exposure, the initial acute inflammatory response is later followed by a chronic sclerosing sialadenitis and resultant xerostomia[92]; glandular loss may be associated with a relative increase in adipose tissue.[93] Minor gland changes include necrosis with squamous metaplasia of the excretory duct and acini, goblet cell metaplasia, and cellular atypia of the ductal epithelium. Such changes should not be mistaken for squamous cell carcinoma. The lobular arrangement of the affected glands, the presence of ductal lumina with intraluminal mucin, or the persistence of occasional mucous cells aids in the proper interpretation.

Chronic (juvenile) recurrent parotiditis shows dilatation of interlobular ducts with marked periductal lymphocytic infiltration. Exocytosis of lymphocytes into the ductal epithelium, which is often hyperplastic, is typical, as is inflammation within the lobules. Resultant atrophy and fibrosis are of variable degrees.[85]

The granulomas of sarcoidosis are typically noncaseating, although central necrosis is occasionally seen.[86] Clinical correlation and special stains help distinguish sarcoidosis from mycobacterial and fungal infection. Furthermore, Wegener's granulomatosis must also be considered. The diagnosis of head and neck Wegener's granulomatosis can be difficult. In one study, vasculitis, necrosis, and granulomatous inflammation were seen together in only 16% of biopsy specimens from head and neck cases of Wegener's granulomatosis.[94] Necrotizing arteritis is the fundamental feature of Wegener's granulomatosis. Elastic stains may aid in identifying remnants of vessels in tissue damaged by inflammation and necrosis.[95]

Treatment and Prognosis. In cases of chronic obstructive sialadenitis encountered by the surgical pathologist, the affected gland generally has been removed surgically, which is curative. Treatment of sialadenitis secondary to infection or associated with a systemic disorder (e.g., sarcoidosis) should be directed at the underlying cause.

Sjögren's Syndrome and Myoepithelial Sialadenitis

Given the intimate association of myoepithelial sialadenitis (MESA), or benign lymphoepithelial lesion (BLEL), with Sjögren's syndrome (SS), it is appropriate to include these unique salivary gland lesions under the heading of Sjögren's syndrome. It is important to remember that although most patients with SS develop MESA, many cases occur in individuals without the clinical findings of SS.[96, 97] SS is an autoimmune disease characterized by the progressive lymphocytic infiltration and destruction of exocrine glands, particularly the salivary and lacrimal. Although the current diagnostic criteria of SS are somewhat controversial,[98] the characteristic symptomatology is xerostomia and xerophthalmia. These findings are attributable to exocrine gland destruction with resultant decreased saliva and tear production. The disease occurs in primary and secondary forms. Xerostomia and xerophthalmia in the absence of another connective tissue disease is termed primary Sjögren's syndrome,[99] previously referred to as Mikulicz's disease or sicca syndrome.[100] Secondary SS occurs in association with another connective tissue disease, such as rheumatoid arthritis, systemic lupus erythematosus, scleroderma, polymyositis, or polyarteritis.[100] Autoantibodies SS-A/Ro and SS-B/La are found with increased frequency in patients with secondary and primary SS, respectively.[95] The lymphocytic infiltrate of the salivary glands is commonly associated with changes in the salivary ducts, producing a characteristic histologic appearance known as MESA, or BLEL. The pathogenesis of this latter group of lesions is not known.

Clinical Features. Up to 90% of patients with SS are females. The average age at diagnosis is 50 years; SS is uncommon in patients under the age of 20 and may rarely occur in children.[101] In the major glands, 85% of cases involve the parotid gland and the remaining affect the submandibular gland. Sublingual gland involvement is rare but has been described.[102] The principal clinical symptoms are due to dryness of the eyes and mouth, resulting in keratoconjunctivitis[103] and difficulty with speaking and swallowing of food. Patients are at risk for candidal stomatitis, rapidly progressive dental caries, and periodontal disease.[95, 104]

Many patients present with firm, diffuse enlargement of the salivary glands, which is usually but not always bilateral; rarely there may be bilateral multicystic disease.[104a] Induration of the glands without enlargement may be evident early in the course of the disease.[96] These changes are usually painless or associated with slight tenderness.

A typical sialographic feature of the affected parotid is the formation of punctate cavitary defects filled with radiopaque contrast medium, described as a "fruit-laden, branchless tree." This characteristic appearance is believed to be due to leakage of the contrast material through the weakened salivary gland ducts.[105]

Pathologic Features. The microscopic hallmark of SS is a lymphocytic sialadenitis. Progressive lymphocytic infiltration leads to acinar loss. There is some ductal preservation with epithelial proliferation to form characteristic epimyoepithelial islands, the essential histologic feature of MESA or BLEL. Immunohistochemistry has shown that both ductal and myoepithelial cells participate in the formation of these lesions.[106] The parotid tail or labial salivary glands are commonly biopsied for diagnosis of Sjögren's syndrome. The early histopathologic changes are similar in both sites,[107] although epimyoepithelial islands are not typically encountered in the minor salivary glands of the lip. Early in disease, focal aggregates of lymphocytes are seen in parenchymal lobules with associated acinar involution. A focus score of greater than one focus ($\geq$50 lymphocytes) per 4 mm^2 is considered to be diagnostic of the disease.[108] As the inflammation progresses, partial and then total parenchymal loss becomes evident, and the lymphocytic infiltrate dominates. Lymphoid follicles with germinal centers are common, although they vary in a given case from scant to extensive.[109] Plasma cells are inconspicuous in the early phases of the disease but may become prominent in later stages. Rarely, a few granulomas may be found in a minor gland biopsy specimen; this finding should not be taken as evidence of sarcoidosis. In later stages, epithelial and myoepithelial duct cells proliferate predominantly in the major glands and show metaplastic changes, producing the epimyoepithelial islands characteristic of myoepithelial sialadenitis (Fig. 6–4A).[110] Occasionally, cystic change may be seen and rarely it may be prominent. Interlobular septa are typically preserved; thus, the affected gland maintains a lobular architecture.[109] One recent report described prominent sebaceous differentiation.[111] Rarely, Sjögren-like chronic inflammatory infiltrates can be seen in patients with other types of connective tissue diseases without the clinical findings typical for SS.

Differential Diagnosis. The differential diagnosis includes nonspecific chronic sialadenitis, lymphoepithelial carcinoma, HIV-associated salivary lymphoepithelial cysts, and lymphoma. Distinction from nonspecific chronic sialadenitis is not difficult. MESA exhibits a much more pronounced and uniform lymphocytic infiltrate than chronic sialadenitis. Moreover, epimyoepithelial islands and germinal centers are not usually seen in chronic sialadenitis. Distinguishing the labial gland lesions of SS from nonspecific sialadenitis can be more problematic. Adherence to the focus score criteria will usually allow adequate differentiation of nonspecific inflammation from the lesions of SS.

Lymphoepithelial carcinoma should not be mistaken for MESA. This distinction can be complicated by the presence of MESA-like areas within lymphoepithelial carcinoma. Moreover, lymphoepithelial carcinoma may evolve in the setting of a pre-existing MESA. Thus, it is important that any case of MESA be carefully examined for areas of carcinoma. In MESA, the epithelial cells making up the myoepithelial lesions lack atypia, necrosis, and mitotic activity. In addition, the proliferating islands are usually small to moderately sized and are well circumscribed. Carcinomas, in comparison, tend to have larger and more irregular islands or collections of tumor cells and, in addition, may have a sheet-like growth pattern. In contrast with MESA, carcinomas exhibit nuclear atypia with irregular chromatin; also, mitotic activity and necrosis may be seen. An infiltrative or destructive pattern of growth is indicative of carcinoma.

Patients positive for HIV with persistent generalized lymphadenopathy may also develop lymphoid hyperplasia of the salivary glands, usually involving the parotid. This process frequently involves proliferation of the ductal elements, often with cystic change and myoepithelial islands similar to those seen in MESA. The HIV lesions tend to be cystic while MESA tends to form more solid lesions. A careful history and clinical evaluation will usually resolve this differential in problematic cases.

Finally, the distinction between MESA and malignant lymphoma can be problematic, especially in its early stage, and may be difficult to diagnose by light microscopy alone. Immunohistochemical and molecular biology techniques are necessary in this situation to demonstrate the monoclonality typical of lymphoma. We require monoclonality and morphologic evidence of a clonal population before making a diagnosis of an early lymphoma (Fig. 6–4B, C). Please refer to Chapter 12 for additional information.

Treatment and Prognosis. Patients with MESA and no evidence of an autoimmune disease should be followed carefully, as some, but not all, will subsequently develop an autoimmune disease. Patients with SS and MESA have an incurable disease. Therefore, treatment is directed toward symptomatic relief. Patients with SS have a 43.8 times higher risk for developing non-Hodgkin's lymphoma than age-matched control subjects.[112] Lymphomas may develop within MESA or within lymph nodes at other sites. Patients with MESA but without SS are also at an increased risk of developing a lymphoma. Progressive unilateral swelling in an enlarged parotid gland in a patient with SS, especially in older females, is suggestive of lymphoma.[113] The developing malignancy is usually a low-grade, monocytoid B-cell lymphoma.[114]

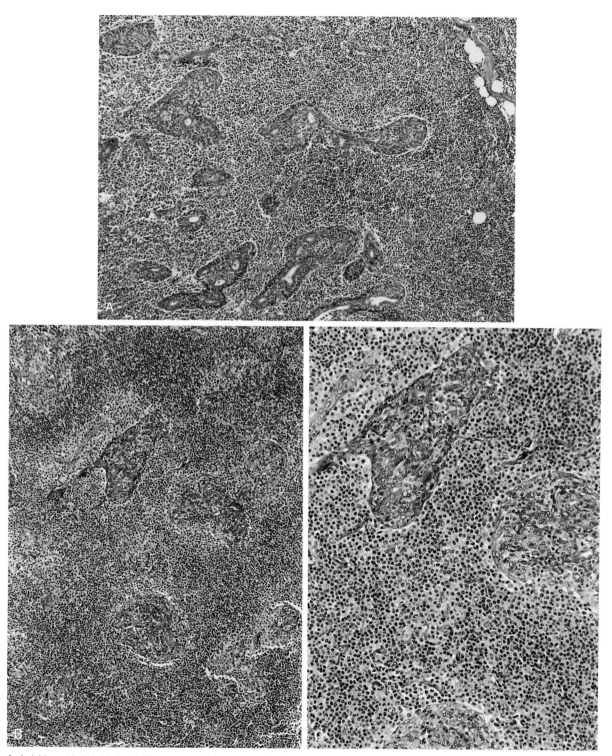

Figure 6–4. *A,* Myoepithelial sialadenitis. There are multiple epimyoepithelial islands, several of which have residual ductal lumina. These islands are surrounded by normal-appearing lymphocytes, which also focally infiltrate the epimyoepithelial islands. *B,* Early low-grade lymphoma. Note numerous myoepithelial islands surrounded by collections of monomorphic medium-sized lymphocytes that contain abundant pale cytoplasm and uniform nuclei. *C,* Higher power detail of *B.* Note epimyoepithelial islands surrounded by a uniform lymphoid population. A monoclonal population of cells was demonstrated using molecular techniques.

Sialolithiasis

Sialolithiasis is a common cause of salivary gland disease with a prevalence rate of approximately 1.2%.[115] Stones occur as a result of calcification of an intraluminal organic nidus such as dried secretion, bacterial colonies, or cellular debris. Ductal inflammation as well as increased viscosity and stasis of saliva have been suggested as predisposing factors.[116] Up to 10% of affected individuals exhibited generalized stone formation in the urinary tract, bile duct system, and salivary glands.[117] Lithiasis is the most common cause of acute and chronic infections involving the major salivary glands.[118] Sequelae of long-standing calculi include chronic sialadenitis, duct dilatation, and gland atrophy.

Clinical Features. Eighty percent of major gland sialoliths occur in the submandibular (Wharton's) duct.[117] The increased viscosity of submandibular saliva and the upward, curved path of the submandibular duct predispose to stone formation in this gland.[119] Twenty percent of stones occur in the parotid (Stensen's) duct[117];

rarely, stones are encountered in the sublingual gland. Minor gland lithiasis occasionally occurs and is most frequently seen in the upper lip and buccal mucosa.[120, 121] Lithiasis is typically unilateral, although occasional patients may present with bilateral or multiple gland involvement.[122] Affected ducts may contain several stones. Stones preferentially affect men, with a peak incidence in the fourth and fifth decades.[117] Up to 4% of cases occur in individuals younger than 20 years of age.[117]

Sialolithiasis is typically diagnosed on clinical and radiographic features. Presenting symptomatology, the result of ductal obstruction, includes episodic swelling and postprandial pain. Fever may accompany secondary acute bacterial infection. Sialolithiasis of minor glands is usually asymptomatic, presenting as a small, firm nodule. Radiography is useful in imaging stones, although 20% and 80% of submandibular and parotid stones, respectively, are radiolucent.[117] Moreover, intraparenchymal sialoliths may be difficult to demonstrate.[120]

Pathologic Features. Sialoliths vary from microscopic to 6.4 cm in diameter.[123] They range from white to yellowish to tan with a smooth or rough surface and may be friable. In cross section, stones frequently exhibit concentric laminations. Microscopically, the ductal epithelium of the affected salivary gland is usually compressed and commonly shows squamous, oncocytic, or mucous cell metaplasia. These metaplastic changes may mimic tumor if sampled via fine needle aspiration.[124] Without treatment for sialolithiasis, recurrent retrograde infection of the gland is common.

Long-standing disease with retention of secretions leads to chronic obstructive sialadenitis. Histologic changes include periductal and lobular chronic inflammatory cell infiltrates, occasional acute inflammation, ductal dilatation, and parenchymal atrophy with scarring. It is important to remember that stones may occur secondarily in association with neoplasms such as acinic cell carcinoma and mucoepidermoid carcinoma,[120] as well as other conditions such as HIV infection.[122]

Treatment and Prognosis. Treatment includes antibiotics in the case of secondary infection and surgical removal of impacted stones. Shock wave lithotripsy also has been used with success.[125] Recurrent or recalcitrant stones with resultant recurring chronic sialadenitis may warrant excision of the affected gland.

Sialadenosis

In contrast with the primary hormonal control of other major gastrointestinal accessory glands, principal regulation of major salivary gland function is via the autonomic nervous system.[126] Through incompletely understood mechanisms, dysregulation of autonomic control may lead to a benign form of salivary gland enlargement called *sialadenosis*.[127] Many conditions have been implicated in the development of sialadenosis, all presumably mediating their effect through the influence of the autonomic nervous system. Reported associations include obesity, starvation, anorexia nervosa, bulimia, starch ingestion, alcoholism, diabetes mellitus, celiac and liver disease, acromegaly, catecholamine excess, and heavy metal intoxication, among others.[128, 129]

Clinical Features. Clinically, sialadenosis presents as painless, recurrent, bilateral (rarely unilateral) swelling of the parotid glands. The peak incidence is in the fifth and sixth decades; there is no apparent gender predilection.[130] The clinical differential diagnosis includes other causes of bilateral salivary gland enlargement, such as sarcoidosis, Sjögren's syndrome, tuberculosis, malignant lymphoma, sialadenitis, gout, and Graves' disease.

Pathologic Features. Microscopically, glands appear essentially normal aside from increased acinar diameter and cytoplasmic changes. Principally, as a result of cellular hypertrophy, the diameter of acini may be two to three times the expected diameter.[130, 131] Hyperplasia has also been implicated in the enlargement process.[128, 132] Individual acinar cells are swollen and appear basophilic (granular form) or translucent (honeycombed or vacuolated pattern). Inflam-

mation is not a feature of sialadenosis. If the disease persists, there is eventual atrophy of the parenchyma with fatty replacement.[128] Fine needle aspiration biopsy has been used successfully to diagnose this lesion.[133]

Treatment and Prognosis. Treatment should be directed toward amelioration of the underlying cause or associated medical condition. Swelling secondary to drugs or hormonal imbalance may resolve if the drug is stopped or if the imbalance is corrected; however, the sialadenosis secondary to cirrhosis, endocrine disorders such as diabetes, or neurogenic abnormalities is resistant to treatment.[134] In bulimia, cessation of vomiting is usually associated with decrease in the size of the affected salivary glands.[129] Standard therapy frequently includes salivary substitutes and sialagogues; surgery may be necessary in cases that are refractory to other forms of therapy.

PRIMARY CYSTIC DISEASE

Primary cystic lesions of the major salivary glands are unusual; neoplasms are largely responsible for cystic change involving the major glands. Thus, the initial obligation of the surgical pathologist when confronted with a cystic salivary gland lesion is to exclude neoplasia (e.g., acinic cell carcinoma, mucoepidermoid carcinoma). However, when encountered in the major glands, primary cystic disease typically occurs in the parotid gland, accounting for 2% to 5% of all parotid lesions.[135] In contrast, primary cystic and pseudocystic lesions are extremely common in the minor salivary glands.

Minor Salivary Glands

Mucocele

Clinical Features. Mucoceles (*mucus extravasation phenomenon*) are the most commonly encountered salivary gland lesions, with a prevalence of 1.4 per 1000 persons.[136] They are pseudocysts resulting from the rupture of minor salivary gland ducts with mucus extravasation into adjacent soft tissue. Proteolytic enzymes may play a role in the pathogenesis of these lesions.[137] Though usually presenting in the first three decades of life, these lesions may be encountered in persons of any age. The lower lip is the most common site of involvement. Mucoceles may arise virtually anywhere within the oral cavity; sites naturally devoid of minor salivary glands, such as the gingiva, are the exception. Often there is a clinical history of trauma to the area.[138] Mucoceles are painless, raised, translucent to bluish-white, soft, fluctuant masses. Superficial lesions appear vesicular; deeper lesions are covered by normal-appearing mucosa.

Pathologic Features. Microscopically, mucoceles show central degenerative spaces, without epithelial linings, which are frequently surrounded by granulation tissue (Fig. 6–5). Variable amounts of eosinophilic extracellular mucin are present in these spaces and can be highlighted on mucicarmine stain. Inflammatory cells, particularly mucin-laden macrophages with vacuolated cytoplasm, are present within the peripheral granulation tissue and pooled mucus. "Feeder" ducts may be evident at the base of the lesion. Adjacent intact minor salivary glands, if present, can exhibit infiltration by inflammatory cells. Rarely, mucoceles may be located so superficially that they simulate subepithelial blistering disease (e.g., bullous lichen planus, mucous membrane pemphigoid) clinically and microscopically.[139] The presence of minor salivary gland acini or ducts in the area of the superficial blister and the finding of adjacent normal surface epithelium supports the diagnosis of a superficial mucocele, as does positive mucicarmine staining.

Treatment and Prognosis. Treatment is excision of the mucocele and the surrounding minor salivary glands. The mucocele may recur if the suspect gland is not completely removed.

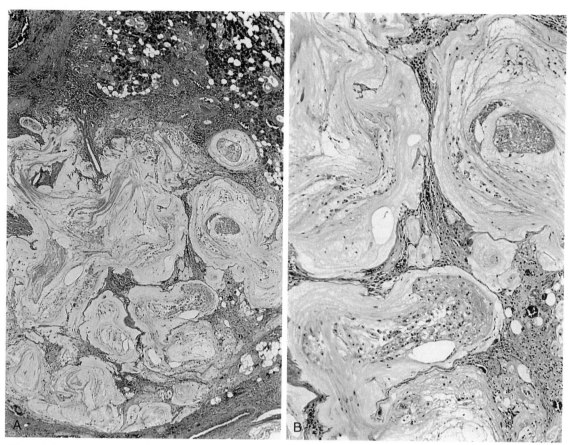

Figure 6–5. Mucocele (mucus extravasation phenomenon). *A,* Multiple pools of extravasated mucin material are seen adjacent to salivary gland tissue. *B,* Higher power detail of the mucin pools, which contain a few macrophages and inflammatory cells.

Mucus Retention Cyst

Clinical Features. *Mucus retention cysts,* or *sialocysts,* though closely related to mucocele, are much less common. Some authors consider mucus retention cysts as a subtype of mucocele[140]; however, it is our preference to separate these two processes, as their pathophysiology is somewhat different. Mucous retention cysts are most commonly seen in the parotid gland where they are known as *salivary duct cysts;* these cysts may also be encountered in minor salivary glands (Fig. 6–6*A,* see p. 338).[141] Representing true cysts with epithelial linings, they develop as a consequence of duct obstruction. The cause of obstruction is typically not detectable, although occasionally a microlith or inspissated secretion may be seen. Patients are usually older than those affected by mucocele; the average age was 45 years in one study.[142] Retention cysts typically occur at sites away from the lip[143] and an antecedent history of trauma is not typical.[142]

Pathologic Features. Generally unicystic, lesions rarely may be multicystic or show ectasia of the adjacent ducts.[143] Retention cysts exhibit a lining epithelium that is composed of cuboidal to columnar cells (apocrine-like snouting may be present), although mucous cells and squamous epithelium may be seen (Fig. 6–6*B,* see p. 338). The epithelial basement membrane of the cyst may appear thickened and the surrounding stroma loose and edematous. Less commonly, oncocytoid change and proliferative papillary changes of the epithelium are encountered. When such are present, these cysts have been referred to as *reactive oncocytoid cysts* and *mucopapillary cysts.*[142]

Retention cysts must be distinguished from true neoplasms of minor salivary gland origin, such as mucoepidermoid carcinoma, inverted ductal papilloma,[144] sialadenoma papilliferum,[145] intraductal papilloma, and cystadenoma.[146, 147] The presence of mucous cells, especially when hyperplastic, in benign cysts can make separation from mucoepidermoid carcinoma difficult. Distinction is based on proliferative activity of mucoepidermoid carcinoma as evidenced by increased cell stratification and expansive growth. Sialadenoma papilliferum and inverted ductal papillomas are both associated with greater degrees of epithelial proliferation than one typically finds in retention cysts and, in addition, the former is associated with a surface papillary component while in the latter the epithelial proliferation is growing down into a dilated duct. The distinction from cystadenoma may be, admittedly, subjective; it is our preference to classify cysts with proliferative papillary changes as papillary cystadenomas if they are multilocular and as intraductal papilloma if they are unicystic.

Treatment and Prognosis. These cysts are treated by complete but conservative surgical excision. They should not recur if completely excised.

Major Salivary Glands

Cystic lesions of the major salivary glands are relatively rare and constitute no more than 5% of primary parotid lesions. Etiologies of cystic disease are diverse, and for classification these may be divided broadly into primary and secondary forms. Aside from salivary duct cysts (retention cysts) and AIDS-related parotid cysts, primary forms of cystic disease are unusual and include benign lymphoepithelial cysts, branchial cleft cysts,[148–150] dermoid cysts,[151, 152] keratinous cysts,[153] and polycystic (dysgenetic) disease of the parotid glands.[154, 155]

Salivary Duct Cysts

Clinical Features. *Salivary duct cysts,* or *sialocysts,* usually arise in the parotid gland. Similar in pathogenesis and histology to mucus retention cysts (see earlier discussion) of minor gland origin, *salivary duct cysts* represent true cysts with epithelial linings. Though these cysts develop as a consequence of duct obstruction, the cause of obstruction is typically not detectable. Patients most commonly present in the fifth decade of life with a slowly enlarging, painless, mass-like lesion.

Pathologic Features. Generally unilocular, lesions rarely may be multicystic or show ectasia of the adjacent ducts. Metaplasia of the epithelial lining is common; cuboidal or columnar, squamous, mucous (goblet), and clear cells may be seen. Focal epithelial proliferations into the cyst lumen may occur and must be distinguished, as in minor salivary gland lesions, from neoplasia. The primary differential diagnostic considerations are cystadenoma and low-grade mucoepidermoid carcinoma and a unicystic acinic cell carcinoma. Distinguishing between the first two entities has already been discussed (see under mucus retention cyst). Finding a focally thickened mucosal lining with papillary projections and periodic acid–Schiff (PAS)–positive, diastase-resistant cytoplasmic granules will allow classification of an unicystic lesion as an acinic cell carcinoma. The absence of lymphoid infiltrates, along with clinical features, serves to distinguish salivary duct cysts, with or without proliferative changes, from Warthin's tumor and branchial cleft cysts. Secondary development of neoplasia within such cysts is very rare.

Treatment and Prognosis. These cysts are treated by complete but conservative surgical excision. They should not recur if completely excised.

Ranula

Clinical Features. *Ranula* (meaning "frog-like" in Latin) is a clinical variant of mucocele that presents as a large swelling in the floor of the mouth. Contrasting mucoceles, ranulas represent a mucus extravasation phenomenon of *major* salivary gland origin. Occurring principally from the sublingual gland, they arise from excretory duct disruption. A minority of lesions may extend through the geniohyoglossus (mylohyoid) muscle and deeper soft tissue to produce a submental or lateral neck swelling termed *plunging* or *cervical ranula.*[156] Occasionally, they may extend into the mediastinum. In contrast with minor salivary gland mucoceles, ranulas produce larger, more noticeable swelling that typically causes minimal discomfort; rarely, however, they can lead to airway compromise. Clinically, cervical ranulas may simulate bursae, angiomas (cystic hygroma), and other potential midline submental-neck lesions such as dermoid cyst, lymphadenopathy, and hematoma. If an associated intraoral ranula is lacking, the diagnostic difficulty of cervical ranula is greatly enhanced.[157] Affected individuals are generally children or young adults. The mean age of patients in one clinical review of "plunging" ranula was 8 years.[158] Reported cases of congenital ranula are attributable to in utero obstruction of a functioning sublingual gland.[159]

Pathologic Features. Microscopically, the appearance is similar to mucocele, although foamy histiocytes tend to be particularly prominent in the pseudocyst wall and inflammatory cells may be inconspicuous.[156] Biopsy of a lateral neck presentation may consist only of amorphous material with rare inflammatory cells. Identifying the amorphous material as mucin will help establish the correct diagnosis.

Treatment and Prognosis. Since recurrence is the rule with simple excision, the treatment for ranula is complete excision of the lesion including the involved sublingual gland.

Acquired Immunodeficiency Syndrome–Related Parotid Cysts

Kaposi's sarcoma, candidal or herpetic oropharyngitis, and cervical lymphadenopathy are the three most common presenting head and neck complaints for HIV infection.[160–164] Less commonly, patients with AIDS develop cystic and solid intraparotid tumors which have been referred to as either cystic benign lymphoepithelial lesion, or benign lymphoepithelial lesion (BLEL) in AIDS, or AIDS-related parotid cysts (ARPC).[165–178] The term ARPC is recommended, as the other terminology may cloud the distinctions between BLEL and AIDS, two clinically and prognostically different entities.

Clinical Features. Patients typically present with unilateral or bilateral painless enlarging masses; imaging studies reveal that bilaterality is the rule rather than the exception, even when the involvement clinically appears unilateral.[167–168] Cervical lymphadenopathy and nasopharyngeal swelling commonly accompany the parotid findings.

Pathologic Features. ARPC appears as cystic spaces lined by squamous epithelium, accompanied by abundant reactive lymphoid stroma (Fig. 6–7, see p. 339). Florid follicular hyperplasia, loss of mantle zone lymphocytes, and follicle lysis can be seen. The lesions may have an encapsulated, segmented appearance, or the inflammatory infiltrate can extend into the parotid parenchyma without encapsulation. Epimyoepithelial islands, identical to those seen in BLEL, can often be observed. Warthin-Finkeldey type multinucleated giant cells may also be seen within involved lymph nodes.

As far as the relationship between ARPC, BLEL, and SS goes, the majority of patients with ARPC have no autoimmune symptomatology and lack serum autoimmune antibodies. The prevailing theory is that ARPC are the result of AIDS-related hyperplastic adenopathy (persistent generalized lymphadenopathy) of periparotid or intraparotid lymph nodes causing obstruction, squamous metaplasia, and cystification of intranodal ducts. However, a recent study by Ihrler and colleagues did not support this theory.[178] They found that lymphoid infiltrates commonly affect parotid parenchyma, inducing striated duct basal cell hyperplasia, which results in BLEL-like morphologic changes. The early changes consisted of periductal lymphoid infiltrates, whereas later changes included intensification of inflammatory infiltrates, ductal cell hyperplasia, lymphoepithelial island formation, and cystification.

A small, distinct subgroup of AIDS patients also have Sjögren's-type symptoms of xerostomia, xerophthalmia, and arthritic pain[165, 166, 171, 172, 179]; however, autoantibodies (antinuclear antibodies) have been identified in only one of all the reported patients.[171] Labial biopsies of minor salivary glands have revealed, for some patients, severe sialadenitis on par with that seen in Sjögren's disease. Nonetheless, although ARPC and the BLEL of SS share similar histologic features, their underlying pathophysiology is different and therefore warrants separate clinical and pathologic designations.

Differential Diagnosis. There can be significant morphologic overlap between the individual features of ARPC and BLEL; obviously there is an enormous clinical impact from this differential diagnosis, as ARPC may herald the diagnosis of HIV infection. Epimyoepithelial islands, a prominent feature of BLEL, may also be observed in ARPC. Warthin-Finkeldey–type multinucleated giant cells are more often seen in ARPC but are occasionally seen in BLEL. BLEL also tends to be less cystic and generally more solid, although cystic change has been observed in 3% of BLEL.[180]

Benign lymphoepithelial cysts may also be included in the differential diagnosis. These lesions, of disputed origin, appear as unilocular simple cysts within intraparotid lymph nodes. They are usually lined by keratinizing squamous epithelium, less frequently by columnar, cuboidal, ciliated, or mucinous epithelium, and there is a prominent lymphoid infiltrate in their walls. The adjacent salivary parenchyma is usually normal, and epimyoepithelial islands are not seen.

Cystadenomata, discussed in a later section, are rare benign multicystic tumors that need to be considered in the differential diagnosis of ARPC. The lymphoid infiltrate is usually lacking in cystadenoma, and, unlike in ARPC, there are frequent intraluminal papillary projections. Other potentially cystic neoplasms (e.g., papillocystic acinic cell carcinoma, low-grade mucoepidermoid carcinoma, Warthin's tumor, cystadenocarcinoma) can be distin-

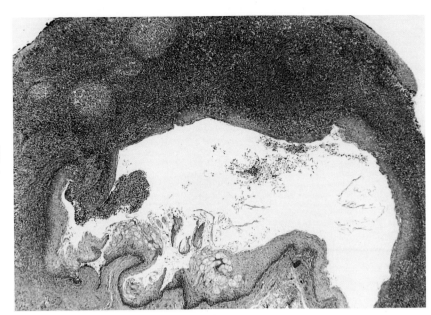

Figure 6–8. Benign lymphoepithelial cyst. The cyst lining is stratified squamous epithelium, which is surrounded almost completely by a dense lymphoid infiltrate containing several reactive lymphoid follicles.

guished from ARPC by careful examination of the histologic constituents.

Treatment and Prognosis. An established radiologic and cytologic diagnosis of ARPC obviates the need for surgical excision. Patients treated by fine needle aspiration may develop recollection of cyst fluid and may require periodic fine needle aspiration.[176]

Benign Lymphoepithelial Cyst

Clinical Features. These rare lesions have in the past been erroneously termed "branchial" cysts. This terminology is misleading, since the probable origin of these lesions is from intra-lymph nodal salivary gland inclusions, as proposed by Bernier and Bhaskar.[181] However, there are still proponents of origin from the branchial apparatus.[182] Without distinctive clinical features, these lesions arise primarily in adults, presenting as painless masses. They have a predilection for men (1.6 to 2.9 : 1) in many series[182]; however, Olsen et al.[183] reported a 5 : 1 female to male ratio for intraparotid cysts and an equal sex incidence for periparotid cysts.

The average age of presentation is in the mid-40s to early 50s with a range in several series of 13 to 81 years.[182, 183] Rare cases have been associated with facial paralysis. The vast majority of lymphoepithelial cysts are unilateral; however, rare patients present with bilateral involvement.[182, 183] The cysts measure up to 6 cm in diameter (average 2.5 cm), are well circumscribed, and generally present within and around the parotid gland. Histologically similar lesions may occur within the mucosa of the oral cavity.[184]

Pathologic Features. Grossly, the cysts are well circumscribed and predominantly unilocular; a multilocular presentation is unusual. The cyst content is variable, ranging from fluid to mucoid to yellow-white and caseous in appearance. The luminal surface is frequently granular. Microscopically, the typical lesion is an encapsulated smooth-walled cyst, free of internal papillae, lined by a stratified squamous epithelium, although cuboidal, columnar, mucous, and sebaceous cells may be present (Fig. 6–8).[185] The epithelium may acquire a "mucoepidermoid" appearance.[186] The cyst wall exhibits dense lymphoid tissue composed of small lymphocytes, plasma cells, germinal centers, and a surrounding thick band of collagen. The nodal origin of the lesion can frequently be demonstrated by the persistence of subcapsular or medullary sinusoids. However, a nodal origin cannot be postulated for the intraoral lesions.

Benign lymphoepithelial cysts must be distinguished from cystic BLEL, Warthin's tumor, low-grade mucoepidermoid carcinoma, true branchial cleft cyst, and a simple keratinous cyst. Distinction from BLEL may be difficult. BLEL contains characteristic epimyoepithelial islands and hyaline basement membrane–like material and typically lacks features of a lymph node. Warthin's tumor is identified by its characteristic double-layered papillary oncocytic epithelium. Features favoring benign lymphoepithelial cyst over low-grade mucoepidermoid carcinoma include lack of mucous cells, the presence of prominent lymphoid stroma, and lack of complex architectural growth.[186] True branchial cleft cysts occurring within the parotid gland are very rare, and their identification is aided by the presence of medial extension or a stalk of attachment to the ear canal or pharyngeal wall.

Branchial Cleft and Other Congenital Cysts

True branchial cleft cysts within the major glands are very rare; however, a few cases within the parotid gland have been reported.[148–150] Branchial cleft cysts and sinuses, vestigial remnants of the branchial apparatus, typically represent remnants of the second or third branchial groove and occur in the lateral neck. Remnants of the first branchial groove, presenting within and adjacent to the parotid gland, constitute less than 1% of all branchial anomalies. Clinical correlation is necessary to make this diagnosis. Histologically, lesions occurring within salivary gland appear identical to branchial cleft cysts present elsewhere. Since the microscopic appearance may be indistinguishable from benign lymphoepithelial cyst, the presence of an accompanying sinus tract or stalk serves to identify the branchial cleft origin.

Rarely, *epidermoid, dermoid,* or unusual *congenital cysts* occur within or adjacent to the major salivary glands.[187–189] Dermoid cysts generally occur mid-line in the floor of the mouth. Distinction from epidermoid cysts is based on the presence of skin adnexa in dermoid cysts. The mid-line location and the lack of a lymphoid infiltrate, moreover, aids in distinguishing dermoid cysts from branchial cleft remnants.

Miscellaneous Non-neoplastic Cystic Lesions

Secondary forms of cystic change may accompany any obstructive process (e.g., calculi), with or without superimposed infection, resulting in inflammation of and damage to the salivary gland ducts. Surgical intervention and trauma have been implicated in the development of secondary cysts and sialoceles.[190, 191] The latter are usually superficial, soft, and filled with saliva. Primary inflammatory processes, as seen in SS and HIV infection, may have a similar effect, leading to cystic degeneration.[192]

Other oddities include gaseous cysts of Stensen's duct, described in glassblowers and musicians,[193] echinococcal cysts in the parotid and submandibular glands,[194, 195] and pneumoparotid.[196]

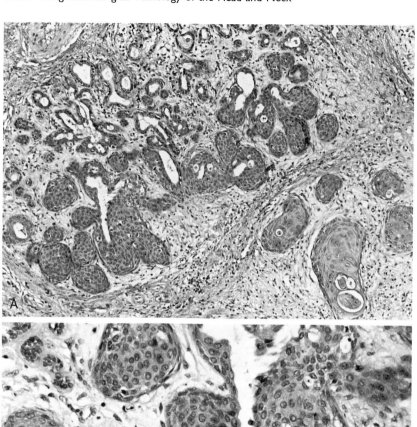

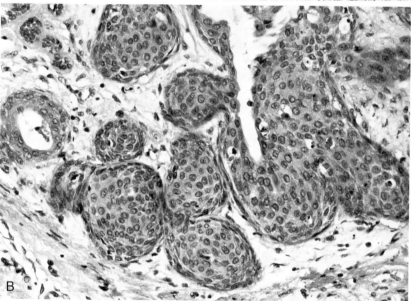

Figure 6–9. Necrotizing sialometaplasia. *A,* The normal salivary gland lobular architecture has been retained; however, there is marked acinar atrophy with replacement by islands of squamous metaplasia. *B,* Higher power detail demonstrating uniform smooth-edged nests of squamous epithelium with several residual ductal lumina. This latter feature is important in separating this lesion from squamous cell carcinoma.

Cystic lesions occurring in proximity to the parotid may be mistaken for primary parotid disease. Most keratinous (epidermoid) cysts presenting as parotid lesions truly arise in the dermis or hypocutis of the skin superficial to the parotid gland.[197] All non-neoplastic cysts should be amenable to limited surgical excision.[198]

TUMOR-LIKE LESIONS

Necrotizing Sialometaplasia

Clinical Features. Necrotizing sialometaplasia (NSM) is a benign, self-healing, necrotizing, variably ulcerative, reactive inflammatory condition of unknown cause. Trauma or some other cause of vascular compromise has been implicated as the most likely etiology for NSM.[199–201] It is also associated with long-term intubation complicated by herpetic infection of the trachea[202, 203] and with local anesthetic injection.[204] It typically arises in the minor salivary glands of the oral cavity, usually involving the palate (77% of patients).[199] NSM less frequently occurs in the major salivary glands (8.7%)[199] and rarely involves the seromucinous glands of the nasopharynx, nose, paranasal sinuses, larynx, and trachea.[199–215] A similar process

has also been described in the breast, skin, and lung,[216–218] and rare cases have been described in dogs.[219] NSM was initially described as a clinicopathologic entity by Abrams and colleagues[210] in 1973, and, although it is a benign process, it may clinically and pathologically simulate a mucoepidermoid or squamous carcinoma, leading to misdiagnosis and overtreatment.[199, 200, 208–210]

The majority of intraoral cases present with ulceration, but in its early stages, NSM may be nonulcerating and simulate a neoplasm due to soft tissue swelling. The ulcer is usually small, with an average size of 1.8 cm (range, 0.7–5 cm in greatest dimension) and may be bilateral (12% of cases).[199] These are usually painful lesions (63%) and patients may also present with numbness (13%); slightly less than one quarter of patients are asymptomatic. Rarely, palatal bone may be involved by this process. The average age of presentation is 45.9 years (range, 1.5–83 years), the male to female ratio is approximately 2:1, and the average duration of symptoms is 3 weeks, with an upper range of up to 6 months.[199]

Pathologic Features and Differential Diagnosis. Histologically, NSM is characterized by various degrees of lobular necrosis and sialadenitis intermixed with squamous metaplasia of excretory ducts and acini (Fig. 6–9). In minor salivary gland or seromucinous gland sites, one may also see pseudoepitheliomatous hyperplasia of

Text continued on page 349

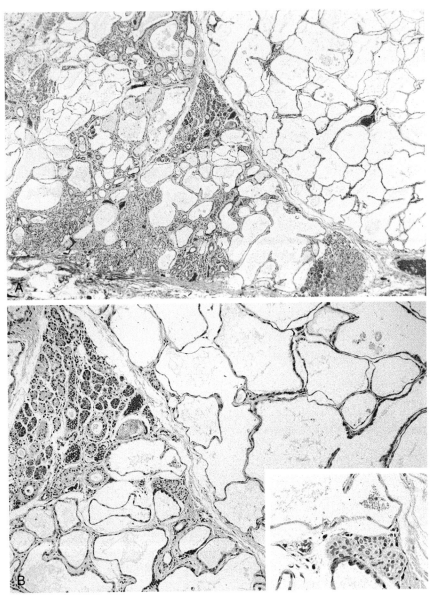

Figure 6–2. Polycystic disease. *A*, Multiple honeycomb-like cystic spaces are replacing portions of salivary gland lobules to different degrees. *B*, Higher power detail. The cystic spaces are lined by a thin layer of flattened epithelium. Focally, a few cells are reactive *(inset)*.

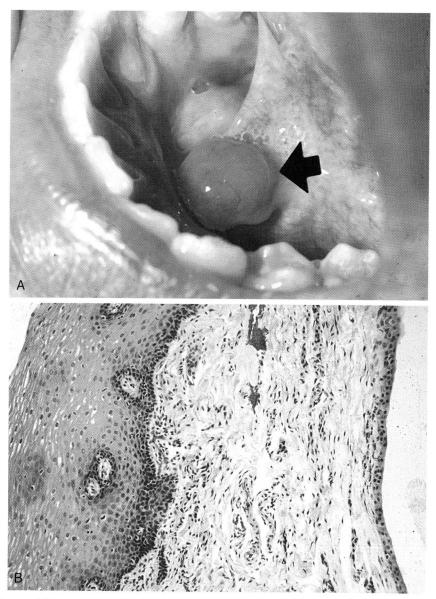

Figure 6–6. Mucus retention cyst. *A,* Note nodular swelling *(arrow)* covered by a thin, somewhat translucent mucosa. (Courtesy of Dr. Jerry Bouquot.) *B,* The submucosal cyst is lined by a thin uniform cuboidal to columnar epithelium *(right side).*

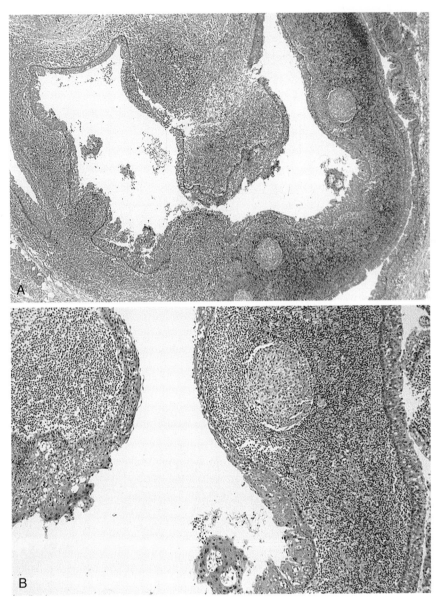

Figure 6–7. AIDS-related parotid cyst. *A,* There is a dilated cyst surrounded by a dense lymphoid stroma containing numerous lymphoid follicles. *B,* Higher power detail. The cyst lining is composed of a bland stratified squamous and columnar epithelium.

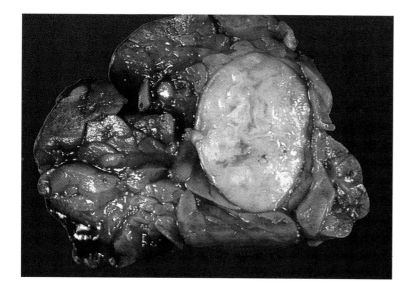

Figure 6–11. Benign mixed tumor of the submandibular gland demonstrating a firm, whitish-tan, well-encapsulated mass.

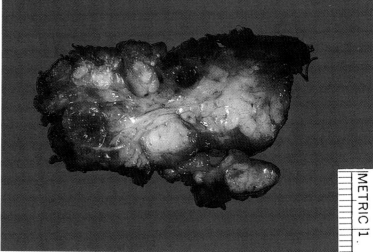

Figure 6–12. Recurrent mixed tumor. There are multiple, oval nodules of whitish-tan tumor in this parotid gland typical of a recurrence.

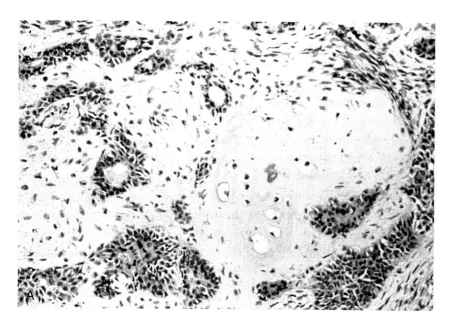

Figure 6–13. A, Mixed tumor with prominent cartilaginous differentiation and surrounding ducts and myoepithelial cells.

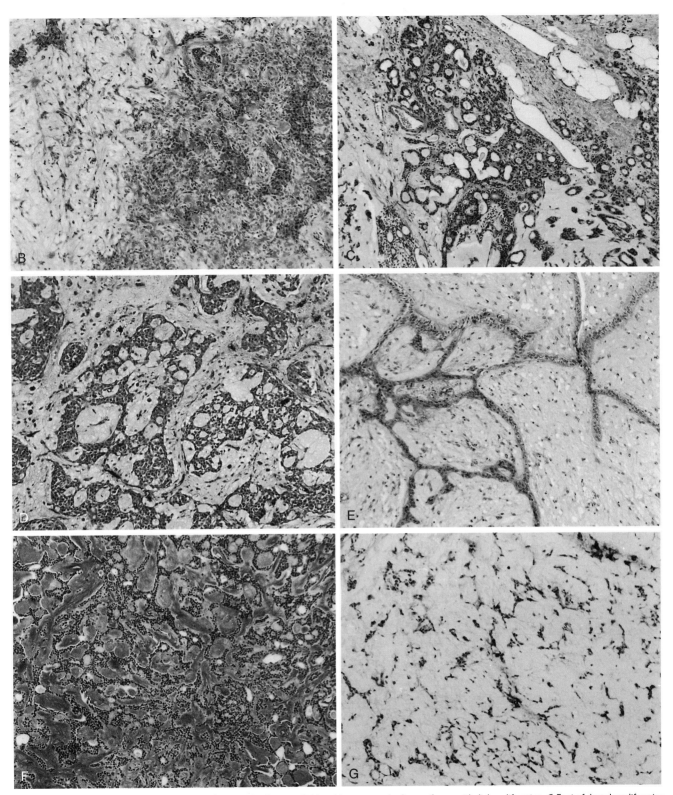

Figure 6–13 *Continued. B–G,* Various patterns in benign mixed tumor. *B,* Myxoid stroma and a focus of myoepithelial proliferation. *C,* Foci of ductal proliferation. *D,* A loose lattice-work of myoepithelial cells in a myxoid stroma. *E,* Thin delicate cords of myoepithelial cells in a loose myxoid stroma. *F,* Interconnecting cords of myoepithelial cells with focal ductal differentiation in a densely hyalinized background. *G,* Diffuse myxoid change with scattered, stellate-appearing modified myoepithelial cells.

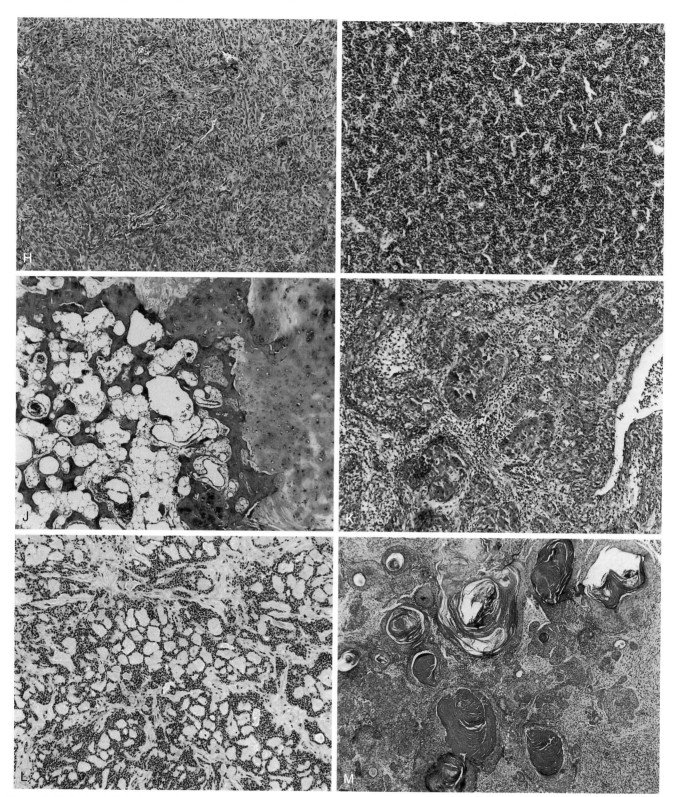

Figure 6–13 *Continued. H–M,* Additional patterns of benign mixed tumor. *H,* An extremely cellular area of myoepithelial proliferation. *I,* Densely packed interconnecting cords of modified myoepithelial cells. *J,* Focus of osseous metaplasia and cartilage. *K,* Foci of oncocytic metaplasia. *L,* Adenoid cystic carcinoma–like changes. *M,* Focus of prominent squamous metaplasia.

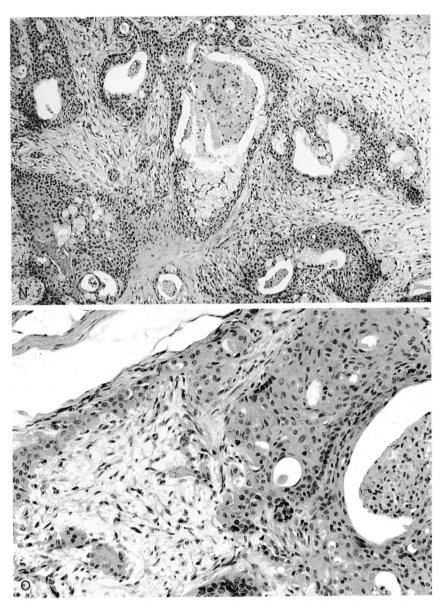

Figure 6–13 *Continued.* *N,* Benign mixed tumor with foci of prominent mucoepidermoid metaplasia. *O,* Detail from an adjacent area of part *N* demonstrating areas of ductal differentiation with peripheral plasmacytoid myoepithelial cells. Plasmacytoid myoepithelial cells are not found in mucoepidermoid carcinoma, thereby confirming the diagnosis of mixed tumor. In addition, the stroma is more cellular than one finds in a mucoepidermoid carcinoma.

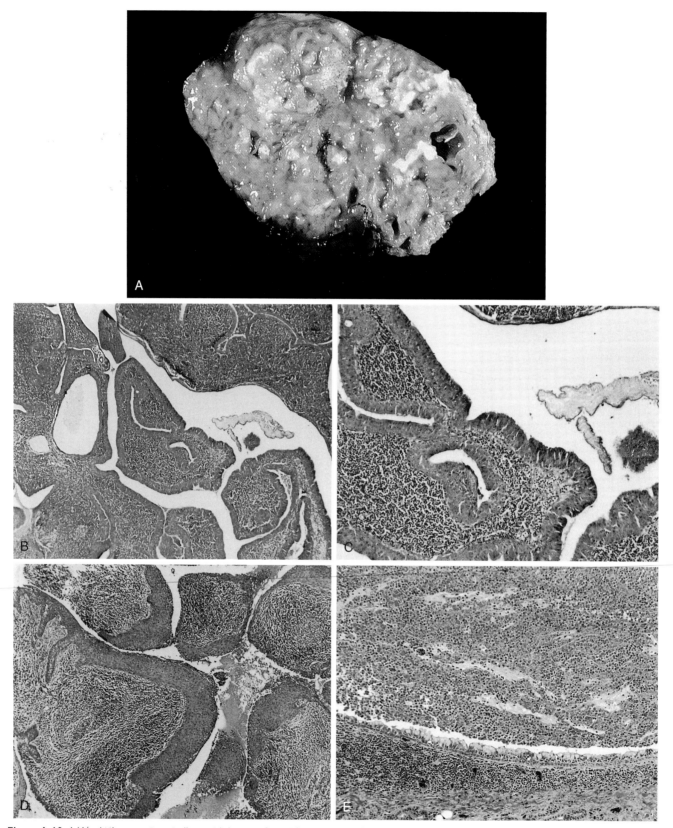

Figure 6–19. *A,* Warthin's tumor is typically tannish-brown, often with cystic spaces. In addition, this tumor demonstrates areas of degeneration and necrosis (yellowish foci). *B–E,* Warthin's tumor is composed of papillary fronds lined by two layers of oncocytic epithelium surrounded by lymphoid stroma *(B and C).* Occasionally, foci of prominent squamous metaplasia *(D)* and/or of mucinous metaplasia *(E)* may be seen within this tumor. These foci may cause diagnostic confusion with mucoepidermoid carcinoma in a fine needle aspiration biopsy specimen.

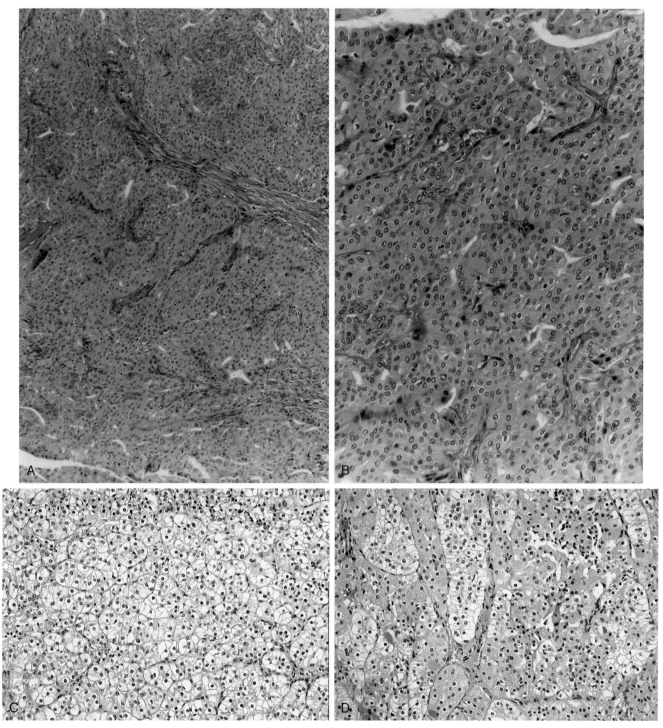

Figure 6–24. *A* and *B,* Oncocytoma is composed of a sheet of oncocytic cells with uniform, predominantly centrally located nuclei and abundant eosinophilic cytoplasm. Clear cell oncocytoma composed predominantly of sheets of clear cells *(C)* with focal areas containing typical oncocytic cells *(D)*.

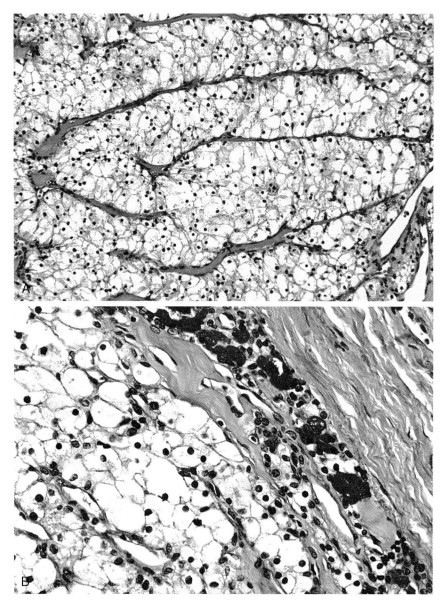

Figure 6–31. Acinic cell carcinoma, clear cell variant. *A,* The majority of this tumor (>98%) was composed of sheets of clear cells with slightly pleomorphic, eccentrically located nuclei and abundant clear cytoplasm. *B,* Periodic acid–Schiff (PAS) stain. Note detail of clear cells *(left).* Very focally within the sheets of clear cells and at the periphery of a few of the sheets were cells with abundant, slightly purplish granular cytoplasm that stained positive with a diastase-treated PAS stain, confirming the diagnosis of acinic cell carcinoma.

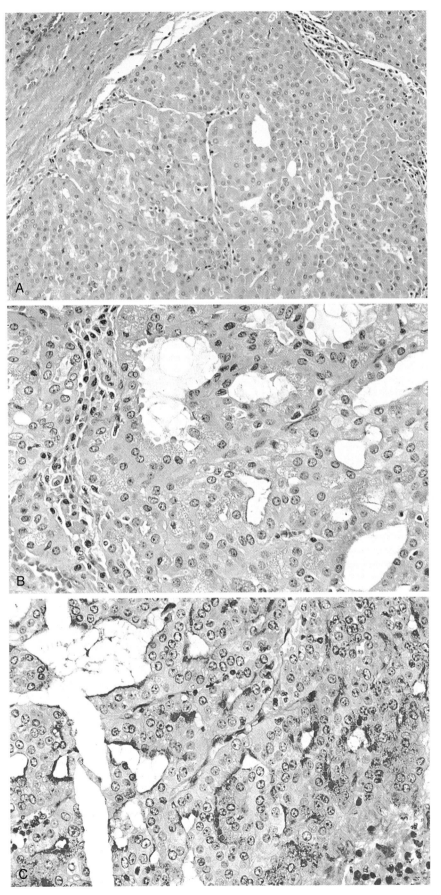

Figure 6–33. Acinic cell carcinoma, oncocytic variant. A, The majority of this tumor was composed of sheets of typical oncocytic cells with bland nuclei and abundant eosinophilic cytoplasm. B, Focally, the tumor had slightly more pleomorphic nuclei, cystic change, and, in addition to areas of eosinophilic cytoplasm, a grayish-purple cytoplasmic granularity was noted. C, A diastase-treated periodic acid–Schiff (PAS) stain demonstrated numerous fine PAS-positive cytoplasmic granules toward the luminal side of the tumor cells, supporting the diagnosis of the oncocytic variant of acinic cell carcinoma. Electron microscopy (not shown) confirmed the presence of both mitochondria and zymogen granules.

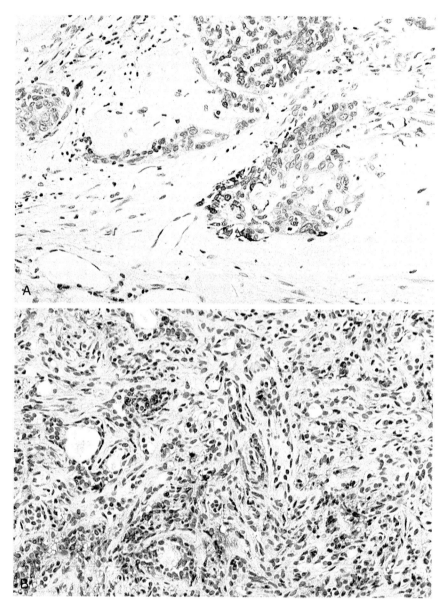

Figure 6–36. Glial fibrillary acidic protein immunohistochemical stain. *A*, Polymorphous low-grade adenocarcinoma. There was only focal epithelial staining; no staining was seen in the stroma. *B*, Cellular mixed tumor. There was staining in the myoepithelial stromal cells as well as focal ductal staining. The stromal staining confirms the diagnosis of mixed tumor.

the overlying surface epithelium. Extremely early lesions may have lobules that demonstrate complete or partial necrosis with minimal or almost no inflammation; occasionally, mucin pooling within the areas of necrosis and granulation tissue may be seen. As this process evolves, one usually finds areas of lobular necrosis associated with acute and chronic inflammation and histiocytes involving the areas of necrosis as well as in the interlobular septa; occasionally, early foci of squamous metaplasia may be present. Older lesions have well-developed squamous metaplasia and usually have a greater degree of inflammation, edema, and fibrosis; foci of necrosis may not be present at this stage, since they may have already healed.

The main differential diagnostic considerations are with squamous cell carcinoma and mucoepidermoid carcinoma. The uniformity and bland cytologic appearance of the squamous cells arranged in a lobular fashion and the location of residual ductal lumina in one or more of these squamous nests strongly support a benign metaplastic process.[200] Also, the lack of incorporated mucous cells in the squamous epithelium can help distinguish it from mucoepidermoid carcinoma. A history of previous surgery or trauma is helpful; however, not all cases of NSM will be associated with an obvious etiology. Occasionally, severe regenerative atypia may accompany NSM, making it difficult to distinguish this process from neoplastic involvement of seromucinous glands with 100% certainty.[220] One can usually separate NSM from tumor extension down excretory ducts by looking for smooth-edged squamous nests arranged in a lobular fashion with residual ductal lumina and by demonstrating extension of the atypical epithelial population from the overlying mucosa.

Treatment and Prognosis. The treatment is observation only, as NSM will heal spontaneously without therapeutic intervention. NSM may arise in association with a benign or malignant lesion.[199, 200] Because of the latter association, close follow-up is necessary until the lesion heals completely. This will usually occur within 5 to 6 weeks.[199]

Sclerosing Polycystic Adenosis

Sclerosing polycystic adenosis is a recently described rare pseudoneoplastic reactive inflammatory process somewhat similar to sclerosing adenosis of the breast. It was first reported in 1996 by Smith and colleagues,[199] who described a series of nine patients from the Armed Forces Institute of Pathology (AFIP). Since this initial report, there have been only two other series, bringing the total number of cases in the literature to 18.[221, 222]

Clinical Features. Patients ranged in age from 12 to 63 years (mean 29.4 years), with a male to female ratio of 2:7. Sixteen cases presented in the parotid gland and two in the submandibular gland. Presenting symptoms ranged from 10 days to 2 years. Patients typically presented with a slow-growing mass; three had, in addition, pain or a "tingling" sensation.

Pathologic Features. Grossly, most tumors were firm or rubbery, were well circumscribed, and were embedded in normal salivary gland; five were multinodular. Tumors ranged in size from 1 to 7 cm in greatest dimension and had cut surfaces that were pale and glistening; a few had tiny visible cysts, 1 to 2 mm in diameter. Microscopically, all tumors were similar. They were unencapsulated and consisted of multiple, densely sclerotic, irregularly defined lobules composed of abundant hyalinized collagen surrounding areas of ductal cystic change. Hyperplasia of ductal and acinar elements with areas of apocrine-like metaplasia were typical (Fig. 6–10). In addition, mucin-containing cells, squamous cells, and ballooned cells occasionally lined ducts and cystic spaces. The intraluminal epithelial proliferation infrequently formed a cribriform pattern, some of which was associated with nesting basement membrane–like material, similar to collagenous spherulosis of the breast. Occasionally, foci of prominent acinar proliferation were seen to a degree that mimicked acinic cell carcinoma (Fig. 6–10C, D). Although focally there were atypical areas, the normal lobular architecture was always

maintained. Eosinophilic intracytoplasmic zymogen granules were seen in some of the acinar-type cells. A chronic inflammatory infiltrate ranging from sparse to dense was associated with the epithelial proliferation. The epithelial lining of occasional ducts was partially or completely denuded and replaced by xanthomatous macrophages. We have seen a patient with a parotid case, with a prominent benign lipomatous component.

Immunohistochemistry demonstrated preservation of the normal lobular structure and positive staining of the tubuloacinar elements with keratin, whereas myoepithelial markers, S100, and smooth muscle actin were found in the flattened myoepithelial cells surrounding ductal and acinar structures (Fig. 6–10E, F).[221]

Differential Diagnosis. Differential diagnosis consists of polycystic (dysgenetic) disease, sclerosing sialadenitis, pleomorphic adenoma, and a carcinoma. The former consists of a diffusely honeycombed, lattice-like network of cysts with inspissated intracystic secretions replacing the normal parenchyma, with only small clusters of residual acini. Unlike sclerosing polycystic adenosis, fibrosis is not prominent and ductal and acinar proliferation is not seen. Sclerosing sialadenitis has prominent fibrosis with varying degrees of chronic inflammation; however, unlike sclerosing polycystic adenosis, the fibrosis does not form nodules and the salivary gland parenchyma is atrophic without ductal or acinar hyperplasia. The proliferation of ducts with surrounding basement membrane may appear like a pleomorphic adenoma. The lobulated growth pattern and a definite mesenchymal component weigh against that diagnosis. The acinic cell and ductal proliferation also suggests a diagnosis of acinic cell carcinoma or of an adenocarcinoma. However, the lobular architecture is always maintained, the atypical nests are rimmed by myoepithelial cells, and the invasive, destructive growth of a carcinoma is lacking.

Treatment and Prognosis. Until more cases with longer follow-up are available, treatment should consist of complete surgical excision with good surgical margins. Follow-up information is available in the AFIP series of six cases (mean, 43 months; range, 7 months to 9 years) and for two of the cases reported by Donath and Seifert.[223] To date, four cases have recurred; one patient had a single recurrence at 4 years 8 months, a second had multiple recurrences over a 9-year period,[221] and two patients had recurrences at 8 years.[223] The other two patients reported in Donath and Seifert's series were alive without evidence of disease at unknown lengths of time.[223] In addition, none of the five cases reported by Batsakis has recurred.[222]

NEOPLASMS
Classification

Over the past 40 years, our knowledge of salivary gland pathology, including the classification and behavior of many of the tumors, has been evolving. The first AFIP salivary gland atlas of tumor pathology was published in 1954. It listed five specific types of benign tumors and four types of carcinomas, including six subtypes of adenocarcinoma (Table 6–1).[224] Over the next 40 years, the classification schemes have increased in complexity (Tables 6–2 through 6–5).[225–228] In 1972, the World Health Organization (WHO) published its first classification of salivary gland tumors (Table 6–2).[225] This introduced the term *monomorphic adenoma,* changed the term *papillary cystadenoma lymphomatosum* to *adenolymphoma* and changed *acinic cell adenocarcinoma* to *acinic cell tumor.* Two years later, Thackray and Lucas published the second AFIP atlas of tumor pathology.[226] Their classification scheme was similar to the WHO classification (Table 6–3). Thackray and Lucas additionally defined other specific types of monomorphic adenomas, including the *clear cell adenoma,* which was later reclassified as epithelial-myoepithelial carcinoma in the most recent WHO classification, and they added malignant lymphoepithelial lesion to the carcinoma category.

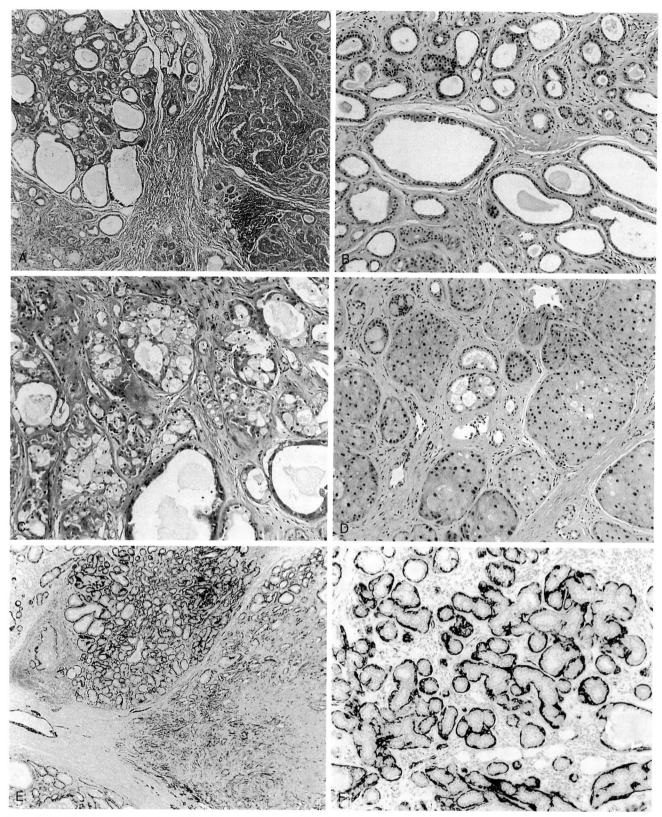

Figure 6–10. Sclerosing polycystic adenosis. The lobular architecture of the salivary gland is maintained *(A and E).* The lobules are composed of hyalinized collagen surrounding cystically dilated ducts *(B and C),* as well as foci of acinar cell proliferation *(C and D). E* and *F* show smooth muscle actin immunohistochemical stains, which demonstrate maintenance of the normal lobular architecture. A myoepithelial cell layer is seen surrounding virtually every one of the proliferating ducts, similar to sclerosing adenosis of the breast.

Table 6–1. Classification of Salivary Gland Neoplasms by Foote and Frazell (1954)

Benign
  Mixed tumor
  Papillary cystadenomata lymphomatosa
  Oxyphil adenoma
  Sebaceous cell adenoma
  Benign lymphoepithelial lesion
  Unclassified
Malignant
  Malignant mixed tumor
  Mucoepidermoid tumor
  Squamous cell carcinoma
  Adenocarcinoma
    Adenoid cystic
    Trabecular or solid
    Anaplastic
    Mucous cell
    Pseudoadamantine
    Acinic cell
  Unclassified

From Foote FW Jr, Frazell EL: Atlas of Tumor Pathology. Tumors of the Major Salivary Glands. 1st Series, Fascicle 11, Washington, DC: Armed Forces Institute of Pathology, 1954.

In 1991, the WHO published its revised classification of salivary gland tumors, greatly expanding the number of different tumor types (Table 6–4).[227] The adenolymphoma was again renamed, this time as Warthin tumor; canalicular adenoma was separated out from basal cell adenoma; and the ductal papillomas, benign myoepithelioma, and cystadenoma were added to the adenoma category. Acinic cell and mucoepidermoid "tumors" were definitively included in the carcinoma category, finally recognizing that all of these tumors have the ability to metastasize. The most significant new addition to the carcinoma group was polymorphous low-grade adenocarcinoma. Additional new tumors include sebaceous carcinoma, basal cell adenocarcinoma, epithelial-myoepithelial carcinoma, salivary duct carcinoma, small cell and undifferentiated carcinomas, oncocytic carcinoma, and malignant myoepithelioma.

In 1996, the most recent AFIP atlas of salivary gland tumor pathology, written by Ellis and Auclair, was published.[228] Their clas-

Table 6–2. Classification of Salivary Gland Neoplasms by the World Health Organization (1972)

Epithelial tumors
  Adenomas
    Pleomorphic adenoma
    Monomorphic adenoma
      Adenolymphoma
      Oxyphilic adenoma
      Other
  Mucoepidermoid tumor
  Acinic cell tumor
  Carcinomas
    Adenoid cystic carcinoma
    Adenocarcinoma
    Epidermoid carcinoma
    Undifferentiated carcinoma
    Carcinoma in pleomorphic adenoma
Nonepithelial tumors
Unclassified tumors
Allied conditions
  Benign lymphoepithelial lesion
  Sialosis
  Oncocytosis

From Thackray AC, Sobin LH: Histological Typing of Salivary Gland Tumours. International Histological Classification of Tumours No 7. Geneva: World Health Organization, 1972.

Table 6–3. Classification of Salivary Gland Neoplasms by Thackray and Lucas (1974)

Adenomas
  Pleomorphic adenoma
  Monomorphic adenoma
    Adenolymphoma
    Oxyphilic adenoma
    Tubular adenoma
    Clear cell adenoma
    Basal cell adenoma
    Trabecular adenoma
    Sebaceous adenoma
    Sebaceous lymphadenoma
Mucoepidermoid tumor
Acinic cell tumor
Carcinomas
  Adenoid cystic carcinoma
  Adenocarcinoma
  Epidermoid carcinoma
  Undifferentiated carcinoma
  Carcinoma in pleomorphic adenoma
  Malignant lymphoepithelial lesion
Connective tissue and other tumors
  Benign
    Hemangioma
    Lymphangioma
    Lipoma
    Neurinoma
  Sarcoma
  Lymphoma
Metastatic tumors

From Thackray AC, Lucas RB: Tumors of the Major Salivary Glands. Atlas of Tumor Pathology, 2nd Series, Fascicle 10, Washington, DC: Armed Forces Institute of Pathology, 1974.

sification system was almost identical to the recent WHO system, with only a few differences (Table 6–5). They clarified the group of tumors classified under the term *carcinoma in pleomorphic adenoma* by subdividing the malignant mixed tumor group into three entities: the more common carcinoma ex pleomorphic adenoma and the much rarer carcinosarcoma and metastasizing mixed tumor. In addition, they included a separate category of clear cell carcinoma that was distinct and different from epithelial-myoepithelial carcinoma and they placed the sebaceous lymphadenoma group of neoplasms into the category of "lymphadenomas," which encompassed tumors with and without sebaceous differentiation.

Benign and Malignant Mixed Tumors

Benign Pleomorphic Adenoma (Benign Mixed Tumor)

Clinical Features. Pleomorphic adenomas (PA) represent the most common of all salivary tumors, accounting for 60% to 70% of all parotid tumors, 40% to 60% of submandibular tumors, and 40% to 70% of all minor salivary neoplasia.[229–233] The only published data on incidence found an annual rate of approximately 2.4 to 3.05 per 100,000 persons.[234, 235] PA also may arise in the nasal cavity, larynx, and paranasal sinuses.[236–238] They occur over a wide age range, from the first to tenth decades of life, with a peak in the third to fourth decades.[233] Table 6–6 is modified from the AFIP consultation series, which is skewed toward more unusual cases and reveals the site distribution for PA.

Parotid tumors usually arise within the superficial lobe, but 10% may occur in the deep lobe, or from an accessory parotid gland. The palate and lip are the two most common minor salivary gland sites. PA may arise within more esoteric sites such as salivary heterotopia in cervical lymph nodes; soft tissue of the neck, upper and lower limbs, axilla, and trunk; mandible; lung; breast; sellar region;

Table 6–4. Revised Classification of Salivary Gland Neoplasms by the World Health Organization (1991)

Adenomas
   Pleomorphic adenoma
   Myoepithelioma (myoepithelial adenoma)
   Basal cell adenoma
   Warthin's tumor (adenolymphoma)
   Oncocytoma (oncocytic adenoma)
   Canalicular adenoma
   Sebaceous adenoma
   Ductal papilloma
      Inverted ductal papilloma
      Intraductal papilloma
      Sialadenoma papilliferum
   Cystadenoma
      Papillary cystadenoma
      Mucinous cystadenoma
Carcinomas
   Acinic cell carcinoma
   Mucoepidermoid carcinoma
   Adenoid cystic carcinoma
   Polymorphous low-grade adenocarcinoma (terminal duct adenocarcinoma)
   Epithelial-myoepithelial carcinoma
   Basal cell adenocarcinoma
   Sebaceous carcinoma
   Papillary cystadenocarcinoma
   Mucinous adenocarcinoma
   Oncocytic carcinoma
   Salivary duct carcinoma
   Adenocarcinoma
   Malignant myoepithelioma (myoepithelial carcinoma)
   Carcinoma in pleomorphic adenoma (malignant mixed tumor)
   Squamous cell carcinoma
   Small cell carcinoma
   Undifferentiated carcinoma
   Other carcinomas
Nonepithelial tumors
Malignant lymphomas
Secondary tumors
Unclassified tumors
Tumor-like lesions
   Sialadenosis
   Oncocytosis
   Necrotizing sialometaplasia (salivary gland infarction)
   Benign lymphoepithelial lesion
   Salivary gland cysts
   Chronic sclerosing sialadenitis of submandibular gland (Küttner tumor)
   Cystic lymphoid hyperplasia in acquired immunodeficiency syndrome

From Seifert G, Sobin LH: Histological Typing of Salivary Gland Tumours. World Health Organization International Histological Classification of Tumours, 2nd ed. New York: Springer-Verlag, 1991.

lacrimal gland and sac; and ear and mediastinum.[239–248] In the skin, they are referred to as chondroid syringomas.

Pleomorphic adenomas are also among the most common salivary tumors capable of metachronous or synchronous occurrence with other salivary neoplasms, especially with Warthin's tumors.[249] Regarding gender predominance, data from civilian sources reveal a female to male ratio of 1.9 : 1.[233] In the major salivary gland, PA present as a firm, mobile, painless mass. Deep lobe parotid tumors are not palpable but may present as an intraoral mass that distends the parapharyngeal space. Minor salivary PA usually present as painless submucosal swellings. Most tumors range from 2 to 6 cm in greatest diameter; however, rare tumors measuring up to 26 cm (6.85 kg) have been reported.[250]

Pathologic Features. On gross examination, PA are bosselated with variable gray-blue, gritty cut surfaces, gelatinous-like foci, and soft tan-gray areas (Fig. 6–11, see p. 340). Necrotic or cystic regions may be seen in larger tumors. They are characteristically circumscribed and noninfiltrating, although "pod-like" peripheral exten-

sions may be occasionally appreciated on gross examination. Recurrent tumors pathognomonically appear as multifocal soft tissue masses and are frequently chondromyxoid in appearance (Fig. 6–12, see p. 340).

Microscopically, PA are a histologically diverse group of tumors composed of a mixture of epithelial and mesenchymal elements (Fig. 6–13, see pp. 340–343). The content and preponderance of both components varies, hence the appellation "pleomorphic" or "mixed." Characteristically, the boundary between the epithelial and mesenchymal components is blurred by the proliferation of myoepithelial or modified myoepithelial cells, which are usually abundant in both areas. The epithelial constituent forms ductal structures composed of large, bland cuboidal cells with vacuolated nuclei surrounded by thickened collars of myoepithelial cells. These latter cells are recognizable by their condensed, smaller, darker nuclei with flattened or triangular shapes and variably eosinophilic to clear cytoplasm. Solid areas of nonlumen-producing epithelial cells admixed with myoepithelial cells can be seen. Crystalloids, including collagenous material, tyrosine-rich crystals, which form flower-like structures, and oxalate-like crystals, may be present.[233] The myoepi-

Table 6–5. Classification of Salivary Gland Neoplasms by Ellis and Auclair (1996)

Benign epithelial neoplasms
   Mixed tumor (pleomorphic adenoma)
   Myoepithelioma
   Warthin's tumor
   Basal cell adenoma
   Canalicular adenoma
   Oncocytoma
   Cystadenoma
   Ductal papillomas
      Sialadenoma papilliferum
      Inverted ductal papilloma
      Intraductal papilloma
   Lymphadenomas and sebaceous adenomas
   Sialoblastoma
Malignant epithelial neoplasms
   Mucoepidermoid carcinoma
   Adenocarcinoma
   Acinic cell adenocarcinoma
   Adenoid cystic carcinoma
   Polymorphous low-grade adenocarcinoma
   Malignant mixed tumors
      Carcinoma ex mixed tumor
      Carcinosarcoma
      Metastasizing mixed tumor
   Squamous cell carcinoma
   Basal cell adenocarcinoma
   Epithelial-myoepithelial carcinoma
   Clear cell adenocarcinoma
   Cystadenocarcinoma
   Undifferentiated carcinomas
      Small cell undifferentiated carcinoma
      Large cell undifferentiated carcinoma
      Lymphoepithelial carcinoma
   Oncocytic carcinoma
   Salivary duct carcinoma
   Sebaceous adenocarcinoma and lymphadenocarcinoma
   Myoepithelial carcinoma
   Adenosquamous carcinoma
   Mucinous adenocarcinoma
Mesenchymal neoplasms
   Benign
   Sarcomas
Malignant lymphomas
Metastatic tumors
Non-neoplastic tumor-like conditions

From Ellis GL, Auclair PL: Atlas of Tumor Pathology. Tumors of the Salivary Glands, 3rd Series, Fascicle 17, Washington, DC: Armed Forces Institute of Pathology, 1996.

Table 6–6. Anatomic Distribution of 6880 Cases of Pleomorphic Adenoma from the Armed Forces Institute of Pathology

	Cases	
Anatomic Site	Number	%
Major Sites		
Parotid	4359	63.4
Submandibular	657	9.5
Sublingual	10	0.1
Neck nodes	89	1.3
Minor Sites		
Palate	711	10.3
Lip	297	4.3
Tongue	16	0.2
Cheek	126	1.8
Floor of mouth	7	0.1
Tonsil/oropharynx	38	0.6
Retromolar	3	—
Other	79	1.1
Not Stated	488	7.1

Modified from Waldron CA: Mixed tumor (pleomorphic adenoma) and myoepithelioma. In: Ellis GL, Auclair PL, Gnepp DR (eds): Surgical Pathology of the Salivary Glands. Philadelphia: WB Saunders, 1991: 165–186.

thelial cells produce the mesenchymal component, which may be myxoid, cartilaginous, or hyalinized. The myoepithelial cells may also have a spindled, plasmacytoid (hyaline cell), polygonal, or clear cell appearance.[251] A prominent spindle cell component may have a schwannoma-like palisading growth pattern. Plasmacytoid myoepithelial cells are round to oval with eccentric nuclei and dense eosinophilic cytoplasm. These may form sheets and small islands within hyalinized stroma.

Approximately 25% of PA demonstrate foci of squamous metaplasia, which may be associated with foci of necrosis. Diffuse squamous metaplasia is uncommon; however, its presence may lead to diagnostic problems.[252–254] Also, occasional tumors have areas of sebaceous metaplasia, oncocytic metaplasia, clear cell change, mucoepidermoid-type metaplasia (Fig. 6–13N, O, see p. 343) and adenoid cystic carcinoma–like foci. Rarely, a PA will have foci of intratumor vascular invasion. In the United States, this finding is extremely rare. One of us (DRG) has observed this twice over the past 25 years. However, in South Africa, this phenomenon appears to be more frequent, with 8.9% of intraoral PA demonstrating vascular invasion.[254a] To date, metastatic disease, increased recurrence, or aggressive behavior has not been associated with vascular invasion.

Myxoid-predominant PA have a tendency toward greater pod-like growth and therefore are more likely to "spill" during surgery. Chondroid differentiation tends to be less prominent than the myxoid component. This chondroid stroma is the only tissue that is relatively specific for PA, and when seen it usually rules out other benign salivary tumors. Occasional tumors may have minimal to abundant lipomatous stroma. A prominent hyalinized component has been noted to correlate with long-standing tumors, or those that subsequently undergo malignant progression.[255] Auclair and Ellis studied 65 pleomorphic adenomas, 9 of which (13.8%) went on to malignant degeneration. They found that the presence of prominent hyalinized stroma correlated ($P < 0.5$) with malignant progression.[255]

Necrosis is usually found more frequently in malignant tumors, but PA may, on occasion, exhibit prominent central necrosis and still follow a benign course.[256] The necrosis may be the result of ischemic infarction and clinically can be associated with abrupt onset of pain. The cellularity of PA may vary considerably from acellular tumors, usually composed of a myxoid component (Fig. 6–13G, see p. 341), to tumors with extreme cellularity with solid sheets of densely

packed modified myoepithelial tumor cells (see Fig. 6–13H, I, see p. 342). These latter tumors are referred to as *cellular mixed tumors.*

True multicentric PA is a rare phenomenon.[257–259] Most major salivary PA are relatively well circumscribed, or encapsulated; occasional tumors may not have a capsule or may be only partially encapsulated. These tumors frequently grow by broad-based or "pod-like" extensions through the capsule; true invasion is not seen. Minor salivary gland PA characteristically lack encapsulation and may incorporate normal host tissue as they expand; destructive invasive growth is not seen. Examination of a PA should include a careful search of the tumor periphery to ensure circumscription. Smooth tumor nodules discrete from the main tumor body speak for the aforementioned pod-like growth pattern, which is distinct from tumor invasion. Tumor invasion is seen as irregular broad-based angulated tumor tongues that jut out from the main mass. In the absence of invasive, destructive overgrowth of benign tumor elements or destructive growth through the capsule, a moderate degree of nuclear atypia and an increased mitotic rate may be tolerated without warranting the diagnosis of carcinoma ex pleomorphic adenoma (see next section).

Differential Diagnosis. The differential diagnosis of a minor salivary gland PA includes polymorphous low-grade adenocarcinoma (PLGA) and adenoid cystic carcinoma (AdCC). Sharply "punched-out" cribriform-type glands are characteristic for AdCC but may also be seen with PLGA and PA. In fact, PA, PLGA and AdCC may be indistinguishable from one another on a limited biopsy specimen. On the resection specimen, the absence of infiltration and perineural invasion also rules out PLGA and AdCC. Squamous metaplasia or chondroid metaplasia, when seen, speaks for PA. Also, proliferative markers and glial fibrillary acidic protein are helpful with this differential diagnosis (see discussion under polymorphous low-grade adenocarcinoma).

Squamous cell carcinoma or mucoepidermoid carcinoma can enter the differential diagnosis in a limited biopsy sample of a pleomorphic adenoma with squamous or mucoepidermoid metaplasia. This is especially so when the lesion occurs in a minor salivary gland site, such as the palate, where tumors have a tendency to be more cellular and lack cartilaginous differentiation. Finding plasmacytoid myoepithelial cells supports the diagnosis of PA and eliminates mucoepidermoid carcinoma and squamous carcinoma from diagnostic consideration.

The luminal cells of PA express cytokeratins, epithelial membrane antigen (EMA), and carcinoembryonic antigen (CEA) to a variable degree. The myoepithelial cells express vimentin, S100, glial fibrillary acid protein (GFAP), desmin, and smooth muscle markers such as HHF-35, calponin, and smooth muscle myosin.[260–262] Light microscopic examination rather than immunohistochemistry is, however, infinitely more useful in distinguishing PA from other salivary tumors. Immunohistochemistry may aid in distinguishing salivary versus non-salivary lesions; for example, expression of cytokeratin, GFAP, and HHF-35 might aid in distinguishing PA from non-salivary tumors such as extraskeletal chondrosarcoma.

Treatment and Prognosis. The majority of pleomorphic adenomas are cured by surgical excision with negative margins. Superficial parotidectomy is the treatment of choice for PA superficial to the facial nerve. Total parotidectomy with preservation of the facial nerve is necessary for deep lobe tumors.[263] The recurrence rate after these procedures is less than 5%.[264–267] Recurrences result from transection of the finger-like or pod-like tumor projections. It has been noted that pleomorphic adenomas with a high stromal chondroid/myxoid content have a greater recurrence rate than predominantly cellular, epithelial tumors.[255, 265] The former tumors have more obvious pseudopods and thinner capsules. Recurrences may be single, but are more characteristically multiple (see Fig. 6–12). Myssiorrek and colleagues noted that the interval to recurrence was somewhat predictive.[264] Patients with more than one recurrence tended to have their first recurrence earlier (mean, 47 months) than patients who were cured after re-excision of their only recurrence (mean, 105 months). In a similar vein, MacGregor and associates noted that PAs that ultimately recurred were more likely to have their initial onset prior to the age of 30.[265] Other series have indicated that younger patients tend to develop recurrences more often than older ones.[268] Most investigators report a 10% to 18% incidence of further recurrence after surgery of the first recurrence (range, 5%–60%).[268] Radiation has been used to treat recurrences, but its utility is still uncertain.[269]

Primary mixed tumors of soft tissue origin appear to behave more aggressively than their salivary gland counterparts. Kilpatrick and coauthors[243] described 19 tumors arising in the soft tissues. Clinical follow-up was available in 10 of these cases; two patients developed metastases to regional lymph nodes 20 years after diagnosis and one to regional lymph nodes and the lung (both noted at initial diagnosis).

Malignant Mixed Tumor

The term *malignant mixed tumor* (MMT) includes three different clinical pathologic entities: carcinoma arising in a benign mixed tumor (carcinoma ex pleomorphic adenoma [Ca-ex-PA]), carcinosarcoma, and metastasizing mixed tumor. Alternatively, the term MMT has been used as a synonym for Ca-ex-PA, as Ca-ex-PA accounts for the vast majority of MMT, whereas carcinosarcoma and metastasizing mixed tumor account for only a very small percentage of tumors in this group. The latest World Health Classification (WHO) scheme uses MMT and Ca-ex-PA interchangeably. Because of potential diagnostic confusion, we prefer to use the term MMT in its broader context and refer specifically to each tumor type when rendering a diagnosis. Many large series of Ca-ex-PAs have been reported and recently summarized.[270] MMTs account for approximately 3.6% of all salivary tumors (range, 0.9%–14%), 12% of all salivary malignancies (range, 2.8%–42.4%), and 6.2% of all mixed tumors (range, 1.9%–23.3%).

Carcinoma ex Pleomorphic Adenoma

Clinical Features. Ca-ex-PA is defined as a mixed tumor in which an epithelial malignancy is present. This group accounts for well over 95% of all MMT.[270–272] Ca-ex-PA most frequently arises in the parotid but may also originate from the submandibular gland and minor salivary sites, most commonly the palate. Presentation with synchronous multiglandular Ca-ex-PA is rare.[273] Tumors occur at any age; they rarely present prior to the age of 2 and are usually seen in the sixth or seventh decade of life, approximately one decade later than in patients with pleomorphic adenomas. Although many Ca-ex-PAs are the result of the accumulation of genetic instabilities in long-standing pleomorphic adenomas, some tumors, such as those arising in young patients, or in patients with a short history of pre-existing tumor, are presumed to have arisen de novo. The most typical history is that of a long-standing mass with rapid growth over the previous 3- to 6-month period; however, a significant proportion of patients present with a clinical history of less than 3 years.[270, 274] Patients frequently complain of a painless mass; but pain, facial nerve palsy, and skin fixation may also occur.

Pathologic Features. The average size of Ca-ex-PA is more than twice that of its benign counterpart, ranging from 1.5 to 25 cm in greatest diameter.[272, 275] Large pleomorphic adenomas, densely hyalinized tumors, and tumors with prominent necrosis should raise the suspicion of malignancy and require extensive sectioning. Grossly, Ca-ex-PAs are usually poorly circumscribed and many are extensively infiltrative. Occasional tumors, however, are well circumscribed, scar-like, or completely encapsulated.[275, 276] Tumors are usually hard and have a white to tan-gray cut surface. The proportion of benign to malignant components can be quite variable, and occasionally extensive sampling is necessary to demonstrate the benign component.

The malignant component is most commonly a poorly differentiated adenocarcinoma (salivary duct type or not otherwise speci-

fied) or undifferentiated carcinoma; however, virtually any form of carcinoma (e.g., mucoepidermoid, clear cell or myoepithelial carcinoma[277]) may be found as the malignant component (Fig. 6–14).[270] Sometimes no histologically benign remnant can be found; if there is clinicopathologic documentation of a previously excised benign mixed tumor at that site, then the malignancy can also be classified as a Ca-ex-PA. An infiltrative, destructive growth pattern is the most reliable criterion for the diagnosis of carcinoma ex mixed tumor. Nuclear hyperchromasia and pleomorphism are frequent, although occasional tumors may demonstrate minimal atypia. This latter feature (tumor grade) has a positive correlation with prognosis (see later discussion). Necrosis is frequent and mitoses are usually easy to find. Ca-ex-PAs should be subclassified into noninvasive, minimally invasive ($\leq$1.5 mm penetration of the malignant component into extracapsular tissue) and invasive ($>$1.5 mm of invasion), as the former two groups have an excellent prognosis whereas the latter group has a more guarded prognosis.

Noninvasive Ca-ex-PAs are also referred to as carcinoma in situ arising in a benign mixed tumor. They range from focal to diffuse or multifocal areas with carcinoma that overgrows and replaces many of the benign elements. Occasionally, tumor cells will replace the inner ductal layer, leaving the normal peripherally located myoepithelial layer intact. The distinction between noninvasive and invasive tumors is based on destructive invasion through the capsule into peritumoral tissues.

Differential Diagnosis. The differential diagnosis is usually with other salivary malignancies, such as adenoid cystic carcinoma, salivary duct carcinoma, and polymorphous low-grade adenocarcinoma, as all of these tumors may have areas of extensive hyalinization. Finding remnants of benign pleomorphic adenoma with the myxoid, the chondroid, or the bland ductal/myoepithelial components should allow for the proper classification of Ca-ex-PA. Also, carcinomas may rarely arise in a histologically benign adenoma (monomorphic adenoma) and must be differentiated from Ca-ex-PA because they appear to have, in initial studies, a more favorable prognosis.[278] From a practical standpoint, the most important differential diagnosis is between minimally invasive Ca-ex-PA and the more typical invasive Ca-ex-PA. This distinction has prognostic significance and affects decisions regarding the need for lymph node dissection and adjuvant radiotherapy (see later discussion).

Treatment and Prognosis. In general, the recommended therapy is wide local excision. Contiguous lymph node dissection and adjuvant radiation therapy is recommended for widely invasive tumors. If the carcinomatous component is histologically less aggressive (see later discussion) or minimally invasive, and if the tumor is adequately excised, then adjuvant radiation therapy may not be necessary.

As a group, Ca-ex-PAs are extremely aggressive malignancies, and approximately 40% to 50% of patients develop one or more recurrences.[270, 272, 274] The metastatic rate varies with each series; up to 70% of patients develop local or distant metastasis.[279] Metastatic sites, in order of frequency, are lung, bone (especially spine), abdomen, and central nervous system.[272, 280] Patients with noninvasive or minimally invasive Ca-ex-PA have an excellent prognosis, similar to that in patients with typical benign mixed tumor (see later discussion). Ca-ex-PA with capsular penetration of more than 1.5 mm is associated with a poor prognosis; survival rates at 5, 10, 15, and 20 years range from 25% to 65%, 24% to 50%, 10% to 35%, and 0% to 38%, respectively.[272, 274, 275, 279, 280] Therefore, it is important to designate those CA-ex-PAs that are confined within the capsule and those invading through the capsule as noninvasive or invasive, respectively, and to differentiate within the latter group between widely invasive versus minimally invasive tumors.

Tortoledo and associates reviewed their experience with 37 patients and found that no patient with less than 8 mm invasion from the capsule died from the tumor, whereas all patients with invasion greater than 9 mm beyond the capsule ultimately died of disease.[275] The local recurrence rate also correlated with extent of invasion; a local recurrence rate of 70.5% was found for tumors with invasion

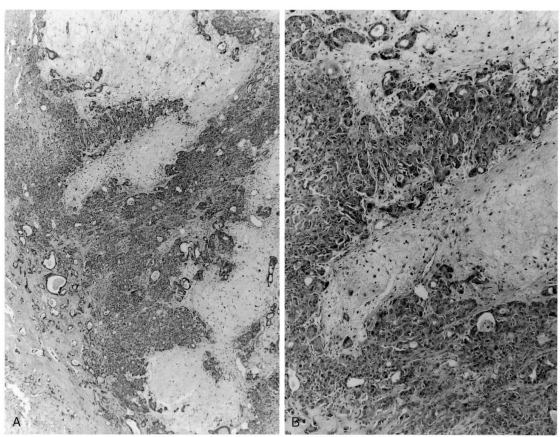

Figure 6–14. Carcinoma ex pleomorphic adenoma, noninvasive type. *A,* Note myxoid/cartilaginous foci with focal stromal hyalinization intermixed with numerous ducts and myoepithelial cells. *B,* A focus of adenocarcinoma is seen surrounding the cartilage. This focus is composed of infiltrating tumor cells with a moderate degree of pleomorphism with focal back-to-back gland formation. This tumor did not invade through the capsule and therefore is classified as the "noninvasive" type of carcinoma ex pleomorphic adenoma.

beyond 6 mm from the capsule, as compared with 16.6% for tumors with invasion of less than 6 mm. The improved prognosis for minimally invasive tumors has been confirmed by Brandwein et al.[276] in a series of 12 noninvasive and minimally invasive Ca-ex-PAs: all 8 minimally invasive Ca-ex-PAs (invasion beyond the capsule of ≤1.5 mm) were recurrence free for periods ranging from 1 to 4 years (mean, 2.5 years). Lewis and Olsen[281] have also recently confirmed that extent of invasion is an important prognosticator. Tumor size and grade are also significant prognosticators. Tortoledo et al.[275] correlated 5-year survival rates with histologic subtype of the carcinoma component: there was a 30% survival rate for undifferentiated carcinomas, 50% for myoepithelial carcinomas, 62% for ductal carcinomas, and 96% for terminal duct carcinomas.

One would expect the carcinomatous elements to be more radiosensitive than the mesenchymal myxoid/chondroid components. Anecdotally, we have seen one case of Ca-ex-PA treated by resection and radiation therapy, in which the patient was plagued by multiple intramandibular recurrences. Paradoxically, the recurrences were not of Ca-ex-PA, but of the histologically benign myxoid component present in the initial tumor.

Chromosomal Changes. Abnormalities in chromosome 8 are most commonly encountered in benign and malignant mixed tumors, indicative of an early event in the genesis of mixed tumors. Bullerdiek et al.[282] performed G-banding analysis on 220 pleomorphic adenomas and found abnormalities in half the tumors. Balanced rearrangements were seen at 8q12 (25%) and 12q13-15 (13%). Interestingly, patients with 8q12 rearrangements were younger and had tumors with a greater stromal content than patients with tumors of normal karyotype or 12q13-15 rearrangements. Microsatellite analysis of CA-ex-PA has revealed that chromosomal loss (loss of heterozygosity) is common to 8q, in both benign and malignant

mixed tumors, suggesting the presence of a tumor suppressor gene on the long arm of chromosome 8. Loss of heterozygosity at 12q was also seen in CA-ex-PA.[283]

Mark et al.[284] studied benign and malignant mixed tumors by G-banding and fluorescent in situ hybridization and found translocations in pleomorphic adenomas, in most cases involving 8q, around the 8q12 region. One Ca-ex-PA revealed a rearrangement at 8q with a breakpoint at q12. Rao et al.[285] found chromosomal gains at 8q23-24 and 12q13-15 by fluorescent comparative genomic hybridization in one case of Ca-ex-PA, corresponding with overexpression of myc (8q24), cyclin D kinase 4 (CDK4), and MDM2 (12q13-15). CDK4 inactivates cyclin D kinase, preventing Rb phosphorylation and MDM2 complexes to wild-type 53; both these changes abrogate G_1 arrest and apoptosis.

Carcinosarcoma

Clinical Features. Carcinosarcoma is composed of a mixture of carcinomatous and sarcomatous elements. Unlike Ca-ex-PA, in which only the carcinomatous elements may metastasize, both carcinomatous and sarcomatous elements of carcinosarcoma may metastasize. Parenthetically, a pure chondrosarcoma apocryphally arising in a "benign mixed tumor" has been reported.[286] Carcinosarcoma is extremely rare, with slightly over 40 cases reported to date.[270, 287–291] Two thirds have arisen in the parotid, approximately 19% in the submandibular glands, and 14% in the palate. One case has been reported in the tongue.[287] The mean age at presentation was 58 years with a range of 14 to 87 years. A number of patients have had a history of recurrent pleomorphic adenoma.[288]

Pathologic Features. Chondrosarcoma and osteosarcoma elements are the most common sarcomatous elements, and moderate to

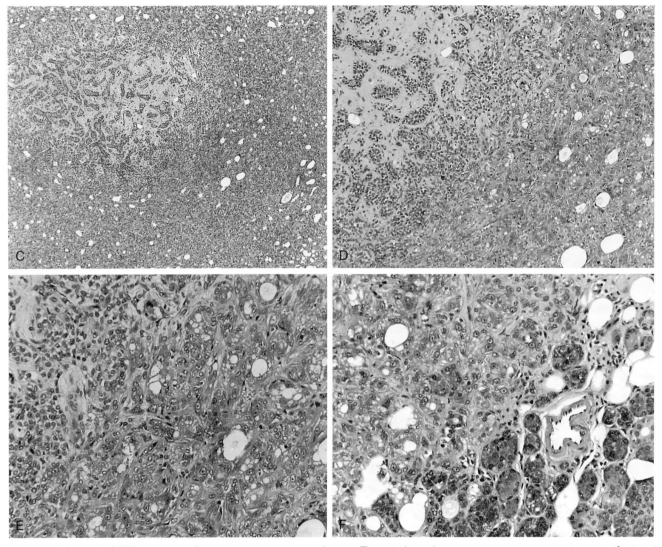

Figure 6–14 *Continued. C–F,* This is a minimally invasive carcinoma ex mixed tumor. The typical mixed tumor portions are seen at various magnifications in the left side of parts *C* and *D* and in part *E.* The carcinoma portion is seen in the right half of the three figures. It is composed of cells that are larger than the normal myoepithelial cells with a moderate degree of pleomorphism and very prominent nucleoli. *F* demonstrates a portion of carcinoma infiltrating focally into adjacent parotid tissue. The distance of infiltration was less than 1.5 mm from the capsule. Therefore, this tumor is classified as a "minimally invasive" carcinoma ex pleomorphic adenoma.

poorly differentiated ductal carcinoma or an undifferentiated carcinoma is the most common carcinomatous component (Fig. 6–15). Local tissue infiltration and destruction are characteristic of this neoplasm.

Treatment and Prognosis. Treatment is wide surgical excision combined with radiation therapy. Almost 60% of patients die of local recurrence or metastatic disease (lungs, bones, central nervous system) usually within a 30-month period.[288–290]

Metastasizing Mixed Tumor

Clinical and Pathologic Features. The metastasizing mixed tumor is the least common of the three types of MMT. To date, approximately 30 cases have been described in the literature, with over three quarters of the tumors arising in the parotid gland, 13% in the submandibular gland, and 9% in the palate.[270, 292–296] Characteristically, the primary salivary gland tumor and its metastasis are composed of the typical mixture of benign-appearing epithelial and mesenchymal components of a mixed tumor (Fig. 6–16). The histologic type is nonpredictive of the tumor's ability to metastasize: mitotic figures and nuclear pleomorphism may be seen, but the tumor is not overtly histologically malignant. These tumors are characterized by

multiple local recurrences and a long interval (1.5 to 55 years) between the primary tumor and the development of metastasis.

It has been postulated that multiple recurrences and surgical procedures allow for some tumors to gain venous access and "benignly" metastasize. Many cases are found to have a normal diploid complement.[293] Karyotypic chromosomal analysis and fluorescent in situ hybridization in one such tumor has revealed numerous translocations, including unbalanced rearrangements of chromosomes 1-13 and 9-21 and monosomy 22, which differ from the typical balanced 8q or 12q translocations seen in pleomorphic adenomas.[294] This suggests that more than happenstance will allow a mixed tumor to gain venous access.

Immunohistochemistry. The greatest utility of immunohistochemistry for salivary neoplasia is in distinguishing primary salivary from nonsalivary gland tumors. One may need to distinguish a metastasizing mixed tumor or carcinosarcoma from a primary soft tissue sarcoma. Also, rare mixed tumors have originated in the soft tissue.[297] The findings of epithelial markers such as keratin within the chondromyxoid stroma, contractile smooth muscle elements, (HHF-35, smooth muscle actin, calponin), or glial fibrillary acidic protein within the myoepithelial cells are features unique to salivary neoplasia and can be helpful in the differential diagnosis.

Treatment and Prognosis. The treatment of choice is surgical excision with aggressive treatment of distant metastases. Half of the tumors metastasize to bone, 30% to the lung, and 30% to the lymph nodes; rarely, tumors metastasize to other body sites. Forty percent of patients died with disease, usually from distant metastases; 47% were alive and well, and 13% were alive with disease.[270]

Myoepithelioma

Benign Myoepithelioma

Myoepithelioma is a tumor composed entirely or predominantly of myoepithelial cells. It represents one extreme in the histologic spectrum of pleomorphic adenoma.[298–304] Criteria to distinguish a mixed tumor with a predominance of myoepithelial cells from a myoepithelioma are largely subjective. Some authors do not accept any ductal differentiation in a myoepithelioma,[305] whereas others do not allow any more than one duct per medium-power field, or no more than one cluster of ducts.[299, 306] We allow up to 5% of the tumor to be composed of ductal epithelium in a myoepithelioma; if there is

greater than 5% ductal differentiation, then it is our preference to designate these tumors as mixed tumors with a myoepithelial predominance. If chondroid or osteoid foci are found, we feel a diagnosis of mixed tumor is appropriate, although some authors allow focal chondroid differentiation.[302]

Clinical Features. Myoepitheliomas occur infrequently, accounting for 0.3%[307] to 1.5%[305] of salivary gland neoplasms and for 2.2% to 5.7% of all major or minor benign salivary gland tumors, respectively.[305] However, with the recent expansion of the histologic range of myoepithelioma, this diagnosis has become more frequent.[301, 302] Since the initial use of the term *myoepithelioma* by Sheldon in 1943,[298] more than 200 cases have been reported.[299–311] Of these cases, approximately 48% occurred in the parotid gland, 10% in the submandibular gland, and 42% in the minor salivary glands or in seromucinous gland sites including the nasal cavity and larynx. Two thirds of the minor gland tumors occurred in the palate. Tumors with the same morphology have also been described in the skin,[312, 312a] lung, and breast, and rare tumors have been described to arise primarily in the soft tissues.[312a, 313] There has been no significant predilection for occurrence in either sex. The patients have ranged in age from 6 to 85 years with a mean age in the early to mid-40s.[305, 309] Similar to most benign salivary gland tumors, myo-

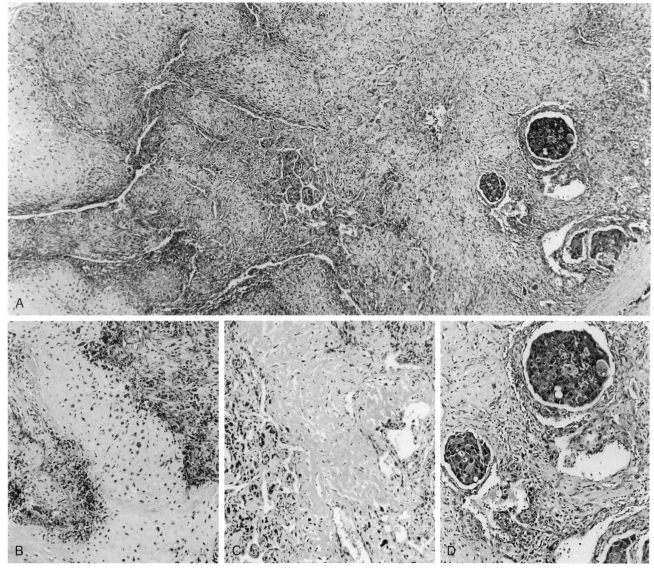

Figure 6–15. Carcinosarcoma. The tumor is composed predominantly of a high-grade sarcoma with small foci of carcinoma (A, right side). Foci of chondrosarcoma were noted (B), as were foci of osteosarcoma (C). A detail of the carcinoma component (D) demonstrates nests of pleomorphic carcinoma cells.

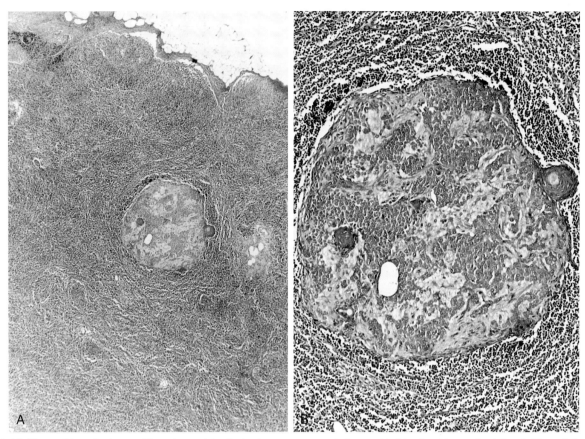

Figure 6–16. Metastasizing mixed tumor. There is a nodule of mixed tumor composed of myoepithelial cells with very focal ductal differentiation, myxoid stroma, and focal squamous differentiation surrounded by the lymphoid cells of this lymph node. A, Low-power picture demonstrating the capsule of the lymph node (top) with a subcapsular sinus and the metastatic tumor nodule. B, A high-power detail of this metastasizing mixed tumor.

epitheliomas most often present as slowly enlarging, asymptomatic masses.

Pathologic Features. Myoepithelioma is a well-circumscribed or encapsulated tumor. It is composed of variable proportions of spindle-shaped, plasmacytoid, polygonal epithelioid, and, rarely, clear[300, 301] myoepithelial or modified myoepithelial cells commonly arranged in sheets, irregular collections, nests, interconnecting trabeculae, or ribbons. Nuclear pleomorphism is usually minimal; however, similar to mixed tumors, a mild to moderate degree of nuclear pleomorphism or atypia may be noted in occasional tumors. Stroma may be minimal or abundant and is usually acellular and mucoid, myxoid, or hyalinized.

Microscopically, myoepitheliomas fall into five patterns: spindle cell type, plasmacytoid cell type, reticular type, clear cell type, and a combination of these types (Fig. 6–17). The spindle cell pattern occurs most frequently and has a predilection for the parotid glands of older individuals.[303] These tumors are often very cellular, with little intervening fibrous tissue or ground substance, and may be multinodular. The spindle cells are usually arranged in sheets, fascicles, or a swirling interdigitating pattern. The plasmacytoid type has a predilection for the palate of younger individuals[303] and may be arranged in sheets; however, it is often less cellular, and the cells may be arranged in groups separated by an abundant, loose, myxoid matrix that is predominantly hyaluronic acid. The plasmacytoid cells, sometimes referred to as hyaline cells, are round, oval, or polyhedral with glassy eosinophilic cytoplasm and eccentric nuclei. The reticular type is composed of interconnecting trabeculae of myoepithelial cells similar to focal areas typically seen in benign mixed tumors. However, the prominent myxochondroid components of benign mixed tumor are lacking. The clear cell type is the rarest variant and is composed of a bland uniform population of epithelioid tumor

cells with moderate amounts of clear cytoplasm. Combinations of these patterns frequently may be present within the same tumor. Rarely, foci of oncocytic metaplasia[313a, 313b] and other tumor combinations such as a myoepithelioma and a basal cell adenoma may be found.

Benign myoepitheliomas of the parotid gland are typically encapsulated, but those arising in the palate or in other minor salivary or seromucinous gland sites are circumscribed but not usually encapsulated. The chondroid and osteoid-like matrix commonly seen in mixed tumors is not seen in myoepitheliomas, although very focal areas of ductal differentiation may be present (<5%). Positive staining for cytokeratin and muscle-specific actin, smooth muscle actin, calponin, or S100 protein confirms the myoepithelial nature of the tumor, although there may be considerable variability of staining within the same tumor and between different tumors. Glial fibrillary acidic protein often stains tumor components but in a more variable fashion, and vimentin is also frequently expressed. However it is important to remember that some tumors, especially the plasmacytoid variant, may not express myoepithelial markers in vivo,[308] although they do express them in vitro.[314]

Differential Diagnosis. Various benign mesenchymal neoplasms, such as fibroma, fibrous histiocytoma, leiomyoma, and schwannoma, may be considered in the histologic differential diagnosis of the spindle cell type of myoepithelioma. Rarely, Kaposi's sarcoma may have focal areas that resemble spindle cell myoepithelioma. Immunohistochemistry or electron microscopy may be necessary to accurately identify the myoepithelial nature of the neoplasm. Of these tumors, only myoepithelioma would be expected to express cytokeratin, muscle-specific or smooth muscle actin, calponin, and S100 protein. Ultrastructural identification of desmosomes, cytoplasmic microfilament arrays with or without dense bodies, pinocytotic vesicles, and basal lamina separating tumor cells from adjacent connective tissue should also help establish the tumor cells as myoepithelial. Plasmacytoma may be confused with the plasmacytoid type of myoepithelioma, although the nuclear morphology of the two is different. The differential diagnosis of the clear cell variant includes any salivary gland tumor that may have clear cytoplasm (e.g., acinic cell carcinoma, oncocytoma, clear cell carcinoma, mucoepidermoid carcinoma, metastatic renal cell carcinoma). Of the tumors in the differential diagnosis, only a malignant myoepithelioma (including the clear cell variant) and an epithelial-myoepithelial carcinoma would show positive immunohistochemical staining of the tumor cells for cytokeratin, muscle-specific or smooth muscle actin, calponin, and S100 protein. The malignant myoepithelioma and its clear cell variant are more invasive, usually, but not always, with a much greater degree of cytologic atypia than their benign counterpart, whereas the epithelial-myoepithelial carcinoma, unlike a benign clear cell myoepithelioma, has a biphasic growth pattern.

Treatment and Prognosis. Since benign myoepitheliomas are considered to represent one extreme of the histologic spectrum of mixed tumor, the treatment and prognosis are essentially the same as for benign mixed tumor. Patients with these tumors should be treated by a complete excision that ensures a tumor-free margin; in minor gland sites, this will usually involve surgical excision with a rim of normal surrounding tissue.

Malignant Myoepithelioma

Clinical and Pathologic Features. Most myoepitheliomas behave in a benign fashion, with a very minimal tendency for recurrence. They have lower recurrence rates than do mixed tumors with only occasional recurrences reported.[305] Occasional myoepitheliomas, however, have been reported to behave in a locally aggressive or malignant fashion.[305, 309, 315–319] Most of these have been spindle cell myoepitheliomas, although rare atypical plasmacytoid tumors or clear cell tumors have been reported.[305, 318] These *malignant myoepitheliomas*, which are also known as *myoepithelial carcinomas*, have a cellular make-up similar to benign myoepithelioma (see earlier discussion) and, in addition, are characterized histologically by cellular atypia or an infiltrative growth pattern, often with prominent necrosis and mitotic activity, and are capable of metastasis (Fig. 6–18). Occasional tumors may demonstrate focal squamous differentiation[305] or clear cytoplasm. If a clear cell tumor has a focal biphasic pattern with intercalated duct–like structures surrounded by clear cells, we prefer to classify it as an epithelial-myoepithelial carcinoma rather than as a clear cell malignant myoepithelioma. Malignant myoepithelioma may also be the malignant component of a carcinoma ex mixed tumor.[315, 320]

Based on combined data from a recent review of 35 cases from the literature and the AFIP,[305] 25 cases from Memorial Sloan-Kettering Cancer Center,[315] and a series of 10 cases from the Beijing

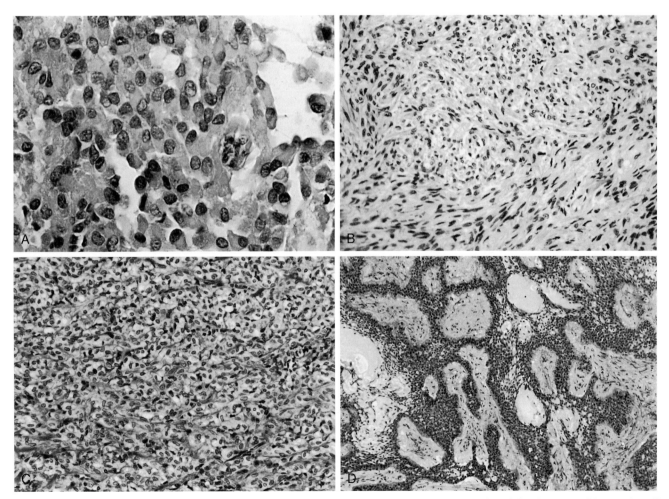

Figure 6–17. The four patterns of benign myoepithelioma: the typical plasmacytoid pattern contains eccentric nuclei and abundant eosinophilic cytoplasm (A); the spindle cell pattern is made up of a uniform population of interlacing bundles of spindle cells with moderate amounts of light eosinophilic cytoplasm (B); the clear cell variant is composed of a somewhat uniform sheet of cells with a moderate amount of clear cytoplasm (C); and the reticular type is composed of numerous interconnecting ribbons of myoepithelial cells (D).

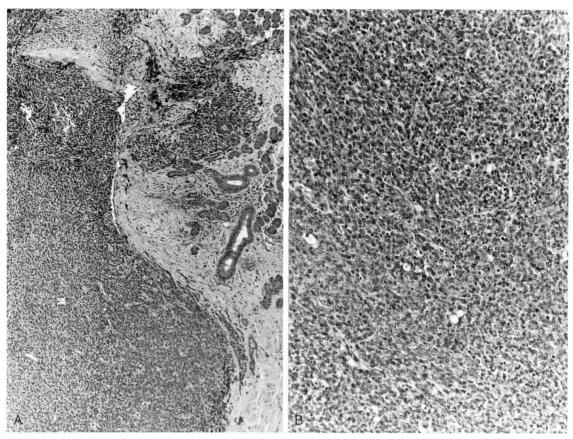

Figure 6–18. Malignant myoepithelioma. There is a poorly circumscribed tumor that is infiltrating adjacent salivary tissue *(A)*. The tumor is composed of a sheet of pleomorphic, plump to spindled tumor cells with minimal cytoplasm *(B)*. This tumor stained for cytokeratin and muscle-specific actin confirming its myoepithelial nature (not illustrated).

Medical University,[321] 64% (45 cases) arose in the parotid gland, 23% (16 cases) arose in the minor salivary or seromucinous glands (most frequently the palate and including one case each in the larynx, maxillary sinus, and base of the tongue), and 11% (8 cases) arose in the submandibular gland. The site was not given for one case. Other authors have also reported rare tumors arising in the maxillary sinus.[315, 322, 323] Patients' age ranged from 14 to 86 years with a mean in the sixth decade, and there was a similar sex distribution in two series[305, 315] and a 4:1 male:female ratio in the other.[321] Tumors ranged in size from 2 to 20 cm in greatest dimension, were usually unencapsulated, and had a gray-white cut surface.

Malignant myoepitheliomas frequently but not always express at least focal reactivity to keratin, S100, smooth muscle actin, muscle specific actin, vimentin, calponin, and glial fibrillary acidic protein; expression of epithelial and myoepithelial differentiation immunohistochemically will allow proper classification of an otherwise undifferentiated sarcoma or clear cell myoepithelioma. Ultrastructural demonstration of myoepithelial differentiation, that is, intracytoplasmic intermediate filaments with dense bodies, extracellular basement membrane material, and junctional complexes, will help establish the diagnosis of an otherwise poorly differentiated malignant neoplasm as a myoepithelial carcinoma. We require keratin positivity together with positive staining for one or more myoepithelial markers or ultrastructural confirmation before a diagnosis of malignant myoepithelioma is made.

Treatment and Prognosis. These tumors should be considered intermediate- to high-grade neoplasms. Treatment consists of wide surgical excision combined with radiation. Sixty-three percent[322] of 46 tumors with follow-up recurred, with frequent multiple recurrences (five of these patients had no additional follow-up information available). Twenty-eight percent of patients (13 patients) died from their disease, 20% (9 patients) were living with disease,

33% (15 patients) were free of disease, 37% (17 patients) developed distant metastases most frequently to the lung, and 8.7% (4 patients) died of unrelated causes.[301, 315, 321]

Warthin's Tumor (Papillary Cystadenoma Lymphomatosum)

Warthin's tumor, also referred to as papillary cystadenoma lymphomatosum, is the second most frequent benign tumor arising in the parotid gland after benign mixed tumor. It has also been referred to in the literature as "adenolymphoma"[324, 325]; however, we prefer not to use this term, as it may give the mistaken impression that one is dealing with a lymphoma.

Clinical Features. Warthin's tumor is a slow-growing, commonly cystic neoplasm that arises almost exclusively in the parotid gland, frequently in its lower portion over the angle of the mandible. Occasional tumors (2.7% to 12%)[326] may arise in extraparotid locations, most frequently in periparotid lymph nodes in the area of the parotid tail or in the upper neck, where it can mimic a lymph node metastasis.[327, 328] Rare tumors with a similar histologic appearance have been reported in the oral cavity,[329] larynx,[329] lacrimal gland,[330] or nasopharynx.[331] A few tumors have been reported in the submandibular gland,[329, 332] but good histologic documentation of a true intraparenchymal submandibular Warthin's tumor is not available.[333]

Patients typically present with swelling with only an occasional patient complaining of pain. The average annual incidence rate for the United States (Jefferson County, Alabama) is 1.43 per 100,000 persons.[334] Warthin's tumor accounts for 4% to 15% of all salivary gland epithelial tumors[333, 335] and represents 4% to 10% of all parotid tumors, with an occasional series showing relative frequencies as high as 30%.[336, 337] Warthin's tumor has a peak incidence in the fifth to seventh decades of life with patients in one review ranging in age between 2.5 and 92 years.[338] It is considered to be more common in males than females, with earlier studies demonstrating male:female ratios of up to 10:1.[338] However, several more recent reports have demonstrated a more equal sex distribution.[336, 337, 339, 340] There appears to be a definite positive association between Warthin's tumor and cigarette smoking[337, 340–343] as well as a history of radiation exposure, with an increasing incidence of these tumors associated with increasing radiation exposure.[344, 345] Recent reports have noted an increasing incidence of this neoplasm in the general population, whereas the incidence of other salivary gland neoplasms has remained constant.[341] The increased incidence of this tumor and its increasing frequency in women, are thought to be related to increased tobacco use among women.[339]

Warthin's tumor arises principally in the white population and is much less frequent in Asian, Hispanic, and black populations,[338, 340] although one recent series has documented an increasing incidence in African Americans.[340] It is the most common salivary gland tumor to present with multifocal or bilateral involvement, with 5% to 14% of patients presenting with bilateral masses, 25% of which present simultaneously and 75% metachronously.[346]

Pathologic Features. Warthin's tumors, on gross examination, present as round to oval, well-circumscribed masses that are typically encapsulated. Their cut surfaces range from a brown to tan-white color, depending on the relative percentage of oncocytic epithelium to lymphoid stroma. These tumors contain a variable number of cysts that exude yellowish, mucoid, brown to clear fluid and, rarely, semisolid caseous material (Fig. 6–19A, see p. 344).[336, 338] Most tumors measure 2 to 4 cm in diameter, but occasional tumors may be over 12 cm in greatest dimension.[347]

The histologic appearance of Warthin's tumor is distinctive and pathognomonic. The tumor is composed of varying proportions of lymphoid stroma and epithelium, with the latter characterized by epithelium-lined cystic spaces, often with numerous papillary projections and containing homogeneous eosinophilic, granular material (Fig. 6–19B, C, see p. 344). The epithelial lining of the cystic spaces and papillae are composed of two layers of oncocytic cells: an inner row of tall columnar cells with central or luminally located nuclei and an outer layer of cuboidal and polygonal cells. The cytoplasm in both layers is usually granular and intensely eosinophilic due to abundant mitochondria, a classic characteristic of this neoplasm. Frequently, scattered mucin-secreting cells and foci with squamous metaplasia are seen (Fig. 6–19D, E). These may be found together, and rarely one or both components may be abundant.[335, 348] During frozen section examination or with fine needle aspiration biopsy, the latter cell types may result in a false-positive diagnosis of mucoepidermoid or squamous cell carcinoma, especially if the squamous elements are associated with reactive atypia.

The lymphoid stroma is always benign and reactive (with rare exceptions, see later discussion), with frequent follicle formation often containing germinal centers. Rarely, tumors will exhibit a foreign body giant cell reaction with cholesterol clefts and granulomas,[335, 348] and sebaceous differentiation may be found.[349] The proportion of epithelial to lymphoid component is variable from tumor to tumor and within the same tumor, leading some investigators to subclassify this neoplasm into four groups: (1) *typical type* with an epithelial component of 50% (77% of tumors), (2) *stroma poor* with an epithelial component of 70% to 80% (13.5% of tumors), (3) *stroma rich* with an epithelial component of 20% to 30% (2% of tumors), and (4) a *metaplastic type* with large areas of squamous metaplasia (7.5 of tumors).[348]

Malignancy developing in Warthin's tumor is an extremely rare event representing less than 1% of Warthin's tumors in several large series.[348, 350, 351] Carcinomas and lymphomas occur with approximately equal frequency; squamous cell carcinoma, mucoepidermoid carcinoma, undifferentiated carcinoma, adenocarcinoma (oncocytic and other types), and other carcinomas have been reported;[333, 348, 350–353, 353a] Seifert reported a patient with bilateral

mucoepidermoid carcinomas arising in association with bilateral Warthin's tumors.[354] Destructive growth with associated desmoplasia is a strong indicator of malignancy. Atypia by itself is worrisome, although occasional benign Warthin's tumors, especially the metaplastic subtype, may exhibit a significant degree of cytologic atypia.

Several theories on the pathogenesis of Warthin's tumor have been advocated. The most popular of these contends that the tumor develops from heterotopic salivary gland epithelium present in preexisting intraparotid or periparotid lymph nodes.[333, 338, 350, 355, 356] Other authors have suggested, however, that these tumors result from an adenomatous or metaplastic epithelial proliferation with secondary lymphocytic infiltration.[333, 338, 350, 355, 357] Epstein-Barr virus appears to have some role in the pathogenesis of Warthin's tumor.[358, 359] The virus has been found in tumor epithelium, especially in patients with multifocal or bilateral lesions,[352] and there appears to be a higher frequency of autoimmune disorders in patients with Warthin's tumor than in patients with mixed tumors or in healthy subjects.

Differential Diagnosis. The histologic pattern of this neoplasm is so characteristic that other tumors usually do not need to be considered in the differential diagnosis. Rarely, however, other tumors may come under diagnostic consideration. Oncocytic papillary cystadenoma has a similar epithelial component, but unlike Warthin's tumor, it is found more frequently in minor gland sites than in the parotid gland and it lacks the characteristic lymphoid component. Infarcted Warthin's tumors, those with necrosis, and those with prominent squamous or mucinous metaplasia may be accompanied by fibrosis and a significant degree of cytologic atypia. The destructive, infiltrative growth characteristic of malignancy is, however, lacking. In problematic cases, additional tissue sampling usually will help establish proper classification.

Treatment and Prognosis. The recommended treatment is superficial parotidectomy with preservation of the facial nerve plus good operative exposure to exclude multifocal disease, especially in periparotid lymph nodes. To reduce the risk of facial nerve damage, some observers recommend enucleation whenever feasible.[333, 360, 361] Earlier studies have demonstrated recurrence rates as high as 25%, most likely due to multifocal disease, but the majority of recent studies document rates of 2% or less.[333] Similar results are achieved by investigators using enucleation.[360]

Carcinomas arising in Warthin's tumor are extremely rare and of such varying histologic type that only minimal information is available as to prognosis. These were most recently reviewed by Ellis and Auclair,[333] who noted that 33% of tumors metastasized to regional lymph nodes and one tumor metastasized distantly.

Basal Cell Adenoma and Adenocarcinoma

Basal Cell Adenoma

Basal cell adenoma (BCA) as defined by the WHO is a distinctive, benign neoplasm composed of isomorphic basaloid cells organized with a prominent basal cell layer and distinct basement membrane–like material. BCA lacks the myxochondroid stromal component of a pleomorphic adenoma.[362] Kleinsasser and Klein first established BCA as a specific entity in 1967.[363] Since that time, there has been disagreement about the spectrum of tumors belonging to this group and about their proper designation. Many series in the 1970s and 1980s classified these tumors with other non-mixed tumors, including canalicular adenomas, into the category of "monomorphic adenomas." Therefore, it is difficult to obtain precise demographic information on these tumors. In 1991, the WHO separately classified BCA and canalicular adenoma (see Table 6–4), a practice with which we concur.

Clinical Features. BCA accounts for 1% to 2% of all salivary gland epithelial tumors.[362, 364] Over 80% of BCAs arise in the major salivary glands, the majority occurring in the parotid gland. Less frequently, these tumors may be found in minor gland sites, with the upper lip being the most common site, followed by the buccal mucosa.[364] In addition, BCA has been reported at sites of periparotid or cervical intranodal ectopic salivary gland[365] and intranasally.[366]

Basal cell adenomas arise almost exclusively in adults. The average age of patients with BCA is 57.7 years,[364] more than a decade older than the average age of patients with pleomorphic adenoma.[367] A recent report describes three very unusual cases of congenital BCA.[368] We feel, however, that these examples are most appropriately classified under the spectrum of sialoblastoma rather than as a special type of BCA (see sialoblastoma section). There is a 2 : 1 female predominance for most BCAs, although the membranous variant has an equal male : female distribution.[363, 364, 369, 370] Clinically indistinguishable from pleomorphic adenoma, the typical case of BCA presents as a mobile superficial parotid tumor.

Pathologic Features. Except for some of the membranous type of BCAs, which have a multifocal or multinodular growth pattern, BCAs are round to oval, well-encapsulated, soft to firm neoplasms. Most tumors measure less than 3 cm, although diameters up to 8 cm have been described.[364] On cut section, they are typically uniform and solid without necrosis. However, occasional cysts filled with brown mucinous material may be present. Tumors vary from grayish-white to light brown to pink, and their appearance often simulates an enlarged lymph node.[371]

Microscopically, BCAs are benign tumors composed of relatively isomorphic basaloid cells, a conspicuous basal cell layer, and distinctive basement membrane–like material. Most tumors are well circumscribed and encapsulated, although any of the subtypes may have a multinodular microscopic pattern. BCAs lack the characteristic myxochondroid matrix of pleomorphic adenoma. Based on architecture, basal cell adenomas may be divided into four subtypes: solid, trabecular, tubular, and membranous (Fig. 6–20). Although the solid variant appears most frequently, individual tumors commonly display several architectural growth patterns. The distinctive basaloid cells that make up these tumors have two histologic phenotypes. The first cell type, found peripherally, frequently in a palisading arrangement within the cell nests and cords, is a small cuboidal or columnar cell, with round, deeply staining nuclei and little discernible cytoplasm. The second cell type is larger with modest cytoplasm, indistinct cell borders, and a pale-staining oval nucleus; moreover, nuclei may exhibit small eosinophilic nucleoli. Larger cells predominate centrally within the epithelial nests, sheets, and trabeculae. Focal clear cell change, though unusual, may be present; these cells are glycogen negative by PAS stain.[369] Spindled myoepithelial cells are occasionally found in the stroma of a few tumors surrounding the basaloid tumor nests. Rarely, sebaceous[371] and oncocytic[371a] differentiation may be found.

Hallmarking the **solid variant** of BCA are neoplastic cells growing in solid epithelial sheets, broad bands, or islands with peripheral palisading. Of significant diagnostic aid are distinctive basosquamous whorls present centrally within the cellular nests. Cells in these whorls, or eddies, acquire a squamoid appearance and occasionally show frank maturation to keratinizing squamous cells with pearl formation. Although minute luminal structures can be present in solid cell masses,[372] ductal structures are not usually obvious in this variant. Cystic change, however, may be encountered. Stroma is scanty and frequently hyalinized. Slightly irregular to round foci with hyalinized basement membrane–like material may be found within tumor islands, which may communicate with similar extracellular material at the periphery of the tumor nodules. Rarely, mitoses and apoptotic cells may be encountered. Perineural encroachment by tumor cells has been described and is not necessarily an indication of malignancy[373]; however, definitive perineural invasion strongly argues for a diagnosis of basal cell adenocarcinoma.

In the **trabecular** subtype, tumor cells grow as thin trabeculae and cords separated by strands of vascularized stroma. Neoplastic cells have the same appearance as those seen in the solid variant. In occasional tumors, focal microcystic stromal change imparts an ameloblastoma-like appearance.[371] Rare tumors with a trabecular pattern will have a richly cellular stroma composed of modified myoepithelial cells at the periphery of and between the tumor cords.[374]

In the **tubular** type, which is the least frequent variant, ductal structures are a prominent feature. Lumina lined by cuboidal cells are surrounded by one or more layers of basaloid cells. Proteinaceous eosinophilic material is present within ductal lumina. Not uncommonly, trabecular and ductal patterns are encountered together. This has led some investigators to consider the tubular and trabecular variants as a single tubulotrabecular type.[370]

The **membranous** form of BCA, also known as the dermal anlage tumor, has been separated from the other variants because of its particular clinical associations with a tumor diathesis and its histology.[375] Affected patients have a propensity to develop membranous BCAs, multiple dermal cylindromas (turban tumors), trichoepitheliomas, eccrine spiradenomas, trichilemmomas, and basal cell epitheliomas.[370] However, the majority of membranous basal cell adenomas occur independent of this association. Contrasting the other subtypes, membranous basal cell adenoma tends to be multilobulated or multinodular and is often not encapsulated. This explains the high recurrence rates of 25% to 37%, similar to that encountered with dermal cylindroma.

Histologically, membranous BCA is strikingly similar to dermal cylindroma. Cellular nests and/or trabeculae are surrounded, characteristically, by a thick collar of eosinophilic hyaline basement membrane–like material. Similar PAS-positive material is present as intraepithelial droplets or globules, which often coalesce within the cellular nests.

Ultrastructurally, abundant stromal and intercellular reduplicated, multilayered basal laminae are seen corresponding to the hyaline basement membrane material evident histologically and so particularly prominent in the membranous variant.[372, 375] Several cell types have been demonstrated by electron microscopy, including centrally placed squamous cells, basally located secretory cells, intermediate cells, and peripheral myoepithelial-like cells.[372] The tubular variant contains luminal cells with microvillous surface specialization, terminal junctional complexes, and occasional secretory granules corresponding to ductal differentiation.[366, 372]

Immunohistochemical staining is nonspecific, variable, and somewhat dependent on histologic subtype. The solid variant shows high molecular weight cytokeratin positivity centrally and negativity peripherally; this observation is congruent with central squamous differentiation.[376] Positive staining for CEA, apical or cytoplasmic or both, may be seen in luminal cells in areas of ductal differentiation.[377, 378] Myoepithelial-like cells that stain positive for muscle-specific actin may be present throughout, although they tend to concentrate peripherally within cell nests. Staining for S100 protein is inconsistent but is typically located in the peripheral cells adjacent to connective tissue stroma.[370] Zarbo and coauthors[378a] studied 14 basal cell adenomas with three sensitive, smooth-muscle markers (α-smooth muscle actin, smooth muscle myosin heavy chain, and calponin). They found that 13 stained with all three markers, usually at the periphery of nests or trabeculae.

Differential Diagnosis. The most problematic and significant consideration in the differential diagnosis is adenoid cystic carcinoma. BCA may have areas closely simulating adenoid cystic carcinoma. Distinction is based on coexistent areas typical of BCA (e.g., typical solid pattern areas), the encapsulated, noninvasive growth pattern of basal cell adenoma, the lack of perineural invasion, and the more bland tumor cell population. The distinctive basosquamous whorls of BCA are helpful, as squamous differentiation is not usually encountered in adenoid cystic carcinoma. Also, the cribriform pattern typical of adenoid cystic carcinoma is infrequent in BCA.

Separation from basal cell adenocarcinoma is predominantly architectural, as the cellular composition of these two tumors is similar. These low-grade carcinomas exhibit invasive, unencapsulated growth into adjacent soft tissue, often with associated perineural or vascular invasion. In addition, Nagao et al.[379] recently noted that proliferation rates of greater than 5% using Ki-67 immunohistochemistry support a diagnosis of basal cell adenocarcinoma, whereas rates under 2.7% are more characteristic of BCA.

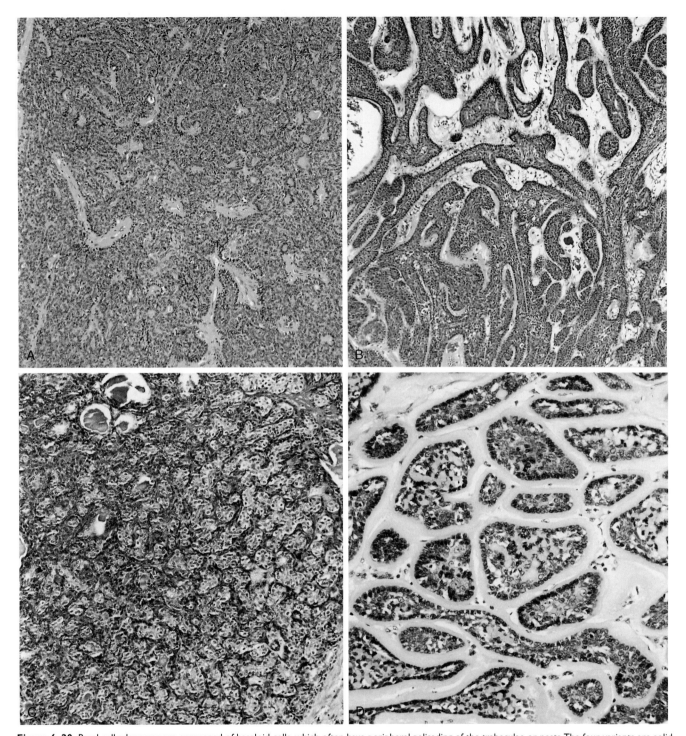

Figure 6–20. Basal cell adenomas are composed of basaloid cells, which often have peripheral palisading of the trabeculae or nests. The four variants are solid (A), trabecular (B), tubular (C), and membranous (D).

Distinction from high-grade carcinoma with basaloid cells is based on the noninvasive growth pattern, lack of mitotic figures, and absence of apoptotic cells in BCA. Cellular pleomorphic adenomas are distinguished by the presence of characteristic myxochondroid stroma, whereas canalicular adenomas can be distinguished by their double row of low columnar or cuboidal cells arranged in parallel branching cords. In addition, myoepithelial differentiation is not seen in canalicular adenoma.

Treatment and Prognosis. These benign tumors are amenable to conservative resection (e.g., superficial parotidectomy). However, recurrence may develop in a significant percentage of patients (25%) with the membranous variant of BCA.[370] Although exceedingly rare,

malignant transformation of BCA has been reported.[380] Adenoid cystic carcinoma,[371, 381] basal cell adenocarcinoma,[382] adenocarcinoma (not otherwise specified) and salivary duct carcinoma[383] have been described to arise in association with BCA.

Basal Cell Adenocarcinoma

Clinical Features. Although prior reports[384–387] described isolated cases of malignant "basal cell" and "basaloid" tumors of salivary gland origin, Ellis and Wiscovitch[388] clearly established basal cell adenocarcinoma (BCAC) as a distinct type of low-grade carcinoma of salivary gland origin. Considered the malignant counterpart of basal cell adenoma, with which it shares demographic and histologic features, BCAC may arise either de novo or from a pre-existing basal cell adenoma.[389] These tumors account for 1.6% of all salivary gland tumors and 2.9% of malignant salivary gland neoplasms.[390] Almost 90% of cases arise in the parotid gland, where they account for 0.6% of parotid tumors[391] and up to 5% of primary parotid carcinomas.[390, 392] Less commonly, they occur within the submandibular gland,[388] minor salivary glands, or sinonasal tract,[393, 394] and rarely may arise in the sublingual gland.[395]

No gender predominance has been noted. BCAC occurs over a wide age range (third to tenth decades), with a mean age at diagnosis of 60 years. The majority of BCAC arise de novo; however, slightly less than one quarter of cases have been documented to arise in its benign counterpart, the basal cell adenoma.[396] The presenting manifestations are nonspecific and include a parotid or submandibular mass and, occasionally, pain. Facial nerve involvement was not encountered in two reported series.[388, 396] Association with concurrent skin adnexal tumors (especially eccrine cylindromas and trichoepitheliomas) has been noted in 14% of patients with BCAC,[396] which is less frequent than the association of concurrent basal cell adenomas and adnexal tumors (25%–35%).

Pathologic Features. BCAC ranges in size from 0.7 to 7.0 cm with a mean size in two series of 2.4 and 3.4 cm.[391, 396] BCAC mimics the architectural patterns of basal cell adenoma: solid, membranous, trabecular or tubular patterns. The solid pattern, most commonly encountered, has predominantly confluent tumor islands with areas of palisading basaloid cells. The membranous pattern has closely approximated nests or single islands surrounded by hyaline basement membrane material, which may also be found within the islands, forming a jigsaw puzzle–like pattern (Fig. 6–21). The trabecular pattern forms interconnecting ribbons or cords of tumor with occasional glandular spaces. These glandular spaces are more open and pronounced in the tubular pattern. Low-power scanning of BCAC reveals the standard features of aggressive neoplasia: infiltration into or destructive overgrowth of surrounding tissue, possible necrosis, and perineural or vascular invasion (Fig. 6–21A, D. Multicentricity can rarely be seen in major salivary gland BCAC. Basement membrane hyaline can be quite prominent in the trabecular, membranous, and tubular patterns. Hyaline material is deposited and dissects between cells resulting in a "pseudocribriforming" pattern (see differential diagnosis). Nuclear palisading is frequent at the periphery of the infiltrating nests and islands. Squamous differentiation with keratin pearls can be seen toward the center of the islands. Spindled myoepithelial cells may be present and are usually located at the periphery of the tumor islands. Cells within the center of islands may have a loose and discohesive stellate reticulin ameloblastoma-like pattern.

Cytologically, BCAC is composed of basaloid cells with oval to round nuclei and high nuclear-to-cytoplasmic ratios. Mitotic figures and cellular pleomorphism may be marked, although tumors frequently have minimal atypia, with the diagnosis of carcinoma being based on invasive growth or perineural or vascular invasion. Perineural and vascular invasion are common and, when present in an otherwise typical basal cell adenoma, should lead to the diagnosis of BCAC being given serious consideration. An unusual tumor may warrant a diagnosis of BCAC on mitotic activity alone. Ellis and Auclair consider a mitotic count greater than 4 or 5 per 10 high-power fields to be an indication of malignancy.[392] This is supported in the recent report by Nagao et al.,[391] who found in their series of basal cell adenomas and BCACs that all basaloid tumors with mitotic rates over 4 per 10 high-power fields were carcinomas.

Ultrastructurally, BCAC appears similar to basal cell adenoma; both ductal and myoepithelial cells are encountered.[397, 398] Amorphous deposition of basal lamina is found between cells and around groups of cells. True glandular differentiation with apical vacuoles and microvilli is sparse.[397] Immunohistochemistry is currently of no aid in distinguishing BCAC from basal cell adenoma, as these two neoplasms have similar immunophenotypes.[398, 399] DNA ploidy studies on isolated cases of BCAC have reported both diploid and

aneuploid results,[397, 400] whereas p53 mutations and expression of epidermal growth factor are found in 55% and 27%, respectively, of tumors.[391]

Differential Diagnosis. The differential diagnosis of BCAC includes basaloid-squamous cell carcinoma (BSC), adenoid cystic carcinoma (AdCC), and basal cell adenoma (BCA). An infiltrating cribriforming pattern, palisading cells, and hyaline deposits are common to BCAC, BSC, and AdCC. The need to distinguish BSC from BCAC arises only when BCAC originates in minor salivary sites. Cribriform formation is common to both BSC and BCAC, and both BSC and BCAC may express vimentin with a "dot-like" cytoplasmic distribution[395, 399] as well as squamous differentiation. One can unequivocally distinguish BSC from BCAC by identifying overlying squamous carcinoma in situ or a superficially located squamous carcinoma. In addition, the mitotic activity in BSC is far greater than one finds in BCAC, whereas an ameloblastoma-like stellate reticulin pattern is only seen in BCAC.

Although the cribriform-like pattern of AdCC is only rarely encountered in BCAC, distinction from adenoid cystic carcinoma, particularly the solid variant, can be challenging. The cells of AdCC tend to be more uniform, smaller, more angulated, and more hyperchromatic than the cells of BCAC. The dual cell population, typical of BCAC, is not conspicuous in adenoid cystic carcinoma. One can distinguish BCAC from AdCC by identifying squamous differentiation and areas with a stellate reticulin ameloblastoma-like pattern. Vimentin may be a helpful diagnostic adjunct, as AdCC may have diffuse vimentin expression, whereas BCAC may have a "dot-like" cytoplasmic distribution.

The trabecular, solid, and tubular variants of basal cell adenoma, which also have a propensity to arise in the parotid gland, usually can be distinguished from BCAC by encapsulation of the former. However, the membranous variant of BCA may cause diagnostic difficulty, as it is frequently unencapsulated and may grow in a multifocal fashion. Similarities between the membranous variant of BCA and BCAC include histology, lack of encapsulation, and nearly equal recurrence rates. We feel that mitotic rates greater than 4 per 10 high-power fields or an invasive destructive pattern of growth into adjacent tissues or perineural or vascular invasion is necessary to establish a diagnosis of BCAC. In addition, quantification of cycling cells may be helpful. In a recent study of 11 BCACs and 9 BCAs, Ki-67 rates over 5% strongly indicated malignancy.[391]

Rarely, other tumors need to be considered in the differential diagnosis of BCAC. Polymorphous low-grade adenocarcinoma generally arises in association with minor salivary glands; such an origin is exceedingly rare for BCAC. Additionally, the former exhibits a variety of growth patterns foreign to BCAC, such as a single-file pattern, as seen in lobular carcinoma of the breast. Distinction from pleomorphic adenoma, in particular those with a multicentric growth pattern, is based on lack of characteristic chondromyxoid stroma. High-grade basaloid malignancies, such as neuroendocrine carcinoma, exhibit mitotic activity, apoptosis, and necrosis beyond that seen in BCAC. Immunohistochemistry is helpful in establishing a diagnosis of neuroendocrine carcinoma. Distinction from skin-based basal cell carcinoma relies on clinical features.

Treatment and Prognosis. BCAC is optimally treated by wide surgical resection with negative margins. With adequate resection, additional therapy is not warranted, but adjuvant radiotherapy may be used for cases with close or positive resection margins. Elective neck dissection is not warranted. Reported cases of major salivary BCAC with clinical follow-up reveal a low-grade malignant biology.[388, 391, 395, 396, 401, 402] The general impression is that major salivary BCAC is less aggressive than adenoid cystic carcinoma. Muller and Barnes[396] culled 45 cases of BCAC with clinical follow-up from the literature, which demonstrated a local recurrence rate of 37%, local metastatic rate of 8%, and distant metastatic rate of 4%; disease-related mortality occurred in 2% of patients. In addition, Nagao et al.[391] recently reported 11 cases, 10 with follow-up: 50% of tumors recurred, none metastasized, and there were no deaths from tumor. Minor salivary or seromucinous gland BCAC

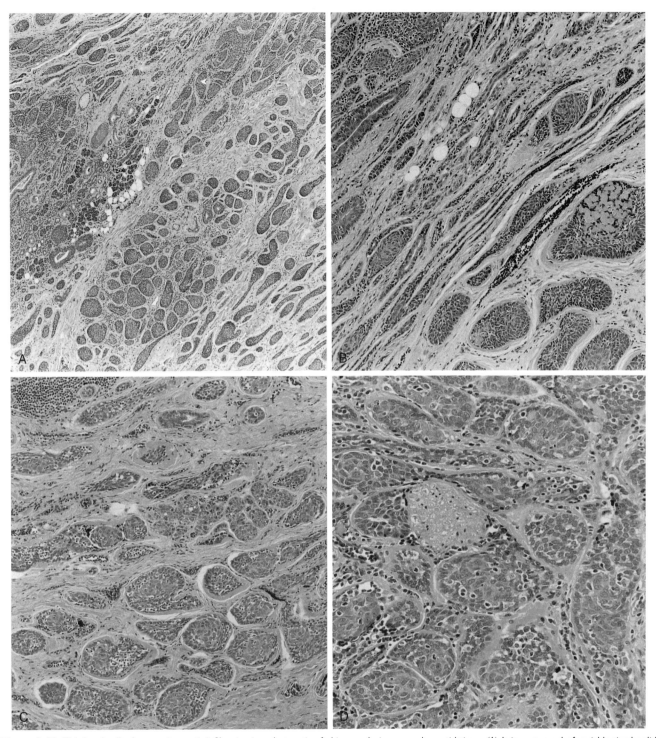

Figure 6–21. This basal cell adenocarcinoma is infiltrating in a destructive fashion, replacing normal parotid tissue *(A)*. It is composed of variably sized, solid nests of bland basaloid cells, similar to basal cell adenoma, some of which have peripheral palisading and are surrounded by basement membrane material (membranous pattern) *(B, C)*. In addition, there is focal basement membrane production within tumor nests *(B)*. A focus of perineural invasion is seen *(D)*.

have a more aggressive course owing to tumor stage at presentation and the inherent poorer resectability of minor salivary gland tumors. Four of 12 patients reported by Fonseca and Soares with intraoral or sinonasal BCAC died of disease within 4 to 7 years.[393]

Canalicular Adenoma

Until the recent WHO classification in 1991, canalicular adenoma was classified as a variant of basal cell adenoma (BCA) or mono-

morphic adenoma (see Tables 6–2 through 6–4). There are, however, sufficient clinicopathologic and histologic differences between BCA and canalicular adenoma to warrant separate classification.

Clinical Features. Canalicular adenomas are benign neoplasms that arise almost exclusively from the minor salivary glands of the oral cavity, where they account for 4% to 6% of minor salivary gland tumors.[403, 404] These tumors commonly affect older patients, with a peak incidence in the seventh decade.[403] The average age of incidence varies from 60 to 67 years.[405, 406] Females are more commonly affected than males. The female-to-male ratio according to different studies ranges from 1.2:1 to 1.8:1.[405–407] Clinically, canalicular adenoma presents as a slow-growing, asymptomatic, mobile nodule, most commonly arising in the upper lip (73% to 100% of cases in reported series[404, 406, 407]). It is the second most common upper lip salivary gland tumor after benign mixed tumor.[403] In decreasing frequency of occurrence, these tumors may occasionally arise in the buccal mucosa, lower lip, palate, and major salivary glands.[403, 408, 409] Rarely, canalicular adenoma may present with multiple clinically palpable nodules, with one report of 13 discrete nodules in the upper lip and anterior buccal mucosa.[409] Metachronous tumors may also be seen.[409]

The mass is usually small at the time of diagnosis, with a mean diameter of 1.7 cm.[406] The overlying mucosa is normally intact; occasionally, it is slightly bluish, mimicking a mucocele.[409]

Pathologic Features. The microscopic appearance of canalicular adenoma is characteristic (Fig. 6–22). These tumors are usually circumscribed or encapsulated and are composed of interconnecting strands or cords of uniform, single, cuboidal to columnar cells, usually with scant to moderate amounts of eosinophilic cytoplasm, oval nuclei with diffuse granular nuclear chromatin, and indistinct borders that form parallel columns, producing long canaliculi with scattered duct-like or gland-like structures. These cords may alternately separate and come together forming a "beads on a string" arrangement. Occasional foci may contain widened cellular areas between the parallel columns composed of slightly smaller polygonal cells. Because of the absence of myoepithelial cells (see later discussion), the epithelial cells are sharply demarcated from the surrounding stroma. Cellular pleomorphism is minimal, and mitoses, if present, are rare. In addition, occasional tumors will have papillary projections into the cystic spaces.[410] Rare psammoma bodies, scattered mucinous or oncocytic cells, and areas with cystic change may be found.[410] The stroma separating parallel rows of cells is delicate, well vascularized, commonly mucoid, and sparsely cellular. Multifocal microscopic foci of canalicular adenoma are common (22% in one series of 49 patients[407]); in these cases, the main tumor frequently is encapsulated, whereas the smaller foci often are not.[406, 409]

Ultrastructural and immunohistochemical studies confirm the ductal nature of the tumor cells.[410, 411] The tumor cells stain for cytokeratin and S100 and very focally for glial fibrillary acidic protein. Smooth muscle actin, calponin, and smooth muscle myosin heavy chain are not found in canalicular adenoma.[378a, 403, 411] Myoepithelial cells are *not* usually a part of this tumor,[378a, 410] although one report did demonstrate myoepithelial-like cells adjacent to the capsule of one tumor.[412]

Differential Diagnosis. The differential diagnosis consists of BCA, polymorphous low-grade adenocarcinoma, adenoid cystic carcinoma, and, rarely, pleomorphic adenoma. Parallel rows of tumor cells are not usually a feature of BCA, and their presence should allow appropriate classification. However, occasional tumors may have overlapping histologic features with BCA, making further subclassification impossible.[404] Immunohistochemistry should be helpful, as BCA, unlike canalicular adenoma, frequently has myoepithelial cells that stain with appropriate markers. Also, rarely, both BCA and canalicular adenoma may occur in the same patient.[404] Polymorphous low-grade adenocarcinoma and adenoid cystic carcinoma also do not have large areas with parallel rows of tumor. In addition they, unlike canalicular adenoma, infiltrate adjacent tissues in a destructive fashion, are frequently associated with perineural invasion, and may have myoepithelial cells that can be demonstrated immunohistochemically. Pleomorphic adenomas, unlike canalicular adenomas, will frequently have cartilaginous foci and myoepithelial cells. In addition, the border between the epithelial elements and myxoid matrix within pleomorphic adenoma is "blurred" by myoepithelial cells. This is different from the "sharp" border between the tubules and canaliculi and matrix of canalicular adenoma.

Treatment and Prognosis. Treatment is complete surgical excision. Recurrence after surgical removal is rare and most likely is due to multifocality rather than true recurrence.

Benign and Malignant Oncocytic Tumors

Clinical Features

Major Salivary Glands

Oncocytic tumors are relatively rare, representing 1.6% of 13,749 primary epithelial salivary gland tumors and 1.9% of over 8000 parotid consultations received at the AFIP.[413] The major salivary glands were the dominant site, accounting for 86% of 226 cases (200 benign and 26 malignant). In general practice, oncocytomas represent 1% or less of all parotid tumors. Benign tumors are 5 to 16 times more common than their malignant counterpart.[413–415] In a series of 68 patients with oncocytic salivary tumors, 84% occurred in the parotid, 11% in the submandibular gland, and 5% were incidental findings within cervical lymph nodes.[415] There is no gender pre-

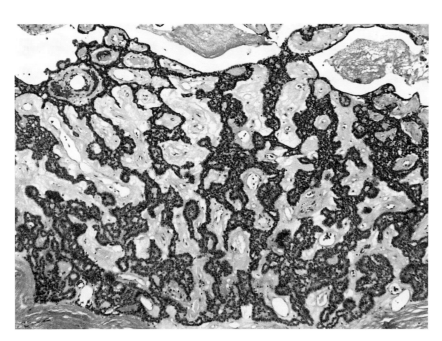

Figure 6–22. Canalicular adenoma is made up of double rows of interconnecting and branching cords of tumor composed of bland, basaloid, cuboidal to columnar cells. The surrounding stroma is acellular with very sparse collagen production.

dilection for these tumors,[415, 416] and most patients present with unilateral painless masses. Oncocytomas are rare in patients younger than 50 years of age, with a peak incidence in the seventh to ninth decades.[414] A history of previous radiation exposure has been documented in 20% of patients with oncocytic tumors; these patients tend to present with oncocytomas two decades earlier than the mean (43 versus 63 years).[415] One report also mentions a familial association with oncocytosis.[417] Oncocytomas may be multifocal or bilateral[418] and in up to 7% of cases, they may be associated with diffuse oncocytosis rather than single tumor nodules.[415, 419–421]

Most oncocytic carcinomas, also referred to as malignant oncocytomas, arise in the parotid gland, with about 10% arising in the submandibular gland. To date, slightly over 50 cases have been reported.[413–415, 422–430] The average age is about 60 years (29–91 years) and there is a 2 : 1 male predominance.[414, 424] The most common clinical presentation is that of a slow-growing mass often associated with pain or facial paralysis.

On gross examination, parotid or submandibular oncocytomas may appear as single, small, well-circumscribed, brown tumors that may have central star-like fibrosis and occasional cyst formation. Oncocytomas may also occur as part of a generalized process, oncocytosis, in which the entire gland undergoes multifocal oncocytic metaplasia and hyperplasia.[415, 417, 431, 432] In this case, the glandular architecture is entirely replaced by multiple brown-tan nodules, some of which may have central scarring, with one or more dominant tumor nodules that overgrow and distort the normal architecture. Oncocytic carcinomas range from well circumscribed to widely invasive.

Minor Salivary or Seromucinous Gland Sites

Larynx. The clinicopathologic features of minor salivary or seromucinous gland oncocytic tumors are sufficiently distinctive from major salivary tumors to warrant separate discussion. Laryngeal oncocytic lesions produce polypoid masses, most often involving the supraglottis. Rather than being a true neoplastic process, laryngeal oncocytic lesions, referred to as papillary oncocytic cystadenomata, are the result of oncocytic metaplasia and hyperplasia of seromucinous glands, with prominent cyst formation. They have been appropriately likened to extraparotid Warthin's tumors. At the other end of the spectrum, predominantly solid oncocytomas have *not* been reported in the larynx. The clinicopathologic features of laryngeal oncocytic lesions are discussed in Chapter 5.

Oral Cavity. A small fraction (5%) of all oncocytic lesions arise in the oral cavity; the palate and cheek are the most common sites.[413] These lesions may span the spectrum from oncocytic papillary cystic tumors (oncocytic papillary cystadenomas) with a variable degree of lymphocytic infiltrate[433, 434] to more solid oncocytomas.[435–437] An association of parotid Warthin's tumors and oral oncocytic papillary cystadenomas has been reported.[434] These lesions may occur on the lips, buccal mucosa, tonsillar fossa, or palate. They form submucosal circumscribed swellings; only one case has been documented as locally invasive.[437]

Sinonasal Cavity. Oncocytic processes from this anatomic site are classified as variations of oncocytic schneiderian (cylindrical cell) papilloma, as discussed in Chapter 3, or as seromucinous gland neoplasia. Unlike major salivary gland oncocytomas, which are usually benign tumors, sinonasal oncocytic tumors have a greater tendency toward local aggression. A few cases of unequivocally benign oncocytoma or pleomorphic adenomas with extensive oncocytic metaplasia have been reported.[438–440] These tumors have a propensity for the lower septum or vestibule. Oncocytic tumors of the superior nasal cavity may also originate from the lacrimal apparatus.[441]

A number of sinonasal oncocytic tumors have shown histologic evidence of local invasion from the onset.[441–445] These tumors occur with a male preponderance (5 : 3) and most are diagnosed after the fifth decade of life. They are generally larger than benign tumors and more clinically aggressive, with a propensity to affect the maxilla or nasal cavity.

Pathologic Features

Oncocytic lesions of the salivary gland are classified as acinar and ductal metaplasia, oncocytosis (nodular or diffuse), oncocytoma (benign or malignant), or tumors with oncocytic metaplasia (e.g., oncocytic mixed tumor, oncocytic mucoepidermoid carcinoma). Oncocytic change of ductal and acinar epithelial cells is termed oncocytic metaplasia (Fig. 6–23A, B). This process is unusual in persons under 50 and becomes more frequent with increasing age. Oncocytosis is the replacement of normal portions of the salivary gland with oncocytes. These may diffusely replace normal parenchyma (diffuse oncocytosis) or more typically produce multiple nodules (oncocytic hyperplasia or nodular oncocytosis). Rarely, the cytoplasm is clear and is termed clear cell oncocytosis (Fig. 6–23C, D). One recent case of oncocytic metaplasia and hyperplasia of the nasopharynx demonstrated prominent melanin pigmentation within the oncocytes.[446]

The distinction between a large hyperplastic nodule and oncocytoma is sometimes difficult and often arbitrary. Usually, an oncocytoma presents as a mass lesion, is larger than other adjacent hyperplastic nodules, and is well circumscribed with at least a partially formed capsule. Most benign oncocytic tumors are solid, with a variable cystic component (Fig. 6–24A, B, see p. 345). The oncocytes form organoid nests and trabeculae with very occasional ducts. Rarely, a papillary cystic tumor will be composed completely of oncocytes. We prefer, as do others,[415] to classify tumors with papillary cystic growth as an oncocytic type of cystadenoma. Cytologically, oncocytes are most frequently cuboidal, with abundant bright pink granular cytoplasm, and have decreased nuclear-to-cytoplasmic ratios when compared with normal parotid ductal cells. They can also have a columnar shape, in which case the nuclear-to-cytoplasmic ratio remains relatively normal. Oncocytic nuclei are typically very round and centrally placed; the nucleoli may be single and prominent.

Focal clear cell change may be seen, with rare tumors being composed almost entirely of clear cells that contain glycogen.[447–450] These latter tumors are referred to as clear cell oncocytomas (Fig. 6–24C, D, see p. 345). Foci of sebaceous and squamous differentiation as well as "pyknocytes," oncocytes with shrunken condensed nuclei, may be found.[415] Occasional tumors may have areas of chronic inflammation. The presence of tall oncocytes with tapered ends, binucleated cuboidal oncocytes, and pyknocytes may be useful in distinguishing oncocytomas from other salivary neoplasms (see later discussion). All tumors that have perineural invasion should be considered potentially malignant. Tumor hyalinization can be present, entrapping nodules of oncocytes and giving a false impression of invasion. Likewise, oncocytomas may be hypervascular with dilated vessels, giving the false effect of vascular invasion, and a rare tumor may be immunoreactive for prostate-specific antigen.[451]

Patients with oncocytic carcinoma typically present with a single or multinodular unencapsulated gray-brown mass.[414] The tumor cells are usually more pleomorphic than their benign counterpart; nuclei are often centrally located and contain large irregular nucleoli, although occasional cases may lack significant atypia.[426, 430] Invasive growth into adjacent tissues is characteristic; scattered mitotic figures and perineural invasion are frequent and foci of necrosis may be found (Fig. 6–25).

Virtually any salivary gland lesion may contain foci of oncocytes; however, this component is usually localized and does not usually cause diagnostic confusion. Although uncommon, the two tumors that most frequently have prominent oncocytic metaplasia are mucoepidermoid carcinoma and benign mixed tumor. Both of these tumors may have areas of prominent oncocytic metaplasia, accounting for 90% or more of the tumor mass. Careful histologic sampling reveals both components and allows for proper classification. Recently, a unique oncocytic lipoadenoma of the submandibular gland was reported.[452]

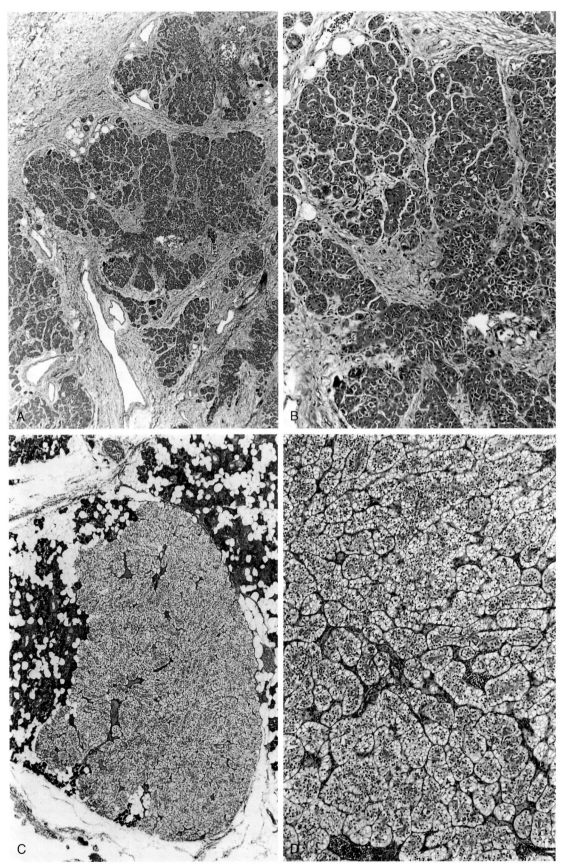

Figure 6–23. A and B, Diffuse oncocytic metaplasia. The normal acini are totally replaced by oncocytic cells with abundant eosinophilic cytoplasm. C and D, Nodular clear cell oncocytosis. This nodule is circumscribed but unencapsulated and replaces the normal serous tissue and fat (C). There are numerous nests of uniform cells with abundant clear cytoplasm (D). This process is usually multifocal and does not destroy the normal anatomic arrangement of the gland.

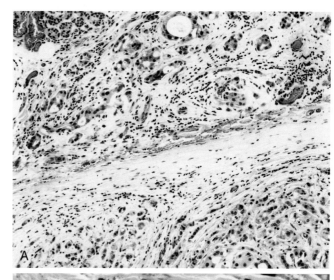

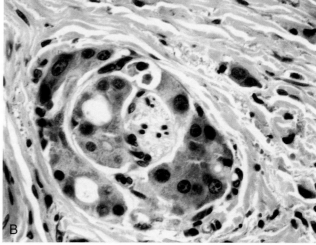

Figure 6–25. Oncocytic carcinoma. This is a destructive infiltrating tumor *(A)* composed of numerous irregular small nests of pleomorphic oncocytic cells with abundant eosinophilic *(B)* to vesicular cytoplasm *(C)*. Nucleoli are prominent *(C)*, there is focal perineural invasion *(B)*, and some of the tumor nests demonstrate lumina.

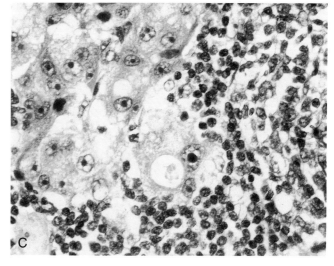

Differential Diagnosis

Most oncocytomas will not cause any diagnostic difficulty. Rarely, clear cell change within oncocytes may cause diagnostic confusion, as clear cell oncocytoma may resemble acinic cell carcinoma. This is illustrated by the cases of oncocytoma described by Brandwein and Huvos,[415] and the case of bilateral clear cell oncocytoma that was published by Nelson and colleagues as bilateral acinic cell carcinoma.[447] An association between clear cell oncocytosis, prior facial radiotherapy, bilateral multifocal disease, and recurrence after parotidectomy has been seen.[413, 415, 448] Ultrastructural examination has shown that glycogen accumulation is responsible for this clear cell change.[449, 450] The extent of the clear cell component relates to the degree of glycogen extraction, which occurs during fixation. Careful light microscopic examination usually reveals focal areas with typical eosinophilic oncocytes scattered among the clear oncocytes (see Fig. 6–24*D*, p. 345). Oncocytosis of the surrounding parotid gland is also very common; it produces a "checkerboard" pattern of parotid adipose tissue and oncocytic nodules. This finding may also be helpful in establishing the diagnosis of oncocytoma, as opposed to other clear cell entities. Also, rarely, "oncocytoid" artifact secondary to electrocautery may cause diagnostic confusion with oncocytoma or oncocytosis.[453]

The main pathologic considerations in the differential diagnosis in addition to acinic cell carcinoma are clear cell carcinoma, mucoepidermoid carcinoma, and metastatic renal cell carcinoma. The balloon cell variant of melanoma is also a "clear cell" tumor that may metastasize to periparotid lymph nodes. Identification of tapered oncocytes, binuclear oncocytes, pink granular cytoplasm, and surrounding parotid oncocytosis is very helpful in establishing the correct diagnosis.

Acinic cell carcinoma can lack the characteristic cytoplasmic basophilic granularity and rarely may have oncocytic cytoplasm. The nuclei of acinic cell carcinoma typically are eccentrically placed and bean-shaped. The zymogen granules of acinic cell carcinoma are positive with digested-PAS staining, while oncocytes are positive for PAS but negative with digested-PAS. Phosphotungstic acid hematoxylin stain, incubated for 48 hours (rather than the standard overnight incubation), is also helpful; the mitochondria appear as cytoplasmic blue granules under oil immersion microscopy. In difficult cases, electron microscopy is the final arbitrator in distinguishing mitochondria from zymogen granules. Mucoepidermoid carcinoma (MEC) may also resemble oncocytoma as the keratinizing cells may have an oncocytoid appearance. The intermediate cells and mucin-producing cells of MEC can resemble clear oncocytes. MECs are frequently cystic and may grow in solid sheets and infiltrating tumor islands, rather than in nests and trabeculae, as oncocytomas do. When cysts are seen in MEC, mucinous goblet cells are easily identified and establish the diagnosis. Unlike oncocytoma, MEC will be positive for intracellular mucicarmine material. Rarely, MEC will undergo prominent oncocytic metaplasia, with the mucoepidermoid component being the minor component.[454] Thorough histologic sampling demonstrates both components and allows proper classification.

The group of clear cell carcinomas are usually low-grade salivary malignancies. They may appear encapsulated at major salivary sites, or have an infiltrating margin. Some evidence of ductal differentiation is usually present in the epithelial-myoepithelial type of clear cell carcinoma and diffuse areas of dense hyalinization are seen in hyalinizing clear cell carcinoma. These latter features are not found in oncocytoma. Also, scattered cells with typical eosinophilic granular cytoplasm are not seen in the clear cell carcinomas. Cytologically, the nuclei of clear cell carcinoma are more pleomorphic, peripherally placed, and triangular or condensed, unlike the round centrally placed nuclei of oncocytomas. Like oncocytomas, many clear cell carcinomas have cytoplasmic glycogen and are PAS-positive and digested-PAS-negative, hence their previous name "glycogen rich adenomas." Electron microscopy may rarely be necessary to establish the appropriate diagnosis.

Metastatic renal cell carcinoma, while also a "clear cell neoplasm," has greater cellular pleomorphism and is associated with hemorrhage and rich vascularity, features not present in clear cell oncocytoma. Rare mixed tumors may have a prominent oncocytic component. Adequate histologic sampling and finding foci of typical mixed tumor will allow this separation. Last, granular cell tumor can occur along any nerve trunk and has been reported in the parotid.[455] As an eosinophilic tumor, this too should be considered in the differential diagnosis of oncocytoma.

In the sinonasal tract, the differential diagnosis of oncocytic tumors includes oncocytic cylindrical cell papilloma, moderately differentiated neuroendocrine carcinoma and low-grade intestinal type adenocarcinoma. Oncocytic cylindrical cell papilloma has areas of a characteristic papillary architecture lined with a pseudostratified columnar epithelium producing a lace-like cribriform pattern with numerous intramucosal microcysts. Goblet cells are frequently present in oncocytic cylindrical cell papilloma but not in oncocytoma. Neuroendocrine tumors may also appear oncocytoid and have mixed on-

cocytic features. Immunohistochemistry will usually allow separation, as neuroendocrine tumors will frequently have dot-like perinuclear staining for low molecular weight cytokeratin and stain for some of the neuroendocrine markers, including synaptophysin, chromogranin, and leu-7. Ultrastructural examination from the postoperative resection can definitively distinguish an oncocytoma from a neuroendocrine tumor if immunohistochemistry is inconclusive. Last, low-grade intestinal type adenocarcinoma may have an oncocytoid appearance. Evidence of heterogeneous elements (e.g., mucinous differentiation, papillary structures) and a greater degree of cytologic atypia can be helpful in establishing this diagnosis.

Treatment and Prognosis

The majority of parotid and submandibular oncocytomas behave in a benign fashion after complete surgical resection, even if rare aggressive features such as perineural invasion have been identified.[413] Local recurrence of an oncocytoma is unusual and often the result of persistent multifocal oncocytosis in the remaining deep parotid lobe.[413]

Most malignant parotid or submandibular oncocytomas are high-grade neoplasms with frequent recurrences and metastatic spread. They should be treated by wide local excision. Adjuvant radiation therapy should be strongly considered and the appropriate neck should be treated either surgically or with radiation. These tumors are often locally aggressive and infiltrative[425, 456, 457] and can metastasize, either to cervical lymph nodes or in a widespread fashion to the central nervous system, bone, liver, and lung.[413, 425–428, 458, 459] Although many of these reports have short follow-up periods, some papers have documented a protracted course with single or multiple local recurrences and distant metastases.[422, 425–427, 443] In a recent review of 37 cases with follow-up, almost 85% of malignant oncocytomas developed regional or distant metastases and 32% developed local recurrence.[422] Four of eight patients with follow-up in Goode and Corio's review died of disease,[426] and the average survival for patients with metastasizing tumors was 3.8 years.[415] Distant metastasis is a poor prognostic sign, with all patients dying of disease.[424] Tumor-related mortality may occur up to a decade after the original diagnosis. Félix et al.[429] were able to correlate malignant appearance and behavior for two cases with tumor aneuploidy, while seven benign control oncocytomas were diploid. Malignant parotid and submandibular oncocytomas usually appear aggressive from the onset; only rarely is there evidence of pre-existing benign oncocytoma or oncocytosis.[425, 448]

Locally invasive sinonasal oncocytic tumors appear to follow a low-grade malignant course with multiple recurrences. Three of eight patients[442, 443] developed recurrent disease 3 to 7 years after initial diagnosis. Two of these patients had multiple recurrences—one at 3 and 10 years, the other at 5 and 7 years. Both of these patients were disease-free 1 year after treatment of the second recurrence. It appears that recurrent disease remains localized, with no attributable deaths due to disease. One patient, for whom limited information was available, did develop locoregional metastatic disease.[445]

Ductal Papillomas

Primary papillary tumors arising from the salivary gland ductal system are rare lesions and are classified, in decreasing order of incidence,[460] into three distinct tumor types: (1) intraductal papilloma, (2) sialadenoma papilliferum, which is analogous to syringocystadenoma papilliferum of the sweat glands, and (3) inverted ductal papilloma.

Intraductal Papilloma

Clinical Features. This is a rare, infrequently reported tumor that is more likely to occur in the ducts of minor salivary glands especially of the lip, and, in decreasing order of frequency, has been

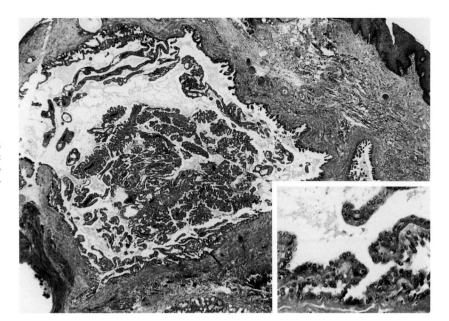

Figure 6–26. Intraductal papilloma. This tumor has numerous papillary fronds projecting into the cystic lumen. These fronds are covered by bland cuboidal to columnar epithelium *(inset)*. (Courtesy of Dr. Gary Ellis, Armed Forces Institute of Pathology.)

found in the palate, buccal mucosa, parotid gland duct, and submandibular gland duct[460–463]; one case has also been reported in the nasal cavity[464] and one in the sublingual gland.[464a] Of the three types of salivary gland ductal papillomas, intraductal papilloma accounted for slightly over 50% of 45 papillomas on file at the AFIP.[460] Clinically, intraductal papillomas present as small, asymptomatic submucosal masses, usually ranging up to 2.0 cm in greatest dimension[463]; they commonly occur in the fifth and sixth decades (mean age, 54 years; range, 29–77 years).[460]

Pathologic Features. Intraductal papillomas are well circumscribed or encapsulated, *unicystic* tumors with luminal papillary proliferation that partially or completely fills a dilated portion of an excretory duct. Microscopically, the papilloma arises from the surface of a dilated salivary gland duct and, unlike inverted papilloma or sialadenoma papilliferum, is usually located away from the orifice. The intraductal papilloma is unicystic and is usually composed of numerous papillary fronds that extend from the duct wall into the cystic lumen. The projections have delicate fibrovascular cores and are covered by a uniform, bland, cuboidal, or columnar and occasional mucinous epithelium similar to the lining of the cystically dilated salivary duct (Fig. 6–26).[460] The proliferating fronds do not extend out of the salivary duct. If the process involves more than one duct, it is best classified as a cystadenoma.

Differential Diagnosis. The differential diagnosis consists of a papillary cystadenoma, papillary changes due to duct obstruction, low-grade papillary cystic acinic cell carcinoma, and mucoepidermoid carcinoma. Whether intraductal papilloma is a separate and distinct entity from papillary cystadenoma or whether it falls within its spectrum still has to be resolved. Papillary cystadenomas are multicystic by definition, whereas intraductal papillomas are always unicystic. Salivary gland duct blockage is frequently associated with ductal dilation and epithelial proliferation in the ductal segment proximal to the obstruction.[465] However, the hyperplasia is not as extensive and lacks the complexity of an intraductal papilloma. Rarely, acinic cell and mucoepidermoid carcinomas may present as unicystic neoplasms. The complex papillary architecture with delicate fibrovascular cores of intraductal papilloma is lacking, and the presence of acinic cells in the former and of squamous, clear, and mucin-containing cells in the latter should allow for proper classification.

Treatment and Prognosis. Treatment is simple excision. These tumors do not recur. However, one case report described a papillary adenocarcinoma possibly arising from a parotid intraductal papilloma.[466] A second report described an intraductal papillary adenocarcinoma with an associated invasive component, which could possibly represent the malignant counterpart of an intraductal papilloma.[464a]

Sialadenoma Papilliferum

Clinical Features. Sialadenoma papilliferum is an exophytic tumor with multiple papillary surface fronds and deeper duct-like structures that are usually in continuity with the surface epithelium.[467] This tumor was first described by Abrams and Finck[468] in 1969. Since that time, slightly over 50 salivary gland cases have been reported.[463, 468–475] The frequency of sialadenoma papilliferum in the literature varies from 0.6% to 2% of benign salivary gland tumors.[460, 469–471] Although this tumor can arise in the major salivary gland ducts and has been reported in the parotid gland,[460, 468] sialadenoma papilliferum is much more common in the minor glands of the mouth, particularly the palate (85% of tumors)[463]; it has also been reported in the esophagus.[476]

All patients are adults (mean age, 62 years; range, 32–87 years) and there is a slight male predisposition.[463] Intraoral tumors are usually less than 1 cm in diameter but have reached over 2.5 cm in greatest dimension.[460] The largest reported case was the parotid tumor in Abrams and Finck's original report, which reached 7.5 cm in greatest dimension.[468] Sialadenoma papilliferum occurs near or at the orifice of a salivary gland excretory duct and presents as a well-circumscribed painless papillary, verrucoid surface lesion. Clinically, it is commonly misdiagnosed as squamous papilloma.

Pathologic Features. Microscopically, the tumor has exophytic and endophytic components (Fig. 6–27). The outer portion is a typical papilloma with broad-based finger-like projections supported with delicate fibrous connective tissue cores extending above the level of the adjacent mucosa for a distance of up to 1 cm.[463] The covering epithelium of the fronds is stratified squamous, which may be hyperkeratotic or parakeratotic. A mixed inflammatory cell infiltrate composed of lymphocytes, plasma cells, and neutrophils is usually present in this component of the lesion. The deeper endophytic component is unencapsulated and composed of glands or branching, occasionally tortuous ducts that may be cystic and are continuous with the interpapillary clefts of the surface component. Some of the ducts may be dilated and show intraluminal papillary projections. The epithelial lining of the ducts and cysts is usually composed of a double layer of cells, a tall columnar luminal cell, and a cuboidal or flattened basal cell layer. Both cell types are brightly eosinophilic with oncocytic features and are consistent with interlobular and excretory duct epithelium.[463] Occasionally, mucocytes may be seen in-

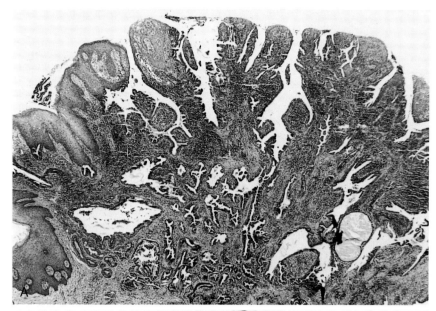

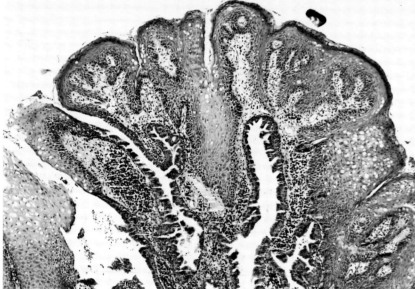

Figure 6–27. Sialadenoma papilliferum demonstrating the typical exophytic papillary surface and deeper ductal components *(A)*. The bland surface squamous epithelium communicates with the underlying columnar epithelium lining the ductal structures *(B)*. (Courtesy of Dr. Gary Ellis, Armed Forces Institute of Pathology.)

termixed with the ductal epithelium and inflammatory cells are frequently present in the stroma.

The differential diagnosis includes squamous papilloma, verrucous carcinoma, papillary cystadenoma, and mucoepidermoid carcinoma. The former two lack the deeper glandular or ductal portion of sialadenoma papilliferum, whereas the latter two lack the papillary surface component.

Treatment and Prognosis. Complete surgical excision is usually curative. Only one tumor has recurred following local excision; this was treated by re-excision.

Inverted Ductal Papilloma

Clinical Features. Inverted ductal papilloma is the rarest of the three types of ductal papilloma. Slightly more than 20 cases have been reported.[460, 463, 470, 477–480] A review of the limited number of cases in the literature shows that they occur in the minor salivary glands of adults with a mean age of 50 years (range, 32–66 years).[463] There is no sex predilection. The lip and buccal mucosa are more frequently involved (88%), but this tumor may occasionally arise in other oral sites. Clinically, inverted ductal papilloma presents as an asymptomatic, firm, submucosal nodule and does not usually exceed

1.5 cm in diameter. Like sialadenoma papilliferum, it occurs near the orifice of salivary ducts.

Pathologic Features. Histologically, inverted ductal papilloma is a well-circumscribed luminal papillary proliferation arising at the junction of a salivary excretory duct with the oral mucosa. Depending on the plane of section, the tumor may communicate with the surface epithelium through a narrow pore or be located just below the overlying mucosal surface. Inverted papilloma grows as a nodular, often spherical mass pushing into the lamina propria. It is composed of basaloid and stratified squamous epithelium, usually without keratin surrounding fibrovascular cores extending in a broad, bulbous papillary pattern from a luminal surface and usually filling the lumen (Fig. 6–28). Cleft-like spaces between papillary fronds frequently may be seen. The epithelial cells are uniform with only minimal if any atypia and mitotic figures are usually inconspicuous. In addition, the papillary fronds are often covered with cuboidal or columnar duct cells and occasional scattered mucous cells may be found in all levels of the epithelium.

Differential diagnosis consists predominantly of mucoepidermoid carcinoma, since both lesions characteristically are composed of squamous and mucin-secreting cells. However, these tumors can be differentiated by the lack of circumscription, frequent multicystic growth pattern, multinodular growth, and tumor infiltration that are characteristic of mucoepidermoid carcinoma.

Treatment and Prognosis. Inverted ductal papillomas are treated with surgical excision, which is curative; they do not recur. Although these tumors have some histologic similarity to sinonasal inverted squamous papillomas, there is no associated risk of malignant transformation, as is seen with the nasal tumors.

Mucoepidermoid Carcinoma

Clinical Features. Mucoepidermoid carcinoma (MEC) has an annual incidence of 0.44 per 100,000 persons.[481] It accounts for 2.8% to 15.5% of all salivary gland tumors, 12% to 29% of malignant salivary gland tumors, and 6.5% to 41% of minor salivary gland tumors, representing the most common type of malignant minor salivary gland tumor in most series.[482–485] However, the relative frequency of MEC in the United Kingdom (12% of malignant salivary gland tumors) is much lower than in the United States (29%) or in Germany (21.6%).[482–484] Fifty-three percent to slightly over 56% occur in the major salivary glands, with 85% to 88% occurring in the parotid gland, 8% to 13% occurring in the submandibular gland, and 2% to 4% involving the sublingual gland.[482, 483] In the minor salivary glands, MEC most commonly arises on the palate, but a significant number may also be found in the retromolar area, the floor of the mouth, the buccal mucosa, the lip, and the tongue.[482, 485]

MEC may also rarely arise primarily within the body of the mandible or maxilla, where it is the most common central salivary gland tumor of the jaws.[486] They also may occasionally arise from heterotopic intra–lymph nodal salivary gland tissue, the larynx, lacrimal gland, nose, paranasal sinuses, lung, and trachea.[487, 488] MEC is most frequently seen in the 35- to 65-year-old age group but may be found at any age. It is the most common malignant salivary gland tumor to arise in children and adolescents under 20 years of age[489–491] and is unusual in the first decade of life. MEC has a slight predilection for women, with approximately 60% of tumors arising in women.[482]

The most common etiologic factor that has been implicated in the development of mucoepidermoid carcinomas is radiation, with as many as 44% of patients with a history of a radiation-associated adenocarcinoma developing a MEC. Latency periods in this group ranged from 7 to 32 years.[492–494] Recently, Land et al.[495] reviewed data on 145 major and minor salivary gland tumors from atomic bomb survivors exposed to radiation from Hiroshima and Nagasaki and found an increased relative risk of 9.3 for patients with mucoepidermoid carcinoma, with the proportion of MECs increasing with increasing dose of radiation. There was also a slightly lower increased relative risk for Warthin's tumor, but not for other neoplasms. Two children with acute lymphoblastic leukemia treated with multiagent chemotherapy and prophylactic cranial irradiation developed MEC at 6 and 7 years, respectively, after successful treatment of leukemia.[495a]

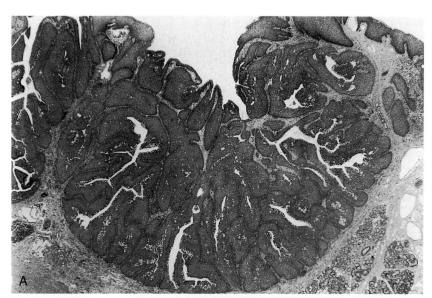

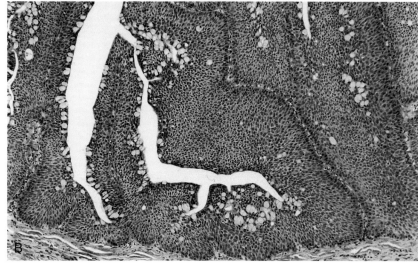

Figure 6–28. Inverting ductal papilloma. This tumor is continuous with the overlying surface epithelium and grows in an inverting pattern, forming a smooth-edged, broad-based mass *(A)*. It is composed of immature squamous or basaloid epithelium, frequently with cuboidal or columnar cells at its junction with the lumen. In addition, numerous mucinous goblet cells are often intermixed with the basaloid and squamous cells *(B)*.

Mucoepidermoid carcinomas typically present as slowly growing (up to 40 years), firm masses clinically indistinguishable from the more common pleomorphic adenoma.[494] Pain is unusual and more often associated with high-grade tumors. In one large series, high-grade mucoepidermoid carcinoma was the carcinoma most often associated with facial nerve palsy.[496]

Pathologic Features. On gross examination, MEC may appear circumscribed, but it is seldom encapsulated. High-grade tumors have poorly defined margins and may be associated with fixation to the adjacent skin and soft tissues. The cut surface ranges from gray to tan-yellow to pink, and cystic features are common and may be prominent.[482] The tumors usually range in size from 1 to 4 cm in greatest dimension; however, occasional patients may present with larger tumors (over 12 cm).[482]

Microscopically, mucoepidermoid carcinomas are composed of varying proportions of epidermoid cells, mucus-secreting cells, and "intermediate" cells, which are cells of intermediate differentiation between the other two cell types (Fig. 6–29). Intermediate cells include the smaller basal cells as well as larger cells that are differentiating toward squamous and mucin-secreting cells. Clear cells, many of which contain glycogen or mucin or both, are present in most mucoepidermoid carcinomas and often are a prominent feature. Tumors, especially low-grade neoplasms, frequently have distinct columnar cells containing intracellular mucin (goblet-like cells). Epidermoid cells have abundant eosinophilic cytoplasm and are occasionally associated with keratin production, including pearl formation. Rarely, keratin production may be prominent. These tumors show great variability in the composition of cell types. Cellular pleomorphism and atypia may be found and range from minimal to severe. Necrosis, prominent mitotic activity, neural invasion, and, rarely, a prominent lymphoid reaction may be seen. Occasional MECs will be associated with a prominent oncocytic component and are referred to as the oncocytic

variant.[497, 498] Rare MECs may be associated with dense sclerosis, obfuscating the diagnosis,[499] and an occasional tumor may arise within a salivary duct cyst.[500]

These tumors are histologically classified into low-, intermediate-, and high-grade. Suggested grading criteria have included the relative proportion of cell types, the degree of tumor invasiveness, anaplasia, the pattern of invasion, the degree of maturation of the various cellular components, mitotic rates, presence or absence of necrosis, neural or vascular invasion, and the proportion of tumor composed of cystic spaces relative to solid growth.[496, 501–505]

Low-grade tumors commonly develop a nesting pattern with multiple well-circumscribed squamous nests containing numerous clear cells, some of which contain intracytoplasmic mucin (Fig. 6–29A, B). Many low-grade tumors, especially in the minor salivary glands, contain a prominent mucin-secreting component composed of columnar cells lining cystic spaces (Fig. 6–29C). Nuclear atypia, mitotic activity, and an infiltrative growth pattern are not usually features of low-grade tumors. *Intermediate-grade tumors* are less cystic and show a greater tendency to form larger, more irregular nests or sheets of squamous cells and often have a more prominent intermediate cell population (Fig. 6–29D, E). A minor degree of nuclear atypia and mitotic activity may be present, and a small infiltrative component is usually noted. *High-grade tumors* are predominantly solid with greater degrees of atypia; they are usually very similar to squamous cell carcinoma. These are infiltrative tumors with scant mucin production that may require careful search and special stains for identification of intracellular mucin (Fig. 6–29F).

Grading MEC is subjective with different criteria used in various series.[496, 501–505] Recently Auclair, Goode, and Ellis established more uniform and reproducible histologic criteria (Table 6–7) that correlated with clinical outcome.[501, 505] The histopathologic features that were most useful in indicating aggressive behavior were a cys-

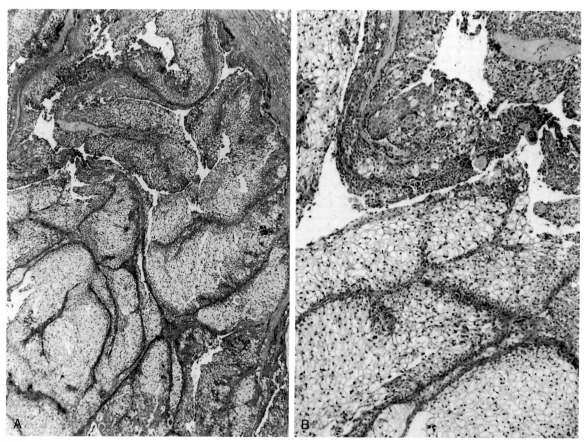

Figure 6–29. *A* and *B*, Low-grade mucoepidermoid carcinoma demonstrating irregular nests of clear cells with focal squamous differentiation (*B*, top portion).

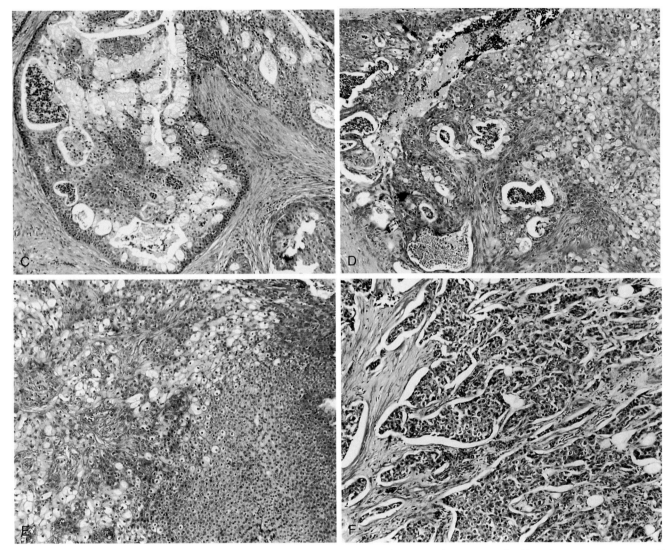

Figure 6–29 *Continued. C–F,* Various patterns in mucoepidermoid carcinoma. *C,* A low-grade tumor with cystic spaces lined by columnar, mucin-secreting cells and focally by squamous epithelium. *D* and *E* demonstrate intermediate-grade tumors with prominent clear cell change. In addition, areas of squamous differentiation *(D)* and a sheet of intermediate cells *(E, right half)* are seen. High-grade tumor *(F)* is composed of poorly differentiated, irregular nests of infiltrating tumor cells. This tumor demonstrated only very focal mucinous differentiation.

Table 6–7. Grading Parameters and Point Values for Mucoepidermoid Carcinoma

Parameter	Point Value
Cystic component of <20%	+2
Neural invasion	+2
Necrosis	+3
Four or more mitoses per 10 HPF	+3
Anaplasia	+4

Grade	Point Score
Low	0–4
Intermediate	5–6
High	7–14

HPF, high-power fields.

Modified from Ellis GL, Auclair PL: Atlas of Tumor Pathology: Tumors of the Salivary Glands, 3rd series, fascicle 17. Washington, DC: Armed Forces Institute of Pathology, 1996:155–175.

tic component of less than 20% of tumor area, 4 or more mitotic figures per 10 high-power fields, nerve invasion, tumor necrosis, and the presence of cellular anaplasia (cellular and nuclear pleomorphism, increased nuclear-to-cytoplasmic ratios, prominent or multiple nucleoli, and hyperchromasia). Each of these parameters was assigned a point value and the total sum of points for the five variables determined the tumor grade (see Table 6–7). In our experience, this scheme tends to "downgrade" MEC. We propose that additional grading parameters (vascular/lymphatic invasion, aggressive pattern of infiltration) be included.

Differential Diagnosis. The differential diagnosis consists of necrotizing sialometaplasia (NSM), cystadenoma and cystadenocarcinoma, metastatic squamous carcinoma (for high-grade tumors), sebaceous carcinoma and other clear cell tumors, adenosquamous carcinoma, and, rarely, pleomorphic adenoma. NSM can rarely simulate low-grade MEC; however, NSM retains the lobular architecture of the normal gland and has smooth-edged cell nests. It lacks the cystic growth typical of low-grade MEC, and intermediate-type cells are not found. In both cystadenoma and cystadenocarcinoma there is usually less stroma between the cysts as compared with MEC, there is usually a papillary component, and the squamous component typical of MEC is not seen. Metastatic squamous carcinoma typically has more keratin production than MEC and it does not contain any cells with intracellular mucin, whereas high-grade MEC will always contain at least a few mucin-containing cells. Sebaceous carcinoma and other clear cell carcinomas do not usually contain intracellular mucin material in the clear cell population and they lack intermediate-type cells and goblet cells. Adenosquamous carcinoma is in the differential primarily for minor gland tumors. It can usually be separated from MEC because these tumors have two distinctly separate components, squamous and glandular, while in MEC the squamous and mucinous components are usually intimately associated with each other in the same tumor nests. Rarely, a mixed tumor may have areas of prominent mucoepidermoid metaplasia (see Fig. 6–13N, O) or have MEC arise as the malignant component of a carcinoma ex mixed tumor. Careful histologic sampling will allow separation from the latter while the absence of destructive overgrowth of normal tissues and the presence of stromal myoepithelial cells will allow separation from the former.

Treatment and Prognosis. Prognosis is a function of the histologic grade, adequacy of excision, and clinical staging (see Appendix). Complete surgical excision is the treatment of choice for MEC. Adequate excision is important in all grades of tumor, with much higher recurrence rates reported with positive surgical margins (on the order of 50% for low- and intermediate-grade tumors and slightly over 80% for high-grade tumors).[506] The frozen section assessment of MEC surgical margins may be difficult because of ductal hyperplasia and squamous metaplasia in salivary gland tissue adjacent to the tumor and because microscopic islands of tumor may extend beyond the grossly discernible tumor mass. Radiation therapy should be added in high-grade tumors and in patients with residual microscopic disease at the surgical margins. In patients with low-grade tumors, the survival rate is 90% to 100%; with the exception of submandibular gland tumors, these tumors rarely recur or metastasize. Recent data from the AFIP indicated that 5% of major gland and 2.5% of minor gland low-grade MECs metastasized to regional lymph nodes or resulted in death. This may be explained by tumor stage at presentation. The metastatic rate for high-grade tumors was 55% for the major glands and 80% for those of minor salivary gland origin.[482] Metastatic, recurrence, and death rates for patients with low-grade submandibular gland tumors were 13%, 9%, and 13%, respectively.[482] Several patients in this latter series with small (low stage) low-grade tumors with adequate treatment inexplicably died of disease. Spiro et al.[496] also found more frequent metastases with submandibular gland MEC than from other major gland sites. Therefore, any tumor of the submandibular gland, irrespective of grade, should be treated aggressively.[505] Survival is better with tumors arising in younger patients and among females, whereas survival is adversely affected in patients over 60 years of age.[507] Intermediate- and high-grade tumors have a greater tendency to infiltrate, recur, and metastasize, with reported cure rates at 5, 10, and 15 years of 49%, 42%, and 33%, respectively.[496] In a recent study, Plambeck et al.[508] reported 5- and 10-year survival rates of 91.9% and 89.5%, respectively, regardless of tumor grade. Stage appeared to be a better prognosticator: all patients who died had stage 3 or 4 disease, and 5- and 10-year survival rates for this group were 63.5% and 52%, respectively. Suzuki et al.[509] recently found that MECs that overexpressed HER-2/neu had lower 5-year survival rates than tumors with weak expression (25% vs 89%).

Acinic Cell Carcinoma

The WHO Tumor Classification defines acinic cell carcinoma (ACC) as "a malignant epithelial neoplasm that demonstrates some cytological differentiation toward (serous) acinar cells."[510] This definition is conceptually incomplete, as ultrastructural and immunohistochemical studies have clearly illustrated *multi-directional differentiation* toward acinar, ductal, and myoepithelial elements.[511–514] ACC is better defined as a primary salivary gland neoplasm demonstrating differentiation toward the terminal (interca-

lated) duct–acinar unit and exhibiting one or more of the recognized histologic patterns.

Clinical Features. ACC accounts for 7% to 17.5%[515–518] of malignant salivary gland tumors. The parotid gland, the most common primary site, is involved in up to 90% of cases.[518, 519] Moreover, ACC constitutes 10% to 30%[518, 520, 521] of primary malignant parotid gland tumors. The minor salivary glands are the second most common site of occurrence,[518, 522] with the majority involving the upper lip or vestibule, buccal mucosa, and palate.[523, 524] The submandibular and sublingual glands are less commonly involved.[518, 522] Unusual sites of origin include ectopic salivary gland,[525] lacrimal gland,[526] nasal cavity,[520, 527] mandible,[520, 528] larynx,[529, 530] trachea,[531, 532] lung,[533] vallecula,[533a] and, least frequently, breast.[534]

The reported age range for patients with ACC is 3 to 91 years,[518] with a female-to-male ratio of approximately 2 : 1.[520, 535–537] Patients present with nearly equal frequency from the third through the seventh decades of life.[518] Interestingly, the average age at diagnosis, 38 to 46 years, is nearly a decade younger than in patients with other parotid malignancies.[538] After mucoepidermoid carcinoma, ACC is the second most common malignant salivary gland neoplasm occurring in childhood.[539]

After Warthin's tumor and pleomorphic adenoma, ACC is the third most common bilateral salivary gland tumor, and it is the most frequent malignant tumor to present bilaterally.[540] Multifocal presentation of ACC is described as well.[537] No well-established clinical associations for ACC exist, although single reports have documented ACC in patients with ataxia-telangiectasia,[541] Sjögren's syndrome,[542] and oculocerebrorenal syndrome.[543] One report documents a familial occurrence.[543a]

Nearly all patients present with a mass. The reported interval between development of symptoms and diagnosis has ranged from 1 month to 40 years,[544, 545] although most patients have symptoms for less than 1 year.[545] Hemorrhage into the tumor can result in sudden clinical enlargement of the presenting mass. Associated pain and tenderness may occur in up to 50% of patients and is not necessarily an adverse prognostic indicator.[545] Evidence of facial nerve involvement with paresis or paralysis, present in 3% to 7.5% of patients, was found to be an ominous prognostic sign in one study.[545] However, another series found that clinical pain and fixation, but not cranial nerve VII weakness, were associated with a poor prognosis.[546]

Pathologic Features. Grossly, the typical ACC is an intraparenchymal, circumscribed, tan-gray, rubbery mass. Though generally less than 3 cm in greatest dimension, diameters up to 22 cm have been recorded.[547] Neoplasms with marked lymphocytic infiltration may resemble a lymph node, and gross cystic change may be present. Recurrent tumors are characterized by a multinodular appearance.[546] Dedifferentiated ACCs, a rare high-grade variant, are grossly bosselated tumors that exhibit ill-defined borders and typically infiltrate adjacent soft tissue and bone.[548]

The variable histologic appearance of ACC coupled with its relatively uncommon occurrence account for the diagnostic difficulties engendered by this tumor. ACC is the most common salivary gland neoplasm encountered in consultation by one author (DRG). Diagnostically, the microcystic and less common variants can be particularly troublesome. The four principal histologic types are solid, microcystic, papillary-cystic, and follicular (Fig. 6–30).[510, 545, 549] Spectrums exist between these growth patterns, and tumors commonly exhibit a mixture of patterns.

On initial low-power examination,[528] the growth pattern of large nests and lobules with little intervening stroma and a basophilic hue allows one to suspect a diagnosis of ACC. However, one should not totally depend on the cytoplasmic basophilia to suspect ACC, as zymogen-poor ACC may appear more eosinophilic or clear (see later discussion). ACCs characteristically grow as solid sheets of serous cells, frequently arranged in organoid groupings separated by thin fibrous septa. Prominent lymphoid infiltrates, present in up to one third of ACCs,[546] are another potential clue to the diagnosis at scanning magnification. A delicate fibrous pseudocapsule may en-

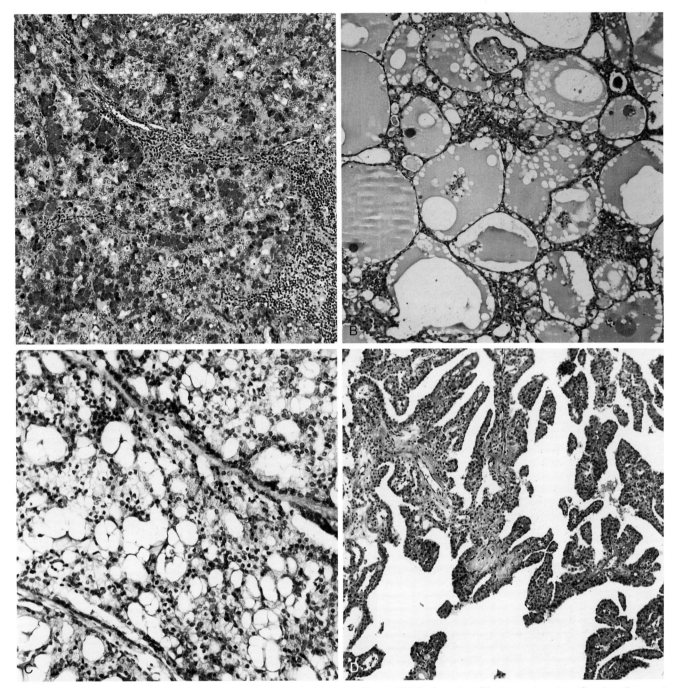

Figure 6–30. Acinic cell carcinoma: solid pattern with a prominent lymphocytic infiltrate *(A)*, follicular variant *(B)*, microcystic variant *(C)*, and papillary cystic variant *(D)*.

close smaller tumors, and psammoma body–like calcifications may be present.[549]

The *solid variant* or "classic" ACC is composed of well-differentiated serous acinar cells notable for the prominent basophilic to gray granularity of their cytoplasm (Fig. 6–30A). The zymogen granules are the packaged secretory product of acinar cells. These granules range from extremely fine to moderately coarse[550] and show diastase-resistant PAS positivity and mucicarmine negativity. Individual cells are polygonal with conspicuous cytoplasmic borders. Nuclei are small and uniform. Foci of nonspecific glandular cells may be present. In such areas, cell borders become indistinct, imparting a syncytial appearance to the tumor cells. These cells stain eosinophilic to amphophilic, cytoplasmic granules are sparse to absent, and nuclei may appear mildly enlarged and vesicular. Cellular

atypia and mitotic figures, if present, are generally found in these areas. Scattered tumor cells may have vacuolated, foamy cytoplasm. Perineural and vascular invasion are not typical features of ACC. If either is present, a higher grade malignancy should be suspected.

The *microcystic variant* of ACC, featuring prominent cellular vacuolization and intercellular cystic change, has a characteristic "lattice-like"[528] or "fenestrated"[546] appearance (Fig. 6–30C). Contrasting the acinar differentiation of the solid variant, microcystic ACC recapitulates the terminal (intercalated) duct–acinar unit. Ductal-type and acinar-type cells usually intermingle to varying degrees. The inconsistent presence of acinar cells explains the marked variation in staining intensity and consistency with PAS staining for zymogen granules in microcystic ACC. Zymogen granules may be difficult to demonstrate and are usually found at least focally after careful searching. Resembling intercalated duct cells of non-neoplastic salivary gland, ductal cells are generally cuboidal with limited amphophilic or eosinophilic cytoplasm and with distinct borders. Nuclei, as with acinar cells, are usually uniform and bland, but rarely may demonstrate mild pleomorphism and atypia. Intercellular microcysts and vacuolated cells may contain mucicarmine-positive material, which can, on occasion, be abundant.[535, 550] Moreover, intracytoplasmic mucicarminophilic cytoplasmic granules have been noted.[533, 550] Ultrastructurally, both dense zymogen-like granules and light mucus-type granules have been shown in ACC.[512]

Spiro[520] and Abrams[549] first described the *papillocystic* and *follicular variants* of ACC, respectively. These patterns may coexist with the solid and microcystic patterns, aiding in the recognition of these tumors as ACC. Cellular features are similar to those encountered in the solid and microcystic patterns; mucicarmine-positive material may also be prominent in this variant. Batsakis[551] proposed two forms of genesis for the papillocystic pattern of ACC: retrogressive and neoplastic. The end-stage of the former is a unilocular cyst with attenuated and swollen neoplastic cells accompanied by papillary excrescences (Fig. 6–30D). The follicular pattern appears to be an exaggerated acinar-microcystic pattern in which dilated acini are lined by a flattened epithelium and contain watery or colloid-like material (Fig. 6–30B).[551] Focal clear cell change in ACC is common and likely degenerative in nature.[528, 551, 552] Occasional tumors exhibit such extensive clear cell change (in greater than 90% of tumor cells) that we feel it is appropriate to designate these tumors as the *clear cell* variant of ACC (Fig. 6–31, see p. 346).[553]

Other described variants of ACC include *dedifferentiated, oncocytic, hybrid* tumors and the recently separated *well-differentiated ACC with lymphoid stroma.* The well-differentiated ACC with lymphoid stroma is an acinic cell carcinoma with a better prognosis than the conventional ACC. It is defined as a well-circumscribed to encapsulated tumor with a solid or microcystic pattern in which the tumor cells are *all* surrounded by and intermingled with a prominent lymphoid response.[554] *Dedifferentiated* ACC[555, 556] exhibits areas of low-grade acinic cell carcinoma and areas of dedifferentiated high-grade adenocarcinoma or undifferentiated carcinoma within the same tumor (Fig. 6–32). One recent case was associated with an undifferentiated spindle cell neoplasm.[557] Vascular or lymphatic space invasion and regional lymph node metastases are common in the dedifferentiated tumors. Oncocytic change in ACC may obfuscate the diagnosis (Fig. 6–33, see p. 347).[550, 558] We have seen several tumors with extensive oncocytic change in which a diagnosis of oncocytoma was entertained. In one, a heavy lymphoid infiltrate raised the suspicion of ACC. Diastase-resistant PAS–positive granules with ultrastructural confirmation was useful in establishing the presence of secretory or zymogen granules in such tumors (Fig. 6–33C).[559]

Multiple examples of unusual hybrid tumors combining ACC with various other tumor types have been described, including terminal duct carcinoma with acinous cell differentiation,[560] ACC ex mixed tumor,[561] ACC combined with salivary duct carcinoma,[562] and ACC combined with mucoepidermoid carcinoma.[563]

Differential Diagnosis. The differential diagnosis of the solid variant of ACC is limited; however, these tumors may so closely re-

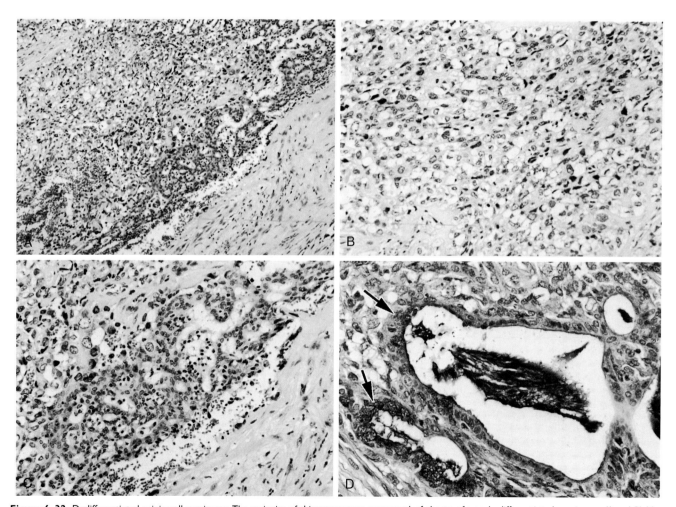

Figure 6–32. Dedifferentiated acinic cell carcinoma. The majority of this tumor was composed of sheets of poorly differentiated carcinoma *(A and B).* Very focally, small foci of cells with a microcystic pattern composed of uniform intercalated duct–type cuboidal cells were seen *(A, lower portion of tumor and C, middle).* These contained diastase-resistant periodic acid–Schiff (PAS) positive cytoplasmic granules *(D, arrows).* The bland cuboidal cells and positive PAS staining confirmed the presence of the acinic cell component in this tumor. The poorly differentiated carcinoma component did not stain with PAS.

capitulate normal salivary gland, both architecturally and cytologically, that a diagnosis of sialadenitis or sialadenosis is considered, especially on frozen section examination. The lack of intercalated, striated, and excretory ducts and normal lobular architecture, however, aids in recognizing the neoplastic nature.[564] Microcystic ACC is often mistaken for mucoepidermoid carcinoma due to the prominent mucicarmine positivity of many of the microcysts. The absence of goblet cells and a squamous element distinguishes ACC from mucoepidermoid carcinoma. Furthermore, in ACC mucicarminophilic material is frequently extracellular and nuclei tend to be more bland, uniform, and peripherally located. The papillocystic variant of ACC must be distinguished from papillary cystadenocarcinoma. The presence of recognizable ACC or zymogen granules by PAS staining or ultrastructural examination may be essential in making this distinction. Finding areas with a population of somewhat uniform intercalated duct–like cells is supportive of a diagnosis of ACC. The follicular variant is a potential mimic of follicular carcinoma of the thyroid. Thyroglobulin staining is of potential aid in this situation, though we have never encountered such a need. Other patterns of ACC are usually present, allowing for proper classification. Clear cell oncocytoma and primary or metastatic clear cell carcinoma may be diagnostic considerations in the face of extensive clear cell change, although, in our experience, rare single cells with diastase-resistant PAS–positive granules can still be identified in the clear cell variant of ACC (see Fig. 6–31). In clear cell oncocytoma, nuclei are usually more central and uniform, whereas the clear cell ACC have more peripherally located and slightly more pleomorphic nuclei.

By electron microscopic examination, ACCs may display multidirectional differentiation toward acinar, ductal, and myoepithelial elements.[512, 513] Zymogen granules appear as membrane-limited, round bodies containing a flocculent material of low electron density.[552] Granule density is fixation dependent.[565]

Immunohistochemistry is of little practical aid in diagnosis, due in part to differing antigen expression between the same and differing histologic types of ACC.[514, 566] Cells exhibiting acinar differentiation may stain positively for amylase,[566] lactoferrin,[511] and vasoactive intestinal polypeptide[514] and negatively for keratin[511, 513]; however, keratin, epithelial membrane antigen, and CEA[514, 567] positivity is seen in luminal lining cells of the ductal elements in the cystic/follicular foci.[511] Normal serous acini are frequently immunoreactive for amylase; however, amylase is found in only occasional acinic cell carcinomas and is therefore not useful in establishing this diagnosis.[566]

Treatment and Prognosis. Surgical excision with clear margins is the goal of treatment. For the majority of parotid tumors, superficial lobectomy[538, 545, 550] is adequate, although some have advocated total parotidectomy.[535, 537, 544] For neoplasms involving the deep lobe, however, total parotidectomy is warranted. Elective neck dissection is not indicated.[535, 544, 545, 550] Recurrences tend to be multiple and require rigorous surgical re-excision.[549, 550] Most studies suggest that radiation therapy is of little utility in the treatment of ACC.[535, 546, 550]

Acinic cell carcinoma is capable of a notoriously protracted clinical course. Disease-free and determinate survival curves do not level off until after a decade.[546] Five-year determinate survival ranges from 76% to 90%. Survival drops to between 44% and 67% beyond 15 years.[520, 521, 536, 546, 550] Expected rates of recurrence, metastasis, and mortality with modern surgical therapy approximate 30%, 13%, and 13%, respectively.[546] Patients may succumb to progressive locoregional or metastatic disease. The latter may be by lymphatic or hematogenous spread or both.[536] Lung and bone are the most common sites of hematogenous spread. Long-term survival is possible after documentation of metastatic disease.

Efforts to histologically identify those tumors that will ultimately behave aggressively have generally been disappointing.[545, 549] Some have noted a trend toward aggressive behavior in tumors with increased mitotic activity, cellular atyp-

ia,[517, 536, 537, 546, 550] and desmoplasia.[546] Lewis and coworkers, in particular, found a strong positive correlation between increased mitotic activity and aggressive behavior that is corroborated by recent MIB-1 studies.[545, 568, 569] Others, moreover,[516, 519, 551] have described some success in prognostically grading ACC. These efforts aside, the relative rarity of ACC, the biologic progression of histologically bland tumors, and the lack of standardized criteria make clinically relevant grading of these tumors difficult at best. Recently, Michal et al.[554] reported on a well-differentiated variant that is surrounded completely by lymphoid stroma, which has a better prognosis than conventional tumors. These tumors had a low mitotic index and all 12 patients in their series remained well without evidence of disease with follow-up periods averaging just under 7 years (range 19 months to 14 years). Determining whether this trend will continue requires additional cases with longer follow-up.

Conflicting results have been reported using ploidy in predicting outcome in ACC. El-Naggar[570] noted an association between aneuploidy and poor outcome. Others, however, have found the majority of ACCs to be diploid,[517, 571] and have concluded that ploidy is of little utility. Moreover, Timon[572] concluded that neither S-phase values nor mean argyrophilic nucleolar organizing region (AgNOR) counts allow separation of ACC for prognostic purposes.

In our experience, and as reported by others,[520, 521, 545, 550] clinical stage at presentation gives the most prognostic information. Accordingly, metastases,[520, 521, 550] large size,[520, 545] deep lobe parotid involvement,[520, 550] and multinodularity[545] all have been associated with a poor clinical outcome. Finally, *dedifferentiated* ACC carries a poor prognosis and warrants treatment afforded for high-grade carcinomas.

Adenoid Cystic Carcinoma

Clinical Features. Adenoid cystic carcinoma (AdCC) occurs over a very wide age range, from the first to the ninth decades of life, but with a preponderance in the fourth to seventh decades.[573–576] The female-to-male ratio is approximately 3:2.[577] There is considerable geographic variation in the incidence of AdCC. In England and Western Europe and in the older literature, it is the most common malignant intraoral salivary gland tumor. However, in the contemporary United States, mucoepidermoid carcinoma, polymorphous low-grade adenocarcinoma, and other tumors are more frequently encountered.[577–579]

Typically AdCC is a slow-growing, widely infiltrative tumor with a tendency for perineural spread. Patients present with pain and a mass that may have evolved over years. Mucosal ulceration, especially of the palate, is common. Occasional tumors present with intracranial involvement, closely mimicking a meningioma clinically and radiographically, and, rarely, a tumor may have an occult presentation.[578–581] Table 6–8 represents a compilation of tumor sites for AdCC derived from over 1600 cases.[574–576, 582, 583] The parotid gland, palate, submandibular gland, and sinonasal tract are the most commonly affected upper aerodigestive tract sites; minor salivary gland or seromucinous gland sites are more frequently involved than the major salivary glands combined (Table 6–8).

After squamous carcinoma, AdCC is the second most frequent malignant tumor of the trachea; 45.5% of patients had tumors in the upper trachea. The male-to-female ratio is almost equal and the average age at presentation is between 45 and 60 years (range, 15–80 years).[584] Histologically similar tumors can also be found at other sites, including the external ear, lacrimal glands, esophagus, breast, prostate, cervix, ovary, Bartholin's gland, lung, and skin.[585–590]

Pathologic Features. Grossly, these tumors are firm and gray-white. They are frequently locally invasive but can appear as subtle scar-like lesions. Smaller tumors may be circumscribed or, rarely, encapsulated. They have a tendency to extend along nerves, and "skip lesions" may be seen considerable distances away from the main tumor mass. Rarely, tumors will present in an occult fashion involving interlobar septa without a definitive mass.[581]

Table 6–8. Distribution of Sites for Adenoid Cystic Carcinoma of the Upper Aerodigestive Tract

Site	Cases	
	Number	%
Parotid gland	336	21.0
Palate	271	17.0
Other site, not stated	242	15.0
Submandibular gland	210	13.0
Sinonasal, nasopharynx	184	11.0
Tongue, floor of mouth	129	8.0
Tonsil, pharynx	69	4.3
Lip	53	3.3
Buccal	44	2.7
Sublingual gland	30	1.8
Retromolar trigone	21	1.3
Gingiva	10	0.6
Larynx/trachea	10	0.6
Lacrimal gland	5	0.3
Total	**1614**	

Data from Spiro and Huvos,[574] Conley and Casler,[575] Garden et al.,[576] Kim et al.,[582] and Auclair et al.[583]

The WHO classification schema divides AdCC into the following microscopic patterns: tubular, cribriform (glandular), and solid (Fig. 6–34).[591] The cribriform is the most frequent, while the solid pattern is the least frequent pattern observed. Adenoid cystic carcinomas are composed of cells of two types: ductal cells and abluminal myoepithelial cells.

Cytologically, AdCC is composed of a somewhat uniform, bland population of cells with oval basophilic nuclei with homogeneous chromatin distribution, and usually with little cytoplasm, reminiscent of basal cell carcinoma of the skin. The nuclei are frequently angulated and may rarely have coarse chromatin and prominent nucleoli. Although these latter two features are more likely in the solid, high-grade tumors, high-grade cytology may occasionally be seen with intermediate-grade tumors.

A mixture of patterns is common to AdCC; classification is made according to the predominant pattern. However, if a tumor has more than 30% of the solid pattern, it is classified as the solid variant. The tubular pattern (well-differentiated or grade I) is characterized by slender tubules, solid cords, and glandular structures infiltrating a well-hyalinized background (Fig. 6–34B, C). These are composed of myoepithelial cells often surrounding central luminal forming epithelial structures. The cribriform pattern (moderately differentiated or grade II) is characterized by invasive tumor islands with multiple "holes" (pseudocysts or pseudolumina) punched out in a "Swiss cheese" or sieve-like pattern (Fig. 6–34A). The pseudolumina are sharply demarcated from the surrounding cells and may contain a "rind" of dense pink basement membrane material and central blue mucopolysaccharides, or they may be entirely filled by the basement membrane material (see Fig. 6–34).[592] They are not true glandular lumina, lacking microvilli and apical junctional complexes,[593] but attest to the productivity of AdCC tumor cells, which make type IV collagen, laminin, chondroitin sulfate, and fibronectin. True lumina are scattered between the pseudocysts and are surrounded by myoepithelial cells. These lumina are much smaller than the pseudocystic spaces and are lined by cuboidal cells similar to those seen in normal salivary gland intercalated ducts. The solid pattern (poorly differentiated or grade III) consists of large islands of carcinoma composed predominantly of myoepithelial cells with infrequent true lumina lined by cuboidal epithelial cells, with only occasional punctuation by pseudocysts (Fig. 6–34D). A temporal progression in tumor grade may be observed.[594] Perineural spread is a feature common to all patterns. Mitotic figures and apoptotic cells are occasionally present in intermediate-grade tumors and are common to high-grade AdCC. Necrosis is seen, usually only in the solid pattern. Recently four adenoid cystic carcinomas were reported to be associated with a "dedifferentiated" high-grade component, similar to that seen rarely in acinic cell carcinoma.[595, 595a] Two patients presented with both components (typical AdCC and a poorly differentiated carcinoma) at initial presentation; the poorly differentiated component of the other two was associated with recurrences at 4 and 10 years, respectively.

One should be reluctant to diagnose AdCC on a limited biopsy, especially in the absence of definite tumor infiltration. The cribriform pattern so typical of AdCC may also be seen, rarely, in basal cell adenomas, in mixed tumors, and in polymorphous low-grade adenocarcinomas. The diagnosis of minor salivary gland tumors on limited biopsy material is especially challenging, as benign minor salivary tumors are rarely encapsulated but are well circumscribed.

The basement membrane material in the pseudolumina is PAS- and alcian blue–positive and reacts with antibodies against type IV collagen.[592] Cytokeratins and glandular epithelial markers (CEA, EMA) are positive in AdCC, especially in areas of ductular differentiation. The pseudocystic areas tend not to express these markers. S100 will stain the tumor diffusely, whereas smooth muscle actin and GFAP will accentuate the myoepithelial (abluminal) component.[596, 597]

Differential Diagnosis. Low- or intermediate-grade (tubular and cribriform patterns) tumors must be distinguished from basal cell adenoma and polymorphous low-grade adenocarcinoma (PLGA). Typically these tumors are "misdiagnosed" as AdCC, rather than the converse. Tumor infiltration and the presence of perineural invasion are the most important features to distinguish AdCC from basal cell adenoma, as the latter are circumscribed or encapsulated tumors lacking perineural invasion. However, with a limited biopsy, it may be literally impossible to differentiate between these tumors, as the bland cytology, myoepithelial-epithelial relationship, and tubular and cribriforming patterns can be features of both tumors. AdCC-like foci can also be seen in benign mixed tumor and may present diagnostic difficulty with limited biopsy material. Also we have seen one typical AdCC that had a small focus of cartilaginous metaplasia. Typical plasmacytoid myoepithelial cells are common in benign mixed tumor and are not seen in AdCC. Squamous metaplasia can be seen in basal cell adenoma and pleomorphic adenoma; it is an extremely rare and focal finding in AdCC and so may serve as a hint that one is not looking at AdCC.

The distinction between PLGA and AdCC is more challenging. Both PLGA and AdCC have similar patterns (cribriform, solid, and tubular) and a tendency for local infiltration and perineural spread. The cell types and the epithelial-myoepithelial relationship are thought to be common to both tumors; however, Prasad et al.,[597a] using three smooth muscle markers (α-smooth muscle actin, smooth muscle myosin heavy chain, and calponin), stained the myoepithelial cells in all AdCCs, while all the PLGAs examined were negative. A "polymorphous" or variegated architecture characterizes PLGA, whereas AdCC has a more limited range of histologic patterns with no more than three patterns: solid, tubular, and cribriform growth. In addition, foci of papillary growth and areas of single-file single cell infiltration are characteristic of PLGA but not of AdCC. Basophilic pools of glycosaminoglycans are frequent in AdCC and are not typical of PLGA. By contrast, at low power, PLGA will reveal a "steel gray" type of stromal background.[598] PLGAs may form solid areas, but they lack the overall high-grade "feel" (coarse chromatin, increased mitotic figures, apoptosis, and necrosis) associated with solid AdCC.

If mitotic figures are easily found, then PLGA becomes an unlikely possibility, although occasional mitoses may be noted. Commensurate with this, the MIB-1 proliferative index, which reflects expression of the cell cycle–associated antigen Ki-67, may be helpful. Skalova et al.[599] studied 21 PLGAs and 20 AdCCs and found that PLGAs had a mean proliferative index of 2.4%, while AdCC had a mean value of 21.4%; no overlap in MIB-1 index values was seen between both groups. Epithelial membrane antigen and polyclonal CEA may assist in distinguishing these tumors. Gnepp et al.[600] have shown that EMA and CEA can stain an equal proportion of luminal cells in AdCC. In contrast, the tumor cells of PLGA were found to have dissimilar expressions of EMA and CEA; the majority of tumor cells were reactive to EMA, and usually only a small minority of tumor cells reacted with polyclonal CEA. However, as the number of cases examined was small, further studies are necessary to confirm this finding.

Basaloid squamous carcinoma (BSC) also enters into the differential diagnosis of solid AdCC in minor salivary or seromucinous gland sites. Both tumors may produce basement membrane–like material and have cribriform and solid areas. The basement membrane material secreted by BSC tends to dissect between tumor cells, rather than to form crisp cribriform spaces as seen in AdCC. Necrosis and basaloid cells (ovoid with high nuclear-to-cytoplasmic ratio), with prominent nucleoli and coarse chromatin, can be seen in both tumors, although single-cell necrosis, a brisk mitotic rate, and a greater degree of nuclear atypia are much more frequent in BSC. One can distinguish BSC from solid AdCC by identifying focal keratinization, attachment to the rete pegs, or the presence of a surface squamous dysplasia/carcinoma-in-situ component or a superficially located invasive squamous carcinoma. In addition, true lumina are found in AdCC, whereas they are not seen in BSC.

Gnepp and Heffner found areas of surface mucosal origin, some of which were associated with surface mucosal in situ changes, in 58% of sinonasal AdCC.[601] The mucosal carcinoma in situ changes were not squamous in origin, as is seen in BSC, but were similar to the deeper tumor epithelium. Both BSC and AdCC can express cytokeratin and S100, but solid AdCC may express vimentin diffusely and retain some myoepithelial smooth muscle antigenicity such as GFAP and smooth muscle actin. BSC may also ex-

press vimentin, and when it does it has a "dot-like" cytoplasmic distribution.

Basal cell adenocarcinoma (BCAC) may also enter into the differential diagnosis of intermediate- or high-grade AdCC, especially for parotid tumors. An infiltrating cribriforming pattern, palisading basaloid cells, and hyaline deposition are features that may be common to both BCAC and AdCC. BCAC are usually composed of a blander population of tumor cells than AdCC. In addition, BCAC may have a "jig-saw puzzle"–type pattern of discrete "interlocking" tumor islands. The cells in the center of these islands can be discohesive and loosely aggregated, reminiscent of the stellate reticulum pattern seen in some ameloblastomas. Squamous differentiation and this latter pattern are not seen in AdCC and when present help distinguish BCAC from AdCC.

Treatment and Prognosis. Wide surgical resection with negative margins is the standard primary therapy. Adjuvant radiation therapy is usually indicated for most tumors; however, some would argue that well-resected T1 AdCC may not require adjuvant radiation therapy. Primary conventional radiotherapy has never been shown to provide sufficient local disease control. However, there are emerging data suggesting that neutron therapy, which involves larger particles of greater energy, can achieve reasonable local control as a primary therapeutic modality.[602, 603, 603a] Adoptive immunotherapy in combination with chemoradiotherapy has recently shown promising results.[604] Larger series with more patients are necessary to confirm these preliminary data.

AdCC has been noted to have a greater local recurrence rate when compared with other malignant salivary tumors (p = .0059).[605] This propensity for local recurrence (up to 62%) is high-

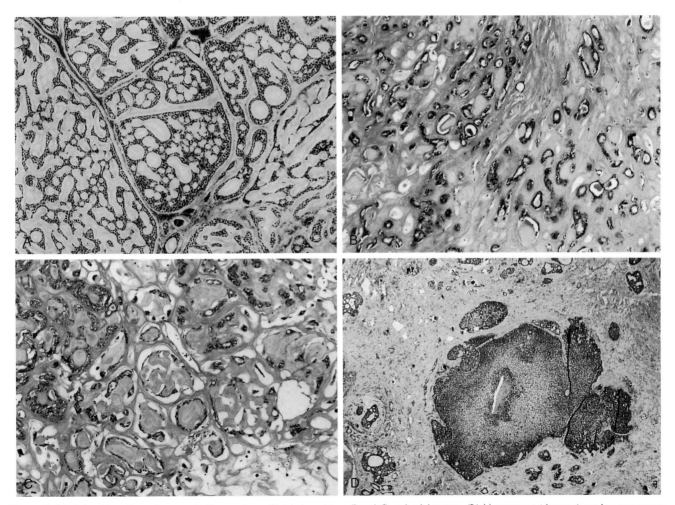

Figure 6–34. Adenoid cystic carcinoma: cribriform pattern *(A)*, tubular pattern *(B and C)*, and solid pattern *(D)*. Note areas with prominent basement membrane deposition *(A–C)*.

est within the first 5 years, but a significant number of patients will develop local recurrence after 10, 15, and 20 years.[576, 599, 600] Actuarial local control rates at 5, 10, and 15 years of 95%, 86%, and 79%, respectively, have been reported.[576] Distant metastases are much more frequent than local lymph node metastases. The rate of developing distant metastasis is 40% to 50% for all AdCC,[574, 576, 606] and these may occur from 10 to 108 months (median 96) after initial diagnosis. Approximately 3% to 8% of patients have metastases at initial presentation.[607] Tumors most frequently metastasize to lung and less frequently to bone and soft tissues. Rarely, an adenoid cystic carcinoma of the maxillary sinuses may metastasize to cervical nodes before the primary tumor is detected.[607] Distant metastasis usually occurs in conjunction with local recurrence but may develop in the absence of locoregional disease[576, 608]; it was the most common type of treatment failure in one recent series.[608]

Spiro reported disease-free intervals, after adequate primary therapy, from 1 month to 19 years (median 36 months) and disease-free intervals of greater than 10 years in 9 of 113 patients (8%).[606] Survival with distant metastases was less than 3 years in 54%, but more than 10 years (with a maximum of 16 years) in 10% of patients. A recent series from M.D. Anderson Cancer Center of 160 patients using consistent surgical and radiation therapy in 87.5% of patients yielded disease-specific survival rates at 5, 10, and 15 years of 89.0%, 67.4%, and 39.6% respectively.[608] Treatment failure was documented in 37% of patients ranging from 2 months to 19 years. Eight percent failed locoregionally only, 22% only failed distantly, and 7% had both locoregional and distant failures. Major (named) nerve invasion, positive margins, and solid histologic features predicted treatment failures, whereas nodal metastases, major nerve involvement, solid histologic features, and four or more symptoms present at diagnosis were associated with increased disease mortality.

Surgical prognosticators in other series include tumor grade, stage, site, nerve involvement, and resection margins. A number of studies confirm that the grading system, based on pattern of differentiation and tumor stage, correlates with survival for AdCC.[609–614] Regarding grade as a prognosticator, the cumulative survival rates at 5, 10, and 15 years are 92%, 65%, and 14%, respectively, for grade I tumors, 76%, 26%, and 5% for grade II tumors, and 39%, 26%, and 5% for grade III tumors.[610] Tumor site is another important prognosticator: generally major salivary sites have a more favorable outcome than minor salivary gland sites.[574, 575] Adenoid cystic carcinomas of the trachea have a better prognosis than their counterpart in the upper respiratory tract, with 5-year survival rates ranging between 66% and 100% and 10-year survival rates ranging between 50% and 75%. These data are summarized in a recent review by Azar et al.[584] Sites such as the sinonasal tract are inherently less resectable and have the worst prognosis.[575] Spiro and Huvos have shown that tumor stage is a better prognostic discriminator than tumor grade.[574] This fact has been underappreciated, as AdCCs are not commonly encountered as stage I tumors. Patients with stage I tumors had a lower rate of local recurrence (23%) than that for patients with tumors of stages II through IV (60%). Their cumulative 10-year survival rates per stage were 75% (stage I), 43% (stage II), and 15% (stage III/IV). Histologic grade did have survival impact early in the disease course: one third of recurrences were evident within 1 year for intermediate- or high-grade tumors, whereas only 14% of low-grade tumors recurred in 1 year.

Garden et al.[576] reported on 83 patients (42%) with microscopic positive margins and 55 patients (28%) with close margins (defined as 5 mm or less) or uncertain margins. Perineural spread was seen in 69% of cases and invasion of a major (named) nerve occurred in 28% of patients. Local recurrences developed in 18% of patients with positive margins as compared with 9% of patients with close or uncertain margins, and 5% of patients with negative margins (p = .02). Patients with major (named) nerve involvement had a crude failure rate of 18% (10 of 55) as compared with 9% (13 of 143) of patients without major nerve involvement (p = .02).

Dedifferentiated AdCCs are aggressive tumors and should be treated with aggressive surgery and adjuvant modalities, including radiation therapy. Two of the four patients died after developing the dedifferentiated component, one at 9 months and one at 15 months from recurrent and metastatic disease.[595, 595a] Although additional cases are necessary to confirm the initial report, it appears that patients with this tumor have a guarded prognosis.

DNA ploidy has shown promise as a prognosticator and may be especially helpful in the preoperative planning phase. Franzen et al.[614] studied 51 AdCCs and found that 39 tumors were diploid and 12 were aneuploid. Grade III AdCC was more often associated with aneuploidy than were grade I or II tumors (p = .011) and ploidy also correlated with clinical stage (p = .011). They found that the combination of S phase greater than 6% plus aneuploidy is a sensitive predictor of treatment failure.[614] Recently Franchi et al. found that E-cadherin expression was a prognostic marker for disease-free interval and survival in AdCC, independent of clinical stage and other histopathologic parameters.[615] Reduced expression correlated with shorter disease-free intervals and actual survival rates. Mean argyrophilic nucleolar organizing region (AgNOR) counts have been found to correlate with histologic grade,[616] and Vulahula et al.[617] have found that high AgNOR counts may be predictive of metastases. In addition, Xie et al.[618] found that the percentage of tumor nuclei with more than one nucleolar organizing region correlated with treatment failure.

Molecular genetic studies have shown that a progression in tumor grade is associated with the accumulated loss of tumor suppressor genes. $p53$ mutations appear to be a late event in the histogenesis of AdCC and are more involved with tumor progression and recurrence. Loss-of-heterozygosity analyses derived from microdissections of varying grades of AdCC within the same tumor reveal that the number of mutations at either the $p53$ or Rb gene is greater in higher grade foci than in lower grade foci. The higher grade foci may contain additional mutations as compared with lower grade foci.[619]

Polymorphous Low-Grade Adenocarcinoma

Polymorphous low-grade adenocarcinoma (PLGA) of the salivary gland is a recently described form of adenocarcinoma. It was reported almost simultaneously in 1983 by two independent groups. Freedman and Lumerman[620] described 12 distinctive tumors, which they termed *lobular carcinoma,* and 1 month later Batsakis et al.[621] independently published a report on a group of similar tumors they termed *terminal duct carcinoma.* Approximately 6 months after their initial publication, Evans and Batsakis[622] published a second series of 14 tumors that were histologically similar to the previous two series, coining the term *polymorphous low-grade adenocarcinoma.* Since these early descriptions, well over 400 tumors have been described in the literature, with the overwhelming majority arising in minor salivary gland sites.[620–645, 645a]

Clinical Features. PLGA is the second most common intraoral malignant salivary gland neoplasm, after mucoepidermoid carcinoma, accounting for 26% of carcinomas.[628] Approximately 60% of the cases have involved the palate, with most of the others arising in various other intraoral sites. Seventeen PLGAs have involved major salivary glands, including one case each in the submandibular and sublingual glands; three arose in the nasal cavity, one of which was associated with an undifferentiated carcinoma; and two have been described in the nasopharynx.[627, 629, 631, 633–635, 637, 639, 645a] We have seen one case in the larynx infiltrating extralaryngeal soft tissue. In addition, three cases have been described in the lacrimal gland,[642] nine cases have been reported as the malignant component of carcinoma ex mixed tumor in one series,[643] and one paper reported two patients with simultaneous multifocal intraoral PLGAs.[644] Approximately two thirds of the tumors have occurred in females, with most arising in patients in the fifth through eighth decades of life. However, like many salivary gland tumors, there is a wide age range of occurrence, ranging from 16 to 94 years. To date, only one tumor has been reported in the pediatric population.[645] Patients usually present with firm, elevated, painless, nonulcerated masses that range from 0.6 to 6 cm in maximum dimension.

Pathologic Features. Histologically, PLGAs are characterized by an infiltrative growth pattern, histologic blandness, cytologic uniformity, and cellular organizational diversity. Tumor cells are usually small and uniform, with bland, minimally hyperchromatic nuclei, inconspicuous to slightly enlarged nucleoli, and scant to moderately abundant, clear to eosinophilic cytoplasm (Fig. 6–35). Mitoses may be present but are usually sparse. Atypical mitotic figures are usually not found. These tumors are unencapsulated and may be well circumscribed; however, foci of infiltrative growth into adjacent normal tissue are seen in almost every case (Fig. 6–35A, B). In occasional cases, tumors are well circumscribed and multiple sections will be necessary to demonstrate foci of tumor invasion. Tumors commonly invade adjacent soft tissue and salivary gland lobules and may infiltrate adjacent bone; perineural growth is common and is as frequent in PLGA as in adenoid cystic carcinoma. The overlying surface epithelium is usually intact but may be ulcerated.

The tumor cells are arranged in varied patterns, ranging from sheets, interconnecting cords, small tubules, solid islands, ducts, cystic and cribriform areas, to other foci having a single-file pattern (Fig. 6–35C–E). Foci of oncocytic or clear cell change, squamous or mucinous metaplasia, or areas with papillary change may be found. Necrosis is usually not seen unless associated with overlying surface ulceration. The intervening stroma is usually minimal; however, occasional tumors may have areas with more abundant hyaline or mucohyaline material. Crystalloids similar to those found in mixed tumors have occasionally been observed.[646, 647]

Differential Diagnosis. Most PLGAs will not cause diagnostic difficulty if careful attention is paid to the lack of pleomorphism, organizational diversity, and arrangement of the tumor cells. However, occasional tumors, especially in a small biopsy specimen, may be confused with adenoid cystic carcinoma (AdCC) or a cellular mixed tumor. The diversity of growth patterns and lack of angulated, dark-staining tumor cells support the diagnosis of PLGA and usually allow separation from AdCC. Several years ago, Gnepp et al.[624] published a small series suggesting that differences in staining patterns of epithelial membrane antigen (EMA) and polyclonal carcinoembryonic antigen (CEA) helped with this differential diagnosis. The staining patterns of these antigens were almost identical and limited to true lumina in AdCC. However, they were different in PLGA with focal luminal staining with CEA whereas EMA stained both luminal and nonluminal cells. A similar differential staining pattern was found in a recent series of PLGA with these two antibodies.[630] Recently Prasad and coauthors[597a, 648] demonstrated that new smooth muscle markers (calponin and smooth muscle myosin heavy chains) might be helpful in this differential diagnosis, as they were positive in all eight AdCCs and negative in all 27 PLGAs studied. Not all PLGAs are devoid of myoepithelial markers. Araujo et al.,[648a] using muscle-specific actin, documented staining in three of 30 tumors. In addition, there have been two recent studies indicating that proliferative rates (Ki-67) for PLGA and AdCC are quite different, with little or no overlap in their ranges.[626, 649] AdCC usually has rates greater than 10% (mean values 21.4% for all tumors in one study and 20.5% for low-grade tumors, 54% for high-grade tumors in the other) vs less than 6.4% (mean values 1.6% and 2.4%) for PLGA. Additional studies are necessary to confirm and refine these preliminary data, as greater proliferative rates (average 7%) for PLGA have been reported by others.[630]

The majority of mixed tumors will have at least a focal mesenchymal-like component consisting of cartilage or a myxoid background or both and foci with plasmacytoid myoepithelial cells, allowing proper classification. Typical benign plasmacytoid myoepithelial cells and myxochondroid areas are not usually found in PLGA, although some tumors will contain spindle-shaped cells that express a myoepithelial phenotype. However, one author (DRG) has

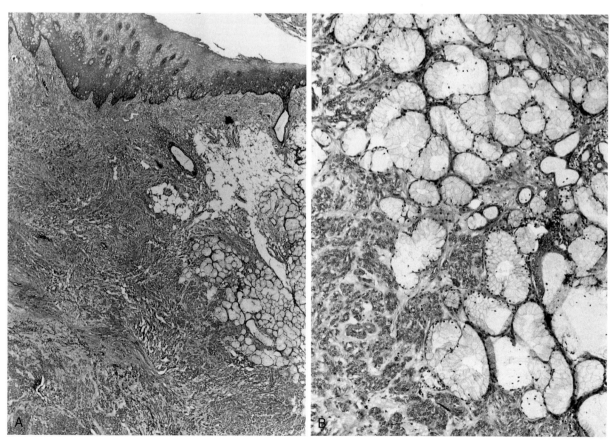

Figure 6–35. *A* and *B,* Polymorphous, low-grade adenocarcinoma of the palate demonstrating peripheral destructive, invasive overgrowth of adjacent mucinous acini.

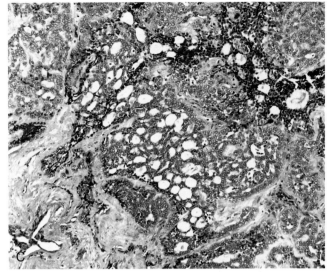

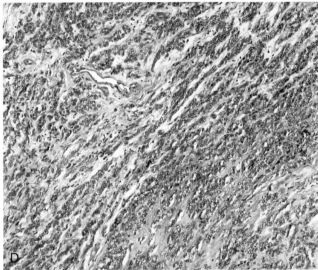

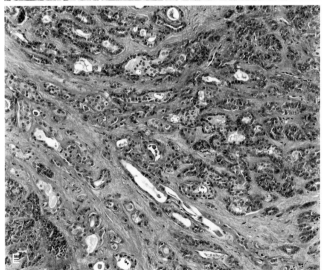

Figure 6–35 *Continued. C–E,* Polymorphous, low-grade adenocarcinoma is composed of bland basaloid cells arranged in varied growth patterns: cribriform areas *(C),* solid nests with foci having a single-file growth pattern *(D),* and ductal structures *(E).*

seen a recent case in consultation that did have a very focal area with plasmacytoid-type cellular differentiation in PLGA. In addition, although many minor salivary gland mixed tumors are not encapsulated, they are well circumscribed and grow in a broad-based pushing fashion. They lack the peripheral infiltrating growth typical of PLGA. However, occasional mixed tumors may cause diagnostic difficulty when they have irregular pushing margins that are difficult to discern from an invasive growth pattern. Rarely, a PLGA appears deceptively benign and may grow with pushing margins, with invasion seen only focally in one of four or five histologic sections. Therefore, one needs to exercise care when dealing with limited biopsy material or with cellular mixed tumors that have irregular margins.

Staining with glial fibrillary acidic protein (GFAP) may be helpful with this latter differential diagnosis. GFAP was expressed only focally in two PLGAs (14%) in a recent study and was localized only to the epithelial component (Fig. 6–36A, see p. 348).[625] In contrast, 93% of mixed tumors expressed GFAP in a focal or diffuse fashion (Fig. 6–36B). Occasional cellular mixed tumors may not stain at all or may only demonstrate epithelial positivity for GFAP.[625] Focal staining by this antibody in PLGA has also been documented in several other series.[630, 632] Positive staining in mesenchymal-like cells or diffuse staining in the epithelial or myoepithelial component equates with a diagnosis of mixed tumor, while a negative study or focal staining only in the epithelial component is supportive but not diagnostic of PLGA. Therefore, in the latter instance, other histologic criteria need to be utilized to establish the proper diagnosis.

Some authors include low-grade papillary adenocarcinomas arising in the palate as a subtype of PLGA.[650] These tumors are histologically different and distinctive from polymorphous low-grade adenocarcinoma because they lack the pleomorphic growth patterns and contain almost exclusively papillary and cystic structures (PLGA may have papillary-cystic foci, but the predominant growth pattern is not papillary). They are also more aggressive biologically and therefore are more properly classified under the designation of papillary cystadenocarcinoma, which we prefer, or low-grade papillary adenocarcinoma.

Rarely, a lobular carcinoma of the breast metastasizes to the oral cavity, simulating PLGA. Good clinical history and histologic comparison with the breast primary tumor helps establish the correct diagnosis.[650a]

Treatment and Prognosis. Treatment consists of wide local surgical excision with possible adjuvant radiation therapy for inadequate margins or for recurrent tumors, although the literature indicates that the majority of recurrences are controlled by surgical re-excision only.[632] A lymph node dissection should be added for those patients with cervical lymphadenopathy. The overall survival rate for PLGA is excellent. It behaves in an indolent fashion, but may locally recur in 9% to 17% of patients.[632, 640] In addition, 0% to 9% of patients in the largest reported series (164 cases) and in a recent literature review (204 cases, 116 with follow-up), respectively, developed cervical lymph node metastases,[632, 640] and two patients developed pulmonary metastases.[632, 651] To date, only three patients have died from PLGA, two had direct extension to adjacent vital structures and the third, in addition to a local recurrence, developed pulmonary metastases.[632, 651] A fourth person died with, but not due to, tumor. This person was treated by incisional biopsy only and refused any additional therapy.[632] In addition, there is one case in which orbital and multiple skin metastases, including non-head and neck sites, developed 15 years after initial presentation[652] and two patients who developed histologic transformation to a higher grade neoplasm after recurrences and radiation therapy 17 and 26 years, after initial surgery.[653]

When PLGA occurs as the malignant component of a carcinoma ex mixed tumor, it also carries a better prognosis than that for other types of carcinoma arising in association with a benign mixed tumor.[643]

Clear Cell Carcinoma

The clear cell carcinomas of the salivary gland are a group of uncommon neoplasms containing a significant proportion of tumor cells with clear cytoplasm that do not fit into other categories of carcinoma. Evidence accumulating over the past decade indicates that this group of clear cell carcinomas is really a heterogeneous collection of neoplasms, the majority of which fall within the spectrum of epithelial-myoepithelial carcinoma. However, as more experience with this group of neoplasms has accumulated, another subtype of primary clear cell carcinoma, distinct from epithelial-myoepithelial carcinoma, was recently described.[654] Hyalinizing clear cell carcinoma is a low-grade carcinoma characterized by nests of clear cells in a densely hyalinizing stroma. As increasing evidence accumulates, we think that additional subtypes of clear cell carcinoma, distinct from epithelial-myoepithelial and hyalinizing clear cell carcinoma, will be described.[655] If a primary clear cell carcinoma does not have any of the characteristics of epithelial-myoepithelial carcinoma or of hyalinizing clear cell carcinoma, then it would be appropriate to classify it as clear cell carcinoma, not otherwise specified.

Over the years, the clear cell carcinomas have been reported under a variety of names including adenomyoepithelioma, clear cell or tubular solid adenoma, monomorphic clear cell tumor, glycogen-rich adenoma and adenocarcinoma, clear cell carcinoma, and salivary duct carcinoma.[656]

Epithelial-Myoepithelial Carcinoma

Clinical Features. In 1972, Donath et al.[657] described eight cases of a previously unrecognized clear-cell tumor of salivary gland origin, which they termed *epithelial-myoepithelial carcinoma.* However, it was not until 1982 that Corio and colleagues introduced this neoplasm into the English language literature.[658] Epithelial-myoepithelial carcinoma (EMCa) is a rare tumor, accounting for approximately 0.5% to 1% of salivary gland neoplasms.[656-660] It occurs most often in older individuals, usually in the sixth and seventh decades of life; rarely, tumors will arise in the pediatric population[656] with one tumor reported in an 8-year-old.[661] Approximately 60% of tumors arise in women.[660] About 80% occur in the parotid gland, with the remaining cases distributed almost equally between the submandibular and minor salivary glands (most commonly palate); rare tumors arise in the sublingual gland.[656, 662] Occasionally EMCa will arise in upper respiratory tract sites such as the larynx, maxillary sinus, or nose. Similar tumors have been reported in the trachea and lung,[663, 664] lacrimal gland,[665] and the breast, where they have been called *adenomyoepithelioma.*[660] Patients typically present with slowly enlarging masses, usually without other symptomatology, but pain and facial nerve weakness have been reported in occasional patients.

Pathologic Features. Grossly, EMCas are well-delineated and firm and may have areas of infiltration into adjacent tissue. They range in size up to 12 cm in greatest dimension,[666] although the average tumor size is 2 to 3 cm.[660] Histologically, these tumors are often well circumscribed and may have a single or multinodular growth pattern, usually surrounded, at least partially, by a thick fibrous capsule. Careful observation often demonstrates tumor nests invading through the capsule into adjacent parenchyma.

Histologically, these are biphasic tumors with islands, large nests, or sheets of tumor cells composed of scattered small ducts lined by cuboidal epithelium similar to normal intercalated ducts. The ducts are immediately surrounded by varying numbers of clear cells that often, in turn, are surrounded by dense hyalinized basement membrane material (Fig. 6–37A–C). Occasionally, columnar cells and small foci of early squamous metaplasia may be seen proliferating within ductal structures. In very rare tumors, areas with a spindle cell population of tumor cells (spindle cell myoepithelial cells) instead of clear myoepithelial cells may be found around the ductal component. The clear cell component may also be arranged in solid nests or sheets (Fig. 6–37D, E). The proportion and arrangement of nodular aggregates of the biphasic component and sheets of clear cells are quite variable from tumor to tumor. In occasional tumors, the clear cell component may predominate and the more typical biphasic portions of the neoplasm may not be readily apparent. If *any* areas of the biphasic tumor population are present, we prefer to classify this tumor as an epithelial-myoepithelial carcinoma rather than, as some authors do, diagnosing those with a minimal ductal component and a myoepithelial phenotype as clear cell malignant myoepithelioma.[667] If there is no ductal differentiation and the tumor has a myoepithelial phenotype, it is appropriate to classify it as a malignant clear cell myoepithelioma. If a tumor is composed of sheets of clear cells without ductal differentiation or a myoepithelial phenotype, it is best classified as a clear cell carcinoma.

Nuclear atypia is usually minimal, but occasional tumors can demonstrate a moderate degree of cellular and nuclear atypia.[666] Recently, one patient with a dedifferentiated epithelial-myoepithelial carcinoma was reported.[667a] The patient had a rapidly growing parotid mass, which was composed of areas of typical EMCa (<20%) and an undifferentiated carcinoma (>80%) with prominent perineural and vascular invasion. Mitotic figures are not usually prominent (<2 per 10 high-power fields), although occasional tumors will have a mitotic rate as high as 10 per 10 high-power fields.[656] Areas of necrosis may also be seen. The clear cell component contains abundant glycogen and ultrastructurally as well as immunohistochemically it has characteristics of myoepithelial differentiation. The ductal lumina may, on occasion, contain mucinous material; however, intracellular mucin is not present in the clear cell component or in the ductal epithelial cells. Perineural invasion and, less frequently, intravascular growth may be found. Occasional tumors may have adenoid cystic–like foci.

Differential Diagnosis. The differential diagnosis consists of other salivary gland tumors with clear cell foci, including benign mixed tumor, clear cell oncocytoma, clear cell myoepithelioma, sebaceous adenoma and carcinoma, acinic cell carcinoma, mucoepidermoid carcinoma, hyalinizing clear cell carcinoma (see next section), polymorphous low-grade adenocarcinoma, and metastatic renal cell carcinoma. Careful histologic sampling will identify the true nature of benign mixed tumor and polymorphous low-grade adenocarcinoma, as the clear cell changes in these neoplasms are seen only focally. Histologic sampling will also allow separation from clear cell oncocytoma; foci of typical oncocytoma can usually be found intermixed with the clear cells and, in addition, the biphasic growth pattern is not seen in oncocytoma. Oncocytosis is also commonly seen in parotid parenchyma adjacent to an oncocytoma.

Clear cell myoepithelioma is an extremely rare tumor. It is well circumscribed or encapsulated, is composed of a more uniform and blander population of tumor cells with less nuclear pleomorphism than is typically seen in EMCa, and it usually has lesser amounts of clear cytoplasm. Sebaceous adenoma and carcinoma have a foamy, vacuolated cytoplasm compared with the completely clear cytoplasm of EMCa, and myoepithelial markers are uniformly negative. In addition, cytoplasmic vacuoles in sebaceous neoplasms frequently make numerous small indentations on the nucleus. This feature is not seen in EMCa. Mucoepidermoid carcinoma, unlike EMCa, will have intermediate and clear cells, some of which contain intracellular mucin, and acinic cell carcinoma lacks the biphasic growth pattern and has at least a few cells with diastase-resistant PAS–positive, fine cytoplasmic granules. Metastatic renal cell carcinoma has a much more prominent vascular background than is typically seen in EMCa and lacks the biphasic growth of EMCa. In addition, renal cell carcinoma characteristically has greater nuclear pleomorphism and atypia and does not stain with myoepithelial immunohistochemical markers. Rezende and coworkers[667b] examined three primary clear cell salivary gland carcinomas and 12 clear cell renal carcinomas (six primary and six metastatic).[667b] They found that all three salivary tumors stained for high molecular weight cytokeratin (keratin 903) and carcinoembryonic antigen, whereas all 12 renal carcinomas had completely negative findings. Hyalinizing

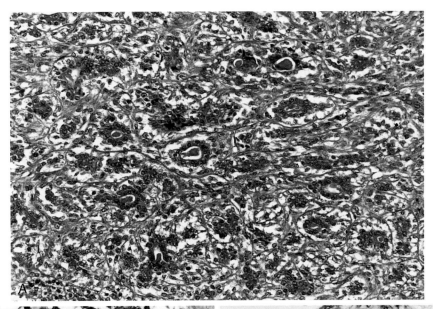

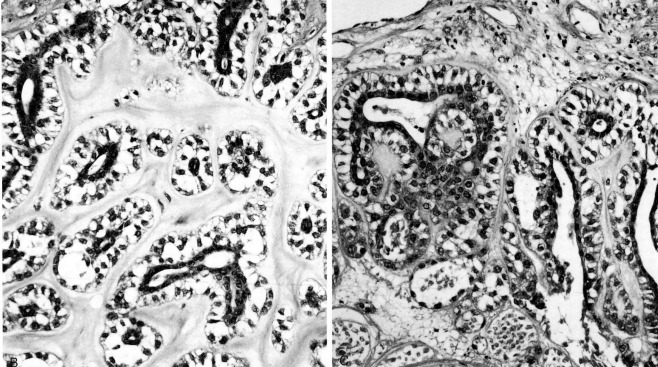

Figure 6–37. *A,* Epithelial myoepithelial carcinoma demonstrating tightly packed nests of tumor composed of intercalated duct–like structures surrounded by clear myoepithelial cells. Prominent basement membrane material frequently surrounds tumor nests *(B).* A more complex geometric arrangement may be seen *(C).*

clear cell carcinoma lacks the biphasic growth pattern and, unlike EMCa, has prominent areas with thin cords of clear cells in an amyloid-like stroma. In addition, all myoepithelial immunohistochemical markers are usually negative (see later discussion).

Treatment and Prognosis. Wide surgical excision is the treatment of choice for this neoplasm. Even with complete excision, however, recurrence and distant metastasis may cause difficulty.[668] To date, available data are insufficient to determine the efficacy of adjuvant postoperative radiotherapy.

This tumor should be considered a low- to intermediate-grade neoplasm. Up to 50% of patients in the reported series (mean, 30%[660]) have developed tumor recurrence, with as many as six episodes of recurrence having been reported in a single patient. Most recurrences develop within 5 years, but intervals up to 9 years have

been observed.[666] Metastases have involved regional lymph nodes (18% of patients), with hematogenous spread seen in 8% to 10% of patients, usually to lung and kidney.[660] Five- and 10-year survival rates are 87% and 67.5%, respectively.[660] Most investigators have been unable to relate any histologic variables with prognosis; however, Fonseca and Soares,[666] in a recent series of 22 tumors, found that nuclear atypia in more than 20% of the tumor was the only variable that correlated with prognosis.

Hyalinizing Clear Cell Carcinoma

Clinical Features. Hyalinizing clear cell carcinoma is a recently recognized subtype of clear cell carcinoma of the salivary glands.[654, 669–671] It is a distinctive tumor characterized by a densely hyalinized stroma and a lack of myoepithelial differentiation. Approximately 80% of the tumors arise in the minor salivary glands of the oral cavity, usually involving the submucosa of the palate or tongue. It may also occur in the parotid gland or larynx and rarely may arise within the mandible or maxilla.[672] Approximately 75% of patients are women. Patients typically presented with a painless mass that had been present for months to several years. One patient presented initially with a cervical lymph node metastasis.[654]

Pathologic Features. Hyalinizing clear cell carcinoma is characterized by dense fibrous stroma, often having an amyloid-like feel, surrounding cords, nests, sheets, and trabeculae of tumor cells. The predominant tumor cell population is characterized by a round to polygonal shape with abundant clear, PAS-positive cytoplasm (Fig. 6–38). The nuclei are centrally located, with mild pleomorphism and inconspicuous nucleoli. Small areas in many tumors contain cells with eosinophilic cytoplasm and very localized areas in occasional tumors will demonstrate squamous differentiation. Focal perineural invasion is seen; vascular invasion is not found. The clear cells are mucicarmine-negative, and all myoepithelial markers, including S100, smooth muscle actin, and muscle-specific actin, were negative. Ultrastructural studies also have not demonstrated any evidence of myoepithelial differentiation. Two reported tumors have demonstrated very focal ductal differentiation with scant extracellular mucin, and two others contained a few clear cells with intracellular mucin droplets. In addition, several tumors have had a prominent lymphoid infiltrate.

The differential diagnosis is similar to epithelial-myoepithelial carcinoma (see earlier discussion).

Treatment and Prognosis. The treatment is surgical, with complete excision being the goal. The prognosis is generally good. Two of the patients in the series by Milchgrub et al.[654] presented with cervical lymph node metastases, whereas Tang et al.[671] reported a case with multiple recurrences. None of the 10 patients with follow-up in the series by Milchgrub et al. developed additional metastases or local recurrence. However, long-term follow-up on patients with this tumor is not currently available. It would seem from the initial reported cases that this is a very low-grade carcinoma with indolent behavior.

Salivary Duct Carcinoma

Salivary duct carcinoma (SDC) is a clinicopathologically distinct salivary tumor that was originally recognized by Kleinsasser in 1968[673] and gained wider recognition in the mid- to late 1980s. Since its initial introduction, the term *salivary duct carcinoma* has been used in a more generic sense by many observers for any primary adenocarcinoma demonstrating focal ductal differentiation. Although many tumors originate from the salivary duct system, this term should be reserved *only* for tumors that histologically resemble ductal carcinomas of the breast.

Clinical Features. Since its initial description,[673] more than 150 cases have been described,[674–697] although it is our experience that this tumor is more common than its incidence in the literature indicates. There is a distinct male predominance of at least 4 : 1, and most patients present after the age of 50. Patients typically present with a history of recent onset and rapid growth of a mass that may be painful and fluctuate in size. Occasional patients have longer clinical histories, and facial paresis may be present. The parotid gland is the most common site of origin, but submandibular[674, 675, 694] and sublingual gland tumors,[676] minor salivary gland tumors,[676–680] and maxillary and laryngeal cases have been reported.[681, 682]

Pathologic Features. Grossly, tumors can be of variable size ranging up to 7 cm.[683] They are usually firm, solid, tan, white, or gray, with a variable cystic component. Infiltration in the surrounding parenchyma is usually obvious, but occasional tumors may appear to be circumscribed. SDC may also arise as the malignant component of a carcinoma ex pleomorphic adenoma, so that grossly the features of a pleomorphic adenoma (myxoid, chondroid, or tan soft elements) may also be present. Microscopically, SDC can be subclassified as either high-grade or low-grade, infiltrative or predominantly (>90%) intraductal.

The high-grade, infiltrative tumor was the entity first recognized and reported, as it is the most commonly encountered, representing greater than 90% of cases. High-grade SDC resembles grade 2 and 3 intraductal and infiltrating breast ductal carcinoma, both architecturally and cytologically (Fig. 6–39). Comedonecrosis within

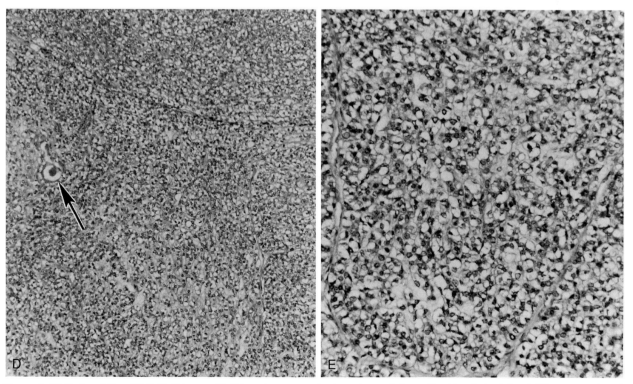

Figure 6–37 *Continued. D* and *E,* Epithelial myoepithelial carcinoma may also have sheets of clear cells with only focal ductal differentiation *(arrow).*

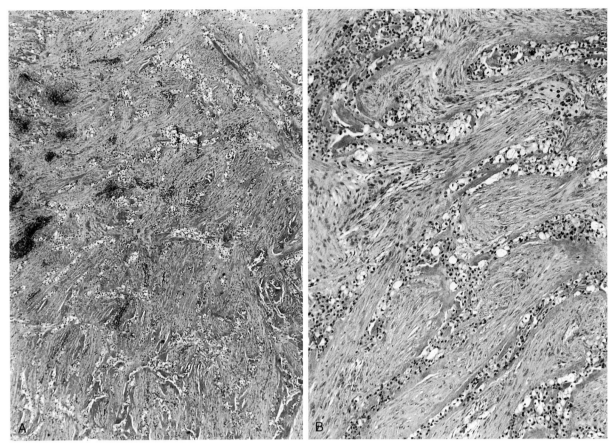

Figure 6–38. Hyalinizing clear cell carcinoma (A, B) composed of infiltrating thin cords of bland clear cells in a fibroblastic hyaline stroma.

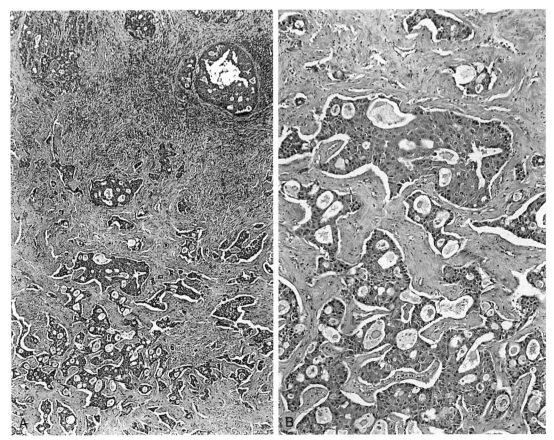

Figure 6–39. Salivary duct carcinoma, high-grade type (A, B), composed of numerous irregular nests of infiltrating tumor in a desmoplastic background. The tumor cells demonstrate moderate atypia with areas of cribriforming similar to ductal carcinoma of the breast (B).

ducts, "Roman bridge" formation, and an intraductal cribriform pattern are typically seen. As with breast, the ductal lesions may be multifocal within the gland. The tumor infiltrates with a cribriform pattern or its infiltration (or metastasis) may totally recapitulate the "intraductal comedonecrotic pattern" seen within salivary ducts. Papillary and solid areas may be seen with psammoma bodies, as well as focal evidence of squamous differentiation. Perineural spread (60% of cases) and intravascular tumor emboli (31% of cases) are common.

Cytologically, these cells have abundant light pink cytoplasm and large pleomorphic nuclei with prominent nucleoli and coarse chromatin. Rarely, keratinization and even squamous pearls may be seen. The cytoplasm may also be densely eosinophilic and granular with an oncocytic appearance and prominent cytoplasmic membranes. Mitotic figures are usually abundant. Goblet cells are not seen within SDC, a feature that can be helpful in the differential diagnosis (see later discussion). These tumors may have prominent intracellular and intraductal mucin secretions. Rare tumors may have a prominent spindle cell or sarcomatoid (metaplastic) growth pattern similar to that in metaplastic ductal carcinomas of the breast.[698]

The cytologically low-grade variant was recognized and reported by Delgado et al.,[684] and Tatemoto[685] in 1996. Unlike the more frequent and familiar high-grade tumors, low-grade SDC has smaller cells with finely dispersed chromatin and small nucleoli, and may have apocrine-type cytoplasmic microvacuoles, which may in-

dent the nuclear contour (Fig. 6–40). The cytoplasm may contain fine yellow to brown pigment and cytoplasmic membranes may be indistinct. The papillae can contain fibrovascular cores. Mitotic figures are negligible and necrosis is minimal. These tumors are strongly and diffusely S100-positive (Fig. 6–40, *inset*), whereas the high-grade variant is usually S100-negative.

There have been some reports to suggest that purely intraductal or minimally invasive SDC may be associated with an improved prognosis.[686–689] Therefore, it is important to indicate this possibility in the surgical report. Purely intraductal SDC (either high-grade or low-grade) will have epithelial hyperplasia, "Roman bridge" formation, micropapillary and tuft formation, and comedonecrosis (in the case of high-grade SDC). The intraductal lesions may be seen in multiple, enlarged, adjacent ducts, resulting in a crowded appearance. In a purely intraductal tumor, the surrounding basement membrane and fibrous tissue of the large ducts is still intact and discernible.

Differential Diagnosis. The differential diagnosis for high-grade SDC includes the papillary cystic and microcystic variants of acinic cell carcinoma (ACC), metastatic squamous carcinoma, metastatic breast carcinoma, melanoma, mucoepidermoid carcinoma, oncocytic carcinoma, and mucus-producing papillary adenocarcinoma.

The papillary cystic and microcystic variants of ACC are usually composed of a blander cell population than high-grade SDC. The tumor cells are much less pleomorphic, demonstrate only mini-

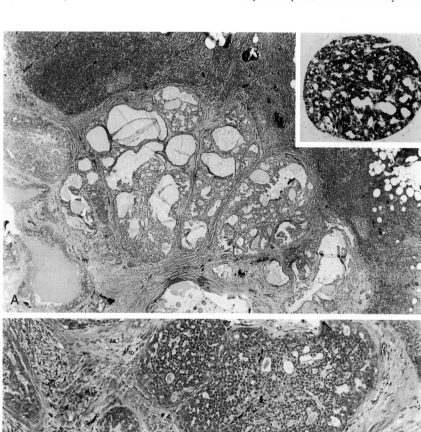

Figure 6–40. Salivary duct carcinoma, low-grade type. This tumor is growing in a broad-based pushing fashion and has a prominent cystic component *(A)*. It is composed of bland tumor cells (grade I nuclei) arranged in solid and cribriform patterns without necrosis *(B)*. An S100 immunohistochemical stain was diffusely positive *(inset)*, confirming the diagnosis.

mal atypia, and have nucleoli that, unlike SDC, are usually small and inconspicuous. In addition, diastase-resistant PAS–positive diastase-resistant granules are found at least focally in ACC.

Despite a superficial resemblance to squamous carcinoma, this diagnosis can be discarded as soon as the infiltrating cribriform pattern is recognized. Squamous carcinoma may have a "glandular" component secondary to irradiation or artifact (acanthomatous pseudoglands), but the appearance of these glands differs from the "crisp" rounded appearance of the cribriform pattern.

Salivary duct carcinoma resembles ductal carcinoma of the breast, which can rarely metastasize to parotid lymph nodes. Therefore, the possibility of a primary breast carcinoma should be considered anytime SDC is diagnosed in a woman. Identification of dysplastic changes or in situ changes in nearby ducts supports a primary origin. Moreover, primary SDC is only rarely estrogen positive (less than 3% of cases) and when positive it usually stains much less than 25% of tumor cell nuclei.[693–697] Therefore, if an in situ component is not found and estrogen receptors are seen in more than 25% of tumor nuclei, the possibility of a metastasis from a breast primary should be given strong consideration.

Metastatic melanoma with an epithelioid pattern, or anaplastic lymphoma, should be considered if one encounters a predominantly solid SDC. An immunohistochemical panel (vimentin, cytokeratin, HMB-45, leukocyte common antigen, and CD 30 [Ki-1]) will be helpful as SDC will be cytokeratin positive and negative for HMB-45, leukocyte common antigen, and CD 30. Goblet cells are not seen with infiltrating duct carcinoma (aside from goblet cell metaplasia within ducts), although intraductal and intracytoplasmic mucin material may be observed, thus ruling out mucoepidermoid carcinoma and mucus-producing papillary adenocarcinoma.

Salivary duct carcinoma may have an oncocytic appearance, raising the possibility of oncocytic carcinoma, an extremely rare neoplasm. Although SDC and oncocytic carcinoma are both composed of large epithelioid cells, the latter has rounder nuclei and a greater amount of cytoplasm. Phosphotungstic acid hematoxylin stain (incubated for 48 hours) or ultrastructural examination, or both, will be most helpful in making this distinction. A phosphotungstic acid hematoxylin stain will reveal intracytoplasmic fine blue granules indicative of mitochondria; ultrastructural examination even on formalin-fixed paraffin-embedded tissue will confirm the presence of multiple mitochondria, albeit poorly preserved.

The differential diagnosis of low-grade SDC consists of predominantly the papillary cystic and microcystic variants of ACC and polymorphous low-grade adenocarcinoma (PLGA). Papillary cystic and microcystic ACC contains vacuolated cells, similar to the microvacuolated cells of low-grade SDC, and may have cystic spaces lined by bland to mildly atypical tumor cells. However, the vacuoles of the latter are smaller and refractile and are associated with yellow to brown pigment, whereas PAS-positive diastase-resistant fine cytoplasmic granules will be found in the former. The pigment in low-grade SDC may also stain with the PAS stain. Ultrastructural study will confirm zymogen granules in ACC. PLGA can be distinguished from low-grade SDC by its distinctive neurotropism and infiltrative lobular, trabecular, and tubular patterns.

Treatment and Prognosis. High-grade SDC is one of the most aggressive salivary malignancies and therefore should be treated by wide surgical excision combined with radiation and possibly chemotherapy. In addition, because of the high risk of cervical nodal metastases (59%) the neck should be treated with a lymph node dissection or with radiation. Barnes and colleagues compiled 104 cases of SDC from the literature, concluding that 33% of reported patients developed local recurrence and 46% developed distant metastasis.[673, 674, 679, 683, 686–688, 690–692] Sites for distant metastasis (in decreasing order of occurrence) include lungs, bones, liver, brain, and skin. Sixty-five percent of patients died of disease, between 5 months and 10 years, usually within 4 years of diagnosis. The clinical course is characterized by distant metastases early in the course of the disease.

For low-grade, in situ, or minimally invasive tumors, wide resection with negative margins is recommended. Adjuvant therapy

can be withheld, with "watchful waiting." Estrogen receptor positivity is an infrequent finding,[675, 693] so anti-estrogen adjuvant therapy is generally not an option.

Few positive prognosticators have emerged from clinicopathologic studies, most likely because of the overwhelmingly aggressive nature of SDC. Small tumor size, absence of perineural or lymphatic invasion, lack of cervical metastases, and tumor diploidy have failed to predict the few patients with long disease-free survival. However, it has been suggested that carcinomas that remain entirely intraductal, or those with minimal infiltration into the adjacent parenchyma, may have a favorable prognosis. Of the four patients reported to have purely intraductal SDC, two were disease free after 3 and 5 years,[687, 688] one developed infiltrating carcinoma after 1 year, and another experienced local recurrences after 5 and 8 years.[688] Two patients with predominantly (>90%) intraductal SDC were disease free at 2 and 3 years.[676] So while the prognosis of purely or predominantly intraductal SDC may be relatively favorable, as with intraductal breast carcinoma, there remains a definite possibility of recurrence or disease progression.

Of the six patients reported by Delgado et al. with low-grade SDC, all were disease free at 2 to 12 years of follow-up (mean, 7 years). Of the two patients in Brandwein et al.[674] original report with long disease-free survivals, one could be classified as having low-grade SDC (Case #7) and was disease free after 5½ years' follow-up. Barnes et al.[683] found that low-grade nuclei did correlate with a tendency toward euploidy but, paradoxically, also correlated with a tendency for lymphatic metastasis. To date, the low-grade variant appears to have a much better prognosis than the higher grade variant. However, data on additional cases are necessary to confirm this trend.

Undifferentiated Carcinoma

As a group, undifferentiated carcinomas of the salivary glands are uncommon neoplasms. These tumors lack light microscopic features that permit more definitive classification. Undifferentiated carcinomas are separated into small and large cell types. A size of 30 microns has been used, by some, as a point of division to distinguish small from large cells. A subtype of undifferentiated large cell carcinoma is recognized, *lymphoepithelial carcinoma,* which has a prominent lymphoid stroma and is histologically identical to the similarly named neoplasms of the nasopharynx. These latter tumors have an association with Epstein-Barr virus infection and exhibit a marked racial predilection for Southern Chinese and Eskimos.

Small Cell Carcinoma

Small cell carcinoma (SmCC) has been reported in several sites throughout the head and neck, including the salivary glands, larynx, nasal cavity and paranasal sinuses, oral cavity, pharynx, and cervical esophagus.[699] SmCC of the salivary glands is a malignant tumor with histologic, ultrastructural, and immunohistochemical features similar to SmCC of the lung.[700] In 1972, Koss et al.[701] described 14 minor salivary gland tumors that were histologically similar to pulmonary small cell carcinoma. This series of tumors differed from pulmonary SmCC in that a better prognosis was noted and occasional foci of ductal differentiation were present. Four of 14 patients survived longer than 5 years. Subsequent reports have confirmed a survival advantage for SmCC of the salivary gland relative to SmCC of the lung.

Small cell carcinomas are rare primary salivary gland tumors. Although accounting for less than 1% of all salivary gland tumors,[699, 702–704] SmCC constitutes 2.8%[701] and 1.8%[705] of all minor and major salivary gland malignancies, respectively. Greater than 80% of major gland cases arise in the parotid gland.[706]

Histologic, ultrastructural, and immunohistochemical studies have documented multidirectional differentiation in salivary gland SmCC.[701, 703, 705, 707] Tumor cells have a tendency to exhibit either ductal or neuroendocrine characteristics, although squamous, myoepithelial, and exocrine differentiation have all been described. Several authorities[700, 703] recognize two types of salivary gland SmCC: small cell ductal carcinoma and small cell neuroendocrine carcinoma. However, Gnepp and Wick[705] demonstrated immunohistochemically that neuroendocrine characteristics can be found in most, if not all, salivary gland SmCCs. Thus, we question the validity of separate subtypes. Tumors with and without demonstrable neuroendocrine differentiation appear to have a better prognosis than pulmonary SmCC.[702]

Clinical Features. Typically, patients present with a painless, rapidly growing mass[10] of less than 3 months' duration.[702, 703, 708–710] Most patients present during the fifth to seventh decade of life; however, tumors have been found in patients 5 to 86 years of age.[699, 706, 708] SmCC is slightly more common in men (1.6:1).[699] Unlike SmCC in other body sites, endocrine syndromes do not typically occur in association with these tumors.

Pathologic Features. Grossly, major gland SmCC is a multilobulated, poorly circumscribed tumor that infiltrates adjacent soft tissues[702, 709]; less commonly, neoplasms are well circumscribed. Tumors are white to grayish; necrosis and hemorrhage are common. SmCC is composed of sheets, ribbons, or nests of tumor cells within a variably fibrous stroma. Tumor cells are as large or slightly larger (1.5 to 2 times) than lymphocytes, and round to oval with scant eosinophilic cytoplasm, although fusiform and larger polygonal cells may be present (Fig. 6–41). Nuclear chromatin is evenly dispersed and varies from finely granular to coarsely clumped. Pyknotic nuclei, nuclear molding, and crush artifact are common. Nucleoli, if present, are inconspicuous. Mitotic figures may be numerous; up to 4 mitotic figures per high-power field is not unusual. Squamous differentiation[701, 707, 711] is well described in SmCC. Positive Grimelius' impregnation[711] has been reported; nevertheless, argentaffin and argyrophil stains are of little utility.[702] Intracellular glycogen is not demonstrable (PAS-negative).[703] Vascular and perineural invasion are common.

Many tumors exhibit very focal areas of ductal differentiation by light microscopy. One hybrid tumor has been described with both well-developed ductal and small cell components.[699] Areas of SmCC may be seen to arise from the basilar ductal epithelium.[709]

Nonetheless, ultrastructural and neuroendocrine immunohistochemical studies may be necessary to identify areas of ductal or neuroendocrine differentiation. Ultrastructurally, ductal forms of SmCC exhibit cells with poorly formed desmosomes,[706, 707] myofilament-like structures, and tonofilaments.[704] Only 30% of tumors[705] exhibit membrane-bound neurosecretory, dense core granules (≤150 nm) in cytoplasmic dendritic processes.[703, 709, 710, 712]

Immunohistochemically, SmCC is positive for cytokeratin, which may manifest as punctate, paranuclear staining,[712] and the majority of cases are positive for EMA.[705] Although most tumors will exhibit positivity for NSE, only 30% of cases are positive for synaptophysin or chromogranin or both.[705, 707, 710, 712]

Differential Diagnosis. Small cell carcinoma of the salivary glands must be distinguished from metastatic carcinoma. Pulmonary SmCC has been reported to manifest initially with metastases to the parotid gland.[713] Kraemer et al.[703] required that the following conditions be met prior to diagnosing primary salivary gland SmCC. First, there should be no history of lung cancer or current evidence of a pulmonary tumor. Second, there should be no prior history of cutaneous neuroendocrine carcinoma (Merkel cell carcinoma) in which invasion of or metastases to the salivary gland cannot be clinically excluded. Both SmCC of salivary glands and Merkel cell carcinoma have been reported to be cytokeratin 20 (CK 20)–positive.[714] Thus, CK 20 may be an useful adjunct in distinguishing SmCC of salivary gland from metastatic pulmonary SmCC (CK 20–negative). Clinical history, moreover, is useful in excluding metastatic basaloid squamous cell carcinoma and malignant melanoma or direct invasion by cutaneous basal cell carcinoma. SmCC tends to show more crush artifact than any of these tumors. Immunohistochemical staining for cytokeratin, S100 protein, and HMB-45 separates SmCC from malignant melanoma.

Clear evidence of epithelial differentiation, such as ductal differentiation, aids in distinguishing SmCC from malignant lymphoma. Moreover, the nuclear characteristics of SmCC differ from malignant lymphoma. Nuclei in SmCC exhibit more finely stippled chromatin with smoother nuclear contours relative to malignant lymphoma. Immunohistochemical staining for cytokeratin and leukocyte common antigen is useful in difficult cases. The vast major-

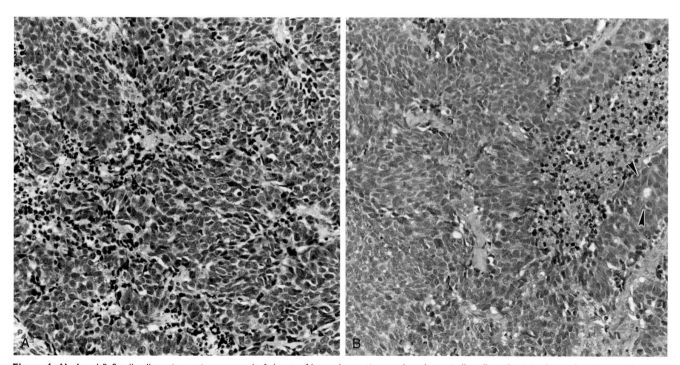

Figure 6–41. A and B, Small cell carcinoma is composed of sheets of hyperchromatic round, oval to spindly cells with minimal cytoplasm, inconspicuous or absent nucleoli, and focal necrosis (B). One rosette-like structure is present (arrowheads).

ity of salivary gland SmCCs are cytokeratin–positive; staining is commonly punctate and paranuclear in character.

Distinction from solid-type adenoid cystic carcinoma (AdCC) may be problematic. Like SmCC, solid AdCC can grow in sheets and nests and exhibit prominent mitotic activity. Focal areas of cribriform architecture, as seen in typical AdCC, are especially helpful, since they are not present in SmCC, and the paranuclear CK positivity of SmCC is not seen in AdCC. Moreover, although neuron-specific enolase positivity may be seen in AdCC, neither chromogranin nor synaptophysin positivity is expected.

Recently, primary primitive neuroectodermal tumor (PNET) of the parotid gland has been reported that potentially may mimic SmCC.[715] Rosette formation and MIC2 immunohistochemical positivity supports a diagnosis of PNET. Homer-Wright rosettes have been described in SmCC of the parotid gland.[710] It is possible that such tumors actually represented primary PNET of the salivary gland.[715]

Rarely, carcinoid tumors may arise in the parotid.[716, 717] These are lower grade neuroendocrine tumors with more cytoplasm, less atypia, and a more organoid growth pattern.

Treatment and Prognosis. The treatment of choice is wide local excision and ipsilateral cervical lymphadenectomy. Adjuvant chemotherapy or radiation therapy, or both, may be warranted. SmCC of the salivary glands may metastasize to cervical lymph nodes and other sites including the liver, central nervous system, and mediastinum. Although salivary gland SmCC does not metastasize as frequently as pulmonary SmCC, locoregional metastases are present at diagnosis in up to 50% of cases.[701] SmCC arising in the major or minor glands has a better prognosis than pulmonary or laryngeal SmCC. The 2- and 5-year survival rates for small cell carcinomas arising in the major salivary glands are 70% and 46%, respectively,[702] whereas those arising in the larynx are only 16% and 5%, respectively.[718]

Large Cell Undifferentiated Carcinoma

Large cell undifferentiated carcinoma (LCUC) represents a group of high-grade malignant epithelial tumors that are too poorly differentiated to permit classification into any other group of carcinoma.[700] Meaningful demographics of LCUC are difficult to determine. Aside from the rarity of LCUC, studies have lacked uniform diagnostic criteria and several have not segregated the data into small- versus large-cell variants.[719]

Clinical Features. Although one study found two thirds of patients with LCUC presenting in the fourth to fifth decade of life, the majority of cases in the AFIP Tumor Registry presented in the seventh and eighth decades of life (age range, 40–96 years).[699] LCUC accounts for approximately 1% of epithelial salivary gland neoplasms.[708, 719, 720] The majority involve the parotid gland; up to 25% of cases arise in the submandibular gland. A rare case of minor salivary LCUC has been reported.[721] Men and women appear to be equally affected. Unlike the lymphoepithelial type of undifferentiated carcinoma, no association with Epstein-Barr virus infection or racial predilection has been found.[706]

Patients typically present with a rapidly growing mass of short duration. Tumors are firm and often fixed due to the infiltration of surrounding tissues. Infiltration of skin with ulceration is frequent. Seventh cranial nerve and palpable cervical node involvement are common at presentation, and invasion of bone may be seen.

Pathologic Features. Grossly, LCUC is usually poorly encapsulated and markedly invasive into skin and soft tissues. Tumors are solid with a grayish-white cut surface. Areas of necrosis and hemorrhage may be prominent. Microscopically, LCUC, by definition, is too poorly differentiated to allow more specific classification. A few authors, however, allow very minor foci of more recognizable forms of carcinoma.[722, 723] The tumor cells are large, greater than 30 microns, and generally polygonal. Abundant eosinophilic, granular cytoplasm is common, although clear cell areas[719] may be present. Nuclei are vesicular and round, usually with one or more prominent

nucleoli. Spindle cells and tumor giant cells (anaplastic/bizarre or osteoclastic-like)[724] are also possible features of LCUC. Tumor cells, often appearing loosely cohesive, form sheets, trabeculae, or thin cords that are separated by fibrovascular stroma. Mitotic activity is usually brisk, up to or in excess of 15 mitotic figures per 10 high-power fields. Hemorrhage and necrosis may be noted, and perineural or vascular invasion is common. Lymphoplasmacytic infiltrates may be present, although they are typically sparse to patchy and are not as extensive as those encountered in lymphoepithelial carcinoma. Cytoplasmic glycogen is demonstrable in some tumors by PAS staining.

Ultrastructurally, tumor cells may exhibit squamous or glandular differentiation, the former as tonofilaments, the latter as intracellular mucin vacuoles. Neuroendocrine differentiation is rare; neurosecretory granules have been described in one case of LCUC.[708] With immunohistochemistry, LCUC stains positively for cytokeratin and may show focal staining for EMA and CEA.[725] Of possible significance, p53 overexpression has been detected in tumor cells in two of three cases studied.[726]

Differential Diagnosis. In establishing the diagnosis, metastatic tumors must be excluded. In one study of 22 undifferentiated carcinomas of the salivary glands, 8 cases were determined to represent metastases.[727] Metastatic poorly differentiated forms of adenocarcinoma, squamous cell carcinoma, melanoma, and undifferentiated carcinoma, such as nasopharyngeal carcinoma, may simulate primary LCUC. Limited foci of mucin production may be found in LCUC and do not obviate this diagnosis.[721] Squamous differentiation, particularly if prominent, should raise the suspicion of metastatic disease. Histologically, metastatic melanoma can mimic LCUC. In both, tumor cells commonly have pleomorphic nuclei, prominent nucleoli, and the potential to spindle morphologically. Immunohistochemical staining for cytokeratin, S100, and HMB-45 distinguishes these tumors. Separating LCUC from large-cell lymphoma in difficult cases is aided by staining for cytokeratin, leukocyte common antigen, CD 20, and CD 30.

Primary tumors resembling LCUC include poorly differentiated adenocarcinoma, mucoepidermoid, and squamous carcinoma. Readily apparent ductal or tubular formation or mucin production favors a diagnosis of adenocarcinoma, not otherwise specified. The presence of neoplastic goblet cells strongly suggests a diagnosis of mucoepidermoid carcinoma. In such a case, a diligent effort should be made to look for squamous differentiation, either keratinization, intercellular bridges, or intermediate cells. As mentioned, prominent squamous differentiation should raise the suspicion of metastasis. Limited or rare foci of glandular or squamous change do not preclude the diagnosis of LCUC. Extensive spindle cell areas may simulate sarcoma. Immunohistochemically, significant positivity for cytokeratin or EMA essentially precludes a diagnosis of sarcoma. Auclair et al.[728] reclassified five putative salivary gland sarcomas as *anaplastic spindled carcinomas* on the basis of keratin or EMA positivity.

Interestingly, undifferentiated carcinoma may arise in association with a variety of benign and malignant neoplasms. These tumors include pleomorphic adenoma,[724] salivary duct carcinoma, acinic cell carcinoma, and polymorphous low-grade carcinoma.[729] In one study,[719] undifferentiated carcinoma accounted for 56% of carcinomas arising in association with pleomorphic adenoma. We have seen undifferentiated carcinoma arise in association with acinic cell carcinoma[730] and salivary duct carcinoma. The infiltrating component of salivary duct carcinoma may have an undifferentiated pattern that overgrows the diagnostic ductal component.[731] Thus, when considering a diagnosis of LCUC, an effort should be made to exclude an underlying or associated neoplasm. Finally, embryonal carcinoma is a very rare neoplasm of childhood that may simulate LCUC.[732]

Treatment and Prognosis. Wide local excision and aggressive radiotherapy are the treatments of choice. Follow-up data are minimal. Moreover, little distinction in therapy and follow-up has been made for large- versus small-cell types of undifferentiated carcinoma. Nevertheless, these tumors are aggressive with local recurrences, regional nodal metastases, and distant metastases developing in more than half the patients. More than 60% of affected patients die of their disease.[708] Tumor size correlates with behavior: patients with tumors exceeding 4 cm had a mean survival time of 7.7 months, with all patients dying from disease, whereas patients with tumors less than 4 cm had a mean survival of 46 months, with 50% dying of their disease.[708]

Lymphoepithelial Carcinoma

Lymphoepithelial carcinoma (LEC) , also referred to as malignant lymphoepithelial lesion or undifferentiated carcinoma with lymphoid stroma,[700] is considered the malignant counterpart of benign lymphoepithelial lesion. Hilderman initially described these tumors in 1962.[733] LEC is a rare tumor and accounts for 0.4% of all salivary gland neoplasms in the AFIP Tumor Registry.[706] These tumors are histologically indistinguishable from the similarly named neoplasms of nasopharyngeal origin.

Clinical Features. The tumors show a marked racial predilection for Eskimos (prompting the designation *Eskimoma*) and Southern Chinese individuals.[734–736] Approximately 75% of reported cases have occurred in these two groups.[737] A familial association has also been described.[738, 739] The parotid gland is affected in over 90% of cases, although several submandibular tumors have been reported in Cantonese individuals.[736] One case of an intraoral LEC of presumed minor salivary gland origin has been reported.[740] The median age of affected persons is 39 years (range, 10–86 years) and there is a 3 : 2 female predominance.[737]

These tumors may arise de novo or in the setting of a preceding or concurrent benign lymphoepithelial lesion.[734, 741] An association with the latter is encountered in up to 33% of patients.[736] There is no association with Sjögren's syndrome (SS) or malignant lymphoma.[735, 742] We recently saw a case in an AIDS patient. As with LEC of nasopharyngeal origin, Epstein-Barr virus (EBV) has been strongly implicated in the oncogenesis of these tumors. In addition to elevated serum titers of anti-EBV antibodies in some patients, EBV genome and mRNA have been demonstrated in tumor cells via in situ hybridization techniques.[743–746] Most EBV-related tumors have been in Asian patients, however, occasional tumors in white patients may be associated with EBV.[747] Conversely, epithelial cells in benign lymphoepithelial lesion appear negative for EBV infection.[745]

Patients present with an indurated mass of variable duration. Not uncommonly, the history is of a long-standing mass with a recent, rapid increase in size. Associated pain and discomfort are common and facial nerve palsy is seen in up to 20% of cases.[748] Cervical lymph node involvement is present in 41% of patients at presentation, although many of these nodal metastases are clinically occult.[736, 749]

Pathologic Features. Tumors present as solid masses ranging from 1 to 10 cm in diameter.[707] On cut section, they may appear either encapsulated or infiltrative and are cream-colored to yellowish-gray with possible hemorrhagic foci. Microscopically, these tumors are defined as undifferentiated carcinomas intimately intermingled with a dense lymphoid stroma (Fig. 6–42). They are composed of sheets, strands, or irregular nests that may interconnect and are surrounded by a benign, dense lymphoid stroma. Tumor cells are large and polygonal or slightly spindled with vesicular nuclei. Syncytial nests of tumor cells are typical, characterized by overlapping nuclei and indistinct cell borders. Reactive histiocytes have been reported to impart a "starry sky" pattern within syncytial nests.[736] Tumor cell cytoplasm may be relatively abundant and slightly amphophilic, particularly in polygonal cells. Nuclear chromatin is coarse or clumped. Nucleoli are prominent and commonly multiple.

By definition, tumors are undifferentiated, although rare foci of keratinization have been described in an otherwise typical LEC. Ultrastructural evidence of squamous cell differentiation in the form of cytoplasmic tonofilaments has been identified.[748, 749] Glandular differentiation is not present and mucicarmine staining is negative. Perineural invasion is present in at least 50% of cases.[736] Mitotic activity is variable, ranging from an average of 2 to greater than 40 mitoses per 10 high-power fields.[736] Atypical epithelial changes may be present in non-neoplastic ducts adjacent to the tumor, supporting the concept that these tumors arise from lining epithelium of the salivary ducts. In a minority of cases, areas of a coexistent or underlying benign lymphoepithelial lesion with typical benign-appearing epimyoepithelial islands may be present.

Immunohistochemically, neoplastic cells are cytokeratin-positive. Overexpression of p53 oncoprotein has been reported in these cells, as well as increased staining for Ki-67.[745] These markers may aid in distinguishing LEC from benign lymphoepithelial lesion (BLEL).

Differential Diagnosis. The differential diagnosis of LEC includes BLEL, metastatic tumors, and malignant lymphoma. Distinc-

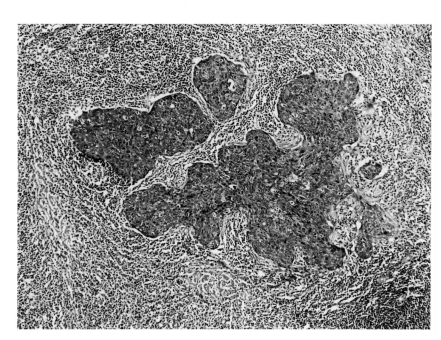

Figure 6–42. Lymphoepithelial carcinoma composed of irregular nests of pleomorphic carcinoma cells surrounded by an abundant lymphoid stroma.

tion from BLEL is based on the malignant cytologic features, anaplasia and mitotic activity, and the infiltrative growth pattern of LEC. Given the potentially identical histology, immunohistochemistry, and ultrastructure of nasopharyngeal carcinoma, clinical evaluation for a possible nasopharyngeal primary should be made in all patients with LEC of presumed salivary gland origin. Metastatic amelanotic melanoma and squamous cell carcinoma are common secondaries to the parotid gland. The former may be separated from LEC by its cytokeratin-negative, S100-positive, and HMB-45-positive immunophenotype. Metastatic squamous cell carcinoma lacks the intimate architectural intermingling of epithelial and lymphoid elements. Co-existent benign lymphoepithelial lesion supports the diagnosis of LEC. In equivocal cases, history and clinical evaluation will aid in excluding metastatic tumors. Immunohistochemically, separation from malignant lymphoma can be made through the use of appropriate lymphoid markers, such as leukocyte common antigen, CD20, Leu-M1 (CD15), and CD30.

Treatment and Prognosis. Appropriate therapy for LEC includes complete surgical excision with negative surgical margins and adjuvant radiation therapy.[750, 751] As with LEC of nasopharyngeal origin, salivary LEC appears, at least in some cases, to be particularly radiosensitive.[750, 751] Given the high incidence of regional metastases, treatment of the cervical lymphatic chain, either surgically or with radiation therapy, is warranted in all cases. Prognosis correlates with initial stage of disease. Advanced stage disease has a poor prognosis. These tumors have been reported to have higher mitotic rates, necrosis, and greater anaplasia. Reported overall 5-year survival rates vary widely and are likely sullied by early reports of high mortality in patients receiving suboptimal treatment. Five-year survival rates of 66% to 80%[746, 750] have been achieved with a combination of surgery and radiation therapy. Up to 20% of patients, nevertheless, will develop local recurrence or distant metastases within 3 years of diagnosis.[706]

Sebaceous Lesions

Sebaceous glands are commonly found in the parotid (10% to 42% of glands) and are found less frequently in the submandibular glands (5% to 6% of glands) using standard surgical pathology sampling techniques (see Fig. 6-1); however, they are only rarely seen in the sublingual gland or in parotid area lymph nodes.[752–757] Intraoral sebaceous glands, known as Fordyce's granules, are commonly found in approximately 80% of individuals, most frequently on the buccal mucosa or vermilion border of the upper lip.[758]

Salivary gland sebaceous neoplasms are classified histologically into five categories: sebaceous adenoma, sebaceous lymphadenoma, sebaceous carcinoma, sebaceous lymphadenocarcinoma, and sebaceous differentiation in other tumors. Although sebaceous differentiation in the parotid and submandibular glands is relatively common, sebaceous neoplasms in these locations are extremely rare. Approximately 149 primary sebaceous tumors of salivary gland origin have been reported in the world literature: 24 sebaceous adenomas, 40 sebaceous lymphadenomas, 29 sebaceous carcinomas, 3 sebaceous lymphadenocarcinomas, and 53 sebaceous lesions associated with other tumors.[752, 753, 756, 759]

Unlike sebaceous neoplasms of the skin, which are associated with an increased risk of developing visceral, predominantly colonic, carcinomas,[760, 761] it would appear that there is no increased risk of developing a visceral carcinoma in patients with a salivary gland sebaceous tumor.

Sebaceous Adenoma

Clinical Features. The sebaceous adenoma is a rare, benign tumor that accounts for 0.1% of all salivary gland neoplasms and slightly less than 0.5% of all salivary adenomas.[762] The mean age at initial clinical presentation is 58 years (range, 22–90 years); the male-to-female ratio is approximately 1.6:1.[752, 753] Twelve of 24

reported tumors arose in the parotid gland, 4 in the buccal mucosa, 2 in the submandibular gland, and 3 in the area of the lower molars or retromolar region. The site of origin is not available for three tumors.

Pathologic Features. These adenomas range in size from 0.4 to 3.0 cm in diameter. On gross examination, the tumors are commonly encapsulated or sharply circumscribed, and they vary from grayish-white to pinkish-white to yellow or yellowish-gray. These tumors are composed of sebaceous cell nests, often with areas of squamous differentiation with minimal atypia and pleomorphism and no tendency to invade local structures (Fig. 6-43). Many tumors are microcystic or composed predominantly of ectatic salivary ducts with focal sebaceous differentiation. The sebaceous glands varied markedly in size and in tortuosity and are frequently embedded in a fibrous stroma. Occasional adenomas demonstrate marked oncocytic metaplasia, and histiocytes or foreign body giant cells, or both (22% of adenomas), can be seen focally. Lymphoid follicles, cytologic atypia, cellular necrosis, and mitoses are usually not observed in sebaceous adenomas.

Sebaceous adenomas may be confused histologically with low-grade mucoepidermoid carcinomas. This differential diagnosis is discussed in the sebaceous lymphadenoma section.

Treatment and Prognosis. Treatment consists of complete surgical excision. These tumors should not recur.

Sebaceous Lymphadenoma

The sebaceous lymphadenoma is a rare, benign tumor composed of well-differentiated, variably shaped nests of sebaceous glands and ducts within a background of lymphocytes and lymphoid follicles. There is minimal cytologic atypia and no tendency to invade local structures. These tumors appear to arise from intralymph nodal sebaceous nests in a fashion similar to Warthin's tumors arising from intranodal ectopic salivary gland tissue.[752, 753, 756]

Clinical Features. Approximately 75% of patients are first diagnosed in the sixth to eighth decade of life (range, 25–89 years), with no gender predominance. Patients typically present with a mass. Thirty-seven of the 40 reported tumors occurred in or around the parotid gland, and one tumor occurred in the anterior midline of the neck. The site was not stated in two patients.

Pathologic Features. Tumors have ranged from 1.3 to 6.0 cm in greatest dimension. Sebaceous lymphadenomas are usually encapsulated, but rarely may be incompletely encapsulated or unencapsulated. They can be solid (Fig. 6-44), multicystic, or unicystic masses that range from yellow to yellow-white to pink-tan or gray. Sebum or cheesy material is commonly found in many of the cysts.

The majority of tumors are composed of variably sized sebaceous glands admixed with salivary ducts in a diffuse lymphoid background (Fig. 6-45). Others consist mainly of lymphocytes and lymphoid follicles surrounding salivary ducts with only occasional sebaceous glands. Histiocytes and foreign body giant cell inflammatory reactions caused by extravasated sebum are commonly observed. By definition, all tumors have a lymphoid background, and about one half have well-developed lymphoid follicles. In addition, tumors may contain small areas of identifiable residual lymph node. Focal necrosis has been observed in only one tumor.

Forty-three percent of sebaceous lymphadenomas are associated with a foreign body inflammatory reaction to extravasated sebum. This foreign body reaction can be helpful in differentiating these tumors from mucoepidermoid carcinoma (MEC). Mucoepidermoid carcinoma frequently is cystic and may contain nests of clear cells, but foreign body inflammation is unusual in that malignancy. In addition, unlike MEC, which contains intracellular mucin in some clear cells, mucin positivity is never found in the clear sebaceous cells. However, intracellular and extracellular mucin may occasionally be found within ducts adjacent to sebaceous cells.

Treatment and Prognosis. Complete surgical excision is the treatment of choice. These tumors should not recur if properly excised.

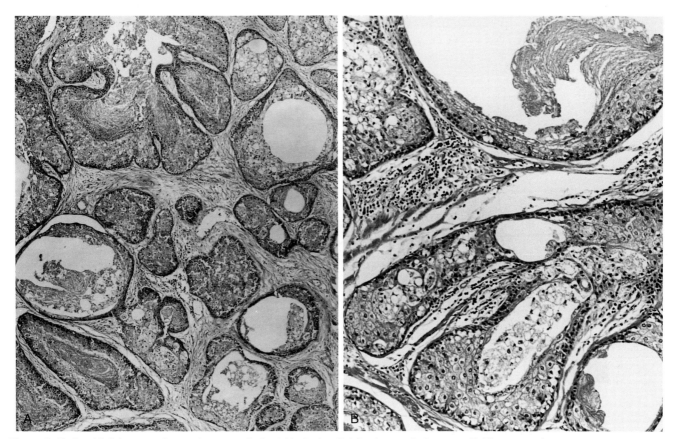

Figure 6–43. *A* and *B,* Sebaceous adenoma is composed of variably sized, well-defined nests of sebaceous cells. There is a multicystic component containing holocrine secretory material.

Sebaceous Carcinoma

Sebaceous carcinoma is a malignant tumor composed predominantly of sebaceous cells of varying maturity that are arranged in sheets or nests, or both, with different degrees of pleomorphism, nuclear atypia, and invasiveness.

Clinical Features. There is a biphasic age distribution with peak incidence in the third decade and the seventh and eighth decades of life (age range, 17–93 years).[752, 753, 756] The male-to-female incidence is almost equal. Twenty-seven of the 29 reported tumors arose in the parotid gland, 1 from the oral cavity, and 1 from the vallecula. Patients most frequently present with a painful mass with varying degrees of facial nerve paralysis and occasional fixation to the skin.

Pathologic Features. Sebaceous carcinomas have ranged from 0.6 to 8.5 cm in greatest dimension and vary from yellow, tan-white, grayish-white, white, to pale pink. Tumors are well circumscribed or partially encapsulated, with pushing or locally infiltrating margins. Cellular pleomorphism and cytologic atypia are uniformly present and are much more prevalent than in sebaceous adenomas. Tumor cells may be arranged in multiple large foci or in sheets and have hyperchromatic nuclei surround by abundant clear to eosinophilic cytoplasm (Fig. 6–46). Areas of cellular necrosis and fibrosis are commonly found. Perineural invasion has been observed in more than 20% of tumors, whereas vascular invasion is extremely infrequent. Rare oncocytes and foreign body giant cells with histiocytes may be observed, but lymphoid tissue with follicles or subcapsular sinuses is not seen.

Treatment and Prognosis. The treatment of choice is wide surgical excision for low-grade and low-stage carcinomas. Adjunctive radiation therapy is recommended for higher-stage and higher-grade tumors. The overall 5-year survival rate is 62%, slightly less than the survival rate for similar tumors arising in the skin and orbit (84.5%).[763] The longest recorded survival, 13 years, occurred in a patient who was 22 years old at the time of diagnosis; however, be-

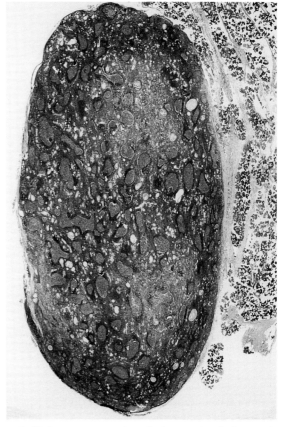

Figure 6–44. Low-power overview of sebaceous lymphadenoma demonstrating an encapsulated tumor with numerous prominent lymphoid follicles and microcystic spaces.

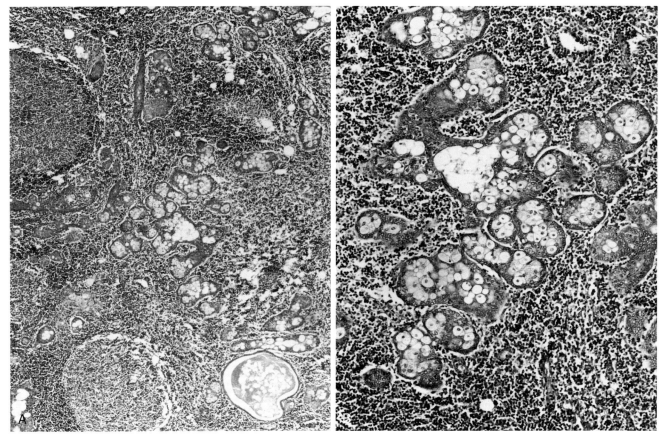

Figure 6–45. *A* and *B,* This sebaceous lymphadenoma is composed of numerous variably shaped sebaceous glands and small ductal cysts surrounded by a prominent lymphoid stroma containing numerous germinal centers.

cause of insufficient data, it is not yet possible to predict whether the survival rates differ between younger and older patients.

Sebaceous Lymphadenocarcinoma

Sebaceous lymphadenocarcinoma is the malignant counterpart of sebaceous lymphadenoma and represents carcinoma arising in a sebaceous lymphadenoma. It is the rarest sebaceous tumor of the salivary glands. To date, only three have been reported.[752–754]

Clinical Features. All three patients were in their seventh decade; two patients were male and one female. The tumors arose within the parotid gland or in periparotid lymph nodes. Patients had histories of a mass, two of which were present for more than 20 years.

Pathologic Features. Tumor color varies from yellow-tan to gray. These carcinomas are focally encapsulated, locally invasive with foci of sebaceous lymphadenoma intermixed with or adjacent to regions of pleomorphic carcinoma cells exhibiting varying degrees of invasiveness (Fig. 6–47). The malignant portion has ranged from sebaceous carcinoma to sheets of poorly differentiated carcinoma, with areas of ductal differentiation, adenoid cystic carcinoma–like areas, or epithelial-myoepithelial carcinoma (Fig. 6–47C, D). Perineural invasion was present in one tumor. Collections of histiocytes have been present in two cases, whereas a foreign body giant cell reaction was found in one tumor. Oncocytes have not been described. Cellular atypia is not observed in the sebaceous lymphadenoma portion of the tumor.

Treatment and Prognosis. Appropriate therapy consists of wide local excision with possible adjuvant radiation therapy if tumors are clinically aggressive. Available follow-up information is minimal, but pulmonary metastasis did occur in one patient.

Sebaceous Lesions Associated with Other Salivary Gland Neoplasms

Fifty-three salivary gland tumors with sebaceous differentiation that do not fall into one of the four previously discussed categories of sebaceous neoplasia have been described in the literature.[753, 756, 764] Thirteen mixed tumors and six carcinomas ex mixed tumor were associated with sebaceous differentiation.[753] Eleven mucoepidermoid carcinomas, 3 oncocytomas, and 15 Warthin's tumors had foci of sebaceous differentiation. One of the Warthin's tumors was associated with the development of a carcinoma.[753] Additionally, single examples of sebaceous differentiation have been reported in adenoid cystic carcinoma, acinic cell carcinoma, basal cell adenoma, a basal cell adenoma from which arose an adenoid cystic carcinoma, and an oral adenocarcinoma.[756] We have additionally observed sebaceous foci in several mixed tumors, in one oncocytoma, and in a myoepithelial carcinoma.

Cystadenoma and Cystadenocarcinoma

Cystadenoma

Clinical Features. Cystadenoma is a benign cystic epithelial neoplasm that frequently contains epithelium-lined papillary projections into the cystic spaces. It represents 0.7% to 8.1% of all benign salivary tumors,[765, 766] 4.1% of all benign epithelial salivary gland tumors reviewed at the AFIP since 1985,[767] and 0.7% of benign parotid tumors in a recent series based on the new WHO classification (see Table 6–4).[768] These tumors occur most frequently in the major glands, with almost 65% arising in the major salivary glands (parotid gland, 57.7%; submandibular gland, 6.6%; and sublingual gland,

0.5%); 10.7% arise in the lip, 8.2% in the cheek, 7.1% involve the palate, and 9.1% other intraoral sites.[766] These tumors represent 7% of minor gland and 3.1% of major gland benign tumors.[767] Cystadenoma can also arise in the larynx or in the sinonasal area.[769] They occur more frequently in females, with a female-to-male ratio ranging from 2:1 to 3:1 in two series.[765, 767] The mean patient age is approximately 57 years (range, 12–89 years),[767] with the greatest prevalence between the sixth and eighth decades of life.[766] Cystadenoma is asymptomatic and presents as a small, slowly enlarging nodule, usually less than 1 cm in greatest dimension, in the minor salivary glands[765]; tumors in the major glands tend to be larger.

Pathologic Features. The diagnostic histologic criteria of cystadenoma are controversial. These tumors are usually multicystic and well circumscribed and may be encapsulated; occasional unicystic tumors have been described. We prefer to designate all unicystic lesions with papillary intraluminal projections as intraductal papillomas rather than as unicystic cystadenomas. The number and size of the cystic structures vary between tumors. The epithelial lining of the cysts also varies within and between tumors, from thin to thick, often with intraluminal papillary projections. Epithelium can be cuboidal, flat, columnar or, rarely, squamous, with bland, uniform nuclei (Fig. 6–48). Occasional tumors have areas of solid epithelial proliferation. Mitotic activity is rare and cellular atypia is not usually seen in this neoplasm. Oncocytic or mucinous changes of the epithelial lining may be present and, occasionally, may be prominent. If the latter changes are dominant, tumors should appropriately be termed oncocytic or mucinous cystadenomas. Up to 55% of cystadenomas have a chronic inflammatory infiltrate,[765] which on occasion can be marked,[766, 770] with a density similar to that seen in Warthin's tumor.[770] Because of variations in histologic features, some cystadenomas have been called *duct ectasia, salivary duct cyst, oncocytic papillary cystadenoma, papillary mucous cystadenoma,* and *papillary hyperplasia.*[765]

Differential Diagnosis. Differential diagnosis consists of a simple cyst, duct ectasia, polycystic (dysgenetic) disease, Warthin's tumor, intraductal papilloma, low-grade mucoepidermoid carcinoma, the papillary cystic variant of acinic cell carcinoma, and cystadenocarcinoma. Both duct ectasia and a simple cyst have a smooth epithelial lining without papillary intraluminal projections. In addition, duct ectasia, unlike cystadenoma, usually involves several ductal segments and is often associated with fibrosis, atrophy of the adjacent salivary gland, and chronic inflammation. Polycystic disease is extremely rare and involves the entire salivary gland more diffusely than does the well-circumscribed cystadenoma. The oncocytic variant of papillary cystadenoma has similar epithelial features to a Warthin's tumor; however, the characteristic lymphoid component is lacking. Intraductal papilloma has overlapping histologic features with cystadenoma. Whether intraductal papilloma is a separate and distinct entity from papillary cystadenoma or whether it falls within its spectrum has yet to be resolved. As mentioned, we prefer to define papillary cystadenoma as multicystic and intraductal papilloma as unicystic. If the process involves more than one duct, it is best classified as a cystadenoma.

Low-grade mucoepidermoid carcinoma (MEC) shares some histologic characteristics with cystadenoma. One can distinguish it from cystadenoma by paying close attention to the non-cystic component of the tumor. The papillae in MEC, when present, are more irregular and complex than those found in cystadenoma. Solid "budding" islands of tumor are frequent in MEC; these are not usually found in cystadenoma. Also, the intermediate cells so characteristic of MEC are not found in cystadenoma. The papillary cystic variant of acinic cell carcinoma (ACC) may be difficult to separate from cystadenoma. Finding areas with more typical ACC patterns or diastase-resistant PAS–positive fine cytoplasmic granularity will confirm the diagnosis of ACC. In addition, the rare examples of ACC with a pure papillary cystic pattern, unlike papillary cystadenoma, are usually composed of an uniform population of cuboidal intercalated duct–like cells and have foci with more complex epithelial proliferation with cribriform-like or microcystic architecture. Cystadenocarcinoma has a greater degree

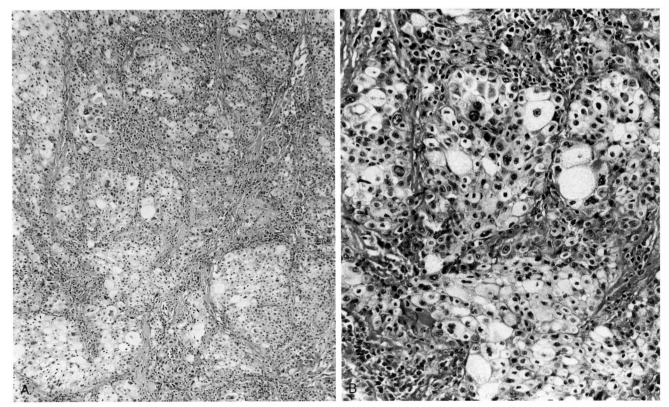

Figure 6–46. *A* and *B,* Sebaceous carcinoma composed of sheets of pleomorphic hyperchromatic sebaceous cells with prominent nucleoli and varying amounts of finely vacuolated clear cytoplasm.

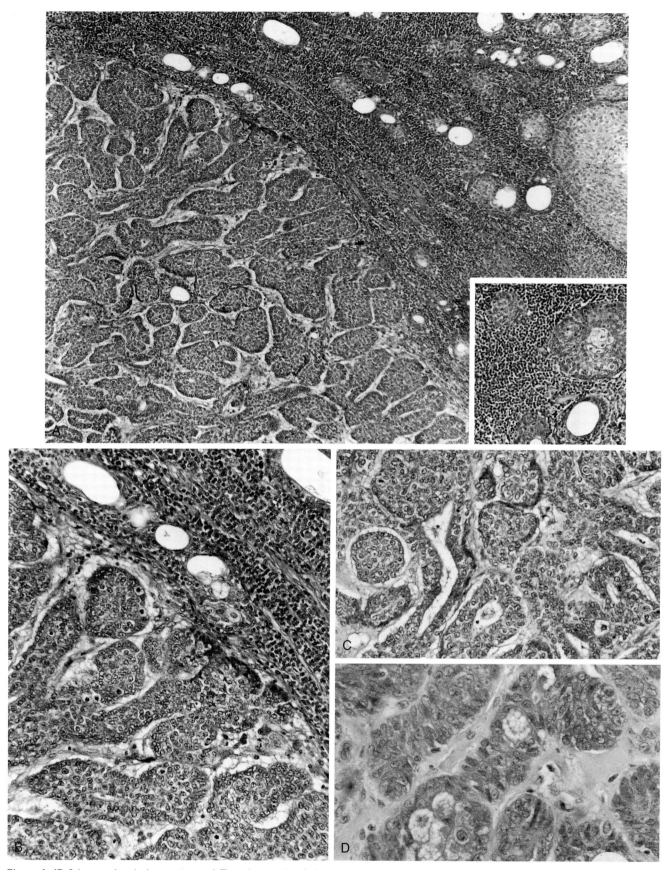

Figure 6–47. Sebaceous lymphadenocarcinoma. *A,* The sebaceous lymphadenoma component is in the upper right and the carcinoma is in the lower left. The inset details the sebaceous lymphadenoma with a squamous nest containing central sebaceous differentiation and a small cyst, both of which are surrounded by lymphoid cells. *B,* Detail of the junction of the sebaceous lymphadenoma and carcinoma component. The carcinoma is composed of nests of poorly differentiated carcinoma cells with areas of ductal differentiation *(C)* and focal sebaceous differentiation *(D).*

of cellular and nuclear atypia than cystadenoma, and foci of invasion can be found.

Treatment and Prognosis. These lesions are successfully treated with conservative but complete surgical excision, which is usually curative.[767]

Cystadenocarcinoma

Cystadenocarcinomas are a distinct, morphologically diverse group of epithelial tumors characterized by invasive growth and cystic structures lined by epithelium, often arranged in a papillary growth pattern without histologic characteristics of other recognizable forms of salivary gland carcinoma that may form cystic structures, such as ACC, mucoepidermoid carcinoma, or polymorphous low-grade adenocarcinoma.[771, 772] Terms previously used for cystadenocarcinoma in the literature include malignant papillary cystadenoma, mucus-producing adenopapillary carcinoma, low-grade papillary adenocarcinoma of the palate, and papillary adenocarcinoma.[773] We include the low-grade papillary adenocarcinoma of the palate reported by Mills et al.[774] in the cystadenocarcinoma group, rather than as a variant of polymorphous low-grade adenocarcinoma.[775]

Clinical Features. Cystadenocarcinomas are rare neoplasms and have only recently been included in the new WHO salivary gland tumor classification as a specific type of carcinoma (see Table 6–4). Because of their rarity and differences of classification in various series, specific data on clinical features are sparse. Of 79 tumors reported from the two largest series (57 cases from AFIP and 22 from China), 65% were from the parotid glands, 2.5% were from the sublingual glands, 1% were from the submandibular glands, and 32% were from the minor glands (lip 10%, palate 9%, buccal mucosa 9%, tongue 3%, retromolar area 1%).[772, 776] Of 22 additional reported cases of minor gland involvement, 82% involved the palate.[777] Labial mucosa, buccal mucosa, and lingual mucosa lesions

have also been reported. Patient ages have ranged from 5 to 87 years, with peak prevalence in the sixth decade, except in China, where the average age at diagnosis is 37 years, with 59% of cases occurring in patients less than 39 years of age.[776] Sixty percent of patients were male.[772, 776, 777]

This tumor typically presents as a gradually enlarging, asymptomatic mass, sometimes with surface ulceration, and in one series 32% of patients had pain.[776] One recent case report additionally documented a sublingual gland tumor presenting as a ranula.[778]

Pathologic Features. Tumors ranged from 0.4 to 10 cm in greatest dimension, with an average size of 2.4 and 2.2 cm in the major and minor salivary glands, respectively.[772, 776] Grossly, they are circumscribed, unencapsulated, cystic, white-gray masses containing clear to brownish, occasionally mucoid fluid. All tumors demonstrate infiltrative growth, often associated with a desmoplastic reaction. The cysts frequently interconnect and vary in size within a given tumor, ranging from microscopic to 3 cm in diameter.[772, 773] Many cysts had ruptured and were associated with inflammatory reactions. Seventy-five percent of cases contain prominent areas of papillary growth, with most of the remaining tumors demonstrating occasional or focal papillary growth.[772] A cystic pattern without papillary intraluminal projections was uncommon.[772] The papillary morphology varies from simple linear strands to complex structures with branching fibrovascular cores. Areas of solid tumor growth were seen in 16 of the AFIP tumors (28% of cases) and 6 cases demonstrated focal comedo-type necrosis.[772]

These tumors are cytologically diverse. Cells lining the cystic spaces are most frequently simple cuboidal in nature, similar to intercalated duct epithelium, but they also were lined by columnar, simple squamous, and mucus-secreting cells (Fig. 6–49); stratified squamous epithelium was not found. In addition, areas containing cells with clear or oncocytic cytoplasm or hobnailing were seen. Nuclear pleomorphism and atypia vary from minimal to moderate in

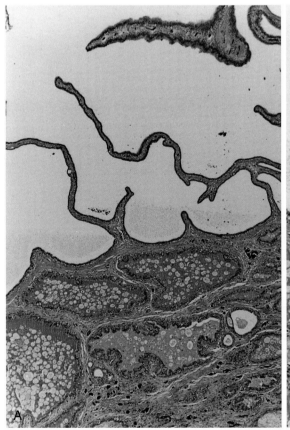
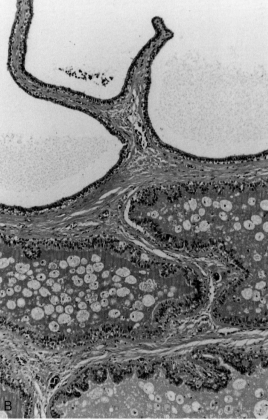

Figure 6–48. This papillary cystadenoma is a multicystic tumor composed of delicate fronds projecting into the cystic lumina *(A)*. The fronds contain vascular cores lined by bland columnar and cuboidal epithelium *(B)*.

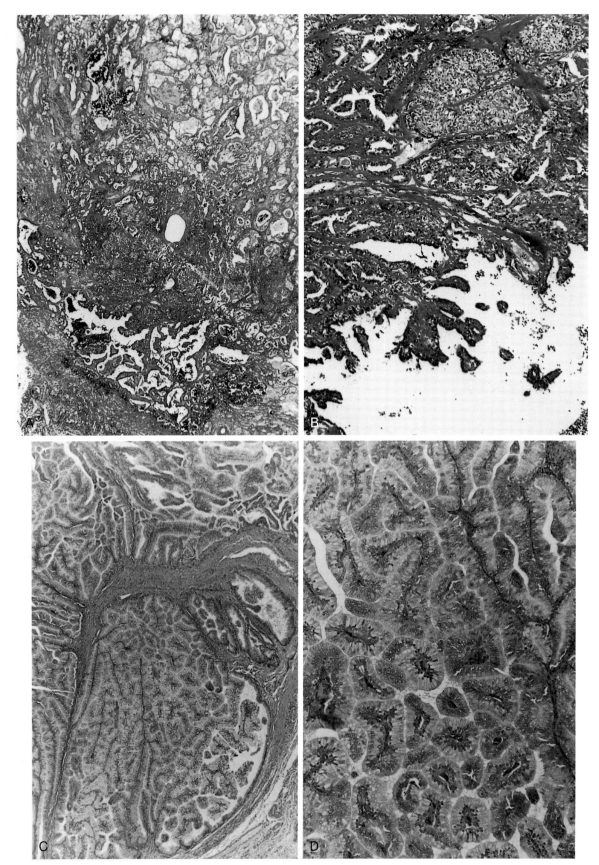

Figure 6–49. *A* and *B,* This low-grade papillary cystadenocarcinoma is composed of numerous cystic spaces with focal areas of papillary projections into cystic spaces. Focally, solid islands of tumor *(B)* are invading into the adjacent fibrous stroma. The cells are somewhat uniform and have minimal atypia. Because of lack of atypia and pleomorphism, this tumor is classified as low grade. *C* and *D,* Mucinous papillary cystadenocarcinoma, high grade. This multicystic tumor is composed of tightly packed intraluminal projections of tall, mucin-producing, columnar cells with a moderate degree of cytologic atypia.

the AFIP series and from minimal to severe in the series from China. We have observed, as have others,[779] rare high-grade tumors with severe nuclear atypia and pleomorphism. Mitotic figures range from none to as many as 30 per 10 high-power fields.[772] Extracellular mucin material was identified in 75% of the AFIP tumors, while perineural invasion and psammoma bodies are occasionally noted.[772]

Differential Diagnosis. Differential diagnosis consists of cystadenoma, polymorphous low-grade adenocarcinoma (PLGA), mucoepidermoid carcinoma (MEC), the papillary cystic variant of acinic cell carcinoma (ACC), and salivary duct carcinoma (SDC). Cystadenomas can be separated from cystadenocarcinoma by their lack of stromal invasion. Polymorphous low-grade adenocarcinoma may have focal areas with papillary cystic growth similar to cystadenocarcinoma but, in addition, it has a much more varied architectural arrangement composed of "basaloid" cells arranged in nests, cords, ducts, and cribriform patterns. In addition, perineural invasion is common in PLGA and is infrequent in cystadenocarcinoma.

Low-grade MEC frequently has papillary cystic foci. It can usually be differentiated from cystadenocarcinoma by finding mixtures of mucinous and epidermoid cells lining the cysts, by finding solid areas with focal mucinous differentiation between the cysts, and by the presence of intermediate cells. Intermediate cells are not found in cystadenocarcinoma, and squamous differentiation is unusual and, when present, is usually seen focally without stratification.

The papillary cystic variant of ACC may cause diagnostic confusion with cystadenocarcinoma. Finding areas of more typical ACC (solid, follicular, or microcystic) or diastase-resistant PAS–positive fine cytoplasmic granularity will confirm the diagnosis of ACC. Last, both high- and low-grade salivary duct carcinoma may have papillary cystic foci. Tumor cells in high-grade SDC frequently are larger than those found in cystadenocarcinoma and have more pleomorphic nuclei, often with prominent nucleoli and abundant eosinophilic cytoplasm. In addition, high-grade SDCs have more frequent areas of necrosis and higher mitotic rates. Both high- and low-grade SDC are often arranged in patterns typical of intraductal breast carcinoma with cribriform formation and luminal bridging.

Treatment and Prognosis. The majority of the tumors are low- to moderate-grade neoplasms; however, occasional tumors are high-grade. The prognosis with cystadenocarcinomas varies depending on the grade and the clinical stage of the tumor, with neoplasms of lower grade and clinical stage having a much better prognosis than those of higher stage and grade. Treatment should, therefore, be based on the grade and stage of the tumor. Wide surgical excision with good margins is appropriate for low- and intermediate-grade tumors, together with a neck dissection if lymphadenopathy is detected. For high-grade and advanced-stage tumors, adjuvant radiation therapy should be added.

Due to their rarity, only limited follow-up information is available in the literature. Data were available in 40 patients from the AFIP series.[772] All patients were free of tumor and alive (36 patients) or died from other causes (4 patients) at a mean follow-up interval of 59 months. Three patients (7.5%) developed local recurrence, whereas three others had metastatic adenocarcinoma in regional lymph nodes at initial presentation, and one patient developed regional nodal metastasis at 55 months, for an overall rate of metastasis of 10%. In addition, 18% of patients had a history of or developed a second primary malignancy, usually at distant sites.

Mostofi et al.[777] found a local recurrence rate of 27% and a cervical lymph nodal metastatic rate of almost 23% for 22 minor gland tumors. In addition, one patient with a lymph node metastasis also developed distant metastasis to the lung and vertebrae and expired from disease 20 years after initial diagnosis.[777, 780] Chen[776] divided the 22 papillary cystadenocarcinomas into high or low grades and was able to correlate the frequency of recurrence and lymph node metastasis with tumor grade. Eight of 12 (67%) high-grade tumors recurred, whereas only 2 of 10 (20%) low-grade tumors recurred. In addition, three patients with high-grade tumors developed lymph

node metastases and three died from their disease at 6 months, 4 years, and 9 years. None of the patients with low-grade tumors developed metastases and all were alive without evidence of disease.

Primary Squamous Cell Carcinoma

Primary squamous cell or epidermoid carcinoma (SCC) of the parotid and submandibular glands are extremely rare neoplasms. The incidence of primary parotid SCC is variable, ranging from 0.3% to 8.9% of all parotid tumors and between 2.1% and 11.4% of submandibular gland tumors.[781–785] The lower figures (<1%) for the parotid are probably more accurate, as the incidence, in our experience, is frequently overestimated as a result of the inadvertent inclusion of tumor metastases to the parotid gland. For a parotid tumor to be considered primary, one must exclude metastatic SCC from skin of the upper face and scalp, or, less commonly, from the upper aerodigestive tract. Direct extension from the external auditory canal or overlying skin SCC[786] must also be excluded, as well as other primary parotid tumors that have a squamous appearance, namely high-grade mucoepidermoid carcinoma and salivary duct carcinoma. For primary submandibular SCC, one must rule out direct extension from a floor-of-mouth SCC; metastatic carcinoma is much less likely to occur. Rarely, SCC will arise in an accessory parotid duct or in the sublingual gland.[784] Occasional SCCs arise from minor salivary ducts. These tumors have not received any attention in the literature and are treated as routine upper aerodigestive tract SCCs.

Clinical Features. Few published series have addressed the issue of primary parotid SCC[781, 783, 785, 787] and there are even fewer reports that illustrate the histology. Almost 90% of cases involve the parotid gland, usually the superficial lobe, with most of the remaining cases arising in the submandibular gland.[785, 788] A male predominance is seen, and most cases occur during or after the fifth decade, although rare tumors have occurred in the pediatric population.[789] An association with previous irradiation has been noted.[783, 785, 788] Presenting signs and symptoms include a mass, with or without pain, and facial nerve paralysis.

Pathologic Features. Histologically, salivary gland squamous carcinoma appears similar to other upper aerodigestive tract SCC. There is a tendency toward better differentiation and keratinization, and less than 10% of tumors are poorly differentiated.[788] In situ ductal dysplasia can be seen[786, 790] and is helpful in establishing a diagnosis of a primary neoplasm; however, its absence does not obviate the possibility of a primary tumor. As mentioned, one is obliged to sample the tumor generously and perform mucin stains, which are uniformly negative.

The differential diagnosis includes metastatic SCC, which is much more frequent than a primary squamous carcinoma, mucoepidermoid carcinoma, and also salivary duct carcinoma and oncocytic carcinoma, both of which can occasionally have an epithelioid or squamoid appearance. Careful histologic sampling will allow separation from the latter two diagnostic considerations, as more typical areas will be found allowing proper classification. Intracellular mucin positivity will help confirm the diagnosis of a mucoepidermoid carcinoma, and a careful history should rule out a metastasis.

Rarely, a squamous cell carcinoma may be the carcinoma component of a carcinoma ex mixed tumor or the malignant component of a carcinoma arising in a Warthin's tumor.[791, 792] Careful sampling should identify all tumor components and allow proper classification. Lymphoepithelial carcinoma has a unique, nonkeratinized immature appearance with abundant lymphoid stroma, which is easily distinguished from primary SCC.

We recently saw an unfortunate case of primary parotid SCC with extensive perineural spread. This patient presented with a dermal SCC and slight facial nerve palsy. As his parotid imaging studies were negative, the dermatologist erroneously concluded that the dermal SCC was unrelated to the facial nerve palsy, and commenced Mohs' surgery. The patient underwent 3 days' worth of Mohs' surgery, without achieving negative margins. He was transferred to our institution where a parotidectomy and temporal bone resection were performed. A 1-cm SCC was present in the deep lobe of the parotid. Extensive perineural spread was found, thereby explaining the dermal satellite as well as the failure to obtain clear resection margins. Of note, the surrounding skin did not reveal actinic damage, which speaks against the possibility of a dermal primary.

Treatment and Prognosis. Patients have been treated either with primary surgery or combined surgery and radiation. Survival and course is dictated, as with almost all salivary tumors, by tumor stage and grade. Elective neck dissection appears warranted, as there is a significant rate of lymphatic spread. Gaughan reported a 50% survival rate at 5 years[783] and the Memorial Sloan-Kettering group reported survival rates at 5, 10, 15, and 20 years to be 21%, 15%, 13%, and 10, respectively.[785]

Colloid Carcinoma

Clinical Features. Primary colloid or mucinous carcinoma of the salivary glands is an extremely rare neoplasm. We prefer to use the term *colloid* rather than *mucinous,* as the latter term may also be used for any carcinoma with abundant mucus production. Colloid carcinomas have been reported in many areas of the body, including the gastrointestinal tract, breast, paranasal sinuses, eyelid, and skin. Only 11 cases with salivary gland involvement have been reported to date.[793–796] Patients' ages have ranged from 42 to 86 years (mean, 69.5 years) and the tumor was slightly more common in females, with a male-to-female ratio of 5:6. Older patients are mostly female, whereas younger patients are male. The most frequent presenting symptom is a mass of 1 to 12 months' duration, although one patient had an 11-year history and one patient had a "long" history of a slowly enlarging mass. Tumors range from 2.5 to 4.0 cm in greatest dimension. Six of the 11 cases originated in the minor salivary glands, 2 in the parotid gland, 2 in the submandibular gland, and 1 in the sublingual gland.

Pathologic Features. We define salivary gland colloid carcinoma in a fashion similar to the definition used in the breast as a tumor usually having good circumscription with a soft gelatinous gross appearance that contains large lakes or pools of contiguous extracellular mucin in direct contact with the stroma. The mucin lakes surround malignant epithelium, which may form glands, solid nests, single cells, or, occasionally, mucin-containing signet ring cells (Fig. 6–50). Until we have a better understanding of the range and biologic behavior of colloid carcinomas arising in the salivary glands, tumors with malignant epithelium lining any portions of the cystic spaces are best classified as mucinous cystadenocarcinoma rather than as colloid carcinomas, since the biology of these two patterns in the breast differs.[797]

Differential Diagnosis. Differential diagnosis includes mucinous cystadenocarcinoma, metastatic tumor, and mucin extravasation phenomenon. The first has cystic areas with tumor epithelium against fibrous stroma, rather than pools of mucin between the stroma and tumor cells. A metastasis can be ruled out by careful clinical history and evaluation. Mucin extravasation phenomenon contains pools of interstitial mucin, often with inflammatory changes and areas of fibrosis. Unlike colloid carcinoma, neoplastic epithelium is not found within the mucin pools.

Treatment and Prognosis. All reported cases were treated with surgical resection and four also received postoperative radiation therapy. Clinical follow-up is available for nine patients. Four patients died from recurrent or metastatic disease at 12, 34, 36, and 72 months after their initial diagnosis. Two patients were alive with recurrent or metastatic disease at 42 and 72 months. One patient died secondary to a metastatic pancreatic carcinoma at 3 years without evidence of colloid carcinoma; another patient died from metastatic endometrial carcinoma 29 months after diagnosis with no evidence

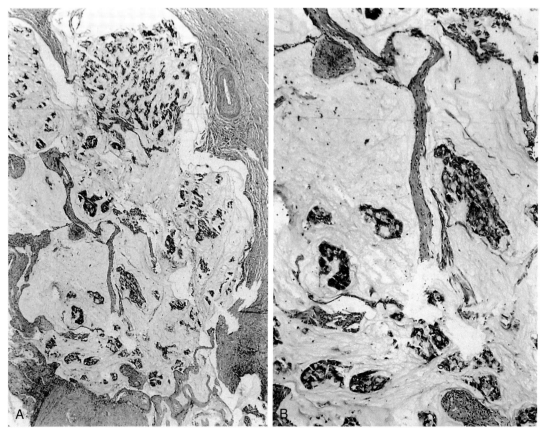

Figure 6–50. Colloid carcinoma composed of multiple pools of mucin in a fibrous stroma *(A),* which surrounds atypical pleomorphic carcinoma cells *(B).*

of colloid carcinoma; and one patient was alive at 56 months with unknown disease status. Two of the patients who died from tumor had regional lymph node involvement at the time of diagnosis, and one had an incompletely excised tumor.

From the preceding, one can conclude that primary colloid carcinoma of the salivary glands is an aggressive tumor with a significant risk of local recurrence and metastasis.

Adenocarcinoma, Not Otherwise Specified

Clinical Features. Adenocarcinoma, not otherwise specified is a group of salivary gland carcinomas with ductal or glandular differentiation that do not have sufficient histologic features compatible with any of the currently recognized categories of salivary gland carcinoma to allow for a more specific designation other than "not otherwise specified." These are uncommon but not rare tumors. Approximately two thirds involve the minor salivary or seromucinous glands of the upper respiratory tract, and one third involve the major salivary glands.[798] At the AFIP, this group of neoplasms accounts for 9% of salivary gland tumors and 16.8% of all salivary gland malignancies since 1985.[799] The relative frequency of these tumors is quite variable in the literature, ranging from 1.9% to 11.8% of salivary gland tumors, but they usually rank as one of the three most common types of malignant salivary gland tumors.[800] In a recent series of parotid tumors reclassified according to the new WHO (see Table 6–4), adenocarcinoma not otherwise specified represented 2.7% of all epithelial tumors and 17.8% of malignant epithelial tumors.[801]

At the AFIP, these tumors are slightly more common in women than in men, with an average age at presentation of 58 years (range, 10–93 years). Other series have demonstrated a slight male predominance.[798, 802] Approximately 60% occur in the major salivary glands with 90% of these arising in the parotid gland and 10% in the submandibular gland[799]; occasional cases have been reported in the sublingual gland.[800] Forty percent arose in the minor glands in decreasing order of frequency: the palate (usually hard palate), buccal mucosa, and upper and lower lips. Tumors may present as asymptomatic or painful masses; fixation to adjacent or deeper tissues is frequent.[799]

Pathologic Features. Tumors frequently range in size up to 10 cm in greatest dimension and may have circumscribed or infiltrating borders.[800] Grossly, these tumors are firm with cut surfaces ranging from white to whitish-yellow; areas of necrosis may be seen.[799] The adenocarcinomas are composed only of a few cell types arranged in an endless variety of growth patterns with areas of glandular or ductal differentiation that do not resemble any of the known ("named") types of salivary gland carcinoma. Tumors are classified as low-, intermediate-, or high-grade using criteria similar to those used for adenocarcinomas in other anatomic areas.

Treatment and Prognosis. Treatment is wide local excision for low-grade and low-stage tumors, whereas intermediate- or high-grade tumors with positive or close margins, or advanced-stage tumors should be treated more aggressively with wide surgical excision and adjuvant radiation therapy. In addition, for high-grade tumors, the appropriate neck area should be treated with radiation or neck dissection. Referral for neutron beam therapy is a therapeutic option for inoperable cases.

Information on the biologic behavior of adenocarcinoma not otherwise specified is sparse. Only two series with sufficient number of cases are available.[798, 802] Since these are older series that were published before the recent 1991 WHO classification of salivary gland tumors, some of their tumors would most probably be reclassified as newly recognized variants of salivary gland carcinoma. In addition to the major and minor salivary glands, cases from upper respiratory sites were also included. Despite these limitations, the data in the two series are the best currently available.[799] Matsuba et al.[802] recorded a median survival for the 54 patients in their series of 4 years. They found that survival was dependent on tumor location,

with oral cavity tumors having a more favorable prognosis (approximately 76% at 10 years) than those of the parotid (26% at 10 years) or submandibular glands. In addition, patients with low-grade tumors had lower rates of distant and cervical lymph node metastasis and greater disease-free intervals. Cervical lymph node metastases developed in 23% of patients, with 73% dying within 3 years; distant metastases developed in 37% of patients, with 93% dying within 3 years. These authors concluded that tumor grade did not significantly affect overall patient survival which was similar for well, moderately, and poorly differentiated tumors (approximately 25% at 10 years).

Spiro et al.[798] found that grade and, especially, tumor stage were important prognostic indicators in their series of 204 patients. Recurrence was more frequent in patients with high-grade tumors and there was good correlation with survival: grade 1, 2, and 3 tumors had 69%, 46%, and 8% 5-year and 54%, 31%, and 3% 15-year survival rates, respectively. The most accurate predictor of outcome appeared to be clinical stage, with stage I, II, and III tumors having 15-year cure rates of 67%, 35%, and 8%, respectively. Patients with tumors of the oral cavity had better survival rates (56% at 5 years) than those seen in patients with tumors of the parotid gland (45% at 5 years), who, in turn, had better survival rates than those in patients with tumors arising in the submandibular gland (13% at 5 years). Twenty-six percent of patients developed distant metastases, which were more frequent in previously treated patients or in those with high-grade tumors.

Congenital Tumors Including Sialoblastoma

The most frequent neonatal or congenital salivary gland tumor to arise in a major salivary gland is a hemangioma. Other neoplasms are uncommon in this population and include teratoma, hamartoma, sialoblastoma, and "adult type" salivary gland tumors such as mixed tumor, sebaceous adenoma, mucoepidermoid carcinoma, adenoid cystic carcinoma, poorly differentiated carcinoma, epithelial-myoepithelial carcinoma, and adenocarcinoma.[803, 804] We prefer to use the proposed classification scheme of Batsakis et al.[805] for congenital and neonatal tumors: (1) neoplasms fulfilling criteria for a specific salivary gland tumor (e.g., pleomorphic adenoma) should be classified as such; (2) neoplasms not classifiable according to the criteria used for adult tumors should be called sialoblastoma with the additional qualifier of benign or malignant; (3) criteria for defining histologic evidence of malignancy are similar to those for adult tumors and include vascular or neural invasion and the presence of cytologic atypia beyond that expected for embryonic epithelium. Batsakis et al.[805] have stated that invasive growth without the latter findings is less reliable, since invasion is intrinsic to embryonic epithelium; however, we have seen one case in which the invasive pattern correlated with multiple recurrences and tumor progression.[806]

Sialoblastoma was first reported in 1966 by Vawter and Tefft,[807] who used the term *embryoma*. Since that time, there have been multiple terms applied to describe this group of tumors, including congenital basal cell adenoma, basaloid adenoma, monomorphic adenoma, congenital hybrid basal cell adenoma–adenoid cystic carcinoma, low-grade basaloid carcinoma, adenoid cystic carcinoma, and sialoblastoma.[803, 806, 808] In their case report, Taylor et al.[809] drew an analogy between this tumor and others with a blastomatous appearance, suggesting the term *sialoblastoma*.

Some observers prefer to separately classify these congenital tumors into basal cell adenoma and hybrid basal cell–adenoid cystic carcinoma in addition to a separate category of sialoblastoma; however, these authors concede that sialoblastoma and basal cell adenoma are similar and have overlapping histologic features.[803] Because of these overlapping and varied histologic features, the rarity of these neoplasms, and the lack of in-depth experience at any single institution, it is our preference to combine all congenital basaloid tumors into one group termed sialoblastoma. As more experience is accrued, we may be able to subdivide this group into meaningful subcategories. For now we would like to suggest using a classification scheme as follows: well-differentiated (grade 1), including the basal cell subtype as well as tumors without cytologic atypia or invasive growth; moderately differentiated (grade 2), including cases with invasive growth, greater cytologic atypia, and necrosis but without definitive evidence of malignancy (no neural or vascular invasion or metastatic spread); and poorly differentiated (grade 3), tumors that have definite evidence of malignancy.

Clinical and Pathologic Features. To date there have been approximately 23 tumors reported that fit into the broad definition of sialoblastoma.[803–808] Sialoblastomas arise almost exclusively in the major glands, over 80% involve the parotid and the remainder the submandibular gland. They are slightly more common in females than in males. Sialoblastoma arises almost exclusively in the perinatal period, with one tumor presenting in a 32-month-old[810]; additionally, Daley and Dardick[811] reported a somewhat similar-appearing neoplasm in an adult. Grossly, these tumors range up to 15 cm in greatest dimension[809] and are usually encapsulated or at least well circumscribed, but they may be locally infiltrative. Microscopically these tumors try to recapitulate embryonic development of the major salivary glands, with their histologic patterns reflecting the various stages of phenotypic expression and differentiation.[805] Sialoblastomas frequently have variable histologic patterns within the same tumor and in different tumors. This consists of solid, multinodular nests and sheet-like collections of primitive-appearing epithelial cells with a basaloid morphology focally forming ducts and duct-like structures, which may have peripheral palisading (Fig. 6–51). The primitive nest-like pattern is frequently destructive and aids in separating this tumor from adenoid cystic carcinoma and basal cell adenoma or adenocarcinoma. Basal cell adenoma does not exhibit destructive growth, whereas adenoid cystic or basal cell adenocarcinoma grows in a less destructive pattern. Cribriform areas

similar to those in adenoid cystic carcinoma may be found and areas of spindling have been noted. Sebaceous cell clusters as well as nests of myoepithelial cells and foci with squamous differentiation have been described.[803] Occasional acinar differentiation may also be seen. This latter feature, together with more embryonic-type histology, will help separate sialoblastoma from hamartoma, which usually has much more prominent acinar differentiation and mature elements.

The nuclei in sialoblastoma are round to oval, usually with minimal to moderate amounts of cytoplasm. Nuclear pleomorphism is variable, as is the presence of nucleoli. Necrosis may be present and is more frequent in malignant tumors. Surrounding the nests and collections of epithelium, there is a loose mesenchyme, which often has an embryonic appearance.[804] Mitoses are frequently found and may be plentiful; atypical mitoses are not usually seen.

Anti-keratin antibodies stain the ductal elements and occasional cells in the solid islands, whereas anti-actin stains many of the abluminal cells; anti-S100 stains both ductal and abluminal elements.[806, 808, 809]

Treatment and Prognosis. Complete surgical excision with negative margins is the treatment of choice.[806, 808] Adjuvant chemotherapy and radiotherapy have been tried, but the limited number of cases hampers assessment of these modalities.[803, 806] The limited number of cases and short follow-up of reported cases also preclude making definitive conclusions about biologic behavior, although published data do indicate that sialoblastoma can be locally aggressive and malignant. Five of the 23 reported cases have recurred, several multiple times, or had local persistence of disease, and two cases developed regional lymph node metastases.[803, 806, 809, 812] Progression of tumor grade with recurrence and increasing mitotic rates has been seen.[806] One patient had four recurrences with inoperative tumor extending into the skull at 43 months.[809] Low-grade tumors

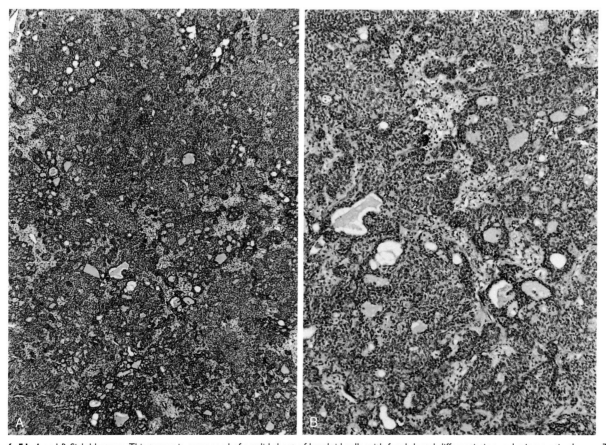

Figure 6–51. *A* and *B*, Sialoblastoma. This tumor is composed of a solid sheet of basaloid cells with focal ductal differentiation and microcystic change. Tumor cells are fairly uniform with minimal cytoplasm and only slight pleomorphism. Portions of this tumor are growing in solid sheets, whereas other areas are arranged in more of a nesting pattern.

appear to be less aggressive than higher grade tumors, with only one recurrence in eight tumors.[803]

Metastasis to Major Salivary Glands

Clinical and Pathologic Features. Metastatic involvement of the major salivary glands or of the lymph nodes adjacent to the major salivary glands is a frequent occurrence, accounting for one third of all metastases to head and neck sites in one epidemiologic investigation.[813] The parotid glands contain 3 to 32 (average 20) intraglandular lymph nodes that are interconnected by a plexus of lymph vessels, which drain the skin from the side of the head above the parotid gland, the orbital region, and the nose, upper lip, external auditory canal, eustachian tube, and tympanic membrane.[814, 815] In contrast, the submandibular or sublingual glands proper do not contain any intraparenchymal lymph nodes.

Metastases to the parotid region and submandibular gland is a fairly common phenomenon, with an incidence most frequently ranging between 1% and 4% of salivary gland neoplasms in various published series.[815] There is considerable variability in incidence, but metastases account for an average of slightly over 16% of malignant tumors (range, 3%–72%).[815] Approximately 90% of metastases involve the parotid region, with the remainder involving the submandibular gland. Metastases to the sublingual gland have not been reported to date. Squamous cell carcinoma and malignant melanoma are the most common neoplasms metastasizing to the major salivary gland area, accounting for 60% and 14.5% of cases, respectively.[815] Eighty-five percent to 88% of tumors with known primary sites metastasizing to the parotid area originate in the head and neck region, with 84% to 89% of the head and neck primaries arising from skin sites.[815, 816] Twelve percent to 15% of the parotid metastases had primary locations in non-head and neck sites, most commonly originating in the lung, kidney (Fig. 6–52), and breast.[815, 816] Other sites of primaries include, in decreasing order of incidence, the colorectum, prostate gland, skin, stomach, uterus, and pancreas. The opposite was true in the submandibular gland, with 85% of tumors arising in infraclavicular primary sites, the most common of which were also the breast, kidney, and lung.[815]

The most frequent age at diagnosis for metastases to the major salivary glands is the seventh decade, but it ranges from infancy to the tenth decade of life. Patients are usually over 50 years of age (85%) and there is an approximately 2:1 male-to-female ratio.[817] Patients usually present with an unilateral mass. In most cases, the primary tumor is known; however, occasionally, the metastasis is the initial presentation of disease,[818, 819] and, rarely, bilateral involvement may be seen.[818]

Treatment and Prognosis. Treatment should consist of complete surgical excision with a modified cervical lymph node dissection for patients with palpable disease or evidence of nodal involvement by imaging.[820] The addition of adjuvant radiation therapy is controversial, with variable recommendations. The primary location and tumor type will influence final therapeutic recommendations. If there has been tumor spillage or if there is residual microscopic disease, then postoperative radiation therapy is suggested by some authors,[820] whereas others recommend combination surgery and radiotherapy for all patients with metastatic carcinoma of the skin.[821]

It is difficult to generalize about prognosis due to the different tumor types and variable primary locations one encounters. For most tumors, metastatic disease implies a poorer prognosis for a given primary tumor. If the metastasis is from an infraclavicular primary and is only one of many metastatic deposits, the prognosis is usually poor. However, if the metastasis is only a single focus, local control of the primary tumor and metastasis is possible.[817]

Patients with head and neck skin primaries that metastasized to the parotid area have a better prognosis if the tumor is confined to the lymph nodes than if the parotid parenchyma is involved (8% vs 79% local recurrence rates).[822] The overall rate of disease control in the parotid area in a recent series of 77 patients with carcinoma of

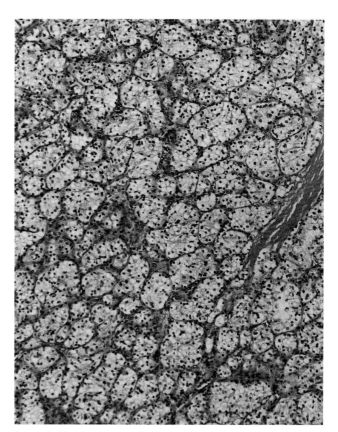

Figure 6–52. Metastatic renal cell carcinoma composed of variably sized nests of clear cells with slight nuclear pleomorphism and a prominent vascular background.

the skin and parotid metastases was 82% at 5 years, with an overall 5-year survival rate of 54%.[821] Patients with head and neck mucosal primaries have a very poor prognosis, with only 1 of 10 patients alive and disease free at 5 years.[816] Ironically, patients with malignant melanoma involving the parotid have a better prognosis if no primary site is found.[823] In a series of 19 patients, there were 6 with no known primary. Five of these were disease free at a mean of 4.2 years (range, 14 months to 7.5 years) and one patient died of disease at 17 months. Extraparotid primary melanomas were found in the other 13 cases (10 cutaneous and 3 mucosal). All but one of these patients were disease free at follow-up: nine died of melanoma (mean 2.6 years, range 10 months to 5 years) and the other three had metastatic disease (mean 4.3 years, range 3 to 6 years); only one patient was disease free at 2 years.

Central Salivary Gland Tumors of the Maxilla and Mandible

Rarely, salivary gland tumors arise primarily within the jaws. To accept a tumor as primary and central in origin, there must be no evidence of a primary lesion within the salivary glands or at any other site. Radiologic evidence of bone destruction, integrity of cortical bone, and a definitive diagnosis of a salivary gland neoplasm are also necessary to confirm central origin.[824, 825] These tumors may arise from ectopic salivary gland tissue from a developmental abnormality, from seromucinous glands displaced from the maxillary sinus, or from neoplastic transformation of the lining of an odontogenic cyst.[826, 827]

Clinical Features. Approximately 75% of these tumors occur in the mandible, while 25% involve the maxilla; at least 30% are associated with a dental cyst or an impacted tooth.[824] The mean age at presentation is 48 years (range, 1–85 years) with a very slight female predilection.[824] Jaw swelling is the most frequent presenting symptom, but, in decreasing order of frequency, pain, trismus, paraesthesia, mobile teeth, and drainage or hemorrhage may also occur.

Pathologic Features. The most common intraosseous salivary gland tumor in the largest review of 138 tumors[824] is mucoepidermoid carcinoma, accounting for 65% of tumors; adenoid cystic carcinoma (18%), carcinoma ex mixed tumor (4%), adenocarcinoma (4%), benign mixed tumor (4%), acinic cell carcinoma (4%), and monomorphic adenoma (1%) were also reported. In addition, hyalinizing clear cell carcinoma has been reported to arise within the jaws.[828]

Differential diagnosis for mucoepidermoid carcinoma (MEC) in this location consists of glandular odontogenic cyst, also known as sialo-odontogenic or mucoepidermoid cyst, clear cell odontogenic carcinoma, metastatic renal cell carcinoma, and calcifying epithelial odontogenic tumor. There is some overlap in the histologic features of the glandular odontogenic cyst and mucoepidermoid carcinoma. These can be separated by paying attention to the lining of glandular odontogenic cyst, which is thinner and does not demonstrate areas of thickening or microcystic change, as does an MEC. Clear cell odontogenic carcinoma and metastatic renal cell carcinoma both lack intracellular mucin and a squamous component, whereas calcifying epithelial odontogenic tumor will have foci with amyloid-like stromal material.

Treatment and Prognosis. Complete surgical excision is the treatment of choice, with radical excision offering a better chance for cure than more conservative procedures such as marginal resection, enucleation, or curettage.[824] For mucoepidermoid carcinoma, the recurrence rates with conservative and radical therapy were 40% and 13%, respectively[824]; 9% of patients died from their disease.[825] Within each histologic tumor type, there appears to be no correlation between tumor grade and prognosis. However, the histologic type of carcinoma is significant, with 50% of patients with adenoid cystic carcinoma having metastatic disease, whereas in the mucoepidermoid carcinoma group, the metastatic rate was 9%.[824]

Mesenchymal Neoplasms

Nonepithelial tumors, excluding lymphoid neoplasms, account for 1.9% to 4.7% of salivary gland tumors[829–832] with benign lesions being more common than sarcomas. The ratio of benign to malignant mesenchymal neoplasms varies from series to series, ranging from 18:1 to 2.4:1.[830, 831] Greater than 85% of soft tissue neoplasms involve the parotid gland, over 10% arise in the submandibular gland, and only a rare tumor involves the sublingual gland.

Vascular tumors are the most common benign mesenchymal neoplasm, representing almost 40% of the benign tumors.[830, 831] Seventy-five percent to 80% of vascular neoplasms are hemangiomas, with the greatest incidence occurring in the first decade of life (Fig. 6–53). The majority of the other vascular tumors are lymphangiomas, with an occasional hemangiopericytoma being reported. Other types of benign soft tissue neoplasms arising in the major salivary glands include neural tumors, most frequently schwannoma and neurofibroma, with a rare meningioma[831]; fibrous tumors, most frequently nodular fasciitis, fibrous histiocytoma, and fibromatosis with an occasional myxoma, myofibromatosis, fibroma, solitary fibrous tumor[833, 834] or inflammatory pseudotumor[835]; lipomas including the pleomorphic variety[836]; and miscellaneous other tumors including granular cell tumor,[837] angiomyoma, glomangioma, giant cell tumor, and osteochondroma.

Salivary gland *sarcomas* arise in an older population than their benign soft tissue counterparts. They are rare tumors, accounting for only 0.3% of salivary gland tumors.[832] Virtually any type of sarcoma may arise primarily in the salivary gland (Table 6–9).[831, 838, 839] In the largest published series, hemangiopericytoma, malignant schwannoma, fibrosarcoma, and malignant fibrous histiocytoma were the most common neoplasms, accounting for 16%, 15%, 14%, and 11% of reported sarcomas, respectively.[838] These are aggressive neoplasms, with 40% to 64% of patients developing recurrences and 38% to 64% developing metastases (usually hematogenous), and the mortality rate is 36% to 64%, usually within 3 years of diagnosis.[838, 839] The most successful treatment is wide surgical excision or surgery combined with radiation. For more specific information about each tumor, the reader is referred to the excellent text on soft tissue tumors by Enzinger and Weiss.[840]

Hybrid Tumors

A hybrid tumor is defined as a salivary neoplasm composed of two or more disparate patterns that are not included in each other's histologic realm. For instance, tumors with features of both mucoepidermoid carcinoma and adenoid cystic carcinoma, or acinic cell and cribriform salivary duct carcinoma, are examples of hybrid tumors. There is presently no other nomenclature with which to adequately describe these types of tumors. The disparity inherent to hybrid tumors comes from the fact that each element differentiates toward distinctly different salivary elements: for example, excretory duct versus acini or excretory duct versus intercalated duct. Shared foci of phenotypic differentiation may be seen within salivary tumors; these cases would not be considered hybrid tumors. For instance, Grenko and colleagues have described adenoid cystic carcinomas with foci of epithelial-myoepithelial carcinoma–like differentiation, and vice versa.[841] Both of these tumors are composed of ductal and myoepithelial elements, and presumably it is a matter of degree of local gene expression that dictates the histologic phenotype. Therefore, these tumors would not be considered as hybrid tumors, but as variations in differentiation.[841, 842] By this definition, tumors with patterns of both canalicular and basal cell adenoma, or adenoid cystic carcinoma and basal cell adenocarcinoma, would also not be considered hybrid tumors. Also, hybrid tumors would not show evidence of evolution from one entity to another. For instance, a tumor with features of mucoepidermoid carcinoma and pleomorphic adenoma is not a hybrid tumor and is better classified as mucoepidermoid carcinoma ex pleomorphic adenoma.

The term "hybrid tumor" has also been used in conjunction with sialoblastomas. These tumors represent a clinicopathologically distinct category,[843, 844] usually diagnosed prior to the age of 1 year, with a basaloid cytology and varying degrees of maturation and invasiveness. A tumor with features of basal cell adenoma and adenoid cystic carcinoma in a child under the age of 1 year is better classified as a sialoblastoma; the different histologic pattern here again would be an example of differentiation towards similar histologic elements. Last, a hybrid tumor should be distinguished from a "collision tumor," which is the physical intermingling of two tumors, each with a physically distinct site of origin. We have recently seen liposarcoma metastasize to the thyroid gland. A papillary thyroid carcinoma had engrafted itself upon the liposarcoma; this is an ideal example of a collision tumor.

There are but few examples of salivary hybrid tumors in the literature.[845–848] Seifert and Donath[845] estimated that hybrid tumors accounted for less than 0.1% of all salivary tumors. Two of their cases (a parotid Warthin's tumor and a sebaceous gland lymphadenoma, and a parotid cribriform salivary duct carcinoma and an acinic cell carcinoma) satisfy this definition of hybrid tumor. Dreyer et al.[846] also reported a parotid hybrid tumor with both Warthin's tumor and sebaceous lymphadenoma. Evans and Cruickshank[847] illustrate a sebaceous carcinoma that occurred in conjunction with mucoepidermoid carcinoma. Kamio et al.[848] reported a palatal tumor with both cribriform salivary duct carcinomatous and adenoid cystic carcinomatous elements. They showed acceptable immunohistochemical distinctions between the two elements, confirming the multiclonality of these tumors: the salivary duct carcinoma expressed p53 and c-erbB-2 protein, whereas the adenoid cystic carcinomatous elements were negative. Snyder and Paulino[848a] described a similar tumor arising in the submandibular gland. Croitoru et al.[848b] described three tumors that qualified as hybrid carcinomas using our

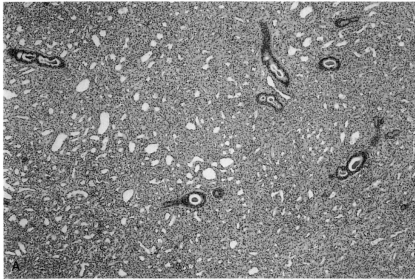

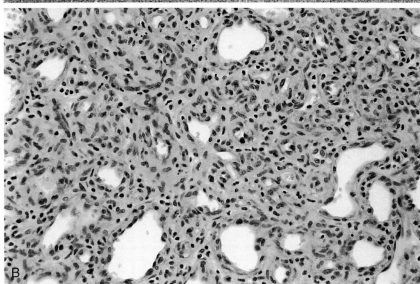

Figure 6–53. *A* and *B,* Infantile hemangioma. The normal parenchyma has been totally replaced by a cellular hemangioma composed of proliferating immature, closely packed capillaries. Scattered residual salivary ducts are still visible *(A)*.

definition: one was an adenoid cystic and mucoepidermoid carcinoma; the second was an epithelial-myoepithelial and salivary duct carcinoma, and the third was a mixture of adenoid cystic and salivary duct carcinoma. All told, more experience is necessary with salivary hybrid tumors before this group can be better characterized.

Treatment and prognosis should be based on the most poorly differentiated (highest grade) component of the hybrid tumor.

Miscellaneous Lesions

Giant Cell Tumor

Extraosseous giant cell tumors composed of osteoclastic-type giant cells have been described in many parts of the body including the soft tissue, pancreas, thyroid gland, liver, breast, ovary, kidney, urinary bladder, lung, colon, heart, and skin, and recently in the salivary gland.[849] Approximately 16 salivary gland tumors with prominent areas of osteoclastic type giant cells have been reported in the literature.[849–855] Three were histologically malignant,[850, 853] at least five were associated with carcinoma ex mixed tumor or an adenocarcinoma,[851, 853] and one was associated with a carcinosarcoma.[852] All but two cases arose in the parotid gland, and these two were in the submandibular gland. Male-to-female ratios are slightly over 3 : 1

and the average age at tumor presentation is 61 years (range, 28–92 years).

The giant cell portion of these tumors is similar to giant cell tumor of bone, consisting of vascular stroma with round to spindled mononuclear cells and scattered multinucleated giant cells containing 5 to 30 nuclei. Generally the giant cells are distributed fairly uniformly throughout the giant cell portion of the tumor but there may be variability from field to field (Fig. 6–54). The mononuclear cells are usually bland but occasionally may exhibit a mild or moderate degree of cytologic atypia. Osteoid, bone and occasionally cartilage may be found.

Due to the rarity of these lesions, the other different tumor components associated with the giant cell tumor, and the short follow-up periods reported, one cannot accurately access the biologic behavior of these neoplasms. Until more information becomes available, treatment and prognosis should be based on degree of atypia, local aggressiveness and other types of coexisting neoplastic proliferation, if present.

Primitive Neuroectodermal Tumor

Primitive neuroectodermal tumor (PNET) is a rare tumor found in children and young adults, commonly in the gluteal region, thighs,

Table 6–9. Salivary Gland Sarcomas*

Tumor Type	Cases (number)		
	Armed Forces Institute of Pathology Registry[838]	*M.D. Anderson Cancer Center Registry[839]*	*University of Hamburg Registry[830]*
Hemangiopericytoma	14	—	—
Malignant schwannoma	13	2	2
Fibrosarcoma	12	2	—
Malignant fibrous histiocytoma	9	3	4
Rhabdomysarcoma	7	2	2
Angiosarcoma	5	—	—
Synovial sarcoma	4	—	—
Kaposi's sarcoma	3	3†	—
Leiomyosarcoma	3	—	—
Liposarcoma	2	—	—
Alveolar soft part sarcoma	2	—	—
Epithelioid sarcoma	1	—	—
Extraosseous chondrosarcoma	1	—	—
Osteosarcoma	—	2	—
Malignant hemangioendothelioma	—	—	1
Sarcoma, poorly differentiated	9	—	—
Total	**85**	**14**	**9**

*Excluding lymphomas.
†Arose in intraparotid lymph nodes.

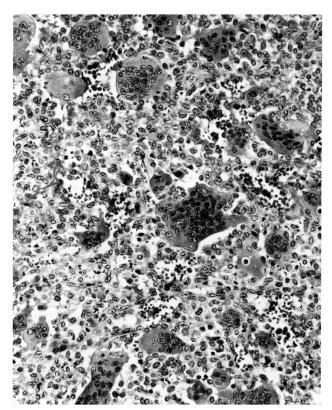

Figure 6–54. Giant cell tumor. There are numerous variably sized multinucleated giant cells in a background of mononuclear cells. (Courtesy of Dr. Gary Ellis, Armed Forces Institute of Pathology.)

shoulder, and arms.[856] In the head and neck area, these tumors have been described in the maxilla, orbit, and soft tissues of the neck.[857] The first two cases of primary parotid primitive neuroectodermal tumor have recently been described in a 45- and 60-year-old male and female, respectively.[857]

Histologically, tumor cells are small and round or oval with minimal cytoplasm and clumped chromatin. Rosettes are frequently found and mitoses vary from moderate to numerous. Differential diagnosis includes small cell carcinoma. Prominent rosette formation and MIC2 positivity support a diagnosis of PNET.

In general, PNETs are highly aggressive tumors requiring a combined treatment approach consisting of surgery, radiation, and chemotherapy. Unfortunately, no follow-up was available on the two parotid cases.

SPECIAL TECHNIQUES: FINE NEEDLE ASPIRATION BIOPSY AND FROZEN SECTION DIAGNOSIS

Fine Needle Aspiration Biopsy

Fine needle aspiration (FNA) is an office procedure that can provide clinicians with rapid, nonsurgical diagnoses. The head and neck is uniquely suited for FNA, as most of the structures are readily palpable and accessible during an office visit. FNA can be performed at the initial consultation, rather than delaying the procedure for ultrasonographically or computed tomographically guided aspiration. Correlation of the clinical impression, cytodiagnosis, and radiographic imaging can then begin to guide the surgeon along treatment pathways. It can be used both as a diagnostic test and as a screening tool to triage patients into different treatment groups, such as surgical vs medical management vs following without intervention.[858] FNA biopsy is useful in establishing whether a given lesion is neoplastic or inflammatory, is a lymphoma or an epithelial malignancy, or represents a metastasis or a primary tumor.[859] Unnecessary surgery can be avoided in approximately one third of cases[860] especially in (1) patients whose salivary gland lesion is part of a more generalized disease process, (2) patients with inflammatory lesions in which a clinical suspicion of malignancy is low, (3) patients in poor health who are not good operative candidates, (4) patients with metastasis to a salivary gland or adjacent lymph node, and (5) patients with some evidence of lymphoproliferative disease.[861]

Every technique, however, has its limitations. Air drying is a common artifact with clinician-prepared slides and results in loss of chromatin detail and decreased readability. It has been shown that the diagnostic yield for FNAs is improved when the cytologist is present to prepare the specimens and assess the specimen for adequacy. For FNA, as well as other areas of pathology, sampling problems, lack of architecture, and specimen adequacy can severely limit the diagnostic yield. A number of series have examined the diagnostic accuracy of salivary FNA,[862–865] with false-positive and false-negative rates ranging from 1% to 14%. The rate of correctly establishing a diagnosis as benign or malignant ranges from 81% to 98% in most recent reports; however, a specific diagnosis can be made only in approximately 60% to 75% of cases.[860]

Certain "diagnostic couples" may be indistinguishable from one another on FNA. For instance, pleomorphic adenoma and adenoid cystic carcinoma are both common to salivary glands. Although chondroid differentiation or squamous differentiation can distinguish pleomorphic adenoma from adenoid cystic carcinoma, there is sufficient histologic overlap (epithelial-myoepithelial ductular components, basement membrane–like hyalinization) that distinction between the two may be impossible on FNA and must await histologic examination. Another diagnostic salivary couple would be low- to intermediate-grade mucoepidermoid carcinoma and a reactive ductular process such as necrotizing sialometaplasia. Large salivary ducts may undergo squamous or goblet cell metaplasia after obstruction or ischemic damage. Cytologically, this process may be indistinguishable from low/intermediate-grade mucoepidermoid carcinoma. Intraparotid lymph node is a common source for parotid FNA; the differential diagnosis between hyperplastic lymph node and lymphoma may also cause difficulties.

We feel that the FNA biopsy is a useful diagnostic test that aids the clinician's decision-making processes and helps to optimize patient care. Best results will be obtained with experienced pathologists reading the cases and when the cytologist or cytotechnician is present to prepare and screen the specimen. Also, correlating FNA results with radiographic and clinical impression usually will assure greater accuracy.

Frozen Section Examination

When considering all head and neck neoplasia, the accuracy of frozen section diagnoses of salivary gland lesions is the most controversial. A review of 2460 frozen sections from 24 series revealed an overall accuracy rate for a benign or malignant diagnosis, excluding deferred diagnoses, of 96.3%.[866–871] The false-positive rate (benign tumors initially diagnosed as malignant) was 1.1%, false-negative rate (malignant tumors initially diagnosed as benign) was 2.6%, and 2% of cases were deferred. If one subdivides the salivary gland lesions into benign and malignant groups, it becomes apparent that the accuracy rate of 98.7%, excluding deferred diagnoses, is excellent for the benign lesions, which constitute 80% of the frozen sections. But in the malignant tumor group, the accuracy rate of 85.9% is suboptimal. The most common benign tumor overdiagnosed as malignant was benign mixed tumor, which was frequently called mucoepidermoid carcinoma or adenoid cystic carcinoma.[866] Oncocytoma, monomorphic adenoma, Warthin's tumor, benign lymphoepithelial lesion, a lymphoepithelial cyst, and a case of sarcoidosis have also caused difficulty.[867–872]

Mucoepidermoid carcinoma is the malignancy most frequently associated with a false-negative benign frozen section diagnosis, whereas acinic cell carcinoma, adenoid cystic carcinoma, malignant mixed tumor, and an occasional lymphoma have also caused difficulty. Many of these false-negative errors have been caused by poor sampling, either by the surgeon or by the pathologist. The variable histologic appearance of many salivary gland tumors is well known, making inadequate sampling a special diagnostic problem. Sections must include the tumor, capsule, and adjacent tissue to evaluate the tumor's local invasiveness and its relationship to the capsule. Sections should never be taken from only the middle of the tumor.

If the tumor appears completely encapsulated and uniform on gross examination, and the initial frozen section contains a benign tumor with a classic histology, then a specific diagnosis can be rendered. If the tumor is multifocal, invasive, or appears necrotic, the

tumor should be carefully sampled with two or more frozen sections before a specific diagnosis is rendered. Multinodularity can be seen in some benign lesions such as recurrent mixed tumors, oncocytoma, the membranous type of basal cell adenoma, and canalicular adenoma.[873, 874] In difficult cases, often the only information the surgeon needs to plan a surgical approach is whether a given tumor is benign or malignant; a more specific histologic diagnosis is not necessary.

We believe, as do others,[875] that it is possible to accurately perform frozen section diagnoses on salivary gland lesions. Several years ago, one of us (DRG) reviewed 301 frozen sections performed by 66 pathologists at four different institutions, including 162 benign tumors, 72 malignant tumors, and 67 benign non-neoplastic lesions.[866] An accuracy rate for all benign and malignant diagnoses of 98%, excluding deferred diagnoses, was reported. The false-positive rate was 0.7% and the false-negative rate was 1.3%. This compares favorably with accuracy rates for published series of frozen section diagnoses from other regions of the body.[872] The accuracy rate for the malignant group was just under 95%, a value that is slightly less than that expected for frozen sections from other areas of the body.[872] These results are nevertheless within an acceptable range of accuracy. From the preceding, one can conclude that it is possible to accurately diagnose salivary gland neoplasms at frozen section. However, the literature does indicate that caution should be exercised when dealing with malignant tumors. Therefore, it is important to remember that a therapeutic decision should never be made on the basis of a frozen section diagnosis alone, but always in conjunction with the clinical findings.

TUMORS OF THE LACRIMAL GLAND AND SAC

The lacrimal gland develops from invaginations of epithelial buds of the basal conjunctiva and is not fully developed until the third or fourth year of life.[876] The gland is not truly encapsulated and is composed of mixed serous and mucinous acini. It is divided into two lobes by a portion of the levator palpebrae muscle aponeurosis, forming the orbital and palpebral lobes. Although the superficial palpebral lobe is one third to one half the size of the deeper orbital lobe, a disproportionately higher number of lacrimal gland neoplasms arise in the orbital lobe.[877] Accessory lacrimal glands are often found in the substantia propria of the conjunctiva[876] and ectopic lacrimal gland tissue (choristoma) has been reported in the cornea, intraorbital tissues, and lower eye lid; one case was intraocular.[878]

The lacrimal drainage system transports tears to the nasal cavity; it is composed of the puncta, the lacrimal canaliculi, the lacrimal sac, and the nasolacrimal duct. The canaliculi are tubular structures lined by nonkeratinizing squamous epithelium, whereas the sac is lined by a stratified columnar epithelium that may be ciliated and contains scattered goblet cells. The nasolacrimal duct is lined by ciliated respiratory epithelium containing goblet cells.[876, 879] Mixed serous and mucinous glands are frequently found in the soft tissue just underneath or deep to lacrimal sac epithelium, and serous glands with rare mucinous cells may be seen beneath the nasolacrimal duct.[880]

Clinical Features. Lacrimal gland lesions account for 5.5% of patients who present to their physician with an orbital problem,[881] while in two large series (Table 6–10), tumors of the lacrimal gland and sac account for 1.4% of biopsied masses arising in the eye and ocular adnexa, including the eyelid and conjunctiva.[876] Lacrimal gland tumors are approximately twice as frequent as those arising in the lacrimal sac. The histologic classification of five recent series of lacrimal gland tumors is summarized in Table 6–11. Tumors of the lacrimal glands are similar to those arising in the salivary glands except for Warthin's tumor, which is common in the major salivary glands but is virtually never found in the lacrimal glands, with only one well-documented case reported to date.[882] Lacrimal tumors arise

Table 6–10. Tumors of the Eye and Ocular Adnexa

Location of Tumor	Cases (number)	
	Armed Forces Institute of Ophthalmic Pathology Registry	Brazilian Registry of Ophthalmic Pathology
Eyelid	846	869
Conjunctiva	1258	476
Retina	268	150
Uvea	760	148
Lacrimal gland	53	18
Lacrimal sac	33	9
Orbit	396	182
Optic nerve	34	17
Total	3648	1869

Modified from McLean IW, Burnier MN, Zimmerman LE, Jakobiec FA: Atlas of Tumor Pathology: Tumors of the Eye and Ocular Adnexa, 3rd series, fascicle 12. Washington, DC: Armed Forces Institute of Pathology, 1994:214–232.

in all age ranges with the average age at presentation varying dependent on tumor type.[883] Patients with adenoid cystic carcinoma (AdCC) (average age of 39.4 years) and benign mixed tumor (average age of 40.8 years) tended to be younger than those with malignant mixed tumors (average age of 53 years)[883] and adenocarcinoma (mean age of 60 years).[884] These differences in age of presentation are supported in other series.[885] Patients with inflammatory pseudotumors frequently present with orbital pain accompanied by swelling, redness, ptosis, proptosis, and mobility restriction.[886] Patients with lacrimal gland carcinomas more frequently present with pain than do patients with adenomas (15% vs 72%).[887]

Lacrimal sac tumors are usually primary and of epithelial origin; metastatic tumors confined to the sac are exceedingly rare, with metastases usually involving adjacent structures (eyelid, orbit, paranasal sinuses, or nose).[876] Lacrimal sac masses involve patients of all ages. However, average age of onset varies with histologic type: carcinomas are found in older patients, with a mean of 58 years of age (range, 16–89), whereas benign papillomas are seen in younger patients, with a mean of 44 years and a range of 9 to 88 years.[879] The most frequent presenting signs and symptoms are epiphora (53%), recurrent dacryocystitis (38%) and/or a lacrimal sac mass (36%).[879] Due to their slow growth, papillomas often masquerade as a chronic dacryocystitis; the combination of pain and hemorrhage is frequently associated with a lacrimal sac malignancy.

Pathologic Features. Fifty-five percent of lacrimal gland tumors have an inflammatory origin, 28% are epithelial neoplasms, 14% are reactive or malignant lymphoproliferative processes, and approximately 2% to 3% are soft tissue tumors or cysts.[884, 888, 889] Epithelial neoplasms cover the full range of pathology found in the major salivary glands (see Table 6–11).[876, 881, 883–885, 888–901] The ratio of benign to malignant epithelial tumors is 1:1, but there is considerable variation from series to series, most likely due to referral patterns.[876, 881, 883, 884, 888, 889] The most common epithelial tumors are benign mixed tumors (52% of all epithelial tumors), adenoid cystic carcinomas (25% of all epithelial tumors), and carcinoma ex mixed tumors (9% of all epithelial tumors) (see Table 6–11). Mucoepidermoid carcinoma, acinic cell carcinoma, and epithelial-myoepithelial carcinoma do occur in the lacrimal gland,[897, 900, 901] but with a much lower frequency than is seen in major or minor salivary gland sites. Only six cases of mucoepidermoid carcinoma and no cases of acinic cell carcinoma were observed in seven recent series that included 478 epithelial lacrimal gland tumors.[876, 881, 883–885, 888, 889] Only one example of an epithelial-myoepithelial carcinoma has been reported to date, and this was as the malignant component of a carcinoma ex mixed tumor.[901] Metastases to the lacrimal glands are also extremely infrequent, with only three occurrences reported in these same series.

When they do occur, the most likely primary sites are breast and lung.[884]

Overall, 55% of lacrimal sac tumors are malignant, with 62% to 94% in various series (mean 73%) being epithelial in origin, excluding reactive inflammatory processes (inflammatory pseudotumors) (Table 6–12).[879] Thirty-eight percent to 87% (mean, 53%) of the epithelial tumors are carcinomas, representing, in decreasing order of frequency, squamous cell carcinoma, transitional cell carcinoma (nonkeratinizing squamous carcinoma), adenoid cystic and mucoepidermoid carcinoma, adenocarcinoma and oncocytic carcinoma, and poorly differentiated carcinoma (Table 6–13).[879] Rarely, other types of carcinoma have been reported; Karim et al.[902] have described an eccrine adenocarcinoma.

Twenty-five percent to 28% of lacrimal sac tumors are papillomas, including exophytic, inverting, and mixed types, and the remaining epithelial tumors are adenomas, most of which have an oncocytic phenotype with occasional mixed tumors (see Table 6–13).[876, 879, 903] The papillomas may be covered with squamous cells, stratified columnar epithelium with goblet cells, or a mixture of these cell types. The remaining 6% to 28% of the lacrimal sac tumors in various series[879] are nonepithelial and most frequently mesenchymal in origin, with benign fibrous histiocytoma being the most common,[903] followed in frequency by lymphoproliferative lesions (either benign reactive lesions or lymphoma) and melanoma (see Table 6–12). Rarely, acquired melanosis of the conjunctiva may spread into the lacrimal sac.[904] Dermoid and epidermoid cysts may occur[905] and occasional mucoceles have been described.[906]

Treatment and Prognosis. The treatment for lacrimal gland tumors varies with the diagnosis and clinical extent of disease. Tumors found by radiologic and clinical examination to be inflammatory or to have a lymphoid pattern should be treated with antibiotics and steroids after a careful search to rule out granulomatous disease or sarcoidosis if they are of recent onset and have inflammatory symptoms.[889] These inflammatory pseudotumors, including the sclerosing variant, may also be treated with limited surgical excision or debulking with excellent results.[886] Long-standing, painless lesions present for greater than 10 months should undergo an FNA biopsy and, if insufficient for diagnosis, an open biopsy to rule out lymphoma. Lesions with an epithelial appearance on radiographic studies (round or globular with smooth edges or infiltration) should undergo dacryoadenectomy with complete removal of the tumor. This should be done without a previous biopsy, as the risk of recurrence for benign mixed tumor is significantly greater with a presurgical biopsy, 0% to 3% vs 32% at 5 years. However, recurrences can usually be minimized after preoperative biopsy by performing a lateral orbitotomy, total dacryoadenectomy, and removal of the biopsy tract.[887]

Malignant tumors with positive margins can be managed by reexcision, preferably by macroscopic removal of tumor or by orbital exenteration followed by radiotherapy.[889] The extent of surgery is somewhat controversial, with differing opinions for the more invasive lesions, as one recent series failed to demonstrate improved survival with extensive versus more limited local excision.[889] Therefore, one should thoroughly discuss all surgical options, as well as potential benefits and risks, with the patient before committing to a management plan. In addition, a recent report has indicated a favorable response for two patients with advanced AdCC treated with preoperative neoadjuvant intracarotid chemotherapy using cisplatin and intravenous doxorubicin hydrochloride, combined with postoperative radiation augmented by intravenous cisplatin and doxorubicin.[899] Others also feel that intra-arterial chemotherapy is a rational treatment choice for AdCC.[898]

Malignant lacrimal gland tumors have recurrence rates of 52% to 63% and a metastatic rate of 26% to 50%.[884, 885] Adenoid cystic carcinomas have the highest recurrence rates; in one series all 12 patients developed recurrences.[884] Prominent basaloid differentiation (solid growth pattern) in an AdCC is associated with a reduction in disease-free survival (10% at 4 years with a basaloid pattern vs approximately 72% without this pattern) and higher recurrence rates

Table 6–11. Lacrimal Gland Tumors

Type	Cases (number)					
	Cullen Eye Institute[884]	Wills Eye Hospital[888]	Shanghai Medical University[883]*	Armed Forces Institute of Pathology[876]	R.E. Kennedy[881]	Total Number (and %) of Epithelial Tumors
Inflammatory						
Chronic dacryoadenitis	43	71			12	
Reactive lymphoid hyperplasia	13					
Sarcoidosis/ granulomatous	13	18				
Lipogranuloma	2					
Dacryops	4	8				
Acute		1				
Epithelial Tumors						392
Benign mixed tumor	17	17	140	19	12	205 (52)
Adenoid cystic carcinoma	12	2	68	13	3	98 (25)
Adenocarcinoma	2	3	3	2	2	12 (3)
Carcinoma ex mixed tumor	6		25	5		36 (9)
Metastatic carcinoma	3					3 (0.8)
Mucoepidermoid carcinoma		2	2			4 (1)
Undifferentiated carcinoma			20			20 (5)
Polymorphous low-grade adenocarcinoma			3			3 (0.8)
Malignant lymphoepithelial lesion			3			3 (0.8)
Spindle cell carcinoma			1			1
Papillary adenocarcinoma			2			2
Sebaceous carcinoma			2			2
Myoepithelioma			2			2
Carcinosarcoma	1		1			
Lymphoid						
Malignant lymphoma	4	6		5		
Benign lymphoid hyperplasia		12		7	12	
Atypical lymphoid hyperplasia		1				
Benign lympho-epithelial lesion				1		
Plasmacytoma				1		
Nonepithelial Tumors						
Lipoma		1				
Cysts					4	
Total	120	142	272	53	45	

*Epithelial tumors only.

Table 6–12. Lacrimal Sac Tumors

Type	Cases (number)
Epithelial	271
Benign	74
Malignant	197
Mesenchymal	53
Benign	22
Malignant	31
Lymphoid/reticulosis	28
Melanoma	15
Neural	3
Pseudotumor inflammation	54
Total	**424**

*Data from Stefanyszyn MA, Hidayat AA, Pe'er JJ, Flanagan JC: Lacrimal sac tumors. Ophthal Plast Reconstr Surg 1994;10:169–184.

(69% with a predominant basaloid pattern [>50% of the tumor] vs 26% without this pattern).[885] Similarly, in an earlier study, Gamel and Font[895] found median survival times and 5-year survival rates with and without the basaloid pattern of 3 and 8 years and 21% and 71%, respectively.

Lacrimal gland AdCC may rarely arise in children and teenagers and appears to have a better prognosis than similar tumors arising in the adult population. Tellado et al.[891] reported 11 tumors in children and found median survival times in children to be more than twice the survival times associated with AdCC in patients of all ages (5 years in the general population vs greater than 10 years in children). Children also had much better 15-year survival rates than the general population (58% vs 12%) and appeared to have lower grade tumors, with only two tumors having greater than 25% of a basaloid cell (solid) population, which may account, in part, for their better prognosis.

The treatment of epithelial lacrimal sac tumors is complete surgical removal with wide excision for malignant tumors; radiation therapy should also be added for most malignant epithelial lesions, with the possible exception of low-grade mucoepidermoid carcinoma.[879, 905, 907] Extension of tumor down the nasolacrimal duct has caused a significant number of recurrences and therapeutic failures. Therefore, a lateral rhinostomy should be performed in all premalig-

Table 6–13. Lacrimal Sac Epithelial Tumors

Type	Cases (number)
Benign Tumors	
Papilloma	32
Squamous	19
Transitional	13
Oncocytoma	4
Benign mixed tumor	2
Total benign	**38**
Malignant Tumors	
Papilloma with carcinoma	6
Carcinoma	38
Squamous cell carcinoma	22
Transitional cell carcinoma	5
Mucoepidermoid carcinoma	3
Adenoid cystic carcinoma	3
Adenocarcinoma	2
Oncocytic adenocarcinoma	2
Poorly differentiated carcinoma	1
Total malignant	**44**

nant and malignant epithelial lesions with a tendency for intraepithelial or intraductal spread.[879] However, in cases of lymphoma, radiation therapy with the possible addition of chemotherapy is the preferred mode of therapy.[908] Inverting papillomas may be locally invasive and, if not completely excised, may recur. Carcinomas recur in up to 40% of patients and frequently invade surrounding structures[876]; they also metastasize to regional lymph nodes in approximately 27% of patients and may spread to distant sites (9.1% of patients).[896] Patients treated with wide excision and lateral rhinotomy have a recurrence rate of 12.5%, whereas patients treated only with lacrimal sac excision have a recurrence rate of 43.7%.[905] Mortality rates are a function of the tumor stage and type, with rates averaging 37.5%.

Papillary squamous tumors have the best prognosis, with a mortality of 13.6%; squamous cell carcinoma has a mortality rate of 50%; adenocarcinoma has a 66.6% mortality rate; and transitional cell carcinoma has a 100% mortality rate.[905] In the nonepithelial group, fibrous histiocytoma has a good prognosis with complete excision, the prognosis of lymphoma depends on classification and stage, and malignant melanoma has a dismal prognosis, even with aggressive therapy.[882]

REFERENCES

Embryology

1. Banerjee SD, Cohn RH, Bernfield MR: Basal lamina of embryonic salivary epithelia: Production by the epithelium and role in maintaining lobular morphology. J Cell Biol 1977;73:445–463.
2. Sanders EJ: The roles of epithelial-mesenchymal cell interactions in developmental processes. Biochem Cell Biol 1988;66:530–540.
3. Seifert G, Miehlke A, Haubrich J, Chilla R: Diseases of the Salivary Glands: Pathology, Diagnosis, Treatment, Facial Nerve Surgery. Stuttgart, Georg Thieme Verlag, 1986:24–26.
4. Martinez-Madrigal F, Micheau C: Histology of the major salivary glands. Am J Surg Pathol 1989;13:879–899.
5. Silvers AR, Som PM: Salivary glands. In: Yousem DM (ed): Head and neck imaging. Radiol Clin North Am 1998;36:941–966.

Anatomy

6. Martinez-Madrigal F, Bosq J, Casiraghi O: Major salivary glands. In: Sternberg SS (ed): Histology for Pathologists, 2nd ed. Philadelphia: Lippincott-Raven, 1997:405–429.
7. Ellis GL, Auclair PL: The normal salivary gland. In: Ellis GL, Auclair PL, Gnepp DR (eds): Surgical Pathology of the Salivary Glands. Philadelphia: WB Saunders, 1991:1–26.
8. Dardick I: Histogenesis and morphogenesis of salivary gland tumors. In: Ellis GL, Auclair PL, Gnepp DR (eds): Surgical Pathology of the Salivary Glands. Philadelphia: WB Saunders, 1991:108–128.
9. Silver AR, Som PM: Salivary glands. Radiol Clin North Am 1998;36:941–966.
10. Gnepp DR: Sebaceous neoplasms of salivary gland origin: A review. Pathol Annu 1983;18 (part 1):71–102.
11. Takeda Y: Melanocytes in the human parotid gland. Pathol Internat 1997;47:581–583.
12. Feind CR: The head and neck. In: Haagensen CD, Feind CR, Herter FP, Slanetz CA Jr, Weinberg FA (eds): The Lymphatics in Cancer. Philadelphia: WB Saunders, 1972:63–66.
13. Gnepp DR: Metastatic disease to the major salivary glands. In: Ellis GL, Auclair PL, Gnepp DR (eds): Surgical Pathology of the Salivary Glands. Philadelphia: WB Saunders, 1991:560–69.
14. Toh H, Kodama J, Fujuda J, et al: Incidence and histology of human accessory parotid glands. Anat Rec 1993;236:589–590.
14a. Takeda Y: Existence and distribution of melanocytes and HMB-45–positive cells in the human minor salivary glands. Pathol Int 2000;50:15–19.

Developmental Disorders

15. Myers MA, Youngberg RA, Bauman JM: Congenital absence of the major salivary glands and impaired lacrimal secretion in a child: Case report. J Am Dent Assoc 1994;125:210–212.

16. Wiedemann H: Salivary gland disorders and heredity. Am J Med Genet 1997;68:222–224.
17. Codjambopoulo VP, Ender-Griepekoven I, Broy H: Bilaterale Doppelanlage der Glandula submandibularis und des Submandibularisganges. Fortschr Rontgenstr 1992;157:185–186.
18. Pownell PH, Brown OE, Pransky SM, Manning SC: Congenital abnormalities of the submandibular duct. Int J Pediatr Otorhinolaryngol 1992;24:161–169.
19. Hoggins GS, Hutton JB: Congenital sublingual cystic swellings due to imperforate salivary ducts. Two case reports. Oral Surg Oral Med Oral Pathol 1974;37:370–373.
20. Shiang EL, Holmes L: The lacrimo-auriculo-dento-digital syndrome. Pediatr 1977;59:927–930.
21. Harada H, Morimatsu M, Kusukawa J, Kameyama T: A hamartoma-like mass on the palate? A possible discussion regarding the components of a pigmented naevus and hyperplastic salivary gland. J Laryngol Otol 1997;111:296–299.
22. Tang TT, Glicklich M, Siegesmund KA, et al: Neonatal cystic choristoma in submandibular salivary gland simulating cystic hygroma. Arch Pathol Lab Med 1979;103:536–539.
23. Dehner LP, Valbuena L, Perez-Atayde A, et al: Salivary gland anlage tumor ("congenital pleomorphic adenoma"). A clinicopathologic, immunohistochemical and ultrastructural study of nine cases. Am J Surg Pathol 1994;18:25–36.
24. Lassaletta-Atienza L, Lopez-Rios F, Martin G, et al: Salivary gland heterotopia in the lower neck: A report of five cases. Int J Pediatr Otorhinolaryngol 1998;43:153–161.
25. Hinni ML, Beatty CW: Salivary gland choristoma of the middle ear: Report of a case and review of the literature. Ear Nose Throat J 1996;75:422–424.
26. Saeger KL, Gruskin P, Carberry JN: Salivary gland choristoma of the middle ear. Arch Pathol Lab Med 1982;106:39–40.
27. Perry BP, Scher RL, Gray L, et al: Pathologic quiz case 1: Salivary gland choristoma of the middle ear. Arch Otolaryngol Head Neck Surg 1998;124:714, 716.
28. Warnock GR, Jensen JL, Kratochvil JL: Developmental diseases. In: Ellis GL, Auclair PL, Gnepp DR (eds): Surgical Pathology of the Salivary Glands. Philadelphia: WB Saunders, 1991:10–25.
29. Marshall JN, Soo G, Coakley FV: Ectopic salivary gland in the posterior triangle of the neck. J Laryngol Otol 1995;109:669–670.
30. Afanas'ev VV, Starodubtsev VS: Salivary gland heterotopia in the bone tissue of the mandible. Stomatologiia (Mosk) 1995;74:69–70.
31. Bouquot JE, Gnepp DR, Dardick I, Hietanen JHP: Intraosseous salivary tissue: Jawbone examples of choristomas, hamartomas, embryonic rests and inflammatory entrapment. Another histogenetic source for intraosseous adenocarcinoma. Oral Surg Oral Med Oral Pathol Oral Radiol Endod 2000; in press.
32. Moskow BS, Baden E: Gingival salivary gland choristoma. Report of a case. J Clin Periodontol 1986;13:720–724.
33. Ledesma-Montes C, Fernandez-Lopez R, Garces-Ortiz M, et al: Gingival salivary gland choristoma. A case report. J Periodontol 1998;69:1164–1166
34. Tatter SB, Edgar MA, Klibanski A, Swearingen B: Symptomatic salivary-rest cyst of the sella turcica. Acta Neurochir 1995;135:150–153.
35. Cameselle-Teijeiro J, Varela-Duran J: Intrathyroid salivary gland–type tissue in multinodular goiter. Virchows Arch 1994;425:331–334.
36. Feigin GA, Robinson B, Marchevsky A: Mixed tumor of the mediastinum. Arch Pathol Lab Med 1986;110:80–81.
37. Weitzner S: Ectopic salivary gland tissue in submucosa of rectum. Dis Colon Rectum 1983;26:814–817.
38. Marwah S, Berman ML: Ectopic salivary gland in the vulva (choristoma): Report of a case and review of the literature. Obstet Gynecol 1980;56:389–391.
39. Dikman SH, Toker C: Seromucinous gland ectopia within the prostate stroma. J Urol 1973;109:852–854.
40. Sevila A, Morell A, Navas J, et al: Orifices at the lower neck: Heterotopic salivary glands. Dermatol 1997;194:360–361.
41. Goodman RS, Daly JF, Valensi Q: Heterotopic salivary tissue and branchial cleft sinus. Laryngoscope 1981;91:260–264.
42. Stingle WH, Priebe CJ Jr: Ectopic salivary gland and sinus in the lower neck. Ann Otol Rhinol Laryngol 1974;83:379–381.
43. Joseph MP, Goodman ML, Pilch BZ, et al: Heterotopic cervical salivary gland tissue in a family with probable branchio-otorenal syndrome. Head Neck Surg 1986;8:456–462..
44. Shinohara M, Ikebe T, Nakamura S, et al: Multiple pleomorphic adenomas arising in the parotid and submandibular lymph nodes. Br J Oral Maxillofac Surg 1996;34:515–519.
45. Surana R, Moloney R, Fitzgerald RJ: Tumours of heterotopic salivary tissue in the upper cervical region in children. Surg Oncol 1993;2:133–136.
46. Mair IW, Elverland HH, Knudsen OS: Heterotopic salivary pleomorphic adenoma. J Otolaryngol 1978;7:158–60.
47. Pesavento G, Ferlito A: Benign mixed tumour of heterotopic salivary gland tissue in upper neck. Report of a case with a review of the literature on heterotopic salivary gland tissue. J Laryngol Otol 1976;90:577–584.
48. Brandwein MS, Huvos AG: Oncocytic tumors of major salivary glands. A study of 68 cases with follow-up of 44 patients. Am J Surg Pathol 1991;15:514–528.
49. Bondi R, Nardi P, Urso C: Endomandibular acinic cell carcinoma. Appl Pathol 1989;7:260–264.
50. Perzin KH, Livolsi VA: Acinic cell carcinoma arising in ectopic salivary gland tissue. Cancer 1980;45:967–972.
51. Magliulo G, Vingolo GM, Cristofari P, Natale AS: Primary adenoid cystic carcinoma of the middle ear and mastoid. Acta Otorhinolaryngol Belg 1993;47:39–42.
52. Cawson RA, Gleeson MJ, Eveson JW: The pathology and surgery of the salivary glands. Oxford: ISIS Medical Media, 1997:22–32.
53. Seifert G, Thomsen ST, Donath K: Bilateral dysgenetic polycystic parotid glands: Morphological analysis and differential diagnosis of a rare disease of salivary glands. Virchows Arch A Pathol Anat Histopathol 1981;390:273–288.
54. Seifert G: Mucoepidermoid carcinoma in a salivary duct cyst of the parotid gland. Contribution to the development of tumours in salivary gland cysts. Pathol Res Pract 1996;192:1211–1217.
55. Garcia S, Martini F, Caces F, et al: Maladie polykystique des glandes salivaires: Description d'une atteinte des glandes sous-maxillaires. Ann Pathol 1998;18:58–60.
56. Batsakis JG, Bruner JM, Luna MA: Polycystic (dysgenetic) disease of the parotid glands. Arch Otolaryngol Head Neck Surg 1988;114:1146–1148.
57. Dobson CM, Ellis HA: Polycystic disease of the parotid glands: Case report of a rare entity and review of the literature. Histopathol 1987;11:953–961.
58. Ficarra G, Sapp JP, Christensen RE, et al: Dysgenetic polycystic disease of the parotid gland: Report of a case. J Oral Maxillofac Surg 1996;54:1246–1249.
59. Seifert G, Miehlke A, Haubrich J, Chilla R: Diseases of the Salivary Glands: Pathology, Diagnosis, Treatment, Facial Nerve Surgery. Stuttgart: Georg Thieme Verlag, 1986:63–70.
60. Giansanti JS, Baker GO, Waldron CA: Intraoral, mucinous, minor salivary gland lesions presenting clinically as tumors. Oral Surg Oral Med Oral Pathol 1971;32:918–922.
61. Barrett AW, Speight PM: Adenomatoid hyperplasia of oral minor salivary glands. Oral Surg Oral Med Oral Pathol Oral Radiol Endod 1995;79:482–487.
62. Ellis AL, Auclair PL: Atlas of Tumor Pathology: Tumors of the Salivary Glands. Washington DC: Armed Forces Institute of Pathology, 1996:437–438.
63. Buchner A, Merrell PW, Carpenter WM, Leider AS: Adenomatoid hyperplasia of minor salivary glands. Oral Surg Oral Med Oral Pathol 1991;71:583–587.
64. Arafat A, Brannon RB, Ellis GL: Adenomatoid hyperplasia of mucous salivary glands. Oral Surg Oral Med Oral Pathol 1981;52:51–55.
65. Aufdemorte TB, Ramzy I, Holt GR, et al: Focal adenomatoid hyperplasia of salivary glands. A differential diagnostic problem in fine needle aspiration biopsy. Acta Cytologica 1985;29:23–28.

Infectious Sialadenitis

66. Wells DH: Suppuration of the submandibular salivary glands in the neonate. Am J Dis Child 1975;129:628–630.
67. Ungkanont K, Kolatat T, Tantinikorn W: Neonatal suppurative submandibular sialadenitis: A rare clinical entity. Int J Pediatr Otorhinolaryngol 1998;43:141–145.
68. Chitre VV, Premchandra DJ: Recurrent parotitis. Arch Dis Childhood 1997;77:359–363.
69. Giglio MS, Landaeta M, Pinto ME: Microbiology of recurrent parotitis. Pediatr Infect Dis J 1997;16:386–390.
70. Seifert G, Miehlke A, Haubrich J, Chilla R: Diseases of the Salivary

Glands: Pathology, Diagnosis, Treatment, Facial Nerve Surgery. Stuttgart: Georg Thieme Verlag, 1986:110–163.

71. Rieu PN, van den Broek P, Pruszczynski M, et al: Atypical mycobacterial infection of the parotid gland. J Pediatr Surg 1990;25:483–486.

72. Rowe-Jones JM, Vowles R, Leighton SE, Freedman AR: Diffuse tuberculous parotitis. J Laryngol Otol 1992;106:1094–1095.

73. Werning J: Infections and systemic diseases. In: Ellis GL, Auclair PL, Gnepp DR (eds): Surgical Pathology of the Salivary Glands. Philadelphia: WB Saunders, 1991:39–59.

74. O'Connell JE, George MK, Speculand B, Pahor AL: Mycobacterial infection of the parotid gland: An unusual cause of parotid swelling. J Laryngol Otol 1993;107:561–564.

75. Guneri EA, Ikiz AO, Atabey N, et al: Polymerase chain reaction in the diagnosis of parotid gland tuberculosis. J Laryngol Otol 1998;112:494–496.

76. Brill SJ, Gilfillan RF: Acute parotitis associated with influenza type A: A report of twelve cases. N Engl J Med 1977;296:1391–1392.

77. Gelfand MS, Cleveland KO, Lancaster D, et al: Adenovirus parotitis in patients with AIDS. Clin Infect Dis 1994;19:1045–1048.

78. Wagner RP, Tian H, McPherson MJ, et al: AIDS-associated infections in salivary glands: Autopsy survey of 60 cases. Clin Infect Dis 1996;22:369–371.

79. Raab SS, Thomas PA, Cohen MB: Fine-needle aspiration biopsy of salivary gland mycoses. Diagn Cytopathol 1994;11:286–290.

80. Scott GB, Buck BE, Leterman JG, et al: Acquired immunodeficiency syndrome in infants. N Engl J Med 1984;310:76–81.

Chronic Sialadenitis, Sjögren's Syndrome, and Myoepithelial Sialadenitis

81. Bates D, O'Brien CJ, Tikaram K, Painter DM: Parotid and submandibular sialadenitis treated by salivary gland excision. Aust N Z J Surg 1998;68:120–124.

82. Alexander C, Bader JB, Schaefer A, et al: Intermediate and long-term side effects of high-dose radioiodine therapy for thyroid carcinoma. J Nucl Med 1998;39:1551–1554.

83. Seifert G, Miehlke A, Haubrich J, Chilla R: Sialadenitis. In: Diseases of the Salivary Glands: Pathology, Diagnosis, Treatment, Facial Nerve Surgery. Stuttgart: Georg Thieme Verlag, 1986:110–163.

84. Wiedemann HR: Salivary gland disorders and heredity. Am J Med Genet 1997;68:222–224.

85. Ericson S, Zetterlund B, Ohman J: Recurrent parotitis and sialectasis in childhood: Clinical, radiologic, immunologic, bacteriologic, and histologic study. Ann Otol Rhinol Laryngol 1991;100:527–535.

86. Van der Walt JD, Leake J: Granulomatous sialadenitis of the minor salivary glands. A clinicopathological study of 57 cases. Histopathol 1987;11:131–144.

87. Kavanaug AF, Huston DP: Wegener's granulomatosis presenting with unilateral parotid enlargement. Am J Med 1988;85:741–742.

88. Giglio MS, Landaeta M, Pinto ME: Microbiology of recurrent parotitis. Pediatr Infect Dis J 1997;16:386–390.

89. Eversole LR, Sabes WR: Minor salivary gland duct changes due to obstruction. Arch Otolaryngol 1971;94:19–24.

90. Harrison JD, Epivatianos A, Bhatia SN: Role of microliths in the etiology of chronic submandibular sialadenitis: A clinicopathological investigation of 154 cases. Histopathol 1997;31:237–251.

91. Rasanen O, Jokinen K, Dammert K: Sclerosing inflammation of the submandibular salivary gland (Küttner tumour). Acta Otolaryngol 1972;74:297–301.

92. Fajardo FE, Berthrong M: Radiation injury in surgical pathology. Part III. Salivary glands, pancreas and skin. Am J Surg Pathol 1981;5:279–296.

93. Harrington AC, Stasko T: Radiation-induced adiposis of the parotid. J Dermatol Surg Oncol 1994;20:246–250.

94. Devaney KO, Travis WD, Hoffman G, et al: Interpretation of head and neck biopsies in Wegener's granulomatosis. A pathologic study of 126 biopsies in 70 patients. Am J Surg Pathol 1990;14:555–564.

95. Cawson RA, Gleeson MJ, Everson JW: Sialadenitis. In: Pathology and Surgery of the Salivary Glands. Oxford: ISIS Medical Media, 1997: 33–63.

96. Daniels TE: Benign lymphoepithelial lesions and Sjogren's syndrome. In: Ellis GL, Auclair PL, Gnepp DR (eds): Surgical Pathology of the Salivary Glands. Philadelphia: WB Saunders, 1991:83–106.

97. Ostberg Y: The clinical picture of benign lympho-epithelial lesion. Clin Otolaryngol Allied Sciences 1983;8:381–390.

98. Fox RI, Tornwall J, Maruyama T, Stern M: Evolving concepts of diagnosis, pathogenesis, and therapy of Sjögren's syndrome. Curr Opin Rheumatol 1998;10:446–456.

99. Moutsopoules HM, Mann DL, Johnson AH, et al: Genetic differences between primary and secondary sicca syndrome. N Engl J Med 1979;301:761–763.

100. Bloch KJ, Buchanan WW, Whol MJ, et al: Sjögren's syndrome: A clinical, pathological, and serological study of sixty-two cases. Med 1992;71:386–401.

101. Chudwin DS, Daniels TE, Wara DW, et al: Spectrum of Sjögren syndrome in children. J Pediatr 1981;98:213–217.

102. Anavi Y, Mintz S: Benign lymphoepithelial lesion of the sublingual gland. J Oral Maxillofac Surg 1992;50:1111–1113.

103. Whitcher JP: Clinical diagnosis of the dry eye. Int Ophthalmol Clin 1987;27:7–24.

104. Daniels TE, Silverman S, Michalski JP, et al: The oral component of Sjögren's syndrome. Oral Surg Oral Med Oral Pathol 1975;39:875–885.

104a. Ahmad I, Ray J, Cullen RJ, Shortridge RT: Bilateral and multicystic major salivary gland disease: A rare presentation of primary Sjögren's syndrome. J Laryngol Otol 1998;112:1196–1198.

105. Som PM, Shugar JM, Train JS, et al: Manifestations of parotid gland enlargement: Radiographic, pathologic, and clinical correlations. Part I. The autoimmune pseudosialectasis. Radiol 1981;141:415–419.

106. Dardick I, van Nostrand AW, Rippstein P, et al: Characterization of epimyoepithelial islands in benign lymphoepithelial lesions of major salivary gland: An immunohistochemical and ultrastructural study. Head Neck Surg 1988;10:168–178.

107. Chisholm DM, Waterhouse JP, Mason DK: Lymphocytic sialadenitis in the major and minor glands: A correlation in postmortem subjects. J Clin Pathol 1970;23:690–694.

108. Chisholm DM, Mason DK: Labial salivary gland biopsy in Sjögren's syndrome. J Clin Pathol 1968;21:656–660.

109. Ellis GL, Auclair PL: Tumor-Like Conditions. In: Tumors of the Salivary Glands, 3rd series. Washington, DC: Armed Forces Institute of Pathology, 1996:411–413.

110. Batsakis JG: Lymphoepithelial lesion and Sjögren's syndrome. Ann Otol Rhinol Laryngol 1987;96:354–355.

111. Ide F, Shimoyama T, Horie N, et al: Benign lymphoepithelial lesion of the parotid gland with sebaceous differentiation. Oral Surg Oral Med Oral Pathol Oral Radiol Endod 1999;87:721–724.

112. Kassan SS, Thomas TL, Moutsopoudos HM, et al: Increased risk of lymphoma in sicca syndrome. Ann Intern Med 1978;89:888–892.

113. Sciubba JJ, Auclair PL, Ellis GL: Malignant lymphoma. In: Ellis GL, Auclair PL, Gnepp DR (eds): Surgical Pathology of the Salivary Glands. Philadelphia: WB Saunders, 1991:528–543.

114. Shin SS, Sheibani K, Fishleder A, et al: Monocytoid B-cell lymphoma in patients with Sjögren's syndrome: A clinicopathologic study of 13 patients. Hum Pathol 1991;22:422–430.

Sialolithiasis

115. Rauch S, Gorlin RJ: Diseases of the salivary glands. In: Gorlin RJ, Goldman HM (eds): Oral Pathology. St Louis, Mosby, p 962, 1970.

116. Shafer WG, Hine MK, Levy BM: A Textbook of Oral Pathology, 4th ed. Philadelphia: WB Saunders, 1983:557.

117. Iro H, Zenk J, Benzel W: Minimally invasive therapy for sialolithiasis—the state of the art. Otolaryngol Head Neck 1995;9:3–48.

118. Epker BN: Obstructive and inflammatory diseases of the major salivary glands. Oral Surg Oral Med Oral Pathol 1972;33:2–27.

119. Seifert G, Miehlke A, Haubrich J, Chilla R: Diseases of the Salivary Glands: Pathology, Diagnosis, Treatment, Facial Nerve Surgery. Stuttgart: Georg Thieme Verlag, 1986:110.

120. Raymond AK, Batsakis JG: Pathology consultation: Angiolithiasis and sialolithiasis in the head and neck. Ann Otol Rhinol Laryngol 1992;101:455–457.

121. Jensen JL, Howell FV, Rick GM, et al: Minor salivary gland calculi. A clinicopathologic study of forty-seven new cases. Oral Surg Oral Med Oral Pathol 1979;47:44–50.

122. Ottaviani F, Galli A, Lucia MB, et al: Bilateral parotid sialolithiasis in a patient with acquired immunodificiency syndrome and immunoglobulin G multiple myeloma. Oral Surg Oral Med Oral Pathol 1997;83:552–554.

123. Mustard TA: Calculus of unusual size in Wharton's duct. Br Dent J 1945;79:129–132.

124. Stanley MW, Bardales RH, Beneke J, et al: Sialolithiasis: Differential

diagnostic problems in fine-needle aspiration cytology. Am J Clin Pathol 1996;106:229–233.

125. Iro H, Zenk J, Waldfahrer F, et al: Extracorporeal shock wave lithotripsy of parotid stones: Results of a prospective clinical trial. Ann Otol Rhinol Laryngol 1998;107:860–864.

Sialadenosis

126. Kutchai HC: Gastrointestinal secretions. In: Berne RM, Levy MN (eds): Physiology. St. Louis: CV Mosby, 1988:687.

127. Donath K, Spillner M, Seifert G: The influence of the autonomic nervous system on the ultrastructure of the parotid acinar cells. Experimental contribution to the neurohormonal sialadenosis. Virchows Arch A Pathol Anat Histol 1974;364:15–33.

128. Batsakis JG: Pathology consultation. Sialadenosis. Ann Otol Rhinol Laryngol 1988;97:94–95.

129. Coleman H, Altini M, Nayler S, et al: Sialadenosis: A presenting sign in bulimia. Head Neck 1998;20:758–762.

130. Seifert G, Miehlke A, Haubrich J, Chilla R: Diseases of the Salivary Glands: Pathology, Diagnosis, Treatment, Facial Nerve Surgery. Stuttgart: Georg Thieme Verlag, 1986:78–84.

131. Donath K, Seifert G: Ultrastructural studies of the parotid glands in sialadenosis. Virchows Arch A Pathol Anat Histol 1975;365:119–135.

132. Chisholm DM, Adi MM, Ervine IM, Ogden GR: Cell deletion by apoptosis during regression of rat parotid sialadenosis. Virchows Arch 1995;427:181–186.

133. Ascoli V, Albedi FM, De Blasiis R, Nardi F: Sialadenosis of the parotid gland: Report of four cases diagnosed by fine-needle aspiration cytology. Diagn Cytopathol 1993;9:151–155.

134. Ellis AL, Auclair PL: Atlas of Tumor Pathology: Tumors of the Salivary Glands, 3rd Series, Fascicle 17. Washington DC: Armed Forces Institute of Pathology, 1996:434–435.

Primary Cystic Disease

135. Work WP: Cysts and congenital lesions of the parotid gland. Otolaryngol Clin North Am 1977;10:339–343.

136. Bouquot JE, Gundlach KKH: Odd lips: the prevalence of common lip lesions in 23616 white Americans over 35 years of age. Quintessence Int 1987;18:277–284.

137. Azuma M, Tamatani T, Fukui K, et al: Proteolytic enzymes in salivary extravasation mucoceles. J Oral Pathol Med 1995;24:299–302.

138. Standish SM, Shafer WG: Mucus retention phenomenon. J Oral Surg 1959;17:15–22.

139. Eveson JW: Superficial mucoceles: Pitfall in clinical and microscopic diagnosis. Oral Surg Oral Med Oral Pathol 1988;66:318–322.

140. Seifert G: Mucoepidermoid carcinoma in a salivary duct cyst of the parotid gland. Contribution to the development of tumours in salivary gland cysts. Pathol Res Pract 1996;192:1211–1217.

141. Koudelka BM: Obstructive disorders. In: Ellis GL, Auclair PL, Gnepp DR (eds): Surgical Pathology of the Salivary Glands. Philadelphia: WB Saunders, 1991:26–38.

142. Eversole LR: Oral sialocysts. Arch Otolaryngol Head Neck Surg 1987;113:51–56.

143. Southam JC: Mucous retention cysts of the oral mucosa. J Oral Pathol 1974;3:197–202.

144. White DK, Miller AS, McDaniel RK, et al: Inverted ductal papilloma: A distinctive lesion of minor salivary gland. Cancer 1982;49:519–524.

145. Abrams AM, Finck FM: Sialadenoma papilliferum: A previously unreported salivary gland tumor. Cancer 1969;24:1057–1063.

146. Kerpel SM: The papillary cystadenoma of minor salivary gland origin. Oral Surg Oral Med Oral Pathol 1978;46:820–826.

147. Wilson DF, MacEntree MI: Papillary cystadenoma of minor salivary gland origin. Oral Surg Oral Med Oral Pathol 1974;37:915–918.

148. Sobieski EJ, Kleinhenz RRJ, Metheny J: Branchiogenic cyst within the parotid gland. Arch Otolaryngol 1965;82:395–397.

149. Miglets AW: Parotid branchial cleft cyst with facial paralysis. Arch Otolaryngol 1975;101:637–638.

150. Work WP: Cysts and congenital lesions of the parotid gland. Otolaryngol Clin North Am 1977;10:339–343.

151. Meyer I: Dermoid cysts (dermoids) of the floor of the mouth. Oral Surg Oral Med Oral Pathol 1955;8:1149–1164.

152. Link JF, McKean TW: Dermoid cysts: Report of case. J Oral Surg 1965;23:451–455.

153. Pieterse AS, Seymout AE: Parotid cysts: An analysis of 16 cases and suggested classification. Pathology 1981;13:225–234.

154. Seifert G, Thomsen ST, Donath K: Bilateral dysgenetic polycystic parotid glands: Morphological analysis and differential diagnosis of a rare disease of salivary glands. Virchows Arch A Pathol Anat Histopathol 1981;390:273–288.

155. Batsakis JG, Bruner JM, Luna MA: Polycystic (dysgenetic) disease of the parotid glands. Arch Otolaryngol Head Neck Surg 1988;114:1146–1148.

156. Batsakis JG, McClatchey KD: Pathology consultation: Cervical ranulas. Ann Otol Rhinol Laryngol 1988;97:561–562.

157. Langlois NE, Kolhe P: Plunging ranula: A case report and a literature review. Hum Pathol 1992;23:1306–1308.

158. Matt BH, Crockett DM: Plunging ranula in an infant. Otolaryngol Head Neck Surg 1988;99:330–333.

159. Redpath TH: Congenital ranula. Oral Surg Oral Med Oral Pathol 1969;28:542–542.

160. Abemayor E, Calcaterra T: Kaposi's sarcoma and AIDS. An update with emphasis on its head and neck manifestation. Arch Otolaryngol 1983;109:536–542.

161. Lozada F, Silverman S, Migliorati CA, et al: Oral manifestations of tumor and opportunistic infections in AIDS: Findings in 53 homosexual men with Kaposi's sarcoma. Oral Surg 1983;56:491–494.

162. Marcusen DC, Sooy CD: Otolaryngologic and head and neck manifestations of AIDS. Laryngoscope 1985;95:401–405.

163. Phelan JA, Saltzman BR, Freidland GH, et al: Oral findings in AIDS patients. Oral Surg Oral Med Oral Pathol 1987;64:50–56.

164. Silverman S, Migliorati CA, Lozarda-Nur F, et al: Oral findings in people with or at high risk for AIDS: A study of 375 homosexual males. JADA 1986;112:187–192.

165. Couderc LJ, D'Agay MF, Danon F, et al: Sicca complex and infection with HIV. Arch Intern Med 1987;147:898–901.

166. Finfer MD, Schinella RA, Rothstein SG, et al: Cystic parotid lesions in patients at risk for AIDS. Arch Otolaryngol Head Neck Surg 1988;114:1290–1294.

167. Shugar JM, Som PM, Jacobson AL, et al: Multicentric parotid cysts and cervical adenopathy in AIDS patients. A newly recognized entity: CT and MR manifestations. Laryngoscope 1988;98:772–775.

168. Tunkel DE, Loury MC, Fox CH, et al: Bilateral parotid enlargement in HIV seropositive patients. Laryngoscope 1989;99:590–595.

169. Ryan JR, Ioachim HL, Marmer J, et al: AIDS-related lymphadenopathies presenting in the salivary gland lymph nodes. Arch Otolaryngol 1985;111:554–556.

170. Smith FB, Rajdeo H, Panesar N, et al: Benign lymphoepithelial lesion of the parotid gland in intravenous drug users. Arch Pathol Lab Med 1988;112:742–745.

171. Schoidt M, Greenspan D, Levy JA, et al: Does HIV cause salivary gland disease? AIDS 1989;3:819–822.

172. Ulirisch RC, Jaffe ES: Sjögren's syndrome-like illness associated with the AIDS-related complex. Hum Pathol 1987;18:1063–1068.

173. De Vries EJ, Kapadia SB, Johnson JT, et al: Salivary gland lymphoproliferative disease in AIDS. Otolaryngol Head Neck Surg 1988;99:59–62.

174. D'Agay MF, de Roquancourt A, Peuchmaur M, et al: Cystic benign lymphoepithelial lesion of the salivary glands in HIV positive patients. Report of two cases with immunohistochemical study. Virchows Arch A Pathol Anat Histopathol 1990;417:353–356.

175. Ferraro FJ Jr, Rush BF Jr, Ruark D, Oleske J: Enucleation of parotid lymphoepithelial cyst in patients who are human immunodeficiency virus positive. Surg Gynecol Obstet 1993;177:524–526.

176. Sperling NM, Lin PT, Lucente FE. Cystic parotid masses in HIV infection. Head Neck 1990;12:337–341.

177. Som PM, Brandwein MS, Silvers A, et al: Nodal inclusion cysts of the parotid gland and parapharyngeal space: A discussion of lymphoepithelial, AIDS-related parotid, and branchial cysts, cystic Warthin's tumors, and cysts in Sjögren's syndrome. Laryngoscope 1995;105:1122–1128.

178. Ihrler S, Zietz C, Riederer A, et al: HIV-related parotid lymphoepithelial cysts. Immunohistochemistry and 3-D reconstruction of surgical and autopsy material with special reference to formal pathogenesis. Virchows Arch A Pathol Anat Histopathol 1996;429:139–147.

179. Van Vooren JP, Farber CM, Daelemans P, et al: Acute Sjögren-like syndrome as the first manifestation of a generalized CMV infection in a patient with AIDS. J Laryngol Otol 1995;109:1113–1114.

180. Daniels TE: Benign lymphoepithelial lesion and Sjögren's syndrome. In: Ellis G, Auclair P, Gnepp DR (eds): Surgical Pathology of the Salivary Glands. Philadelphia: WB Saunders, 1991:83–106.

181. Bernier JL, Bhaskar SN: Lymphoepithelial lesions of salivary glands. Cancer 1958;11:1156–1178.

182. Jenson JL: Idiopathic diseases. In: Ellis GL, Auclair PL, Gnepp DR (eds): Surgical Pathology of the Salivary Glands. Philadelphia: WB Saunders, 1991:60–82.

183. Olsen KD, Maragos NE, Weiland LH: First branchial cleft anomalies. Laryngoscope 1980;90:423–436.

184. Buchner A, Hansen LS: Lymphoepithelial cysts of the oral cavity: A clinicopathologic study of thirty-eight cases. Oral Surg Oral Med Oral Pathol 1980;50:441–449.

185. Gnepp DR, Sporck FT: Benign lymphoepithelial parotid cyst with sebaceous differentiation-cystic sebaceous lymphadenoma. Am J Clin Pathol 1980;74:683–687.

186. Weidner N, Geisinger KR, Sterling RT, et al: Benign lymphoepithelial cysts of the parotid gland: A histologic, cytologic, and ultrastructural study. Am J Clin Pathol 1986;85:395–401.

187. Turetschek K, Hospadka H, Steiner E: Case report. Epidermoid cyst of the floor of the mouth: Diagnostic imaging by sonography, computed tomography and magnetic resonance imaging. Br J Radiol 1995;68:205–207.

188. Ohishi M, Ishii T, Shinohara M, et al: Dermoid cyst of the floor of the mouth: Lateral teratoid cyst with sinus tract in an infant. Oral Surg Oral Med Oral Pathol 1985;60:191–194.

189. Addante RR: Congenital cystic dilatation of the submandibular duct. Oral Surg Oral Med Oral Pathol 1984;58:656–658.

190. Tunkel DE, Furin MJ: Salivary cysts following parotid duct translocation for sialorrhea. Otolaryngol Head Neck Surg 1991;105:127–129.

191. Avery BS: A sialocele and unusual parotid fistula—a case report. Br J Oral Surg 1980;18:40–44.

192. Pratt LW: Cystic lesions of the parotid region. J Maine Med Assoc 1965;56:21–23.

193. Saunders HF: Pneumonparotitis. N Engl J Med 1973;289:698.

194. Altman MM, Gutman D: Echinococcus of the parotid gland. J Laryngol Otol 1966;80:409–411.

195. Onerci M, Turan E, Ruacan S: Submandibular hydatid cyst. A case report. J Craniomaxillofacial Surg 1991;19:359–361.

196. Alcalde RE, Ueyama Y, Lim DJ, Matsumura T: Pneumoparotid: Report of a case. J Oral Maxillofac Surg 1998;56:676–680.

197. Richardson GS, Clairmont AA, Erickson ER: Cystic lesions of the parotid gland. Plast Reconstr Surg 1978;61:364–370.

198. Ethell AT: A rare 'parotid tumour.' J Laryngol Otol 1979;93:741–744.

Necrotizing Sialometaplasia

199. Brannon RB, Fowler CB, Hartman KS: Necrotizing sialometaplasia: A clinicopathologic study of sixty-nine cases and review of the literature. Oral Surg Oral Med Oral Pathol 1991;72:317–325.

200. Gnepp DR: Warthin tumor exhibiting sebaceous differentiation and necrotizing sialometaplasia. Virchows Arch A Pathol Anat Histopathol 1981;391:267–273.

201. Dardick I, Jeans MTD, Sinnott NM, et al: Salivary gland components involved in the formation of squamous metaplasia. Am J Pathol 1985;119:33–43.

202. Ben-Izhak O, Ben-Arieh Y: Necrotizing squamous metaplasia in herpetic tracheitis following prolonged intubation: A lesion similar to necrotizing sialometaplasia. Histopathol 1993;22:265–269.

203. Ben-Izhak O, Ben-Arieh Y: Necrotizing sialometaplasia of the larynx [letter to the editor]. Am J Clin Pathol 1995;105:251–252.

204. Shigematsu H, Shigematsu Y, Noguchi Y, Fujita K: Experimental study on necrotizing sialometaplasia of the palate in rats: Role of local anesthetic injections. Int J Oral Maxillofac Surg 1996;25:239–241.

205. Sneige N, Batsakis JG: Necrotizing sialometaplasia. Ann Otol Rhinol Laryngol 1992;101:282–284.

206. Jensen JL: Idiopathic diseases. In: Ellis GL, Auclair PL, Gnepp DR (eds): Surgical Pathology of the Salivary Glands. Philadelphia: WB Saunders, 1991:60–82.

207. Romagosa V, Bella MR, Truchero C, Moya J: Necrotizing sialometaplasia (adenometaplasia) of the trachea. Histopathol 1992;21:280–282.

208. Littman CD: Necrotizing sialometaplasia (adenometaplasia) of the trachea. Histopathol 1993;298–299.

209. Russell JD, Glover GW, Friedmann I: View from beneath: Pathology in focus, necrotizing sialometaplasia. J Laryngol Otol 1992;106:569–571.

210. Abrams AM, Melrose RJ, Howell FV: Necrotizing sialometaplasia: A disease simulating malignancy. Cancer 1973;32:130–135.

211. Maisel RH, Johnston WH, Anderson HA, et al: Necrotizing sialometaplasia involving the nasal cavity. Laryngoscope 1977;87:429–434.

212. Walker GK, Fechner RE, Johns ME, et al: Necrotizing sialometaplasia of the larynx secondary to atheroscleromatous embolization. Am J Clin Pathol 1982;77:221–223.

213. Batsakis JG, Manning JT: Necrotizing sialometaplasia of major salivary glands. J Laryngol Otol 1987;101:962–966.

214. Anneroth G, Hansen LS: Necrotizing sialometaplasia: The relationship of its pathogenesis to its clinical characteristics. Int J Oral Surg 1982;11:283–291.

215. Ratnatunga N, Edussuriya B: Necrotizing adenometaplasia (sialometaplasia) of the nasopharynx. Ceylon Med J 1994;39:107–108.

216. Hurt MA, Diaz-Arias AA, Rosenholtz MJ, et al: Post-traumatic lobular squamous metaplasia of breast. An unusual pseudocarcinomatous metaplasia resembling squamous (necrotizing) sialometaplasia of the salivary gland. Mod Pathol 1988;1:385–390.

217. Metcalf JS, Maize JC: Squamous syringometaplasia in lobular paniculitis and pyoderma gangrenosum. Am J Dermatopathol 1990;12:141–149.

218. Zschoch H: Mucous gland infarct with squamous metaplasia in the lung. A rare site of so called necrotizing sialometaplasia. Pathologe 1992;13:45–48.

219. Brooks DG, Hottinger HA, Dunstan RW: Canine necrotizing sialometaplasia: A case report and review of the literature. J Am Anim Hosp Assoc 1995;31:21–25.

220. Gnepp DR: Frozen sections. In: Gnepp DR (ed): Pathology of the Head and Neck. New York: Churchill Livingstone, 1988:1–24.

Sclerosing Polycystic Adenosis

221. Smith BC, Ellis GL, Slater LJ, Foss RD: Sclerosing polycystic adenosis of major salivary glands: A clinicopathologic analysis of nine cases. Am J Surg Pathol 1996;20:161–170.

222. Batsakis J: Sclerosing polycystic adenosis: Newly recognized salivary gland lesion—a form of chronic sialadenitis? Adv Anat Pathol 1996;3:298–304.

223. Donath K, Seifert G: Sklerosierende polyzystische Sialadenopathie: Eine seltene nichttumorose Erkrankung. Pathologe 1997;18:368–373.

Classification

224. Foote FW Jr, Frazell EL: Atlas of Tumor Pathology. Tumors of the Major Salivary Glands, 1st Series, Fascicle 11. Washington, DC: Armed Forces Institute of Pathology, 1954.

225. Thackray AC, Sobin LH: Histological Typing of Salivary Gland Tumours. International Histological Classification of Tumours No 7. Geneva: World Health Organization, 1972.

226. Thackray AC, Lucas RB: Tumors of the Major Salivary Glands. Atlas of Tumor Pathology, 2nd series, Fascicle 10. Washington, DC: Armed Forces Institute of Pathology, 1974.

227. Seifert G, Sobin LH: Histological Typing of Salivary Gland Tumours. World Health Organization International Histological Classification of Tumours, 2nd ed. New York: Springer-Verlag, 1991.

228. Ellis GL, Auclair PL: Atlas of Tumor Pathology. Tumors of the Salivary Gland, 3rd Series, Fascicle 17. Washington, DC: Armed Forces Institute of Pathology, 1996.

Benign Mixed Tumors

229. Eveson JW, Cawson RA: Salivary gland tumors: A review of 2410 cases with particular reference to histologic types, site, age, and sex distribution. J Pathol 1985;146:51–58.

230. Spiro RH: Salivary neoplasms: Overview of a 35 year experience with 2,807 patients. Head Neck Surg 1986;8:177–184.

231. Eneroth CM: Salivary gland tumors in the parotid gland, submandibular gland and the palate region. Cancer 1971;27:1415–1418.

232. Waldron CA, El-Mofty S, Gnepp DR: Tumors of the intraoral minor salivary glands: A demographic and histologic study of 426 cases. Oral Surg Oral Med Oral Pathol 1988;66:323–333.

233. Waldron CA: Mixed tumor (pleomorphic adenoma) and myoepithelioma. In: Ellis GL, Auclair PL, Gnepp DR (eds): Surgical Pathology of the Salivary Glands. Philadelphia: WB Saunders, 1991:165–186.

234. Bouquot JE, Kurland LT, Weiland LH: Primary salivary epithelial neoplasms in the Rochester, Minnesota population [abstract]. J Dent Res 1979;58:419.

235. Pinkston JA, Cole P: Incidence rates of salivary gland tumors: Results

from a population-based study. Otolaryngol Head Neck Surg 1999;120:834–840.

236. Compagno J, Wong RT: Intranasal mixed tumors. Am J Clin Pathol 1977;68:213–218.

237. Berenholz L, Kessler A, Segal S: Massive pleomorphic adenoma of the maxillary sinus: A case report. Int J Oral Maxillofac Surg 1998;27:372–373.

238. Heffner DK: Sinonasal and laryngeal salivary gland lesions. In: Ellis GL, Auclair PL, Gnepp DR (eds): Surgical Pathology of the Salivary Glands. Philadelphia: WB Saunders, 1991:544–559.

239. Pesavento G, Ferlito A: Benign mixed tumor of heterotopic salivary gland tissue in upper neck. Report of a case with review of the literature on heterotopic salivary gland tissue. J Laryngol 1976;90:577–584.

240. Shinohara M, Ikebe T, Nakamura S, et al: Multiple pleomorphic adenomas arising in the parotid and submandibular lymph nodes. Br J Oral Maxillofac Surg 1996;34:515–519.

241. Feigin GA, Robinson B, Marchevsky A: Mixed tumor of the mediastinum. Arch Pathol Lab Med 1986;110:80–81.

242. Asai S, Tang X, Ohta Y, Tsutsumi Y: Myoepithelial carcinoma in pleomorphic adenoma of salivary gland type, occurring in the mandible of an infant. Pathol Int 1995;45:677–683.

243. Kilpatrick SE, Hitchcock MG, Kraus MD, et al: Mixed tumors and myoepitheliomas of soft tissue: A clinicopathologic study of 19 cases with a unifying concept. Am J Surg Pathol 1997;21:13–22.

244. Surana R, Moloney R, Fitzgerald RJ: Tumours of heterotopic salivary tissue in the upper cervical region in children. Surg Oncol 1993;2:133–136.

245. Moran CA: Primary salivary gland–type tumors of the lung. Semin Diagn Pathol 1995;12:106–122.

246. Hampton TA, Scheithauer BW, Rojiani AM, et al: Salivary gland–like tumors of the sellar region. Am J Surg Pathol 1997;21:424–434.

247. Rose GE, Wright JE: Pleomorphic adenoma of the lacrimal gland. Br J Ophthalmol 1992;76:395–400.

248. Cuadros CL, Ryan SS, Miller RE: Benign mixed tumor (pleomorphic adenoma) of the breast: Ultrastructural study and review of the literature. J Surg Oncol 1987;36:58–63.

249. Seifert G, Donath K: Multiple tumours of the salivary glands—terminology and nomenclature. Eur J Cancer B Oral Oncol 1996;32:3–7.

250. Buenting JE, Smith TL, Holmes DK: Giant pleomorphic adenoma of the parotid gland: Case report and review of the literature. Ear Nose Throat J 1998;77:634–640.

251. Lomax-Smith JD, Azzopardi JG: The hyaline cell: A distinctive feature of "mixed" salivary tumours. Histopathol 1978;2:77–92.

252. Dardick I, van Nostrand AWP, Phillips MJ: Histogenesis of salivary gland pleomorphic adenoma (mixed tumor) with an evaluation of the role of the myoepithelial cell. Hum Pathol 1982;3:60–75.

253. Donath K, Seifert G: Tumour-simulating squamous cell metaplasia (SCM) in necrotic areas of salivary gland tumours. Pathol Res Pract 1997;193:689–693.

254. Lam KY, Ng IOL, Chan GSW: Palatal pleomorphic adenoma with florid squamous metaplasia: A potential diagnostic pitfall. J Oral Pathol Med 1998;27:407–410.

254a. Coleman H, Altini M: Intravascular tumour in intra-oral pleomorphic adenomas: A diagnostic and therapeutic dilemma. Histopathol 1999;35:439–444.

255. Auclair PL, Ellis GL: Atypical features in salivary gland mixed tumors: Their relationship to malignant transformation. Mod Pathol 1996;9:652–657.

256. Allen CM, Damm D, Neville B, et al: Necrosis in benign salivary gland neoplasms. Not necessarily a sign of malignant transformation. Oral Surg Oral Med Oral Pathol 1994;78:455–461.

257. Batsakis JG: Recurrent mixed tumors. Ann Otol Rhinol Laryngol 1986;95:543–544.

258. Gnepp DR, Schroeder W, Heffner D: Synchronous tumors arising in a single major salivary gland. Cancer 1989;63:1219–1224.

259. Ishikawa N, Hashimoto K: Bilateral pleomorphic adenoma of the parotid gland. J Otolaryngol 1998;27:94–96.

260. Oguchi N, Hirano T, Asano G: Immunohistopathological properties of cytoskeletal proteins and extracellular matrix components in pleomorphic adenomas of salivary glands. Nippon Jibiinkoka Gakkai Kaiho 1993;96:780–786.

261. Savera AT, Gown AM, Zarbo RJ: Immunolocalization of three novel smooth muscle specific proteins in salivary gland pleomorphic adenoma: Assessment of the morphogenetic role of myoepithelium. Mod Pathol 1997;10:1093–1100.

262. Mori M, Yamada K, Tanaka T, Okada Y: Multiple expression of kera-

tins, vimentin, and S-100 protein in pleomorphic salivary adenomas. Virchows Arch B Cell Pathol Incl Mol Pathol 1990;58:435–444.

263. Patel N, Poole A: Recurrent benign parotid tumours: The lesson not learnt yet? Aust N Z J Surg 1998;68:562–564.

264. Myssiorek D, Ruah CB, Hybels RL: Recurrent pleomorphic adenomas of the parotid gland. Head Neck 1990;12:332–336.

265. McGregor AD, Burgoyne M, Tan KC: Recurrent pleomorphic salivary adenoma: The relevance of age at first presentation. Br J Plast Surg 1988;41:177–181.

266. Henriksson G, Westrin KM, Carlsoo B, Silfversward C: Recurrent primary pleomorphic adenomas of salivary gland origin: Intrasurgical rupture, histopathologic features, and pseudopodia. Cancer 1998;82:617–620.

267. Renehan A, Gleave EN, Hancock BD, et al: Long term follow up of over 1000 patients with salivary gland tumours treated in a single centre. Br J Surg 1996;83:1750–1754.

268. Laskawi R, Schott T, Schröder M: Recurrent pleomorphic adenomas of the parotid gland: Clinical evaluation and long-term follow-up. Br J Oral Maxillofac Surg 1998;36:48–51.

269. Yugueros P, Goellner JR, Petty PM, Woods JE: Treating recurrence of parotid benign pleomorphic adenomas. Ann Plast Surg 1998;40:573–576.

Malignant Mixed Tumors

270. Gnepp DR: Malignant mixed tumors of the salivary glands: A review. Pathol Annu (part 1) 1993;28:279–328.

271. Spiro RH, Huvos AG, Strong EW: Malignant mixed tumor of salivary origin: A clinicopathologic study of 146 cases. Cancer 1977;39:388–396.

272. Foote FW Jr, Frazell EL: Tumors of the major salivary glands. Cancer 1953;6:1065–1133.

273. McGrath MH: Malignant transformation in concurrent benign mixed tumors of the parotid and submaxillary glands. Plast Reconstr Surg 1980;65:676–678.

274. LiVolsi VA, Perzin KH: Malignant mixed tumors arising in salivary glands I. Carcinomas arising in benign mixed tumors: A clinicopathologic study. Cancer 1977;39:2209–2230.

275. Tortoledo ME, Luna MA, Batsakis JG: Carcinomas ex pleomorphic adenoma and malignant mixed tumors. Arch Otolaryngol 1984;110:172–176.

276. Brandwein M, Huvos AG, Dardick I, et al: Noninvasive and minimally invasive carcinoma ex mixed tumor. A clinicopathologic and ploidy study of 12 patients with major salivary tumors of low (or no?) malignant potential. Oral Surg Oral Med Oral Pathol Oral Radiol Endod 1996;81:655–664.

277. Klijanienko J, El-Naggar AK, Servois V, et al: Mucoepidermoid carcinoma ex pleomorphic adenoma: Nonspecific preoperative cytologic findings in six cases. Cancer 1998;84:231–234.

278. Luna MA, Batsakis JG, Tortoledo ME, del Junco GW: Carcinomas ex monomorphic adenoma of salivary glands. J Laryngol Otol 1989;103:756–759.

279. Gerughty RM, Scofield HH, Brown FM, Hennigar GR: Malignant mixed tumors of salivary gland origin. Cancer 1969;24:471–486.

280. Thomas WH, Coppola ED: Distant metastases from mixed tumors of the salivary glands. Am J Surg 1965;109:724–730.

281. Lewis JE, Olsen KD: Carcinoma-ex-pleomorphic adenoma: Pathologic analysis of 73 cases. Mod Pathol 1998;11:121A.

282. Bullerdiek J, Wobst G, Meyer-Bolte K: Cytogenetic subtyping of 220 salivary gland pleomorphic adenomas: Correlation to occurrences, histologic subtype, and in vitro cellular behavior. Cancer Genet Cytogenet 1993;65:27–31.

283. Gillenwater A, Hurr K, Wolf P, et al: Microsatellite alterations at chromosome 8q loci in pleomorphic adenoma. Otolaryngol Head Neck Surg 1997;117:448–452.

284. Mark HF, Hanna I, Gnepp DR: Cytogenetic analysis of salivary gland type tumors. Oral Surg Oral Med Oral Pathol Oral Radiol Endod 1996;82:187–192.

285. Rao PH, Murty VV, Louie DC, Chaganti RSK: Nonsyntenic amplification of MYC with CDK4 and MDM2 in a malignant mixed tumor of salivary gland. Cancer Genet Cytogenet 1998;105:160–163.

286. Bocklage T, Feddersen R: Unusual mesenchymal and mixed tumors of the salivary gland. An immunohistochemical and flow cytometric analysis of three cases. Arch Pathol Lab Med 1995;119:69–74.

287. Takata T, Nikai H, Ogawa I, Ijuhin N: Ultrastructural and immunohis-

tochemical observations of a true malignant mixed tumor (carcinosarcoma) of the tongue. J Oral Pathol Med 1990;19:261–265.

288. Stephen J, Batsakis JG, Luna MA, et al: True malignant mixed tumors (carcinosarcoma) of salivary glands. Oral Surg Oral Med Oral Pathol 1986;61:597–602.

289. Garner SL, Robinson RA, Maves MD, Barnes CH: Salivary gland carcinosarcoma: True malignant mixed tumor. Ann Otol Rhinol Laryngol 1989;98:611–614.

290. Alvarez-Canas C, Rodilla IG: True malignant mixed tumor (carcinosarcoma) of the parotid gland. Report of a case with immunohistochemical study. Oral Surg Oral Med Oral Pathol Oral Radiol Endod 1996;81:454–458.

291. Julie C, Aidan D, Arkwright S, et al: Carcinosarcome de la glande sous-maxillaire. Ann Pathol 1997;17:35–37.

292. Gnepp DR, Wenig GM: Malignant mixed tumors: In: Ellis GL, Auclair PL, Gnepp DR (eds): Surgical Pathology of the Salivary Glands. Philadelphia: WB Saunders, 1991:350–368.

293. Wenig BM, Hitchcock CL, Ellis GL, Gnepp DR: Metastasizing mixed tumor of salivary glands. A clinicopathologic and flow cytometric analysis. Am J Surg Pathol 1992;16:845–858.

294. Jin Y, Jin C, Arheden K, et al: Unbalanced chromosomal rearrangements in a metastasizing salivary gland tumor with benign histology. Cancer Genet Cytogenet 1998;102:59–64.

295. Hoorweg JJ, Hilgers FJM, Keus RB, et al: Metastasizing pleomorphic adenoma: A report of three cases. Eur J Surg Oncol 1998;24:452–455.

296. Goodisson DW, Buff RGM, Creedon AJ, et al: A case of metastasizing pleomorphic adenoma. Oral Med Oral Surg Oral Pathol Oral Radiol Endod 1999;87:341–345.

297. Kilpatrick SE, Hitchcock MG, Kraus MD, et al: Mixed tumors and myoepitheliomas of soft tissue: A clinicopathologic study of 19 cases with a unifying concept. Am J Surg Pathol 1997;21:13–22.

Myoepithelioma

298. Sheldon WH: So-called mixed tumors of the salivary glands. Arch Pathol 1943;35:1–20.

299. Barnes L, Appel BN, Perez H, et al: Myoepithelioma of the head and neck: Case report and review. J Surg Oncol 1985;28:21–28.

300. Dardick I, Van Nostrand AWF: Myoepithelial cells in salivary gland tumors—revisited. Head Neck Surg 1985;7:395–408.

301. Dardick I, Cavell S, Boivin M, et al: Salivary gland myoepithelioma variants: Histological, ultrastructural and immunocytological features. Virchows Arch A Pathol Anat Histopathol 1989;416:25–42.

302. Dardick I, Thomas MJ, Van Nostrand AWP: Myoepithelioma: New concepts of histology and classification—a light and electron microscopic study. Ultrastruct Pathol 1989;13:187–224.

303. Lins JEW, Gnepp DR: Myoepithelioma of the palate in a child. Int J Pediatr Otorhinolaryngol 1986;11:5–13.

304. Sciubba JJ, Brannon R: Myoepithelioma of salivary glands: Report of 23 cases. Cancer 1982;47:562–572.

305. Ellis GL, Auclair PL: Atlas of Tumor Pathology Tumors of the Salivary Glands. Washington, DC: Armed Forces Institute of Pathology, 1996:39–153.

306. Waldron CA. Mixed tumor (pleomorphic adenoma) and myoepithelioma. In: Ellis GL, Auclair PL, Gnepp DR (eds): Surgical Pathology of the Salivary Glands. Philadelphia: WB Saunders, 1991:163–186.

307. Seifert G: Oralpathologie I: Pathologie der Speicheldrusen. Berlin: Springer-Verlag, 1996.

308. Franquemont DW, Mills SE: Plasmacytoid monomorphic adenoma of salivary glands. Absence of myogenous differentiation and comparison to spindle cell myoepithelioma. Am J Surg Pathol 1993;17:146–153.

309. Jie W, Qiguang W, Kaihua S, Chengrui B: Quantitative multivariate analysis of myoepithelioma and myoepithelial carcinoma. Int J Oral Maxillofac Surg 1995;24:153–157.

310. Waldron CA, El-Mofty SK, Gnepp DR: Tumors of the intraoral minor salivary glands: A demographic and histopathologic study of 426 cases. Oral Surg Oral Med Oral Pathol 1988;66:323–333.

311. Takai Y, Dardick I, Mackay A, et al: Diagnostic criteria for neoplastic myoepithelial cells in pleomorphic adenomas and myoepitheliomas. Immunocytochemical detection of muscle-specific actin, cytokeratin 14, vimentin, and glial fibrillary acidic protein. Oral Surg Oral Med Oral Pathol Oral Radiol Endod 1995;79:330–341.

312. Fernandez-Figueras M, Puig L, Trias I, et al: Benign myoepithelioma of the skin. Am J Dermatopathol 1998;20:208–212.

312a. Michal M, Miettinem M: Myoepitheliomas of the skin and soft tissues. Report of 12 cases. Virchows Arch 1999;434:393–400.

313. Kilpatrick SE, Hitchcock MG, Kraus MD, et al: Mixed tumors and myoepitheliomas of soft tissue: A clinicopathologic study of 19 cases with a unifying concept. Am J Surg Pathol 1997;21:13–22.

313a. Dardick I, Birek C, Lingen MW, Rowe PE: Differentiation and the cytomorphology of salivary gland tumors with specific reference to oncocytic metaplasia. Oral Surg Oral Med Oral Pathol Oral Radiol Endod 1999;88:691–701.

313b. Skalova A, Michal M, Ryska A, et al. Oncocytic myoepithelioma and pleomorphic adenoma of the salivary glands. Virchows Arch 1999;434:537–546.

314. Jaeger RG, de Oliveira PT, Jaeger MMMJ, de Araujo VC: Expression of smooth-muscle actin in cultured cells from human plasmacytoid myoepithelioma. Oral Surg Oral Med Oral Pathol Oral Radiol Endod 1997;84:663–667.

315. Savera AT, Klimstra DS, Huvos AG: Myoepithelial carcinoma of the salivary glands. A clinicopathologic study of 25 cases. Mod Pathol 1999;12:130A.

316. El-Mofty SK, O'Leary TR, Swanson PE: Malignant myoepithelioma of salivary glands: Clinicopathologic and immunophenotypic features. Review of literature and report of 2 new cases. Int J Surg Pathol 1994;2:133–140.

317. Hsiao CH, Cheng CJ, Yeh KL: Immunohistochemical and ultrastructural study of malignant plasmacytoid myoepithelioma of the maxillary sinus. J Formos Med Assoc 1997;96:209–212.

318. Michal M, Skalova A, Simpson RHW, et al: Clear cell malignant myoepithelioma of the salivary glands. Histopathol 1996;28:309–315.

319. Bombi JA, Alos L, Rey M, et al: Myoepithelial carcinoma arising in a benign myoepithelioma: Immunohistochemical, ultrastructural, and flow-cytometrical study. Diagn Cytopathol 1996;15:415–420.

320. Suzuki H, Inoue K, Fujioka Y, et al: Myoepithelial carcinoma with predominance of plasmacytoid cells arising in a pleomorphic adenoma of the parotid gland. Histopathol 1998;32:86–87.

321. Jie W, Qiguang W, Kaihua S, Chengrui B: Quantitative multivariate analysis of myoepithelioma and myoepithelial carcinoma. Int J Oral Maxillofac Surg 1995;24:153–157.

322. Craadt van Roggen JF, Baatenburg-de Jong RJ, Verschuur HP, et al: Myoepithelial carcinoma (malignant myoepithelioma): First report of an occurrence in the maxillary sinus. Histopathol 1998;32:239–241.

323. Hsiao CH, Cheng C, Yeh K: Immunohistochemical and ultrastructural study of malignant plasmacytoid myoepithelioma of the maxillary sinus. J Formos Med Assoc 1997;96:209–212.

Warthin's Tumor

324. Thackray AC, Sobin LH: Histological Typing of Salivary Gland Tumours. Geneva: World Health Organization, 1972.

325. Seifert G, Sobin LH, et al: Histological Typing of Salivary Gland Tumours, World Health Organization International Histological Classification of Tumours. 2nd ed. New York: Springer-Verlag, 1991.

326. Ellies M, Laskawi R, Arglebe C: Extraglandular Warthin's tumours: Clinical evaluation and long-term follow-up. Br J Oral Maxillofac Surg 1998;36:52–53.

327. Astor FC, Hanft KL, Rooney P, et al: Extraparotid Warthin's tumor: Clinical manifestations, challenges, and controversies. Otolaryngol Head Neck Surg 1996;114:732–735.

328. Sato T, Ishibashi K: Multicentric Warthin tumor of the paraparotid region mimicking lymph node metastases of homolateral oral and oropharyngeal squamous cell carcinoma: Reports of two cases. J Oral Maxillofac Surg 1998;56:75–80.

329. Van der Wal JE, Davids JJ, van der Waal I: Extraparotid Warthin's tumours—report of 10 cases. Br J Oral Maxillofac Surg 1993;31:43–44.

330. Bonavolonta G, Tranfa F, Staibano S, et al: Warthin tumor of the lacrimal gland. Am J Opthalmol 1997;124:857–858.

331. Kristensen S, Tveteras K, Friedmann I, Thomsen P: Nasopharyngeal Warthin's tumour: A metaplastic lesion. J Laryngol Otol 1989;103:616–619.

332. Kukreja HK, Jain HK: Adenolymphoma of submandibular gland. J Laryngol Otol 1971;85:1201–1203.

333. Ellis GL, Auclair PL: Benign epithelial neoplasms. In: Tumors of the Salivary Glands. Washington, DC: Armed Forces Institute of Pathology, 1996:39–153.

334. Pinkston JA, Cole P: Incidence rates of salivary gland tumors: Results from a population-based study. Otolaryngol Head Neck Surg 1999;120:834–840.

335. Eveson JW, Cawson RA: Warthin's tumor (cystadenolymphoma) of

salivary glands: A clinicopathologic investigation of 278 cases. Oral Surg Oral Med Oral Pathol 1986;61:256–262.

336. Kennedy TL: Warthin's tumor: A review indicating no male predominance. Laryngoscope 1983;93:889–891.

337. Monk JS Jr, Church JS: Warthin's tumor: A high incidence and no sex predominance in central Pennsylvania. Arch Otolaryngol Head Neck Surg 1992;118:477–478.

338. Chapnik JS: The controversy of Warthin's tumor. Laryngoscope 1983;93:695–716.

339. Lamelas J, Terry JH, Alfonso AE: Warthin's tumor: Multicentricity and increasing incidence in women. Am J Surg 1987;114:347–351.

340. Yoo GH, Eisele DW, Askin FB, et al: Warthin's tumor: A 40-year experience at the Johns Hopkins Hospital. Laryngoscope 1994;104:799–803.

341. Pinkston JA, Cole P: Cigarette smoking and Warthin's tumor. Am J Epidemiol 1996;144:183–187.

342. Vories AA, Ramirez SG: Warthin's tumor and cigarette smoking. South Med J 1997;90:416–418.

343. Yu GY, Liu XB, Li ZL, Peng X: Smoking and the development of Warthin's tumour of the parotid gland. Br J Oral Maxillofac Surg 1998;36:183–185.

344. Land CE, Saku T, Hayashi Y, et al: Incidence of salivary gland tumors among atomic bomb survivors, 1950–1987. Evaluation of radiation-risk. Radiat Res 1996;146:28–36.

345. Saku T, Hayashi Y, Takahara O, et al: Salivary gland tumors among atomic bomb survivors, 1950–1987. Cancer 1997;79:1465–1475.

346. Gnepp DR, Schroeder W, Heffner D: Synchronous tumors arising in a single major salivary gland. Cancer 1989;63:1219–1224.

347. White RR, Arm RN, Randall P: A large Warthin's tumor of the parotid. Case report. Plast Reconstr Surg 1978;61:452–454.

348. Seifert G, Bull HG, Donath K: Histologic subclassification of the cystadenolymphoma of the parotid gland: Analysis of 275 cases. Virchows Arch A Pathol Anat Histopathol 1980;388:13–38.

349. Gnepp DR: Sebaceous neoplasms of salivary gland origin: A review. Pathol Annu Part 1 1983;18:71–102.

350. Warnock GR: Papillary cystadenoma lymphomatosum (Warthin's tumor). In: Ellis GL, Auclair PL, Gnepp DR (eds): Surgical Pathology of the Salivary Glands. Philadelphia: WB Saunders, 1991:187–201.

351. Seifert G: Karzinome in vorbestehenden Warthin-Tumoren (Zystadenolymphomen) der Parotis: Klassifikation, Pathogenese und Differentialdiagnose. Pathologe 1997;18:359–367.

352. Nagao T, Sugano I, Ishida Y, et al: Mucoepidermoid carcinoma arising in Warthin's tumour of the parotid gland: Report of two cases with histopathological, ultrastructural and immunohistochemical studies. Histopathol 1998;33:379–386.

353. Medeiros LJ, Rizzi R, Lardelli P, Jaffe ES: Malignant lymphoma involving a Warthin's tumor: A case with immunophenotypic and gene rearrangement analysis. Hum Pathol 1990;21:974–977.

353a. Park CK, Manning JT Jr, Battifora H, Medeiros LJ: Follicle center lymphoma and Warthin tumor involving the same anatomic site. Report of two cases and review of the literature. Am J Clin Pathol 2000;113:113–119.

354. Seifert G: Bilateral mucoepidermoid carcinomas arising in bilateral pre-existing Warthin's tumours of the parotid gland. Oral Oncol 1997;33:284–287.

355. Azzopardi JG, Hou LT: The genesis of adenolymphoma. J Pathol Bact 1964;88:213–218.

356. Shinohara M, Nakamura S, Harada T, et al: Warthin's tumor of the parotid glands, adenomatous hyperplasia and oncocytic adenomatous hyperplasia of the intranodal heterotopic salivary glands: A comparative immunohistochemical assessment. Acta Histochem Cytochem 1996;29:17–27.

357. Aguirre JM, Echebarria MA, Martinez-Conde R, et al: Warthin tumor: A new hypothesis concerning its development. Oral Surg Oral Med Oral Pathol Oral Radiol Endod 1998;85:60–63.

358. Santucci M, Gallo O, Calzolari A, Bondi R: Detection of Epstein-Barr viral genome in tumor cells of Warthin's tumor of parotid gland. Am J Clin Pathol 1993;100:662–665.

359. Gallo O: Is Warthin's tumor an Epstein Barr virus–related disease? Int J Cancer 1994;58:756–757.

360. Heller KS, Attie JN: Treatment of Warthin's tumor by enucleation. Am J Surg 1988;156:294–296.

361. Yu GY, Ma DQ, Liu XB, et al: Local excision of the parotid gland in the treatment of Warthin's tumour. Br J Oral Maxillofac Surg 1998;36:186–189.

Basal Cell Adenoma

362. Seifert G, Sobin LH, et al: Histological Typing of Salivary Gland Tumours, 2nd ed. Berlin: Springer-Verlag, 1991:13.

363. Kleinsasser O, Klein HJ: Basalzelladenome der Speicheldrusen. Arch Klin Exp Ohren Nasen Kehlkopfheilk 1967;189:302–316.

364. Kratochvil FJ: Canalicular adenoma and basal cell adenoma. In: Ellis GL, Auclair PL, Gnepp DR (eds): Surgical Pathology of the Salivary Glands. Philadelphia: WB Saunders, 1991:202–224.

365. Luna MA, Tortoledo ME, Allen M: Salivary dermal analogue tumors arising in lymph nodes. Cancer 1987;59:1165–1169.

366. Zarbo RJ, Ricci A, Kowalczyk PD, Carun RW: Intranasal dermal analogue tumor (membraneous basal cell adenoma): Ultrastructure and immunohistochemistry. Arch Otolaryngol 1985;111:333–337.

367. Batsakis JG: Basal cell adenoma of the parotid gland. Cancer 1972;29:226–230.

368. Seifert G, Donath K: The congenital basal cell adenoma of salivary glands. Contribution to the differential diagnosis of congenital salivary gland tumours. Virchows Arch A Pathol Anat Histopathol 1997;430:311–319.

369. Nagao K, Matsuzaki O, Saiga H, et al: Histopathologic studies of basal cell adenoma of the parotid gland. Cancer 1982;50:736–745.

370. Ellis GL, Auclair PL: Tumors of the Salivary Gland. Atlas of Tumor Pathology, 3rd Series, Fascicle 17. Washington, DC: Armed Forces Institute of Pathology, 1996:39–153.

371. Bernacki EG, Batsakis JG, Johns ME: Basal cell adenoma: Distinctive tumor of salivary glands. Arch Otolaryngol 1974;99:84–87.

371a. Dardick I, Birek C, Lingen MW, Rowe PE: Differentiation and the cytomorphology of salivary gland tumors with specific reference to oncocytic metaplasia. Oral Surg Oral Med Oral Pathol Oral Radiol Endod 1999;88:691–701.

372. Joa W, Keh P, Swerdlow MA: Ultrastructure of the basal cell adenoma of the parotid gland. Cancer 1976;37:1322–1333.

373. Strauss M, Abt A, Mahataphongse VP, Conner GH: Basal cell adenoma of the major salivary glands. Report of a case with facial nerve encroachment. Arch Otolaryngol 1981;107:120–124.

374. Dardick I, Daley TD, van Nostrand AWP: Basal cell adenoma with myoepithelial-derived "stroma": A new major salivary gland entity. Head Neck Surg 1986;8:257–267.

375. Headington JT, Bataskis JG, Beals TF, et al: Membranous basal cell adenoma of parotid gland, dermal cylindromas, and trichoepitheliomas: Comparative histochemistry and ultrastructure. Cancer 1977;39:2460–2469.

376. Dardick I, Lytwyn A, Bourne AJ, Byard RW: Trabecular and solid-cribriform types of basal cell adenoma. A morphologic study of two cases of an unusual variant of monomorphic adenoma. Oral Surg Oral Med Oral Pathol 1992;73:75–83.

377. Ogawa I, Nikai H, Takata T, et al: The cellular composition of basal cell adenoma of the parotid gland: An immunohistochemical analysis. Oral Surg Oral Med Oral Pathol 1990;70:619–626.

378. Ferreiro JA: Immunohistochemistry of basal cell adenoma of the major salivary glands. Histopathol 1994;24:539–542.

378a. Zarbo RJ, Prasad AR, Regezi JA, et al: Salivary gland basal cell and canalicular adenomas: Immunohistochemical demonstration of myoepithelial cell participation and morphogenetic considerations. Arch Pathol Lab Med 2000;124:401–405.

379. Nagao T, Sugano I, Ishida Y, et al: Basal cell adenocarcinoma of the salivary glands: Comparison with basal cell adenoma through assessment of cell proliferation, apoptosis, and expression of p53 and bcl-2. Cancer 1998;82:439–447.

380. Klima M, Wolfe K, Johnson PE: Basal cell tumors of the parotid. Arch Otolaryngol 1978;104:111–116.

381. Evans RW, Cruickshank AH: Epithelial Tumours of the Salivary Glands. Philadelphia: WB Saunders, 1970:58–76.

382. Hyma BA, Scheithauer BW, Weiland LH, Irons GB: Membranous basal cell adenoma of the parotid gland: Malignant transformation in a patient with multiple dermal cylindromas. Arch Pathol Lab Med 1988;112:209–211.

383. Nagao T, Sugano I, Ishida Y, et al: Carcinoma in basal cell adenoma of the parotid gland. Pathol Res Pract 1997;193:171–178.

Basal Cell Adenocarcinoma

384. Evans RW, Crickshank AH: Epithelial Tumours of Salivary Glands. Philadelphia: WB Saunders, 1970:58–76.

385. Klima M, Wolfe SK, Johnson PE: Basal cell tumors of the parotid gland. Arch Otolaryngol 1978;104:111–116.

386. Chen KTK: Carcinoma arising in monomorphic adenoma of the salivary gland. Am J Otolaryngol 1985;6:39–41.

387. Murty GE, Welch AR, Soames JV: Basal cell adenocarcinoma of the parotid gland. J Laryngol Otol 1990;104:150–151.

388. Ellis GL, Wiscovitch JG: Basal cell adenocarcinomas of major salivary glands. Oral Surg Oral Med Oral Pathol 1990;69:461–469.

389. Batsakis JG, Luna MA: Basaloid salivary carcinomas. Ann Otol Rhinol Laryngol 1991;100:785–787.

390. Ellis GL, Auclair PL: Atlas of Tumor Pathology: Tumors of the Salivary Glands. Washington, DC: Armed Forces Institute of Pathology, 1996:257–267.

391. Nagao T, Sugano I, Ishida Y, et al: Basal cell adenocarcinoma of the salivary glands: Comparison with basal cell adenoma through assessment of cell proliferation, apoptosis, and expression of p53 and bcl-2. Cancer 1998;82:439–447.

392. Ellis GL, Auclair PL: Basal cell adenocarcinoma. In: Ellis GL, Auclair PL, Gnepp DR (eds): Surgical Pathology of the Salivary Glands. Philadelphia: WB Saunders, 1991:441–454.

393. Fonseca I, Soares J: Basal cell adenocarcinoma of minor salivary and seromucous glands of the head and neck region. Semin Diagn Pathol 1996;13:128–137.

394. Lo AK, Topt JS, Jackson IT, et al: Minor salivary gland basal cell adenocarcinoma of the palate. J Oral Maxillofac Surg 1992;50:531–534.

395. Mima T, Shirasuna K, Kishino M, Matsuya T: Basal cell adenocarcinoma of the sublingual gland: Report of a case. J Oral Maxillofac Surg 1996;54:1121–1123.

396. Muller S, Barnes L: Basal cell adenocarcinoma of the salivary glands. Report of seven cases and review of the literature. Cancer 1996;78:2471–2477.

397. McCluggage G, Sloan J, Cameron S, et al: Basal cell adenocarcinoma of the submandibular gland. Oral Surg Oral Med Oral Pathol Oral Radiol Endod 1995;79:342–350.

398. Quddus MR, Henley JD, Affify AM, et al: Basal cell adenocarcinoma of the salivary gland: An ultrastructural and immunohistochemical study. Oral Surg Oral Med Oral Pathol Oral Radiol Endod 1999;87:845–892.

399. Williams SB, Ellis GL, Auclair PL: Immunohistochemical analysis of basal cell adenocarcinoma. Oral Surg Oral Med Oral Pathol 1993;75:64–69.

400. Moroz K, Ferreira C, Dhurandhar N: Fine needle aspiration of basal cell adenocarcinoma of the parotid gland. Report of a case with assessment of DNA ploidy in aspirates and tissue sections by image analysis. Acta Cytol 1996;40:773–778.

401. Atula T, Klemi PJ, Donath K, et al: Basal cell adenocarcinoma of the parotid gland: A case report and review of the literature. J Laryngol Otol 1993;107:862–864.

402. Gallimore AP, Spraggs PD, Allen JP, Hobsley M: Basaloid carcinomas of salivary glands. Histopathol 1994;24:139–144.

Canalicular Adenoma

403. Ellis GL, Auclair PL: Atlas of Tumor Pathology. Tumors of the Salivary Glands. Washington, DC: Armed Forces Institute of Pathology, 1996:95–103.

404. Waldron CA, El-Mofty SK, Gnepp DR: Tumors of the intraoral minor salivary glands: A demographic and histologic study of 426 cases. Oral Surg Oral Med Oral Pathol 1988;66:323–333.

405. Mintz GA, Abrams AM, Melrose RJ: Monomorphic adenoma of the major and minor salivary glands: Report of 21 cases and review of the literature. Oral Surg Oral Med Oral Pathol 1982;53:375–386.

406. Kratochvil FJ: Canalicular adenoma and basal cell adenoma. In: Ellis GL, Auclair PL, Gnepp DR (eds): Surgical Pathology of the Salivary Glands. Philadelphia: WB Saunders, 1991:202–224.

407. Daley TD, Gardner DG, Smout MS: Canalicular adenoma: Not a basal cell adenoma. Oral Surg Oral Med Oral Pathol 1984;57:181–188.

408. Batsakis JG, Brannon RB, Sciubba JJ: Monomorphic adenoma of major salivary glands. A histologic study of 96 tumours. Clin Otolaryngol 1981;6:129–143.

409. Rousseau A, Mock D, Dover DG, Jordan RCK: Multiple canalicular adenomas: A case report and review of the literature. Oral Surg Oral Med Oral Pathol Oral Radiol Endod 1999;87:346–350.

410. Dardick I: Salivary Gland Tumor Pathology. New York: Igaku-Shoin, 1996:61–67.

411. Ferreiro JA: Immunohistochemical analysis of salivary gland canalicular adenoma. Oral Surg Oral Med Oral Pathol 1994;78:761–765.

412. Guccion JG, Redman RS: Canalicular adenoma of the buccal mucosa: An ultrastructural and histochemical study. Oral Surg Oral Med Oral Pathol 1986;61:173–178.

Benign and Malignant Oncocytic Tumors

413. Auclair PL, Ellis GL, Gnepp DR, et al: Salivary gland neoplasms: General considerations. In: Ellis GL, Auclair PL, Gnepp DR, (eds): Surgical Pathology of the Salivary Glands. Philadelphia: WB Saunders, 1991:135–164.

414. Ellis GL, Auclair PL: Atlas of Tumor Pathology: Tumors of the Salivary Glands. Washington, DC: Armed Forces Institute of Pathology, 1996:103–114, 318–324.

415. Brandwein MS, Huvos AG: Oncocytic tumors of major salivary glands. A study of 68 cases with follow-up of 44 patients. Am J Surg Pathol 1991;15:514–528.

416. Thompson LD, Wenig BM, Ellis GL: Oncocytomas of the submandibular gland. A series of 22 cases and a review of the literature. Cancer 1996;78:2281–2287.

417. Sørensen M, Baunsgaard P, Frederiksen P, Haahr PA: Multifocal adenomatous oncocytic hyperplasia of the parotid gland. (Unusual clear cell variant in two female siblings.) Pathol Res Pract 1986;181:254–257.

418. Gnepp DR, Schroeder W, Heffner D: Synchronous tumors arising in a single major salivary gland. Cancer 1989;63:1219–1224.

419. Deutsch E, Elion A, Zelig S, Ariel I: Synchronous bilateral oncocytoma of the parotid glands. A case report. J Otol Rhinol Laryngol 1984;46:66–68.

420. Boley JO, Robinson DW: Bilateral oxyphilic granular cell adenoma of the parotid. Report of a case. Arch Pathol 1954;58:564–567.

421. Blanck C, Eneroth CM, Jakobsson PA: Bilateral tumors of the parotid gland. Opusc Med Bd 1974;19:30–33.

422. Coli A, Bigotti G, Bartolazzi A: Malignant oncocytoma of the major salivary glands. Report of a post-radiation case. J Exp Clin Cancer Res 1998;17:65–70.

423. Mahnke CG, Janig U, Werner JA: Metastasizing malignant oncocytoma of the submandibular gland. J Laryngol Otol 1998;112:106–109.

424. Nakada M, Nishizaki K, Akagi H, et al: Oncocytic carcinoma of the submandibular gland: A case report and literature review. J Oral Pathol Med 1998;27:225–228.

425. Gray SR, Cornog JL, Sei IS: Oncocytic neoplasms of salivary glands: A report of 15 cases including two malignant oncocytomas. Cancer 1976;38:1306–1317.

426. Goode RK, Corio RL: Oncocytic adenocarcinoma of salivary glands. Oral Surg Oral Med Oral Pathol 1988;65:61–66.

427. Haberman RS, Rodger WA, Haberman PH: Malignant oncocytic adenocarcinoma of the parotid gland with metastasis to bone. Surg Pathol 1990;3:221–226.

428. Sikorowa L: Oncocytoma malignum. Nowotwory 1957;7:125–131.

429. Félix A, Fonseca I, Soares J: Oncocytic tumors of salivary gland type: A study with emphasis on nuclear DNA ploidy. J Surg Oncol 1993;52:217–222.

430. Sugimoto T, Wakizono S, Uemura T, et al: Malignant oncocytoma of the parotid gland: A case report with an immunohistochemical and ultrastructural study. J Laryngol Otol 1993;107:69–74.

431. Vigliani R, Genetta C: Diffuse hyperplastic oncocytosis of the parotid gland. Case report with histochemical observations. Virchows Arch Pathol Anat 1982;397:235–240.

432. Schwartz IS, Feldman M: Diffuse multinodular oncocytoma ("oncocytosis") of the parotid gland. Cancer 1969;23:636–640.

433. Fantasia JE, Miller AS: Papillary cystadenoma lymphomatosum arising in minor salivary glands. Oral Surg 1981;52:411–416.

434. Gaillard A, Nicouleau P, Jacquemaire D, et al: Cystadenolymphomes multiples des parotides et de la levre superieure. Rev Stomatol Chir Maxillofac 1981;82:282–285.

435. Damm DD, White DK, Geissler RH, et al: Benign solid oncocytoma of intraoral minor salivary glands. Oral Surg Oral Med Oral Pathol 1989;67:84–86.

436. Chau MY, Radden BG: Intraoral benign solid oncocytoma. Int J Oral Maxillofac Surg 1986;15:503–506.

437. Briggs J, Evans JNG: Malignant oxyphilic granular cell tumor (oncocytoma) of the palate. Oral Surg 1967;23:796–802.

438. Thomas MR, Ward K, Al Khabori M, et al: Oncocytic mixed nasal tumor. J Laryngol Otol 1993;107:732–734.

439. Buchanan JA, Krolls SO, Sneed WF, et al: Oncocytoma in the nasal vestibule. Otolaryngol Head Neck Surg 1988;99:63–65.

440. Klausen OG, Steinsvåg S, Olofsson J: Oncocytoma presenting as a choanal polyp: A case report. J Otolaryngol 1992;21:196–198.

441. Fayet B, Bernard JA, Zachar D, et al: Oncocytome nasal malin révélé par une mucocèle du sac lacrymal avec hémolacrymie. J Fr Ophtalmol 1990;13:153–158.

442. Martin H, Janda J, Behrbohm H: Lokal invasive Onkozytom der Nasenhohle. Zentralbl Allg Pathol Anat 1990;136:703–706.

443. Johns ME, Batsakis JG, Short CD: Oncocytic and oncocytoid tumors of the salivary glands. Laryngoscope 1973;83:1940–1952.

444. Siwerrsson U, Kindblom LG: Oncocytic carcinoid of the nasal cavity and carcinoid of the lung in a child. Pathol Res Pract 1984;178:562–569.

445. Hamperl H: Das Onkozytom der Speichheldrusen. Z Krebsforsch 1962;64:427–440.

446. Kurihara K, Nakagawa K: Pigmented variant of benign oncocytic lesion of the pharynx. Pathol Int 1997;47:315–317.

447. Nelson DW, Nichols RD, Fine G: Bilateral acinous cell tumors of the parotid gland. Laryngoscope 1978;88:1935–1941.

448. Jensen ML: Multifocal adenomatous oncocytic hyperplasia in parotid glands with metastatic deposits or primary malignant transformation? Pathol Res Pract 1989;185:514–521.

449. Ellis GL: "Clear cell" oncocytoma of the salivary gland. Human Pathol 1988;19:862–867.

450. Davy CL, Dardick I, Hammond E, Thomas MJ: Relationship of clear cell oncocytoma to mitochondrial-rich (typical) oncocytomas of parotid salivary gland. An ultrastructural study. Oral Surg Oral Med Oral Pathol 1994;77:469–469.

451. Holmes GF, Eisele DW, Rosenthal D, et al: PSA immunoreactivity in a parotid oncocytoma: A diagnostic pitfall in discriminating primary parotid neoplasms from metastatic prostate cancer. Diagn Cytopathol 1998;19:221–225.

452. Hirokawa M, Shimizu M, Manabe T, et al: Oncocytic lipoadenoma of the submandibular gland. Human Pathol 1998;29:410–412.

453. Shick PC, Brannon RB: Oncocytoid artifact of the parotid gland. Oral Surg Oral Med Oral Pathol Oral Radiol Endod 1998;86:720–722.

454. Jahan-Parwar, Huberman RM, Donovan DT, et al: Oncocytic mucoepidermoid carcinoma of the salivary glands. Am J Surg Pathol 1999;23:523–529.

455. Said-Al-Naief N, Ivanov K, Jones M, et al: Granular cell tumor of the parotid. Ann Diagn Pathol 1999;3:35–38.

456. Loke YW: Salivary gland tumors in Malaya. Br J Cancer 1967;21:665–674.

457. Johns ME, Regezi JA, Batsakis JG: Oncocytic neoplasms of salivary glands: An ultrastructural study. Laryngoscope 1977;87:262–271.

458. Bauer WH, Bauer JD: Classification of glandular tumors of salivary glands. Study of 143 cases. Arch Pathol 1953;55:328–346.

459. Zajtchuk JT, Patow CA, Hyams VJ: Cervical heterotopic salivary gland neoplasms: A diagnostic dilemma. Otolaryngol Head Neck Surg 1982;90:178–181.

Ductal Papillomas

460. Ellis GL, Auclair PA: Ductal papillomas. In: Ellis GL, Auclair PL, Gnepp DR (eds): Surgical Pathology of the Salivary Glands. Philadelphia: WB Saunders, 1991:238–251.

461. Neville BW, Damm DD, Weir JC, Fantasia JE: Labial salivary gland tumors. Cancer 1988;61:2113–2116.

462. Ishikawa T, Imada S, Ijuhin N: Intraductal papilloma of the anterior lingual salivary gland. Case report and immunohistochemical study. Int J Oral Maxillofac Surg 1993;22:116–117.

463. Ellis AL, Auclair PL: Atlas of Tumor Pathology: Tumors of the Salivary Glands. Washington, DC: Armed Forces Institute of Pathology, 1996:120–130.

464. Saleh HA, Abbarah T: Intraductal papilloma of the minor salivary gland involving the nasal cavity: Is it a distinct histopathologic entity? Otolaryngol Head Neck Surg 1998;118:850–852.

464a. Nagao T, Sugano I, Matsuzaki O, et al: Intraductal papillary tumors of the major salivary glands: Case reports of benign and malignant variants. Arch Pathol Lab Med 2000;124:291–295.

465. Eversole LR, Sabes WR: Minor salivary gland duct changes due to obstruction. Arch Otolaryngol 1971;94:19–24.

466. Shiotani A, Kawaura M, Tanaka Y, et al: Papillary adenocarcinoma possibly arising from an intraductal papilloma of the parotid gland. J Otorhinolaryngol Relat Spec 1994;56:112–115.

467. Seifert G, Sobin LH, Batsakis JG, et al: Histological Typing of Salivary Gland Tumours, 2nd ed. Berlin: Springer-Verlag, 1991.

468. Abrams AM, Finck FM: Sialadenoma papilliferum: A previously unreported salivary gland tumor. Cancer 1969;24:1057–1063.

469. Mitre BK: Sialadenoma papilliferum: Report of a case and review of literature. J Oral Maxillofac Surg 1986;44:469–474.

470. Regezi JA, Lloyd RV, Zarbo RJ, McClatchey KD: Minor salivary gland tumors. A histologic and immunohistochemical study. Cancer 1985;55:108–115.

471. Waldron CA, El-Mofty SK, Gnepp DR: Tumors of the intraoral minor salivary glands: A demographic and histopathologic study of 426 cases. Oral Surg Oral Med Oral Pathol 1988;66:323–333.

472. Maiorano E, Favia G, Ricco R: Sialadenoma papilliferum: An immunohistochemical study of five cases. J Oral Pathol Med 1996;25:336–342.

473. Markopoulos A, Kayavis I, Papanayotou P: Sialadenoma papilliferum of the oral cavity: Report of a case and review of literature. J Oral Maxillofac Surg 1997;55:1181–1184.

474. Asahina I, Abe M: Sialadenoma papilliferum of the hard palate: A case report and review of literature. J Oral Maxillofac Surg 1997;55:1000–1003.

475. Pimentel MTY, Amado ML, Sarandeses AG: Recurrent sialadenoma papilliferum of the buccal mucosa. J Laryngol Otol 1995;109:787–790.

476. Su JM, Hsu H, Hsu P, et al: Sialadenoma papilliferum of the esophagus. Am J Gastroenterol 1998;93:461–462.

477. White DK, Miller AS, McDaniel RK, et al: Inverted duct papilloma: A distinctive lesion of minor salivary glands. Cancer 1982;49:519–524.

478. Hegarty DJ, Hopper C, Speight PM: Inverted ductal papilloma of minor salivary glands. J Oral Pathol Med 1994;23:334–336.

479. Koutlas IG, Jessurun J, Iamaroon A: Immunohistochemical evaluation and in-situ hybridization in a case of oral inverted ductal papilloma. J Oral Maxillofac Surg 1994;52:503–506.

480. de Sousa SOM, Sesso A, de Araujo NS, de Araujo VC: Inverted ductal papilloma of minor salivary gland origin: Morphological aspects and cytokeratin expression. Eur Arch Otorhinolaryngol 1995;252:370–373.

Mucoepidermoid Carcinoma

481. Pinkston JA, Cole P: Incidence rates of salivary gland tumors: Results from a population-based study. Otolaryngol Head Neck Surg 1999;120:834–840.

482. Ellis GL, Auclair PL: Atlas of Tumor Pathology, Tumors of the Salivary Glands. Washington, DC: Armed Forces Institute of Pathology, 1996:155–175, 353–355.

483. Seifert G: Oralpathologie I: Pathologie der Speicheldrusen. Berlin: Springer-Verlag, 1996:503, 527–550.

484. Cawson RA, Gleeson MJ, Eveson JW: Pathology and Surgery of the Salivary Glands. Oxford: ISIS Medical Media, 1997:117–169.

485. Waldron CA, El-Mofty SK, Gnepp DR: Tumors of the intraoral minor salivary glands: A demographic and histologic study of 426 cases. Oral Surg Oral Med Oral Pathol 1988;66:323–333.

486. Brookstone MS, Huvos AG: Central salivary gland tumors of the maxilla and mandible: A clinicopathologic study of 11 cases with an analysis of the literature. J Oral Maxillofac Surg 1992;50:229–236.

487. Wedell B, Burian P, Dahlenfors R, et al: Cytogenetical observations in a mucoepidermoid carcinoma arising from heterotopic intranodal salivary gland tissue. Oncol Reports 1997;4:515–516.

488. Noda S, Sundaresan S, Mendeloff EN: Tracheal mucoepidermoid carcinoma in a 7-year-old child. Ann Thorac Surg 1998;66:928–929.

489. Krolls SO, Trodahl JN, Boyers RC: Salivary gland lesions in children. A survey of 430 cases. Cancer 1972;30:459–469.

490. Castro EB, Huvos AG, Strong EW, Foote FW Jr: Tumors of the major salivary glands in children. Cancer 1972;29:312–317.

491. Seifert G, Okabe H, Caselitz J: Epithelial salivary gland tumors in children and adolescents. Analysis of 80 cases (Salivary Gland Registry 1965–1984). ORL J Otorhinolaryngol Relat Spec 1986;48:137–149.

492. Spitz MR, Batsakis JG: Major salivary gland carcinoma. Descriptive epidemiology and survival of 498 patients. Arch Otolaryngol 1984;110:45–49.

493. Kaste SC, Hedlund G, Pratt CB: Malignant parotid tumors in patients previously treated for childhood cancer: Clinical and imaging findings in eight cases. AJR Am J Roentgenol 1994;162:655–659.

494. Auclair PL, Ellis GL: Mucoepidermoid carcinoma. In: Ellis GL, Auclair PL, Gnepp DR (eds): Surgical Pathology of the Salivary Glands. Philadelphia: WB Saunders, 1991:269–298.

495. Land CE, Saku T, Hayashi Y, et al: Incidence of salivary gland tumors

among atomic bomb survivors, 1950–1987. Evaluation of radiation-related risk. Rad Res 1996;146:28–36.

495a. Prasannan L, Pu A, Hoff P, et al: Parotid carcinoma as a second malignancy after treatment of childhood acute lymphoblastic leukemia. J Pediatr Hematol Oncol 1999;21:535–538.

496. Spiro RH, Huvos AG, Berk R, Strong EW: Mucoepidermoid carcinoma of salivary origin: A clinicopathologic study of 367 cases. Am J Surg 1978;136:461–468.

497. Hamed G, Shmookler BM, Ellis GL, et al: Oncocytic mucoepidermoid carcinoma of the parotid gland. Arch Pathol Lab Med 1994;118:313–314.

498. Jahan-Parwar B, Huberman RM, Donovan DT: Oncocytic mucoepidermoid carcinoma of the salivary glands. Am J Surg Pathol 1999;23:523–529.

499. Muller S, Barnes L, Goodurn WJ Jr: Sclerosing mucoepidermoid carcinoma of the parotid. Oral Surg Oral Med Oral Pathol Oral Radiol Endod 1997;83:685–690.

500. Seifert G: Mucoepidermoid carcinoma in a salivary duct cyst of the parotid. Contribution to the development of tumours in salivary gland cysts. Pathol Res Pract 1996;192:1211–1217.

501. Auclair PL, Goode RK, Ellis GL: Mucoepidermoid carcinoma of intraoral salivary glands. Evaluation and application of grading criteria in 143 cases. Cancer 1992;69:2021–2030.

502. Batsakis JG, Luna MA: Pathologic consultation: Histopathologic grading of salivary gland neoplasms. I. Mucoepidermoid carcinomas. Ann Otol Rhinol Laryngol 1990;99:835–838.

503. Evans HL: Mucoepidermoid carcinoma of salivary glands: A study of 69 cases with special attention to histologic grading. Am J Clin Pathol 1984;81:696–701.

504. Hicks JM, El-Naggar AK, Flaitz CM, et al: Histologic grading of mucoepidermoid carcinoma of major salivary glands in prognosis and survival: A clinicopathologic and flow cytometric investigation. Head Neck 1995;17:89–95.

505. Goode RK, Auclair PL, Ellis AL: Mucoepidermoid carcinoma of the major salivary glands: Clinical and histologic analysis of 234 cases with evaluation of grading criteria. Cancer 1998;82:1217–1224.

506. Healey WV, Perzin KH, Smith L: Mucoepidermoid carcinoma of salivary gland origin. Classification, clinical pathologic correlation, and results of treatment. Cancer 1970;26:368–388.

507. O'Brien CJ, Soong SJ, Herrera GA, et al: Malignant salivary tumors: Analysis of prognostic factors and survival. Head Neck Surg 1986;9:82–92.

508. Plambeck K, Friedrich RE, Heller D, et al: Mucoepidermoid carcinoma of the salivary glands: Clinical data and follow-up of 52 cases. J Cancer Res Clin Oncol 1996;122:177–180.

509. Suzuki M, Ichimiya I, Matsushita F, et al: Histologic features and prognosis of patients with mucoepidermoid carcinoma of the parotid gland. J Laryngol Otol 1998;112:944–947.

Acinic Cell Carcinoma

510. Seifert G, Sobin LH: Histological Typing of Salivary Gland Tumours. World Health Organization International Histological Classification of Tumours, 2nd ed. New York: Springer-Verlag, 1991.

511. Warner TFCS, Seo IS, Azen EA, et al: Immunocytochemistry of acinic cell carcinomas and mixed tumors of salivary glands. Cancer 1985;56:2221–2227.

512. Chaudhry AP, Cutler LS, Leifer C, et al: Histogenesis of acinic cell carcinoma of the major and minor salivary glands: An ultrastructural study. J Pathol 1986;148:307–320.

513. Dardick I, George D, Jeans D, et al: Ultrastructural morphology and cellular differentiation in acinic cell carcinoma. Oral Surg Oral Med Oral Pathol 1987;63:325–334.

514. Takahashi H, Fujita S, Okabe H, et al: Distribution of tissue markers in acinic cell carcinomas of salivary gland. Pathol Res Pract 1992;188:692–700.

515. Spiro RH: Salivary neoplasms: Overview of a 35-year experience with 2,807 patients. Head Neck Surg 1986;8:177–184.

516. Guimaraes DS, Amaral AP, Prado LF, et al: Acinic cell carcinoma of salivary glands: 16 cases with clinicopathologic correlation. J Oral Pathol Med 1989;18:396–399.

517. Hamper K, Mausch HE, Caselitz J, et al: Acinic cell carcinoma of the salivary glands: The prognostic relevance of DNA cytophotometry in a retrospective study of long duration (1965–1987). Oral Surg Oral Med Oral Pathol 1990;69:68–75.

518. Ellis GL, Auclair PL: Acinic cell adenocarcinoma. In: Ellis GL, Auclair PL, Gnepp DR (eds): Surgical Pathology of the Salivary Glands. Philadelphia: WB Saunders, 1991:81–90.

519. Seifert G, Miehlke A Haubrich J, Chilla R: Diseases of the Salivary Glands: Pathology, Diagnosis, Treatment, Facial Nerve Surgery. Stuttgart: Georg Thieme Verlag, 1986:224–230.

520. Spiro RH, Huvos AG, Strong EW: Acinic cell carcinoma of salivary origin: A clinicopathologic study of 67 cases. Cancer 1978;41:924–935.

521. Kane WJ, McCaffrey TV, Olsen KD, Lewis JE: Primary parotid malignancies: A clinical and pathologic review. Arch Otolaryngol Head Neck Surg 1991;117:307–315.

522. Eveson JW, Cawson RA: Salivary gland tumours. A review of 2410 cases with particular reference to histological types, site, age and sex distribution. J Pathol 1985;146:51–58.

523. Chen S-Y, Brannon RB, Miller AS, et al: Acinic cell adenocarcinoma of minor salivary glands. Cancer 1978;42:678–685.

524. Hiratsuka H, Imamura M, Miyakawa A, et al: Acinic cell carcinoma of minor salivary gland origin. Oral Surg Oral Med Oral Pathol 1987;63:704–708.

525. Perzin KH, LiVolsi VA: Acinic cell carcinoma arising in ectopic salivary gland tissue. Cancer 1980;45:967–972.

526. De Rosa G, Zeppa P, Tranfa F, Bonavolonta G: Acinic cell carcinoma arising in a lacrimal gland: First case report. Cancer 1986;57:1988–1991.

527. Perzin KH, Cantor JO, Johannessen JV: Acinic cell carcinoma arising in nasal cavity. Cancer 1981;47:1818–1822.

528. Abrams AM, Melrose RJ: Acinic cell tumors of minor salivary gland origin. Oral Surg Oral Med Oral Pathol 1978;48:220–233.

529. Ferlito A: Histological classification of larynx and hypopharynx cancers and their clinical implications. Pathologic aspects of 2052 malignant neoplasms diagnosed at the ORL Department of Padua University from 1966 to 1976. Acta Otolaryngol Suppl 1976;342:1–88.

530. Squires JE, Mills SE, Cooper PH, et al: Acinic cell carcinoma: Its occurrence in the laryngotracheal junction after thyroid radiation. Arch Pathol Lab Med 1981;105:266–268.

531. Ansari MA, Marchevsky A, Strick L, Mohsenifar Z: Upper airway obstruction secondary to acinic cell carcinoma of the trachea: Use of Nd:YAG laser. Chest 1996;110:1120–1122.

532. Horowitz Z, Kronenberg J: Acinic cell carcinoma of the trachea. Auris Nasus Larynx (Tokyo) 1994;21:193–195.

533. Moran CA, Suster S, Koss MN: Acinic cell carcinoma of the lung: A clinicopathologic, immunohistochemical, and ultrastructural study of five cases. Am J Surg Pathol 1992;16:1039–1050.

533a. Carrat X, Devars F, Deminiere C, et al: Vallecular acinic cell carcinoma in a 9-year-old girl: Report of an unusual case. Int J Pediatr Otorhinolaryngol 2000;52:61–64.

534. Roncaroli F, Lamovcc J, Zidar A, Eusebi V: Acinic cell–like carcinoma of the breast. Virchows Arch 1996;429:69–74.

535. Fox NM, ReMine WH, Woolner LB: Acinic cell carcinoma of the major salivary glands. Am J Surg 1963;106:860–867.

536. Eneroth C-M, Jakobsson PA, Blanck C: Acinic cell carcinoma of the parotid gland. Cancer 1966;19:1761–1772.

537. Batsakis JG, Chinn EK, Weimert TA, et al: Acinic cell carcinoma: A clinicopathologic study of thirty-five cases. J Laryngol Otol 1979;93:325–340.

538. Spafford PD, Mint DK, Hay J: Acinic cell carcinoma of the parotid gland: Review and management. J Otolaryngol 1991;20:262–266.

539. Castro EK, Huvos AG, Strong EW, Feet JW: Tumors of the major salivary glands in children. Cancer 29; 1972:312–317.

540. Gnepp DR, Schroeder W, Heffner D: Synchronous tumors arising in a single salivary gland. Cancer 1989;63:1219–1224.

541. Mock C, Coleman G, Ree JH, et al: Ataxia telangiectasia and acinic cell carcinoma of the parotid gland. J Surg Oncol 1988;39:133–138.

542. Delaney WE, Balogh K Jr: Carcinoma of the parotid gland associated with benign lymphoepithelial lesion (Mikulicz's disease) in Sjögren's syndrome. Cancer 1966;19:853–860.

543. Jones AO, Lam AH, Martin HC: Acinic cell carcinoma of the parotid in children. Australas Radiol 1997;41:44–48.

543a. Depowski PL, Setzen G, Chui A, et al: Familial occurrence of acinic cell carcinoma of the parotid gland. Arch Pathol Lab Med 1999;123:1118–1120.

544. Chong GC, Beahrs OH, Woolner LB: Surgical management of acinic cell carcinoma of the parotid gland. Surg Gynecol Obstet 1974;138:65–68.

545. Ellis GL, Corio RL: Acinic cell carcinoma: A clinicopathologic analysis of 294 cases. Cancer 1983;52:542–549.

546. Lewis JE, Olsen KD, Weiland LH: Acinic cell carcinoma: Clinicopathologic review. Cancer 1991;67:172–179.
547. Angeles-Angeles A, Caballero-Mendoza E, Tapia-Rangel B, et al: Giant acinic cell adenocarcinoma with papillary-cystic pattern of the parotid gland. Rev Invest Clin 1998;50:245–248.
548. Stanley RJ, Weiland LH, Olsen KD, Pearson BW: Dedifferentiated acinic cell (acinous) carcinoma of the parotid gland. Otolaryngol Head Neck Surg 1988;98:155–161.
549. Abrams AM, Cornyn J, Scofield LS: Acinic cell adenocarcinoma of the major salivary glands: A clinicopathologic study of 77 cases. Cancer 1965;18:1145–1162.
550. Perzin KH, LiVolsi VA: Acinic cell carcinomas arising in salivary glands: A clinicopathologic study. Cancer 1979;44:1434–1457.
551. Batsakis JG, Luna MA, El-Naggar AK: Histopathologic grading of salivary gland neoplasms: II. acinic cell carcinomas. Ann Otol Rhinol Laryngol 1990;99:929–933.
552. Echevarria RA: Ultrastructure of the acinic cell carcinoma and clear cell carcinoma of the parotid gland. Cancer 1967;:20:563–571.
553. Gnepp DR, Hanna IT, Chai L: The clear cell variant of acinic cell carcinoma does exist: A review of four cases [abstract]. Oral Surg Oral Med Oral Pathol Oral Radiol Endod (In press).
554. Michal M, Skalova A, Simpson RH, et al: Well-differentiated acinic cell carcinoma of salivary glands associated with lymphoid stroma. Human Pathol 1997;28:595–600.
555. Stanley RJ, Weiland LH, Olsen KD, Pearson BW: Dedifferentiated acinic cell (acinous) carcinoma of the parotid gland. Otolaryngol Head Neck Surg 1988;98:155–161.
556. Henley JD, Geary WA, Jackson CL, et al: Dedifferentiated acinic cell carcinoma of the parotid gland: A distinct rarely described entity. Hum Pathol 1997;28:869–873.
557. Ferreiro JA, Kochar AS: Parotid acinic cell carcinoma with undifferentiated spindle cell transformation. J Laryngol Otol 1994;108:902–904.
558. Crissman JD, Rosenblatt A: Acinous cell carcinoma of the larynx. Arch Pathol Lab Med 1978;102:233–236.
559. Henley JD, Rehan J, Oda D, et al: Oncocytic metaplastic tumors of salivary gland origin [abstract]. Oral Surg Oral Med Oral Pathol Oral Radiol Endod 1997;84:187–188.
560. Batsakis JG, Wozniak KJ, Regezi JA: Acinous cell carcinoma: A histogenetic hypothesis. J Oral Surg 1977;35:904–906.
561. Gnepp DR: Malignant mixed tumors of the salivary glands: A review. Pathol Annu 1993;28(part 1):279–328.
562. Seifert G, Donath K: Hybrid tumours of salivary. Definition and classification of five rare cases. Eur J Cancer B Oral Oncol 1996;32B:251–259.
563. Ballestin C, Lopez-Carreira M, Lopez JI: Combined acinic cell mucoepidermoid carcinoma of the parotid gland. Report of a case with immunohistochemical study. APMIS 1996;104:99–102.
564. Thackray AC, Lucas RB: Tumors of the Major Salivary Glands. Washington, DC: Armed Forces Institute of Pathology, 1974:81–90.
565. Erlandson RA, Tandler B: Ultrastructure of acinic cell carcinoma of the parotid gland. Arch Pathol 1972;93:130–140.
566. Childers EL, Ellis GL, Auclair PL: An immunohistochemical analysis of anti-amylase antibody reactivity in acinic cell adenocarcinoma. Oral Surg Oral Med Oral Pathol Oral Radiol Endod 1996;81:691–694.
567. Abenoza P, Wick MR: Acinic cell carcinoma of salivary glands. An immunohistochemical study. Lab Invest 1985;52:1A.
568. Skalova A, Leivo I, von Boguslawsky K, Saksela E: Cell proliferation correlates with prognosis in acinic cell carcinomas of salivary gland origin. Immunohistochemical study of 30 cases using the MIB 1 antibody in formalin-fixed paraffin sections. J Pathol 1994;173:13–21.
569. Hellquist HB, Sundelin K, Di Bacco A, et al: Tumour growth fraction and apoptosis in salivary gland acinic cell carcinomas. Prognostic implications of Ki-67 and bcl-2 expression and of in-situ end labeling (TUNEL). J Pathol 1997;181:323–329.
570. El-Naggar AK, Batsakis JG, Luna MA, et al: DNA flow cytometry of acinic cell carcinomas of major salivary glands. J Laryngol Otol 1990;104:410–416.
571. Gustafsson H, Lindholm C, Carlsoo B: DNA cytophotometry of acinic cell carcinoma and its relation to prognosis. Acta Oto-Laryngol 1987;104:370–376.
572. Timon CI, Dardick I, Panzarella T, et al: Acinic cell carcinoma of salivary glands. Arch Otolaryngol Head Neck Surg 1994;120:727–733.

Adenoid Cystic Carcinoma

573. Hyams VJ, Batsakis JG, Micheals L: Nonepidermoid epithelial neoplasms of the upper respiratory tract. In: Atlas of Tumor Pathology, Tumors of the upper respiratory tract and ear, 2nd series. Washington, DC: Armed Forces Institute of Pathology, 1986:83–111.
574. Spiro RH, Huvos AG: Stage means more than grade in adenoid cystic carcinoma. Am J Surg 1992;164:623–628.
575. Conley J, Casler JD: Adenoid Cystic Cancer of the Head and Neck. New York: Thieme Medical Publishers, 1991.
576. Garden AS, Weber RS, Morrison WH, et al: The influence of positive margins and nerve invasion in adenoid cystic carcinoma of the head and neck treated with surgery and radiation. Int J Radiat Oncol Biol Phys 1995;32:619–626.
577. Ellis GL, Auclair PL: Atlas of Tumor Pathology, Tumors of the Salivary Glands. Washington, DC: Armed Forces Institute of Pathology, 1996:203–216.
578. Waldron CA, El-Mofty SK, Gnepp DR: Tumors of the intraoral minor salivary glands: A demographic and histologic study of 426 cases. Oral Surg Oral Med Oral Pathol 1988;66:323–333.
579. Eveson JW, Cawson RA: Salivary gland tumors: A review of 2410 cases with particular reference to histologic types, site, age and sex distribution. J Pathol 1985;146:51–58.
580. Brunori A, Scarano P, Iannetti G, Chiappetta F: Dumbbell tumor of the anterior skull base: Meningioma? No, adenoid cystic carcinoma! Surg Neurol 1998;50:470–474.
581. Coup A, Williamson JMS, Curley JWA: Septal, widely infiltrative and clinically occult adenoid cystic carcinoma of the parotid gland. J Laryngol Otol 1997;111:491–492.
582. Kim KH, Sung MW, Chung PS, et al: Adenoid cystic carcinoma of the head and neck. Arch Otolaryngol Head Neck Surg 1994;120:721–726.
583. Auclair PL, Ellis GL, Gnepp DR, et al: Salivary gland neoplasms: General considerations. In: Ellis GL, Auclair PL, Gnepp DR (eds): Surgical Pathology of the Salivary Glands. Philadelphia: WB Saunders, 1991:144–145.
584. Azar T, Abdul-Karim FW, Tucker HM: Adenoid cystic carcinoma of the trachea. Laryngoscope 1998;108:1297–300.
585. Kleer CG, Oberman HA: Adenoid cystic carcinoma of the breast: Value of histologic grading and proliferative activity. Am J Surg Pathol 1998;22:569–575.
586. Eichhorn JH, Scully RE: "Adenoid cystic" and basaloid carcinomas of the ovary: Evidence for a surface epithelial lineage. A report of 12 cases. Mod Pathol 1995;8:731–740.
587. Urso C, Giannini A, Rubino I, Bondi R: Adenoid cystic carcinoma of sweat glands: Report of two cases. Tumori 1991;77:264–267.
588. Cerar A, Jutersek A, Vidmar S: Adenoid cystic carcinoma of the esophagus: A clinicopathologic study of three cases. Cancer 1991;67:2159–2164.
589. Tsukahara Y, Mori A, Fukuta T, et al: Adenoid cystic carcinoma of Bartholin's gland: A clinical, immunohistochemical and ultrastructural study of a case with regard to its histogenesis. Gynecol Obstet Invest 1991;31:110–113.
590. Cohen RJ, Goldberg RD, Verhaart MJS, Cohen M: Adenoid cyst–like carcinoma of the prostate gland. Arch Pathol Lab Med 1993;117:799–801.
591. Seifert G, Sobin LH, et al: World Health Organization International Histological Classification of Tumours: Histological Typing of Salivary Gland Tumours, 2nd ed. Berlin: Springer-Verlag, 1991.
592. Cheng J, Saku T, Okabe H, Furthmayr H: Basement membranes in adenoid cystic carcinoma. Cancer 1992;2631–2640.
593. Tandler B: Ultrastructure of adenoid cystic carcioma of salivary gland origin. Lab Invest 1971;24:504–512.
594. Yamamoto Y, Saka T, Makimoto K, Takahashi H: Histological changes during progression of adenoid cystic carcinoma. J Laryngol Otol 1992;106:1016–1020.
595. Cheuk W, Chan JKC, Ngan RKC: Dedifferentiation in adenoid cystic carcinoma of salivary gland: An uncommon complication associated with an accelerated clinical course. Am J Surg Pathol 1999;23:465–472.
595a. Moles MA, Avila IR, Archilla AR: Dedifferentiation occurring in adenoid cystic carcinoma of the tongue. Oral Surg Oral Med Oral Pathol Oral Radiol Endod 1999;88:177–180.
596. Chen JC, Gnepp DR, Bedrossian CWM: Adenoid cystic of the salivary glands: An immunohistochemical analysis. Oral Surg Oral Med Oral Pathol 1988;65:316–326.
597. Azumi N, Battifora H: The cellular composition of adenoid cystic carcinoma. An immunohistochemical study. Cancer 1987;60:1589–1598.
597a. Prasad AR, Savera AT, Gown AM, Zarbo RJ: The myoepithelial immunophenotype in 135 benign and malignant salivary gland tumors

other than pleomorphic adenoma. Arch Pathol Lab Med 1999;123:801–806.

598. Castle JT, Thompson LDR, Wenig BM, Kessler HP: Polymorphous low-grade adenocarcinoma (PLGA): A clinicopathological study of 164 cases. J Oral Pathol 1998;27:360.

599. Skalova A, Simpson RH, Lehtonen H, Leivo I: Assessment of proliferative activity using the MIB1 antibody help to distinguish polymorphous low grade adenocarcinoma from adenoid cystic carcinoma of salivary glands. Pathol Res Pract 1997;193:695–703.

600. Gnepp DR, Chen JC, Warren C: Polymorphous low grade adenocarcinoma of minor salivary gland: A immunohistochemical and clinicopathologic study. Am J Surg Pathol 1988;12:461–468.

601. Gnepp DR, Heffner DK: Mucosal origin of sinonasal tract adenomatous neoplasms. Mod Pathol 1989;2:365–371.

602. Krull A, Schwarz R, Engenhart R, et al: European results in neutron therapy of malignant salivary gland tumors. Bull Cancer Radiother 1996;83 Suppl:125S–129S.

603. Prott FJ, Haverkamp U, Willich N, et al: Ten years of fast neutron therapy in Munster. Bull Cancer Radiother 1996;83 Suppl:115S–121S.

603a. Douglas JG, Laramore GE, Austin-Seymour M, et al: Treatment of locally advanced adenoid cystic carcinoma of the head and neck with neutron radiotherapy. Int J Radiat Oncol Biol Phys 2000;46:551–557.

604. Ueta E, Osaki T, Yamamoto T, Yoneda K. Induction of differentiation in maxillary adenoid cystic carcinomas by adoptive immunotherapy in combination with chemoradiotherapy. Oral Oncol 1998;34:105–111.

605. Beckhardt RN, Weber RS, Zane R, et al: Minor salivary gland tumors of the palate: Clinical and pathologic correlates of outcome. Laryngoscope 1995;105:1155–1160.

606. Spiro RH: Distant metastasis in adenoid cystic carcinoma of salivary origin. Am J Surg 1997;174:495–498.

607. Warren CJ, Gnepp DR, Rosenblum BN: Adenoid cystic carcinoma metastasizing before detection of the primary lesion. South Med J 1989;82:1277–1280.

608. Fordice J, Kershaw C, El-Naggar A, Goepfert H: Adenoid cystic carcinoma of the head and neck: Predictors of morbidity and mortality. Arch Otolaryngol Head Neck Surg 1999;125:149–152.

609. Matsuba HM, Spector GJ, Thawley SE, et al: Adenoid cystic salivary gland carcinoma: A histopathologic review of treatment failure patients. Cancer 1986;57:519–524.

610. Szanto PA, Luna MA, Tortoledo E, White RA: Histologic grading of adenoid cystic carcinoma of the salivary glands. Cancer 1984;54:1062–1069.

611. Nascimento AG, Amaral ALP, Pradao LAF, et al: ACC of salivary glands: A study of 61 cases with clinicopathologic correlations. Cancer 1986;57:312–319.

612. Perzin KH, Gullane P, Clairmont AC: ACC arising in salivary glands: A correlation of histologic features and clinical course. Cancer 1978;42:265–282.

613. Huang M, Ma D, Sun K, et al : Factors influencing survival rate in adenoid cystic carcinoma of the salivary glands. Int J Oral Maxillofac Surg 1997;26:435–439.

614. Franzen G, Nordgard S, Boysen M, et al: DNA content in adenoid cystic carcinomas. Head Neck 1995;17:49–55.

615. Franchi A, Gallo O, Bocciolini C, et al: Reduced E-cadherin expression correlates with unfavorable prognosis in adenoid cystic carcinoma of salivary glands of the oral cavity. Am J Clin Pathol 1999;111:43–50.

616. Yamamoto Y, Itoh T, Saka T, Takahashi H: Nucleolar organizer regions in adenoid cystic carcinoma of the salivary glands. Eur Arch Otorhinolaryngol 1995;252:176–180.

617. Vuhahula EA, Nikai H, Ogawa I, et al: Correlation between argyrophilic nucleolar organizer region (AgNOR) counts and histologic grades with respect to biologic behavior of salivary adenoid cystic carcinoma. J Oral Pathol Med 1995;24:437–442.

618. Xie X, Nordgard S, Halvorsen TB, et al: Prognostic significance of nucleolar organizer regions in adenoid cystic carcinomas of the head and neck. Arch Otolaryngol Head Neck Surg 1997;123:615–620.

619. Papadaki H, Finkelstein SD, Kounelis S, et al: The role of p53 mutation and protein expression in primary and recurrent adenoid cystic carcinoma. Human Pathol 1996;27:567–572.

Polymorphous Low-Grade Adenocarcinomas

620. Freedman PD, Lumerman H: Lobular carcinoma of intraoral minor salivary gland origin: Report of twelve cases. Oral Surg Oral Med Oral Pathol 1983;56:157–165.

621. Batsakis JG, Pinkston GR, Luna MA, et al: Adenocarcinomas of the oral cavity: A clinicopathologic study of terminal duct carcinomas. J Laryngol Otol 1983;97:825–835.

622. Evans HL, Batsakis JG: Polymorphous low-grade adenocarcinomas of minor salivary glands: A study of 14 cases of a distinctive neoplasm. Cancer 1984;53:935–942.

623. Ellis GL, Auclair PL: Atlas of Tumor Pathology, Tumors of the Salivary Glands. Washington, DC: Armed Forces Institute of Pathology, 1996:216–228, 360–361.

624. Gnepp DR, Chen JC, Warren C: Polymorphous low-grade adenocarcinoma of minor salivary gland: An immunohistochemical and clinicopathologic study. Am J Surg Pathol 1988;12:461–468.

625. Gnepp DR, El-Mofty S: Polymorphous low-grade adenocarcinoma: Glial fibrillary acidic protein staining in the differential diagnosis with cellular mixed tumors. Oral Surg Oral Med Oral Pathol Oral Radiol Endod 1997;83:691–695.

626. Skalova A, Simpson RHW, Lehtonen H, Leivo I: Assessment of proliferative activity using the MIB1 antibody helps to distinguish polymorphous low grade adenocarcinoma from adenoid cystic carcinoma of salivary glands. Pathol Res Pract 1997;193:695–703.

627. Ritland F, Lubensky I, LiVolsi VA: Polymorphous low-grade adenocarcinoma of the parotid salivary gland. Arch Pathol Lab Med 1993;117:1261–1263.

628. Waldron CA, El-Mofty SK, Gnepp DR: Tumors of the intraoral minor salivary glands: A demographic and histologic study of 426 cases. Oral Surg Oral Med Oral Pathol 1988;66:323–333.

629. Wenig BM, Harpaz N, DelBridge C: Polymorphous low-grade adenocarcinoma of seromucous glands of the nasopharynx: A report of a case and a discussion of the morphologic and immunohistochemical features. Am J Clin Pathol 1989;92:104–109.

630. Perez-Ordonez B, Linkov I, Huvos AG: Polymorphous low-grade adenocarcinoma of minor salivary glands: A study of 17 cases with emphasis on cell differentiation. Histopathol 1998;32:521–529.

631. Blanchaert RH, Ord RA, Kumar D: Polymorphous low-grade adenocarcinoma of the sublingual gland. Int J Oral Maxillofac Surg 1998;27:115–117.

632. Castle JT, Thompson LDR, Frommelt RA, et al: Polymorphous low grade adenocarcinoma (PLGA): A clinicopathologic study of 164 cases. Cancer 1999;86:207–219.

633. Kotliar S, Kemp B, Luna MA, et al: Terminal duct adenocarcinoma of the parotid gland: A report of twelve cases and review of the literature. Mod Pathol 1994;7:100A.

634. Miliauskas JR: Polymorphous low-grade (terminal duct) adenocarcinoma of the parotid gland. Histopathol 1991;19:555–557.

635. Haba R, Kobayashi S, Miki H, et al: Polymorphous low-grade adenocarcinoma of submandibular gland origin. Acta Patholog Jpn 1993;43:774–777.

636. Lloreta J, Serrano S, Corominas JM, et al: Polymorphous low-grade adenocarcinoma arising in the nasal cavities with an associated undifferentiated carcinoma. Ultrastruct Pathol 1995;19:365–370.

637. Merchant WJ, Cook MG, Eveson JW: Polymorphous low-grade adenocarcinoma of the parotid gland. Br J Oral Maxillofac Surg 1996;34:328–330.

638. Puxeddu R, Puxeddu P, Parodo G, Faa G: Polymorphous low-grade adenocarcinoma of the parotid gland. Eur J Morphol 1998;36 suppl:262–266.

639. Barak AP, Grobbel MA, Rabaja DR: Polymorphous low-grade adenocarcinoma of the parotid gland. Am J Otolaryngol 1998;19:322–324.

640. Vincent SD, Hammond HL, Finkelstein MW: Clinical and therapeutic features of polymorphous low-grade adenocarcinoma. Oral Surg Oral Med Oral Pathol 1994;77:41–47.

641. Ellis GL, Auclair PL: Atlas of Tumor Pathology: Tumors of the Salivary Glands. Washington, DC: Armed Forces Institute of Pathology, 1996:216–228.

642. Chuo N, Ping-Kuan K, Dryja TP: Histopathological classification of 272 primary epithelial tumors of the lacrimal gland. Chinese Med J 1992;105:481–485.

643. Tortoledo ME, Luna MA, Batsakis JG: Carcinomas ex pleomorphic adenoma and malignant mixed tumors. Arch Otolaryngol 1984;110:172–176.

644. Clayton JR, Pogrel A, Regezi JA: Simultaneous multifocal polymorphous low-grade adenocarcinoma: Report of two cases. Oral Surg Oral Med Oral Pathol Oral Radiol Endod 1995;80:71–77.

645. Minic AJ: Polymorphous low-grade adenocarcinoma of the palate in a 16 year old male patient. Br J Oral Maxillofac Surg 1996;34:540–541.

645a. Lengyel E, Somogyi A, Godery M, et al: Polymorphons low-grade adenocarcinoma of the nasopharynx. Case report and review of the literature. Strahlenther Onkol 2000;176:40–42.

646. Cleveland DB, Cosgrove MM, Martin SE: Tyrosine-rich crystalloids in a fine needle aspirate of a polymorphous low grade adenocarcinoma of a minor salivary gland: A case report. Acta Cytol 1994;38:247–251.

647. Raubenheimer EJ, van Heerden WFP, Thein T: Tyrosine-rich crystalloids in a polymorphous low-grade adenocarcinoma. Oral Med Oral Surg Oral Pathol 1990;70:480–482.

648. Prasad AR, Gown AM, Zarbo RJ: Novel smooth muscle specific proteins in salivary gland tumors. Am J Clin Pathol 1998;109:122A.

648a. Araujo V, Sousa S, Jaeger M, et al: Characterization of the cellular component of polymorphous low-grade adenocarcinoma by immunohistochemistry and electron microscopy. Oral Oncol 1999;35:164–172.

649. Vargus H, Sudilovsky D, Kaplan MJ, et al: Mixed tumor, polymorphous low-grade adenocarcinoma and adenoid cystic carcinoma of the salivary gland: Pathogenic implications and differential diagnosis by Ki-67 (MIB1), BCL2, and S100 immunohistochemistry. Appl Immunohistochem 1997;5:8–16.

650. Mills SE, Garland TA, Allen MS: Low-grade papillary adenocarcinoma of palatal salivary gland origin. Am J Surg Pathol 1984;8:367–374.

650a. Nicol KK, Iskandar SS: Lobular carcinoma of the breast metastatic to the oral cavity mimicking polymorphous low-grade adenocarcinoma of the minor salivary glands. Arch Pathol Lab Med 2000;124:157–159.

651. Tanaka F, Wada H, Inui K, et al: Pulmonary metastasis of polymorphous low-grade adenocarcinoma of the minor salivary gland. Thorac Cardiovasc Surg 1995;43:178–180.

652. Thomas KM, Cumberworth VL, McEwan J: Orbital and skin metastases in a polymorphous low grade adenocarcinoma of the salivary gland. J Laryngol Otol 1995;109:1222–1225.

653. Pelkey TJ, Mills SE: Histologic transformation of polymorphous low-grade adenocarcinoma of salivary gland. Am J Clin Pathol 1999;111:785–791.

Clear Cell Carcinoma

654. Milchgrub S, Gnepp DR, Vuitch FM, et al: Hyalinizing clear cell carcinoma of the salivary gland. Am J Surg Pathol 1994;18:74–82.

655. Shrestha P, Yang LT, Liu BL, et al: Clear cell carcinoma of salivary glands: Immuno-histochemical evaluation of clear tumor cells. Anticancer Res 1994;14:825–836.

656. Ellis AL, Auclair PL: Atlas of Tumor Pathology, Tumors of the Salivary Glands. Washington, DC: Armed Forces Institute of Pathology, 1996:268–289.

657. Donath K, Seifert G, Schmitz R: Zur Ultrastruktur des tubularen Speichelgangcarcinoms: Epithelial-myoepitheliales Schaltstückcarcinom. Virchows Arch A Pathol Anat Histopathol 1972;356:16–31.

658. Corio RL, Sciubba JJ, Brannon RB, Batsakis JG: Epithelial-myoepithelial carcinoma of intercalated duct origin: A clinicopathologic and ultrastructural assessment of sixteen cases. Oral Surg Oral Med Oral Pathol 1982;53:280–287.

659. Daley TD, Wysocki GP, Smout MS, Slinger RP: Epithelial-myoepithelial carcinoma of salivary glands. Oral Surg Oral Med Oral Pathol 1984;57:512–519.

660. Seifert G: Are adenomyoepitheliomas of the breast and epithelial-myoepithelial carcinoma of the salivary glands identical tumors? Virchows Arch 1998;433:285–287.

661. Morinaga S, Hashimoto S, Tezuka F: Epithelial-myoepithelial carcinoma of the parotid gland in a child. Acta Pathol Jpn 1992;42:358–363.

662. Brocheriou C, Auriol M, de Roquancourt A, et al: Carcinome epithelial-myoepithelial des glandes salivaires. Etude de 15 observations et revue de la litterature. Ann Pathol 1991;11:316–325.

663. Wilson RW, Moran CA: Epithelial-myoepithelial carcinoma of the lung: immunohistochemical and ultrastructural observations and review of the literature. Hum Pathol 1997;28:631–635.

664. Shanks JH, Hasleton PS, Curry A, et al: Bronchial epithelial-myoepithelial carcinoma. Histopathol 1998;33:87–94.

665. Ostrowski ML, Font R, Halpern J, et al: Clear cell epithelial-myoepithelial carcinoma arising in pleomorphic adenoma of the lacrimal gland. J Ophthalmol 1994;101:925–930.

666. Fonseca I, Soares J: Epithelial-myoepithelial carcinoma of the salivary glands. A study of 22 cases. Virchows Arch A Pathol Anat Histopathol 1993;422:389–396.

667. Michal M, Skalova A, Simpson RHW, et al: Clear cell malignant myoepithelioma of the salivary glands. Histopathol 1996;28:309–315.

667a. Fonseca I, Felix A, Soares J: Dedifferentiation in salivary gland carcinomas [letter]. Am J Surg Pathol 2000;24:469–471.

667b. Rezende RB, Drachenberg CB, Kumar D, et al: Differential diagnosis between monomorphic clear cell adenocarcinoma of salivary glands and renal (clear) cell carcinoma. Am J Surg Pathol 1999;23:1532–1538.

668. Stiernberg CM, Batsakis JG, Bailey BJ, Clark WD: Epithelial-myoepithelial carcinoma of the parotid gland. Otolaryngol Head Neck Surg 1986;94:240–242.

669. Batsakis JG, El-Naggar AK, Luna MA: Pathology consultation: Hyalinizing clear cell carcinoma of salivary origin. Ann Otol Rhinol Laryngol 1994;103:746–748.

670. Simpson RHW, Sarsfield PTL, Clarke T, et al: Clear cell carcinoma of minor salivary glands. Histopathol 1990;17:433–438.

671. Tang SK, Wan SK, Chan JKC: Hyalinizing clear cell carcinoma of salivary gland: Report of a case with multiple recurrences over 12 years [letter]. Am J Surg Pathol 1995;19:240–242.

672. Berho M, Huvos AG: Central hyalinizing clear cell carcinoma of the mandible and the maxilla a clinicopathologic study of two cases with an analysis of the literature. Hum Pathol 1999;30:101–105.

Salivary Duct Carcinoma

673. Kleinsasser O, Klein HJ, Hubner G: Spiechelgangcarcinoma: Ein den Milchgangcarcinomen der brustdruse Analogiegruppe von Speicheldrusentumoren. Arch Klin Exp Ohre Nasen Kehlkopfheilkd 1968;192:100–115.

674. Brandwein MS, Jagirdar J, Patil J, et al: Salivary duct carcinoma (cribriform salivary carcinoma of excretory ducts). A clinicopathologic and immunohistochemical study of 12 cases. Cancer 1990;65:2307–2314.

675. Lewis JE, McKinney BC, Weiland LH: Salivary duct carcinoma: Clinicopathologic and immunohistochemical review of 26 cases. Cancer 1996;77:223–230.

676. Zohar Y, Shem-Tov, Gal R: Salivary duct carcinoma in major and minor salivary glands: A clinicopathological analysis of four cases. J Craniomaxillofac Surg 1988;16:320–323.

677. Theaker JM: Extramammary Paget's disease of the oral mucosa with in-situ carcinoma of minor salivary gland ducts. Am J Surg Pathol 1988;12:890–895.

678. Yoshimura Y, Tawara K, Yoshigi J, Nagaoka S: Concomitant salivary duct carcinoma of a minor buccal salivary gland and papillary cystadenoma lymphomatosum of a cervical lymph node: Report of a case and review of the literature. J Oral Maxillofac Surg 1995;53:448–453.

679. Pesce C, Colacino R, Buffa P: Duct carcinoma of the minor salivary glands: A case report. J Laryngol Otol 1986;10:611–613.

680. Epivatianos A, Dimitrakopoulos J, Trigonidis G: Intraoral salivary duct carcinoma: A clinicopathological study of four cases and review of the literature. Ann Dent 1995;54:36–40.

681. Ferlito A, Gale N, Hvala H: Laryngeal salivary duct carcinoma. J Laryngol Otol 1981;95:731–738.

682. Kumar RV, Kini L, Bhargava AK, et al: Salivary duct carcinoma. J Surg Oncol 1993;54:193–198.

683. Barnes L, Rao U, Krause J, Contis L, et al: Salivary duct carcinoma. Part I. A clinicopathologic evaluation and DNA image analysis of 13 cases with review of the literature. Oral Surg Oral Med Oral Pathol 1994;78:64–73.

684. Delgado R, Klimstra D, Albores Saavedra J: Low grade salivary duct carcinoma. A distinctive variant with a low grade histology and a predominant intraductal growth pattern. Cancer 1996;78:958–967.

685. Tatemoto Y, Ohno A, Osaki T: Low malignant intraductal carcinoma on the hard palate: A variant of salivary duct carcinoma? Eur J Cancer B Oral Oncol 1996;32:275–277.

686. Delgado R, Vuitch F, Albores-Saavedra J: Salivary duct carcinoma. Cancer 1993;72:1503–1512.

687. Anderson C, Muller R, Piorkowski R, et al: Intraductal carcinoma of major salivary gland. Cancer 1992;69:609–614.

688. Chen KTK: Intraductal carcinoma of the minor salivary glands. J Laryngol Otol 1983;97:189–191.

689. Tortoledo ME, Luna MA, Batsakis JG: Carcinoma–ex-pleomorphic adenoma and malignant mixed tumor. Arch Otolaryngol 1984;110:172–176.

690. Afzelius LE, Cameron WR, Svensson C: Salivary duct carcinoma: A clinicopathologic study. Head Neck 1987;9:151–156.

691. Fayemi AO, Toker C: Salivary duct carcinoma. Arch Otolaryngol 1974;99:366–368.

692. Hui KK, Batsakis JG, Luna MA, et al: Salivary duct adenocarcinoma: A high grade malignancy. J Laryngol Otol 1986;100:105–114.

693. Barnes L, Rao U, Contis L, et al: Salivary duct carcinoma. Part II. Immunohistochemical evaluation of 13 cases for estrogen and progester-

one receptors, cathepsin D, and c-erbB-2 protein. Oral Surg Oral Med Oral Pathol 1994;78:74–80.

694. Martinez-Barba E, Cortes-Guardiola JA, Minguela-Puras A, et al: Salivary duct carcinoma: Clinicopathological and immunohistochemical studies. J Craniomaxillofac Surg 1997;25:328–334.

695. Hellquest HB, Karlsson MG, Nilsson C: Salivary duct carcinoma: A highly aggressive salivary gland tumour with overexpression of c-erbB-2. J Pathol 1994;172:35–44.

696. McKinney B, Lewis J, Weiland L, et al: Salivary duct carcinoma. Clinicopathologic and immunohistochemical review of 26 cases. Mod Pathol 1994;7:100A.

697. Ockner DM, Mills SE, Swanson PE, Wick MR: Salivary duct carcinoma: An immunohistologic comparison with invasive ductal carcinoma of the breast. Mod Pathol 1994;7:100A.

698. Henley J, Seo IF, Dayan D, Gnepp DR: Sarcomatoid salivary duct carcinoma of the parotid gland. Hum Pathol 2000;33:208–213.

Undifferentiated Carcinoma

699. Eversole LR, Gnepp DR, Eversole GM: Undifferentiated carcinoma. In: Ellis GL, Auclair PL, Gnepp DR (eds): Surgical Pathology of the Salivary Glands. Philadelphia: WB Saunders, 1991:422–440.

700. Seifert G, Sobin LH: Histological Typing of Salivary Gland Tumours. World Health Organization International Histological Classification of Tumours, 2nd ed. New York: Springer Verlag, 1991.

701. Koss LC, Spiro RH, Hajdu S: Small cell (oat cell) carcinoma of minor salivary gland origin. Cancer 1972;30:737–741.

702. Gnepp DR, Corio RL, Brannon RB: Small cell carcinoma of the major salivary glands. Cancer 1986;58:705–714.

703. Kraemer BB, Mackay B, Batsakis JG: Small cell carcinomas of the parotid gland: A clinicopathologic study of three cases. Cancer 1983;52:2115–2121.

704. Yaku Y, Kanda T, Yoshihara T, et al: Undifferentiated carcinoma of the parotid gland. Virchows Arch A Path Anat Histopathol 1983;401:89–97.

705. Gnepp DR, Wick MR: Small cell carcinoma of the major salivary glands. An immunohistochemical study. Cancer 1990;66:185–192.

706. Ellis GL, Auclair PL: Atlas of Tumor Pathology: Tumors of the Salivary Glands. Washington, DC: Armed Forces Institute of Pathology, 1996:311–318.

707. Rollins CE, Yost BA, Costa MJ, Vogt PJ: Squamous differentiation in small-cell carcinoma of the parotid gland. Arch Pathol Lab Med 1995;119:183–185.

708. Hui KK, Luna MA, Batsakis JG, et al: Undifferentiated carcinomas of the major salivary glands. Oral Surg Oral Med Oral Pathol 1990;69:76–83.

709. Scher RL, Feldman PS, Levine PA: Small-cell carcinoma of the parotid gland with neuroendocrine features. Arch Otolaryngol Head Neck Surg 1988;114:319–321.

710. Huntrakoon M: Neuroendocrine carcinoma of the parotid gland: A report of two cases with ultrastructural and immunohistochemical studies. Hum Pathol 1987;18:1212–1217.

711. Hayashi Y, Nagamine S, Yanagawa T, et al: Small cell undifferentiated carcinoma of the minor salivary gland containing exocrine, neuroendocrine, and squamous cells. Cancer 1987;60:1583–1588.

712. Brown DH, Illman J, MacMillan C: Small-cell anaplastic carcinoma of the parotid gland. J Otolaryngol 1997;26:332–334.

713. Hisa Y, Tatemoto K: Bilateral parotid gland metastases as the initial manifestation of a small cell carcinoma of the lung. Am J Otolaryngol 1998;19:140–143.

714. Chan JK, Suster S, Wenig BM, et al: Cytokeratin 20 immunoreactivity distinguishes Merkel cell (primary cutaneous neuroendocrine) carcinomas and salivary gland small cell carcinomas from small cell carcinomas of various sites. Am J Surg Pathol 1997;21:226–234.

715. Deb RA, Desai SB, Amonkar PP, et al: Primary primitive neuroectodermal tumour of the parotid gland. Histopathol 1998;33:375–378.

716. Nicod JL: Carcinoide de la parotide. Bull Assoc Franc L'Etude Cancer 1958;45:214–222.

717. Eusebi V, Pileri S, Usellini L, et al: Primary endocrine carcinoma of the parotid salivary gland associated with a lung carcinoid: A possible new association. J Clin Pathol 1982;35:611–616.

718. Gnepp DR, Ferlito A, Hyams: Primary anaplastic small cell (oat cell) carcinoma of the larynx: Review of the literature and report of 18 cases. Cancer 1983;51:1731–1745.

719. Nagao K, Matsuzak O, Saiga H et al: Histopathologic studies of undifferentiated carcinoma of the parotid gland. Cancer 1982;50:1572–1579.

720. Seifert G, Miehlke A, Haubrich J, Chilla R: Diseases of the Salivary Glands: Pathology, Diagnosis, Treatment, Facial Nerve Surgery. Stuttgart: Georg Thieme Verlag, 1986:171.

721. Moore JG, Bocklage T: Fine-needle aspiration biopsy of large-cell undifferentiated carcinoma of the salivary glands: Presentation of two cases, literature review, and differential cytodiagnosis of high-grade salivary gland malignancies. Diagn Cytopathol 1998;19:44–50.

722. Donath K, Seifert G, Sunder-Plassmann E: Ultrastrukturelle Subklassifikation undifferenzierter Parotiscarcinome: Analyse von 11 Fallen. J Cancer Res Clin Oncol 1982;103:75–92.

723. Blanck C, Backstrom A, Eneroth C-M, et al: Poorly differentiated solid parotid carcinoma. Acta Radiol 1974;13:17–31.

724. Balogh K, Wolbarsht RL, Federman M, et al: Carcinoma of the parotid gland with osteoclastlike giant cells. Immunohistochemical and ultrastructural observations. Arch Pathol Lab Med 1985;109:756–761.

725. Lopez JI, Alfaro J, Ballestin C: Undifferentiated carcinoma of parotid gland. J Clin Pathol 1991;44:432–433.

726. Soini Y, Kamel D, Nuorva K, et al: Low p53 protein expression in salivary gland tumours compared with lung carcinomas. Virchows Arch A Path Anat Histopathol 1992;421:415–420.

727. Takata T, Caselitz J, Seifert G: Undifferentiated tumours of salivary glands. Immunocytochemical investigations and differential diagnosis of 22 cases. Pathol Res Pract 1987;182:161–168.

728. Auclair PL, Langloss JM, Weiss SW, et al: Sarcomas and sarcomatoid neoplasms of the major salivary gland regions. Cancer 1986;58:1305–1315.

729. Lloreta J, Serrano S, Corominas JM, et al: Polymorphous low-grade adenocarcinoma arising in the nasal cavities with an associated undifferentiated carcinoma. Ultrastructural Pathol 1995;19:365–370.

730. Henley JD, Geary WA, Jackson CL, et al: Dedifferentiated acinic cell carcinoma of the parotid gland: A distinct rarely described entity. Hum Pathol 1997;28:869–873.

731. Garland TA, Innes DJ Jr, Fechner RE: Salivary duct carcinoma: An analysis of four cases with review of literature. Am J Clin Pathol 1984;81:436–441.

732. Donath K, Seifert G, Lentrodt J: The embryonal carcinoma of the parotid gland: A rare example of an embryonal tumor. Virchows Arch A Path Anat Histopathol 1984;403:425–440.

733. Hilderman WC, Gordon JS, Large HL Jr, et al: Malignant lymphoepithelial lesion with carcinomatous component apparently arising in parotid gland: A malignant counterpart of benign lymphoepithelial lesion? Cancer 1962;15:606–610.

734. Arthaud JB: Anaplastic parotid carcinoma ("malignant lymphoepithelial lesion") in seven Alaskan natives. Am J Clin Pathol 1972;57:275–286.

735. Krishnamurthy S, Lanier AP, Dohan P, et al: Salivary gland cancer in Alaskan natives, 1966–1980. Hum Pathol 1987;18:986–996.

736. Saw D, Lau WH, Ho JH, et al: Malignant lymphoepithelial lesion of the salivary gland. Hum Pathol 1986;17:914–923.

737. Borg MF, Benjamin CS, Morton RP, et al: Malignant lympho-epithelial lesion of the salivary gland: A case report and review of the literature. Australas Radiol 1993;37:288–291.

738. Merrick Y, Albeck H, Nielsen NH, et al: Familial clustering of salivary gland carcinoma in Greenland. Cancer 1986;57:2097–2102.

739. Autio-Harmainen H, Paakko P, Alavaikko M, et al: Familial occurrence of malignant lymphoepithelial lesion of the parotid gland in a Finnish family with dominantly inherited trichoepithelioma. Cancer 1988;61:161–166.

740. Worley NK, Daroca PJ Jr: Lymphoepithelial carcinoma of the minor salivary gland. Arch Otolaryngol Head Neck Surg 1997;123:638–640.

741. Gravanis MB, Giansanti JS: Malignant histopathologic counterpart of the benign lymphoepithelial lesion. Cancer 1970;26:1332–1342.

742. Batsakis JG, Bernacki EG, Rice DH, et al: Malignancy and the benign lymphoepithelial lesion. Laryngoscope 1975;85:389–399.

743. Saemundsen AK, Albeck H, Hansen JP, et al: Epstein-Barr virus in nasopharyngeal and salivary gland carcinomas of Greenland Eskimos. Br J Cancer 1982;46:721–728.

744. Leung SY, Chung LP, Yuen ST, et al: Lymphoepithelial carcinoma of the salivary gland: In-situ detection of Epstein-Barr virus. J Clin Pathol 1995;48:1022–1027.

745. Nagao T, Ishida Y, Sugano I, et al: Epstein-Barr virus–associated undifferentiated carcinoma with lymphoid stroma of the salivary gland in Japanese patients. Comparison with benign lymphoepithelial lesion. Cancer 1996;78:695–703.

746. Sheen TS, Tsai CC, Ko JY, et al: Undifferentiated carcinoma of the major salivary glands. Cancer 1997;80:357–363.

747. Gallo O, Santucci M, Calzolari A, et al: Epstein-Barr virus (EBV) infection and undifferentiated carcinoma of the parotid gland in Caucasian patients. Acta Otolaryngol (Stockh) 1994;114:572–575.

748. Kott ET, Goepfert H, Ayala AG, et al: Lymphoepithelial carcinoma (malignant lymphoepithelial lesion) of the salivary glands. Arch Otolaryngol 1984;110:50–53.

749. Redondo C, Garcia A, Vazquez F: Malignant lymphoepithelial lesion of the parotid gland: Poorly differentiated squamous cell carcinoma with lymphoid stroma. Cancer 1981;48:289–292.

750. Bosch JD, Kudryk WH, Johnson GH: The malignant lymphoepithelial lesion of the salivary glands. J Otolaryngol 1988;17:187–190.

751. Povah WB, Beecroft W, Hodson I, et al: Malignant lympho-epithelial lesion: The Manitoba experience. J Otolaryngol 1984;13:153–159.

Sebaceous Neoplasms

752. Gnepp DR, Brannon R: Sebaceous neoplasms of salivary gland origin, report of 21 cases. Cancer 1984;53:2155–2170.

753. Gnepp DR: Sebaceous neoplasms of salivary gland origin: A review. Pathol Annu 1983;18(Part 1):71–102.

754. Linhartova A: Sebaceous glands in salivary gland tissue. Arch Pathol 1974;98:320–324.

755. Gnepp DR, Sporck FT: Lymphoepithelial cyst with sebaceous differentiation (cystic sebaceous lymphadenoma). Am J Clin Pathol 1980; 74:683–687.

756. Auclair PL, Ellis GL, Gnepp DR: Other benign epithelial neoplasms. In: Ellis GL, Auclair PL, Gnepp DR (eds): Surgical Pathology of the Salivary Glands. Philadelphia: WB Saunders, 1991:252–267.

757. Martinez-Madrigal F, Bosq J, Casiraghi O: Major salivary glands. In: Sternberg SS (ed): Histology for Pathologists, 2nd ed. Philadelphia: Lippincott-Raven 1997:405–429.

758. Neville BW, Damm DD, Allen CM, Bouquot JE: Oral and Maxillofacial Pathology. Philadelphia: WB Saunders, 1995:5–6.

759. Moll ME, Billeret-Lebranchu V, Piquet JJ, Lecomte-Houcke M: Une tumeur parotidienne inhabituelle [An uncommon tumor of parotid gland]. Ann Pathol 1998;18:437–438.

760. Rulon DB, Helwig EB: Multiple sebaceous neoplasms of the skin: An association with multiple visceral carcinomas, especially of the colon. Am J Clin Pathol 1973;60:745–753.

761. Housholder MS, Zeligman I: Sebaceous neoplasms with visceral carcinomas. Arch Derm 1980;116:61–64.

762. Seifert G, Miehlke A, Haubrich J, Chilla R: Diseases of the Salivary Glands: Pathology, Diagnosis, Treatment, Facial Nerve Surgery. Stuttgart: Georg Thieme Verlag, 1986:171, 215, 216.

763. Boniuk M, Zimmerman LE: Sebaceous carcinoma of the eyelid, eyebrow, caruncle, and orbit. Trans Am Acad Ophthal Otolaryngol 1968;72:619–642.

764. Uchibori N, Yoshizaki S, Shamoto M, Takeuchi J: Epidermoid carcinoma arising in parotid adenolymphomatous lesion with microdeposit of amyloid substance. Acta Pathol Jpn 1983;33:141–146.

Cystadenoma and Cystadenocarcinoma

765. Waldron CA, El-Mofty SK, Gnepp DR: Tumors of the intraoral minor salivary glands: A demographic and histopathologic study of 426 cases. Oral Surg Oral Med Oral Pathol 1988;66:323–333.

766. Auclair PL, Ellis GL, Gnepp DR: Other benign epithelial neoplasms. In: Ellis GL, Auclair PL, Gnepp DR (eds): Surgical Pathology of the Salivary Glands. Philadelphia: WB Saunders, 1991:252–268.

767. Ellis GL, Auclair PL: Atlas of Tumor Pathology: Tumors of the Salivary Glands. Washington, DC: Armed Forces Institute of Pathology, 1996:115–122.

768. van der Wal JE, Leverstein H, Snow GB, et al: Parotid gland tumors: Histologic reevaluation and reclassification of 478 cases. Head Neck 1998;20:204–207.

769. Brandwein M, Huvos A: Laryngeal oncocytic cystadenomas. Eight cases and a literature review. Arch Otolaryngol Head Neck Surg 1995;121:1302–1305.

770. Pahl S, Puschel W, Federspil P: Cystadenoma of the parotid with unusual prominent lymphoid stroma. J Laryngol Otol 1997;111:883–885.

771. Ellis GL, Auclair PL Gnepp DR, Goode RK: Other malignant epithelial neoplasms. In: Ellis GL, Auclair PL, Gnepp DR (eds): Surgical Pathology of the Salivary Glands. Philadelphia: WB Saunders, 1991:464–470.

772. Foss RD, Ellis GL, Auclair PL: Salivary gland cystadenocarcinomas: A clinicopathologic study of 57 cases. Am J Surg Pathol 1996;20:1440–1447.

773. Ellis GL, Auclair PL: Atlas of Tumor Pathology: Tumors of the Salivary Glands. Washington, DC: Armed Forces Institute of Pathology, 1996:289–296.

774. Mills SE, Garland TA, Allen MS Jr: Low-grade papillary adenocarcinoma of palatal salivary gland origin. Am J Surg Pathol 1984;8:367–374.

775. Slootweg PJ: Low-grade adenocarcinoma of the oral cavity: Polymorphous or papillary? J Oral Pathol Med 1993;22:327–330.

776. Chen XM: Papillary cystadenocarcinoma of the salivary glands: Clinicopathologic analysis of 22 cases [in Chinese]. Chung Hua Kou Chiang Hsueh Tsa Chih 1990;25:102–104.

777. Mostofi R, Wood RS, Christison W, Talerman A: Low-grade papillary adenocarcinoma of minor salivary glands: Case report and literature review. Oral Surg Oral Med Oral Pathol 1992;73:591–595.

778. Danford M, Eveson JW, Flood TR: Papillary cystadenocarcinoma of the sublingual gland presenting as a ranula. Br J Oral Maxillofac Surg 1992;30:270–272.

779. Pollett A, Perez-Ordonez B, Jordan RCK, Davidson MJ: High-grade papillary cystadenocarcinoma of the tongue. Histopath 1997;31:185–188.

780. Slootweg PJ, Muller H: Low-grade adenocarcinoma of the oral cavity: A comparison between the terminal duct and the papillary type. J Craniomaxillofac Surg 1987;15:359–364.

Primary Squamous Cell Carcinoma

781. Batsakis JG, McClatchey KD, Johns M, et al: Primary squamous cell carcinoma of the parotid gland. Arch Otolaryngol 1976;102:355–357.

782. Batsakis JG: Primary squamous cell carcinoma of the major salivary glands. Ann Otol Rhinol Laryngol 1983;92:97–98.

783. Gaughan RK, Olsen KD, Lewis JE: Primary squamous cell carcinoma of the parotid gland. Arch Otolaryngol Head Neck Surg 1992;118:798–801.

784. Talmi YP, Finkelstein Y, Zohar Y: Invasive squamous cell skin cancer of the major salivary glands. In: Sacristan T, Alvarez-Vicent JJ, Bartual J, et al (eds): Otorhinolaryngology: Head and Neck Surgery. Proceedings of the XIV World Congress of Otorhinolaryngology, Head and Neck Surgery, Madrid, Spain, September 10–15, 1989, Vol II. Amsterdam: Kugler and Ghedini Publications, 1991:2753–2756.

785. Shemen LJ, Huvos AG, Spiro RH: Squamous cell carcinoma of salivary gland origin. Head Neck Surg 1987;9:235–240.

786. Sakurai K, Urade M, Kishimoto H, et al: Primary squamous cell carcinoma of the accessory parotid duct epithelium. Oral Surg Oral Med Oral Pathol Oral Radiol Endod 1998;85:447–451.

787. Sterman BM, Kraus DH, Sebek BA, et al: Primary squamous cell carcinoma of the parotid gland. Laryngoscope 1990;100:146–148.

788. Ellis GL, Auclair PL: Atlas of Tumor Pathology: Tumors of the Salivary Glands. Washington, DC: Armed Forces Institute of Pathology, 1996:155–373.

789. Cartei G, Zorat P, Cartei F, et al: Poorly differentiated squamous cell carcinoma of the parotid gland in a 13-year-old girl [letter]. Med Pediatr Oncol 1998;30:374–375.

790. Leader M, Jass JR: In-situ neoplasia in squamous cell carcinoma of the parotid. A case report. Histopathol 1985;9:325–329.

791. Baker M, Yuzon D, Baker BH: Squamous cell carcinoma arising in benign adenolymphoma (Warthin's tumor) of the parotid gland. J Surg Oncol 1980;15:7–10.

792. Damjanov I, Sneff EM, Delerme AN, et al: Squamous cell carcinoma arising in Warthin's tumor of the parotid gland. Oral Surg Oral Med Oral Pathol 1983;55:286–290.

Colloid Carcinoma

793. Osaki T, Hirota J, Ohno A, Tatemoto Y: Mucinous adenocarcinoma of the submandibular gland. Cancer 1990;66:1796–1801.

794. Gunzl H-J, Donath K, Schmelzle R: Klinik und Pathohistologie muzinoser Adenokarzinome der kleinen Speicheldrusen. Pathologe 1993;14:210–215.

795. Gnepp D, Estalilla O, Henley J, Ellis G: Primary colloid (mucinous) carcinoma of the salivary glands [abstract]. Oral Surg Oral Med Oral Pathol 1997;84:188.

796. Krogdahl AS, Schou C: Mucinous adenocarcinoma of the sublingual gland. J Oral Pathol Med 1997;26:198–200.

797. Sharkey FE, Allred DC, Valente PT: Breast. In: Damjanov I, Linder J (eds): Anderson's Pathology. St Louis: Mosby–Year Book, 1996:2375.

Adenocarcinoma, Not Otherwise Specified

798. Spiro RH, Huvos AG, Strong EW: Adenocarcinoma of salivary origin. Clinicopathologic study of 204 patients. Am J Surg 1982;144:423–431.
799. Ellis GL, Auclair PL: Atlas of Tumor Pathology: Tumors of the Salivary Glands. Washington, DC: Armed Forces Institute of Pathology, 1996:155–373.
800. Auclair PL, Ellis GL: Adenocarcinoma, not otherwise specified. In: Ellis GL, Auclair PL, Gnepp DR (eds): Surgical Pathology of the Salivary Glands. Philadelphia: WB Saunders, 1991:318–332.
801. van der Wal JE, Leverstein H, Snow GB, et al: Parotid gland tumors: Histologic reevaluation and reclassification of 478 cases. Head Neck 1998;20:204–207.
802. Matsuba HM, Mauney M, Simpson JR, et al: Adenocarcinomas of major and minor salivary gland origin: A histopathologic review of treatment failure patterns. Laryngoscope 1988;98:784–788.

Congenital Tumors Including Sialoblastoma

803. Seifert G, Donath K: The congenital basal cell adenoma of salivary glands. Contribution to the differential diagnosis of congenital salivary gland tumours. Virchows Arch A Path Anat Histopathol 1997;430:311–319.
804. Batsakis JG, Frankenthaler R: Pathology consultation: Embryoma (sialoblastoma) of salivary glands. Ann Otol Rhinol Laryngol 1992;101:958–960.
805. Batsakis JG, Mackay B, Ryka AF, Seifert RW: Perinatal salivary gland tumours (embryomas). J Laryngol Otol 1988;102:1007–1011.
806. Brandwein M, Al-Naeif NS, Manwani D, et al: Sialoblastoma: Clinicopathological/immunohistochemical study. Am J Surg Pathol 1999;23:342–348.
807. Vawter GF, Tefft M: Congenital tumors of the parotid gland. Arch Pathol 1966;82:242–245.
808. Hsueh C, Gonzalez-Crussi F: Sialoblastoma: A case report and review of the literature on congenital epithelial tumors of salivary gland origin. Pediatr Pathol 1992;12:205–214, 631.
809. Taylor GP: Case 6: Congenital epithelial tumor of the parotid—sialoblastoma. Pediatr Pathol 1988;8:447–452.
810. Adkins GF: Low grade basaloid adenocarcinoma of the salivary gland in childhood: The so-called hybrid basal cell adenoma–adenoid cystic carcinoma. Pathol 1990;22:187–190.
811. Daley TD, Dardick I: An unusual parotid tumor with histogenetic implications for salivary gland neoplasms. Oral Surg Oral Med Oral Pathol 1983;55:374–381.
812. Simpson PR, Rutledge JC, Schaefer SD, Anderson RC: Congenital hybrid basal cell adenoma–adenoid cystic carcinoma of the salivary gland. Pediatr Pathol 1986;6:199–208.

Metastasis to Major Salivary Glands

813. Bouquot JE, Weiland LH, Kurland LT: Metastases to and from the upper aerodigestive tract in the population of Rochester, Minnesota, 1935–1984. Head Neck 1989;11:212–218.
814. Feind CR: The head and neck. In: Haagensen CD, Feind CR, Herter FP, Slanetz CA Jr, Weinberg FA (eds): The Lymphatics in Cancer. Philadelphia: WB Saunders, 1972:59–230.
815. Gnepp DR: Metastatic disease to the major salivary glands. In: Ellis GL, Auclair PL, Gnepp DR (eds): Surgical Pathology of the Salivary Glands. Philadelphia: WB Saunders, 1991:560–569.
816. Pisani P, Krengli M, Ramponi A, et al: Metastases to parotid gland from cancers of the upper airway and digestive tract. Br J Oral Maxillifac Surg 1998;36:54–57.
817. Ellis GL, Auclair PL: Atlas of Tumor Pathology: Tumors of the Salivary Gland. Washington, DC: Armed Forces Institute of Pathology, 1997:403–410.
818. Hisa Y, Tatemoto K: Bilateral parotid gland metastases as the initial manifestation of a small cell carcinoma of the lung. Am J Otolaryngol 1998;19:140–143.
819. Saiz AD, Sachdev U, Brodman ML, Deligdisch L: Metastatic uterine leiomyosarcoma presenting as a primary sarcoma of the parotid gland. Obstet Gynecol 1998;92:667–668.

820. Malata CM, Camilleri IG, McLean NR, et al: Metastatic tumours of the parotid. Br J Oral Maxillofac Surg 1998;36:190–195.
821. delCharco JO, Mendenhall WM, Parsons JT, et al: Carcinoma of the skin metastatic to the parotid area lymph nodes. Head Neck 1998;20:369–373.
822. Lee K, McKean ME, McGregor IA: Metastatic patterns of squamous carcinoma in the parotid lymph nodes. Br J Plast Surg 1985;38:6–10.
823. Wang BY, Lawson W, Robinson RA, et al: Malignant melanoma of the parotid: Comparison of survival for patients with metastases from known vs unknown primary tumor sites. Arch Otolaryngol Head Neck Surg 1999;125:635–639.

Central Salivary Gland Tumors of the Maxilla and Mandible

824. Brookstone MS, Huvos AG: Central salivary gland tumors of the maxilla and mandible: A clinicopathologic study of 11 cases with an analysis of the literature. J Oral Maxillofac Surg 1992;50:229–236.
825. Waldron CA, Koh ML: Central mucoepidermoid carcinoma of the jaws: Report of four cases with analysis of the literature and discussion of the relationship to mucoepidermoid, sialodontogenic, and glandular odontogenic cysts. J Oral Maxillofac Surg 1990;48:871–877.
826. Ellis GL, Auclair PL: Atlas of Tumor Pathology: Tumors of the Salivary Gland. Washington, DC: Armed Forces Institute of Pathology, 1996:172–175.
827. Bouquot JE, Gnepp DR, Dardick I, Hietanen JHP: Intraosseous salivary tissue: Jawbone examples of choristomas, hamartomas, embryonic rests and inflammatory entrapment. Another histogenetic source for intraosseous adenocarcinoma. Oral Surg Oral Med Oral Pathol Oral Radiol Endod 2000; in press.
828. Berho M, Huvos AG: Central hyalinizing clear cell carcinoma of the mandible and the maxilla: A clinicopathologic study of two cases with an analysis of the literature. Hum Pathol 1999;30:101–105.

Mesenchymal Neoplasms

829. Eneroth CM: Histological and clinical aspects of parotid tumors. Acta Otolaryngol Suppl (Stockh) 1964;191:1–99.
830. Seifert G, Miehlke A, Haubrich J, Chilla R: Diseases of the Salivary Glands: Pathology, Diagnosis, Treatment, Facial Nerve Surgery. Stuttgart: Georg Thieme Verlag, 1986.
831. Auclair PL, Ellis GL, Gnepp DR, et al: Salivary gland neoplasms: General considerations. In: Ellis GL, Auclair PL, Gnepp DR (eds): Surgical Pathology of the Salivary Glands. Philadelphia: WB Saunders, 1991:135–164.
832. Cawson RA, Gleeson MJ, Eveson JW: Pathology and Surgery of the Salivary Glands. Oxford: ISIS Medical Media, 1997:170–190.
833. Guarino M, Giordano F, Pallotti F, Ponzi S: Solitary fibrous tumour of the submandibular gland. Histopathol 1998;32:571–573.
834. Sato J, Asakura K, Yokoyama Y, Satoh M: Solitary fibrous tumor of the parotid gland extending to the parapharyngeal space. Eur Arch Otorhinolaryngol 1998;255:18–21.
835. Williams SB, Foss RD, Ellis GL: Inflammatory pseudotumors of the major salivary glands. Clinicopathologic and immunohistochemical analysis of six cases. Am J Surg Pathol 1992;16:896–902.
836. Graham CT, Roberts AHN, Padel AF: Pleomorphic lipoma of the parotid gland. J Laryngol Otol 1998;112:202–203.
837. Said-Al-Naief N, Ivanov K, Jones M, et al: Granular cell tumor of the parotid. Ann Diagn Pathol 1999;3:35–38.
838. Auclair PL, Langloss JM, Weiss SW, Corio RL: Sarcomas and sarcomatoid neoplasms of the major salivary gland regions: A clinicopathologic and immunohistochemical study of 67 cases and review of the literature. Cancer 1986;58:1305–1315.
839. Luna MA, Tortoledo ME, Ordonez NG, et al: Primary sarcomas of the major salivary glands. Arch Otolaryngol Head Neck Surg 1991;117:302–306.
840. Enzinger FM, Weiss SW: Soft Tissue Tumors, 3rd ed. St Louis: CV Mosby, 1995.

Hybrid Tumors

841. Grenko RT, Abendroth CS, Davis AT, et al: Hybrid tumors or salivary gland tumors sharing common differentiation pathways? Reexamining adenoid cystic and epithelial-myoepithelial carcinomas. Oral Surg Oral Med Oral Pathol Oral Radiol Endod 1998;86:188–195.

842. Hanada T, Hirase H, Ohyama M: Unusual case of myoepithelioma associated with adenoid cystic carcinoma of the parotid gland. Auris Nasus Larynx 1995;22:65–70.

843. Adkins GF: Low grade basaloid adenocarcinoma of salivary gland in childhood: The so called hybrid basal cell adenoma–adenoid cystic carcinoma. Pathol 1990;22:187–190.

844. Simpson PR, Rutledge JC, Shaefer SD, et al: Congenital hybrid basal cell adenoma–adenoid cystic carcinoma of the salivary gland. Pediatr Pathol 1986;6:199–208.

845. Seifert G, Donath K: Hybrid tumours of salivary glands. Definition and classification of five rare cases. Eur J Cancer B Oral Oncol 1996;32B:251–259.

846. Dreyer T, Battmann A, Silberzahn J, et al: Unusual differentiation of a combination tumor of the parotid gland. A case report. Pathol Res Pract 1993;189:577–581.

847. Evans RW, Cruickshank AH: Epithelial Tumors of the Salivary Glands: Major Problems in Pathology. Philadelphia: WB Saunders, 1970:267.

848. Kamio N, Tanaka Y, Mukai M, et al: A hybrid carcinoma: Adenoid cystic carcinoma and salivary duct carcinoma of the salivary gland. An immunohistochemical study. Virchows Arch A Pathol Anat Histopathol 1997;430:495–500.

848a. Snyder ML, Paulino AF: Hybrid carcinoma of the salivary gland: Salivary duct adenocarcinoma–adenoid cystic carcinoma. Histopathology 1999;35:380–383.

848b. Croitoru CM, Suarez PA, Luna MA: Hybrid carcinomas of salivary glands: Report of 4 cases and review of the literature. Arch Pathol Lab Med 1999;123:698–702.

Miscellaneous Lesions

849. Ellis GL, Gnepp DR: Unusual salivary gland tumors. In: Gnepp DR (ed): Pathology of the Head and Neck. New York: Churchill Livingstone, 1988:585–561.

850. Ellis GL, Auclair PL: Atlas of Tumor Pathology: Tumors of the Salivary Gland. Washington, DC: Armed Forces Institute of Pathology, 1996:255–373.

851. Donath K, Seifert G, Roser K: The spectrum of giant cells in tumours of the salivary glands: An analysis of 11 cases. J Oral Pathol Med 1997;26:431–436.

852. Grenko RT, Tytor M, Boeryd B: Giant-cell tumour of the salivary gland with associated carcinosarcoma. Histopathol 1993;23:594–595.

853. Balogh K, Wolbarsht RL, Federman M, O'Hara CJ: Carcinoma of the parotid gland with osteoclastlike giant cells. Immunohistochemical and ultrastructural observations. Arch Pathol Lab Med 1985;109:756–761.

854. Itoh Y, Taniguti Y, Arai K: A case of giant cell tumor of the parotid gland. Ann Plast Surg 1992;28:183–186.

855. Eusebi V, Martin SA, Govoni E, Rosai J: Giant cell tumor of major salivary glands: Report of three cases, one occurring in association with a malignant mixed tumor. Am J Clin Pathol 1984;81:666–675.

856. Enzinger FM, Weiss SW: Soft Tissue Tumors, 3rd ed. St Louis: Mosby–Year Book, 1995:929–964.

857. Deb RA, Desai SB, Amonkar PP, et al: Primary primitive neuroectodermal tumour of the parotid gland. Histopathol 1998;33:375–378.

Special Techniques

858. Raab SS, Sigman JD, Hoffman HT: The utility of parotid gland and level I and level II neck fine-needle aspiration. Arch Pathol Lab Med 1998;122:823–827.

859. Zakowski M: Fine-needle aspiration cytology of tumors: Diagnostic accuracy and potential pitfalls. Cancer Invest 1994;12:505–515.

860. Ellis GL, Auclair PL: Atlas of Tumor Pathology: Tumors of the Salivary Glands. Washington, DC: Armed Forces Institute of Pathology, 1996:441–463.

861. Filopoulos E, Angeli S, Daskalopoulou D, et al: Pre-operative evaluation of parotid tumours by fine needle biopsy. Eur J Surg Oncol 1998;24:180–183.

862. Layfield LJ, Tan P: Fine-needle aspiration of salivary gland lesions. Comparison with frozen sections and histologic findings. Arch Pathol Lab Med 1987;111:346–353.

863. Weinberger MS, Rosenberg WW, Meurer WT, Robbins KT: Fine-needle aspiration of parotid gland lesions. Head Neck 1992;14:483–487.

864. Al-Khafaji BM, Nestok BR, Katz RL: Fine-needle aspiration of 154 parotid masses with histologic correlation: Ten-year experience at the University of Texas M.D. Anderson Cancer Center. Cancer 1998;84:153–159.

865. Chan MK, McGuire LJ, King W, et al: Cytodiagnosis of 112 salivary gland lesions. Correlation with histologic and frozen section diagnosis. Acta Cytol 1992;36:353–363.

866. Gnepp DR, Rader WR, Cramer SF, et al: Accuracy of frozen section diagnosis of the salivary gland. Otolaryngol Head Neck Surg 1987;96:325–330.

867. Cohen MB, Ljung B-ME, Boles R: Salivary gland tumors. Fine-needle aspiration vs. frozen section diagnosis. Arch Otolaryngol Head Neck Surg 1986;112:867–869.

868. Heller KS, Attie JN, Dubner S: Accuracy of frozen section in evaluation of salivary tumors. Am J Surg 1993;166:424–427.

869. Megerian CA, Maniglia AJ: Parotidectomy: A ten year experience with fine needle aspiration and frozen section biopsy correlation. Ear Nose Throat J 1994;73:377–380.

870. Chan MKM, Mcguire LJ, King W, et al: Cytodiagnosis of 112 salivary gland lesions: Correlation with histologic and frozen section diagnosis. Acta Cytol 1992;36:353–363.

871. Zheng JW, Song XY, Nie XG: The accuracy of clinical examination versus frozen section in the diagnosis of parotid masses. J Oral Maxillofac Surg 1997;55:29–31.

872. Gnepp DR: Frozen sections. In: Gnepp DR (ed): Pathology of the Head and Neck. New York, Churchill Livingstone, 1988:1–24.

873. Batsakis JG, Brannon RB, Sciubba JJ: Monomorphic adenomas of major salivary glands: A histologic study of 96 tumors. Clin Otolaryngol 1981;6:129–143.

874. Daley TD: The canalicular adenoma: Considerations on differential diagnosis and treatment. J Oral Maxillofac Surg 1984;42:728–730.

875. Luna MA: Uses, abuses and pitfalls of frozen section diagnoses of diseases of the head and neck. In: Barnes EL (ed): Surgical Pathology of the Head and Neck. New York: Marcel Dekker, 1985:7–22.

Tumors of the Lacrimal Gland and Sac

876. McLean IW, Burnier MN, Zimmerman LE, Jakobiec FA: Atlas of Tumor Pathology: Tumors of the Eye and Ocular Adnexa. Washington, DC: Armed Forces Institute of Pathology, 1994:215–232.

877. Vangveeravong S, Katz SE, Rootman J, White V: Tumors arising in the palpebral lobe of the lacrimal gland. Ophthalmol 1996;103:1606–1612.

878. Sakurai H, Mitsuhashi N, Hayakawa K, et al: Ectopic lacrimal gland of the orbit. J Nucl Med 1997;38:1498–1500.

879. Stefanyszyn MA, Hidayat AA, Pe'er JJ, Flanagan JC: Lacrimal sac tumors. Ophthal Plast Reconstr Surg 1994;10:169–184.

880. Pe'er J, Hidayat AA, Ilsar M, et al: Glandular tumors of the lacrimal sac. Their histopathologic patterns and possible origins. Ophthalmol 1996;103:1601–1605.

881. Kennedy RE: An evaluation of 820 orbital cases. Trans Am Ophthalmol Soc 1984;82:134–156.

882. Bonavolonta G, Tranfa F, Staibano S, et al: Warthin tumor of the lacrimal gland. Am J Ophthalmol 1997;124:857–858.

883. Chuo N, Ping-Kuan K, Dryja TP: Histopathological classification of 272 primary epithelial tumors of the lacrimal gland. Chinese Med J 1992;6:481–485.

884. Font RL, Smith SL, Bryan RG: Malignant epithelial tumors of the lacrimal gland: A clinicopathologic study of 21 cases. Arch Ophthalmol 1998;116:613–616.

885. Wright JE, Rose GE, Garner A: Primary malignant neoplasms of the lacrimal gland. Br J Ophthalmol 1992;76:401–407.

886. Mombaerts I, Schlingemann RO, Goldschmeding R, et al: The surgical management of lacrimal gland pseudotumors. Ophthalmol 1996;103:1619–1627.

887. Rose GE, Wright JE: Pleomorphic adenoma of the lacrimal gland. Br J Ophthalmol 1992;76:395–400.

888. Shields CL, Shields JA: Review of lacrimal gland lesions. Trans Pa Acad Ophthalmol Otolaryngol 1990;42:925–930.

889. Polito E, Leccisotti A: Epithelial malignancies of the lacrimal gland: Survival rates after extensive and conservative therapy. Ann Opthalmol 1993;25:422–426.

890. Heaps RS, Miller NR, Albert DM, et al: Primary adenocarcinoma of the lacrimal gland: A retrospective study. Ophthalmol 1993;100:1856–1860.

891. Tellado MV, McLean IW, Specht CS, Varga J: Adenoid cystic carcinomas of the lacrimal gland in childhood and adolescence. Ophthalmol 1997;104:1622–1625.

892. Katz SE, Rootman J, Dolman PJ, et al: Primary ductal adenocarcinoma of the lacrimal gland. Ophthalmol 1996;103:157–162.
893. Grossniklaus HE, Wojno TH, Wilson MW, Someren AO: Myoepithelioma of the lacrimal gland. Arch Ophthalmol 1997;115:1588–1590.
894. Harvey PA, Parsons MA, Rennie IG: Primary sebaceous carcinoma of lacrimal gland: A previously unreported primary neoplasm. Eye 1994;8:592–595.
895. Gamel JW, Font RL: Adenoid cystic carcinoma of the lacrimal gland: The clinical significance of a basaloid histologic pattern. Hum Pathol 1982;13:219–225.
896. Pecorella I, Garner A: Ostensible oncocytoma of accessory lacrimal glands. Histopathol 1997;30:264–270.
897. Eviatar JA, Hornblass A: Mucoepidermoid carcinoma of the lacrimal gland: 25 cases and a review and update of the literature. Ophthal Plast Reconstr Surg 1993;9:170–181.
898. Goldberg RA: Intra-arterial chemotherapy: A welcome new idea for the management of adenocystic carcinoma of the lacrimal gland. Arch Ophthalmol 1998;116:372–373.
899. Meldrum ML, Tse DT, Benedetto P: Neoadjuvant intracarotid chemotherapy for treatment of advanced adenocystic carcinoma of the lacrimal gland. Arch Ophthalmol 1998;116:315–321.
900. Rosenbaum PS, Mahadevia PS, Goodman LA, Kress Y: Acinic cell carcinoma of the lacrimal gland. Arch Ophthalmol 1995;113:781–785.
901. Ostrowski ML, Font R, Halpern J, et al: Clear cell epithelial-myoepithelial carcinoma arising in pleomorphic adenoma of the lacrimal gland. J Ophthalmol 1994;101:925–930.
902. Karim MM, Inoue M, Minato K, et al: Eccrine adenocarcinoma of the lacrimal sac region. Ophthalmologica 1997;211:44–48.
903. Pe'er JJ, Stefanyszyn M, Hidayat AA: Nonepithelial tumors of the lacrimal sac. Am J Ophthalmol 1994;118:650–658.
904. Kuwabara H, Takeda J: Malignant melanoma of the lacrimal sac with surrounding melanosis. Arch Pathol Lab Med 1997;121:517–519.
905. Ni C, D'Amico DJ, Fan CQ, Kuo PK: Tumors of the lacrimal sac: A clinicopathologic analysis of 82 cases. Int Ophthalmol Clin 1982;22:121–140.
906. Hulka GF, Kulwin DR, Weeks SM, Cotton RT: Congenital lacrimal sac mucoceles with intranasal extension. Otolaryngol Head Neck Surg 1995;113:651–655.
907. Fliss DM, Freeman JL, Hurwitz JJ, Heathcote JG: Mucoepidermoid carcinoma of the lacrimal sac: A report of two cases with observations on the histogenesis. Can J Ophthalmol 1993;28:228–235.
908. Nakamura K, Uehara S, Omagari J, et al: Primary non-Hodgkin's lymphoma of the lacrimal sac: A case report and a review of the literature. Cancer 1997;80:2151–2155.

7 : Pathology of the Thyroid and Parathyroid Glands

Ronald A. DeLellis, Gerardo Guiter, and Barbara J. Weinstein

Diseases of the thyroid and parathyroid glands are among the most common of all endocrine disorders. Affected patients may be relatively asymptomatic or may have evidence of hypofunction, hyperfunction, or a mass lesion. As a group, the diseases of these endocrine glands are of major importance, since most are amenable to highly effective surgical or medical treatment. The purpose of this chapter is to provide an overview of the pathology of the thyroid and parathyroid glands.

THYROID GLAND

Embryology

The thyroid gland is derived from both central and paired lateral anlagen. The central anlage, which gives rise to the thyroglossal duct, the isthmus, and the major portion of each central lobe, develops as a midline diverticulum from the floor of the pharynx at the level of the second pharyngeal pouches late in the fourth week of development.[1, 2] During its subsequent development, the central thyroid anlage becomes solid as it migrates caudally. The developing thyroid remains connected with the oral cavity (foramen cecum) by the thyroglossal duct which eventually becomes obliterated. Remnants of the thyroglossal duct, however, may be found in up to 40% of individuals in the form of the pyramidal lobe. Failure of normal migration of the thyroid anlage may lead to the presence of ectopic thyroid tissue along its entire line of normal descent. Persistence of the thyroglossal duct, on the other hand, may lead to thyroglossal duct cysts or sinus tracts.[3]

The ultimobranchial bodies, which originate from the fourth and fifth pharyngeal pouch complexes, give rise to C cells, solid cell nests, and portions of the lateral thyroids.[4] The progenitors of the C cells, which are derived from the neural crest, migrate to the ultimobranchial bodies prior to their incorporation into the developing thyroid gland.[5]

Anatomy and Physiology

The thyroid gland is a bilobed organ located in the midportion of the neck immediately anterior to the larynx and trachea. The two lobes are joined by the isthmus, which is located just below the level of the cricoid cartilage. The pyramidal lobe, if present, extends from the isthmus superiorly to the anterior aspect of the thyroid cartilage. Gland weight is variable and is dependent, in part, on the amount of iodine in the diet and on a variety of other factors, including sex and hormonal status. In nonendemic goiter regions, the normal gland weighs 15 to 35 g.

The arterial supply is derived from the superior and inferior thyroid arteries. The veins drain into the internal jugular, brachycephalic, and anterior jugular veins. The gland is richly endowed with lymphatic vessels, which connect both lobes via the isthmus. Collecting lymphatics emerge from the gland in proximity to the venous drainage system. The major draining nodes include those in the immediate pericapsular region, the internal jugular chain, the pretracheal, paratracheal, and prelaryngeal areas, the recurrent laryngeal nerve chain, and the retropharyngeal and retroesophageal areas.[6]

The functional unit of the thyroid is the follicle, which is separated from the interstitium by a complete basement membrane (Fig. 7–1, see p.433). Groups of 20 to 30 follicles are organized into lobules, which are separated by thin layers of fibrous connective tissue. The amount of fibrous tissue increases with age. There is considerable variation in the size of the follicles; however, most range from 200 to 300 μm in diameter.[7] The central region of the follicle contains periodic acid–Schiff–positive colloid in which thyroglobulin is stored prior to its intracellular hydrolysis. Calcium oxalate crystals, which are birefringent in polarized light, are often present within the colloid, particularly in the glands of older individuals.

The follicular cells vary considerably in size and shape, depending on their functional status. In general, follicular cells with a columnar shape are considered to be functionally active, whereas those with a flattened shape are relatively inactive. The nucleus is round to ovoid with finely granular chromatin and usually a single small nucleolus. Follicular cells stain positively for thyroglobulin, triiodothyronine (T_3), and thyroxine (T_4). They also contain low molecular weight cytokeratins, vimentin, and epithelial membrane antigen.[8] Ultrastructurally, follicular cells are characterized by apical microvilli, extensively developed cisternae of granular endoplasmic reticulum, moderate numbers of mitochondria, and well-developed Golgi regions. Prominent collections of lysosomes are also evident in the apical cytoplasm, adjacent to areas of active thyroglobulin resorption.[9]

Follicular cells with abundant eosinophilic cytoplasm are referred to as oncocytes, oxyphil cells, Askanazy cells, or Hürthle cells. The term *Hürthle cell,* however, is a misnomer, since the cells that Hürthle described in the dog thyroid were most likely C cells.[10] At the ultrastructural level, oncocytic cells are characterized by the presence of numerous mitochondria.

The aspirated smear from normal thyroid consists of a few three-dimensional groups of cells of variable size and/or monolayered sheets with a honeycomb arrangement. Single follicular cells are also usually present.[11] The nucleus of the follicular cell is central and round with smooth contours and finely punctate chromatin. Nucleoli are usually small. Naked follicular cell nuclei can be distinguished from lymphocytes, since the latter typically have more heterogeneous chromatin and a thin rim of cytoplasm. Colloid stains blue with the May-Grünwald-Giemsa method or variably orange, green, or yellow with the Papanicolaou stain. Degenerated follicular cells have foamy to granular cytoplasm with pyknotic nuclei and may be indistinguishable from histiocytes. Oncocytes typically feature abundant granular eosinophilic cytoplasm with nuclei that are larger than follicular cells and prominent nucleoli. Rarely, ciliated cells and cartilage from the trachea may be seen in thyroid aspirates as well as skeletal muscle, skin, fat, and blood vessels.[12]

In some instances, the thyroid follicular cells may undergo squamous metaplasia. This process is characterized by the presence of compact groups of polygonal cells with eosinophilic cytoplasm. Foci of keratinization and intercellular bridges may also be evident. Metaplastic squamous cells in the thyroid are typically positive for cytokeratins but are negative for calcitonin and thyroglobulin. Foci of squamous metaplasia occur most commonly in the setting of chronic thyroiditis, as discussed in subsequent sections; however, they may also occur in a wide variety of neoplastic and non-neoplastic conditions of the thyroid.

The follicular cells may contain a variety of pigments. Iron deposits may occur as a result of local hemorrhage or, more rarely, as a manifestation of iron storage disease. Lipofuscin deposits occur commonly, particularly in the thyroid glands of older individuals. This pigment is typically periodic acid-Schiff–positive and is also intensely autofluorescent.

Black pigmentation of the thyroid may result from the administration of the tetracycline derivative minocycline.[13] Pigment deposition may occur in normal follicular cells or in benign or neoplastic follicular epithelial cells. The nature of the minocycline pigment, however, is unknown. It has been suggested that the pigment may represent an oxidation product of the drug or a combination of lipofuscin and oxidized minocycline. The accumulation of this pigment has no apparent effect on thyroid function.

Physiology

Synthesis of thyroid hormone begins by active transport of iodine into the follicular cells. Intracellular iodide is oxidized to iodine by peroxidase and is bound to tyrosine to form the hormonally-inactive iodotyrosines monoiodotyrosine and diiodotyrosine.[14] The formation of T_4 results from coupling of two diiodotyrosine molecules, whereas the formation of T_3 results from the coupling of one molecule of monoiodotyrosine and one molecule of diiodotyrosine. The iodothyronine molecules are subsequently incorporated into thyroglobulin. Stimulation of the follicular cells by thyroid-stimulating hormone (TSH) results in the resorption of colloid via the apical aspect of the follicular cell and the subsequent release of T_4 and T_3 at the basal aspect of the cell where they subsequently enter the systemic circulation. The iodotyrosines undergo subsequent intrathyroidal deiodination with recycling of the resulting free iodide.

Thyroid hormone biosynthesis and secretion are tightly controlled by the actions of TSH and thyroid hormone-releasing hormone (TRH) in a classic negative feedback loop.[14] TRH stimulates the synthesis and release of TSH, whereas T_3 and T_4 inhibit these activities. Decreased production of T_3 and T_4 will lead to increased synthesis and secretion of TSH and TRH. Prolonged stimulation of the thyroid by TSH will lead to the development of thyroid hyperplasia.

C Cells

C cells are difficult to identify in hematoxylin-eosin–stained sections, although they sometimes exhibit cytoplasmic clearing.[15] They can be recognized in Diff-Quick–stained smears on the basis of their contents of metachromatic granules.[16] C cells are most reliably identified by immunohistochemical methods using antibodies to calcitonin or chromogranin A (Fig. 7–2, see p. 433). C cells occupy an exclusively intrafollicular position and are separated from the interstitium by the follicular basal lamina and from the colloid by the cytoplasm of adjacent follicular cells.[17] Generally, C cells are present in highest concentrations in a zone that corresponds to the junction of the upper and middle thirds of the lateral lobes. They are generally present as single cells or as small cell clusters. Up to 50 C cells may be present per single low power field in glands from adults. They are present in higher concentrations in the glands of neonates than in those of adults. Rarely, C cell nodules may be encountered in the thyroid glands of older individuals.[18]

The major secretory product of the C cell is calcitonin. The primary transcript of the calcitonin gene gives rise to two different messenger RNAs (mRNAs) by tissue-specific alternative splicing events that produce calcitonin and the calcitonin gene-related peptide mRNAs.[19] The calcitonin gene-related peptide is expressed in thyroid and nervous tissue, but calcitonin is produced in large quantities only in the thyroid gland. In addition to calcitonin, the C cells produce a variety of other peptides, including somatostatin, gastrin-releasing peptide, and thyrotropin-releasing hormone.[8] They also contain biologically active amines, including serotonin. Ultrastructurally, C cells contain membrane-bound secretory granules, which represent sites of storage of calcitonin and other peptides (Fig. 7–3). Type I granules have an average diameter of 280 nm, whereas the type II granules measure 130 nm in average diameter.[20]

Other Components of Normal Thyroid

Solid cell nests, which are remnants of the ultimobranchial bodies, are most commonly found along the central axis of the middle and upper thirds of the lateral lobes, primarily within the interstitium.[21] They are found in approximately 3% of routinely examined thyroids but have been demonstrated in up to 60% of thyroid glands subjected to serial blocking. Most solid cell nests measure up to 0.1 mm in diameter, although occasional nests may measure up to 2 mm (Fig. 7–4, see p. 433). Individual cells are polygonal to oval with elongated nuclei containing finely granular chromatin. A second cell type has a round nucleus with clear cytoplasm. Some of the cells within the nests contain thyroglobulin, while others contain calcitonin.[22]

A variety of other structures may be found within or just adjacent to the thyroid gland. Portions of thymus gland are present in up to 50% of normal thyroid glands studied by serial sectioning techniques.[23] Parathyroid glands may be present just beneath the thyroid capsule or, more rarely, within more central regions of the thyroid.[23] Rarely, intrathyroidal parathyroid tissue may become adenomatous. Paraganglia have also been identified in the capsule of the thyroid and may give rise to true paragangliomas.[24] In addition, groups of mature fat cells, skeletal muscle, and cartilage have been identified in normal thyroid glands.[23]

Congenital Anomalies

Congenital anomalies of the thyroid are uncommon, with a prevalence of 1.4 cases per 1000 with a relative frequency of 49% for cases of dysgenesis (hemiagenesis, agenesis or athyreosis, absent isthmus), 27% for thyroglossal duct remnants, 12% for ectopic thyroids (lingual and pre-epiglottic), and 12% for accessory thyroid tissues.[25]

Failure of development of the thyroid gland (athyreotic cretinism) is the most common cause of sporadic cretinism, occurring in approximately 1 of 4000 newborns.[26] Varying degrees of partial agenesis also occur. Abnormalities in the descent of the thyroid gland lead to varying degrees of ectopia. In many patients with thyroid ectopia, the ectopic tissue is the only thyroid present. Lingual glands are present typically at the base of the tongue, just beneath the foramen cecum.[27] Ectopic thyroid tissue may also occur between the hyoid bone and the cricoid cartilage in the midline (median subhyoid thyroid ectopia). Additional sites of ectopic thyroid tissue include the trachea, larynx, esophagus, soft tissues of the neck, and mediastinum. Rare examples of ectopic thyroid have been reported in the porta hepatis and gallbladder.

Very rarely, one or more normal-appearing thyroid follicles may be present within the soft tissue of the neck or in cervical lymph nodes (so-called "lateral aberrant thyroid").[28, 29] The presence of non-neoplastic thyroid in the soft tissues of the neck can occur as a result of a developmental anomaly (as discussed earlier), as a consequence of surgery or trauma, or as a result of so-called "parasitic" nodules of hyperplastic thyroid tissue in patients with goiter. The presence of normal thyroid follicles in cervical lymph nodes has been a particularly problematic and controversial issue. Thus, while some authors suggest that normal thyroid follicles may very rarely be present in cervical lymph nodes,[29] others indicate that the presence of thyroid tissue in cervical nodes is evidence of metastatic disease in all cases.[30] Typically, metastatic deposits involve multiple lymph nodes. Moreover, the metastatic deposits have nuclear features typical of papillary thyroid carcinoma, as discussed in subse-

Text continued on page 441

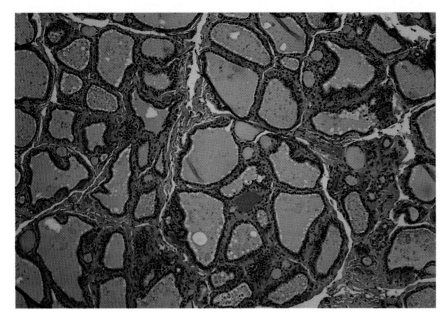

Figure 7–1. Normal thyroid. The follicular cells have a low cuboidal shape, and the colloid is deeply eosinophilic.

Figure 7–2. Normal thyroid stained for calcitonin with the immunoperoxidase technique using diaminobenzidine as the chromogen. The C cells have abundant granular cytoplasm.

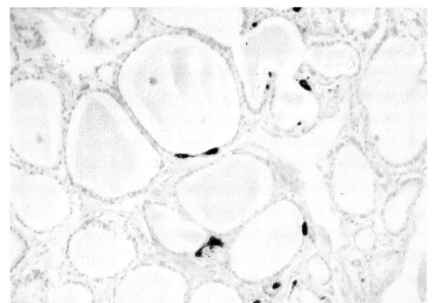

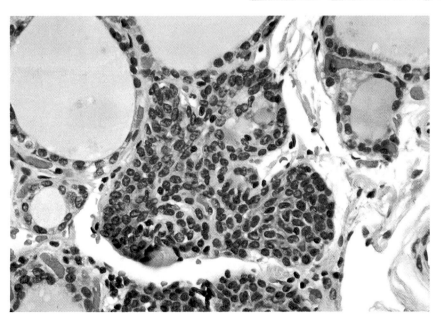

Figure 7–4. Solid cell nest. The individual cells are relatively small with a high nuclear : cytoplasmic ratio.

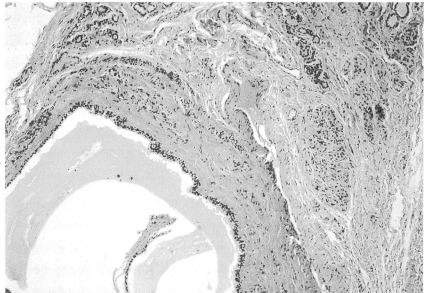

Figure 7–5. Thyroglossal duct cyst. The cyst has a fibrous wall and is lined by a pseudostratified epithelium in this area. A few groups of follicular cells are present at one edge of the cyst.

Figure 7–6. Acute thyroiditis (Papanicolaou's stain of fine needle aspiration biopsy). Numerous neutrophils surround a cluster of follicular cells.

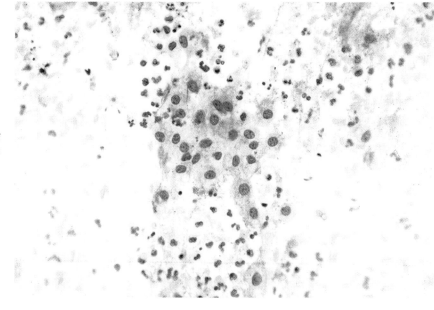

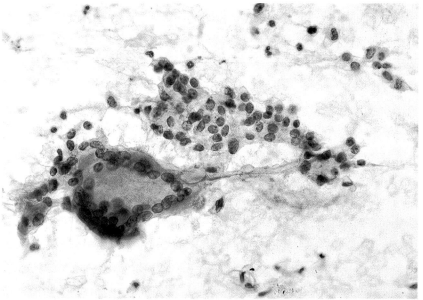

Figure 7–7. Subacute thyroiditis (hematoxylin-eosin stain of fine needle aspiration biopsy). A multinucleate giant cell is present in this field.

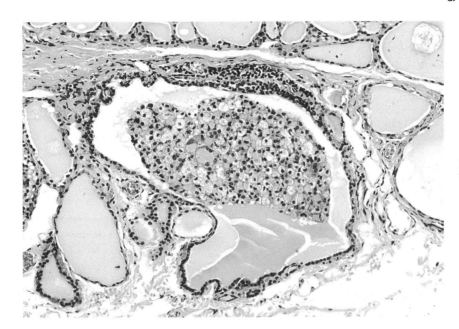

Figure 7–8. Multifocal granulomatous thyroiditis. The follicle contains histiocytes.

Figure 7–10. Hashimoto's thyroiditis. Oncocytes have abundant granular eosinophilic cytoplasm and nuclei with small but distinct nucleoli.

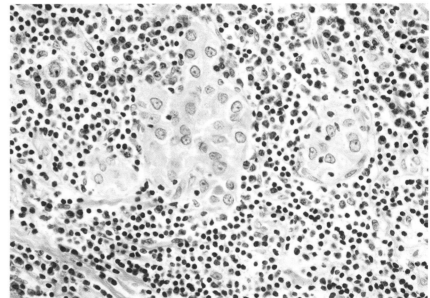

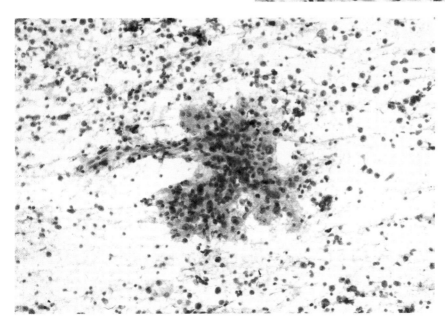

Figure 7–12. Hashimoto's thyroiditis (hematoxylin-eosin stain of fine needle aspiration biopsy). Numerous lymphocytes surround a large group of oncocytes.

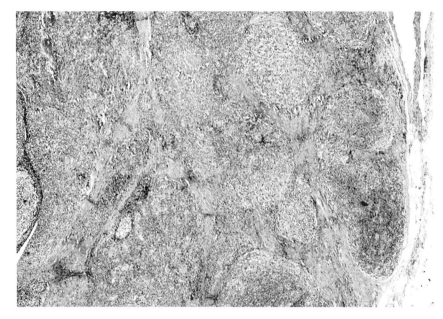

Figure 7–13. Fibrous variant of Hashimoto's disease. The thyroid gland is transected by broad bands of fibrous tissue.

Figure 7–14. Fibrous variant of Hashimoto's disease. A fibrous band separates two nodules of thyroid tissue that exhibit extensive lymphoplasmacytic infiltration and clusters of oncocytes.

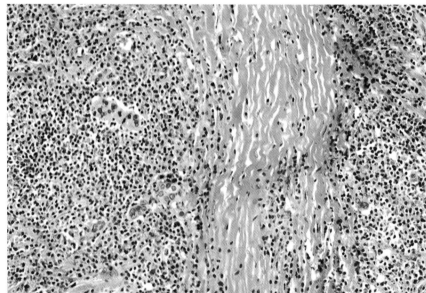

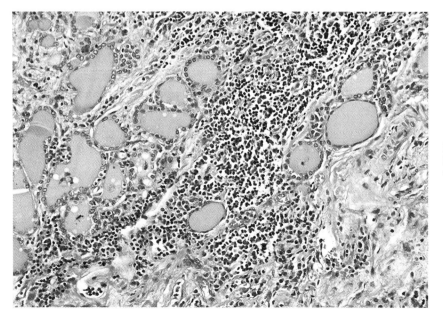

Figure 7–15. Focal, nonspecific, lymphocytic thyroiditis. The follicles are separated by a lymphocytic infiltrate.

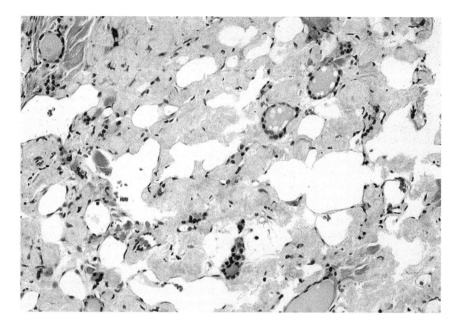

Figure 7–19. Amyloid goiter. The parenchyma is almost completely replaced by amyloid deposits and groups of adipocytes.

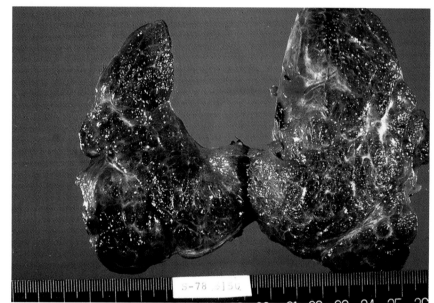

Figure 7–20. Graves' disease. Both lobes of the thyroid are symmetrically enlarged.

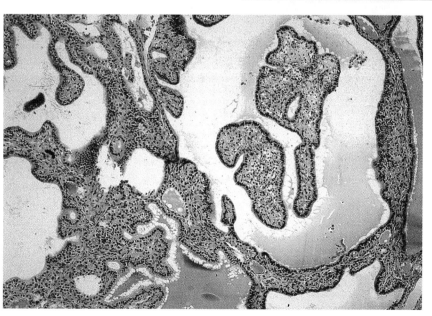

Figure 7–21. Graves' disease (treated). Many of the follicles are lined by papillary projections of hyperplastic follicular cells. Most of the follicles contain pale-staining colloid or are devoid of colloid.

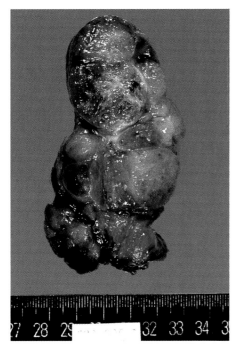

Figure 7–23. Multinodular (nontoxic) goiter. This thyroid lobe is completely replaced by multiple nodules, some of which are partially encapsulated (gross specimen).

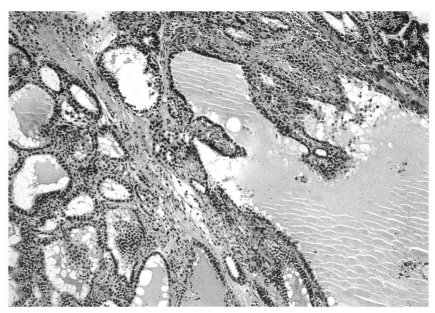

Figure 7–24. Multinodular (nontoxic) goiter. There is considerable variation in follicular size. One follicle is markedly enlarged and is filled with colloid. There are foci of papillary change.

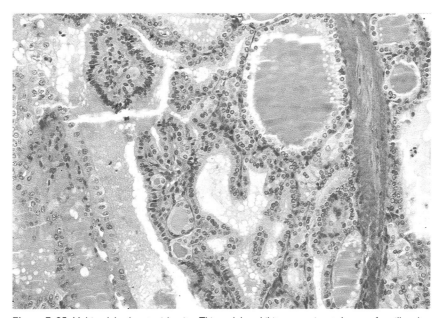

Figure 7–25. Multinodular (nontoxic) goiter. This nodule exhibits a prominent degree of papillary hyperplasia.

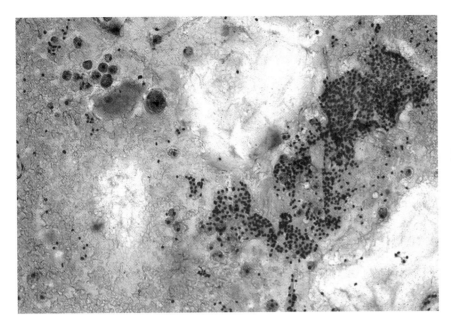

Figure 7–26. Multinodular (nontoxic) goiter (hematoxylin-eosin stain of fine needle aspiration biopsy). This aspirate demonstrates sheets of follicular cells, colloid, and occasional hemosiderin-laden macrophages.

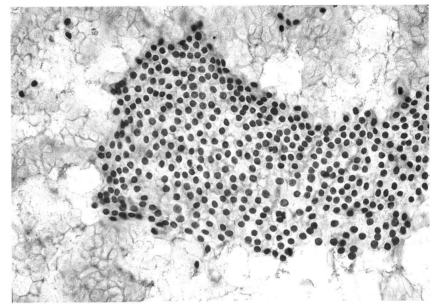

Figure 7–27. Multinodular (nontoxic) goiter (hematoxylin-eosin stain of fine needle aspiration biopsy). A large sheet of follicular cells has a typical honeycomb pattern.

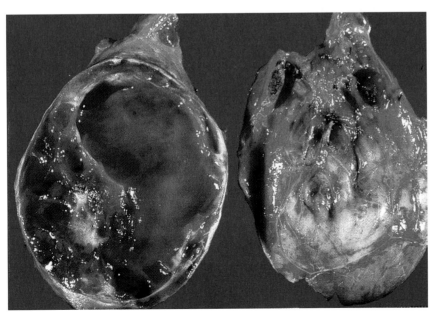

Figure 7–28. Follicular adenoma with extensive recent hemorrhage.

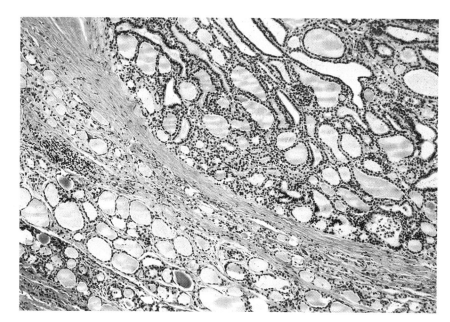

Figure 7–29. Follicular adenoma. The tumor is separated from the adjacent thyroid by a complete fibrous capsule.

Figure 7–30. Follicular adenoma (hematoxylin-eosin stain of fine needle aspiration biopsy). Microfollicles are evident.

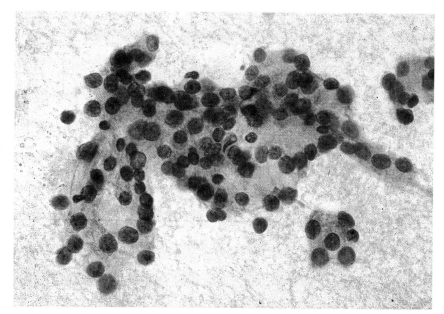

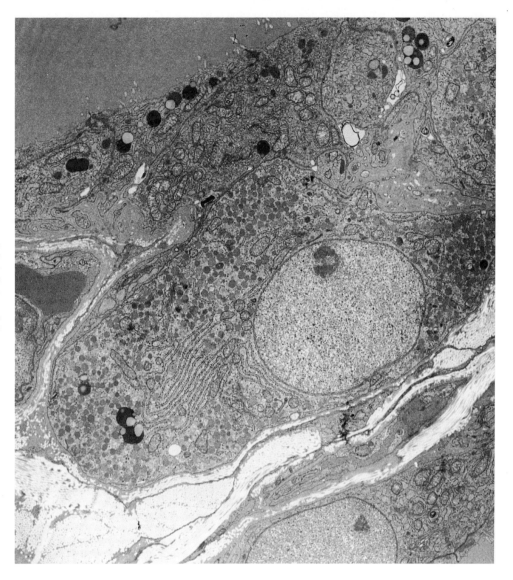

Figure 7–3. Electron micrograph of a C-cell. The cell is filled with membrane-bound, electron-dense secretory granules. The C-cell is separated from the colloid by the follicular cells, which have prominent lysosomes and apical microvilli. A continuous basal lamina separates the C-cell from the interstitium of the gland. (1200× mag.)

quent sections. As noted by LiVolsi,[31] however, "normal appearing thyroid tissue anywhere in lymph nodes lateral to the jugular vein represents metastatic papillary thyroid carcinoma and is not a developmental anomaly."[31]

Persistence of the thyroglossal duct typically presents in children or young adults as a midline cyst (Fig. 7–5, see p. 434).[3, 32] Rupture of the cyst leads to the development of a sinus tract or fistula. Since the duct passes through the body of the hyoid bone, the entire fibrous vestige of the duct, together with the midportion of the hyoid, should be removed to prevent recurrences. The cysts may be lined by cuboidal, ciliated columnar, or squamous epithelium with or without thyroid follicles in the stroma. Microscopic examination may reveal evidence of abscess formation or granulation tissue. Very rarely, thyroid neoplasms, particularly papillary thyroid carcinomas, may arise within remnants of the thyroglossal duct.[33, 34]

Congenital anomalies of the C cells are exceptionally rare. In the DiGeorge syndrome, which is characterized by partial or complete absence of derivatives of the third and fourth branchial pouches, C cells are present in 25% to 50% of cases and are typically reduced in number. The finding that C cells are present in some cases of the complete DiGeorge syndrome suggests an alternative source of these cells, possibly from the endoderm.[35, 36]

Lateral cystic structures in the neck that may contain calcitonin and thyroglobulin most likely represent remnants of the ultimobranchial bodies.[25] The cysts may measure up to 1.5 cm in diameter and consist of three to five thin-walled, multiloculated, mucin-containing cysts with or without associated parathyroid tissue. Some piriform sinus fistulas may also arise from remnants of the ultimobranchial bodies.[37]

Thyroiditis

The term *thyroiditis* refers to a heterogeneous group of inflammatory disorders of the thyroid gland, ranging from acute bacterial infections to chronic autoimmune diseases marked by inflammatory infiltrates and varying degrees of fibrosis. These diseases are most often classified into acute, subacute, and chronic forms, depending on the nature of the inflammatory infiltrates and the course of the disease.

Acute Thyroiditis

Clinical Features and Pathogenesis. Acute thyroiditis is an uncommon inflammatory disease usually due to infection by pyogenic bacteria.[38] Rarely, acute thyroiditis may be caused by fungi, parasites, viruses, and *Pneumocystis carinii,* particularly in immunosuppressed individuals.[39, 40] Pre-existent thyroid disease, especially nodular goiter, has been reported to be present in more than 50% of adult patients with acute thyroiditis. Infectious agents may reach the thyroid via the blood stream, by extension from the oropharynx (piriform sinus), or from the salivary glands.[41] In a recent series of patients with acute thyroiditis, six of six patients had a piriform sinus fistula.[42] Clinical manifestations include the abrupt onset of unilateral anterior neck pain and fever. Patients are usually euthyroid, although rarely there may be a transient elevation of T_4.[38]

Pathologic Features. Grossly, the gland may appear asymmetrically enlarged, with foci of abscess formation. Aspirated material contains degenerated follicular cells, necrotic debris, fibrin, numerous neutrophils, and histiocytes (Fig. 7–6, see p. 434). Rarely, microorganisms can be identified. The differential diagnosis in fine needle aspiration biopsies includes infected thyroglossal duct cysts, cervical infections, the early phases of subacute thyroiditis, and some anaplastic carcinomas which may have abundant acute inflammatory cells.

Treatment and Prognosis. Treatment consists of antibiotics and surgical drainage, if necessary. In those patients with an infected piriform sinus fistula, complete excision of the fistula is essential to prevent recurrent acute thyroiditis.[42] Permanent sequelae of acute thyroiditis are exceptionally rare.

Subacute Granulomatous Thyroiditis

Clinical Features and Pathogenesis. Subacute granulomatous thyroiditis (de Quervain's disease) occurs most commonly in middle-aged women.[43] Typically, there is sudden onset of unilateral anterior neck pain that may radiate to the ear, mandible, or upper chest. Release of T_3 and T_4, due to damage of the follicular epithelium, may induce transient hyperthyroidism. A subsequent hypothyroid phase may occur and may last for several months. Very rarely, permanent hypothyroidism may occur. Physical examination reveals fever, tachycardia, and an irregularly enlarged, firm gland that is painful to palpation. Usual laboratory findings include a normal to slightly elevated white blood cell count and markedly increased erythrocyte sedimentation rate.

This disorder is often preceded by an inflammatory process of the upper respiratory tract and occurs more frequently in summer and fall months. In addition, it is often seen in association with viral illnesses, and rising antibody titers against a variety of viral antigens including mumps, measles, rhinoviruses, adenovirus, and coxsackie virus have been documented.[44] Circulating antibodies against the TSH receptor have been described, although they are most likely the consequence of antigen release during viral infection of the gland.

Pathologic Features and Differential Diagnosis. Grossly, the thyroid is usually asymmetrically enlarged. On cross-section, there may be one or more firm, irregular, yellow-white areas, which may resemble carcinoma grossly. Areas of involvement may vary from several millimeters to more than 2 cm in diameter. Early in the process, there is disruption of thyroid follicles with subsequent release of colloid into the stroma. This results in an inflammatory response dominated initially by neutrophils and microabscess formation and subsequently by a granulomatous process with lymphocytes, histiocytes, and multinucleate giant cells surrounding and engulfing deposits of colloid (colloidophagy) (Fig. 7–7, see p. 434).[45] Ultimately, there is fibrosis, especially in areas of severe tissue destruction.

The differential diagnosis includes multifocal granulomatous (palpation) thyroiditis, sarcoidosis, and tuberculosis, which are discussed in subsequent sections. Larger lesions, particularly in fibrotic phases, may simulate carcinoma grossly.

Treatment and Prognosis. Treatment generally includes aspirin and nonsteroidal anti-inflammatory agents. In some instances, corticosteroids have been used until symptoms disappear and the thyroid mass decreases.[42] Those patients who develop persistent masses are generally treated by surgery to exclude the possibility of malignancy.

Tuberculosis and Sarcoidosis

Granulomatous thyroiditis due to infection with *Mycobacteria* is rare.[46] *Mycobacteria* infection may involve the gland by hematog-

enous dissemination or by direct extension from a contiguous involved lymph node. Typical findings include the presence of necrotizing granulomas with Langhans-type giant cells and variable numbers of acid-fast organisms. Thyroid involvement by sarcoidosis has also been reported.[47]

Multifocal Granulomatous Thyroiditis

The entity known as *multifocal granulomatous thyroiditis,* or *palpation thyroiditis,* was first described by Carney et al.[48] in 1975. It is a common, incidental histologic finding in surgical pathology material and represents a response to trauma as a result of palpation of the thyroid gland. Histologically, it is characterized by loss of follicular epithelium and the presence of mononuclear histiocytes, lymphocytes, plasma cells, and multinucleate giant cells (Fig. 7–8, see p. 435). Palpation thyroiditis is present in 90% of surgically resected thyroid glands, in 10% to 40% of thyroid glands studied at autopsy from hospitalized patients, and in essentially no thyroid glands obtained from forensic autopsies. These findings suggest that multifocal granulomatous thyroiditis is the result of trauma more likely to occur in patients undergoing neck surgery than in patients in the hospital admitted for other reasons or in patients dying outside a hospital.

The differential diagnosis includes subacute granulomatous thyroiditis, C-cell hyperplasia, and solid cell nests. Typically, multifocal granulomatous thyroiditis involves one or several contiguous follicles and is not accompanied by the fibrosis and inflammation that are usually seen in subacute granulomatous thyroiditis. The mononuclear histiocytes may bear a superficial resemblance to hyperplastic C cells; however, C cells can be identified on the basis of their content of calcitonin and chromogranin. The cells making up solid cell nests are typically positive for cytokeratins. Histiocytes in multifocal granulomatous thyroiditis, on the other hand, are typically positive for lysozyme and CD68.

Hashimoto's Thyroiditis

Clinical Features and Pathogenesis. Hashimoto's thyroiditis (struma lymphomatosa) is the most common cause of goitrous hypothyroidism in iodine-sufficient areas. It is considerably more common in women than in men, and most cases occur between the ages of 30 and 50. Most patients present with painless goiter. The prevalence of the disease appears to be increasing in the general population; moreover, Hashimoto's disease occurs with higher prevalence in patients with multiple endocrine neoplasia type 2 (MEN 2); polyneuropathy, organomegaly, endocrinopathy, M-protein, and skin changes (POEMS); and Turner's and Down's syndromes.[49] During the initial phases of the disease, most patients are euthyroid, approximately 20% are hypothyroid, and 5% have evidence of hyperthyroidism.

Hashimoto's thyroiditis is a prototypic autoimmune disorder, and it is one of the triad of thyroid autoimmune disorders that includes Graves' disease and primary atrophic thyroiditis. The process begins with activation of CD4 (helper) T lymphocytes, which may become activated by viruses or bacteria that contain proteins that are similar to thyroid proteins (molecular mimicry).[49] Alternatively, thyroid cells may present their own intracellular antigens to CD4 cells via the expression of MHC class II proteins. The mechanisms of the initial activation of T cells in this setting, however, are unknown.

Activated CD4 cells can stimulate the recruitment of autoreactive B cells into the thyroid.[49] The B cells subsequently produce a variety of antibodies to thyroglobulin, microsomal antigen (peroxidase), and the TSH receptor. Activated CD4 cells also recruit CD8 cells, which may participate in the direct killing of follicular cells. Antibodies against peroxidase, which are present in more than 90% of patients, can fix complement and can induce complement-dependent cytotoxicity. Thyroglobulin antibodies are found in more than 75% of affected patients, but their role in the pathogenesis of the disorder is unknown. Antibodies against the TSH receptor are present in 10% to 15% of patients and appear to be TSH-blocking antibodies.

Hashimoto's thyroiditis is associated with a variety of other autoimmune diseases, including Graves' disease, Sjögren's disease, systemic lupus erythematosus, rheumatoid arthritis, primary adrenocortical insufficiency, type 1 diabetes mellitus, pernicious anemia, and autoimmune oophoritis. Up to 50% of first-degree relatives of patients with Hashimoto's disease have thyroid autoantibodies. There is an association of Hashimoto's disease with certain HLA types, such as HLA-B8 and HLA-DR5 or HLA-D3 (when relatives have a history of Graves') and HLA-DR4. The laboratory diagnosis of Hashimoto's thyroiditis is confirmed by the finding of antithyroid antibodies, particularly antimicrosomal antibodies, in the serum.

Pathologic Features and Differential Diagnosis. Grossly, the gland is enlarged with weights averaging from 40 to 80 g. The enlargement is usually diffuse and symmetric. The gland is typically firm but not hard, and the external surface is smooth and lobulated.[50] Rarely, the inflammatory process can extend into the surrounding muscle, resulting in some adherence of the gland to the muscle, but usually the gland can be dissected easily from the surrounding soft tissues. The cut surface of the gland is pale tan-yellow due to the presence of abundant lymphoid tissue.

Microscopically, the gland is diffusely involved, with some variation from area to area. The dominant feature is a marked lymphoplasmacytic infiltration, with lymphoid follicles containing germinal centers (Fig. 7–9).[51] Small B and T lymphocytes, plasma cells, and immunoblasts surround and extend into thyroid follicles. The thyroid follicles are typically decreased in number and reduced in size, with small lumens and absent or diminished dense pink colloid. Occasional multinucleate giant cells exhibiting colloidophagy may be present in some follicles. The follicular epithelial cells typically reveal widespread oncocytic changes with abundant granular eosinophilic cytoplasm, large nuclei, and prominent nucleoli (Fig. 7–10, see p. 435). Foci of squamous metaplasia with areas of cyst formation are relatively common, and mild degrees of interlobular fibrosis are also evident.

Hyperplastic nodules composed of small follicles with tall columnar oncocytic cells with few inflammatory cells may be present. In some cases, the extent of oncocytic change may be so extensive that the findings may simulate an oncocytic neoplasm. The presence of cells with nuclear enlargement and hyperchromasia and the presence of a fibrous capsule may further suggest the possibility of an oncoyctic neoplasm. However, the presence of a chronic inflamma-

tory infiltrate together with the overall nodular appearance of the gland should suggest the diagnosis of Hashimoto's disease.

Foci of papillary hyperplasia may also be evident in cases of Hashimoto's disease. The presence of cells with nuclear clearing and overlapping may suggest the possibility of papillary thyroid carcinoma (Fig. 7–11). Generally, however, the criteria for making an unequivocal diagnosis of papillary carcinoma in the setting of Hashimoto's thyroiditis are similar to those used when inflammatory changes are absent.[10] An additional problem is the presence of lobules of thyroid tissue (parasitic nodules), which are separated anatomically from the main mass of thyroid tissue. The presence of lymphoid tissue surrounding groups of hyperplastic follicular cells may raise the possibility of metastatic thyroid carcinoma in such instances.

An increased risk of papillary thyroid carcinoma has been reported in patients with Hashimoto's disease, particularly in surgical series,[52] but the relationship has not been proven convincingly. This issue is confounded by the frequent occurrence of chronic thyroiditis adjacent to papillary thyroid carcinomas; however, in many cases, this may represent a nonspecific chronic thyroiditis rather than true Hashimoto's disease. Recent studies have demonstrated that a very high proportion of patients with Hashimoto's disease express the *ret/PTC1* and *ret/PTC3* oncogenes in extracts of thyroid tissue.[53] These observations suggest that some of the nuclear changes observed in Hashimoto's thyroiditis could reflect the development of incipient papillary thyroid carcinomas. Additional studies are required, however, to confirm these observations.

The risk for the development of primary thyroid lymphoma is substantially increased in patients with Hashimoto's disease.[54] The distinction between thyroid lymphomas and Hashimoto's disease is discussed in detail in a subsequent section.

Fine Needle Aspiration Biopsy. Aspirates from Hashimoto's thyroiditis usually reveal scant colloid and abundant cellularity with a combination of epithelial and lymphoid cells in varying proportions (Fig. 7–12, see p. 435).[11, 55] The inflammatory infiltrate typically includes small lymphocytes, plasma cells, follicular center cell types, histiocytes, and multinucleate giant cells.[56] Both stretched fibers, resulting from artifactual distortion of lymphocytes, and lymphoglandular bodies may be prominent.

The epithelial cells are usually present both as tissue fragments and as single cells, and include oncocytic and non-oncocytic follicular cells.[57] Oncocytic cells are large with well-defined, finely granular eosinophilic cytoplasm and hyperchromatic nuclei. Large,

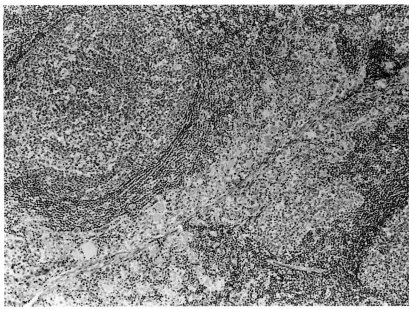

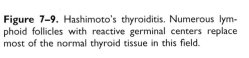

Figure 7–9. Hashimoto's thyroiditis. Numerous lymphoid follicles with reactive germinal centers replace most of the normal thyroid tissue in this field.

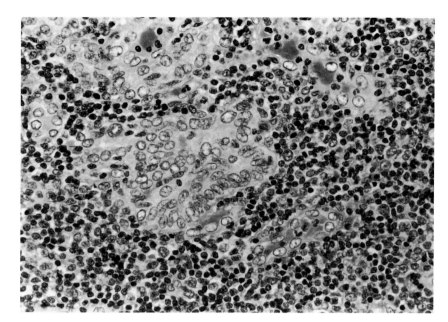

Figure 7–11. Hashimoto's thyroiditis. Groups of follicular cells exhibit nuclear clearing and overlapping.

cherry-red nucleoli, a feature of oncocytic tumors, are not usually present. Non-oncocytic follicular cells may also exhibit some nuclear atypia, and metaplastic squamous cells and flame cells may also be present.[58] In advanced stages, the aspirates reveal scanty cellularity with a small number of lymphoid cells and a few stromal fragments. Psammoma bodies have been reported in rare cases of Hashimoto's thyroiditis.[59]

The differential diagnosis of Hashimoto's thyroiditis includes non-Hodgkin's lymphomas. In lymphomas, the aspirates typically reveal a monomorphic population of atypical lymphoid cells without a significant epithelial component. Immunophenotyping reveals a monoclonal population of lymphoid cells, whereas in Hashimoto's thyroiditis the lymphoid population is polyclonal.

Treatment and Prognosis. Approximately 20% of patients with Hashimoto's disease are hypothyroid at presentation, but the frequency of subsequent hypothyroidism increases at a rate of approximately 4% per year.[49] Patients with associated hypothyroidism are generally treated by thyroid hormone replacement.[42] Thyroidectomy is usually reserved for those patients with compressive symptoms or those in whom a neoplasm is suspected.

Fibrous Variant of Hashimoto's Thyroiditis

Clinical Features and Pathogenesis. The fibrous variant of Hashimoto's thyroiditis was first clearly defined by Katz and Vickery in 1974.[60] Prior to that time, there was confusion in the literature between this entity and Riedel's disease. The fibrous variant occurs in individuals older than those with the classic form of the disease and is somewhat more common in men than in women. Patients usually present with a larger goiter, hypothyroidism, and very high titers of antimicrosomal and antithyroglobulin antibodies. Symptoms of compression, including dysphagia and dyspnea, are not unusual, owing to the large size of the gland.

Pathologic Features and Differential Diagnosis. Grossly, the thyroid is markedly enlarged.[60] The cut surface is tan-yellow and firm because of the presence of extensive fibrosis. Microscopically, thick collagen bands separate lobules of atrophic thyroid follicles (Figs. 7–13 and 7–14, see p. 436). The follicles reveal the usual changes seen in the classic variant of Hashimoto's thyroiditis, including follicular atrophy, oncocytic changes, and marked lymphoplasmacytic infiltration with germinal center formation. In addition, there is extensive squamous metaplasia in which the compo-

nent cells may exhibit minor degrees of cytologic atypia. Occasional cases of the fibrous variant of Hashimoto's disease may contain cystic areas lined by squamous epithelium.[10]

In contrast to Riedel's disease, the gland in the fibrous variant of Hashimoto's disease is not adherent to the surrounding soft tissues of the neck. Moreover, oncocytic changes and squamous metaplasia are not present in Riedel's disease.

Treatment. Generally, total thyroidectomy is performed to alleviate compressive symptoms.

Atrophic Autoimmune Thyroiditis

This entity, which has also been referred to as idiopathic, primary, or nongoitrous myxedema, was thought to represent the end stage of chronic thyroiditis, with the gland showing extensive parenchymal destruction and atrophy with marked fibrosis.[61] Patients with primary myxedema may exhibit serum thyroid-stimulation blocking antibodies. These antibodies block the action of TSH in vitro and may represent an important etiopathogenetic mechanism in this disease. Other antibodies such as thyroid growth–blocking antibody may also participate in the genesis of this disorder. Primary myxedema presents in older patients and is associated with hypothyroidism.

Grossly, the gland is markedly atrophic (2 to 5 g) and appears small and fibrotic in contrast to the thyroid enlargement typical of the fibrous variant of Hashimoto's disease.[62] Microscopically, there is follicular atrophy, squamous metaplasia, lymphoplasmacytic infiltration, and marked fibrosis. Katz and Vickery[60] suggest that there may be a progression from cases of lymphocytic thyroiditis to fibrous proliferation (fibrous variant of Hashimoto's disease) or fibrous atrophy (atrophic autoimmune thyroiditis).

Juvenile Thyroiditis

Juvenile thyroiditis, which occurs predominantly in children and women, is considered to be a variant of Hashimoto's thyroiditis. This entity is thought to be responsible for approximately 40% of cases of goiter in children.[63] Most affected individuals are euthyroid or slightly hypothyroid. Histologically, the thyroid gland contains a moderate amount of lymphoid tissue with germinal centers but with few or no oncocytes. The follicular epithelium is typically cuboidal to columnar and may have papillary infoldings.

Subacute Lymphocytic (Painless) Thyroiditis

Subacute lymphocytic painless thyroiditis is a benign, often self-limited disease of probable autoimmune origin.[64] Most cases have been reported in women, primarily in the postpartum period. Subacute lymphocytic thyroiditis may be seen in association with other autoimmune diseases (such as Sjögren's syndrome, idiopathic Addison's disease, systemic lupus erythematosus, Graves' disease, or Hashimoto's thyroiditis). Serum levels of T_4 and T_3 are usually increased. Thyroid autoantibodies are frequently positive, and their presence can be of value in predicting the occurrence of symptomatic disease and requirement for replacement therapy.

Morphologic features of subacute lymphocytic thyroiditis include focal to diffuse lymphocytic infiltration, mild to moderate follicular destruction, and mild to severe follicular hyperplasia (more common and pronounced in the postpartum type).[64] Usually there are no oncocytic changes or stromal fibrosis. During the recovery phase, there is histologic improvement with well-preserved follicular architecture, absent follicular destruction, and only lymphocytic infiltration with mild epithelial hyperplasia. Histopathologic differences from Hashimoto's thyroiditis include lack of oncocytic metaplasia, minimal follicular atrophy, minimal fibrosis, loss of germinal center formation, and presence of destroyed follicles.

Focal Nonspecific Thyroiditis

This entity, also known as simple chronic thyroiditis, represents the most common subtype of thyroiditis in surgical and autopsy pathologic material.[65] The incidence in autopsy series varies from 15% to 40%. It is more common in women, and its incidence increases with age. Its incidence has increased with the addition of iodine to dietary supplies.[66] Patients have low titers of serum thyroid autoantibodies and are usually euthyroid. Only 10% to 20% of patients have latent subclinical hypothyroidism, and usually the greater the degree of lymphocytic infiltration, the greater the degree of thyroid functional abnormalities. Grossly, there are no abnormalities. Microscopically, there are focal collections of lymphocytes, admixed with plasma cells, usually within the fibrous septa without involvement of the thyroid parenchyma (Fig. 7–15, see p. 436). Follicular epithelial cells do not show oncocytic changes.

Drug-Induced Thyroiditis

Lithium may induce goiter and hypothyroidism after prolonged therapy.[67, 68] Microscopically, there is focal follicular atrophy, lym-

phocytic infiltration, and mild fibrosis. A variety of other drugs, including phenytoin, amiodarone, and bromides, may also be associated with lymphocytic thyroiditis.[69]

Radiation-Induced Thyroid Injury

Radiation-induced abnormalities of the thyroid may result from external radiation or from the administration of ^{131}I or other isotopes. The effects of radiation on the thyroid gland can be divided into acute and chronic phases. In the acute stage following the first few weeks of irradiation, the thyroid reveals vascular congestion, edema, acute inflammation, and follicular disruption. In addition, necrosis of vessel walls, thrombosis, and hemorrhage may be present.[70] Hypothyroidism can occur within a relatively brief time following irradiation and is most likely responsible for the death of thyroid follicular cells. The late development of hypothyroidism following irradiation, on the other hand, may have an autoimmune basis.[70]

In the chronic phase, patients are hypothyroid. The severity of hypothyroidism is generally related to the extent of external irradiation.[70] The incidence of hypothyroidism following the administration of radioactive iodine is apparently less dependent on the total dose of irradiation. Typically, the chronic phases of radiation injury are associated with atrophy and fibrosis of the gland. Microscopically there is follicular atrophy and destruction, fibrosis, lymphocytic infiltration, and squamous or oncocytic metaplasia. Epithelial and stromal cells may reveal nuclear atypia and pleomorphism. Vascular changes, including intimal thickening and fibrosis of vessel walls with surrounding mononuclear inflammatory infiltrates, may be evident (Figs. 7–16 and 7–17).

Extensive studies have been performed on the thyroid glands of children exposed to large doses of irradiation following the Chernobyl catastrophe in the Soviet Union.[71] The most significant isotopes released in the fallout were ^{131}I and other shorter lived iodine isotopes, including ^{132}I and ^{133}I. Absorption of contaminated food and water resulted in extensive internal irradiation of the gland. Additional sources of irradiation resulted from protracted gamma radiation from external sources and from internal exposure to longer lived isotopes, including cesium, strontium, and plutonium.[71]

In the thyroid glands of children with thyroid cancer from this series, the most common finding in the non-neoplastic thyroid was interlobular and perifollicular fibrosis, which was observed in 81% of the cases (see Fig. 7–16).[72] Foci of papillary hyperplasia with pe-

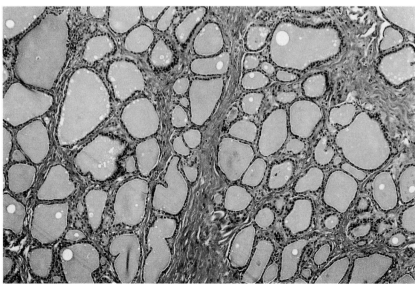

Figure 7–16. Radiation-induced changes. Note prominent perifollicular fibrosis and rare intrafollicular papillary infoldings. (Courtesy of Yuri Nikiforov, MD and Douglas Gnepp, MD.)

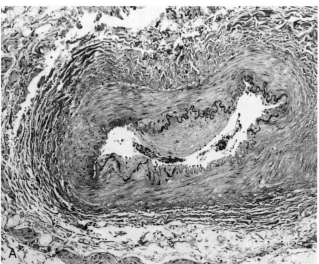 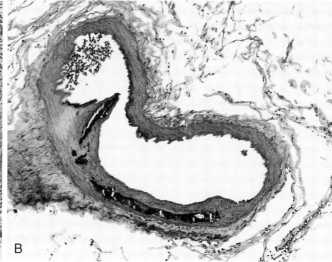

Figure 7–17. Radiation-induced vascular changes in thyroid gland. Note *(A)* focal intimal fibrosis, elastic damage, and calcification and *(B)* prominent calcification of the vascular wall. (Courtesy of Yuri Nikiforov, MD and Douglas Gnepp, MD.)

ripheral scalloping of colloid were found in 79% of cases. Changes in intrathyroidal and perithyroidal arteries, including reduplication and fragmentation of the elastica as well as absence of the elastica, were noted in 73% of the cases (see Fig. 7–17A, B). Calcification of the elastica was also a frequent finding.[71, 73] Approximately two thirds of the glands had irregularly enlarged follicles, which were distended with colloid and desquamated cells. Multiple colloid nodules were identified in approximately one third of the cases. Approximately one third of the glands had areas with mild epithelial nuclear pleomorphism, and lymphocytic infiltrates were observed in 23% of the cases. Foci of squamous metaplasia or oncocytic change were not identified in these cases. In 59 patients with benign diseases, multinodular goiter was present in 48%, adenomatoid nodules in 30%, lymphocytic thyroiditis in 18%, follicular adenoma in 15%, diffuse hyperplasia in 3%, and diffuse hyperplasia with atypia and nodularity in 8%.

Riedel's Disease

Clinical Features and Pathogenesis. Riedel's disease represents a manifestation of the group of systemic fibrosing diseases known as *multifocal idiopathic fibrosclerosis,* which also includes mediastinal and retroperitoneal fibrosis.[74–76] Riedel's disease usually involves the thyroid as well as other structures in the neck, including the parathyroid glands. In one study by Schwaergerle et al.,[77] one third of patients with Riedel's disease reported after 1960 had other fibrosing lesions.[77] This disorder is very rare. A review of the Mayo Clinic experience by Hay[78] revealed only 37 cases among 56,700 thyroidectomies performed between 1920 and 1984. Riedel's disease primarily affects women between the ages of 30 and 60 years. Patients usually present with a history of painless goiter, which may grow and progress to produce symptoms of pressure and compression of surrounding structures.

Most patients are euthyroid unless there is complete fibrosis of the gland. Hyperthyroidism is rare, occurring in less than 5% of patients. In some cases, thyroid autoantibodies may be present in low titers. However, there does not appear to be a direct relationship between Riedel's disease and autoimmune thyroid disease, and previous suggestions that Riedel's may be an autoimmune process are probably incorrect. However, Hashimoto's thyroiditis and Riedel's disease may rarely coexist.[79]

Pathologic Features and Differential Diagnosis. The disease may be unilateral or bilateral. The gland is typically "stony" hard or "woody" and is fixed to adjacent structures. Enlarged cervical lymph

nodes may be present, and this feature, in conjunction with a fixed, hard gland, may lead to a strong clinical suspicion of carcinoma. The diagnosis of this disorder requires an open biopsy. Histologically, hyalinized fibrous tissue replaces the thyroid gland and may extend into the adjacent soft tissues of the neck (Fig. 7–18). The inflammatory infiltrate includes lymphocytes, plasma cells, and variable numbers of eosinophils. Evidence of venulitis may be present. Generally, fine needle aspirates are unsuccessful because of the extensive fibrosis.

The differential diagnosis includes the fibrosing variant of Hashimoto's disease, discussed previously, and fibrous atrophy of the thyroid. In contrast to the latter condition, the gland in Riedel's disease is typically enlarged. Since occasional cases of papillary thyroid carcinoma may be accompanied by extensive fibrosis, tumor should be ruled out by extensive sampling in suspected cases of Riedel's disease. The paucicellular variant of undifferentiated (anaplastic) thyroid carcinoma may also mimic Riedel's disease. This variant of undifferentiated carcinoma appears hypocellular with mild atypia of the spindle cells.[79a]

Treatment and Prognosis. Surgical treatment alone is often insufficient to alleviate the symptoms of compression. Studies by Few et al.[80] suggest that tamoxifen is effective for treatment of this disorder. The mechanisms of action of this drug may be related to the stimulation and release of transforming growth factor-β, which may have a role in the inhibition of fibroblastic proliferation.[80]

Amyloidosis

Amyloid goiter is a rare condition characterized by massive enlargement of the thyroid as a result of the deposition of amyloid fibrils in the interstitium and blood vessels of the gland in patients with primary or secondary amyloidosis.[81] The disease may be unilateral or bilateral and the gland is typically firm, waxy, and yellow-tan on cross-section. The amyloid deposits exhibit Congophilia and green birefringence in polarized light. The follicular cells are typically atrophic, although occasional nuclear enlargement may also be evident (Fig. 7–19, see p. 437). Clusters of mature adipocytes are often present within the amyloid deposits, and, in some cases, a foreign body giant cell reaction may be evident.

As discussed in a subsequent section, occasional cases of medullary thyroid carcinoma may be almost completely replaced by amyloid deposits and may, therefore, simulate an amyloid goiter. Extensive sampling of such cases together with immunostaining for calcitonin are usually sufficient to identify foci of tumor.

Treatment. In patients with massive amyloid goiters, thyroidectomy may be required to relieve compressive symptoms.

Hyperplasia of the Thyroid

Hyperplastic diseases of the thyroid are common entities that are manifested by diffuse or nodular enlargement of the gland. Clinically, enlargement of the thyroid gland by any cause is referred to as *goiter.* Hyperplasia of the thyroid gland may be associated with hyperfunction (Graves' disease), hypofunction (endemic goiter, dyshormonogenic goiter), or normal function (multinodular goiter).

Graves' Disease

The term *thyrotoxicosis* refers to a spectrum of changes that result from exposure of the body to excess quantities of thyroid hormone.[14] Hyperthyroidism refers to syndromes associated with overproduction of thyroid hormones by the thyroid gland. The causes of hyperthyroidism in the order of frequency include Graves' disease, toxic multinodular goiter, and toxic adenoma. It has been estimated that Graves' disease occurs in approximately 0.4% of the population in the United States.

Clinical Features and Pathogenesis. Most patients with Graves' disease (diffuse toxic goiter) present in the third or fourth decades, with a four- to fivefold predominance in women.[14] Clinically, Graves' disease is characterized by diffuse goiter, thyrotoxicosis, infiltrative ophthalmopathy, and infiltrative dermopathy (pretibial myxedema). The disease has an autoimmune origin and is initiated by the presence in the serum of immunoglobulins directed against regions of the plasma membrane of the thyroid follicular cells that contain the thyroid-stimulating hormone (TSH) receptor. This results in stimulation of adenyl cyclase, leading to growth of the thyroid gland, increased vascularity, and secretion of T_3 and T_4. A genetically determined organ-specific defect in suppressor T lymphocytes may be responsible for initiating immunoglobulin production by B lymphocytes.

Pathologic Features and Differential Diagnosis. Typically, the thyroid gland in patients with Graves' disease is diffusely and symmetrically enlarged, with weights ranging from 50 to 150 g (Fig. 7–20, see p. 437). On cross-section, the gland lacks the translucent appearance of normal thyroid but rather appears beefy and red. Microscopically, there is preservation of the normal lobular architecture; however, the follicles appear small and irregularly shaped. This is due to the presence of numerous papillary epithelial infoldings with basally placed nuclei (Fig. 7–21, see p. 437).[82] Follicular cells tend to be tall with focally vacuolated cytoplasm and basally placed nuclei. Occasional oncocytes may be evident. Colloid is scanty, and it typically exhibits a very pale eosinophilic appearance with peripheral scalloping. The stroma may appear slightly fibrotic and occasional lymphoid follicles with active germinal centers may be evident. Very rarely, psammoma bodies might be evident in the papillae and raise the possibility of papillary carcinoma.

The papillary areas in Graves' disease may, on occasion, be confused with those seen in papillary thyroid carcinoma. An important feature to differentiate these entities is the preservation of the lobular architecture in cases of Graves' disease. Moreover, the papillae in Graves' disease tend to be simple and nonbranching, whereas those in papillary carcinoma more often exhibit a branching architecture. While the colloid in Graves' disease tends to be pale and watery, the colloid in cases of papillary carcinoma is often densely stained. In contrast to the basal localization of nuclei in areas of papillary hyperplasia, the nuclei in papillary carcinomas are present in nonbasal areas; moreover, the nuclei in papillary carcinoma are typically overlapped with finely dispersed chromatin, contain grooves, and also may exhibit characteristic inclusions, as discussed in subsequent sections.

The pathology of the gland is affected by specific forms of treatment.[83] In patients treated with potassium iodide, the follicles become filled with colloid, and the follicular cells assume a more cuboidal shape. Following treatment with propylthiouracil, the appearance of the gland is unchanged, presumably owing to the continued stimulation of the gland by TSH. Treatment with radioactive iodine results in fibrosis with follicular atrophy and scattered follicular cells with atypical nuclear features.

Fine Needle Aspiration Biopsies. Aspirates from Graves' disease usually reveal clusters of hyperplastic follicular cells with or without a follicular pattern and scant colloid in a background of abundant red blood cells. Papillae, lymphocytes, and Hürthle cells may be present in variable proportions. The follicular cells exhibit mildly atypical hyperchromatic nuclei and many cytoplasmic vacuoles, which probably represent dilated cisternae of endoplasmic reticulum associated with augmented protein synthesis.[16] These cells, which are called *flame cells,* are not pathognomonic of Graves' disease and may be seen in other entities such as Hashimoto's thyroiditis and nontoxic goiter.[84] They may also be present, in low numbers, in follicular or papillary carcinoma. Pitts and Berry[85] have mentioned their presence in metastatic carcinoma as evidence of a thyroid origin.

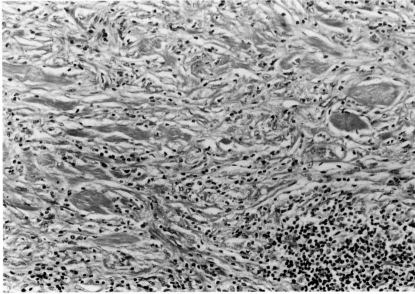

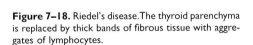

Figure 7–18. Riedel's disease. The thyroid parenchyma is replaced by thick bands of fibrous tissue with aggregates of lymphocytes.

Treatment and Prognosis. The treatment of patients with Graves' disease is controversial. The major agents employed in the chemotherapeutic management of affected patients include drugs of the thioamide class, which inhibit the oxidation and organic binding of iodide.[14] Cessation of treatment, however, leads to a relatively frequent recurrence of thyrotoxicosis. Subtotal thyroidectomy, on the other hand, is associated with recurrent disease in only 10% of cases, but the risk of complications, including permanent hypothyroidism, vocal cord paralysis, and hypoparathyroidism, is relatively high. Radioiodine administration produces the ablative effects of surgery without the immediate operative and postoperative complications of subtotal thyroidectomy. The major disadvantage of radioactive iodine administration, however, is the late development of hypothyroidism. Selection of specific forms of therapy should be tailored to the needs of individual patients.[14]

Goitrous Hypothyroidism and Endemic Goiter

Goitrous hypothyroidism is characterized by an impaired ability to synthesize T_3 and T_4 because of inadequate dietary iodine (endemic goiter), ingestion of drugs that interfere with thyroid hormone synthesis, or enzymatic defects in the biosynthesis of thyroid hormones.[86] As a result of inadequate thyroid hormone production, there is hypersecretion of TSH, which leads to increased thyroid growth and stimulation of thyroid hormone biosynthesis.

The term *endemic goiter* is used when this condition occurs in more than 10% of the population in a defined geographic area.[87] The most important endemic goiter regions include the northern and southern slopes of the Himalayas, the Andean region of South America, the European Alps, mountainous regions of China, central regions of Africa, and, to a lesser extent, the coastal areas of Europe. Low levels of dietary iodine are the major cause of endemic goiter; however, ingestion of natural goitrogens (vegetables of the Brassica family, including cabbage and turnips, which contain high concentrations of thioglucosides) may be responsible for the development of goiter. Cyanoglucosides represent another important group of goitrogens and are found in high concentrations in cassava, maize, bamboo shoots, and sweet potatoes.[87] Flavinoids, which are found in high concentrations in millet, are also goitrogenic. In general, the severity of goiter formation is related to the extent of iodine deficiency. Initially, goiter formation is diffuse, but with repeated episodes of hyperplasia and involution, multiple nodules supervene to produce a diffuse and nodular goiter, similar to that observed in patients with nontoxic nodular goiter.

Endemic goiter can be prevented by the addition of iodine to the diet and by the elimination of goitrogens in foodstuffs. In adults with large goiters, suppression of TSH by the administration of thyroxine can lead to diminished thyroid size. Surgical treatment is reserved for individuals with very large goiters that fail to involute following TSH suppression or those patients in whom malignancy is suspected.[87]

Dyshormonogenic Goiter

Clinical Features and Pathogenesis. Defects in hormone biosynthesis are rare causes of goitrous hypothyroidism (dyshormonogenic goiter).[8] Although goiter may be present at birth, it more commonly develops at 1 to 2 years of age. Most of the enzymatic defects are inherited as autosomal recessive traits. The various defects include those involved in iodide transport, organification, iodotyrosine coupling, iodotyrosine dehalogenase activity, and iodoprotein secretion. Goiters in affected individuals tend to be very large and multinodular.[88, 89]

Pathologic Features and Differential Diagnosis. Typically, the thyroid gland is markedly enlarged and multinodular. On cross-section, individual nodules vary from those that are beefy red to those that are firm and white to gray-tan. Individual nodules may be surrounded by broad bands of fibrous connective tissue.

Histologically, the nodules vary from those with papillary or follicular architectural patterns to those that are predominantly solid

(Fig. 7–22A, B). Generally, the papillae are nonbranching and lack the nuclear features that are typical of papillary carcinomas. The luminal spaces contain little or no colloid. In those nodules with follicular patterns of growth, there may be considerable variation in nuclear size and shape. Other nodules may exhibit more solid growth patterns with pronounced nuclear hyperchromasia and mitotic activity. Because of the atypical cytologic features, the solid appearance of many of the nodules, and the presence of partial fibrous encapsulation, the possibility of malignancy is often entertained, particularly when the clinical history is unavailable.

Very rare examples of follicular carcinoma developing in patients with dyshormonogenic goiter have been reported.[90] The diagnosis of malignancy in this setting should be rendered with particular caution and should be made only when there is evidence of invasion of adjacent normal tissues, metastases, or unequivocal vascular invasion.

Treatment and Prognosis. Treatment of patients with dyshormonogenic goiter includes the administration of thyroxine until the serum TSH becomes normalized. Surgery is indicated in those patients with very large goiters causing physical disfigurement or compressive symptoms. The prognosis is generally excellent for patients with mild enzymatic defects. In patients with severe forms of the disease, both growth retardation and mental retardation occur unless thyroid hormone is replaced very early in the course of the disease.

Nontoxic Nodular Goiter

Clinical Features and Pathogenesis. The term *nontoxic goiter* refers to enlargement of the thyroid gland in the absence of hyperthyroidism or hypothyroidism, inflammatory processes, or neoplasms.[8] Thyroid enlargement may be diffuse or diffuse and nodular. Nontoxic nodular goiter is the most common form of goiter in the United States. With large goiters, displacement or compression of the esophagus and trachea may give rise to dysphagia or dyspnea. Pain may be associated with hemorrhage into one of the nodules. Clinically, the incidence of nontoxic nodular goiter is 3% to 5%.[91] At autopsy, the prevalence of this disorder is substantially higher and is in the range of 30% to 50%.

The development of goiter most likely results from a variety of mechanisms that lead to impairment of T_3 and T_4 production.[14] This leads to increased production of TSH and subsequent stimulation of the thyroid gland. One hypothesis is that the inability to form sufficient T_3 and T_4 represents an inborn error of metabolism that is related to, but not as severe as, that present in patients with dyshormonogenic goiter. The levels of TSH are not substantially increased in individuals with nodular goiter, however. This suggests that levels of TSH may be only minimally or sporadically increased in affected patients. An alternative possibility is that subsets of thyroid follicular cells may be more susceptible to the stimulatory actions of normal levels of TSH. It has also been suggested that there may be a class of thyroid growth-stimulating immunoglobulins that stimulate growth but do not stimulate adenylase activity in patients with nontoxic nodular goiter.

Pathologic Features and Differential Diagnosis. The initial phase of the development of this type of goiter is characterized by diffuse glandular enlargement. There is hyperplasia of follicular cells with the formation of papillary infoldings of the epithelium and scant amounts of colloid. In the phase of involution, the follicles become filled with colloid. Rupture of follicles may lead to inflammation with histiocytes, lymphocytes, and multinucleate giant cells. The disease process is, therefore, characterized by alternating phases of hyperplasia and involution.

Nodular thyroids are typically enlarged, with weights ranging up to 500 g (Fig. 7–23, see p. 438). Typically, the gland is markedly distorted by multiple adenomatous nodules that measure from less than 1 cm to many centimeters in diameter. In some instances, the growth may extend beneath the sternum (substernal goiter). Individual nodules have a remarkable array of histologic appearances. Some may be composed of markedly enlarged follicles that are dis-

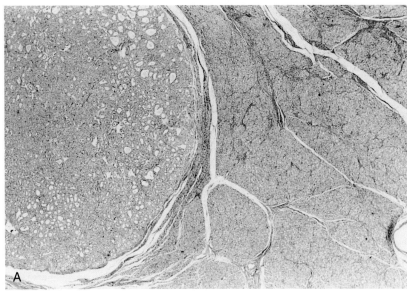

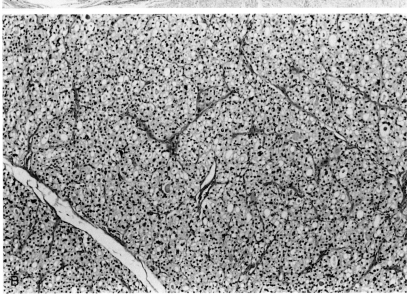

Figure 7–22. *A*, Dyshormonogenic goiter. A thyroid nodule with a microfollicular pattern appears sharply circumscribed. The adjacent thyroid parenchyma has a solid appearance. *B*, Dyshormonogenic goiter. The thyroid gland has a solid appearance without colloid. Occasional nuclei appear hyperchromatic.

tended with colloid (Fig. 7–24, see p. 438), whereas others may have a microfollicular appearance. Other nodules may appear hyperplastic, with papillary formations extending into the follicular spaces (Fig. 7–25, see p. 438). Nodules composed of oncocytes may also occur. Individual nodules are partially demarcated from the adjacent thyroid parenchyma by an incomplete fibrous capsule. In contrast to adenomas, which typically have a uniform follicular architecture, adenomatous nodules are characterized by variation in follicular size. The adjacent thyroid parenchyma is not usually compressed adjacent to adenomatous nodules, in contrast to the compressive effects of adenomas. Degenerative changes including hemorrhage, calcification, and ossification are frequent. Some follicular nodules may undergo complete cystification.

Recent studies employing molecular techniques have revealed that some of the nodules in multinodular goiters may represent clonal proliferations.[92] In the series of cases reported by Apel et al.,[93] seven hyperplastic (adenomatous) nodules were polyclonal and 18 were monoclonal. The adjacent thyroid parenchyma was polyclonal in all cases. Moreover, there were no morphologic differences with respect to cellularity or encapsulation in nodules that were monoclonal or polyclonal.

Fine Needle Aspiration Biopsy. Fine needle aspirates usually reveal an admixture of benign follicular cells, colloid, and inflammatory cells in variable proportions[12, 94–96] (Fig. 7–26, see p. 439). In the initial diffuse hyperplastic stages, aspiration yields numerous

follicular cells and scanty colloid, whereas in phases of involution, smears demonstrate scant cellularity and abundant colloid. The follicular cells are arranged in monolayered sheets and in tissue fragments, with or without a follicular pattern (Fig. 7–27, see p. 439). They have a moderate amount of well-defined cytoplasm and round, regular, uniform nuclei that exhibit polarity. Groups of oncocytes may be evident in some cases. Prominent nucleoli are usually absent, except in the hyperplastic stage.

Hemosiderin-laden macrophages are almost always present in fine needle aspiration biopsies of multinodular goiters. Their nuclei are usually bland but can occasionally exhibit marked degenerative atypia. A few lymphocytes as well as multinucleated giant cells can also be present. Occasionally, hyperinvoluted nodular goiter with old hemorrhage, granulation tissue, and fibrosis yields aspirated material composed of stromal and inflammatory cells in a background of abundant colloid. In these cases, if follicular cells are present, they may possess vacuolated, foamy cytoplasm with small nuclei but large nucleoli, raising the possibility of a neoplastic process.

Treatment and Prognosis. Patients with large multinodular goiters with evidence of compressive symptoms are generally treated by subtotal thyroidectomy. This approach is also used in individuals in whom carcinoma is suspected. In patients with normal or elevated levels of TSH, administration of thyroid hormone may lead to a decrease in the size of the goiter. Radioactive iodine has also been used in some instances.

Thyroid Nodules and Thyroid Cancer: General Considerations

The prevalence of thyroid nodules is dependent on numerous factors, including the age of the population, geographic locale, and the sensitivity of the detection system. In the Framingham study, thyroid nodules were identified clinically in 6.4% of women and 1.5% of men, with a nodule accrual rate of 0.09% per year.[97] The prevalence of thyroid nodules is 5 to 10 times higher in glands studied by ultrasonography and in thyroid glands examined directly at autopsy.[91] Of those nodules that have been surgically removed, 42% to 77% prove to be adenomatous or hyperplastic nodules, 15% to 40% are adenomas, and 8% to 17% are carcinomas, depending on the series. The prevalence of thyroid nodules of all types, including carcinomas, however, is substantially higher in individuals exposed to prior irradiation.

Thyroid cancer accounts for approximately 1% of all cancers diagnosed in the United States, exclusive of carcinomas of the skin.[98] The annual incidence in the United States is approximately 40 cases per million, with a predominance of cases occurring in women. The incidence of thyroid cancer has increased three- to five-fold between 1935 and 1975, based on data from the Connecticut Tumor Registry, but the reasons for this increase are not clear. The prevalence of thyroid cancer is 67 per 100,000 population for females and 23 per 100,000 for males. The death rate for thyroid cancer of all types is approximately four cases per million, or approximately one tenth the incidence rate.

Genetic and environmental factors have been implicated in the development of thyroid cancer.[98, 99] Radiation exposure is a well-known risk factor, and doses in the range of 200 to 500 cGy are associated with the development of thyroid cancer at a rate of 0.5% per year.[100] Radiation exposure in childhood produces a higher risk for the development of thyroid cancer than does radiation exposure in adulthood.[101] In the series of thyroid cancer cases following the Chernobyl nuclear accident, the highest number of patients that subsequently developed cancer was in the group that was less than 1 year of age at the time of exposure, and this number decreased progressively through age 12 years.[71] Chemical carcinogens have been implicated in thyroid carcinogenesis in rodents; however, there are few studies noting this association in humans. Iodine supplementation of the diet is associated with a decreasing risk of follicular carcinoma but a corresponding increasing risk of papillary carcinoma.[98]

The vast majority of benign and malignant thyroid neoplasms are of follicular cell origin. In general, papillary carcinomas and minimally invasive follicular carcinomas are low-grade malignancies with an excellent prognosis, whereas undifferentiated (anaplastic) carcinomas are high-grade malignancies with a very poor prognosis. Widely invasive follicular carcinomas and poorly differentiated carcinomas have a prognosis that is intermediate between these two groups. Tumors of C-cell origin account for 5% to 10% of all thyroid neoplasms, whereas sarcomas and malignant lymphomas account for a small proportion of the cases.

The treatment of thyroid cancer is covered in several recent reviews.[102–104]

Diagnostic Approaches Including Fine Needle Aspiration Biopsy

Numerous modalities have been employed for the preoperative diagnosis of thyroid cancer, including serum thyroglobulin levels, radionuclide scans, and ultrasonography.[105] These techniques, however, have relatively low discriminatory value for the separation of benign and malignant thyroid nodules.

Fine needle aspiration biopsy is the most sensitive, specific, and cost-effective approach for the diagnosis of thyroid nodules. The introduction of this technique has resulted in a decreased rate of thyroid surgery and an increased rate of identifying cancer when surgery is performed.

Gharib and Goellner[106] and Gharib et al.[12] reviewed seven large series comprising more than 18,000 patients who underwent a fine needle aspiration biopsy. The average rate of benign cytologic diagnosis was 69% and the average rate of malignant cytologic diagnosis was 3.5%. The average rates of suspicious and nondiagnostic cytologic results were 10% and 17%, respectively. In general, even with repetitive aspirations performed by experienced physicians, 10% of smears will be nondiagnostic. In approximately 80% of patients, a definitive benign or malignant diagnosis can be offered after a fine needle aspiration biopsy.[106] The false-negative rate can be defined as the percentage of patients with a benign diagnosis by fine needle aspiration biopsy who subsequently had a malignant diagnosis at surgery.

In general, the true false-negative rates vary between 1% and 5%,[106] while the false-positive rate is about 1%.[16] For satisfactory specimens, 1 in 20 to 40 patients with a benign diagnosis by fine needle aspiration biopsy may have a malignant diagnosis after surgery and 1 in 100 patients with a malignant diagnosis may actually have a benign condition.[16, 107] In general, false-negative results are primarily due to inadequate sampling.[108] Therefore, it is important to define stringent criteria to decide whether a specimen is adequate and satisfactory for diagnosis. This is particularly important for cystic lesions, in which smears often exhibit histiocytes with no or few epithelial cells. Other causes of false-negative results include specimens diluted with excess blood,[109] small tumor size,[110] and the presence of occult carcinomas.[111] Medullary carcinoma has been associated with a relatively high false-negative rate.[112]

False-positive results are usually caused by interpretative errors. The most common sources of error include nodular goiter with papillary hyperplasia,[113] Hashimoto's thyroiditis with papillary hyperplasia, and follicular adenomas with artifactual nuclear clearing and nuclear atypia. Each of these conditions may be misinterpreted as papillary carcinoma.[108] The overinterpretation of oncocytic cells in Hashimoto's thyroiditis, goiters, or adenomas also represents a common source of error.[16]

The two most significant limitations of this technique are nondiagnostic aspirates and suspicious results.[114] It is important to emphasize that only 1.1% of patients with unsatisfactory specimens will have a malignant diagnosis after surgery.[115] Currently, fine needle aspiration has an accuracy that is at least comparable to that of frozen section.[116, 117] For papillary carcinoma, the accuracy of fine needle aspiration biopsies, in fact, is superior to that of frozen section.[118] For follicular lesions, although frozen sections can demonstrate capsular or vascular invasion, complete sampling of the lesion at the time of frozen section is impractical. Therefore, many times the frozen section is only reported as follicular neoplasm. Frozen sections, however, may be useful for intraoperative diagnoses and decision-making in patients with unsatisfactory or suspicious fine needle aspiration biopsy diagnoses.[117, 119]

The ultimate goal of any fine needle aspiration biopsy is to provide the pathologist with a specimen in which the material is sufficient to render a cytopathologic diagnosis. Therefore, the specimen should be adequate not only in terms of cellularity but also in thickness, fixation, and staining. It is difficult to generate a definition of adequacy for a thyroid aspirate smear, and different workers have provided different criteria that define an adequate sample. Kini defines it as a specimen with eight to 10 tissue fragments of well-preserved follicular epithelium on at least two slides with a total of six thin smears from six different sites of a given nodule.[11] Following these criteria, the rate of unsatisfactory specimens is 20%.

Other workers have proposed different criteria. Gharib et al.[12] define an adequate specimen as one with six groups of well-preserved follicular cells, each group consisting of 10 or more cells (rate of unsatisfactory smears is 21%). Nguyen et al.[120] proposed as a criterion of adequacy 10 large clusters of follicular cells with 20 cells or more in each cluster, present on all available smears (rate of unsatisfactory smears is 5%). Finally, Hamburger[121] proposed six clusters of cells on each of at least two slides prepared from separate aspirates, with six smears prepared from six different aspirates.[121]

Thyroid Cysts

Cystic lesions of the thyroid gland are common, representing 6% to 35% of all surgically removed solitary thyroid nodules. They usually are the result of degeneration, hemorrhage, or necrosis of an adenomatous nodule. Similar changes may occur in benign or malignant neoplasms, particularly papillary thyroid carcinoma. True primary cysts of the thyroid are exceedingly rare, although cystic degeneration of solid cell nests has been reported. Cystic change occurs more commonly in lesions larger than 4 cm. Fine needle aspiration biopsy is a useful technique, first in identifying thyroid lesions as cysts, and second in detecting malignant cells. Aspirates of many thyroid cysts are often technically insufficient because of poor cellularity. It is therefore essential to assess the adequacy of the specimen to avoid a false-negative diagnosis. Any cyst that recurs or any palpable nodule identified after evacuation of a cyst must be reaspirated to rule out malignancy. However, only 1% of all aspirated cysts prove to be malignant.[115]

Benign Tumors

Clinical Features and Pathogenesis. Follicular adenomas are benign, encapsulated tumors with evidence of follicular cell differentiation. Molecular studies have established that most adenomas have a clonal origin.[91, 122] Adenomas occur predominantly in women and usually present as single, painless nodules that are cold on scan. Hyperfunctional (toxic) adenomas, in contrast, will appear "hot" on thyroid scan. Adenomas may also be multiple, and, in these instances, they may be difficult if not impossible to distinguish from adenomatous nodules. Rarely, patients may present with pain and rapid enlargement of the adenoma due to hemorrhage, which may occur spontaneously or as a consequence of fine needle aspiration biopsy (Fig. 7–28, see p. 439).

Pathologic Features and Differential Diagnosis. Typically, adenomas are expansile, round to ovoid lesions that are separated from the adjacent normal thyroid parenchyma by a thin but complete fibrous capsule (Fig. 7–29, see p. 440), with compression of the adjacent normal thyroid parenchyma. In contrast to follicular carcinomas, follicular adenomas lack evidence of capsular or vascular invasion. Most resected adenomas measure from 1 to 3 cm in diameter, although occasional very large adenomas may occur. They vary from pink-white and red to tan-brown. Foci of hemorrhage, cyst formation, fibrosis, and calcification may be evident. Usually, the pattern of follicular growth is uniform within the adenoma, in contrast to hyperplastic nodules, which commonly exhibit variations in the sizes and shapes of individual follicles.

Adenomas are subclassified according to the predominant pattern of follicular growth. The embryonal (trabecular or solid) adenoma is composed of nests of follicular cells with few or no follicles. Microfollicular (fetal) adenomas are composed of small follicles containing scanty luminal colloid. Simple (normofollicular) adenomas are composed of follicles of approximately the same size as those in the adjacent normal thyroid, whereas macrofollicular adenomas are composed of follicles that are substantially larger than those of the adjacent normal follicles. Follicular adenomas contain both low molecular weight cytokeratins and vimentin. In addition, the cells are positive for thyroglobulin, T_3, and T_4.[123]

Foci of clear cell change may be present throughout the tumor or may be restricted to small groups of follicles. Factors responsible for clear cell change in follicular adenomas include the presence of cytoplasmic vesicles, which may originate from degenerated and cystically dilated mitochondria, or from dilation of the endoplasmic reticulum or Golgi vesicles. In some instances, clear cell change has been traced to the intracellular accumulation of glycogen, lipid, or thyroglobulin. Occasional adenomas may contain cells with a signet ring appearance. The cytoplasmic vacuoles are typically positive for thyroglobulin and may also contain mucin. Such tumors have been referred to as *signet ring adenomas*.[124]

The differential diagnosis includes adenomatous (hyperplastic) nodules, follicular carcinoma, the follicular variant of papillary carcinoma, and the follicular (tubular) variant of medullary carcinoma. Generally, adenomatous nodules exhibit considerable variation in the size of the component follicles, whereas the follicular structure of adenomas tends to be more uniform. Moreover, the capsule surrounding adenomas is complete, while it is often incomplete around adenomatous nodules. The distinction of follicular adenoma from carcinoma depends on the demonstration of capsular or vascular invasion, or both, in the latter. The follicular variant of papillary carcinoma is characterized by a series of nuclear changes, which are detailed in a subsequent section. The follicular (tubular) variant of medullary carcinoma is characterized by the presence of chromogranin or calcitonin within the tumor cells, whereas stains for thyroglobulin are negative.

Fine Needle Aspiration Biopsy. Adenomas with a predominant macrofollicular pattern generally contain abundant colloid and scant cellular components. Follicular cells usually are arranged in monolayered sheets, sometimes with a honeycomb pattern (Fig. 7–30, see p. 440). Occasionally, microfollicles with normal cell size are identified. The cytologic appearance is very similar to that of nodular goiter, making the distinction difficult if not impossible in some instances. Simple (normofollicular) adenomas may reveal aspiration cytology similar to that of normal thyroid tissue, with colloid present in variable amounts. If the adenoma is large, morphology can vary based on the sampling of different areas within the tumor.

Aspirates of cellular adenomas usually contain numerous cells with little or no colloid. Follicular cells are usually grouped in syncytial tissue fragments, with or without a follicular pattern (microfollicular adenoma) or a trabecular pattern (trabecular adenoma). The cells have a small amount of pale cytoplasm and enlarged hyperchromatic nuclei with an altered polarity. Nucleoli are usually inconspicuous. Adenomas cannot be distinguished from carcinomas on the basis of fine needle aspiration biopsy. This subject is discussed in greater detail in the section on follicular carcinoma.

Fine needle aspiration biopsy may lead to a variety of worrisome histologic alterations in adenomas. Distinguishing between true capsular invasion and the changes associated with fine needle aspiration biopsies may be, at times, exceedingly difficult. These changes have been referred to as WHAFFT (worrisome histologic alterations following fine needle aspiration of the thyroid).[50] Acute changes (occurring less than 3 weeks following aspiration) include hemorrhage and granulation tissue with giant cells and hemosiderin-laden macrophages, mitoses, necrosis, nuclear clearing, poorly formed granulomas, capsular distortion, and, rarely, infarction. Generally, the foci of hemorrhage and granulation tissue are linear and are perpendicular to the center of the nodule. Chronic changes, usually occurring between 1 and 6 months after aspiration, include linear fibrosis adjacent to hemosiderin-laden macrophages; oncocytic, spindle cell, and squamous metaplasias; infarction; pseudoinvasion of the capsule; random nuclear atypia; papillary degeneration often associated with cyst formation; and calcification. Foci of pseudoinvasion tend to be linear, and the presence of hemorrhage, hemosiderin deposition, granulation tissue, and the focal and geographic pattern of the lesions favors a fine needle aspiration biopsy–associated change rather than true capsular invasion (Fig. 7–31).

Adenoma Variants

In addition to adenomas composed of small or large follicles, a variety of adenoma variants have been described, including "atypical" adenomas, adenomas with bizarre nuclei, oncocytic adenomas, hyalinizing trabecular adenomas, adenolipomas and adenochondromas, and adenomas with papillary hyperplasia.

Atypical Adenoma

The term *atypical adenoma* was introduced by Hazard and Kenyon[125] to describe adenomas in which there were closely packed

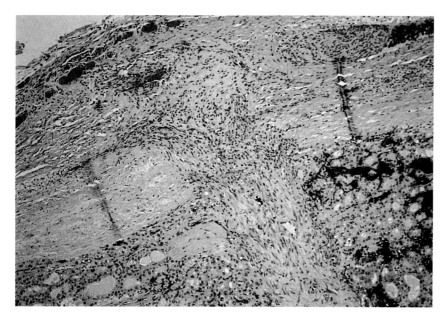

Figure 7–31. Follicular adenoma. A healing needle tract site extends through the capsule into the periphery of the adenoma.

follicles lacking a central lumen, solid columns of cells, sheet-like masses of cells, and areas of spindle cell growth. As a result of this very broad histopathologic definition, many pathologists have used this term indiscriminately for any adenoma with features that deviate from typical or usual adenomas.[10] This approach should be discouraged and, in fact, Rosai et al.[10] have suggested that the term *atypical adenoma* be replaced with the designation *hypercellular adenoma*. In any event, lesions with any atypical features should be examined carefully to rule out evidence of capsular or vascular invasion.

Adenomas with Bizarre Nuclei

Similar to other benign endocrine tumors, follicular adenomas may contain groups of cells with markedly enlarged and hyperchromatic nuclei. Thyroid tumors with these features have been termed *adenomas with bizarre nuclei*.[10] Although the presence of such nuclei may suggest the possibility of malignancy, they occur, in fact, more often in benign than in malignant follicular lesions of the thyroid (Fig. 7–32, see p. 453).

Oncocytic (Hürthle Cell) Adenomas

Oncocytic adenomas are benign tumors composed exclusively or predominantly of oncocytes. The tumors are round to ovoid and are separated from the adjacent thyroid parenchyma by a fibrous capsule. In larger tumors with foci of degenerative changes, groups of oncocytes may become entrapped within the capsule. Such foci should be distinguished from areas of true capsular invasion, as discussed in the section on oncocytic carcinoma. On cross-section, the tumors are dark brown and solid. Oncocytic tumors may undergo needle biopsy–induced or spontaneous infarct-like necrosis.[126, 127]

The pattern of growth is usually follicular (Fig. 7–33) but may be solid (Fig. 7–34, see p. 453) or trabecular. The intrafollicular colloid may be weakly basophilic and may contain psammoma body–like calcifications (see Fig. 7–33). The nuclei are usually large and vesicular with coarsely clumped chromatin and prominent nucleoli, while the cytoplasm is deeply eosinophilic and granular. The granular appearance is due to the presence of numerous mitochondria. Marked swelling of the mitochondria may lead to a clear appearance of the tumor cells (Fig. 7–35, see p. 453).

Text continued on page 468

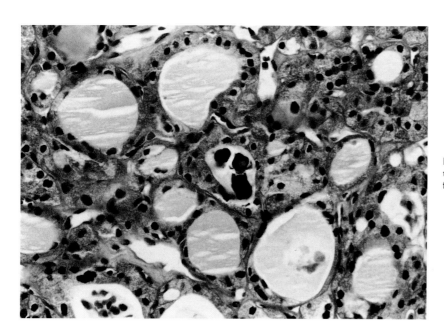

Figure 7–33. Follicular adenoma, oncocytic type. This tumor has a follicular pattern. The colloid in the central follicle is calcified and resembles a psammoma body.

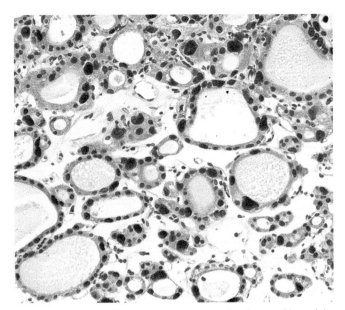

Figure 7–32. Follicular adenoma with bizarre nuclear features. Many of the nuclei in this field are enlarged and hyperchromatic.

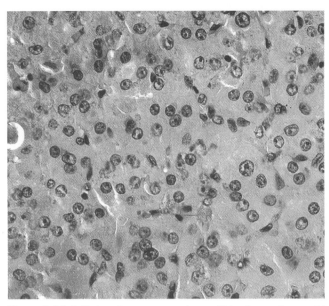

Figure 7–34. Follicular adenoma, oncocytic type. This adenoma has a solid appearance.

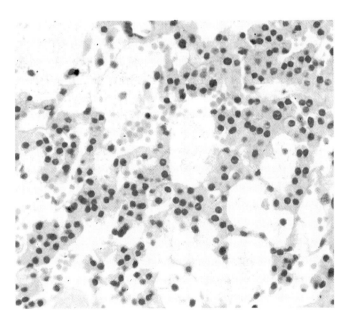

Figure 7–35. Follicular adenoma, oncocytic type. Most of the cells have abundant granular eosinophilic cytoplasm. Some cells, however, have clear cytoplasm.

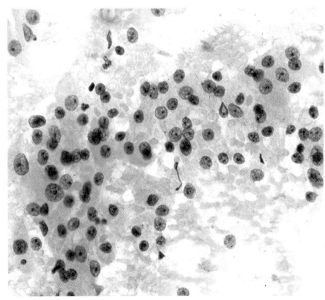

Figure 7–36. Follicular adenoma, oncocytic type (hematoxylin-eosin stain of fine needle aspiration biopsy). The cells have abundant eosinophilic cytoplasm.

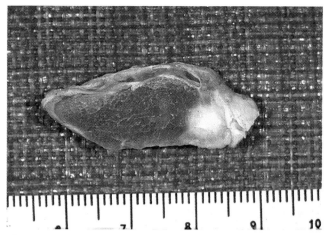

Figure 7–38. Papillary thyroid carcinoma. This microcarcinoma is located just beneath the capsule and has a sclerotic pattern.

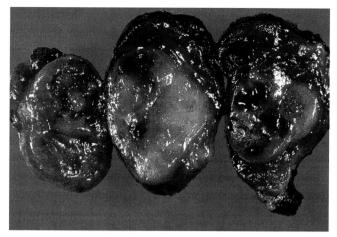

Figure 7–39. Papillary thyroid carcinoma. This tumor is circumscribed but not encapsulated. Foci of cystic change and hemorrhage are evident.

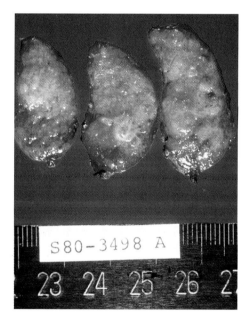

Figure 7–40. Papillary thyroid carcinoma, diffuse sclerosing type. This tumor has replaced the entire lobe of the gland.

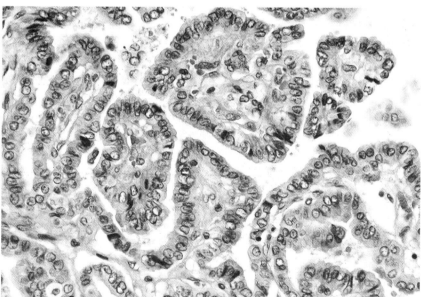

Figure 7–42. Papillary thyroid carcinoma. The nuclei are overlapped and have a ground-glass appearance with grooves.

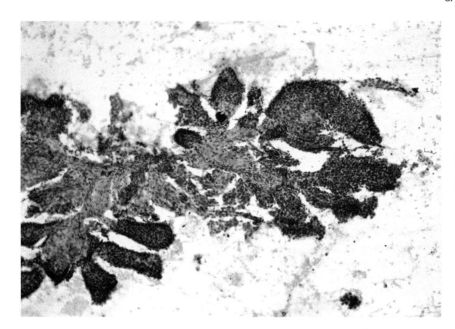

Figure 7–44. Papillary thyroid carcinoma (hematoxylin-eosin stain of fine needle aspiration biopsy). A tissue fragment with a papillary architecture is present.

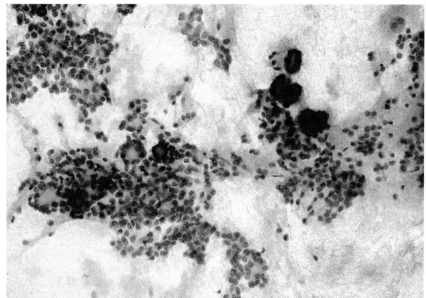

Figure 7–45. Papillary thyroid carcinoma (hematoxylin-eosin stain of fine needle aspiration biopsy). Several psammoma bodies are present.

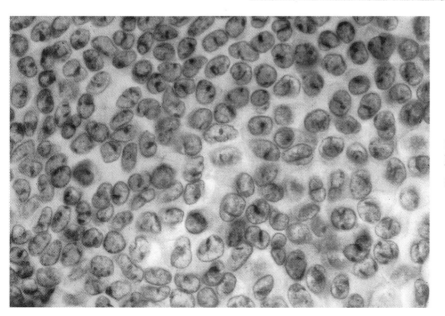

Figure 7–46. Papillary thyroid carcinoma (hematoxylin-eosin stain of fine needle aspiration biopsy). The tumor cells have finely granular chromatin and prominent grooves.

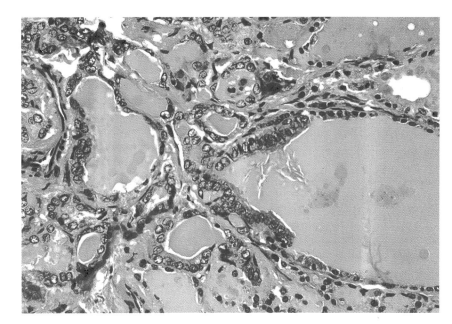

Figure 7–47. Papillary thyroid carcinoma. Nuclear features typical of papillary carcinoma are restricted to a few follicles.

Figure 7–48. Papillary thyroid carcinoma, microcarcinoma type. The tumor is present in a subcapsular location and is associated with considerable fibrosis.

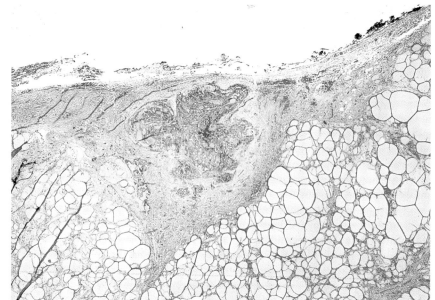

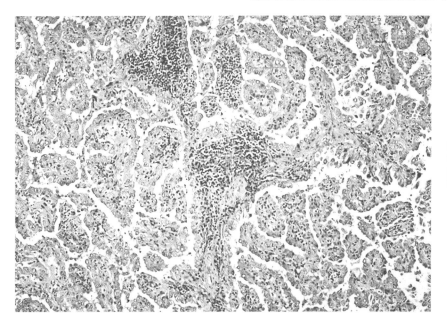

Figure 7–51. Papillary thyroid carcinoma, oncocytic type. The tumor cells have abundant granular eosinophilic cytoplasm. A prominent lymphocytic infiltrate in the stroma is evident.

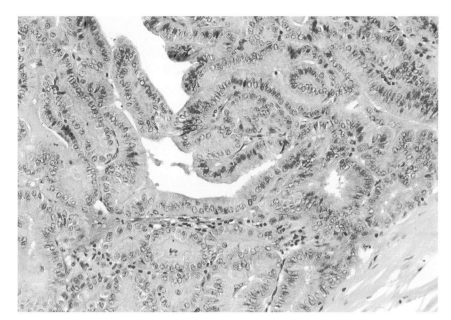

Figure 7–53. Papillary thyroid carcinoma, tall cell variant. The tumor cells are at least twice as tall as they are wide and have abundant eosinophilic cytoplasm.

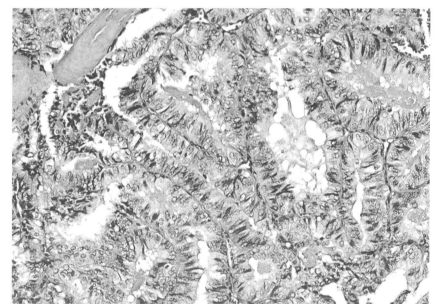

Figure 7–55. Papillary thyroid carcinoma, columnar variant. The tumor cell nuclei are arranged in a pseudostratified pattern.

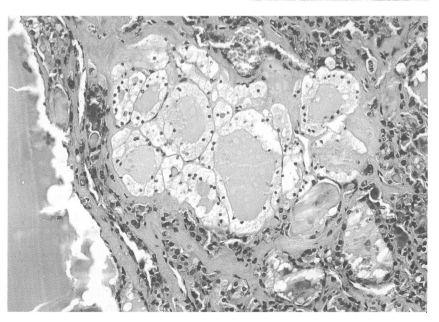

Figure 7–56. Follicular carcinoma. This tumor exhibits focal areas of clear cell change.

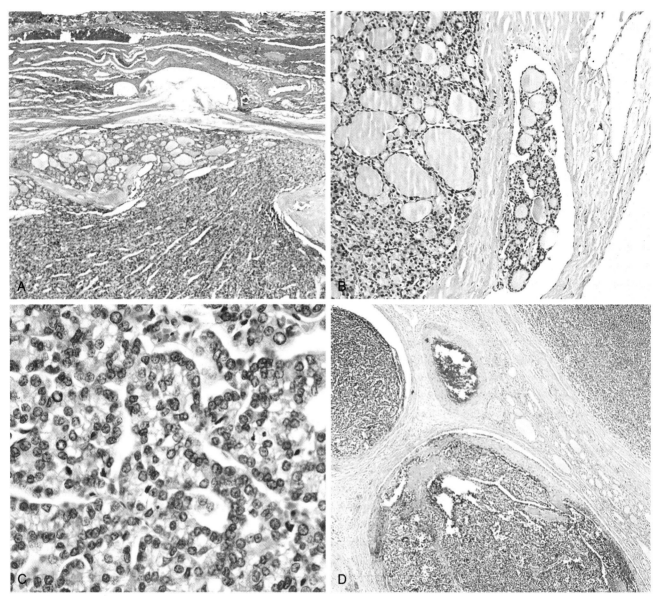

Figure 7–57. Follicular carcinoma. *A,* Minimally invasive follicular carcinoma. The tumor transgresses the connective tissue capsule. *B,* Minimally invasive follicular carcinoma. Tumor is present within a capsular vein and is attached to the venous wall *C,* Widely invasive follicular carcinoma. This tumor has a predominant microfollicular growth pattern. *D,* Widely invasive follicular carcinoma. Multiple areas of vascular invasion are present.

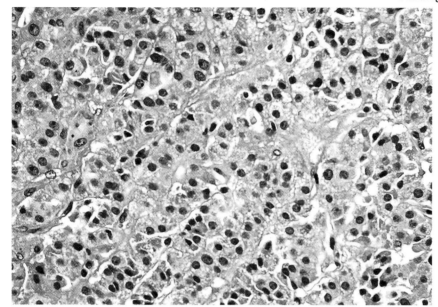

Figure 7–59. Oncocytic carcinoma. This tumor has a mixed solid and trabecular growth pattern.

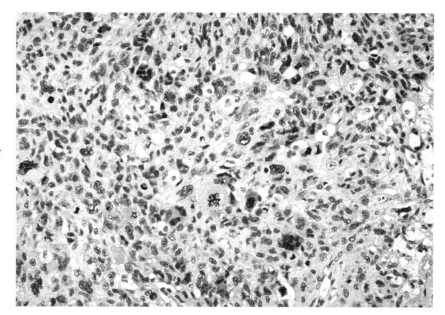

Figure 7–61. Undifferentiated thyroid carcinoma. This tumor is composed of large pleomorphic cells with areas of spindle cell growth.

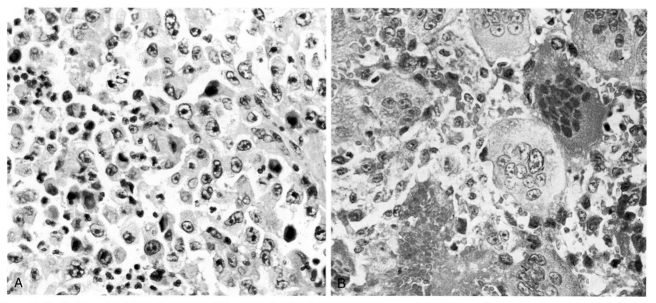

Figure 7–63. Undifferentiated thyroid carcinoma. A, This tumor focally exhibits a hemangioendotheliomatous appearance. B, This tumor contains osteoclast-like giant cells.

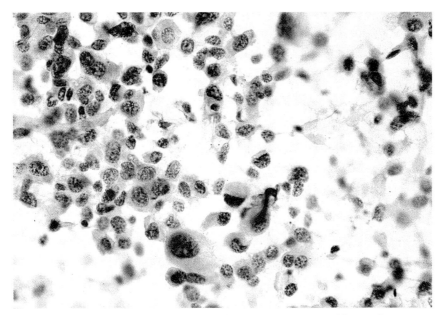

Figure 7–64. Undifferentiated thyroid carcinoma (hematoxylin-eosin stain of fine needle aspiration biopsy). The aspirate contains numerous pleomorphic tumor cells.

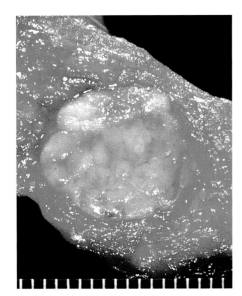

Figure 7–65. Medullary thyroid carcinoma. This tumor from a patient with type 2A multiple endocrine neoplasia has a solid appearance.

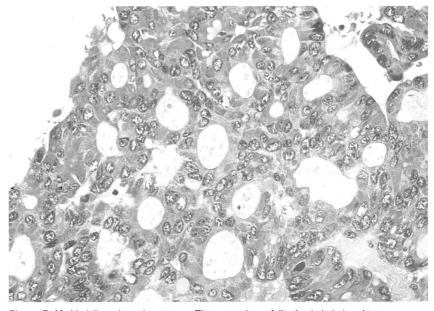

Figure 7–68. Medullary thyroid carcinoma. This tumor has a follicular (tubular) architecture.

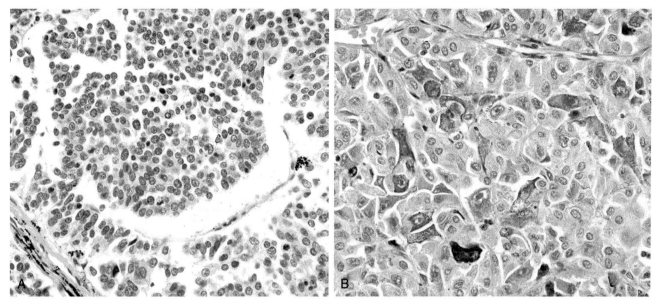

Figure 7–69. Medullary thyroid carcinoma. *A*, This tumor is composed predominantly of small cells. *B*, This tumor contains melanin-rich cells.

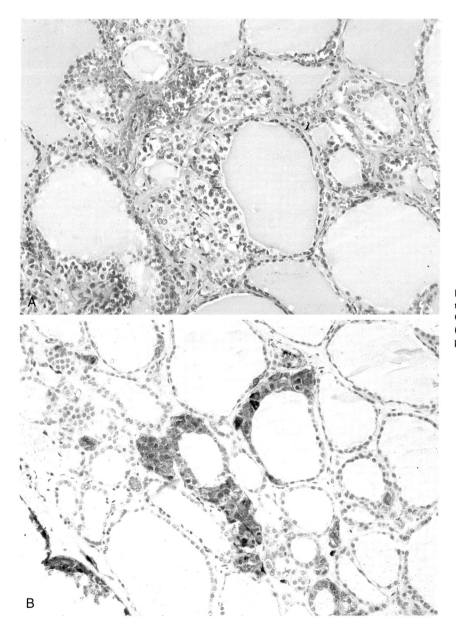

Figure 7–71. *A*, C-cell hyperplasia in a patient with type 2A multiple endocrine neoplasia. The hyperplastic C cells surround individual follicles. *B*, Same case as *A* (immunoperoxidase stain for calcitonin). The hyperplastic C cells contain immunoreactive calcitonin.

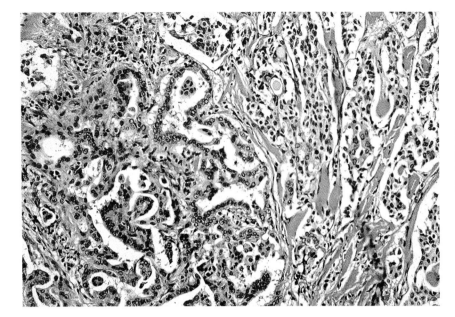

Figure 7–74. Mixed papillary and medullary carcinoma. The papillary component (left) is characterized by cells with relatively clear and overlapping nuclei. The medullary component (right) has a more solid appearance.

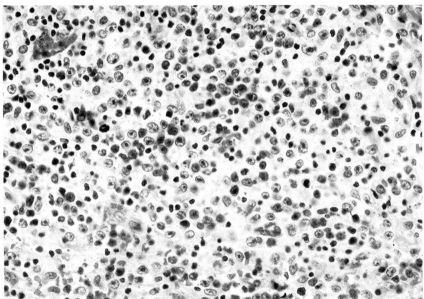

Figure 7–75. Malignant lymphoma. The tumor is composed of cells with immunoblastic features.

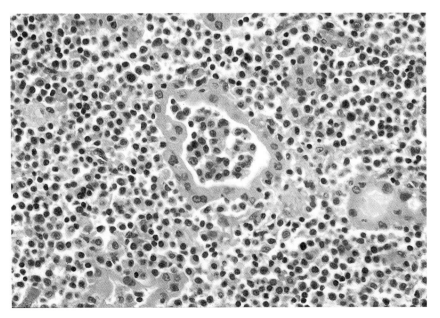

Figure 7–76. Malignant lymphoma. The tumor has the appearance of a low grade mucosa-associated lymphoid tissue lymphoma (MALT) with a characteristic lymphoepithelial lesion.

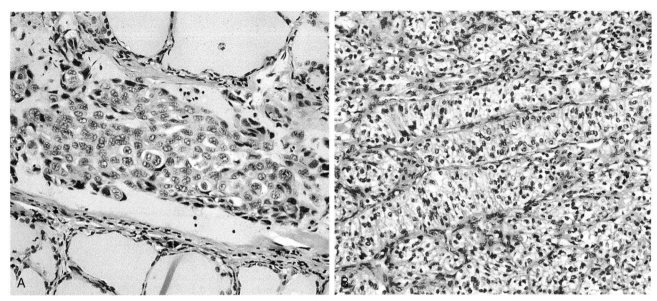

Figure 7–80. Secondary tumors of the thyroid gland. *A,* Metastatic poorly differentiated bronchogenic adenocarcinoma. *B,* Metastatic renal cell carcinoma. The tumor is composed of nests and cords of clear cells. Note the prominent vascular background characteristic of this neoplasm.

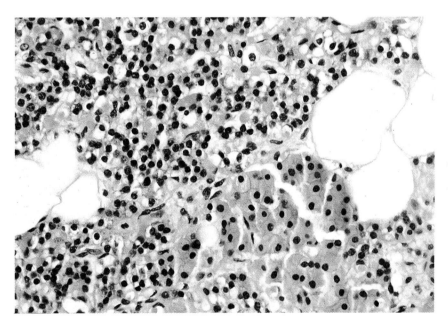

Figure 7–81. Normal adult parathyroid gland. Chief cells have relatively small hyperchromatic nuclei with focally vacuolated cytoplasm. Oncocytes have abundant eosinophilic cytoplasm. A small amount of stroma fat is present in the field.

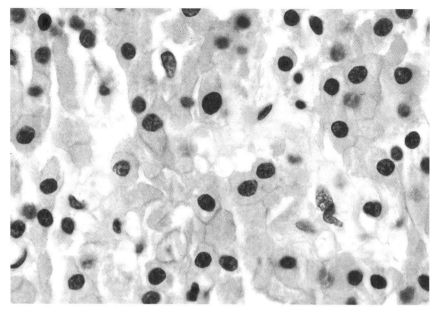

Figure 7–82. Normal adult parathyroid. The oncocytes have abundant granular eosinophilic cytoplasm.

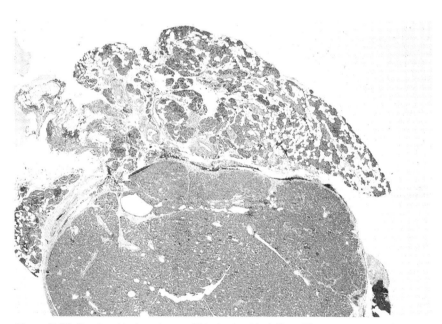

Figure 7–83. Parathyroid microadenoma. This gland weighed 60 mg. The upper portion of the field contains adjacent normocellular parathyroid tissue.

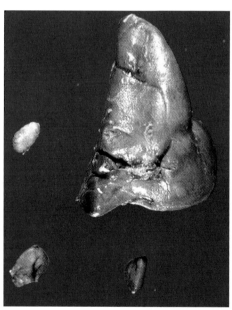

Figure 7–84. Parathyroid adenoma involving the right upper parathyroid gland. The adenoma has a pyramidal shape and lobulated contours (postmortem preparation). The other parathyroid glands are normal. (Courtesy of Prof. Dr. M Stolte, Bayreuth, Germany).

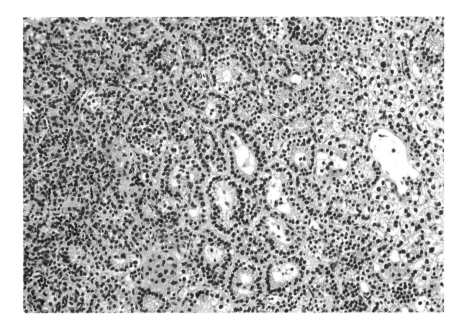

Figure 7–86. Parathyroid adenoma. The chief cells are arranged in tubular (glandular) formations.

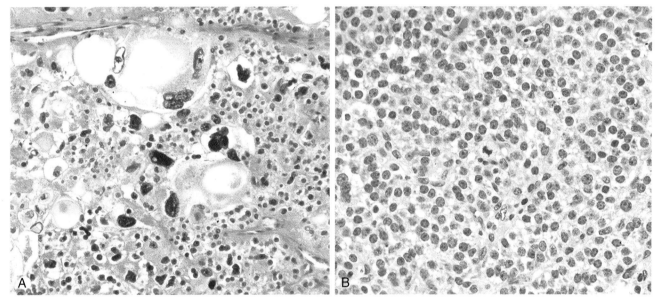

Figure 7–88. Parathyroid adenoma. *A*, Groups of chief cells in this adenoma have enlarged and hyperchromatic nuclei. *B*, Occasional mitotic figures are present in this adenoma.

Figure 7–89. Parathyroid adenoma. The cells in the normal rim of this adenoma have nuclei that are smaller than those in the adenoma and their cytoplasm is extensively vacuolated.

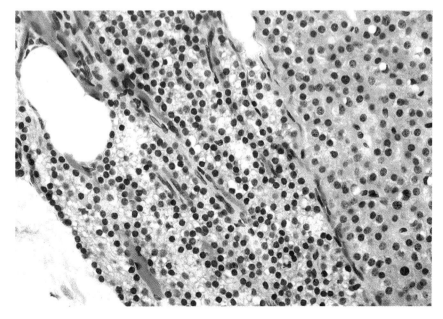

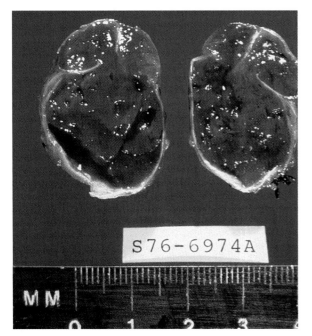

Figure 7–90. Oncocytic parathyroid adenoma. The tumor is red-brown.

Figure 7–91. Oncocytic parathyroid adenoma. The tumor is composed of large cells with abundant granular eosinophilic cytoplasm.

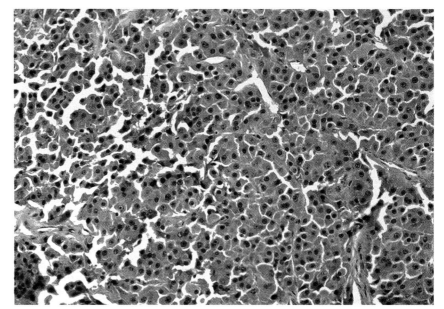

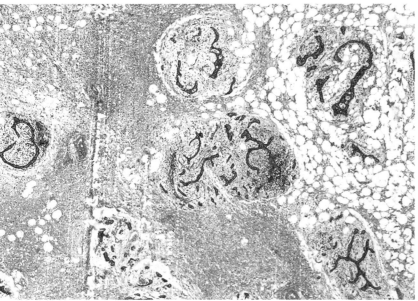

Figure 7–92. Parathyroid lipoadenoma. The stromal component of this tumor is composed of fat and fibromyxoid tissue.

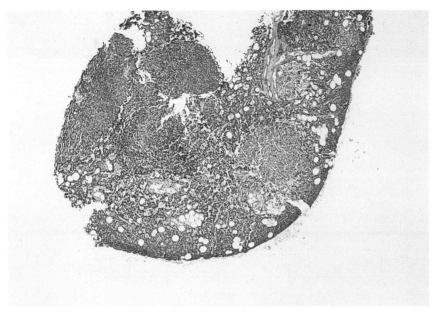

Figure 7–95. Nodular chief cell hyperplasia in a patient with type 1 multiple endocrine neoplasia. The gland contains multiple nodules of chief cells.

Figure 7–96. Nodular chief cell hyperplasia (same case as Figure 7-95). The stroma in the diffusely hyperplastic area contains a few fat cells. The nodular focus is devoid of chief cells.

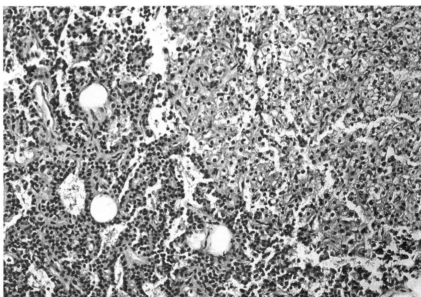

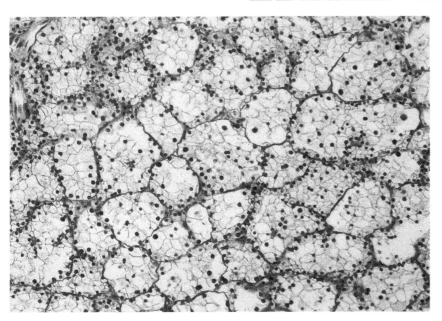

Figure 7–97. Clear cell hyperplasia. The cells have extensively vacuolated cytoplasm.

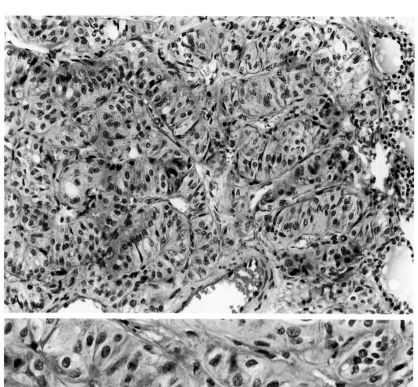

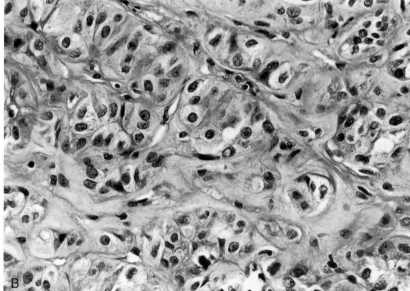

Figure 7–37. Hyalinizing trabecular adenoma. A, The tumor cells are arranged in long branching cords. B, Occasional nuclear pseudoinclusions are evident in this field.

Oncocytic tumors usually yield aspirates with high cellularity and scanty colloid (Fig. 7–36, see p. 453). The smears typically reveal a monomorphic, follicular cell population with cells present singly or in loose clusters with or without a syncytial or follicular arrangement.[11] Lymphocytic infiltrates are generally sparse. The oncocytes are large, oval to polygonal, with well-defined cell borders and abundant granular cytoplasm. In Papanicolaou-stained smears, the cells can be oncocytic, cyanophilic, or amphophilic. The nuclei are usually eccentric, round, sometimes pleomorphic, single or double. Single, large nucleoli are usually present and may be quite prominent (cherry-red macronucleus). Oncocytes are found in oncocytic tumors but occasionally also in non-neoplastic conditions such as Hashimoto's thyroiditis, adenomatous goiter, and Graves' disease, forming non-neoplastic oncocytic nodules.[128]

Features favoring an oncocytic tumor over a non-neoplastic condition with oncocytes are a high percentage (>90%) of oncocytes when compared with all follicular cells. Generally, more than 10% of the oncocytes are single, with three-dimensional syncytial groups, marked nuclear enlargement and pleomorphism, prominent nucleoli, and no inflammatory cells in the background.[58, 129] On the other hand, features that favor a diagnosis of a non-neoplastic nodule in a setting of goiter or Hashimoto's thyroiditis include an ad-

mixture of follicular cells and oncocytes, a spectrum of nuclear changes from normal to reactive to atypical, bland chromatin, small nucleoli, inflammatory background, degenerated follicular cells, and cohesive clusters of cells with a honeycomb pattern.[16]

Hyalinizing Trabecular Adenoma

Hyalinizing trabecular adenomas represent a distinctive adenoma subtype in which there is extensive stromal hyalinization together with intracytoplasmic deposition of intermediate filaments.[130–132] This tumor has also been referred to as paraganglioma-like adenoma of the thyroid.[133] The tumor cells, which are arranged in a trabecular pattern, may have some of the cells inserted perpendicularly into the walls of blood vessels (Fig. 7–37A). Some cases have their component cells arranged in a Zellballen pattern reminiscent of paragangliomas.[133] Nuclei of the tumor cells may have pseudoinclusions and grooves, and some workers have suggested a relationship to papillary thyroid carcinoma (Fig. 7–37B). In fact, psammoma bodies may be present. The patterns of cytokeratin expression have suggested that these tumors may represent peculiar encapsulated variants of papillary carcinoma.[133a] The tumor cells stain positively for thyroglobulin, and some cases have been reported to stain positively for neuron-specific enolase, chromogranin A, neurotensin, and somatostatin.[132] These findings suggest that some hyalinizing trabecular adenomas may have evidence of neuroendocrine differentiation. Although the vast majority of hyalinizing trabecular adenomas are benign, several recent studies have indicated that some may, in fact, represent carcinomas.[134] The differential diagnosis includes medullary thyroid carcinomas, true paraganglioma, and the solid variant of papillary thyroid carcinoma, which are discussed in detail in subsequent sections.

Adenolipoma and Adenochondroma

Adenolipomas are follicular adenomas in which the follicular elements are separated by mature fat cells. The stromal fat most probably arises as a result of metaplasia of connective tissue elements.[135] Similar changes may also occur in normal and hyperplastic thyroid and in papillary carcinomas.[136] The stromal components of adenomas may very rarely undergo cartilaginous metaplasia (adenochondroma).[137]

Adenomas with Papillary Hyperplasia

Adenomas may also exhibit foci of papillary hyperplasia. Typically, the papillary processes are short and point toward the lumina of cystically dilated follicles. The component follicular cells are tall with basally situated, round nuclei. The central regions often appear cystic. Alternatively, these lesions have also been referred to as hyperplastic papillary adenomas.[138]

Treatment of Adenomas

Follicular adenomas and their variants are adequately treated by lobectomy. Indications for surgery include (1) evaluation for possible carcinoma, (2) treatment of toxic (hyperfunctioning) symptoms, (3) resolution of a cosmetic problem, and (4) alleviation of compressive symptoms.[139]

Malignant Tumors

Papillary Thyroid Carcinoma

Clinical Features and Pathogenesis. Papillary thyroid carcinoma (PTC) is, by far, the most common type of thyroid malignancy, with an incidence that is considerably higher than that of follicular tumors in iodine-rich areas. This tumor type occurs in all age groups and accounts for the vast majority of thyroid cancers in childhood.[140] The mean age at diagnosis is 40 years. Most patients present with evidence of a mass lesion within the thyroid gland or with evidence of enlargement of regional lymph nodes. Papillary thyroid carcinoma is two to three times more frequent in females than in males, and there is a well-known relationship between exposure to low-dose radiation and the development of this tumor type. In studies of thyroid glands of children exposed to radiation following the Chernobyl accident, Nikiforov et al.[71] found a high frequency of micropapillary hyperplasia in thyroid tissue adjacent to foci of papillary carcinoma. These findings suggest that micropapillary hyperplasia could represent a precursor of the carcinoma.

The risk of thyroid cancer, particularly of the papillary type, also appears to be increased in familial adenomatous polyposis syndromes, including Gardner's and Cowden's syndromes.[141] Harach et al.[142] have concluded that thyroid tumors associated with familial adenomatous polyposis have a characteristic appearance that permits their distinction from the more common variants of papillary thyroid carcinoma.

Rearrangements of the *ret* and *trk* oncogenes have been implicated in the development of papillary thyroid carcinoma.[99] Both *ret* and *trk* form chimeric oncogenes as a result of fusion of their tyrosine kinase domains with 5′ sequences of different activating genes. The resultant fusion proteins exhibit constitutive tyrosine kinase activity.[143–146] Studies of transgenic mice have demonstrated that thyroid-targeted expression of the *ret*/PTC oncogene leads to the development of thyroid carcinoma with features of papillary carcinoma.[146a] There is also evidence derived from tissue culture studies that *ret*/PTC is directly responsible for the development of the characteristic nuclear changes of papillary carcinoma.[146b] There is considerable variation in the frequency of *ret* rearrangements in different geographic areas and in different age groups, ranging from 3% to 67%.[146c] At least some of these differences may be related to different detection techniques; alternatively, they may point to different pathogenetic mechanisms.

Three major patterns of *ret* rearrangements have been characterized.[143–146] These include fusion with the D105170 locus (*ret*/PTC1), the regulatory unit R1α of protein kinase A (*ret*/PTC2) or with the gene *ele* 1 (*ret*/PTC3). *Ret*/PTC1 and *ret*/PTC3 occur as a result of intrachromosomal inversions of chromosome 10. *Ret*/PTC2 occurs as a result of a t(10;17)(q11.2;q23) translocation that leads to a fusion sequence with the gene encoding R1α of protein kinase A. Several additional variants of the *ret* oncogene have also been reported.[146d,146e]

Ret rearrangements are highly prevalent in pediatric papillary thyroid carcinomas, including those occurring after radiation exposure and those occurring sporadically.[146] The types of *ret*/PTC rearrangements differ between these groups with *ret*/PTC3 occurring more commonly in post-Chernobyl cases (predominantly solid variants of papillary carcinoma). In this series, 79% of the solid variants had a *ret*/PTC3 rearrangement, whereas *ret*/PTC3 was present in only 19% of usual papillary carcinomas. In contrast, *ret*/PTC1 was present in 7% of solid variants and 38% of the usually papillary carcinomas. These findings suggest that different types of *ret* rearrangements confer distinctive phenotypic properties to neoplastic thyroid cells.[146f] There are two separate studies that suggest that papillary thyroid carcinomas with *ret* rearrangements are slow-growing tumors that do not progress toward more aggressive neoplasms.[146g,h]

The *trk* oncogenes are created by a specific rearrangement of the *NTK1* gene, which encodes a receptor for nerve growth factor. The *trk* oncogenes are activated in approximately 20% of papillary thyroid carcinomas. The *c-met* oncogene protein is expressed in a high proportion of papillary thyroid carcinomas, and the overexpression of this protein appears to be correlated with rearrangements of *ret* or *trk*.[99] Mutations of the *ras* oncogene, on the other hand, are uncommon.[99]

Pathologic Features and Differential Diagnosis. Papillary carcinomas vary considerably in size, from those that are barely visible grossly to those that completely replace the thyroid gland. Most average between 2 and 3 cm in diameter and have ill-defined margins, a firm consistency, and a solid to granular white appearance (Figs. 7–38, 7–39, and 7–40, see p. 454). Occasional PTCs may present as encapsulated neoplasms, which may be impossible to distinguish grossly from follicular adenomas.[147] Foci of cystic degeneration are common, both in the primary tumors and in lymph node metastases (Fig. 7–41).

According to the World Health Organization (WHO) classification, PTC is defined as a malignant epithelial tumor showing evidence of follicular cell differentiation, typically with papillary and follicular structures as well as characteristic nuclear changes.[148] The papillae are formed by fibrovascular cores, which are covered by cuboidal to columnar neoplastic epithelial cells (Fig. 7–42, see p. 454). The papillae may be long and branching or may have a parallel orientation. Edema of the fibrovascular cores may result in an appearance similar to that of placental villi. Most papillary thyroid carcinomas also contain neoplastic follicles, which in some cases may form the predominant growth pattern.

The nuclei are round to ovoid with frequent indentations and irregularities, which are responsible for the typical clefted or grooved appearance.[149, 150] Nuclear pseudoinclusions that result from protrusions of the cytoplasm into the nucleus are relatively common.[151] In formalin-fixed paraffin-embedded samples, the nuclei have an "empty" appearance, with apposition of the chromatin along the nuclear membrane.[152–154] This feature results in the characteristic ground-glass or "Orphan Annie" appearance.[155] Small nucleoli are usually present, and they are often adjacent to the nuclear membrane. Even in thin histologic preparations, the nuclei frequently appear overlapped.

The cytoplasm is typically smooth and eosinophilic, and foci of squamous metaplasia are common (Fig. 7–43A). Many of the tumors have an abundant fibrous stroma as well as a lymphoplasmacytic infiltrate.[156] In occasional cases, the prominence of the stroma may suggest a nodular fasciitis-like appearance.[157] A prominent lymphocytic infiltrate may be evident in approximately one third of the cases.

Papillary thyroid carcinomas are usually positive for thyroglobulin and also may stain for T_3 and T_4.[9] The tumor cells typically contain both cytokeratins and vimentin. Generally, papillary carcinomas are positive for both high and low molecular weight keratins, whereas follicular carcinomas are more commonly reactive for low molecular weight keratins only.[158, 159] Using chain-specific keratin monoclonal antibodies against keratin 19, Schelfhout et al.[160] found uniformly positive staining in papillary carcinomas and weak or absent staining in follicular carcinomas. The specificity of cytokeratin 19 as a marker for papillary thyroid carcinoma, however, has been challenged.[160a,160b] Estrogen receptor protein is present in approximately 75% of papillary carcinomas and in 35% of follicular carcinomas.[161]

Psammoma bodies are found in up to 50% of cases and are most common in those tumors with a predominant papillary pattern (see Fig. 7–43B).[147, 162] In some instances, isolated or "naked" psammoma bodies may be identified. Presumably, they represent foci of tumor that have undergone retrogressive changes with the presence of fibrosis and lymphocytic infiltrates.

Multiple foci of papillary thyroid carcinoma involving both lobes of the gland are evident in approximately 20% of cases.[163] These foci most likely represent intrathyroidal lymphatic metastases. The tumors typically spread to draining lymph nodes, which are involved in approximately one third of cases.[147] Vascular invasion is considerably less common and occurs in about 5% of cases. Distant metastases involving lung, bone, or liver develop in less than 15% of cases.

Fine Needle Aspiration Biopsy. Aspirates from papillary carcinomas usually contain abundant cells, which may be grouped in papillary tissue fragments, monolayered sheets, and three-dimensional clusters with or without a follicular pattern (Figs. 7–44, 7–45, and 7–46, see p. 455[11] Papillary fragments, which are found

in 90% of cases,[164, 165] usually reveal a branching pattern with a regular external contour with nuclear palisading. A central vascular stromal core may be present. The cells are usually cuboidal, but they can exhibit any morphology (columnar, polygonal, squamous, or spindle-shaped). The cytoplasm can be moderate to abundant and sometimes dense with well-defined margins, so-called "metaplastic cytoplasm."[166] In about 50% of cases, multiple small cytoplasmic vacuoles are identified.[166]

The nuclei are usually large and overlapping with finely punctate, "dusty to powdery" chromatin and frequent intranuclear cytoplasmic inclusions.[166–169] Another feature that is almost always present in aspirate smears of papillary carcinoma is the nuclear groove, which appears as a cleft-like invagination of the nuclear membrane along the long axis of the nucleus. Nuclear grooves have been identified in 80% of nonpapillary tumors and 55% of non-neoplastic thyroid conditions[169]; however, in nonpapillary tumors, nuclear grooves are present in a low percentage of cells, whereas in papillary carcinomas they are present in usually more than 20% of the cells.

Psammoma bodies are present in approximately 20% of papillary carcinoma aspirates.[169] However, the presence of a rare psammoma body in the absence of other typical features of papillary carcinoma must be interpreted with caution, since they may occur in other entities. "Ropy" colloid strands ("chewing gum" colloid), foamy histiocytes, multinucleate giant cells, and lymphoid cells are occasionally seen in aspirates from papillary carcinoma. Chewing gum colloid is present in about 20% of cases[165] and is quite characteristic of papillary carcinoma.

Papillary fragments may be present in nodular goiter, occasional adenomas and in some cases of Graves' disease.[165] This can appear in aspirate smears in the form of papillary structures with or without stromal cores. However, in these cases, the typical nuclear features of papillary carcinoma are absent. Therefore, papillary clusters in the absence of the other diagnostic features of papillary carcinoma are not sufficient to warrant a diagnosis of papillary carcinoma.

The follicular variant of papillary carcinoma is characterized by three-dimensional cell clusters with or without a follicular pattern together with nuclear features of conventional papillary carcinomas.[170] The tall and clear cell variants have also been described in cytologic preparations.[171]

Cystic changes in papillary carcinoma may cause significant diagnostic problems. In these cases, the smears may be poorly cellular with pronounced degenerative changes due to inflammation,

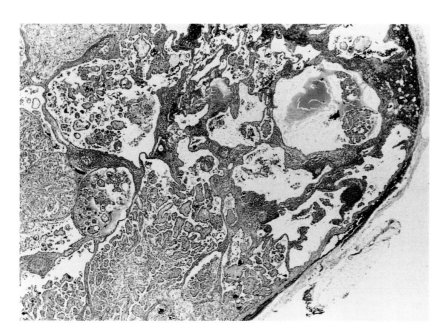

Figure 7–41. Lymph node with metastatic papillary thyroid carcinoma. A typical papillary architecture is present in this field. Areas of cystic change are present.

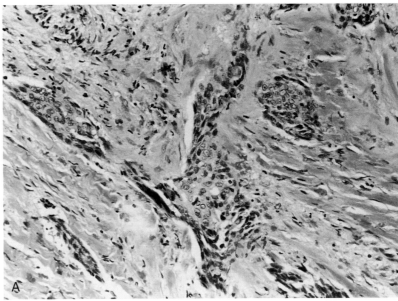

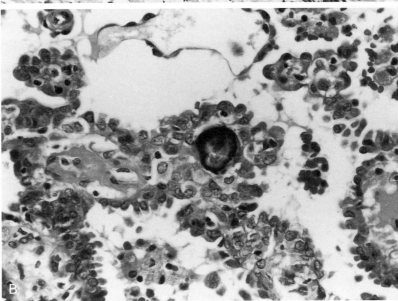

Figure 7–43. Papillary thyroid carcinoma. *A,* This tumor demonstrates extensive squamous metaplasia in addition to a prominent fibrous stroma. *B,* A psammoma body is present in the center of this field.

hemorrhage, and necrosis. If the smear reveals changes suggestive but not diagnostic of papillary carcinoma, a reaspiration of the cyst or any residual nodule within the cyst wall should be performed to confirm the diagnosis.

Occasionally, papillary carcinoma can be seen in association with Hashimoto's thyroiditis, and that occurrence can create diagnostic dilemmas. Moreover, both entities share some cytologic features, such as multinucleated giant cells, lymphocytes, oncocytic cell changes, and occasional squamous metaplasia. However, in the presence of a predominance of epithelial cells arranged in papillary clusters, mature lymphoid cells, and follicular cells with the typical nuclear features of papillary carcinoma, a diagnosis of papillary carcinoma can and should be made.

Variants of Papillary Carcinoma

Microcarcinoma

Papillary microcarcinoma, as defined by the WHO classification, is a papillary carcinoma that measures less than 1 cm in diameter (Figs. 7–47 and 7–48, see p. 456). This variant has been referred to previously as occult or latent papillary carcinoma or occult sclerosing carcinoma (nonencapsulated sclerosing tumor).[148, 172] Since not all small papillary carcinomas are associated with sclerosis, the term

papillary microcarcinoma is preferred. These tumors are very common, with some studies reporting them in up to 35.6% of thyroids examined at autopsy.[173] The frequency of detection is clearly dependent on the extent of histologic sampling. In a recent surgical series of 425 patients with thyroid diseases other than carcinomas of follicular origin, 71 cases (16.7%) had one or more micropapillary carcinomas. Fifty-one of 343 women (14.9%) and 20 of 82 men (24.4%) had occult micropapillary carcinomas.[174]

The most common type of papillary microcarcinoma is characterized by neoplastic follicles in a densely fibrotic stroma. Some of the lesions may be composed of fibrous tissue almost exclusively, with only a few groups of neoplastic cells. In other instances, papillary microcarcinomas without sclerosis may blend imperceptibly with adjacent non-neoplastic follicles. Occasional papillary microcarcinomas may be encapsulated. Although papillary microcarcinomas may metastasize to regional nodes, overall prognosis is excellent.

Encapsulated Type

The *encapsulated variant* of PTC is a papillary tumor that is separated from the adjacent thyroid parenchyma by a fibrous capsule (Fig. 7–49A).[147] They account for up to 10% of all PTCs. Although these tumors were sometimes referred to as papillary adenomas in the past, approximately 25% may metastasize to regional nodes. The prognosis of the encapsulated variant of PTC is excellent.

Follicular Variant

The *follicular variant* of PTC is characterized by a predominant follicular growth pattern (Fig. 7–49B).[175] Follicles often have a tubular configuration with occasional formation of bud-like projections, which most likely represent abortive attempts at the formation of papillae. The colloid is densely eosinophilic and often appears scalloped. Although most follicular variants of papillary carcinoma are not encapsulated, some of these tumors may be surrounded by a fibrous capsule (encapsulated follicular variant).

Macrofollicular Variant

A *macrofollicular variant* of PTC in which follicles are distended with colloid also occurs (Fig. 7–50).[176] These tumors may bear a striking resemblance to adenomatous nodules and have been misdiagnosed frequently as such. Careful search, however, will often demonstrate cellular foci with typical nuclear features of conven-

tional papillary thyroid carcinoma. Abortive papillae may also be evident.

Oncocytic Variant

The oncocytic variant of PTC is rare. The tumors exhibit a prominent papillary growth pattern, which is admixed with follicular solid and trabecular areas. These tumors are characterized by cells having typical nuclear features of PTC with abundant granular eosinophilic cytoplasm (Fig. 7–51, see p. 456).[177, 178] Occasional cases may have a prominent lymphocytic stroma, which may impart a Warthin-like appearance.[179] The prognosis is generally similar to that of the usual PTC.

Solid Variant

The *solid* variant describes a tumor with the typical nuclear features of PTC with a predominant solid growth pattern (Fig. 7–52A).[147] This variant typically may be associated with the presence of fibrous bands and a focal lymphocytic infiltrate and is found more frequently in children. In the series of 83 papillary carcinomas reported by Nikiforov and Gnepp[72] following the Chernobyl disaster, the solid variant was the most common subtype, accounting for 34%

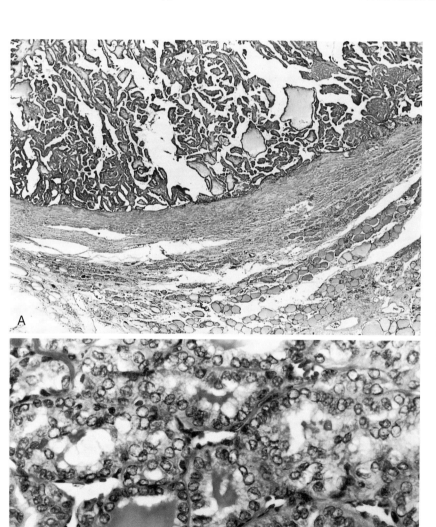

Figure 7–49. A, Papillary thyroid carcinoma, encapsulated variant. This tumor was separated from the adjacent thyroid by a complete fibrous capsule. B, Papillary thyroid carcinoma, follicular variant. The tumor cell nuclei have all the features of typical papillary carcinoma. The colloid appears densely stained.

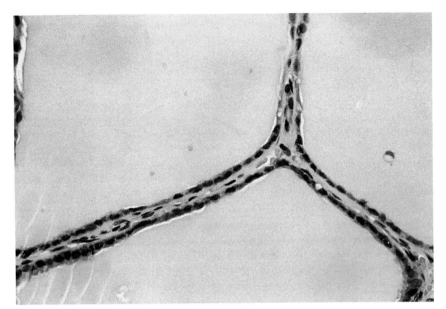

Figure 7–50. Papillary thyroid carcinoma, macrofollicular variant. The follicles in this case are distended by colloid and the surrounding cells appear atrophic. This tumor was present in a cervical lymph node.

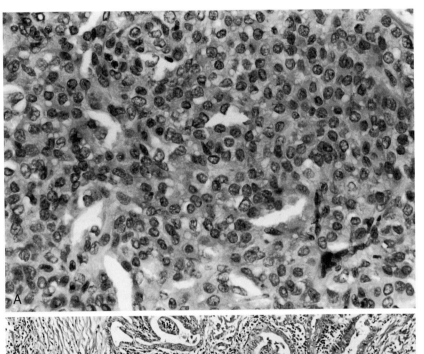

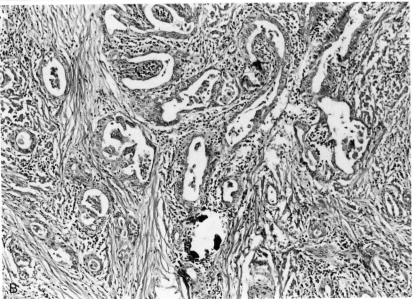

Figure 7–52. Papillary thyroid carcinoma. *A,* Solid variant. This tumor lacks a papillary or follicular pattern. The nuclear features, however, are typical of papillary carcinoma. *B,* Diffuse sclerosing variant. The tumor cells have a squamoid appearance. Psammoma bodies are prominent and the stroma is fibrotic with a lymphocytic infiltrate.

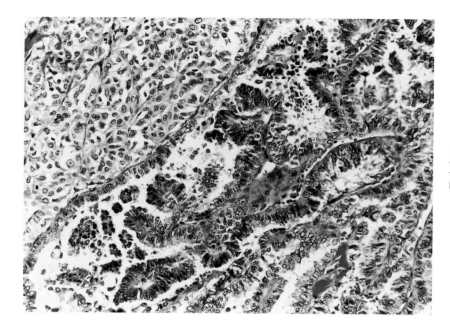

Figure 7–54. Papillary thyroid carcinoma, mixed tall cell and columnar variants with areas of poorly differentiated thyroid carcinoma. This was a large tumor that had extensively invaded the soft tissues of the neck.

of the cases. In a study of 34 papillary carcinomas in patients 7 to 18 years of age (14% with a history of prior irradiation), the solid variant was found in 21%.[180] In children without radiation exposure, the solid variant was found in only 8%.[71] The radiation-induced thyroid tumors were commonly associated with a *ret*/PTC3 rearrangement, whereas sporadic papillary carcinomas were characterized by a high prevalence of *ret*/PTC1 rearrangements, as discussed previously.[146f, 181]

Diffuse Follicular Variant

The *diffuse follicular variant,* which may involve the entire thyroid gland, may be extremely difficult to differentiate from adenomatous goiter.[182] It is an aggressive neoplasm that tends to occur in young patients and is characterized by diffuse involvement of the entire thyroid. There is a high incidence of pulmonary and osseous metastases.

Diffuse Sclerosing Variant

The *diffuse sclerosing variant* is characterized by diffuse involvement of one or both lobes. Typically, neoplastic papillae are present in cleft-like spaces that most likely represent lymphatic channels (Fig. 7–52B). In addition, the tumor cells exhibit extensive squamous metaplasia.[153] Fibrosis and lymphocytic infiltration are prominent and psammoma bodies are numerous. This variant occurs predominantly in children or young adults and is more commonly associated with lymph node and pulmonary metastasis.

Tall Cell Variant

The *tall cell variant* is characterized by tumor cells that are twice as tall as they are wide, occurring in at least 30% of the tumor and with areas of trabecular growth (Figs. 7–53, see p. 457, and 7–54).[170, 183, 184] Foci of extensive lymphocytic infiltration may be apparent in some cases.[185] Although most series indicate that the tumors are generally larger than the usual PTCs and tend to occur in an older age group, studies by Ostrowski and Merino[186] have suggested that these differences may not be statistically significant. However, extrathyroidal extension is significantly more common in the tall cell variant, as compared with papillary carcinomas of the usual type. Moreover, tumor cells in the tall cell variant typically exhibit strong staining for CD15 and epithelial membrane antigen and also exhibit strong positivity with some carcinoembryonic antigen antibodies. These studies support the notion that the tall cell variant

is distinct from papillary thyroid carcinoma of the usual type. Combining data from several series, Burman et al.[187] demonstrated that patients with the tall cell variant had a higher mortality and a higher rate of recurrent or persistent disease, as compared with patients with the usual PTCs. However, the prognosis was comparable to that of the usual PTCs in patients less than 50 years of age. Studies reported by Ruter et al.[188] demonstrated a significantly higher rate of p53 positivity, as determined by immunohistochemistry, than the usual type of papillary carcinoma. However, the stage of the disease was a more accurate prognostic determinant than the p53 status.

Columnar Variant

The *columnar variant* has generally been considered to be an aggressive type of PTC, which is characterized by nuclear stratification and the presence of subnuclear vacuoles (Fig. 7–55, see p. 457).[189] Evans[190] reported a series of four cases of an encapsulated columnar variant in which there was no evidence of recurrence or metastasis. These findings suggest that the presence of a capsule in columnar cell tumors is a feature associated with a good prognosis. Cases with combined tall cell and columnar features have also been reported (see Fig. 7–54).[191]

Dedifferentiated Variant

Dedifferentiated variants of PTC are characterized by the presence of poorly differentiated or undifferentiated carcinoma together with foci of typical PTC or one of its variants (see Fig. 7–54). The prognosis for these tumors is essentially that of the least differentiated component (see Fig. 7–54).

Treatment and Prognosis. The surgical treatment of PTC is controversial. Although some authors recommend lobectomy and isthmusectomy (followed by suppression of thyroid-stimulating hormone [TSH]), others recommend total thyroidectomy with or without ^{131}I treatment. Several studies have failed to demonstrate significant survival differences between these approaches when the tumor measures less than 1 cm in diameter. Mazzaferri and Jhiang,[192] however, have reported a lower mortality rate in a large group of patients treated by near-total thyroidectomy. Proponents of total thyroidectomy argue that this approach provides the opportunity for postoperative radioactive iodine treatment and also permits more accurate monitoring of serum thyroglobulin levels as an index of disease recurrence. For tumors measuring larger than 1 cm in diameter or belonging to one of the more aggressive subtypes, total thyroidectomy is considered to be the procedure of choice by most authors. Most surgeons favor a modified cervical lymph node dissection with preservation of the sternocleidomastoid muscle in patients with lymph node involvement.

The prognosis of papillary thyroid carcinoma is dependent on numerous variables,[140, 193, 193a] and, generally, patients can be stratified into low-risk and high-risk subsets. Several scoring systems have been developed for risk assessment. The AGES scoring system incorporates age, tumor grade, tumor extent, and tumor size.[193] The AMES system, developed by Cady et al.,[194, 195] utilizes age, distant metastases, extrathyroidal invasion and metastases, and primary tumor size. The European Organization for Research and Treatment of Cancer (EORTC) developed a scoring system that includes age, sex, principal cell type, extrathyroidal invasion, and distant metastases.[196] A TNM staging system, which was introduced by the International Union Against Cancer (UICC), has also been used extensively for prognostic assessment.[196–198]

Several generalizations can be made on the basis of these scoring systems. Features associated with high risk include direct extension of tumor into the soft tissues of the neck (extrathyroidal invasion), distant metastases, large size of primary tumor (greater than 5 cm) and age (greater than 41 years of age for males and greater than 51 years of age for females). With respect to tumor size, 20-year mortality rates were 6%, 16%, and 50% for tumors measuring 2 to 3.9 cm, 4 to 6.9 cm, and more than 7 cm, respectively.[193]

The effects of tumor grade on prognosis are controversial. Data from the Mayo Clinic indicate that grade 1 tumors fare considerably better than those with grades 2, 3, or 4 features.[140] Akslen has proposed a grading system based on nuclear atypia, tumor necrosis, and vascular invasion.[198a] In this system, grade 1 tumors included those without any of these features, whereas grade 2 tumors included those with one or more of these features. The risk of thyroid cancer deaths was considerably greater in grade 2 tumors in this study. It should be noted, however, that the vast majority of PTCs are grade 1. Aneuploidy is more common in tumors occurring in elderly patients and in those that are moderately to poorly differentiated and have capsular invasion.[199] Multivariant analyses have demonstrated, however, that age at diagnosis and capsular invasion are more important prognostic factors than aneuploidy.

Histologic variants associated with a worse prognosis than conventional papillary carcinomas include the diffuse sclerosing type, the tall and columnar variants, and the diffuse follicular type. Tumors with foci of poorly differentiated or anaplastic carcinoma are associated with a poor prognosis. The presence of vascular invasion and multicentricity are features that may negatively affect prognosis.

Follicular Carcinoma

Clinical Features and Pathogenesis. Follicular carcinomas are malignant epithelial tumors that show evidence of follicular cell differentiation and do not belong to any of the other distinctive types of thyroid malignancies.[11, 148, 200] They account for approximately 15% of malignant thyroid tumors. The frequency of this tumor type has decreased in recent years, owing primarily to the recognition of the follicular variant of papillary carcinoma.[201] Similar to papillary carcinomas, prior radiation exposure also increases the risk of follicular carcinoma. *Ras* mutations have been found in both follicular adenomas and carcinomas and appear to be more common in those tumors developing in iodine-deficient areas.[99]

Patients with follicular carcinoma are, on average, 10 years older than those with papillary carcinoma. Similar to papillary carcinomas, follicular carcinomas are considerably more common in females than in males.[202] Most patients present with a palpable thyroid nodule, which is usually "cold" on scan. Occasionally, patients may present with distant metastasis involving bone or lung. Follicular carcinomas are subdivided into minimally and widely invasive types.

Pathologic Features and Differential Diagnosis. The gross features of minimally invasive follicular carcinomas do not differ significantly from those of follicular adenomas. However, the cap-

sules of carcinomas often are thicker than those of adenomas.[203] Microscopically, carcinomas may exhibit normofollicular, microfollicular, or macrofollicular features; however, they tend to exhibit a greater tendency for microfollicular, solid, trabecular, or atypical growth patterns.[204] Foci of clear cell change may be evident (Fig. 7–56, see p. 457).

The diagnosis of malignancy rests on the demonstration of capsular or vascular invasion. Accordingly, it is essential to examine multiple sections that include the capsule. If the lesion is sufficiently small, the entire capsular region should be examined. For larger lesions, at least five blocks should be examined. In the presence of areas suspicious for invasion or in cellular and mitotically active lesions, five additional blocks should be examined.[204]

To qualify as capsular invasion, most pathologists require penetration of the entire thickness of the capsule (Fig. 7–57A, see p. 458). Often, this takes the form of a mushroom-like pattern of extension of tumor through the capsule. In cases in which the tumor is present within the capsule but does not extend into the adjacent normal parenchyma, additional levels should be prepared. If additional levels do not reveal full capsular penetration, a diagnosis of follicular carcinoma should not be made.

In some cases, a separate nodule may be present, external to the capsule. Serial sections are required to determine whether there is a connection with the main tumor mass. The demonstration of a connection between the two nodules is indicative of a carcinoma, but the absence of a connection does not completely rule out this possibility. Tangential cuts of the edge of a follicular neoplasm may also simulate capsular invasion, and additional sections may be required to demonstrate that the lesion, is, in fact, invested by an intact capsule.

To qualify for vascular invasion, tumor cells should be present in vessels within or beyond the capsule (Fig. 7–57B, see p. 458). The tumor cells should project into the lumen of the vessel and should conform to the overall shape of the vessel. The intravascular tumor should also be covered at least in part by endothelial cells. The presence of a small group of follicles bulging into a thin-walled vessel within the capsule is insufficient evidence of vascular invasion, particularly when deeper sections fail to reveal unequivocal evidence of vascular invasion.[204]

Artifactual dislodgment of tumor cells into vessels may occur during specimen preparation and sectioning. Typically, the tumor cell clusters in such instances have irregular outlines, are not attached to vascular walls, and are not covered by an endothelial lining.

The diagnosis and nomenclature of minimally invasive follicular carcinomas are controversial. Some have suggested that tumors with capsular invasion should be classified only as "follicular neoplasms of low malignant potential" and that the term "minimally invasive follicular carcinoma" be restricted to tumors with vascular invasion.[204a] This suggestion is based on the observation that tumors with capsular invasion rarely behave as true carcinomas.

Widely invasive carcinomas feature extensive invasion of the adjacent thyroid with multiple foci of capsular and vascular invasion (Figs. 7–57C and 7–57D, see p. 458). These tumors are more likely to exhibit mitotic activity and areas of pleomorphism. Common sites of metastasis include lung, bone, and liver. In contrast to the excellent prognosis of the minimally invasive tumors, the prognosis of widely invasive follicular carcinomas is poor.[202]

Fine Needle Aspiration Biopsy. Follicular carcinomas usually yield aspirates that are cytologically indistinguishable from those of microfollicular adenomas (Fig. 7–58). Smears are very cellular, with colloid present in small amounts. The cells are grouped in a syncytial pattern, with a predominance of microfollicles. Nuclei are crowded with loss of polarity; moreover, they are usually enlarged and hyperchromatic with nucleoli almost always present. In general, the risk of follicular carcinoma is inversely related to the follicle size.[16]

There is considerable overlap in findings of aspiration smears between nodular goiter, follicular adenomas, and follicular carcinomas. Lesions with abundant colloid and few cells—"colloid nodules"—have a low risk of being follicular carcinoma.[12] More than 90% of patients with this type of finding will have a colloid goiter; a few will have a follicular adenoma and, very rarely (1%), a follicular carcinoma. The opposite end of the spectrum is represented by smears with abundant cells with a microfollicular pattern and scanty colloid, that is, a "follicular neoplasm." This type of finding will correspond in approximately 90% of cases to a follicular neoplasm, but only in approximately 20% to 25% of cases to a follicular carcinoma. In between these two ends of the spectrum, there are lesions in which smears reveal abundant cells, but colloid is also present in significant amounts. DeMay designates these intermediate types of lesions as "cellular nodules."[16] They have an intermediate risk of being a follicular neoplasm but a low risk of being a follicular carcinoma. In the intermediate type of smears, features that favor the diagnosis of a goiter include the presence of degenerative changes, including macrophages, foam cells, giant cells with or without hemosiderin, fibrosis, a predominance of medium to large follicles with a honeycomb pattern, and small- to medium-sized follicular cells with occasional slightly pleomorphic nuclei. On the other hand, features that favor a diagnosis of neoplasm over a goiter are high cellularity, a predominant microfollicular pattern, scant colloid, and absence of significant degenerative changes. Features that favor a diagnosis of carcinoma include high cellularity, crowded, disorganized microfollicles, and large atypical nuclei with prominent nucleoli.

Treatment and Prognosis. The prognosis for patients with minimally invasive follicular carcinoma is excellent and is generally similar to that of patients with papillary carcinomas of the usual type.[139] Ten-year survival rates approach 100%. Factors that impact negatively on prognosis include stage at presentation, age greater than 50 years, and the extent of angioinvasion. Thus, young patients with minimally invasive tumors will have excellent prognosis. In contrast, 10-year survival rates in patients with widely invasive tumors are in the range of 25% to 45%.

The treatment of follicular carcinomas, particularly those of the minimally invasive type, is controversial.[139] Some surgeons favor lobectomy with isthmusectomy and suppression of TSH with thyroxine.[205] Other surgeons favor total thyroidectomy with ablation of any remaining thyroid tissue with [131]I. The latter approach also permits the use of serum thyroglobulin measurements to monitor the development of metastases. For patients with widely angioinvasive

tumors, most authors favor total thyroidectomy followed by ^{131}I treatment.

Oncocytic Carcinoma

Clinical Features and Pathogenesis. Although Thompson and coworkers suggested in 1974 that all oncocytic tumors of the thyroid were malignant or potentially malignant,[206] more recent studies have rejected this claim.[127, 206] It is now recognized that oncocytic adenomas exist and that they can be distinguished from oncocytic carcinomas using criteria similar to those used to distinguish follicular adenomas from carcinomas. Thus, oncocytic carcinomas should be defined on the basis of capsular or vascular invasion, as discussed in the section on follicular carcinoma.

Oncocytic carcinomas account for approximately 2% to 3% of all thyroid malignancies and occur more commonly in women, with a female:male ratio of 2:1. On average, patients with oncocytic carcinomas are about a decade older than those with oncocytic adenomas. The clinical presentation does not differ from that of patients with follicular carcinomas of nononcocytic type.

Pathologic Features and Differential Diagnosis. Oncocytic carcinomas are generally larger than oncocytic adenomas, but the size range is considerable. In the series reported by Carcangiu et al.,[127] most of the carcinomas measured more than 5 cm in diameter. Minimally invasive tumors are generally surrounded by a fibrous connective tissue capsule, which makes their distinction from oncocytic adenomas impossible grossly. Widely invasive carcinomas exhibit extensive capsular invasion or may lack a capsule altogether. Multiple nodules of tumor may be present in the adjacent thyroid parenchyma next to the main tumor mass. A subset of tumors may have equivocal features of malignancy (minimal or questionable capsular invasion, a predominantly solid growth pattern, marked nuclear atypia, or extensive necrosis), but these tumors are likely to behave in a benign fashion.[127]

As compared with adenomas, oncocytic carcinomas are more likely to have a solid or trabecular pattern (Fig. 7–59, see p. 459). In one series, only 14% of the carcinomas had a follicular pattern.[127] Additionally, the tumor cells in carcinomas are more likely to have a higher nuclear:cytoplasmic ratio than adenomas, and occasional mitotic figures may also be evident. Foci of clear cell change may be present.[6] The tumors are generally positive for thyroglobulin and cytokeratin, although the intensity of staining is generally less than that of non-oncocytic follicular tumors. A diagnosis of oncocytic carcinoma should be made only when there is evidence of capsular or vascular invasion, and the criteria for these features are the same as those described for follicular neoplasms. Oncocytic carcinomas have a greater propensity for invasion into the surrounding soft tissues than do follicular carcinomas.

Fine Needle Aspiration Biopsy. The distinction between oncocytic adenomas and carcinomas can only be made on the basis of capsular and vascular invasion. While fine needle aspiration biopsies are of value in the diagnosis of an oncocytic neoplasm, surgical excision is mandatory for definitive subclassification. Oncocytic tumors that behave in a malignant fashion tend to have small cells with large pleomorphic nuclei, abnormal chromatin, and multiple prominent nucleoli. In addition, they may show intranuclear cytoplasmic inclusions.

Treatment and Prognosis. Generally, both minimally and widely invasive oncocytic carcinomas are treated by near-total or total thyroidectomy. Radioactive iodine and external irradiation are of questionable value in the postoperative management of patients with these tumors.

As noted previously, oncocytic carcinomas are more likely to invade the soft tissues of the neck than follicular carcinomas. The most common sites of metastasis are lung and bone.[207] Lymph node metastases are more common than in follicular carcinomas and less common than in papillary carcinomas. Overall, the prognosis for oncocytic carcinomas is less favorable than the prognosis for follicular carcinomas. Five-year survival rates are in the range of 50% to 60%.

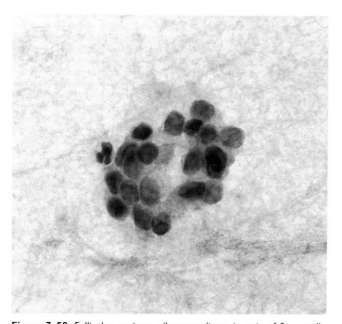

Figure 7–58. Follicular carcinoma (hematoxylin-eosin stain of fine needle aspiration biopsy). The cells exhibit moderate atypia.

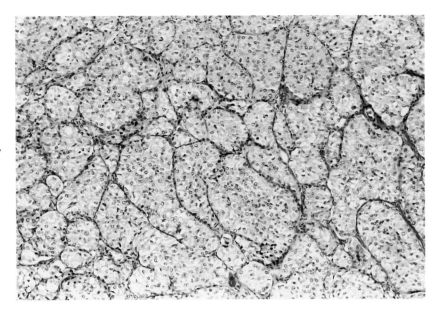

Figure 7–60. Poorly differentiated thyroid carcinoma, insular type. This tumor is composed of large nests (insulae) of tumor cells.

Poorly Differentiated Carcinomas

Clinical Features and Pathogenesis. Poorly differentiated thyroid carcinomas include a heterogeneous group of neoplasms whose behavioral and histologic features are intermediate between well-differentiated and undifferentiated thyroid carcinomas.[208–210] The best described tumor of this group is classified as *insular* carcinoma. The frequency of this tumor type appears to differ in different geographic regions. In central Italy, the tumors account for approximately 4% of all thyroid carcinomas.

There is a slight female predominance, and the median age at diagnosis is 55 years. Most patients present with a thyroid mass of variable duration. Analysis of several series of cases revealed regional metastases in 36% and distant metastases in 26% at presentation.[187]

Pathologic Features and Differential Diagnosis. Grossly, the tumors appear solid and gray-white with foci of necrosis and infiltrative margins.[209] The tumor is characterized by the presence of multiple round to ovoid nests of relatively small cells with high nuclear:cytoplasmic ratios. Most of the tumor cells have a solid growth pattern, but microfollicles containing small deposits of colloid are not uncommon. The tumor exhibits variable numbers of mitoses and foci of necrosis. Tumor cells are typically positive for thyroglobulin and may show focal immunoreactivity for somatostatin. Both vascular and lymphatic metastases are common (Fig. 7–60).

Foci of insular growth may be found occasionally in nonneoplastic thyroid conditions (e.g., dyshormonogenic goiter) and in differentiated thyroid carcinomas, particularly of the papillary type.[211] Some authors have suggested that the presence of an insular component in a differentiated thyroid carcinoma may not necessarily indicate that the tumor will have the usual aggressive behavior of a "pure" insular carcinoma.

The differential diagnosis includes undifferentiated thyroid carcinoma, poorly differentiated follicular carcinoma, and medullary carcinoma. Undifferentiated carcinomas generally feature greater degrees of pleomorphism, mitotic activity, and necrosis. Pilotti et al.[212] studied the distribution of *bcl*-2 and p53 in 22 cases of undifferentiated carcinoma and in 19 cases of poorly differentiated carcinoma. *Bcl*-2 was found in 84% of cases of poorly differentiated carcinoma and in 13% of undifferentiated carcinoma. p53 was found in approximately 50% of the cases in each category; however, differences in patterns of staining were apparent. Although almost all tumor cells were positive for p53 in undifferentiated carcinoma, positive staining was restricted to areas showing active infiltrating growth in the poorly differentiated carcinomas. These studies indicate that immunohistochemical analysis of *bcl*-2 may be useful in

the distinction of poorly differentiated and undifferentiated thyroid carcinomas. Medullary thyroid carcinomas can be distinguished from insular carcinomas on the basis of positive reactions for calcitonin and chromogranin.

Fine Needle Aspiration Biopsy. Aspirate smears from insular carcinomas are usually very cellular.[213] The background reveals numerous red blood cells and scanty colloid.[214] The follicular cells are small and monomorphic and are present predominantly as single cells. In addition, they can be arranged in sheets with or without a microfollicular, papillary, trabecular, or solid pattern. The cytoplasm is scant and without specific features. The nuclei are enlarged and overlap, without prominent variation in size or shape. The chromatin is fine to coarsely granular. Intranuclear cytoplasmic inclusions and nuclear grooves may be present.[215] Occasionally there is marked focal nuclear atypia.

Treatment and Prognosis. Treatment modalities for insular carcinomas are not fully established. For those tumors with a pure insular morphology, treatment approaches similar to those used for undifferentiated carcinomas are generally used. Metastases are common, with the most frequent sites of metastatic disease being regional lymph nodes, liver, and bone. The prognosis for insular carcinoma is poor. In a recent review, 25% of patients had died of their disease, 29% were alive with evidence of disease, 41% had no evidence of disease, and 5% had died with disease.[187]

The prognosis of differentiated thyroid carcinomas with a focal insular pattern is most likely dependent on the extent of the insular component.

Undifferentiated (Anaplastic) Carcinoma

Clinical Features and Pathogenesis. Undifferentiated carcinomas of the thyroid are uncommon tumors that account for a very small proportion of all thyroid malignancies in most large series.[11, 216] The tumors are best described as highly malignant neoplasms that appear wholly or partially undifferentiated by light microscopy but show evidence of epithelial differentiation by immunohistochemistry (presence of cytokeratins) or electron microscopy (desmosomes and tonofilaments).

The tumors occur principally in older adults, with a mean age of approximately 65 years and a female predominance. In some instances, a pre-existing thyroid mass may have been present for many years, and in some instances residual papillary or follicular carcinomas can be identified. The tumors are more frequent in areas of endemic goiter. Undifferentiated carcinomas present most commonly as rapidly enlarging masses with evidence of hoarseness, dyspnea, or dysphagia. Occasional patients may have evidence of distant metastases at presentation. Most patients are euthyroid, but occasional patients have had hypothyroidism or hyperthyroidism. The mechanism of hyperthyroidism is probably related to destruction of the thyroid parenchyma with the release of thyroid hormones into the circulation.

Pathologic Features and Differential Diagnosis. Undifferentiated carcinomas are typically very large tumors with evidence of extensive infiltration of the adjacent soft tissues of the neck. On cross-section, they have a fleshy appearance with foci of necrosis and hemorrhage. The histologic features are highly variable, but three basic patterns have been recognized (Figs. 7–61, see p. 459, 7–62, and 7–63, see p. 459). Tumors composed of round to polygonal cells and resembling nonkeratinizing squamous cell carcinomas have been designated *squamoid* type.[216] Occasional foci of keratinization may also be evident in some cases. The *spindle cell or sarcomatoid variant* is composed of bundles of spindle-shaped cells resembling fibrosarcoma, malignant fibrous histiocytoma, or malignant hemangioendothelioma (Fig. 7–63A). The *giant cell variant* is composed of very large cells with single or multiple hyperchromatic nuclei, some of which may resemble Reed-Sternberg cells. Rare variants containing multiple giant cells with osteoclast-like features also occur (Fig. 7–63B).[217] The *paucicellular variant* of undifferentiated carcinoma is characterized by the presence of acellular fibrous tissue or infarcted tissue with central dystrophic calcification and hypocellular foci with mildly atypical spindle cells admixed with collagen and lymphocytes.[217a] Most cases that were previously classified as anaplastic carcinomas of the small cell type now have been shown to represent malignant lymphomas.

Virtually all types of undifferentiated thyroid carcinoma have evidence of intense mitotic activity, areas of necrosis, and evidence of vascular invasion. Some tumors may contain prominent populations of acute inflammatory cells. Ultrastructurally, poorly developed desmosomes may be evident. Most undifferentiated carcinomas will show positive reactions for both cytokeratins and vimentin[218, 219]; however, keratin immunoreactivity may be both weak and focal. Most studies have revealed absent staining for thyroglobulin except in foci of pre-existing, well-differentiated carcinomas that may be present within the tumors. As noted by Rosai et al.,[277] a diagnosis of undifferentiated carcinoma should be favored when any pleomorphic tumor appears to arise within the thyroid, particularly if the patient is elderly and there is evidence of a residual better differentiated thyroid tumor within the gland. In those instances, the most appropriate interpretation would be undifferentiated malignant tumor, consistent with undifferentiated carcinoma.

The differential diagnosis includes malignant lymphoma, sarcoma, medullary thyroid carcinoma, and metastatic carcinoma. Malignant lymphomas are typically positive for leukocyte common antigen (CD45RO) and other markers of lymphoid differentiation. Sarcomas may arise within the thyroid or may involve the gland secondarily. Typically, sarcomas are positive for vimentin and may also contain cytokeratins. In some instances, it may be impossible, therefore, to differentiate a sarcoma from an undifferentiated carcinoma. However, the treatment of these tumor types is essentially identical. Metastatic carcinomas are discussed in a subsequent section. Medullary carcinomas of the spindle and giant cell types may resemble undifferentiated carcinomas; however, medullary carcinomas are typically positive for chromogranins and calcitonin.

Fine Needle Aspiration Biopsy. Aspirates from anaplastic carcinoma are typically highly cellular; however, in tumors with extensive degenerative change, cellularity may be low (Fig. 7–64, see p. 460). The cells are present singly or in clusters, and there is marked cellular pleomorphism.[11, 221] The cell types include squamoid, giant-cell, and spindle-cell. The nuclei are bizarre and single or multiple. They reveal coarsely clumped chromatin and single or multiple, prominent, irregular nucleoli. Mitotic figures may be numerous. The background smear reveals necrotic debris with tumor diathesis and polymorphonuclear leukocytes. The presence of numerous neutrophils in some aspirates may lead to a mistaken diagnosis of acute thyroiditis.

Treatment and Prognosis. Undifferentiated carcinomas are generally treated by a combination of surgery, external irradiation, and chemotherapy. [131]I treatment is ineffective.

The prognosis for undifferentiated carcinoma is poor, with mean survivals in the range of 7 to 12 months.[216] Most patients die as a direct result of extensive local tumor growth. The tumors also frequently metastasize to regional lymph nodes, and hematogenous metastases are common late in the course of the disease.

Squamous Cell Carcinoma

Clinical Features and Pathogenesis. Pure squamous cell carcinomas of the thyroid, as defined by obvious squamous differentiation and cytologic atypia, are rare.[222] These tumors occur most often in elderly patients who may have a history of pre-existing goiter. The tumors typically grow rapidly and are associated with extensive local invasion. Occasional patients may present with fever, leukocytosis, and hypercalcemia, which may be mediated by the secretion of interleukin-1.[223, 224]

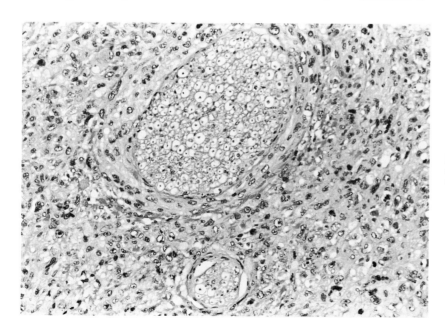

Figure 7–62. Undifferentiated thyroid carcinoma. This tumor extensively invades the soft tissues of the neck with entrapment of large nerves.

Pathologic Features and Differential Diagnosis. Squamous carcinomas are typically large tumors that replace the thyroid extensively. The tumors may show a spectrum of appearances ranging from those which are well differentiated to those which are poorly differentiated. In many cases, the squamous components merge with areas of undifferentiated carcinoma; accordingly, some authors have placed these tumors in the undifferentiated category. Similar to undifferentiated carcinomas, small foci of well-differentiated papillary or follicular carcinoma may be found within squamous carcinomas. This finding supports the view that some squamous carcinomas may arise from metaplastic foci of differentiated thyroid carcinomas, particularly of the papillary type.

Primary squamous cell carcinomas of the thyroid must be distinguished from metastases of squamous cell carcinoma to the thyroid gland and from direct extension of primary squamous carcinomas originating from the larynx or trachea.

Treatment and Prognosis. Treatment is essentially identical to that of undifferentiated thyroid carcinomas. The prognosis is very poor, with most patients dying as a consequence of the effect of local tumor invasion.

Medullary Carcinoma

Clinical Features and Pathogenesis. Medullary carcinoma is a malignant thyroid tumor composed of cells showing evidence of C-cell differentiation and usually containing calcitonin. This tumor type was first described as a distinctive morphologic entity by Horn in 1951.[225] Hazard et al.[226] subsequently defined its major histologic features, including the presence of stromal amyloid, and suggested the name *medullary carcinoma* to describe it. On the basis of similarities to certain solid thyroid tumors in animals and to normal parafollicular cells, Williams[227] suggested that medullary carcinomas were derived from parafollicular cells. With the demonstration of the parafollicular cell origin of calcitonin, subsequent studies demonstrated calcitonin in tumor extracts in serum of affected patients.[228]

These tumors account for 5% to 10% of all thyroid malignancies.[229] They may occur sporadically or as a component of type 2 multiple endocrine neoplasia (MEN) syndromes, which are inherited as autosomal dominant traits.[230] In most large series, sporadic tumors account for approximately 75% of all cases. Results of calcitonin screening studies indicate that sporadic medullary carcinomas may constitute up to 25% of all thyroid cancers found in patients with nodular thyroid disease.[230a] MEN 2A is characterized by medullary thyroid carcinoma, pheochromocytoma, and parathyroid chief cell hyperplasia or adenoma. A second genetically distinct syndrome (MEN 2B) is characterized by medullary thyroid carcinoma, pheochromocytoma, ocular and gastrointestinal ganglioneuromatosis, and skeletal abnormalities. A third category of familial medullary thyroid carcinoma is characterized by the development of thyroid tumors only.

Sporadic medullary carcinomas are principally tumors of middle-aged adults (mean age, 50 years) with a slight female predominance.[231] Generally, patients present with unilateral gland involvement with or without associated nodal metastasis. Patients with MEN 2A–associated medullary carcinomas have a mean age of approximately 20 years, whereas patients with MEN 2B may develop thyroid tumors in childhood. The mean age of patients with familial medullary thyroid carcinoma is approximately 50 years. With the use of biochemical and molecular screening methods, the average age of patients with familial tumors has decreased progressively. In contrast to sporadic tumors, which are usually unilateral, most familial medullary carcinomas are bilateral at presentation.

As discussed in the next section, familial tumors are associated with germline mutations in the *ret* proto-oncogene, whereas somatic mutations of codon 918 have been demonstrated in a subset of sporadic tumors.[230] Sporadic tumors occur with equal frequency in different parts of the world. In rare instances, these tumors may arise in patients with Hashimoto's disease[232] or in patients with long-standing hypercalcemia of diverse etiologies.[233] There are no data to

support a link between the development of these tumors and prior irradiation to the head and neck.

Pathologic Features and Differential Diagnosis. The tumors may vary considerably in size, and although they are sharply circumscribed, they are usually not encapsulated (Fig. 7–65, see p. 460). Tumors measuring less than 1 cm in diameter have been referred to as medullary microcarcinomas or as occult medullary carcinomas.[233a] On cross-section, the tumors are tan to pink, and their consistency can vary from soft to firm. Some tumors may appear grossly fibrotic with small foci of yellow discoloration.

The smaller tumors typically occur at the junctions of the upper and middle thirds of the lateral lobes, corresponding to the areas in which C cells normally predominate. When the tumors become very large, they may replace the entire lobe. Sporadic tumors are generally unilateral, but familial tumors are typically bilateral, multicentric, and associated with C-cell hyperplasia (see section on Familial Medullary Thyroid Carcinoma and C-cell Hyperplasia).

Most sporadic and familial tumors are nonencapsulated and exhibit a solid growth pattern; however, organoid, lobular, trabecular, and insular patterns are also common (Fig. 7–66A to D).[234] Some tumors may also contain follicular structures. Although most tumors appear grossly circumscribed, microscopic evaluation usually demonstrates an infiltrative margin. Individual tumor cells may be round, polygonal, or spindle-shaped with frequent admixtures of these cell types. Nuclei are round to ovoid with speckled chromatin. Binucleate cells may be present as well as variable numbers of giant cells. Nuclear pseudoinclusions, similar to those seen in PTCs, may be prominent. The cytoplasm varies from amphophilic to eosinophilic and, in well-fixed preparations, it may be granular. Occasional tumors may have clear cytoplasm. Mucin-positive vacuoles may be present in the cytoplasm of some tumor cells. Foci of necrosis, mitotic activity, and hemorrhage are more commonly present in larger tumors.

Stromal amyloid deposits are present in approximately 80% of cases (Fig. 7–67). Occasionally, the amyloid deposits may elicit a foreign body giant cell reaction. Additionally, the stroma may appear quite fibrotic with foci of calcification. Rare psammoma bodies may be present.

Numerous variants of medullary thyroid carcinoma have been described, including follicular (tubular) (Fig. 7–68, see p. 460),[235] papillary and pseudopapillary,[236] angiomatous,[237] small cell (Fig. 7–69A, see p. 461),[238] giant cell,[239] clear cell,[240] melanotic (Fig. 7–69B),[241] oncocytic,[242] squamous,[242] amphicrine (Fig. 7–70A) (composite calcitonin- and mucin-producing),[243] and paraganglioma-like (Fig. 7–70B).[244] An encapsulated adenoma-like variant has also been described. Although some workers have considered the encapsulated tumors to represent benign tumors, others have considered them to represent carcinomas (Fig. 7–70B).[245]

Medullary carcinomas of all types are usually positive for low molecular weight cytokeratins, whereas high molecular weight keratins are rarely expressed.[159] Vimentin is variably present, and occasional cases contain subpopulations of neurofilament-positive cells. The tumors are typically positive for markers of neuroendocrine differentiation, including neuron-specific enolase, chromogranins, and synaptophysin.[246] In addition, medullary carcinomas are typically positive for carcinoembryonic antigen. Calcitonin is present in approximately 80% of medullary carcinomas. Those cases which are negative for the peptide may give positive signals with in situ hybridization methods for calcitonin messenger RNA.[247] In addition to calcitonin, medullary carcinomas may contain somatostatin, adrenocorticotropic hormone and pro-opiomelanocortin derivatives, neurotensin, serotonin, and other amines.[9]

Ultrastructurally, medullary carcinomas are characterized by the presence of membrane-bound secretory granules, which represent the sites of storage of calcitonin and other peptide products. The larger granules have an average diameter of 280 nm with moderately electron dense finely granular contents that are closely applied to the limiting membranes of the granules.[248] Smaller granules have an average diameter of 130 nm with more electron dense contents that are

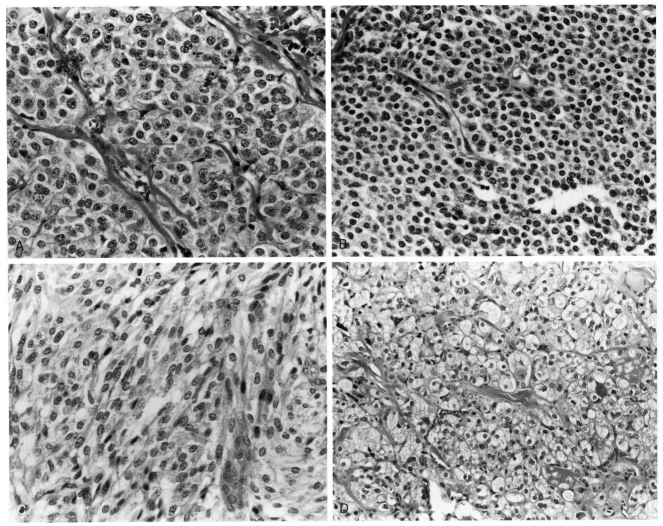

Figure 7–66. Medullary thyroid carcinoma. *A,* This tumor is composed of large nests of cells with abundant granular cytoplasm. *B,* This tumor is composed of sheets of monomorphic cells with central nuclei. *C,* This tumor has a spindle cell growth pattern. *D,* This tumor is composed predominantly of clear cells.

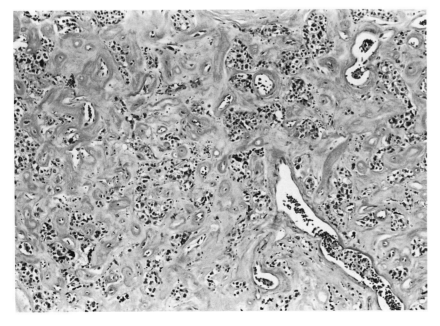

Figure 7–67. Medullary thyroid carcinoma. This tumor contains abundant stromal amyloid deposits.

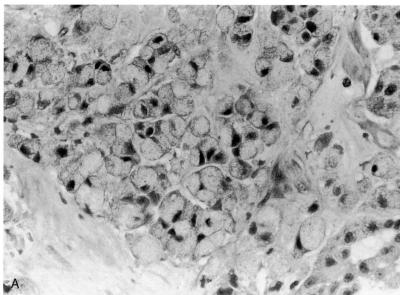

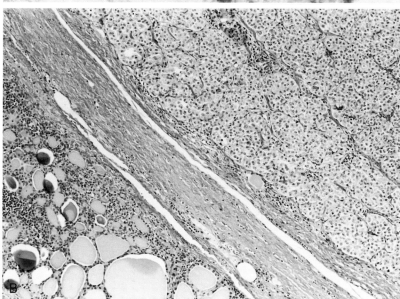

Figure 7–70. Medullary thyroid carcinoma. *A,* This tumor is composed of mucin-rich cells that also contain calcitonin (amphicrine type). *B,* This encapsulated tumor has a paraganglioma-like pattern.

separated from the limiting membranes by a narrow electron lucent space.

Medullary thyroid carcinomas may mimic virtually the entire spectrum of benign and malignant thyroid neoplasms. Occasional tumors may have a papillary or pseudopapillary appearance with nuclear pseudoinclusions and psammoma bodies. However, the papillary variants of medullary carcinoma are positive for calcitonin and chromogranin. Medullary carcinomas may contain neoplastic follicular structures and must, therefore, be distinguished from follicular carcinomas. The follicles in these tumors are typically positive for calcitonin. Entrapped residual normal thyroid follicles are found frequently in medullary carcinomas. In contrast to the neoplastic follicles, the entrapped normal follicles are positive for thyroglobulin (see section on Mixed Medullary and Follicular Cell Tumors).

Medullary carcinomas must also be distinguished from insular carcinomas. The latter tumors are characterized by the presence of solid sheets of tumor cells with occasional microfollicles. They are typically positive for thyroglobulin and their stroma is negative for amyloid. Medullary carcinomas of spindle and giant cell types must also be distinguished from undifferentiated carcinomas. The latter tumors are negative for calcitonin and chromogranin. Medullary carcinomas must also be distinguished from malignant lymphomas,

which are typically positive for leukocyte common antigen and other lymphoid differentiation markers. Medullary carcinomas may have a "plasmacytoid" appearance and must be distinguished from plasmacytomas. The latter tumors may also contain amyloid deposits, but the component cells are usually positive for immunoglobulins.

Eusebi et al.[249] described two cases of small cell thyroid carcinoma that were positive for chromogranin but negative for calcitonin by immunohistochemistry. Both tumors were negative for calcitonin messenger RNA when studied by in situ hybridization. These tumors may represent primary small cell carcinomas of the thyroid and should be separated from the small cell variant of medullary carcinoma.

The hyalinizing trabecular adenoma is typically encapsulated, as are some variants of medullary carcinoma. A trabecular growth pattern may be present in both tumors, and both may exhibit areas of hyalinization. However, the stroma of medullary carcinoma is typically positive for amyloid, whereas that of hyalinizing trabecular adenoma is not. Moreover, hyalinizing trabecular adenomas are negative for calcitonin. Paragangliomas are typically positive for chromogranin in the chief cells while the sustentacular cells are positive for S-100 protein. Oncocytic variants of follicular derived tumors are usually positive for thyroglobulin while oncocytic variants of medullary carcinoma are positive for calcitonin. Occasional intrathyroidal parathyroid adenomas may be mistaken for medullary carcinomas. Parathyroid tumors can be identified on the basis of their positivity for parathyroid hormone and chromogranin A.

Fine Needle Aspiration Biopsy. The broad histologic spectrum displayed by medullary carcinomas is also reflected in fine needle aspiration material.[250] Smears are usually cellular,[251] but the cellularity is inversely related to the amount of amyloid produced by the tumor. Tumor cells are present singly or in loosely cohesive clusters, occasionally with a syncytial arrangement.

Medullary carcinoma cells are usually pleomorphic and four different cell types can be present: small, round cells with vesicular nuclei and a thin rim of cytoplasm (carcinoid-like cells), plump cells with eccentric nuclei and a moderate amount of cytoplasm (plasmacytoid cells), spindle cells with elongated nuclei, and large cells with abundant cytoplasm. Usually there is a mixed cell pattern. If a single cell type predominates, it is most commonly the plasmacytoid type. The nuclei of the tumor usually reveal a salt and pepper distribution of chromatin[16] and an occasional single, prominent nucleolus. Both nuclear cytoplasmic inclusions and nuclear grooves may be present. Mild nuclear pleomorphism with binucleated cells is commonly seen, especially in the plasmacytoid cell type, and mitoses are occasionally present. Severe nuclear atypia with bizarre, multinucleated giant tumor cells are present in a small proportion of cases.

The cytoplasm of medullary carcinoma cells varies from scanty to abundant, and cytoplasmic borders are usually ill-defined. The cytoplasm is generally pale with a fibrillar appearance. A highly characteristic feature of medullary carcinoma is the presence of metachromatic neurosecretory cytoplasmic granules in May-Grünwald-Giemsa–stained smears only. Their incidence varies in different reports from 10% to 85%.[11, 250] Another helpful diagnostic feature is the frequent presence of amyloid as extracellular amorphous material. It has a similar quality to colloid in Papanicolaou-stained smears, and therefore it should be specifically identified with special stains such as Congo red. The identification of amyloid is a helpful feature but is not a pathognomonic feature for the diagnosis of medullary carcinoma, since amyloid can be present in cases of amyloid goiter and plasmacytoma.

The diagnostic accuracy of medullary carcinoma should approach 80%. The eccentric nuclear position, salt-and-pepper chromatin, intranuclear cytoplasmic inclusions, red cytoplasmic granules, and the presence of amyloid are diagnostic. However, diagnosis may be further confirmed by demonstrating calcitonin granules with immunoperoxidase techniques.

Treatment and Prognosis. Both familial and sporadic forms of medullary carcinoma are treated by total thyroidectomy with dis-

section of the central lymph nodes from the region of the hyoid bone to the innominate vein. Generally, a modified lateral node dissection is reserved for patients with jugular nodal metastases. The probability of nodal metastases increases with the size of the primary tumor.[252] In addition to metastases involving the central and lateral cervical nodes, medullary carcinoma may metastasize to a variety of distant sites including lung, bones, and liver. The adrenal glands are also common sites of metastasis, and in patients with MEN 2A and 2B, metastases to pheochromocytomas may be evident.

The 5-year survival rate for patients with these tumors is 60% to 70% and the 10-year survival rate is in the range of 40% to 50%. Patients with small MEN 2A–associated tumors (less than 0.5 cm in diameter) have a greater than 95% 10-year survival rate. The prognosis for patients with MEN 2B–associated medullary carcinomas is more guarded, since these tumors may metastasize early in their course.

The most important prognostic factor is tumor stage. The presence of perithyroidal soft tissue involvement, nodal metastases, and distant metastases is associated with decreased survival probabilities.[253] There are no apparent differences in survival among various histologic patterns of primary tumors. Moreover, there are no significant survival differences based on the presence of bombesin, somatostatin, neurotensin, or S-100 positive cells.[253] Tumors that contain abundant calcitonin immunoreactive cells have been reported to have a better prognosis than calcitonin-poor tumors.[254]

Plasma levels of carcinoembryonic antigen and calcitonin have been used to evaluate the tumor burden in patients with medullary thyroid carcinomas. The finding of persistently elevated carcinoembryonic antigen levels in the face of decreasing calcitonin values has been suggested as a marker of aggressive disease.[255]

Familial Medullary Thyroid Carcinoma and C-Cell Hyperplasia

The familial forms of the tumors are preceded by phases of C-cell hyperplasia that have been identified on the basis of enhanced calcitonin secretory responses to calcium and pentagastrin stimulation tests. C-cell hyperplasia is characterized by increased numbers of C cells within follicular spaces. With further progression, C cells fill and expand follicles to produce nodular C-cell hyperplasia.[231, 248] (Fig. 7–71A, B, see p. 461) Transition of this phase of C-cell growth to medullary thyroid carcinoma is characterized ultrastructurally by extension of C cells through the follicular basement membrane into the interstitium of the thyroid gland (Fig. 7–72). McDermott et al.[256] confirmed these findings using an immunoperoxidase technique for the demonstration of type IV collagen.

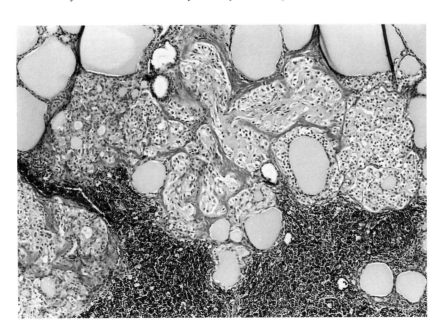

Figure 7–72. Familial medullary thyroid carcinoma in a patient with type 2A multiple endocrine neoplasia. In addition to C-cell hyperplasia, there is an area of medullary carcinoma that has invaded the stroma. The lymphocytes in the lower portion of the field are from a portion of intrathyroidal thymus gland.

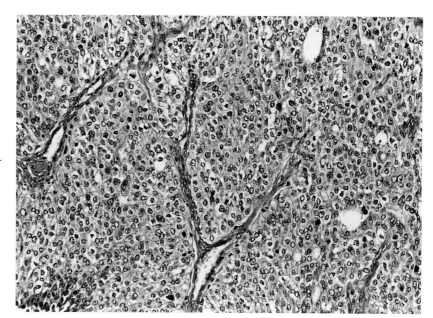

Figure 7–73. Mixed medullary and follicular carcinoma. The tumor has a predominant solid appearance.

The distinction of normal C-cell distribution from the earliest phases of C-cell hyperplasia is difficult.[257] Although initial studies suggested that the presence of 10 C cells per low-power field constituted sufficient evidence for C-cell hyperplasia, more recent studies indicate that this diagnosis should be made when there are at least 50 C cells per low-power field.[258]

C-cell hyperplasia has also been reported in association with hypercalcemic states, in patients with Hashimoto's disease, and adjacent to papillary and follicular carcinomas. This type of C-cell hyperplasia has been referred to as secondary or physiologic C-cell hyperplasia. Perry et al.[259] propose that the C-cell hyperplasia seen in association with MEN 2 syndromes and physiologic C-cell hyperplasia represent distinct histologic and biologic entities. Physiologic C-cell hyperplasia is characterized by increased numbers of normal C cells, which can be distinguished from adjacent follicular cells only on the basis of positive immunostains for calcitonin. Physiologic hyperplasia is usually diffuse rather than nodular. C-cell hyperplasia associated with MEN 2 syndromes is usually both diffuse and nodular and can often be diagnosed on the basis of examination of hematoxylin-eosin–stained sections. Perry et al.[259] stress the fact that C cells in MEN 2 syndromes are frequently dysplastic and propose that this type of hyperplasia be termed "neoplastic" hyperplasia. Cytologic atypia, although present in many cases of MEN 2–associated C-cell proliferation, is not a universal feature of this disorder, however. Kaserer[259a] has reported that some sporadic tumors may occur in the setting of C-cell hyperplasia.

Recent studies have demonstrated the molecular origins of the MEN 2A, MEN 2B, and familial medullary thyroid carcinoma syndromes.[230] Dominant germline mutations in different regions of the *ret* proto-oncogene have been demonstrated in the vast majority of familial cases studied to date. Molecular testing has largely replaced provocative testing of calcitonin secretion for the diagnosis of familial forms of medullary thyroid carcinoma. In addition, somatic mutations of the *ret* proto-oncogene have been demonstrated in a subset of patients with sporadic medullary thyroid carcinomas.

Mixed Medullary and Follicular Cell Tumors

Mixed medullary and follicular tumors are rare tumors that are composed of cells with evidence of C-cell and follicular differentiation and contain calcitonin or other peptides and thyroglobulin. Rarely, mixed tumors may occur in a familial setting.[259b] These tumors, which have also been referred to as *intermediate carcinomas,* must be distinguished from medullary carcinomas with entrapped normal follicles and from the follicular variant of medullary carcinoma.[260]

Such tumors might arise from uncommitted stem cells of the ultimobranchial bodies and could have the potential to differentiate into C cells and follicular cells.

Grossly, these tumors may be partially encapsulated or completely invasive. They frequently have solid and follicular areas with or without foci of cribriform growth (Fig. 7–73). In rare instances, some of the tumors may have a component of indifferent cells, with tubules and cystic structures resembling ultimobranchial remnants. The mixed tumors invariably stain positively for thyroglobulin. In the series of 14 cases reported by Ljungberg et al.,[260] 4 also contained calcitonin, 8 contained somatostatin, and 10 contained neurotensin-immunoreactive cells. Ultrastructurally, some of the cells contain neurosecretory granules of C-cell type, whereas others contain dilated cisternae of endoplasmic reticulum, as would be expected of follicular cells. Tumor cells in regional nodal metastases contained both thyroglobulin and one or more neuropeptides.

Several examples of mixed papillary and medullary carcinoma have also been described (Fig. 7–74, see p. 462).[261] Cells with the morphologic features of papillary carcinoma were thyroglobulin-positive but negative for carcinoembryonic antigen and calcitonin. The medullary carcinoma cells had the reversed immunohistochemical profile. Metastases also show similar mixed features. Whether these tumors arise from a single stem cell or represent collision tumors remains to be determined.

Studies suggest, however, that mixed tumors are not derived from a single stem cell based on differences in *ret* mutations and loss of heterozygosity and on X-chromosome inactivation patterns.[261a, 261b] The follicular structures in mixed tumors are often polyclonal and exhibit hyperplastic rather than neoplastic features. According to their "hostage" hypothesis, entrapped non-neoplastic follicles are stimulated by trophic factors, leading to hyperplastic follicular foci. Acquired genetic defects in follicular cells lead to neoplastic transformation and development of papillary or follicular carcinoma.[261a, 261b]

Malignant Lymphomas

Clinical Features and Pathogenesis. Malignant lymphomas occurring as primary thyroidal tumors account for 1% to 2% of all thyroid malignancies, and most patients present with a rapidly enlarging neck mass.[262] These tumors occur primarily in the sixth decade of life, with a female predominance. Most patients present with evidence of unilateral or bilateral thyroid enlargement with or without associated lymphadenopathy. Occasional patients may present with hoarseness, dyspnea, or dysphagia due to infiltration of the trachea or esophagus by tumor. Thyroid lymphomas are strongly associated with pre-existing Hashimoto's thyroiditis.[263] Most patients are euthyroid, although a subset may have hypothyroidism because of the associated Hashimoto's disease.

Pathologic Features and Differential Diagnosis. Thyroid lymphomas typically present as bulky solid masses that replace all or part of the thyroid gland. When the tumors are large, they may extend directly into the soft tissues of the neck. Regional nodes may or may not be involved. On cross-section, the tumors are white to pale tan. Small foci of necrosis and hemorrhage may be evident, but extensive areas of necrosis, such as those seen in undifferentiated carcinomas, are uncommon.

Most thyroid lymphomas are of B cell type and most have a diffuse architecture, although follicular lymphomas may also occur. Large cell and immunoblastic lymphomas account for the vast majority of primary thyroid lymphomas (Fig. 7–75, see p. 462). These tumors typically infiltrate between the follicles and also invade follicles to produce characteristic lymphoepithelial lesions (Fig. 7–76, see p. 462). Moreover, the lymphoid infiltrate often extends beyond the thyroid to involve the soft tissue of the neck.

Several studies have suggested that thyroid lymphomas share certain histologic and functional similarities with lymphomas arising in mucosa-associated lymphoid tissues (MALT).[264, 265] According to this hypothesis, there is a continuum between chronic lymphocytic thyroiditis, low-grade MALT-type lymphoma, and large cell lymphoma. Involvement of reactive lymphoid follicles by lymphoma cells may be prominent at the peripheries of the tumors. The distinction between severe chronic thyroiditis and follicular colonization by lymphoma may be extremely difficult and may require detailed immunophenotypic and genotypic analyses. Features that favor a diagnosis of lymphoma include involvement of the lumina of thyroid follicles, vascular invasion, and infiltration of lymphocytes beyond the thyroid capsule (see Fig. 7–76, p. 462). However, it should be remembered that invasion of thyroid follicles by lymphoid cells may also occur in Hashimoto's thyroiditis.

The differential diagnosis of malignant lymphoma also includes anaplastic thyroid carcinoma, insular carcinoma, and medullary thyroid carcinoma. Anaplastic thyroid carcinomas are typically positive for cytokeratins, although the extent of staining may be slight.[265] In thyroid lymphomas, occasional entrapped follicular cells will exhibit positive staining for cytokeratins and thyroglobulin. This type of staining should be distinguished from staining of the tumor cell cytoplasm. Thyroid lymphomas, on occasion, may have a vaguely lobular growth pattern, which may raise the possibility of insular carcinoma. This tumor type is typically positive for cytokeratins and thyroglobulin, whereas medullary thyroid carcinomas are positive for cytokeratins and calcitonin.

Fine Needle Aspiration Biopsy. Aspirates from thyroid glands involved by non-Hodgkin's lymphoma are typically highly cellular. The cells are present singly or rarely in small tissue fragments. Generally, there are no germinal center cells or epithelial cells present, and the aspirates reveal a monomorphic lymphoid cell population, usually of large cell type. Karyorrhexis is usually seen, but tumor diathesis is infrequent. The differential diagnosis of non-Hodgkin's lymphoma includes Hashimoto's thyroiditis and undifferentiated carcinoma.[266] Features that favor a diagnosis of lymphoma over Hashimoto's thyroiditis include a monomorphic, monoclonal lymphoid population and absence of plasma cells, phagocytic histiocytes, germinal center cells, and oncocytes. Features that favor a diagnosis of lymphoma over anaplastic carcinoma are lack of cellular cohesion, monomorphic lymphoid population, and occasional presence of lymphoglandular bodies. The diagnosis can be confirmed by appropriate immunohistochemical analyses, as discussed earlier.

Treatment and Prognosis. The role of thyroidectomy in patients with thyroid lymphomas is controversial. Some surgeons favor thyroidectomy in patients with tumors confined to the gland, and others favor biopsy followed by radiotherapy and chemotherapy, depending on the stage of the disease. Survival is dependent upon the

stage of the disease at presentation. Those patients with tumors confined to the gland without involvement of the regional nodes have 5-year survival rates in the range of 80% to 100%. The 10-year survival rates are in the range of 50% for patients treated with chemotherapy and radiotherapy.

Plasmacytoma

Plasma cell neoplasms may arise directly within the thyroid gland or may involve the gland secondarily as a manifestation of multiple myeloma. Primary plasmacytomas typically occur in older individuals, and most commonly arise on a background of chronic lymphocytic thyroiditis.[267, 268] The tumors are composed of mature and immature plasma cells with round nuclei, coarsely clumped chromatin, and generally small nucleoli. Immunophenotypic studies reveal monoclonality of these cells. Amyloid deposits may be present.

The differential diagnosis includes MALT lymphoma, plasma cell granuloma, and medullary thyroid carcinoma. MALT lymphomas may contain a high proportion of plasma cells in addition to small lymphocytes, some of which may appear atypical. In plasma cell granulomas, the plasma cells are typically polyclonal, as discussed subsequently. The nuclei of medullary thyroid carcinoma cells may resemble those of plasma cells, and the stroma of these tumors often contains amyloid. However, the carcinoma cells are typically positive for chromogranin and calcitonin.

Hodgkin's Disease

Hodgkin's disease, usually of the nodular sclerosing type, may rarely arise within the thyroid gland.[269] Secondary involvement of the gland may also occur by direct extension of cervical node disease.[270] The features of Hodgkin's disease in the thyroid are similar to those seen in other sites.

Other Lymphoproliferative and Hematologic Disorders

Langerhans' cell histiocytosis (eosinophilic granuloma) may involve the thyroid gland as a primary disorder or may be a manifestation of systemic disease.[271, 272, 272a] This disorder is characterized by the presence of cells with grooved vesicular nuclei and faintly eosinophilic cytoplasm. Variable numbers of eosinophils are present. The diagnosis can be confirmed by positive immunostains for S-100 protein, lysozyme, CD 1a, and CD 68 and by the presence of Birbeck granules at the ultrastructural level. In patients with disease confined to the thyroid, prognosis is excellent. Patients with a disseminated disease, on the other hand, have a poor prognosis.

Sinus histiocytosis with massive lymphadenopathy (Rosai-Dorfman disease) may rarely occur as a primary thyroid lesion or may involve the thyroid secondarily from involved perithyroidal lymph nodes. On occasion, sinus histiocytosis with massive lymphadenopathy may simulate subacute thyroiditis clinically.[273] The histiocytic cells are characterized by round to ovoid vesicular nuclei with abundant eosinophilic cytoplasm and evidence of phagocytosed lymphocytes (emperipolesis), erythrocytes, or neutrophils. The cells exhibit positivity for S-100 protein, α_1-antichymotrypsin, CD 68, and lysozyme.

Plasma cell granuloma is characterized by the presence of nodular lesions composed of polyclonal plasma cells together with other inflammatory elements. The lesions may infiltrate adjacent tissues, and may, therefore, simulate plasmacytomas. Moreover, plasma cell granulomas may be associated with polyclonal gammopathy.[274]

Rare examples of extramedullary hematopoiesis have also been reported in the thyroid gland.[275]

Mesenchymal Tumors

Clinical Features and Pathogenesis. Both benign and malignant mesenchymal tumors may occur in the thyroid gland. Benign tumors include those of vascular (hemangioma, lymphangioma), muscle (leiomyoma), neural (neurilemmoma), and adipocyte (lipoma) origins.

Sarcomas are malignant tumors of presumed mesenchymal origin.[200] Virtually all types of sarcomas have been reported as primary thyroid malignancies, including osteosarcomas and chondrosarcomas.[276] They constitute a small proportion of primary thyroid malignancies.[277] They tend to occur in older individuals, are rapidly growing, and are usually fatal, owing to extensive local invasion. In this regard, they are similar to undifferentiated carcinomas.

Angiosarcoma is the most common of this group of tumors and it occurs primarily in the endemic goiter regions of Europe.[278] The mean age of affected patients is 60 years and there is a slight male predominance.

Pathologic Features and Differential Diagnosis. Grossly, sarcomas are large tumors that may replace part or all of the thyroid gland. The tumors often have a fleshy appearance with frequent areas of necrosis and hemorrhage. Direct invasion of the soft tissues of the neck is common. Angiosarcomas are commonly hemorrhagic with multiple blood-filled cystic spaces.

Histologically, the tumors vary from those that are solid to those with irregular vascular slits or anastomosing channels lined by large atypical endothelial cells. The tumor cells are usually positive for vimentin, Ulex europaeus, and the factor VIII-related antigen. CD 31 and CD 34 may also be positive. Tumors with epithelioid features may exhibit cytokeratin positivity.[279, 280] Ultrastructurally, Weibel-Palade bodies are present in well-differentiated angiosarcomas. The histologic features of other sarcomas are similar to those described in other sites.[276]

The major differential diagnosis of thyroid sarcomas is undifferentiated carcinoma. Generally, however, undifferentiated carcinomas exhibit evidence of epithelial differentiation as determined by ultrastructural analysis and immunohistochemistry. In some instances, this distinction may be impossible, particularly since some sarcomas may exhibit immunoreactivity for cytokeratins.

Treatment and Prognosis. Treatment usually includes a combination of surgery, radiotherapy, and chemotherapy. Even with these combined approaches, prognosis is very poor and is generally comparable to that of undifferentiated carcinomas.

Unusual Thyroid Tumors

Thymic and related branchial pouch tumors may occur as primary thyroid neoplasms.[281] Thymomas occur most commonly in middle-aged females and probably arise from intrathyroidal thymic remnants. The tumors are generally surrounded by a fibrous capsule with extensions of fibrous tissue into the substance of the neoplasm. They are composed of variable numbers of polygonal to spindle-shaped epithelial cells and lymphocytes (Fig. 7–77A). The differential diagnosis includes undifferentiated carcinoma and malignant lymphoma. Undifferentiated carcinomas lack the lobular pattern that is typical of thymomas and almost always feature cells with pronounced nuclear atypia and prominent mitotic activity. Lymphomas can be excluded by the absence of cytokeratin-positive epithelial elements. The vast majority of intrathyroidal thymomas behave as benign neoplasms.

A separate tumor type that has been recognized recently is the *spindle epithelial tumor with thymus-like differentiation* (SETTLE) (Fig. 7–77B).[281, 282] This tumor occurs primarily in late adolescence. Histologically, the tumor is composed of bundles of spindle-shaped cells that merge into epithelial-type cells and form cords, tubules, or papillae. Glandular structures lined by mucinous or respiratory-type epithelium may also be present. The tumor cells, including the spindle cell elements, are positive for cytokeratins. The differential diagnosis includes undifferentiated carcinoma and teratoma. Undifferentiated carcinomas generally exhibit marked nuclear atypia and high mitotic activity; moreover, they lack the cords, tubules, and papillae that may be seen in SETTLE tumors. Teratomas, on the other hand, are composed of derivatives of all these germ layers. The be-

havior of SETTLE tumors is unpredictable, and delayed metastases may occur many years after excision of the primary tumors.

Carcinomas showing thymus-like differentiation (CASTLE) have also been described. The mean age at onset is approximately 50 years.[281] The CASTLE tumors most commonly involve the lower poles of the thyroid and extend frequently into the adjacent soft tissues of the neck. Typically, tumors present as firm lobulated gray-white masses. Tumor cells are of intermediate to large size with vesicular nuclei, coarsely clumped chromatin, and prominent nucleoli. Foci of squamous differentiation may be apparent (Fig. 7–78). Lobules and cords of tumor cells are usually separated by fibrous septa containing lymphocytes and plasma cells. These features distinguish CASTLE tumors from undifferentiated carcinomas. Nodal metastases occur in approximately 50% of patients with CASTLE tumors, and most patients have relatively long survival periods.

Teratomas of the thyroid are rare tumors that usually arise in the neck and involve the thyroid gland by direct extension. They have been reported both in neonates and in adults.[283] As in other sites, teratomas are composed of derivatives of ectoderm, endoderm, and mesoderm. In neonates and infants, the tumors may attain enormous proportions and typically contain both solid and cystic areas. Although some of the tumors in neonates and infants contain immature elements, the vast majority pursue a benign clinical course. Teratomas in adults occur somewhat more commonly in females than in males. In contrast to their benign behavior in infants, teratomas in adults are most often aggressive neoplasms that pursue a malignant course.[284] Rosai et al.[200] have suggested that thyroid teratomas in adults are not germ cell neoplasms but rather represent malignant neuroepithelial tumors.

Paragangliomas of the thyroid gland are exceptionally rare. These tumors most likely arise from paraganglia that may be present within the capsule of the thyroid.[24, 285] Grossly, they present as encapsulated neoplasms that vary in size from those which are barely visible grossly to those which measure up to 3 cm in diameter. Typically, they are composed of nests of cells separated by a fibrovascular stroma. Paragangliomas contain chief cells and sustentacular cells; however, the sustentacular cells are difficult to visualize in hemotoxylin-eosin–stained sections (Fig. 7–79). Typically, the sustentacular cells are positive for S-100 protein, whereas the chief cells are positive for chromogranin A. Ultrastructurally, the chief cells contain typical membrane-bound neurosecretory granules. The differential diagnosis includes hyalinizing trabecular adenoma, the solid variant of papillary carcinoma, and medullary thyroid carcinoma. The first two tumors are typically positive for cytokeratins and thyroglobulin, and medullary carcinomas are positive for cytokeratins and calcitonin. Paragangliomas, on the other hand, are negative for thyroglobulin, calcitonin, and cytokeratins, but contain S-100–positive cells surrounding the nests of chief cells.

Mucoepidermoid carcinomas rarely may arise in the thyroid gland.[286–288] These tumors have been reported to occur over a wide age range, although most occur in the fifth to seventh decades. They tend to be circumscribed but not encapsulated and are characterized by an admixture of squamous and mucus cells in a solid or cystic pattern. Cribriform areas and foci of necrosis may be evident, and the stroma is typically fibrotic. Mucoepidermoid carcinomas of the thyroid are indolent tumors that tend to metastasize to cervical lymph nodes, a pattern of spread similar to that of papillary carcinoma. This finding, together with the presence of psammoma bodies, suggests a histogenetic link to papillary carcinoma. Miranda et al.[289] reported a follicular variant of papillary carcinoma that contained foci of mucoepidermoid carcinoma. Both components were also identified in foci of extracapsular invasion and in nodal metastases.

Anaplastic transformation has been recorded in an example of a papillary and mucoepidermoid thyroid carcinoma.[290] Although some authors favor an origin from solid cell nests,[286] others postulate a follicular cell origin.[291]

Sclerosing mucoepidermoid carcinoma with eosinophilia typically occurs on a background of Hashimoto's thyroiditis.[292] The tu-

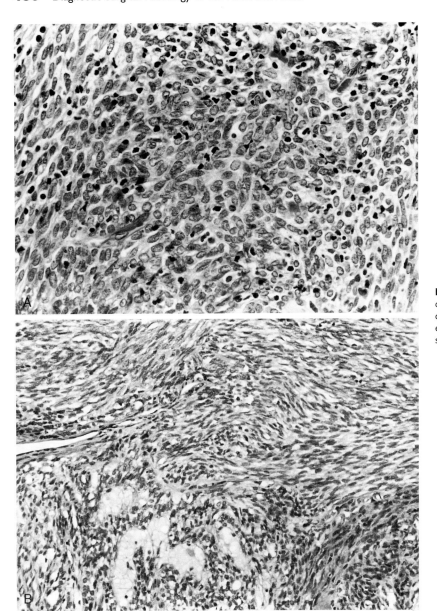

Figure 7–77. *A*, Intrathyroidal thymoma. The tumor is composed of spindle-shaped cells admixed with lymphocytes. *B*, Spindle epithelial tumor with thymus-like differentiation (SETTLE). The tumor is composed primarily of spindle-shaped cells with a few areas of gland formation.

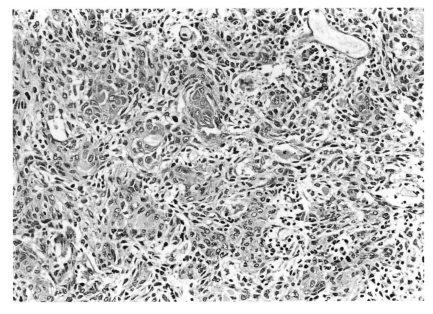

Figure 7–78. Carcinoma showing thymus-like differentiation (CASTLE). The tumor cells have a spindle shape and form pearl-like clusters.

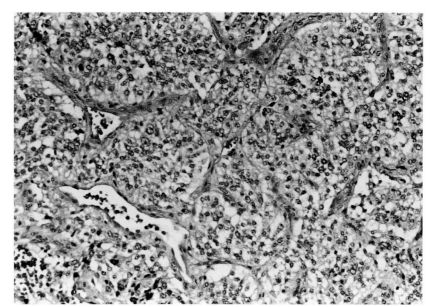

Figure 7–79. Paraganglioma. The tumor is composed of cell nests in a "zellballen" pattern. Sustentacular cells cannot be clearly distinguished in this preparation.

mor is characterized by nests and cords of neoplastic cells embedded in a fibrous stroma containing abundant eosinophils.

Adenosquamous carcinomas of the thyroid are exceptionally rare neoplasms that are probably unrelated to the aforementioned mucoepidermoid carcinomas.[293] Histologically, they are composed of malignant squamous cells with foci of mucin production. Their behavior is identical to that of undifferentiated carcinomas.

Secondary Tumors

Secondary involvement of the thyroid by tumor may occur as a result of direct extension from contiguous structures, such as the larynx, or as a result of hematogenous spread. Autopsy studies have revealed thyroid metastases in up to 20% of patients with disseminated carcinomatosis, with breast, lung, and skin (melanoma) being the most common primary sites (Fig. 7–80A, see p. 463).[294] In a clinical series of 43 cases reported by Nakhjavani et al.,[295] the kidney was the most common primary tumor site (33%), followed by lung (16%), esophagus (9%), uterus (7%), and skin (5%). The mean interval from the diagnosis of the primary tumor to the development of thyroid metastases was 106 months for renal carcinoma, 131 months for carcinoma of the breast, and 132 months for cancer of the uterus. These findings suggest that the appearances of a new thyroid mass in a patient with a known history of previous cancer should be considered as a potential metastatic site.

Metastases from clear cell kidney carcinomas may be extremely difficult to differentiate from primary clear cell tumors of the thyroid (Fig. 7–80B, see p. 463).[294, 296] The latter tend to be single, whereas metastases are more commonly multiple; moreover, metastases tend to have prominent degrees of vascularity. Immunohistochemical staining for thyroglobulin is typically negative in metastatic tumors; however, residual normal follicular cells that can be entrapped within the tumor may be positive.

PARATHYROID GLANDS
Embryology

The parathyroid glands are derivatives of the third and fourth branchial pouches. They are first recognizable at 5 to 6 weeks of development (8 to 9 mm embryonic stage) as thickenings of the anterodorsal branchial pouch epithelium.[2, 297] The inferior parathyroids, together with the thymus, are derived from the third pouch, and they are also referred to as *parathyroid III*. Both the thymus and

parathyroid III have a complex pattern of migration before they assume their final position caudad to the derivation of the fourth pouch. Failure of separation of parathyroid III from the thymus results in its appearance in the lower neck within the thymic tongue, anterior mediastinum, or, rarely, in the posterior mediastinum. Early separation of parathyroid III from the thymus, on the other hand, may result in its final position cephalad to parathyroid IV. Because of these features, parathyroid III may be found from the angle of the jaw to the pericardium. Parathyroid IV, on the other hand, is more constant in its final position. This parathyroid develops from the fourth branchial pouch together with the ultimobranchial body. Typically, parathyroid IV is close to the point at which the inferior thyroid artery crosses the recurrent laryngeal nerve at the cricothyroid junction.

Anatomy and Physiology

Most normal adults have four parathyroid glands, while approximately 13% of normal individuals have more than four and 3% have only three glands.[298] The glands most often appear as flattened, ovoid or bean-shaped structures. They generally measure 4 to 6 mm in length, 2 to 4 mm in width, and 1 to 2 mm in thickness. The average combined weight of the glands is 120 ± 3.5 mg for males and 142 ± 5.2 mg for females, with corresponding parenchymal weights of 82.0 ± 2.6 mg and 88.9 ± 3.9 mg, respectively.[299]

The superior parathyroid glands (IV) are most commonly found within a circumscribed area at a distance of about 1 cm from the intersection of the recurrent laryngeal nerve and the inferior thyroid artery.[300] Occasional glands may be found in the capsule of the thyroid and, rarely, may be present within the substance of the thyroid. The superior parathyroids may, on occasion, be present within the carotid sheath or in the retroesophageal or retropharyngeal space. The inferior parathyroids (III) exhibit considerably more variation in their anatomy than do the superior parathyroids. Sixty-one percent of the inferior parathyroids are inferior, posterior, or lateral to the lower pole of the thyroid, whereas 17% are present high up on the anterior aspect of the thyroid. Other sites for the inferior glands include the thyrothymic ligament, cervical thymus, lower thymus, and lower mediastinum.

The arterial supply of the glands is derived from branches of the superior thyroid artery (parathyroid IV) and inferior thyroid artery (parathyroid III). Venous drainage of the upper glands occurs via the superior or lateral thyroid vein, whereas drainage of the lower glands occurs via the lateral or inferior thyroid vein. Lymphatic drainage originates from a subcapsular plexus into the superior deep cervical, pretracheal, paratracheal, retropharyngeal, and inferior deep cervical nodes.

The parenchymal cells of the parathyroids include chief cells, varying numbers of oncocytes, and transitional oncocytes (Fig. 7–81, see p. 463).[299] The chief cells are generally polyhedral and measure 8 to 10 μm in diameter. The nuclei are round and centrally placed and have coarse chromatin with sharp nuclear membranes. The cytoplasm is faintly eosinophilic and may appear clear or vacuolated. Ultrastructurally, resting chief cells have relatively straight plasma membranes; increased functional activity is associated with greater tortuousity of the membranes. Chief cells contain moderate numbers of mitochondria as well as secretory deposits. Prosecretory granules have an average diameter of 0.2 μm and are located adjacent to the Golgi regions. Mature secretory granules have an average diameter of 0.3 μm. Resting chief cells contain frequent lipid droplets and relatively abundant glycogen.[301]

Oncocytes measure 12 to 20 μm in diameter and have a densely eosinophilic granular cytoplasm (Fig. 7–82, see p. 464). The nuclei tend to be larger and more vesicular than those found in chief cells. Ultrastructurally, oncocytes contain numerous mitochondria with relatively few secretory granules. Transitional oncocytes are smaller and less eosinophilic than oncocytes and contain fewer mitochondria. Oncocytic nodules may be prominent in the parathyroid glands of elderly individuals. The oncocytes appear first at puberty and increase in number with advancing age.

Chief cells contain cytokeratins as their major intermediate filament.[302] Parathyroid hormone may be identified by immunohistochemistry.[302a] An alternative approach to the demonstration of parathyroid hormone is the use of in situ hybridization methods with probes for parathyroid hormone messenger RNA.[303] The chief cells also contain parathyroid hormone secretory protein, which can be demonstrated with antibodies to chromogranin A.[304]

The stromal compartment of the gland includes mature fat cells, blood vessels, and varying amounts of connective tissue, which tends to increase with the age of the individual. Until adolescence, the amount of stromal fat is minimal, although obese children tend to have more stromal fat than lean individuals. The number of fat cells increases until the age of 25 to 30. In older individuals, the amount of fat is determined largely by constitutional factors. Although earlier studies had indicated that adult parathyroids contained approximately 50% stromal fat, more recent analyses have demonstrated a considerably lower stromal fat content. In an autopsy study of normal parathyroids, two thirds of the glands had less than 20% stromal fat, whereas only 9% had more than 40%.[305]

Stromal fat is often irregularly distributed throughout the gland, and polar regions tend to be richer in fat than more central regions. Biopsies from the polar regions, therefore, may give spuriously high stromal fat : parenchymal ratios.

Parathyroid hormone is an 84 amino acid peptide with a molecular weight of 9500.[306] It is encoded by a gene on the short arm of chromosome 11. The hormone is synthesized as a 115 amino acid–containing precursor, pre-pro-parathyroid hormone. This precursor enters the endoplasmic reticulum where the 25 amino acid–containing N-terminal portion of the molecule is cleaved. The resultant intermediary protein, pro-parathyroid hormone, is subsequently transported to the Golgi region where cleavage of the hexapeptide-containing N-terminal segment of the molecule occurs. As a result, pro-parathyroid hormone is converted to parathyroid hormone.

The levels of calcium and phosphorus are controlled by the actions of parathyroid hormone, calcitriol, and calcitonin.[306] Under normal conditions, the concentration of calcium in serum ranges from 9 to 10.5 mg/dL (2.2 to 2.6 mmol/L). In the extracellular fluid, 46% of the calcium is bound to protein, 48% is present as ionized calcium, and the remainder is associated with diffusible ion complexes. The most important regulator of the synthesis and secretion of parathyroid hormone is ionized calcium. Increased levels of ionized calcium inhibit the synthesis of parathyroid hormone, while decreased levels of calcium stimulate its synthesis. Parathyroid hormone maintains serum calcium levels by promoting calcium entry into the blood from bone, kidney, and the gastrointestinal tract. In bone, it stimulates bone resorption and inhibits bone formation. By stimulating renal synthesis of calcitriol, parathyroid hormone favors gastrointestinal absorption of calcium. In the kidney, parathyroid hormone stimulates resorption of calcium, enhances clearance of phosphate, and promotes an increase in the enzyme that is important in the production of active vitamin D.

Hyperparathyroidism

Hyperparathyroidism refers to a metabolic derangement characterized by increased production of parathyroid hormone.[306] Serum calcium may be decreased, increased, or normal, depending on renal function and other factors. In primary hyperparathyroidism, excess parathyroid hormone originates from adenoma, hyperplasia, or carcinoma of the parathyroid glands.[307] Serum calcium levels are characteristically increased, although occasional patients may be normocalcemic. Secondary hyperparathyroidism is an adaptive increase in parathyroid hormone production induced most commonly by the hypocalcemia and hyperphosphatemia of chronic renal failure. Tertiary hyperparathyroidism refers to the development of autonomous parathyroid hyperfunction in patients with secondary hyperparathyroidism.

The incidence of primary hyperparathyroidism has increased dramatically over the past several decades, primarily as a result of the introduction of multiphasic biochemical screening programs.[308] Prior to 1970, most patients with primary hyperparathyroidism presented with renal disease (calculi, nephrocalcinosis) or with bone disease (osteitis fibrosa cystica). Currently, most patients with hyperparathyroidism are either asymptomatic or have relatively mild and nonspecific complaints of lethargy or weakness.

Parathyroid Adenoma

Clinical Features and Pathogenesis. Parathyroid adenomas are benign neoplasms composed of chief cells, oncocytes, transitional oncocytes, or mixtures of these cell types.[309] They are responsible for 80% to 85% of all cases of primary hyperparathyroidism in most series.[310] In some institutions, however, the incidence of adenomas is considerably lower owing to differences in diagnostic criteria and differences in patterns of patient referrals.[311] Although adenomas can occur at any age, most become evident in the fourth decade. They occur more commonly in females, with a female : male ratio of about 3 : 1.

Although early studies using isoenzymes of glucose-6-phosphate dehydrogenase suggested that adenomas represented polyclonal proliferations, more recent studies employing molecular technologies, including X-chromosome inactivation patterns, indicate that they are monoclonal proliferations.[312–315] Clonal deletions of chromosome 11q13 (the site of the MEN 1 gene) occur in 26% to 39% of parathyroid adenomas, whereas mutations of the gene occur in 12% to 22% of cases.[315a] Approximately 5% of adenomas contain an activated form of the PRAD (parathyroid adenoma)-1 oncogene (cyclin D1).[313] The activation of PRAD-1 results from the juxtaposition of the regulatory region of the parathyroid hormone gene on chromosome 11 with the coding region of PRAD-1. This rearrangement results in the overexpression or deregulation of PRAD-1 in the tumor cell, leading to stimulation of cell proliferation.

There are few data relating to the pathogenesis of these tumors. They may occur in association with MEN types 1 and 2, although most parathyroid lesions in these syndromes are currently classified pathologically as hyperplasias. There is also some suggestion that ionizing radiation plays a role in their development. The most common cellular defect in parathyroid adenomas is an increase in the calcium value needed to inhibit secretion of parathyroid hormone (shift in calcium inhibitory set point). This may be attributed in part to decreased numbers of calcium receptors on the plasma membranes of chief cells. Juhlin et al.[316] have generated a series of monoclonal antibodies against a receptor on parathyroid chief cells that is involved in the sensing and gating of calcium. Immunohistochemical studies have revealed intense staining of the parathyroid cells of normal and suppressed glands, but decreased staining in cases of hyperplasia and adenomas.

Pathologic Features and Differential Diagnosis. Approximately 90% of parathyroid adenomas involve the upper or lower glands of the neck, with the remainder occurring in a variety of other sites including the mediastinum, retroesophageal space, or within the thyroid.[309, 310] Rare examples of adenoma have been encountered in the pericardium, vagus nerve, or soft tissues adjacent to the angle of the jaw. Most adenomas involve a single gland, although adenomas occurring in two or more glands have been reported.

Adenomas vary considerably in size, ranging from those measuring less than 6 mm in diameter (microadenomas) to those measuring many centimeters in diameter (Figs. 7–83 and 7–84, see p. 464). There is some correlation between tumor size and symptomatology. In the cases reported by Castleman and Roth,[310] adenomas associated with severe bone disease had an average weight of 10 g, whereas most smaller tumors were less symptomatic. Most adenomas have an ovoid shape, but occasional tumors may be bilobed or even multilobed. The risk of incomplete excision is high in adenomas that are multilobular. Adenomas usually can be dissected easily from the surrounding connective tissue of the neck, unless there has been hemorrhage and cyst formation. On cross-section, adenomas are typically soft and vary in color from tan to orange-brown. Foci of cystic change are common, particularly in large adenomas.

Most adenomas are composed of chief cells arranged in cords and nests, glandular formations, or sheets with frequent admixtures of these patterns (Fig. 7–85). In rare instances, the neoplastic chief cells may be arranged in papillary formations.[317] Gland-like (tubule) formations may contain a colloid-type material similar to that seen in normal thyroid (Fig. 7–86, see p. 465). The colloid may be Congophilic and may exhibit green birefringence, typical of amyloid deposits. Focal calcification of the luminal colloid may also occur.

Neoplastic chief cells are generally larger than those seen in the adjacent normal gland.[319] The cytoplasm is faintly eosinophilic but occasionally appears clear. Nodular aggregates of chief cells with more or less cytoplasm than the bulk of chief cells composing the

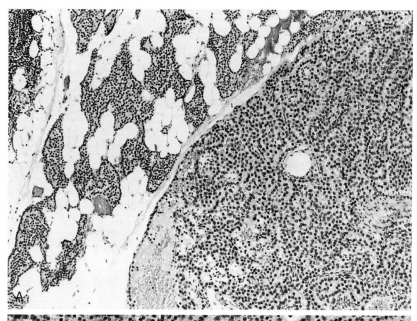

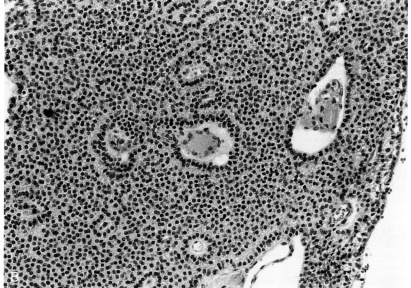

Figure 7–85. *A,* Intrathymic parathyroid adenoma. The adenoma is sharply demarcated from the adjacent rim of normal parathyroid. A small rim of thymus is present in the upper left corner of the field. *B,* Parathyroid adenoma. The chief cells have a palisaded arrangement around blood vessels.

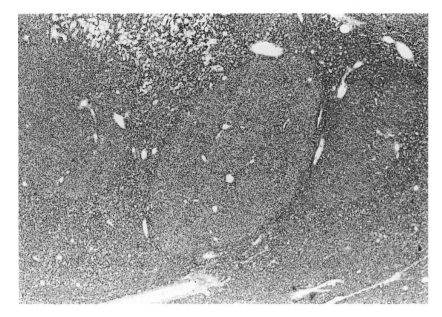

Figure 7–87. Parathyroid adenoma. The neoplastic chief cells are arranged focally in a nodular pattern.

gland are relatively frequent within the tumors (Fig. 7–87). Such nodules often have a higher proliferative fraction than the nonnodular portions of the adenoma.[318]

Nuclei of adenoma cells are generally round and central with dense chromatin and occasional small nucleoli. Enlarged hyperchromatic nuclei may be scattered throughout the gland, and in occasional cases they may form nodular aggregates. In the absence of other features of malignancy, the presence of such atypical cells should not be construed as evidence of malignancy (Fig. 7–88*A*, see p. 465).

Although mitotic activity has been considered to be a criterion of malignancy in parathyroid tumors, Snover and Foucar[320] identified mitoses in 70% of adenomas (Fig. 7–88*B*). Similar findings have been reported by San Juan et al.[321] These findings indicate that mitotic activity may be found in adenomas and, therefore, should not be used as the sole criterion of malignancy.

A rim of non-neoplastic chief cells, representing residual normal gland, is present in 50% to 60% of cases (Fig. 7–89, see p. 465; see also Figs. 7–83, p. 464, and 7–85). The probability of finding a rim of normal parathyroid tissue decreases with increasing size of the adenoma. Typically, the cells within the rim are smaller than adenoma cells, and they frequently contain fat droplets measuring 0.5 to 1.5 mm in diameter.[319] Generally, if fat is present within the adenoma cells, it tends to be more finely dispersed than in the nonneoplastic gland.

Stromal fat deposits may be present within some adenomas. They may be distributed diffusely throughout the adenoma or may be present in small aggregates. Stromal fat may, on occasion, be so abundant that a small biopsy may be misinterpreted as a normal gland. Although the amount of fibrous stroma is generally sparse within an adenoma, occasional adenomas may contain abundant fibrous tissue. Fibrosis most likely represents a degenerative phenomenon and may be accompanied by chronic inflammation and hemosiderin deposition.

Adenoma Variants

Microadenomas measure less than 6 mm in diameter. They can be so small that they may be missed on surgical exploration and frozen section examination. In several reported cases, microadenomas were apparent only after the paraffin-embedded blocks were serially sectioned.[322, 323]

Oncocytic adenomas account for approximately 5% of all parathyroid adenomas. Although initial studies suggested that oncocytic adenomas were nonfunctional, recent studies indicate that they may be associated with hyperparathyroidism.[324, 325] Wolpert et al.[326] have suggested that at least 90% of the cells should be oncocytes before a tumor is considered to be an oncocytic adenoma. On cross-section, oncocytic adenomas are soft and orange-tan to dark brown (Fig. 7–90, see p. 466). Cells may be arranged in cords, nests, tubules, or solid sheets. The component cells have abundant granular eosinophilic cytoplasm, similar to oncocytes in other locations (Fig. 7–91, see p. 466). Ultrastructural studies have confirmed the presence of numerous mitochondria

The *parathyroid lipoadenoma (hamartoma)* is a rare, benign neoplasm characterized by the proliferation of parenchymal and stromal elements (Fig. 7–92, see p. 466).[327, 328] These tumors may be accompanied by signs and symptoms of hyperparathyroidism. Reported cases of lipoadenoma have weighed between 0.5 and 420 g. The stromal compartment of lipoadenomas typically features abundant fibroadipose tissue with areas of myxoid changes and chronic inflammation.

Water clear cell adenomas have also been reported but are exceptionally rare.[328a] The cytologic features of this variant are similar to those described in the section on Primary Clear Cell Hyperplasia.

The term *atypical parathyroid adenoma* has been used to describe adenomas that have some of the features of parathyroid carcinomas but lack evidence of true invasive growth.[329] These include adherence of tumor to adjacent soft tissues, mitotic activity, trabecular growth pattern, and the presence of neoplastic cells in the capsule of the tumor. A diagnosis of atypical adenoma implies that the behavior of the tumor is unpredictable with respect to recurrence and metastasis.

The existence of *double adenomas* is controversial. Verdonk and Edis[330] reported double adenomas in 1.9% of patients with primary hyperparathyroidism. The criteria for inclusion in this category include (1) two enlarged glands, each weighing more than 70 mg and (2) the presence of two normal-sized remaining glands. In this series, 5 of 38 patients with double adenomas had one of the MEN syndromes. Following excision of the double adenomas, 37 patients had normal parathyroid function with a follow-up of almost 5 years, whereas only 1 patient with MEN had persistence of hypercalcemia. These findings indicate that double adenomas may exist, but their distinction from hyperplasia of the pseudoadenomatous type is exceedingly difficult.

Differential Diagnosis. Adenomas must be distinguished from hyperplasias, and knowledge of the surgical findings is essential for this distinction.[331] Close cooperation between the pathologist and surgeon is, therefore, mandatory. In cases of hyperplasia, enlargement of at least two glands is usually apparent grossly. In contrast, most adenomas involve a single gland. Thus, the presence of a single, enlarged gland together with three normal-sized glands is virtually diagnostic of adenoma. Usually, the largest gland is removed first. If a rim of normal or suppressed parathyroid is identified, the enlarged gland in all probability represents an adenoma. However, occasional hyperplastic glands may also have a rim of normal-appearing parathyroid. Accordingly, biopsy of a second gland is necessary for accurate categorization of the case. If the second gland is normal in size, the diagnosis of adenoma is practically assured.

The use of fat stains in the evaluation of parathyroid biopsies is based on the fact that intracellular fat is decreased or absent in hyperfunctioning chief cells, as compared with normal or suppressed chief cells.[319] However, the use of fat stains for this purpose is not without problems, since some hyperfunctioning chief cells may contain fairly abundant intracellular fat. Bondeson et al.[332] examined parathyroid glands from almost 200 cases of hyperparathyroidism with a modified oil red O technique. They concluded that access to two complete glands and the use of fat stains permitted highly reproducible and reliable distinction between cases of hyperplasia and adenoma. The rate of equivocal findings for cases in which two glands were available was 8%. Similar findings have been reported by other groups.[333]

The distinction of parathyroid adenomas from carcinomas and hyperplasias is discussed in subsequent sections. The distinction of parathyroid adenomas from other neoplasms occurring in this region is generally straightforward, since most patients with adenomas will have evidence of hypercalcemia. Occasionally, however, it is difficult to differentiate parathyroid adenomas from follicular and C-cell tumors, since approximately 0.2% of parathyroids are present within the substance of the thyroid gland. Although parathyroid adenomas with a completely follicular pattern are rare, it is not uncommon to find some evidence of follicle formation within a relatively high proportion of adenomas. The difficulty may be compounded by the fact that colloid-like material may be present within parathyroid follicles. Generally, however, parathyroid adenomas contain more glycogen than do tumors of follicular origin, whereas diastase-resistant periodic acid-Schiff–positive material in thyroid follicular cells usually represents colloid or lipofuscin.

Immunohistochemistry is of considerable value in the distinction of follicular and parathyroid neoplasms. Follicular cells are typically positive for thyroglobulin, whereas parathyroid cells are negative for this marker.[9] Chromogranin A, on the other hand, is positive in parathyroid cells but is absent from follicular cells. Antibodies to parathyroid hormone and nucleic acid probes to parathyroid hormone messenger RNA are also of value for the positive identification of parathyroid cells.[302a, 303] Some parathyroid adenomas are difficult to distinguish from medullary thyroid carcinomas. The latter tumors are typically positive for calcitonin, chromogranin A, and carcinoembryonic antigen, whereas parathyroid tumors are positive for chromogranin A only.

Treatment and Prognosis. Parathyroid adenomas are optimally treated by removal of the enlarged gland and usually biopsy of a normal-sized gland. Rates of recurrent disease in patients with these tumors are very low; however, recurrent hyperparathyroidism can occur because of incomplete removal of the adenoma or spillage of tumor tissues at the time of primary surgery.

Parathyroid Carcinoma

Clinical Features and Pathogenesis. Parathyroid carcinoma is a rare neoplasm that accounts for 0.5% to 2% of all cases of hyperparathyroidism.[334] Most cases occur in the fifth or sixth decades, although rare cases have been reported in children. This tumor has a high probability of local recurrence and the potential to metastasize late in its course to regional nodes and distant sites. The sex ratio of patients with parathyroid carcinoma is approximately equal.

Most affected patients have serum calcium levels in excess of 14 mg/dL, although occasional tumors may be nonfunctional.[335] Metabolic complications tend to be more common than in patients with adenomas.

Pathologic Features and Differential Diagnosis. Parathyroid carcinomas present most commonly as ill-defined masses that are densely adherent to the surrounding soft tissues or thyroid gland. Some carcinomas may be completely encapsulated and may be impossible to distinguish from adenomas grossly. In the series of carcinomas reported by Wang and Gaz, the tumors measured 1.5 to 6 cm in diameter (mean 3.0 cm), with a mean weight of 6.7 g.[335] On cross-section, most tumors are firm and gray-white. In patients with recurrent tumors, ill-defined masses of firm gray-tan tumor tissue may be present in and around the operative site.

Parathyroid carcinomas are typically composed of chief cells arranged in solid or trabecular patterns (Fig. 7–93A–F and 7–94). The component cells may differ minimally from those of adenomas; alternatively, they may exhibit considerable pleomorphism. Occasional carcinomas may be composed of oncocytic cells exclusively (Fig. 7–93C).

The microscopic diagnosis of parathyroid carcinoma is often difficult. Some cases may differ minimally from parathyroid adenomas, while others are obviously anaplastic. As described by Schantz and Castleman,[336] the principal diagnostic features for carcinoma included thick fibrous bands, mitotic activity, capsular invasion, and vascular invasion (see Fig. 7–93). With the exception of vascular invasion, however, none of these criteria is absolute. Areas of fibrosis, for example, are not uncommon in large adenomas that have undergone retrogressive changes. Mitotic activity has been identified in a substantial proportion of adenomas, and capsular involvement may be seen in benign lesions. Invasion of the adjacent soft tissues, perineural spaces, or thyroid gland, however, is diagnostic of malignancy (Figs. 7–93 and 7–94).

Bondeson et al.[337] have examined the histopathologic features of a series of 95 neoplasms in which the diagnosis of parathyroid carcinoma had been made. In this series, 56 cases that demonstrated extraglandular invasion or recurrence were classified as definitive carcinomas. The remaining 39 cases were classified as "equivocal." Fibrosis, necrosis, nuclear atypia with macronucleoli, and mitotic figures were more common in the carcinoma group. These variables were positively correlated with an aberrant DNA pattern, as demonstrated by image cytometry. Moreover, the triad of macronucleoli, more than 5 mitoses per 50 high-power fields, and necrosis was associated with aggressive behavior. Mitotic activity was a prognostic factor but was of limited diagnostic significance, since in about half of the cases of carcinoma, the frequency of mitoses did not exceed the values found in benign lesions.

The value of ploidy analysis for the distinction of adenomas and carcinomas using nuclei extracted from paraffin-embedded samples is controversial.[338] Aneuploidy has been recorded in 3% to 25% of adenomas in different published series.[338, 339] A high frequency of aneuploidy has been reported by some authors in carcinomas, but others have found no significant differences.[340] Levin et al.[329] demonstrated, however, that patients with aneuploid carcinomas have a more aggressive clinical course than those with diploid tumors. Using fresh tissue samples, however, Obara et al.[341] demonstrated aneuploidy in 60% of carcinomas, 9% of adenomas, and 50% of hyperplasias.[341]

Proliferative activity in parathyroid adenomas has also been examined with antibodies to Ki-67 (MIB 1). Abbona et al.[342] reported a difference between all carcinomas and adenomas ($P < .05$) with respect to MIB 1 scores. There were no significant differences, however, between nonaggressive carcinomas and adenomas. On the other hand, both mitotic rates and MIB 1 scores of clinically aggressive carcinomas were significantly different from those of adenomas ($P < .01$). Although MIB 1 scores were not useful for the distinction of adenomas from nonaggressive carcinomas, in this study they did provide important prognostic information with respect to predicting aggressive behavior in carcinomas. Vargas et al.[343] have reported

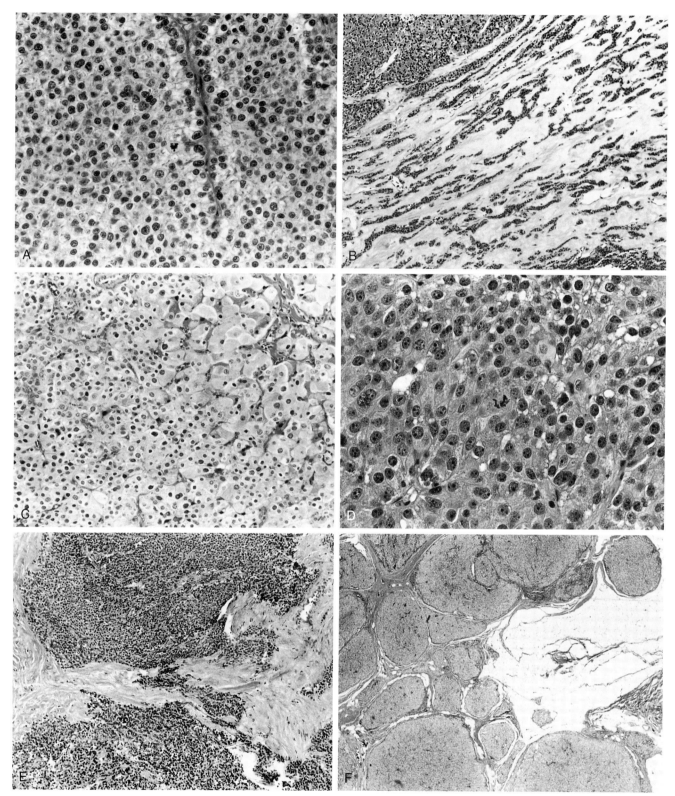

Figure 7–93. Parathyroid carcinoma. *A,* This tumor has a predominant solid growth pattern with an average of 1 mitosis per 10 high-power fields. *B,* This tumor has a predominant trabecular growth pattern with bands of fibrous tissue between tumor cells. *C,* This parathyroid carcinoma is composed of oncocytic cells with abundant granular eosinophilic cytoplasm. *D,* The nuclei in this tumor are enlarged and hyperchromatic with prominent nucleoli. An atypical mitosis is present in the center of the field. *E,* This tumor has extensive areas of banding fibrosis. *F,* Recurrent parathyroid carcinoma. This tumor has extensively invaded the soft tissue of the neck.

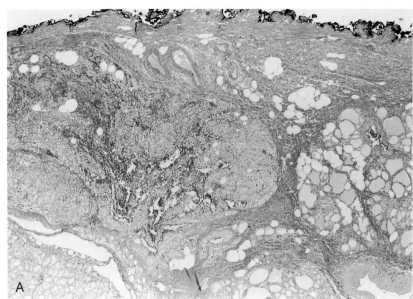

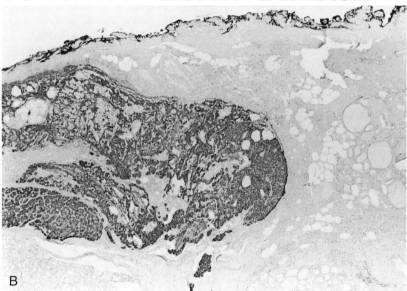

Figure 7–94. Recurrent parathyroid carcinoma invading the thyroid gland. The tumor recurred approximately 2 years after the excision of a large parathyroid adenoma with atypical features. *B,* Same case as *A* stained for chromogranin A. The tumor is strongly stained for chromogranin A while the adjacent thyroid gland is unreactive.

that a tumor proliferative fraction in excess of 40 MIB 1–positive cells per 1000 cells strongly correlates with malignancy. Analyses of p53 and *bcl*-2 by immunohistochemistry, on the other hand, were not useful in making this distinction.[343]

Another approach to the distinction of carcinomas and adenomas has involved the use of antibodies to the retinoblastoma (RB) protein. Cryns et al.[344] have reported an absence of the RB protein in a small series of carcinomas, whereas this protein was present in parathyroid adenomas. Vargas et al.[343] have demonstrated positive staining for RB protein in 100% of parathyroid adenomas; however, 80% of carcinomas were also RB-positive. Farnebo and coworkers[344a] have demonstrated the lack of utility of RB localization for the distinction of parathyroid adenomas and carcinomas.

Treatment and Prognosis. Parathyroid carcinomas are treated optimally by en bloc resections, with removal of the adjacent involved thyroid lobe.[345] Regional lymph node dissection is generally reserved for those patients with documented metastases. Recurrences are usually apparent within 3 to 5 years of primary surgery. Metastatic disease develops in approximately one third of patients, with common sites of involvement including lung, cervical lymph nodes, and liver.

Primary Chief Cell Hyperplasia

Clinical Features and Pathogenesis. The term *primary chief cell hyperplasia* refers to an absolute increase in parenchymal cell mass resulting from a proliferation of chief cells, oncocytes, and transitional oncocytes in multiple parathyroid glands in the absence of a known stimulus for parathyroid hormone hypersecretion.[309] This disease was first recognized as a cause of primary hyperparathyroidism in 1958.[346] Primary chief cell hyperplasia accounts for approximately 15% of all cases of primary hyperparathyroidism and is more common in women than men (3 : 1 ratio).

Approximately 75% of patients with this disorder have apparent sporadic disease and the remainder have isolated familial hyperparathyroidism or one of the MEN syndromes. At least 90% of patients with MEN 1 will have evidence of primary hyperparathyroidism, and 30% to 40% of patients with MEN 2A will have this disorder. Parathyroid proliferative disease does not occur in patients with MEN 2B or familial medullary thyroid carcinoma.

Identification of patients with these syndromes can be accomplished by the use of molecular diagnostic procedures. As discussed in the section on familial medullary thyroid carcinoma, dominant activating germ line mutations have been identified in the *ret* proto-oncogene (10q11.2) in patients with MEN 2A and MEN 2B and familial medullary thyroid carcinoma.[230] The gene for MEN 1, on the other hand, has been localized to chromosome 11q13. This gene contains 10 exons and encodes a ubiquitously expressed 2.8 kb transcript.[347] The predicted 610 amino acid protein product, which has been termed *menin,* exhibits no similarities to any previously known protein. The gene belongs to the tumor suppressor gene family and a variety of loss-of-function mutations have been identified in affected individuals.[347] In patients with MEN 1, an inherited mutation leads to inactivation of one copy of the gene followed by deletion or mutation of the second copy of the gene. Sporadic tumors of the types occurring in MEN 1, by comparison, result from two sequential mutations of the gene in a single somatic cell.[347a]

Approximately 50% to 60% of parathyroid lesions in MEN 1 harbor clonal allelic losses of chromosome 11q13 similar to those described by Larsson in pancreatic tumors from patients with MEN 1.[315, 348] Allelic losses tend to occur in parathyroid lesions that are larger than those without such losses. These findings have suggested that the development of parathyroid lesions in MEN 1 may be preceded by phases of polyclonal hyperplasia without allelic losses and that hyperplasia in these instances might occur as a result of diminished function of the inherited mutant allele. Hyperplasia could result from an abnormal response of parathyroid tissue to physiologic stimuli or to the presence of an abnormal circulating factor. In this regard, Brandi[349] described a circulating mitogen for parathyroid endothelial cells in the sera of MEN 1 patients.

Pathologic Features and Differential Diagnosis. Symmetric enlargement of all glands occurs in about one half of patients with primary chief cell hyperplasia, while the remainder have evidence of asymmetric glandular enlargement.[350, 351] The former pattern of hyperplasia has been termed *classic hyperplasia,* and the latter has been referred to as *pseudoadenomatous hyperplasia. Occult hyperplasia* refers to minimal enlargement of all glands. Total gland weight varies considerably in cases of hyperplasia, with 54% weighing less than 1 g, 28% weighing 1 to 5 g, and 18% weighing 5 to 10 g.

The predominant cell in this form of primary hyperplasia is the chief cell, although variable numbers of oncocytes and transitional oncocytes are also evident. Stromal fat cells are usually markedly reduced. However, because of the regional variations in stromal fat cells, small biopsies of hyperplastic glands may show a relatively high ratio of stromal fat cells to chief cells. The proliferation of chief cells may occur either in a diffuse or in a nodular pattern (Figs. 7–95 and 7–96, see p. 467). The nodular variant is more common and may be particularly evident in the early phase of the disease. Hyperplastic chief cells may be arranged in solid sheets, cords, or follicles. In addition to chief cells, variable numbers of oncocytes and transitional oncocytic cells are also present.

Occasional cases of chief cell hyperplasia have abundant stromal fat cells, and biopsies of such glands may lead to an erroneous diagnosis of a normocellular gland if the pathologist is not aware of the gland size. Strauss et al.[352] introduced the term *lipohyperplasia* to describe hyperplastic glands with abundant stromal fat.

Multifocal aggregates of hyperplastic chief cells may be evident in the soft tissues of the neck or mediastinum in patients with primary hyperparathyroidism.[353] These lesions, which are referred to as *parathyromatosis,* may be responsible for persistent or recurrent hyperparathyroidism in patients treated by subtotal parathyroidectomy for primary chief cell hyperplasia.

Chronic parathyroiditis is rarely found in association with primary chief cell hyperplasia.[354] Although the origin of the lymphocytic infiltration is unknown, it has been suggested that this disorder may have an autoimmune origin. Cystic changes in primary chief cell hyperplasia are uncommon, and, when they occur, they usually involve markedly enlarged hyperplastic glands.[355, 356] An unusual familial variant of primary cystic chief cell hyperplasia has also been reported.

The major differential diagnosis is parathyroid adenoma. As discussed in a previous section, parathyroid adenomas most com-

monly involve a single gland, whereas chief cell hyperplasia involves multiple glands.

Treatment and Prognosis. The treatment of primary chief cell hyperplasia is subtotal parathyroidectomy or total parathyroidectomy with grafting of approximately 100 mg of parathyroid tissue into the forearm.[357] The rate of recurrent hyperparathyroidism in patients treated by subtotal parathyroidectomy is approximately 15%. Cases of recurrent disease may be due to failure to recognize and remove supernumerary or ectopic glands, the presence of parathyromatosis or inadvertent implantation of hyperplastic parathyroid tissue into the soft tissues of the neck. In cases of recurrent disease, proliferation of autografted parathyroid tissue may be extreme enough to simulate malignancy.[358]

Primary Clear Cell Hyperplasia

Clinical Features and Pathogenesis. Primary clear cell hyperplasia is a rare disorder characterized by an absolute increase in parathyroid parenchymal cell mass resulting from a proliferation of vacuolated water-clear (wasserhelle) cells in multiple parathyroid glands in the absence of a known stimulus for parathyroid hormone hypersecretion.[310, 359] There is no apparent familial incidence of the disease, and no known association with any of the MEN syndromes. The degree of hypercalcemia tends to be greater in patients with clear cell hyperplasia than in those with chief cell hyperplasia.

Pathologic Features and Differential Diagnosis. Most patients with primary clear cell hyperplasia have enlargement of all four parathyroid glands. The glands are typically red-brown to brown with foci of cystic change, hemorrhage, and fibrosis.[310] The latter changes tend to involve the largest glands. Upper glands tend to be larger than lower glands.

Clear cell hyperplasia typically involves the glands in a diffuse fashion. Individual cells have multiple, small cytoplasmic vacuoles that are thought to be derived from the Golgi vesicles (Fig. 7–97, see p. 467). The extensive cytoplasmic vacuolization is responsible for the clear cytoplasmic appearance.[360] Nuclei are round to ovoid and moderately hyperchromatic with an eccentrically placed nucleolus.

The differential diagnosis includes parathyroid adenoma, clear cell thyroid tumors and metastases of clear cell carcinoma, particularly of renal origin. The absence of thyroglobulin and calcitonin, which are typically found in follicular and C-cell tumors, respectively, and of parathyroid hormone or chromogranin A, which are typically found in parathyroid lesions, should raise the possibility of metastatic disease.

Secondary Hyperparathyroidism

Clinical Features and Pathogenesis. Secondary hyperparathyroidism refers to an adaptive increase in parathyroid parenchymal mass resulting from a proliferation of chief cells, oncocytes, and transitional oncocytes in multiple parathyroid glands in the presence of a known stimulus to parathyroid hormone secretion, most commonly low levels of ionized calcium in the blood.[306] The most common cause of secondary hyperparathyroidism is chronic renal failure. Other causes include dietary deficiency of vitamin D, other abnormalities of vitamin D metabolism, and pseudohypoparathyroidism. Once the process of parathyroid hyperplasia begins, the set point for the control of parathyroid hormone secretion by ionic calcium rises, and this leads to further parathyroid hyperplasia and hypersecretion of parathyroid hormone.[361] The major clinical manifestations include bone pain and skeletal deformities (renal osteodystrophy), muscle weakness, growth retardation, and extraskeletal calcification.

Although the parathyroid changes that occur in patients with secondary hyperparathyroidism are classified as hyperplasias, molecular studies indicate that some of the proliferations are monoclonal.[362, 363] It is possible that clonal lesions in the setting of secondary hyperplasia may have greater autonomy than polyclonal lesions, but the exact significance of clonal proliferations remains to be determined.

Pathologic Features and Differential Diagnosis. The gross appearance of the glands is generally similar to that seen in patients with primary chief cell hyperplasia.[364, 365] Generally, there is a greater uniformity of gland size than in patients with primary hyperplasia, particularly in early stages of the disease. With prolongation of the stimulus for parathyroid hormone hypersecretion, there is a tendency for a greater degree of variation in gland size. In a large series of cases reported by Roth and Marshall,[365] the weight of the glands varied from 120 mg to 6 g. The earliest change in the glands is a decreased number of fat cells and their replacement by widened cords and nests of chief cells. Typically, the proliferating chief cells are present in diffuse sheets, but other areas may show cord-like, acinar, or trabecular growth patterns. Prominent mitotic activity may be evident. Advanced stages of secondary hyperplasia are characterized by nodular proliferations of chief cells and oncocytes (Fig. 7–98). The proliferation of oncocytic cells may be particularly striking. In some instances, the foci of nodular proliferation may be surrounded by a fibrous capsule. Areas of hemorrhage, calcification, chronic inflammation, and cyst formation may be evident, particularly in large glands.

Parathyromatosis may be responsible for the recurrence of hyperparathyroidism following parathyroidectomy in patents with chronic renal failure.[365a] The etiology of "postsurgical parathyromatosis" is the seeding of parathyroid tissue in the soft tissue of the neck, following surgical manipulation. Parathyromatosis may also occur as a result of developmental dispersion of parathyroid tissue in the neck or mediastinum ("ontogenous parathyromatosis").

The differential diagnosis includes primary chief cell hyperplasia, parathyroid adenoma, and parathyroid carcinoma. Primary and secondary hyperplasia cannot be distinguished on the basis of gross or microscopic examination. The clinical history is essential to make this distinction. As noted in previous sections, parathyroid adenoma typically involves a single gland whereas secondary hyperplasia involves multiple glands. Glands from patients with longstanding secondary hyperplasia may, on occasion, be difficult to distinguish from those with parathyroid carcinoma. The glands from both conditions may exhibit extensive fibrosis and mitotic activity. Hyperplastic glands, however, lack the infiltrative properties of parathyroid carcinomas.

Treatment and Prognosis. Surgical treatment is indicated in cases of secondary hyperplasia when medical management fails to control progressive skeletal symptoms, pruritis, and extraskeletal calcification.[366] Subtotal parathyroidectomy is the treatment of choice. Approximately 50 mg of parathyroid tissue is left in situ in the neck or is autotransplanted into the forearm. Recurrent hyperparathyroidism is generally treated by excision of the parathyroid remnant or the ingrafted tissue. In some instances, the proliferation of autografted tissue may be extreme enough to simulate malignancy.[358]

Tertiary Hyperparathyroidism

The term *tertiary hyperparathyroidism* refers to the development of autonomous parathyroid hyperfunction in patients with previously documented secondary hyperparathyroidism.[367] The mechanisms for the development of tertiary hyperparathyroidism are unknown, although several studies have suggested that it may result from a calcium set point error. According to this hypothesis, the cellular response function is shifted away from normal toward higher calcium concentrations. Parathyroid chief cells, which have higher set points of suppression, increase their biosynthetic and secretory activities and are stimulated to divide even at normal calcium concentrations. This sequence of events leads to an increased parenchymal cell mass. In the series of cases studied by Krause and Hedinger,[368] only 5% of the patients had adenomas. The hyperplasia was predominantly diffuse in 44%, and the remaining patients had nodular hyperplasia. Glands with nodular hyperplasia were larger than those with diffuse hyperplasia.

Patients with tertiary hyperparathyroidism are generally treated by subtotal parathyroidectomy.[366]

Secondary Tumors

Secondary involvement of the parathyroid by tumor may occur by direct extension from adjacent structures such as the thyroid or larynx or by lymphatic and hematogenous spread. In autopsy studies, metastases to the parathyroid glands are found in almost 12% of patients.[369, 370] The most common sites of origin were breast, skin (melanoma), and lung. Hypoparathyroidism resulting from tumorous involvement of these parathyroids is rare.

Parathyroid Cysts

Cystic lesions of the parathyroid glands may develop as a result of degeneration of an adenoma or hyperplastic gland. Other cysts of the

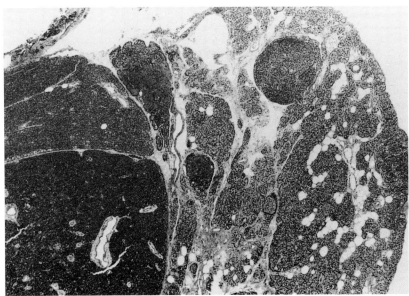

Figure 7–98. Secondary parathyroid hyperplasia. There are multiple nodules composed of chief cells and oncocytes throughout the gland.

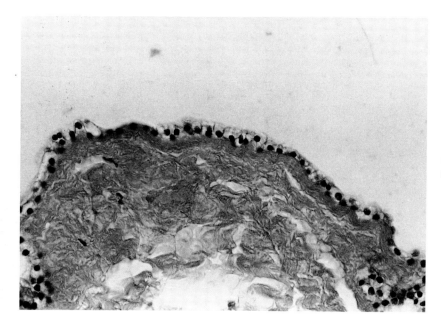

Figure 7–99. Parathyroid cyst. The cyst is lined by glycogen-rich chief cells with a clear appearance.

parathyroid have a developmental origin. Cysts containing thymus and parathyroid are sometimes referred to as third pharyngeal pouch cysts.[371] Parathyroid cysts are loosely attached to the thyroid, and their walls are typically gray-white and translucent.[372, 373] The cyst fluid is usually thin, watery, and straw-colored. One hypothesis for their development suggests that they may represent persistent Kürst-einer's canals, which are found in association with the developing parathyroid. The wall is composed of fibrous connective tissue, and the cysts are usually lined by cuboidal cells of chief cell origin (Fig. 7–99).

Hypoparathyroidism and Pseudohypoparathyroidism

Deficiency of parathyroid hormone results in hypocalcemia, hypocalciuria, and hypophosphatemia. Clinically, hypoparathyroidism is characterized by increased neuromuscular excitability, mental changes, calcifications in the basal ganglia, and lens and cardiac conduction abnormalities. The most common cause of hypoparathyroidism is inadvertent excision or devascularization of the glands during thyroid or parathyroid surgery. Congenital abnormalities involving maldevelopment of the third and fourth pharyngeal pouches (DiGeorge syndrome) may also be associated with neonatal hypoparathyroidism.[374]

Autoimmune processes may involve the parathyroid gland and may result in hypoparathyroidism. In patients with type I polyglandular autoimmune disease, there is evidence of hypoparathyroidism, Addison's disease, and mucocutaneous candidiasis.[375] Affected individuals may also have evidence of insulin-dependent diabetes mellitus, primary hypogonadism, autoimmune thyroid disease, or pernicious anemia. Histologically, autoimmune parathyroid disease is characterized by glandular atrophy and lymphocytic infiltration. Infiltrative processes such as amyloidosis may also involve the parathyroid glands and may give rise to hypoparathyroidism.

Genetic disorders that may be inherited as dominant, recessive, or X-linked traits have also been implicated in the development of some forms of hypoparathyroidism. Some of these disorders have been traced to mutations in the gene encoding parathyroid hormone.

The term *pseudohypoparathyroidism* is used to describe patients with hypocalcemia, hyperphosphatemia, increased plasma levels of parathyroid hormone, and unresponsiveness of target tissues to the effects of parathyroid hormone.[376] Affected patients typically have mental retardation, short stature, multiple defects in bone

development, and soft tissue calcifications. Parathyroid glands in pseudohypoparathyroidism disorder are hyperplastic.[377]

REFERENCES

Embryology, Anatomy, and Physiology

1. Norris EH: The early morphogenesis of the human thyroid gland. *Am J Anat* 1918;24:443–465.
2. Norris EH: The parathyroid glands and lateral thyroid in man: Their morphogenesis, histogenesis, topographic anatomy and prenatal growth. *Contrib Embryol Carneg Inst* 1937;26:247–294.
3. Allard RHB: The thyroglossal cyst. *Head Neck Surg* 1982;5:134–146.
4. Sugiyama S: The embryology of the human thyroid gland including ultimobranchial body and others related. *Ergebn Anat Entwicklungsgesch* 1971;44:3–111.
5. LeDouarin N, Fontain J, LeLievre C: New studies on the neural crest origin of the avain ultimobranchial cells: Interspecific combinations and cytochemical characterization of C-cells based on the uptake of biogenic amine precursors. *Histochemistry* 1974;38:297–305.
6. Rosai J, Carcangiu ML, DeLellis RA: *Tumors of the Thyroid Gland. Atlas of Tumor Pathology.* Washington, DC: Armed Forces Institute of Pathology, 1992:183–193.
7. LiVolsi VA: Thyroid. In: Sternberg SS, ed. *Histology for Pathologists.* New York: Raven Press, 1992:301–310.
8. DeLellis RA: Endocrine tumors. In: Colvin RB, Bhan AK, McCluskey RT, eds. *Diagnostic Immunopathology.* New York: Raven Press, 1995:551–577.
9. Klinck GH, Oertel JE, Winship T: Ultrastructure of normal human thyroid. *Lab Invest* 1970;22:2–22.
10. Rosai J, Carcangiu ML, DeLellis RA: *Tumors of the Thyroid Gland. Atlas of Tumor Pathology.* Washington, DC: Armed Forces Institute of Pathology, 1992:135–160.
11. Kini SR: *Guides to Clinical Aspiration Biopsy: Thyroid.* New York: Igaku-Shoin, 1987.
12. Gharib H, Goellner JR, Johnson DA: Fine needle aspiration cytology of the thyroid: A 12-year experience with 11,000 biopsies. *Clin Lab Med* 1993;13:669–709.
13. Gordon G, Sparano BM, Kramer AW, et al: Thyroid gland pigmentation and minocycline therapy. *Am J Pathol* 1984;117:98–109.
14. Larsen PR, Ingbar SH: The thyroid gland. In: Wilson JD, Foster DW, eds. *Textbook of Endocrinology.* Philadelphia: W.B. Saunders, 1992:357–488.
15. Braunstein H, Stephens CL: Parafollicular cells of human thyroid. *Arch Pathol* 1968;86:659–666.
16. DeMay R: *The Art and Science of Cytopathology.* Chicago: ASCP Press, 1996:703–778.

17. DeLellis RA, Nunnemacher G, Wolfe HJ: C-cell hyperplasia: An ultrastructural analysis. *Lab Invest* 1977;36:237–248.
18. Gibson WC, Peng T-C, Croker BP: C-cell nodules in the adult human thyroid: A common autopsy finding. *Am J Clin Pathol* 1981;75:347–350.
19. MacIntyre I: Calcitonin: Physiology, biosynthesis, secretion, metabolism and mode of action. In: DeGroot LJ, ed. *Endocrinology.* Philadelphia: W.B. Saunders, 1989:892–901.
20. DeLellis RA, May L, Tashjian AH Jr, Wolfe HJ: C-cell granule heterogeneity in man. An ultrastructural immunocytochemical study. *Lab Invest* 1978;38:263–269.
21. Harach HR: Solid cell nests in the thyroid. *J Pathol* 1988;155:191–200.
22. Nadig J, Weber E, Hedinger C: C-cells in vestiges of the ultimobranchial body in human thyroid glands. *Virchows Arch B [Cell Pathol]* 1978;27:189–191.
23. Carpenter GR, Emery JL: Inclusions in the human thyroid. *J Anat* 1976;122:77–89.
24. Zak F, Lawson W: Glomic (paraganglionic) tissue in the larynx and capsule of the thyroid gland. *Mt Sinai J Med* 1972;39:82–90.

Congenital Anomalies

25. Williams ED, Toyn CE, Harach HR: The ultimobranchial and congenital thyroid abnormalities in man. *J Pathol* 1989;159:135–141.
26. Gaby M: The role of thyroid dysgenesis and maldescent in the etiology of sporadic cretinism. *J Pediatr* 1962;60:830–835.
27. Baughman RA: Lingual thyroid and lingual thyroglossal duct remnants. A clinical and histopathological study with review of the literature. *Oral Surg Oral Med Oral Path* 1972;34:781–799.
28. Frantz VK, Forsythe F, Hanford JM, Rogers WM: Lateral aberrant thyroids. *Ann Surg* 1942;115:161–183.
29. Meyer JS, Steinberg LS: Microscopically benign thyroid nodules in cervical lymph nodes. Serial section study of lymph node inclusions and entire thyroid gland in five cases. *Cancer* 1969;24:302–311.
30. Butler JJ, Tulinius H, Ibanez ML, et al: Significance of thyroid tissue in lymph nodes associated with carcinoma of the head, neck or lung. *Cancer* 1967;20:103–112.
31. LiVolsi VA: *Surgical Pathology of the Thyroid.* Philadelphia: W.B. Saunders, 1990, p 9.
32. Solomon JR, Rangecroft L: Thyroglossal duct lesions in childhood. *J Pediatr Surg* 1984;19:555–561.
33. Chen KT: Cytology of thyroglossal cyst papillary carcinoma. *Diagn Cytopathol* 1993;9:318–321.
34. Weiss SD, Orlich CC: Primary papillary carcinoma of a thyroglossal duct cyst. Report of a case and literature review. *Br J Surg* 1991;78:87–89.
35. Palacios J, Gamallo C, Garcia M, Rodriguez JI: Decrease in thyrocalcitonin-containing cells and analysis of other congenital anomalies in 11 patients with DiGeorge anomaly. *Am J Med Genet* 1993;46:641–646.
36. Pueblitz S, Weinberg AG, Albores-Saavedra J: Thyroid C-cells in the DiGeorge anomaly: A quantitative study. *Pediatr Pathol* 1993;13:463–473.
37. Miyauchi A, Matsuzuka F, Kuma K, Katayama S: Piriform sinus fistula and the ultimobranchial body. *Histopathol* 1992;20:221–227.

Thyroiditis

38. Singer PA: Thyroiditis. Acute, subacute and chronic. *Med Clin North Am* 1991;75:61–77.
39. Frank TS, LiVolsi VA, Connor AM: Cytomegalovirus infection of the thyroid in immunocompromised adults. *Yale J Biol Med* 1987;60:1–8.
40. Guttler R, Singer PA, Axline SG, Greaves TS, McGill JJ: *Pneumocystis carinii* thyroiditis. Report of three cases and review of the literature. *Arch Intern Med* 1993;153:393–396.
41. Miyauchi A, Matsuzuka F, Kuma K, Takai S: Piriform sinus fistula: A route of infection in acute suppurative thyroiditis. *Arch Surg* 1981;116:66–69.
42. Iida F, Sugenoya A: *Textbook of Endocrine Surgery.* Philadelphia: W.B. Saunders, 1997.
43. Volpe R, Row VV, Ezrin C: Circulating viral and thyroid antibodies in subacute thyroiditis. *J Clin Endocrinol Metab* 1967;27:1275–1284.
44. Volpe R: Subacute (de Quervain's) thyroiditis. *Clin Endocrinol Metab* 1979;8:81–95.
45. Ofner C, Hittmair A, Kröll I, et al: Fine needle aspiration cytodiagnosis of subacute (de Quervain's) thyroiditis in an endemic goitre area. *Cytopathol* 1994;5:33–40.
46. Sachs MK, Dickinson G, Amazon K: Tuberculous adenitis of the thyroid mimicking subacute thyroiditis. *Am J Med* 1988;85:573–575.
47. Karlish AJ, MacGregor GA: Sarcoidosis, thyroiditis and Addison's disease. *Lancet* 1970;2:330–333.
48. Carney JA, Moore SB, Northcutt RC, et al: Palpation thyroiditis (multifocal granulomatous folliculitis). *Am J Clin Pathol* 1975;64:639–647.
49. Dayan CM, Daniels GH: Chronic autoimmune thyroiditis. *N Engl J Med* 1996;335:99–107.
50. LiVolsi VA, Merino MJ: Worrisome histologic alterations following fine needle aspiration of the thyroid (WHAFFT). *Pathol Annu* 1994;29:99–120.
51. LiVolsi VA: The pathology of autoimmune thyroid disease: A review. *Thyroid* 1994;4:333–339.
52. Dailey ME, Lindsay S, Skahen R: Relation of thyroid membranes to Hashimoto's disease of the thyroid gland. *AMA And Surg* 1955;70:291–297.
53. Wirtschafter A, Schmidt R, Rosen D, et al: Expression of the RET/PTC fusion gene as a marker for papillary carcinoma in Hashimoto's thyroiditis. *Laryngoscope* 1997;107:95–100.
54. Kato I, Tajima K, Suchi T, et al: Chronic thyroiditis as a risk factor for B-cell lymphoma in the thyroid gland. *Jpn J Cancer Res* 1985;76:1085–1090.
55. Jayaram G, Marwaha RK, Gupta RK, et al: Cytomorphologic aspects of thyroiditis: A study of 51 cases with functional, immunologic and ultrasonographic data. *Acta Cytol* 1987;31:687–693.
56. Friedman J, Shimaoka K, Rao U, et al: Diagnosis of chronic lymphocytic thyroiditis (nodular presentation) by needle aspiration. *Acta Cytol* 1981;25:513–522.
57. Poropatich C, Marcus D, Oertel Y: Hashimoto's thyroiditis: Fine needle aspirations of 50 asymptomatic cases. *Diagn Cytopathol* 1994;11:141–145.
58. Gonzalez JL, Wang HH, Ducatman BS: Fine needle aspiration of Hürthle cell lesions. A cytomorphologic approach to diagnosis. *Am J Clin Pathol* 1993;100:231–235.
59. Dugan JM, Atkinson BF, Avitabile A, et al: Psammoma bodies in fine needle aspirate of the thyroid in lymphocytic thyroiditis. *Acta Cytol* 1987;31:330–334.
60. Katz SM, Vickery AL: The fibrous variant of Hashimoto's thyroiditis. *Hum Pathol* 1974;5:161–170.
61. Drexhage HA, Bottazzo GF, Bitensky L, et al: Thyroid growth blocking antibodies in primary myxoedema. *Nature* 1981;289:594–596.
62. Sclare G: The thyroid in myxedema. *J Pathol Bacteriol* 1963;85:263–278.
63. Rallison ML, Dobyns BM, Keating FR, et al: Occurrence and natural history of chronic lymphocytic thyroiditis in childhood. *J Pediatr* 1975;86:675–682.
64. Gluck FB, Nusynowitz ML, Plymate S: Chronic lymphocytic thyroiditis, thyrotoxicosis and low radioactive iodine uptake: Report of four cases. *N Engl J Med* 1975;293:624–628.
65. Kurashima C, Hirokawa K: Focal lymphocytic infiltration in thyroids of elderly people. *Survey Synth Pathol Res* 1985;4:457–466.
66. Weaver DK, Batsakis JG, Nishiyama RH: Relationship of iodine to "lymphocytic goiters". *Arch Surg* 1969;98:183–186.
67. Shopsin B, Shenkman L, Blum L, Hollander CS: Iodine and lithium-induced hypothyroidism. Documentation of synergism. *Am J Med* 1973;55:695–699.
68. Perrild H, Madsen SN, Hansen JE: Irreversible myxedema after lithium carbonate. *Br Med J* 1978;1:1108–1109.
69. Smyrk TC, Goellner JR, Brennan MD, Carney JA: Pathology of the thyroid in amiodarone-associated thyrotoxicosis. *Am J Surg Path* 1987;11:197–204.

Radiation-Induced Thyroid Injury

70. LiVolsi VA: *Surgical Pathology of the Thyroid Gland.* Philadelphia: W.B. Saunders, 1990:164–166.
71. Nikiforov Y, Gnepp DR, Fagin JA: Thyroid lesions in children and adolescents after the Chernobyl disaster: Implications for the study of radiation tumorigenesis. *J Clin Endocrinol Metab* 1996;81:9–14.
72. Nikiforov Y, Gnepp DR: Pediatric thyroid cancer after the Chernobyl disaster. Pathomorphologic study of 84 cases (1991–1992) from the Republic of Belarus. *Cancer* 1994;74:748–766.
73. Nikiforov YE, Heffess SC, Korzenko AV, et al: Characteristics of fol-

licular tumors and non-neoplastic thyroid lesions in children and adolescents exposed to radiation as a result of the Chernobyl disaster. *Cancer* 1995;76:900–909.

Riedel's Disease

74. Nielson HK: Multifocal idiopathic fibrosclerosis: Two cases with simultaneous occurrence of retroperitoneal fibrosis and Riedel's thyroiditis. *Acta Med Scand* 1980;206:119–123.
75. Davies D, Furness P: Riedel's thyroiditis with multiple organ fibrosis. *Thorax* 1984;39:959–960.
76. Wold LE, Weiland LH: Tumefactive fibroinflammatory lesions of the head and neck. *Am J Surg Path* 1983;7:477–482.
77. Schwaegerle SM, Bauer TW, Esselstyn CB Jr: Riedel's thyroiditis. *Am J Clin Pathol* 1988;90:715–722.
78. Hay ID: Thyroiditis: A clinical update. *Mayo Clin Proc* 1985;60:836–843.
79. Taubenberger JK, Merino MJ, Medeiros LJ: A thyroid biopsy with histologic features of both Riedel's thyroiditis and the fibrosing variant of Hashimoto's thyroiditis. *Hum Pathol* 1992;23:1072–1075.
79a. Wan S-K, Chan JKC, Tang S-K: Paucicellular variant of anaplastic thyroid carcinoma: A mimic of Riedel's thyroiditis. *Am J Clin Pathol* 1996;105:388–393.
80. Few J, Thompson NW, Angelos P, et al: Riedel's thyroiditis: Treatment with tamoxifen. *Surgery* 1996;120:993–998.

Amyloidosis

81. Hamed G, Heffess CS, Shmookler BM, Wenig BM: Amyloid goiter: A clinicopathologic study of 14 cases and review of the literature. *Am J Clin Pathol* 1995;104:306–312.

Hyperplasia of the Thyroid

82. Spjut HJ, Warren WD, Ackerman LV: A clinical pathological study of 76 cases of recurrent Graves' disease, toxic (non-exophthalmic) goiter and nontoxic goiter. *Am J Clin Pathol* 1957;27:367–392.
83. Eggen PC, Seljelid R: The histological appearance of hyperfunctioning thyroids following various pre-operative treatments. *Acta Pathol Microbiol Scand* 1973;81:16–20.
84. Friedman M, Shimaoka K, Getaz P: Needle aspiration of 310 thyroid lesions. *Acta Cytol* 1979;23:194–203.
85. Pitts WC, Berry GJ: Marginal vacuoles in metastatic thyroid carcinoma: A case report. *Diagn Cytopathol* 1989;5:200–202.
86. Gaitan E, Nelson NC, Poole GV: Endemic goiter and endemic thyroid disorders. *World J Surg* 1991;15:205–215.
87. Cheung P-SY: Medical and surgical treatment of endemic goiter. In: Clark OH, Dub Q-Y, eds. *Textbook of Endocrine Surgery*. Philadelphia: W.B. Saunders, 1997:15–21.
88. Kennedy JS: The pathology of dyshormonogenetic goiter. *J Pathol* 1969;99:251–264.
89. Matos PS, Bisi H, Medeiros-Nato G: Dyshormonogenetic goitre: A morphological and immunohistochemical study. *Endocrine Pathol* 1994;5:59–65.
90. Vickery AL: The diagnosis of malignancy in dyshormonogenetic goiter. *Clin Endocrinol Metab* 1981;10:317–335.

Non-Toxic Nodular Goiter

91. Mazzaferri E: Management of a solitary thyroid nodule. *N Engl J Med* 1993;328:553–559.
92. Hicks DG, LiVolsi VA, Neidich JA, et al: Clonal analysis of solitary follicular nodules in the thyroid. *Am J Pathol* 1990;137:553–562.
93. Apel RL, Ezzat S, Bapat BV, et al: Clonality of thyroid nodules in sporadic goiter. *Diagn Mol Pathol* 1995;4:113–121.
94. Akerman M, Tennvall J, Biörklund A, et al: Sensitivity and specificity of fine needle aspiration cytology in the diagnosis of tumors of the thyroid gland. *Acta Cytol* 1985;29:850–855.
95. Suen KC: How does one separate cellular follicular lesions of the thyroid by fine needle aspiration biopsy? *Diagn Cytopathol* 1988;4:78–81.
96. Fiorella RM, Isley W, Miller LK, Kragel PJ: Multinodular goiter of the thyroid mimicking malignancy: Diagnostic pitfalls in fine needle aspiration biopsy. *Diagn Cytopathol* 1993;9:351–357.

Thyroid Nodules and Thyroid Carcinoma: General Considerations

97. Vander JB, Gaston EA, Dawber TR: The significance of nontoxic thyroid nodules. Final report of a 15 year study of the incidence of thyroid malignancy. *Ann Intern Med* 1968;69:537–540.
98. Ain KB: Papillary thyroid carcinoma: Etiology, assessment and therapy. *Endocrinol Metab Clin North Am* 1995;24:711–760.
99. Farid NR, Zou M, Shi Y: Genetics of follicular thyroid cancer. *Endocrinol Metab Clin North Am* 1995;24:865–883.
100. Schneider AB: Radiation-induced thyroid tumors. *Endocrinol Metab Clin North Am* 1990;19:495–508.
101. Becker DV, Robbins J, Beebe GW, et al: Childhood thyroid cancer following the Chernobyl accident: A status report. *Endocrinol Metab Clin North Am* 1996;25:197–211.
102. Brierley JD, Tsang RW: External radiation therapy in the treatment of thyroid malignancy. *Endocrinol Metab Clin North Am* 1996;25:141–157.
103. Maxon HR, Smith HS: Radioiodine-131 in the diagnosis and treatment of metastatic well differentiated thyroid cancer. *Endocrinol Metab Clin North Am* 1990;19:685–718.
104. Ross DS: Long-term management of differentiated thyroid cancer. *Endocrinol Metab Clin North Am* 1990;19:719–739.
105. Burch HB: Evaluation and management of the solid thyroid nodule. *Endocrinol Metab Clin North Am* 1995;24:663–710.
106. Gharib H, Goellner JR: Fine needle aspiration biopsy of the thyroid: An appraisal. *Ann Intern Med* 1993;118:282–289.
107. Caruso DR, Mazzaferri EL: Fine needle aspiration biopsy in the management of thyroid nodules. *Endocrinologist* 1991;1:194–198.
108. Caraway NP, Sneige N, Samaan NA: Diagnostic pitfalls in thyroid fine needle aspiration: A review of 394 cases. *Diagn Cytopathol* 1993;9:345–350.
109. Piromalli D, Martelli G, Del Prato I, et al: The role of fine needle aspiration in the diagnosis of thyroid nodules: Analysis of 795 consecutive cases. *J Surg Oncol* 1992;50:247–250.
110. Schmid KW, Lucciarini P, Ladurner D, et al: Papillary carcinoma of the thyroid gland: Analysis of 94 cases with pre-operative fine needle aspiration cytologic examination. *Acta Cytol* 1987;31:591–594.
111. Jayaram G: Fine needle aspiration cytologic study of the solitary thyroid nodule: Profile of 308 cases with histologic correlation. *Acta Cytol* 1985;29:967–973.
112. Dunn JT: When is a thyroid nodule a sporadic medullary carcinoma? *J Clin Endocrinol Metab* 1994;78:824–825.
113. Silverman JF, West RL, Larkin EW, et al: The role of fine needle aspiration biopsy in the rapid diagnosis and management of thyroid neoplasm. *Cancer* 1986;57:1164–1170.
114. Gharib H: Fine needle aspiration biopsy of thyroid nodules: Advantages, limitations and effect. *Mayo Clin Proc* 1994;69:44–49.
115. Ashcraft MW, Van Herle AJ: Management of thyroid nodules. II: Scanning techniques, thyroid suppressive therapy and fine needle aspiration. *Head Neck Surg* 1981;3:297–322.
116. Mazzaferri EL, De Los Santos ET, Rofagha-Keyhani S: Solitary thyroid nodule: Diagnosis and management. *Med Clin North Am* 1988;72:1177–1211.
117. Rodríguez JM, Parrilla P, Sola J, et al: Comparison between preoperative cytology and intraoperative frozen section biopsy in the diagnosis of thyroid nodules. *Br J Surg* 1994;81:1151–1154.
118. Tielens ET, Sherman SI, Hruban RH, et al: Follicular variant of papillary thyroid carcinoma: A clinicopathologic study. *Cancer* 1994;73:424–431.
119. McHenry CR, Rosen IB, Walfish PG, et al: Influence of fine needle aspiration biopsy and frozen section examination on the management of thyroid cancer. *Am J Surg Path* 1993;166:353–356.
120. Nguyen G-K, Ginsberg J, Crockford PM: Fine needle aspiration biopsy cytology of the thyroid: Its value and limitations in the diagnosis and management of solitary thyroid nodules. *Pathol Annu* 1991;26:63–91.
121. Hamburger JI: Diagnosis of thyroid nodules by fine needle biopsy: Use and abuse. *J Clin Endocrinol Metab* 1994;79:335–339.

Benign Tumors

122. Namba H, Matsuo K, Fagin JA: Clonal composition of benign and malignant thyroid tumors. *J Clin Invest* 1990;86:120–125.
123. Davila RM, Bedrossian CW, Silverberg AB: Immunocytochemistry of the thyroid in surgical and cytological specimens. *Arch Pathol Lab Med* 1988;112:51–56.

124. Schröder S, Böcker W: Signet ring cell thyroid tumors. Follicle cell tumors with arrest of folliculogenesis. *Am J Surg Path* 1985;9:619–629.

125. Hazard JB, Kenyon R: Atypical adenoma of the thyroid. *Arch Pathol* 1954;58:554–563.

126. Bronner MP, LiVolsi VA: Oxyphilic (Askanazy/Hürthle cell) tumors of the thyroid. Microscopic features predict biologic behavior. *Surg Pathol* 1988;1:137–150.

127. Carcangiu ML, Bianchi S, Savino D, et al: Follicular Hürthle cell tumors of the thyroid gland. A study of 153 cases. *Cancer* 1991;68:1944–1953.

128. Davidson HG, Campora RG: Thyroid. In: Bibbo M, ed. *Comprehensive Cytopathology.* Philadelphia: W.B. Saunders, 1991:649–670.

129. Ravinsky E, Safneck JR: Fine needle aspirates of follicular lesions of the thyroid glands: The intermediate-type smear. *Acta Cytol* 1990;34:813–820.

130. Carney JA, Ryan J, Goellner JR: Hyalinizing trabecular adenoma of the thyroid gland. *Am J Surg Path* 1987;11:583–591.

131. Sambade C, Sarabando C, Nesland MJ, et al: Hyalinizing trabecular adenoma of the thyroid. Hyalinizing spindle cell tumor of the thyroid with dual differentiation. *Ultrastruct Pathol* 1989;13:275–280.

132. Katoh R, Jasani B, Williams ED: Hyalinizing trabecular adenoma of the thyroid: A report of three cases with immunohistochemical and ultrastructural studies. *Histopathol* 1989;15:211–224.

133. Bronner MP, LiVolsi VA, Jennings TA: PLAT: Paraganglioma-like adenoma of the thyroid. *Surg Pathol* 1988;1:383–389.

133a. Fonseca E, Nesland JM, Sobrinho-Simoes M: Expression of stratified epithelial type cytokeratins in hyalinizing trabecular adenomas supports their relationship with papillary carcinomas of the thyroid. *Histopathol* 1997;31:330–335.

134. Molberg K, Albores-Saavedra J: Hyalinizing trabecular carcinoma of the thyroid gland. *Hum Pathol* 1994;25:192–197.

135. Hjorth L, Thomsen LB, Nielsen VT: Adenolipoma of the thyroid gland. *Histopathol* 1986;10:91–96.

136. Gnepp DR, Ogorzalek JM, Heffess CS: Fat-containing lesions of the thyroid gland. *Am J Surg Path* 1989;13:605–612.

137. Visona A, Pea M, Bozzola L, et al: Follicular adenoma of the thyroid gland with extensive chondroid metaplasia. *Histopathol* 1991;18:278–279.

138. LiVolsi VA: *Surgical Pathology of the Thyroid.* Philadelphia: W.B. Saunders, 1990.

139. Doherty GM: *Textbook of Endocrine Surgery.* Philadelphia: W.B. Saunders, 1997.

Papillary Thyroid Carcinoma

140. McConahey WM, Hay ID, Woolner LB, et al: Papillary thyroid cancer treated at the Mayo Clinic, 1946 through 1970: Initial manifestations, pathologic findings, therapy and outcome. *Mayo Clin Proc* 1986;61:978–996.

141. Rustgi AK: Hereditary gastrointestinal polyposis and nonpolyposis syndromes. *N Engl J Med* 1994;331:1694–1702.

142. Harach HR, Williams GT, Williams ED: Familial adenomatous polyposis-associated thyroid carcinoma: A distinct type of follicular cell neoplasm. *Histopathol* 1994;25:549–561.

143. Donghi R, Sozzi G, Pierotti MA, et al: The oncogene associated with human papillary thyroid carcinoma (PTC) is assigned to chromosome 10q11-q12 in the same region as multiple endocrine neoplasia type 2A (MEN 2A). *Oncogene* 1989;4:521–523.

144. Grieco M, Santoro M, Berlingieri MT, et al: PTC is a novel rearranged form of the *ret* proto-oncogene and is frequently detected *in vivo* in human thyroid papillary carcinomas. *Cell* 1990;60:557–563.

145. Bongarzone I, Pierotti MA, Monzini N, et al: High frequency of activation of tyrosine kinase oncogenes in human papillary thyroid carcinoma. *Oncogene* 1989;4:1457–1462.

146. Sozzi G, Bongarzone I, Miozza M, et al: A t(10;17) translocation creates the *ret*/ptc2 chimeric transforming sequence in papillary thyroid carcinoma. *Genes Chromosomes Cancer* 1994;9:244–250.

146a. Jhiang SM, Sagartz JE, Tong Q, et al: Targeted expression of the *ret*/PTC 1 oncogene induces papillary thyroid carcinomas. *Endocrinol* 1996;137:375–378.

146b. Fischer AH, Bond JA, Taysavang P, et al: Papillary thyroid carcinoma oncogene (*RET*/PTC) alters the nuclear envelope and chromatin structure. *Am J Pathol* 1998;153:1443–1450.

146c. Lam AKY, Montone KT, Nolan KA, LiVolsi VA: *Ret* oncogene activation in papillary thyroid carcinoma: Prevalence and implication of the histological parameters. *Hum Pathol* 1998;29:565–568.

146d. Fugazzola L, Pierotte MA, Vigano E, et al: Molecular and biochemical analysis of *RET*/PTC4, a novel oncogenic rearrangement between RET and ELE 1 genes, in a post-Chernobyl papillary thyroid cancer. *Oncogene* 1996;13:1093–1097.

146e. Klugbauer S, Demidchik EP, Lengfelder E, Rabes HM: Detection of a novel type of RET rearrangement (PTC5) in thyroid carcinomas after Chernobyl and analysis of this involved RET-fused gene RFG5. *Cancer Res* 1998;58:198–203.

146f. Nikiforov YE, Rowland JM, Bove KE, et al: Distinctive pattern of *ret* oncogene rearrangements in morphological variants of radiation induced and sporadic thyroid papillary carcinomas in children. *Cancer Res* 1997;57:1690–1694.

146g. Tallini G, Santoro M, Helie M, et al: RET/PTC oncogene activation defines a subset of papillary thyroid carcinomas lacking evidence of progression to poorly differentiated or undifferentiated tumor phenotypes. *Clinical Cancer Res* 1998;4:287–294.

146h. Soares P, Fonseca E, Wynford-Thomas D, Sobrino-Simoes M: Sporadic *ret*-rearranged papillary carcinoma of the thyroid: A subset of slow-growing, less aggressive thyroid neoplasms? *J Pathol* 1998;185:71–78.

147. Carcangiu ML, Zampi G, Rosai J: Papillary thyroid carcinoma. A study of its many morphologic expressions and clinical correlates. *Pathol Annu* 1985;20(pt. 1):1–44.

148. Hedinger C, Williams ED, Sobin LH: *Histological Typing of Thyroid Tumors. WHO International Histological Classification of Tumors.* New York: Springer-Verlag, 1988.

149. Chan JK, Saw D: The grooved nucleus. A useful diagnostic criterion of papillary carcinoma of the thyroid. *Am J Surg Path* 1986;10:672–679.

150. Deligeorgi-Politi H: Nuclear crease as a cytodiagnostic feature of papillary thyroid carcinoma in fine needle aspiration biopsies. *Diagn Cytopathol* 1987;3:307–310.

151. Oyama T: A histopathological, immunohistochemical and ultrastructural study of intranuclear cytoplasmic inclusions in thyroid papillary carcinoma. *Virchows Arch* 1989;(A)414:91–104.

152. Gray A, Doniach I: Morphology of the nuclei of papillary carcinoma of the thyroid. *Br J Cancer* 1969;23:49–51.

153. Vickery AL: Thyroid papillary carcinoma. *Am J Surg Pathol* 1983;7:797–807.

154. Vickery AL, Carcangiu ML, Johannessen JV, Sobrinho-Simoes M: Papillary carcinoma. *Sem Diagn Pathol* 1985;2:90–100.

155. Hapke MR, Dehner LP: The optically clear nucleus: A reliable sign of papillary carcinoma of the thyroid? *Am J Surg Pathol* 1979;3:31–38.

156. Isarangkul W: Dense fibrosis. Another diagnostic criterion for papillary thyroid carcinoma. *Arch Pathol Lab Med* 1993;117:645–646.

157. Chan JK, Carcangiu ML, Rosai J: Papillary carcinoma of the thyroid with exuberant nodular fasciitis-like stroma, Report of three cases. *Am J Clin Pathol* 1991;95:309–314.

158. Henzen-Logmans SC, Mullink H, Ramaekers FC, et al: Expression of cytokeratins and vimentin in epithelial cells of normal and pathological thyroid tissue. *Virchows Arch A (Pathol Anat) Histopathol* 1987;410:347–354.

159. Miettinen M, Franssila K, Lehto VP, et al: Expression of intermediate filament proteins in thyroid gland and thyroid tumors. *Lab Invest* 1984;50:262–270.

160. Schelfhout LJ, Van Muijen GNP, Fleuren GP: Expression of keratin 19 distinguishes papillary thyroid carcinomas from follicular carcinoma and follicular thyroid adenoma. *Am J Clin Pathol* 1989;92:654–658.

160a. Miettinen M, Kovatich AJ, Karkkainen P: Keratin subsets in papillary and follicular thyroid lesions. A paraffin section analysis with diagnostic implications. *Virchocus Arch* 1997;430:239–245.

160b. Kragsterman B, Grimelius L, Wallin G, et al: Cytokeratin 19 expression in papillary thyroid carcinoma. *Appl Immunohistochem Mol Morphol* 1999;7:181–195.

161. Diaz NM, Mazoujian G, Wick M: Estrogen receptor protein in thyroid neoplasms. An immunohistochemical analysis of papillary carcinoma, follicular carcinoma and follicular adenoma. *Arch Pathol Lab Med* 1991;115:1203–1207.

162. Johannessen JV, Sobrinho-Simoes M: The origin and significance of thyroid psammoma bodies. *Lab Invest* 1980;43:287–296.

163. Meissner WA, Adler A: Papillary carcinoma of the thyroid. A study of the pattern in 226 patients. *Arch Pathol* 1958;66:518–525.

164. Akhtar M, Ashraf-Ali M, Huq M, Bakry M: Fine needle aspiration biopsy of papillary thyroid carcinoma: Cytologic, histologic and ultrastructural correlations. *Diagn Cytopathol* 1991;7:373–379.

165. Kaur A, Jayaram G: Thyroid tumors: Cytomorphology of papillary carcinoma. *Diagn Cytopathol* 1991;7:469–472.

166. Miller TR, Bottles K, Holly EA, et al: A stepwise logistic regression analysis of papillary carcinoma of the thyroid. *Acta Cytol* 1986;30:285–293.

167. Basu D, Jayaram G: A logistic model for thyroid lesions. *Diagn Cytopathol* 1992;8:23–27.

168. Christ ML, Hasa J: Intranuclear cytoplasmic inclusions (invaginations) in thyroid aspirations: Frequency and specificity. *Acta Cytol* 1989;23:327–331.

169. Francis IM, Das DK, Sheikh ZA, et al: Role of nuclear grooves in the diagnosis of papillary thyroid carcinoma. A quantitative assessment on fine needle aspiration smears. *Acta Cytol* 1995;39:409–415.

170. Harach RH, Zusman SB: Cytopathology of the tall cell variant of thyroid papillary carcinoma. *Acta Cytol* 1992;36:895–899.

171. Kaw YT: Fine needle aspiration cytology of the tall cell variant of papillary carcinoma of the thyroid. *Acta Cytol* 1994;38:282–283.

172. Klinck GH, Winship T: Occult sclerosing carcinoma of the thyroid. *Cancer* 1955;8:701–706.

173. Harach HR, Franssila KO, Wasenuis VM: Occult papillary carcinoma of the thyroid. A "normal" finding in Finland. A systematic autopsy study. *Cancer* 1985;56:531–538.

174. Fink A, Tomlinson G, Freeman JL, et al: Occult micropapillary carcinoma associated with benign follicular thyroid disease and unrelated thyroid neoplasms. *Mod Pathol* 1996;9:816–820.

175. Chem KT, Rosai J: Follicular variant of thyroid papillary carcinoma. A clinicopathologic study of six cases. *Am J Surg Pathol* 1977;1:123–130.

176. Albores-Saavedra J, Gould E, Vardaman C, Vuitch F: The macrofollicular variant of papillary thyroid carcinoma. A study of 17 cases. *Hum Pathol* 1991;22:1195–1205.

177. Sobrinho-Simoes M, Nesland M, Holm JR, et al: Hürthle cell and mitochondrion-rich papillary carcinomas of the thyroid: An ultrastructural and immunocytochemical study. *Ultrastruct Pathol* 1985;8:131–142.

178. Berho M, Suster S: The oncocytic variant of papillary carcinoma of the thyroid: A clinicopathologic study of 15 cases. *Hum Pathol* 1997;28:47–53.

179. Apel RL, Asa SL, LiVolsi VA: Papillary Hürthle cell carcinoma with lymphocytic stroma. "Warthin-like" tumor of the thyroid. *Am J Surg Pathol* 1995;19:810–814.

180. Peters SB, Chatten I, LiVolsi VA: Pediatric papillary thyroid carcinoma. *Mod Pathol* 1994;7:55A.

181. Nikiforov YE, Rowland JM, Monforte-Munoz H, Fagin JA: Comparative morphologic and molecular genetic analysis of radiation-induced and sporadic thyroid papillary carcinoma in children. *Mod Pathol* 1997;10:51A.

182. Sobrinho-Simoes M, Soares J, Carneiro F, Limbert E: Diffuse follicular variant of papillary carcinoma of the thyroid: Report of eight cases of a distinctive aggressive type of thyroid tumor. *Surg Pathol* 1990;3:189–203.

183. Hawk WA, Hazard JB: The many appearances of papillary carcinoma of the thyroid. *Cleve Clin Q* 1976;43:207–215.

184. Johnson TL, Lloyd RV, Thompson NW, et al: Prognostic implication of the tall cell variant of papillary thyroid carcinoma. *Am J Surg Pathol* 1988;12:22–27.

185. Ozaki O, Ito K, Mimura T, et al: Papillary carcinoma of the thyroid. Tall cell variant with extensive lymphocyte infiltration. *Am J Surg Path* 1996;20:695–698.

186. Ostrowski ML, Merino MJ: Tall cell variant of papillary thyroid carcinoma. A reassessment and immunohistochemical study with comparison to the usual type of papillary carcinoma of the thyroid. *Am J Surg Pathol* 1996;20:964–974.

187. Burman KD, Ringel MD, Wartofsky L: Unusual types of thyroid neoplasms. *Endocrinol Metab Clin North Am* 1996;25:49–68.

188. Ruter A, Dreifus J, Jones M, et al: Overexpression of p53 in tall cell variants of papillary thyroid carcinoma. *Surgery* 1996;120:1046–1050.

189. Ferreiro JA, Hay ID, Lloyd RV: Columnar cell carcinoma of the thyroid. Report of three additional cases. *Hum Pathol* 1996;27:1156–1160.

190. Evans HL: Encapsulated columnar cell neoplasms of the thyroid. A report of four cases suggesting a favorable prognosis. *Am J Surg Pathol* 1996;20:1205–1211.

191. Akslen LA, Varhaug JE: Thyroid carcinoma with mixed tall-cell and columnar-cell features. *Am J Clin Pathol* 1990;94:442–445.

192. Mazzaferri EL, Jhiang SM: Long term impact of initial surgical and medical therapy on papillary and follicular thyroid cancer. *Am J Med* 1994;97:418–428.

193. Hay ID: Papillary thyroid carcinoma. *Endocrinol Clin North Am* 1990;19:545–576.

193a. Woolner LB, Beahrs OH, Black BM, et al: Classification and prognosis of thyroid carcinoma. A study of 885 cases observed in a 30-year period. *Am J Surg* 1961;102:354–387.

194. Cady B, Sedgwick CE, Meissner WA, et al: Risk factor analysis in differentiated thyroid cancer. *Cancer* 1979;43:810–820.

195. Cady B, Rossi R, Silverman M, et al: Further evidence of the validity of risk group definition in differentiated thyroid carcinoma. *Surgery* 1985;98:1171–1178.

196. Byar DP, Green SB, Dor P, et al: A prognostic index for thyroid carcinoma: A study of the EORTC thyroid cancer cooperative group. *Eur J Cancer* 1979;15:1033–1041.

197. Wittekind C, Sobin LH: *TNM Classification of Malignant Tumours,* 5th ed. New York: Wiley-Liss, 1997.

198. American Joint Commission on Cancer: *AJCC Cancer Staging Manual,* 5th ed. Philadelphia: Lippincott-Raven, 1997.

198a. Akslen LA: Prognostic importance of histologic grading in papillary thyroid carcinoma. *Cancer* 1993;72:2680–2685.

199. Joensuu H, Klemi P, Eerola E, Tuominen J: Influence of cellular DNA content on survival in differentiated thyroid cancer. *Cancer* 1986;58:2462–2467.

Follicular Carcinoma

200. Rosai ML, Carcangiu ML, DeLellis RA: *Tumors of the Thyroid Gland. Atlas of Tumor Pathology.* Washington, DC: Armed Forces Institute of Pathology, 1992:49–64.

201. Grebe SK, Hay ID: Follicular thyroid cancer. *Endocrinol Metab Clin North Am* 1995;24:761–801.

202. Lang W, Choritz H, Hundeshagen H: Risk factors in follicular thyroid carcinomas. A retrospective follow-up study covering a 14 year period with emphasis on morphological findings. *Am J Surg Pathol* 1986;10:246–255.

203. Evans HL: Follicular neoplasms of the thyroid. A study of 44 cases followed for a minimum of ten years with emphasis on differential diagnosis. *Cancer* 1984;54:535–540.

204. Franssila KO, Ackerman LV, Brown CL, Hedinger CE: Follicular carcinoma. *Semin Diagn Pathol* 1985;2:101–122.

204a. Carcangiu ML: Minimally invasive follicular carcinoma. *Endocrin Pathol* 1997;8:231–234.

205. Cooper DS, Schneyer CR: Follicular and Hürthle cell carcinoma of the thyroid. *Endocrinol Metab Clin North Am* 1990;19:577–591.

Oncocytic Carcinoma

206. Thompson NW, Dunn EL, Batsakis JG, Nishiyama RH: Hürthle cell lesions of the thyroid gland. *Surg Gynecol Obstet* 1974;139:555–560.

207. Tollefsen HR, Shah JP, Huvos AG: Hürthle cell carcinoma of the thyroid. *Am J Surg* 1975;130:390–394.

Poorly Differentiated Carcinoma

208. Sakamoto A, Kasai N, Sugano H: Poorly differentiated carcinoma of the thyroid. A clinicopathologic entity for a high risk group of papillary and follicular carcinomas. *Cancer* 1983;52:1849–1855.

209. Carcangiu ML, Zampi G, Rosai J: Poorly differentiated ("insular") thyroid carcinoma. A reinterpretation of Langhans' "wuchernde Struma." *Am J Surg Pathol* 1984;8:655–668.

210. Papotti M, Botto Micca F, Favero A, et al: Poorly differentiated thyroid carcinomas with primordial cell component. A group of aggressive lesions sharing insular, trabecular and solid patterns. *Am J Surg Pathol* 1993;17:291–301.

211. Ashfaq R, Vuitch F, Delgado R, Albores-Saavedra J: Papillary and follicular carcinomas with an insular component. *Cancer* 1994;73:416–423.

212. Pilotti S, Collini P, DelBo R, et al: A novel panel of antibodies that segregates immunocytochemically poorly-differentiated carcinoma from undifferentiated carcinoma of the thyroid gland. *Am J Surg Pathol* 1994;18:1054–1064.

213. Sironi M, Collini P, Cantaboni A: Fine needle aspiration cytology of insular thyroid carcinoma: A report of four cases. *Acta Cytol* 1992;36:435–439.

214. Pietribiasi F, Sapino A, Papotti M, Bussolati G: Cytologic features of

poorly differentiated "insular" carcinoma of the thyroid, as revealed by fine needle aspiration biopsy. *Am J Clin Pathol* 1990;94:687–692.

215. Zakowski MF, Schlesinger K, Mizrachi HH: Cytologic features of poorly differentiated "insular" carcinoma of the thyroid. A case report. *Acta Cytol* 1992;36:523–526.

Undifferentiated (Anaplastic) Carcinoma

216. Rosai J, Saxen EA, Woolner L: Undifferentiated and poorly differentiated carcinoma. *Semin Diagn Pathol* 1985;2:123–136.
217. Hashimoto H, Koga S, Watanabe H, Enjoji M: Undifferentiated carcinoma of the thyroid gland with osteoclast-like giant cells. *Acta Pathol Jpn* 1980;30:323–334.
217a. Wan S-K, Chan JKC, Tang S-K: Paucicellular variant of anaplastic thyroid carcinoma. A mimic of Riedel's thyroiditis. *Am J Clin Pathol* 1996;105:388–393.
218. Hurlimann J, Gardiol D, Scazziga B: Immunohistology of anaplastic thyroid carcinoma. A study of 43 cases. *Histopathology* 1987;11:567–580.
219. Ordonez NG, El-Naggar AK, Hickey RC, Samaan NA: Anaplastic thyroid carcinoma. Immunocytochemical study of 32 cases. *Am J Clin Pathol* 1991;96:15–24.
220. Rosai J: *Ackerman's Surgical Pathology.* St. Louis: Mosby–Year Book, 1996.
221. Atkinson BF: Fine needle aspiration of the thyroid. *Monogr Pathol* 1993;35:166–199.

Squamous Cell Carcinoma

222. Simpson WJ, Carruthers J: Squamous cell carcinoma of the thyroid gland. *Am J Surg* 1988;156:44–46.
223. Saito K, Kuratomi Y, Yamamoto K, et al: Primary squamous cell carcinoma of the thyroid associated with marked leukocytosis and hypercalcemia. *Cancer* 1981;48:2080–2083.
224. Sato K, Fujii Y, Ono M, et al: Production of interleukin-1 alpha-like factor and colony stimulating factor by a squamous cell carcinoma of the thyroid (T3 M-5) derived from a patient with hypercalcemia and leukocytosis. *Cancer Res* 1987;47:6474–6480.

Medullary Carcinoma and C-Cell Hyperplasia

225. Horn RC: Carcinoma of the thyroid. Description of a distinctive morphological variant and report of seven cases. *Cancer* 1951;4:697–707.
226. Hazard JB, Hawke WA, Crile G: Medullary (solid) carcinoma of the thyroid: A clinicopathological entity. *J Clin Endocrinol Metab* 1959;19:152–161.
227. Williams ED: Histogenesis of medullary carcinoma of the thyroid. *J Clin Pathol* 1966;19:114–118.
228. Bussolati G, Pearse AGE: Immunofluorescent localization of calcitonin in the 'C'-cells of the dog and pig thyroid. *J Endocrinol* 1967;37:205–209.
229. Sizemore GW: Medullary carcinoma of the thyroid gland. *Semin Oncol* 1987;14:306–314.
230. DeLellis RA: Multiple endocrine neoplasia syndromes revisited. Clinical, morphological and molecular features. *Lab Invest* 1995;72:494–505.
230a. Rieu M, Lame M-C, Richard A, et al: Prevalence of sporadic medullary thyroid carcinoma: The importance of routine measurement of serum calcitonin in the diagnostic evaluation of thyroid nodules. *Clin Endocrinol* 1995;42:453–460.
231. Rosai J, Carcangiu ML, DeLellis RA: *Tumors of the Thyroid Gland. Atlas of Tumor Pathology.* Washington, DC: Armed Forces Institute of Pathology, 1992:207–258.
232. Weiss LM, Weinberg DS, Warhol MJ: Medullary carcinoma arising in a thyroid with Hashimoto's disease. *Am J Clin Pathol* 1983;80:534–538.
233. LiVolsi VA, Feind CR: Incidental medullary thyroid carcinoma in sporadic hyperparathyroidism. An expansion of the concept of C-cell hyperplasia. *Am J Clin Pathol* 1979;71:595–599.
233a. Mizukami Y, Kurumaya H, Nonomura A, et al: Sporadic medullary microcarcinoma of the thyroid. *Histopathology* 1992;21:375–377.
234. Papotti M, Sambataro D, Pecchioni C, Bussolati G: The pathology of medullary carcinoma of the thyroid: Review of the literature and personal experience of 62 cases. *Endocrine Pathol* 1996;7:1–20.

235. Harach HR, Williams ED: Glandular (tubular and follicular) variants of medullary carcinoma of the thyroid. *Histopathology* 1983;7:83–97.
236. Kakudo K, Miyauchi A, Yakai SI, et al: C-cell carcinoma of the thyroid, papillary type. *Acta Pathol Jpn* 1979;29:653–659.
237. Papotti M, Sapino A, Abbona G, et al: Pseudoangiosarcomatous features in medullary carcinoma of the thyroid. *Int J Surg Pathol* 1995;3:29–36.
238. Mendelsohn G, Baylin SB, Bigner SH, et al: Anaplastic variants of medullary thyroid carcinoma. A light microscopic and immunohistochemical study. *Am J Surg Pathol* 1980;4:333–341.
239. Kakudo K, Miyauchi A, Ogihara T, et al: Medullary carcinoma of the thyroid. Giant cell type. *Arch Pathol Lab Med* 1978;102:445–447.
240. Landon G, Ordonez NG: Clear cell variant of medullary carcinoma of the thyroid. *Hum Pathol* 1985;16:844–847.
241. Marcus JN, Dise CA, LiVolsi VA: Melanin production in a medullary thyroid carcinoma. *Cancer* 1982;49:2518–2526.
242. Dominguez-Malagon H, Delgado-Chavez R, Torres-Najera M, et al: Oxyphil and squamous variants of medullary thyroid carcinoma. *Cancer* 1989;63:1183–1188.
243. Golouh R, Us-Krasovec M, Auersperg M, et al: Amphicrine-composite calcitonin and mucin-producing carcinoma of the thyroid. *Ultrastruct Pathol* 1985;8:197–206.
244. Huss LJ, Mendelsohn G: Medullary carcinoma of the thyroid gland: An encapsulated variant resembling the hyalinizing trabecular (paraganglioma-like) adenoma of thyroid. *Mod Pathol* 1990;3:581–585.
245. Mendelsohn G, Oertel J: Encapsulated medullary thyroid carcinoma [abstract]. *Lab Invest* 1981;44:43A.
246. Holm R, Sobrinho-Simoes M, Nesland JM, et al: Medullary carcinoma of the thyroid gland: An immunocytochemical study. *Ultrastruct Pathol* 1985;8:25–41.
247. Zajac JD, Penschow J, Mason T, et al: Identification of calcitonin and calcitonin gene-related peptide messenger RNA in medullary thyroid carcinoma by hybridization histochemistry. *J Clin Endocrinol Metab* 1986;62:1037–1043.
248. DeLellis RA, Wolfe HJ: The pathobiology of the human calcitonin (C)-cell. A review. *Pathol Annu* 1981;16:25–52.
249. Eusebi V, Damiani S, Riva C, et al: Calcitonin-free oat cell carcinoma of the thyroid gland. *Virchows Arch A (Pathol Anat) Histopathol* 1990;417:267–271.
250. Bose S, Kapila K, Verma K: Medullary carcinoma of the thyroid: A cytological immunocytochemical and ultrastructural study. *Diagn Cytopathol* 1992;8:28–32.
251. Mendoca ME, Ramos S, Soares J: Medullary carcinoma of the thyroid: A re-evaluation of the cytological criteria of diagnosis. *Cytopathology* 1991;2:93–102.
252. Bigner SH, Cox EB, Mendelsohn G, et al: Medullary carcinoma of the thyroid in the multiple endocrine neoplasia IIA syndrome. *Am J Surg Pathol* 1981;5:459–472.
253. Schroder S, Bocker W, Baisch H, et al: Prognostic factors in medullary thyroid carcinomas. Survival in relation to age, sex, stage, histology, immunocytochemistry and DNA content. *Cancer* 1988;61:806–816.
254. Lippman SM, Mendelsohn G, Trump DL, et al: The prognostic and biological significance of cellular heterogeneity in medullary thyroid carcinoma: A study of calcitonin, L-dopa decarboxylase and histaminase. *J Clin Endocrinol Metab* 1982;54:233–240.
255. Mendelsohn G, Wells SA, Baylin SB: Relationship of tissue carcinoembryonic antigen and calcitonin to tumor virulence in medullary thyroid carcinoma. An immunohistochemical study in early, localized and virulent disseminated stages of disease. *Cancer* 1984;54:657–662.
256. McDermott MB, Swanson PE, Wick MR: Immunostains for collagen type IV discriminate between C-cell hyperplasia and microscopic medullary carcinoma in multiple endocrine neoplasia, type 2A. *Hum Pathol* 1995;26:1308–1312.
257. DeLellis RA: The pathology of medullary thyroid carcinoma and its precursors. In: LiVolsi VA, DeLellis RA, eds. *Pathobiology of the Parathyroid and Thyroid Glands.* Baltimore: Williams & Wilkins, 1993:72–102.
258. Albores-Saavedra J, Monforte H, Nadji M, Morales AR: C-cell hyperplasia in thyroid tissue adjacent to follicular cell tumors. *Hum Pathol* 1988;19:795–799.
259. Perry A, Molberg K, Albores-Saavedra J: Physiologic versus neoplastic C-cell hyperplasia of the thyroid. Separation of distinct histologic and biologic entities. *Cancer* 1996;77:750–756.
259a. Kaserer K, Schenba C, Neuhold N, et al: C-cell hyperplasia and medullary thyroid carcinoma in patients routinely screened for serum calcitonin. *Am J Surg Pathol* 1998;22:722–728.

259b. Mizukami Y, Michigishi T, Nonomura A, et al: Mixed medullary-follicular carcinoma of the thyroid occurring in familial form. *Histopathology* 1993;284–289.

260. Ljungberg O, Bondeson L, Bondeson AG: Differentiated thyroid carcinoma, intermediate type: A new tumor entity with features of follicular and parafollicular cell carcinoma. *Hum Pathol* 1984;15:218–228.

261. Albores-Saavedra J, De la Mora TG, De la Torra-Rendon F, Gould E: Mixed medullary papillary carcinoma of the thyroid: A previously unrecognized variant of thyroid carcinoma. *Hum Pathol* 1990;21:1151–1155.

261a. Volante M, Papotti M, Roth J, et al: Mixed medullary-follicular carcinoma: Molecular evidence for a dual origin of tumor components. *Am J Pathol* 1999;155:1499–1509.

261b. Matias-Guin X: Mixed medullary and follicular carcinoma of the thyroid: On the search for its histogenesis. *Am J Pathol* 1999;155:1413–1418.

Malignant Lymphoma, Plasmacytoma, Lymphoproliferative, and Hematologic Diseases

262. Freeman C, Berg JW, Cutler SJ: Occurrence and prognosis of extranodal lymphomas. *Cancer* 1972;29:252–260.

263. Williams ED: Malignant lymphoma of the thyroid. *Clin Endocrinol Metab* 1981;10:379–389.

264. Anscombe AM, Wright DH: Primary malignant lymphoma of the thyroid: A tumor of mucosa-associated lymphoid tissue: Review of seventy-six cases. *Histopathology* 1985;9:81–97.

265. Aozasa K, Inoue A, Yoshimura H, et al: Intermediate lymphocytic lymphoma of the thyroid. An immunologic and immunohistologic study. *Cancer* 1986;57:1762–1767.

266. Das DK, Gupta SK, Francis IM, Ahmed MS: Fine needle aspiration cytology diagnosis of non-hodgkin lymphoma of thyroid: A report of four cases. *Diagn Cytopathol* 1993;9:639–645.

267. Aozasa K, Inoue A, Yashimura, et al: Plasmacytoma of the thyroid gland. *Cancer* 1986;58:105–110.

268. Rubin J, Johnson JJ, Killeen R, Barnes L: Extramedullary plasmacytoma of the thyroid associated with a serum monoclonal gammopathy. *Arch Otolaryngol Head Neck Surg* 1990;116:855–859.

269. Compagno J, Oertel JE: Malignant lymphoma and other lymphoproliferative disorders of the thyroid gland. A clinicopathologic study of 245 cases. *Am J Clin Pathol* 1980;74:1–11.

270. Feigin GA, Buss DH, Paschal B, et al: Hodgkin's disease manifested as a thyroid nodule. *Hum Pathol* 1982;13:774–776.

271. Coode PE, Shaikh MU: Histiocytosis X of the thyroid masquerading as thyroid carcinoma. *Hum Pathol* 1988;19:239–241.

272. Thompson LDR, Wenig BM, Adair CF, et al: Langerhans cell histiocytosis of the thyroid gland. A series of seven cases and a review of the literature. *Mod Pathol* 1996;9:145–149.

272a. Saiz E, Bakotic BW: Isolated Langerhans histiocytosis of the thyroid: A report of two cases with nuclear imaging–pathologic correlations. *Ann Diagn Pathol* 2000;4:23–28.

273. Larkin DF, Dervan PA, Munnelly J, Finucane J: Sinus histiocytosis with massive lymphadenopathy simulating subacute thyroiditis. *Hum Pathol* 1986;17:321–324.

274. Yapp R, Linder J, Schenken JR, Karrer FW: Plasma cell granuloma of the thyroid. *Hum Pathol* 1985;16:848–850.

275. Schmid C, Beham A, Seewan HL: Extramedullary haematopoiesis in the thyroid gland. *Histopathology* 1989;15:423–425.

Mesenchymal Tumors

276. Shin W-Y, Aftalion B, Hotchkiss E, et al: Ultrastructure of a primary fibrosarcoma of the human thyroid gland. *Cancer* 1979;44:584–591.

277. Rosai J, Carcangui ML, DeLellis RA: *Tumors of the Thyroid Gland. Atlas of Tumor Pathology.* Washington, DC: Armed Forces Institute of Pathology, 1992:259–265.

278. Egloff B: The hemangioendothelioma of the thyroid. *Virchows Arch (A) Pathol Anat Histopathology* 1983;400:119–142.

279. Tanda F, Massarelli G, Bosincu L, Cossu V: Angiosarcoma of the thyroid: A light, electron microscopic and histoimmunological study. *Hum Pathol* 1988;19:742–745.

280. Ruchti C, Gerber HA, Schaffner T: Factor VIII-related antigen in malignant hemangioendothelioma of the thyroid: Additional evidence for the endothelial origin of this tumor. *Am J Clin Pathol* 1984;82:474–480.

Unusual Thyroid and Secondary Tumors

281. Chan JK, Rosai J: Tumors of the neck showing thymic or related branchial pouch differentiation, a unifying concept. *Hum Pathol* 1991;22:349–367.

282. DeLellis RA, Tischler AS, Wolfe HJ: Multidirectional differentiation in neuroendocrine neoplasms. *J Histochem Cytochem* 1984;32:899–904.

283. Fisher JE, Cooney DR, Voorhess ML, Jewett TC: Teratoma of the thyroid gland in infancy. Review of the literature and two case reports. *J Surg Oncol* 1982;21:135–140.

284. Kimler SC, Muth WF: Primary malignant teratoma of the thyroid: Case report and literature review of cervical teratomas in adults. *Cancer* 1978;42:311–317.

285. Buss DH, Marshall RB, Baird FG, Myers RT: Paraganglioma of the thyroid gland. *Am J Surg Pathol* 1980;4:589–593.

286. Wenig BM, Adair CF, Heffess CS: Primary mucoepidermoid carcinoma of the thyroid gland: A report of six cases and a review of the literature of a follicular epithelial-derived tumor. *Hum Pathol* 1995;26:1099–1108.

287. Franssila KO, Harach HR, Wasenius VM: Mucoepidermoid carcinoma of the thyroid. *Histopathology* 1984;8:847–860.

288. Harach HR, Day ES, deStrizic NA: Mucoepidermoid carcinoma of the thyroid. Report of a case with immunohistochemical studies. *Medicina* 1986;46:213–216.

289. Miranda RN, Myint MA, Gnepp DR: Composite follicular variant of papillary carcinoma and mucoepidermoid carcinoma of the thyroid. Report of a case and review of the literature. *Am J Surg Pathol* 1995;19:1209–1215.

290. Cameselle-Teijeiro J, Febles-Perez C, Sobrinho-Simoes M: Papillary and mucoepidermoid carcinoma of the thyroid with anaplastic transformation. A case report with histologic and immunohistochemical findings that support a provocative histogenetic hypothesis. *Pathol Res Pract* 1995;191:1214–1221.

291. Cameselle-Teijeiro J: Mucoepidermoid carcinoma and solid cell nests of the thyroid (correspondence). *Hum Pathol* 1996;27:861–863.

292. Chan JK, Albores-Saavedra J, Battifora H, et al: Sclerosing mucoepidermoid carcinoma of the thyroid with eosinophilia. A distinctive low grade malignancy arising from the metaplastic follicles of Hashimoto's thyroiditis. *Am J Surg Path* 1991;15:438–448.

293. Bakri K, Shimaoka K, Rao U, Tsukada Y: Adenosquamous carcinoma of the thyroid after radiotherapy for Hodgkin's disease. A case report and review. *Cancer* 1983;52:465–470.

294. Ivy HK: Cancer metastatic to the thyroid. A diagnostic problem. *Mayo Clin Proc* 1984;59:856–859.

295. Nakhjavani M, Gharib H, Goellner JR, van Heerden JA: Metastasis to the thyroid gland. A report of 43 cases. *Cancer* 1997;79:574–578.

296. Carcangiu ML, Sibley RK, Rosai J: Clear cell change in primary thyroid tumors. A study of 38 cases. *Am J Surg Pathol* 1985;9:705–722.

Parathyroid Glands: Embryology, Anatomy, and Physiology

297. Gilmour JR: The embryology of the parathyroid glands, the thymus, and certain associated rudiments. *J Pathol* 1937;45:507–522.

298. Akerström G, Malmaeus J, Bergström R: Surgical anatomy of human parathyroid glands. *Surgery* 1984;95:14–21.

299. Grimelius L, Akerström G, Johansson H, Bergström R: Anatomy and histopathology of human parathyroid glands. *Pathol Annu* 1981;16(pt 2):1–24.

300. Wang C: The anatomic basis of parathyroid surgery. *Ann Surg* 1976;183:271–275.

301. Abu-Jawdeh GM, Roth SI: Parathyroid glands. In: Sternberg SS, ed. *Histology for Pathologists.* New York: Raven Press, 1992:11–20.

302. Miettinen M, Franssila K, Lehto V-P, et al: Expression of intermediate filament proteins in thyroid gland and thyroid tumors. *Lab Invest* 1984;50:262–270.

302a. Tomika T: Immunocytochemical staining patterns for parathyroid hormone and chromogranin in parathyroid hyperplasia, adenoma and carcinoma. *Endocrin Pathol* 1999;10:145–156.

303. Stork PJ, Herteaux C, Frazier R, et al: Expression and distribution of parathyroid hormone and parathyroid hormone messenger RNA in pathological conditions of the parathyroid. *Lab Invest* 1989;60:92A.

304. Wilson BS, Lloyd RV: Detection of chromogranin in neuroendocrine cells with a monoclonal antibody. *Am J Pathol* 1984;115:458–468.

305. Dufour DR, Wilkerson SY: The normal parathyroid revisited: Percentage of stromal fat. *Hum Pathol* 1982;13:717–721.

306. Aurbach GD, Marx SJ, Spiegel AM: Parathyroid hormone, calcitonin and the calciferols. In: Wilson JD, Foster DW, eds. *Textbook of Endocrinology.* Philadelphia: W.B. Saunders, 1992:1397–1476.

Hyperparathyroidism

307. Mallette LE: The functional and pathological spectrum of parathyroid abnormalities in hyperparathyroidism. In: Bilezekian JP, Marcus R, Levine MA, eds. *The Parathyroids. Basic and Clinical Concepts.* New York: Raven Press, 1994:423–455.
308. Palmër M, Jakobsson S, Akerström G, Ljunghall S: Prevalence of hypercalcemia in a health survey: A 14 year follow-up study of serum calcium values. *Eur J Clin Invest* 1988;18:39–46.

Parathyroid Adenoma

309. DeLellis RA: *Tumors of the Parathyroid Gland. Atlas of Tumor Pathology.* Washington, DC: Armed Forces Institute of Pathology, 1993.
310. Castleman B, Roth SI: *Tumors of the Parathyroid Glands. Atlas of Tumor Pathology.* Washington, DC: Armed Forces Institute of Pathology, 1978.
311. Ghandur-Mnaymneh L, Kimura N: The parathyroid adenoma. A histopathologic definition with a study of 172 cases of primary hyperparathyroidism. *Am J Pathol* 1984;115:70–83.
312. Jackson CE, Cerny JC, Block M, Fialkow PJ: Probable clonal origin of aldosteronomas versus multicellular origin of parathyroid adenomas. *Surgery* 1982;92:875–879.
313. Arnold A: Molecular mechanisms of parathyroid neoplasia. *Endocrinol Metab Clin North Am* 1994;23:93–107.
314. Arnold A, Staunton CE, Kim HG, et al: Monoclonality and abnormal parathyroid hormone genes in parathyroid adenomas. *N Engl J Med* 1988;318:658–662.
315. Friedman E, Sakaguchi A, Bale AE, et al: Clonality of parathyroid tumors in familial multiple endocrine neoplasia type 1. *N Engl J Med* 1989;321:213–218.
315a. Komminoth P: Review: Multiple endocrine neoplasia type 1, sporadic neuroendocrine tumors and MENIN. *Diagn Mol Pathol* 1999;8:107–112.
316. Juhlin C, Akerström G, Klaraskog L, et al: Monoclonal antiparathyroid hormone antibodies revealing defect expression of a calcium receptor mechanism in hyperparathyroidism. *World J Surg* 1988;12:552–558.
317. Sahin A, Robinson RA: Papillae formation in parathyroid adenoma. A source of possible diagnostic error. *Arch Pathol Lab Med* 1988;112:99–100.
318. Loda M, Lipman J, Cukor B, et al: Nodular foci in parathyroid adenomas and hyperplasias. An immunohistochemical analysis of proliferative activity. *Hum Pathol* 1994;25:1050–1056.
319. Roth SI, Gallagher MJ: The rapid identification of "normal" parathyroid glands by the presence of intracellular fat. *Am J Pathol* 1976;84:521–528.
320. Snover DC, Foucar K: Mitotic activity in benign parathyroid disease. *Am J Clin Pathol* 1981;75:345–347.
321. San Juan J, Monteagudo C, Fraker D, et al: Significance of mitotic activity and other morphologic parameters in parathyroid adenomas and their correlation with clinical behavior. *Am J Clin Pathol* 1989;112:99–100.
322. Liechty RD, Teter A, Suba EJ: The tiny parathyroid adenoma. *Surgery* 1986;100:1048–1052.
323. Rasbach DA, Monchik JM, Geelhoed GW, Harrison TS: Solitary parathyroid microadenoma. *Surgery* 1984;96:1092–1098.
324. Ordonez NG, Ibanez ML, Mackay B, et al: Functioning oxyphil cell adenomas of parathyroid gland: Immunoperoxidase evidence of hormonal activity in oxyphil cells. *Am J Clin Pathol* 1982;78:681–689.
325. Bedetti CD, Dekker A, Watson CG: Functioning oxyphil cell adenoma of the parathyroid glands. A clinicopathologic study of 10 patients with hyperparathyroidism. *Hum Pathol* 1984;15:1121–1126.
326. Wolpert HR, Vickery AL, Wang CA: Functioning oxyphil cell adenomas of the parathyroid glands. A study of 15 cases. *Am J Surg Path* 1989;13:500–504.
327. Abul-Haj SK, Conklin H, Hewitt WC: Functioning lipoadenoma of the parathyroid gland: Report of a unique case. *N Engl J Med* 1962;266:121–123.
328. LeGolvan DP, Moore BP, Nishiyama RH: Parathyroid hamartoma. Report of two cases and review of the literature. *Am J Clin Pathol* 1977;67:31–35.

328a. Grenko RT, Anderson KM, Kauffman GA, Abt AB: Water clear cell adenoma of the parathyroid: A case report with immunohistochemistry and election microscopy. *Arch Pathol Lab Med* 1995;119:1072–1074.
329. Levin KE, Chew KL, Ljung BM, et al: Deoxyribonucleic acid cytometry helps identify parathyroid carcinomas. *J Clin Endocrinol Metab* 1988;67:779–784.
330. Verdonk CA, Edis AJ: Parathyroid "double adenomas": Fact or fiction? *Surgery* 1981;90:523–526.
331. Carney JA: Pathology of hyperparathyroidism. A practical approach. In: LiVolsi VA, DeLellis RA, eds. *Pathobiology of the Parathyroid and Thyroid Glands.* Baltimore: Williams & Wilkins, 1993:34–62.
332. Bondeson AG, Bondeson L, Ljungberg O, Tibblin S: Fat staining in parathyroid disease: Diagnostic value and impact on surgical strategy. Clinicopathologic study of 191 cases. *Hum Pathol* 1985;16:1255–1263.
333. Clarke MR, Hoover WW, Carty SE, et al: Atypical fat staining patterns in hyperparathyroidism. *Int J Surg Pathol* 1996;3:163–168.

Parathyroid Carcinoma

334. Shane E: Parathyroid carcinoma. In: Bilezekian JP, Marcus R, Levine MA, eds. *The Parathyroids. Basic and Clinical Concepts.* New York: Raven Press, 1994:575–582.
335. Wang CA, Gaz RD: Natural history of parathyroid carcinoma. Diagnosis, treatment and results. *Am J Surg* 1985;149:522–527.
336. Schantz A, Castleman B: Parathyroid carcinoma: A study of 70 patients. *Cancer* 1973;31:600–605.
337. Bondeson L, Sandelin K, Grimelius L: Histopathological variables and DNA cytometry in parathyroid carcinoma. *Am J Surg Pathol* 1993;17:820–829.
338. Mallette LE: DNA quantitation in the study of parathyroid lesions. A review. *Am J Clin Pathol* 1992;98:305–311.
339. Joensuu H, Klemi PJ: DNA aneuploidy in adenomas of endocrine organs. *Am J Pathol* 1988;132:145–151.
340. Harlow S, Roth SI, Bauer K, Marshall RB: Flow cytometric DNA analysis of normal and pathological parathyroid glands. *Mod Pathol* 1991;4:310–315.
341. Obara T, Fujimoto Y, Kanaji Y, et al: Flow cytometric DNA analysis of parathyroid tumors. Implication of aneuploidy for pathologic and biologic classification. *Cancer* 1990;66:1555–1562.
342. Abbona GC, Papotti M, Gasparri G, Bussolati G: Proliferative activity in parathyroid tumors as detected by Ki-67 immunostaining. *Hum Pathol* 1995;26:135–138.
343. Vargas MP, Vargas HI, Kleiner DE, Merino MJ: The role of prognostic markers (MIB-1, RB,bcl-2) in the diagnosis of parathyroid tumors. *Mod Pathol* 1997;10:12–17.
344. Cryns VL, Thor A, Xu H-J, et al: Loss of the retinoblastoma tumor suppressor gene in parathyroid carcinoma. *N Engl J Med* 1994;330:757–761.
344a. Farnebo F, Auer G, Farnebo LO, et al: Evaluation of retinoblastoma and Ki-67 immunostaining as diagnostic markers of benign and malignant parathyroid disease. *World J Surg* 1999;23:68–74.
345. Tibbin SAG, Bergenfelz AOJ: Surgical approach to primary hyperparathyroidism. In: Clark OH, Duk QY, eds. *Textbook of Endocrine Surgery.* Philadelphia: W.B. Saunders, 1997:365–371.

Primary Hyperplasia

346. Cope O, Keynes WM, Roth SI, Castleman B: Primary chief cell hyperplasia of the parathyroid glands: A new entity in the surgery of hyperparathyroidism. *Ann Surg* 1958;148:375–388.
347. Chandrasekharappa SC, Guru SC, Manickam P, et al: Positional cloning of the gene for multiple endocrine neoplasia—type I. *Science* 1997;276:404–407.
347a. Lubensky IA, Debelenko LV, Zhuang G, et al: Allelic deletions on chromosome 11q13 in multiple tumors from individual MEN 1 patients. *Cancer Res* 1996;56:5272–5278.
348. Larsson C, Friedman E: Localization and identification of the multiple endocrine neoplasia type 1 disease gene. *Endocrinol Metab Clin North Am* 1994;23:67–79.
349. Brandi ML: Multiple endocrine neoplasia type 1: General features and new insights into etiology. *J Endocrinol Investig* 1991;14:61–72.
350. Black WC, Haff RC: The surgical pathology of parathyroid chief cell hyperplasia. *Am J Clin Pathol* 1970;53:565–579.
351. Akerström G, Bergström R, Grimeluis L, et al: Relation between

changes in clinical and histopathological features of primary hyperparathyroidism. *World J Surg* 1986;10:696–702.

352. Strauss FH, Kaplan EL, Nishiyama RH, Bigos ST: Five cases of parathyroid lipohyperplasia. *Surgery* 1983;94:901–905.

353. Reddick RL, Costa JC, Marx SJ: Parathyroid hyperplasia and parathyromatosis. *Lancet* 1977;1:549.

354. Bondeson AG, Bondeson L, Ljungberg O: Chronic parathyroiditis associated with parathyroid hyperplasia and hyperparathyroidism. *Am J Surg Pathol* 1984;8:211–215.

355. Mallette LE: Management of hyperparathyroidism in the multiple endocrine neoplasia syndromes and other familial endocrinopathies. *Endocrinol Metab Clin North Am* 1994;23:19–36.

356. Fallon MD, Haines JW, Teitelbaum SL: Cystic parathyroid gland hyperplasia: Hyperparathyroidism presenting as a neck mass. *Am J Clin Pathol* 1982;77:104–107.

357. Al-Sobhi S, Clark OH: Parathyroid hyperplasia: Parathyroidectomy. In: Clark OH, Duk Q-Y, eds. *Textbook of Endocrine Surgery.* Philadelphia: W.B. Saunders, 1997:372–379.

358. Klempa I, Frei U, Röttger P, et al: Parathyroid autografts—morphology and function: Six years' experience with parathyroid autotransplantation in uremic patients. *World J Surg* 1984;8:540–544.

359. Albright F, Bloomberg E, Castleman B, Churchill ED: Hyperparathyroidism due to diffuse hyperplasia of all parathyroid glands rather than adenoma of one. Clinical study on three such cases. *Arch Intern Med* 1934;54:315–329.

360. Roth SI: The ultrastructure of primary water-clear cell hyperplasia of the parathyroid glands. *Am J Pathol* 1970;61:233–248.

Secondary and Tertiary Hyperparathyroidism

361. Salusky IB, Ramirez JA, Coburn JW: The real osteodystrophies. In: DeGroot LJ, ed. *Endocrinology,* 3rd ed. Philadelphia: W.B. Saunders, 1995.

362. Falchetti A, Bale AE, Amorosi A, et al: Progress of uremic hyperparathyroidism involves allelic loss on chromosome 11. *J Clin Endocrinol Metab* 1993;76:139–144.

363. Shan L, Nakamura M, Nakamura Y, et al: Comparative analysis of clonality and pathology in primary and secondary hyperparathyroidism. *Virchows Arch* 1997;430:247–251.

364. Pappenheimer AM, Wilens SL: Enlargement of the parathyroid glands in renal disease. *Am J Pathol* 1935;11:73–91.

365. Roth SI, Marshall RB: Pathology and ultrastructure of the human parathyroid glands in chronic renal failure. *Arch Intern Med* 1969;124:397–407.

365a. Stehman-Breen C, Muirhead N, Thorning D, Sherrard D: Secondary hyperparathyroidism complicated by parathyromatosis. *Am J Kidney Dis* 1996;28:502–507.

366. Sancho JJ, Sitges-Serra A: Surgical approach to secondary hyperparathyroidism. In: Clark OH, ed. *Textbook of Endocrine Surgery.* Philadelphia: W.B. Saunders, 1997:403–409.

367. St. Goar WT: Case records of the Massachusetts General Hospital (Case 29-1963). *N Engl J Med* 1963;268:943–953.

368. Krause MW, Hedinger CE: Pathologic study of parathyroid glands in tertiary hyperparathyroidism. *Hum Pathol* 1985;16:772–784.

Secondary Tumors and Cysts

369. Horwitz CA, Myers WP, Foote FW: Secondary malignant tumors of the parathyroid glands. Report of two cases with associated hypoparathyroidism. *Am J Med* 1972;52:797–808.

370. de la Monte S, Hutchins GM, Moore GW: Endocrine organ metastases from breast carcinoma. *Am J Pathol* 1984;114:131–136.

371. Wick MR: Mediastinal cysts and intrathoracic thyroid tumors. *Semin Diagn Pathol* 1990;7:285–294.

372. Wang C, Vickery AL, Maloof F: Large parathyroid cysts mimicking thyroid nodules. *Ann Surg* 1972;175:448–453.

373. Calandra DB, Shah KH, Prinz RA, et al: Parathyroid cysts: A report of 11 cases including two associated with hyperparathyroid crisis. *Surgery* 1983;94:887–892.

Hypoparathyroidism and Pseudohypoparathyroidism

374. Conley ME, Beckwich JB, Mancer JF, Tenckhoff L: The spectrum of the DiGeorge syndrome. *J Pediatr* 1979;94:883–890.

375. Whyte MP: Autoimmune aspects of hypoparathyroidism. In: Bilezikian JP, Levine MA, Marcus R, eds. *The Parathyroids.* New York: Raven Press. 1994;753–764.

376. Levine MA, Schwindinger WF, Downs RW, Moses AM: Pseudoparathyroidism. Clinical, biochemical and molecular features. In: Bilezikian JP, ed. *The Parathyroids.* New York: Raven Press. 1994:781–800.

377. Mann JP, Alterman S, Hills AG: Albright's hereditary osteodystrophy comprising pseudohypoparathyroidism and pseudopseudohypoparathyroidism. *Ann Intern Med* 1962;56:315–342.

8 Soft Tissue and Bone Lesions

Samir K. El-Mofty and Michael Kyriakos

An encyclopedic discourse on all soft tissue and bone tumor or tumor-like conditions that may occur in the head and neck region, defined here as any anatomic location above the level of the clavicle, is beyond the scope of this chapter. However, some anomalies, including chordoma, embryonal rhabdomyosarcoma, spindle cell lipoma, and the benign neural tumors, occur relatively frequently in this region and, as in the case of fibromatosis colli, are even specific to the region. Others, including osteosarcoma, osteoblastoma, chondrosarcoma, and chondroblastoma, are relatively uncommon but produce significant histologic diagnostic problems when they do occur.

In this chapter we describe the clinical and radiologic manifestations, location, gross and histologic appearance, treatment, and therapeutic outcomes of some of the major bone and soft tissue lesions that affect this region. It is not our purpose to provide extensive descriptions on the gamut of histologic patterns that many of those lesions may assume; rather, their general histomorphology is given and, where appropriate, the important differential diagnostic features. For more detailed and expanded coverage of the individual lesions, and for those not discussed here, the reader is directed to the monographs and articles referenced in the general bibliography section on the clinical and pathologic aspects of bone and soft tissue lesions both in general, as well as for those in the head and neck region.[1–42]

SOFT TISSUE LESIONS

Fibrous Tissue Tumors and Tumor-Like Lesions

Fibrosarcoma

Fibrosarcoma was formerly considered the most common of the soft tissue sarcomas, but with better definition of lesions such as the fibromatoses and malignant fibrous histiocytoma, the number of tumors designated as fibrosarcoma has been considerably reduced.[43] In some reviews, from one third to one half of cases previously diagnosed as fibrosarcoma were found to represent other diagnostic categories.[44, 45]

Clinical Features. Fibrosarcoma occurs in all age groups, but most commonly affects adults between 40 and 70 years of age.[43–47] Congenital or infantile fibrosarcomas are defined in the World Health Organization classification as those that occur in patients less than 5 years of age. However, most are discovered at birth or within the first year of life.[5, 46–50] In general, male patients account for approximately 60% of fibrosarcomas.[44–47] Of 123 patients with fibrosarcoma of the head and neck region, 24% were under 21 years of age.[51, 52]

The head and neck is involved in 2% to 20% of cases of fibrosarcoma,[43, 44, 46, 47, 51, 53, 54] and 13% to 19% of infantile and congenital cases.[46, 47, 49] The most common sites within this region include the face, neck, scalp, paranasal sinuses, mandible, and larynx, with rare examples in the nasal cavity, nasopharynx, and intraoral region.[51, 52, 55–60]

Fibrosarcoma usually develops as a slowly growing, painless mass that may be present for several years. It takes origin from either the superficial fascial connective tissue or the deep subcutaneous tissue; in the head and neck, however, it may be deeply situated.[45, 55]

Pathologic Features. The tumor may appear well circumscribed and on section is firm, gray-white, and lobulated.[8, 45] In infants and young children it tends to be more friable and less well circumscribed.[44, 46] Areas of necrosis and hemorrhage are present in the less well differentiated tumors. Tumor size is dependent on location, with the more superficial tumors in the range of from 3.0 to 4.0 cm, whereas the deeper tumors are larger.[44–47]

Microscopically, fibrosarcoma is composed of spindle-shaped cells arranged in intersecting fascicles, which, in the well-differentiated tumors, create a characteristic herringbone pattern (Fig. 8–1A, see p. 507).[8, 44, 45, 47] Nuclei are tapered and usually uniform without significant atypia (Fig. 8–1B, see p. 507); the presence of many large and atypical bizarre tumor giant cells excludes the diagnosis of fibrosarcoma. The cytoplasm tends to be ill-defined, with poorly formed cell borders. Reticulin and collagen production is most prominent in the well-differentiated tumors and may lead to hyalinized areas with wide separation of the tumor cells.[8, 44, 47] In less well-differentiated tumors there is a decreased amount of stromal collagen, with increased cellularity and crowding of the cells, and a greater tendency to necrosis.[8, 44, 47] In these tumors, the cells are less uniform, being less often spindle-shaped with greater cell-to-cell variation in size than in the well-differentiated tumors, and there is increased mitotic activity. Congenital or infantile fibrosarcomas tend to be less differentiated with loss of the herringbone pattern, contain cells that are rounder and less spindle-shaped, have a decreased amount of collagen and a greater degree of vascularity than those in adults,[44, 46] and contain foci of necrosis (Fig. 8–2, see p. 508).

Fibrosarcoma lends itself to histologic grading based on its degree of differentiation, and may be classified as well, moderately, or poorly differentiated, or given a numerical grade, I to IV, with grade IV indicating the least degree of differentiation. Most fibrosarcomas are moderately differentiated, grades II to III.[44, 45, 47] In adults, this grading system has prognostic implications, as it correlates with the incidence of local recurrence, metastases, and survival, the better differentiated tumors having the best prognosis.[8, 43, 45, 53, 54]

Electron microscopically, fibrosarcomas contain fibroblasts as well as occasional myofibroblasts.[61, 62] Immunohistochemical stains are of little diagnostic help except in a negative sense, as the cells are reactive only for vimentin and not for markers present in other tumor types.[56] Cytogenetic analysis has demonstrated gains (trisomies) in chromosomes 8, 11, 17, and 20 in infantile fibrosarcomas, but not in those in adults.[58, 63]

Differential Diagnosis. A diagnosis of fibrosarcoma based on a small biopsy sample may prove incorrect because other sarcomas, such as synovial sarcoma, malignant peripheral nerve sheath tumor, malignant fibrous histiocytoma, and rhabdomyosarcoma, may contain fibroblastic or spindle cell foci that mimic fibrosarcoma.[56]

Smith et al.[64] described six cases of a spindle cell tumor that they designated as myofibrosarcoma. The tumor occurred in the head and neck region of children, 7.5 to 18 years of age, and had the light microscopic appearance of a fibrosarcoma with a herringbone pattern and abundant collagen, but also with storiform foci and areas of pleomorphic, high-grade tumor. By electron microscopy the cells lacked skeletal muscle features and appeared to be myofibroblastic; immunohistochemically, the tumor cells stained with smooth muscle markers. Four of the six patients died of tumor, one with metastases, while two were alive 13 months and 8 years after excision of the tumor.

The histologic separation of fibrosarcoma from the more common benign fibromatoses, as well as from benign and reactive fibroblastic lesions, is a major problem. This is especially true when dealing with childhood fibrous lesions. Indeed, the distinction between a cellular fibromatosis with increased mitotic activity and a fibrosarcoma may be impossible.[49, 65] The finding of significant mitotic activity, nuclear atypia, and foci of necrosis are factors that favor a diagnosis of fibrosarcoma. Some reports on head and neck fibrosarcoma may be misleading because of their inclusion of cases of infiltrative fibromatosis under the heading of low-grade fibrosarcoma.[50, 52] Although locally aggressive, fibromatosis, unlike fibrosarcoma, does not metastasize.

Treatment and Prognosis. Wide local excision is the therapy of choice for fibrosarcoma. Recurrence rates range from 25% to 75%, with the higher rates for tumors that are poorly differentiated, larger than 5.0 cm, and present at the surgical margins of excision.[43, 51, 57] Approximately 50% of patients with fibrosarcoma develop distant metastases, some developing more than 20 years after therapy.[43, 45] In head and neck fibrosarcomas, distant metastases are reported in 20% to 25% of cases.[51, 52, 55] The metastatic rate increases with increasing tumor grade.[43, 51] However, Fu and Perzin[60] found that only 1 of their 10 patients with nasal cavity, paranasal sinus, or nasopharyngeal fibrosarcoma developed metastases. Regional lymph node involvement occurs in less than 10% of cases, with some series containing no examples of lymph node metastases[8, 45, 52, 53, 55]; prophylactic radical lymph node dissection has no place in the treatment of fibrosarcoma.

Overall 5- and 10-year survival rates for fibrosarcomas of all anatomic sites range from 50% to 60%.[8, 45, 53] In the report of head and neck fibrosarcoma by Swain et al.,[55] 12 of 16 patients with well-differentiated tumors who were adequately treated for cure survived, but only one of five patients with poorly differentiated tumors did so. Those patients with superficial tumors, which tended to be better differentiated, had the best prognosis. Fibrosarcomas of the head and neck appear to have a poorer prognosis than those of extremity origin, despite the fact that most are well-differentiated.[51, 53] This probably reflects the limited type of resection possible in this region with resultant positive surgical margins.[51, 60]

Unlike adult fibrosarcoma, the prognosis in children cannot be predicted on the basis of the tumor's histology.[5, 46, 47] In general, fibrosarcomas in children have a more favorable prognosis, than those in adults, with 5-year survival rates as high as 80% to 85%, despite local recurrence rates of up to 50% after wide local excision.[5, 46, 47] Few patients with childhood fibrosarcoma have died of metastatic disease,[46, 47, 49, 50, 66] with reported metastatic rates of from 0% to 10%.[5, 46, 47, 49, 50] The younger the child, the more favorable the prognosis.[47] However, this may reflect the inclusion of cases of locally aggressive, non-metastasizing fibromatosis that is difficult to distinguish from fibrosarcoma in this age group (see Infantile Fibromatosis section). Older children (older than 10 years) have the less favorable survival rates of adults.[5, 47]

Fibromatosis

The fibromatoses are a diverse group of non-metastasizing, locally invasive fibroblastic or myofibroblastic lesions, many of which tend to recur after resection.[67, 68] They arise in a wide variety of anatomic locations and in all age groups; however, some occur exclusively or predominantly in infants and young children, whereas others are more frequent in adults, leading to their broad classification as in-

fantile or juvenile fibromatoses, and adult fibromatoses (i.e., those occurring in patients over the age of 20 years).[67, 69]

As a group, the adult forms are more common than the juvenile types. However, one should not view this classification as a strict division, as some of the "adult" fibromatoses, such as the desmoid lesions, also occur in young children, and, conversely, some of the infantile and juvenile types, such as myofibromatosis, are also encountered in adults. Unfortunately, the generic designation of infantile or juvenile fibromatosis has been used by some authors as a specific histologic diagnosis for any fibromatosis in a child, without further amplification, resulting in a sea of terminologic confusion. To designate a patient as having a juvenile or infantile fibromatosis is of little value without an indication as to the specific type present. If a tumor in a young child has the light microscopic features of an adult-type desmoid, then it should be designated as such and not as a "juvenile fibromatosis." If a lesion in a child is histologically acceptable as a fibromatosis, and it cannot be placed within any of the specific infantile/juvenile categories, then it should be designated as a desmoid type fibromatosis. We avoid the use of such terms as aggressive fibromatosis or fibrosarcoma-like fibromatosis (see Infantile/Juvenile Fibromatosis section).

The head and neck region may be the site of origin for a variety of fibromatoses, only a few of which are described here; the reader is referred to the excellent reviews and articles in the bibliography for more comprehensive coverage.[66–69]

Desmoid Fibromatosis (Desmoid Tumor)

The desmoid fibromatoses are arbitrarily divided into those that arise in the anterior abdominal wall and those located elsewhere, the "extra-abdominal" desmoids, also designated as "aggressive" fibromatoses.[67, 69, 70] All, regardless of site, are also known simply as a desmoid tumor and are histologically identical.

Clinical Features. Desmoids occur in people of all ages, from infants to patients in the eighth decade of life, but most patients are in the third or fourth decades of life.[8, 67, 69–78] Unlike abdominal desmoids, which are unusual in those under 20 years of age, approximately 15% to 30% of extra-abdominal lesions occur in children.[5, 67, 68, 70, 75, 79, 80] In a series of 34 head and neck desmoids, patients ranged from 18 months to 72 years of age; 30 of the patients developed their lesion by age 50 years.[78] In another series of head and neck cases, patients ranged from newborn to 70 years with 25% younger than 15 years of age.[76] Fibromatosis of the oral and paraoral tissues most often occurs in young patients, most of whom are in the first decade of life.[79, 80]

Although abdominal wall desmoids are far more frequent in women,[68] there is less of a sex difference in the extra-abdominal lesions, with some series showing a female preponderance while in others men were equally affected.[8, 67–71, 74, 76, 78, 81]

The head and neck region accounts for approximately 10% to 30% of all desmoid cases.[67, 68, 77–79, 81–83] Among 367 cases accessioned at the Armed Forces Institute of Pathology (AFIP), 35 (10%) were so located.[8]

Within the head and neck, 40% to 85% of desmoid tumors occur in the neck, usually the upper neck[78]; other reported sites include the face, scalp, oral and nasal cavities, paranasal sinuses, tongue, submandibular and submental areas, orbit and infraorbital regions, cheek, parotid region, tonsillar area, nasopharynx, gingiva, lip, and floor of mouth.[8, 73, 76, 78–82, 84] The supraclavicular fossa is also a common location, either as a primary site, or from secondary involvement by desmoids extending upward from the shoulder-girdle area.[8, 70, 78, 80]

Clinically, desmoids are firm to hard masses that may be tender or painful, although most are painless.[70, 72, 74, 76, 77, 79, 83] Most enlarge slowly, but those in the head and neck may develop rapidly.[76, 78] Desmoids also develop in surgical scars and in sites that received prior radiation therapy[8, 67, 75, 85]; multicentric lesions occur,[74, 86, 87] as do familial cases.[88] There is an increased incidence of desmoid tumors in patients with Gardner's syndrome, in which the

Text continued on page 515

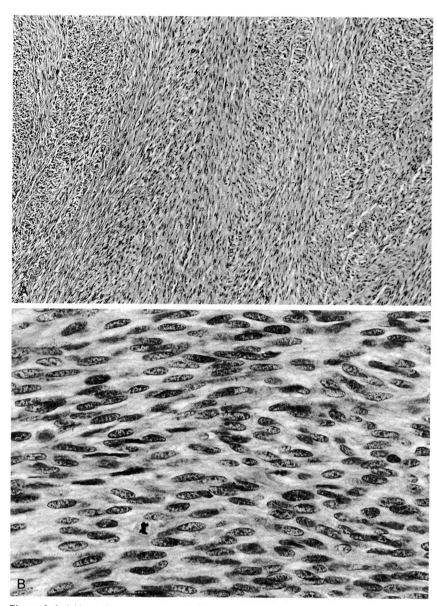

Figure 8–1. *A,* Herringbone pattern in well-differentiated adult fibrosarcoma. Even at this low power, mitotic figures are easily seen. *B,* Compact area in adult fibrosarcoma shows uniform, tapered-cell nuclei without significant atypia. Cell boundaries are indistinct. A mitotic figure is seen.

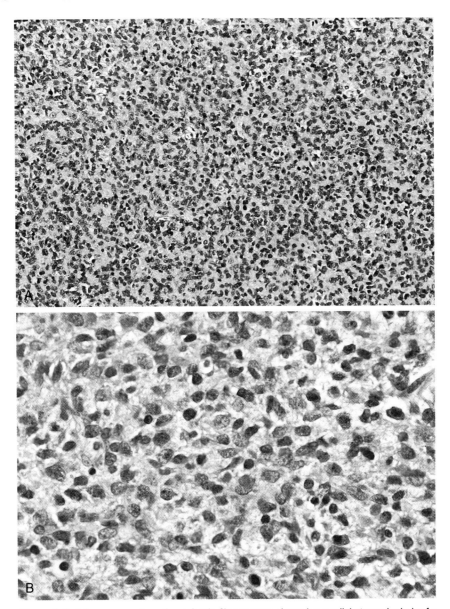

Figure 8–2. A, Low power view of an infantile fibrosarcoma shows hypercellularity and a lack of a herringbone pattern. B, Cells of infantile fibrosarcoma have round to oval nuclei, with less cytoplasm and collagen formation than in adult fibrosarcoma.

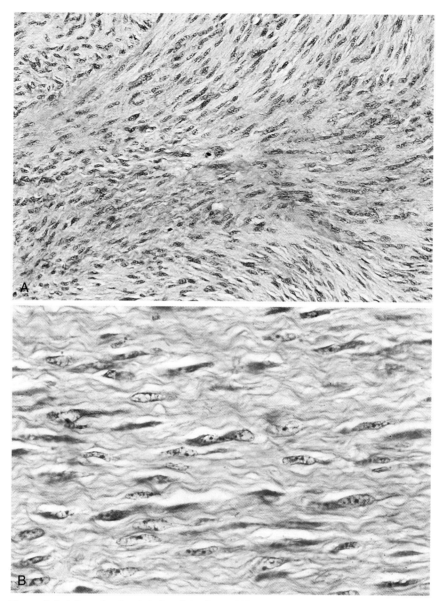

Figure 8–3. *A*, Example of a relatively cellular desmoid fibromatosis with cells arranged in interlacing fascicles. Such lesions must be distinguished from well-differentiated fibrosarcoma. *B*, High-power view of a desmoid fibromatosis shows cells with uniform spindled nuclei, well separated by relatively abundant collagen fibers. Mitotic activity is absent.

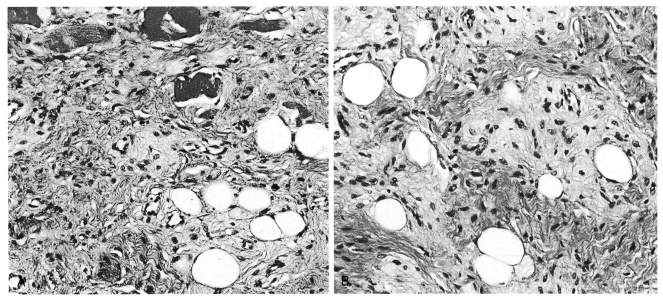

Figure 8–4. *A,* Infantile desmoid fibromatosis shows infiltration and replacement of skeletal muscle by mature fibroblasts, with collagen formation, as well as fat- and light-staining myxoid areas. *B,* Higher-power view of infantile desmoid fibromatosis shows collagenous areas and fat mixed with myxoid foci containing immature fibroblasts.

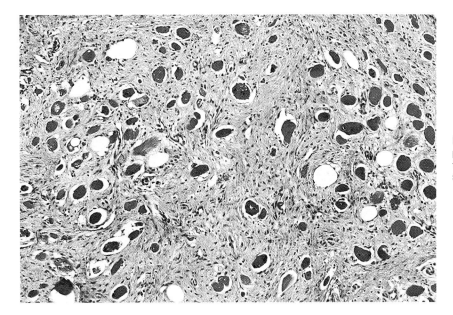

Figure 8–5. Fibromatosis colli. Muscle is partially replaced by fibrous tissue that dissects between and entraps individual muscle fibers, which show various stages of degeneration.

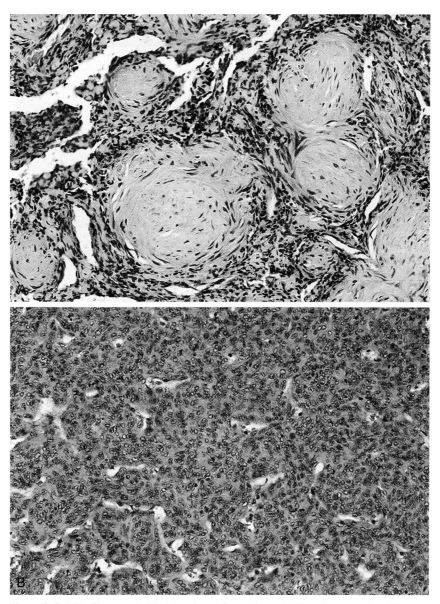

Figure 8–6. *A,* Myofibromatosis. Nodular whorls of smooth muscle–like cells are enveloped by compact, immature-appearing stromal cells associated with slit-like vascular spaces. *B,* Myofibromatosis. Hemangiopericytomatous focus composed of round to oval cells with indistinct cytoplasmic borders, interspersed with slit-like vascular spaces.

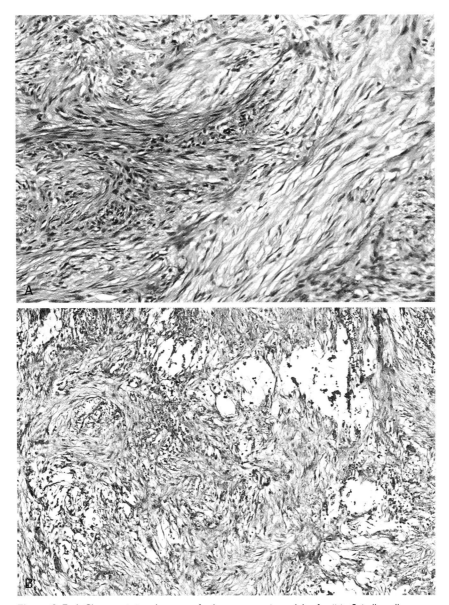

Figure 8–7. *A,* Characteristic, edematous, feathery pattern in nodular fasciitis. Spindle cells are arranged in sweeping fascicles. *B,* Loose arrangement of spindle cells in nodular fasciitis. Irregular cystic spaces, containing extravasated red blood cells, are present. The spaces contain hyaluronic acid.

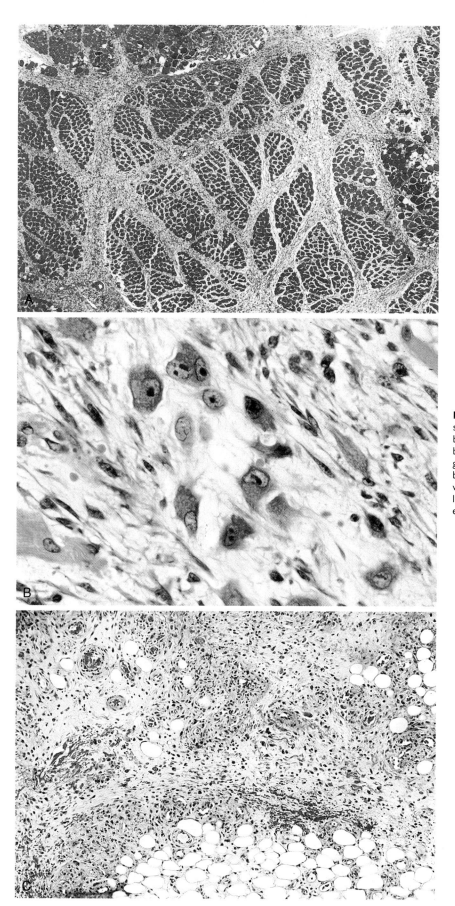

Figure 8–8. *A,* Low-power view of proliferative myositis shows a checkerboard-like pattern created by fibrous proliferation encasing muscle bundles. *B,* Large, basophilic cells, with a superficial resemblance to ganglion cells, are loosely scattered within the myxoid fibrous septae in proliferative myositis. *C,* Low-power view of proliferative fasciitis shows fibrovascular proliferation involving the fascia, associated with a proliferation of oval to pyramidal cells.

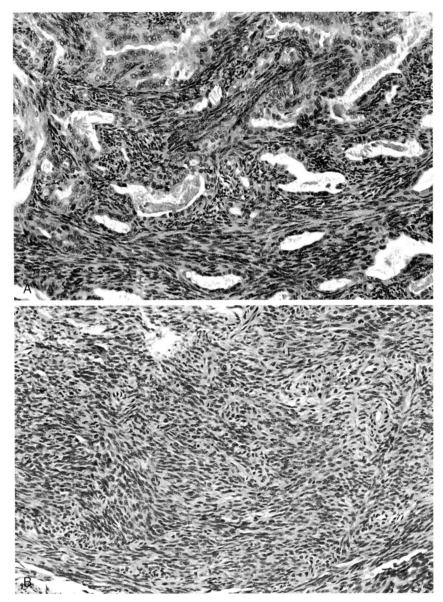

Figure 8–9. *A*, Biphasic synovial sarcoma characterized by intimate mixture of pale, epithelial-like cells forming glands within a spindle cell stroma. Some glandular spaces contain blue, mucinous material. *B*, Monophasic synovial sarcoma composed only of fibrosarcomatous spindle cell elements. The diagnosis of synovial sarcoma would depend on the demonstration of epithelial features in the cells by electron microscopy or immunohistochemistry.

desmoid lesion may develop either prior to or after the appearance of the intestinal polyps.[67, 68, 71, 72]

Pathologic Features. Grossly, desmoids are gray-white, whorled or trabeculated masses, usually with ill-defined margins,[67, 70, 76, 77, 79] that develop within muscle, aponeurotic tissue, or fascia.[8, 77, 83] They infiltrate skeletal muscle and microscopically extend beyond it to advance along the fascia,[70, 77, 83] such that the histologic extent may be several centimeters beyond the grossly visible limit,[68] an important consideration if adequate surgical excision is to be achieved. In desmoids of the sinonasal tract, destructive infiltration of bone is common.[81]

Microscopically, desmoids are composed of mature, uniform, spindle-shaped cells, arranged in interlacing bands and fascicles, surrounded and separated by a variable amount of collagenous stroma (Fig. 8–3, see p. 509).[67, 70, 77, 78, 82, 83] The lesion invades muscle and tendon, separating and pushing aside muscle fibers, many of which undergo atrophy and disappear. The cellularity varies from hypocellular hyalinized foci, which are sometimes myxoid, to compact cellular regions.[70, 78] The cells lack pleomorphism (see Fig. 8–3B), and mitoses are not common but may be more frequent in childhood lesions.[67, 70, 77–79, 82, 83] The lack of pleomorphism and significant mitotic activity helps distinguish the usual adult desmoid from fibrosarcoma, although at times a very cellular fibromatosis that contains a few mitotic figures may be difficult or impossible to distinguish from a well-differentiated fibrosarcoma.[49, 65, 69] Aggregates of lymphocytes are frequently present at the peripheral margin of a desmoid and may help distinguish it from reactive fibrosis, which lacks such aggregates.

By electron microscopy, desmoids contain both fibroblasts and myofibroblasts, the latter at times being the dominant cells.[86, 89] Approximately 50% of desmoid tumors show chromosomal abnormalities, with deletion of the long arm of chromosome 5 the most frequent structural abnormality, as well as trisomies for chromosomes 8 and 20.[90, 91] Molecular genetic analysis of female patients with desmoid tumors demonstrated nonrandom inactivation of the X chromosome consistent with a clonal process, indicating that these lesions are neoplastic and not reactive.[92]

Treatment and Prognosis. The major difficulty encountered in the treatment of desmoid tumor is its high rate of local recurrence, from 19% to 77%, following excision, with multiple recurrences not uncommon.[67, 68, 70, 72, 74, 75, 78, 79–83, 86] In the head and neck region, local recurrence develops in 50% to 70% of patients.[76, 78, 81] Here, the recurrence rate is higher for those in the neck (60%) than for other sites, and it is less than 25% for oral and sinonasal lesions.[81] As might be expected, recurrence rates depend on the adequacy of the original resection, with recurrences in up to 90% of those cases treated by lesional or marginal resection.[74] In most recurrences, the initial resection was usually incomplete.[75, 76, 78, 83] Even with wide resections, recurrences are reported in 19% to 40% of cases.[76, 77] Most recurrences develop within 2 years of the original operation.[8, 70, 72, 74] However, it should be emphasized that not all desmoids with positive surgical margins recur.[93]

Although desmoids are non-metastasizing lesions, patients have died from local invasion of vital structures in the neck, tracheal compression, or mediastinal extension.[60, 67, 75, 77, 78] Death from desmoid fibromatosis is not common, however.

Desmoids have also been successfully treated with a variety of medications, including nonsteroidal anti-inflammatory agents, ascorbic acid, progesterone, tamoxifen, and colchicine.[71, 94–96] High-dose external radiation therapy for either inoperable or recurrent lesions, or as a surgical adjuvant for large primary tumors, has also been successfully employed, yielding complete or partial responses in from approximately 65% to 90% of cases.[67, 70, 73, 78, 93, 97, 98]

Chemotherapeutic agents have been employed to reduce tumor size preoperatively; for treatment of tumors not amenable to surgical attack; and for recurrent tumors, with objective responses in the majority of patients, some of whom have achieved complete tumor regression.[82, 99, 100]

Infantile and Juvenile Fibromatosis (Juvenile Aggressive Fibromatosis, Infantile Desmoid Fibromatosis, Congenital Fibrosarcoma-Like Fibromatosis)

A variety of specific fibromatoses occur in children that have well-defined clinical presentations and anatomic locations and histomorphology. Unfortunately, all too often the occurrence of a benign fibroblastic lesion in a child leads to its appellation as an "infantile" or "juvenile" fibromatosis simply because of the patient's age, the terms used in a diagnostic sense rather than more properly as nonspecific terms for the broad range of fibromatoses that occur in childhood.[101] Any fibromatosis that cannot be assigned to a specific diagnostic category should be designated as a musculoaponeurotic fibromatosis, regardless of the age of the patient.

The histology of these nonspecific childhood lesions may be identical to that in adults, or have a more cellular or immature appearance, and be more mitotically active to the degree that their distinction from infantile or juvenile fibrosarcoma is a major problem. Use of the term *aggressive*, which is frequently appended to these lesions,[102–109] is an unnecessary redundancy, as all of the usual fibromatoses, with the notable exception of fibromatosis colli, are locally aggressive lesions with diffuse destructive infiltration of soft tissue, muscle, or bone, and a high incidence of local recurrence. Although we have some sympathy for the term "fibrosarcoma-like fibromatosis" as an appellation for some of the highly cellular, mitotically active fibroblastic lesions that occur in children,[67] we prefer not to use it as it may be prone to being misinterpreted as a true fibrosarcoma. Unfortunately, one frequently cannot determine in many of these lesions whether it is a fibrosarcoma or a fibromatosis.[49, 66, 68]

Our discussion of these nonspecific childhood forms of fibromatoses in a separate section, apart from the desmoid tumors, may thus seem contradictory. However, as much of the literature on these lesions exists under the designations of infantile, juvenile, or aggressive fibromatosis, it is appropriate to provide a summary of their features as they occur in the head and neck. The terms *juvenile* or *infantile* fibromatosis are used almost exclusively in this section as the designation for these nonspecific fibromatoses but only as a convenience, reflecting their use by reports in the literature.

Clinical Features. One third of juvenile fibromatoses occur in the head and neck,[5, 8, 66, 110] with approximately 50% of congenital fibromatoses in this site.[66, 111, 112] Two thirds of oral and paraoral fibromatoses occur in the first decade of life.[79] Most cases of so-called aggressive fibromatosis occur within the first 2 years of life,[67, 102–104] with occasional cases in older children.[103, 105, 108, 112–114] A particular histologic variant, infantile desmoid fibromatosis, usually occurs during the first 3 years of life,[67, 115, 116] with only rare cases in older children.[8]

As with most fibromatoses, the presenting symptom is that of a firm to hard mass that is usually painless,[76, 79, 102, 107, 113] but on occasion may be painful.[79, 109] Although slow growth is usual for most fibromatoses, those in the head and neck may develop in a matter of a few weeks to a few months.[76, 79, 84, 108, 114, 117, 118]

Virtually every site in the head and neck region has been involved, with the most common sites being the soft tissues of the neck,[76, 110, 119] the submandibular and paramandibular region,[76, 102, 103, 108, 109, 114, 115, 117, 118] the tongue,[79, 106, 110, 112] the parotid region,[79, 103, 107, 110] and the cheek.[76, 79, 103] Other reported sites include the face[76, 110]; nasal and paranasal region[104]; paranasal sinus[76]; lower eyelid and infraorbital region[84, 113]; alveolus[79, 84, 109, 110, 114]; floor of mouth[79, 116]; tonsillar and retromolar region[79, 104, 109, 110]; lip[76, 79]; nasopharynx[79, 104]; palate[79, 109]; larynx[116]; scalp[110]; and infratemporal region.[76]

Pathologic Features. The childhood head and neck lesions do not differ in their gross appearance from those in adults, being firm, hard to rubbery, nonencapsulated masses that infiltrate soft tissue and muscle,[66, 84, 102, 103, 107, 108, 113–115] with invasion of adjacent bone frequently found.[79, 102, 103, 105, 109, 114, 115, 117] Many are less than 5.0 cm in size,[76, 79, 102, 106, 108, 113, 114, 116] but those of greater size occur,[79, 103, 105, 107, 114, 118, 119] some as large as 14 cm.[103]

Histologically, nonspecific fibromatosis of childhood is morphologically diverse. One form in very young children, usually infants, has been designated as diffuse or mesenchymal and is considered to be the infantile type of desmoid tumor. It is composed of immature, round to oval mesenchymal cells that are haphazardly arranged in a myxoid stroma associated with skeletal muscle fibers and, at times, abundant fat (Fig. 8–4, see p. 510).[8, 67, 79, 106, 115, 119] Other infantile and juvenile fibromatoses are densely cellular, with interlacing fascicles or whorls of spindle-shaped, mitotically active cells. Slit-like vascular spaces are frequently found within the centers of the fascicles. Still others are less cellular with a more abundant collagenous stroma and resemble the adult form of desmoid tumor. All of these lesions are infiltrative with involvement of skeletal muscle and may extend along the fascia and aponeurosis and invade bone.

Treatment and Prognosis. The histology of most of these childhood fibromatoses is not predictive of future aggressive behavior.[5, 8, 66] Following surgical excision, local recurrence develops in 25% to 40% of cases,[79, 109, 113] and usually occurs within a matter of a few months after excision,[79, 109, 113] although several years may elapse before it becomes manifest.[66] Inadequate excision with positive surgical margins is associated, as it is in adult desmoid tumors, with a high incidence of local recurrence, but this is not an invariable event, as some incompletely excised lesions have not recurred.[105, 110, 115, 116] A higher incidence of local recurrence is reported for lesions that contain more slit-like blood vessels or a high proportion of immature mesenchymal cells.[119] Spontaneous regression following biopsy is also reported.[8, 102, 115]

Rare cases of death due to direct invasion of vital structures has occurred.[101] Although metastases are reported from examples of "aggressive" fibromatosis, this violates the basic definition of a fibromatosis as a non-metastasizing lesion and such lesions must be considered as fibrosarcomas.[76] Such occurrences emphasize our inability, based on current methodology, to clearly distinguish some of the fibromatoses from congenital infantile or juvenile fibrosarcoma.[66] In debatable cases, it appears preferable to diagnose the lesion as a fibrosarcoma, with an explanation that despite such a diagnosis the lesion may not clinically behave as a malignancy. Indeed, from a clinical point of view, the overwhelming majority of these nonspecific fibromatoses in the head and neck region, regardless of their histology, ultimately are cured by surgical means.[8, 66, 79, 102, 103, 105, 109, 110, 113–115]

Fibromatosis Colli (Sternocleidomastoid Tumor)

Fibromatosis colli, also known as sternocleidomastoid tumor (SCMT), is the most common of the juvenile fibromatoses.[66] SCMT is unique among the fibromatoses not only in its selectivity for the sternocleidomastoid muscle but also for its lack of extension beyond the muscle. As a result, some prefer to consider SCMT separately from the fibromatoses as some form of benign fibrous proliferation.[8, 54]

Clinically, the most significant manifestation of SCMT is its ability to produce a torticollis ("wry-neck"). There are several forms of torticollis, including congenital and acquired varieties, that may be caused by neurologic, traumatic, infectious, or neoplastic conditions, and SCMT is only one such cause. Unfortunately, in the literature torticollis is frequently equated with SCMT, when it is only the clinical result of that condition. Furthermore, not all cases of SCMT result in clinical torticollis; the incidence of SCMT as a cause of congenital torticollis varies from 14% to 23% of cases.[120] In a review of 624 cases of infantile torticollis, Cheng et al.[121] found 35% to be associated with SCMT.

Clinical Features. SCMT is rarely discovered at birth but usually becomes evident within the following several weeks, the mean time to development being 3.0 to 3.5 weeks.[122–128] In a study of

7835 infants, SCMT was found in 30 (0.4%).[127] A history of difficult labor or breech presentation is present in 40% to 50% of cases, but whether birth trauma is involved in the pathogenesis of the lesion is unknown[120, 122, 123, 125–128]; SCMT has occurred in children delivered by cesarean section.[123, 125, 128]

An SCMT develops as an olive-shaped or oval tumor mass within the lower third of the sternocleidomastoid muscle, in either its sternal or clavicular heads, and frequently both[128, 129]; the mastoid insertion is rarely involved.[66, 126] The lesion may be so inconspicuous that it is overlooked by the child's parents and is discovered only during a well-baby examination.[127] The tumor slowly increases in size for a few months and then, in most cases, gradually regresses and disappears in 4 to 6 months.[66, 121, 127, 130] SCMT is usually movable, may be somewhat tender, and, as stated previously, may be associated with torticollis. In the presence of torticollis the head is tilted toward the side of the involved muscle, and the face is turned away from the affected side. There is no statistical difference in terms of the side affected[122]; rarely, the condition is bilateral.[122] As the tumor grows, asymmetry of the face and head (plagiocephaly) may develop.[120, 124, 127, 129] A 14% incidence of ipsilateral congenital dislocation of the hip has been reported in patients with muscular torticollis.[130] Hip dysplasia associated with congenital torticollis was found in 11% to 14% of cases, but an SCMT was present in only a minority of the patients.[129, 131] Computed tomography or sonography may allow a confident diagnosis, in the appropriate clinical setting, by localizing a neck mass to the sternocleidomastoid muscle.[122]

Pathologic Features. In those children with SCMT who require surgery, the tumor consists of a firm, spindle-shaped, 0.5 to 3.0 cm mass that has a glistening, white, tendon-like appearance, located within the belly of the muscle.[66, 123, 125, 126] Microscopically, one sees replacement of muscle fibers, which are in various stages of degeneration, by immature-appearing cellular fibrous tissue (Fig. 8–5, see p. 510).[66, 123, 125, 126] Mitoses are rare,[66] and hemosiderin pigment, a marker of possible previous trauma, may be detected; however, it is never a prominent feature, and has been noted to be absent by some authors.[66, 125, 126] In older children, the fibrous tissue is eventually replaced by noncellular, collagenous scar-like tissue in which are scattered remnants of muscle fibers.[66] The fibrosis is either focal or diffusely present in the muscle but does not extend beyond its borders. The process may resemble a desmoid tumor,[124] however, the latter is more cellular than SCMT and its cells are in broad sheets or fascicles, rather than the less defined proliferation of fibrous tissue in SCMT, and it lacks the large areas of noncellular collagen that occurs in SCMT. The relatively large numbers of entrapped individual muscle fibers in SCMT (see Fig. 8–5) also differs from desmoid tumor, which tends to push aside muscle fibers.[54] The lack of extension of SCMT beyond the boundaries of the muscle is also in sharp contrast with the usual diffuse infiltrative behavior of desmoid tumor.

The importance of fibromatosis colli also lies in not confusing it with the infantile desmoid tumor of soft tissue,[8, 67] an infiltrative, destructive lesion that requires excision (see previous section). Radiologic studies to exclude the diagnosis of fibromatosis colli should be done whenever dealing with a cervical soft tissue mass in a child.

Treatment and Prognosis. The proper treatment for SCMT is controversial, with some advocating early surgical intervention in infants, and others proposing the use of conservative physical therapy.[120, 122, 124, 125, 129, 131] Because over 80% of these tumors that develop in infants spontaneously regress, operative management is usually not required,[120, 121, 127] surgical intervention being reserved for those patients with persistent and deforming torticollis or for those who develop progressive torticollis at an older age.[128]

Myofibromatosis (Congenital Generalized Fibromatosis; Infantile Myofibromatosis)

Among congenital mesenchymal tumors, Kauffman and Stout[112] found the fibromatoses to be second in incidence only to vascular tumors. Of the solitary fibromatoses in their study, 50% arose in the head and neck area. A similar distribution was found by Coffin and Dehner[132] among 190 soft tissue tumors in the first year of life, where fibroblastic-myofibroblastic lesions accounted for 27% of the cases. The lesion previously designated as congenital generalized or congenital solitary fibromatosis,[101] and now more commonly referred to as infantile myofibromatosis,[133] is the most frequent of the fibromatoses in infancy.[111, 134]

Myofibroma, as its name implies, is a myofibroblastic lesion that usually arises in the subcutaneous tissue or muscle. It usually occurs as multiple lesions widely distributed over the body, including the bones, but without visceral involvement; or in a generalized form that also involves the viscera.[66, 101, 112, 135–139] Some authors have used the terms *multiple, diffuse,* or *generalized* to refer either to cases in which more than one lesion is present or to those in which there is visceral involvement, causing some terminologic confusion. We prefer the classification of Rosenberg et al.,[66] who divided their cases into multiple and visceral forms, *multiple* designating those tumors that involve the skin, subcutaneous tissue, muscle, or bone and *visceral* for cases in which there is organ involvement.

As the histomorphology of the multiple forms became better recognized, it was found that a solitary form also existed that usually occurs in either the skin or subcutaneous tissue, or as an isolated skeletal lesion.[140–153] Indeed, in some series the solitary form is the most common type encountered.[133]

Clinical Features. The lesions of myofibromatosis are almost always present at birth or noted shortly thereafter, although new lesions may subsequently develop.[66, 133, 138] Approximately 70% to 90% of cases are found within the first two decades of life.[111, 133, 134, 143, 144, 146, 154] However, similar lesions have also been found in adults, with some patients in the seventh and eighth decades of life.[66, 133, 134, 138, 141–143, 146–148, 150, 151, 153, 154] The visceral forms of the disease, however, apparently occur only in newborns or neonates, while the adult or juvenile cases tend to be solitary. Familial cases have been reported, with either an autosomal recessive, or an autosomal dominant transmission with reduced penetrance suggested as the mode of inheritance.[133, 135, 147]

The superficial lesions involve the skin and subcutaneous tissue and appear as firm to rubbery, well-delimited nodules[142, 151, 154] that may be solitary or multiple, with some patients having as many as 100 lesions widely distributed over the body surface.[66, 67] The more superficial nodules may have a purplish hue and simulate a hemangioma.[133, 154] The nodules are small, usually less than 3.0 cm, but some as large as 9.0 cm are reported.[111, 133, 134, 138, 141–143] Intramuscular lesions tend to be well circumscribed, and may even shell out easily at the time of operation, but occasionally appear to infiltrate the soft tissue.[66, 67, 133, 155] Both the superficial and intramuscular varieties may contain central necrotic foci, some with calcification.[66, 67, 133, 138, 139] Intraosseous lesions, which may occur in any bone, are radiolucent and, in older lesions, frequently have a sclerotic border. Bone involvement is quite common in both the multiple and visceral forms of the disease, occurring in over 60% of those with multiple lesions and in almost half of those with visceral lesions.[66, 156, 157] Bone lesions associated with the multiple or visceral forms of the disease usually occur in the metaphysis of the long bones,[133, 146, 156] whereas solitary bone lesions most frequently occur in the craniofacial bones with only occasional cases in the long bones.[137, 144, 146, 148, 149, 153]

Infantile myofibromatosis occurs in any area of the body, with a predilection for the head and neck, trunk, extremities, and shoulder girdle region.[66, 67, 132, 138] Within the head and neck, cases are reported in the scalp, orbit, parotid region, tongue, larynx, eyelid, retromolar region, buccal mucosa, nasal ala, face, sublingual region, subretinal fundus, gingiva, eyebrow, anterior floor of mouth, mandible, and ear canal.[133, 135, 136, 138, 140–143, 145, 147, 148, 150, 151, 153, 155, 158] At the AFIP, the head and neck region was involved in 16 of 45 solitary lesions (36%), with the scalp and skull involved in 6, the forehead and orbit in 5, the cheek-parotid region in 2, and the neck in 3 patients;

at least 4 of 16 patients with multicentric lesions also had head and neck involvement, and 4 other patients with generalized disease had lesions widely distributed over the body surface, presumably also including the head and neck region.[133]

Pathologic Features. Histologically, in contrast to desmoid tumors, the spindle-shaped mesenchymal cells of myofibroma have a more immature appearance than the cells of desmoid tumor. The lesion frequently has a distinct zonal growth pattern, with the periphery composed of spindle-shaped fibroblastic cells and plump smooth muscle-like cells arranged in bands, whorls, or fascicles (Fig. 8–6A, see p. 511). These cells may merge with the smooth muscle in the walls of adjacent blood vessels, or actually invade into their lumens. Hyalin or chondroid-like hypocellular foci may alternate with more cellular areas. The more central region of the lesion may show bland necrosis and focal or diffuse calcification, such necrosis being unique among the fibromatoses. The central zone may contain polyhedral cells with somewhat pleomorphic nuclei and often has a prominent vascular pattern, with slit-like spaces, creating a hemangiopericytoma-like appearance (Fig. 8–6B, see p. 511). Mitotic figures vary from numerous to scant or absent.[66, 67, 133, 135, 138, 139, 141–143, 150, 151, 159] In some cases, this usual zonal pattern is reversed.[141] Because of the occasional occurrence of cells with pleomorphic nuclei, increased mitotic activity, vascular invasion, and hemangiopericytomatous-like vascular pattern, some cases of myofibroma have been misdiagnosed as malignant.[141, 143, 151]

Myofibromatosis has been extensively studied by electron microscopy,[136, 140, 141, 144, 147, 149, 151, 152] with most studies showing the component cells to be predominantly myofibroblasts with fibroblasts and smooth muscle cells also present. Immunohistochemical studies[135, 141–145, 149, 152, 159] correlate with these findings, with the spindle cells being reactive for vimentin, smooth muscle actin, and muscle-specific actin. Desmin reactivity, although reported in one study,[143] has been uniformly absent, the lone exception later attributed to the use of a nonspecific antibody.[141, 152] It has been postulated that the lesions of myofibromatosis originate from undifferentiated cells with the capacity to differentiate into several cell types[140]; or from cells with features intermediate between myofibroblasts, glomus cells, and pericytes[151]; or from vascular subintimal mesenchymal or smooth muscle cells.[159] It has been proposed that infantile myofibromatosis is closely related to congenital or infantile hemangiopericytoma, as both lesions share many clinical, anatomic, and histologic features, such that the more histologically immature appearing infantile hemangiopericytoma may represent only an earlier stage in the development of myofibroma.[111, 160, 161]

Treatment and Prognosis. Most infants with visceral myofibromatosis die shortly after birth, although survival for months to years has been reported in a few cases.[66, 67, 133, 134, 156] Patients with pulmonary lesions have an especially grim prognosis.[156–158] In a review by Rosenberg et al.,[66] two of four patients without lung involvement survived, but only 2 of 11 with pulmonary lesions did so. In contrast, only 1 of 16 patients without visceral lesions died, with death in the single patient due to a cervical lesion that expanded into the spinal canal. Most of the nonvisceral solitary or multiple lesions, including bone lesions, eventually undergo spontaneous regression.[66, 134–136, 138] Local recurrence of solitary lesions following excision is reported but is uncommon.[111, 133, 134, 138, 141, 145, 152]

Pseudosarcomatous Fibrous Lesions (Nodular Fasciitis, Cranial Fasciitis, Proliferative Fasciitis, Proliferative Myositis)

A group of benign reactive fibrous lesions exist that are frequently misdiagnosed as malignant because of their cellularity, content of atypical cells, and high mitotic activity.[162–166] These "pseudosarcomas" include nodular fasciitis, proliferative fasciitis, and proliferative myositis, and of these, only nodular fasciitis occurs with any frequency in the head and neck region. In one national cancer registry, slightly over 10% of cases histologically classified as sarcomas were, upon review, reclassified as benign, and in this latter group approximately 60% of the cases consisted of one of these pseudosarcomatous fibrous lesions.[167]

Nodular Fasciitis

Nodular fasciitis has been designated by a variety of terms, including subcutaneous pseudosarcomatous fibromatosis, to infiltrative fasciitis, pseudosarcomatous fasciitis, and proliferative fasciitis. Because the last term is now used for another of the pseudosarcomas (see later discussion), we use *nodular fasciitis* for the lesion discussed here.

Clinical Features. Nodular fasciitis is the most frequent of the pseudosarcomatous fibrous lesions and occurs in patients from newborn to over 80 years of age; most are adults with mean and median age range between 38 and 44 years.[163, 169–173] From 40% to 50% of cases occur in patients between 20 and 40 years of age[169, 174]; it is uncommon in those older than 50 years of age.[175]

Nodular fasciitis may involve any portion of the body, including the deep soft tissues and visceral organs[170, 174]; however, approximately one half of all cases occur in the superficial soft tissues of the upper extremities, the forearm being the single most common site.[8, 167–170, 172–175] The head and neck region accounts for approximately 5% to 20% of cases.[8, 68, 172–176] In a review by Meister et al.[168] of seven large series of nodular fasciitis, 191 of 1269 cases (15%) were in the head and neck region, with the range in these series from 0% to 19%. The head and neck is the most common site in children, accounting for approximately 50% of cases.[8]

Clinically, nodular fasciitis develops as a mass that is occasionally painful or tender. Characteristically, it grows rapidly and is present for less than 1 month in over half of the patients[8, 168, 173, 174, 177, 178]; it is uncommon for symptoms to be present for more than 1 year.[168, 174, 178] In most cases, the lesion arises from the superficial fascia and grows into the subcutaneous tissue as a round to oval, well-circumscribed nodule, although at times it may appear to be poorly delimited and infiltrative. Some lesions grow primarily along the fascia, whereas others extend into the underlying muscle.[8, 168] The nodule is rarely larger than 5.0 cm, with most between 1.0 and 3.0 cm.[8, 168, 172–174]

Nodular fasciitis may occur anywhere within the head and neck region, but the neck, face, and forehead are the most common sites.[174–177] Other locations include the trachea, hypopharynx, parotid gland, masseter muscle, conjunctiva, and orbit.[169–171, 175–180] In the face, the lesions most often occur within the subcutaneous tissue close to bone prominences, such as the angle and inferior border of the mandible, the zygomatic arch, and the anterior mandible.[181] Intraoral lesions are extremely rare, with reported cases arising in the buccal mucosa, labial mucosa, tongue, palate, and alveolar ridge.[174, 176, 177, 181–185]

Small- to medium-sized arteries and veins are also the sites of origin of nodular fasciitis (intravascular fasciitis), with the head and neck region second only to the upper extremity as a location for this variant.[166, 176] Here, the scalp, face, neck, labial mucosa, mucobuccal fold, and buccal mucosa have been involved.[166, 186, 187] The lesion of intravascular fasciitis is small, ranging from 0.6 to 2.5 cm.[166, 186, 187]

Pathologic Features. Nodular fasciitis has a wide range of histologic patterns,[174] but all have certain features in common (Fig. 8–7, see p. 512). These consist of long fascicles of slender, spindle-shaped, fibroblast-like cells arranged in curved, whorled, or S-shaped patterns (see Fig. 8–7A). A storiform configuration may be present similar to that in fibrohistiocytic lesions.[172, 175] The fascicles are loosely arranged, being separated by a myxoid stroma that creates a characteristically edematous or "feathery" appearance (see Fig. 8–7A).[8, 174] Cells with prominent nucleoli and a more oval to round shape may also occur. Although some degree of cellular atypia may be found, and a high mitotic rate is not uncommon, bizarre pleomorphic cells are not present and the mitotic figures are not

atypical.[174] Frequently present, and a helpful diagnostic feature, are extravasated red blood cells that either diffusely insinuate between the stromal cells or are arranged in clusters within microscopic cystic spaces that contain grayish-blue hyaluronidase-sensitive acid mucopolysaccharide (see Fig. 8–7B).[168, 174] Inflammatory cells, mainly lymphocytes, are scattered throughout the lesion but are not numerous; multinucleated giant cells may be found,[172, 173, 175] as well as foci of cartilaginous and osseous metaplasia.[163, 175] Nodular fasciitis is quite vascular, frequently with capillaries arranged in a fan-like or radial array at its periphery.[174]

Intravascular fasciitis may be confused with a malignant tumor because of the infiltration of blood vessels associated with soft tissue involvement. The soft tissue component may so overshadow the vascular component that special stains are required to identify the involved blood vessels.[166, 184, 187] In addition to the usual pattern of nodular fasciitis, multinucleated histiocytes occur in this lesion, but not ganglion-type giant cells.[166, 187]

By electron microscopy, the spindle cells in nodular fasciitis are myofibroblasts.[178, 182, 184] Immunohistochemically, these cells are reactive for vimentin, smooth muscle actin, and muscle-specific actin, but negative for S-100 protein and desmin.[172, 178, 180]

Differential Diagnosis. Owing to its cellularity and amount of myxoid stroma, nodular fasciitis may simulate a variety of other lesions. The clinical features of rapid development, size less than 5.0 cm, and location in the superficial soft tissue are factors that favor a benign process. Histologically, the lesion lacks the pleomorphism, bizarre cells, and atypical mitotic activity of malignant fibrous histiocytoma, or the heterogeneous cell content and associated epidermal hyperplasia of cutaneous atypical fibrous histiocytoma. It also lacks the compact cellularity of either desmoid fibromatosis or fibrosarcoma, or the fascicular pattern of leiomyosarcoma with its more eosinophilic spindle cells having blunt-ended (cigar-shaped) nuclei. The absence of S-100 protein separates nodular fasciitis from benign nerve sheath tumors.

Treatment and Prognosis. Local excision, even at times incomplete excision, is curative in almost all cases of nodular fasciitis, with less than 5% of patients developing a local recurrence.[168, 173, 174, 181]

Cranial Fasciitis

Cranial fasciitis[188, 189] is an uncommon subtype of nodular fasciitis with a few cases reported in the English-language medical literature.[188–197] The lesion develops rapidly and arises from the deep layers of the scalp, most frequently in the temporal, parietal, or temporoparietal areas. Although one case was reported in the skull base with an associated intracranial mass, its atypical location casts some doubt on whether it should be considered a cranial fasciitis.[194] Patients have ranged in age from newborn to 11 years (mean 3.6 years; median 2.5 years).

Cranial fasciitis develops as a mass that may be as large as 10.0 cm[188, 194] but is usually 3.0 to 4.5 cm in maximum dimension.[189, 190–193, 196, 197] In the majority of cases, the outer table of the cranial bone is involved such that origin from the periosteum is a possibility. The lesion may erode through the inner table to involve the dura.[188, 191, 192] Histologically, cranial fasciitis is identical to nodular fasciitis. Simple excision has been curative in all cases, even in those incompletely excised.

Proliferative Myositis and Proliferative Fasciitis

Proliferative myositis and proliferative fasciitis are both benign reactive myofibroblastic, pseudosarcomatous lesions that are histologically closely related to nodular fasciitis and may be considered as variants of that lesion.[198] The term *proliferative fasciitis* was previously used as a synonym for nodular fasciitis but is now restricted to the lesion described here.[162] Both proliferative myositis and proliferative fasciitis are less common than nodular fasciitis.

Clinical Features. Proliferative fasciitis and myositis occur almost exclusively in adults from 40 to 60 years of age[162-164, 199-201] and, unlike nodular fasciitis, rarely develop in children.[202] Both have a rapid clinical onset, evolving over a period of only a few weeks[162-164]; pain and tenderness may occur, especially in proliferative fasciitis.[162, 164]

Proliferative myositis develops within skeletal muscle, usually in the upper arm and shoulder.[163, 164] It varies from 1.0 to 6.0 cm and grossly appears as poorly demarcated, scar-like tissue within the muscle.[164] The head and neck is an uncommon site,[163, 201, 202] with only 4 of the 33 cases (12%) reported from the AFIP located in this area; three of these were within the sternocleidomastoid muscle, and one in the neck.[164]

Proliferative fasciitis also rarely occurs in the head and neck, with the extremities, especially the forearm and thigh, the most commonly involved sites.[162] Of 53 cases reported from the AFIP, only 1 involved the head[162]; the face was involved in one of eight cases reported by Kitano et al.,[165] and Ushigome et al.[201] reported one case in the mandibular region. The lesion arises between the muscle and the subcutaneous tissue and infiltrates along the superficial fascia and the fibrous septa that extend into the subcutaneous tissue. Not all cases involve the fascia, with some found exclusively in the subcutaneous fat.[8] Mixed forms exist where muscle, fascia, and subcutaneous tissue are all involved.[162, 163]

Pathologic Features. Histologically, both proliferative myositis and fasciitis show a proliferation of spindle-shaped cells as seen in nodular fasciitis (Fig. 8-8, see p. 513). In proliferative myositis, this spindle cell fibroblastic proliferation surrounds and separates large groups of muscle fibers, creating a checkerboard-like pattern (see Fig. 8-8A). The distinguishing feature that separates proliferative myositis and fasciitis from conventional nodular fasciitis is the presence of large cells that have an abundant basophilic cytoplasm, and a nucleus with one to two prominent nucleoli, which superficially gives them the appearance of ganglion cells (see Fig. 8-8B); however, Nissl substance is absent.[162-164] Such cells may also be confused with rhabdomyoblasts, but their lack of striations and their basophilic, rather than eosinophilic, cytoplasm serves to distinguish them from the latter, as does their lack of myoglobin or desmin by immunohistochemistry.[8, 200-202] A myxoid background (see Fig. 8-8B), as in nodular fasciitis, is also present, and cartilaginous and osseous foci may be found.[163, 175]

The rare cases that occur in childhood may differ histologically from those in adults, being more cellular, less infiltrative, and less myxoid, occasionally showing the presence of neutrophils, and lacking the slender fibroblasts found in the adult forms.[202]

By electron microscopy the cells of proliferative myositis and proliferative fasciitis have fibroblastic or myofibroblastic features.[199-202] Some authors postulate that the cells arise from perivascular cells and represent activated pericytes.[199, 200]

Treatment and Prognosis. Despite their histologic appearance and infiltrative character, proliferative myositis and proliferative fasciitis are self-limited reactive lesions with no tendency to recur following local excision.

Synovial Sarcoma

Synovial sarcoma (SS) predominantly affects young adults, two thirds of whom are younger than 40 years of age, with most patients in the third decade of life.[203-205] Most commonly, SS is found in the vicinity of large joints and bursae, with 75% to 95% in the extremities. Despite its name, SS rarely arises from synovial membranes, with only about 10% actually involving joint spaces.[204-206] Indeed, SS may occur in areas that are anatomically devoid of synovioblastic tissue such as the abdominal wall, pelvis, and the head and neck region.[203, 206-210] Although there are many individual case reports of SS involving the head and neck,[208, 211-315] probably less than 150 cases are reported in the English-language medical literature.[211, 214, 216] The incidence in the head and neck in most reported series has varied from 0% to 16%.[8, 214, 217-221]

Among 345 cases accessioned at the AFIP, 31 occurred in the head and neck.[8]

Clinical Features. The mean age for patients with SS of the head and neck varies from 25 to 30 years, with a range from 7 to 63 years.[206, 207, 214, 215, 222] The patients tend to be younger than those with SS at other sites.[207, 220, 223-225]

Within the head and neck, SS is most commonly a hypopharyngeal or parapharyngeal tumor, although virtually any site may be affected, including the superior aspect of the neck just beneath the mandible,[226] the prevertebral area from the base of the skull to the hypopharynx, the anterior neck along the borders of the sternocleidomastoid muscle, and orofacial and laryngeal sites.[206, 210, 215, 226]

Clinically, patients with head and neck SS usually present because of a painless mass; about 20% have pain.[206-208, 211-214, 216, 226-228] Occasionally, dysphagia, dyspnea, or hoarseness may be the initial complaint because of tumor pressure on the hypopharynx and larynx.[206, 209, 211-213, 215, 222, 226] In contrast to patients with synovial sarcomas of other sites, in whom symptoms may be present for several years,[203, 204] those with head and neck lesions usually seek medical attention within a year of onset of their symptoms.[206-208]

Synovial sarcomas in the head and neck average approximately 5.0 cm in size with a range from 1.0 to 12.0 cm.[8, 206-209, 212-214, 218, 220, 227, 228] They are firm to rubbery, well-circumscribed, spherical or micronodular tumors with a pseudocapsule. Cystic and hemorrhagic foci may be present.[8, 206] Calcification is radiologically evident in 30% to 40% of synovial sarcomas in the extremities,[203, 204] and may be so extensive as to justify the appellation of calcifying synovial sarcoma. None of the 32 patients reported under this designation had tumors in the head and neck region.[229]

Pathologic Features. Histologically, classic SS is characterized by a biphasic pattern consisting of tightly compacted fibroblast-like spindle cells among which are scattered pale, epithelial-like cells that are arranged in either glandular formations, compact nests, or cleft-like spaces (Fig. 8-9A, see p. 514).[204, 205, 220, 221, 223, 230] The spindle cell areas may resemble fibrosarcoma. Mast cells are numerous,[206] and hyalinized scar-like areas may be quite prominent; microcalcification occurs in 30% to 60% of cases,[203, 206] and, rarely, osteoid and bone formation may be found.[231] Synovial sarcoma may be quite vascular, with the vascular pattern frequently having a hemangiopericytoma-like pattern.[8, 232]

The epithelial-like cells may be cuboidal or tall and columnar and form papillary projections that extend into cleft-like spaces. These glandular formations may be so well differentiated that they simulate metastatic adenocarcinoma.[233] The gland-like spaces and clefts contain a mucin-like material that stains with periodic acid-Schiff (PAS), mucicarmine, and alcian blue stains and is resistant to hyaluronidase digestion.[206, 209, 230, 232] The spindle cells elaborate a stromal mucin, which is eliminated by hyaluronidase.[206]

The relative proportion of spindle cells to epithelial-like cells varies from case to case and even within the same lesion.[205] The spindle cell areas are preponderant in most lesions, and many sections may have to be examined before epithelial-like cells are found. A small biopsy might lack epithelial-like foci and the tumor may be interpreted as either a fibrosarcoma or other type of spindle cell tumor.

Monophasic forms of SS exist that consist entirely of spindle or epithelial-like cells (Fig. 8-9B, see p. 514),[232] although the epithelial monophasic form is quite rare and may reflect a biphasic tumor with a predominant epithelial component.[8]

Cytogenetic analysis of SS has demonstrated a specific reciprocal chromosomal translocation involving chromosomes X and 18 (X;18) in approximately 75% of both biphasic and monophasic cases.[234-236]

The spindle cells of both biphasic and monophasic SS express vimentin; less commonly the epithelial-like cells also are reactive for this marker. Of more significance, however, is that the epithelial markers cytokeratin and epithelial membrane antigen are found not only in the epithelial and, to a lesser degree, spindle cell components of biphasic tumors, but also in a smaller percentage of monophasic spindle cell tumors; one or both of these markers are present in SS in roughly 90% of cases.[214, 219, 221, 225, 237, 238] The cytokeratin component may be chain-specific.[239, 240] Some synovial sarcomas contain cells that express S-100 protein,[219, 221, 237, 241, 241] and CD99.[243, 244] Significantly, the cells of normal synovium do not stain for cytokeratin.

Electron microscopic studies of SS have demonstrated epithelial features not only in the epithelial-like cells but also in the spindle cell component.[217, 221, 225, 237, 245] SS probably originates from undifferentiated or pluripotential cells that have the capacity to differentiate either toward fibroblast-like or epithelial-like cells,[206, 210] thus explaining the occurrence of these tumors in locations within the head and neck that are devoid of synovial tissue.

Differential Diagnosis. Distinction between biphasic SS and most other soft tissue sarcomas generally poses no great histologic problem. However, poorly differentiated SS and malignant hemangiopericytoma may be difficult to separate owing to the pericytomatous vascular pattern present in both tumors.[8] Hemangiopericytoma lacks positivity for cytokeratin or epithelial membrane antigen and, in most cases, contains cells reactive for CD34, an antigen absent in SS.[3] Epithelioid sarcoma may also mimic an epithelial dominant SS and contains cells that are reactive for cytokeratin and epithelial membrane antigen, but its cells are reactive for CD34.[5, 25] The clinical presentation of epithelioid sarcoma also differs from SS by its superficial location, usually in the upper extremity, tendency to ulcerate the skin, and rarity in the head and neck.[25] Unlike SS, epithelioid sarcoma apparently lacks cytokeratin 7.[239, 240]

It may be impossible to distinguish, by routine sections, monophasic SS from other spindle cell–prominent lesions such as malignant peripheral nerve sheath tumor (MPNST), fibrosarcoma, and leiomyosarcoma. Immunohistochemical stains are especially useful in this regard, with the lack of epithelial marker reactivity in fibrosarcoma and the lack of muscle markers (desmin, muscle-specific antigen, smooth muscle antigen) in SS and their presence in leiomyosarcoma. Although a small number of synovial sarcomas are S-100 protein positive, this reaction is never diffuse or very strong, whereas S-100 protein is found in over 50% of cases of MPNST.[3] The latter tumor also lacks epithelial differentiation except in the very rare glandular schwannoma.[241] Electron microscopy of MPNST demonstrates schwannian differentiation that is absent in SS. The simultaneous presence of cytokeratin, epithelial membrane antigen, and S-100 protein, as occurs in SS, has not been found in MPNST.[242]

Treatment and Prognosis. Therapy for SS is primarily surgical; however, owing to the inability to do extensive radical removal in the head and neck region, local recurrence rates are relatively high, ranging from 25% to 26%.[208, 212] Postoperative radiation therapy may reduce the rate of local recurrence[212]; chemotherapy has also been shown to produce beneficial effects in SS in the limited number of patients reported to date.[246] In general, SS pursues a protracted course with some patients developing metastases up to 20 years after initial therapy.[8, 203, 204] Some believe that all patients, if followed for a sufficient time, will develop metastatic disease.[204] There does not appear to be any correlation between histologic features and survival, with the exception that calcifying synovial sarcoma appears to have a better prognosis than the usual synovial sarcoma.[229] Most studies show no differences in survival between the biphasic and monophasic subtypes.[223, 224] Tumor size is probably the most important single prognostic determinant, with tumors less than 5.0 cm in maximum size having a better prognosis than those of larger size.[206, 218, 220, 224, 232, 246] The extent of the tumor and the presence of positive resection margins also influences survival.[220, 247] Synovial sarcoma of the tongue may have a better prognosis than those in other head and neck locations.[227]

Although most metastases are blood-borne, about 10% to 20% of patients have regional lymph node metastases; however, radical lymph node dissection is not advocated in the absence of lymphadenopathy.[203, 213] Metastases from biphasic tumors have either a bi-

phasic or a monophasic pattern, whereas metastases from monophasic tumors are monophasic.[232]

Five-year survival rates for SS range from 3% to 69% with most series reporting rates of 40% to 50%; lower 10-year survival rates reflect the late appearance of metastases.[8, 203, 205, 206, 208, 220, 232] Five-year survival rates for head and neck lesions do not differ significantly from those for synovial sarcomas at other sites.[206, 215]

Peripheral Nerve Sheath Tumors

The two most common benign tumors of peripheral nerves are neurilemoma (schwannoma) and neurofibroma. Although the Schwann cell is believed by most authors to be the cell of origin for both of these tumors[248–250] they are sufficiently distinctive, both clinically and pathologically, that they are usually easily separable. It is believed that the mesodermally derived perineural fibroblasts participate with Schwann cells in the formation of these tumors.[248, 249, 251, 252] The neoplastic cells in these tumors have the capacity to form a variety of tissues including bone, cartilage, fat, muscle, collagen, and even glands.[248, 253] Such a diversity of tissues is seen most commonly in the malignant neurogenous tumors.

Neurilemoma and neurofibroma should not be confused with the "traumatic" neuroma that develops following some form of tissue injury.[248, 250] These firm, rubbery, tender or painful masses result from an exaggeration of the normal repair process and are not neoplasms. They are composed of a tangle of regenerating axons interwoven with Schwann cells in a fibrous stroma. They rarely produce symptoms until they assume sufficient size to be clinically evident.

The head and neck region is the most common location for both neurilemoma and neurofibroma. An increased relative risk for development of head and neck peripheral nerve sheath tumors has been reported in patients exposed to low-dose radiation for the treatment of tinea capitis during childhood.[254] The latent period ranged from 6 to 29 years (mean 17.6 years); the majority of the tumors were schwannomas.

Neurilemoma (Schwannoma)

Clinical Features. Neurilemomas develop from the neural sheath of peripheral motor, sensory, sympathetic, and cranial nerves, the exceptions being the optic and olfactory cranial nerves that lack Schwann cell sheaths.[250, 255, 257] Approximately 25% to 45% of neurilemomas occur in the head and neck region.[255, 257–260] The majority of these arise in the central nervous system, particularly in the acoustic nerve. Of the 138 neurilemomas outside the central nervous system area, 52 (38%) were in the head and neck region.[257]

Cervical neurilemomas are divided into medial and lateral groups.[261] The lateral tumors arise from the cervical nerve trunks and the cervical and brachial plexus; the medial tumors arise from cranial nerves (IX–XII) and the cervical sympathetic chain. These latter tumors frequently manifest clinically as parapharyngeal tumors.[261] However, any nerve, small or large, may be involved.

Almost every anatomic site in the head and neck has been involved by neurilemoma, including the soft tissues of the face, especially the preauricular region, the forehead, orbit, scalp, lip, maxilla, mandible, floor of mouth, tongue, paranasal sinus, nasal fossa, parotid gland, nasopharynx, and larynx.[256, 262, 263–266] Tumors that arise from the cervical nerve trunks may extend through the spinal foramen into the spinal cord; such lesions are termed *dumbbell tumors*.[261, 264] Parapharyngeal lesions may present as bulging tonsillar or retrotonsillar masses.[264]

Patients are usually in the third to fourth decades of life[248, 249, 256–258, 263, 264, 267] but no age group is exempt, from infants to patients over 80 years of age. Women are affected more often than men in ratios of 3:2 to 2:1.[249, 259, 263, 264]

Most patients complain of a painless mass without neurologic symptoms.[267] The tumors may produce pressure symptoms as they

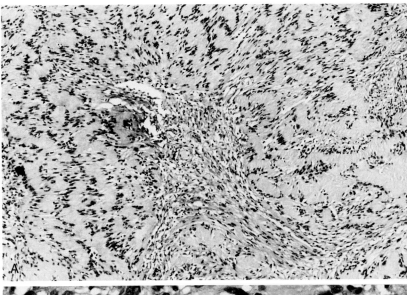

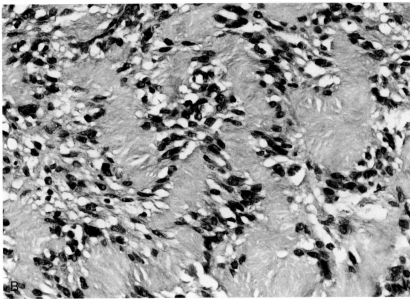

Figure 8–10. *A,* Schwannoma with a dominant Antoni A component. An Antoni B area is seen in the center of the field. *B,* Palisaded schwannoma cells producing organoid structures (Verocay body).

enlarge, especially those within the confined anatomic regions of the head and neck.[249, 255–257, 263] Vocal cord dysfunction, hoarseness, cough, breathing difficulty, and, rarely, Horner's syndrome may occur depending on the specific anatomic region affected.[257, 261] An interesting, but inconsistent, clinical finding in vagus nerve schwannomas is sporadic cough elicited by manual pressure on the tumor.[268]

The lesions are slow-growing and may be present for several years before the patient seeks medical attention. A correct preoperative diagnosis of neurilemoma is rarely made[256, 260]; however, the magnetic resonance visualization of a solitary, fusiform neck mass that appears to arise from neural tissue is strongly suggestive of a schwannoma, particularly if a vascular tumor is excluded by angiography.[269]

Neurilemomas, in contrast to neurofibromas, are usually sharply circumscribed and encapsulated with an oval, round, or fusiform shape.[248–250] When in a large nerve trunk, they are usually movable laterally, but not in a vertical direction. In the soft tissues, a nerve may not be recognizable. The tumors are usually small, most are less than 5.0 cm, but lesions up to 10.0 cm have occurred in the head and neck region.[255, 256, 258, 263, 264] Neurilemomas that arise in a major nerve trunk may be dissected free without impairing the nerve, since nerve fibers are not part of the tumor. Multiple neurile-

momas may occur, and such patients are frequently found to also have associated multiple neurofibromas.[250]

Pathologic Features. The tumor is tan-gray to white and frequently has a watery or slimy consistency. Cystic degeneration and hemorrhage are not uncommon.[249, 250]

The typical neurilemoma has a biphasic histologic pattern composed of compact cellular regions, the Antoni A areas, mixed with loosely arranged hypocellular regions, the Antoni B areas (Fig. 8–10A).[248, 250] The relative proportions of these regions varies from tumor to tumor, and some are found in which one of these regions may form the entire lesion. Most neurilemomas, however, will contain both Antoni A and Antoni B foci. The Antoni A regions are composed of bipolar spindle-shaped Schwann cells that have oval to elongate nuclei and fibrillar eosinophilic cytoplasm that may fuse to form hyaline masses. These cells characteristically are aligned into interweaving fascicles or are so arranged that their nuclei are juxtaposed in rows, creating the classic palisading pattern of this tumor. However, a similar palisading pattern may be found in other lesions, such as smooth muscle tumors, and while highly suggestive of a neurogenous lesion it is not in itself diagnostic. The Schwann cells may also group themselves to create organoid structures, the Verocay bodies, that are similar in appearance to tactile corpuscles (Fig. 8–10B). Mitotic figures are either absent or rare.

Neurilemomas are quite vascular, accounting for the large hemorrhagic foci noted in some. Large blood vessels with densely hyalinized walls are quite common and are characteristic of neurilemomas. Neurites are not present within the substance of the tumor. Occasional neurilemomas are found in which the cells are hyperchromatic and take on bizarre nuclear configurations. These are termed "ancient" neurilemomas, with the cell changes reflecting degeneration.[270-271] Cellular atypia in neurogenous tumors is not evidence of malignancy. An unsettled issue is the relationship between the Schwann cells and the perineural fibroblasts in the formation of these tumors, with some authors believing that these are actual functional variants of the same cell.[251, 252]

Neurilemomas stain strongly with antibodies to S-100 protein. This stain may be used to distinguish the more cellular neurilemomas from smooth muscle tumors, with which they may be confused, but which are negative for S-100 protein.[272, 273]

Two variants of neurilemoma designated "cellular schwannoma" and "plexiform neurilemoma" are important to recognize since they may be mistaken for sarcoma.[274, 275] Cellular schwannoma is composed predominantly of highly cellular Antoni A areas with hyperchromatic nuclei and a moderate degree of mitotic activity. Plexiform neurilemoma show multinodular growth pattern[274] and tend to be extremely cellular.[275]

Treatment and Prognosis. Following simple local excision, neurilemomas rarely recur.[248, 249, 264, 265] In Conley's 76 patients, only two developed a recurrence.[256] Neurilemomas virtually never undergo malignant degeneration.

Neurofibroma

Clinical Features. Neurofibroma may occur as a solitary lesion or as multiple tumors in cases of neurofibromatosis (von Recklinghausen's disease). Neurofibromas tend to occur at an earlier age than do neurilemomas, usually in patients from 20 to 40 years of age,[8] with an approximately equal sex incidence. The tumor is uncommon in children or adolescents.[276] In a review of 139 neurogenic tumors in patients from newborn to 20 years of age, 60 neurofibromas occurred in 41 patients, 20 of which were in the head and neck area. Twelve of the 41 patients had neurofibromatosis.[276]

Neurofibromas are somewhat more common than neurilemomas, but this probably reflects the inclusion within reports of patients with associated neurofibromatosis. Solitary neurofibromas limited to the head and neck area are rare.[255, 257] Among 13 neurogenous tumors of the face and neck reported by Katz and associates, 11 were neurilemomas and two were neurofibromas.[267]

Neurofibromas generally arise in the subcutaneous tissue as small 2.0 to 4.0 cm nodules. In the skin they may produce protuberant, sagging, disfiguring masses.[277] Within the head and neck region, they are more frequently seen in the head area, unlike neurilemomas for which the lateral cervical area is the most common site.[265] In patients with neurofibromatosis, the neurofibromas that occur in the head and neck area are most commonly located in the orbital region and midlateral aspect of the neck.[278] As with neurilemomas, neurofibromas also take origin from a variety of locations in the head and neck, including the nasopharynx, paranasal sinuses, hypopharynx, larynx, tongue, floor of mouth, vagus nerve, salivary gland, and buccal area.[262, 265-267] In the tongue, which is a common site, macroglossia may result from infiltration by the neurofibroma.[265] Neurofibromas have also developed in areas that received previous radiation therapy.[248]

When in the superficial soft tissues, neurofibromas are usually ill-defined and unencapsulated, but when within the deeper soft tissues or in a major nerve, they are better circumscribed and appear encapsulated.[248-250, 265] In large nerve trunks they may also form irregular fusiform swellings, creating a tangled, worm-like mass. The finding of such a plexiform neurofibroma is tantamount to a diagnosis of von Recklinghausen's disease.[250]

Pathologic Features. On gross examination, neurofibromas tend to be softer than neurilemomas and, on cut surface, have a gray-white glistening appearance. The tumor feels slimy and may be quite gelatinous. This gelatinous quality may be so exaggerated as to suggest the diagnosis of myxoma.[250, 279] When associated with a large nerve, the nerve is seen to course through the tumor and is such an integral part of it that it cannot be dissected free of the tumor.[249]

Histologically, neurofibroma contains a mixture of cells, which vary from spindle-shaped to stellate, and whose nuclei tend to be elongated and at times wavy or twisted (Fig. 8–11).[248, 249, 279, 280] Scattered lymphocytes and mast cells are also present, the mast cells being far more common than in neurilemomas. Short collagen fibers are present and are arranged in bundles or nodular arrays. Unlike neurilemomas, neurites are present within the substance of the tumor, although without special stains they may be difficult to see. The tumor matrix is loose and appears edematous, with the cells being widely separated within it. This matrix stains strongly for acid mucopolysaccharide, unlike the weak or negative reaction given by the matrix of neurilemomas.[250, 279] Plexiform neurofibromas may contain large areas of normal nerve lying within the mucoid matrix and between the spindle-shaped tumor cells. The biphasic pattern of Antoni A and Antoni B areas is usually absent, as is the conspicuous vascularity of neurilemoma. However, some neurofibromas contain areas that re-

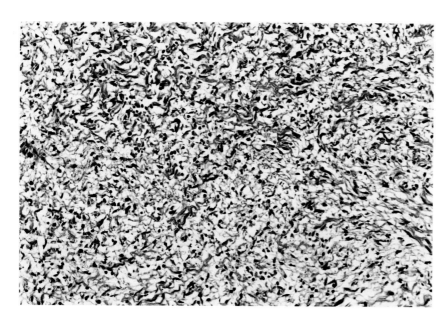

Figure 8–11. Neurofibroma, elongated cells with wavy nuclei interspersed with collagen bundles. Numerous lymphocytes and mast cells are present.

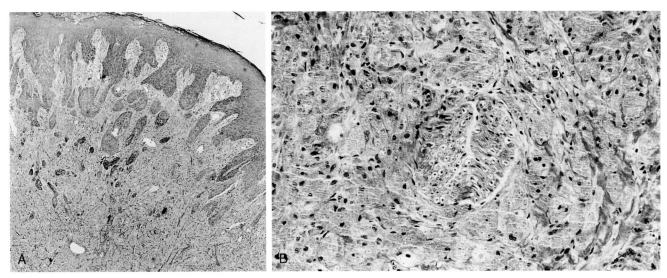

Figure 8–12. Granular cell tumor of the tongue. The surface epithelium shows pseudoepitheliomatous hyperplasia. *B*, Higher magnification showing cells with granular cytoplasm and small dark nuclei arranged concentrically around a peripheral nerve.

semble neurilemoma to such a degree that a clear histologic distinction between the two tumors is not always possible.[250, 279]

Mitoses are scarce in the usual neurofibroma. Indeed, the presence of more than an occasional mitotic figure in several high-power microscopic fields should suggest the possibility of malignancy. Focal cellular pleomorphism, which may occur in these tumors, is not an indication of malignancy when it is unassociated with mitotic activity.[250, 279] Neurofibromas, like neurilemomas, also stain positively for S-100 protein, although the intensity of the reaction and the number of cells that stain is not as great as in neurilemomas.[272, 273] Rare and unusual neurofibromas are described with a variety of different histologic patterns including epithelioid, pacinian, and pigmented; these neurofibromas are described in detail elsewhere.[8, 250]

Treatment and Prognosis. Solitary neurofibroma, like solitary neurilemoma, has a low incidence of recurrence following local excision.[250, 263] Malignant development in a solitary neurofibroma is not common; however, patients with neurofibromatosis do have a significant risk of developing malignant neurogenous tumors. This is discussed in the next section.

Granular Cell Tumor

Described by Abrikossoff in 1926, granular cell tumor was initially assumed to be of striated muscle origin and was known for many years as *granular cell myoblastoma*. The histogenesis of this neoplasm has been the subject of considerable controversy, but most investigators now believe it to be of neural origin. Electron microscopic and immunohistochemical investigations have added support to the neural (Schwann cell) theory of origin.[281]

Clinical Features. Granular cell tumor originates in a variety of tissues, particularly the skin and mucus membranes, most notably of the upper aerodigestive tract; 20% arise in the tongue.[281] As a rule, the lesions present as solitary, painless nodules in the dermis, subcutis, or submucosa. In the tongue they commonly involve its intrinsic muscles. Laryngeal tumors may be associated with hoarseness. Tumors affecting multiple sites are reported in 10% to 15% of the cases.[8, 282]

Granular cell tumors occur in patients of any age but are most common in persons in the fourth to sixth decade of life and are rare in children.[8, 282] However, several laryngeal tumors have been described in children under 12 years of age.[283] The tumor is more common in women than men and black patients far outnumber whites.[8, 284]

Pathologic Features. Microscopically, granular cell tumor is distinctive, consisting of large, uniform, polyhedral cells with eosinophilic granular cytoplasm. The nucleus is small, hyperchromatic, and centrally or eccentrically located (Fig. 8–12). The tumor cells form sheets, nests, and cords. Although the tumor is almost always benign, it tends to have undefined borders and may be infiltrative. A characteristic feature of the dermal and submucosal tumors is to be associated with acanthosis and pseudoepitheliomatous hyperplasia of the overlying squamous epithelium (see Fig. 8–12*A*). This feature can be so remarkable that it is mistaken for squamous cell carcinoma.[8, 281, 285] Another characteristic histologic feature that may also be of histogenetic significance is the close association of the granular cells and peripheral nerves. Frequently, the granular cells are concentrically arranged about the remnants of small peripheral nerves (see Fig. 8–12*B*).

With immunohistochemical staining, the tumor cells show positive reactivity to neural markers including S-100 protein, Leu 7, neuron-specific enolase, and myelin basic protein.[286–288] The tumor cells, however, do not react to glial fibrillary acidic protein or to the neurofilament proteins.[289, 290] Ultrastructurally, granular cell tumors show a highly characteristic picture. Typically, the intracellular granules are membrane-bound autophagic vacuoles that contain cellular debris including mitochondria, fragmented endoplasmic reticulum, and myelin figures.[291, 292]

Treatment and Prognosis. Treatment of granular cell tumor is excision. Recurrence may follow incomplete removal.

Malignant Granular Cell Tumor

Malignant granular cell tumors are exceedingly rare: only 35 cases have so far been described in the English-language literature.[293] These typically present with recent rapid growth in a tumor of long duration. Malignant granular cell tumors have not been observed in children and most are large, measuring more than 4 cm.[293] Like the benign tumor, the malignant counterpart occurs much more commonly in females.

The microscopic features of malignant granular cell tumor resemble those of the benign tumor. Therefore, some observers advocate the restriction of malignant diagnosis to only those cases that show distant metastasis.[294] Features that are reported to be associated with malignant behavior include marked nuclear pleomorphism, excessive mitosis, and necrosis.[8, 281, 293, 294] The ultrastructural features and the immunohistochemical characteristics are similar to those of the benign type.[8, 293, 294]

Malignant Peripheral Nerve Sheath Tumor (Malignant Schwannoma, Neurosarcoma)

Malignant tumors of peripheral nerve have been designated as malignant schwannomas. This is somewhat confusing in that *schwannoma* is used as a synonym for *neurilemoma,* a tumor that virtually never becomes malignant. Furthermore, some of these malignant neurogenous tumors histologically resemble fibrosarcoma, for which the term *neurofibrosarcoma* has been used.[295] However, many of these malignant neural lesions tend to be undifferentiated or pleomorphic with little to suggest either Schwann cell differentiation or fibrosarcoma. Currently, *malignant peripheral nerve sheath tumor* (MPNST) is used to designate these tumors. The lesions usually show variable degrees of Schwann cells, perineural, and fibroblastic differentiation.

We restrict the diagnosis of MPNST to tumors that clearly arise within a nerve, contain histologic areas of neurofibroma, or develop in a patient with von Recklinghausen's disease. The percentage of patients with von Recklinghausen's disease who develop a malignant neurogenous tumor has ranged from 5% to 30%.[296, 297] MPNST is not common, accounting for no more than 5% to 10% of all sarcomas.[298, 299] They are far less frequent than benign peripheral nerve tumors, making up only about 2% to 12% of neural sheath tumors.[300, 301] In the head and neck, they have a similar frequency.[264]

Several reports have confirmed the development of MPNST at previously irradiated sites.[302–304] In one study the latency period varied from 5 to 29 years, with a mean of 16.9 years.[302] The malignant lesion occurred equally in patients with and without neurofibromatosis.

Clinical Features. Malignant neural tumors found in association with von Recklinghausen's disease develop in patients 20 to 50 years of age (mean approximately 30 years), but patients who develop spontaneous neurosarcomas are about 10 to 15 years older.[296, 300, 302, 305, 306] Of 16 malignant peripheral nerve sheath tumors occurring in children and adolescents, who ranged in age from 6 months to 18 years (mean 16 years), 7 (44%) had neurofibromatosis.[276] There was no difference in the mean or age range of those children with and without neurofibromatosis. The head and neck was the presenting site in four cases, with the others in the trunk (10 cases) and extremities (2 cases).

Women are more commonly affected in those few reports that mention MPNST in the head and neck, but the number of patients in these reports is few.[264, 266, 296]

The most common clinical complaint in patients with neurosarcoma is the presence of a swelling or a mass that is painful in about one half of the cases.[296, 302, 306, 307] Paresthesia, muscle atrophy, and weakness may be present, depending on whether a major nerve trunk is involved.[296, 307] Patients with von Recklinghausen's disease may indicate that the lesion had been present for many years prior to its sudden enlargement.[296] Rapid growth in a known neurofibroma or the spontaneous development of a rapidly growing soft-tissue mass, associated with pain, in a patient with von Recklinghausen's disease is highly suggestive of malignancy.

Most neurogenic sarcomas develop in the extremities or the trunk.[296, 300, 302, 306, 307] Despite being a frequent site for benign neurogenous tumors, the head and neck region is not a common location for these malignant tumors, accounting for only 6% to 19% of all cases.[296, 302, 306, 308] In most series, less than 10% of neurosarcomas occur in this area. The tumors that develop in patients with von Recklinghausen's disease tend to be centrally located in the trunk, pelvic, and shoulder regions, with fewer tumors in the extremities or head and neck.[305, 307]

In the head and neck, MPNSTs are found in a variety of locations, including the brachial plexus, vagus and other cranial nerves, lateral and posterior neck, cheek, pharynx, larynx, supraclavicular area, maxilla, mandible, upper lip, parotid region, nose, parapharyngeal area, paranasal sinuses, and nasopharynx.[256, 264–267, 308, 309]

Pathologic Features. When a major nerve is affected, the tumor frequently forms a fusiform or nodular swelling that diffusely infiltrates the nerve.[296, 306, 307] It also extends into the surrounding soft tissue and contains areas of hemorrhage and necrosis. Few neurosarcomas are small[300, 307, 308]; their sizes vary from 5 cm to greater than 10.0 cm.[300] In patients with von Recklinghausen's disease, the tumors arise not only in major nerve trunks but in areas of pre-existing neurofibromas, from areas adjacent to major nerves, and in areas where a major nerve could not be identified.[296]

Microscopically, neurosarcomas have fields composed of spindle cells arranged in interlacing fascicles with a herringbone pattern as in fibrosarcoma.[250, 306, 307] Unlike fibrosarcoma, the hyperchromatic nuclei are twisted and show various degrees of pleomorphism. The stroma is fibrotic or myxomatous. Commonly densely cellular fascicles alternate with hypocellular myxoid zones where the parallel orientation of the cells is lacking (Fig. 8–13). Mitoses are frequent, usually one or more per high-power field, and foci of hemorrhage and necrosis are also common.[250, 300, 305, 307] On a purely histologic basis, these "neurofibrosarcomas" are indistinguishable from the usual soft-tissue fibrosarcoma. Undifferentiated pleomorphic sarcomas may also arise within peripheral nerves. These contain bizarre giant cells and polygonal mononuclear cells with hyperchromatic nuclei.[296, 300, 305] Pleomorphic tumors are noted by some to develop more frequently in patients with von Recklinghausen's disease, but others report them to be more common in patients without this disease.[296, 300, 305] Neurosarcomas developing in areas that had received prior radiation therapy are usually of the pleomorphic type.[305]

Metaplastic elements, such as malignant osteoid and cartilage, as well as areas of liposarcoma and rhabdomyosarcoma may occur in MPNST.[250, 296, 300, 302, 307] Tumors with rhabdomyosarcomatous differentiation have been termed malignant "Triton" tumors.[253, 310] In a review of 36 cases, Brooks et al.[310] found that this variant of neurogenic sarcoma occurs in young adults (mean age 35 years) and is evenly distributed between male and female patients. The majority of cases, over 70%, are associated with von Reckinghausen's neurofibromatosis. In this group, there is a male predominance and the patients are younger than those who develop sporadic tumors, which tended to occur in older females. In both patient groups, the head and neck and the trunk were the most common sites of origin. The neurofibromatosis-associated Triton tumors were three times as common in the head and neck as in the trunk.[310]

In a review of 10 malignant Triton tumors of the head and neck, the most common location was the neck (5 cases); the face and paranasal sinuses were sites for 2 cases each, and 1 arose in the temporal area.[311]

Benign peripheral nerve tumors with striated muscle also occur, and these have been variously called neuromuscular hamartoma, benign Triton tumor, or neuromuscular choristoma.[280, 312] One of the two patients reported by Bonneau and Brochu had the lesion in the supraclavicular fossa. In their review of the literature, they found six cases, three of which arose in the brachial plexus and, with the exception of one patient who was 14 years old, all the tumors were in children under 2 years of age.[280]

Although stains for S-100 protein are positive in almost all benign neural tumors, neurosarcomas are less frequently positive. Approximately half to two thirds of these tumors will be positive for S-100 protein, but the intensity of the reaction is not great, and usually only a few tumor cells are stained.[272, 273] However, Wick et al.,[313] using two other neural markers, myelin basic protein and Leu-7, in addition to S-100 protein, found that 68% of 62 malignant peripheral nerve tumors expressed at least one of these three determinants.

Because of the poorly differentiated nature of many of these neurosarcomas, electron microscopy has not been very successful in differentiating them from other soft-tissue spindle cell tumors,[272, 273] although some tumors with the light microscopic features of malignant fibrous histiocytoma have been successfully diagnosed as malignant neural tumors by electron microscopy.[314] A MPNST may show the same features as benign nerve sheath tumor. Most significantly the tumor cells elaborate branched cytoplasmic processes covered by basal lamina.

Treatment and Prognosis. Neurosarcomas are highly malignant lesions with recurrences following local excision in from 50% to 80% of patients.[296, 300, 305, 306] Patients with von Recklinghausen's disease who develop neurosarcoma have a poor prognosis, with 5-year survival rates of 15% to 30%, in contrast to patients with de novo lesions for whom the 5-year survival rates range from 50% to 75%.[296, 300, 305, 307] Recurrences and metastases from these tumors may occur as late as 5 and 10 years after therapy.[300, 307] Local recurrence of MPNST in patients with von Recklinghausen's disease is indicative of a grave prognosis, with almost all such patients dying of their disease.[305] Small tumors, less than 5.0 cm, have a better prognosis than larger lesions.[302] There is no apparent correlation of survival with the grade of the tumor or its mitotic rate. Malignant "Triton" tumors have a poor prognosis, and radiation-induced neurosarcomas are almost always fatal.[253, 305] In a review of 10 malignant Triton tumors of the head and neck, Bhatt et al.[311] found that those of the head had a lower grade histology and were less clinically aggressive than those in the neck. The latter were more commonly associated with neurofibromatosis.

Data on tumors arising in the head and neck are scarce. In Conley and Janecka's series of 14 patients with head and neck malignant neural tumors, 12 died within 3 years, and the other 2 patients were alive and free of disease at 1 and 4 years after therapy.[256] Patients with head and neck neurosarcomas are said to have a poorer prognosis than those with extremity tumors.[302] This outcome might be attributable to the difficulty of achieving wide excision of the lesion with tumor-free margins in the head and neck, owing to the proximity of vital structures. When radical tumor removal is not possible, excision combined with high-dose radiation therapy was found to be effective.[302]

Malignant Peripheral Neuroectodermal Tumor and Extraskeletal Ewing's Sarcoma

Malignant peripheral neuroectodermal tumor (PNET) and extraskeletal Ewing's sarcoma (EES) infrequently occur in the head and neck region; however, their cytomorphology overlaps that of other tumors that may be encountered here, such as embryonal rhabdomyosarcoma, lymphocytic lymphoma, mesenchymal chondrosarcoma, and metastatic small cell carcinoma. PNET and EES share a variety of demographic, clinical, morphologic, and cytogenetic features to the degree that some believe they are members of the same family of tumors, differing only in the extent of their cytologic differentiation.

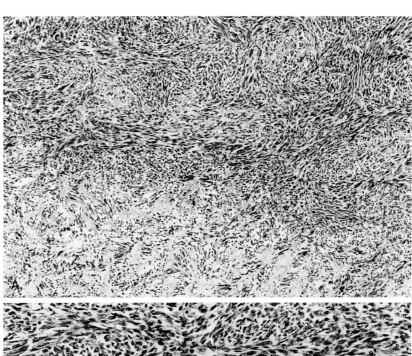
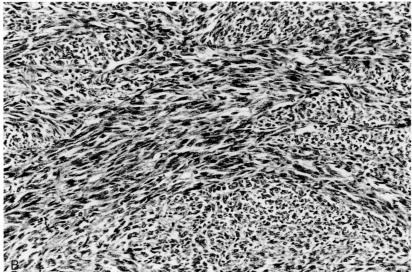

Figure 8–13. *A,* Malignant peripheral nerve sheath tumor. Densely cellular fascicles alternating with less cellular areas. *B,* Higher magnification showing hyperchromatic and twisted nuclei.

The histologic and biologic relationship between these lesions has been well reviewed by others.[315, 316]

Malignant Peripheral Neuroectodermal Tumor

Peripheral neuroectodermal tumor was first described by Stout[317] as an ulnar nerve tumor, composed of small cells that formed rosettes that he termed *malignant neuroectodermal tumor of peripheral nerve*. Similar tumors were subsequently also found within the soft tissues unrelated to a nerve. A variety of diagnostic labels have been applied to these tumors, with malignant peripheral neuroectodermal tumor (MPNET) now most frequently used.[25] Here, we use the shorthand designation, peripheral neuroectodermal tumor (PNET).

Clinical Features. PNET primarily affects children and young adults, with 90% of patients younger than 30 years of age and 75% younger than 20 years; mean and median ages are approximately 15 years.[25] The tumor usually manifests as a mass that commonly is painful. If a major nerve is involved, secondary neurologic symptoms may be present.[317, 318] The duration of symptoms is short, usually less than 6 months. Unlike classic neuroblastoma, which histologically resembles PNET, serum catecholamine levels are seldom elevated.[318, 319–323]

In the soft tissues, PNET has a predilection for the trunk, especially the paraspinal and chest wall regions, which account for almost half of all cases.[25] The head and neck region is involved in approximately 5% of cases. Here, the neck is the most common site, with the orbit and face occasionally being involved.[320, 322, 324–335]

Despite the usual short clinical history, PNET is generally a large tumor, with 80% greater than 5.0 cm and some as large as 40 cm.[25, 326] Those in the head and neck range from 2.0 to 6.0 cm.[325, 327, 328, 330, 333]

Pathologic Features. Grossly, the tumor is multinodular or lobular and may appear well circumscribed. On section, it is soft, fleshy, gray-white to tan with frequent foci of hemorrhage and necrosis.[318, 319, 326, 328–330]

Histologically, PNET is composed of sheet-like masses of loosely cohesive small, round to oval or slightly elongated cells with similarly shaped nuclei (Fig. 8–14*A*, see p. 527). The latter may have grooves or infoldings, with a coarse or clumped chromatin that is uniformly or irregularly distributed. Nucleoli are usually small or absent, and the cytoplasm is scant and ill-defined. Fibrovascular septa may divide the tumor into nests or lobules.[25, 318, 324, 326, 328–331] Some cases of so-called large cell or atypical Ewing's sarcoma that are more pleomorphic and have a coarse chromatin pattern and prominent nucleoli are probably examples of PNET.[319, 332, 336]

Neural differentiation at the light microscopic level may be evidenced by the presence of rosettes. These may be of the Homer-Wright type, called "pseudorosettes" by some (Fig. 8–14*B*, see p. 527), which have a central core of interdigitating cytoplasmic projections,[318, 321, 322, 324, 336, 337] or the less common "true" rosettes of the Flexner-Wintersteiner type (Fig. 8–14*C*, see p. 527) in which the cytoplasmic projections are arranged about a central, well-defined lumen.[322, 324, 337] Ganglion cells and Schwann-like spindle cells may rarely occur.[318, 319, 332, 336, 337] Mitoses are frequent and focal necrosis may be present. Stains for glycogen are positive in approximately 50% of cases.[25]

Although the foregoing description applies to most cases of PNET, some have a completely undifferentiated histologic appearance that resembles Ewing's sarcoma, being composed of small cells with uniform nuclei that have a powdery and evenly distributed chromatin,[321, 324, 329, 332, 337, 338] with no evidence of neural differentiation. In such cases, electron microscopic or immunohistochemical evidence of neural differentiation is required to distinguish the tumor from Ewing's sarcoma.

By electron microscopy, the cells of PNET contain abundant cytoplasmic organelles; glycogen, which may be abundant; and, in the majority of cases, dense core neurosecretory granules; microtubules and intermediate filaments may also be present. Characteristically, the cells possess interdigitating cytoplasmic processes.

A basal lamina is usually absent, but cell junctions of different types are formed, including desmosome or desmosome-like forms.[25, 324, 330, 331, 334, 337, 339]

Differential Diagnosis. Among the immunohistochemical markers of neural differentiation used to establish a diagnosis of PNET, reactivity for the enzyme neuron specific enolase (NSE) has been the most commonly studied; approximately 90% of PNET cases contain NSE-positive cells.[25] Indeed, some authors require positive reactivity for this enzyme as part of their criteria for the diagnosis of PNET.[320, 326, 337] However, NSE is not a specific marker for neural differentiation, being found in a number of non-neural lesions.[340, 341] Reactivity for other neural markers, including synaptophysin, neurofilament protein, Leu-7 antigen, S-100 protein, and chromogranin, have been found, respectively, in 46%, 41%, 40%, 36%, and 22%, of cases of PNET.[25] Some authors require reactivity for at least two neural markers before a diagnosis of PNET is accepted if this is the only evidence for such a diagnosis.[321] Reactivity for vimentin is present in 75% of cases, in contrast to its absence in almost all cases of neuroblastoma.[25]

The recent introduction of antibodies that recognize the pseudoautosomal gene product p30/32^{MIC2} (CD99) has proved useful in establishing the diagnosis of PNET,[332, 342–346] as approximately 90% of cases are positive.[25] Although this gene product is also present in Ewing's sarcoma, it is absent in neuroblastoma. However, experience with these antibodies established their nonspecificity for PNET and Ewing's sarcoma has become evident since CD99 was found in a wide range of divergent tumors, including such small, blue cell tumors as rhabdomyosarcoma, lymphoblastic lymphoma, small cell osteosarcoma, and mesenchymal chondrosarcoma.[3, 343, 347–350] PNET lacks leukocyte common antigen (CD45), which is present in almost all malignant lymphocytic lymphomas.

Significantly, PNET shares with bone and soft tissue Ewing's sarcoma the chromosomal translocation (11;22)(q24;q12).[323, 350–352] This translocation forms gene fusions (EWS/FLI-1; EWS/ERG) that result in the production of a hybrid protein that can be detected using reverse transcriptase-polymerase reactions.[349, 354] The fusion product was found in 95% to 100% of cases of PNET and Ewing's sarcoma and was thought to be specific to these tumors.[349, 354] However, it has also been found in some polyphenotypic small cell tumors as well as rhabdomyosarcoma.[355]

Cases of embryonal rhabdomyosarcoma (ERMS), especially the more primitive forms that lack acidophilic rhabdomyoblasts or cells with cross-striations, may be difficult to distinguish from PNET by light microscopy. This is a major problem in the head and neck area, a common site for ERMS. Compounding this problem are those examples of ERMS that are reported reactive for CD99, Leu-7, and NSE.[25] However, PNET lacks desmin and muscle-specific actin, markers for muscle differentiation that are present in most rhabdomyosarcomas, and the cells of PNET lack the electron microscopic features of skeletal muscle differentiation present in ERMS.

Lymphoblastic and non-cleaved small-cell lymphoma may both mimic PNET when rosettes are histologically absent. Electron microscopy easily separates these tumors from PNET.[25] Although some lymphoblastic lymphomas are immunohistochemically reactive for CD99,[348] the presence of leukocyte common antigen in lymphoma, provided antigen retrieval techniques are used for paraffin embedded tissue, helps distinguish these tumors.[356, 357] Markers for B and T cells are also useful in distinguishing lymphoma from PNET or Ewing's sarcoma,[348] as is electron microscopy.[25] Mesenchymal chondrosarcoma is distinguished from PNET or Ewing's tumor by its content of chondroid or cartilaginous islands.

Treatment and Prognosis. PNET is a highly malignant tumor with mortality rates in some series of 60% to 85%,[25, 321, 324, 328–330, 337, 350] with an average time till death of 18 months. In the head and neck region, some long-term survivors are reported who were treated with a combination of surgery, radiation, and chemotherapy.[325, 331, 334, 335]

Text continued on page 539

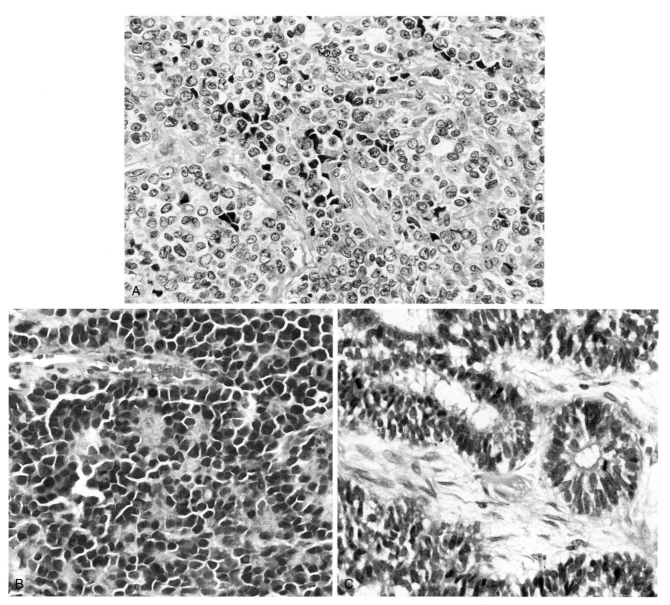

Figure 8–14. *A*, Malignant peripheral neuroectodermal tumor (PNET) shows proliferation of small cells with scant cytoplasm. Nuclei vary somewhat in size and shape, some with small nucleoli. Smaller cells with dense hyperchromatic nuclei are present, similar to the dark cells of Ewing's sarcoma. *B*, Neural differentiation in this PNET is evident by the formation of Homer-Wright pseudorosettes, with central neurofibrillary material. *C*, Example of PNET showing Flexner-Wintersteiner true rosettes, with a central well-defined lumen.

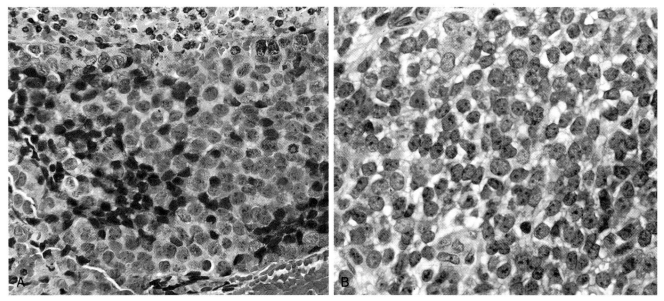

Figure 8–15. *A,* Ewing's sarcoma. Uniform small cells with little to no visible cytoplasm. Nuclei are round with uniformly distributed, powdery chromatin. Scattered smaller dark cells with hyperchromatic dense nuclei are also present. *B,* Ewing's sarcoma. Cells have somewhat coarser chromatin than the cells shown in part *A* and small nucleoli are present. Some cells have a vacuolated, clear cytoplasm due to the presence of glycogen.

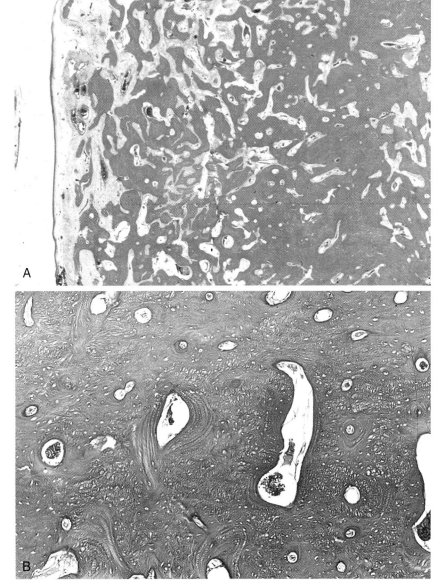

Figure 8–25. *A,* Osteoma of frontal sinus. Compact and trabecular bone is present beneath intact mucosa at the left of the field. *B,* Compact cortical-type bone of the osteoma shown in part *A* contains haversian systems.

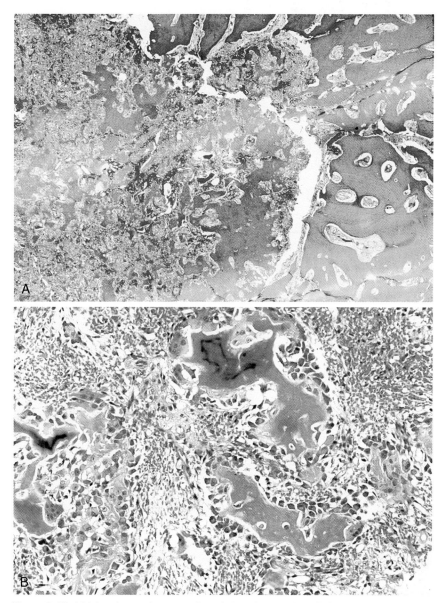

Figure 8–27. *A,* Nidus of osteoid osteoma abuts thickened mature bone. *B,* Osteoid trabeculae, some partially calcified, within the nidus of an osteoid osteoma. The trabeculae are rimmed by plump osteoblasts with occasional osteoclasts. The stroma is hemorrhagic.

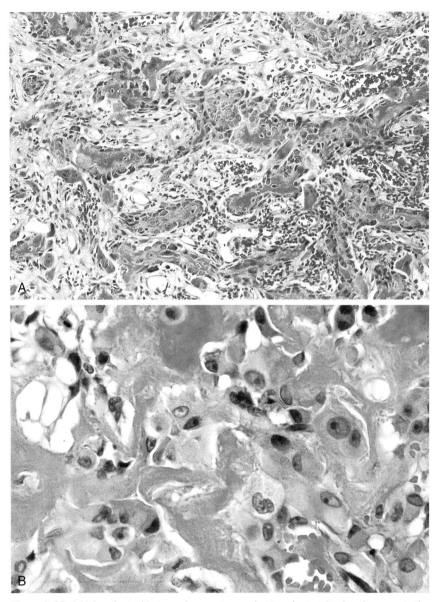

Figure 8–29. *A,* Nidus of osteoblastoma shows active production of osteoid trabeculae, some in the early stage of bone formation. The trabeculae are lined by enlarged osteoblasts with occasional osteoclasts. Numerous dilated capillaries are present in the stroma. *B,* Large epithelioid osteoblasts, in osteoblastoma, have abundant cytoplasm and large nuclei containing prominent nucleoli. Formation of lace-like osteoid is seen.

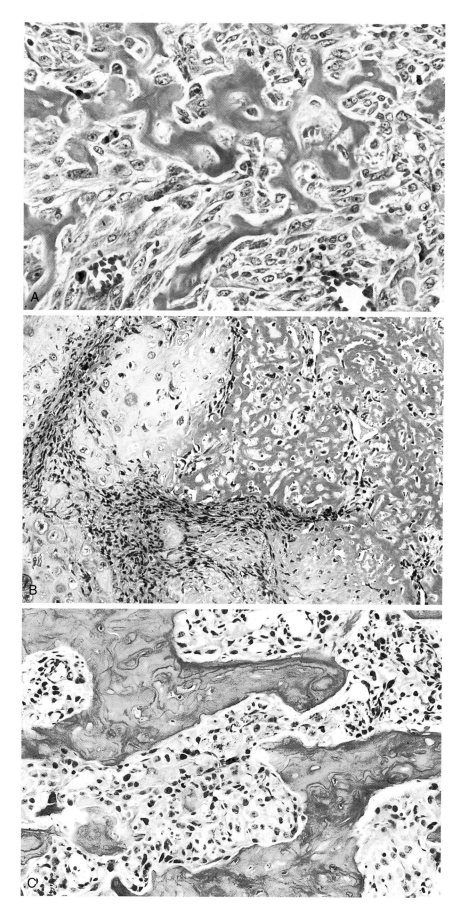

Figure 8–30. *A,* Osteosarcoma. Lace-like streamers of pink osteoid produced by malignant stromal cells (osteoblasts). *B,* Area in a conventional osteosarcoma shows a combination of osteoid, malignant cartilage, and spindle cell fibrous zones. *C,* Conventional osteosarcoma shows trabeculae of irregular tumor bone. Malignant osteoblasts fill the space between the trabeculae. Compare with the osteoblastoma shown in Figure 8–29*A.*

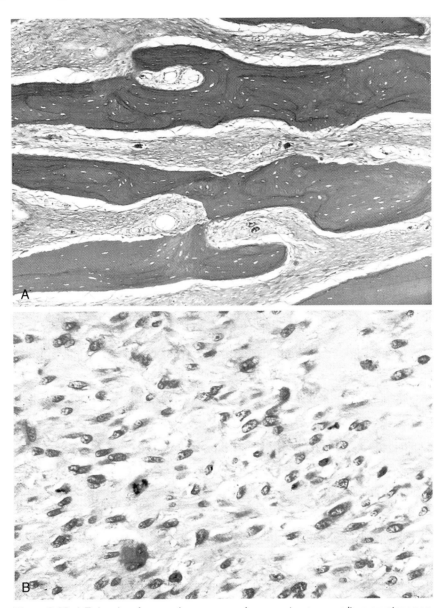

Figure 8–33. *A,* Trabeculae of parosteal osteosarcoma have prominent cement lines, creating a pagetoid appearance. The tumor lacks the abundant stromal cells filling the spaces between trabeculae, as found in conventional osteosarcoma. *B,* Fibrous stroma of parosteal osteosarcoma contains cells with ill-defined cytoplasmic limits and oval to round nuclei, with mild atypia. A few mitotic figures are present. The cells are separated by strands of collagen.

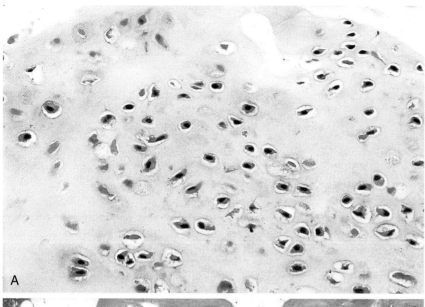

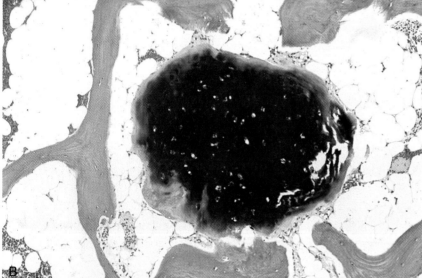

Figure 8–34. *A*, Enchondroma shows small, uniform chondrocytes whose nuclei are densely hyperchromatic (ink-dot) without a visible chromatin pattern. Cells are well separated from each other. *B*, An island of hyaline cartilage in an enchondroma is separated from the adjacent bone trabeculae by a zone of normal marrow tissue. This pattern of growth contrasts with that of chondrosarcoma shown in Figure 8–40*C*.

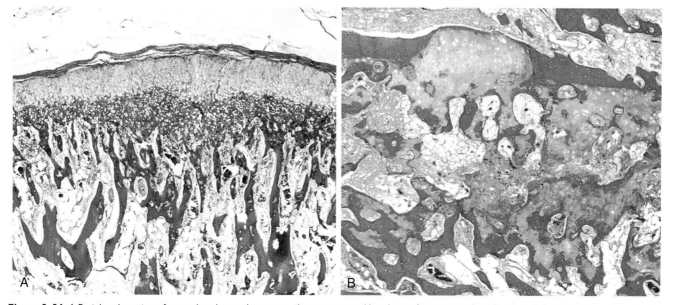

Figure 8–36. *A*, Peripheral portion of osteochondroma shows a cartilage cap covered by a layer of periosteum (perichondrium). Active enchondral ossification is present, with widely dilated capillaries present at the base of the cartilage. The marrow is filled with fat. *B*, Bone within osteochondroma shows persistence of partially ossified hyaline cartilage within the centers of the trabeculae.

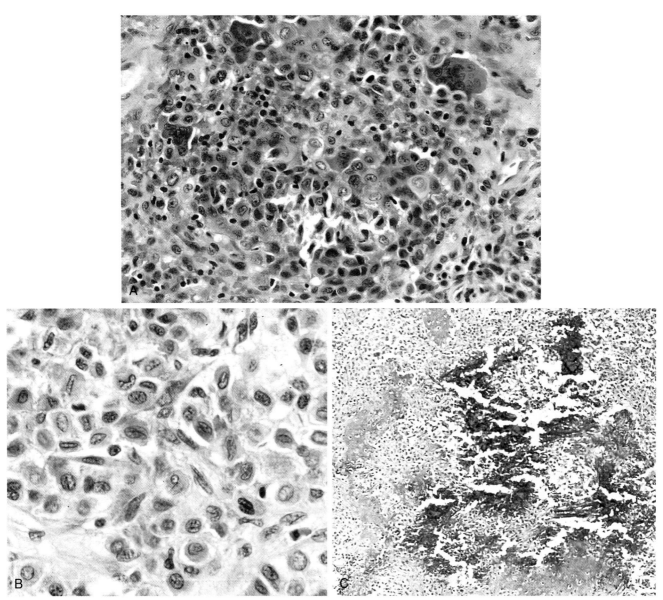

Figure 8–38. *A*, Chondroblastoma. Tumor contains compact mononuclear cells with densely eosinophilic cytoplasm and well-defined borders. Osteoclast-type giant cells are also present. *B*, Convoluted and grooved nuclei are present in some cells of this chondroblastoma. Such cells may resemble those of eosinophilic granuloma. *C*, Focus of dystrophic calcification in chondroblastoma. At the periphery of the focus, islands of pink chondroid are present.

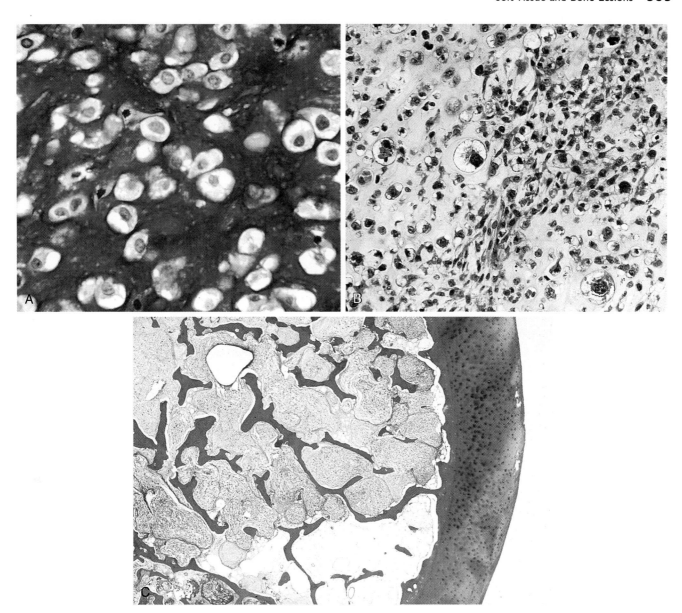

Figure 8–40. *A,* Low-grade chondrosarcoma. The tumor cells are of greater size than normal chondrocytes, with larger, open-faced nuclei that have a uniform, fine chromatin pattern. Several mitotic figures are present, an uncommon finding in most chondrosarcomas. *B,* High-grade chondrosarcoma. Hypercellular tumor contains pleomorphic cells, some with large bizarre nuclei. A few cells are spindle-shaped. *C,* Growth pattern of chondrosarcoma shows infiltration between existing normal bone, resulting in trabeculae that are closely abutted and surrounded by tumor.

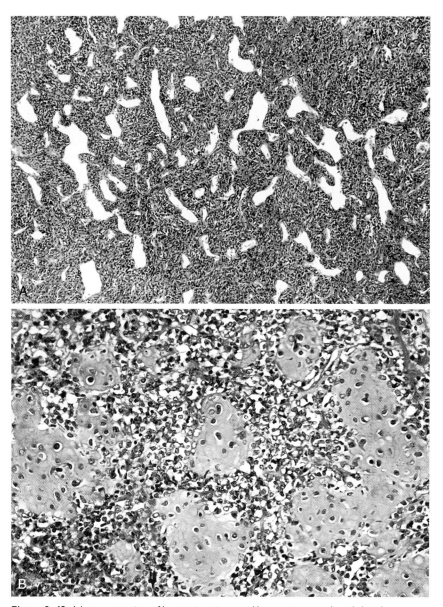

Figure 8–42. *A,* Low-power view of hemangiopericytoma-like area in mesenchymal chondrosarcoma. Tightly compacted small blue cells surround and bulge into gaping vascular spaces. *B,* Islands of chondroid surrounded by small tumor cells in mesenchymal chondrosarcoma. Nuclei of the "chondrocytes" within lacunar spaces resemble the nuclei of the stromal tumor cells.

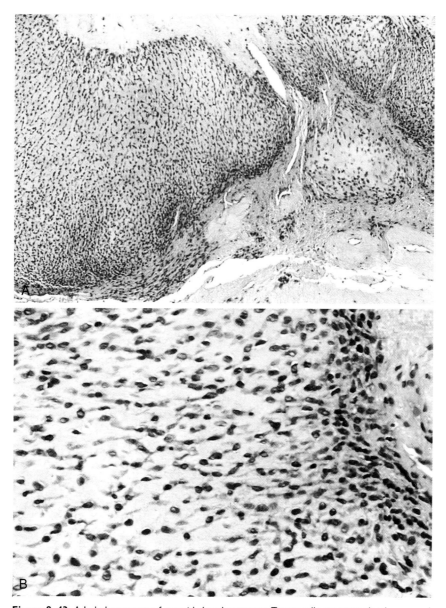

Figure 8–43. *A*, Lobular pattern of myxoid chondrosarcoma. Tumor cells are more closely arranged at the periphery of the lobules. *B*, Radial, cord-like arrangement of tumor cells in myxoid chondrosarcoma. Cells are embedded in grayish myxoid stroma.

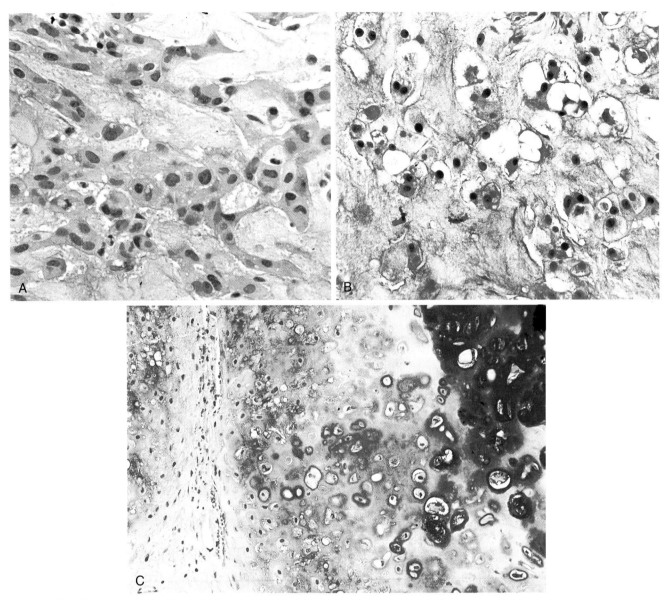

Figure 8–45. *A,* Chordoma. Strands of epithelial-like cells, with abundant eosinophilic cytoplasm, reside in a blue-gray mucinous stroma. *B,* Area of chordoma with tumor cells showing cytoplasmic vacuolation with the formation of multivacuolated physaliferous cells. *C,* Chondroid chordoma. Chordoma cells to the left of the field merge into a nodule of hyaline-appearing cartilage with low-grade malignant features.

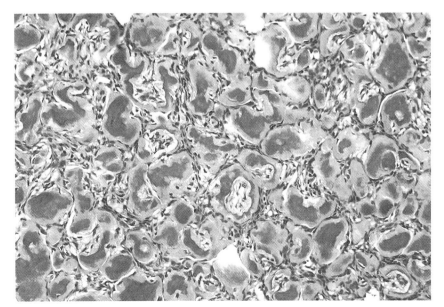

Figure 8–51. Psammomatoid ossifying fibroma, uniform small ossicles (psammomatoid bodies) in cellular stroma.

Extraskeletal Ewing's Sarcoma

The existence of an extraskeletal form of Ewing's sarcoma (EES) was established by Angervall and Enzinger in 1975,[358] although Tefft et al.[359] had previously reported a small number of cases in the paravertebral soft tissues. Extraskeletal Ewing's tumor is morphologically identical to the osseous form, and may cytologically overlap other small blue cell tumors, including PNET. Indeed, some cases of EES reported in the older medical literature would now be diagnosed as PNET because of the presence of features, such as rosettes or neurosecretory granules, indicative of neural differentiation.[332, 339, 360] Ewing's sarcoma and PNET have in common the (11;22)(q24;q12) chromosomal transposition,[323, 351–353] and reactivity for CD99.[332, 342, 344]

Clinical Features. EES most commonly occurs in adolescents and young adults, although newborns and patients over 80 years of age are reported. These tumors occur in somewhat older patients than does either PNET or skeletal Ewing's sarcoma, with mean patient ages ranging from 19 to 26 years (median 16 to 20 years).[358, 361, 362–364]

The trunk, especially the paravertebral region, and the extremities are the most common locations for EES, although it also occurs in a wide variety of other soft tissue sites with only 5% to 12% of cases occurring in the head and neck.[360, 361, 363, 365, 366] In the head and neck region, the soft tissue of the neck is the most common site, with other locations including the nasal fossa, nose, eyelid, scalp, and orbit.[350, 358, 359, 360, 363, 365, 366–373]

Extraskeletal Ewing's sarcoma grows rapidly and may be painful or tender.[358, 362, 364] It is usually deeply situated within skeletal muscle, although it may arise in the superficial cutaneous or subcutaneous tissue.[358, 362, 364, 374] The deep tumors may become attached to underlying bone and elicit a periosteal reaction that may radiologically suggest an intraosseous origin. Before a diagnosis of EES is accepted, careful radiologic examination of the adjacent bone should be done to rule out the possibility of a primary skeletal Ewing's sarcoma with soft tissue extension.[371]

Pathologic Features. Grossly, EES is usually a soft, friable, gray-white mass whose cut surface contains necrotic and hemorrhagic zones. Most exceed 5.0 cm, and even in the limited confines of the head and neck, tumors as large as 14 cm and 20 cm are reported.[366, 367, 372]

Extraskeletal Ewing's sarcoma is histologically identical to its skeletal counterpart,[358, 364] consisting of small, closely packed, oval to round cells arranged in broad fields separated by fibrous septa. Nuclei are oval to round, with a fine, powdery, uniformly distributed chromatin and at times a small, uniform nucleolus (Fig. 8–15, see p. 528). The cytoplasm is scanty and ill-defined but may be vacuolated because of the presence of glycogen, which is present in the majority of cases (see Fig. 8–15B). Areas of necrosis, containing ghost tumor cell remnants, are quite frequent. Despite its rapid clinical evolution, mitotic figures are not common. Cells with small, hyperchromatic, dense nuclei and scant cytoplasm, so called "dark cells," may be found scattered throughout the tumor (see Fig. 8–15A). Definitive rosettes are not found in EES, and their presence would indicate, in the proper clinical setting, that the tumor is a PNET. Although the cell nuclei in EES are more homogeneous than those of PNET, lacking infoldings, irregularities, or coarse chromatin, some examples of PNET exist in which the light microscopic cytology completely mimics that of Ewing's sarcoma and only by electron microscopy or immunohistochemistry can evidence of neural differentiation be demonstrated.[447, 450, 455, 458, 472–476]

The electron microscopic pattern of EES also parallels that of skeletal Ewing's sarcoma. Cytoplasmic glycogen is found in almost all cases, frequently in large pools, and the cells show, in contrast to PNET, a general lack of organelles, the cells having an undifferentiated appearance. The cytoplasmic processes, neurosecretory granules, and microtubules, as in the cells of PNET, are absent.[360, 362, 363, 365, 375] Immunohistochemically, the cells of EES are vimentin positive and, in some cases, may show reactivity for NSE.

However, owing to the nonspecific nature of this enzyme, we do not classify such a tumor as being neural on this basis alone and require other immunohistochemical or electron microscopic features of neural differentiation to be present before ruling out a diagnosis of EES. Despite the number of cases of EES that prove to be PNET when extensively analyzed by either electron microscopy or immunohistochemistry, we do not mean to imply that a true EES does not exist; however, we restrict the diagnosis of EES to a lesion that shows no evidence of neural differentiation by either light or electron microscopy, or by immunohistochemistry.

Treatment and Prognosis. Although early reports of EES indicated a poor prognosis, subsequent studies of patients who received combination treatment modalities with radiation and chemotherapy, in addition to surgical resection, indicate that the majority of patients can be salvaged, including those with head and neck tumors, with 5-year survival rates of from 48% to 64%.[321, 350, 358, 361, 363, 365, 376] Whether Ewing's sarcoma has a better prognosis than PNET is an unsettled issue, with some believing this to be the case,[321, 329, 376–381] while others report no prognostic differences between these two tumors.[350, 360, 382–384] These results may be the reflection of the different criteria used by investigators to classify a tumor as either a PNET or an EES.

Paragangliomas

Paraganglionic tissue of the head and neck embryologically derives from the neural crest, develops in the paravertebral region in association with the arterial vessels and cranial nerves of the ontogenetic gill arches, and is associated with the autonomic nervous system.[385, 386]

Cells of the paraganglia are capable of producing and storing vasoactive and neurotransmitter substances, such as the catecholamines norepinephrine and epinephrine, as well as a variety of hormones, including serotonin, gastrin, and somatostatin. The catecholamines are stored in cytoplasmic neurosecretory granules that may be seen by electron microscopy. Tumors of extra-adrenal paraganglionic tissue usually do not give a positive chromaffin reaction and therefore were termed *nonchromaffin paragangliomas*.[386, 387] However, by the use of more sensitive methods such as formaldehyde-induced fluorescence, catecholamines can be demonstrated in the extra-adrenal paraganglionic tumors. Therefore, the term *nonchromaffin* should no longer be used as a prefix for these tumors.[385, 387] Similarly, the term *glomus tumor*, which is frequently used as an appellation for tumors of the paraganglionic system, is not accurate. True glomus tumors are mainly located in the skin and superficial soft tissues of the extremities and have no relationship to the tumors of the paraganglia.[387]

A practical classification of the paraganglionic system was established to clarify an area previously noted for its diverse terminology. This classification is based on location and divides the paraganglia into branchiomeric, intravagal, aorticosympathetic, and visceral-autonomic groups.[385] The branchiomeric group contains many tumors that are located in the head and neck and includes the jugulotympanic, intercarotid, orbital, nasal, subclavian, laryngeal, coronary, aorticopulmonary, and pulmonary paraganglia. Although not a member of the branchiomeric paraganglia, tumors of the intravagal paraganglia are usually included with this group for the sake of discussion. In this section tumors of the carotid body and intravagal paraganglia are discussed. The clinically important jugulotympanic tumors are more appropriately discussed as part of the tumors of the middle ear.

Carotid Body Paraganglioma (Carotid Body Tumor)

The normal carotid body is found at the bifurcation of the common carotid artery as an adherent, 5.0 to 6.0 mm, pink mass on the adventitia of the medial side of the vessel.[385, 386, 388] It is supplied by blood vessels of the external carotid artery and has a sensory nerve supply via the glossopharyngeal nerve.[386, 388] The carotid body is a chemoreceptor that monitors and responds to changes in blood oxygen, carbon dioxide, and pH levels.[387, 388] Tumors of this organ have previously been termed *chemodectomas.* The function of the other paraganglia, such as the intravagal or jugulotympanic is not defined, and because no chemoreceptor function is known for these, *chemodectoma* is not an accurate general designation for tumors of this system.[387]

The normal carotid body is composed of nests of epithelial cells, the chief cells, that originate from the neural crest.[385-388] These cells are arranged in clusters, forming the so-called Zellballen. They have a finely granular eosinophilic cytoplasm, and the cell nests are surrounded by thin, richly vascular fibrous septa, which are best demonstrated by reticulin stains. Between the chief cells are Schwann-like sustentacular cells that are difficult to identify by light microscopy but are identified by electron microscopy and immunohistochemically.[387] The function of these sustentacular cells is not established, but they are intimately associated with the chief cells. The chief cells contain the argyrophilic neurosecretory granules that contain catecholamines.[385]

Clinical Features. Carotid body tumors, namely carotid body paragangliomas, are the most common tumors of the head and neck paraganglia, constituting between 60% and 67% of the total.[8, 389, 390] Despite over 600 reported cases,[391] it should be remembered that these are still uncommon lesions. Only 69 paragangliomas of the head and neck were found in over 600,000 operations (0.12%) at Memorial Hospital, New York, and only 1 in 13,400 autopsies.[390] They are thought to be more common in patients who live at high altitudes.[385]

Paragangliomas occur at all ages, from children to patients in the ninth decade of life, but the mean age is between 45 and 50 years.[388, 390, 392-395, 396] A female predominance has been found in several series,[388, 392, 395, 397] whereas some have found an almost equal sex incidence.[390, 393, 394] Enzinger and Weiss claim that the male-to-female incidence is about equal, except for a higher female incidence in those patients living at high altitudes.[8]

Carotid body paragangliomas manifest themselves as slowly growing, painless neck masses located beneath the anterior edge of the sternocleidomastoid muscle just lateral to the tip of the hyoid bone.[386, 388-390, 393, 395, 397] They may expand upward into the neck or, occasionally, bulge into the pharynx.[386] Owing to compression of adjacent cranial or sympathetic nerves, hoarseness, vocal cord paralysis, and dysphagia are noted.[385, 386, 388, 390, 393] The lesions usually have long duration with an average of 2 to 8 years; some are present for as long as 47 years.[390, 392, 395, 396] Occasionally, however, symptoms are present for only a few weeks.[388, 394, 395]

Between 2% and 10% of patients have bilateral tumors, either simultaneously or consequentially.[388, 394, 395] Parry et al.[395] state that such patients are younger than those with unilateral tumors. Carotid body paragangliomas are rarely functional[386, 389-391] but may occur along with jugulotympanic or intravagal paragangliomas, or with pheochromocytoma,[391, 394] in association with medullary carcinomas of the thyroid, and in patients with neurofibromatosis.[8] Occasional cases occur in families and appear to be transmitted as an autosomal dominant trait. Up to one third of familial tumors are bilateral.[395] The familial form accounts for 7% to 9% of paragangliomas in the head and neck. Multiple tumors occur in 25% to 48% of the cases, including both synchronous and metachronous tumors.[397, 398] An association between carotid body paraganglioma, parathyroid adenomas, and hyperplasia has been reported.[399] It is suggested that such an association may represent another variable expression of the multiple endocrine neoplasia syndrome.[399]

The association of extra-adrenal paraganglioma, particularly those of the head and neck, with gastric leiomyosarcoma and pulmonary chondroma has been termed *Carney's triad.* The triad is rare and occurs predominantly in young girls.[400, 401] The coexistence of two of the three stigmata of this syndrome is evident in at least 20% of cases.[402]

On physical examination, the carotid body tumor may be movable from side to side, but not in a vertical direction, and may trans-

mit the arterial pulse.[386, 389, 393] The diagnosis may almost always be established preoperatively by selective angiography, which shows a vascular mass at the carotid artery bifurcation.[391, 393, 397] Preoperative biopsy of such a mass has no place in the management of these lesions because of the potential for severe hemorrhage.[389, 391, 397]

Pathologic Features. Grossly, the tumors vary from 2.0 to 9.0 cm, with most being about 4.0 cm. in greatest dimension.[386, 388, 390, 392-394, 396] They are well circumscribed, appear encapsulated, and are firm, reddish gray to brown, and quite vascular.

Histologically, carotid body paragangliomas closely replicate the morphology of the normal carotid body (Fig. 8–16A).[385, 386, 388] The nests of chief cells tend to be somewhat larger than normal,[386, 403] and areas may occur where the cells are spindle-shaped ("sarcomatoid foci"); other areas may be so highly vascular that they are suggestive of an angioma[385, 386, 396] or hemangiopericytoma.[386, 388, 403] Most tumor cells have a bland appearance, but it is not uncommon to find scattered large pleomorphic cells with hyperchromatic nuclei.[386, 388, 403] Mitotic activity is not common and is usually absent. The tumor cells have an abundant clear to finely granular eosinophilic cytoplasm, and cell nests are set off by reticulin fibers.[8, 385, 396] Occasionally, the cells are arranged in short ribbons or cords that are divided and compressed by extensive fibrous bands.[8, 403] A capsule may not be present, and infiltration of the tumor cells into the adventitia of the adjacent artery is seen.[396] By electron microscopy, the tumor cells contain neurosecretory granules[385, 387, 394, 403] and, at the light microscope level, are argyrophilic but argentaffin-negative with silver stains.[8, 390] Sustentacular cells are usually demonstratable in carotid body tumors.[8, 387, 403]

In an immunohistochemical study of 11 head and neck paragangliomas, 9 of which were carotid body tumors, Warren et al.[404] found that all stained intensely for neuron-specific enolase and some contained a variety of hormones such as serotonin, leu-enkephalin, substance P, vasoactive intestinal peptide, gastrin, somatostatin, vasopressin, melanocyte-stimulating hormone, and calcitonin. Sustentacular cells are demonstrated with antisera to S-100 protein (Fig. 8–16B).[8]

The histologic differential diagnosis from metastatic thyroid medullary carcinoma is important. The lack of reactivity with antibodies to cytokeratin, carcinoembryonic antigen, and calcitonin, in addition to the presence of sustentacular cells favors the diagnosis of paraganglioma over medullary thyroid carcinoma.

Treatment and Prognosis. Surgical therapy is the essential method of treatment for carotid body tumors. If the tumor is completely removed, recurrences are uncommon, occurring in about 10% of cases.[388, 390] The operative mortality rate has decreased over the years with improved techniques for vascular grafting and bypass procedures. The rate of occurrence of cerebrovascular accidents following operation has also been dramatically reduced by these techniques.[388, 397]

The incidence of malignant carotid body tumors has varied in the literature from 1.5% to 50%.[388, 390, 394-396] Such a wide discrepancy in incidence is caused by the variable criteria used to determine malignancy in these tumors. The higher figures were based on the histologic presence of pleomorphic cells and local invasion, criteria that are unreliable in predicting malignant behavior. The only reliable criterion for establishing the malignancy of a paraganglioma is the presence of either local lymph node involvement, distant metastases, or extensive local invasion. When these more stringent guidelines are used, fewer than 10% of paragangliomas are reported as malignant and most likely the true rate is less than 5%.[388, 394-397] However, metastatic rates as high as 12.5% have been reported.[405] The evolution of metastatic disease may be quite slow, with metastases developing from 3 to 16 years after diagnosis with some patients developing metastases up to 35 years after their original therapy.[385, 386, 393, 395] Of the cases that metastasize, involvement of regional lymph nodes is as frequent as metastasis to distant sites.[388, 395] Bone and lung are the main sites for distant metastasis.

Recent studies have suggested a possible role for immunohistochemical stains in prediction of malignant behavior of paragan-

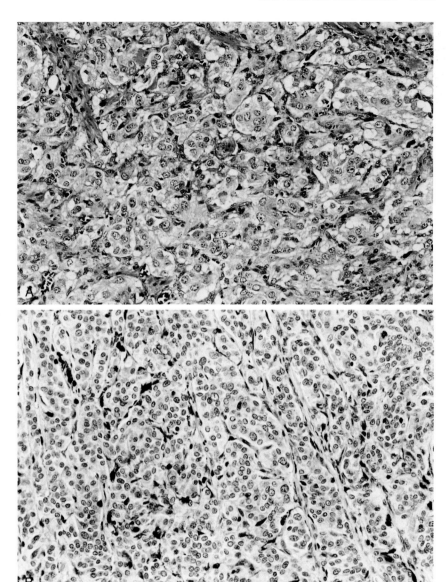

Figure 8–16. *A,* Carotid body paraganglioma showing the characteristic nesting pattern of the chief cells (Zellballen). *B,* Sustentacular cells are positively stained with antibodies to S-100 protein.

glioma. Achilles et al.[406] indicate that clinically malignant extraadrenal paragangliomas lack S-100 positive sustentacular cells. Other studies have shown a decrease in the expression of neuropeptides in malignant paraganglioma.[407] Barnes and Taylor[408] found no apparent relationship between the DNA content of paraganglioma cells and their malignant potential.

Intravagal Paraganglioma

Intravagal paragangliomas arise from nests of paraganglionic tissue located within or adjacent to the vagus nerve, most commonly at the level of the ganglion nodosum, which may itself be replaced by tumor.[385, 409] However, intravagal paragangliomas may be located at any point along the cervical path of the vagus nerve.[409]

Clinical Features. Women are more commonly affected than men, and patient ages parallel those for carotid body lesions, with a mean age of approximately 50 years (range, 18 to 71 years).[385, 390, 396] The tumor usually manifests as a painless neck mass, although a case was reported in which severe pain was the predominant presentation.[410] The tumors arise behind the angle of the mandible and not infrequently bulge into the pharynx to produce dysphagia.[8, 385, 396, 411–413] Tumor compression of the adjacent nerves may produce symptoms such as weakness of the tongue,

vocal cord paralysis, hoarseness, or even Horner's syndrome.[8, 389, 390, 411, 413] Angiography shows a vascular mass situated above the carotid bifurcation, a finding virtually diagnostic of this tumor.[390, 411]

As with carotid body tumors, the duration of symptoms is usually long, about 4 years.[390, 411, 413] Only one functional intravagal paraganglioma has been reported.[409]

Intravagal paragangliomas are less common than either carotid body or jugulotympanic paragangliomas. A recent review yielded 145 cases reported in the English-language medical literature.[415] Although familial examples exist, these are much rarer than familial carotid body tumors. Kahn[414] reported only the second such case in 1976, and Chaudhry et al.[409] found only four such cases. Intravagal paragangliomas have been found in association with other head and neck paragangliomas[409, 414]; multicentricity in nonfamilial cases occurs in 28% of cases.[415]

Pathologic Features. Grossly, intravagal paragangliomas appear well circumscribed, but they may extend upward into the base of the skull and range in size from 2.0 to 6.0 cm.[390, 396] Histologically, intravagal paragangliomas differ only slightly from carotid body paragangliomas, with perhaps more abundant fibrous septa that compress the chief cells.[385, 412] Nerve fibers and ganglion cells may be seen because of the tumor's close association with the vagus nerve and the ganglion nodosum.[385] Only a few of these tumors have been examined by electron microscopy, with sustentacular cells seen in some studies and not in others.[409, 414] Immunohistochemical staining characteristics are similar to those of the carotid body paraganglioma.

Treatment and Prognosis. As with carotid body tumors, surgical excision is the treatment of choice for intravagal paraganglioma. In Lack's series of 13 cases,[390] a resection was done in 12, with follow-up available in 11. Of these, 8 patients were alive and well for an average of 7 years (range, 6 months to 16 years). Two patients were alive with residual tumor, 2 and 15 years later, and one patient died of unrelated causes 14 years after therapy.

Malignant vagal paragangliomas are reported to be more frequent than malignant carotid body tumors.[403, 409, 412, 414] In the review by Chaudhry,[409] 13 of the 72 intravagal paragangliomas (18%) had metastasized, only four of these to distant sites, whereas the remainder involved only regional lymph nodes.

Lymphangioma and Cystic Hygroma

Of lesions of the lymphatic system, only lymphangioma and cystic hygroma are encountered frequently in the head and neck region. Whether these are true tumors or represent malformations or hamartomas is still debated, but this issue is of no clinical consequence, and the lesions are treated here as true tumors.[8]

Lymphangiomas accounted for 26% of 228 vascular tumors in children and adolescents.[416] Of those, 53% occurred in the head and neck. A frequency of five cases per 3000 admissions to a children's hospital has been reported.[417]

The terminology of these lesions has caused some confusion in the past, but basically they are divided into three morphologic types: capillary (lymphangioma circumscriptum), cavernous (lymphangioma cavernosum), and cystic (cystic hygroma).[8, 417, 418]

Lymphangioma circumscriptum is clinically the least significant and usually is confined to the superficial skin or the mucous membrane, forming small vesicle-like lesions.[419, 420] They are usually asymptomatic, although they may produce symptoms by being irritated. They are cutaneous tumors and will not be further considered here except to say that they may occur in conjunction with the other two forms of lymphangioma.

The separation of cavernous lymphangioma from cystic hygroma is valid only in the clinical sense, as histopathologically the lesions are similar.[421] The distinctive gross pattern that separates the two is primarily based on the location and the quality of the surrounding soft tissue.[417, 422] If the surrounding soft tissue, as in the neck, is loose and permits expansion of the lesion, the cavernous lymphatic tumor will expand into the typical gross multicystic appearance of a hygroma.

Clinical Features. Approximately two thirds of lymphangiomas are present or noted shortly after birth, and 80% to 95% are present by the end of the second year of life.[415–418, 423–426] Cystic hygroma may also be detected in utero by ultrasonography. It has been shown that these cases are commonly associated with Turner's syndrome.[8] In most series there is no significant sex difference, or only a slight male predominance.

Lymphangiomas occur in a variety of body locations, including the retroperitoneum, mesentery, groin, extremities, chest wall, mediastinum, and within viscera.[415, 424] The head and neck region, however, accounts for between 40% and 70% of all lesions.[8]

The cavernous form of lymphangioma is found most frequently in the tongue, cheek, floor of mouth, lips, and nose. Cystic hygroma is most common in the neck,[417, 418, 424] frequently located in the posterior triangle lying behind the sternomastoid muscle; it is less common in the anterior cervical triangle.[423] However, as it enlarges it may extend into the anterior compartment, upward into the cheek or parotid region, or down into the mediastinum or axilla.[421] Of 34 cases of cervicofacial cystic hygroma, 21 were located cephalad to the hyoid bone.[427] The tongue is the most frequently involved intraoral site, with most of the tumors involving the anterior two thirds, although the base of the tongue is occasionally involved.[422, 428] The tumor produces macroglossia and is the single most common cause of this condition.[428] Lymphangiomas of the tongue are also associated with cystic lymphangiomas located at other sites.[422, 428] However, lymphangiomas may vary from localized pinhead-sized single vesicles to extensive and diffuse lesions that infiltrate the entire tongue, causing nodularity of the surface with vesicle-like projections.[422, 428] The tongue may be enlarged to such an extent that it cannot be placed in the mouth.[422, 428]

Most children with lymphangioma are brought to the physician's attention because the parents notice a mass that had slowly enlarged.[417, 418, 421] Occasionally, however, because of the marked size that some of these tumors attain, especially cystic hygromas, the child may develop signs of respiratory distress, difficulty in swallowing, or difficulty in nursing with regurgitation.[415, 417, 421, 423, 426] These problems are rare, however, and most patients are asymptomatic.[424, 425] Cystic hygroma located superior to the hyoid bone are more likely to cause dysphagia or airway compromise than those inferior to it.[427]

Cavernous lymphangiomas vary from millimeter-sized lesions to those of several centimeters[420, 422, 424] and may be well circumscribed or diffusely invasive, involving subcutaneous tissue and underlying muscle. They extend by budding along fascial planes, great vessels, or nerve trunks to form ill-defined spongy and compressible masses.[8, 424] When the skin is involved, they may produce bluish bulges. Cystic hygromas vary from a single soft mass with a smooth round contour to lobulated, multicystic masses.[418, 423] Their walls are thin, and, unless there has been previous infection, they will transilluminate.[418] The individual cysts communicate with each other such that accidental rupture of any one of them will cause collapse of the entire mass, thus masking the limits of its extension.[421] Cystic hygromas in the neck have room to expand, owing to the loose areolar type connective tissue in this region and, like cavernous lymphangioma, also extend along the great vessels and nerves and between muscle groups by finger-like projections.[417, 423, 424] These projections may be easily overlooked at operation and serve as a focus for recurrence. Cystic hygromas vary from 1.0 cm to 30.0 cm with a mean size of 8.0 cm.[426] They usually contain clear, serous-type fluid.[418, 423]

Pathologic Features. As mentioned, cavernous lymphangioma and cystic hygroma are histologically similar and consist of dilated, thin-walled sinuses that are filled with eosinophilic, acellular lymph fluid.[419, 420] These spaces are lined by flat endothelial cells[418, 421, 423] and vary from small (capillary) to large (cavernous), much in the same way that a hemangioma may contain small or large channels.[417] The intervening stroma may be quite scanty, with closely packed channels, or it may be more abundant, with the spaces separated by stroma. This stroma varies from a loose myxomatous lace-like material to areas with dense hyalinization.[417, 419, 423] When there has been previous infection, the stroma is markedly increased.[586] Scattered lymphoid aggregates are found, occasionally in the form of germinal follicles, and wisps of smooth muscle fibers may also be present (Fig. 8–17).[8, 418]

Treatment and Prognosis. Surgical therapy, with as wide an excision as possible while preserving cosmetic function, is the best approach to these lesions.[415, 417, 421, 424] Staged excisions may be necessary to avoid mutilating surgery for these benign but troublesome tumors. Recently carbon dioxide laser photocoagulation has been used with success in the management of tongue and superficial lingual lymphangiomas.[429, 430] Lymphangiomas are radioresistant, and the use of radiation therapy in infants and young children is to be avoided whenever possible.[418, 425, 426] Despite their benign nature, surgical management is difficult, especially for the cavernous lymphangioma, because of its tendency to spread along vital structures and the subsequent high incidence of recurrence. There was no recurrence in any case thought to be completely excised.[415] Most recurrences appear within 1 year, many within 6 months.[426] Among 27 excisions of head and neck cystic hygromas in children, Adeyemi[431] reported a 22% recurrence rate.

Mortality rates are between 3% and 7%, with the largest lesions having the higher mortality rates.[415, 417, 418, 423–425] In Barrand and Freeman's series of nine "massive" infiltrating hygromas,[432] four of eight patients operated upon died. Most deaths have been postoperative. Lymphangiomas, especially intraoral ones, are prone to infection and may suddenly increase in size because of this, with life-threatening consequences.[425]

Lipoma, Lipomatosis, and Liposarcoma

Lipoma

Lipoma is the most common soft-tissue tumor[8, 433] but its true incidence is difficult to assess, as many patients have small asymptomatic masses and never seek medical attention. In a series of 1331 benign soft-tissue tumors, lipomas made up 48% of the total cases.[434] It is only when the tumor reaches such a size that it is either cosmetically distracting or impinges on vital structures that the patient seeks attention. There are few published reports in which large numbers of patients with adipose tumors are described,[435, 436] as pathologists and clinicians have not been stimulated by this prosaic tumor, and usually only individual case reports are published when the lipoma arises in unusual locations. Allen's excellent monograph on adipose tumors, however, describes over 40 varieties of benign mesenchymal lesions in which fat is a prominent or major component.[437] In addition, recent descriptions of lipomas with histologic features that may mimic or be confused with liposarcoma have stimulated a renewed interest in the common lipoma.

Clinical Features. Lipomas tend to occur in obese patients or those with recent weight gain.[8, 435] Approximately 60% to 75% of these patients are women[435, 437–439] in the fifth to sixth decades of life.[435, 437, 438] However, in his extensive review of lipomas of the oral cavity, Hatziotis found that of 125 recorded cases in which the sex of the patient was mentioned, 68 (54%) were males.[438] The tumor is uncommon in the first two decades of life and is rarely found in children.[8, 433, 435–437, 439] Lipoma is usually a solitary, painless mass that gradually increases in size or becomes stationary after a period of growth.

Most lipomas are between 1.0 cm and 5.0 cm in maximum dimension,[8, 437] but, depending on location, they may reach enormous size, 50 to 60 cm, and weigh many kilograms.[8, 436, 437] Lipoma is a soft, freely movable mass that almost always arises in the subcuta-

neous tissue.[437, 439] The most common sites include the shoulder, arms, and trunk.[8, 433, 437, 439] The head and neck region accounts for approximately 15% to 20% of all cases, with the neck being more commonly affected than the head; the face and scalp are rarely involved.[8, 435] Oral cavity lipomas are rare, accounting for only 1% to 2% of all benign tumors in this site.[438] The cheek was the most common site in the 145 oral lipomas reported by Hatziotis, accounting for 46 cases, whereas the tongue was the site in 28, the floor of the mouth in 21, the buccal sulcus and vestibule in 18, the palate in 13, the lips in 9, and the gingiva in 8, with two sites not stated.[438] Pharyngeal lipomas are equally rare. In the neck and oral cavity, the tumor may be pedunculated or sessile.[438] Lipomas also rarely occur in the larynx, tonsil, maxillary antrum, and jaw bones.[440–444]

It should be remembered that lipomas are usually superficially located, in contrast to the malignant tumor of adipose tissue, liposarcoma, which arises in the deep soft tissue and which is rarely superficial. This is an important clinical point for distinguishing between these two tumors. Deeply situated intramuscular and intermuscular lipomas, however, do occur, but these are usually found in the distal extremities and shoulder region and are quite rare in the muscles of the head and neck.[437, 445]

Pathologic Features. Grossly, lipomas are smooth, well-circumscribed, round to oval encapsulated masses. The cut surface varies from yellow to orange and is greasy to the touch. The tumors may be lobulated.[8, 437] Microscopically, there is a thin fibrous capsule from which delicate septa extend into the substance of the tumor, separating it into lobules that are composed of mature adipose cells (Fig. 8–18A). The presence of a fibrous capsule serves to distinguish a lipoma from a simple aggregation of fat.[436] Scattered myxoid areas may be found, and small foci of fat necrosis, probably the result of minor trauma, are occasionally seen within the lobules. Electron microscopic studies have shown that the cells of lipoma are morphologically similar to the cells of normal mature adipose tissue.[446] Cytogenetic studies of lipoma suggest that a chromosomal translocation, t(3;12) may be a characteristic features of this tumor.[447]

Multiple lipomas occur in 1% to 7% of cases, at times in patients with a family history of multiple lipomas. Multiple lipomas also occur in patients with neurofibromatosis and in those with the multiple endocrine neoplasia syndrome.[433, 437] These multiple conventional fatty tumors must be distinguished from angiolipoma, which is frequently multiple but rarely occurs in the head and neck.

Treatment and Prognosis. True lipomas rarely recur (1% to 2%) after adequate local excision.[8, 437] Such an occurrence should raise the clinical suspicion of liposarcoma, especially if the tumor is

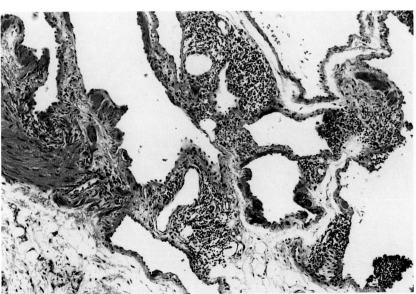

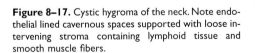

Figure 8–17. Cystic hygroma of the neck. Note endothelial lined cavernous spaces supported with loose intervening stroma containing lymphoid tissue and smooth muscle fibers.

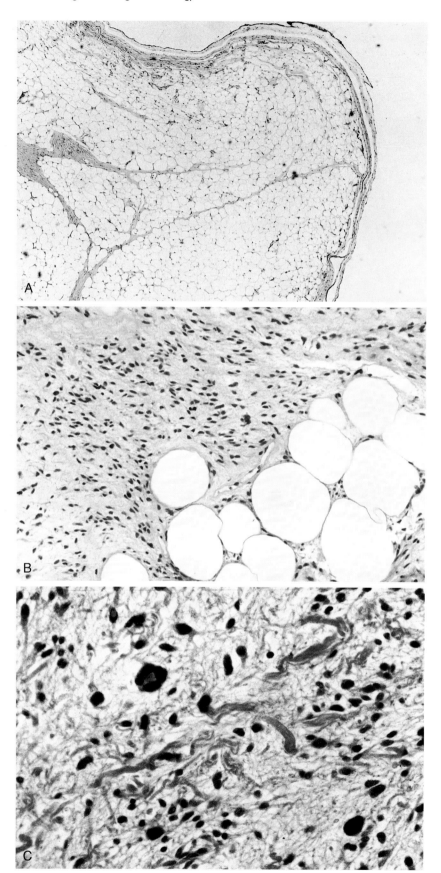

Figure 8–18. *A,* Lipoma. Lobules of mature adipocytes separated by delicate septa extending from a thin fibrous capsule. *B,* Spindle cell lipoma showing areas of mature fat cells interspersed with bland spindle cells in a myxoid stroma. The numerous small cells with round nuclei are mast cells. *C,* Pleomorphic lipoma. Cells with atypical, hyperchromatic, multiple nuclei are present. A multinuclear floret-like cell is seen.

not superficially located. Two subvariants of lipoma are frequently found in the posterior neck and histologically may be confused with liposarcoma: spindle cell lipoma, and pleomorphic lipoma (see subsequent discussion).

Spindle Cell Lipoma

Clinical Features. Unlike the usual lipoma, spindle cell lipoma is far more common in men than women, with over 90% of cases in men. In the 114 patients reported from the Armed Forces Institute of Pathology (AFIP), 104 (91%) were men.[448] The lesion is uncommon in patients younger than 40 years of age; the mean age is between 55 and 60 years, with a range of 24 to 81 years.[448–450] Almost all of these tumors are located in the subcutaneous tissue of the upper back, shoulder, or neck. Spindle cell lipoma is extremely rare in the upper aerodigestive tract. Single examples are reported in the hard palate,[451] floor of mouth,[452] tongue,[453] and larynx.[454] Some spindle cell lipomas extend from the deep subcutaneous tissue to involve the fascia and underlying muscle.[448, 449]

Pathologic Features. Spindle cell lipomas range in size from 1 to 13 cm, with a median size between 4 cm and 5 cm.[437, 448–450] Grossly, they resemble an ordinary lipoma, being circumscribed and encapsulated, although the deep lesions may appear infiltrative,[448, 449] and they may at times have gray-white gelatinous foci.[437, 448, 449] Microscopically, the lesion consists of varying proportions of bland-appearing, elongated, spindle cells; fat cells; bundles of birefringent collagen; and a myxoid stroma. Mast cells may be quite common (Fig. 8–18B). In some of the tumors, the spindle cells make up almost the entire lesion, with only a few scattered fat cells seen, but others show the usual pattern of a conventional lipoma with only a few small foci of spindle cells. The spindle cells and the collagen bands may at first suggest a diagnosis of neurilemoma, neurofibroma, hemangiopericytoma, or smooth muscle tumor.[448–450] At times, scattered multivacuolated cells with hyperchromatic and atypical nuclei are present. These, combined with the mucoid matrix, may simulate a sclerosing or myxoid liposarcoma.[437, 449, 450] Mitotic activity, however, is rare in spindle cell lipomas, and its superficial location should serve as a clue to its benign nature. Spindle cell lipomas also lack lipoblasts, pools of mucinous material, and a diffuse plexiform capillary network as found in some liposarcomas.[437, 448, 449] The atypical cells in spindle cell lipoma may reflect a transitional-type lesion from a pure spindle cell lipoma to the closely related entity, pleomorphic lipoma.[437, 449, 450]

Electron microscopic studies have been done on only a few examples of spindle cell lipoma, with the spindle cells thought to represent fibroblasts or fibroblast-like cells analogous to the stellate mesenchymal cells seen in primitive fat lobules.[448, 450]

Treatment and Prognosis. None of the 63 cases reported by Enzinger and Harvey,[448] for which adequate follow-up information was available, had recurrences following surgical excision, and neither did any of the 14 patients reported by Angervall et al.[449] Allen,[437] however, noted a recurrence 3 years after therapy in 1 of 10 patients. The concern for spindle cell lipoma is, as for pleomorphic lipoma, that it not be confused with liposarcoma.

Pleomorphic Lipoma

Pleomorphic lipoma, a benign tumor of adipose tissue, is the most likely to be histologically misdiagnosed as liposarcoma because of its content of atypical lipoblasts.[455] Although some differences of opinion exist as to what type of lesion should be designated as a pleomorphic lipoma,[455, 456] its general histologic features are well described.[455, 457]

Clinical Features. Patient age and anatomic distribution of pleomorphic lipoma are similar to those for spindle cell lipoma, a finding that is not surprising, because adipose lesions containing elements of both tumor types exist.[437, 449, 450] Pleomorphic lipoma occurs almost exclusively in adults, with a mean patient age between 50 and 70 years.[437, 455, 456] They are rare in patients less than 40

years of age, with only two of Shmookler and Enzinger's 48 patients in that age group.[455] In three publications, the percentage of male patients ranged from 57% to 89%.[437, 455, 457]

In most instances, patients complain of a slowly growing mass that may be present for many years. In some, however, the mass rapidly enlarges within only a few weeks.[455] Approximately 80% of the lesions occur in the neck, shoulder, and upper back. In Shmookler and Enzinger's series of 48 patients,[455] the neck was the site of origin in 24 patients, with 15 of these in the posterior neck. A case of pleomorphic lipoma was reported in the tongue.[458]

The tumors arise from the subcutaneous tissue as well as from within muscle, with the former more common. The intramuscular lesions are more common in the extremities, especially in the thigh.[457] The subcutaneous lesions are usually well circumscribed, being partially or completely encapsulated, whereas the intramuscular tumors may have an infiltrative appearance. In either location, tumors as large as 29 cm have been recorded, although most are in the 5.0 cm to 10.0 cm range.[455–457] Subcutaneous tumors are usually smaller than the intramuscular lesions.

Pathologic Features. Histologically, pleomorphic lipomas are characterized by the presence of variegated cells, consisting of multivacuolated lipoblasts with atypical nuclei, mixed with hyperchromatic, multinucleated cells. These latter cells have nuclei arranged in a peripheral wreath-like pattern about a central core of eosinophilic cytoplasm and have been called *floret-like* cells (Fig. 8–18C).[444, 455] The nuclei tend to overlap and blend together. The number of floret cells varies from case to case, being abundant in some and rare in others.[455] Whether their presence is essential to the diagnosis[437] is debated, with Evans et al.[456] noting them in only one third of their cases. In addition to floret cells, mononuclear cells of various sizes, with hyperchromatic and atypical nuclei, are also found. Between these atypical cells are mature fat cells and bands of birefringent collagen.[455] In up to one quarter of the cases, focal areas are present with the features of spindle cell lipoma.[455] Myxoid areas within the collagen bands, or between the cells, are also common. Mast cells and lymphocytes are also present; mitoses are uncommon.

The histologic distinction between pleomorphic lipoma and liposarcoma may be difficult to make.[455, 456] Indeed, 65% of the pleomorphic lipomas that were received in consultation at the AFIP were diagnosed as liposarcoma by the submitting pathologists.[455] The site of the lesion may well be the deciding factor in determining whether one is dealing with a liposarcoma or a benign adipose tumor.

Treatment and Prognosis. Patients with pleomorphic lipomas arising in the subcutaneous tissue do well, with only rare recurrences reported despite less than adequate excision.[455, 456] There is some difference of opinion about whether the intramuscular lesions should be designated as benign. Although Evans et al.[456] reported a local recurrence rate of close to 70% for intramuscular lesions, no tumor recurred after total excision. Shmookler and Enzinger, however, claim that some recurrences are less differentiated than the initial tumor and are fully malignant, and preferred to regard the intramuscular tumors as low-grade liposarcomas.[455] In Kindblom's series, 9 of the 21 tumors recurred during follow-up intervals of 6 months to 25 years. Five of these nine were subcutaneous, and the other four were intermuscular or intramuscular tumors. The single lesion in the neck recurred four times.[457]

Lipoblastomatosis and Lipomatosis

Lipoblastomatosis is an infiltrative but benign neoplasm of adipose tissue. The tumor occurs exclusively during infancy and early childhood. It infiltrates the subcutaneous tissue and underlying muscles of the extremities.[8] Boys are more commonly affected than girls. A review of the English medical literature for the last 10 years shows two cases reported in the neck,[459, 460] and another involved the face and neck.[461] Microscopically, the lesions are composed of lobules of immature fat cells separated by connective tissue septa and areas of loose myxoid matrix. The lobules are composed of lipoblasts in different stages of maturation. Lipoblastomas are clinically and histologically identical to lipoblastomatosis, yet they are circumscribed and confined to the subcutis.

A peculiar distribution of fatty tissue about the cervical region may be encountered by the head and neck surgeon. This entity, termed *Madelung's disease, cervical lipomatosis,* or *symmetric cervical lipomatosis,* is a striking condition that causes gross deformity of the head and neck region by producing a cervical distribution of fat resembling a horse-collar.[462, 463] It is characterized by the gradual deposit of nontender adipose tissue in a superficial location about the neck, postauricular area, and suboccipital and parotid regions.[437, 462, 463] These subcutaneous deposits are nonencapsulated and poorly circumscribed, with tongue-like extensions of the fat between muscle groups. The deposits consist of mature fat with an increased amount of fibrous tissue.[437] Patients are middle-aged men frequently with a history of alcoholism and liver disease.[437, 462, 463] They usually complain of the gross cosmetic deformity, although some patients seek medical attention because of respiratory distress caused by airway compression by the fatty masses.[437, 463] The larynx has been involved by extension of the fat through the thyrohyoid membrane into the false cord.[464] Excision of the fatty masses may be necessary, although the lack of clearly defined surgical tissue planes makes dissection difficult.[445, 462, 463] The condition may improve with abstinence from alcohol.[8, 437]

Liposarcoma

Liposarcoma is among the most common adult soft-tissue sarcomas, although the reported incidence varies greatly from institution to institution, varying from 5% to 30% of all soft-tissue sarcomas.[465] With the establishment of malignant fibrous histiocytoma as a distinct entity, this tumor has, in some institutions, equaled or surpassed liposarcoma as the most common sarcoma of adults.[8] Furthermore, with the recent descriptions of spindle cell lipoma and pleomorphic lipoma, benign tumors that may be histologically confused with liposarcoma, some lesions previously diagnosed as liposarcoma will no doubt, upon review, be reclassified as one or the other of these tumors.[455, 456] Indeed, in some series, one half of the lesions previously designated as liposarcoma were, upon review, placed in some other diagnostic category.[465, 466] It should be remembered that liposarcomas are still relatively rare tumors and are estimated to account for 10% to 25% of primary fat-containing neoplasms.[434, 436, 437, 443] In other studies, the frequency of liposarcoma was 1.5% to 2.5% of lipomas.[434, 436, 437] For all practical purposes, liposarcomas arise de novo and not from pre-existing lipomas.

Clinical Features. Most patients with liposarcoma are adults in the fourth to sixth decades of life, with a mean patient age of about 50 years.[466–467] Liposarcomas in children are rare. In a survey from the AFIP, Shmookler and Enzinger found only 17 examples in children in their collection of 2500 liposarcomas. Many cases reported as liposarcoma in children probably represent benign lipoblastoma.[473, 475] A diagnosis of liposarcoma in a child younger than 5 years of age should be viewed with skepticism.[437, 468]

Unlike lipomas, which are more common in women, roughly 55% to 60% of liposarcoma cases occur in men.[466–468] This male prevalence also holds true for liposarcomas of the head and neck region; almost two thirds of the patients with liposarcomas in this region have been males.[469, 470]

In general, liposarcomas originate from the deep soft tissues and, unlike lipomas, rarely arise in the subcutaneous tissue.[8, 437] They usually occur between major muscle groups, with the most frequent locations being the thigh, retroperitoneum, inguinal region, shoulder area, and buttocks.[8, 467, 468] The head and neck region is involved in only 2% to 6% of cases.[8, 437, 471]

McCulloch et al.[472] reviewed 76 cases of liposarcoma of the head and neck reported in the world literature from 1911 to 1990. Patients ranged in age from 6 months to 90 years, with a mean age of 42 years; the majority were in the fourth to sixth decades of life.

Most liposarcomas in the head and neck are located in the neck; other sites include the cheek, forehead, scalp, orbit, floor of mouth,

soft palate, pharynx, meninges, larynx, nasopharynx, paranasal sinuses, nasal cavity, supraclavicular fossa, maxilla, mandible, and mastoid.[443, 469–471, 473, 474]

As with other soft-tissue sarcomas, liposarcomas are usually nodular masses that appear well circumscribed. In the head and neck area, they are usually smaller than those in such areas as the thigh or retroperitoneum, where lesions weighing many thousands of grams may occur,[468] although liposarcomas as large as 15 cm in greatest dimension have been reported in the head and neck region.[470]

Pathologic Features. Depending on the histologic variety of liposarcoma, the tumors may vary grossly from those that resemble a benign lipoma, being soft, greasy, and bright yellow, to myxoid tumors with a white-gray translucent surface that feels slimy.[437, 466] Mucoid material may freely drip from the surface of such tumors. Other liposarcomas, however, may have a gross appearance that does not differ from other types of sarcomas.

Histologically, liposarcoma is a tumor composed of lipoblasts. However, the number of lipoblasts may vary considerably among the histologic subtypes of liposarcoma. Furthermore, the presence of lipoblasts per se does not establish a tumor as a liposarcoma because these cells, or cells that simulate them, are also found in reactive conditions involving fat and in benign lipoblastoma of childhood,[437, 475] and in other malignant tumors such as malignant fibrous histiocytoma and osteosarcoma.[8] The correct diagnosis depends on the finding of other cellular constituents as well as the overall pattern of the lesion.

Lipoblasts are divided into univacuolated and multivacuolated types.[437] In the univacuolated form, the cells are smaller than mature adipose cells and have a signet-ring appearance produced by a single, large, and sharply delimited cytoplasmic fat vacuole that pushes the nucleus against the cell membrane and deforms it into a demilune shape.[437] These univacuolated lipoblasts may be confused with the cells of a signet-ring lymphoma or, more commonly, with the cells of a mucin-producing adenocarcinoma. Multivacuolated lipoblasts have a central hyperchromatic nucleus that is frequently large and bizarre in shape. The cytoplasm contains several large or small fat vacuoles that are characteristically well defined and that indent or scallop the nucleus (Fig. 8–19A).

Liposarcomas are divided into four major histologic varieties: a well-differentiated type, which is further classified into a lipoma-like and sclerosing forms; a myxoid type; a round cell type; and a pleomorphic type. There are also mixed tumors that contain various combinations of the four types.[466, 468] A dedifferentiated form of liposarcoma has also been described that consists of areas of well-differentiated liposarcoma juxtaposed to foci of poorly differentiated spindle-cell sarcomas.[465]

Well-differentiated liposarcoma accounts for 20% to 30% of cases.[437, 465, 466] The lipoma-like variety, as its name implies, histologically closely resembles a simple lipoma except for the focal occurrence of regions in which hyperchromatic and bizarre lipoblasts are found (see Fig. 18–19A). It is this form of liposarcoma that may be underdiagnosed as a lipoma if sufficient sampling of the lesion is not done. The true nature of the "lipoma" may become evident only when it recurs despite what was thought to be adequate local excision. In Kindblom's series, 10 of the 26 well-differentiated liposarcomas were originally diagnosed as lipoma until microscopic examination of the recurrent tumors established the correct diagnosis.[466, 471] On the other hand, atypical adipose tumors of the subcutaneous tissue, designated as well-differentiated liposarcoma, and which may occur in the head and neck area, behave as benign neoplasms and are not known to metastasize. These tumors have been designated *atypical lipomas* by Kindblom,[466] a title later endorsed by several investigators[8, 465, 476] and recently incorporated into the World Health Organization classification of soft tissue tumors.[477] In these tumors, location rather than histomorphology is the best predictor of behavior.

Myxoid liposarcoma is the most common histologic type, accounting for 35% to 50% of liposarcomas at all sites.[437, 465, 468] It is characterized by widely separated, monomorphic fusiform or stellate cells residing in a mucoid stroma rich in hyaluronic acid. Pools or lakes of this material are frequently present. A diagnostically important feature is the presence of a delicate plexiform capillary network that serves to separate liposarcoma (Fig. 8–19B) from the essentially avascular soft-tissue myxoma with which it may be confused.[437, 465, 468] Cell pleomorphism and significant mitotic activity are not features of myxoid liposarcoma, and lipoblasts may at times be difficult to find in some cases.

Round cell liposarcoma is considered by some to be a variant of the myxoid type, although foci of myxoid liposarcoma are present in less than half of the cases.[465] The tumor is composed of round to oval cells that have a fine, multivacuolated cytoplasm and a central round nucleus that may be hyperchromatic but usually is not markedly atypical (Fig. 8–19C). Mitoses are not common. Round cell liposarcoma makes up about 10% to 15% of all liposarcomas.[437, 466, 468] Myxoid and round cell liposarcomas are currently considered as one group of lesions, "myxoid/round cell liposarcoma," with a continuum of grades from pure myxoid (low grade) to pure round cell (high grade). The intermediate grade shows transitional features. Behavior can be related to the round cell component.[478]

Pleomorphic liposarcoma is the most anaplastic of the liposarcomas and accounts for 10% to 25% of cases.[437, 465, 468] It contains an abundant mix of tumor giant cells that have a dense, glassy eosinophilic cytoplasm and bizarre lipoblasts (Fig. 8–19D). Numerous abnormal mitotic figures are present throughout the tumor. Pleomorphic liposarcoma may be difficult or impossible to distinguish from pleomorphic malignant fibrous histiocytoma.[8, 479] Malignant fibrous histiocytoma may contain lipoblast-like cells, and there may be a

histologic overlap between these two tumor entities such that they are not distinguishable at the light microscopic level.

Recurrent liposarcomas may have a histologic appearance that differs from the original primary tumor, containing components of other liposarcoma subtypes or, more important from a diagnostic standpoint, features of other sarcomas such as malignant fibrous histiocytoma, hemangiopericytoma, or unclassified spindle cell sarcoma.[480]

Electron microscopic studies of liposarcoma have dealt mainly with the myxoid variety. Here, the prevailing view is that the tumor roughly recapitulates the embryonic development of white fat,[446, 481, 482] although some have suggested origin from brown fat.[483]

Myxoid liposarcoma is the most common variety found in the head and neck region. In the 35 cases reported by Baden and Newman, 71% were myxoid, 14% round cell, and 9% liposarcomas with a mixture of subtypes.[469]

Treatment and Prognosis. Surgical therapy remains the main form of treatment, although postoperative radiation therapy may be beneficial, especially for the well-differentiated and myxoid variants that appear to respond best to such therapy.[467, 484]

Prognosis for liposarcoma is directly correlated with the histologic appearance of the tumor.[437, 465, 468] The overall 5-year survival rate is roughly 45% to 65%. The well-differentiated and myxoid tumors have excellent 5-year survival rates of 75% to 100% despite local recurrence rates that have ranged between 50% and 100% in some series.[437, 465, 466, 468] Pleomorphic liposarcoma has a poorer prognosis, with 5-year survival rates of from 0% to 21%. Round cell liposarcoma has only a slightly better prognosis, with 5-year sur-

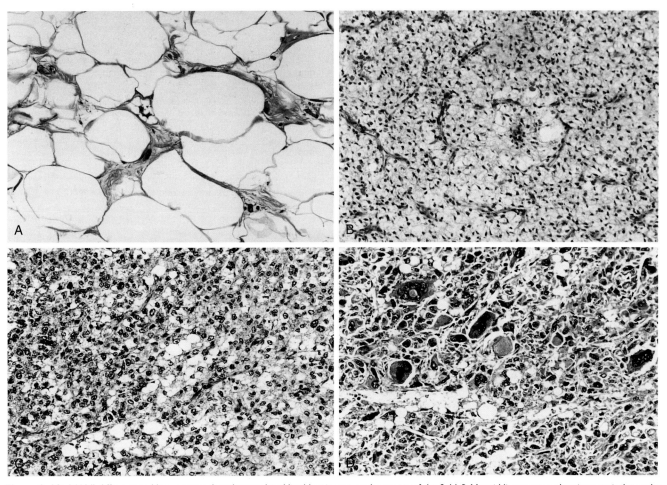

Figure 8–19. *A,* Well-differentiated liposarcoma. A multivacuolated lipoblast is seen at the center of the field. *B,* Myxoid liposarcoma showing a typical vascular pattern. A small amount of intercellular mucoid material is identified. *C,* Round cell liposarcoma. Note small round cells with uniform hyperchromatic nuclei and vacuolated or granular cytoplasm. *D,* Pleomorphic liposarcoma. Note numerous bizarre tumor giant cells and lipoblasts.

vival rates of 18% to 27%. Local recurrence rates for these latter two liposarcomas have been between 75% and 80%.[437, 465, 466, 468] The well-differentiated tumors tend to recur locally before there is evidence of distant metastases. Indeed, metastases from well-differentiated liposarcomas are extremely rare. Metastases from the other liposarcomas are usually via the blood stream, with the lungs the most commonly involved site. Lymph nodes are only rarely involved. Of the 35 patients with head and neck liposarcomas listed by Baden and Newman, 10 were lost to follow-up. In the remaining 25 cases, 2 patients died of causes unrelated to their tumor; 14 patients died of tumor, 8 were alive and well for more than 5 years, and 1 was alive with tumor at 11 years. In the eight patients free of tumor, six had a well-differentiated "myxoid" type and two had a mixed liposarcoma. The patient alive with tumor also had a well-differentiated myxoid tumor.[469]

Rhabdomyoma and Rhabdomyosarcoma

Rhabdomyoma

Rhabdomyoma of the soft tissue is a benign tumor that accounts for only 1% to 2% of tumors with skeletal muscle differentiation, the remainder being rhabdomyosarcomas.[485] Rhabdomyomas are uncommon, with less than 100 cases reported.[486, 487] Among 5844 soft-tissue tumors, only 1 was diagnosed as rhabdomyoma.[488] Despite this rarity, rhabdomyomas are discussed here not only because they have a predilection to occur in the head and neck but also because they must be differentiated from the more common, and more clinically significant, rhabdomyosarcoma that also occurs frequently in this anatomic location.

The glycogen-containing lesion of the heart, also designated as "rhabdomyoma," is most likely a hamartoma and has no relationship to the tumors described here. The cardiac lesion is associated with the tuberous sclerosis syndrome, but the soft-tissue rhabdomyoma is not.[489]

Soft tissue rhabdomyomas are divided into two histologic forms, the adult and fetal varieties.[485] Roughly an equal number of cases of each type have been reported.

Clinical Features. Adult rhabdomyoma occurs principally in patients with a mean age between 50 and 55 years (range, 8 to 82).[486, 488, 490–493]

Fetal rhabdomyoma also occurs over a broad age span, from newborns to patients over 60 years of age.[486, 488, 491] On average, however, the patients are younger than those with adult rhabdomyomas, with a mean age of 22 to 26 years.[486, 488]

Adult rhabdomyoma is four to five times more frequent in male than in female patients.[486, 494] Almost an equal number of male and female patients with fetal rhabdomyoma are reported; however, this includes women with genital tract lesions. If these are excluded, there is a male prevalence in fetal rhabdomyomas, similar to that in the adult variety; this also holds true for fetal rhabdomyomas of the head and neck.[486, 495]

Adult rhabdomyomas occur almost exclusively in the head and neck.[486] In the review by Konrad et al.[488], only 3 of 49 reported cases arose outside the head and neck area. The most common sites include the pharynx (including the nasopharynx, oropharynx, and hypopharynx), larynx, soft tissues of the neck, and intraoral sites including the lip, tongue, base of tongue, submandibular and sublingual areas, floor of mouth, tonsil, soft palate, buccal mucosa, and orbit.[496–508] In contrast to the common occurrence of rhabdomyosarcoma in the orbit, Knowles and Jakobiec[502] reported the first documented example of orbital rhabdomyoma in 1975 and rejected, as undocumented, five previously reported cases. Few rhabdomyomas have actually been found within skeletal muscle such as the sternocleidomastoid and sternohyoid muscles[501, 503] and the intrinsic muscles of the tongue.[496] A total of 11 multicentric adult rhabdomyomas have been reported, all but one of which have been in men.[487, 503, 509] These may be simultaneous or develop asynchro-

nously several years apart. All of these multicentric lesions have been in the head and neck and were found in patients older than 50 years of age, with one exception in a 32-year-old man.

Fetal rhabdomyomas are also principally found in the head and neck but, as stated earlier, they also occur in the female genital region.[485, 486, 492] Excluding the latter, between 70% and 75% of fetal rhabdomyomas arise in the head and neck[486, 495, 510] with other sites including the axilla, chest wall, stomach, anus, abdominal wall, and thigh.[485–488, 490, 510, 511] Within the head and neck, the posterior auricular region is the most common location; other sites include the orbit, nose, face, neck, tongue, soft palate, base of tongue, parotid region, larynx, and nasopharynx.[486] Rare examples of multicentric fetal rhabdomyomas are reported.[486]

Rhabdomyomas are slowly growing lesions that may be present for many years, some patients having noted a mass for up to 50 years.[486, 489, 497, 501, 504]

Pathologic Features. Grossly, the adult form appears to be well circumscribed or even encapsulated,[494, 511] but the fetal type may be less well defined and appear infiltrative.[8, 485, 486, 491, 495, 502] The adult type varies from a few millimeters to 15 cm in diameter,[486, 488, 493, 494, 497] whereas fetal rhabdomyomas tend to be somewhat smaller, ranging from 1.5 to 8.0 cm in greatest dimension.[485, 486, 495]

Histologically, the adult tumor is more easily recognized. It consists of a uniform aggregation of large, oval to round cells, that have an abundant granular eosinophilic cytoplasm containing large amounts of glycogen, causing it to appear vacuolated in routine sections, creating so-called spider-web cells.[8, 489, 494, 500] Nuclei are uniform and either central or eccentric (Fig. 8–20A). Intracytoplasmic crystalline-like or rod-shaped bodies are found, which electron microscopic studies have shown to be hypertrophic Z-band material that resembles that seen in nemaline myopathy.[486, 489, 491, 500, 501] By electron microscopy, thick and thin myofilaments and large mitochondria are also found.[8, 488, 497–500, 505, 506, 508, 512]

Despite the apparent mature differentiation of the cells, cross-striations are difficult to find in routine hematoxylin-eosin–stained sections, but a careful search will yield at least some cells with striations. Mitotic figures are rare. Owing to the granularity of their cytoplasm, the cells have been confused with those of granular cell tumor. However, the cells of the latter tumor lack cross-striations, and although they contain intracytoplasmic periodic acid-Schiff–positive material, this is diastase-resistant and not glycogen. They also lack the thick and thin myofilaments of skeletal muscle cells.[489, 499, 500] The cells of granular cell tumor stain positively for S-100 protein, whereas those of rhabdomyoma do not,[513, 514] the latter are reactive for the muscle markers desmin and myoglobin.[512]

Fetal rhabdomyomas are histologically less uniform than the adult tumors. They tend to arise in the subcutaneous tissue or within the superficial soft tissues.[8, 485, 511] They are composed of immature-appearing skeletal muscle fibers, in various stages of differentiation, mixed with mesenchymal-type cells that vary from small oval to round cells to larger cells with bipolar tapering cytoplasmic extensions (Fig. 8–20B).[8, 486, 511] Cross-striations are present but, like the adult form, the number of cells with striations varies considerably. The most mature cells are found at the periphery of the lesion (Fig. 8–20C).[485, 509] Both cell types are loosely arranged in bands that are haphazardly arranged within a myxoid stroma that contains hyaluronic acid and gives the lesion an overall edematous appearance[485, 486]; mitoses are scarce. di Sant'Agnese and Knowles divide fetal rhabdomyomas into two groups: a fetal "myxoid" type, which is the same as the tumor originally described by Dehner and Enzinger,[485] and a fetal "cellular" variant. They found a total of four such cellular tumors among the 28 fetal rhabdomyomas in the literature, and 6 of their own 15 new cases were of this type. In this variety, the myxoid stroma is either lacking or sparse, and there is a preponderance of thin, elongated spindle cells that are arranged in a herringbone or palisaded pattern.[486] Mild nuclear pleomorphism may be seen in the cells of this cellular form. Occasional ribbon- and strap-shaped cells are also present, but cross-striations are difficult to

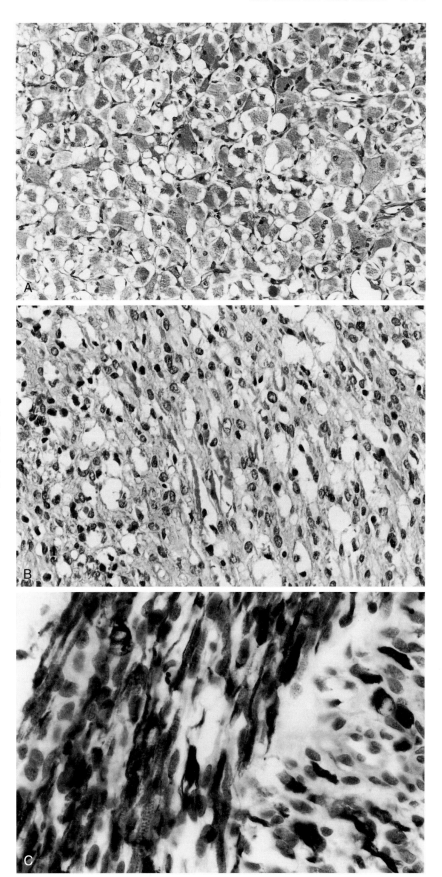

Figure 8–20. *A,* Adult rhabdomyoma. Note large round cells with abundant granular vacuolated cytoplasm and uniform, predominantly eccentric nuclei. *B,* Fetal rhabdomyoma. Note pleomorphic population of mesenchymal-type cells varying from small round to larger cells with bipolar, tapering, cytoplasmic extensions. *C,* Fetal rhabdomyoma, with desmin immunostain accentuating the cross striations in some of the elongated cells at the periphery of the lesion.

find. Crotty, Nakhleh, and Dehner[515] reported two cases of the cellular rhabdomyoma in the buccal tissue of a 2.5-year-old girl and an 8-year-old girl. The authors proposed that the cellular rhabdomyoma is distinct from the classic fetal rhabdomyoma and may represent a more differentiated tumor they termed *juvenile rhabdomyoma.* Gardner and Corio[510] question whether the myxoid stroma must be present in the so-called fetal "myxoid" variant and believe that there are cases, one of which they report, in which the patterns of both forms of fetal rhabdomyoma blend with each other.

Few cases of fetal rhabdomyoma have been studied by electron microscopy, but the cells of these tumors also show skeletal muscle differentiation, as in the adult form[485, 488, 511]; however, they lack the Z-band hypertrophy seen in the latter.[506, 512] Fetal rhabdomyoma is immunohistochemically analogous to adult rhabdomyoma, with the cells reactive for desmin and myoglobin.[512, 516]

Differential Diagnosis. Although adult rhabdomyoma is histologically easily separated from rhabdomyosarcoma, the fetal variety may be confused with this malignant tumor. Indeed, as suggested by Dehner and Enzinger,[485] this distinction may be quite subtle. The superficial location of rhabdomyoma, versus the usually deeply situated rhabdomyosarcoma; the lack of necrosis and significant cell pleomorphism; the maturation of the tumor cells toward the periphery (Fig. 8–20*C*); and the scarcity of mitotic activity are all points in favor of the diagnosis of rhabdomyoma.[8, 485, 486, 509, 511]

Treatment and Prognosis. Local recurrences of adult rhabdomyoma are rare after excision,[490, 492, 500, 502, 507] but some patients have had several recurrences.[490, 507] Only one fetal rhabdomyoma has been reported to recur, and this tumor was located in the neck.[488] Metastases have never been reported from rhabdomyomas.

Based on their finding of two rhabdomyomas in a patient with the basal cell nevus syndrome, Dahl et al.[511] believe that the fetal rhabdomyoma is a malformation and not a neoplasm. Dehner and Enzinger,[485] in their original description of fetal rhabdomyoma, also raised the possibility that the lesion was hamartomatous.

Rhabdomyosarcoma

Since the late 1970s, rhabdomyosarcoma has been the sarcoma that has received the most clinical interest, as evidenced by the extensive number of publications on the subject that have appeared during this time. Among the factors that contribute to this interest is the highly aggressive nature of rhabdomyosarcoma and its propensity to affect children and young adults, with all the emotional impact that such a situation engenders among physicians and parents alike. In addition, rhabdomyosarcoma is the sarcoma that has responded best to improved methods in radiation therapy and chemotherapy to the extent that its previous poor prognosis has been replaced by the hope that the majority of patients may now be cured.[517] The various reports from the Intergroup Rhabdomyosarcoma Study group (IRS) that are referred to in this chapter serve as models of what a cooperative effort among pathologists, surgeons, radiation therapists, and oncologists can accomplish.

Rhabdomyosarcoma is the most common sarcoma in children, accounting for approximately one half of the malignant soft-tissue tumors in this group and 4% to 8% of all malignant lesions in those younger than 15 years of age.[517–522] Overall, rhabdomyosarcoma accounts for 8% to 20% of sarcomas in patients of all ages.[521–525]

There are four principal varieties of rhabdomyosarcoma: embryonal (ERMS), alveolar (ARMS), pleomorphic (PRMS), and botryoid. The botryoid variety, however, is considered a variant of ERMS with a characteristic gross appearance.[526] It grows beneath mucosal surfaces of body cavities and forms grape-like polypoid masses. A compact round-cell rhabdomyosarcoma with scant myogenesis, originally classified as ERMS, was recently included in the ARMS category despite its lack of classical alveolar architecture.[519] The reclassification was based on cytologic as well as prognostic considerations. Because the embryonal, botryoid, and alveolar tumors occur predominantly in children, whereas the pleomorphic tumor is most common in elderly adults, the general term *juvenile*

rhabdomyosarcoma has been used by some to designate the first three tumors and *adult rhabdomyosarcoma* as a synonym for the pleomorphic tumors.[527, 528] Although it is true that these tumors are more common in certain age groups, any one of them may occur in patients of any age.

Clinical Features. Approximately two thirds of patients with childhood rhabdomyosarcoma are younger than 10 years of age.[517] Alveolar rhabdomyosarcoma tends to occur in slightly older patients, with a mean age of 15 to 20 years.[529] At the Armed Forces Institute of Pathology (AFIP), the median age for 440 patients with ERMS was 8 years and the median age for 118 patients with ARMS was 16 years.[8] Less than 10% of pleomorphic rhabdomyosarcomas occur in children[523]; the mean age for this tumor is 50 to 55 years.[526] Newborns account for 2% to 3% of patients with rhabdomyosarcoma.[8]

Males account for roughly 55% to 70% of patients.[528, 530–534] In some reports, however, there is no significant sex difference.[532] Black patients are less commonly affected than white patients[524, 531, 532, 534–536]; in some studies whites are affected three times more commonly than blacks.[8, 518]

The distribution of tumor types depends on the anatomic region involved. In children, the head and neck accounts for 30% to 50% of cases, whereas the genitourinary tract and the extremities each account for about 20% of the total.[517, 520, 522, 537] Within the head and neck region, ERMS is most common,[522, 531, 534, 537–540] whereas the alveolar and pleomorphic tumors are more common in the extremities.[523, 525, 529, 538]

Most rhabdomyosarcomas have no direct association with skeletal muscle but arise instead from between muscle groups or directly from the deep connective soft tissue. For the most part they grow rapidly, such that symptoms are usually present for less than a year,[525, 526, 531, 534, 541, 542] although isolated cases are encountered in which it is claimed that symptoms were present for several years.[524]

In the head and neck region, the orbital region is the most common site for rhabdomyosarcoma. Of 246 rhabdomyosarcomas of the head and neck at the AFIP, 44% were located in the orbit, eyelid, or skull, and this region accounted for almost 20% of all rhabdomyosarcomas on file, second only to paratesticular lesions in occurrence. The remaining head and neck rhabdomyosarcomas involved the nasal cavity, nasopharynx, palate, mouth, and pharynx in 30%; the paranasal sinuses, cheek, and neck in 19%; and the ear and mastoid in 7%.[8]

Li and Fraumeni[543] found some evidence of a familial association of malignancies in patients with rhabdomyosarcomas, with a higher incidence of soft-tissue sarcomas in siblings of these patients, as well as a higher incidence of other tumors, which tended to occur at a young age, in their relatives. Now known as the Li-Fraumeni syndrome, this is an autosomal dominant disorder that predisposes individuals to multiple forms of cancer, including breast carcinoma, soft tissue sarcoma, osteosarcoma, leukemia, and adrenal cortical carcinoma. These diverse tumor types occur at unusually early ages compared with their usual age of onset. A germ cell line mutation of tumor suppressor gene p53 is found in a majority of family members with the Li-Fraumeni syndrome.[544, 545] An increased incidence of brain tumors and adrenocortical carcinoma has been noted by others in relatives of those with rhabdomyosarcomas, as well as a purported incidence of rhabdomyosarcoma in patients with neurofibromatosis.[521]

Patients with head and neck rhabdomyosarcomas demonstrate a variety of presenting symptoms that are dependent on the anatomic location of the tumors. Those with orbital tumors almost always have exophthalmos that is of rapid onset and progressive.[531, 534, 536] Middle ear tumors may manifest as otitis media with pain and ear drainage, at times bloody, or the presence of granulation-type tissue or a polyp in the external auditory canal.[524, 531, 546] Nasal and nasopharyngeal tumors may cause breathing difficulty, nasal stuffiness, or nasal bleeding.[547] Polypoid masses may be found in these locations.[548] Neurologic symptoms, including facial nerve paralysis, is produced by lesions arising in the mastoid and nasopharynx.[549] The duration of symptoms is usually less than 1 year, and most last less than 6 months.[526, 531, 535, 541] In the series reported by Masson and Soule,[524] only 6 of 88 patients had symptoms for longer than 1 year; one patient had symptoms for 5.5 years.

Pathologic Features. In the IRS, 57% of the rhabdomyosarcomas were embryonal, 19% were alveolar, 6% were botryoid, and 1% were pleomorphic.[522] These figures closely parallel the distribution noted at the AFIP, an institution that has a large number of consultation cases involving patients of all ages.[550]

Although the finding of cross-striations in a malignant-appearing small cell soft-tissue tumor, in the proper clinical setting, is unequivocal evidence of rhabdomyosarcoma, whether or not a tumor is determined to have such cells very much depends on the diligence and skill of the pathologist. An extensive search of many sections may be required before striated tumor cells are found.[541] Furthermore, the likelihood of misinterpretation of cytoplasmic artifacts for actual striations increases with the pathologist's desire to prove that the tumor is a rhabdomyosarcoma.

Embryonal Rhabdomyosarcoma. Histologically, embryonal rhabdomyosarcomas vary considerably, from very primitive-appearing lesions with virtually no evidence of muscle differentiation, to those that contain numerous strap-shaped cells with cross-striations.[8, 525–527, 530, 554] The overall pattern has been likened to the embryologic stage of normal muscle development found between the third and tenth weeks of gestation.[530] Most tumors consist of small, spindle-shaped cells with tapering bipolar cytoplasmic extensions, mixed with small, round to oval cells, which are not much larger than lymphocytes or small monocytes, with little or no visible cytoplasm (Fig. 8–21A). With maturation, these latter cells accumulate an intensely eosinophilic cytoplasm (Fig. 8–21B). Such "rhabdomyoblasts" may be scarce, but if present they are an important diagnostic feature. Trichrome stains are helpful in locating these cells, as their cytoplasm stains brightly red with these stains.[8] Mitoses are frequent in ERMS. The tumor commonly has a loose myxoid matrix, which contains acid mucopolysaccharide, in which the tumor cells are widely dispersed (see Fig. 8–21A).

In some embryonal rhabdomyosarcomas, the tumor is composed of closely packed spindle cells, with eosinophilic fibrillary cytoplasm, arranged in fascicles or bands such that the tumor resembles a fibrosarcoma or a leiomyosarcoma (leiomyomatous rhabdomyosarcoma). Intercellular collagen is present and may be abundant.[520, 562, 563] It predominantly affects male children and has a predilection to involve the paratesticular area; however, 6 of 21 cases from the German-Italian Cooperative Soft Tissue Sarcoma Study occurred in the head and neck.[562] The prognosis in spindle cell rhabdomyosarcoma is believed to be better than that in the classical form.[563]

The cells of ERMS, like those of all rhabdomyosarcomas, contain glycogen, although not every cell will stain using the periodic acid-Schiff method. The cells located at the periphery of the tumor will most consistently stain for glycogen. The presence of cytoplasmic glycogen in small, oval to round tumor cells is similar to what is found in extraskeletal Ewing's sarcoma or peripheral neuroectodermal tumor. Indeed, by light microscopy and routine stains, the differential diagnosis between ERMS and these tumors may be impossible to make. In general, striated cells are found in approximately one third of embryonal rhabdomyosarcomas, with reported figures from 15% to 60%.[8, 524, 526, 528, 530, 536, 540, 542, 564]

Some embryonal rhabdomyosarcomas are termed *well-differentiated* because they contain numerous spindle-shaped or tubular cells with cross-striations (Fig. 8–21C).[542] Still others describe "pleomorphic" foci within otherwise typical embryonal tumors that contain cells with large, irregular, and atypical nuclei, as would be seen in an adult PRMS.[8] In the botryoid rhabdomyosarcomas, there is an exaggeration of the myxoid matrix such that it comes to form the major component of the tumor. The central portions of these tumors are characteristically hypocellular, and there is a tendency of the tumor cells to aggregate in a narrow band at their periphery just beneath the overlying mucosa or body cavity lining. This *cambium layer* is distinctive to this form of rhabdomyosarcoma.[8, 526, 527]

Alveolar Rhabdomyosarcoma. In its fully developed form, ARMS is histologically characterized by tumor cells arranged in ill-defined groups or nests separated by fibrous bands. Within the center of these nests, the cells are loosely cohesive, forming spaces which, under low-power microscopic examination, mimic pulmonary alveolar spaces (Fig. 8–22A).[529, 538, 554] The peripheral cells of these nests rest on the fibrous trabeculae, being attached by tapered strands of cytoplasm. Free-floating tumor cells, 15 to 30 mm in diameter, are found within the alveolar spaces, along with smaller cells similar to those in ERMS (Fig. 8–22B). Large, multinucleated giant cells, up to 200 μm in diameter, with a wreath-like arrangement of nuclei and a granular eosinophilic cytoplasm, are commonly found floating within these spaces. In other portions of the tumor, the cells may be either compact or loosely arranged but without evidence of space formation, creating regions indistinguishable from ERMS. Strap-shaped and tadpole-shaped rhabdomyoblasts, and spider-web cells produced by cytoplasmic vacuolization, may be found but are less common than in the embryonal form. Striated cells are present in about 30% of cases but may be difficult to find.[8, 529, 538, 564] Mitotic figures are usually plentiful.

A characteristic chromosomal translocation t(2;13)(q14,q37) is commonly found in alveolar rhabdomyosarcoma.[8] Solid variants of alveolar rhabdomyosarcoma are described. They lack an alveolar pattern and are composed of densely packed masses of tumor cells resembling the round cells seen in ERMS.[8] Alveolar features are seen in most cases in association with the solid areas.

As would be expected from their microscopic description, rhabdomyosarcomas exist that contain varying proportions of both alveolar and embryonal patterns.[528, 529] Such tumors are either diagnosed as mixed rhabdomyosarcomas or designated by the dominant pattern.

Pleomorphic Rhabdomyosarcoma. This rhabdomyosarcoma, which is uncommon in the head and neck area[535, 565] was formerly considered to be the most common rhabdomyosarcoma. However, with the increasing awareness by pathologists of the histologic parameters of both the embryonal and alveolar types, PRMS is now the least frequent of the rhabdomyosarcomas. Furthermore, many pleomorphic tumors previously diagnosed as rhabdomyosarcoma are examples of malignant fibrous histiocytoma,[566] a tumor that frequently has a pleomorphic and anaplastic microscopic appearance and that occurs in similar patients, namely elderly adults[523, 530, 567] and in similar locations, the extremities, as PRMS.[8, 566] The diagnosis of PRMS should be restricted to those tumors with cells showing unequivocal cross-striations, contain myoglobin, or, by electron microscopy, show evidence of myogenic differentiation.[568] Because this tumor arises within large muscle groups in the extremities,[523, 527, 550, 567] care must be exercised not to confuse degenerating and abnormal-appearing muscle cells, which still retain their striations, with actual tumor cells.

Based on older descriptions, PRMS is composed of numerous anaplastic cells, many with irregular bizarre configurations.[523, 567] Numerous large, multinucleated tumor giant cells, which have a bright eosinophilic glassy cytoplasm, are present. Tadpole-shaped, racquet-shaped, and strap-shaped cells are seen (Fig. 8–23). Mitotic figures are frequent, many of which are abnormal, and necrosis is common. Striated cells are reported in the literature in 7% to 100% of cases.[523, 526, 528, 567]

Electron microscopic examination may be helpful in making a specific diagnosis in those situations in which the light microscopic diagnosis is in doubt.[551, 552] The presence of both the thick and thin myofilaments, myosin and actin, or of actual Z-band material is diagnostic of skeletal muscle differentiation.[551, 553] However, even these studies may fail to provide the evidence needed for a diagnosis of rhabdomyosarcoma.[553, 554] Owing to the inherent sampling problems associated with electron microscopy, the area of tumor that is most differentiated may be missed. Furthermore, the tumor cells may be so primitive that they do not contain morphologic features of

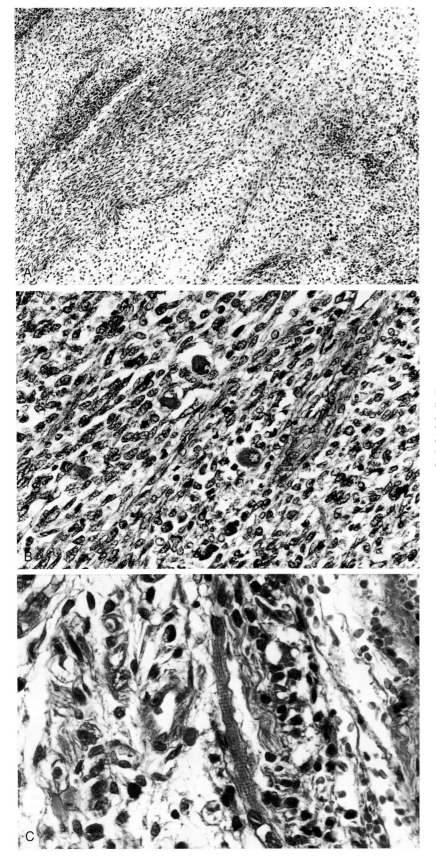

Figure 8–21. *A,* Embryonal rhabdomyosarcoma. Note small, spindle-shaped cells mixed with small round cells. Areas of loose myxoid matrix are evident and alternate with a hypercellular zone. *B,* Embryonal rhabdomyosarcoma, with higher magnification showing rhabdomyoblastic cells (center of field). *C,* Embryonal rhabdomyosarcoma. A large tubular cell with cross-striation is shown.

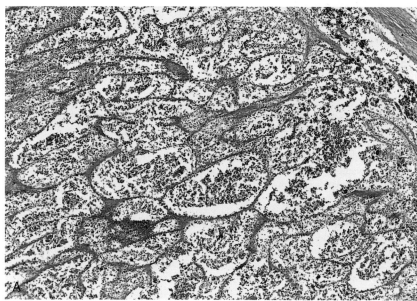

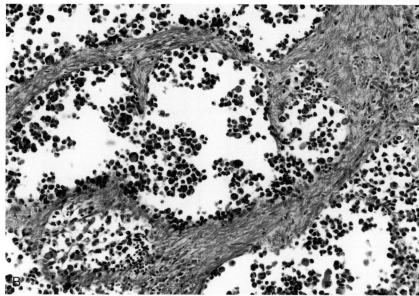

Figure 8–22. *A,* Alveolar rhabdomyosarcoma, low magnification, showing the typical alveolar pattern. *B,* Higher magnification of sample shown in part *A,* showing peripheral cells attached to fibrous trabeculae while free-floating tumor cells are found within the alveolar spaces.

skeletal muscle differentiation. In an electron microscopic study of 31 rhabdomyosarcomas, Mierau and Favara[551] found 13 that contained specific morphologic features, either myofilaments or Z-bands, to establish a diagnosis. However, in 17 tumors even the most differentiated cells lacked specific myoblastic characteristics. In a survey of the literature, these authors found that in only about one half of the tumors considered to be rhabdomyosarcomas did electron microscopy verify the diagnosis.

Immunohistochemical techniques are of great help in the diagnosis of these tumors. The demonstration of such cell constituents as desmin, myosin, muscle specific actin, and myoglobin has allowed tumors to be categorized as having myogenous differentiation. Tsokos et al.[555] reported the results in 23 rhabdomyosarcomas, 11 alveolar and 12 embryonal, immunologically stained for myosin, myoglobin, and several creatine kinase isoenzymes. Myosin was found in a higher percentage of the tumors, being present in all 11 alveolar lesions and 10 of the 12 embryonal lesions, whereas myoglobin was found in 10 of 11 alveolar tumors and 5 of the 11 embryonal tumors tested. Because myosin is also found in smooth muscle cells, myoglobin is considered the more specific marker for skeletal muscle differentiation.

Several investigations have shown that desmin staining is the most sensitive indicator of rhabdomyosarcoma.[556, 557] In a study sponsored by the Intergroup Rhabdomyosarcoma Study, staining of frozen sections shows even greater sensitivity than either formalin- or alcohol-fixed sections. The proportion of desmin-positive cells was higher in alcohol-fixed than formalin-fixed sections.[558] In the same study, myoglobin and creatine kinase (MM isoenzyme) were less sensitive markers.[558] However, desmin and cytoplasmic intermediate filaments are present in both smooth and skeletal muscle fibers.

More recently, the protein product of the skeletal muscle myogenesis gene *MyoD1* has been used with success as a marker for rhabdomyosarcoma cells.[559, 560] The detection of *MyoD1* RNA and protein was found to be highly sensitive and specific for rhabdomyosarcoma.[559, 560] In tumors that express *MyoD1,* deletions in chromosome 11 were associated with ERMS differentiation, whereas those without chromosome deletions showed alveolar histology.[559]

It should be noted that some non-myogenous tumor cells that infiltrated skeletal muscle, such as cells from breast carcinoma, melanoma, and lymphoma, also stained for myoglobin, as did other cells identified as histiocytes.[561] These spurious results are thought to be due to nonspecific adsorption or ingestion of released myoglobin from damaged normal muscle cells, or to represent some form of fixation artifact. Hence positive immunohistochemical staining for myogenic markers in a small cell tumor infiltrating and destroying muscle must be interpreted with care.

Treatment and Prognosis. The IRS developed a clinical grouping or staging classification that is both simple and useful in coordinating reports and end results from various institutions. This consists of four groups and is based on the extent of the tumor and whether it is totally resected.[521, 522] Patients in group I are those with localized tumors that are completely resected; group II includes patients whose tumors have been completely resected grossly but in whom there is microscopic residual tumor; group III contains patients in whom gross tumor is still present after resection, or in whom only a biopsy is done; and group IV is used to designate patients with distant metastases. It should be emphasized that the group in which a patient is placed very much depends on the aggressiveness, or lack of it, of the surgeon. For instance, a patient with an orbital tumor for which a resection is done may be placed into group I or II. However, if the surgeon decides only to biopsy the tumor and treat the patient with chemotherapy and radiation therapy, such a patient would be categorized as a group III patient. Despite this potential for variability, survival rates correlate with this clinical grouping; group I patients have the best prognosis, and those in group IV the least favorable outlook. In reported series, roughly 15% of patients are in group I, 25% in group II, 40% in group III, and 20% in group IV.[517, 521]

In the past, rhabdomyosarcoma carried an extremely poor prognosis, with only 10% to 15% of patients surviving,[517, 520, 524, 530, 569] although some reports indicated better survival rates of about 30% to 35%, depending on the type of rhabdomyosarcoma involved.[523, 533, 537] Alveolar rhabdomyosarcoma had the worst prognosis, with a 5-year survival rate of only 5%, with most patients dying within a year of diagnosis.[524, 525, 529, 537, 538, 550] Embryonal rhabdomyosarcoma had a slightly better prognosis with 5-year survival rates of 10% to 20%.[525, 542, 550] Pleomorphic rhabdomyosarcomas had a better prognosis than the childhood cases, with 5-year survival rates of approximately 30% to 35%.[523, 550, 567]

This overall poor prognosis applied equally to rhabdomyosarcomas of the head and neck, with the exception of orbital tumors, which tend to remain localized and have a lower rate of local recurrence and a relatively low incidence of lymph node metastases.[521, 522, 531, 537, 570] In the review by Dito and Batsakis of head and neck rhabdomyosarcomas, local recurrence developed in 85 of 116 patients (73%) with nonorbital tumors, but in only 25 of 54 (46%) with orbital involvement. The overall 3-year survival rate in their

patients was 16%, but the 5-year survival rate was only 6%. The average survival for all patients was 17 months.[531]

These historically poor survival statistics have dramatically changed since the introduction and use of radiation therapy and multidrug chemotherapy for treatment so that long-term survival figures in the 85% to 95% range are now reported. Prognosis depends less on tumor type than on extent of the tumor.[528, 533, 535] In a retrospective study of 60 children with rhabdomyosarcoma of the head and neck treated at the Children's Hospital of Philadelphia between 1970 and 1987, the overall death rate decreased from 50% in the period of 1970 to 1971 to 23% in the period of 1980 to 1987.[571] These results illustrate the effect of improved management protocols.

Radical and mutilating surgery for the treatment of head and neck rhabdomyosarcoma has been largely replaced by the use of radiation and chemotherapy. Surgical therapy is used to excise small, readily accessible tumors or to reduce tumor bulk.[521] This is followed by intense treatment with the other two modalities.[565] Chemotherapy itself can reduce tumor size to an extent that a large nonresectable tumor may become amenable to resection.[572]

An important finding of the IRS was the fact that tumors originating in so-called parameningeal sites, which include the ear and mastoid, nasopharynx, paranasal sinuses, and parapharyngeal areas, have a propensity to extend into the central nervous system.[569, 573–575] Tefft and associates reported that of 57 tumors originating in these areas, 20 patients (35%) developed meningeal extension that, despite therapy, was almost uniformly fatal.[569, 573] About half of these patients had received inadequate radiation therapy and all such therapy had been delayed. The treatment protocol was modified in 1977 to begin early radiation therapy with the addition of periodic intrathecal and standard chemotherapy.[809] As a result of this more intense therapy, the complete remission rate improved to 76%, and the percentage of patients that were tumor free or alive at 3 years was 57% and 68%, respectively, compared to 33% and 41% in those treated before 1977.[576]

The overall survival data from the IRS indicate 5-year survival rates for patients in group I as 81% to 93%; for those in group II as 72%; for those in group III as 52%; and for those in group IV 20%. The overall 5-year tumor-free survival rate was estimated to be 55%.[577] The best survival was in patients with orbital tumors. The estimated percentage of patients surviving 5 years was, in decreasing order, by primary site: orbit 89%, genitourinary 74%, head and neck excluding orbit and parameningeal sites 55%, extremities 47%, parameningeal sites 47%, trunk 45%, and retroperitoneum 34%.[577]

Although prolongation of survival is now reported, the long-term effects of the radiation and chemotherapy regimens, especially

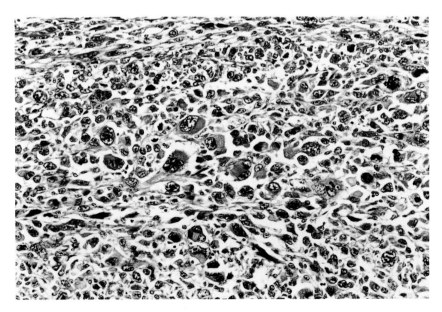

Figure 8–23. Pleomorphic rhabdomyosarcoma. Note anaplastic cells with bizarre nuclear features. Several are multinucleated with bright eosinophilic cytoplasm. Elongated, strap-shaped, and tadpole-shaped cells are also present.

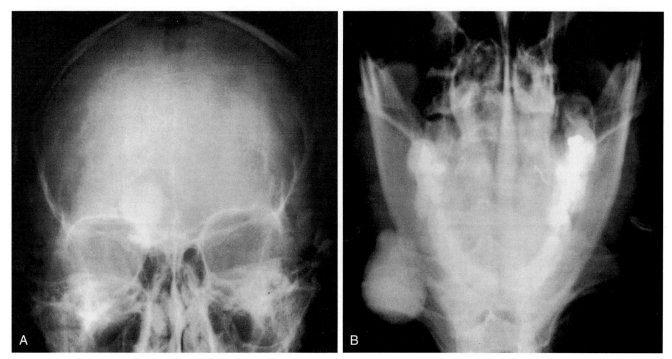

Figure 8–24. A, Radiograph of the skull shows a well-circumscribed, diffusely dense, ovoid "ivory" osteoma in the right frontal sinus. B, Radiographic view of the mandible shows a homogeneously dense, slightly lobulated mass adherent to the cortex, consistent with a surface-based osteoma.

in young children, await future evaluation. However, that such questions are even asked is a tribute to the successful efforts made in the treatment of this aggressive and formerly highly fatal tumor.

BONE

Benign Bone Tumors

Osteoma

Osteoma occurs almost exclusively in the head and neck region, only rarely developing elsewhere. Its reported incidence varies considerably, being dependent on the population studied and ranging from 0.002% in patients attending an otolaryngologic clinic to 3.0% among patients with sinonasal inflammatory disease.[578] The true incidence is unknown, however, as only approximately 10% of osteomas are symptomatic.[579]

Clinical Features. Osteomas are most frequently diagnosed in the second to fourth decades of life, being uncommon in the first decade. The average patient age has varied from 25 to 35 years.[579, 580] Paranasal sinus osteomas are more common in male patients.[12, 579, 580]

Osteoma frequently is an incidental finding in radiologic evaluations of the head and neck for other problems.[578, 580, 581] Symptoms may be quite diverse depending on the lesion's location, and include chronic sinusitis, local pain, headache, nasal obstruction, a painful or painless mass, exophthalmos, focal facial asymmetry, difficulty opening the mouth, meningitis, and hearing loss or a sensation of ear plugging.[578–586]

The most common site of origin is the paranasal sinuses,[578–580, 582, 583, 587] with the frontal sinus (Fig. 8–24A) the most frequent location,[578–580] and the ethmoid, maxillary, and sphenoid sinuses involved in descending order of frequency.[580, 582] Osteomas also arise from either the inner or the outer tables of the cranial bones,[35, 38, 588] including the mastoid and middle ear,[584, 586] and the jaw bones (Fig. 8–24B), especially the mandible.[35, 588–592] Extraskeletal osteomas occur in the buccal mucosa,[585] tongue,[593] and nasal cavity.[582] However, these are not true neoplasms and are termed *choristomas.*[33]

Radiologically, osteoma typically appears as a dense, opaque, sharply defined mass that is usually broad based[578, 580, 582–585, 587–589] and ranges from less than 1.0 cm to 8.5 cm in maximum size.[578, 582, 584, 589] An important clinical feature of head and neck osteomas is their association with Gardner's syndrome and familial adenomatosis coli.[581, 588, 590–592] In this association, the osteomas tend to be multiple and most frequently arise in the mandible, especially at the mandibular angle,[588, 590, 592] and in the maxilla.[591] Osteomas may be the first manifestation of these syndromes and occur up to 10 years prior to the discovery of the intestinal polyps.[581, 590]

Pathologic Features. Histologically, most osteomas are composed of hard, dense, compact lamellar bone, similar to cortical bone, in which haversian systems are present (Fig. 8–25, see p. 528). Cement lines may be prominent with densely stained, parallel accretion lines at the peripheral margin. These so-called "ivory" or "compact" osteomas have little stroma, and that which is present consists of bland fibrous tissue. Osteomas may also be composed predominantly of mature lamellar trabecular bone between which fat and marrow elements are found.[19, 31, 578, 582, 583] Osteomas on the surfaces of the bones forming the paranasal sinuses bulge into the sinus cavity, covered by sinus mucosa.

Treatment and Prognosis. Osteomas found incidentally in asymptomatic patients need not be removed, as follow-up studies frequently have shown no increase in size over several years' duration.[579] For symptomatic lesions, local excision is curative in almost all cases,[579, 581, 582] although rare recurrences after several years are reported.[579, 581, 582, 585]

Osteoid Osteoma

Clinical Features. Most patients with osteoid osteoma are in the second decade of life, with approximately 75% between the ages of 5 and 30 years; mean and median ages range from 12 to 17 years.[32, 35, 38, 594, 595] Males outnumber female patients in a ratio of 2 : 1 to 3 : 1[32, 35, 38, 594]; in spinal osteoid osteomas this ratio is 6 : 1.[595]

In the head and neck, the cervical spine is the most common site,[595–602] with other locations including the mandible,[38, 603, 604] maxilla,[604, 605] and various skull bones.[604, 606–609] Overall, however, osteoid osteoma is uncommon in the head and neck. Among 861 cases in four series, only 18 (2.1%) were so situated.[19, 32, 35, 38] In the spine, the tumor usually arises from the posterior elements, with the base of the transverse process, the lamina, and the pedicle the most common sites; the vertebral body is only rarely involved.[595–598]

Pain is virtually a universal symptom in patients with osteoid osteoma, only rare cases being painless.[597] The pain is usually most severe at night and is frequently dramatically relieved by aspirin. Patients with cervical spine involvement may have limitation of neck movement, or a scoliosis associated with torticollis. Neurologic symptoms and signs with reflex changes and muscle atrophy also occur.[595, 597–601] In the absence of abnormal radiologic studies, the duration of symptoms prior to diagnosis may be quite long, with some patients having symptoms for several years.[595, 597–601] Patients have been referred for psychiatric evaluation because of their persistent complaint of unexplained pain.[597, 607] Osteoid osteoma should be considered in any young patient who has persistent neck pain or painful scoliosis, and appropriate radiologic studies should be instituted.

Conventional radiographs of osteoid osteoma in its active, proliferative phase show a lucent, round to oval area, the nidus, surrounded by a zone of dense bone (Fig. 8–26). The size of the lesion is determined by the size of the nidus, not including the surrounding sclerotic bone. Although most osteoid osteomas are 1.0 cm or less in maximum size, some authors have accepted lesions as large as 1.5 cm to 2.0 cm as osteoid osteoma.[610–613] This radiologic pattern, combined with the clinical presentation, is virtually diagnostic of osteoid osteoma. However, routine radiologic studies may either fail to show the lesion, or show a lesion without the typical pattern.[595–602, 609, 610] Bone scans are the most sensitive method for discovering the lesion, with increased radionuclide uptake found in all cases[597–602, 610]; tomograms or computed tomographic (CT) scans are also more sensitive and accurate than routine radiographs for locating the lesion and showing its extent.[600–602] Over time, the nidus becomes increasingly calcified and ossified and eventually may become completely opaque.

The nidus may be located within the cancellous bone or the cortex or beneath the periosteum.[35, 603, 611, 614] An intracortical location is most frequent and here the nidus expands to reach the periosteum, where it induces the production of extensive, and highly dense, new bone that surrounds and extends for a considerable distance on either side of the nidus.[611, 613] Osteoid osteomas confined to the spongiosa may have little or no reactive bone about them, a situation often found in vertebral based lesions.[610]

Pathologic Features. In its active growth phase, where there is considerable vascularity, osteoid osteoma grossly appears as a discrete, round to oval lesion marked by a cherry-red or reddish-brown color.[613, 615] In this phase it is quite granular and friable and is easily displaced from the adjacent bone.[615] In its mature phase, where there is more calcification and bone production, the lesion is hard and gritty and blends with the bone around it.

Histologically, the nidus consists of active new bone, in various stages of maturity, within a loose fibrous stroma that contains numerous dilated thin walled blood vessels (Fig. 8–27, see p. 529).[31, 38, 604, 611–613, 615] Seams of osteoid are present that are lined by plump osteoblasts lacking pleomorphism or atypia (see Fig. 8–27B). Occasionally, osteoblasts are found that have large, hyperchromatic nuclei in association with brisk, but normal, mitotic activity.[31] The osteoid gradually undergoes calcification and conversion to woven and mature bone. Active osteoclastic activity is also present so that one may find simultaneous new bone production and bone resorption, which eventually results in bone that has a mosaic, pagetoid appearance.[38, 611, 613]

In some lesions, the nidus consists entirely of osteoid arranged in broad sheets with focal calcification; other lesions contain calcium and woven bone. The center is usually the most highly mineralized portion of the lesion. The periphery of the nidus may have mature bone trabeculae that forms an anastomotic or interlacing network that fuses with either the normal cortical bone or, if present, adjacent sclerotic compact bone. In intramedullary osteoid osteoma that lack adjacent compact bone, the nidus is separated from the adjacent cancellous bone by a zone of vascular connective tissue.

Differential Diagnosis. The distinction between osteoid osteoma and osteoblastoma cannot be made on the basis of histology alone, as both tumors are morphologically similar. Osteoblastoma is larger than osteoid osteoma, usually greater than 2.0 cm in maximum size and, unlike osteoid osteoma which has a limited growth potential and rarely exceeds 1.0 cm, is a progressive and expansive lesion. Clinically, the pain associated with osteoblastoma is also less often relieved by aspirin. Osteoid osteoma is distinguished from osteosarcoma by its radiologic pattern, strict histologic circumscription, and lack of significant cytologic atypia, abnormal mitotic figures, or malignant cartilage.

Treatment and Prognosis. Almost all osteoid osteomas are cured by complete en bloc excision of the nidus.[604] Although some patients are cured even when no nidus is histologically found, recurrences may develop in such individuals.[604] Recent innovations have involved the destruction of the nidus by percutaneous drilling or the use of radiofrequency techniques.[616, 617]

Osteoblastoma

Among osteoblastomas, the reported incidence in the head and neck has varied from 13% to 26%.[32, 35, 38]

Clinical Features. Approximately 75% to 90% of osteoblastomas occur in patients younger than 30 years of age, with only occasional cases in older patients.[32, 35, 38, 618–625]

In the head and neck, the cervical spine is the most common location[35, 38, 618–621, 626–632]; other sites include the facial and skull bones[618, 620–622, 624, 630, 633] including the temporal bone,[622, 631, 633, 634] occipital bone,[622, 632, 635] ethmoid,[622, 631, 636] frontal,[633, 637] and sphenoid bones[623, 629]; the orbit/supraorbital region[630, 633, 638]; mandible[38, 625, 633, 639–643]; and maxilla.[618, 620, 625, 630, 633, 644]

The incidence of skull involvement among all cases of osteoblastoma has varied from 2% to 20%.[34, 622, 633, 636, 642] In the vertebrae, osteoblastoma arises mainly from the posterior elements[19, 619, 627, 645]; origin from the vertebral body is uncommon.[619, 645]

Patients with osteoblastoma are almost always symptomatic, with pain present in approximately 90% or more of

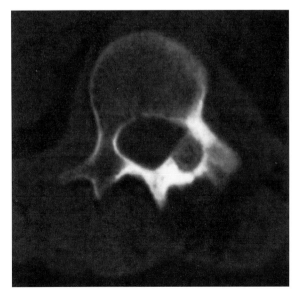

Figure 8–26. Osteoid osteoma of vertebra. Computed tomographic (CT) scan shows a relatively large, lucent area (nidus), containing a small central zone of calcification in the pedicle. The adjacent bone shows markedly increased density.

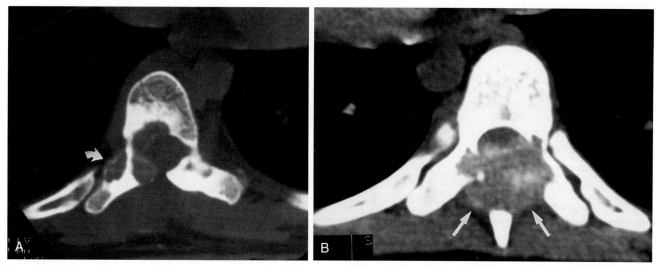

Figure 8–28. *A,* Osteoblastoma involving posterior elements of vertebra. Computed tomographic scan shows an expansive lesion, with an intact shell of bone *(arrow),* similar to that seen in an aneurysmal bone cyst. *B,* Another view of the lesion shown in part *A (arrows)* shows its aggressive appearance with destruction of bone and growth into the spinal canal.

cases.[618, 619, 621, 627, 629, 640, 641, 643] In the jaw bones, osteoblastoma may present as a swelling[625, 639, 644] that may be painless.[625, 640] Osteoblastomas of the spine and base of skull frequently produce neurologic symptoms because of their extension into the spinal canal.[618, 619, 624, 629, 632] Those in the cervical vertebrae may, similar to osteoid osteoma, be associated with scoliosis and torticollis.[624, 626, 627] Symptoms may be present for as short a time as 1 to 2 months[621, 625, 640] or for several years prior to diagnosis, especially in patients with spinal lesions in whom plain radiographs often fail to demonstrate the lesion. However, even osteoblastomas of the jaw have been present for long periods prior to diagnosis.[618, 620, 624, 625, 627, 640]

Radiologically, osteoblastoma is usually a lucent, well-circumscribed, expansive defect (Fig. 8–28)[621, 625, 629, 633, 635] that may contain focal calcification and radiopaque areas.[621, 625, 629, 635, 644] Cortical destruction may occur and be associated with periostitis and expansion into the soft tissue (see Fig. 8–28*B*) such that the radiologic pattern suggests an aggressive process.[618, 621] Plain radiographs may not demonstrate the lesion,[619, 626, 627] especially in vertebral cases, but bone scans are invariably positive and are a sensitive and accurate means of finding the lesion.[619, 626, 627] CT scans are also of great value in determining the precise location and extent of the lesion.[627, 629]

Osteoblastoma may have a periosteal, cortical, or medullary location, with the latter most frequent; however, a periosteal location is more common for osteoblastomas in the facial and cranial bones, especially the maxilla.[641, 644] Intracortical osteoblastoma is associated with surrounding sclerotic bone,[630, 645] which is absent in medullary lesions.[630]

The nidus of osteoblastoma is greater than 2.0 cm, with most ranging from 4 to 7 cm in maximum size.[31, 38, 646] Unlike osteoblastoma of the long bones, which seldom extends into the soft tissue, vertebral osteoblastoma frequently spreads into the epidural space and into the paraspinal tissues and may extend to involve adjacent vertebrae.[619]

Pathologic Features. On gross examination, osteoblastoma appears fairly well delimited within either the cortex or cancellous bone. The tumor is hemorrhagic, is purple to reddish-brown, and has a gritty or granular consistency with occasional cystic regions.[19, 31, 38, 645] Within the head and neck, osteoblastoma may reach a surprisingly large size (>5 cm),[621, 622, 637, 641] with vertebral lesions as large as 15 cm reported.[618]

The basic histologic pattern of osteoblastoma is similar to that of osteoid osteoma (Fig. 8–29, see p. 530), consisting of a well-vascularized connective tissue stroma, containing widely dilated capillaries, in which there is active production of osteoid and primitive woven bone.[19, 38, 630, 645, 646] However, there is considerable variation in this pattern from tumor to tumor. In the less mature lesion, there is an abundance of connective tissue stroma in which osteoclast-type giant cells and small foci of osteoid are present, some in a lace-like pattern. With maturation there is progressive mineralization of the osteoid with conversion to trabeculae of coarse woven bone, rimmed by plump osteoblasts. The trabeculae may fuse to form an anastomosing, net-like pattern. The osteoblasts usually lack any significant atypia, having round to oval, regular nuclei, often with prominent nucleoli. Mitotic activity is infrequent.

The most mature portion of osteoblastoma is located at its periphery, where lamellar bone is found. Here, the interface between the tumor and the adjacent normal bone is usually sharp, with little or no evidence of infiltration into the normal bone.

Osteoclasts are present and are frequently found to be actively resorbing (remodeling) the newly formed bone trabeculae. The combination of bone production and resorption leads to the formation of pagetoid-appearing bone with prominent cement lines.[19, 35] Some osteoblastomas contain large sheets of osteoid with little or no stroma and few osteoblasts. The intertrabecular stroma in osteoblastoma is loosely arranged with its content of thin-walled blood vessels and lacks the crowding and sheet-like grouping of atypical cells that occurs in osteosarcoma.

Rare osteoblastomas contain an abundant number of large cells, with bizarre, atypical, hyperchromatic nuclei and large nucleoli. In combination with osteoid and bone production, such a lesion may easily be histologically confused with conventional osteosarcoma. However, these "pseudosarcomatous" tumors lack significant mitotic activity, an important distinguishing feature from osteosarcoma in which mitotic figures are frequent and commonly abnormal.[31, 645, 647]

The relationship between what has been described as "malignant osteoblastoma",[648] and the lesion designated as "aggressive osteoblastoma"[646] is unclear. Common to these tumors is the presence of numerous large, epithelioid-like osteoblasts that rim the bone trabeculae or are focally arranged in large sheets (see Fig. 8–29*B*). Numerous osteoclast-type giant cells are also present. Highly calcified tumor bone, intensely stained with hematoxylin and termed *spiculated tumor bone* was found in the cases.[648]

Both aggressive osteoblastoma and malignant osteoblastoma may focally contain areas that cannot be distinguished histologically from osteosarcoma, but an important feature is their lack of atypical mitotic figures, necrosis, malignant cartilage, or peripheral permeation at the interface between the lesion and the adjacent normal cancellous bone.

Complicating this issue, Bertoni and associates reported examples of osteosarcoma that histologically resembled osteoblastoma[631, 649] and suggested that these were similar to the lesions described as malignant and aggressive osteoblastoma. Although both aggressive and malignant osteoblastoma were reported to have a greater tendency than conventional osteoblastoma for local recurrence, other investigators have not found this to be the case.[618, 621]

Differential Diagnosis. The histologic distinction between osteoblastoma and osteosarcoma is one of the most difficult diagnostic problems in orthopedic tumor pathology. The problem is compounded by the fact that osteoblastoma may, on occasion, have an aggressive-appearing radiologic pattern,[618, 621] and osteosarcoma may contain foci that are histologically indistinguishable from osteoblastoma.[631, 650, 651] With an adequate amount of tissue, the most critical histologic feature that allows separation of osteoblastoma from an osteoblastoma-like osteosarcoma is the sharp, noninfiltrative margin found in osteoblastoma, in contrast to the characteristically peripheral infiltrative pattern of osteosarcoma. However, when only small biopsy specimens are available, the peripheral margin may not be represented and it may not be possible to distinguish between these two tumors.[618, 621, 631, 651] Conventional osteoblastic osteosarcoma is distinguished from osteoblastoma by its atypical, pleomorphic stromal cells and osteoblasts with their sheet-like intertrabecular grouping, atypical mitotic figures, necrosis, and malignant cartilaginous areas. Although osteoblastoma lacks cartilage in most cases, foci of mature or immature chondroid may occur; but unlike the cartilage in osteosarcoma, this chondroid lacks cytologic atypia.[652]

The distinction between osteoid osteoma and osteoblastoma is not possible histologically, and the diagnosis rests on the size of the lesion and the clinical setting. Osteoid osteoma is rarely larger than 1.5 cm and, unlike osteoblastoma, is rarely progressive.[645] Although the pain associated with osteoblastoma may, as in osteoid osteoma, be more prevalent at night, it is rarely as sharply intense as in the osteoid osteoma and not as frequently relieved by aspirin.[19, 31, 35] Osteoblastoma is far more frequent in the vertebrae, jaw bones, and skull than is osteoid osteoma.[34] In the jaw bones, it may be difficult, on histologic grounds alone, to distinguish osteoblastoma from cementoblastoma.[640, 642] The latter is an odontogenic tumor that is intimately associated with the cementum of the tooth root.[33]

Treatment and Prognosis. Complete en bloc resection of osteoblastoma is almost always curative[618]; depending on its location, however, this is not always possible, and marginal resection or curettage procedures must be used. In such cases, local recurrence rates of 10% to 20% are reported.[618, 621, 625, 640, 643] Death due to local extension of the tumor may occur,[618] as well as from surgical complications of its treatment.[621, 627] Malignant transformation of osteoblastoma is reported that usually, but not always, occurs only after local recurrence.[618, 651, 653, 654] However, some of these cases may represent an underdiagnosed osteoblastoma-like osteosarcoma.[631, 649]

Osteosarcoma

General Features

Approximately 80% to 85% of osteosarcomas arise in the long bones; they are relatively infrequent in the head and neck area. Among 5155 cases of osteosarcoma in seven large series, only 336 (6.5%) involved the skull, mandible or maxilla, facial bones, or cervical vertebrae.[19, 32, 35, 38, 655–657]

Osteosarcoma may arise secondarily to some underlying condition, the most frequent of which include Paget's disease, usually in the polyostotic form[658, 659]; fibrous dysplasia, also most frequently in the polyostotic form[660, 661]; bone infarct[662]; and irradiated bone.[663] The craniofacial region is the most common site for osteo-

sarcoma arising on the basis of pre-existing fibrous dysplasia.[660, 661] Osteosarcoma has been associated with loss of function of the tumor suppressor retinoblastoma *(Rb)* gene,[664, 665] being the most frequent second malignancy to develop in patients with the inherited form of retinoblastoma[664]; however, *Rb* gene alteration has also been found in osteosarcoma unassociated with retinoblastoma.[664, 666]

Clinical Features. Osteosarcoma occurs in patients of all ages, from children less than 5 years of age[667, 668] to adults in the tenth decade of life[32]; however, 70% to 95% of patients are in the first two decades of life, with a peak incidence in the second decade.[19, 32, 35, 38] At Memorial Hospital, 10% of all osteosarcomas occurred in patients older than 60 years of age, over one half of whom had some underlying condition such as Paget's disease.[669] Older patients (>50 years of age) have a higher incidence of craniofacial involvement than younger patients, this site accounting for from 13% to 33% of osteosarcomas in this age group.[669, 670] In general, osteosarcoma is more common in male patients, in ratios of 1.3:1 to 2:1.[19, 32, 35, 38]

Approximately 80% of all osteosarcomas are of the conventional intramedullary type. Radiologically, these osteosarcomas have an aggressive appearance with extensive cancellous and cortical bone destruction with tumor extension into the soft tissues. Depending on the proportion of bone produced by the tumor, it will appear either totally lytic or densely sclerotic or, in the majority of cases, have a mixed lytic-sclerotic pattern.[31, 34, 38]

Pathologic Features. On gross examination, there is good correlation with the radiologic pattern with extensive bone destruction being present and, in over 90% of cases, an associated soft tissue mass.[31, 671] The tumor's appearance and consistency varies considerably depending on the proportion of cartilage, fibrous tissue, and bone present. It may be pink to gray-white with a "fish-flesh" appearance, or gray to blue-gray, associated with firm, white fibrous nodular masses. In tumors with abundant bone production, the tumor may be quite hard and require a saw to section. Yellow to yellow-white calcific foci are usually found throughout the lesion, as well as areas of hemorrhage, necrosis, and cystic change. In most osteosarcomas, even those with abundant bone formation, the peripheral soft tissue margins usually contain highly cellular regions that are soft enough to section with a scalpel blade and it is from such regions that tissue should be obtained whenever frozen section biopsy material is needed.[671]

Histologically, osteosarcoma is defined as a tumor characterized by the direct formation of osteoid or primitive woven bone by malignant tumor stromal cells (Fig. 8–30, see p. 531).[12, 19, 31, 38, 672] It is important to emphasize that the finding of unequivocal osteoid or tumor bone formed by malignant-appearing stromal cells establishes the diagnosis of osteosarcoma regardless of the quantity of this material present. The pattern and amount of this tumor osteoid or bone varies considerably, not only from tumor to tumor but also from area to area within the tumor. Osteoid may be found as thin, eosinophilic strands of hyalin-like material interspersed between the malignant stromal cells, producing a "lace-like" pattern (see Fig. 8–30A). These strands may fuse to form larger, irregular seams or trabeculae. The osteoid may also occur in broad sheet-like masses in which the malignant stromal cells become "choked off" and eventually disappear. Of diagnostic importance, the osteoid trabeculae are not rimmed by an orderly proliferation of osteoblasts as in benign reactive bone. Also unlike reactive new bone formation, where the stroma between the bone trabeculae contains dilated capillaries and loosely arranged bland stromal cells, in osteosarcoma this space is usually packed with malignant stromal cells (see Fig. 8–30C). Under polarized light, osteoid has a woven or mat-like appearance, unlike the more orderly longitudinal fiber array found in collagen.[31] However, at times, the light microscopic distinction between collagen and osteoid may be problematic, with the diagnosis dependent on the experience of the pathologist. To convert to bone, osteoid must undergo calcification such that the presence of fine granules of calcification within the eosinophilic strands or trabeculae is a helpful clue to the diagnosis of osteoid.

A further histologic problem is distinguishing osteoid from chondroid. Contrary to common belief, chondroid, like osteoid, stains pink with conventional hematoxylin-eosin stains, and not blue as associated with hyalin cartilage.[31] Chondroid usually occurs as well-defined islands, usually sharply set off from the surrounding cellular stroma, and has a less fibrillar appearance than does osteoid.[31]

Immunohistochemical stains for the noncollagenous bone proteins osteocalcin and osteonectin have been used in an attempt to distinguish osteosarcoma from other malignant bone tumors. Although osteonectin is found in osteosarcoma, its presence in a variety of other tumors makes it unreliable as a diagnostic marker.[673–676] Reactivity for osteocalcin has been used by some authors for distinguishing osteosarcoma from malignant fibrous histiocytoma and fibrosarcoma, but it was found to occur in chondroblasts as well.[677, 678]

As the osteoid in osteosarcoma becomes calcified to form tumor bone, it may be deposited on residual normal trabeculae. This tumor bone has an irregular appearance, is strongly hematoxylinophilic, and, by polarized light, has a woven or basket-weave pattern unlike the uniform lamellar pattern of normal bone. Within this tumor bone, the now incorporated stromal cells (malignant osteoblasts) lie within lacunar spaces. These "osteocytes" have small, hyperchromatic and irregularly shaped nuclei.

Although the majority of osteosarcomas produce an abundance of osteoid and tumor bone and are thus classified as osteoblastic, others contain a predominance of malignant cartilage (chondroblastic type), or fibrous, spindle cell areas (fibrosarcomatous/fibrohistiocytic type) where osteoid or tumor bone may be scarce and require examination of many sections to find. In recent years, a variety of other histologic subtypes of osteosarcoma have been reported, including chondroblastoma-like[679]; chondromyxoid fibroma-like[31]; osteoblastoma-like[680]; clear cell[681]; epithelioid[682–684]; and malignant fibrous histiocytoma-like[658, 663, 669, 685, 686]; however, with the exception of the latter subtype, all the others are exceptionally rare.

The abundant tumor bone produced by osteoblastic osteosarcoma may be so extensive that it crowds out much of the intervening stroma such that it may be difficult to find stromal cells directly producing osteoid or bone. Despite this, the general permeative growth pattern and the quality and abundance of this irregular tumor bone serve to establish the diagnosis of osteosarcoma.[31, 671] Chondroblastic osteosarcomas contain an abundance of malignant-appearing chondroid and cartilage, arranged in lobules or islands, with cells within lacunar spaces.[687] The periphery of the lobules tend to be more cellular and the cells frequently assume spindle shapes. Calcification with enchondral ossification may be present. Fibrosarcomatous osteosarcoma contains large areas composed of spindle cells that may assume a herringbone pattern indistinguishable from fibrosarcoma. Fibrohistiocytic osteosarcomas have abundant large, pleomorphic tumor cells with bizarre enlarged nuclei, as well as abnormal spindle-shaped cells. Multinucleated tumor giant cells with an abundant glassy eosinophilic cytoplasm are frequent, as are smaller histiocyte-like cells having a fine granular cytoplasm. A storiform pattern may be found in the spindle cell areas, the overall pattern appearing identical to that of soft tissue malignant fibrous histiocytoma. Biopsy tissue from any of these three histologic varieties of osteosarcoma may not contain obvious osteoid or tumor bone, and the diagnosis of osteosarcoma must be presumptive pending examination of a resection specimen. Most conventional intramedullary osteosarcomas express a wide spectrum of histologic patterns[31, 38] and contain a mixture of elements, from areas showing osteoid or tumor bone to those with cartilaginous, fibrosarcomatous, or fibrohistiocytic foci (see Fig. 8–30B, see p. 531).

In all forms of osteosarcoma, one finds a permeative growth pattern with tumor percolating between and entrapping existing normal bone trabeculae. Upward of one quarter of osteosarcomas contain scattered benign osteoclast-type giant cells,[31, 671, 687–689] which at times may be so numerous as to simulate a giant cell tumor (GCT). Such cells may be frequent in osteosarcomas arising in

Paget's disease.[659, 688] Distinguishing a GCT with bone formation from an osteoclast-rich osteosarcoma may be difficult, especially on biopsy tissue.[31, 671, 687–689] However, with adequate tissue, the bone in true GCT is frequently at the periphery of the lesion, rather than scattered haphazardly throughout the tumor as in osteosarcoma, and it is rimmed by an orderly array of plump osteoblasts as in reactive bone, versus the unlined bone of conventional osteosarcoma. Malignant cartilage is absent in GCT, and osteoclast-rich osteosarcoma will invariably have foci diagnostic of conventional osteosarcoma elsewhere in its substance. Osteosarcomas that arise in association with Paget's disease or in irradiated bone are most frequently of the fibrosarcomatous or fibrohistiocytic type,[658, 663, 690] as are those osteosarcomas that occur in patients over the age of 60 years.[669]

Mitotic activity is easily found in all forms of conventional osteosarcoma, with frequent abnormal forms.[671, 687] The absence of mitotic activity should give one pause in making a diagnosis of osteosarcoma, and suggests the possibility of a pseudosarcomatous tumor.[31] Hemorrhage and necrosis are also frequent. Such spontaneous necrosis may involve 40% to 70% of the total tumor area.[691, 692] The degree of tumor necrosis induced by chemotherapy has been correlated with prognosis,[692–694] with patients classified as "good" responders when the necrosis involves 90% or more of the tumor and "poor" responders when there is a lesser degree of necrosis[694, 695]; patients with a good therapeutic response have significantly better 5-year survival rates.[692, 693, 696] However, these data are based almost entirely on the results obtained for appendicular osteosarcomas[696] and may not apply to those in the head and neck region owing to the inability here to perform extensive surgical removal of the tumor and the technical problem of delivering adequate chemotherapy in this region.[695, 697]

Although some experienced bone tumor pathologists attempt to grade conventional intramedullary osteosarcomas,[689, 698, 699] the extensive variability from area to area that exists in the majority of these tumors makes such grading suspect, as well as the fact that, with the exception of the "well-differentiated" intraosseous form of osteosarcoma, grading appears to have little or no prognostic value.

By electron microscopy,[700–704] a variety of cell types are found in osteosarcoma, including fibroblasts, myofibroblasts, chondroblasts, osteoblasts, multinucleated giant cells, histiocytes, and primitive undifferentiated mesenchymal cells. A characteristic finding in the tumor cells is an abundance of a dilated, anastomosing rough endoplasmic reticulum associated with an intercellular matrix of collagen that contains needle-shaped hydroxyapatite crystals. Cytoplasmic glycogen and lipid droplets may also be found.

Osteosarcoma of the Skull

Among the 5155 osteosarcomas in our review, the bones of the skull, exclusive of the maxilla and mandible, were the site of origin in only 72 cases (1.4%). In up to one half of cranial osteosarcomas, the tumor arises secondary to some underlying condition, most commonly Paget's disease, fibrous dysplasia, or in irradiated bone.[704–710]

Clinical Features. Although patients as young as 2 years of age and those in the ninth decade of life are reported, most patients are in the fourth and fifth decades of life, an older age than for those with osteosarcoma of the appendicular skeleton.[704–706, 711–713] This reflects the component of patients with cranial osteosarcoma that have Paget's disease or radiation sarcoma, conditions that most often occur in older patients. Such secondary osteosarcomas occur in patients approximately 20 to 30 years older than those with primary cranial osteosarcoma.[704, 705] Unlike the male dominance in osteosarcoma of the long bones, the male:female ratio in osteosarcoma of the skull is roughly equal.[704–706, 712, 713]

Any of the skull bones may be involved, with reported cases in the calvarium[704, 705] and skull base[705, 714]; the occipital,[706, 712, 715, 716] parietal,[706, 708, 712, 717] frontal,[707, 710, 717] and temporal bones[706, 707, 712]; the orbit[706, 710, 717]; the ethmoid,[706, 712, 713] sphenoid,[706, 707, 712] and maxillary sinuses[713]; the nasal fossa[706, 713, 717]; the zygoma[706, 718]; and the sella area.[704, 709, 719] In some cases, the tumor may be so large that its exact site of origin cannot be established.[713, 714, 720]

Clinically, the dominant complaint is that of a painless mass or bulge,[704, 705, 714, 720] although cranial nerve symptoms, epistaxis, and eye displacement may occur, reflecting the location of the tumor.[704, 705] Most cases are diagnosed within 6 months of the onset of symptoms.[704, 705, 713]

Pathologic Features. Osteoblastic osteosarcoma is the most common type encountered in the skull,[704, 705, 711, 713] but chondroblastic,[705, 713] fibroblastic,[704, 706, 712, 713] fibrohistiocytic,[705, 706] small cell,[1023, 1028] telangiectatic,[704, 705, 712] and well-differentiated[716] subtypes also occur.

Treatment and Prognosis. In a review of 201 patients with craniofacial osteosarcoma, 61 of whom had cranial lesions, it was found that the best overall and disease-free survival rates were associated with complete surgical removal of the tumor and the use of chemotherapy, the latter improving survival even in those patients with incomplete resections.[721]

The prognosis for osteosarcoma of the skull and facial bones is generally poor, with the reported results influenced by the number of secondary osteosarcomas in the series. The 5-year survival rate is approximately 10%[706, 711, 713, 718] with only a few long-term survivors[704, 705]; metastases develop in approximately 45% of cases.[704, 711, 713] Patients with osteosarcoma secondary to Paget's disease have a very poor prognosis, with almost all dying of tumor.[704, 705]

Osteosarcoma of the Jaw Bones

Clinical Features. The jaw bones were involved in 255 (4.9%) of the 5155 cases of osteosarcoma in our review, with 135 in the maxilla (2.6%) and 120 in the mandible (2.3%). The ratio of mandibular to maxillary cases varies in the literature, with the mandible accounting for 44% to 73% of cases and the maxilla for 27% to 56%.[722–730] Within the mandible, the body is the most common location, accounting for 55% to 75% of cases[722, 725, 730]; the angle is involved in 8% to 20% of cases[722–725]; the ramus in 8% to 15%[722, 723, 725]; and the symphysis in 10% to 15%.[722–725, 731] In the maxilla, the alveolar ridge is the most common site,[722–725, 730] with the antrum,[722, 723, 725] anterior midline,[725] and hard palate[723, 732] also involved.

Although cases occur in children,[722–725, 733] this is uncommon; most patients are in the third to fourth decades of life, generally one decade older than patients with appendicular osteosarcoma.

Clinically, the majority of patients complain of a swelling or a mass that is often, but not always, painless; pain alone may also occur.[722, 723, 725, 726, 729–731, 734] Numbness or paresthesia of the lip or chin reflects tumor involvement of the inferior alveolar nerve and is an important clue to the diagnosis of an aggressive lesion.[722, 730] Loosening of the teeth may be the first or even dominant manifestation of the disease[723, 725, 726, 729, 732, 734, 735] such that the dentist may be the one whom the patient first sees for medical attention. Other symptoms include nasal obstruction, epistaxis, or visual disturbances secondary to antral involvement.[726] Although a history of symptoms for as long as 30 years is recorded,[730] most patients seek medical attention within 6 months of the onset of symptoms.[722, 729]

Osteosarcoma of the jaw bones has developed as a consequence of predisposing conditions, the most common of which is prior radiation therapy to the region; such a history is present in approximately 10% of cases.[722, 723, 726, 732, 735] The tumor has also developed secondary to Paget's disease,[723, 732, 735] fibrous dysplasia,[732, 734, 735] retinoblastoma,[735] and chronic osteomyelitis.[732]

Radiologically, osteosarcoma of the jaw has a purely lytic and destructive pattern (Fig. 8–31A) in 35% to 45% of cases; a sclerotic pattern in 5% to 65% of cases; and a mixed pattern of lysis and sclerosis in 22% to 50% of cases.[722–724] A sunburst pattern, with radiating spicules of bone (Fig. 8–31B) is considered a characteristic feature of osteosarcoma of the jaw, especially in mandibular lesions[723, 725, 726, 728, 730, 731]; however, it is not frequent, occurring

in 7% to 27% of cases.[723, 725, 726, 728, 730] Extraosseous soft tissue extension is radiologically evident in 30% to 100% of cases.[722–724] An important radiologic feature of osteosarcoma of the jaws is symmetric widening of the periodontal membrane space that may also be associated with loss of the lamina dura (see Fig. 8–31B). Although not specific for osteosarcoma, its occurrence is suggestive of an aggressive process.[725, 727, 730, 731]

Pathologic Features. Osteosarcomas of the jaw bone have ranged from 2 to 10 cm in maximum size.[722, 723, 736, 737] The histologic type has varied in different series, some reporting a predominance of osteoblastic tumors,[722, 730, 731, 734] and others reporting a chondroblastic[723, 724, 726] or fibroblastic[737] predominance. In addition to parosteal and periosteal osteosarcomas (see subsequent discussion), examples of telangiectatic,[727, 736] small cell,[738, 739] well-differentiated,[740] and high-grade surface[724] osteosarcoma are reported.

Treatment and Prognosis. Intralesional or marginal excision of osteosarcoma of the jaw leads to local recurrence in 36% to 100% of cases[722, 723, 727, 730, 731, 733]; such recurrences carry a poor prognosis,[722, 723] as most patients die from local recurrence.[723, 726, 731] The rate of local recurrence in maxillary osteosarcoma has varied from 29% to 60% and in mandibular lesions from 43% to 66%.[723, 730, 734] Distant metastases occur, although there is considerable variation in the literature as to its incidence, with reported rates of 6% to 52%.[723, 725, 726, 729, 730, 734] Metastases from mandibular osteosarcoma are more frequent than from maxillary lesions, with the incidence in mandibular lesions ranging from 33% to 71% of cases, and for maxillary lesions from 13% to 20%.[729, 730, 734]

Overall 5-year survival rates range from 23% to 47%, with most series reporting rates of 35% to 45%.[722, 723, 725, 726, 730, 731] Radical excision yields the best prognosis,[723] with 5-year survival rates for maxillary lesions of 25% to 63% and for mandibular lesions of 24% to 71%.[725, 730, 733, 734] Some authors express the view that mandibular lesions have a better prognosis than maxillary tumors.[725]

Vertebral Osteosarcoma

The vertebral column was the site of origin in 116 (2.3%) of the 5155 conventional osteosarcomas in our survey. Of these cases, the cervical vertebrae were the least common site, accounting for only 9 cases.

Clinical Features. Most vertebral osteosarcomas arise secondary to some other condition, most notably Paget's disease or following radiation therapy to the region, de novo cases being uncommon.[741–745] In 1994, Kebudi et al.[746] found only 45 cases of vertebral osteosarcoma in the absence of Paget's disease or radiation therapy in the American and European medical literature since 1904. Despite the high incidence of spinal involvement in Paget's disease, the actual occurrence of vertebral osteosarcoma in such patients is quite uncommon.[743, 747]

Patients with vertebral osteosarcoma have ranged from 3 to 70 years of age[742, 743, 747] and are older, on average, than those with appendicular osteosarcoma,[742, 743] reflecting the inclusion of older adults with Paget's disease and radiation-induced tumors. Virtually all patients with vertebral osteosarcoma present because of pain that is frequently associated with neurologic symptoms, sensory as well as motor.[742, 743, 744–749] Those with osteosarcoma of the cervical vertebrae may have pain that radiates into the upper extremity.[745, 746, 749] The presence of a palpable mass is uncommon.[742, 746]

Radiologically, vertebral osteosarcoma is a destructive, usually nonexpansive lesion with soft tissue extension found in the majority of cases (Fig. 8–32).[742–745, 747–749] Within the vertebra, the body is involved in almost all cases,[742, 743, 745, 746, 748] although the tumor frequently extends to involve the posterior elements as well; primary origin from the posterior elements is uncommon.[742, 743, 744]

Pathologic Features. Most cases of vertebral osteosarcoma are osteoblastic, although chondroblastic, fibroblastic, and fibrohistiocytic subtypes occur.[742, 743, 745, 748, 749] Distinguishing osteoblastoma from osteosarcoma is a major problem, as cases of vertebral

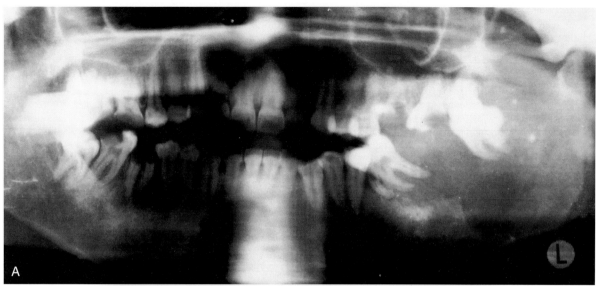

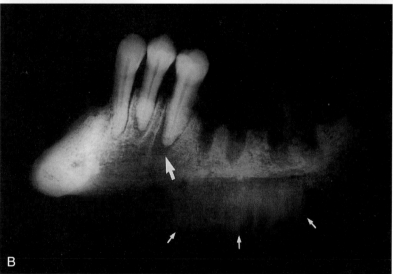

Figure 8–31. *A,* Osteosarcoma of the mandible. Large, predominantly osteolytic, aggressive-appearing lesion involves the left hemimandible. The tumor has destroyed the cortex superiorly, with marked displacement and distortion of the teeth. *B,* Specimen radiograph of a mandibular osteosarcoma shows the canine tooth *(left)* and first and second premolars. There is widening of the periodontal membrane space *(large arrow)* associated with loss of the lamina dura. Spiculated, extraosseous tumor expansion is present *(small arrows).*

osteosarcoma have been misdiagnosed as osteoblastoma on biopsy tissue.[743, 744, 745] Perhaps contributing to this problem is the knowledge that the spine is a common site for osteoblastoma but an uncommon location for osteosarcoma. As mentioned earlier, the most helpful histologic feature that separates osteoblastoma from osteosarcoma is the peripheral permeative pattern in osteosarcoma, in contrast to the sharp interface of the nidus of osteoblastoma with the host bone at its periphery. Rare cases will be found where the distinction between these tumors may be histologically impossible, and only the course of the disease unmasks the true nature of the lesion.

Treatment and Prognosis. The prognosis in vertebral osteosarcoma is dismal, with almost all patients dying of tumor, usually within 1 year of diagnosis.[742, 743, 746, 748] This no doubt reflects the difficulty in adequately resecting tumors in this region. In none of the 10 patients with vertebral osteosarcoma treated at Memorial Hospital could the tumor be completely resected.[743] Of 27 patients with vertebral osteosarcoma reported from the Mayo Clinic, there was only 1 survivor (3.7%); all those with cervical vertebral lesions died.[742] The poor prognosis in vertebral osteosarcoma may also be a reflection of the number of older patients with Paget's disease or radiation-induced tumors. However, the prognosis in the 45 patients

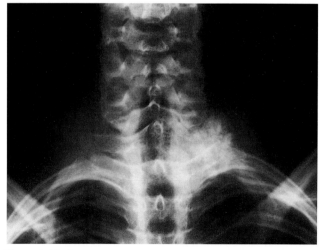

Figure 8–32. Osteosarcoma arising from C7 shows sclerotic and spiculated tumor bone associated with destruction of the left half of the vertebra.

with primary vertebral osteosarcoma reported by Kebudi et al.[746] was also poor, with 36 (80%) dead of tumor, 2 (4.4%) alive with tumor, and only 7 (15%) alive without tumor, only two of whom were long-term survivors.

Parosteal Osteosarcoma

Parosteal osteosarcoma affects the long bones in approximately 95% of cases, with the femur involved in the majority of cases. Among 226 cases of parosteal osteosarcoma at the Mayo clinic, only 1, a mandibular lesion, was located in the head and neck region.[750] In the head and neck region, the mandible and maxilla have been the most common sites of involvement,[751–757] in addition to the cranial bones.[757–759]

Clinical Features. Patients with parosteal osteosarcoma are generally older than those with conventional osteosarcoma, with 80% older than 20 years of age; most patients are in the third and fourth decades of life.[32, 750, 760]

In the head and neck, a painless swelling is the most common symptom, although the lesion may be tender.[751, 753, 756, 757–759] The tumor typically grows slowly and although in some patients the tumor is detected within a few days to several months of symptom onset,[753, 759] other patients have had a mass for as long as 10 years prior to diagnosis.[751, 759]

Parosteal osteosarcoma arises on the surface of the bone and forms a coarsely lobulated or bosselated, usually broad-based mass that rests on and bulges from the cortical surface.[761–763] Radiologically, the underlying cortex is frequently thickened, and a radiolucent cleavage-plane may be seen between the tumor and the underlying cortex. The base of the lesion is usually more densely ossified than the periphery. Radiolucent zones may be found within the tumor that represent either entrapped normal soft tissue, low-grade cartilage or fibrous tissue, or areas of dedifferentiated tumor.[750] Occasionally, invasion into the underlying bone is seen.[759] The central portion of parosteal osteosarcoma is not in direct continuity with the medullary cavity of the underlying bone.

Even in the confined space of the head and neck, some parosteal osteosarcomas have been as large as 16 cm, although most are between 3 cm and 5 cm.[751, 752, 753, 757–759]

Pathologic Features. Grossly, parosteal osteosarcoma appears well-delimited and typically grows to envelop the external aspect of the bone.[761, 762, 764] Medullary involvement is infrequent and its development appears correlated with the length of time that the tumor has been present, with long-standing tumors eventually invading into and through the underlying cortex.[750, 761, 765] The frequency of the latter varies from 1.3% to 59%.[750, 760, 765]

A fibrous capsule or a cartilaginous cap may be found at the tumor's peripheral margin.[763] Despite this seeming gross circumscription, microscopically, the tumor invades and incorporates the adjacent skeletal muscle and fat within its substance.[760, 766] The consistency of the tumor varies depending on the proportion of fibrous, osseous, and cartilaginous tissue present.[761, 762, 766] The periphery may be soft and fleshy and easily cut with a scalpel, but the basal portion is usually hard, requiring a saw to section. Here, the cut surface shows white to yellow-white chalk-like areas of calcification and ossification.[38, 752] In long-standing tumors, the entire lesion may be rock hard due to extensive bone formation.

Histologically, parosteal osteosarcoma may be difficult to diagnose, especially on small biopsy specimens, if careful attention is not given to the clinical and radiologic features (Fig. 8–33, see p. 532). The stromal and osseous elements in parosteal osteosarcoma usually lack clear evidence of cytologic malignancy, or that which is present may be so scarce as to require many sections to discover.[763, 764, 766] The tumor is composed of a fibrous stroma in which reside irregular spicules and trabeculae of bone (see Fig. 8–33A).[760, 764, 765] The stroma varies in its cellularity; some cases are relatively hypocellular with the stroma containing abundant collagen separating bland-appearing spindle cells (see Fig. 8–33B)[760, 761, 765]; in others the stroma is more cellular, containing

plumper and more atypical cells creating a fibrosarcoma-like pattern.[760, 763, 765] Mitotic figures may be scarce and require extensive search to find.[760, 763] The bone trabeculae are irregular, being of woven or lamellar type, and frequently arranged in parallel arrays (see Fig. 8–33A). Unlike conventional osteosarcoma, the trabeculae may be rimmed by a layer of plump but benign-appearing osteoblasts.[31, 760, 766] In other areas, the bone arises directly by metaplastic transformation of the fibrous stroma as in fibrous dysplasia.[31, 763] It is at the peripheral margin of the tumor that one finds more cellular zones composed of primitive-appearing cells that have enlarged and irregular nuclei, and which form osteoid.[38, 764, 765] Here, direct invasion of skeletal muscle and fat is found. The base of the lesion consists of densely compact woven or lamellar bone in contrast to its more fibrous, spindle-cell peripheral component. Cartilaginous foci, of variable size, occur in 50% to 80% of cases.[750, 761, 763, 764, 766] These foci may have cytologic features of low-grade chondrosarcoma, with increased cellularity and atypia, and show enchondral ossification. The amount of cartilage varies from tumor to tumor, but it is never the dominant element as it is in periosteal osteosarcoma.

Foci of dedifferentiation in which areas of high-grade sarcoma, usually malignant fibrous histiocytoma, fibrosarcoma, or conventional osteosarcoma are found, may occur in an otherwise typical parosteal osteosarcoma. Such dedifferentiated areas usually develop only after several local recurrences, but may be found at the time of initial presentation.[750, 755, 763, 765–768] The incidence of dedifferentiation varies from 16% to 43%[750, 767, 768]; dedifferentiated lesions have occurred in the head and neck region.[756]

In the literature, some osteosarcomas listed as parosteal type have been histologically graded numerically from I to III, a grade III lesion being an overtly malignant tumor with features of conventional osteosarcoma.[19, 761, 765] However, such a tumor is best classified as a high-grade surface osteosarcoma,[769] rather than a parosteal osteosarcoma, as it has a considerably worse prognosis than true parosteal osteosarcoma.

Differential Diagnosis. The differential diagnosis of parosteal osteosarcoma includes sessile osteochondroma, myositis ossificans, and periosteal osteosarcoma. Unlike parosteal osteosarcoma, the radiologic pattern of osteochondroma shows continuity between the lesion and the underlying parent bone. Histologically, osteochondroma has a cartilage cap composed of benign rather than malignant cartilage; the cancellous bone is of lamellar type, and the central portion of the lesion contains marrow fat or hematopoietic elements and lacks the fibrous stroma of parosteal osteosarcoma. Periosteal osteosarcoma has more abundant and more atypical cartilage than parosteal osteosarcoma, and its spindle cell elements are larger and more atypical than the spindle cells of parosteal osteosarcoma. Essentially, periosteal osteosarcoma is a high-grade surface chondroblastic osteosarcoma, in contrast to the low-grade fibro-osseous character of parosteal osteosarcoma.

Myositis ossificans is the lesion most likely to be histologically confused with parosteal osteosarcoma. The clinical situation may enable one to easily separate the two conditions provided there is a history of recent trauma to the involved site followed by the rapid appearance of a soft tissue mass that gradually ossifies over time. However, such a history may be lacking, the patient complaining only of a slowly enlarging mass. Radiologically, myositis ossificans usually appears separate from the underlying bone, although in some long-standing cases it may continue to grow and ultimately attach itself to the bone and thus radiologically simulate parosteal osteosarcoma. The classic histologic feature of myositis ossificans is its zonal pattern in which the periphery of the growing lesion shows the most mature degree of bone differentiation with the more central and basal aspects composed of a stroma of immature, and sometimes atypical, cells in which there is primitive (woven) bone production. This contrasts with parosteal osteosarcoma in which the periphery of the lesion shows the least mature elements and the basal or central regions contain more mature bone. In the fully developed form of myositis, the lesion may become totally ossified, being composed of mature compact lamellar bone such as to resemble an osteoma; such a degree of organization is never found in parosteal osteosarcoma.

Treatment and Prognosis. In general, parosteal osteosarcoma has an excellent prognosis following complete surgical excision, with a 5-year survival rate of approximately 80%. However, 10-year survival rates are somewhat lower owing to the appearance of late metastases in some patients.[750] The course of parosteal osteosarcoma in the head and neck region is not well established because of its rarity, with only a few reports containing long-term follow-up information.[754, 756, 759] At the time of these reports, however, almost all of the patients were alive and well.[753, 754, 756–759] Dedifferentiated parosteal osteosarcoma has a poor prognosis with metastases in approximately 50% of patients at 5 years.[750, 767] Whenever possible, a wide local complete excision should be done for parosteal osteosarcoma to prevent local recurrence and the possibility of dedifferentiation.[750]

Periosteal Osteosarcoma

Periosteal osteosarcoma is a subperiosteal surface-based tumor[770] that occurs in the long bones in over 95% of cases. Location in the head and neck is rare. In the Netherlands' series of 17 cases, only 1, a mandibular lesion, was in the head and neck region[32]; in 26 cases at the Mayo Clinic, none arose in the head and neck.[38] Only individual case reports of mandibular[771–773] and maxillary periosteal osteosarcoma[774] are reported.

Clinical Features. The age range for periosteal osteosarcoma is quite broad, with approximately 60% to 75% of patients in the second decade of life; it is uncommon in the first decade. In the few head and neck cases, patients have ranged from 20 to 65 years of age.[32, 34, 771–775] Periosteal osteosarcomas of the mandible and maxilla are usually small, ranging from 2.7 to 3.5 cm.[771–774]

Although the radiologic appearance of periosteal osteosarcoma in the long bones usually shows a radiating pattern of osseous spicules that extend outward from the cortex,[770, 775–777] the few cases reported in the jaws have not, with an occasional exception,[773] demonstrated this pattern.

Pathologic Features. On gross examination, periosteal osteosarcoma rests on a thickened cortex, which may be minimally invaded by the tumor,[770, 776, 778] and appears well delimited by the periosteum. On section, the periphery of the tumor is soft and well-rounded and has a distinct chondroid appearance with glistening gray to gray-white lobules that contain white to yellow streaks of calcification or ossification.[770–772, 774, 776]

Microscopically, periosteal osteosarcoma consists of lobules of high-grade malignant cartilage that are separated by spindle-shaped mesenchymal cells in which eosinophilic lace-like ribbons of osteoid are found.[770] However, these osteoid areas may be quite sparse and difficult to find and are best seen at the peripheral growing margin of the lesion.[770, 775, 777, 778] In some cases, fibroblastic or even osteoblastic foci may be found and even predominate, such that the tumor may be difficult to distinguish from a conventional high-grade surface osteosarcoma.[776, 777]

Differential Diagnosis. Unlike parosteal osteosarcoma, large seams of parallel-oriented osteoid or tumor bone do not occur in periosteal osteosarcoma, nor does it have the abundant fibroblastic stroma of parosteal osteosarcoma.

The scarcity of osteoid in some cases of periosteal osteosarcoma has led to diagnostic confusion with juxtacortical chondrosarcoma, a problem further compounded by the fact that the eosinophilic ribbons that occur in periosteal osteosarcoma are considered by some as representing collagen and not osteoid.[778, 779] In contrast to periosteal osteosarcoma, however, juxtacortical chondrosarcoma is composed of low-grade hyaline cartilage and lacks atypical spindle cell elements.

Treatment and Prognosis. In the long bones, periosteal osteosarcoma has a prognosis that is intermediate between that of parosteal osteosarcoma and conventional osteosarcoma, with a lower incidence of metastases than conventional osteosarcoma.[774, 775–777] The few patients with periosteal osteosarcoma of the jaw were all alive and well at the time of the reports.[771–774]

Extraskeletal Osteosarcoma

Extraskeletal osteosarcoma accounts for only 2% to 5% of all osteosarcomas.[780–783]

Clinical Features. Unlike its intraosseous counterpart, extraskeletal osteosarcoma occurs in older patients: The mean and median age is in the sixth decade of life[780, 782, 784–786] with some patients in the ninth decade of life[784–786]; only 5% to 10% of patients are younger than 30 years of age.[784–786]

The majority of extraskeletal osteosarcomas occur in the lower extremity,[780, 785, 786] with the head and neck region involved in less than 5% of cases.[780, 785] Here, extraskeletal osteosarcoma has occurred in the soft tissues of the face[784, 785]; neck[785, 786]; floor of the orbit[787]; larynx[788]; and tongue.[783] Extraskeletal osteosarcoma has developed secondary to previous radiation therapy,[789] including cases in the head and neck.[787, 790]

Pathologic Features and Differential Diagnosis. With only rare exceptions,[791] extraskeletal osteosarcomas are high-grade lesions whose varied morphologic pattern mirrors that of conventional intraosseous osteosarcoma.[781, 784] However, other malignant epithelial and mesenchymal tumors may contain focal bone formation and pose diagnostic problems,[789] as may the surface osteosarcomas of bone, parosteal, periosteal, and high-grade osteosarcoma that invade soft tissue. Before a diagnosis of extraskeletal osteosarcoma is made, therefore, other soft tissue tumors with bone formation must be excluded and radiologic studies done to exclude origin from adjacent bone.

Important in the differential diagnosis is the distinction of extraskeletal osteosarcoma from myositis ossificans. In its fully developed and mature form, myositis ossificans is composed of compact lamellar bone residing within a fibrous stroma, resembling an osteoma. However, in its evolving early stages, the central portion of myositis ossificans contains immature stromal fibroblasts and myofibroblasts, which may show nuclear atypia, frequent mitotic figures, and florid new bone and osteoid formation such that it may be impossible to distinguish it from extraskeletal osteosarcoma when only small biopsy tissue is available. The well-delimited mature, new bone formation at the peripheral margin of a more mature myositis ossificans is in contrast to the invasive, anaplastic, spindle-cell periphery of extraskeletal osteosarcoma that lacks bone maturation. It is imperative that when there is a strong clinical likelihood that the lesion represents a developing myositis ossificans, the pathologist be made aware of such information.

Treatment and Prognosis. Extraskeletal osteosarcoma is highly aggressive, with a high incidence of local recurrence following surgical excision and distant metastases,[781, 784–786, 792] with most patients dying of tumor within 2 to 3 years of diagnosis.[782, 786]

Benign Cartilaginous Tumors

Chondroma (Enchondroma)

Chondromas are rare in the head and neck region. In over 10,000 bone lesions at the Mayo Clinic, there were no cases of enchondroma in the jaw or facial bones.[38] Among 1243 chondromas in four large series, only 4 (0.32%) were in the head and neck region.[19, 32, 35, 38]

Clinical Features. Most patients with chondromas are in the second to fourth decades of life[35, 38]; those with head and neck lesions have ranged in age from the first to the eighth decade of life.[793–795] Chondromas of the head and neck are reported in patients in Ollier's disease and Maffucci's syndrome.[794, 796–798]

Chondromas may develop within bone or the soft tissues. Those in the cranial bones usually originate in the base of the skull, with origin in the sella, clivus, parasellar area, and posterior fossa.[794, 796–800] Other sites include the nasal cartilage,[801, 802] cervical vertebrae,[795, 803–805] soft palate,[806, 807] paranasal sinuses,[800–802] nasopharynx,[802, 808] region of the foramen magnum,[793] eustachian tube,[799] tongue,[806, 807, 809] gingiva,[806, 810] cheek and buccal mucosa,[806, 807, 811] and larynx.[812–815] Soft tissue chondromas of the oral cavity are believed to be choristomas rather than true neoplasms.[33]

Chondromas of the cervical spine frequently cause cord or nerve compression with neurologic impairment, including Horner's syndrome; respiratory difficulty may be produced by direct pressure on airway passages.[793, 795, 803–805] Intracranial chondromas produce a variety of signs and symptoms due to compression of cranial nerves, with resulting nerve palsies, or from increased intracranial pressure, with headache, diplopia, visual loss, tinnitus, hearing loss, and facial numbness among the most frequent, as well as pituitary dysfunction and optic nerve atrophy.[794, 796–800] Laryngeal chondromas are most frequently associated with hoarseness or dyspnea.[812–815] Owing to the slow growth of chondromas, it is not uncommon for patients either to know of the presence of a mass or to have symptoms for several years prior to diagnosis.[794, 797, 799–800, 804, 805, 813]

Pathologic Features. Grossly, enchondromas consist of blue-white to blue-gray cartilage with white to yellow foci of calcification. The surface is translucent and has a distinct lobular configuration. Histologically, most chondromas consist of lobules of hyaline cartilage with chondrocytes within well-formed lacunae.[11, 38] The chondrocytes are small, with indistinct cytoplasmic borders; nuclei are typically small, round, and densely hyperchromatic (Fig. 8–34A, see p. 533). Occasional binucleate cells may be found but are not numerous. Calcified foci are frequently present. In these areas, the lacunar spaces and the chondrocytes are enlarged, with irregular plump nuclei. Such calcified areas with their enlarged and atypical cells in chondromas should be taken into consideration in evaluating a cartilaginous lesion for the possibility of chondrosarcoma.

The cartilage lobules are found in nests between the cancellous bone trabeculae and separated from them by a clear zone (Fig. 8–34B, see p. 533). The periphery of the individual islands of cartilage may show encasement by woven or lamellar bone,[810] a sign of slow growth, usually indicating a benign process. In contrast to chondrosarcoma, there is no infiltration of the intertrabecular marrow spaces with entrapment of the bone trabeculae, or of cortical haversian system invasion.

The degree of cellularity varies considerably and those in children and adolescents may be quite hypercellular and contain plump and irregular chondrocytes such as to resemble low-grade chondrosarcoma. In adults, occasional chondromas may have chondrocytes that have large, open-faced nuclei, with a visible chromatin pattern, and binucleate cells that are easily found to such a degree that chondrosarcoma is suggested. In such cases, a radiologic pattern that shows an absence of cortical destruction or of soft tissue extension are important points that favor a benign diagnosis. Those chondromas in Ollier's disease and Maffucci's syndrome may be more cellular than conventional chondromas, contain atypical nuclei and binucleated chondrocytes, and have a more myxoid stroma, all features that suggest low-grade chondrosarcoma.[39] Again, the radiologic appearance is of critical importance in distinguishing such lesions from chondrosarcoma. Mitoses are extremely rare to nonexistent in chondroma, and the finding of more than a rare mitotic figure indicates a high probability that the tumor is malignant.[11]

The occurrence of malignant transformation of chondroma is much debated, with some authors claiming that all chondrosarcomas arise from pre-existing chondromas,[11] while others claim to find no evidence of a pre-existing chondroma in their chondrosarcoma cases.[39] However, it is well accepted that patients with Ollier's disease and Maffucci's syndrome have a high risk of malignant change in their enchondromas, with a reported incidence that varies from 12% to 50%.[38, 817–820]

The histologic distinction between chondroma and high-grade chondrosarcoma presents no difficulty, although its distinction from

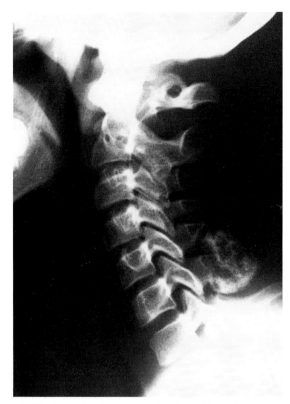

Figure 8–35. Osteochondroma. Lateral radiographic of the spine shows a lobulated, calcified mass rising from the spinous process of C6, without bone destruction or a soft tissue mass.

well-differentiated chondrosarcoma is among the most difficult problems in orthopedic pathology.[816] Indeed, in the head and neck region, some cartilaginous tumors are found where this separation is not possible. The occurrence of individual chondrocyte necrosis, numerous binucleated cells, occasional mitotic figures, and enlarged plump chondrocytes with visible nuclear chromatin are all features that favor a diagnosis of chondrosarcoma, as is invasion of intertrabecular marrow spaces and cortical bone.[819, 820] However, biopsy tissue specimens may not show these features, and the diagnosis will depend on the experience of the examining pathologist. In the head and neck we believe that all symptomatic cartilage lesions should be considered and treated as chondrosarcoma.

Osteochondroma

Less than 1% of all osteochondromas occur within the head and neck region; among 2381 cases listed in four series,[19, 32, 35, 38] only 14 were in the head and neck. Solitary osteochondroma occurs in patients in the second decade of life, the majority less than 20 years of age.[32, 35, 38] In the head and neck, however, spinal and mandibular osteochondromas occur later in life, patients usually being 40 years of age or older, with some in the sixth or seventh decades of life.[821–834] Osteochondromas have developed following external radiation therapy, especially in children.[835–837] In the head and neck region, the cervical spine is the most common location[32, 35, 38, 822–827, 829, 831, 838–844]; almost one half of patients with cervical spine involvement have osteochondromas in other bones.[842] Other reported sites include the mandible,[821, 828, 830, 832–834, 838] maxilla,[32, 834, 846] and, rarely, the cranial bones, especially from the skull base.[19, 838, 847, 848] However, some of the tumors reported as examples of osteochondroma of the skull base may represent chondromas or well-differentiated chondrosarcomas.[847, 848] In the spine, osteochondroma is almost always situated in the posterior elements (Fig. 8–35) with only rare examples arising anteriorly from the vertebral body.[824, 843] In the mandible, the coronoid area and condyle are the most frequent sites.[828, 830, 832, 833]

Symptoms caused by osteochondroma depend on its location: vertebral osteochondromas may cause a variety of neurologic deficits associated with spinal cord compression.[824, 827, 831, 839–845] Pressure from spinal osteochondromas may cause dysphagia and vocal cord paralysis,[826] as well as carotid, subclavian, and vertebral artery compression.[826, 843] Mandibular lesions may produce facial asymmetry, malocclusion, or difficulty in opening the mouth.[828, 830, 832–834] If sufficiently superficially located, a painful or painless mass may be found on physical examination.[822, 824, 827, 830, 840, 843]

Because of the anatomic complexity of the head and neck region, routine radiographs may not demonstrate the osteochondroma, especially those involving the vertebrae,[826, 844] such that symptoms may be present for relatively long periods before the diagnosis is established.[826, 840, 841, 844, 845]

Pathologic Features. Osteochondroma may be a pedunculated or sessile mass protruding from the parent bone—its cortex is in direct continuity with the cortex of the affected bone, being enveloped by its periosteum.[838] Externally, it is covered by a cartilaginous cap that is either smooth and uniform, or irregular and bosselated with a cauliflower-like appearance.[38, 838] The cartilage cap in adults is generally either only a few millimeters in thickness or completely absent, the latter the result of loss from wear and tear abrasion; in children and adolescents the cap may be several centimeters thick.[19, 38] In an adult the development of secondary chondrosarcoma arising in an osteochondroma results in cartilage that is several centimeters thick, usually greater than 2.0 cm, and such a finding is strongly indicative of malignancy.[19, 35, 849]

In the confined space of the head and neck, osteochondroma are usually small. In the spine, they are generally 2.0 to 3.0 cm in maximum size,[822, 831, 839, 841, 845] but even here those as large as 7.0 cm are reported.[822, 840] Mandibular lesions range from 2.0 to 6.0 cm.[821, 833, 834]

Although osteochondroma is predominantly composed of cancellous bone, its growth is by enchondral ossification of its cartilaginous cap, similar to that which occurs at the epiphyseal growth plate. As such, the growth of an osteochondroma parallels that of the remainder of the skeletal system. When the parent bone in which the osteochondroma occurs ceases its growth, so does the osteochondroma. An increase in the size of a known osteochondroma in a skeletally mature individual is highly suspicious of secondary malignant change.

Histologically, the cartilage cap of osteochondroma is composed of hyaline cartilage whose chondrocytes usually have a single, small, dark nucleus and rest within individual lacunae (Fig. 8–36, see p. 533). Binucleate chondrocytes are numerous in young patients and are not an indication of chondrosarcoma, as would be suggested in adult lesions. In actively growing osteochondromas, the chondrocytes align themselves in closely opposed parallel columns with increasing size of the lacunar spaces as they approach the interface with the underlying cancellous bone. If bone growth has ceased, however, the chondrocytes are noncolumnated and are widely spaced from each other. The junction of the cartilage with the cancellous bone resembles that of a normal epiphyseal growth plate; the cartilage becomes calcified, is invaded by small blood vessels, and undergoes enchondral ossification with the formation of mature bone trabeculae (see Fig. 8–36A). However, bone trabeculae containing persistent central cores of nonossified or partially ossified cartilage may be found within the deeper portions of the lesion (see Fig. 8–36B). Fatty marrow, with or without hematopoietic elements, is also present within the cancellous portion of the osteochondroma, an important distinction from parosteal osteosarcoma in which marrow elements are not present. If bone growth has ceased, the cartilage-bone interface appears quiescent without evidence of vascular invasion or enchondral ossification.

Treatment and Prognosis. Local excision is curative in almost all cases, provided the entire lesion, with its periosteal membrane, is removed.[838] Although malignant tumors, such as malignant

fibrous histiocytoma or osteosarcoma, are reported to arise in solitary osteochondroma,[850, 851] the most frequent secondary malignant tumor is chondrosarcoma.[849] In adults, the finding of a thick cartilage cap, increased cellularity, frequent binucleated chondrocytes, enlarged chondrocyte nuclei with a visible chromatin pattern, and occasional mitotic figures, are all features of secondary chondrosarcoma. The incidence of malignant change in a solitary osteochondroma ranges in the literature from 1% to 4%.[849] However, the true incidence is unknown, as many osteochondromas are asymptomatic and never come to medical attention. The incidence of malignant change in multiple osteochondromatosis is higher then in the solitary form, with incidence rates varying from 2% to 25%.[38, 849, 852] Death secondary to spinal cord compression by osteochondroma has occurred.[831, 841]

Chondroblastoma

Many of the reported series dealing with chondroblastoma either lack any examples within the head and neck region or report an incidence of less than 1% at this site.[32, 35, 853] In the Mayo Clinic series of 495 cases, however, 6.9% were located in the skull or facial bones.[854]

Clinical Features. Approximatley 60% to 75% of chondroblastomas occur in the second decade of life, with mean and median ages ranging from 17 to 22 years.[35, 38, 855, 856] patients with chondroblastoma of the skull or facial bones are older, however,[857, 858] with mean and median ages in the fourth decade.[854, 855, 859, 860] In the Mayo Clinic series, 83% of the cases in the head and neck region were in patients older than 30 years of age.[854, 859]

Within the head and neck, chondroblastoma has occurred in the mandible,[854–856, 858, 859] maxilla,[857, 861, 862] cervical vertebra,[856, 863, 864] parietal bone,[854, 858, 859, 865] and occipital bone,[862] but the most frequently involved site is the temporal bone.[854, 855, 858–860, 862, 865–869] In a review of 44 cases of chondroblastoma of the cranial bones, 33 were in the neurocranium, with the temporal bone involved in 32 of these cases.[869]

In general, 80% to 95% of patients with chondroblastoma of any site present because of pain,[853, 855, 870] which may be associated with local swelling.[855, 856, 870] Patients with temporal bone involvement frequently have associated ear symptoms, including hearing loss,[855, 859, 860, 867–869] sensation of ear plugging,[855, 859, 860, 866, 867, 869] tinnitus,[855, 859, 860, 867–869] otalgia,[860, 867] and dizziness or vertigo[855, 859, 860, 867]; seizures also occur.[859, 860] Patients with vertebral chondroblastoma may have neck stiffness and neurologic symptoms.[863] Many patients seek medical attention within a few weeks to months of the onset of their symptoms,[857, 861, 865, 866, 867, 869] but others have symptoms for several years prior to diagnosis.[858, 865, 867, 868]

Radiologically, chondroblastoma has ranged from 1 cm to 19 cm[855, 856] but most commonly is about 4 cm in maximum size.[855, 856, 858, 870] It is usually a round or oval lytic lesion sharply delimited from the adjacent normal bone[855–857, 859] and may be bordered by a sclerotic rim.[855, 856, 858] In the head and neck region, however, it is often not as well delimited and may have an aggressive appearance (Fig. 8–37) with destruction of cortical bone.[859, 863, 866, 867] Focal calcification (see Fig. 8–37B) is apparent in 35% to 50% of cases.[855, 856]

Pathologic Features. Curettage specimens of chondroblastoma consist of friable, reddish-brown to gray fragments that may contain flecks of calcium; hemorrhagic cystic regions may be present.[858, 871, 872]

Histologically, chondroblastoma is characterized by broad areas of round, oval, or polyhedral chondroblasts that have well-defined cytoplasmic borders; the cytoplasm usually is densely eosinophilic (Fig. 8–38A, see p. 534). Nuclei are round, oval, or reniform and frequently are indented or cleaved (Fig. 8–38B); one or two small nucleoli may be present.[31, 858, 871, 872] Cells with enlarged, hyperchromatic nuclei may occur and are more frequently found in chondroblastomas of the head and neck than in other sites.[854, 855]

Mitotic activity is found in approximately 75% of cases but is usually not abundant, with only one to two mitotic figures per 10 high power fields.[854–856] Multinucleated osteoclast-type giant cells occur in 15% to 73% of cases (Fig. 8–38A, see p. 534).[854, 856, 859]

Characteristic foci of individual cell necrosis occur and are associated with dystrophic calcification (Fig. 8–38C, see p. 534) that may form a lace-like arrangement about the individual necrotic cells, creating a chicken-wire pattern. Such dystrophic calcification occurs in approximately 30% to 67% of cases.[854–856, 859] Islands of pink chondroid (see Fig. 8–38C) are present in 90% to 97% of cases[854–856] and its presence is taken by some as essential for the diagnosis.[858] In chondroblastomas of the head and neck, however, chondroid material is less frequently found than it is in the long bones, and in some cases may be quite scarce.[854, 859, 867]

Epithelioid-like cells are found in from 10% to 15% of cases[854, 855] and are most prominent in chondroblastomas of the head and neck.[854] Hemosiderin-laden tumor cells and macrophages ("pigmented cells") occur in 80% to 90% of head and neck cases.[854, 859] Cystic, hemorrhagic foci that simulate aneurysmal bone cyst are found in 15% to 40% of cases[853, 854–856, 872]; such lesions have been called *cystic chondroblastomas*.[872] Hyaline cartilage with enchondral ossification may be found, as well as foci of osteoid and mature bone.[19, 854, 858]

Differential Diagnosis. Although the diagnosis of chondroblastoma does not require immunohistochemical stains, the chondroblasts are positive for S-100 protein[856, 873] and lack reactivity for macrophage markers. Aberrant cytokeratin reactivity has been found in the cells of chondroblastoma.[856, 873]

Because of the presence of osteoclast-type giant cells, a diagnosis of giant cell tumor may be considered, but chondroid tissue and hyaline cartilage are not found in true giant-cell tumor. Because of the rare occurrence of bone formation in chondroblastoma, osteoblastoma may enter the differential diagnosis, but osteoblastoma has a more florid production of osteoid and bone and only rarely contains cartilage. The stroma of osteoblastoma is also more vascular, containing thin-walled dilated capillaries, and the stromal cells lack the dense eosinophilic cytoplasm and cleaved nuclei of the chondroblasts of chondroblastoma. The histiocytes of eosinophilic granuloma, with their eosinophilic cytoplasm and cleaved nuclei, may appear similar to the chondroblasts of chondroblastoma, and they also contain S-100 protein. However, the cells of eosinophilic granuloma are reactive for CD1a and lack the chondroid and dystrophic calcification found in chondroblastoma.

Clear cell chondrosarcoma,[874] a tumor that mainly involves the long bones but has also been reported in the maxilla and skull,[875, 876] may pose a problem in histologic diagnosis. This sarcoma contains chondroblast-like cells and scattered osteoclast-type giant cells and chicken-wire-type calcification. However, the cells of clear cell chondrosarcoma have an abundant clear cytoplasm, with distinct cytoplasmic borders, unlike the densely eosinophilic cytoplasm of the cells of chondroblastoma. In addition, small areas of ossification are scattered throughout clear cell chondrosarcoma and, in approximately 50% of the cases, areas of conventional chondrosarcoma are present.[874]

Treatment and Prognosis. Therapy for chondroblastoma consists primarily of surgical curettage. Local recurrence following such therapy occurs in approximately 15% of cases,[853, 855, 856, 860, 870] with time to recurrence ranging from 5 months to 8 years.[853, 855] Recurrences are cured by further conservative surgical procedures in almost all cases. Locally aggressive behavior and even metastases and death has been reported in rare cases of chondroblastoma,[854, 855, 873, 877] including a patient with cervical spine chondroblastoma who died because of direct invasion of the mediastinum.[864] Malignant change secondary to radiation therapy is reported in chondroblastoma as well as spontaneous malignant transformation.[858, 878–880]

Chondrosarcoma

General Features

Among a total of 2235 cases of chondrosarcoma in four series, 127 (5.7%) were in the head and neck region, with the incidence among the individual series varying from 4.2% to 6.7%.[19, 32, 35, 38]

Clinical Features. In contrast to osteosarcoma, chondrosarcoma is uncommon in the first two decades of life,[881] with most patients in the fourth to sixth decades.[32, 35, 38] In head and neck cases, the mean and median patient ages range from 35 to 45 years,[882–888]

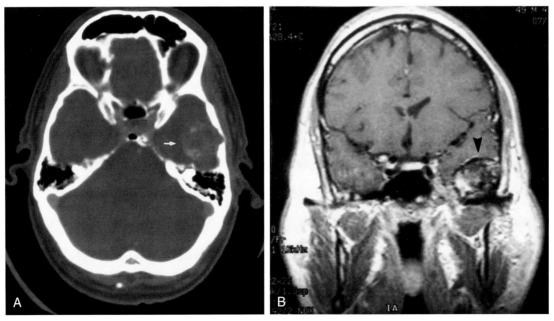

Figure 8–37. A, Chondroblastoma. Axial computed tomographic image shows a tumor (*arrow*) arising from the temporal bone. The matrix of the tumor appears calcific and there is partial destruction of the cortical bone. B, Coronal magnetic resonance image shows the tumor (*arrowhead*) arising from the floor of the temporal bone with extension into the middle cranial fossa. Calcium deposits (black) are scattered throughout the tumor.

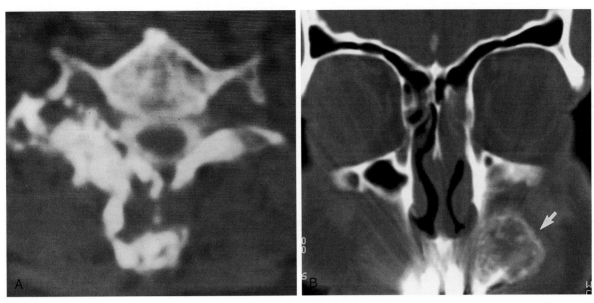

Figure 8–39. A, Chondrosarcoma of vertebrae. Axial computed tomographic image shows destruction of the right posterior elements of the vertebral body with extensive calcification. B, Low-grade chondrosarcoma of the left maxilla. Note the well-defined expansive, relatively benign-appearing lesion, with spotty calcification (arrow).

although patients younger than 20 years of age are reported.[882–886, 889]

Chondrosarcoma has occurred in virtually every site within the head and neck region, with the most common locations being the maxilla,[881, 882, 888–893] mandible,[882, 883, 888, 889, 892] base of the skull,[887, 892, 894–896] cervical vertebrae,[19, 32, 35, 38, 884, 888, 889, 892, 897] and nasal cavity and nasal septum.[38, 882, 883, 886, 888, 890, 891, 898] Less common sites include the paranasal sinuses,[882, 883, 888, 890, 892] orbit and retrobulbar region,[881, 888, 889, 892] bones of the cranium,[29, 32, 881, 883, 885, 888, 889, 899] hyoid bone,[38, 892] and nasopharynx.[892, 900] Chondrosarcoma of the larynx is discussed separately. Chondrosarcomas in the head and neck region that occur in children are prone to involve the nasal cavity, paranasal sinuses, and facial bones.[881, 882, 906]

In the head and neck, patient symptoms are nonspecific and vary from the presence of a painful or painless mass to headache, hearing loss, and neurologic problems, depending on tumor location.[882, 884, 888, 895, 896] The duration of symptoms has ranged from a few months to 35 years prior to diagnosis.[882, 897] Chondrosarcomas of the head and neck have occurred in patients with Ollier's disease[896] and Maffucci's syndrome.[882, 899]

Radiologically, chondrosarcoma has the features of an aggressive destructive lesion in almost all cases (Fig. 8–39), with evident calcification in 45% to 80% of cases.[34, 882, 884, 885, 894, 901] Those chondrosarcomas with an extensive myxoid component frequently lack calcification.[885] Base of skull chondrosarcomas cannot be radiologically distinguished from chordoma.[887, 901]

Chondrosarcomas often attain a large size prior to diagnosis, even in the limited anatomic space of the head and neck. They may be relatively large, with those greater than 10.0 cm reported[882, 897, 900]; one spinal chondrosarcoma reached a size of 22 cm prior to diagnosis.[897]

Pathologic Features. On gross examination, erosion of the cortex with soft tissue extension is almost always present, an important feature distinguishing chondrosarcoma from enchondroma.[902] On section, chondrosarcoma has a lobular, blue-gray to gray-white, translucent, glistening surface.[35, 38, 904] Although firm, they are usually easily cut with a scalpel, except for those areas that appear as yellow to yellow-white flecks or spicules of dense calcification or ossification.[35, 902–904] Soft, gelatinous, myxoid foci may exist and even predominate in some cases.[35, 38, 902, 903] Necrosis within the center of the lobules is common.[34, 904]

Histologically, chondrosarcoma usually contains an abundant amount of hyaline-type cartilage with lacunae containing round to oval cells that have enlarged nuclei possessing a clearly visible chromatin pattern (Fig. 8–40A, see p. 535). The cells may occur in clusters or be haphazardly arranged in broad sheets. In general, chondrosarcomas are hypercellular with increasing cellularity in the more poorly differentiated tumors (Fig. 8–40B). Numerous binucleated cells and tumor cells with large, single or multiple nuclei may be found. The occurrence of binucleated cells should not, of itself, be taken as evidence of malignancy, as even the most histologically bland appearing chondroma may contain occasional binucleated cells. In chondrosarcoma, however, such cells are much more frequent, being most numerous in the more poorly differentiated tumors. High-grade chondrosarcomas have increased numbers of pleomorphic cells with large atypical bizarre nuclei, and foci containing atypical spindle-shaped cells may also be present (see Fig. 8–40B).[31, 35, 38, 902, 904, 905] Although the finding of mitotic activity in a cartilaginous tumor is an excellent indication of malignancy, even high-grade chondrosarcomas may lack this feature.[902, 906] The lobules of chondrosarcoma usually lack the peripheral encasement by woven or lamellar bone that frequently occurs in chondromas,[11, 907] although in long-standing, well-differentiated chondrosarcoma one may find some bone formation at the peripheral margin of occasional lobules.

Both benign and malignant cartilage tumors contain areas of calcification. Within and adjacent to such areas, the chondrocytes are enlarged and may have hyperchromatic irregular nuclei.[902, 906] It is important not to evaluate such areas when trying to determine whether the lesion is cytologically benign or malignant. However, the finding of individual cell necrosis within areas not marred by calcification or degeneration is an important clue to the diagnosis of chondrosarcoma.[31] Calcified cartilage, be it benign or malignant, may undergo ossification. This bone forms directly on the cartilage and may histologically appear quite normal, even when the pre-existing cartilage has high-grade malignant features. Myxoid degeneration of the stroma, with a vacuolated to bubbly appearance, is a common feature in chondrosarcoma. This may be quite extensive, with the cells widely separated within the myxoid matrix and arranged in loose strands or cords. Here the tumor cells may have a vacuolated cytoplasm.

Chondrosarcoma infiltrates between existing normal bone trabeculae and directly abuts and surrounds them (Fig. 8–40C, see

p. 535), unlike the pattern in enchondroma where the islands of cartilage remain apart from the trabecular bone, separated from it by a clear zone of loose fibrous tissue. Chondrosarcoma causes endosteal erosion and invades the cortex, filling the haversian canals, and it extends into the soft tissue, features not found in enchondroma.[11, 907, 908] The cartilage associated with Ollier's disease and Maffucci's syndrome may be hypercellular, with a haphazard distribution of cells that frequently reside in a myxoid stroma and demonstrate nuclear atypia, such that care must be exercised to avoid an overdiagnosis of chondrosarcoma. Recourse to the clinical situation and the absence of an aggressive radiologic appearance in such lesions is helpful in avoiding this error.

A variety of systems have been employed for the grading of chondrosarcoma,[38, 902, 904, 905, 908] with emphasis on such items as nuclear morphology, mitotic activity, and degree of cellularity, usually dividing the tumors into three or four grades (I-IV). Most chondrosarcomas are well to moderately differentiated (grade I and II) tumors that contain an abundance of hyalin-like cartilage, although myxoid or mucinous foci of degeneration may be present.[902, 905] Most chondrosarcomas in the head and neck region are well-differentiated (grade I) tumors,[882, 884, 887, 888, 890] although here too myxoid change may be found,[882, 885] especially in temporal bone lesions.[885] Poorly differentiated (grade III) chondrosarcomas are uncommon, regardless of anatomic location.

Differential Diagnosis. Despite the foregoing histologic description, the diagnosis of chondrosarcoma may be among the most difficult problems in orthopedic tumor pathology. The diagnosis of high-grade, poorly differentiated chondrosarcoma usually poses no difficulty, but a low-grade, well-differentiated chondrosarcoma may often be impossible, based on histology alone, to distinguish from a benign enchondroma.[11, 903, 905] The occurrence of chondrocytes with enlarged atypical nuclei having a distinct chromatin pattern, and individual cell necrosis, while good indicators of malignancy, may be absent in small biopsy specimens, the cartilage resembling that of enchondroma. In addition, enchondromas may contain some cells with enlarged, open-faced nuclei as in chondrosarcoma. It is important in cases in which the histologic pattern is not clear-cut, to assess other parameters, including the clinical presentation, location, and radiologic appearance, to determine whether the lesion is malignant. It should be noted that enchondroma of the jaw and facial bones is extremely rare—at the Mayo Clinic, no enchondroma of these sites was found in over 10,000 tumor cases—such that any clinically symptomatic cartilage lesion in this area is probably best considered malignant.[882]

The histologic distinction between a chondroblastic osteosarcoma, with its abundant malignant cartilaginous component, and chondrosarcoma may also be quite difficult when dealing with only small biopsy samples. Although bone formation occurs in chondrosarcoma, it does so on the framework of a pre-existing cartilage matrix and not, as in osteosarcoma, directly by malignant stromal cells. However, biopsy specimens may miss the latter areas, sampling only malignant cartilage. In such cases, the correct diagnosis may be made only after examination of the entire resection specimen.

Rare cases of clear cell chondrosarcoma[909] have been reported in the head and neck region.[910, 911] This form of chondrosarcoma is characterized by the presence of large cells, with a clear to granular cytoplasm and well-defined cell borders, interspersed with osteoclast-type giant cells and small spicules of bone or osteoid. These clear cell tumors may frequently contain small foci of conventional chondrosarcoma.[909] Osteoclast-type giant cells are not a feature of conventional chondrosarcoma.

Dedifferentiated chondrosarcoma[912] may develop following the local recurrence of a previous low-grade chondrosarcoma or arise de novo. It occurs predominantly in the long bones and is characterized by the occurrence of lobules or islands of low-grade malignant cartilage, or normal-appearing hyaline cartilage, that are juxtaposed to sarcomatous spindle cell foci that most often have the feature of either fibrosarcoma or malignant fibrous histiocytoma, but at times may show osteosarcomatous, rhabdomyosarcomatous, or

angiosarcomatous differentiation.[913–916] Since spindle cell areas also occur in high-grade chondrosarcomas, it is important that the diagnosis of dedifferentiated chondrosarcoma, which has an exceedingly poor prognosis, not be made in the presence of high-grade malignant cartilage. Dedifferentiated chondrosarcoma has been reported in the supraorbital region.[892]

Since chondrosarcoma may exhibit a myxoid stroma in which the tumor cells are widely separated and may contain cytoplasmic vacuoles, the distinction between it and chordoma becomes important, especially in those chondrosarcomas arising in the base of the skull, which are frequently myxoid. The problem is further compounded by the not infrequent occurrence of cartilaginous foci in chordomas of the base of skull. Such *chondroid chordomas* may be impossible to distinguish from true chondrosarcoma by routine light microscopy, requiring immunohistochemical or electron microscopic studies for their distinction (see Chordoma section).

Treatment and Prognosis. Prognosis in chondrosarcoma depends primarily on the ability to adequately excise the tumor, always a problem in the restricted confines of the head and neck. Positive surgical margins result in an increased incidence of local recurrence[888] and classification of the lesion to a higher grade. Well-differentiated chondrosarcomas have a low incidence of metastatic disease and a relatively good prognosis.[884, 888, 890, 904, 916] The 5-year survival rate for chondrosarcoma of the head and neck has varied from 43% to 95%.[881, 882, 888, 917, 918] Although considered to be a radioresistant tumor, with some exceptions noted,[919] proton beam therapy has been successfully used in the treatment of head and neck chondrosarcoma.[917, 918, 920] Chondrosarcoma of the head and neck region usually grows slowly and may cause death by uncontrolled local spread.[882, 885, 888, 889, 894] Metastases are not common, with some series having no patients who developed metastatic disease,[882, 885, 890] while others report a metastatic rate of 8% to 18%.[888–890]

Chondrosarcoma of the Larynx

Less than 1% of laryngeal tumors are sarcomas,[921] with chondrosarcoma the most common of these.[922–925]

Clinical Features. Patients with laryngeal chondrosarcoma are usually between 40 and 70 years of age; only rarely does the tumor occur in people younger than 30 years of age.[32, 921, 925–931]

Chondrosarcoma has been reported in almost every site within the laryngeal region, including the supraglottic and subglottic regions,[926] the arytenoid,[928, 932] the vocal cord,[928] the epiglottis,[929, 933] the hyoid bone,[932] and the corniculate.[929] However, 70% to 90% of cases arise from the cricoid cartilage, especially the posterior or lateral cricoid,[921, 925, 927–931, 934] with the thyroid cartilage accounting for an additional 10% to 25% of cases.[921, 925, 927–929, 931, 932, 935]

Symptoms reflect the presence of a mass lesion that obstructs the airway, compresses or involves the vocal cord, or compresses the adjacent esophagus, with hoarseness, dysphagia and dyspnea being most frequent.[925, 926, 928] A cervical mass may be found on palpation.[925, 926] Although some patients are reported to have had symptoms for as long as 10 or more years, most are diagnosed within 1 year of symptom onset.[925, 926, 928]

Laryngeal chondrosarcomas vary considerably in size, with lesions as large as 4 to 13 cm reported.[925, 927, 933, 936] Most often they appear as smooth, rounded, soft to hard, submucosal masses.[926, 929] The tumor is usually discovered prior to the occurrence of any invasion beyond the confines of the larynx,[923, 929] although in some series such extension was frequent.[927] Radiologic analysis of the larynx (Fig. 8–41) demonstrates the presence of tumor that, in almost all cases, will characteristically show coarse or stippled calcifications.[926, 927, 929] Computed tomography (see Fig. 8–41B) accurately reflects the site and extent of the lesion.

Pathologic Features. Histologically, the vast majority of laryngeal chondrosarcomas are well differentiated (low-grade) hyaline tumors[925–927]; however, examples of dedifferentiated,[922, 923, 927, 937, 938] myxoid,[930, 936] and high-grade chondrosarcomas are reported[935, 938] as are rare radiation-induced chondrosarcomas.[939]

The diagnosis of laryngeal chondrosarcoma may pose significant problems, since the tumor is frequently submucosal and obtaining representative biopsy tissue by endoscopy may be difficult, and its well-differentiated hyaline pattern makes the distinction from benign chondroma frequently impossible.[924, 940] Indeed, it is not uncommon for the biopsy tissue to be interpreted as a benign chondroma,[924, 928, 934, 940] and the lesion excised, only to have it recur years later as a histologically overt chondrosarcoma.[921, 924, 940] The occurrence of a true chondroma of the larynx is quite rare, however,

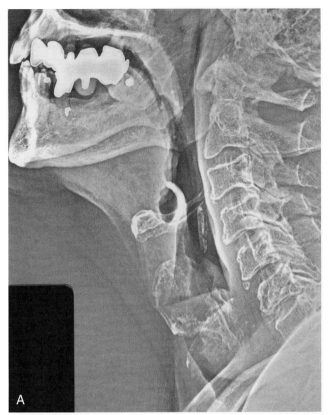

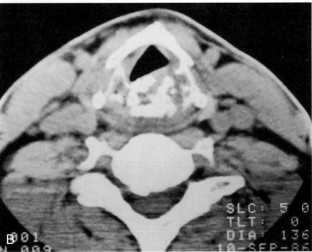

Figure 8–41. *A,* Laryngeal chondrosarcoma. Lateral xeroradiograph shows a large calcified mass anterior to the C4 to C6 vertebral bodies. The pattern and shape of the calcification is abnormal and not that of normal laryngeal cartilage. *B,* Computed tomographic scan of the larynx shows scattered disorganized calcification posteriorly, with an associated soft tissue mass. The anterior component impinges on and narrows the laryngeal airway.

as over 90% of all laryngeal cartilaginous tumors are chondrosarcomas.[922, 925] Any symptomatic cartilage lesion of the larynx is best diagnosed and treated as a chondrosarcoma despite the presence of a bland histologic appearance.

Treatment and Prognosis. Although total laryngectomy for laryngeal chondrosarcoma may be curative, the usual slow growth of this tumor[925, 926, 928, 935] has led to the use of conservative resection for its management.[924, 925, 928, 941] Such a therapeutic approach yields an incidence of local recurrence in 40% to 80% of cases,[925, 928, 941] although the time to recurrence may be many years, in some instances as long as 20 to 30 years.[924–926, 931, 935, 941] Total laryngectomy seems best reserved for those few cases of high-grade chondrosarcoma.[925, 928] Laryngeal chondrosarcoma may cause death due to local extension,[925, 934, 941] but metastases, most commonly to the lungs, occur in 8% to 14% of cases despite the well-differentiated nature of the tumor.[928–931, 933, 935, 937, 940, 941] At the Mayo Clinic, the overall 5- and 10-year survival rates were 90% and 81%, respectively, with disease-free survival rates of 68% and 54% at these intervals.[925]

Mesenchymal Chondrosarcoma

Mesenchymal chondrosarcoma (MC) accounts for 3% to 5% of all chondrosarcomas.[19, 31, 35, 38] The tumor may arise either within bone or from the soft tissues. One third to one half of MC are extraosseous in origin.[942–945] The head and neck region is a relatively common location for MC, accounting for 20% to 30% of cases.[944, 945]

Clinical Features. Although congenital examples of MC are reported,[946] as well as cases in patients older than 80 years of age,[38, 942, 944, 945, 947, 948] most patients are in the second to third decades of life[35, 38, 942, 944, 945, 948] with mean and median ages of 20 to 30 years.[32, 35, 943, 944, 948, 949, 950]

In the head and neck, the mandible[942, 945, 947, 948, 951] and maxilla[942, 944, 945, 948, 952–954] are the most frequent sites, with the maxilla less commonly involved than the mandible. Other sites include the orbit,[942, 945, 949, 955] nasopharynx,[942, 945] ethmoid sinus,[956, 957] maxillary sinus,[957] parapharyngeal-tonsillar area,[958] soft tissue of the face and neck,[32, 942, 943, 950, 952, 959] cerebellum,[947] bones of the skull,[942, 944, 945, 947] and the cervical vertebrae.[945, 950, 952, 960]

Symptoms are nonspecific, with pain, swelling, or an evident mass.[945, 948] The duration of symptoms is quite variable, with patients having symptoms for as long as 10 years or for only a few days or weeks.[945, 948]

Radiologically, intraosseous MC appears similar to conventional chondrosarcoma, being lytic with or without matrix calcification.[942, 945, 948] Those of soft tissue origin appear as a mass that frequently contains calcification.[945]

Pathologic Features. Grossly, MC has a gray, gray-white, or pink surface and is soft, firm, or even hard. Nodules of blue-gray cartilage may be visible, and almost all cases contain white to yellow-white areas of calcification or ossification.[35, 38, 942, 944, 961] In the head and neck, MC varies from 3 cm to 7 cm in maximum size.[951, 952, 957, 958]

Histologically (Fig. 8–42, see p. 536), soft tissue and skeletal mesenchymal chondrosarcomas are identical, showing a biphasic pattern of undifferentiated-appearing stromal cells that exist in combination with islands of cartilage.[35, 38, 942–944, 961] The stromal cells, usually arranged in broad expanses, are small with little cytoplasm and have hyperchromatic, round to spindle-shaped nuclei.[35, 38, 943, 962] The cells are fairly uniform without significant pleomorphism and resemble the cells of Ewing's sarcoma. Mitoses may be either frequent or difficult to find. An abundant, thin-walled, vascular network is diffusely present among the stromal cells, which protrude into the vascular lumens, creating a pattern of staghorn-shaped spaces similar to those in hemangiopericytoma (see Fig. 8–42A).[35, 38, 942–944] An abundant reticulin fiber network is found about the stromal cells.[942, 961]

The cartilage in MC may be so abundant that it is easily found in random sections of the tumor, or so scarce that numerous sections are required for its discovery.[35, 952, 957] The islands of cartilage tend to be small and cytologically resemble either normal hyalin cartilage or low-grade chondrosarcoma (see Fig. 8–42B, see p. 536).[35, 38, 942, 943, 961, 962] The interface between the stromal cells and the cartilage is usually quite sharp, although there are cases in which this transition is gradual.[942, 943, 962] The cartilage may show calcification and foci of enchondral ossification.[35, 38, 942, 943, 952, 962]

By electron microscopy, the stromal cells of MC have a primitive mesenchymal appearance with a transition to cells that show cartilaginous differentiation; cytoplasmic glycogen is either absent or scant.[953, 963] Immunohistochemically, the stromal cells are reactive for vimentin[950, 960] but lack S-100 protein which, however, is found in the cells of the cartilage islands.[964] Reactivity of the tumor cells for CD99 (p30/32^MIC2), using antibody 013 with antigen retrieval techniques, is found in the stromal cells with absent or focal weak reactivity in the cells of the cartilaginous foci.[965] Cytogenetic studies of MC have shown a chromosomal translocation, t(11;22)(q24;q12), similar to that which occurs in Ewing's sarcoma.[966, 967]

Differential Diagnosis. The histologic differential diagnosis of MC includes Ewing's sarcoma, malignant peripheral neuroectodermal tumor (MPNET), hemangiopericytoma, small cell osteosarcoma, and dedifferentiated chondrosarcoma. When adequate tissue is present, the distinction between Ewing's sarcoma and MC poses no great difficulty, as Ewing's sarcoma lacks the reticulin meshwork and vascular pattern of MC, usually has a moderate to abundant amount of cytoplasmic glycogen, and, most important, lacks cartilaginous foci. However, small biopsy specimens may only contain the undifferentiated small cell component that is morphologically similar in both tumors, and the cells of both tumors may be positive for CD99. In such cases, the distinction between these two tumors may be impossible by light microscopy without examination of the entire resected tumor. Unlike the relatively high incidence of MC in the head and neck, less than 5% of Ewing's sarcomas occur in this region.[25, 34, 35, 38]

Malignant peripheral neuroectodermal tumor is also only infrequently found in the head and neck region (see earlier). The nuclei of the small cells of this tumor tend to be more irregular and pleomorphic than those of MC, and the tumor may show evidence of neural differentiation by the presence of rosettes. Although the cells of MPNET are immunohistochemically reactive for CD99, they may be positive for S-100 protein, which is absent in MC. Most important, the cells of MPNET are also reactive for a variety of other neural markers,[25] and the tumor lacks cartilage formation.

Small cell osteosarcoma is distinguished from MC by the presence of lace-like osteoid strands or tumor bone produced by its cells. Although bone may be found in MC, it arises from enchondral ossification of the cartilage islands and is not formed directly by the stromal cells. Dedifferentiated chondrosarcoma may simulate MC with lobules of normal or low-grade chondrosarcoma juxtaposed to spindle-shaped stromal cells; however, these spindle cells are large and pleomorphic with highly atypical nuclei, in contrast to the uniform nuclei of the small cells of MC. The stromal areas in dedifferentiated chondrosarcoma may have the pattern of fibrosarcoma, malignant fibrous histiocytoma, or even osteosarcoma, as opposed to the uniformly undifferentiated appearance of the cells of MC. A history of prior removal of a low-grade chondrosarcoma also helps separate these two tumors. Hemangiopericytoma is distinguished from MC by its lack of cartilage and positive immunohistochemical staining for CD34.

Treatment and Prognosis. The clinical course of MC is quite variable, with some patients experiencing early metastases and death, whereas others have a protracted clinical course with long-term survival. Metastases or local recurrence have occurred more than 10 years after treatment, and in some cases as long as 20 years after.[942, 945, 952, 954] Metastases, most commonly to the lungs but also to regional or distant lymph nodes and bones,[944, 945] may develop after several local recurrences[942] or in the absence of local recurrence.[945] The rate of metastases from MC of all sites varies from

45% to 75%,[943, 945, 947] with overall 5-year survival rates ranging from 40% to 55%[944, 945, 962]; 10-year survival rates are lower secondary to the development of late metastases. In the head and neck, death from tumor has occurred in 35% to 80% of cases.[943, 944, 947, 950, 954]

Extraskeletal Myxoid Chondrosarcoma

Extraskeletal myxoid chondrosarcoma (ESMC) accounts for 6% to 12% of all chondrosarcomas.[19, 32]

Clinical Features. In a review of 114 cases of ESMC of all sites,[25] patients ranged in age from 1 to 92 years; approximately 70% were equal to or older than 40 years of age, with mean and median ages in the fifth decade of life.[25, 968–970] In ESMC of the head and neck, patients have ranged in age from 9 to 68 years.[971] Clinically, ESMC usually develops as a slowly growing mass that may be painful or painless and may be present for many years; in patients with head and neck tumors, symptoms have been present for 1 week[972] to as long as 10 years.[968, 971]

Extraskeletal myxoid chondrosarcoma is predominantly a tumor of the extremities, with the head and neck region involved in only approximately 5% of cases.[25] Here, the tumor has been reported in the tongue,[973] nasal cavity,[968, 969] neck,[25, 968, 969] scalp,[971] chin,[974] maxillary sinus,[32, 972] larynx,[32] nasal septum,[32] and falx.[975]

Pathologic Features. Grossly, ESMC appears as a soft, lobular or multilobular mass with a gelatinous, mucoid, gray-white surface. Areas of cystic degeneration and hemorrhage are frequent.[25] The tumor is usually deeply located between or within skeletal muscle, although cases in the subcutaneous tissue occur.[8, 25] In the head and neck, tumors have ranged in size from 1 to 29 cm.[968, 971, 972, 974]

Histologically, the cells of ESMC are arranged in multiple lobules (Fig. 8–43A, see p. 537) that have an abundant myxoid stroma. The tumor cells are polygonal and spindle or stellate and have round to oval, bland nuclei and a scant to moderate amount of deeply eosinophilic cytoplasm that may be vacuolated (Fig. 8–43B). This vacuolization may be singular, pushing the nucleus to the side, creating signet-ring cells or, when multiple, cells that resemble the physaliferous cells of chordoma.[968, 969, 976] In the center of the lobules the cells are loosely arranged, with some forming small nests or clusters, whereas those toward the periphery assume a radial pattern of columns, cords, or strands (see Fig. 8–43B).[969, 970, 977] Rarely, larger cells are found that have a more abundant cytoplasm and resemble epithelioid cells; these may have dense, cytoplasmic inclusions forming rhabdoid-like cells.[968, 969, 976] Some have a decreased amount of stroma and are more cellular than usual.[969, 970] Actual chondroid or cartilage formation is uncommon in ESMC,[698, 970, 978] as is mitotic activity.[968, 969, 978, 979]

The tumor cells stain for cytoplasmic glycogen,[969, 976, 978] while the myxoid stroma is strongly positive with alcian blue, colloidal iron, and mucicarmine stains. The results of prior treatment with hyaluronidase on these stromal staining reactions has varied in the literature, with some studies indicating either total or partial elimination of the reaction,[968, 978] and others that the reaction was hyaluronidase-resistant.[8, 969, 980]

The tumor cells of ESMC are positive for S-100 protein and vimentin and lack cytokeratin and epithelial membrane antigen.[978, 980–982] By electron microscopy, the cells show evidence of cartilaginous differentiation. A prominent feature is the presence of a dilated, well-formed, rough endoplasmic reticulum with a dense granular matrix. The cells have a well-formed Golgi apparatus, lipid droplets, pinocytotic vesicles, glycogen, aggregates of microfilaments, and scalloped irregular cytoplasmic borders with long and short cytoplasmic processes. Desmosome-like junctions and a focal basal lamina are also present. A characteristic feature, found in approximately one third of the cases, is the presence of parallel microtubules within the cisternae of the rough endoplasmic reticulum.[970, 980, 981–984] Cytogenetic studies of ESMC show a nonrandom chromosomal translocation.[983, 984]

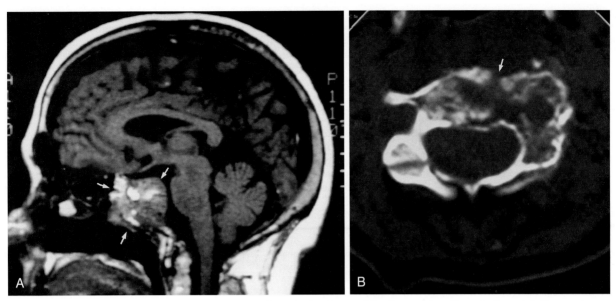

Figure 8–44. *A*, Sagittal magnetic resonance image shows large chordoma that has destroyed the clivus and the sella turcica (*arrows*). *B*, Computed tomographic image of cervical chordoma shows expansive lytic destruction of the body of C2 with fracture anteriorly (*arrow*).

Differential Diagnosis. A diagnosis of ESMC should be made only after ruling out an osseous origin, despite the fact that intraosseous chondrosarcomas are infrequently of pure myxoid type. In the head and neck region, the most important histologic differential diagnosis involves chordoma. Both tumors contain cells disposed within a myxoid stroma, growing in rows or cords, with cytoplasmic vacuolization, which stain for S-100 protein. Indeed, some examples of ESMC were designated as "chordoid" sarcomas before it was recognized that they were unrelated to chordoma.[968, 970–975] The cells of chordoma, in contrast to those of ESMC, are reactive for cytokeratin and epithelial membrane antigen.

Chondroid syringoma of the skin and mixed tumor of salivary gland origin may also be histologically difficult to distinguish from ESMC. However, these tumors are superficially located and contain tubular, acinar, or duct-like structures. Most important, their cells are cytokeratin positive and, by electron microscopy cells with epithelial and myoepithelial features are found. Myxoid liposarcoma, another tumor with a myxoid stroma, has stellate and spindle cells with cytoplasmic vacuoles (lipoblasts) that are S-100 positive, but, unlike in ESMC, the cells are not arranged in cords or strands, and they lack glycogen. Myxoid liposarcoma also has a prominent plexiform capillary pattern that is absent in ESMC.

Treatment and Prognosis. Although long considered a less aggressive tumor than conventional chondrosarcoma, long-term follow-up studies of ESMC have indicated its fully malignant nature, with metastases developing in some patients more than 10 years after diagnosis.[25, 968, 977, 979, 982]

The prognosis for patients with head and neck tumors is unclear, owing to the lack of long-term follow-up data.[968, 970–975] Among eight patients on whom information is available, six were alive and well 2 months to 2 years following therapy.[968, 970, 972–975] One was well 12 months following treatment of a local recurrence that developed 10 months after operation.[975] Two patients died of disease, one due to local recurrence at 5 months.[968] The other, a 9-year old boy who had had a scalp mass since birth, died of pulmonary metastases; the diagnosis of ESMC was made only at autopsy.[971]

Chordoma

Chordomas are divided into three broad categories based on anatomic location: those that arise in the spheno-occipital area, those in the sacrococcygeal region, and those that involve the remainder of the vertebral column.

Chordomas arise from remnants of the ectodermally derived embryonic notochord and may develop anywhere along the tract of this structure. The cephalad portion of the embryonic notochord pursues a convoluted course from which dendritic tracts penetrate the cranial bone anlage to ramify beneath the nasopharyngeal mucosa and extend into the parapharyngeal space and anteriorly into the future region of the paranasal sinuses.[985–990] By the fifth week of embryonic development, the notochord becomes encased by the anlage of the bones of the skull and vertebral column and gradually disappears, although microscopic vestiges of this notochord persist and are found in 0.5% to 2% of autopsies.[986, 988, 991–993] These vestiges are most commonly found in the midline in the spheno-occipital synchondrosis but are also found in the maxilla and mandible.[990] In the adult, the nucleus pulposus of the intervertebral disc represents the remnant of the primitive notochord; however, chordomas arise not from the nucleus pulposus, but from the vestigial remnants, as the anatomic location of these tumors roughly parallels the site frequency of occurrence of these remnants along the craniospinal axis.[989, 992, 994]

Clinical Features. The tumor most frequently occurs in patients in the fifth to sixth decade of life. This is true for vertebral chordomas, but patients with cranial lesions are somewhat younger, with mean and median ages ranging from 35 to 53 years.[32, 35, 38, 995–1002] The age range for chordoma is quite broad, however, with cases in children,[1003–1007] some less than 1 year of age,[985, 1007] to patients in the eighth decade of life.[32, 38, 999]

In three series, containing a total of 489 chordomas, 248 (51%) were sacrococcygeal, 93 (19%) were vertebral, and 148 (30%) were spheno-occipital.[19, 32, 38] In other reports, the spheno-occipital region has accounted for 16% to 36% of cases.[32, 993, 995, 988, 1001, 1008] Within the cranial area, the clivus and parasellar area is the most frequent location.[32, 995, 998, 1001, 1003, 1004, 1006, 1008–1010] Cranial chordomas tend to arise in the basiocciput along the clivus at or inferior to the spheno-occipital synchondrosis, or in the basisphenoid along the upper clivus (Fig. 8–44*A*). They are most often situated in the midline but may be lateral and extend ventrally toward the nasopharynx, nasal cavity, and paranasal sinuses or through the foramen magnum. Approximately 40% of vertebral chordomas are cervical,[32, 996, 1001, 1003, 1008–1012] being approximately equally distributed among the cervical vertebrae as to location, with two or more vertebral bodies involved in more than one half of the cases.[1012] Vertebral chordomas are most commonly located anteriorly in the body (Fig. 8–44B)[1012, 1013] but may also involve the posterior elements.[993] Chordomas in children and young adults in the first and second decades of life occur most frequently in the spheno-occipital region.[1003, 1006, 1007]

Cranial chordomas arising in other than these two major sites are exceptional, with rare cases in the nasopharynx,[988, 1014–1016] paranasal sinuses,[987, 988, 1016] parotid region,[1014] petrous bone,[1010] nasal cavity,[1015, 1016] soft palate, hard palate, and alveolar ridge.[1015]

The most common symptoms caused by cranial chordomas are headache[997–1000, 1002, 1017–1019] and visual disturbances,[998, 1017, 1018] including diplopia,[995, 998, 1000, 1002, 1003, 1016–1019] the latter frequently due to cranial nerve palsy,[997–1002, 1018] with the sixth cranial nerve the most commonly affected because of its proximity to the clivus, a major site of origin for cranial chordoma.[998, 1000, 1018, 1019] Vertebral chordoma usually produces pain with associated neurologic symptoms[1001, 1011, 1018]; dysphagia may occur due to esophageal compression.[1016, 1018] Nasal obstruction or the presence of a nasopharyngeal mass[988, 1018] may be present from ventral extension of a cranial-based lesion.[997, 1016, 1017] The duration of symptoms prior to diagnosis may be quite short, 1 month or less,[32, 995, 999, 1001, 1006] or many years, some patients having symptoms for as long as 14 to 16 years.[32, 995, 998, 999, 1001, 1002]

Plain radiographs of the head and neck region may not always demonstrate the lesion,[995, 1001] but with CT and MRI examinations, the site and extent of the tumor is usually clearly shown (see Fig. 8–44). The lesion may appear lytic,[32, 1011] or have sclerotic foci.[999, 1001, 1002, 1005, 1018, 1020] Chordoma destroys and erodes bone[999, 1001, 1002, 1005, 1018, 1020] and frequently produces an extraosseous soft tissue mass.[993, 1005] The disc space and adjacent vertebral body may be involved.[1013, 1020] Matrix calcification is radiologically evident in 30% to 70% of cases.[32, 995, 999, 1001, 1002, 1005, 1013, 1018–1020]

Pathologic Features. Cranial chordomas vary from pea-sized to those that fill the entire middle cranial fossa.[1001, 1021] Vertebral chordomas are intermediate in size and range from 1 to 10 cm (mean 5.0 cm).[996] Chordomas are expansive tumors that characteristically are usually somewhat lobulated and may have an encephaloid appearance with a variable texture depending on the amount of chondroid or mucinous material they produce.[994, 995, 1001, 1011, 1021–1023] They are characteristically gelatinous, translucent gray to blue-gray with focal areas of hemorrhage and cyst formation.[35, 1001, 1011, 1021, 1024] The highly mucinous lesions are soft and even semiliquid, whereas those with abundant chondroid are firm and solid.[35, 994, 1011, 1021] Vertebral chordomas almost always have an associated extraosseous component that may appear delimited by a pseudocapsule.[990, 1011, 1021, 1023, 1024] This soft tissue extension frequently involves the intraspinous space, as well as adjacent vertebrae with destruction of the intervertebral disc space.[1011, 1012, 1020] This latter feature is in contrast to the situation with metastatic carcinoma, which may histologically be easily confused with chordoma that does not classically produce intervertebral disc destruction.[1020] Cranial chordomas may erode the dura and penetrate into the brain[31, 1020, 1021] or extend ventrally into the nasopharynx, nasal cavity, or paranasal sinuses[992, 1008, 1014, 1017, 1018, 1021] or posteriorly through the foramen magnum.[998]

Histologically, most chordomas have a distinct lobular configuration produced by criss-crossing fibrous septa.[35, 995, 1001, 1011, 1022, 1023] The lobules consist of either solid masses of tumor cells or pools of mucin in which reside tissue fragments and individual tumor cells.[1001, 1011, 1021] The cells have stellate, polygonal, or spindle shapes and an eosinophilic, fairly abundant vacuolated cytoplasm (Fig. 8–45A, B, see p. 538).[35, 995, 1001] Nuclei are plump and oval, with a diffuse chromatin pattern and a small nucleolus. Some cells have an epithelioid appearance resembling carcinoma cells.[1011, 1022] Binucleated and a few multinucleated forms may also be found, as well as atypical hyperchromatic pleomorphic cells.[35, 995–997, 1001, 1003, 1004, 1016, 1022, 1023, 1025] In some areas, the cells may form compact spindle cell foci resem-

bling fibrosarcoma.[993] With the accumulation of intracellular mucin, the cytoplasmic vacuoles enlarge and merge, pushing the nucleus to the periphery, creating signet-ring cells.[995, 1011, 1022] Larger cells, with central nuclei and an abundant vacuolated and reticulated cytoplasm, are termed *physaliferous cells* (see Fig. 8–45B).[31, 35, 1001, 1011, 1021, 1023] Although characteristic of chordoma, these latter cells are rarely predominant.[31, 38, 995, 1021, 1023] In most chordomas, mitotic activity is either absent or scarce.[995, 1001, 1011, 1021, 1022, 1024]

Spindle cell sarcomatous regions may develop in chordoma either following radiation therapy[1026] or de novo, representing the so-called "dedifferentiated" chordoma.[998, 1025, 1027] These regions may have the appearance of malignant fibrous histiocytoma, fibrosarcoma, chondrosarcoma, or osteosarcoma.[38, 995, 998, 1011, 1021, 1022, 1026, 1027] Chordomas in children may have compact, sarcomatoid foci, including the presence of rhabdoid-like cells.[996, 1004, 1028] Such foci may so dominate the histologic pattern that the tumor can be distinguished from other spindle-cell neoplasms only by immunohistochemical or electron microscopic means.[1003]

In 1973, Heffelfinger et al.[995] described chordomas that contained hyaline-type chondroid or cartilaginous tissue with tumor cells residing within lacunar spaces (Fig. 8–45C, see p. 538). The amount of this cartilaginous matrix varied from tumor to tumor, with some having a predominance of chordomatous tissue and others an equal amount of both elements, and, in a smaller number of cases, the cartilaginous foci predominated such that the lesion was indistinguishable from either chondroma or chondrosarcoma, with only focal regions of conventional chordoma being present. The authors designated such a cartilage-containing chordoma as a "chondroid chordoma." Numerous subsequent examples of this variant have been published.[997, 998, 1001, 1006, 1010, 1014, 1029–1035, 1038] Almost all such tumors occur in the spheno-occipital region[995]; only a few examples have been reported in the spinal column, including the cervical vertebrae.[1036, 1037]

Among 208 cases of cranial chordomas reported in six series, 61 (29.3%) had chondromatous features, with a range of 14.3% to 41.7%.[995, 997, 998, 1001, 1006, 1024] The variability in percentages may be attributed to the fact that a diagnosis of cranial chordoma may be based on only small biopsy specimens that may not contain any cartilaginous elements. Similarly, some chordomas with an abundant cartilaginous component may be misdiagnosed as a chondrosarcoma.[997] Indeed, some authors, using immunohistochemical stains, claimed that chondroid chordoma did not exist and that all such tumors were in reality low-grade chondrosarcomas.[1032, 1033] However, others, using similar techniques, have verified the histologic validity of chondroid chordoma.[1010, 1030, 1031, 1034, 1036, 1037]

By electron microscopy, chordoma contains cells that resemble those of the developing notochord,[995, 1039] with undifferentiated-appearing stellate cells, physaliferous cells, and cells with features intermediate or transitional between these cell types. The cells themselves show the presence of desmosomes, tonofilaments, a well-developed Golgi apparatus, intermediate filaments, a dilated rough endoplasmic reticulum that frequently surrounds or is in alternating arrays with mitochondria, parallel arrays of crystalline structures of microtubules within the endoplasmic reticulum, pinocytotic vesicles, and abundant cytoplasmic glycogen.[1004, 1010, 1029, 1038, 1040, 1041] Similar fine structural features are present in chondroid chordoma.[1010, 1029, 1038, 1040, 1041] The cytoplasmic vacuoles consist of either dilated endoplasmic reticulum or, in physaliferous cells, cytoplasmic invaginations or herniations of extracellular interstitial material.[1010, 1029, 1038, 1040, 1041]

Immunohistochemically, all chordomas contain cytokeratin-positive cells,[1031–1034, 1037, 1042–1044] and reactivity for epithelial membrane antigen (EMA) is present in 83% to 100% of cases.[1030–1034, 1037, 1042–1044] S-100 protein occurs in 44% to 100% of cases,[1030, 1031, 1033, 1034, 1037, 1042–1044] and vimentin in almost all cases,[1030, 1033, 1034, 1037, 1043, 1044] with only rare exceptions.[1031] Among 99 cases for which there are data on carcinoembryonic antigen, reactivity was present in 33 cases (33%).[1030, 1031, 1033, 1034, 1037, 1044] Neuron-specific enolase has been found in 80% to 100% of cases[1033, 1037] and Leu-7 antigen in 35%.[1037] These immunohistochemical results roughly parallel those found in notochordal tissue, where reactivity for cytokeratin, EMA, S-100 protein, and neuron-specific enolase is found.[1032, 1037, 1042] In chordomas exhibiting anaplastic or sarcomatous foci, cytokeratin and EMA reactivity may be absent in such areas.[1025, 1026] Results using antibodies to glial fibrillary acidic protein have varied, with some studies finding no reactivity,[1044] and others reporting positivity in 57% to 100% of cases.[1045, 1046] These discrepant results probably reflect the different types of antibody employed.[1047]

Chondroid chordomas exhibit a immunohistochemical phenotype similar to that of conventional chordoma, with positive results for cytokeratin and EMA, including those cells within the cartilaginous areas of the tumor.[1010, 1030, 1031, 1037, 1041] Those tumors diagnosed by light microscopy as chondroid chordomas, but which lacked reactivity for cytokeratin or EMA, thus forming the basis for the claim that chondroid chordoma did not exist, must be viewed, in light of the abundant immunohistochemical and electron microscopic evidence subsequently established, to have been chondrosarcomas with myxoid change.

Differential Diagnosis. Histologically, the distinction between chondrosarcoma and chondroid chordoma may be difficult on routine hematoxylin-eosin–stained sections. This is especially true for those chondrosarcomas that arise from the base of the skull, which tend to have a myxoid stroma. A biopsy specimen taken from a lesion in this location and which shows only cartilaginous tissue may well represent a chondroid chordoma. Although the cells of chondrosarcoma contain S-100 protein, they lack cytokeratin[1035–1037, 1042, 1043] and epithelial membrane antigen.[1032, 1035, 1037, 1042, 1043] Immunohistochemical stains for cytokeratin and EMA should be performed even for non-myxoid hyaline cartilaginous lesions of the base of the skull to rule out chondroid chordoma.

Metastatic carcinoma, especially that producing intracellular or extracellular mucin and involving the vertebrae, may also be difficult to distinguish from chordoma on the basis of biopsy tissue. In both conditions, the tumor cells are positive for cytokeratin and EMA and, like chordoma, some carcinomas may express vimentin and S-100 protein.[1047, 1048] Although most metastatic carcinomas are usually more pleomorphic than chordoma, this is not always the case, since some chordomas may contain pleomorphic cells. Hence, in some cases the distinction between these tumors cannot be made on morphologic or immunohistochemical grounds alone; only the clinical assessment can determine the true nature of the lesion. Radiologically, the involvement of adjacent vertebrae by the tumor would favor the diagnosis of chordoma.

Chordomas located in unusual sites, such as the paranasal sinuses or soft palate, have been misdiagnosed on biopsy tissue as salivary gland tumors,[987, 992, 1015] especially mixed tumor with its myxochondroid or chondroid component. However, the morphologic diversity of mixed tumor with its tubular and ductal structures and variety of cell forms should make the distinction from chordoma fairly easy when sufficient tissue is available.[1049] Although both tumors share immunohistochemical reactivity for cytokeratin, vimentin, S-100 protein, and glial fibrillary acidic protein, chordoma cells lack the reactivity for smooth muscle actin found in the myoepithelial cells of mixed tumor.[1049]

Treatment and Prognosis. The incidence of metastatic disease from chordomas of all sites varies from 3.6% to 58.3%.[32, 995, 1003, 1018, 1022, 1024] The metastases may involve regional lymph nodes[1033, 1017] or be systemic.[1003, 1004, 1017] Among 274 patients with cranial chordoma and follow-up data reported in 10 series, 18 (6.6%) developed metastatic disease,[995, 997, 998, 1000, 1001, 1009, 1016, 1028] with an incidence in the individual reports varying from 0% to 57%. Vertebral chordomas have a high metastatic rate; among 91 patients on whom data are available, 27 (29.7%) developed metastatic disease,[996, 1001, 1009, 1011, 1024]

with the incidence in some series as high as 60% to 80%.[1009, 1011] Metastases may develop late in the clinical course, in some cases as long as 8 to 10 years after therapy.[1008, 1011, 1036]

The mortality rate for cranial chordomas treated with surgical and conventional radiation therapy has ranged from 33% to 100%.[997, 998, 1000, 1002, 1006, 1014, 1016, 1017, 1050] With the use of proton beam therapy, however, 5-year local control rates of approximately 80% are reported.[1028, 1051, 1052] To date, vertebral chordomas still have a poor prognosis, with mortality rates of 75% to 80% and few patients disease-free at 5 years.[1001, 1011] Among chordomas in general, patients younger than 40 years of age may have a better prognosis than older patients,[998, 1034] although some investigators find no difference in terms of age.[997, 1011] Female patients are reported to have a worse prognosis than male patients.[997] Chordomas of the maxillary sinus appear to be more indolent, with few deaths due to tumor.[987] Recent studies indicate a better prognosis for chordomas that demonstrate positivity for estrogen and progesterone receptors.[1053] Childhood chordomas are considered to be more aggressive, with a poorer overall prognosis than adult types,[1003, 1004, 1007] with some exceptions reported.[1006, 1023]

The results of follow-up studies in chondroid chordoma have varied, with some reports indicating either an overall better prognosis,[995, 1024] or no difference compared with conventional chordoma.[997, 1010] This variability is probably due to the inclusion in some series of cases of chondrosarcoma misdiagnosed as chondroid chordoma. In a series from the Massachusetts General Hospital, 40% of the cranial chondrosarcomas had been misdiagnosed as chondroid or nonchondroid chordomas; the prognosis for chondrosarcoma was found to be significantly better than that for chordoma.[997] Some investigators have attributed the better prognosis in chondroid chordoma to age effect, finding that those patients with chondroid chordoma are younger and thus have a better prognosis.[998, 1034] Indeed, it is claimed that the histologic distinction between chondroid chordoma and chondrosarcoma of the base of the skull is of no importance, as the prognosis for both is age-dependent, with no survival difference between them.[1034]

FIBRO-OSSEOUS LESIONS OF THE CRANIOFACIAL SKELETON

A group of lesions affecting the craniofacial skeleton and characterized microscopically by fibrous stroma containing various combinations of bone and cementum-like material fall under the general rubric *benign fibro-osseous lesions*. They include a wide variety of lesions of developmental, dysplastic, and neoplastic origins with differing clinical and radiographic presentation and behavior. Because of the histologic similarities between these diverse diseases, proper diagnosis requires correlation of history, clinical, and radiographic findings. In the absence of this information, the pathologist can seldom be more specific than to report that the condition in question represents a benign fibro-osseous lesion.

The more important types of craniofacial fibro-osseous lesions will be discussed here.

Fibrous Dysplasia

Fibrous dysplasia (FD) is a skeletal anomaly in which normal bone is replaced and distorted by poorly organized and inadequately mineralized, immature, woven bone and fibrous connective tissue. The disease may affect a single bone (monostotic) or multiple bones (polyostotic). Polyostotic fibrous dysplasia is less common, occurring in only 25% to 30% of cases.[19, 1054] A few of these cases (about 3%) may also be associated with skin pigmentation and endocrine abnormalities, a condition known as the McCune-Albright syndrome. The syndrome is much more common in females.[19, 1054]

Clinical Features. The craniofacial skeleton may be involved in either of the two types of FD. Polyostotic FD exhibits various degrees of severity. In its milder form, only a few bones localized to one region of the body are affected, usually asymmetrically. In its more severe forms, almost all of the skeleton is involved. In more than half of the cases, the femur, tibia, fibula, ribs, and humerus are affected. In addition, in 40% to 50% of individuals with polyostotic FD, the disease is detected in the base of the skull and other sites in the craniofacial skeleton.[1054] In monostotic fibrous dysplasia, which constitutes 70% to 75% of all fibrous dysplasias, the ribs, femur, and tibia are the most commonly involved bones.[1055] In 20% to 25% of monostotic fibrous dysplasia, the bones of the skull are affected, particularly the maxilla and mandible. The molar and premolar area is the most favored site.[19, 40, 1054, 1055] In monostotic fibrous dysplasia of the skull, the pathologic process is not always limited to one bone, but may extend by continuity across suture lines to involve adjacent bones.[40] Thus, the commonly used notation *monostotic* is not always accurate.

Fibrous dysplasia appears to be a disorder of growing bones. Most cases are initially identified in children and adolescents. Up to 83% of patients affected by craniofacial fibrous dysplasia are diagnosed within the first two decades of life. However, milder lesions may present later in life.[19, 40, 1054, 1055] Whereas monostotic FD occurs with equal frequency in both males and females, polyostotic FD is more common in females, with a female : male ratio of 3 : 1.[1056, 1057]

Swelling of the facial bones is the first sign in the majority of cases. In contrast, pain is the most frequent symptom in extracranial FD and is occasionally due to pathologic fracture.[1058, 1059] Diffuse thickening of the bones with involvement of the paranasal sinuses, orbits, and foramina of the skull base can produce a variety of symptoms, including headache, visual loss, proptosis, diplopia, hearing loss, anosmia, nasal obstruction, epistaxis, epiphora, mucocele, and sinusitis.[1058] Temporal bone involvement with occlusion of bony canals may result in cholesteatoma formation.[1059]

Biochemical abnormalities are rare in monostotic FD. Elevation of alkaline phosphatase is encountered in 70% of patients with polyostotic disease.[1060] The degree of elevation may be commensurate with the extent of the disease. In more severe cases, urinary hydroxyproline is also elevated. However, most patients have normal blood calcium and phosphate levels.[1057, 1061]

A range of endocrinopathies accompany polyostotic FD in the McCune-Albright syndrome,[1062] the most common of which is sexual precocity in female subjects, sometimes as early as the first months of life.[1057] The second most commonly associated endocrinopathy is hyperthyroidism. Other hormonal abnormalities include acromegaly,[1063] hyperprolactinemia,[1064] hyperparathyroidism,[1065] gynecomastia,[1066] and Cushing's syndrome.[1067]

Rarely, intramuscular myxoma has been reported in association with the polyostotic FD, a condition known as the Mazabraud's syndrome.[1068-1072] Only 26 such cases have so far been reported. Of these, six were associated with the McCune-Albright syndrome. The myxomas often occur as multiple tumors and tend to be located in the vicinity of the affected bone.[1071, 1072]

The radiographic appearance of FD has been classified into three types[1058, 1073]: pagetoid or "ground glass," sclerotic, and cystic. Variations in the relative amount of bone to fibrous tissue contents influence the radiographic appearance. The sclerotic feature is seen when bone exceeds the fibrous tissue. The reverse is true in cystic-appearing lesions. Regardless of their types, the lesions almost always have ill-defined borders, which blend imperceptibly into the adjacent normal bone.[40, 1057] The affected bones expand and the cortical bone becomes considerably thinned. Lesions involving the craniofacial bones tend to be sclerotic or "ground glass" in appearance. Paranasal sinuses may become obliterated, and displacement of the orbit is a common feature (Fig. 8–46, see p. 538).[1055, 1058] Computed tomographic scans may be useful in evaluating the skull base foramina.[1058]

Pathologic Features. Grossly, the affected bone is rubbery, compressible, grayish white tissue that has a gritty texture when cut with a scalpel. Microscopically, normal bone is replaced with a cellular fibroblastic stroma containing variable amounts of randomly

arranged irregular, usually delicate, bone trabeculae. The trabeculae are not connected to one another. They often assume curvilinear forms resembling Chinese script letters (Fig. 8–47A).[19, 1054, 1057, 1058, 1074, 1075] Typically, the bone trabeculae in fibrous dysplasia are immature, woven in type, and rich in osteoids and lack osteoblastic rimming (Fig. 8–47B). The osteocytic lacunae are wider than normal. Osteoclasts are occasionally present and mitoses are rare.

It has been suggested that the bone in fibrous dysplasia of the craniofacial skeleton, unlike that in long bones, may undergo matu-

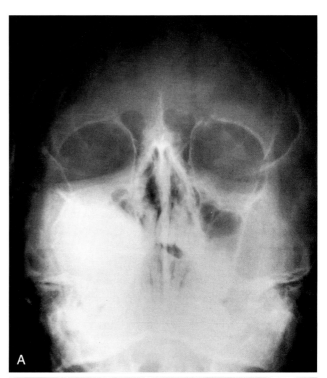

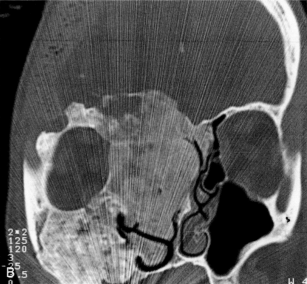

Figure 8–46. *A,* Fibrous dysplasia of the maxilla. Waters' view radiograph shows a diffusely sclerotic right maxilla. Although the features of the lesion are not completely defined in this single projection, the combination of sclerosis without bone destruction and the location in the maxillary bone suggest fibrous dysplasia. *B,* Fibrous dysplasia. A coronal computed tomographic scan shows a homogeneous sclerotic lesion that occupies the right maxilla, both ethmoids, completely obliterating the air cells with extension to the sphenoid and causing orbital displacement. The right nasal turbinates are obscured.

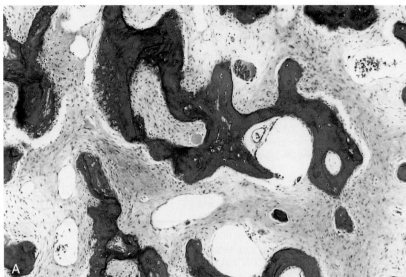

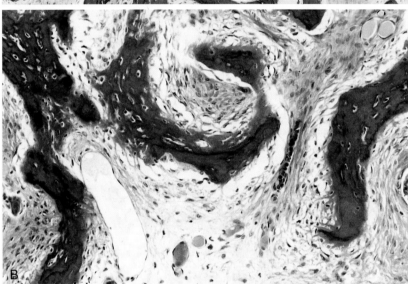

Figure 8–47. *A,* Fibrous dysplasia. Bone trabeculae form irregular structures resembling Chinese script letters. *B,* Higher magnification of immature woven bone in fibrous dysplasia. There is a lack of osteoblastic rimming.

ration to lamellar bone.[1074, 1075] This feature has been demonstrated in serial biopsies showing progressive maturation to a lesion consisting of lamellar bone in a moderately cellular fibrous stroma. The bony trabeculae in the "mature" lesions tend to be parallel to one another.[40, 1074, 1075]

Treatment and Prognosis. Treatment of fibrous dysplasia is exclusively surgical but is not always indicated. Solitary small lesions may remain asymptomatic and static, thus requiring no treatment.[1058] In the past, surgical intervention was delayed as long as possible until after puberty with the hope that the disease would become quiescent.[1054, 1057, 1058, 1074, 1075] Because of multiple reports of persistence in later years, however, it is now recommended that surgery be performed as soon as the lesion becomes marked, with progressive deformity, pain, or interference with function.[1057] Simple contouring of facial or skull bones back to normal dimensions has proved quite effective. About one fourth of the patients so treated will require repeated operations because of recurrence of bony enlargement.[40, 1057, 1074, 1075] Partial excision followed by grafting with normal autologous bone[1057, 1076] or acrylic implant[1057] may achieve a reduction in the rate of recurrence.

Malignant degeneration has been reported in a few cases of fibrous dysplasia, most of which were osteosarcomas or, less frequently, fibrosarcoma and chondrosarcoma.[1057, 1058, 1074, 1075] The majority of these cases were in patients who have received radiation therapy for fibrous dysplasia. In 13 patients who previously received radiation therapy for treatment of craniofacial fibrous dysplasia, 11 malignancies occurred in that region.[1058, 1077] There was no significant difference in the lag time between those who did and those who did not receive radiation and eventually developed sarcoma. The mean interval between diagnosis of FD and development of malignancy was 13.5 years. The overall rate of malignant change is 0.5% (1/200 patients) if left untreated.[1057, 1058, 1078, 1079] This rate increases 400-fold in patients who have received radiotherapy.[1057, 1058, 1078, 1080] Because of this risk, radiation therapy for fibrous dysplasia is now definitely contraindicated. As a consequence of abandonment of radiation therapy as a treatment modality for FD, more recent investigations show more cases of spontaneous sarcomatous changes unrelated to radiation exposure than those following radiation. Of 15 patients who had both fibrous dysplasia and osteosarcoma at Memorial Sloan Kettering Center, only one had a previous history of radiation.[19, 1080] Significantly, in some patients, the initial diagnosis of fibrous dysplasia was made simultaneously with the discovery of the sarcoma.

Sarcomatous transformation is signaled by clinical and radiographic signs, including rapid growth, pain, invasion into cortical bone with an associated soft tissue mass, and elevation of alkaline phosphatase level.[40, 1056–1058, 1074, 1075] It is prudent to keep patients with FD under long-term follow-up and any patient showing clinical or radiographic evidence of change after a long period should be subjected to an adequate biopsy to rule out sarcomatous change.

Ossifying Fibroma

The term *ossifying fibroma* is used to describe a benign bone-producing fibrous neoplasm of the skeleton. Lesions that may differ in their clinical presentation, site of predilection, sex and age distribution, and microscopic appearance have been included under the umbrella diagnosis of ossifying fibroma. Ossifying fibroma of the craniofacial skeleton are separated into four clinicopathologic entities. Familiarity with the distinct entities of ossifying fibroma is not merely of academic interest but also can be of value in distinguishing them from other fibro-osseous and non-fibro-osseous bone lesions, and thus influence the proper management and the outcome of treatment.

Ossifying Fibroma of Odontogenic Origin (Cemento-Ossifying Fibroma)

Ossifying fibroma of odontogenic origin is a benign jaw lesion that has been variously called ossifying fibroma, cementifying fibroma, and cemento-ossifying fibroma. The last is the designation used in the recent World Health Organization (WHO) classification.[1085] The tumor is limited to the tooth-bearing area of the mandible and maxilla.[40, 1074, 1075] The neoplastic cells elaborate bone and cementum and hence the belief that they derive from the progenitor cells of the periodontal ligament,[1081] cells that are capable of dual differentiation into osteoblasts and cementoblasts. Cemento-ossifying fibromas (COF), which have also been termed *periodontomas* by some authors,[28] are distinctive jaw lesions that should not be confused with lesions termed *ossifying fibroma,* which occur in other parts of the skeleton.[1074, 1075, 1085]

Clinical Features. COF most frequently presents clinically as a painless expansion of the jaw. A few cases may be discovered on routine radiographic examination. It affects the mandible much more commonly than the maxilla.[1082] The peak age of incidence is the third and fourth decades, but the lesion may be seen in patients of a wide age range. There is a definite female predilection, with a female : male ratio high as 5 : 1.[1082]

Radiographically, the tumor is well defined and unilocular; it may be radiolucent or show various degrees of opacification, depending on the relative amount of calcified material present (Fig. 8–48).[40, 1074, 1082, 1083] Large mandibular lesions may cause a characteristic thinning and downward "bowing" of the inferior border.[40] Displacement of adjacent teeth may be seen, and less frequently root resorption may occur.[1074, 1082] The tumor may attain a very large size if not adequately treated. On surgical exploration, the lesion is well demarcated from the surrounding bone and can be easily shelled out from its bony bed,[1074, 1082] and some lesions may have a definite capsule. This demarcation from the surrounding tissue is an important feature in distinguishing COF from FD.

Pathologic Features. Microscopically, the lesions are composed of fibrous connective tissue stroma containing calcified

structures. The connective tissue usually shows dense cellularity and sparse collagen fibers. The cells are fibroblastic and commonly show hyperchromatic nuclei. The calcified structures are composed of irregular trabeculae of osteoid or bone and lobulated basophilic masses of cementum or cementum-like tissue (Fig. 8–49).[1074, 1082, 1084] These structures bear resemblance to cementicles found in normal periodontal membrane.[1082, 1084] They may coalesce and form anastomosing trabeculae with curvilinear configuration, which may be acellular.

Polarized light microscopy reveals both woven and lamellar bone. The cementum or cementum-like tissue is usually woven and may show a characteristic quilted pattern.[1082, 1084] Osteoblastic rimming is focally present.[1084] Osteoclast-like multinucleated cells are encountered in some lesions.

Treatment and Prognosis. Most lesions grow slowly, and conservative surgical excision is the treatment of choice. Some lesions may be removed from the jaw with relative ease by curettage. Untreated tumors could attain massive size and may require en bloc resection. Sarcomatous transformation of cemento-ossifying fibroma has not been documented.[1074, 1082, 1084]

Juvenile Active Ossifying Fibroma

Also known as juvenile aggressive ossifying fibroma[1085] and trabecular desmo-osteoblastoma,[28] juvenile active ossifying fibroma (JAOF) is a relatively rare lesion, defined in the WHO histologic classification of odontogenic tumors[1085] as an actively growing lesion, well demarcated from surrounding bone, that is composed of cell-rich fibrous tissue containing bundles of cellular osteoid and bone trabeculae without osteoblastic rimming.

Clinical Features. The great majority of the patients are children and adolescents.[40, 1074, 1075, 1085-1087] Only 20% of the patients are over 15 years of age.[1086] Males and females are equally affected.[40, 28, 1074, 1085-1087] The maxilla and the mandible are the dominant sites of incidence. Occurrence in the maxilla is slightly more frequent than in the mandible. Origin in extragnathic locations is extremely rare.[40, 1086, 1087]

Clinically, JAOF is often characterized by a progressive and sometimes rapid expansion of the affected area; pain is a rare symptom. In the maxilla, obstruction of the nasal passages and epistaxis may be present. Radiographically, the tumor may be fairly well demarcated. Depending on the amount of calcified tissue produced, the lesion will show varying degrees of radiolucency or radiopacity.[28, 1074] Ground-glass appearance has been described.[28, 1086]

Pathologic Features. Microscopically, JAOF has a characteristic loose structure. The stroma is cell-rich, with spindle or polyhedral cells that produce little collagen.[28, 1074, 1075, 1087] Cellular, immature osteoids form strands that may be long and slender or plump. These structures have been likened to paint brush strokes (Fig. 8–50A). The immature cellular osteoid is not always easily distinguished from the cellular stroma.[28, 1074, 1075, 1085] Irregular mineralization takes place at the center of the strands. Maturation to lamellar bone is not observed. Local aggregates of osteoclastic giant cells are invariably present in the stroma (Fig. 8–50B). Mitotic activity of the stromal cells may be present but is never numerous.

Treatment and Prognosis. The clinical course of JAOF is characterized by infrequent recurrence following conservative excision. One or more recurrences were observed in 3 of 10 patients reported by Slootweg et al.[1087] Eventual complete cure could be achieved in those cases without resorting to radical surgical intervention.

Psammomatoid Ossifying Fibroma

Psammomatoid ossifying fibroma (PSOF) is a lesion that affects the extragnathic craniofacial bones, particularly centered on the periorbital, frontal, and ethmoid bones. PSOF was initially described by Gogl as early as 1949 under the designation *psammomatoid fibroma*

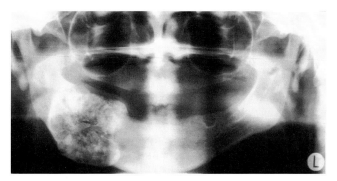

Figure 8–48. Ossifying fibroma of the mandible, panoramic radiograph showing large expansive lesion of the right mandible. The tumor is well defined with corticated borders.

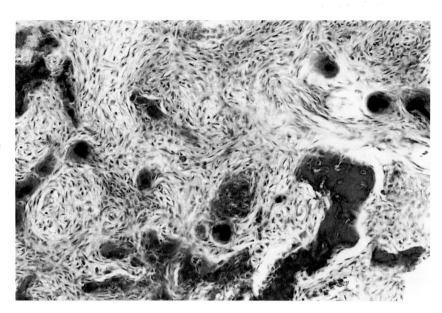

Figure 8–49. Ossifying fibroma. Note trabeculae of bone and cementum-like structures in a hypercellular stroma.

of the nose and paranasal sinuses.[1088] Margo, in 1985,[1089] described PSOF as a distinctive solitary fibro-osseous lesion of young individuals that affects the orbit and shows distinguishing histologic features. PSOF was also reported under the designation *juvenile active ossifying fibroma* by Johnson et al.[22] and *juvenile ossifying fibroma with psammoma-like ossicles*[1087] and *psammous desmo-osteoblastoma* by Makek.[28] PSOF is not classified under osseous tumors of the jaws in the Armed Forces Institute of Pathology (AFIP) Atlas of Tumor Pathology,[1090] nor has it been considered a gnathic tumor in the WHO histologic classification of odontogenic tumors.[1085] PSOF is more likely a separate histopathologic entity than a variant of the gnathic cemento-ossifying fibroma, as suggested by Slootweg et al.[1091] Production of cementum by a benign bone tumor of the orbital bones is highly unlikely.

Clinical Features. Afflicted individuals tend to be young, although the average age of incidence has varied in different studies from 17.8 to 22.6 years.[22, 1087, 1089, 1092, 1093] In general, patients with PSOF are a few years older than those with JAOF. But, as in the case of JAOF, there is no sex predilection.

The greatest majority of the reported cases of PSOF originated in the paranasal sinuses, particularly frontal and ethmoid.[22, 28, 1093] About 10% have been reported in the calvarium.[22] Makek[28] in his review indicated that 7% of the cases occurred in the mandible. These were more likely cemento-ossifying fibromas with prominent spheroid cemental components with some histologic similarities.

A case of PSOF is clinically manifested as bone expansion that may involve the orbital or the nasal bones and sinuses. The eye and sinonasal involvement may result in proptosis, with visual complaints including blindness, nasal obstruction, headache, ptosis, papilledema, and disturbances in ocular mobility.[22, 1089, 1093]

Radiographic examination shows a round, well-defined, sometimes corticated osteolytic lesion with a cystic appearance.[1089, 1091, 1093] Sclerotic changes are evident in the lesion and a plain skull film may show a ground-glass appearance.[1094] In computed tomographic scans set on bone window, the lesions appear less dense than normal bone.[1094] The lesions may range in size from 2 to 8 cm in diameter.[1089] PSOF may appear multiloculated on CT scans. It is stated that in the facial skeleton a well-circumscribed expansile mass with a thick wall of bone density on CT scan and enhancement of this area on post contrast MR image is strongly suggestive of psammomatoid ossifying fibroma.[1095]

Pathologic Features. On gross examination, the tumor is described as yellowish, white and gritty. On light microscopic examination, the tumor is significant for multiple round uniform small ossicles (psammomatoid bodies) embedded in a relatively cellular stroma composed of uniform, stellate, and spindle shaped cells (Fig. 8–51, see p. 538).[1089, 1091, 1096] Occasionally, shrunken cells become embedded in the calcified matrix of the ossicles. The psammomatoid bodies are basophilic and bear superficial resemblance to dental cementum, but may have an osteoid rim.[22, 1089] Because of a superficial resemblance between these ossicles and the cementum spheres of the odontogenic ossifying fibroma, the lesion has occasionally been mislabeled cemento-ossifying fibroma, implying an odontogenic origin which, as mentioned above, is rather unlikely in extragnathic bone.[1092] Mitotic activity is extremely rare in the stromal cells. At the periphery of the lesion, the ossicles seem to coalesce and form irregular thin bony trabeculae that may become thicker, with numerous reversal lines resembling Paget's bone.[1089] A shell of normal bone is usually present and may show osteoclastic resorption endosteally associated with osteoblastic activity on the periosteal surface.[1089]

Treatment and Prognosis. Surgical excision is the treatment of choice, although recurrence even after definitive surgery is not unusual, and, in some cases, multiple recurrences over a long follow-up period is reported.[1089, 1097]

Extragnathic Ossifying Fibroma of the Skull

The cranial bones may, on rare occasions, harbor ossifying fibromas that are histologically distinct from the above-mentioned entities. The tumors are generally composed of immature and mature bone trabeculae in a fibrous stroma without evidence of psammomatoid or cementoid features. Such tumors have been reported in the frontal, parietal, temporal, sphenoid, and occipital bones.[1098–1101] The majority of the patients are in their second and third decades and there is no gender predilection. A few of the tumors were complicated by intracranial extension.[1098]

Clinical presentations include local swelling, pain, headache, motor disorders, exophthalmus, diplopia, and mild spastic hemiparesis.[1098, 1099] The duration of the symptoms ranges from 1 to 10 years with a median of 3.2 years.[1098–1100] Radiographic examination shows well-defined osteolytic lesions with variable opacities. Microscopically, the tumors have well-defined borders and are composed of irregular trabeculae of bone in a cellular fibrous connective tissue stroma. The trabeculae of bone may be lamellar or woven in character or may show contribution of the two types. Osteoblastic rimming is commonly seen on the bone trabeculae.

Treatment and Prognosis. Surgical excision is the treatment of choice. Recurrence is usually due to incomplete removal.

Cemento-Osseous Dysplasia

Cemento-osseous dysplasia of the jaws consists of non-neoplastic fibro-osseous lesions and is commonly seen. Two types are well recognized, *periapical cemento-osseous dysplasia* (cementoma), and *florid cemento-osseous dysplasia*. These two entities should ideally be identified clinically and radiographically, and it would be uncommon to receive surgical specimens from them. Indeed, surgical intervention is contraindicated, especially in the case of florid cemento-osseous dysplasia, because even a simple biopsy or dental extraction may result in local infection, pain, and a complicated clinical course.[40, 1074, 1075]

Periapical Cemental Dysplasia (Periapical Cementoma)

Periapical cemental dysplasia is a relatively common condition, particularly in middle-aged black women. It is non-neoplastic, presumably a dysplastic disorder. The anterior mandibular teeth are more often involved by asymptomatic, periapical radiolucencies, which in older lesions become heavily calcified. In their early stages, the lesions are radiolucent and may be confused with periapical inflammatory disease. Treatment is not required.[33, 40]

Florid Cemento-Osseous Dysplasia

Florid cemento-osseous dysplasia is infrequently seen and has been reported under various alternative designations. This condition usually presents in middle-aged or elderly black women and radiographically is characterized by extensive sclerotic areas, often involving the posterior quadrants of the mandible and maxilla symmetrically.[40, 1102]

Periapical cemental dysplasia and florid cemento-osseous dysplasia are microscopically analogous and are composed of proliferating fibrous connective tissue stroma containing foci of cementum. Osteoid or bone are invariably present as well (Fig. 8–52). More advanced lesions show an increase in mineralization. In florid cemento-osseous dysplasia, large sclerotic masses are formed that are hypocellular and extremely dense with little marrow spaces and few haversian systems (see Fig. 8–52).[40, 1102]

GIANT CELL LESIONS OF THE CRANIOFACIAL SKELETON

Giant cell lesions of the craniofacial skeleton are a group of heterogeneous clinical entities affecting the skull bones that share common microscopic features. Histologically, they are composed of

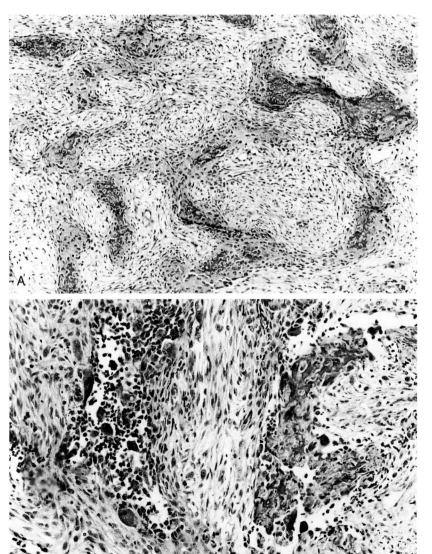

Figure 8–50. *A,* Juvenile active ossifying fibroma. The lesion is composed of cellular immature osteoid trabeculae in a spindle cell–rich stroma. *B,* Juvenile active ossifying fibroma. Note focal aggregates of osteoclast-like giant cells.

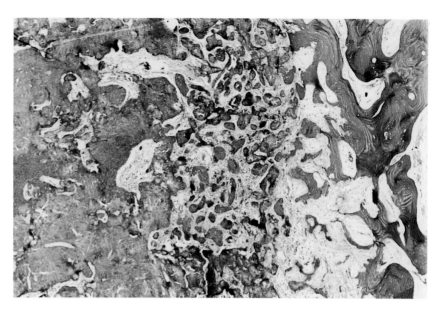

Figure 8–52. Cemento-osseous dysplasia. The lesion is well demarcated from the jaw bone *(right)*. Bone trabeculae and cementum-like tissue are present at the periphery *(center)*. Increased mineralization leads to formation of dense sclerotic masses at the center of the lesion *(left)*.

multinucleated osteoclastic giant cells and mononuclear, spindle-shaped and polygonal cells in a vascular stroma with little or no collagen fibers.

These entities include giant cell granuloma, giant cell tumor, aneurysmal bone cyst, cherubism, and brown tumors associated with hyperparathyroidism.

Giant Cell Granuloma

Giant cell granuloma (GCG) is a common lesion. It affects predominantly but not exclusively the jaws. It is also known as giant cell reparative granuloma. For 100 years following Paget's description of giant cell tumors of long bones,[1103] the jaw lesions were considered identical. It was not until 1953 that Jaffe,[1104] observing their invariably benign clinical course, suggested that the jaw lesions are not true neoplasms and coined the term *giant cell reparative granuloma.* There is little evidence that the lesion represents a reparative process, and indeed some show aggressive behavior similar to that of a true neoplasm. The term *reparative* has been dropped by the majority of pathologists.[33, 1105] Controversy still exists concerning the relationship of giant cell tumor (GCT) and GCG. Whether or not "true" giant cell tumors occur in the jaws is uncertain. This topic is discussed later.

Clinical Features. GCG can occur at any age, but the majority present before the age of 30 years. There is a distinct gender predilection, with 65% of cases affecting females. The mandible is a more common site of occurrence than the maxilla, with more than 70% of the cases occurring in the mandible. The anterior part of the mandible is a favorable site, and lesions commonly cross the midline.[33, 1106, 1107] The majority of the giant cell granulomas of the jaws present as painless expansion of bone or are detected on routine radiographic examination. The lesions appear as a well-defined radiolucency, which may be either unilocular or multilocular. They are generally uncorticated and may vary considerably in size (Fig. 8–53A).[1106, 1107]

Pathologic Features. Microscopically, giant cell granuloma of the jaws are unencapsulated and are composed of multinucleated osteoclast-like giant cells dispersed in a richly vascular stroma with little collagen deposition (Fig. 8–53B).[33, 1105, 1107] Two types of stromal cells are identified, a spindle-shaped fibroblastic cell and a polygonal macrophage-like cell. The giant cells may be focally aggregated or are evenly dispersed in the lesions.[33, 1105, 1107, 1108] These cells may vary considerably in size from one case to another, and the number of nuclei per cell also varies from few to several dozen.

While at the periphery of the lesion endothelial lined capillaries are present, the vasculature in the main part of the lesion is in the form of sinusoidal spaces that are not lined with endothelial cells.[1105] Hemosiderin granules and focal areas of ossification may be present. The histologic features of giant cell granuloma of the jaws is very similar and may be identical to those seen in giant cell tumor, cherubism, and brown tumors of hyperparathyroidism (see later).

Treatment and Prognosis. Giant cell granuloma of the jaws is usually treated by curettage. Previous studies have reported recurrence rates that vary between 11% and 35%.[33, 1109, 1110] Recurrent lesions often respond to further curettage. The long-term prognosis is good and distant metastases do not develop. Correlation of the histopathologic features with clinical behavior remains debatable, but lesions showing large, uniformly distributed giant cells are believed to behave more aggressively and show a higher frequency of recurrence.[1109, 1110] In these cases, marginal resection may be required for a cure.

Giant Cell Tumor

Clinical Features. Giant cell tumor is an uncommon bone neoplasm that occurs chiefly in the ends of long bones. Giant cell tumors (GCT) are rarely encountered in the skull, where they preferentially occur in the sphenoid and temporal bones.[19, 1111, 1112] In the Mayo Clinic series of 546 cases of GCT, only 4 tumors occurred in the skull, 3 cases involved the sphenoid, and 1 involved the temporal bone.[1111] Of 265 GCT of bone described by Huvos,[19] 3 cases involved the craniofacial bones in patients with Paget's disease. GCTs associated with Paget's disease affect the craniofacial bones more frequently than other bones (Fig. 8–54). About 100 cases of GCT have been reported in patients with Paget's disease and about 50% of the tumors occurred in the skull.[1113]

Involvement of the jaws with GCT outside Paget's disease is debatable, but aggressive giant cell lesions that are characterized by pain, rapid growth, and cortical perforation and show marked tendency to recur after treatment may be examples of "true" giant cell tumors.[33, 1110, 1114]

In a review of 15 giant cell tumors of the skull by Bertoni et al.[1112] the patient ages range from 8 to 78 years (mean 36.5). One third of the patients in this study were older than 50 years, an age group slightly older than the patients with GCT of long bones. The female:male ratio was 2 to 1. In 11 patients, the sphenoid bone was involved. The frontal, temporal, and occipital bones were sites for the other four tumors. One patient had Paget's disease. The duration of the symptoms ranged from weeks to several years and included headache, visual disturbances including blindness, memory loss, and dysphasia in addition to pain and swelling.

Radiographically, the giant cell tumors of the skull are radiolucent without any matrix mineralization. The margins are poorly defined and irregular. Soft tissue masses may frequently be associated with bone destruction. Lesions of the sphenoid bone may present with soft tissue masses in the sella turcica, posterior nasopharynx, ethmoid sinuses, and orbit.[1112]

Pathologic Features. Microscopically, GCT are composed of multinucleated giant cells and round spindle-shaped mononuclear cells. There is similarity in the size of the nuclei of the mononuclear and multinuclear giant cells. Little or no collagen is found in the stroma. Sinusoidal vascular spaces rather than endothelial lined capillaries are present throughout the lesions. The giant cells may be either diffuse or focally clustered. Areas of distinctly spindle-shaped fibroblastic cells devoid of giant cells may be present.[19, 1108, 1112] Typical mitotic figures are consistently present and vary in number between different tumors. Atypical mitoses are not identified. Permeation of surrounding bone marrow spaces may be seen in some cases.

In a comparative histomorphometric study on GCT and GCG, Auclair et al.[1108] found statistically significant differences between the two lesions with regard to stromal cellularity, even distribution of giant cells, number of nuclei in the giant cells, presence of tumor

necrosis, and presence of inflammatory cells. GCT were more cellular and have larger giant cells with more nuclei per cell (Fig. 8–55). The giant cells tended to be more evenly dispersed and there was prominent necrosis and inflammatory reaction. On the other hand, there were no significant differences in regard to presence of hemorrhage, hemosiderin deposits, prominence of osteoid, and focal areas of spindle-shaped cells. In this study, 26% of the giant cell tumors were histologically similar to most giant cell granulomas and 10% of the giant cell granulomas were histologically similar to most giant cell tumors.

Treatment and Prognosis. GCT of the skull bones can be very aggressive, and, because of its location, adequate excision is not always possible. Postoperative radiation therapy is used with some success in achieving local control.[1112]

Aneurysmal Bone Cyst

Clinical Features. Aneurysmal bone cyst (ABC) is a distinct pathologic entity that was first identified by Jaffe and Lichtenstein in 1942.[1115] ABC is a benign cystic lesion of undetermined neoplastic potential. Most authors consider it a reactive vascular malformation. The malignant transformation of rare cases of ABC[1116] and its frequent recurrence after curettage may argue for a neoplastic nature.[1116, 1117] ABC is a lesion of growing bones. Approximately

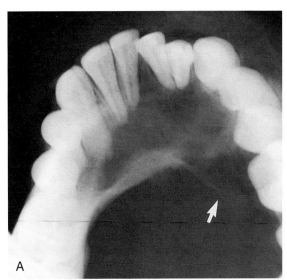

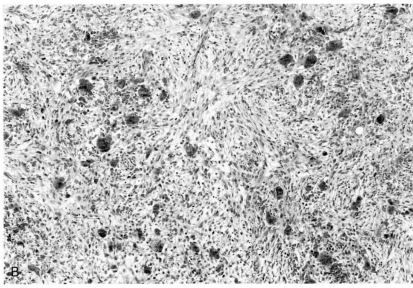

Figure 8–53. *A,* Occlusal radiograph showing giant cell granuloma involving the anterior aspect of the mandible and crossing the symphysis. The lesion is osteolytic and has caused thinning of the posterior cortex of bone *(arrow)* and anterior displacement of the teeth. *B,* Giant cell granuloma. Osteoclast-like giant cells are focally aggregated. The stroma is composed of spindle-shaped and polygonal mononuclear cells with very little collagen deposition.

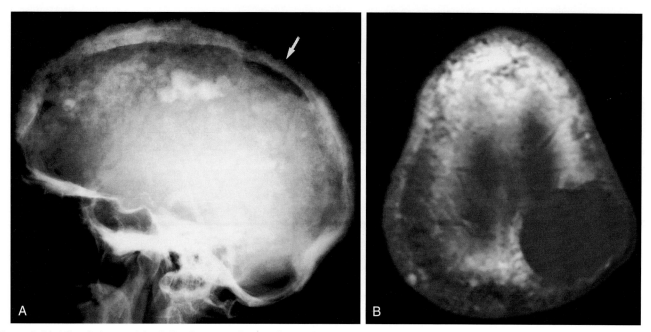

Figure 8–54. *A,* Paget's disease of the skull with associated giant cell tumor. Lateral view of the skull shows characteristic features of Paget's disease with thickening of the diploe and the inner and outer tables of the frontal and parietal bones. Characteristic round sclerotic densities, so-called cotton wool exudates, are present. At the parietal-temporal bone junction, there is an ill-defined osteolytic lesion *(arrow)* that appears to have thinned the inner table. *B,* Computed tomographic scan of the skull shows a large, well-defined round lytic lesion, consistent with giant cell tumor in the midst of Paget's disease.

80% occur in patients who are younger than 20 and almost all patients are under 30 years of age. The peak incidence is in the second decade.[19, 1111, 1118] Although some published series show a female predilection, equal gender ratios are more commonly reported.[19, 1118] ABC may affect any bone, but, judging from reported cases, the craniofacial bones, the vertebral column, and the flat bones of the pelvis are the most common sites. Of the long bones, the femur and tibia are more likely to be involved. In the skull, the jaws are much more frequently affected than the other bones, with somewhat more predilection for the mandible than the maxilla.[1119–1121] In a review of 44 cases of jaw ABC, the ratio of the mandibular to the maxillary cases was 3:2.[1119] In the extragnathic skull, involvement of the frontal, orbital, temporal, and occipital bones have all been reported.[19, 1122–1126]

Aneurysmal bone cyst presents in two clinicopathologic forms: either as a primary lesion or as a secondary lesion aris-

ing in other neoplastic and some non-neoplastic osseous conditions.[19, 1111, 1127, 1128] At least 30% of ABCs are considered to be secondary.[1127, 1128] ABC-like areas are found in various benign conditions, including giant cell tumor, giant cell granuloma, chondroblastoma, chondromyxoid fibroma, osteoblastoma, fibrous dysplasia, and ossifying fibroma. Malignant bone tumors may contain benign aneurysmal bone cyst–like areas.[19, 1111, 1123, 1127–1129] A secondary ABC shows sudden expansion, which has been likened to "blow out," in a pre-existing lesion of bone. Pain and swelling are the two most common clinical features. In a large series of ABCs,[1118] 50% of the patients complained of pain, 25% had both pain and swelling, and the remaining 25% had a mass or swelling without pain. The duration of the symptoms varies from days to months. In the craniofacial skeleton, the deformity of ABC is usually obvious, and on palpation the mass is found to be firm and bony. In this anatomic location, a variety of symptoms may be elicited, in-

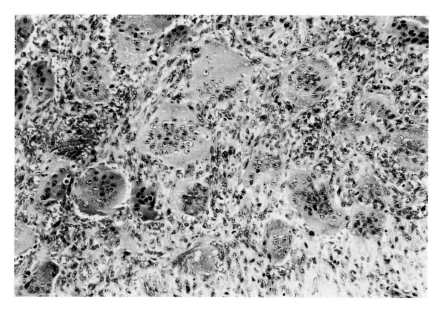

Figure 8–55. Giant cell lesion of the maxilla with clinical and histologic features suggestive of a giant cell tumor. The giant cells are larger with more numerous nuclei than the ones commonly seen in giant cell granuloma.

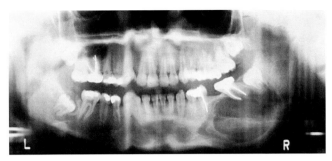

Figure 8–56. Panoramic radiograph showing aneurysmal bone cyst of the right mandible. The lesion is expansive, well-defined, and unilocular.

cluding blurred vision, proptosis, and blindness.[1130] In the jaw cases, numbness of the lower lip, temporomandibular joint pain, trismus, and displacement of teeth with malocclusion may all be manifested.[1118, 1120, 1122] Radiographically, ABC generally presents as a benign yet rapidly growing cystic lesion (Fig. 8–56). It more frequently is unilocular and less frequently is multilocular, even with a "soap bubble" appearance.[19, 1120, 1121, 1127] The fast rate of growth of the lesion can be well demonstrated in serial radiographs.[19] This characteristic rapid expansion may also lead to loss of cortication and even to loss of marginal definition and regularity. A thin cortical shell is usually well demonstrated by computed tomographic (CT) scan even if not obvious in plain radiographs.[1121] Fluid levels are also seen in CT scans. Magnetic resonance imaging is superior to CT scan in determining the extent of the tumor within the bone.[1131]

Pathologic Features. When the lesion is exposed at surgery, the surgeon often observes welling of non-clotted blood in the bony cavity without spurting.[19, 1111] Grossly, the cut section of the lesion appears spongy or honeycomb-like.[19]

Microscopically, the lesion is designated primary or classic ABC if the typical microscopic features are represented throughout the entire specimen. However, when the ABC also has another bone tumor, benign or malignant, the diagnosis of secondary ABC should be rendered. As mentioned previously, about 30% of ABCs are secondary lesions.[1128] Typically, microscopic examination reveals dilated blood, sinusoidal spaces of various sizes that are mostly non-endothelial lined. The surrounding stroma bears close resemblance to giant cell granuloma (GCG) and is composed of spindle-shaped and polygonal macrophage-like cells and multinucleated osteoclastic giant cells interspersed with small vascular spaces (Fig. 8–57).

Reactive osteoid and woven bone, in addition to hemosiderin deposits, are common features. The walls of the dilated sinusoidal spaces do not contain smooth muscle or elastic elements and thus do not mimic blood vessels.[1119–1121]

Treatment and Prognosis. Curettage is the form of therapy that is often utilized and has been associated with high recurrence rate. Rates varying from 21% to 44% have been observed.[1119, 1132, 1133] A recurrence rate of 19% has been reported for ABC of the jaws.[1119] Several factors are suggested as possible risk factors for recurrence, including age of patient, location of lesion,[1133] size of lesion,[1132] and increased mitotic activity.[1134] However, incomplete surgical removal is probably the most important single factor.[1119, 1134]

Cherubism

Clinical Features. Cherubism is a hereditary disease transmitted as an autosomal dominant trait with variable degrees of penetrance in females (50–70%), but with 100% penetrance in males.[1135, 1136] Expressivity varies in different patients. The disease is characterized by bilateral expansion of the jaws caused by giant cell lesions that histologically resemble giant cell granuloma. Expansion of the jaws begins to be noticeable within the first few years of life, becomes progressively larger until puberty, and gradually resolves by middle age. Initially, the lesions may present unilaterally, but they eventually involve both sides of the mandible, particularly at the molar coronoid area. In the maxilla, the tuberosity is involved first but anterior and orbital extensions may follow. A grading system (grade I–IV) for the extent of involvement of the jaws has been proposed.[1137, 1138] The bony expansion is painless and hard. Cortical erosion can occur, which may result in soft tissue extension.[1139, 1140] A blue-gray alveolar ridge swelling can be seen in this case.[1139, 1141] Expansion of the mandible and maxilla leads to facial fullness and occasional encroachment on the orbital bones, producing up-turned eyes in the affected children and resulting in the cherubic appearance from which the disease's name was derived. Involvement of other sites in the skeleton has infrequently been noted, especially in the ribs and long bones.[1141, 1142]

Radiographically, the lesions are expansile and radiolucent, with well-demarcated outlines.[1143, 1144] They may be unilocular but are typically multilocular (Fig. 8–58).[19, 33, 1135, 1137, 1139] The presence of bilateral expansile multilocular radiolucency of the jaws, not involving the condyles in a child, is almost diagnostic of cherubism.[33, 1135, 1137, 1139] Many of the developing teeth may be af-

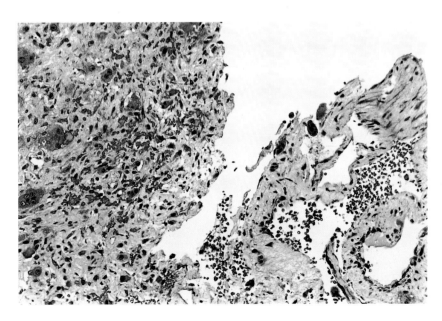

Figure 8–57. Aneurysmal bone cyst of the mandible. Wide sinusoidal spaces are not lined with endothelial cells. The stroma bears close resemblance to giant cell granuloma.

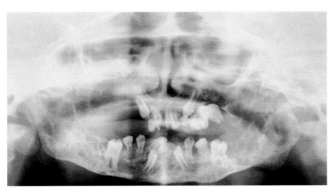

Figure 8–58. Panoramic radiograph of a case of cherubism showing expansive multilocular radiolucent lesions involving mandible and maxilla bilaterally.

fected by the growing lesions, including by misplacement, loss, noneruption, and root resorption.[33, 1135, 1137]

Pathologic Features. The microscopic findings of the lesions in cherubism are essentially similar to giant cell granuloma (see previous discussion).[19, 33] The vascular stroma in cherubism tends to be more loosely arranged, however. The giant cells are few and tend to be small and focally aggregated (Fig. 8–59A).[33, 1135, 1137, 1139]

Eosinophilic cuff-like perivascular deposits are characteristic features of cherubism (Fig. 8–59B), but they are not always present.[33, 1135, 1136, 1139] Hemosiderin deposits and metaplastic bone formation are also noted.

Treatment and Prognosis. Since the pathologic process in cherubism is self-limiting and can even be reversed by age, treatment is dictated by cosmetic and functional needs. Curettage and contouring of bone are the treatments of choice.[33, 1139] Some cases of cherubism show active disease persisting into adult life and cases that showed rapid regrowth after surgical intervention have been reported.[33, 1139, 1142, 1145]

An association between cherubism and Noonan's syndrome, also known as pseudo-Turner's syndrome, has been reported.[33, 1146–1148] The nature and site of the mutations in these two rare syndromes are not as yet known; however, the association may suggest that the mutated genes are probably closely linked.

Brown Tumor of Hyperparathyroidism

Brown tumor is an osseous lesion that develops in bones affected by primary or secondary hyperparathyroidism, as a component of a metabolic bone disease known as osteitis, fibrosa, cystica generalisata, or von Recklinghausen's disease of bone. Brown tumor is cur-

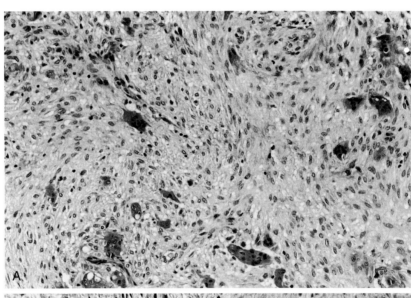
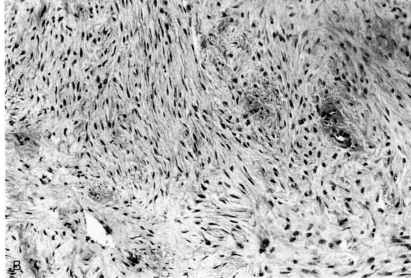

Figure 8–59. *A,* Cherubism. Note sparse giant cells in a background of spindle-shaped and mononuclear cells. *B,* A field showing spindle-shaped cells with characteristic perivascular eosinophilic cuff-like deposits.

rently less frequently encountered since a diagnosis of hyperparathyroidism is now often made on the basis of an elevated serum calcium level in asymptomatic adults.[1149, 1150]

Clinical Features. The lesions may be solitary or multifocal They commonly affect the mandible, clavicle, ribs, and pelvis.[33] In the craniofacial skeletal, the involvement of maxilla, temporal bone, nasal cavity, and paranasal sinuses is noteworthy.[19] Involvement of the orbital bones has also been reported.[1151]

Radiographically, brown tumor is a well-defined lytic lesion that usually causes expansion of the affected bone. It generally assumes a cystic appearance which may be multilocular.[1152] In addition, other associated radiographic signs of hyperparathyroidism are usually present, including subperiosteal resorption, particularly of the phalanges of the index and middle finger, and generalized osteopenia.[33, 1152, 1153] A characteristic radiographic feature in the jaws is the generalized loss of lamina dura surrounding the roots of teeth.

Pathologic Features. Brown tumor of hyperparathyroidism is histologically identical to central giant cell granuloma. It is characterized by intensely vascular fibroblastic stroma serving as background for numerous osteoclast-like multinucleated giant cells. Hemosiderin deposits are common. The vascularity of the lesion and the hemosiderin content impart the color for which the lesion is named.[1153] Some brown tumors, particularly those associated with the metabolic bone disease resulting from chronic renal failure and known as renal osteodystrophy, may be more cellular, with production of reactive trabeculae of woven bone.[33]

Treatment and Prognosis. Treatment is aimed at correction of hyperparathyroidism and management of the metabolic bone disease. Complete resolution of the giant cell lesions is reported to occur within 6 months after removal of a parathyroid adenoma.[1154]

ACKNOWLEDGMENTS

The authors express their appreciation to Dr. William G. Totty, Department of Radiology, Washington University School of Medicine, and Dr. Murali Sundaran, Department of Radiology, St. Louis University School of Medicine, for their help in interpretation of the illustrated radiologic studies, and to Dr. Louis P. Dehner, Department of Pathology, Washington University School of Medicine, for allowing the use of his histologic material to illustrate some of the pediatric soft tissue cases in this chapter.

REFERENCES

Introduction and General Considerations

1. Angervall L, Kindblom L-G: Principles for pathologic-anatomic diagnosis and classification of soft-tissue sarcomas. *Clin Orthop* 1993;289:9–18.
2. Ayala AG, Ro JY, Fanning CV, et al: Core needle biopsy and fine-needle aspiration in the diagnosis of bone and soft-tissue lesions. *Hematol Oncol Clin North Am* 1995;9:633–651.
3. Brooks JSJ: Immunohistochemistry in the differential diagnosis of soft tissue tumors. In: Weiss SW, Brooks JSJ, eds. *Soft Tissue Tumors.* Baltimore: Williams & Wilkins, 1996:65–128.
4. Calonje E, Fletcher CDM: Immunohistochemistry and DNA flow cytometry in soft-tissue sarcomas. *Hematol Oncol Clin North Am* 1995;9:657–674.
5. Coffin CM, Dehner LP, O'Shea PA: *Pediatric Soft Tissue Tumors: A Clinical, Pathological, and Therapeutic Approach.* Baltimore: Williams & Wilkins, 1997.
6. Cooper JE, Allen PW: Low-grade sarcomas. *Pathol Annu* 1990;25(part 2):1–18.
7. Elias AD: Chemotherapy for soft-tissue sarcomas. Clin Orthop 1993;289:94–105.
8. Enzinger FM, Weiss SW: *Soft Tissue Tumors,* 3rd ed. St. Louis: Mosby-Year Book, 1995.
9. Erlandson RA, Rosai J: A realistic approach to the use of electron microscopy and other ancillary diagnostic techniques in surgical pathology. *Am J Surg Pathol* 1995;19:247–250.
10. Farhood AI, Hajdu SI, Shiu MH, et al: Soft tissue sarcomas of the head and neck in adults. *Am J Surg* 1990;160:365–369.
11. Fechner RE, Huvos AG, Mirra JM, et al: A symposium on the pathology of bone tumors. *Pathol Annu* 1984;19(part 1):125–194.
12. Fechner RE, Mills SE: Tumors of the bones and joints. In: *Atlas of Tumor Pathology,* 3rd series, fascicle 8. Washington DC: Armed Forces Institute of Pathology, 1993.
13. Figueiredo MTA, Marques LA, Campos-Filho N: Soft-tissue sarcomas of the head and neck in adults and children: Experience at a single institution with a review of literature. Int J Cancer 1988;41(2):198–200.
14. Fisher C: The value of electromicroscopy and immunohistochemistry in the diagnosis of soft tissue sarcomas: A study of 200 cases. *Histopathology* 1990;16:44154.
15. Fletcher CDM, McKee PH: *Pathobiology of Soft Tissue Tumours.* Edinburgh: Churchill Livingstone, 1990.
16. Goodlad JR, Fletcher CDM: Recent developments in soft tissue tumours. *Histopathology* 1995;27:103–20.
17. Guillou L, Coindre J-M, Bonichon F, et al: Comparative study of the National Cancer Institute and French Federation of Cancer Centers Sarcoma Group grading systems in a population of 410 adult patients with soft tissue sarcoma. *J Clin Oncol* 1997;15:350–362.
18. Harms D, Schmidt D: *Soft Tissue Tumors.* Berlin: Springer-Verlag, 1995.
19. Huvos AG: *Bone Tumors: Diagnosis, Treatment, and Prognosis,* 2nd ed. Philadelphia: WB Saunders, 1991.
20. Jaffe HL: *Tumors and Tumorous Conditions of the Bones and Joints.* Philadelphia: Lea & Febiger, 1958.
21. Jensen OM, Høgh J. Østgaard SE, et al: Histopathological grading of soft tissue tumours. Prognostic significance in a prospective study of 278 consecutive cases. *J Pathol* 1991;163:19–24.
22. Johnson LC, Youseffi M, Viah TN, et al: Juvenile active ossifying fibroma: Its nature dynamics and origin. *Acta Otolaryngol* 1991;488(suppl):1–40.
23. Kempson RL, Hendrickson MR: An approach to the diagnosis of soft tissue tumors. In: Weiss SW, Brooks JSJ, eds. *Soft Tissue Tumors.* Baltimore: Williams & Wilkins, 1996:1–36.
24. Kraus DH, Dubner S, Harrison LB, et al: Prognostic factors for recurrence and survival in head and neck soft tissue sarcomas. *Cancer* 1994;74:697–702.
25. Kyriakos M, Coffin CM, Swanson PE: Diagnostic challenges in soft tissue pathology: A clinicopathologic review of selected lesions. In: Weidner N, ed. *The Difficult Diagnosis in Surgical Pathology.* Philadelphia: WB Saunders, 1996:680–765.
26. Lyos AT, Goepfert H, Luna MA, et al: Soft tissue sarcoma of the head and neck in children and adolescents. *Cancer* 1996;77:193–200.
27. Mackay B: Electron microscopy of soft tissue tumours. In: Fletcher CDM, McKee PH, eds. *Pathology of Soft Tissue Tumors.* Edinburgh: Churchill Livingstone, 1990:199–220.
28. Makek M: *Clinical Pathology of Fibro-osteo-cemental Lesions of the Craniofacial and Jaw Bones.* Basel: Karger, 1983.
29. McCarthy EF: *Differential Diagnosis in Pathology: Bone and Joint Disorders.* New York: Igaku-Shoin, 1996.
30. Miettinen M: Immunohistochemistry of soft-tissue tumors: Possibilities and limitations in surgical pathology. *Pathol Annu* 1990;25(part 1):1–36.
31. Mirra JM: *Bone Tumors: Clinical, Radiologic, and Pathologic Correlations.* Philadelphia: Lea & Febiger, 1989.
32. Mulder JD, Kroon HM, Schütte HE, et al: *Radiologic Atlas of Bone Tumors.* Amsterdam: Elsevier, 1993.
33. Nevill BW, Damm DD, Allen CM, et al: *Oral and Maxillofacial Pathology.* Philadelphia: WB Saunders, 1995.
34. Resnick D, Kyriakos M, Greenway GD: Tumors and tumor-like lesions of bone: Imaging and pathology of specific lesions. In: Resnick D, ed. *Diagnosis of Bone and Joint Disorders,* 3rd ed, vol. 6. Philadelphia: WB Saunders, 1995.
35. Schajowicz F: *Tumors and Tumorlike Lesions of Bone: Pathology, Radiology, and Treatment,* 2nd ed. New York: Springer-Verlag, 1994.
36. Tran LM, Mark R, Meier R, et al: Sarcomas of the head and neck. Prognostic factors and treatment strategies. *Cancer* 1992;70:169–177.
37. Unni KK: *Bone Tumors.* Edinburgh: Churchill Livingstone, 1988.

38. Unni KK: *Dahlin's Bone Tumors: General Aspects and Data on 11,087 Cases,* 5th ed. Philadelphia: Lippincott-Raven, 1996.
39. Unni KK, Dahlin DC: Premalignant tumors and conditions of bone. *Am J Surg* Pathol 1979;3:47–60.
40. Waldron CA: Fibro-osseous lesions of the jaws. *J Oral Maxillofac Surg* 1985;43:249–262.
41. Wanebo HJ, Koness RJ, MacFarlane JK, et al: Head and neck sarcomas: Report of the head and neck sarcoma registry. *Head Neck* 1992;14:1–7.
42. Weiss SW, Brooks JSJ: *Soft Tissue Tumors.* Baltimore: Williams & Wilkins, 1996.

Soft Tissue Lesions

Lesions of Fibrous Tissue

Fibrosarcoma

43. Scott SM, Reiman HM, Pritchard DJ, et al: Soft tissue fibrosarcoma. A clinicopathologic study of 132 cases. *Cancer* 1989;64:925–931.
44. Iwasaki H, Enjoji M: Infantile and adult fibrosarcomas of the soft tissues. *Acta Pathol Jpn* 1979;29:377–388.
45. Pritchard DJ, Soule EH, Taylor WF, et al: Fibrosarcoma: A clinicopathologic and statistical study of 199 tumors of the soft tissues of the extremities and trunk. *Cancer* 1974;33:888–897.
46. Chung EB, Enzinger FM: Infantile fibrosarcoma. *Cancer* 1976; 38:729–739.
47. Soule EH, Pritchard DJ: Fibrosarcoma in infants and children. *Cancer* 1977;40:1711–1721.
48. Coffin CM, Dehner LP: Fibroblastic-myofibroblastic tumors in children and adolescents: A clinicopathologic study of 108 examples in 103 patients. Pediatr Pathol 1991;11:559–588.
49. Coffin CM, Jaszcz W, O'Shea PA, et al: So-called congenital-infantile fibrosarcoma: Does it exist and what is it? Pediatr Pathol 1994; 14:133–150.
50. Balsaver AM, Butler JJ, Martin RG: Congenital fibrosarcoma. *Cancer* 1967;20:1607–1616.
51. Mark RJ, Sercarz JA, Tran L, et al: Fibrosarcoma of the head and neck. *Arch Otolaryngol Head Neck Surg* 1991;117:396–401.
52. Conley J, Stout AP, Healey WV: Clinicopathologic analysis of eighty-four patients with an original diagnosis of fibrosarcoma of the head and neck. *Am J Surg* 1967;114:564–569.
53. Das Gupta TK: *Tumors of the Soft Tissues.* Norwalk, CT: Appleton-Century-Crofts, 1983.
54. Batsakis JG: *Tumors of the Head and Neck: Clinical and Pathological Considerations,* 2nd ed. Baltimore: Williams & Wilkins, 1979.
55. Swain RE, Sessions DG, Ogura JH: Fibrosarcoma of the head and neck: A clinical analysis of forty cases. *Ann Otol* 1974;83:439–444.
56. Heffner DK, Gnepp DR: Sinonasal fibrosarcomas, malignant schwannomas, and "Triton" tumors. A clinicopathologic study of 67 cases. *Cancer* 1992;70:1089–1101.
57. Rockley TJ, Liu KC: Fibrosarcoma of the nose and paranasal sinuses. *J Laryngol Otol* 1986;100:1417–1420.
58. Mandahl N, Heim S, Rydholm A, et al: Nonrandom numerical chromosome aberrations (+8, +11, +17, +20) in infantile fibrosarcoma. *Cancer Genet Cytogenet* 1989;40:137–139.
59. Davies DG: Fibrosarcoma and pseudosarcoma of the larynx. *J Laryngol Otol* 1969;83:423–434.
60. Fu Y-S, Perzin KH: Nonepithelial tumors of the nasal cavity, paranasal sinuses, and nasopharynx. A clinicopathologic study. VI. Fibrous tissue tumors (fibroma, fibromatosis, fibrosarcoma). *Cancer* 1976; 37:2912–2928.
61. Churg AM, Kahn LB: Myofibroblasts and related cells in malignant fibrous and fibrohistiocytic tumors. *Hum Pathol* 1977;8:205–218.
62. Lagacé R, Schürch W, Seemayer TA: Myofibroblasts in soft tissue sarcomas. *Virchows Arch (Pathol Anat)* 1980;389a:1–11.
63. Schofield DE, Fletcher JA, Grier HE, et al: Fibrosarcoma in infants and children: Application of new techniques. *Am J Surg Pathol* 1994;18:14–24.
64. Smith DM, Mahmoud HH, Jenkins JJ, et al: Myofibrosarcoma of the head and neck in children. *Pediatr Pathol Lab Med* 1995;15:403–418.
65. Fisher C: Fibromatosis and fibrosarcoma in infancy and childhood. *Eur J Cancer* 1996;32a:2094–2100.
66. Rosenberg HS, Stenback WA, Sojut HJ: The fibromatoses of infancy and childhood. In: Rosenberg HS, Bolande RP, eds. *Perspectives in Pediatric Pathology.* Chicago: Year Book Medical Publishers 1978;4:269–348.

Fibromatosis

67. Allen PW: The fibromatoses: A clinicopathologic classification based on 140 cases. *Am J Surg Pathol* 1977;1:255;305–321.
68. Mackenzie DH: The fibromatoses: A clinicopathological concept. *Br Med J* 1972;4:277–281.
69. Mackenzie DH: The differential diagnosis of fibroblastic disorders. Oxford: Blackwell Scientific Publications, 1970.
70. Enzinger FM, Shiraki M: Musculo-aponeurotic fibromatosis of the shoulder girdle (extra-abdominal desmoid): Analysis of thirty cases followed up to ten or more years. Cancer 1967;20:1131–1140.
71. Jones IT, Jagelman DG, Fazio VW, et al: Desmoid tumors in familial polyposis coli. *Ann Surg* 1986;204:94–97.
72. Khorsand J, Karakousis CP: Desmoid tumors and their management. *Am J Surg* 1985;149:215–218.
73. Kiel KD, Suit HD: Radiation therapy in the treatment of aggressive fibromatoses (desmoid tumors). *Cancer* 1984;54:2051–2055.
74. Rock MG, Pritchard DJ, Reiman HM, et al: Extra-abdominal desmoid tumors. *J Bone Joint Surg Am* 1984;66:1369–1374.
75. Cole NM, Guiss LW: Extra-abdominal desmoid tumors. *Arch Surg* 1969;98:530–533.
76. Conley J, Healey WV, Stout AP: Fibromatosis of the head and neck. *Am J Surg* 1966;112:609–614.
77. Das Gupta TK, Brasfield RD, O'Hara J: Extra-abdominal desmoids: A clinicopathological study. *Ann Surg* 1969;170:109–121.
78. Masson JK, Soule EH: Desmoid tumors of the head and neck. *Am J Surg* 1966;112:615–622.
79. Fowler CB, Hartman KS, Brannon RB: Fibromatosis of the oral and paraoral region. *Oral Surg Oral Med Oral Pathol* 1994;77: 373–386.
80. Vally IM, Altini M: Fibromatoses of the oral and paraoral soft tissues and jaws. Review of the literature and report of 12 new cases. *Oral Surg Oral Med Oral Pathol* 1990;69:191–198.
81. Gnepp DR, Henley J, Weiss S, et al: Desmoid fibromatosis of the sinonasal tract and nasopharynx. *Cancer* 1996;78:2572–2579.
82. Ayala AG, Ro JY, Goepfert H, et al: Desmoid fibromatosis: A clinicopathologic study of 25 children. *Semin Diagn Pathol* 1986;3:138–150.
83. Hunt RTN, Morgan HC, Ackerman LV: Principles in the management of extra-abdominal desmoids. *Cancer* 1960;13:825–836.
84. Zachariades N, Papanicolaou S: Juvenile fibromatosis. *J Craniomaxillofac Surg* 1988;16:130–135.
85. Ben-Izhak O, Kuten A, Pery M, et al: Fibromatosis (desmoid tumor) following radiation therapy for Hodgkin's disease. *Arch Pathol Lab Med* 1994;118:815–818.
86. Fletcher CDM, Stirling RW, Smith MA, et al: Multicentric extra-abdominal 'myofibromatosis': Report of a case with ultrastructural findings. *Histopathology* 1986;10:713–724.
87. Fong Y, Rosen PP, Brennan MF: Multifocal desmoids. Surgery 1993;114:902–906.
88. Zayid I, Dihmis C: Familial multicentric fibromatosis—desmoids: A report of three cases in a Jordanian family. *Cancer* 1969;24:786–795.
89. Navas-Palacios JJ.: The fibromatoses: An ultrastructural study of 31 cases. *Pathol Res Pract* 1983;176:158–175.
90. Bridge JA, Meloni AM, Neff JR, et al: Deletion 5q in desmoid tumor and fluorescence in situ hybridization for chromosome 8 and/or 20 copy number. *Cancer Genet Cytogenet* 1996;92:150–151.
91. Qi H, Dal Cin P, Hernández JM, et al: Trisomies 8 and 20 in desmoid tumors. *Cancer Genet Cytogenet* 1996;92:147–149.
92. Li M, Cordon-Cardo C, Gerald WL, et al: Desmoid fibromatosis is a clonal process. *Hum Pathol* 1996;27:939–943.
93. Miralbell R, Suit HD, Mankin HJ: Fibromatoses: From postsurgical surveillance to combined surgery and radiation therapy. *Int J Radiat Oncol Biol Phys* 1990;18:535–540.
94. Dominguez-Malagon HR, Alfeiran-Ruiz A, Chavarria-Xicotencatl P, et al: Clinical and cellular effects of colchicine in fibromatosis. *Cancer* 1992;69:2478–2483.
95. Klein WA, Miller HH, Anderson M: The use of indomethacin, sulindac, and tamoxifen for the treatment of desmoid tumors associated with familial polyposis. *Cancer* 1987;60:2863–2868.
96. Lanari A: Effect of progesterone on desmoid tumors (aggressive fibromatosis). *N Engl J Med* 1983;309:1523.
97. Leibel SA, Wara WM, Hill DR: Desmoid tumors: Local control and patterns of relapse following radiation therapy. *Int J Radiat Oncol Biol Phys* 1983;9:1167–1171.
98. Sherman NE, Romsdahl M, Evans H, et al: Desmoid tumors: A 20-year radiotherapy experience. *Int J Radiat Oncol Biol Phys* 1990;19:37–40.

99. Patel SR, Evans HL, Benjamin RS: Combination chemotherapy in adult desmoid tumors. *Cancer* 1993;72:3244–3247.

100. Weiss AJ, Lackman RD: Low-dose chemotherapy of desmoid tumors. *Cancer* 1989;64:1192–1194.

101. Stout AP: Juvenile fibromatosis. *Cancer* 1954;7:953–978.

102. Hoffman CD, Levant BA, Hall RK: Aggressive infantile fibromatosis: Report of a case undergoing spontaneous regression. *J Oral Maxillofac Surg* 1993;51:1043–1047.

103. Thompson DH, Khan A, Gonzalez C, et al: Juvenile aggressive fibromatosis: Report of three cases and review of the literature. *Ear Nose Throat J* 1991;70:462–468.

104. Naidu RK, Aviv JE, Lawson W, et al: Aggressive juvenile fibromatosis involving the paranasal sinuses. *Otolaryngol Head Neck Surg* 1991;104:549–552.

105. Tagawa T, Ohse S, Hirano Y, et al: Aggressive infantile fibromatosis of the submandibular region. *Int J Oral Maxillofac Surg* 1989;18:264–265.

106. Shah AC, Katz RL: Infantile aggressive fibromatosis of the base of the tongue. *Otolaryngol Head Neck Surg* 1988;98:346–349.

107. Fata JJ, Rabuzzi DD: Aggressive juvenile fibromatosis presenting as a parotid mass. *Ear Nose Throat J* 1988;67:680–686.

108. Peede LF Jr, Epker BN: Aggressive juvenile fibromatosis involving the mandible: Surgical excision with immediate reconstruction. *Oral Surg Oral Med Oral Pathol* 1977;43:651–657.

109. Wilkins SA Jr, Waldron CA, Mathews WH, et al: Aggresive fibromatosis of the head and neck. *Am J Surg* 1975;130:412–415.

110. Dehner LP, Askin FB: Tumors of fibrous tissue origin in childhood: A clinicopathologic study of cutaneous and soft tissue neoplasms in 66 children. *Cancer* 1976;38:888–900.

111. Coffin CM, Dehner LP: Fibroblastic-myofibroblastic tumors in children and adolescents: A clinicopathologic study of 108 examples in 103 patients. *Pediatr Pathol* 1991;11:569–588.

112. Kauffman SL, Stout AP: Congenital mesenchymal tumors. *Cancer* 1965;18:460–476.

113. Hidayat AA, Font RL: Juvenile fibromatosis of the periorbital region and eyelid. A clinicopathologic study of six cases. *Arch Ophthalmol* 1980;98:280–285.

114. Melrose RJ, Abrams AM: Juvenile fibromatosis affecting the jaws: Report of three cases. *Oral Surg Oral Med Oral Pathol* 1980;49:317–324.

115. Carr RJ, Zaki GA, Leader MB, et al: Infantile fibromatosis with involvement of the mandible. *Br J Oral Maxillofac Surg* 1992;30:257–262.

116. Takagi M, Ishikawa G: Fibrous tumor of infancy: Report of a case originating in the oral cavity. *J Oral Pathol* 1973;2:293–300.

117. Rodu B, Weathers DR, Campbell WG Jr: Aggressive fibromatosis involving the paramandibular soft tissues. *Oral Surg Oral Med Oral Pathol* 1981;52:395–403.

118. Goepfert H, Cangir A, Ayala AG, et al: Preoperative chemotherapy and surgical resection for aggressive fibromatosis of the head and neck: A case report. 1978;86:656–658.

119. Schmidt D, Klinge P, Leuschner I, et al: Infantile desmoid-type fibromatosis. Morphological features correlate with biological behaviour. *J Pathol* 1991;164:315–319.

120. Hulbert KF: Congenital torticollis. *J Bone Joint Surg Br* 1950;32:50–59.

121. Cheng JCY, Au AWY: Infantile torticollis: A review of 624 cases. *J Pediatr Orthop* 1994;14:802–808.

122. Thomsen JR, Koltai PJ: Sternomastoid tumor of infancy. *Ann Otol Rhinol Laryngol* 1989;98:955–959.

123. Tom LWC, Handler SD, Wetmore RF, et al: The sternocleiodomastoid tumor of infancy. *Int J Pediatr Otorhinolaryngol* 1987;13:245–255.

124. Armstrong D, Pickrell K, Fetter B, et al: Torticollis: An analysis of 271 cases. *Plast Reconstr Surg* 1965;35:14–25.

125. Chandler FA: Muscular torticollis. *J Bone Joint Surg Am* 1948;38:566–588.

126. Fitzsimmons HJ: Congenital torticollis. Review of the pathological aspects. *N Engl J Med* 1933;209:66–71.

127. Coventry MB, Harris LE: Congenital muscular torticollis in infancy. Some observations regarding treatment. *J Bone Joint Surg Am* 1959;41:815–822.

128. Macdonald D: Sternomastoid tumour and muscular torticollis. *J Bone Joint Surg Br* 1969;51:432–443.

129. Binder H, Eng GD, Gaiser JF, et al: Congenital muscular torticollis: Results of conservative management with long-term follow-up in 85 cases. *Arch Phys Med Rehabil* 1987;68:222–225.

130. Iwahara T, Ikeda A: On the ipsilateral involvement of congenital muscular torticollis and congenital dislocation of the hip. *J Jpn Orthop Assoc* 1962;35:1221–1226.

131. Morrison DL, MacEwen GD: Congenital muscular torticollis: Observations regarding clinical findings, associated conditions, and results of treatment. *J Pediatr Orthop* 1982;2:500–505.

132. Coffin CM, Dehner LP: Soft tissue tumors in first year of life: A report of 190 cases. *Pediatr Pathol* 1990;10:509–526.

133. Chung EB, Enzinger FM: Infantile myofibromatosis. *Cancer* 1981;48:1807–1818.

134. Wiswell TE, Davis J, Cunningham BE, et al: Infantile myofibromatosis: The most common fibrous tumor of infancy. *J Pediatr Surg* 1988;23:314–318.

135. Bračko M, Cindro L, Golouh R: Familial occurrence of infantile myofibromatosis. *Cancer* 1992;69:1294–1299.

136. Dimmick JE, Wood WS: Congenital multiple fibromatosis. *Am J Dermatopathol* 1983;5:289–295.

137. Kindblom L-G, Angervall L: Congenital solitary fibromatosis of the skeleton. Case report of a variant of congenital generalized fibromatosis. *Cancer* 1978;41:636–640.

138. Briselli MF, Soule EH, Gilchrist GS: Congenital fibromatosis: Report of 18 cases of solitary and 4 cases of multiple tumors. *Mayo Clin Proc* 1980;55:554–562.

139. Kindblom L-G, Termén G, Säve-Soderbergh J, et al: Congenital solitary fibromatosis of soft tissue, a variant of congenital generalized fibromatosis. *Acta Pathol Microbiol Scand* 1977;85:640–648.

140. Aneiros J, Martinez de Victoria J, Redondo E, et al: Infantile myofibromatosis: Histogenesis. *Histopathology* 1987;11:1223–1224.

141. Beham A, Badve S, Suster S, et al: Solitary myofibroma in adults: Clinicopathological analysis of a series. *Histopathology* 1993;22:335–341.

142. Daimaru Y, Hashimoto H, Enjoji M: Myofibromatosis in adults (adult counterpart of infantile myofibromatosis). *Am J Surg Pathol* 1989;13:859–865.

143. Fletcher CDM, Achu P, Van Noorden S, et al: Infantile myofibromatosis: A light microscopic, histochemical and immunohistochemical study suggesting true smooth muscle differentiation. *Histopathology* 1987;11:245–258.

144. Hasegawa T, Hirose T, Seki K, et al: Solitary infantile myofibromatosis of bone. An immunohistochemical and ultrastructural study. *Am J Surg Pathol* 1993;17:308–313.

145. Hogan SF, Salassa JR: Recurrent adult myofibromatosis. A case report. *Am J Clin Pathol* 1992;97:810–814.

146. Inwards CY, Unni KK, Beabout JW, et al: Solitary congenital fibromatosis (infantile myofibromatosis) of bone. *Am J Surg Pathol* 1991;15:935–941.

147. Jennings TA, Duray PH, Collins FS, et al: Infantile myofibromatosis. Evidence for an autosomal-dominant disorder. *Am J Surg Pathol* 1984;8:529–538.

148. Matthews MS, Tabor MW, Thompson SH, et al: Infantile myofibromatosis of the mandible. *J Oral Maxillofac Surg* 1990;48:884–889.

149. Mizobuchi K, Yoshino T, Ikehara I, et al: Infantile myofibromatosis: Report of two cases. *Acta Pathol Jpn* 1986;36:1411–1418.

150. Sleeman DJ, Eveson JW: Solitary infantile myofibromatosis. *Br J Oral Maxillofac Surg* 1991;29:277–278.

151. Smith KJ, Skelton HG, Barrett TL, et al: Cutaneous myofibroma. *Mod Pathol* 1989;2:603–609.

152. Speight PM, Dayan D, Fletcher CDM: Adult and infantile myofibromatosis: A report of three cases affecting the oral cavity. *J Oral Pathol Med* 1991;20:380–384.

153. Vigneswaran N, Boyd DL, Waldron CA: Solitary infantile myofibromatosis of the mandible. Report of three cases. *Oral Surg Oral Med Oral Pathol* 1992;73:84–88.

154. Wolfe JT, III, Cooper PH: Solitary cutaneous "infantile" myofibroma in a 49-year-old woman. *Hum Pathol* 1990;21:562–564.

155. Baer JW, Radkowski MA: Congenital multiple fibromatosis: A case report with review of the world literature. *AJR* 1973;118:200–205.

156. Brill PW, Yandow DR, Langer LO, et al: Congenital generalized fibromatosis. Case report and literature review. *Pediatr Radiol* 1982;12:269–278.

157. Soper JR, De Silva M: Infantile myofibromatosis: A radiological review. *Pediatr Radiol* 1993;23:189–194.

158. Roggli VL, Kim H-S, Hawkins E: Congenital generalized fibromatosis with visceral involvement. A case report. *Cancer* 1980;45:954–960.

159. Coffin CM, Neilson KA, Ingels S, et al: Congenital generalized myo-

fibromatosis: A disseminated angiocentric myofibromatosis. *Pediatr Pathol* 1995;15:571–587.

160. Mentzel T, Calonje E, Nascimento AG, et al: Infantile hemangiopericytoma versus infantile myofibromatosis. Study of a series suggesting a continuous spectrum of infantile myofibroblastic lesions. *Am J Surg Pathol* 1994;18:922–930.

161. Variend S, Bax NMA, Van Gorp J: Are infantile myofibromatosis, congenital fibrosarcoma, and congenital haemangiopericytoma histogenetically related? *Histopathology* 1995;26:57–62.

Pseudosarcomatous Fibrous Lesions

162. Chung EB, Enzinger FM: Proliferative fasciitis. *Cancer* 1975; 36:1450–1458.

163. Dahl I, Angervall L: Pseudosarcomatous proliferative lesions of soft tissue with or without bone formation. *Acta Pathol Microbiol Scand* 1977;85:577–589.

164. Enzinger FM, Dulcy F: Proliferative myositis. Report of thirty-three cases. *Cancer* 1967;20:2213–2223.

165. Kitano M, Iwasaki H, Enjoji M: Proliferative fasciitis. A variant of nodular fasciitis. *Acta Pathol Jpn* 1977;27:485–493.

166. Patchefsky AS, Enzinger FM: Intravascular fasciitis: A report of 17 cases. *Am J Surg Pathol* 1981;5:29–36.

167. Dahl I, Angervall L: Pseudosarcomatous lesions of the soft tissues reported as sarcoma during a 6-year period (1958–1963). *Acta Pathol Microbiol Scand* 1977;85:917–930.

168. Meister P, Bückmann F-W, Konrad E: Nodular fasciitis (analysis of 100 cases and review of the literature). *Pathol Res Pract* 1978;162:133–165.

169. Kleinstiver BJ, Rodriquez HA: Nodular fasciitis: A study of forty-five cases and review of the literature. *J Bone Joint Surg Am* 1968;50:1204–1212.

170. Stout AP: Pseudosarcomatous fasciitis in children. *Cancer* 1961; 14:1216–1212.

171. Dahl I, Jarlstedt J: Nodular fasciitis in the head and neck. A clinicopathological study of 18 cases. *Acta Otolaryngol* 1980;90:152–159.

172. Montgomery EA, Meis JM: Nodular fasciitis. Its morphologic spectrum and immunohistochemical profile. *Am J Surg Pathol* 1991; 15:942–948.

173. Shimizu S, Hashimoto H, Enjoji M: Nodular fasciitis: An analysis of 250 patients. *Pathology* 1984;16:161–166.

174. Allen PW: Nodular fascitis. *Pathology* 1972;4:9–26.

175. Bernstein KE, Lattes R: Nodular (pseudosarcomatous) fasciitis, a nonrecurrent lesion: Clinicopathologic study of 134 cases. *Cancer* 1982;49:1668–1678.

176. Batsakis JG, El-Naggar AK: Pseudosarcomatous proliferative lesions of soft tissues. *Ann Otol Rhinol Laryngol* 1994;103:578–582.

177. DiNardo LJ, Wetmore RF, Potsic WP: Nodular fasciitis of the head and neck in children. *Arch Otolaryngol Head Neck Surg* 1991;117:1001–1002.

178. Fischer JR, Abdul-Karim FW, Robinson RA: Intraparotid nodular fasciitis. *Arch Pathol Lab Med* 1989;113:1276–1278.

179. Chen KTK, Bauer V: Nodular fasciitis presenting as parotid tumor. *Am J Otolaryngol* 1987;8:179–181.

180. Shlomi B, Mintz S, Jossiphov J, et al: Immunohistochemical analysis of a case of intraoral nodular fasciitis. *J Oral Maxillofac Surg* 1994;52:323–326.

181. Werning JT: Nodular fasciitis of the orofacial region. *Oral Surg* 1979;48:441–446.

182. Bodner L, Dayan D: Nodular fasciitis of the oral mucosa: Light and electron microscopy study. *Head Neck* 1991;13:434–438.

183. Davies HT, Bradley N, Bowerman JE: Oral nodular fasciitis. *Br J Oral Maxillofac Surg* 1989;27:147–151.

184. Kawana T, Yamamoto H, Deguchi A, et al: Nodular fasciitis of the upper labial fascia: Cytometric and ultrastructural studies. *Int J Oral Maxillofac Surg* 1986;15:464–468.

185. Mostofi RS, Soltani K, Beste L, et al: Intraoral periosteal nodular fasciitis. *Int J Oral Maxillofac Surg* 1987;16:505–509.

186. Freedman PD, Lumerman H: Intravascular fasciitis: Report of two cases and review of the literature. *Oral Surg* 1986;62:549–554.

187. Kahn MA, Weathers DR, Johnson DM: Intravascular fasciitis: A case report of an intraoral location. *J Oral Pathol* 1987;16:303–306.

188. Lauer DH, Enzinger FM: Cranial fasciitis of childhood. *Cancer* 1980;45:401–406.

189. Barohn RJ, Kasdon DL: Cranial fasciitis: Nodular fasciitis of the head. *Surg Neurol* 1980;13:283–285.

190. Coates DB, Faught P, Sadove AM: Cranial fasciitis of childhood. *Plast Reconstr Surg* 1990;85:602–605.

191. Hunter NS, Bulas DI, Chadduck WM, et al: Cranial fasciitis of childhood. *Pediatr Radiol* 1993;23:398–399.

192. Inamura T, Takeshita I, Nishio S, et al: Cranial fasciitis: Case report. *Neurosurgery* 1991;28:888–889.

193. Kumon Y, Sakaki S, Sakoh M, et al: Cranial fasciitis of childhood: A case report. *Surg Neurol* 1992 38:68–72.

194. Mollejo M, Milán JM, Ballestin C, et al: Cranial fasciitis of childhood with reactive periostitis. *Surg Neurol* 1990;33:146–149.

195. Patterson JW, Moran SL, Konerding H: Cranial fasciitis. *Arch Dermatol* 1989;125:674–678.

196. Ringsted J, Ladefoged C, Bjerre P: Cranial fasciitis of childhood. *Acta Neuropathol (Berl)* 1985;66:337–339.

197. Sato Y, Kitamura T, Suganuma Y, et al: Cranial fasciitis of childhood: A case report. *Eur J Pediatr Surg* 1993;3:107–109.

198. Meister P, Konrad EA, Buckman FW: Nodular fasciitis and proliferative myositis as variants of one disease entity. *Invest Cell Pathol* 1979;2:277–281.

199. Diaz-Flores L, Herrera AIM, Montelongo RG, et al: Proliferative fasciitis: Ultrastructure and histogenesis. *J Cutan Pathol* 1989;16: 85–92.

200. El-Jabbour JN, Bennett MH, Burke MM, et al: Proliferative myositis. An immunohistochemical and ultrastructural study. *Am J Surg Pathol* 1991;15:654–659.

201. Ushigome S, Takakuwa T, Takagi M, et al: Proliferative myositis and fasciitis. Report of five cases with an ultrastructural and immunohistochemical study. *Acta Pathol Jpn* 1986;26:963–971.

202. Meis JM, Enzinger FM: Proliferative fasciitis and myositis of childhood. *Am J Surg Pathol* 1992;16:364–372.

Synovial Sarcoma

203. Cadman NL, Soule EH, Kelly PJ: Synovial sarcoma. An analysis of 134 tumors. Cancer 1965;18:613–627.

204. Stout AP, Lattes R: Tumors of the soft tissues. In: *Atlas of Tumor Pathology*, 2nd series, fascicle I. Washington DC: Armed Forces Institute of Pathology, 1967.

205. Mackenzie DH: Monophasic synovial sarcoma: A histological entity? *Histopathology* 1977;1:151–157.

206. Roth JA, Enzinger FM, Tannenbam M: Synovial sarcoma of the neck: A follow up study of 24 cases. *Cancer* 1975;35:1243–1253.

207. Lockey MW: Rare tumors of the ear, nose and throat: Synovial sarcoma of the head and neck. *South Med J* 1976;69:316–320.

208. Amble FR, Olsen KD, Nascimento AG, et al: Head and neck synovial cell sarcoma. *Otolaryngol Head Neck Surg* 1992;107:631–637.

209. Chew KK, Sethi DS, Stanley RE, et al: View from beneath: Pathology in focus. Synovial sarcoma of hypopharynx. *J Laryngol Otol* 1992;106:285–287.

210. Nunez-Alonso C, Gashti EN, Christ ML: Maxillofacial synovial sarcoma: Light- and electron-microscopic study of two cases. *Am J Surg Pathol* 1979;3:23–30.

211. Bukachevsky RP, Pincus RL, Shechtman FG, et al: Synovial sarcoma of the head and neck. *Head Neck* 1992;14:44–48.

212. Mamelle G, Richard J, Luboinski B, et al: Synovial sarcoma of the head and neck: An account of four cases and review of the literature. *Eur J Surg Oncol* 1986;12:347–349.

213. Moore DM, Berke GS: Synovial sarcoma of the head and neck. *Arch Otolaryngol Head Neck Surg* 1987;113:311–333.

214. Pai S, Chinoy RF, Pradhan SA, et al: Head and neck synovial sarcomas. *J Surg Oncol* 1993;54:82–86.

215. Shmookler BM, Enzinger FM, Brannon RB: Orofacial synovial sarcoma. *Cancer* 1982;50:269–276.

216. Morland B, Cox G, Randall C, et al: Synovial sarcoma of the larynx in a child: Case report and histological appearances. *Med Pediatr Oncol* 1994;23:64–68.

217. Dardick I, Ramjohn S, Thomas MJ, et al: Synovial sarcoma. Interrelationship of the biphasic and monophasic subtypes. *Pathol Res Pract* 1991;187:871–885.

218. Ladenstein R, Treuner J, Koscielniak E, et al: Synovial sarcoma of childhood and adolescence. Report of the German CWS-81 study. *Cancer* 1993;71:3647–3655.

219. Lopes JM, Bjerkehagen B, Holm R, et al: Immunohistochemical profile of synovial sarcoma with emphasis on the epithelial-type differentiation. A study of 49 primary tumours, recurrences and metastases. *Pathol Res Pract* 1994;190:168–177.

220. Oda Y, Hashimoto H, Tsuneyoshi M, et al: Survival in synovial sarcoma. A multivariate study of prognostic factors with special emphasis on the comparison between early death and long-term survival. *Am J Surg Pathol* 1993;17:35–44.

221. Ordóñez NG, Mahfouz SM, Mackay B: Synovial sarcoma: An immunohistochemical and ultrastructural study. *Hum Pathol* 1990;21:733–749.

222. Jacobs LA, Weaver AW, Synovial sarcoma of the head and neck. *Am J Surg* 1974;128:527–529.

223. Cagle LA, Mirra JM, Storm FK, et al: Histologic features relating to prognosis in synovial sarcoma. *Cancer* 1987;59:1810–1814.

224. El-Naggar AK, Ayala AG, Abdul-Karim FW, et al: Synovial sarcoma. A DNA flow cytometric study. *Cancer* 1990;65:2295–3000.

225. Fisher C: Synovial sarcoma: Ultrastructural and immunohistochemical features of epithelial differentiation in monophasic and biphasic tumors. *Hum Pathol* 1986;17:996–1008.

226. Harrison EG Jr, Black BM, Devine KD: Synovial sarcoma primary in the neck. *Arch Pathol* 1961;71:137–141.

227. Carrillo R, El-Naggar AK, Rodriguez-Peralto JL, et al: Synovial sarcoma of the tongue: Case report and review of the literature. *J Oral Maxillofac Surg* 1992;50:904–906.

228. Miloro M, Quinn PD, Stewart JC: Monophasic spindle cell synovial sarcoma of the head and neck: Report of two cases and review of the literature. *J Oral Maxillofac Surg* 1994;52:309–313.

229. Varela-Duran J, Enzinger FM: Calcifying synovial sarcoma. *Cancer* 1982;50:345–352.

230. Carrillo R, Rodriguez-Peralto JL, Batsakis JG: Synovial sarcomas of the head and neck. *Ann Otol Rhinol Laryngol* 1992;101:367–370.

231. Milchgrub S, Ghandur-Mnaymneh L, Dorfman HD, et al: Synovial sarcoma with extensive osteoid and bone formation. *Am J Surg Pathol* 1993;17:357–363.

232. Hajdu SI, Shiu MH, Fortner JG: Tendosynovial sarcoma: A clinicopathological study of 136 cases. *Cancer* 1977;39:1201–1207.

233. Farris KB, Reed RJ: Monophasic, glandular, synovial sarcomas and carcinomas of the soft tissues. *Arch Pathol Lab Med* 1982;106:129–132.

234. Limon J, Mrozek K, Mandahl N, et al: Cytogenetics of synovial sarcoma: Presentation of ten new cases and review of the literature. *Genes Chromosome Cancer* 1991;3:338–345.

235. Smith S, Reeves BR, Wong L, et al: A consistent chromosome translocation in synovial sarcoma. *Cancer Genet Cytogenet* 1987;26:179–180.

236. Turc-Carel C, Cin PD, Limon J, et al: Translocation X;18 in synovial sarcoma. *Cancer Genet Cytogenet* 1986;23:93.

237. Dickersin GR: Synovial sarcoma: A review and update, with emphasis on the ultrastructural characterization of the nonglandular component. *Ultrastruct Pathol* 1991;15:379–402.

238. Salisbury JR, Isaacson PG: Synovial sarcoma: An immunohistochemical study. *J Pathol* 1985;147:49–57.

239. Hazelbag HM, Mooi WJ, Fleuren GJ, et al: Chain-specific keratin profile of epithelioid soft-tissue sarcomas. An immunohistochemical study on synovial sarcoma and epithelioid sarcoma. *Appl Immunohistochem* 1996;4:176–183.

240. Miettinen M: Keratin subsets in spindle cell sarcomas. Keratins are widespread but synovial sarcoma contains a distinctive keratin polypeptide pattern and desmoplakins. *Am J Pathol* 1991;138:505–513.

241. Fisher C, Schofield JB: S-100 protein positive synovial sarcoma. *Histopathology* 1991;19:375–377.

242. Guillou L, Wadden C, Kraus MD, et al: S-100 protein reactivity in synovial sarcomas: A potentially frequent diagnostic pitfall. Immunohistochemical analysis of 100 cases. *Appl Immunohistochem* 1996;4:167–175.

243. Dei Tos AP, Wadden C, Calonje E, et al: Immunohistochemical demonstration of glycoprotein p30/32^{MIC2} (CD99) in synovial sarcoma. A potential cause of diagnostic confusion. *Appl Immunohistochem* 1995;3:168–173.

244. Renshaw AA: 013 (CD99) in spindle cell tumors. Reactivity with hemangiopericytoma, solitary fibrous tumor, synovial sarcoma, and meningioma but rarely with sarcomatoid mesothelioma. *Appl Immunohistochem* 1995;3:250–256.

245. Lopes JM, Bjerkehagen B, Sobrinho-Simoes M, et al: The ultrastructural spectrum of synovial sarcomas: A study of the epithelial type differentiation of primary tumors, recurrences, and metastases. *Ultrastruct Pathol* 1993;17:137–151.

246. Rosen G, Forscher C, Lowenbraun S, et al: Synovial sarcoma. Uniform response of metastases to high dose ifosfamide. *Cancer* 1994;73:2506–2511.

247. Singer S, Baldini EH, Demetri GD, et al: Synovial sarcoma: Prognostic significance of tumor size, margin of resection, and mitotic activity for survival. *J Clin Oncol* 1996;14:1201–1208.

Peripheral Nerve Tumors

248. Abell MR, Hart WR, Olson JR: Tumors of the peripheral nervous system. *Hum Pathol* 1970;1:503–551.

249. Asbury AK, Johnson PC: *Pathology of Peripheral Nerve.* Philadelphia: WB Saunders, 1978:206–226.

250. Harkin JC, Reed RJ: Tumors of the peripheral nervous system. In: *Atlas of Tumor Pathology,* 2nd series, fascicle 3. Washington, DC: Armed Forces Institute of Pathology, 1969.

251. Lassmann H, Jurecka W, Lassmann G, et al: Different types of benign nerve sheath tumors: Light microscopy, electron microscopy and autoradiography. *Virchows Arch (Pathol Anat)* 1977;375(a):197–210.

252. Lazarus SS, Trombetta LD: Ultrastructural identification of a benign perineural cell tumor. *Cancer* 1978;41:1823–1829.

253. Woodruff JM, Chernik NL, Smith MC, et al: Peripheral nerve tumors with rhabdomyosarcomatous differentiation (malignant triton tumors). *Cancer* 1973;32:426–439.

254. Ron E, Modan B, Boice JD Jr, et al: Tumors of the brain and nervous system after radiotherapy in childhood. *N Engl J Med* 1988;319:1033–1039.

255. Conley JJ: Neurogenous tumors in the neck. *Arch Otolaryngol* 1955;61:167–180.

256. Conley J, Janecka IP: Neurilemmoma of the head and neck. *Trans Am Acad Ophthalmol Otol* 1975;80:459–464.

257. Gore DO, Rankow R, Hanford JM: Parapharyngeal neurilemmoma. *Surg Gynecol Obstet* 1956;103:193–201.

258. Dahl I, Hagmar B, Idvall I: Benign solitary neurilemoma (schwannoma). *Acta Pathol Microbiol Immunol Scand* 1984;92:91–101.

259. Putney FJ, Moran JJ, Thomas GK: Neurogenic tumors of the head and neck. *Laryngoscope* 74:1037–1059.

260. Whitaker WG, Droulias C: Benign encapsulated neurilemoma: A report of 76 cases. *Am J Surg* 1976;42:675–678.

261. Daly JF, Roesler HK: Neurilemmoma of the cervical sympathetic chain. *Arch Otolaryngol* 1963;77:262–267.

262. Hillstrom RP, Zarbo RJ, Jacobs JR: Nerve sheath tumors of the paranasal sinuses: Electron microscopy and histopathologic diagnosis. *Otolaryngol Head Neck Surg* 1990;102:257–263.

263. Das Gupta TK, Brasfield RD, Strong EW, et al: Benign solitary schwannomas (neurilemomas). *Cancer* 1969;24:355–366.

264. Kragh LV, Soule EH, Masson JK: Benign and malignant neurilemmomas of the head and neck. *Surg Gynecol Obstet* 1960;111:211–218.

265. Oberman HA, Sullenger G: Neurogenous tumors of the head and neck. *Cancer* 1967;20:1992–2001.

266. Perzin KH, Panyu H, Wechter S: Nonepithelial tumors of the nasal cavity, paranasal sinuses and nasopharynx: A clinicopathologic study. XII: Schwann cell tumors (neurilemoma, neurofibroma, malignant schwannoma). *Cancer* 1982;50:2193–2202.

267. Katz AD, Passy V, Kaplan L: Neurogenous neoplasms of major nerves of face and neck. *Arch Surg* 1971;103:51–56.

268. St. Pierre S, Theriault R, Laclerc JE: Schwannomas of the vagus in the head and neck. *J Otolaryngol* 1985;14:167–170.

269. Toriumi DM, Atiyah RA, Murad T, et al: Extracranial neurogenic tumors of the head and neck. *Otolaryngol Clin North Am* 1986;19:609–617.

270. Ackerman LV, Taylor FH: Neurogenous tumors within the thorax: A clinicopathological evaluation of forty-eight cases. *Cancer* 1951;4:669–691.

271. Dahl I: Ancient neurilemmoma (schwannoma). *Acta Pathol Microbiol Scand* 1977;85:812–818.

272. Stefansson K, Wollmann R, Jerkovic M: S-100 protein in soft-tissue tumors derived from schwann cells and melanocytes. *Am J Pathol* 1982;106:261–268.

273. Weiss SW, Langloss JM, Enzinger FM: Value of S-100 protein in the diagnosis of soft tissue tumors with particular reference to benign and malignant schwann cell tumors. *Lab Invest* 1993;49:299–308.

274. Woodruff JM, Godwin TA, Erlandson RA, et al: Cellular schwannoma. A variety of schwannoma sometimes mistaken for a malignant tumor. *Am J Surg Pathol* 1981;5:733–744.

275. Woodruff JM, Marshall ML, Godwin TA, et al: Plexiform (multinod-

ular) schwannoma. A tumor simulating the plexiform neurofibroma. *Am J Surg Pathol* 1983;5:691–697.

276. Coffin CM, Dehner LP: Peripheral neurogenic tumors of the soft tissues in children and adolescents: A clinicopathologic study of 139 cases. *Pediatr Pathol* 1989;9:387–407.

277. Kragh LV, Soule EH, Masson JK: Neurofibromatosis (von Recklinghausen's disease) of the head and neck: Cosmetic and reconstructive aspects. *Plast Reconstruct Surg* 1960;25:565–573.

278. Davis WB, Edgerton MT, Hoffmeister SF: Neurofibromatosis of the head and neck. *Plast Reconstruct Surg* 1954;14:186–199.

279. Allen PW: Myxoid tumors of soft tissues (part 1). *Pathol Annu* 1980;15:133–192.

280. Bonneau R, Brochu P: Neuromuscular choristoma: A clinicopathologic study of two cases. *Am J Surg Pathol* 1983;7:521–528.

Granular Cell Tumor

281. McFarland M, Abaza N, El-Mofty SK: Mouth, teeth and pharynx. In: Damjano V, Linder J, eds. *Andersons Pathology,* 10th ed. St. Louis: Mosby, 1996:1593.

282. Collins BM, Jones AC: Multiple granular cell tumors of the oral cavity: Report of a case and review of literature. *J Oral Maxillofac Surg* 1995;53:707–711.

283. Conley SF, Milbrath MM, Beste DJ: Pediatric laryngeal granular cell tumor. *J Otoloaryngeal* 1992;21:450–453.

284. Garancis JC, Komorowsky RA, Kuzma FG: Granular cell myoblastoma. *Cancer* 1970;25:542–550.

285. Vae SF III, Hudson R: Granular cell myoblastoma. *Am J Clin Pathol* 1969;52:208–211.

286. Mazur MT, Shultz JJ, Myers JL: Granular cell tumor: Immunohistochemical analysis of 21 benign tumors and one malignant tumor. *Arch Pathol Lab Med* 1990;114:692–696.

287. Okada H, Yamamoto H, Kawanga T, et al: Granular cell tumor of the tongue: An electron microscopic and immunohistochemical study. *J Nihon Univ School Dentistry* 1990;32:35–43.

288. Mittal KR, True LD: Origin of granules in granular cell tumor: Intracellular myelin formation with autodigestion. *Arch Pathol Lab Med* 1988;112:302–303.

289. Miettinen M, Lehtonen E, Lehtola H, et al: Histogenesis of granular cell tumor: An immunohistological and ultrastructural study. *J Pathol* 1984;142:221–229.

290. Mukai M: Immunohistochemical localization of S-100 protein and peripheral nerve myelin proteins (P2 protein and PO-protein) in granular cell tumors. *Am J Pathol* 1983;112:139–146.

291. Sobel HJ, Marquet E, Schwartz R: Is schwannoma related to granular cell myoblastoma? *Arch Pathol* 1973;95:396–401.

292. Sobel HJ, Schwartz R, Marquet E: Light and electron microscopic study of the origin of granular cell myoblastoma. *J Pathol* 1973;109:101–111.

293. Simsir A, Osborne BM, Greenebaum E: Malignant granular cell tumor: A case report and review of the recent literature. *Hum Pathol* 1996;27:853–858.

294. Jardines L, Cheung L, LiVolsi V, et al: Malignant granular cell tumors: Report of 2 case and review of the literature. *Surgery* 1994;116:49–54.

Malignant Peripheral Nerve Sheath Tumor

295. Storm FK, Eilber FR, Mirra J, et al: Neurofibrosarcoma. *Cancer* 1980;45:126–129.

296. D'Agostino AN, Soule EH, Miller RH: Sarcomas of the peripheral nerves and somatic soft tissues associated with multiple neurofibromatosis (von Recklinghausen's disease). *Cancer* 1963;16:1015–1027.

297. Das Gupta TK, Brasfield RD: Von Recklinghausen's disease. *CA* 1971;21:174–183.

298. Enjoji M, Hashimoto H, Tsuneyoshi M, et al: Malignant fibrous histiocytoma. A clinicopathologic study of 130 cases. *Acta Pathol Jpn* 1980;30:727–741.

299. Krall RA, Kostianovsky M, Patchefsky AS: Synovial sarcoma. A clinical, pathological, and ultrastructural study of 26 cases supporting the recognition of a monophasic variant. *Am J Surg Pathol* 1981;5:137–151.

300. Ghosh BC, Ghosh L, Huvos AG, et al: Malignant schwannoma: A clinicopathologic study. *Cancer* 1973;31:184–190.

301. Trojanowski JQ, Kleinman GM, Proppe KH: Malignant tumors of nerve sheath origin. *Cancer* 1980;46:1202–1212.

302. Ducatman BS, Scheithauer BW, Piepgras DG, et al: Malignant peripheral nerve sheath tumors. A clinicopathologic study of 120 cases. *Cancer* 1986;57:2006–2021.

303. Foley KM, Woodruff JM, Ellis FT, et al: Radiation-induced malignant and atypical peripheral nerve sheath tumors. *Ann Neurol* 1980;7:311–318.

304. Ducatman BS, Scheithauer BW: Postirradiation neurofibrosarcoma. *Cancer* 1983;51:1028–1033.

305. Sordillo PP, Helson L, Hajdu SI, et al: Malignant schwannoma: Clinical characteristics, survival, and response to therapy. *Cancer* 1981;47:2503–2509.

306. Tsuneyoshi M, Enjoji M: Primary malignant peripheral nerve tumors (malignant schwannomas): A clinicopathologic and electron microscopic study. *Acta Pathol Jpn* 1979;29:363–375.

307. Guccion JG, Enzinger FM: Malignant schwannoma associated with von Recklinghausen's neurofibromatosis. *Virchows Arch (Pathol Anat)* 1979;383:43–57.

308. Das Gupta TK, Brasfield RD: Solitary malignant schwannoma. *Ann Surg* 1970;171:419–428.

309. Bailet JW, Abemayor E, Andrews JC, et al: Malignant nerve sheath tumors of the head and neck: A combined experience from two university hospitals. *Laryngoscope* 1991;101:1044–1049.

310. Brooks JSJ, Freeman M, Enterline HT: Malignant "triton" tumors. Natural history and immunohistochemistry of nine new cases with literature review. *Cancer* 1985;55:2543–2549.

311. Bhatt S, Graeme-Cook F, Joseph MP, et al: Malignant triton tumor of the head and neck. *Otolaryngol Head Neck Surg* 1991;105:738–742.

312. Markel SF, Enzinger FM: Neuromuscular hamartoma: A benign Triton tumor composed of mature neural and striated muscle elements. *Cancer* 1982;49:140–144.

313. Wick MR, Swanson PE, Scheithauer BW, et al: Malignant peripheral nerve sheath tumor: An immunohistochemical study of 62 cases. *Am J Clin Pathol* 1987;87:425–433.

314. Herrera GA, Reimann EF, Salinas JA, et al: Malignant schwannomas presenting as malignant fibrous histiocytomas. *Ultrastruct Pathol* 1982;3:253–261.

Malignant Peripheral Neuroectodermal Tumor and Extraskeletal Ewing's Sarcoma

315. Dehner LP: Primitive neuroectodermal tumor and Ewing's sarcoma. *Am J Surg Pathol* 1993;17:1–13.

316. Tsokos M: Peripheral primitive neuroectodermal tumors. Diagnosis, classification, and prognosis. *Perspect Pediatr Pathol* 1992;16:27–98.

317. Stout AP: A tumor of the ulnar nerve. *Proc NY Pathol Soc* 1918;18:2–12.

318. Bolen JW, Thorning D: Peripheral neuroepithelioma: A light and electron microscopic study. *Cancer* 1980;46:2456–2462.

319. Hasegawa T, Hirose T, Kudo E, et al: Atypical primitive neuroectodermal tumors. Comparative light and electron microscopic and immunohistochemical studies on peripheral neuroepitheliomas and Ewing's sarcomas. *Acta Pathol Jpn* 1991;41:444–454.

320. Jürgens H, Bier V, Harms D, et al: Malignant peripheral neuroectodermal tumors. A retrospective analysis of 42 patients. *Cancer* 1988;61:349–357.

321. Schmidt D, Herrmann C, Jürgens H, et al: Malignant peripheral neuroectodermal tumor and its necessary distinction from Ewing's sarcoma. A report from the Kiel Pediatric Tumor Registry. *Cancer* 1991;68:2251–2259.

322. Voss BL, Pysher TJ, Humphrey GB: Peripheral neuroepithelioma in childhood. *Cancer* 1984;54:3059–3064.

323. Whang-Peng J, Triche TJ, Knutsen T, et al: Chromosome translocation in peripheral neuroepithelioma. *N Engl J Med* 1984;311:584–585.

324. Cavazzana AO, Ninfo V, Roberts J, et al: Peripheral neuroepithelioma: A light microscopic, immunocytochemical, and ultrastructural study. *Mod Pathol* 1992;5:71–78.

325. Chowdhury K, Manoukian JJ, Rochon L, et al: Extracranial primitive neuroectodermal tumor of the head and neck. *Arch Orolaryngol Head Neck Surg* 1990;116:475–478.

326. Coffin CM, Dehner LP: Peripheral neurogenic tumors of the soft tissues in children and adolescents. A clinicopathologic study of 139 cases. *Pediatr Pathol* 1989;9:387–407.

327. Hachitanda Y, Tsuneyoshi M, Enjoji M, et al: Congenital primitive neuroectodermal tumor with epithelial and glial differentiation. An ul-

trastructural and immunohistochemical study. *Arch Pathol Lab Med* 1990;114:101–105.

328. Hashimoto H, Enjoji M, Nakajima T, et al: Malignant neuroepithelioma (peripheral neuroblastoma): A clinicopathologic study of 15 cases. *Am J Surg Pathol* 1983;7:309–318.

329. Kushner BH, Hajdu SI, Gulati SC, et al: Extracranial primitive neuroectodermal tumors. The Memorial Sloan-Kettering Cancer Center experience. *Cancer* 1991;67:1825–1829.

330. Llombart-Bosch A, Terrier-Lacombe J, Peydro-Olaya A, et al: Peripheral neuroectodermal sarcoma of soft tissue (peripheral neuroepithelioma): A pathologic study of ten cases with differential diagnosis regarding other small, round-cell sarcomas. *Hum Pathol* 1989;20:273–280.

331. Schmidt D, Harms D, Burdach S: Malignant peripheral neuroectodermal tumours of childhood and adolescence. *Virchows Arch A Pathol Anat Histopathol* 1985;406:351–356.

332. Shishikura A, Ushigome S, Shimoda T: Primitive neuroectodermal tumors of bone and soft tissue: Histological subclassification and clinicopathologic correlations. *Acta Pathol Jpn* 1993;43:176–186.

333. Shuangshoti S: Primitive neuroectodermal (neuroepithelial) tumour of soft tissue of the neck in a child: Demonstration of neuronal and neuroglial differentiaion. *Histopathology* 1986;10:651–658.

334. Swanson PE, Jaszcz W, Nakhleh RE, et al: Peripheral primitive neuroectodermal tumors. A flow cytometric analysis with immunohistochemical and ultrastructural observations. *Arch Pathol Lab Med* 1992;116:1202–1208.

335. Wilson WB, Roloff J, Wilson HL: Primary peripheral neuroepithelioma of the orbit with intracranial extension. *Cancer* 1988;62:2595–2601.

336. Ushigome S, Shimoda T, Nikaido T, et al: Histopathologic diagnostic and histogenetic problems in malignant soft tissue tumors. Reassessment of malignant fibrous histiocytoma, epithelioid sarcoma, malignant rhabdoid tumor, and neuroectodermal tumor. *Acta Pathol Jpn* 1992;42:691–706.

337. Marina NM, Etcubanas E, Parham DM, et al: Peripheral primitive neuroectodermal tumor (peripheral neuroepithelioma) in children: A review of the St. Jude experience and controversies in diagnosis and management. *Cancer* 1989;64:1952–1960.

338. Schmidt D, Mackay B, Ayala AG: Ewing's sarcoma with neuroblastoma-like features. *Ultrastruct Pathol* 1982;3:143–151.

339. Mierau GW: Extraskeletal Ewing's sarcoma (peripheral neuroepithelioma). *Ultrastruct Pathol* 1985;9:91–98.

340. Leader M, Collins M, Patel J, et al: Antineuron specific enolase staining reactions in sarcomas and carcinomas: Its lack of neuroendocrine specificity. *J Clin Pathol* 1986;39:1186–1192.

341. Haimoto H, Takahashi Y, Koshikawa T, et al: Immunohistochemical localization of γ-enolase in normal human tissues other than nervous and neuroendocrine tissues. *Lab Invest* 1985;52:257–263.

342. Ambros IM, Ambros PF, Strehl S, et al: MIC2 is a specific marker for Ewing's sarcoma and peripheral primitive neuroectodermal tumors. Evidence for a common histogenesis of Ewing's sarcoma and peripheral primitive neuroectodermal tumors from MIC2 expression and specific chromosome aberration. *Cancer* 1991;67:1886–1893.

343. Devaney K, Abbondanzo SL, Shekitka KM, et al: MIC2 detection in tumors of bone and adjacent soft tissues. *Clin Orthop* 1995;310:176–187.

344. Fellinger EJ, Garin-Chesa P, Triche TJ, et al: Immunohistochemical analysis of Ewing's sarcoma cell surface antigen p30/32^{MIC2}. *Am J Pathol* 1991;139:317–325.

345. Hamilton G, Fellinger EJ, Schratter I, et al: Characterization of a human endocrine tissue and tumor-associated Ewing's sarcoma antigen. *Cancer Res* 1988;48:6127–6131.

346. Weidner N, Tjoe J: Immunohistochemical profile of monoclonal antibody 013: Antibody that recognizes glycoprotein p30/32^{MIC2} and is useful in diagnosing Ewing's sarcoma and peripheral neuroepithelioma. *Am J Surg Pathol* 1994;18:486–494.

347. Stevenson AJ, Chatten J, Bertoni F, et al: CD99 (p 30/32^{MIC2}) neuroectodermal/Ewing's sarcoma antigen as an immunohistochemical marker. Review of more than 600 tumors and the literature experience. *Appl Immunohistochem* 1994;2:231–240.

348. Riopel M, Dickman PS, Link MP, et al: MIC2 analysis in pediatric lymphomas and leukemias. *Hum Pathol* 1994;25:396–399.

349. Scotlandi K, Serra M, Marara MC, et al: Immunostaining of p30/32^{MIC2} antigen and molecular detection of EWS rearrangements for the diagnosis of Ewing's sarcoma and peripheral neuroectodermal tumor. *Hum Pathol* 1996;27:408–416.

350. Siebenrock KA, Nascimento AG, Rock MG: Comparison of soft tissue Ewing's sarcoma and peripheral neuroectodermal tumor. *Clin Orthop* 1996;329:288–299.

351. Gorman PA, Malone M, Pritchard J, et al: Cytogenetic analysis of primitive neuroectodermal tumors. Absence of the t(11;22) in two of three cases and a review of the literature. *Cancer Genet Cytogenet* 1991;51:13–22.

352. Stephenson CF, Bridge JA, Sandberg AA: Cytogenetic and pathologic aspects of Ewing's sarcoma and neuroectodermal tumors. *Hum Pathol* 1992;23:1270–1277.

353. Turc-Carel C, Aurias A, Mugneret F, et al: Chromosomes in Ewing's sarcoma. I. An evaluation of 85 cases and remarkable consistency of t(11;22)(q24;q12). *Cancer Genet Cytogenet* 1988;32:229–238.

354. Delattre O, Zucman J, Melot T, et al: The Ewing family of tumors: A subgroup of small-round- cell tumors defined by specific chimeric transcripts. *N Engl J Med* 1994;331:294–299.

355. Thorner P, Squire J, Chilton-MacNeill S, et al: Is the EWS/FLI-1 fusion transcript specific for Ewing sarcoma and peripheral primitive neuroectodermal tumor? A report of four cases showing this transcript in a wider range of tumor types. *Am J Pathol* 1996;148:1125–1138.

356. Weidner N: Anti-CD45 [letter to the editor]. *Am J Surg Pathol* 1995;19:733–734.

357. Parham DM: Anti-CD45 [letter to the editor]. *Am J Surg Pathol* 1995;19:732–733.

358. Angervall L, Enzinger FM: Extraskeletal neoplasm resembling Ewing's sarcoma. *Cancer* 1975;36:240–251.

359. Tefft M, Vawter GF, Mitus A: Paravertebral "round cell" tumors in children. *Radiology* 1969;92:1501–1509.

360. Shimada H, Newton WA Jr, Soule EH, et al: Pathologic features of extraosseous Ewing's sarcoma: A report from the Intergroup Rhabdomyosarcoma study. *Hum Pathol* 1988;19:442–453.

361. Stuart-Harris R, Wills EJ, Philips J, et al: Extraskeletal Ewing's sarcoma: A clincal, morphological and ultrastructural analysis of five cases with a review of the literature. *Eur J Cancer* 1986;22:393–400.

362. Hashimoto H, Tsuneyoshi M, Daimaru Y, et al: Extraskeletal Ewing's sarcoma. A clinicopathologic and electron microscopic analysis of 8 cases. *Acta Pathol Jpn* 1985;35:1087–1098.

363. Kinsella TJ, Triche TJ, Dickman PS, et al: Extraskeletal Ewing's sarcoma: Results of combined modality treatment. *J Clin Oncol* 1983;1:489–495.

364. Meister P, Gokel JM: Extraskeletal Ewing's sarcoma. *Virchows Arch A Pathol Anat Histopathol* 1978;378:173–179.

365. Pontius KI, Sebek BA: Extraskeletal Ewing's sarcoma arising in the nasal fossa. Light- and electron-microscopic observations. *Am J Clin Pathol* 1981;75:410–415.

366. Lim TC, Tan WTL, Lee YS: Congenital extraskeletal Ewing's sarcoma of the face: A case report. *Head Neck* 1994;16:75–78.

367. Gustafson RO, Maragos NE, Reiman HM: Extraskeletal Ewing's sarcoma occurring as a mass in the neck. *Otolaryngol Head Neck Surg* 1982;90:491–493.

368. Hara S, Ishii E, Tanaka S, et al: A monoclonal antibody specifically reactive with Ewing's sarcoma. *Br J Cancer* 1989;60:875–879.

369. Howard DJ, Daniels HA: Ewing's sarcoma of the nose. *Ear Nose Throat J* 1993;72:277–279.

370. Lane S, Ironside JW: Extra-skeletal Ewing's sarcoma of the nasal fossa. *J Laryngol Otol* 1990;104:570–573.

371. Rose JS, Hermann G, Mendelson DS, et al: Extraskeletal Ewing sarcoma with computed tomography correlation. *Skeletal Radiol* 1983;9:234–237.

372. Rud NP, Reiman HM, Pritchard DJ, et al: Extraosseous Ewing's sarcoma. A study of 42 cases. *Cancer* 1989;64:1548–1553.

373. Suster S, Ronnen M, Huszar M: Extraskeletal Ewing's sarcoma of the scalp. *Pediatr Dermatol* 1988;5:123–126.

374. Peters MS, Reiman HM, Muller SA: Cutaneous extraskeletal Ewing's sarcoma. *J Cutan Pathol* 1985;12:476–485.

375. Navas-Palacios JJ, Aparicio-Duque R, Valdes MD: On the histogenesis of Ewing's sarcoma: An ultrastructural, immunohistochemical, and cytochemical study. Cancer 1984;53:1882–1901.

376. Granowetter L: Ewing's sarcoma and extracranial primitive neuroectodermal tumors. *Curr Opin Oncol* 1992;4:696–703.

377. Harms D, Schmidt D: Critical commentary to "Cytogenetics of Askin's tumor." *Pathol Res Pract* 1993;189:242–244.

378. Hartman KR, Triche TJ, Kinsella TJ, et al: Prognostic value of histopathology in Ewing's sarcoma. Long-term follow-up of distal extremity primary tumors. *Cancer* 1991;67:163–171.

379. Rousselin B, Vanel D, Terrier-Lacombe MJ, et al: Clinical and radio-

logic analysis of 13 cases of primary neuroectodermal tumors of bone. *Skeletal Radiol* 1989;18:115–120.

380. Tsuneyoshi M, Yokoyama R, Hashimoto H, et al: Comparative study of neuroectodermal tumor and Ewing's sarcoma of the bone. Histopathologic, immunohistochemical and ultrastructural features. *Acta Pathol Jpn* 1989;39:573–581.

381. Brinkhuis M, Wijnaendts LCD, van der Linden JC, et al: Peripheral primitive neuroectodermal tumour and extra-osseous Ewing's sarcoma: A histologic, immunohistochemical and DNA flow cytometric study. *Virchows Arch* 1995;425:611–616.

382. Ladanyi M, Heinemann FS, Huvos AG, et al: Neural differentiation in small round cell tumors of bone and soft tissue with the translocation t(11;22)(q24;q12): An immunohistochemical study of 11 cases. *Hum Pathol* 1990;21:1245–1251.

383. Miser JS, Kinsella TJ, Triche TJ, et al: Treatment of peripheral neuroepithelioma in children and young adults. *J Clin Oncol* 1987;5:1752–1758.

384. Pinto A, Grant LH, Hayes FA, et al: Immunohistochemical expression of neuron-specific enolase and Leu 7 in Ewing's sarcoma of bone. *Cancer* 1989;64:1266–1273.

Paragangliomna

385. Glenner GG, Grimley PM: Tumors of the extra-adrenal paraganglion system (including chemoreceptors). In: *Atlas of Tumor Pathology,* 2nd series, fascicle 9. Washington, DC: Armed Forces Institute of Pathology, 1974.

386. ReMine WH, Weiland LH, ReMine SG: Carotid body tumors: Chemodectomas. *Curr Probl Cancer* 1978;11:1–27.

387. Grimley PM, Glenner GG: Histology and ultrastructure of carotid body paragangliomas: Comparison with the normal gland. *Cancer* 1967;20:1473–1488.

388. Shamblin WR, ReMine WH, Sheps SG, et al: Carotid body tumor (chemodectoma)—clinicopathologic analysis of ninety cases. *Am J Surg* 1971;122:732–739.

389. Irons GB, Weiland LH, Brown WL: Paragangliomas of the neck: Clinical and pathologic analysis of 116 cases. *Surg Clin North Am* 1977;57:575–583.

390. Lack EE, Cubilla AL, Woodruff JM, et al: Paragangliomas of the head and neck region: A clinical study of 69 patients. *Cancer* 1977;39:397–409.

391. Farr HW: Carotid body tumors: A 40-year study. *CA* 1980;30:260–265.

392. Gaylis H, Mieny CJ: The incidence of malignancy in carotid body tumours. *Br J Surg* 1977;64:885–889.

393. Lees CD, Levine HL, Beven EG, et al: Tumors of the carotid body: Experience with 41 operative cases. *Am J Surg* 1981;142:362–365.

394. Merino MJ, Livolsi VA: Malignant carotid body tumors: Report of two cases and review of the literature. *Cancer* 1981;47:1403–1414.

395. Parry DM, Li FP, Strong LC, et al: Carotid body tumors in humans: Genetics and epidemiology. *J Natl Cancer Inst* 1982;68:573–578.

396. Oberman HA, Holtz F, Sheffer LA, et al: Chemodectomas (nonchromaffin paragangliomas) of the head and neck: A clinicopathologic study. *Cancer* 1968;21:838–851.

397. Padberg FT Jr, Cady B, Persson AV: Carotid body tumor: The Lahey Clinic experience. *Am J Surg* 1983;145:526–528.

398. Hodge KM, Byers RM, Peters LJ: Paragangliomas of the head and neck. *Arch Otolaryngol Head Neck Surg* 1988;114:872–877.

399. Steely WM, Davies RS, Brigham RA: Carotid body tumor and hyperparathyroidism. A case report and review of the literature. *Am Surg* 1987;53:337–338.

400. Raafat F, Salman WD, Roberts K, et al: Carney's triad: Gastric leiomyosarcoma, pulmonary chondroma and extra-adrenal paraganglioma in young females. *Histopathology* 1986;10:1325–1333.

401. Carney JA: The triad of gastric epithelioid leiomyosarcoma, pulmonary chondroma and functioning extra-adrenal paraganglioma: Five-year review. *Medicine* 1983;62:159–169.

402. Acha T, Picazo B, Garcia-Martin FJ, et al: Carney's triad: Apropos of a new case. *Med Pediatr Oncol* 2994; 22:216–220.

403. Lack EE, Cubilla AL, Woodruff JM: Paragangliomas of the head and neck region: A pathologic study of tumors from 71 patients. *Hum Pathol* 1979;10:191–218.

404. Warren WH, Memoli VA, Gould VE: Immunohistochemical and ultrastructural analysis of paragangliomas of the head and neck [abstract]. *Lab Invest* 1984;50:66a.

405. Zbaren P, Lehmann W: Carotid body paraganglioma with metastases. *Laryngoscope* 1985;95:450–454.

406. Achilles E, Padberg B-C, Holl K, et al: Immunocytochemistry of paragangliomas: Value of staining for S-100 protein and glial fibrillary acid protein in diagnosis and prognosis. *Histopathology* 1991;18:453–458.

407. Linnoila RI, Lack EE, Steinberg SM, et al: Decreased expression of neuropeptides in malignant paragangliomas: An immunohistochemical study. *Hum Pathol* 1988;19:41–50.

408. Barnes L, Taylor SR: Carotid body paragangliomas: A clinicopathologic and DNA analysis of 13 tumors. *Arch Otolaryngol Head Neck Surg* 1990;116:447–453.

409. Chaudhry AP, Haar JG, Koul A, et al: A nonfunctioning paraganglioma of vagus nerve: An ultrastructural study. *Cancer* 1979;43:1689–1701.

410. Warwick-Brown NP, Richards AES, Cheesman AD: Glomus vagale: An unusual presentation. *J Laryngol Otol* 1986;100:1205–1208.

411. Palacios E: Chemodectomas of the head and neck. *AJR* 1970;110:129–140.

412. Someren A, Karcioglu Z: Malignant vagal paraganglioma: Report of a case and review of literature. *Am J Clin Pathol* 1977;68:400–408.

413. Spector GJ, Ciralsky RH, Ogura JH: Glomus tumors in the head and neck: III. Analysis of clinical manifestations. *Ann Otol Rhinol Laryngol* 1975;84:73–79.

414. Kahn LB: Vagal body tumor (nonchromaffin paraganglioma, chemodectoma, and carotid body-like tumor) with cervical node metastasis and familial association: Ultrastructural study and review. *Cancer* 1976;38:2367–2377.

415. Davidson J, Gullane P: Glomus vagale tumors. *Otolaryngol Head Neck Surg* 1988;99:66–70.

Lymphangioma and Cystic Hygroma

416. Coffin CM, Dehner LP: Vascular tumors in children and adolescents: A clinicopathologic study of 228 tumors in 222 patients. *Pathol Annu* 1993;28(pt 1):97–120.

417. Bill AH Jr, Sumner DS: A unified concept of lymphangioma and cystic hygroma. *Surg Gynecol Obstet* 1965;120:79–86.

418. Watson WL, McCarthy WD: Blood and lymph vessel tumors. A report of 1,056 cases. *Surg Gynecol Obstet* 1940;71:569–588.

419. Flanagan BP, Helwig EB: Cutaneous lymphangioma. *Arch Dermatol* 1977;113:24–30.

420. Peachey RDG, Whimster IW: Lymphangioma of skin. A review of 65 cases. *Br J Dermatol* 1970;83:519–527.

421. Lynn HB: Cystic hygroma. *Surg Clin North Am* 1963;43:1157–1163.

422. Litzow TJ, Lash H: Lymphangiomas of the tongue. *Mayo Clinic Proc* 1961;36:229–234.

423. Gross RE, Goeringer CF: Cystic hygroma of the neck. Report of twenty-seven cases. *Surg Gynecol Obstet* 1939;69:48–60.

424. Harkins GA, Sabiston DC: Lymphangioma in infancy and childhood. *Surgery* 1960;47:811–822.

425. Ninh TN, Ninh TX: Cystic hygroma in children: A report of 126 cases. *J Pediatr Surg* 9:191–195.

426. Stromberg BV, Weeks PM, Wray RC Jr: Treatment of cystic hygroma. *South Med J* 1976;69:1333–1335.

427. Ricciardelli EJ, Richardson MA: Cervicofacial cystic hygroma. *Arch Otolaryngol Head Neck Surg* 1991;117:546–553.

428. Dinerman WS, Myers EN: Lymphangiomatous macroglossia. *Laryngoscope* 1976;86:291–296.

429. Balakrishnan A, Bailey CM: Lymphangioma of the tongue. A review of pathogenesis, treatment and the use of surface laser photocoagulation. *J Laryngol Otol* 1991;105:924–930.

430. Dixon JA, Davis RK, Gilbertson JJ: Laser photocoagulation of vascular malformations of the tongue. *Laryngoscope* 1986;96:537–541.

431. Adeyemi SD: Management of cystic hygroma of the head and neck in Lagos, Nigeria; a 10-year experience. *Int J Pediatr Otorhinolaryngol* 1992;23:245–251.

432. Barrand KG, Freeman NV: Massive infiltrating cystic hygroma of the neck in infancy. *Arch Dis Child* 1973;48:523–531.

Lipoma, Lipomatosis, and Liposarcoma

433. Brasfield RD, Das Gupta TK: Soft tissue tumors: Benign tumors of adipose tissue. *CA* 1969;19:3–7.

434. Myhre-Jensen O: A consecutive 7-year series of 1331 benign soft tissue tumours. *Acta Orthoped Scand* 1981;52:287–293.

435. Adair FE, Pack GT, Farrior JH: Lipomas. *Am J Cancer* 1932. 16:1104–1120.

436. Geschickter CF: Lipoid tumors. *Am J Cancer* 1934;21:617–641.

437. Allen PW: *Tumors and Proliferations of Adipose Tissue. A Clinicopathologic Approach.* New York: Masson Publishing USA, 1981.

438. Hatziotis J Ch: Lipoma of the oral cavity. *Oral Surg* 1971;31:511–524.

439. Wakeley C, Somerville P: Lipomas. *Lancet* 1952;2:995–999.

440. Toppozada HH, Shehata MA, Maher AI: Lipoma of the pharynx (a report of four cases). *J Laryngol Otol* 1973;87:787–793.

441. Tsunoda A: Lipoma in the peri-tonsillar space. *J Laryngol Otol* 1994;108:693–695.

442. To WH, Yeung KH: Intra-osseous lipoma of the maxillary tuberosity. *Br J Oral Maxillofac Surg* 1992;30:122–124.

443. Fu Y-S, Perzin KH: Non-epithelial tumors of the nasal cavity, paranasal sinuses and nasopharynx: A clinicopathologic study. VIII. Adipose tissue tumors (lipoma and liposarcoma). *Cancer* 1977;40:1314–1317.

444. Seldin HM, Seldin DS, Rakower W, et al: Lipomas of the oral cavity: Report of 26 cases. *J Oral Surg* 1967;25:270–274.

445. Kindblom L-G, Angervall L, Stener B, et al: Intermuscular and intramuscular lipomas and hibernomas: A clinical, roentgenologic, histologic, and prognostic study of 46 cases. *Cancer* 1974;33:754–762.

446. Fu YS, Parker FG, Kaye GI, et al: Ultrastructure of benign and malignant adipose tissue tumors (part 1). *Pathol Annu* 1980;15:67–89.

447. Tuc-Carel C, Cin PD, Rao U, et al: Cytogenetic studies of adipose tissue tumors. I. A benign lipoma with reciprocal translocation t(3;12)(q28;q14). *Cancer Genet Cytogenet* 1986;23:283–289.

448. Enzinger FM, Harvey DA: Spindle cell lipoma. *Cancer* 1975; 36:1852–1859.

449. Angervall L, Dahl I, Kindblom L-G, et al: Spindle cell lipoma. *Acta Pathol Microbiol Scand* 1976;84:477–487.

450. Bolen JW, Thorning D: Spindle-cell lipoma: A clinical, light- and electron-microscopical study. *Am J Surg Pathol* 1981;5:435–444.

451. Christopoulos P, Nicolatou O, Patrikiou A: Oral spindle cell lipoma. Report of a case. *Int J Oral Maxillofac Surg* 1989;18:208–209.

452. McDaniel RK, Newland JR, Chiles DG: Intraoral spindle cell lipoma: Case report with correlated light and electron microscopy. *Oral Surg Oral Med Oral Pathol* 1984;57:52–57.

453. Lombardi T, Odell EW: Spindle cell lipoma of the oral cavity: Report of a case. *J Oral Pathol Med* 1994;23:237–239.

454. Fechner RE: Spindle cell lipoma. *Arch Otolaryngol* 1984;110:766–769.

455. Shmookler BM, Enzinger FM: Pleomorphic lipoma: A benign tumor simulating liposarcoma. A clinicopathologic analysis of 48 cases. *Cancer* 1981;47:126–133.

456. Evans HL, Soule EH, Winkelmann RK: Atypical lipoma, atypical intramuscular lipoma, and well differentiated retroperitoneal liposarcoma: A reappraisal of 30 cases formerly classified as well differentiated liposarcoma. *Cancer* 1979;43:574–584.

457. Kindblom L-G, Angervall L, Fassina AS: Atypical lipoma. *Acta Pathol Microbiol Immunol Scand* 1982;90:27–36.

458. Guillou L, Dehon A, Charlin B, Madarnas P. Pleomorphic lipoma of the tongue: Case report and literature review. *J Otolaryngol* 1986;15:313–316.

459. Duhaime A-C, Chatten J, Schut L, et al: Cervical lipoblastomatosis with intraspinal extension and transformation to mature fat in a child. *Childs Nerv Syst* 1987;3:304–306.

460. Mitchell CD: Cervical lipoblastomatosis. *Med Pediatr Oncol* 1985;13:381–383.

461. Hoehn JG, Yalamanchi BA, Pilon V: Benign lipoblastomatosis: Report of a case involving the face and neck. *Reconstr Surg* 1984;73:455–458.

462. Schuler FA III, Graham JK, Horton CE: Benign symmetrical lipomatosis (Madelung's disease): Case report. *Plast Reconstr Surg* 1976;57:662–665.

463. Taylor LM, Beahrs OH, Fontana RS: Benign symmetric lipomatosis. *Mayo Clinic Proc* 1961;36:96–100.

464. Moretti JA, Miller D: Laryngeal involvement in benign symmetric lipomatosis. *Arch Otolaryngol* 1973;97:495–496.

465. Evans HL: Liposarcoma: A study of 55 cases with a reassessment of its classification. *Am J Surg Pathol* 1979;3:507–523.

466. Kindblom L-G, Angervall L, Svendsen P: Liposarcoma: A clinicopathologic, radiographic and prognostic study. *Acta Pathol Microbiol Scand* (Suppl) 1975;253:1–71.

467. Brasfield RD, Das Gupta TK: Liposarcoma. *CA* 1970;20:3–9.

468. Enzinger FM, Winslow DJ: Liposarcoma: A study of 103 cases. *Virchows Arch* 1962;335:367–388.

469. Baden E, Newman R: Liposarcoma of the oropharyngeal region: Review of the literature and report of two cases. *Oral Surg* 1977;44:889–902.

470. Saunders JR, Jaques DA, Casterline PF, et al: Liposarcomas of the head and neck: A review of the literature and addition of four cases. *Cancer* 1979;43:162–168.

471. Kindblom L-G, Angervall L, Jarlstedt J: Liposarcoma of the neck: A clinicopathologic study of 4 cases. *Cancer* 1978;42:774–780.

472. McCulloch TM, Makielski KH, McNutt MA: Head and neck liposarcoma. A histopathologic reevaluation of reported cases. *Arch Otolaryngol Head Neck Surg* 1992;118:1045–1049.

473. Shmookler BM, Enzinger FM: Liposarcoma occurring in children: An analysis of 17 cases and review of the literature. *Cancer* 1983;52:567–574.

474. Wenig BM, Weiss SW, Gnepp DR: Laryngeal and hypopharyngeal liposarcoma. A clinicopathologic study of 10 cases with a comparison to soft-tissue counterparts. *Am J Surg Pathol* 1990;14:134–144.

475. Chung EB, Enzinger FM: Benign lipoblastomatosis. An analysis of 35 cases. *Cancer* 1973;32:482–492.

476. Stewart MG, Schwartz MR, Alford BR. Atypical and malignant lipomatous lesions of the head and neck. *Arch Otolaryngol Head Neck Surg* 1994;120:1151–1155.

477. Weiss SW, Sobin LH: *World Health Organization International Classification of Soft Tissue Tumours: Histological Typing of Soft Tissue Tumours,* 2nd ed. Berlin: Springer-Verlag, 1994.

478. Weiss SW: Lipomatous tumors. In: Weiss SW, Brooks JS, eds. *Soft Tissue Tumors.* Baltimore: Williams & Wilkins, 1996:207–239.

479. Enzinger F: *Management of Primary Bone and Soft Tissue Tumors.* Chicago: Year Book Medical Publishers, 1977:454–455.

480. Snover DC, Sumner HW, Dehner LP: Variability of histologic pattern in recurrent soft tissue sarcomas originally diagnosed as liposarcoma. *Cancer* 1982;49:1005–1015.

481. Battifora H, Nunez-Alonso C: Myxoid liposarcoma: Study of ten cases. *Ultrastruct Pathol* 1980;1:157–169.

482. Bolen JW, Thorning D: Benign lipoblastoma and myxoid liposarcoma: A comparative light- and electron-microscopic study. *Am J Surg Pathol* 1980;4:163–174.

483. Lagacé R, Jacob S, Seemayer TA: Myxoid liposarcoma. An electron microscopic study: Biologic and histogenetic considerations. *Virchows Arch (Pathol Anat)* 1979;384a:159–172.

484. Edland RW: Liposarcoma: A retrospective study of fifteen cases: A review of the literature and a discussion of radiosensitivity. *AJR* 1968;103:778–791.

Rhabdomyoma

485. Dehner LP, Enzinger FM: Fetal rhabdomyoma: An analysis of nine cases. *Cancer* 1972;30:160–166.

486. di Sant'Agnese PA, Knowles DM II: Extracardiac rhabdomyoma: A clinicopathologic study and review of the literature. *Cancer* 1980;46:780–789.

487. Gardner DG, Corio RL: Multifocal adult rhabdomyoma. *Oral Surg* 1983;56:76–78.

488. Konrad EA, Meister P, Hübner G: Extracardiac rhabdomyoma: Report of different types with light microscopic and ultrastructural studies. *Cancer* 1982;49:898–907.

489. Moran JJ, Enterline HT: Benign rhabdomyoma of the pharynx: A case report, review of the literature, and comparison with cardiac rhabdomyoma. *Am J Clin Patholl* 1964;42:174–181.

490. Corio RL, Lewis DM: Intraoral rhabdomyomas. *Oral Surg* 1979;48:525–531.

491. Gold JH, Bossen EH: Benign vaginal rhabdomyoma: A light and electron microscopic study. *Cancer* 1976;37:2283–2294.

492. Scrivner D, Meyer JS: Multifocal recurrent adult rhabdomyoma. *Cancer* 1980;46:790–795.

493. Tanner NSB, Carter RL, Clifford P: Pharyngeal rhabdomyoma: An unusual presentation. *J Laryngol Otol* 1978;92:1029–1036.

494. Kapadia SB, Meis JM, Frisman DM, Ellis GL, Heffner DK, Hyams VJ: Adult rhabdomyoma of the head and neck: A clinicopathologic and immunophenotypic study. *Hum Pathol* 1993;24:608–617.

495. Kapadia SB, Meis JM, Frisman DM, Ellis GL, Heffner DK: Fetal rhabdomyoma of the head and neck: A clinicopathologic and immunophenotypic study of 24 cases. *Hum Pathol* 1993;24:754–765.

496. Boysen M, Scott H, Hovig T, Wetteland J, Kolbenstvedt A: Rhab-

domyoma of the tongue: Report of a case with light microscopic, ultrastructural and immunohistochemical observations. *J Laryngol Otol* 1988;102:1185–1186.

497. Albrechtsen R, Ebbesen F, Pedersen SV: Extracardiac rhabdomyoma: Light and electron microscopic studies of two cases in the mandibular area, with a review of previous reports. *Acta Otolaryngol* 1974;78:458–464.

498. Bagby RA, Packer JT, Iglesias RG: Rhabdomyoma of the larynx. *Arch Otolaryngol* 1976;102:101–103.

499. Battifora HA, Eisenstein R, Schild JA: Rhabdomyoma of larynx. Ultrastructural study and comparison with granular cell tumors (myoblastoma). *Cancer* 1969;23:183–190.

500. Czernobilsky B, Cornog JL, Enterline HT: Rhabdomyoma: Report of a case with ultrastructural and histochemical studies. *Am J Clin Pathol* 1968;49:782–789.

501. Goldman RL: Multicentric benign rhabdomyoma of skeletal muscle. *Cancer* 1963;16:1609–1613.

502. Knowles DM II, Jakobiec FA: Rhabdomyoma of the orbit. *Am J Ophthalmol* 1975;80:1011–1018.

503. Ross CF: Rhabdomyoma of sternomastoid. *J Pathol Bacteriol* 1968;95:556–558.

504. Schlosnagle DC, Kratochvil FJ, Weathers DR, et al: Intraoral multifocal adult rhabdomyoma: Report of a case and review of the literature. *Arch Pathol Lab Med* 1983;107:638–642.

505. Tandler B, Rossi EP, Stein M, et al: Rhabdomyoma of the lip: Light and electron microscopical observations. *Arch Pathol* 1970;89:118–127.

506. Warner TFCS, Goell W, Sundharadas M, et al: Adult rhabdomyoma: Ultrastructure and immunocytochemistry. *Arch Pathol Lab Med* 1981;105:608–611.

507. Winther LK: Rhabdomyoma of the hypopharynx and larynx: Report of two cases and a review of the literature. *J Laryngol Otol* 1976;90:1041–1051.

508. Wyatt RB, Schochet SS, McCormick WF: Rhabdomyoma: Light and electron microscopic study of a case with intranuclear inclusions. *Arch Otolaryngol* 1970;92:32–39.

509. Shemen L, Spiro R, Tuazon R. Multifocal adult rhabdomyomas of the head and neck. *Head Neck* 1992;14:395–400.

510. Gardner DG, Corio RL: Fetal rhabdomyoma of the tongue, with a discussion of the two histologic variants of this tumor. *Oral Surg* 1983;56:293–300.

511. Dahl I, Angervall L, Säve-Söderbergh J: Foetal rhabdomyoma: Case report of a patient with two tumors. *Acta Pathol Microbiol Scand* 1976;84:107–112.

512. Helliwell TR, Sissons MCJ, Stoney PJ, Ashworth MT. Immunochemistry and electron microscopy of head and neck rhabdomyoma. *J Clin Pathol* 1988;41:1058–1063.

513. Nakajima T, Watanabe S, Sato Y, et al: An immunoperoxidase study of S-100 protein distribution in normal and neoplastic tissues. *Am J Surg Pathol* 1982;6:715–727.

514. Stefansson K, Wollmann R, Jerkovic M: S-100 protein in soft-tissue tumors derived from schwann cells and melanocytes. *Am J Pathol* 1982;106:261–268.

515. Crotty PL, Nakhleh RE, Dehner LP: Juvenile rhabdomyoma. An intermediate form of skeletal muscle tumor in children. *Arch Pathol Lab Med* 1993;117:43–47.

516. Eusebi V, Ceccarelli C, Daniele E, Collina G, Viale G, Mancini AM. Extracardiac rhabdomyoma: An immunocytochemical study and review of the literature. *Appl Pathol* 1988;6:197–207.

Rhabdomyosarcoma

517. Sutow WW: Childhood rhabdomyosarcoma. In: *Malignant Solid Tumors in Children. A Review.* New York: Raven Press, 1981:129–147.

518. Agamanolis DP, Dasu S, Krill CE Jr: Tumors of skeletal muscle. *Hum Pathol* 1986;17:778–795.

519. Tsokos M, Webber BL, Parham DM, et al: Rhabdomyosarcoma. A new classification scheme related to prognosis. *Arch Pathol Lab Med* 1992;116:847–855.

520. Bale PM, Reye RDK: Rhabdomyosarcoma in childhood. *Pathology* 1975;7:101–111.

521. Maurer HM, Donaldson M, Gehan EA, et al: Rhabdomyosarcoma in childhood and adolescence. *Curr Probl Cancer* 1978;2:1–35.

522. Maurer HM, Moon T, Donaldson M, et al: The Intergroup Rhabdomyosarcoma Study: A preliminary report. *Cancer* 1977;40:2015–2026.

523. Keyhani A, Booher RJ: Pleomorphic rhabdomyosarcoma. *Cancer* 1968;22:956–967.

524. Masson JK, Soule EH: Embryonal rhabdomyosarcoma of the head and neck. Report on eighty-eight cases. *Am J Surg* 1965;110:585–591.

525. Soule EH, Geitz M, Henderson ED: Embryonal rhabdomyosarcoma of the limbs and limb-girdles: A clinicopathologic study of 61 cases. *Cancer* 1969;23:1336–1346.

526. Horn RC Jr, Enterline HT: Rhabdomyosarcoma: A clinicopathological study and classification of 39 cases. *Cancer* 1958;11:181–199.

527. Stout AP, Lattes R: Tumors of the soft tissues. In: *Atlas of Tumor Pathology*, 2nd series, fascicle I. Washington, DC: Armed Forces Institute of Pathology, 1967.

528. Bale PM, Parsons RE, Stevens MM: Diagnosis and behavior of juvenile rhabdomyosarcoma. *Hum Pathol* 1983;14:596–611.

529. Enterline HT, Horn RC Jr: Alveolar rhabdomyosarcoma: A distinctive tumor type. *Am J Clin Pathol* 1958;29:356–366.

530. Patton RB, Horn RC Jr: Rhabdomyosarcoma: Clinical and pathological features and comparison with human fetal and embryonal skeletal muscle. *Surgery* 1962;52:572–584.

531. Dito WR, Batsakis JG: Rhabdomyosarcoma of the head and neck: An appraisal of the biologic behavior in 170 cases. *Arch Surg* 1962;84:582–588.

532. Feldman BA: Rhabdomyosarcoma of the head and neck. *Laryngoscope* 1982;92:424–440.

533. Flamant F, Hill C: The improvement in survival associated with combined chemotherapy in childhood rhabdomyosarcoma: A historical comparison of 345 patients in the same center. *Cancer* 1984;53:2417–2421.

534. Jones IS, Reese AB, Krout J: Orbital rhabdomyosarcoma: An analysis of sixty-two cases. *Trans Am Ophthalmol Soc* 1965;63:223–255.

535. Newman AN, Rice DH: Rhabdomyosarcoma of the head and neck. *Laryngoscope* 1984;94:234–276.

536. Porterfield JF, Zimmerman LE: Rhabdomyosarcoma of the orbit: A clinicopathologic study of 55 cases. *Virchows Arch (Pathol Anat)* 1962;335:329–344.

537. Sutow WW, Sullivan MP, Ried HL, et al: Prognosis in childhood rhabdomyosarcoma. *Cancer* 1970;25:1384–1390.

538. Enzinger FM, Shiraki M: Alveolar rhabdomyosarcoma: An analysis of 110 cases. *Cancer* 24:18–31.

539. Gaiger AM, Soule EH, Newton WA Jr: Pathology of rhabdomyosarcoma: Experience of the Intergroup Rhabdomyosarcoma Study, 1972–78. *Natl Cancer Inst Monogr* 1981;56:19–27.

540. Lloyd RV, Hajdu SI, Knapper WH: Embryonal rhabdomyosarcoma in adults. *Cancer* 1983;51:557–565.

541. Stobbe GD, Dargeon HW: Embryonal rhabdomyosarcoma of the head and neck in children and adolescents. *Cancer* 1950;3:826–836.

542. Lawrence W Jr, Jegge G, Foote FW Jr: Embryonal rhabdomyosarcoma: A clinicopathological study. *Cancer* 1964;17:361–376.

543. Li FP, Fraumeni JF Jr: Rhabdomyosarcoma in children: Epidemiologic study and identification of a familial cancer syndrome. *J Natl Cancer Inst* 1969;43:1365–1373.

544. Soussi T, Leblanc T, Baruchel A, et al: Germline mutations of the p53 tumor-suppressor gene in cancer-prone families: A review. *Nouv Rev Fr Hematol* 1993;35:33–36.

545. Malkin D: p53 and the Li-Fraumeni syndrome. *Cancer Genet Cytogenet* 1993;66:83–92.

546. Deutsch M, Felder H: Rhabdomyosarcoma of the ear-mastoid. *Laryngoscope* 1974;84:586–592.

547. Canalis RF, Jenkins HA, Hemenway WG, et al: Nasopharyngeal rhabdomyosarcoma: A clinical perspective. *Arch Otolaryngol* 1978;104:122–126.

548. Prior JT, Stoner LR: Sarcoma botryoides of the nasopharynx. *Cancer* 10:957–964.

549. Fleischer AS, Koslow M, Rovit RL: Neurological manifestations of primary rhabdomyosarcoma of the head and neck in children. *J Neurosurg* 1975;43:207–214.

550. Enzinger FM: Recent trends in soft tissue pathology. In: *Tumors of Bone and Soft Tissue.* Chicago: Year Book Medical Publishers, 1965:315–332.

551. Mierau GW, Favara BE: Rhabdomyosarcoma in children: Ultrastructural study of 31 cases. *Cancer* 1980;46:2035–2040.

552. Bundtzen JL, Norback DH: The ultrastructure of poorly differentiated rhabdomyosarcomas: A case report and literature review. *Hum Pathol* 1982;13:301–313.

553. Morales AR, Fine G, Horn RC Jr: Rhabdomyosarcoma: An ultrastructural appraisal. *Pathol Annu* 1972;7:81–106.

554. Gonzalez-Crussi F, Black-Schaffer S: Rhabdomyosarcoma of infancy and childhood: Problems of morphologic classification. *Am J Surg Pathol* 1979;3:157–171.
555. Tsokos M, Howard R, Costa J: Immunohistochemical study of alveolar and embryonal rhabdomyosarcoma. *Lab Invest* 1983;48: 148–155.
556. Kodet R: Rhabdomyosarcoma in childhood. An immunohistological analysis with myoglobin, desmin and vimentin. *Pathol Res Pract* 1989;185:207–213.
557. Eusebi V, Ceccarelli C, Gorza L, et al: Immunocytochemistry of rhabdomyosarcoma. The use of four different markers. *Am J Surg Pathol* 1986;10:293–299.
558. Parham DM, Webber B, Holt H, et al: Immunohistochemical study of childhood rhabdomyosarcomas and related neoplasms. Results of an Intergroup Rhabdomyosarcoma Study project. *Cancer* 1991;67:3072–3080.
559. Scrable H, Witte D, Shimada H, et al: Molecular differential pathology of rhabdomyosarcoma. *Genes Chromosom Cancer* 1989;1: 23–35.
560. Dias P, Parham DM, Shapiro DN, et al: Myogenic regulatory protein (MyoD1) expression in childhood solid tumors: Diagnostic utility in rhabdomyosarcoma. Am J Pathol 1990;137:1283–1291.
561. Eusebi V, Bondi A, Rosai J: Immunohistochemical localization of myoglobin in nonmuscular cells. *Am J Surg Pathol* 1984;8: 51–55.
562. Cavazzana AO, Schmidt D, Ninfo V, et al: Spindle cell rhabdomyosarcoma. A prognostically favorable variant of rhabdomyosarcoma. *Am J Surg Pathol* 1992;16:229–235.
563. Leuschner I, Newton WA Jr, Schmidt D, et al: Spindle cell variants of embryonal rhabdomyosarcoma in the paratesticular region. A report of the Intergroup Rhabdomyosarcoma Study. *Am J Surg Pathol* 1993;17:221–230.
564. Kahn HJ, Yeger H, Kassim O, et al: Immunohistochemical and electron microscopic assessment of childhood rhabdomyosarcoma: Increased frequency of diagnosis over routine histologic methods. *Cancer* 1983;51:1897–1903.
565. Raney RB Jr, Donaldson MH, Sutow WW, et al: Special considerations related to primary site in rhabdomyosarcoma: Experience of the Intergroup Rhabdomyosarcoma Study, 1972–1976. *Natl Cancer Inst Monogr* 1981;56:69–74.
566. Weiss SW, Enzinger FM: Malignant fibrous histiocytoma. An analysis of 200 cases. *Cancer* 1978;41:2250–2266.
567. Linscheid RL, Soule EH, Henderson ED: Pleomorphic rhabdomyosarcomata of the extremities and limb girdles. A clinicopathological study. *J Bone Joint Surg (Am)* 1965;47:715–726.
568. Kodet R, Newton WA Jr, Hamoudi AB, et al: Childhood rhabdomyosarcoma with anaplastic (pleomorphic) features. A report of the Intergroup Rhabdomyosarcoma Study. *Am J Surg Pathol* 1993;17:443–453.
569. Tefft M, Fernandez C, Donaldson M, et al: Incidence of meningeal involvement by rhabdomyosarcoma of the head and neck in children: A report of the Intergroup Rhabdomyosarcoma Study (IRS). *Cancer* 1978;42:253–258.
570. Lawrence W Jr, Hays DM, Moon TE: Lymphatic metastasis with childhood rhabdomyosarcoma. *Cancer* 1977;39:556–559.
571. Anderson GJ, Tom LWC, Womer RB, et al: Rhabdomyosarcoma of the head and neck in children. *Arch Otolaryngol Head Neck Surg* 1990;116:428–431.
572. Exelby PR: Surgery of soft tissue sarcomas in children. *Natl Cancer Inst Monogr* 1981;56:153–157.
573. Gerson JM, Jaffe N, Donaldson MH, et al: Meningeal seeding from rhabdomyosarcoma of the head and neck with base of the skull invasion: Recognition of the clinical evolution and suggestions for management. *Med Pediatr Oncol* 1978;5:137–144.
574. Raney RB: Spinal cord drop metastases from head and neck rhabdomyosarcoma: Proceedings of the Tumor Board of the Children's Hospital of Philadelphia. *Med Pediatr Oncol* 1978;4:3–9.
575. Shimada H, Newton WA Jr, Soule EH, et al: Pathology of fatal rhabdomyosarcoma: Intergroup Rhabdomyosarcoma Study IRS I and II. *Lab Invest* 1984;50:12a.
576. Raney RB, Jr., Tefft M, Newton WA, et al: Improved prognosis with intensive treatment in children with cranial soft tissue sarcomas arising in nonorbital parameningeal sites. A report from the Intergroup Rhabdomyosarcoma Study. *Cancer* 1987;59:147–155.
577. Maurer HM, Beltangady M, Gehan EA, et al: Intergroup Rhabdomyosarcoma Study-I. A final report. *Cancer* 1988;61:209–220.

Bone Lesions

Benign Bone Tumors

Osteoma

578. Earwaker J: Paranasal sinus osteomas: A review of 46 cases. *Skeletal Radiol* 1993;22:417–423.
579. Boysen M: Osteomas of the paranasal sinuses. *J Otolaryngol* 1978;7:366–370.
580. Samy LL, Mostafa H: Osteomata of the nose and paranasal sinuses with a report of twenty one cases. *J Laryngol Otol* 1971;85:449–469.
581. Smith ME, Calcaterra TC: Frontal sinus osteoma. *Ann Otol Rhinol Laryngol* 1989;98:896–900.
582. Fu Y-S, Perzin KH: Non-epithelial tumors of the nasal cavity, paranasal sinuses, and nasopharynx: A clinicopathologic study. II. Osseous and fibro-osseous lesions, including osteoma, fibrous dysplasia, ossifying fibroma, osteoblastoma, giant cell tumor, and osteosarcoma. *Cancer* 1974;33:1289–1305.
583. Mikaelian DO, Lewis WJ, Behringer WH: Primary osteoma of the sphenoid sinus. *Laryngoscope* 1976;86:728–733.
584. Probst LE, Shankar L, Fox R: Osteoma of the mastoid bone. *J Otolaryngol* 1991;20:228–230.
585. Long DE, Koutnik AW: Recurrent intraoral osseous choristoma. Report of a case. *Oral Surg Oral Med Oral Pathol* 1991;72:337–339.
586. Cremers CWRJ: Osteoma of the middle ear. *J Laryngol Otol* 1985;99:383–386.
587. Dolan KD, Babin RW, Smoker WRK: Osteoma of the sphenoidal sinus. *Skeletal Radiol* 1982;8:233–234.
588. Chang CH, Piatt ED, Thomas KE, et al: Bone abnormalities in Gardner's syndrome. *AJR* 1968;103:645–652.
589. Moshref M, Ebrahimi B, Hafez MT: Periosteal compact osteoma. *Oral Surg* 1984;58:743.
590. Perniciaro C: Gardner's syndrome. *Dermatol Clin* 1995;13:51–56.
591. Yuasa K, Yonetsu K, Kanda S, et al: Computed tomography of the jaws in familial adenomatosis coli. *Oral Surg Oral Med Oral Pathol* 1993;76:251–255.
592. Takeuchi T, Takenoshita Y, Kubo K, et al: Natural course of jaw lesions in patients with familial adenomatosis coli (Gardner's syndrome). *Int J Oral Maxillofac Surg* 1993;22:226–230.
593. Tohill MJ, Green JG, Cohen DM: Intraoral osseous and cartilaginous choristomas: Report of three cases and review of the literature. *Oral Surg Oral Med Oral Pathol* 1987;63:506–510.

Osteoid Osteoma

594. Loizaga JM, Calvo M, Lopez Barea F, et al: Osteoblastoma and osteoid osteoma. Clinical and morphological features of 162 cases. *Pathol Res Pract* 1993;189:33–41.
595. Zwimpfer TJ, Tucker WS, Faulkner JF: Ostoeid osteoma of the cervical spine: Case reports and literature review. *Can J Surg* 1982;25:637–641.
596. Fielding JW, Keim HA, Hawkins RJ, et al: Osteoid osteoma of the cervical spine. *Clin Orthop* 1977;128:163–164.
597. Pettine KA, Klassen RA: Osteoid-osteoma and osteoblastoma of the spine. *J Bone Joint Surg Am* 1986;68:354–361.
598. Maiuri F, Signorelli C, Lavano A, et al: Osteoid osteomas of the spine. *Surg Neurol* 1986;25:375–380.
599. Goldstein GS, Dawson EG, Batzdorf U: Cervical osteoid osteoma: A cause of chronic upper back pain. *Clin Orthop Rel Res* 1977;129:177–180.
600. Bucci NM, Feldenzer JA, Phillips WA, et al: Atlanto-axial rotational limitation secondary to osteoid osteoma of the axis. Case report. *J Neurosurg* 1989;70:129–131.
601. Jones DA: Osteoid osteoma of the atlas. *J Bone Joint Surg Br* 1987;69:149.
602. Gamba JL, Martinez S, Apple J, et al: Computed tomography of axial skeletal osteoid osteomas. *AJR* 1984;142:769–772.
603. Foss EL, Dockerty MB, Good CA: Osteoid osteoma of the mandible. Report of a case. *Cancer* 1955;8:592–594.
604. Jackson RP, Reckling FW, Mantz FA: Osteoid osteoma and osteoblastoma. Similar histologic lesions with different natural histories. *Clin Orthop* 1977;128:303–313.
605. Van Der Wall I, Greebe RB, Elias EA: Benign osteoblastoma or osteoid osteoma of the maxilla. Report of a case. *Int J Oral Surg* 1983;12:355–358.

606. Wilder WM, Dowling EA, Brogdon BG: Osteoid osteoma of the mastoid tip. *Skeletal Radiol* 1995;24:551–552.

607. Prabhakar B, Reddy DR, Dayananda B, et al: Osteoid osteoma of the skull. *J Bone Joint Surg Br* 1972;54:146–148.

608. Debois V, van den Bergh R: Benign tumors of the cranial vault. A report of 12 cases. *Clin Neurol Neurosurg* 1979;81:1–12.

609. Neff S, Hansen K, Domanowski GF, et al: Cryptic osteoid osteoma of the cranium: Case report. *Neurosurgery* 1990;27:820–821.

610. Swee RG, McLeod RA, Beabout JW: Osteoid osteoma. Detection, diagnosis, and localization. *Radiology* 1979;130:117–123.

611. Schajowicz F, Lemos C: Osteoid osteoma and osteoblastoma. Closely related entities of osteoblastic derivation. *Acta Orthop Scand* 1970;41:272–291.

612. Byers PD: Solitary benign osteoblastic lesions of bone. Osteoid osteoma and benign osteoblastoma. *Cancer* 1968;22:43–57.

613. de Souza Dias L, Frost HM: Osteoid osteoma–osteoblastoma. *Cancer* 1974;33:1075–1081.

614. Tanaka C, Fujiwara Y, Yamamuro T, et al: Intraperiosteal osteoid osteoma. A case report. *Clin Orthop* 1983;175:190–192.

615. Golding JSR: The natural history of osteoid osteoma with a report of twenty cases. *J Bone Joint Surg Br* 1954;36:218–229.

616. Rosenthal DI, Alexander A,Rosenberg AE, et al: Ablation of osteoid osteomas with a percutaneously placed electrode: A new procedure. *Radiology* 1992;183:29–33.

617. Assoun J, Railhac J-J, Bonnevialle P, et al: Osteoid osteoma: Percutaneous resection with CT guidance. *Radiology* 1993;188:541–547.

Osteoblastoma

618. Lucas DR, Unni KK, McLeod RA, et al: Osteoblastoma: Clinicopathologic study of 306 cases. *Hum Pathol* 1994;25:117–134.

619. Janin Y, Epstein JA, Carras R, et al: Osteoid osteomas and osteoblastomas of the spine. *Neurosurgery* 1981;8:31–38.

620. Loizaga JM, Calvo M, Lopez Barea F, et al: Osteoblastoma and osteoid osteoma. Clinical and morphological features of 162 cases. *Pathol Res Pract* 1993;189:33–41.

621. Rocca CD, Huvos AG: Osteoblastoma: Varied histological presentations with a benign clinical course. An analysis of 55 cases. *Am J Surg Pathol* 1996;20:841–850.

622. Berciano J, Perez-López JL, Fernández F, et al: Voluminous benign osteoblastoma of the skull. *Surg Neurol* 1983;20:383–386.

623. Ciappetta P, Salvati M, Raco A, et al: Benign osteoblastoma of the sphenoid bone. *Neurochirurgia* 1991;34:97–100.

624. Goel A, Bhayani R, Nagpal RD: Massive benign osteoblastoma of the clivus and atlas. *Br J Neurosurg* 1994;8:483–486.

625. El-Mofty S, Refai H: Benign ostoeblastoma of the maxilla. *J Oral Maxillofac Surg* 1989;47:60–64.

626. Mohan V, Sabri T, Marklund T, et al: Clinicoradiological diagnosis of benign osteoblastoma of the spine in children. *Arch Orthop Trauma Surg* 1991;110:260–264.

627. Kirwan E O'G, Hutton PAN, Pozo JL, et al: Osteoid osteoma and benign osteoblastoma of the spine. Clinical presentation and treatment. *J Bone Joint Surg Br* 1984;66:21–26.

628. Nguyen VD, Hersh M: A rare bone tumor in an unusual location: Osteoblastoma of the vertebral body. *Comput Med Image Graph* 1992;16:11–16.

629. Kroon HM, Schurmans J: Osteoblastoma: Clinical and radiologic findings in 98 new cases. *Radiology* 1990;175:783–790.

630. Schajowicz F, Lemos C: Osteoid osteoma and osteoblastoma. Closely related entities of osteoblastic derivation. *Acta Orthop Scand* 1970;41:272–291.

631. Bertoni F, Unni KK, McLeod RA, et al: Osteosarcoma resembling osteoblastoma. *Cancer* 1985;55:416–426.

632. Doron Y, Gruszkiewicz J, Gelli B, et al: Benign osteoblastoma of vertebral column and skull. *Surg Neurol* 1977;7:86–90.

633. Tom LWC, Lowry LD, Quinn-Bogard A: Benign osteoblastoma of the maxillary sinus. *Otolaryngol Head Neck Surg* 1980;88:397–402.

634. Khashaba A, De Donato G, Vassallo G, et al: Benign osteoblastoma of the mastoid part of the temporal bone: Case report. *J Laryngol Otol* 1995;109:565–568.

635. Banerjee AK, Kak VK: Benign osteoblastoma of the occipital bone. *Ear Nose Throat J* 1991;70:215–216.

636. Freedman SR: Benign osteoblastoma of the ethmoid bone. Report of a case. *Am J Clin Pathol* 1975;63:391–396.

637. Williams RN, Boop WC Jr: Benign osteoblastoma of the skull. Case report. *J Neurosurg* 1974;41:769–772.

638. Leone CR Jr, Lawton AW, Leone RT: Benign osteoblastoma of the orbit. *Ophthalmology* 1988;95:1554–1558.

639. Greer RO Jr, Berman DN: Osteoblastoma of the jaws: Current concepts and differential diagnosis. *J Oral Surg* 1978;36:304–307.

640. Smith RA, Hansen LS, Resnick D, et al: Comparison of the osteoblastoma in gnathic and extragnathic sites. *Oral Surg* 1982;54:285–298.

641. Chatterji P, Purohit GN, Bikaner INR: Benign osteoblastoma of the maxilla (periosteal). *J Laryngol Otol* 1978;92:337–345.

642. Fechner RE: Problematic lesions of the craniofacial bones. *Am J Surg Pathol* 1989;13:17–30.

643. Weinberg S, Katsikeris N, Pharoah M: Osteoblastoma of the mandibular condyle: Review of the literature and report of a case. *J Oral Maxillofac Surg* 1987;45:350–355.

644. Kent JN, Castro HF, Girotti WR: Benign osteoblastoma of the maxilla. Case report and review of the literature. *Oral Pathol* 1969;27:209–219.

645. McLeod RA, Dahlin DC, Beabout JW: The spectrum of osteoblastoma. *AJR* 1976;126:321–335.

646. Dorfman HD, Weiss SW: Borderline osteoblastic tumors: Problems in the differential diagnosis of aggressive osteoblastoma and low-grade osteosarcoma. *Semin Diagn Pathol* 1984;1:215–234.

647. Mirra JM, Kendrick RA, Kendrick RE: Pseudomalignant osteoblastoma versus arrested osteosarcoma. A case report. *Cancer* 1976;37:2005–2014.

648. Schajowicz F, Lemos C: Malignant osteoblastoma. *J Bone Joint Surg Br* 1976;58:202–211.

649. Bertoni F, Bacchini P, Donati D, et al: Osteoblastoma-like osteosarcoma. The Rizzoli Institute experience. *Mod Pathol* 1993;6:707–716.

650. Mitchell ML, Ackerman LV: Metastatic and pseudomalignant osteoblastoma: A report of two unusual cases. *Skeletal Radiol* 1986;15:213–218.

651. Merryweather R, Middlemiss JH, Sanerkin NG: Malignant transformation of osteoblastoma. *J Bone Joint Surg Br* 1980;62:381–384.

652. Bertoni F, Unni KK, Lucas DR, et al: Osteoblastoma with cartilaginous matrix. An unusual morphologic presentation in 18 cases. *Am J Surg Pathol* 1993;17:69–74.

653. Figarella-Branger D, Perez-Castillo M, Garbe L, et al: Malignant transformation of an osteoblastoma of the skull: An exceptional occurrence. *J Neurosurg* 1991;75:138–142.

654. Beyer WF, Kühn H: Can an osteoblastoma become malignant? *Virchows Arch Pathol Anat* 1985;408:297–305.

Malignant Bone Tumors

Osteosarcoma

655. Campanacci M, Cervellati G: Osteosarcoma. A review of 345 cases. *Ital J Orthop Traumatol* 1975;1:5–22.

656. Harvei S, Solheim Ø: The prognosis in osteosarcoma. Norwegian national data. *Cancer* 1981;48:1719–1723.

657. Uribe-Botero G, Russell WO, Sutow WW, et al: Primary osteosarcoma of bone. A clinicopathologic investigation of 243 cases, with necropsy studies in 54. *Am J Clin Pathol* 1977;67:427–435.

658. Huvos AG, Butler A, Bretsky SS: Osteogenic sarcoma associated with Paget's disease of bone. A clinicopathologic study of 65 patients. *Cancer* 1983;52:1489–1495.

659. Schajowicz F, Araujo ES, Berenstein M: Sarcoma complicating Paget's disease of bone. A clinicopathological study of 62 cases. *J Bone Joint Surg Br* 1983;65:299–307.

660. Present D, Bertoni F, Enneking WF: Osteosarcoma of the mandible arising in fibrous dysplasia. A case report. *Clin Orthop* 1986;204:238–244.

661. Taconis WK: Osteosarcoma in fibrous dysplasia. *Skeletal Radiol* 1988;17:163–170.

662. Torres FX, Kyriakos, M: Bone infarct-associated osteosarcoma. *Cancer* 1992;70:2418–2430.

663. Huvos AG, Woodard HQ, Cahan WG, et al: Postradiation osteogenic sarcoma of bone and soft tissues. A clinicopathologic study of 66 patients. *Cancer* 1985;55:1244–1255.

664. Benedict WF, Xu H-J, Hu S-X, et al: Role of the retinoblastoma gene in the initiation and progression of human cancer. *J Clin Invest* 1990;85:988–993.

665. Benedict WF, Fung Y-KT, Murphree AL: The gene responsible for the development of retinoblastoma and osteosarcoma. *Cancer* 1988;62:1691–1694.

666. Araki N, Uchida A, Kimura T, et al: Involvement of the retinoblas-

toma gene in primary osteosarcomas and other bone and soft-tissue tumors. *Clin Orthop* 1991;270:271–277.

667. Kozakewich H, Perez-Atayde AR, Goorin AM, et al: Osteosarcoma in young children. *Cancer* 1991;67:638–642.

668. Luiz CPJ, Kharusi WA, Sethu AU, et al: Osteosarcoma in a 26-month-old girl. *Cancer* 1992;70:894–896.

669. Huvos AG: Osteogenic sarcoma of bones and soft tissues in older persons. A clinicopathologic analysis of 117 patients older than 60 years. *Cancer* 1986;57:1442–1449.

670. deSantos LA, Rosengren J-E, Wooten WB, et al: Osteogenic sarcoma after the age of 50: A radiographic evaluation. *AJR* 1978;131:481–484.

671. Dahlin DC: Pathology of osteosarcoma. *Clin Orthop* 1975;111:23–32.

672. McKenna RJ, Schwinn CP, Soong KY, et al: Sarcomata of the osteogenic series (osteosarcoma, fibrosarcoma, chondrosarcoma, parosteal osteogenic sarcoma, and sarcomata arising in abnormal bone). An analysis of 552 cases. *J Bone Joint Surg Am* 1966;48:1–26.

673. Bosse A, Vollmer E, Böcker W, et al: The impact of osteonectin for differential diagnosis of bone tumors. An immunohistochemical approach. *Pathol Res Pract* 1990;186:651–657.

674. Serra M, Morini MC, Scotlandi K, et al: Evaluation of osteonectin as a diagnostic marker of osteogenic bone tumors. *Hum Pathol* 1992;23:1326–1331.

675. Schulz A, Jundt G, Berghauser K-H, et al: Immunohistochemical study of osteonectin in various types of osteosarcoma. *Am J Pathol* 1988;132:233–238.

676. Park Y-K, Yang MH, Park HR: The impact of osteonectin for differential diagnosis of osteogenic bone tumors: An immunohistochemical and in situ hybridization approach. *Skeletal Radiol* 1996;25:13–17.

677. Hasegawa T, Hirose T, Kudo E, et al: Immunophenotypic heterogeneity in osteosarcomas. *Hum Pathol* 1991;22:583–590.

678. Ushigome S, Shimoda T, Fukunaga M, et al: Immunocytochemical aspects of the differential diagnosis of osteosarcoma and malignant fibrous histiocytoma. *Surg Pathol* 1988;1:347–357.

679. Schajowicz F, de Prospero JD, Cosentino E: Case report 641. Chondroblastoma-like osteosarcoma. *Skeletal Radiol* 1990;19:603–606.

680. Bertoni F, Bacchini P, Donati D, et al: Osteoblastoma-like osteosarcoma. The Rizzoli Institute experience. *Mod Pathol* 1993;6:707–716.

681. Povysil C, Matejovsky Z, Zidkova H: Osteosarcoma with a clear-cell component. *Virchows Arch (A)* 1988;412:273–279.

682. Hasegawa T, Shibata T, Hirose T, et al: Osteosarcoma with epithelioid features. An immunohistochemical study. *Arch Pathol Lab Med* 1993;117:295–298.

683. Kramer K, Hicks DG, Palis J, et al: Epithelioid osteosarcoma of bone. Immunocytochemical evidence suggesting divergent epithelial and mesenchymal differentiation in a primary osseous neoplasm. *Cancer* 1993;71:2977–2982.

684. Yoshida H, Yumoto T, Adachi H, et al: Osteosarcoma with prominent epithelioid features. *Acta Pathol Jpn* 1989;39:439–445.

685. Ballance WA, Jr., Mendelsohn G, Carter JR, et al: Osteogenic sarcoma. Malignant fibrous histiocytoma subtype. *Cancer* 1988;62:763–771.

686. Yoshida H, Yumoto T, Minamizaki T: Osteosarcoma with features mimicking malignant fibrous histiocytoma. *Virchows Arch (A)* 1992;421:229–238.

687. Dahlin DC, Unni KK: Osteosarcoma of bone and its important recognizable varieties. *Am J Surg Pathol* 1977;1:61–72.

688. Troup JB, Dahlin DC, Conventry MB: The significance of giant cells in osteogenic sarcoma: Do they indicate a relationship between osteogenic sarcoma and giant cell tumor of bone? *Mayo Clin Proc* 1960;35:179–186.

689. Unni KK: Osteosarcoma of bone. In: Unni KK , ed. *Bone Tumors.* Edinburgh: Churchill Livingstone, 1988:107–133.

690. Wiklund TA, Blomqvist CP, Raty J, et al: Postirradiation sarcoma. Analysis of a nationwide cancer registry material. *Cancer* 1991;68:524–531.

691. Bjornsson J, Inwards CY, Wold LE, et al: Prognostic significance of spontaneous tumour necrosis in osteosarcoma. *Virchows Arch (A)* 1993;423:195–199.

692. von Hochstetter AR: Spontaneous necrosis in osteosarcomas. *Virchows Arch (A)* 1990;417:5–8.

693. Petrilli AS, Gentil FC, Epelman S, et al: Increased survival, limb preservation, and prognostic factors for osteosarcoma. *Cancer* 1991;68:733–737.

694. Raymond AK, Chawla SP, Carrasco CH, et al: Osteosarcoma chemo-

therapy effect: a prognostic factor. *Semin Diagn Pathol* 1987;4:212–236.

695. Raymond AK, Ayala AG: Specimen management after osteosarcoma chemotherapy. In: Unni KK, ed. *Bone Tumors.* Churchill Livingstone, 1988:157–181.

696. Glasser DB, Lane JM, Huvos AG, et al: Survival, prognosis, and therapeutic response in osteogenic sarcoma. The Memorial Hospital experience. *Cancer* 1992;69:698–708.

697. Simone JV, Meyer WH, Link MP: Osteosarcoma: Good news despite crude tools. *J Clin Oncol* 1992;10:1–2.

698. Price CHG: The grading of osteogenic sarcoma. *Br J Cancer* 1952;6:46–68.

699. Meister P, Konrad E, Lob G, et al: Osteosarcoma: Histological evaluation and grading. *Arch Orthop Trauma Surg* 1979;94:91–98.

700. Ferguson RJ, Yunis EJ: The ultrastructure of human osteosarcoma. A study of nine cases. *Clin Orthop* 1978;131:234–246.

701. Reddick RL, Michelitch HJ, Levin AM, et al: Osteogenic sarcoma. A study of the ultrastructure. *Cancer* 1980;45:64–71.

702. Grundmann E, Roessner A, Immenkamp M: Tumor cell types in osteosarcoma as revealed by electron microscopy. Implications for histogenesis and subclassification. *Virchows Arch B (Cell Pathol)* 1981;36:257–273.

703. Garbe LR, Monges GM, Pellegrin EM, et al: Ultrastructural study of osteosarcomas. *Hum Pathol* 1981;12:891–896.

704. Salvati M, Ciappetta P, Raco A: Osteosarcoma of the skull. Clinical remarks on 19 cases. *Cancer* 1993;71:2210–2216.

705. Huvos AG, Sundaresan N, Bretsky SS, et al: Osteogenic sarcoma of the skull. A clinicopathologic study of 19 patients. *Cancer* 1985;56:1214–1221.

706. Nora FE, Unni KK, Pritchard DJ, et al: Osteosarcoma of extragnathic craniofacial bones. *Mayo Clin Proc* 1983;58:268–272.

707. Tanaka S, Nishio S, Morioka T, et al: Radiation-induced osteosarcoma of the sphenoid bone. *Neurosurgery* 1989;25:640–643.

708. Kornreich L, Grunebaum M, Ziv N, et al: Osteogenic sarcoma of the calvarium in children: CT manifestations. *Neuroradiology* 1988;30:439–441.

709. Amine ARC, Sugar O: Suprasellar osteogenic sarcoma following radiation for pituitary adenoma. Case report. *J Neurosurg* 1976;44:88–91.

710. Vener J, Rice DH, Newman AN: Osteosarcoma and chondrosarcoma of the head and neck. *Laryngoscopy* 1984;94:240–242.

711. Caron AS, Hajdu SI, Strong EW: Osteogenic sarcoma of the facial and cranial bones. A review of forty-three cases. *Am J Surg* 1971;122:719–725.

712. Lee Y-Y, Tassel PV, Nauert C, et al: Craniofacial osteosarcomas: Plain film, CT, and MR findings in 46 cases. *AJNR* 1988;9:379–385.

713. Fu Y-S, Perzin KH: Non-epithelial tumors of the nasal cavity, paranasal sinuses, and nasopharynx: A clinicopathologic study. II Osseous and fibro-osseous lesions, including osteoma, fibrous dysplasia, ossifying fibroma, osteoblastoma, giant cell tumor, and osteosarcoma. *Cancer* 1974;33:1289–1305.

714. Wang YC, Shih CJ, Leu FJ, et al: Primary osteogenic sarcoma of the skull: Case report. *Neurosurgery* 1981; 9:307–310.

715. Sim FH, Unni KK, Beabout JW, et al: Osteosarcoma with small cells simulating Ewing's tumor. *J Bone Joint Surg Am* 1979;61:207–215.

716. Kurt A-M, Unni KK, McLeod RA, et al: Low-grade intraosseous osteosarcoma. Cancer 1990;65:1418–1428.

717. Mark RJ, Sercarz JA, Tran L, et al: Osteogenic sarcoma of the head and neck. The UCLA experience. *Arch Otolaryngol Head Neck Surg* 1991;117:761–766.

718. Benson JE, Goske M, Han JS, et al: Primary osteogenic sarcoma of the calvaria. *AJNR* 1984;5:810–813.

719. Reichenthal E, Cohen ML, Manor R, et al: Primary osteogenic sarcoma of the sellar region. Case report. *J Neurosurg* 1981;55:299–302.

720. Shramek JK, Kassner EG, White SS: MR appearance of osteogenic sarcoma of the calvaria. *AJR* 1992;158:661–662.

721. Smeele LE, Kostense PJ, van der Waal I, et al: Effect of chemotherapy on survival of craniofacial osteosarcoma: A systematic review of 201 patients. *J Clin Oncol* 1997;15:363–367.

722. Bertoni F, Dallera P, Bacchini P, et al: The Istituto Rizzoli-Beretta experience with osteosarcoma of the jaw. *Cancer* 1991;68:1555–1563.

723. Clark JL, Unni KK, Dahlin DC, et al: Osteosarcoma of the jaw. *Cancer* 1983;51:2311–2316.

724. Lee Y-Y, Tassel PV, Nauert C, et al: Craniofacial osteosarcomas: Plain film, CT, and MR findings in 46 cases. *AJNR* 1988;9:379–385.

725. Garrington GE, Scofield HH, Cornyn J, et al: Osteosarcoma of the jaws. Analysis of 56 cases. *Cancer* 1967;20:377–391.

726. Kragh LV, Dahlin DC, Erich JB: Osteogenic sarcoma of the jaws and facial bones. *Am J Surg* 1958;96:496–505.

727. Regezi JA, Zarbo RJ, McClatchey KD, et al: Osteosarcomas and chondrosarcomas of the jaws: Immunohistochemical correlations. *Oral Surg Oral Med Oral Pathol* 1987;64:302–307.

728. Adekeye EO, Chau KK, Edwards MB, et al: Osteosarcoma of the jaws: A series from Kaduna, Nigeria. *Int J Oral Maxillofac Surg* 1987;16:205–213.

729. Russ JE, Jesse RH: Management of osteosarcoma of the maxilla and mandible. *Am J Surg* 1980;140:572–576.

730. Slootweg PJ, Müller H: Osteosarcoma of the jaw bones. *J Maxillofac Surg* 1985;13:158–166.

731. Lindqvist C, Teppo L, Sane J, et al: Osteosarcoma of the mandible: Analysis of nine cases. *J Oral Maxillofac Surg* 1986;44:759–764.

732. Eustace S, Svojanen J, Marianacci E, et al: Osteosarcoma of the hard palate. *Skeletal Radiol* 1995;24:392–394.

733. Russ JE, Jesse RH: Management of osteosarcoma of the maxilla and mandible. *Am J Surg* 1980;140:572–576.

734. Caron AS, Hajdu SI, Strong EW: Osteogenic sarcoma of the facial and cranial bones. A review of forty-three cases. *Am J Surg* 1971;122:719–725.

735. Li Volsi VA: Osteogenic sarcoma of the maxilla. *Arch Otolaryngol* 1977;103:485–488.

736. Chan CW, Kung TM, Ma L: Telangiectatic osteosarcoma of the mandible. *Cancer* 1986;58:2110–2115.

737. Forteza G, Colmenero B, López-Barea F: Osteogenic sarcoma of the maxilla and mandible. *Oral Surg Oral Med Oral Pathol* 1986;62:179–184.

738. Giangaspero F, Stracca V, Visona A, et al: Small-cell osteosarcoma of the mandible. Case report. *Appl Pathol* 1984;2:28–31.

739. Edeiken J, Raymond AK, Ayala AG, et al: Small-cell osteosarcoma. *Skeletal Radiol* 1987;16:621–628.

740. Kurt A-M, Unni KK, McLeod RA, et al: Low-grade intraosseous osteosarcoma. *Cancer* 1990;65:1418–1428.

741. Miller TT, Abdelwahab IF, Hermann G, et al: Case report 735: Vertebral osteosarcoma. *Skeletal Radiol* 1992;21:277–279.

742. Shives TC, Dahlin DC, Sim FH, et al: Osteosarcoma of the spine. *J Bone Joint Surg Am* 1986;68:660–668.

743. Barwick KW, Huvos AG, Smith J: Primary osteogenic sarcoma of the vertebral column. A clinicopathologic correlation of ten patients. *Cancer* 1980;46:595–604.

744. Fielding JW, Fietti VG, Hughes JEO, et al: Primary osteogenic sarcoma of the cervical spine. A case report. *J Bone Joint Surg Am* 1976;58:892–894.

745. Marsh HO, Choi C-B: Primary osteogenic sarcoma of the cervical spine originally mistaken for benign osteoblastoma. A case report. *J Bone Joint Surg Am* 1970;52:1467–1471.

746. Kebudi R, Ayan I, Darendeliler E, et al: Primary osteosarcoma of the cervical spine: A pediatric case report and review of the literature. *Med Pediatr Oncol* 1994;23:162–165.

747. Patel DV, Hammer RA, Levin B, et al: Primary osteogenic sarcoma of the spine. *Skeletal Radiol* 1984;12:276–279.

748. Mnaymneh W, Brown M, Tejada F, et al: Primary osteogenic sarcoma of the second cervical vertebra. Case report. *J Bone Joint Surg Am* 1979;61:460–462.

749. Miled KB, Siala M, Hamza Kh.R, et al: Primary osteosarcoma of the cervical spine: One case. *J Neuroradiol* 1988;15:294–300.

750. Okada K, Frassica FJ, Sim FH, et al: Parosteal osteosarcoma. A clinicopathological study. *J Bone Joint Surg Am* 1994;76:366–378.

751. Banerjee SC: Juxtacortical osteosarcoma of mandible: Review of literature and report of case. *J Oral Surg* 1981;39:535–538.

752. Bras JM, Donner R, van der Kwast WAM, et al: Juxtacortical osteogenic sarcoma of the jaws. Review of the literature and report of a case. *Oral Surg* 1980;50:535–544

753. Solomon MP, Biernacki J, Slippen M, et al: Parosteal osteogenic sarcoma of the mandible. Existence masked by diffuse periodontal inflammation. *Arch Otolaryngol* 1975;101:754–760.

754. Som M, Peimer R: Juxtacortical osteogenic sarcoma of the mandible. *Arch Otolaryngol* 1961;74:532–536.

755. Roca AN, Smith JL Jr, Jing B-S: Osteosarcoma and parosteal osteogenic sarcoma of the maxilla and mandible: Study of 20 cases. *Am J Clin Pathol* 1970;54:625–636.

756. Millar BG, Browne RM, Flood TR: Juxtacortical osteosarcoma of the jaws. *Br J Oral Maxillofac Surg* 1990;28:73–79.

757. Iemoto Y, Ushigome S, Ikegami M, et al: Case report 648: Parosteal osteosarcoma arising from the right temporal bone. *Skeletal Radiol* 1991;20:59–61.

758. Marks MP, Marks SC, Segall HD, et al: Case report 420: Parosteal osteosarcoma. *Skeletal Radiol* 1987;16:246–251.

759. Kumar R, Moser RP Jr, Madewell JE, et al: Parosteal osteogenic sarcoma arising in cranial bones: Clinical and radiologic features in eight patients. *AJR* 1990;155:113–117.

760. Unni KK, Dahlin DC, Beabout JW, et al: Parosteal osteogenic sarcoma. *Cancer* 1976;37:2466–2475.

761. Ahuja SC, Villacin AB, Smith J, et al: Juxtacortical (parosteal) osteogenic sarcoma. Histologic grading and prognosis. *J Bone Joint Surg Am* 1977;59:632–647.

762. Smith J, Ahuja SC, Huvos AG, et al: Parosteal (juxtacortical) osteogenic sarcoma. A roentgenological study of 30 patients. *J Can Assoc Radiol* 1978;29:167–174.

763. Van Der Heul RO, Von Ronnen JR: Juxtacortical osteosarcoma. Diagnosis, differential diagnosis, treatment, and an analysis of eighty cases. *J Bone Joint Surg Am* 1967;49:415–439.

764. Dwinnell LA, Dahlin DC, Ghormley RK: Parosteal (juxtacortical) osteogenic sarcoma. *J Bone Joint Surg Am* 1954;36:732–744.

765. Campanacci M, Picci P, Gherlinzoni F, et al: Parosteal osteosarcoma. *J Bone Joint Surg Br* 1984;66:313–321.

766. Copeland MM, Geschickter CF: The treatment of parosteal osteoma of bone. *Surg Gynecol Obstet* 1959;108:537–548.

767. Sheth DS, Yasko AW, Raymond AK, et al: Conventional and dedifferentiated parosteal osteosarcoma. Diagnosis, treatment, and outcome. *Cancer* 1996;78:2136–2145.

768. Wold LE, Unni KK, Beabout JW, et al: Dedifferentiated parosteal osteosarcoma. *J Bone Joint Surg Am* 1984;66:53–59.

769. Wold LE, Unni KK, Beabout JW, et al: High-grade surface osteosarcomas. *Am J Surg Pathol* 1984;8:181–186.

770. Unni KK, Dahlin DC, Beabout JW: Periosteal osteogenic sarcoma. *Cancer* 1976;37:2476–2485.

771. Zarbo RJ, Regezi JA, Baker SR: Periosteal osteogenic sarcoma of the mandible. *Oral Surg* 1984;57:643–647.

772. Minić AJ: Periosteal osteosarcoma of the mandible. *Int J Oral Maxillofac Surg* 1995;24:226–228.

773. Bras JM, Donner R, van der Kwast AM, et al: Juxtacortical osteogenic sarcoma of the jaws. Review of the literature and report of a case. *Oral Surg* 1980;50:535–544.

774. Patterson A, Greer RO Jr, Howard D: Periosteal osteosarcoma of the maxilla: A case report and review of literature. *J Oral Maxillofac Surg* 1990;48:522–526.

775. Ritts GD, Pritchard DJ, Unni KK, et al: Periosteal osteosarcoma. *Clin Orthop* 1987;219:299–307.

776. Spjut HJ, Ayala AG, de Santos LA, et al: *Periosteal Osteosarcoma: Management of Primary Bone and Soft Tissue Tumors.* Chicago: Year Book Medical Publishers, 1977:79–95.

777. Bertoni F, Boriani S, Laus M, et al: Periosteal chondrosarcoma and periosteal osteosarcoma: Two distinct entities. *J Bone Joint Surg Br* 1982;64:370–376.

778. Schajowicz F, McGuire MH, Araujo ES, et al: Osteosarcomas arising on the surfaces of long bones. *J Bone Joint Surg Am* 1988;70:555–564.

779. Schajowicz F: Juxtacortical chondrosarcoma. *J Bone Joint Surg Br* 1977;59:473–480.

780. Lorentzon R, Larsson S-E, Boquist L: Extra-osseous osteosarcoma. A clinical and histopathological study of four cases. *J Bone Joint Surg Br* 1979;61:205–208.

781. Allan CJ, Soule EH: Osteogenic sarcoma of the somatic soft tissues. Clinicopathologic study of 26 cases and review of literature. *Cancer* 1971;27:1121–1133.

782. Rao U, Cheng A, Didolkar MS: Extraosseous osteogenic sarcoma. Clinicopathological study of eight cases and review of literature. *Cancer* 1978;41:1488–1496.

783. Loyzaga JM, Machin PF, Sala J: Osteogenic sarcoma of the tongue. Case report and review of the literature. *Pathol Res Pract* 1996;192:75–78.

784. Sordillo PP, Hajdu SI, Magill GB, et al: Extraosseous osteogenic sarcoma. A review of 48 patients. *Cancer* 1983;51:727–734.

785. Chung EB, Enzinger FM: Extraskeletal osteosarcoma. *Cancer* 1987;60:1132–1142.

786. Lee JSY, Fetsch JF, Wasdhal DA, et al: A review of 40 patients with extraskeletal osteosarcoma. *Cancer* 1995;76:2253–2259.

787. Kauffman SL, Stout AP: Extraskeletal osteogenic sarcomas and chondrosarcomas in children. *Cancer* 1963;16:432–439.

788. Dahm LJ, Schaefer SD, Carder HM, et al: Osteosarcoma of the soft tissue of the larynx. Report of a case with light and electron microscopic studies. *Cancer* 1978;42:2343–2351.

789. Laskin WB, Silverman TA, Enzinger FM: Postradiation soft tissue sarcomas: An analysis of 53 cases. *Cancer* 1988;62:2330–2340.

790. Hasson J, Hartman KS, Milikow E, et al: Thorotrast-induced extraskeletal osteosarcoma of the cervical region. Report of a case. *Cancer* 1975;36:1827–1833.

791. Yi ES, Shmookler BM, Malawer MM, et al: Well-differentiated extraskeletal osteosarcoma. A soft-tissue homologue of parosteal osteosarcoma. *Arch Pathol Lab Med* 1991;115:906–909.

792. Bane BL, Evans HL, Ro JY, et al: Extraskeletal osteosarcoma. A clinicopathologic review of 26 cases. *Cancer* 1990;65:2762–2770.

Benign Cartilaginous Tumors

Chondroma

793. Sharma V, Newton G: Chondroma in the foramen magnum. *Clin Pediatr* 1990;29:478.

794. Miki K, Kawamoto K, Kawamura Y, et al: A rare case of Maffucci's syndrome combined with tuberculum sellae enchondroma, pituitary adenoma and thyroid adenoma. *Acta Neurochir* 1987;87:79–85.

795. Lozes G, Fawaz A, Perper H, et al: Chondroma of the cervical spine. Case report. *J Neurosurg* 1987;66:128–130.

796. Traflet RF, Babaria AR, Barolat G, et al: Intracranial chondroma in a patient with Ollier's disease. Case report. *J Neurosurg* 1989;70:274–276.

797. Chakrabortty S, Tamaki N, Kondoh T, et al: Maffucci's syndrome associated with intracranial enchondroma and aneurysm: Case report. *Surg Neurol* 1991;36:216–220.

798. Ghogawala Z, Moore M, Strand R, et al: Clival chondroma in a child with Ollier's disease. Case report. *Pediatr Neurosurg* 1991–1992;17:53–56.

799. Ikeda K, Kikuta N, Sasaki Y, et al: Extracranial chondroma of the skull base. *Arch Otorhinolaryngol* 1987;243:424–428.

800. Krayenbühl H, Yasargil MG: Chondromas. *Prog Neurol Surg* 1975;6:435–463.

801. Tomich CE, Hutton CE: Chondroma of the anterior nasal spine. *J Oral Surg* 1976;34:911–915.

802. Fu Y-S, Perzin KH: Non-epithelial tumors of the nasal cavity, paranasal sinuses, and nasopharynx: A clinicopathologic study. III. Cartilaginous tumors (chondroma, chondrosarcoma). *Cancer* 1974;34:453–463.

803. Willis BK, Heilbrun MP: Enchondroma of the cervical spine. *Neurosurgery* 1986;19:437–440.

804. Bell MS: Benign cartilaginous tumours of the spine. A report of one case together with a review of the literature. *Br J Surg* 1971;58:707–711.

805. Antic B, Roganovic Z, Tadic R, et al: Chondroma of the cervical spine canal. Case report. *J Neurosurg Sci* 1992;36:239–241.

806. Ünal T, Ertürk S: Cartilaginous choristoma of the gingiva. Report of two cases; review of the literature of both gingival choristomas and intraoral chondromas. *Ann Dent* 1994;53:19–27.

807. Chou L, Hansen LS, Daniels TE: Choristomas of the oral cavity: A review. *Oral Surg Oral Med Oral Pathol* 1991;72:584–593.

808. Timmis P: Chondroma of nasopharynx. *J Laryngol Otol* 1959;73:383–387.

809. Munro JM, Pal Singh MP: Chondroma of the tongue. Report of a case and a consideration of the histogenesis of such lesions. *Arch Pathol Lab Med* 1990;114:541–542.

810. Tosios K, Laskaris G, Eveson J, et al: Benign cartilaginous tumor of the gingiva. A case report. *Int J Oral Maxillofac Surg* 1993;22:231–233.

811. Blum MR, Danford M, Speight PM: Soft tissue chondroma of the cheek. *J Oral Pathol Med* 1993;22:334–336.

812. Neel HB III, Unni KK: Cartilaginous tumors of the larynx: A series of 33 patients. *Otolaryngol Head Neck Surg* 1982;90:201–207.

813. Tiwari RM, Snow GB, Balm AJM, et al: Cartilagenous tumours of the larynx. *J Laryngol Otol* 1987;101:266–275.

814. Devaney KO, Ferlito A, Silver CE: Cartilaginous tumors of the larynx. *Ann Otol Rhinol Laryngol* 1995;104:251–255.

815. Hyams VJ, Rabuzzi DD: Cartilaginous tumors of the larynx. *Laryngoscope* 1970;80:755–767.

816. Mirra JM, Gold R, Downs J, et al: A new histologic approach to the differentiation of enchondroma and chondrosarcoma of the bones. A clinicopathologic analysis of 51 cases. *Clin Orthop* 1985;201:214–237.

817. Cook PL, Evans PG: Chondrosarcoma of the skull in Maffucci's syndrome. *Br J Radiol* 1977;50:833–836.

818. Lewis RJ, Ketcham AS: Maffucci's syndrome: Functional and neoplastic significance. Case report and review of the literature. *J Bone Joint Surg Am* 1973;55:1465–1479.

819. Liu J, Hudkins PG, Swee RG, et al: Bone sarcomas associated with Ollier's disease. *Cancer* 1987;59:1376–1385.

820. Schwartz HS, Zimmerman NB, Simon MA, et al: The malignant potential of enchondromatosis. *J Bone Joint Surg Am* 1987;69:269–274.

Osteochondroma

821. Levine MH, Chessen J, McCarthy WD: Osteochondroma of the coronoid process of the mandible. Report of a case and review of the literature. *N Engl J Med* 1957;257:374–376.

822. Fielding JW, Ratzan S: Osteochondroma of the cervical spine. *J Bone Joint Surg Am* 1973;55:640–641.

823. Wu KK, Guise ER: Osteochondroma of the atlas: A case report. *Clin Orthop* 1978;136:160–162.

824. Nielsen OG, Gadegaard L, Fogh A: Osteochondroma of the cervical spine. *J Laryngol Otol* 1986;100:733–736.

825. Tajima K, Nishida J, Yamazaki K, et al: Case report 545. Osteochondroma (osteocartilagenous exostosis) cervical spine with spinal cord compression. *Skeletal Radiol* 1989;18:306–309.

826. Albrecht S, Crutchfield JS, SeGall GK: On spinal osteochondromas. *J Neurosurg* 1992;77:247–252.

827. Morard M, de Preux J: Solitary osteochondroma presenting as a neck mass with spinal cord compression syndrome. *Surg Neurol* 1992;37:402–405.

828. Kerscher A, Piette E, Tideman H, et al: Osteochondroma of the coronoid process of the mandible. Report of a case and review of the literature. *Oral Surg Oral Med Oral Pathol* 1993;75:559–564.

829. Morikawa M, Numaguchi Y, Soliman JA: Osteochondroma of the cervical spine. MR findings. *Clin Imaging* 1995;19:275–278.

830. Loftus MJ, Bennett JA, Fantasia JE: Osteochondroma of the mandibular condyles. Report of three cases and review of the literature. *Oral Surg* 1986;61:221–226.

831. Rose EF, Fekete A: Odontoid osteochondroma causing sudden death. Report of a case and review of the literature. *Am J Clin Pathol* 1964;42:606–609.

832. Brady FA, Sapp JP, Christensen RE: Extracondylar osteochondromas of the jaws. *Oral Surg* 1978;46:658–668.

833. Allan JH, Scott J: Osteochondroma of the mandible. *Oral Surg* 1974;37:556–565.

834. James RB, Alexander RW, Traver JG Jr: Osteochondroma of the mandibular coronoid process. Report of a case. *Oral Surg* 1974;37:189–195.

835. Cole ARC, Darte JMM: Osteochondromata following irradiation in children. *Pediatrics* 1963;32:285–288.

836. Katzman H, Waugh T, Berdon W: Skeletal changes following irradiation of childhood tumors. *J Bone Joint Surg Am* 1969;51:825–842, 1004.

837. Pogrund H, Yosipovitch Z: Osteochondroma following irradiation. Case report and review of the literature. *Isr J Med Sci* 1976;12:154–157.

838. Meyerding HW: Exostosis. *Radiology* 1927;8:282–288.

839. MacGee EE: Osteochondroma of the cervical spine: A cause of transient quadriplegia. *Neurosurgery* 1979;4:259–260.

840. Fanney D, Tehranzadeh J, Quencer RM, et al: Case report 415. Osteochondroma of the cervical spine. *Skeletal Radiol* 1987;16:170–174.

841. Chiurco AA: Multiple exostoses of bone with fatal spinal cord compression. Report of a case and brief review of the literature. *Neurology* 1970;20:275–278.

842. Cohn RS, Fielding JW: Osteochondroma of the cervical spine. *J Pediatr Surg* 1986;21:997–999.

843. Scher N, Panje WR: Osteochondroma presenting as a neck mass: A case report. *Laryngoscope* 1988;98:550–553.

844. Cooke RS, Cumming WJK, Cowie RA: Osteochondroma of the cervical spine: Case report and review of the literature. *Br J Neurosurg* 1994;8:359–363.

845. Linkowski GD, Tsai FY, Recher L, et al: Solitary osteochondroma with spinal cord compression. *Surg Neurol* 1985;23:388–390.

846. Traub DJ, Marco WP, Eisenberg E, et al: Osteochondroma of the max-

illary sinus: Report of a case. *J Oral Maxillofac Surg* 1990;48:752–755.

847. Fon G, Sage MR: Osteochondroma of the clivus. *Australas Radiol* 1979;23:46–53.

848. List CF: Osteochondromas arising from the base of the skull. *Surg Gynecol Obstet* 1943;76:480–492.

849. Garrison RC, Unni KK, McLeod RA, et al: Chondrosarcoma arising in osteochondroma. *Cancer* 1982;49:1890–1897.

850. Anderson RL Jr, Popowitz L, Li JKH: An unusual sarcoma arising in a solitary osteochondroma. *J Bone Joint Surg Am* 1969;51:1199–1204.

851. Schweitzer G, Pirie D: Osteosarcoma arising in a solitary osteochondroma. *S Afr Med J* 1971;45:810–811.

852. Solomon L: Chondrosarcoma in hereditary multiple exostosis. *S Afr Med J* 1974;48:671–676.

Chondroblastoma

853. Springfield DS, Capanna R, Gherlinzoni F, et al: Chondroblastoma. A review of seventy cases. *J Bone Joint Surg Am* 1985;67:748–755.

854. Kurt A-M, Unni KK, Sim FH, et al: Chondroblastoma of bone. *Hum Pathol* 1989;20:965–976.

855. Turcotte RE, Kurt A-M, Sim FH, et al: Chondroblastoma. *Hum Pathol* 1993;24:944–949.

856. Edel G, Ueda Y, Nakanishi J, et al: Chondroblastoma of bone. A clinical, radiological, light and immunohistochemical study. *Virchows Arch A Pathol Anat Histopathol* 1992;421:355–366.

857. Al-Dewachi HS, Al-Naib N, Sangal BC: Benign chondroblastoma of the maxilla: A case report and review of chondroblastomas in cranial bones. *Br J Oral Surg* 1980;18:150–156.

858. Dahlin DC, Ivins JC: Benign chondroblastoma. A study of 125 cases. *Cancer* 1972;30:401–413.

859. Bertoni F, Unni KK, Beabout JW, et al: Chondroblastoma of the skull and facial bones. *Am J Clin Pathol* 1987;88:1–9.

860. Varvares MA, Cheney ML, Ceisler E, et al: Chondroblastoma of the temporal bone. Case report and literature review. *Ann Otol Rhinol Laryngol* 1992;101:763–769.

861. Martinez-Madrigal F, Vanel D, Luboinski B, et al: Case report 670. Chondroblastoma maxillary sinus. *Skeletal Radiol* 1991;20:299–301.

862. Blaauw G, Prick JJW, Versteege C: Chondroblastoma of the temporal bone. *Neurosurgery* 1988;22:1102–1107.

863. Howe JW, Baumgard S, Yochum TR, et al: Case report 449. Chondroblastoma involving C5 and C6. *Skeletal Radiol* 1988;17:52–55.

864. Hoeffel JC, Brasse F, Schmitt M, et al: About one case of vertebral chondroblastoma. *Pediatr Radiol* 1987;17:392–396.

865. Denko JV, Krauel LH: Benign chondroblastoma of bone. An unusual localization in temporal bone. *Arch Pathol* 1955;59:710–711.

866. Cares HL, Terplan K: Chondroblastoma of the skull. Case report. *J Neurosurg* 1971;35:614–618.

867. Harner SG, Cody DTR, Dahlin DC: Benign chondroblastoma of the temporal bone. *Otolaryngol Head Neck Surg* 1979;87:229–236.

868. Horn KL, Hankinson H, Nagel B, et al: Surgical management of chondroblastoma of the temporal bone. *Otolaryngol Head Neck Surg* 1990;102:264–269.

869. Leong HK, Cong PY, Sinniah R: Temporal bone chondroblastoma: Big and small. *J Laryngol Otol* 1994;108:1115–1119.

870. Bloem JL, Mulder JD: Chondroblastoma: A clinical and radiological study of 104 cases. *Skeletal Radiol* 1985;14:1–9.

871. Jaffe HL, Lichtenstein L: Benign chondroblastoma of bone. A reinterpretation of the so-called calcifying or chondromatous giant cell tumor. *Am J Pathol* 1942;18:969–991.

872. Schajowicz F, Gallardo H: Epiphyseal chondroblastoma of bone. A clinico-pathological study of sixty-nine cases. *J Bone Joint Surg (Br)* 1970;53:205–226.

873. Semmelink HJF, Pruszczynski M, Tilburg AW-V, et al: Cytokeratin expression in chondroblastomas. *Histopathology* 1990;16:257–263.

874. Unni KK, Dahlin DC, Beabout JW, et al: Chondrosarcoma: Clear-cell variant. A report of sixteen cases. *J Bone Joint Surg Am* 1976;58:676–683.

875. Slootweg PJ: Clear-cell chondrosarcoma of the maxilla. *Oral Surg* 1980;50:233–237.

876. Bjornsson J, Unni KK, Dahlin DC, et al: Clear cell chondrosarcoma of bone. Observations in 47 cases. *Am J Surg Pathol* 1984;8:223–230.

877. Kyriakos M, Land VJ, Penning HL, et al: Metastatic chondroblastoma: Report of a fatal case with a review of the literature on atypical, aggressive, and malignant chondroblastoma. *Cancer* 1985;55:1770–1789.

878. Hatcher CH, Campbell JC: Benign chondroblastoma of bone. Its histologic variations and a report of late sarcoma in the site of one. *Bull Hosp Jt Dis* 1951;12:411–430.

879. Sirsat MV, Doctor VM: Benign chondroblastoma of bone. Report of a case of malignant transformation. *J Bone Joint Surg Br* 1970;52:741–745.

880. Reyes CV, Kathuria S: Recurrent and aggressive chondroblastoma of the pelvis with late malignant neoplastic changes. *Am J Surg Pathol* 1979;3:449–455.

Malignant Cartilaginous Tumors

Chondrosarcoma

881. Huvos AG, Marcove RC: Chondrosarcoma in the young. A clinicopathologic analysis of 79 patients younger than 21 years of age. *Am J Surg Pathol* 1987;11:930–942.

882. Saito K, Unni KK, Wollan PC, et al: Chondrosarcoma of the jaw and facial bones. *Cancer* 1995;76:1550–1558.

883. Burkey BB, Hoffman HT, Baker SR, et al: Chondrosarcoma of the head and neck. *Laryngoscope* 1990;100:1301–1305.

884. Shives TC, McLeod RA, Unni KK, et al: Chondrosarcoma of the spine. *J Bone Joint Surg Am* 1989;71:1158–1165.

885. Coltrera MD, Googe PB, Harrist TJ, et al: Chondrosarcoma of the temporal bone. Diagnosis and treatment of 13 cases and review of the literature. *Cancer* 1986;58:2689–2696.

886. Nishizawa S, Fukaya T, Inouye K: Chondrosarcoma of the nasal septum: A report of an uncommon lesion. *Laryngoscope* 1984;94:550–553.

887. Stapleton SR, Wilkins PR, Archer DJ, et al: Chondrosarcoma of the skull base: A series of eight cases. *Neurosurgery* 1993;32:348–356.

888. Ruark DS, Schlehaider UK, Shah JP: Chondrosarcomas of the head and neck. *World J Surg* 1992;16:1010–1016.

889. Arlen M, Tollefsen HR, Huvos AG, et al: Chondrosarcoma of the head and neck. *Am J Surg* 1970;120:456–460.

890. Fu Y-S, Perzin KH: Non-epithelial tumors of the nasal cavity, paranasal sinuses, and nasopharynx: A clinicopathologic study III. Cartilaginous tumors (chondroma, chondrosarcoma). *Cancer* 1974;34:453–463.

891. Kragh LV, Dahlin DC, Erich JB: Cartilaginous tumors of the jaws and facial regions. *Am J Surg* 1960;99:852–856.

892. Finn DG, Goepfert H, Batsakis JG: Chondrosarcoma of the head and neck. *Laryngoscope* 1984;94:1539–1544.

893. Sato K, Nukaga H, Horikoshi T: Chondrosarcoma of the jaws and facial skeleton: A review of the Japanese literature. *J Oral Surg* 1977;35:892–897.

894. Boorstein JM, Spizarny DL: Case report 476. Chondrosarcoma of base of skull (CBS). *Skeletal Radiol* 1988;17:208–211.

895. Barnes L, Kapadia SB: The biology and pathology of selected skull base tumors. *J Neurooncol* 1994;20:213–240.

896. Grossman RI, Davis KR: Cranial computed tomographic appearance of chondrosarcoma of the base of the skull. *Radiology* 1981;141:403–408.

897. Camins MB, Duncan AW, Smith J, et al: Chondrosarcoma of the spine. *Spine* 1978;3:202–209.

898. Nishimura Y, Amano Y, Ogasawara H: Chondrosarcoma of the nasal septum: surgical considerations on Le Fort I osteotomy. *Eur Arch Otorhinolaryngol* 1993;250:59–62.

899. Cook PL, Evans PG: Chondrosarcoma of the skull in Maffucci's syndrome. *Br J Radiol* 1977;50:833–836.

900. Chou P, Mehta S, Gonzalez-Crussi F: Chondrosarcoma of the head in children. *Pediatr Pathol* 1990;10:945–958.

901. Brown E, Hug EB, Weber AL: Chondrosarcoma of the skull base. *Neuroimaging Clin North Am* 1994;4:529–541.

902. O'Neal LW, Ackerman LV: Chondrosarcoma of bone. *Cancer* 1952;5:551–577.

903. Barnes R, Catto M: Chondrosarcoma of bone. *J Bone Joint Surg Br* 1966;48:729–764.

904. Evans HL, Ayala AG, Romsdahl MM: Prognostic factors in chondrosarcoma of bone. A clinicopathologic analysis with emphasis on histologic grading. *Cancer* 1977;40:818–831.

905. Dahlin DC, Salvador AH: Chondrosarcoma of bones of the hands and feet: A study of 30 cases. *Cancer* 1974;34:755–760.

906. Lichtenstein L, Jaffe HL: Chondrosarcoma of bone. *Am J Pathol* 1943;19:553–589.

907. Mirra JM, Gold R, Downs J, et al: A new histologic approach to the

differentiation of enchondroma and chondrosarcoma of the bones. A clinicopathologic analylsis of 51 cases. *Clin Orthop Rel Res* 1985;201:214–237.

908. Sanerkin NG: The diagnosis and grading of chondrosarcoma of bone. A combined cytologic and histologic approach. *Cancer* 1980;45:582–594.

909. Unni KK, Dahlin DC, Beabout JW, et al: Chondrosarcoma: Clear-cell variant. A report of sixteen cases. *J Bone Joint Surg Am* 1976;58:676–683.

910. Bjornsson J, Unni KK, Dahlin DC, et al: Clear cell chondrosarcoma of bone: Observations in 47 cases. *Am J Surg Pathol* 1984;8:223–230.

911. Slootweg PJ: Clear-cell chondrosarcoma of the maxilla. *Oral Surg* 1980;50:233–237.

912. Dahlin DC, Beabout JW: Dedifferentiation of low-grade chondrosarcomas. *Cancer* 1971;28:461–466.

913. McCarthy EF, Dorfman HD: Chondrosarcoma of bone with dedifferentiation: A study of eighteen cases. *Hum Pathol* 1982;13:36–40.

914. Johnson S, Tetu B, Ayala AG, et al: Chondrosarcoma with additional mesenchymal component (dedifferentiated chondrosarcoma) I. A clinicopathologic study of 26 cases. *Cancer* 1986;58:278–286.

915. Frassica FJ, Unni KK, Beabout JW, et al: Dedifferentiated chondrosarcoma. A report of clinicopathological features and treatment of seventy-eight cases. *J Bone Joint Surg Am* 1986;68:1197–1205.

916. Reith JD, Bauer TW, Fischler DF, et al: Dedifferentiated chondrosarcoma with rhabdomyosarcomatous differentiation. *Am J Surg Pathol* 1996;20:293–298.

917. Castro JR, Linstadt DE, Bahary J-P, et al: Experience in charged particle irradiation of tumors of the skull base: 1977–1992. *Int J Radiat Oncol Biol Phys* 1994;29:647–655.

918. Hug EB, Munzenrider JE: Charged particle therapy for base of skull tumors: Past accomplishments and future challenges. *Int J Radiat Oncol Biol Phys* 1994;29:911–912.

919. McNaney D, Lindberg RD, Ayala AG, et al: Fifteen year radiotherapy experience with chondrosarcoma of bone. *Int J Radiat Oncol Biol Phys* 1982;8:187–190.

920. Austin-Seymour M, Munzenrider J, Goitein M, et al: Fractionated proton radiation therapy of chordoma and low-grade chondrosarcoma of the base of the skull. *J Neurosurg* 1989;70:13–17.

921. Gorenstein A, Neel HB, III, Weiland LH, et al: Sarcomas of the larynx. *Arch Otolaryngol* 1980;106:8–12.

922. Bleiweiss IJ, Kaneko M: Chondrosarcoma of the larynx with additional malignant mesenchymal component (dedifferentiated chondrosarcoma). *Am J Surg Pathol* 1988;12:314–320.

923. Nicolai P, Sasaki CT, Ferlito A, et al: Laryngeal chondrosarcoma: Incidence, pathology, biological behavior, and treatment. *Ann Otol Rhinol Laryngol* 1990;99:515–523.

924. Bogdan CJ, Maniglia AJ, Eliachar I, et al: Chondrosarcoma of the larynx: Challenges in diagnosis and management. *Head Neck* 1994;16:127–134.

925. Lewis JE, Olsen KD, Inwards CY: Cartilaginous tumors of the larynx: Clinicopathologic review of 47 cases. *Ann Otol Rhinol Laryngol* 1997;106:94–100.

926. Neel HB, III, Unni KK: Cartilaginous tumors of the larynx: A series of 33 patients. *Otolaryngol Head Neck Surg* 1982;90:201–207.

927. Brandwein M, Moore S, Som P, et al: Laryngeal chondrosarcomas: A clinicopathologic study of 11 cases including two "dedifferentiated" chondrosarcomas. *Laryngoscope* 1992;102:858–867.

928. Lavertu P, Tucker HM: Chondrosarcoma of the larynx. Case report and management philosophy. *Ann Otol Rhinol Laryngol* 1984;93:452–456.

929. Ferlito A, Nicolai P, Montaguti A, et al: Chondrosarcoma of the larynx: Review of the literature and report of three cases. *Am J Otolaryngol* 1984;5:350–359.

930. Moran CA, Suster S, Carter D: Laryngeal chondrosarcomas. *Arch Pathol Lab Med* 1993;117:914–917.

931. Hyams VJ, Rabuzzi DD: Cartilaginous tumors of the larynx. *Laryngoscope* 1970;80:755–767.

932. Finn DG, Goepfert H, Batsakis JG: Chondrosarcoma of the head and neck. *Laryngoscope* 1984;94:1539–1544.

933. Jacobs RD, Stayboldt C, Harris JP: Chondrosarcoma of the epiglottis with regional and distant metastasis. *Laryngoscope* 1989;99:861–864.

934. Eriksen HE, Greisen O, Hjorth L: Chondrosarcoma of the larynx. *J Otorhinolaryngol* 1986;48:270–274.

935. Huizenga C, Balogh K: Cartilaginous tumors of the larynx. A clinicopathologic study of 10 new cases and a review of the literature. *Cancer* 1970;26:201–210.

936. Wilkinson AH III, Beckford NS, Babin RW, et al: Extraskeletal myxoid chondrosarcoma of the epiglottis: Case report and a review of the literature. *Otolaryngol Head Neck Surg* 1991;104:257–260.

937. Nakayama M, Brandenburg JH, Hafez GR: Dedifferentiated chondrosarcoma of the larynx with regional and distant metastases. *Ann Otol Rhinol Laryngol* 1993;102:785–791.

938. Devaney KO, Ferlito A, Silver CE: Cartilaginous tumors of the larynx. *Ann Otol Rhinol Laryngol* 1995;104:251–255.

939. Glaubiger DL, Casler JD, Garrett WL, et al: Chondrosarcoma of the larynx after radiation treatment for vocal cord cancer. *Cancer* 1991;68:1828–1831.

940. Koka VN, Veber F, Haguet J-F, et al: Chondrosarcoma of the larynx. *J Laryngol Otol* 1995;109:168–170.

941. Batsakis JG, Raymond AK: Cartilage tumors of the larynx. *South Med J* 1988;81:481–484.

942. Salvador AH, Beabout JW, Dahlin DC: Mesenchymal chondrosarcoma: Observations on 30 new cases. *Cancer* 1971;28:605–615.

943. Guccion JG, Font RL, Enzinger FM, et al: Extraskeletal mesenchymal chondrosarcoma. *Arch Pathol* 1973;95:336–340.

944. Huvos AG, Rosen G, Dabska M, et al: Mesenchymal chondrosarcoma: A clinicopathologic analysis of 35 patients with emphasis on treatment. *Cancer* 1983;51:1230–1237.

945. Nakashima Y, Unni KK, Shives TC, et al: Mesenchymal chondrosarcoma of bone and soft tissue: A review of 111 cases. *Cancer* 1986;57:2444–2453.

946. Roland NJ, Khine MM, Clarke R, et al: A rare congenital intranasal polyp: Mesenchymal chondrosarcoma of the nasal region. *J Laryngol Otol* 1992;106:1081–1083.

947. Harwood AR, Krajbich JI, Fornasier VL: Mesenchymal chondrosarcoma: A report of 17 cases. *Clin Orthop* 1981;Jul-Aug(158):144–148.

948. Takahashi K, Sato K, Kanazawa H, et al: Mesenchymal chondrosarcoma of the jaw: Report of a case and review of 41 cases in the literature. *Head Neck* 1993;15:459–464.

949. Jacobs JL, Merriam JC, Chadburn A, et al: Mesenchymal chondrosarcoma of the orbit. Report of three new cases and review of the literature. *Cancer* 1994;73:399–405.

950. Rushing EJ, Armonda RA, Ansari Q, et al: Mesenchymal chondrosarcoma. A clinicopathologic and flow cytometric study of 13 cases presenting in the central nervous system. *Cancer* 1996;77:1884–1891.

951. Hollins RR, Lydiatt DD, Markin RS, et al: Mesenchymal chondrosarcoma: A case report. *J Oral Maxillofac Surg* 1987;45:72–75.

952. Dahlin DC, Henderson ED: Mesenchymal chondrosarcoma. Further observations on a new entity. *Cancer* 1962;15:410–417.

953. Mikata A, Iri H, Inuyama Y: Mesenchymal chondrosarcoma: A case report with an ultrastructural study and review of Japanese literatures. *Arch Pathol Jpn* 1977;27:93–109.

954. Bottrill ID, Wood S, Barrett Lee P, et al: Mesenchymal chondrosarcoma of the maxilla. *J Laryngol Otol* 1994;108:785–787.

955. Bagchi M, Husain N, Goel MM, et al: Extraskeletal mesenchymal chondrosarcoma of the orbit. *Cancer* 1993;72:2224–2226.

956. Takimoto T, Kato H, Yamashima T, et al: Mesenchymal chondrosarcoma of the ethmoid sinus. *ORL* 1989;51:369–374.

957. Bloch DM, Bragoli AJ, Collins DN, et al: Mesenchymal chondrosarcomas of the head and neck. *J Laryngol Otol* 1979;93:405–412.

958. Gomersall LN, Needham G: Case report: Mesenchymal chondrosarcoma occurring in the parapharyngeal space. *Clin Radiol* 1990;42:359–361.

959. Shapeero LG, Vanel D, Couanet D, et al: Extraskeletal mesenchymal chondrosarcoma. *Radiology* 1993;186:819–826.

960. Ranjan A, Chacko G, Joseph T, et al: Intraspinal mesenchymal chondrosarcoma. Case report. *J Neurosurg* 1994;80:928–930.

961. Bertoni F, Picci P, Bacchini P, et al: Mesenchymal chondrosarcoma of bone and soft tissues. *Cancer* 1983;52:533 541.

962. Dabska M, Huvos AG: Mesenchymal chondrosarcoma in the young. A clinicopathologic study of 19 patients with explanation of histogenesis. *Virch Arch A Pathol Anat* 1983;399:89–104.

963. Fu Y-S, Kay S: A comparative ultrastructural study of mesenchymal chondrosarcoma and myxoid chondrosarcoma. *Cancer* 1974;33:1531–1542.

964. Swanson PE, Lillemoe TJ, Manivel JC, et al: Mesenchymal chondrosarcoma. An immunohistochemical study. *Arch Pathol Lab Med* 1990;114:943–948.

965. Granter SR, Renshaw AA, Fletcher CDM, et al: CD99 reactivity in mesenchymal chondrosarcoma. *Hum Pathol* 1996;27:1273–1276.

966. Dobin SM, Donner LR, Speights VO Jr: Mesenchymal chondrosar-

coma. A cytogenetic, immunohistochemical and ultrastructural study. *Cancer Genet Cytogenet* 1995;83:56–60.

967. Sainati L, Scapinello A, Montaldi A, et al: A mesenchymal chondrosarcoma of a child with the reciprocal translocation (11;22)(q24;q12). *Cancer Genet Cytogenet* 1993;71:144–147.

968. Tsuneyoshi M, Enjoji M, Iwasaki H, et al: Extraskeletal myxoid chondrosarcoma. A clinicopathologic and electron microscopic study. *Acta Pathol Jpn* 1981;31:439–447.

969. Enzinger FM, Shiraki M: Extraskeletal myxoid chondrosarcoma. An analysis of 34 cases. *Hum Pathol* 1972;3:421–435.

970. Dardick I, Lgacé R, Carlier MT, et al: Chordoid sarcoma (extraskeletal myxoid chondrosarcoma). A light and electron microscope study. *Virchows Arch (Pathol Anat)* 1983;399:61–78.

971. Jessurun J, Rojas ME, Albores-Saavedra J: Congenital extraskeletal embryonal chondrosarcoma. Case report. *J Bone Joint Surg Am* 1982;64:293–296.

972. Jawad J, Lang J, Leader M, et al: Extraskeletal myxoid chondrosarcoma of the maxillary sinus. *J Laryngol Otol* 1991;105:676–677.

973. Goldenberg RR, Cohen P, Steinlauf P: Chondrosarcoma of the extraskeletal soft tissues. A report of seven cases and review of the literature. *J Bone Joint Surg Am* 1967;49:1487–1507.

974. Liu-Shindo M, Rice DH, Sherrod AE: Extraskeletal myxoid chondrosarcoma of the head and neck: A case report. *Otolaryngol Head Neck Surg* 1989;101:485–488.

975. Salcman M, Scholtz H, Kristt D, et al: Extraskeletal myxoid chondrosarcoma of the falx. *Neurosurgery* 1992;31:344–348.

976. Martin RF, Melnick PJ, Warner NE, et al: Chordoid sarcoma. *Am J Clin Pathol* 1973;59:623–635.

977. Weiss SW: Ultrastructure of the so-called "chordoid sarcoma." Evidence supporting cartilagenous differentiation. *Cancer* 1976;37:300–306.

978. Fletcher CDM, Powell G, McKee PH: Extraskeletal myxoid chondrosarcoma: a histochemical and immunohistochemical study. *Histopathology* 1986;10:489–499.

979. Saleh G, Evans HL, Ro JY, et al: Extraskeletal myxoid chondrosarcoma. A clinicopathologic study of ten patients with long-term follow-up. *Cancer* 1992;70:2827–2830.

980. Insabato L, Terracciano LM, Boscaino A, et al: Extraskeletal myxoid chondrosarcoma with intranuclear vacuoles and microtubular aggregates in the rough endoplasmic reticulum. Report of a case with fine needle aspiration and electron microscopy. *Acta Cytol* 1990;34:858–862.

981. Wick MR, Burgess JH, Manivel JC: A reassessment of "chordoid sarcoma." Ultrastructural and immunohistochemical comparison with chordoma and skeletal myxoid chondorsarcoma. *Mod Pathol* 1988;1:433–443.

982. Suzuki T, Kaneko H, Kojima K, et al: Extraskeletal myxoid chondrosarcoma characterized by microtubular aggregates in the rough endoplasmic reticulum and tubulin immunoreactivity. *J Pathol* 1988;156:51–57.

983. Sciot R, Dal Cin P, Fletcher C, et al: t(9;22) (q22–31;q11–12) is a consistent marker of extraskeletal myxoid chondrosarcoma: Evaluation of three cases. *Mod Pathol* 1995;8:765–768.

984. Hirabayashi Y, Ishida T, Yoshida MA, et al: Translocation (9;22) (q22;q12). A recurrent chromosome abnormality in extraskeletal myxoid chondrosarcoma. *Cancer Genet Cytogenet* 1995;81:33–37.

985. Krayenbühl H, Yasargil MG: Cranial chordomas. *Prog Neurol Surg* 1975;6:380–434.

986. Salisbury JR: The pathology of the human notochord. *J Pathol* 1993;171:253–255.

987. Shugar JMA, Som PM, Krespi YP, et al: Primary chordoma of the maxillary sinus. *Laryngoscope* 1980;90:1825–1830.

988. Wright D: Nasopharyngeal and cervical chordoma: Some aspects of their development and treatment. *J Laryngol Otol* 1967;81:1337–1355.

989. Horwitz T: Chordal ectopia and its possible relation to chordoma. *Arch Pathol* 1941;31:354–362.

990. Utne JR, Pugh DG: The roentgenologic aspects of chordoma. *AJR* 1955;74:593–608.

991. Ulich TR, Mirra JM: Ecchordosis physaliphora vertebralis. *Clin Orthop Rel Res* 1982;163:282–289.

992. Berryhill BH, Armstrong BW: Extracranial presentation of craniocervical chordoma. *Laryngoscope* 1984;94:1063–1065.

993. Windeyer BW: Chordoma. *Proc R Soc Med* 1959;52:1088–1100.

994. Mills RP: Chordomas of the skull base. *J Royal Soc Med* 1984;77:10–16.

995. Heffelfinger MJ, Dahlin DC, MacCarty CS, et al: Chordomas and cartilaginous tumors at the skull base. *Cancer* 1973;32:410–420.

996. Bjornsson J, Wold LE, Ebersold MJ, et al: Chordoma of the mobile spine. A cliniocopathologic analysis of 40 patients. *Cancer* 1993;71:735–740.

997. O'Connell JX, Renard LG, Liebsch NJ, et al: Base of skull chordoma. A correlative study of histologic and clinical features of 62 cases. *Cancer* 1994;74:2261–2267.

998. Forsyth PA, Cascino TL, Shaw EG, et al: Intracranial chordomas: A clinicopathological and prognostic study of 51 cases. *J Neurosurg* 1993;78:741–747.

999. Kendall BE, Lee BCP: Cranial chordomas. *Br J Radiol* 1977;50:687–698.

1000. Raffel C, Wright DC, Gutin PH, et al: Cranial chordomas: Clinical presentation and results of operative and radiation therapy in twenty-six patients. *Neurosurgery* 1985;17:703–710.

1001. Eriksson B, Gunterberg B, Kindblom L-G: Chordoma. A clincopathologic and prognostic study of a Swedish national series. *Acta Orthop Scand* 1981;52:49–58.

1002. Mizerny BR, Kost KM: Chordoma of the cranial base: The McGill experience. *J Otolaryngol* 1995;24:14–19.

1003. Coffin CM, Swanson PE, Wick MR, et al: Chordoma in childhood and adolescence. A clinicopathologic analysis of 12 cases. *Arch Pathol Lab Med* 1993;117:927–933.

1004. Kaneko Y, Sato Y, Iwaki T, et al: Chordoma in early childhood: A clinicopathological study. *Neurosurgery* 1991;29:442–446.

1005. Yadav YR, Kak VK, Khosla VK, et al: Cranial chordoma in the first decade. *Clin Neurol Neurosurg* 1992;94:241–246.

1006. Wold LE, Laws ER, Jr: Cranial chordomas in children and young adults. *J Neurosurg* 1983;59:1043–1047.

1007. Matsumoto J, Towbin RB, Ball WS Jr.: Cranial chordomas in infancy and childhood. A report of two cases and review of the literature. *Pediatr Radiol* 1989;20:28–32.

1008. Chetiyawardana AD: Chordoma: Results of treatment. *Clin Radiol* 1984;35:159–161.

1009. Higinbotham NL, Phillips RF, Farr HW, et al: Chordoma. Thirty-five-year study at Memorial Hospital. *Cancer* 1967;20:1841–1850.

1010. Jeffrey PB, Biava CG, Davis RL: Chondroid chordoma. A hyalinized chordoma without cartilaginous differentiation. *Am J Clin Pathol* 1995;103:271–279.

1011. Sundaresan N, Galicich JH, Chu FCH, et al: Spinal chordomas. *J Neurosurg* 1979;50:312–319.

1012. Stoker DJ, Pringle J: Case report 205: Chordoma of mid-cervical spine. *Skeletal Radiol* 1982;8:306–310.

1013. Meyer JE, Lepke RA, Lindfors KK, et al: Chordomas: Their CT appearance in the cervical, thoracic, and lumbar spine. *Radiology* 1984;153:693–696.

1014. Richter HJ, Jr, Batsakis JG, Boles R: Chordomas: Nasopharyngeal presentation and atypical long survival. *Ann Otol* 1975;84:327–332.

1015. Berdal P, Myhre E: Cranial chordomas involving the paranasal sinuses. *J Laryngol Otol* 1964;78:906–919.

1016. Perzin KH, Pushparaj N: Nonepithelial tumors of the nasal cavity, paranasal sinuses, and nasopharynx. A clinicopathologic study. XIV: Chordomas. *Cancer* 1986;57:784–796.

1017. Campbell WM, McDonald TJ, Unni KK, et al: Nasal and paranasal presentations of chordomas. *Laryngoscope* 1980;90:612–618.

1018. Kamrin RP, Potanos JN, Pool JL: An evaluation of the diagnosis and treatment of chordoma. *J Neurol Neurosurg Psychiatry* 1964;27:157–165.

1019. Larson TC III, Houser OW, Laws ER Jr: Imaging of cranial chordomas. *Mayo Clin Proc* 1987;62:886–893.

1020. Firooznia H, Pinto RS, Lin JP, et al: Chordoma: Radiologic evaluation of 20 cases. *AJR* 1976;127:797–805.

1021. Mindell ER: Chordoma. *J Bone Joint Surg Am* 1981;63:501–505.

1022. Volpe R, Mazabraud A: A clinicopathologic review of 25 cases of chordoma (a pleomorphic and metastasizing neoplasm). *Am J Surg Pathol* 1983;7:161–170.

1023. Dahlin DC, MacCarty CS: Chordoma. A study of fifty-nine cases. *Cancer* 1952;5:1170–1178.

1024. Rich TA, Schiller A, Suit HD, et al: Clinical and pathologic review of 48 cases of chordoma. *Cancer* 1985;56:182–187.

1025. Tomlinson FH, Scheithauer BW, Forsythe PA, et al: Sarcomatous transformation in cranial chordoma. *Neurosurgery* 1992;31:13–18.

1026. Fukuda T, Aihara T, Ban S, et al: Sacrococcygeal chordoma with a malignant spindle cell component: A report of two autopsy cases with a review of the literature. *Acta Pathol Jpn* 1992;42:448–453.

1027. Meis JM, Raymond AK, Evans HL, et al: "Dedifferentiated" chordoma: A clinicopathologic and immunohistochemical study of three cases. *Am J Surg Pathol* 1987;11:516–525.

1028. Nielsen GP, Rosenberg AE, Liebsch NJ: Chordoma of the base of skull in children and adolescents: A clinicopathologic study of 35 cases. *Mod Pathol* 1996;9:11a.

1029. Rutherfoord GS, Davies AG: Chordomas—ultrastructure and immunohistochemistry: A report based on the examination of six cases. *Histopathology* 1987;11:775–787.

1030. Abenoza P, Sibley RK: Chordoma: An immunohistologic study. *Hum Pathol* 1986;17:744–747.

1031. Meis JM, Giraldo AA: Chordoma: An immunohistochemical study of 20 cases. *Arch Pathol Lab Med* 1988;112:553–556.

1032. Brooks JJ, LiVolsi VA, Trojanowski JQ: Does chondroid chordoma exist? *Acta Neuropathol* 1987;72:229–235.

1033. Walker WP, Landas SK, Bromley CM, et al: Immunohistochemical distinction of classic and chondroid chordomas. *Mod Pathol* 1991;4:661–666.

1034. Mitchell A, Scheithauer BW, Unni KK, et al: Chordoma and chondroid neoplasms of the spheno-occiput: An immunohistochemical study of 41 cases with prognostic and nosologic implications. *Cancer* 1993;72:2943–2949.

1035. Ishida T, Dorfman HD: Chondroid chordoma versus low-grade chondrosarcoma of the base of the skull: Can immunohistochemistry resolve the controversy? *J Neurooncol* 1994;18:199–206.

1036. Wojno KJ, Hruban RH, Garin-Chesa P, et al: Chondroid chordomas and low-grade chondrosarcomas of the craniospinal axis: An immunohistochemical analysis of 17 cases. *Am J Surg Pathol* 1992;16:1144–1152.

1037. Rosenberg AE, Brown GA, Bhan AK, et al: Chondroid chordoma—a variant of chordoma: A morphologic and immunohistochemical study. *Am J Clin Pathol* 1994;101:36–41.

1038. Persson S, Kindblom L-G, Angervall L: Classical and chondroid chordoma. A light-microscopic, histochemical, ultrastructural and immunohistochemical analysis of the various cell types. *Pathol Res Pract* 1991;187:828–838.

1039. Murad TM, Murthy MSN: Ultrastructure of a chordoma. *Cancer* 1970;25:1204–1215.

1040. Valderrama E, Kahn LB, Lipper S, et al: Chondroid chordoma: Electron-microscopic study of two cases. *Am J Surg Pathol* 1983;7:625–632.

1041. Mierau GW, Weeks DA: Chondroid chordoma. *Ultrastruct Pathol* 1987;11:731–737.

1042. Salisbury JR, Isaacson PG: Demonstration of cytokeratins and an epithelial membrane antigen in chordomas and human fetal notochord. *Am J Surg Pathol* 1985;9:791–797.

1043. Coindre J-M, Rivel J, Trojani M, et al: Immunohistological study in chordomas. *J Pathol* 1986;150:61–63.

1044. Coffin CM, Swanson PE, Wick MR, et al: An immunohistochemical comparison of chordoma with renal cell carcinoma, colorectal adenocarcinoma, and myxopapillary ependymoma: A potential diagnostic dilemma in the diminutive biopsy. *Mod Pathol* 1993;6:531–538.

1045. Kasantikul V, Shuangshoti S: Positivity to glial fibrillary acidic protein in bone, cartilage, and chordoma. *J Surg Oncol* 1989;41:22–26.

1046. Wittchow R, Landas SK: Glial fibrillary acidic protein expression in pleomorphic adenoma, chordoma, and astrocytoma: A comparison of three antibodies. *Arch Pathol Lab Med* 1991;115:1030–1033.

1047. Azumi N, Battifora H: The distribution of vimentin and keratin in epithelial and nonepithelial neoplasms: A comprehensive immunohistochemical study on formalin- and alcohol-fixed tumors. *Am J Clin Pathol* 1987;88:286–296.

1048. Herrera GA, Turbat-Herrera EA, Lott RL: S-100 protein expression by primary and metastatic adenocarcinomas. *Am J Clin Pathol* 1988;89:168–176.

1049. Ellis GL, Auclair PL: Tumors of the salivary glands. In: *Atlas of Tumor Pathology*, 3rd series, fascicle 17. Washington DC: Armed Forces Institute of Pathology, 1996.

1050. Magrini SM, Papi MG, Marletta F, et al: Chordoma: Natural history, treatment and prognosis. The Florence radiotherapy department experience (1956–1990) and a critical review of the literature. *Acta Oncol* 1992;31:847–851.

1051. Tai PTH, Craighead P, Bagdon F: Optimization of radiotherapy for patients with cranial chordoma: A review of dose-response ratios for photon techniques. *Cancer* 1995;75:749–756.

1052. Austin-Seymour M, Munzenrider J, Goitein M, et al: Fractionated proton radiation therapy of chordoma and low-grade chondrosarcoma of the base of the skull. *J Neurosurg* 1989;70:13–17.

1053. Keel SB, Koerner FC, Efird JT, et al: Estrogen and progesterone receptor status and disease specific survival in skull base chordomas. *Mod Pathol* 1996;9:8a.

1054. Barnes L, Peel RL, Verbin RS et al: Diseases of the bones and joints. In Barnes L, ed. *Surgical Pathology of the Head and Neck*, vol 2. New York: Marcel Dekker, 1985:921.

1055. hier Kransdorf MJ, Moser RP, Gilkey FW: Fibrous dysplasia. *Radiographics* 1990;10(3):519–37.

1056. Ross DA, Sasaki CT: Pathology of tumors of the cranial base. *Clin Plastic Surg* 1995;22(3):407–416.

1057. Stomporo BE, Wolf P, Haghighi P: Fibrous dysplasia of bone. *Am Family Physician* 1989;39(3):179–184.

1058. Barat M, Rybak LP, Mann JL: Fibrous dysplasia masquerading as chronic maxillary sinusitis. *Ear Nose Throat J* 1989;68(1):42–46.

1059. Ramsey EH, Strong WE, Frazell LE: Fibrous dysplasia of the craniofacial bone. *Am J Surg* 1968;116:542–546.

1060. Van Horn PE, Dahlia DC, Bickel WH: Fibrous dysplasia: A clinical pathologic study of orthopedic surgical cases. *Proc Mayo Clin* 1963;38:175–189.

1061. Cole DE, Fraser FC, Glorieux FH et al: Panostotic fibrous dysplasia: A congenital disorder of bone with unusual facial appearance, bone fragility, hyperphosphatasemia, and hypophosphatemia. *Am J Med Genet* 1983;14:725–735.

1062. Covanah SFW, Dons RF: McCune-Albright Syndrome: How many endocrinopathies can one patient have. *Southern Med J* 1993;86(3):364–367.

1063. Nakagawa H, Nagasaka A, Sugiura T et al: Gigantism associated with McCune-Albright's syndrome. *Horm Metab Res* 1985;17:522–527.

1064. Chung KF, Alaghband-Zadeh J, Guz A: Acromegaly and hyperprolactinemia in McCune-Albright syndrome. *Am J Dis Child* 1983;137:134–136.

1065. Firat D, Stutzman L: Fibrous dysplasia of the bone: Review of 24 cases. *Am J Med* 1968;44:421–429.

1066. McKusik VA: *Mendilian Inheritance in Man*, 9th ed. Johns Hopkins Univ Press 1990:766–768.

1067. Aarskog D, Tveteraas E: McCune-Albright's Syndrome following adrenadectomy for Cushing's syndrome in infancy. *J Pediatr* 1968;73:89–96.

1068. Aoki T, Kouho H, Hisoaka M et al: Intramuscular myxoma with fibrous dysplasia: A report of two cases with review of literature. *Pathol Int* 1995;45:165–171.

1069. Mazabraud A, Semat P, Roze R: A propos de l'association de fibromyxomes de tissues mous a la dysplasie Libreus des os. *Presse Med* 1967;75:2223–2228.

1070. Logel RJ: Recurrent intramuscular myxoma associated with Albright's syndrome. *J Bone Joint Surg* 1976;58:a565–568.

1071. Prayson MA, Leeson MC: Soft tissue myxomas and fibrous dysplasia of bone: A case report and review of literature. *Clin Orthoped Relat Res* 1993;291:222–228.

1072. Gianoutsos MP, Thomson JF, Marsden FW: Mazabraud's syndrome: Intramuscular myxoma associated with fibrous dysplasia of bone. *Aust NZ J Surg* 1990;60:825–828.

1073. Fries JW: The Roentgen features of fibrous dysplasia of the skull and facial bone: A critical analysis of 39 pathologically proven cases. *Am J Roent Rad Ther Nuc Med* 1957;77:71–88.

1074. Waldron CA: Fibro-osseous lesions of the jaws. *J Oral Maxillofac Surg* 1993;51:828–835.

1075. Waldron CA: Fibro-osseous lesions of the jaws. *J Oral Maxillofac Surg* 1985;43:249–262.

1076. Moore AT, Buncic JR, Munro IR: Fibrous dysyplasia of the orbit in childhood. Clinical features and Management. *Ophthalmology* 1985;92:12–20.

1077. Chen YR, Fairholm D: Fronto-orbito-sphenoidal fibrous dysplasia. *Ann Plast Surg* 1985;15:190–203.

1078. Edgerton TM, Persing AJ, Jane AJ: Surgical treatment of fibrous dysplasia. *Ann Surg* 1985;202:459–479.

1079. Schwartz DT, Alpert M: The malignant transformation of fibrous dysplasia. *Am J Med Sci* 1964;247:35–54.

1080. Taconis WK: Osteosarcoma in fibrous dysplasia. *Skeletal Radiol* 1988;17:163–170.

1081. Hamner JE, Scofield HH, Cornyn J: Benign fibro-osseous lesions of periodontal ligament origin. *Cancer* 1968;22:861.

1082. Eversole LR, Leider AS, Nelson K: Ossifying fibroma: A clinicopathologic study of 64 cases. *Oral Surg Oral Med Oral Pathol* 1985;60:505–511.

1083. Eversole LR, Merell PW, Strub D: Radiographic characteristics of central ossifying fibroma. *Oral Surg Oral Med Oral Pathol* 1985;59:522–527.

1084. Sciubba JJ, Younai F: Ossifying fibroma of the mandible and maxilla. Review of 18 cases. *J Oral Pathol Med* 1989;18:315–321.

1085. Kramer IRH, Pindborg JJ, Shear M, eds: *Histologic Typing of Odontogenic Tumors*. Berlin: Springer-Verlag, 1992.

1086. Slootweg PJ, Müller H: Juvenile ossifying fibroma: Report of 4 cases. *J Craniomaxfac Surg* 1990;18:125–129.

1087. Slootweg PJ, Panders AK, Koopman R, et al: Juvenile ossifying fibroma: An analysis of 33 cases with emphasis on histopathological aspects. *J Oral Pathol Med* 1994;23:385–388.

1088. Gogl H: Das Psammo-osteoid-fibroma der Nase und ihrer Nebenhöhlen. *Monatsschr F Ohrenheilk Lar Rhin* 1949;83:1–10.

1089. Margo CE, Ragsdale BD, Perman KI, et al: Psammomatoid (juvenile) ossifying fibroma of the orbit. *Ophthalmology* 1985;92:150–159.

1090. Hoffman S, Jacouby J, Kroll SO: Intraosseus and parosteal tumors of the jaws. In: *Atlas of Tumor Pathology,* 2nd series, fascile 24. Washington, DC: Armed Forces Institute of Pathology, 1987.

1091. Slootweg PJ, Panders AK, Nikkels PGJ: Psammomatoid ossifying fibroma of the paranasal sinus. An exragnathic variant of cemento-ossifying fibroma. *J Cranio Maxillo-facial Surg* 1993;21:294–297.

1092. Bertrand B, Eloy PH, Cornelis JP, et al: Juvenile aggressive cemento-ossifying fibroma: Case report and review of literature. *Laryngoscope* 1993;103:1385–1390.

1093. Margo CE, Weiss A, Habal MB: Psammomatoid ossifying fibroma. *Arch Ophthalmol* 1986;104:1347–1351.

1094. Shields JA, Nelson LB, Brown JF, et al: Clinical computed tomographic and histopathologic characteristics of juvenile ossifying fibroma with orbital involvement. *Am J Ophthal* 1983;96:650–653.

1095. Han MH, Chang KH, Lee CH, et al: Sinonasal psammomatoid ossifying fibroma: CT and MR manifestations. *AJNR* 1991;12:25–30.

1096. Storkel S, Wilfried W, Makek MS: Psammomous desmo-osteoblastoma: Ultrastructural and immunohistochemical evidence for an osteogenic histogenesis. *Virchows Arch* 1987;411:561–568.

1097. Marvel JB, March MA, Catlin JJ: Ossifying fibroma of the mid-face and paranasal sinuses: Diagnostic and therapeutic considerations. *Otolaryngeal Head Neck Surg* 1991;104:803–808.

1098. Artico M, Cervoni L, Salvati M, et al: Ossifying fibroma of the skull: Clinical and therapeutic study. *Tumori* 1994;80:64–67.

1099. Nakagawa K, Takasato Y, Ito Y, et al: Ossifying fibroma involving the paranasal sinus orbit, anterior cranial fossa: Case report. *Neurosurgery* 1995;36:1192–1195.

1100. Binath O, Erashin Y, Coskun S, et al: Ossifying fibroma of the occipital bone. *Clin Neurol Neurosurg* 1995;97:47–49.

1101. Zappia JJ, LaRovere MJ, Telian SA: Massive ossifying fibroma of the temporal bone. *Otolaryngeal Head Neck Surg* 1990;103:480–483.

1102. Melrose RJ, Abrams AM, Mills BG: Florid osseous dysplasia. *Oral Surg Oral Med Oral Pathol* 1976;41:62–81.

Giant Cell Lesions

1103. Paget J: *Lectures on Surgical Pathology*. London: Longmans, 1853.

1104. Jaffe HL: Giant cell reparative granuloma, traumatic bone and fibrous dysplasia of the jaw bones. *Oral Surg Oral Med Oral Pathol* 1953;6:159–175.

1105. El-Mofty SK, Osdoby P: Growth behavior and lineage of isolated and cultured cells derived from giant cell granuloma of the mandible. *J Oral Pathol* 1985;14:539–552.

1106. Bhashkar SM, Bernier JL, Goldby F: Aneurysmal bone cyst and other giant cell lesions of the jaws. *Oral Surg* 1959;17:30–41.

1107. Waldron CA, Shafer WG: The central giant cell reparative granuloma of the jaws: An analysis of 38 cases. *Am J Clin Pathol* 1966;45:437–447.

1108. Auclair PL, Kratochvil FJ, Slater LJ, et al: A clinical and histomorphologic comparison of the central giant cell granuloma and giant cell tumor. *Oral Surg Oral Med Oral Pathol* 1988;66:197–208.

1109. Ficarra G, Kaban LB, Hansen L: Central giant cell lesions of the mandible and maxilla: A clinicopathologic and cytometric study. *Oral Surg Oral Med Oral Pathol* 1987;64:44–49.

1110. Whitaker SB, Waldron CA: Central giant cell lesions of the jaws. *Oral Surg Oral Med Oral Pathol* 1993;75:199–208.

1111. Dahlin DC, Unni KK: *Bone Tumors, General Aspects, and Data on 8,542 Cases.* 4th ed. Springfield, IL: Charles C Thomas, 1986.

1112. Bertoni F, Unni KK, Beabout JW, et al: Giant cell tumors of the skull. *Cancer* 1992;70:1124–1132.

1113. Mirra JM: Paget's disease. In: Mirra JM, Picci P, Gold RH, eds. *Bone Tumors: Radiologic and Pathologic Correlations,* VII. Philadelphia: Lea & Febiger, 1989:925–940.

1114. Chuong R, Kaban L, Kozakewich H, et al: Central giant cell lesions of the jaws: A clinicopathologic study. *J Oral Maxillofacial Surg* 1986;44:708–713.

1115. Jaffe HL, Lichtenstein L: Solitary unicameral bone cyst. *Arch Surg* 1942;46:1004–1025.

1116. Kyriakos M, Hardy D: Malignant transformation of aneurysmal bone cyst, with an analysis of the literature. *Cancer* 1991;68:1770–1780.

1117. Morton KS: Aneurysmal bone cyst: A review of 26 cases. *Can J Surg* 1986;29:110–115.

1118. Vergel De Dios AM, Bond JR, Shives TC, et al: Aneurysmal bone cyst: A clinicopathologic study of 238 cases. *Cancer* 1992;69:2921–2931.

1119. Gingell JC, Levy BA, Beckerman T, et al: Aneurysmal bone cyst. *J Oral Maxillofac Surg* 1984;42:527–534.

1120. Toljanic JA, Lechewski E, Huvos AG, et al: Aneurysmal bone cysts of the jaws: A case study and review of literature. *Oral Surg Oral Med Oral Pathol* 1987;64:72–77.

1121. Trent C, Byl FM: Aneurysmal bone cyst of the mandible. *Ann Otol Rhino Laryngol* 1993;102:917–923.

1122. Citardi M, Janjua T, Abrahams JJ, et al: Orbitoethmoidal aneurysmal bone cyst. *Otolaryngeal Head Neck Surg* 1996;114:466–470.

1123. Lucarelli MJ, Bilyk JR, Shore JW, et al: Aneurysmal bone cyst of the orbit associated with fibrous dysplasia. *Plast Reconstruct Surg* 1995;96:440–445.

1124. Shah GV, Doctor MR, Shah PS: Aneurysmal bone cyst of the temporal bone: MR findings. *AJNR*. 1995;16:763–766.

1125. Bilge T, Coban O, Ozden B, et al: Aneurysmal bone in cyst of the occipital bone. *Surg Neurol* 1983;20:227–230.

1126. Burns-Cox CJ, Higgins AT: Aneurysmal bone cyst of the frontal bone. *J Bone Joint Surg* (Br) 1969;51:344–345.

1127. Kershisnik M, Batsakis JG: Aneurysmal bone cysts of the jaws. *Ann Otol Rhinol Laryngol* 1994;103:164–165.

1128. Martinez V, Sisson HA: Aneurysmal bone cyst. A review of 123 cases including primary lesions and those secondary to other bone pathology. *Cancer* 1988;61:2291–2304.

1129. Svensson B, Isacsson G: Benign osteoblastoma associated with aneurysmal bone cyst of the mandibular ramus and condyle. *Oral Surg Oral Med Oral Pathol* 1993;76:433–436.

1130. Yee RD, Cogan DG, Thorp TR, et al: Optic nerve compression due to aneurysmal bone cyst. *Arch Ophthalmol* 1977;95:2176–2179.

1131. Zimmer WD, Berquist TH, Sim FH, et al: Magnetic resonance imaging of aneurysmal bone cyst. *Mayo Clinic Proc* 1984;59:633–636.

1132. Biesecker LJ, Marcove RL, Huvos AG, et al: Aneurysmal bone cyst: A clinicopathologic study of 66 cases. *Cancer* 1970;26:615–625.

1133. Tillman BP, Dahlin DC, Lipscomb PR.: Aneurysmal bone cyst: An analysis of 95 cases. *Mayo Clinic Proc* 1968;43:478–495.

1134. Ruiter DJ, Van Rijssel TG, Van Der Veld EA: Aneurysmal bone cyst: A clinicopathologic study of 105 cases. *Cancer* 1977;39:2237–2239.

1135. Kaugar GE, Niamtu III J, Svirsky JA.: Cherubism: Diagnosis, treatment, and comparison with central giant cell granulomas and giant cell tumors. *Oral Surg Oral Med Oral Pathol* 1992;73:369–374.

1136. Peters WJN: Cherubism: A study of 20 cases from one family. *Oral Surg Oral Med Oral Pathol* 1979;47:307–311.

1137. Ayoub AF, El-Mofty S: Cherubism: Report of an aggressive case and review of literature. *J Oral Maxillofac Surg* 1993;51:702–705.

1138. Arnott DJ: Cherubism an initial unilateral presentation. *Br J Oral Surg* 1979;16:38–46.

1139. Koury ME, Stella JP, Epkar BN: Vascular transformation in cherubism. *Oral Surg Oral Med Oral Pathol* 1993;76:20–27.

1140. Weldon L, Cozzi G: Report of case. *J Oral Surg* 1974;32:57–59.

1141. Wayman JB: Cherubism: Report of three cases. *Br J Oral Surg* 1978;16:47–56.

1142. Thompson JW: Cherubism: Familial fibrous dysplasia of the jaws. *Br J Plast Surg* 1959;12:89–103.

1143. Cornelius EA, McClendon JL: Cherubism: Hereditary fibrous dysplasia of the jaws. Rontgenographic features. *Am J Roentgenol Radium Ther Nucl Med* 1969;106:136–143.

1144. Hitomi G, Nishide N, Mitsui K: Cherubism: Diagnostic images and review of literature in Japan. *Oral Surg Oral Med Oral Pathol* 1996;81:623–628.

1145. Hamner JE, Ketcham AS: Cherubism: An analysis of treatment. *Cancer* 1969;23:1133–1143.
1146. Dunlap C, Neville B, Vickers R, et al: The Noonan syndrome-Cherubism association. *Oral Surg Oral Med Oral Pathol* 1989;67:698–705.
1147. Betts NJ, Stewart JCB, Fonseca RJ, et al: Multiple central giant cell lesions with a Noonan-like phenotype. *Oral Surg Oral Med Oral Pathol* 1993;76:601–707.
1148. Addante RR, Breen GH: Cherubism in a patient with Noonan's syndrome. *J Oral Maxillofoc Surg* 1996;54:210–213.
1149. Petti GH: Hyperparathyroidism. *Otolaryngol Clin North Am* 1990;23:339–355.
1150. Parisien M, Silverberg SJ, Shane E, et al: Bone diseases in primary hyperparathyroidism. *Endocrinol Metabol Clin North Am* 1990; 19:19–34.
1151. Levin MR, Chu A, Abdul-Karim FW: Brown tumor and secondary hyperparathyroidism. *Arch Ophthalmol* 1991;109:847–849.
1152. Ayala AG, RO JY, Raymond AK: Bone tumors. In: Damjanov I, Linder J, ed. *Andersons Pathology,* 10th ed. St. Louis: Mosby, 1996:2531–2573.
1153. McFarland M, Abaza NA, El-Mofty S: Mouth, teeth, and pharynx. In: Damjanov I, Linder J, ed. *Andersons Pathology,* 10th ed. St. Louis: Mosby, 1996:1563–1615.
1154. Knezevic G, Uglesic V, Kabler P, et al: Primary hyperparathyroidism: Evaluation of different treatments of jaw lesions based on case reports. *Br J Oral Maxillofac Surg* 1991;29:185–188.

9 ⋮ Odontogenic Cysts and Tumors

Brad W. Neville, Douglas D. Damm, and Carl M. Allen

Odontogenic cysts and tumors represent a surprisingly diverse group of pathologic lesions of the jaws and overlying soft tissues. A basic understanding of the histology and embryology of tooth formation can help in understanding the development and histopathology of these lesions.

Tooth formation is a complex process that involves both epithelium and connective tissues.[1, 2] There are three major tissue components involved in odontogenesis: the enamel organ, the dental papilla, and the dental follicle. The enamel organ is an epithelial structure that is derived from oral ectoderm. The dental papilla and dental follicle are connective tissue structures that are considered ectomesenchymal in nature because they are also partly derived from cells from the neural crest.

For each tooth, odontogenesis begins with the downward proliferation from the oral surface mucosa of epithelium known as the *dental lamina*. This epithelium gives rise to the enamel organ, a cap-shaped structure that subsequently evolves into a bell shape corresponding to the future shape of the crown of the tooth (Fig. 9–1A). After the formation of the enamel organ, the cord of dental lamina epithelium from the surface mucosa will normally fragment and degenerate. However, small islands of this epithelium (rests of the dental lamina) will remain after tooth formation and may be found within the gingival soft tissues and superficial alveolar bone. These primitive dental lamina remnants are believed to be capable of giving rise to several types of developmental odontogenic cysts and tumors.

The enamel organ has four layers of epithelium. The innermost lining layer (on the inside of the "bell") is known as the *inner enamel epithelium* and will become the ameloblastic layer that forms the tooth enamel (Fig. 9–1B). Adjacent to this is a flattened row of epithelial cells known as the *stratum intermedium*. Next is a broad layer of loosely arranged cells known as the *stellate reticulum*. The outermost layer of the enamel organ is called the *outer enamel epithelium*.

Surrounding the enamel organ is loose connective tissue known as the *dental follicle*. Filling the inside of the bell-shaped enamel organ is immature connective tissue known as the *dental papilla*. Contact with the enamel organ epithelium induces the differentiation of a peripheral layer of specialized cells in the dental papilla, which are known as *odontoblasts*. The odontoblasts are the dentin-forming cells and are located adjacent and parallel to the ameloblasts. As the odontoblasts begin to form the dentin of the tooth, they in turn induce the ameloblasts to begin enamel formation.

After crown formation has begun, a thin layer of enamel organ epithelium (Hertwig's root sheath) will proliferate downward and provide the stimulus for odontoblastic differentiation in the root area of the tooth. This epithelial extension later becomes fragmented, but will leave behind small nests of epithelial cells (rests of Malassez) in the periodontal ligament. The rests of Malassez are believed to be the source of epithelium for most periapical cysts but generally are not believed to give rise to odontogenic neoplasms, except possibly for the rare squamous odontogenic tumor.

For the purposes of this chapter, we have used a modified version of the classification scheme for odontogenic cysts and tumors published by the World Health Organization (WHO).[3, 4] The odontogenic cysts are listed in Table 9–1 and the classification of odontogenic tumors is given in Table 9–2.

ODONTOGENIC CYSTS
Dentigerous Cyst (Follicular Cyst)

Tooth enamel is an ectodermally derived structure that is formed by specialized epithelium known as the *enamel organ*. After enamel formation is completed, the enamel organ epithelium atrophies to form a thin, flattened layer of cells that covers the enamel of the unerupted tooth.[5] This layer of epithelium is then known as the *reduced enamel epithelium* (Fig. 9–2). In the normal sequence of events, this reduced enamel epithelium later merges with the surface epithelium and forms the initial gingival crevicular epithelium of the newly erupted tooth.

Before tooth eruption, if fluid accumulates between the reduced enamel epithelium and the crown of the tooth, a cyst will be formed that is known as a *dentigerous* or *follicular cyst*. The dentigerous cyst is the most common developmental odontogenic cyst, making up about 20% of all epithelium-lined cysts of the jaws.[6–9]

Clinical Features. By definition, a dentigerous cyst occurs in association with an unerupted tooth. As logic would dictate, such cysts are most common around impacted teeth, especially mandibular third molars.[6, 10] Maxillary third molars and maxillary cuspids are also frequent sites. However, dentigerous cysts may occur in association with virtually any tooth, including supernumerary teeth and odontomas.[11] Dentigerous cysts arising around unerupted deciduous teeth are distinctly rare.[12, 13]

Although they may occur at any age, dentigerous cysts are most commonly diagnosed in teenagers and young adults.[6, 10] There is a slight male predilection, and their prevalence appears to be higher in whites than blacks. Most dentigerous cysts are small, asymptomatic lesions that are discovered on routine radiographs. Some dentigerous cysts may grow to considerable size and produce bony expansion that is usually painless, unless secondarily infected. However, any particularly large "dentigerous" radiolucency should clinically raise the suspicion of a more aggressive odontogenic lesion such as an odontogenic keratocyst or ameloblastoma.

Radiographically, the dentigerous cyst presents as a well-defined unilocular radiolucency, often with a sclerotic border (Fig. 9–3).[6, 10] Because the epithelial lining is derived from the reduced enamel epithelium, this radiolucency typically surrounds just the crown of the tooth, with the crown projecting into the cyst lumen (*central* variety) (Fig. 9–4). In the *lateral* variety, the cyst develops laterally along the tooth root and partially surrounds the crown. This variety is most commonly associated with mesioangular impacted mandibular third molars. In the *circumferential* variety, the cyst surrounds the crown but also extends down along the root surface, as if the tooth were erupting through the center of the cyst. Some dentigerous cysts may result in considerable displacement of the involved tooth. In addition, larger cysts can cause resorption of adjacent erupted teeth.

The radiographic distinction between an enlarged dental follicle and a small dentigerous cyst can be difficult and rather arbi-

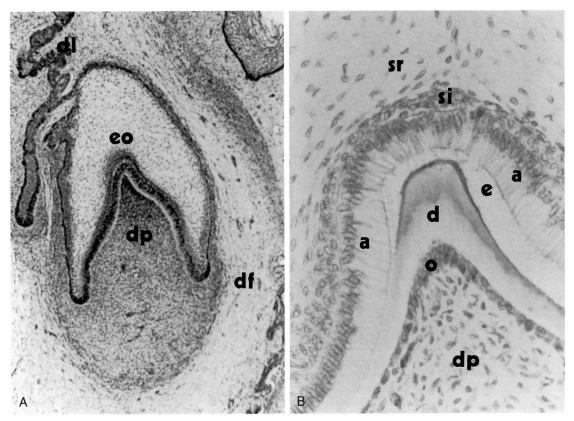

Figure 9–1. Low-power *(A)* and high-power *(B)* views of the bell stage of odontogenesis. a, ameloblasts; d, early dentin formation; df, dental follicle; dl, dental lamina; dp, dental papilla; e, early enamel matrix formation; eo, enamel organ; o, odontoblasts; si, stratum intermedium; sr, stellate reticulum. *(A* courtesy of Dr. Rudy Melfi; *B* courtesy of Dr. William Ries.)

trary.[14, 15] Generally, any pericoronal radiolucency that is larger than 3 to 4 mm in diameter is considered suggestive of cyst formation. However, the radiographic appearance alone cannot be considered diagnostic for a dentigerous cyst, since odontogenic keratocysts, ameloblastomas, and other odontogenic tumors can have an identical appearance. For this reason, biopsy is mandated for all significant pericoronal radiolucencies to confirm the diagnosis.

Pathologic Features. The microscopic appearance of the dentigerous cyst is variable, and clinical correlation is often necessary to definitively establish the diagnosis. If the cyst is not inflamed, it is usually lined by a thin, flattened layer of nonkeratinizing epithelium without rete ridge formation (Fig. 9–5*A*, see p. 607).[10] Because the wall of the cyst is derived from the dental follicle, it is characteristically composed of loose fibrous connective tissue that often contains scattered odontogenic epithelial rests. Sometimes these rests undergo dystrophic calcification.

If a dentigerous cyst becomes secondarily inflamed, the epithelial lining may become thicker and form rete ridges (Fig. 9–5*B*, see p. 607). The wall of an inflamed dentigerous cyst is often more densely collagenized.

Focal mucin-producing cells are often found in the epithelial lining (Fig. 9–6, see p. 607).[16] Although such mucous cells are usu-

Table 9–1. Odontogenic Cysts

Developmental
1. Dentigerous cyst
2. Eruption cyst
3. Odontogenic keratocyst
4. Orthokeratinized odontogenic cyst
5. Gingival cyst of the newborn
6. Gingival cyst of the adult
7. Lateral periodontal cyst
8. Glandular odontogenic cyst
Inflammatory
1. Periapical cyst
2. Residual cyst
Carcinoma arising in odontogenic cysts

Table 9–2. Odontogenic Tumors

Tumors of odontogenic epithelium without odontogenic ectomesenchyme
1. Ameloblastoma
  a. Malignant ameloblastoma
  b. Ameloblastic carcinoma
2. Calcifying epithelial odontogenic tumor
3. Squamous odontogenic tumor
4. Clear cell odontogenic carcinoma
5. Primary de novo intraosseous carcinoma
6. Intraosseous mucoepidermoid carcinoma
Tumors of odontogenic epithelium with odontogenic ectomesenchyme with or without dental hard tissue formation
1. Ameloblastic fibroma
  a. Ameloblastic fibrosarcoma
2. Ameloblastic fibro-odontoma
3. Odontoameloblastoma
4. Adenomatoid odontogenic tumor
5. Calcifying odontogenic cyst
6. Odontoma
Tumors of odontogenic ectomesenchyme with or without included odontogenic epithelium
1. Central odontogenic fibroma
2. Peripheral odontogenic fibroma
3. Granular cell odontogenic tumor
4. Odontogenic myxoma

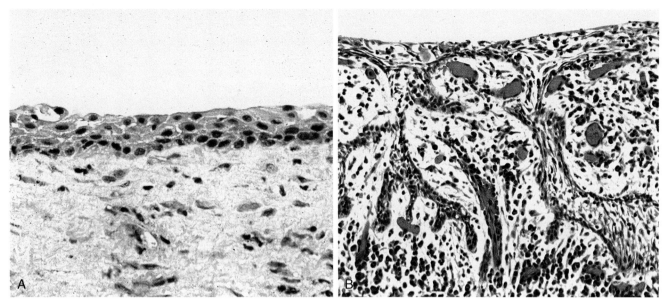

Figure 9–5. *A*, Dentigerous cyst lined by a thin layer of non-keratinizing stratified squamous epithelium. *B*, A secondarily inflamed dentigerous cyst showing irregular proliferation of rete ridges. A mostly chronic inflammatory infiltrate is present in the cyst wall.

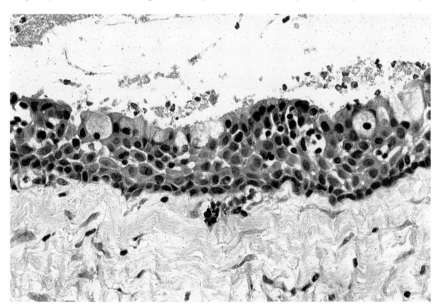

Figure 9–6. Dentigerous cyst. Scattered mucin-producing cells along the surface layer of the epithelium.

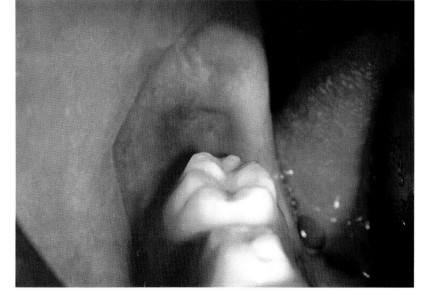

Figure 9–7. Eruption cyst. Seven-year-old male with a bluish swelling of the posterior right mandibular ridge overlying the erupting mandibular first permanent molar.

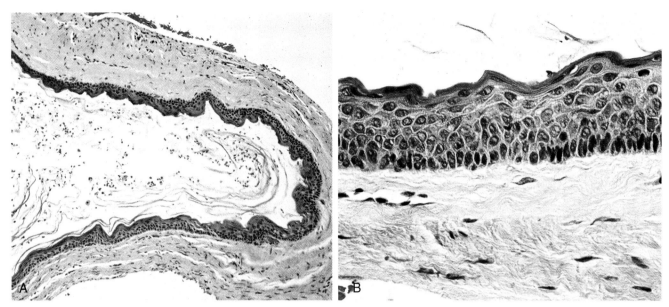

Figure 9–10. Odontogenic keratocyst. *A*, Low-power photomicrograph showing a cyst lined by stratified squamous epithelium of uniform thickness. Desquamated keratin can be seen within the cyst lumen. *B*, High-power view of the epithelial lining showing a palisaded cuboidal to columnar basal cell layer and a corrugated parakeratinized surface.

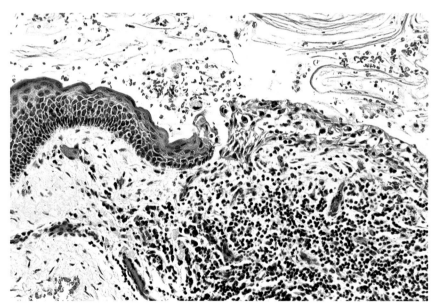

Figure 9–11. Odontogenic keratocyst. Classic odontogenic keratocyst lining is seen on the left side of this photomicrograph, but inflammation has altered the epithelium on the right side, resulting in a nonspecific histopathologic appearance.

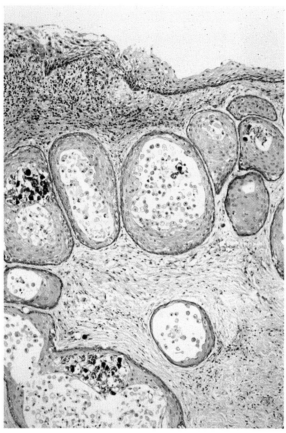

Figure 9–13. Odontogenic keratocyst. Extensive daughter cyst formation in the wall of an odontogenic keratocyst from a patient with the nevoid basal cell carcinoma syndrome. Areas of dystrophic calcification can also be seen.

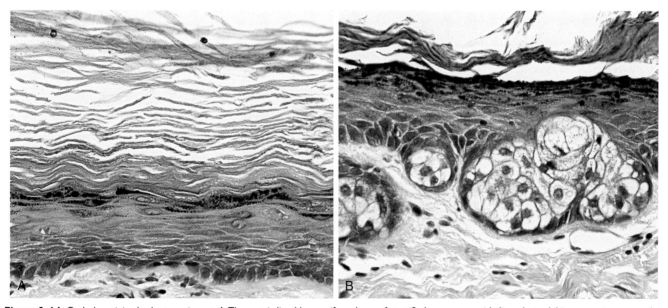

Figure 9–14. Orthokeratinized odontogenic cyst. A, The cyst is lined by a uniform layer of stratified squamous epithelium that exhibits a prominent granular cell layer and abundant orthokeratin production. B, On rare occasions, focal sebaceous glands may be seen along the basal cell layer.

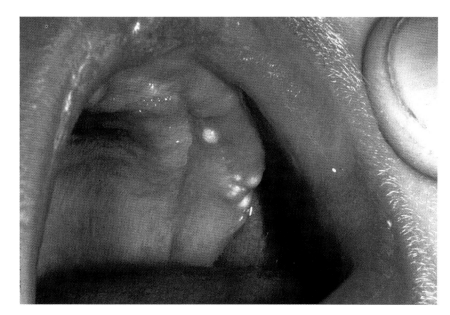

Figure 9–15. Gingival cysts of the newborn. Multiple, small, pearl-like papules on the alveolar ridge of a newborn infant. (From Neville BW, Damm DD, Allen CM, Bouquot JE: *Oral & Maxillofacial Pathology,* Philadelphia: W.B. Saunders, 1995.)

Figure 9–16. Gingival cysts of the newborn. A small keratin-filled cyst is seen within the lamina propria. Adjacent odontogenic epithelial rests (rests of the dental lamina) are evident.

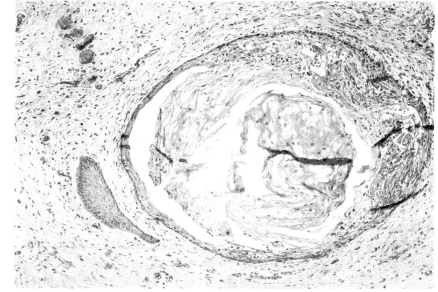

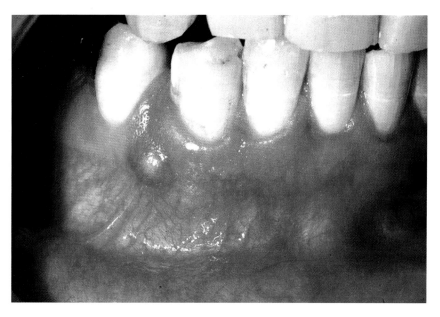

Figure 9–17. Gingival cyst of the adult. Dome-shaped bluish swelling on the gingival mucosa between the right mandibular canine and first premolar.

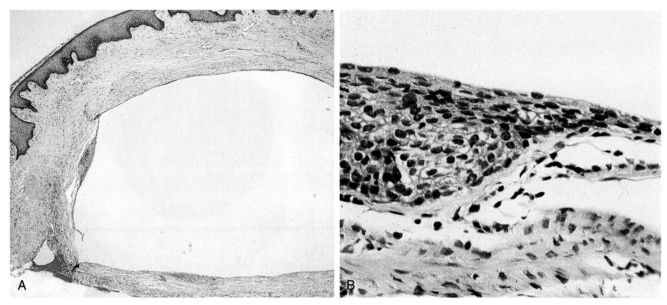

Figure 9–18. Gingival cyst of the adult. *A,* Low-power view showing a cyst with a thin epithelial lining. *B,* High-power view showing the thin epithelial lining on the right and a thickened plaque on the left with glycogen-rich clear cells.

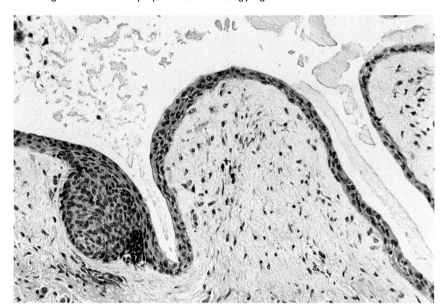

Figure 9–20. Lateral periodontal cyst. The cyst is lined by a thin layer of epithelium with a focal nodular thickening.

Figure 9–21. Lateral periodontal cyst. A "botryoid odontogenic cyst" showing multiple cystic spaces lined by thin epithelium with nodular thickenings.

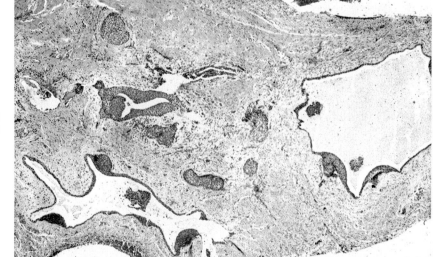

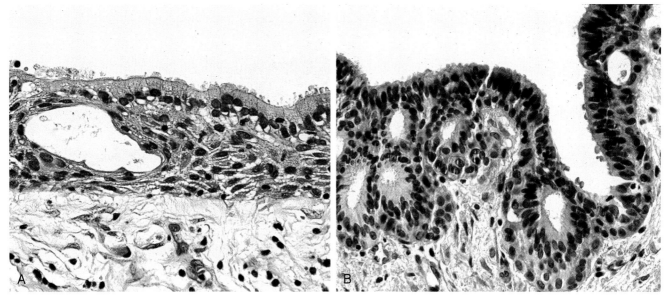

Figure 9–23. Glandular odontogenic cyst. *A,* Stratified squamous epithelial lining that exhibits ciliated columnar cells on the surface. *B,* The epithelium contains prominent gland-like spaces that are also lined by columnar cells.

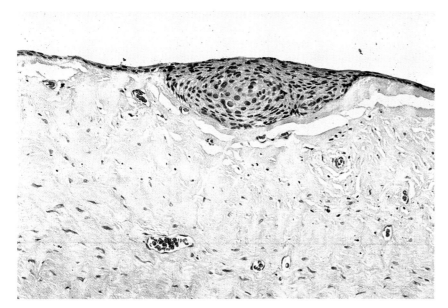

Figure 9–24. Glandular odontogenic cyst. This area of the cyst shown in Figure 9–23*A* shows a thin lining with a nodular thickening suggestive of a lateral periodontal cyst.

Figure 9–26. Periapical cyst. Low-power view showing a cyst lined by an irregular and proliferative layer of stratified squamous epithelium. *Inset:* High-power view showing arcading of the rete ridges and scattered inflammatory cells within the epithelium and cyst wall.

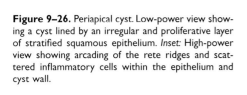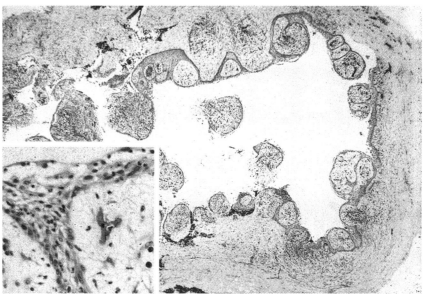

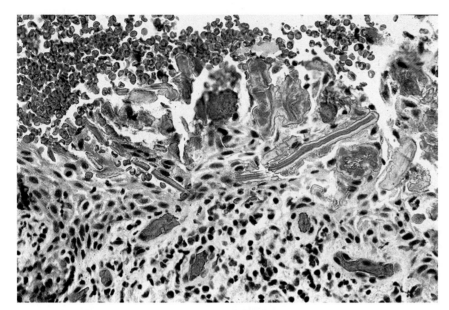

Figure 9–27. Periapical cyst. Rushton bodies in the lining of a periapical cyst.

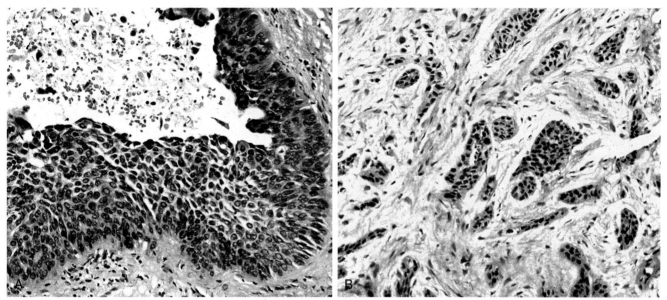

Figure 9–29. Squamous cell carcinoma arising in a dentigerous cyst. *A,* The cystic lining demonstrates severe epithelial dysplasia. *B,* Islands of invasive squamous cell carcinoma can be seen infiltrating into the cyst wall.

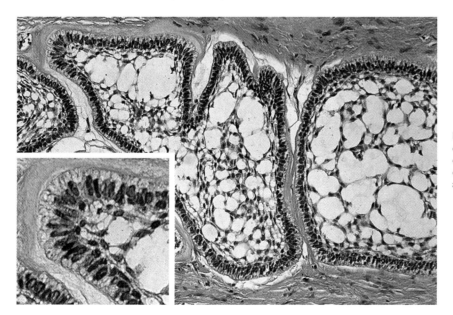

Figure 9–31. Follicular ameloblastoma. Islands of odontogenic epithelium interspersed within mature collagenous connective tissue. *Inset:* Increased magnification showing peripheral columnar differentiation and reverse polarization of the islands.

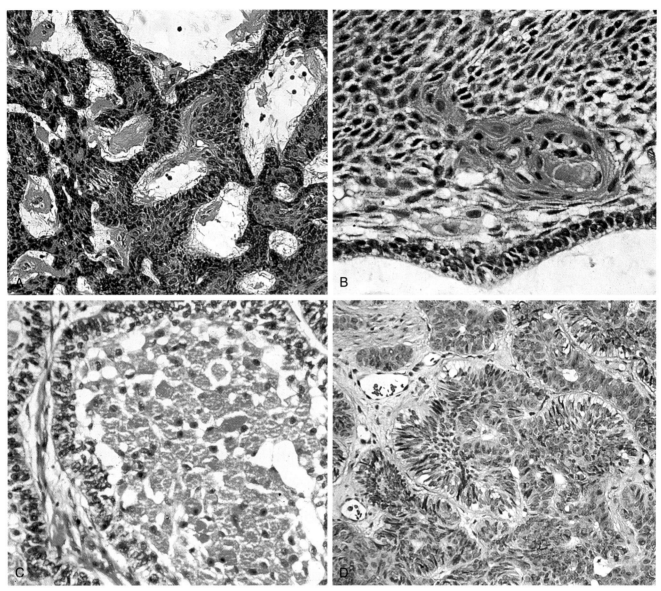

Figure 9–32. *A,* Plexiform ameloblastoma. Long interconnecting strands and cords of odontogenic epithelium that appear to surround central areas of supporting stroma. *B,* Follicular ameloblastoma, acanthomatous variant. Island of ameloblastoma in which the central portion demonstrates squamous differentiation. *C,* Follicular ameloblastoma, granular cell variant. Follicular ameloblastoma in which the central portion of each island contains cells that demonstrate abundant eosinophilic and granular cytoplasm. *D,* Plexiform ameloblastoma, basal cell variant. Interconnecting strands and cords of ameloblastic epithelium that exhibits basophilic nuclei and little cytoplasm.

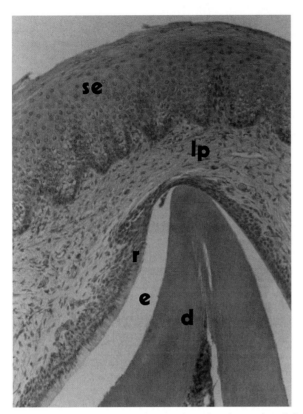

Figure 9–2. Medium-power view showing the reduced enamel epithelium covering a tooth just prior to eruption. d, dentin; e, enamel space (enamel is lost during decalcification); lp, lamina propria; r, reduced enamel epithelium; se, surface epithelium. (Courtesy of Dr. William Ries.)

chromatism. The nuclei may demonstrate polarization away from the basement membrane (reverse polarization), and the superficial epithelial layers may become loosely arranged and resemble the stellate reticulum of the enamel organ. In the odontogenic keratocyst, the epithelium is uniform in nature, usually four to eight cells thick. The basilar layer consists of a palisaded row of cuboidal to columnar cells that may demonstrate hyperchromatism. Characteristically, a corrugated or wavy layer of parakeratin is produced on the epithelial surface and desquamated keratin may be found in the cyst lumen.

Some lesions submitted as dentigerous cysts are partially lined by a thin, fragmented layer of eosinophilic columnar cells that represents the post-functional ameloblastic layer. It is probable that most of these lesions do not technically represent true cysts but just hyperplastic connective tissue dental follicles.[14] Although the lining cells in these cases may be columnar, they do not exhibit nuclear hyperchromatism or other features suggestive of ameloblastomatous transformation. In other instances, one may see follicle-like connective tissue that is only focally or partially lined by a thin, fragmented layer of squamoid epithelium. The pathologist is at a disadvantage in such cases, because it is impossible microscopically to determine whether this epithelium-lined connective tissue was a true fluid-filled sac around the tooth versus a normal or hyperplastic connective tissue follicle. Clinical correlation in such cases is important; if the surgeon clinically describes a cystic lesion, then the diagnosis of dentigerous cyst can often be supported.[19–21] However, more importantly in such cases, the pathologist can rule out the possibility of a more aggressive lesion such as an ameloblastoma or odontogenic keratocyst.

Treatment and Prognosis. Most dentigerous cysts are treated by enucleation along with removal of the associated tooth. If it is important to save the tooth, it may be possible to remove only a portion of the cyst and then aid eruption of the tooth via orthodontic measures.[22] Particularly large dentigerous cysts can sometimes be treated by marsupialization (with biopsy to confirm the diagnosis), which can allow shrinkage of the lesion prior to total removal.

The prognosis for the dentigerous cyst is excellent and the lesion almost never recurs. A rare complication is the development of an ameloblastoma from the cyst lining or from odontogenic epithelial rests within the cyst wall.[23] Also, on occasion a squamous cell carcinoma will arise from a dentigerous cyst lining.[24–26] Many investigators believe that some intraosseous mucoepidermoid carcinomas arise from mucous cells in a dentigerous cyst.[17, 18] For these reasons, careful microscopic examination of all dentigerous cysts is necessary.

ally an incidental finding, they are believed to be the most likely source for the rare intraosseous mucoepidermoid carcinoma of the jaws.[17, 18] Rarely, ciliated epithelial cells will be found. Such findings are indicative of the multipotentiality of odontogenic epithelium.

Differential Diagnosis. The two most significant lesions to distinguish from a dentigerous cyst are the cystic ameloblastoma and the odontogenic keratocyst. In the cystic ameloblastoma, the basilar cells become columnar and demonstrate prominent nuclear hyper-

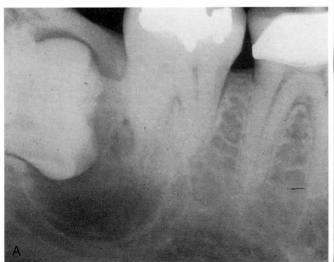
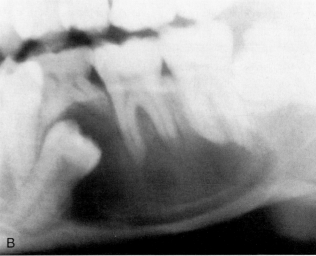

Figure 9–3. Dentigerous cyst. A, Well-circumscribed radiolucency associated with the crown of an impacted mandibular third molar. B, Large dentigerous cyst associated with an impacted mandibular second premolar. (A courtesy of Dr. Brent Klinger; B courtesy of Dr. Cornelious Slaton.)

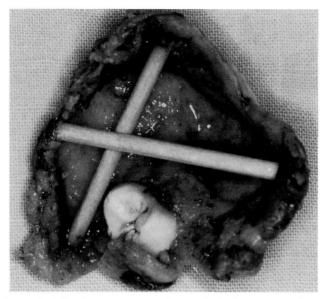

Figure 9–4. Dentigerous cyst. Gross photograph of a dentigerous cyst being held open by two sticks. The tooth crown projects into the cyst lumen.

Eruption Cyst (Eruption Hematoma)

The eruption cyst is a soft tissue variant of the dentigerous cyst.[27, 28] It arises from accumulation of cystic fluid or hemorrhage or both between the crown of an erupting tooth and the surrounding dental follicle.

Clinical Features. The eruption cyst presents as a dome-shaped swelling of the alveolar mucosa overlying an erupting tooth. It characteristically has a translucent, bluish hue due to the collection of cystic fluid and hemorrhage within the follicular sac (Fig. 9–7). Most cases occur in children under the age of 10 years. Although such lesions can occur in association with any erupting tooth, they are most common in the mandibular molar region.

Pathologic Features. Eruption cysts are rarely submitted for microscopic examination. Most such specimens consist of the excised roof of the lesion, which has been removed to allow tooth eruption. The surface of the specimen is covered by normal alveolar mucosa. The deep margin is lined by a thin layer of nonkeratinizing stratified squamous epithelium, which represents the roof of the cyst. A variable amount of inflammation may be present.

Treatment and Prognosis. Most eruption cysts do not require treatment because they usually rupture and allow the tooth to come into place. If tooth eruption appears to be impeded by the lesion, the cyst can be unroofed, which usually allows the tooth to erupt.

Odontogenic Keratocyst

The odontogenic keratocyst is a distinctive histopathologic type of developmental odontogenic cyst that was first described by Philipsen in 1956.[29] It is believed to arise from remnants of dental lamina epithelium. Recognition of this cyst is important for three reasons: (1) the odontogenic keratocyst often tends to act more aggressively than other odontogenic cysts; (2) the odontogenic keratocyst has a higher recurrence rate than other odontogenic cysts; and (3) the odontogenic keratocyst is the specific type of odontogenic cyst that sometimes may be associated with the nevoid basal cell carcinoma syndrome. The odontogenic keratocyst is estimated to make up 8% to 11% of all odontogenic cysts.[30–33]

Clinical Features. The odontogenic keratocyst can occur anywhere within the jaws, and examples have even been reported within the gingival soft tissues.[34, 35] Approximately 65% to 75% of cases are seen in the mandible, with a predilection for the molar/ramus

area.[31–33, 36–40] Frequently, the cyst will occur in association with an impacted tooth, thus mimicking a dentigerous cyst. Odontogenic keratocysts may also clinically mimic other cysts of the jaws, such as the lateral periodontal cyst,[41, 42] periapical cyst,[43, 44] and nasopalatine duct cyst.[45, 46] Some examples of the so-called "globulomaxillary cyst" (which is no longer considered to be a true entity) will turn out to be odontogenic keratocysts when examined microscopically.[47, 48]

The odontogenic keratocyst can occur at any age, but approximately 60% of all cases are diagnosed between the ages of 10 and 40 years. In his series of 312 cysts, Brannon[33] found a mean age of 37 years 9 months. The peak prevalence was in the second and third decades of life, with only 15% of the cases occurring past the age of 60 years. Woolgar et al.[49] reviewed 682 odontogenic keratocysts from 522 patients and found a mean age of 40.4 years for patients with single, nonrecurrent cysts and 26.2 years for patients with multiple cysts or the nevoid basal cell carcinoma syndrome. Although odontogenic keratocysts of the anterior midline maxillary region are uncommon, they usually occur in much older individuals with a mean age of nearly 70 years.[46] The reason for the surprising age difference in this particular subset of odontogenic keratocysts is unknown.

Smaller lesions are usually asymptomatic and are often discovered only during a routine radiographic examination. Larger cysts may result in clinical expansion and palpable thinning of the overlying cortical plate of bone. Occasional odontogenic keratocysts will be associated with pain or drainage, but even extremely large cysts may not cause any symptoms. On radiographic examination, a small odontogenic keratocyst usually presents as a well-circumscribed unilocular radiolucency that often demonstrates a sclerotic border (Fig. 9–8A). Larger cysts may take on a multilocular appearance, especially those lesions that occur in the mandibular molar/ramus region (Fig. 9–8B).

In the older literature, the term *primordial cyst* was used to describe a cyst that occurred in the place where a tooth should have developed (Fig. 9–9).[50] Presumably, the occurrence of such cysts was due to degeneration of the enamel organ prior to the formation of any mineralized tooth structure. However, microscopic examination of such clinical lesions almost always reveals features of an odontogenic keratocyst. For a while these two terms were sometimes used synonymously because odontogenic keratocysts are believed to arise from the dental lamina, or dental "primordium."[30] However, the term *odontogenic keratocyst* is today the preferred designation for such lesions if they show the characteristic microscopic features described in the next section. It is uncertain whether there are any true examples of a clinical primordial cyst (i.e, a cyst occurring in the place of a tooth) that is not an odontogenic keratocyst; however, if such lesions do exist, they must be exceedingly rare.[51]

Pathologic Features. On gross examination, the odontogenic keratocyst often demonstrates a thin, friable wall. The cyst lumen may be filled with clear fluid or a creamy to cheesy keratinaceous material. However, this keratinaceous material is not specific for the odontogenic keratocyst, since other odontogenic cysts may be filled with similar semisolid keratin-like products.

The odontogenic keratocyst is lined by a uniform layer of stratified squamous epithelium that ranges from four to eight cells in thickness (Fig. 9–10, see p. 608).[30, 51–53] This epithelium is usually devoid of rete ridges and sometimes may separate from the fibrous connective tissue wall. The basal layer consists of a palisaded row of cuboidal to columnar cells that are often hyperchromatic. Characteristically, a corrugated or wavy layer of parakeratin is produced on the epithelial surface and abundant desquamated keratin may be found in the cyst lumen. On occasion, focal areas of orthokeratinization may be seen in addition to the more typical parakeratinization.

The wall of the cyst often contains odontogenic epithelial rests and may demonstrate the formation of smaller satellite or "daughter" cysts. In rare instances, cartilage has been reported in the wall of an odontogenic keratocyst.[54]

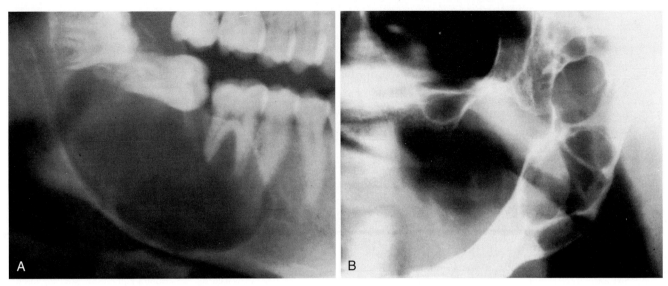

Figure 9–8. Odontogenic keratocyst. *A,* Unilocular radiolucency of the right mandible. *B,* Large multilocular radiolucency of the left mandibular ramus. (*A* courtesy of Dr. A. Paul King; *B* courtesy of Dr. Samuel McKenna)

Although the odontogenic keratocyst is developmental in origin, it may become secondarily inflamed.[36, 53, 55] If this occurs, the inflamed portion of the lining epithelium will lose its characteristic features and may become irregular and proliferative in nature with the formation of rete ridges (Fig. 9–11, see p. 608). In such cases, the diagnosis depends on a thorough examination of the entire cyst with the identification of characteristic features in noninflamed and nonaltered areas of the lining.

Differential Diagnosis. Although the production of keratin gives the lesion its name, keratinization should not be considered the sine qua non of the odontogenic keratocyst. Some keratocysts may produce only a thin layer of parakeratin on the epithelial surface without any significant accumulation in the lumen. Such cases are easily misdiagnosed as a dentigerous cyst, periapical cyst, or other jaw cyst depending on the clinical history. The presence of a palisaded cuboidal/columnar basal cell layer and a wavy, corrugated epithelial surface are more consistent and reliable microscopic features in making the diagnosis of odontogenic keratocyst.

In addition, not every cyst of the jaws that keratinizes is an odontogenic keratocyst. The orthokeratinized odontogenic cyst also exhibits keratin production, but orthokeratin is seen rather than parakeratin.[56–58] Also, orthokeratinized odontogenic cysts do not demonstrate a palisaded basal cell layer or a corrugated epithelial surface.

Treatment and Prognosis. Since the diagnosis may not be known or suspected prior to initial surgery, many odontogenic keratocysts are first treated with enucleation and curettage in a manner similar to treatment of other cysts of the jaws. However, the odontogenic keratocyst has a high recurrence rate that has been estimated in the range of 25% to 30%.[30, 51] For this reason, peripheral ostectomy with a bone bur is often recommended if the diagnosis is known or suspected preoperatively. If the cyst has broken through the cortical plate and is adherent to the overlying mucosa, excision of this mucosa may be indicated.[37] On occasion, a particularly large and aggressive keratocyst may finally require resection and bone grafting.[59, 60]

Some clinicians prefer to use chemical cautery of the bony cavity or intraluminal injection of Carnoy's solution to free the cyst from the bony wall and allow easier removal with a lower recurrence rate.[61] Others have advocated insertion of a polyethylene drainage tube into large keratocysts after cystotomy and incisional biopsy to allow decompression and subsequent reduction in the size of the cystic cavity.[62] Such decompression treatment results in thickening of the cyst lining, allowing easier removal with an apparently lower recurrence rate.

Except for their high recurrence rate and potential for significant bone destruction, the prognosis for the odontogenic keratocyst is generally good. Although most recurrences are seen within several years of the initial surgery, recurrences may not become manifest until 10 or more years after the initial diagnosis. Therefore, longterm follow-up is mandated. Malignant transformation has been reported but is quite rare.[63–66]

Although most odontogenic keratocysts occur as isolated lesions, they sometimes are a component of the nevoid basal cell carcinoma syndrome, or Gorlin syndrome.[49, 51, 67, 68] Affected patients frequently will develop multiple keratocysts (Fig. 9–12). Gorlin syndrome is an autosomal dominant inherited disorder with a wide variety of clinical manifestations. Affected individuals may demonstrate frontal and temporoparietal bossing, hypertelorism, and mandibular prognathism. Other frequent skeletal anomalies include bifid ribs and lamellar calcification of the falx cerebri. The most significant clinical feature is the tendency to develop multiple basal cell carcinomas that may affect both exposed and non-sun-exposed areas

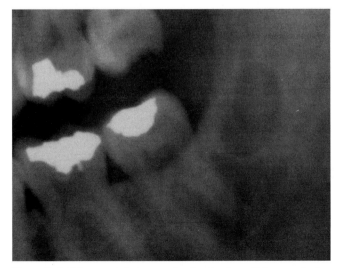

Figure 9–9. Odontogenic keratocyst. Small unilocular radiolucency distal to the left mandibular second molar. Since the third molar never developed in this area, this lesion fulfills the clinical criteria for a "primordial cyst." However, microscopic examination revealed an odontogenic keratocyst.

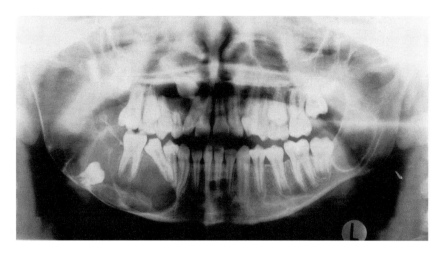

Figure 9–12. Nevoid basal cell carcinoma syndrome. Multiple odontogenic keratocysts involving the right posterior mandible, left posterior mandible, and right maxilla. (Courtesy of Dr. Richard DeChamplain.)

of the skin. Pitting defects on the palms and soles can be found in nearly two thirds of affected patients.

Odontogenic keratocysts are a common finding in patients with Gorlin syndrome, and these cysts are usually the first manifestation that leads to the diagnosis. For this reason, any patient with an odontogenic keratocyst should be evaluated for this condition. Although the cysts in patients with Gorlin syndrome cannot definitely be distinguished microscopically from those not associated with the syndrome, they often demonstrate more epithelial proliferation and daughter cyst formation in the cyst wall (Fig. 9–13, see p. 609).[69] Foci of calcification also appear to be more common in syndrome cysts.[52, 69]

Orthokeratinized Odontogenic Cyst

In addition to the odontogenic keratocyst that produces parakeratin, it has been recognized for many years that other odontogenic cysts may produce orthokeratin. In the past, these lesions have been referred to as the orthokeratinized variant of the odontogenic keratocyst. However, since these lesions are clinically and microscopically different from the more common odontogenic keratocyst, we prefer to designate them as orthokeratinized odontogenic cysts. These orthokeratinized odontogenic cysts represent 12% to 13% of keratinizing odontogenic cysts.[70, 71]

Clinical Features. Orthokeratinized odontogenic cysts predominantly occur in teenagers and young adults, with one study finding that 86% of the patients were between the second and fifth decades of life.[70] There is a male predilection, with 61% to 76% of reported cases in men.[70, 71] The lesion occurs twice as often in the mandible than the maxilla, with a tendency to involve the posterior areas of the jaws. Approximately 75% of all cases are associated with an impacted tooth, thereby clinically mimicking a dentigerous cyst.

The orthokeratinized odontogenic cyst usually presents radiographically as a unilocular radiolucency, but occasional examples will be multilocular. The size can vary from less than 1 cm in diameter to large lesions that are 7 cm or greater. The lesion is frequently asymptomatic and discovered only on routine radiographic examination; however, some cases are associated with pain or swelling.

Pathologic Features. Orthokeratinized odontogenic cysts are lined by a thin, uniform layer of stratified squamous epithelium that is usually four to eight cells thick (Fig. 9–14A, see p. 609). The basal layer usually consists of a row of flattened to cuboidal cells with infrequent rete ridge formation. Orthokeratin is produced on the epithelial surface and is associated with a subjacent granular cell layer. Abundant desquamated keratin may be found in the cyst lumen. Some cysts may show focal parakeratin production, but other features of odontogenic keratocyst are not observed. On rare occasions, focal sebaceous glands may be found in orthokeratinized odontogenic cysts (Fig. 9–14B).[72]

Differential Diagnosis. The most important lesion to distinguish from the orthokeratinized odontogenic cyst is the true odontogenic keratocyst. However, the odontogenic keratocyst exhibits a palisaded basal layer of cuboidal to columnar cells that is often hyperchromatic. A corrugated or wavy layer of parakeratin is produced on the epithelial surface and no granular cell layer should be present.

Treatment and Prognosis. Orthokeratinized odontogenic cysts are usually treated by enucleation and curettage. Unlike the odontogenic keratocyst, recurrence is rare, having been reported in about 3% of cases.[70–72] In addition, the orthokeratinized odontogenic cyst has not been associated with the nevoid basal cell carcinoma syndrome. This further underscores the importance of distinguishing this lesion from the odontogenic keratocyst.

Gingival (Alveolar) Cysts of the Newborn

Gingival cysts of the newborn are small keratin-filled cysts that are found on the alveolar mucosa of newborn infants. They arise from remnants of the dental lamina epithelium.[73–76] Such cysts are quite common, having been reported in up to half of all newborns.[76]

Clinical Features. Gingival cysts of the newborn present as small white pearl-like papules along the alveolar mucosa (Fig. 9–15, see p. 610). Multiple cysts are often seen that are usually 2 to 3 mm in diameter.[74] Lesions are more common on the maxillary arch than the mandibular arch.

Pathologic Features. Although rarely examined microscopically, the gingival cyst of the newborn will show a lining of stratified squamous epithelium.[74, 75] The cyst lumen is filled with desquamated parakeratin (Fig. 9–16).

Treatment and Prognosis. No treatment is required for these asymptomatic lesions since they will disappear on their own accord. In most instances, it is believed that the cyst ruptures and spills out its keratin contents, which allows healing to occur. These cysts are rarely seen after 3 months of age.

Gingival Cyst of the Adult

The gingival cyst of the adult is an uncommon developmental odontogenic cyst that occurs on the gingiva or alveolar mucosa. In Shear's study, it constituted only 0.5% of all cysts in the jaws.[77] The gingival cyst of the adult represents the peripheral counterpart of the lateral periodontal cyst and is believed to arise from rests of the dental lamina epithelium.[78–80] Although the gingival cyst of the newborn also arises from these same cell rests, the gingival cyst of the adult is considered a separate, distinct entity.

Clinical Features. The gingival cyst of the adult most commonly occurs in middle-aged and older adults, with a peak prevalence in the fifth and sixth decades of life.[78–81] For unknown reasons, it shows a striking predilection for the mandibular canine and premolar region, with nearly 75% of cases found there. Maxillary examples also are seen, most commonly around the canine and premolars as well as the lateral incisor area. The lesion is almost always seen on the facial aspect of the gingiva, rather than on the lingual side.

The gingival cyst of the adult appears as a painless, dome-shaped swelling that is usually 0.5 cm or less in size, although occasional cysts may be slightly larger (Fig. 9–17, see p. 610). It often has a bluish, translucent hue due to its fluid contents. In some instances, the cyst may cause "cupping-out" resorption of the underlying alveolar bone, but this may not be evident on radiographic examination. Sometimes such a lesion may actually appear to be partially within soft tissue and partially within bone, raising the question as to whether it would be better classified as a lateral periodontal cyst. However, since the lateral periodontal cyst and the gingival cyst of the adult are actually the same lesion, this question is only academic.

Pathologic Features. The gingival cyst of the adult is lined by a thin, flattened layer of epithelium that often appears to be only one to two cells thick (Fig. 9–18, see p. 611).[79–81] Sometimes this lining is so thin that the lesion is easily missed or is mistaken for the endothelial lining of a dilated blood vessel. Often one can see focal thickened plaques along the epithelial lining. These thickenings usually contain glycogen-rich cells with a clear cytoplasm.

Differential Diagnosis. On occasion, peripheral examples of odontogenic keratocyst will occur within the gingival soft tissues. However, these cysts are lined by a thicker, uniform layer of epithelium that is four to eight cells thick with a palisaded basal layer of cuboidal to columnar cells. In addition, a corrugated or wavy layer of parakeratin is produced on the epithelial surface, and desquamated keratin is often found in the cyst lumen.

Treatment and Prognosis. The gingival cyst of the adult is treated by excisional biopsy. The prognosis is excellent and the lesion should not recur.[82]

Lateral Periodontal Cyst (Botryoid Odontogenic Cyst)

The lateral periodontal cyst is a developmental odontogenic cyst that typically occurs along the lateral root surface of a tooth. It is believed to arise from remnants of the dental lamina epithelium within the alveolar bone.[83–85] The lateral periodontal cyst represents the intrabony counterpart of the gingival cyst of the adult, differing only by its location within bone. It accounts for less than 2% of all epithelium-lined jaw cysts.[86]

In the past, the term *lateral periodontal cyst* has been used to describe a variety of cysts that may be found in a lateral periodontal location, especially laterally positioned radicular cysts and odontogenic keratocysts.[87] However, the lateral periodontal cyst should be distinguished from these other lesions because of its distinctive clinical and histopathologic features.

Clinical Features. The lateral periodontal cyst usually occurs in middle-aged and older adults.[85, 88–91] The lesion is typically asymptomatic and is often discovered during routine radiographic examination. Larger examples may produce a painless expansion of the area. Like the gingival cyst of the adult, the lesion shows a striking predilection for the mandibular canine/premolar region. Maxillary examples are most frequent in the canine/lateral incisor area. Radiographically, the lesion typically presents as a well-circumscribed, unilocular radiolucency located lateral to the roots of vital teeth (Fig. 9–19).

Occasionally, the lesion may be polycystic and exhibit a multilocular appearance on the radiograph or the gross specimen. Because this polycystic variant resembles a cluster of grapes, it is often called a *botryoid odontogenic cyst*.[92–95]

Pathologic Features. The cyst is lined by a thin layer of epithelium that is only one to three cells thick in most areas.[85, 88, 96] Fo-

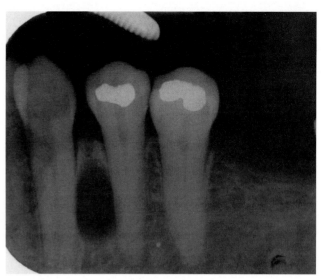

Figure 9–19. Lateral periodontal cyst. Well-circumscribed radiolucency located between the roots of the left mandibular canine and first premolar. (Courtesy of Dr. James Tankersley.)

cal nodular epithelial thickenings are often found along the cyst lining microscopically (Fig. 9–20, see p. 611). These thickenings may exhibit a "swirling" appearance and frequently contain numerous glycogen-rich cells with a clear cytoplasm. Islands of similar-appearing clear cells may be found in the cyst wall and are believed to be rests of the dental lamina. Botryoid odontogenic cysts will show multiple, separate cystic spaces (Fig. 9–21, see p. 611).[92–95]

Differential Diagnosis. Because of its characteristic clinical and microscopic features, diagnosis of the lateral periodontal cyst is usually not difficult. The glandular odontogenic cyst may show focal areas that are identical to the lateral periodontal cyst. However, the glandular odontogenic cyst will also show areas with cuboidal/columnar lining cells, gland-like spaces, and mucin production.

Treatment and Prognosis. The lateral periodontal cyst is treated by conservative surgical enucleation, and recurrence is unusual. Because of their polycystic nature, there is a greater possibility for recurrence with botryoid examples.[93–95]

Glandular Odontogenic Cyst (Sialo-odontogenic Cyst; Mucoepidermoid Cyst; Polymorphous Odontogenic Cyst)

The glandular odontogenic cyst is a rare and recently recognized form of odontogenic cyst.[97–100] Although it is generally accepted as being of odontogenic origin, it also demonstrates glandular features such as the presence of cuboidal/columnar cells, mucin production, and cilia—presumably an indication of the pluripotentiality of odontogenic epithelium.

Clinical Features. The glandular odontogenic cyst most commonly occurs in middle-aged and older adults, although cases have also been reported in teenagers.[101, 102] It shows a striking predilection for the anterior mandible, with many cases crossing the midline (Fig. 9–22). Maxillary examples are less common, but also usually occur in the anterior region.

The size of the cyst can vary from less than 1 cm in diameter to large destructive lesions that may involve most of the jaw. The most common clinical complaint is swelling, although some cases may be associated with pain or paresthesia. Radiographically, the lesion presents as either a unilocular or multilocular radiolucency, usually with well-defined borders.

Pathologic Features. The cyst is lined by stratified squamous epithelium that is variable in thickness.[99] However, the superficial layer characteristically consists of a row of cuboidal to columnar

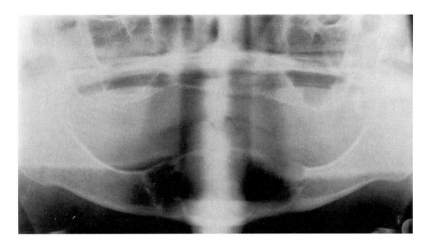

Figure 9–22. Glandular odontogenic cyst. Large multilocular radiolucency of the anterior midline mandible. (Courtesy of Dr. Joseph Carlisle.)

cells, sometimes with the presence of cilia (Fig. 9–23, see p. 612). This surface layer is often irregular and somewhat papillary. Pools of mucicarmine-positive material can be found within the epithelium and are often surrounded by similar cuboidal/columnar cells. Mucous cells may also be found. In some areas, the squamous epithelial cells may form swirling spherical aggregates reminiscent of those seen in the developmental lateral periodontal cyst (Fig. 9–24, see p. 612). This latter finding lends strong support to the belief that these cysts are of odontogenic origin.

Differential Diagnosis. There is similarity and overlap between the microscopic features of the glandular odontogenic cyst and those of a predominantly cystic intraosseous mucoepidermoid carcinoma.[103] However, the epithelial lining of the glandular odontogenic cyst is typically thinner and does not show evidence of the more solid or microcystic epithelial proliferations seen in mucoepidermoid carcinoma. In addition, mucoepidermoid carcinomas do not show the swirling spherical aggregates that are often seen in the glandular odontogenic cyst. Because these aggregates are also a prominent feature of the lateral periodontal cyst, it is possible to microscopically confuse the glandular odontogenic cyst with this entity—particularly the multilocular variant of lateral periodontal cyst known as a *botryoid odontogenic cyst.* However, the lateral periodontal cyst does not exhibit the cuboidal/columnar surface cells and mucin pools.

Treatment and Prognosis. Most glandular odontogenic cysts have been treated by enucleation or curettage. However, a high recurrence rate of around 30% has been noted. For this reason, some authors have suggested that en bloc resection may be a more appropriate therapy for many of these lesions.[101]

Periapical Cyst (Radicular Cyst; Apical Periodontal Cyst)

The periapical cyst is an inflammatory cyst that develops in association with a non-vital tooth. When the pulp of a tooth undergoes necrosis due to caries or other trauma, a granulation tissue response known as a *periapical granuloma* may develop around the root apex as a defensive reaction to bacteria and toxic products from the root canal. If this inflammation persists, it may stimulate proliferation of epithelium about the root to form a cyst. In most instances, the source of this epithelium is believed to be from the rests of Malassez, which are remnants of odontogenic epithelium found within the periodontal ligament along the tooth root. In some instances, the cystic epithelium may originate from the gingival crevicular epithelium, sinus mucosa, or the lining of a fistulous tract.[104] The periapical cyst is the most common odontogenic cyst and accounts for approximately half of all jaw cysts.[105–107]

Clinical Features. Periapical cysts occur in patients over a wide age range, but they are most frequent in young adults.[107–109] It is rare for such cysts to develop in association with deciduous teeth.[110, 111] Periapical cysts are most common in the anterior maxillary area, especially in association with the lateral incisor teeth. However, cysts associated with the deciduous teeth occur more often in the mandible.

Because the periapical cyst is associated with a non-vital tooth, the patient may present with current or prior symptoms of tenderness, pain, swelling, or drainage in the affected area. However, many periapical cysts are asymptomatic, being discovered only during routine radiographic examination.[104, 107] The radiograph shows a radiolucent area of bone destruction that is typically located at the root apex and is associated with loss of the lamina dura—the thin layer of more radiopaque bone that normally surrounds the tooth root (Fig. 9–25A). The radiolucency may appear either well-defined or poorly circumscribed, and resorption of a portion of the root apex is not unusual. Most periapical cysts are 2 cm or less in size, although occasional lesions may demonstrate dramatic enlargement with destruction of a significant portion of the jaw.

A variant of the periapical cyst known as a *lateral radicular cyst* may occur along the side of a tooth rather than at the apex, presumably due to a lateral canal from the non-vital pulp (Fig. 9–25B).[104] Similar laterally positioned cysts also may develop from communication with a deep periodontal pocket. Although such cysts may appear radiographically similar to the developmental lateral periodontal cyst, they should be distinguished as being inflammatory in etiology.

When a non-vital tooth is extracted, periapical inflammatory tissue that is not curetted from the socket may give rise to another variant known as a *residual periapical cyst.*[104] Such a lesion usually presents as a well-circumscribed radiolucency in the extraction site. Older residual periapical cysts may sometimes develop dystrophic calcification, resulting in a central area of radiopacity within the lesion on the radiograph.[112]

Pathologic Features. On gross examination, an intact periapical cyst often exhibits a thick wall surrounding the cystic lumen. However, because many of these lesions are friable or incompletely formed when they are curetted out, they are frequently submitted in multiple fragments, which belies the cystic nature of the lesion. Intact cysts may contain a brownish fluid due to breakdown of blood.[107] Shimmering crystals of cholesterol may also be found within the lumen. Some periapical cysts will demonstrate bright yellow zones within the cyst wall; microscopically, these areas correspond to collections of lipid-laden foamy macrophages.

The periapical cyst (and its variants) are lined by stratified squamous epithelium that is often irregular and proliferative in nature with arcading of the rete ridges (Fig. 9–26, see p. 612).[107] Polymorphonuclear leukocytes are frequently seen migrating into the epithelial lining.[113] Because the epithelium may exhibit extensive areas of ulceration, some periapical cysts may show only focal remnants of an epithelial lining. Mucous cells have been identified in up

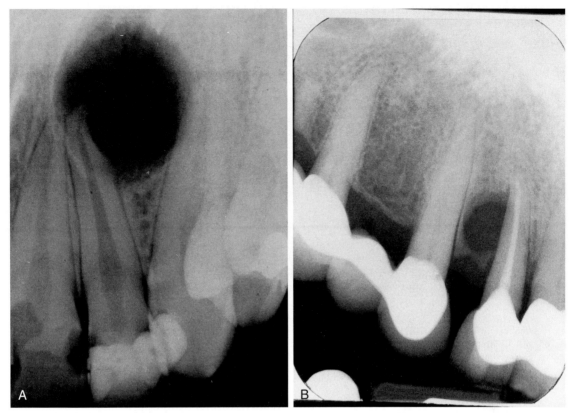

Figure 9–25. *A,* Periapical cyst. Well-circumscribed radiolucency located at the apex of the maxillary left lateral incisor. Associated root resorption is evident. (Courtesy of Dr. Richard SoJourner.) *B,* Lateral radicular cyst. Well-circumscribed radiolucency located lateral to the root of the right maxillary lateral incisor, which has already undergone root canal therapy. (Courtesy of Dr. Larry Durand.)

to 40% of periapical cysts; these cells are usually found along the surface layer and vary from occasional scattered cells to a continuous row.[114] In rare instances, these mucous cells may be associated with ciliated cells.

The cyst wall is composed of fibrous connective tissue with a variable inflammatory cell infiltrate that may include lymphocytes, plasma cells, neutrophils, histiocytes, and occasional eosinophils. Many periapical cysts contain cholesterol clefts that are associated with a foreign body giant cell reaction. Areas of hemorrhage and subsequent hemosiderin pigment are also frequent findings.

Occasionally, the epithelium will contain linear and hairpin-shaped hyaline bodies known as *Rushton bodies* (Fig. 9–27, see p. 613).[115] These structures are typically eosinophilic in color, but may exhibit basophilic mineralization. They appear to be brittle in nature, since they are often fragmented on histopathologic sections. The pathogenesis of Rushton bodies is uncertain. Some investigators believe they are of vascular origin and originate from thrombosed capillaries; others have suggested they represent a type of keratin or enamel cuticle.[107, 116, 117]

Differential Diagnosis. Although the degree of inflammation within the lesion may suggest the diagnosis of a periapical cyst, the histopathologic findings are not specific. Other developmental odontogenic cysts (e.g., dentigerous cysts and odontogenic keratocysts) can have a similar microscopic pattern if secondary inflammation is present. Therefore, clinical correlation and careful microscopic examination of the entire cystic lining are necessary to ensure the correct diagnosis.

Treatment and Prognosis. The treatment of periapical cysts usually involves either root canal therapy or extraction of the associated tooth. If the tooth is extracted, the cyst should be curetted and submitted for histopathologic examination to confirm the diagnosis. If root canal therapy is performed in an effort to save the tooth, it is important for the clinician to follow the lesion radiographically for subsequent bone fill-in. If the lesion does not resolve after root canal

therapy, then periapical surgery (including apicoectomy with retrograde amalgam placement) and biopsy may be indicated.

Carcinoma Arising in Odontogenic Cysts

Carcinomatous transformation of the epithelial lining of an odontogenic cyst is rare. However, such malignancies may represent 1% to 2% of all carcinomas seen in some oral and maxillofacial pathology services.[118]

Clinical Features. Although carcinomas arising within odontogenic cysts may occur over a wide age range, they are most frequently seen in older adults.[119–124] Most examples have been reported in association with residual periapical cysts and dentigerous cysts (Fig. 9–28). There have been a few well-documented cases of carcinoma arising in an odontogenic keratocyst.[125–127] However, some reported examples do not appear to have been associated with true parakeratinizing odontogenic keratocysts, but rather with orthokeratinized odontogenic cysts.[122, 128]

The most commonly reported symptoms are pain and swelling; however, some cases are asymptomatic and the diagnosis is made during microscopic examination of a "routine" odontogenic cyst. The radiographic features may mimic any odontogenic cyst, although the area of bone destruction is often more irregular and ragged in nature.

Pathologic Features. Most carcinomas arising from odontogenic cysts are well-differentiated squamous cell carcinomas.[120] Dysplastic changes may be found within the cystic epithelial lining along with islands of invasive carcinoma in the cyst wall (Fig. 9–29, see p. 613). In some examples, one may be able to find a transition from normal cystic epithelium to carcinoma.

Treatment and Prognosis. The treatment and prognosis of the patient with a carcinoma arising from an odontogenic cyst is similar to other oral carcinomas and depends on the size and extent of the

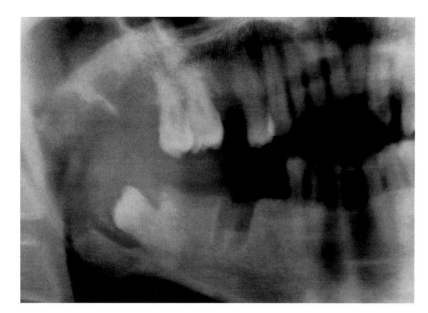

Figure 9–28. Squamous cell carcinoma arising in a dentigerous cyst. There is a large, destructive radiolucency of the right mandibular ramus that is associated with an impacted third molar. (Courtesy of Dr. Ramesh Narang.)

tumor. Surgical management typically involves en bloc excision or radical resection, often with adjunctive radiation therapy. Although relatively few cases have been reported, the 5-year survival rate appears to be approximately 50%.[120, 121] Metastases to regional lymph nodes have been reported but appear uncommon.[120]

ODONTOGENIC TUMORS

Tumors of Odontogenic Epithelium Without Odontogenic Ectomesenchyme

Ameloblastoma

Although relatively rare, ameloblastoma is the most common true neoplasm of odontogenic origin, with a prevalence equal to or exceeding the combined total of all other odontogenic tumors. The tumor appears to arise most frequently from rests of primitive dental lamina that are located in the gingiva, in the alveolar bone above the level of the teeth apices, and in the follicular walls of unerupted teeth. Other possible sources of origin include the gingival surface epithelium and the lining of odontogenic cysts.

The developing enamel organ demonstrates three cell types: ameloblasts, stellate reticulum, and stratum intermedium. The tumor cells seen within ameloblastoma mimic ameloblasts and stellate re-

ticulum but fail to exhibit any areas that resemble stratum intermedium. This missing portion of the enamel organ is thought to be responsible for the inability of the ameloblastoma to demonstrate enamel formation.

Conventional Ameloblastoma

Clinical Features. Prior to a recent profile of 3677 cases of ameloblastoma, the last comprehensive review was performed in 1955.[129, 130] These thorough studies produced data with significant agreement. At the time of diagnosis, the average age of patients with ameloblastoma is 35.9 years; but the peak prevalence drops to 27.7 years if restricted to those discovered in developing countries. Less than 2% are discovered prior to the age of 10 years, and the oldest age at time of diagnosis is 92 years. There is no strong racial predilection.

Approximately 85% of ameloblastomas arise in the mandible, with the majority occurring in the molar/ramus area. Maxillary tumors also develop most frequently in the molar region but occasionally may be seen in the anterior regions, maxillary sinus, or nasal cavity.[131] Except for the desmoplastic variant, ameloblastomas are radiolucent, with approximately 50% being unilocular (Fig. 9–30A). When loculated, the divisions may be large and like a soap bubble in appearance or small and honeycombed (Fig. 9–30B). Cor-

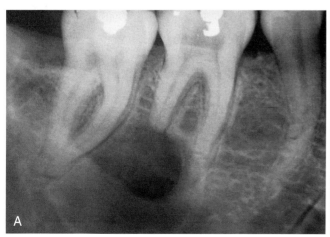
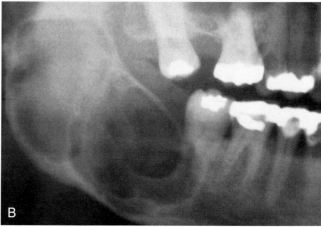

Figure 9–30. Ameloblastoma. *A,* Well-defined unilocular radiolucency of the posterior mandible that is associated with adjacent root resorption of the permanent first molar. Biopsy revealed conventional follicular ameloblastoma. *B,* Well-defined multilocular radiolucency of the posterior mandible on the right side. Biopsy revealed conventional follicular ameloblastoma.

tical expansion and tooth resorption or displacement are relatively common. The borders may be circumscribed or ill-defined.

Pathologic Features. Conventional ameloblastomas are solid infiltrating tumors but demonstrate frequent tendency to undergo cystic change. The cysts may be small and grossly undetectable or large and prominent. Histopathologically, the tumor exhibits significant diversity but typically is arranged into either a follicular or plexiform pattern.

In *follicular ameloblastoma,* islands of odontogenic epithelium are interspersed within a stroma of mature collagenous connective tissue (Fig. 9–31, see p. 613).[132] Upon closer examination, the islands reveal peripheral cells that exhibit columnar differentiation and reverse polarization (nuclei oriented away from the basement membrane with cytoplasmic clearing adjacent to the stroma) (Fig. 9–31*inset*). The central portion of the islands contains loosely arranged epithelial cells that resemble stellate reticulum of the developing enamel organ. The central portion frequently appears edematous and exhibits microcyst formation. The cyst formation and enlargement within individual islands are responsible for the polycystic pattern of growth that is common in the follicular pattern of ameloblastoma.

In *plexiform ameloblastoma,* the odontogenic epithelium is arranged into long strands and cords that often appear to surround central areas of supporting stroma (Fig. 9–32*A*, see p. 614). Upon close examination, the tumor will reveal columnar cells exhibiting reverse polarization surrounding loosely arranged stellate reticulum-like epithelium. In addition to the interconnecting epithelial cords, sheets of tumor cells may be seen. In contrast to the follicular variant, cyst formation is uncommon. The tumor is supported by mature collagenous stroma that may be loose and vascular in areas.

In many lesions, the central areas of the tumor islands demonstrate other patterns, providing the ameloblastoma with histopathologic diversity. The most common variation involves squamous differentiation of the central portion of the tumor islands and is termed *acanthomatous ameloblastoma* (Fig. 9–32*B*, see p. 614). On rare occasions, extensive keratin pearl formation is noted within the islands and has led to the variant named *keratoameloblastoma.*[133, 134] Likewise, in the *granular cell ameloblastoma,* the central portion of the tumor islands exhibits cells that demonstrate abundant granular eosinophilic cytoplasm (Fig. 9–32*C*).[135] Finally, the central portion of the islands of *basal cell ameloblastoma* exhibits darkly basophilic nuclei that demonstrate little cytoplasm and resemble those seen in basal cell carcinoma (Fig. 9–32*D*). Two or more of these patterns of differentiation may be present within an individual tumor. Of all the alternative patterns mentioned, only the acanthomatous pattern occurs with any regularity (11.3%). The final histopathologic diagnosis is guided by the dominant pattern present within the tumor; any impact on the prognosis is difficult to ascertain because of the small number of cases reported with these unusual patterns of differentiation.

One additional pattern warrants separation and further discussion. The *desmoplastic ameloblastoma* is named because of the extremely dense collagenized stroma that supports the tumor.[136–138] Histochemical evaluation of perifollicular collagen suggests the dense stroma is not scar tissue but represents active de novo synthesis of extracellular matrix proteins. The epithelial component is arranged into numerous small, widely scattered compressed islands and cords of spindle-shaped and polygonal epithelial cells (Fig. 9–33, see p. 625). The periphery of the small islands typically is lined by cuboidal cells that occasionally are hyperchromatic. Peripheral columnar cells exhibiting reverse polarization are difficult to demonstrate but usually can be found in occasional islands. Cystic formation within the islands is common. The tumor typically promotes formation of new bone and penetrates the surrounding trabeculae of bone, typically resulting in a mixed radiolucency that radiographically suggests the possibility of a fibro-osseous lesion. In contrast to more typical ameloblastomas, the desmoplastic variant frequents the maxilla and the anterior regions of the jaws.

Differential Diagnosis. The differential diagnosis of ameloblastoma must include any odontogenic tumor that exhibits columnar differentiation and reverse polarization. Within the walls of follicular tissue (dental follicle or dentigerous cyst), numerous rests of dental lamina frequently can be seen. On occasion, rare islands may demonstrate focal columnar differentiation and reverse polarization. Isolated foci do not represent neoplasia and must not be overdiagnosed.[139]

The calcifying odontogenic cyst presents as a solid or predominantly cystic lesion that frequently demonstrates columnar cells with reverse polarization. However, the presence of numerous eosinophilic ghost cells and focal calcifications within the neoplastic islands and cystic lining mitigate against the diagnosis of ameloblastoma. The adenomatoid odontogenic tumor also exhibits extensive columnar differentiation, but close examination reveals duct-like structures in which the nuclei of the cells orient toward the basement membrane and therefore do not demonstrate reverse polarization.

On occasion, the acanthomatous variant of follicular ameloblastoma may demonstrate only focal areas of columnar differentiation and can closely resemble squamous odontogenic tumor. In these instances, the islands of ameloblastoma exhibit peripheral hyperchromatic nuclei that are absent in squamous odontogenic tumor; the possible scarcity of these diagnostic areas confirms the necessity of a thorough search for definitive ameloblastic differentiation.

The WHO type of odontogenic fibroma may demonstrate significant numbers of small odontogenic epithelial islands within a background of fibrous connective tissue, which could be confused with a desmoplastic ameloblastoma. However, the desmoplastic ameloblastoma will show focal areas of columnar differentiation of the peripheral epithelial cells with reverse polarization.

Treatment and Prognosis. Conventional ameloblastoma infiltrates into surrounding bone and extends beyond the apparent radiographic boundaries seen on plain radiographs. The rates of recurrence reported in various reviews are diverse and range from 20% to 90%.[140–142] In a recent review of 3677 cases, the recurrence rate after conservative therapy (34.7%) appears to be approximately twice that associated with radical therapy (17.3%).[129] In addition, the time to clinical evidence of recurrence after conservative therapy is shorter. In planning treatment, the tumor size, location, histopathologic features, and clinical/radiographic presentation should be taken into consideration.

Treatment with curettage may leave small islands of tumor within the bone. Marginal or en bloc resection is the most widely used form of therapy, with many surgeons advocating margins of excision that extend at least 1 cm past the radiographic limits of the tumor.

Some investigators have suggested that children under the age of 10 should not undergo radical surgery. In elderly patients, extensive surgery may not be warranted, depending on the patient's life expectancy and the anticipated time to recurrence. Multilocular ameloblastomas exhibit a higher recurrence rate than unilocular lesions. Maxillary ameloblastomas usually require radical surgery, because the bony architecture does little to impede tumor invasion and close proximity of vital structures in this area makes recurrence potentially dangerous. More conservative therapy of mandibular ameloblastomas often can be considered because of easier radiographic evaluation of the surgical site and the distance to vital structures. Perineural invasion along the inferior alveolar nerve has not been reported.

Review of 3677 cases reveals that the overall recurrence rate of conventional ameloblastoma is 22.7%.[129] Close to half of all recurrences become clinically evident more than 5 years after the initial surgical procedure, with one report documenting a recurrence interval of 33 years. Lifelong follow-up is strongly recommended. Rare malignant transformation has been observed.

Unicystic Ameloblastoma

Clinical Features. Unicystic ameloblastoma is considered at best an in situ or superficially invasive form of ameloblastoma and accounts for 6% of reported cases of ameloblastoma.[143–148] The lesion consists of a single cystic structure that typically presents similar to a dentigerous cyst but may be seen unassociated with an impacted tooth. Radiographically, the lesions present as unilocular or

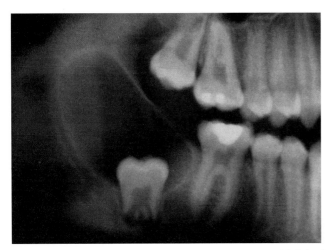

Figure 9–34. Unicystic ameloblastoma, intramural variant. Well-defined pericoronal radiolucency associated with the mandibular permanent second molar on the right side in a 14-year-old female. (Courtesy of Dr. Robert Coles.)

multilocular radiolucencies (Fig. 9–34). Unicystic ameloblastomas are most frequently found in younger patients with an average age at diagnosis of 22.1 years, as compared with 35.9 years for conventional ameloblastomas. Close to half of the cases are discovered during the second decade. Several different variants are seen and have an impact on the therapy and long-term prognosis.

Pathologic Features. *Luminal unicystic ameloblastoma* is a unilocular cyst-like lesion that is lined by epithelium that exhibits columnar differentiation and reverse polarization of the basal cell layer. The basal cell layer is hyperchromatic and contrasts to the remainder of the epithelium that is loose and eosinophilic (Fig. 9–35A, see p. 625). The connective tissue adjacent to the lining epithelium often exhibits a uniform, thin, band-like area of hyalinization. No intraluminal or intramural extension by tumor should be found after thorough examination of the specimen.

Intraluminal unicystic ameloblastoma is a unilocular cyst-like lesion that exhibits one or more nodules of ameloblastoma projecting into the lumen. Thorough examination of the specimen will not reveal extension into the surrounding connective tissue wall. On occasion, this form of unicystic ameloblastoma can produce an intraluminal plexiform pattern of odontogenic epithelium that lacks typical ameloblastomatous differentiation and has been termed *plexiform unicystic ameloblastoma.* The proliferative epithelium often resembles the hyperplastic lining of inflammatory odontogenic cysts and consists of interconnecting cords supported by a delicate and vascular connective tissue stroma (Fig. 9–35B, see p. 625).

The final pattern is superficially invasive and termed *intramural unicystic ameloblastoma.* This unilocular cyst-like lesion exhibits ameloblastomatous invasion into the underlying connective tissue wall of the cyst. The extent and depth of the infiltrative growth may vary considerably; therefore, careful and extensive sampling is necessary to determine the extent of the tumor. Ameloblastomatous involvement of the lining epithelium may or may not be present.

Differential Diagnosis. A number of odontogenic cysts may be confused with unicystic ameloblastoma. Dentigerous cysts frequently present similar clinical and radiographic patterns but lack the hyperchromatic basal cell layer exhibiting columnar differentiation and reverse polarization. Plexiform unicystic ameloblastomas often demonstrate areas that closely resemble the proliferative epithelium of periapical cysts, but these latter cysts are associated with the apices of non-vital teeth, typically reveal a significant inflammatory infiltrate, and usually do not demonstrate the polypoid intracystic growth pattern typical of plexiform unicystic ameloblastoma. Odontogenic keratocysts do exhibit a hyperchromatic and palisaded basal cell layer but lack basilar reverse polarization and the looseness of the suprabasilar epithelium.

As mentioned previously, calcifying odontogenic cyst, adenomatoid odontogenic tumor, and prominent intramural rests of dental lamina should be ruled out. Although similar in appearance, the calcifying odontogenic cyst exhibits numerous eosinophilic ghost cells and focal calcifications. The adenomatoid odontogenic tumor reveals numerous duct-like structures that do not demonstrate reverse polarization. Rarely, rests of dental lamina may reveal focal columnar differentiation and reverse polarization, but these isolated foci do not represent neoplasia.

The diagnosis of unicystic ameloblastoma requires microscopic examination of the entire surgical specimen; definitive diagnosis upon incisional biopsy is not possible. An incisional biopsy of a large cyst within a conventional follicular ameloblastoma often is indistinguishable histopathologically from a luminal unicystic ameloblastoma. Pathologists must resist definitive diagnosis prior to complete removal, at which time thorough evaluation for invasion can be performed.

Treatment and Prognosis. In the luminal and intraluminal variants of unicystic ameloblastoma, the tumor is confined by the fibrous connective tissue wall of the cyst. With complete enucleation of the cyst, recurrence is not expected. By definition, the intramural variant demonstrates invasion of the connective tissue wall. When invasion of the wall is discovered upon histopathologic examination, additional therapy beyond cyst enucleation is recommended; however, some surgeons prefer to await recurrence prior to additional intervention.[149] The aggressiveness of the additional therapy depends on the depth of invasion. This judgment should be made from clinicopathologic correlation at the time of therapy.

Review of reported cases of unicystic ameloblastoma reveals a recurrence rate of 13.7%.[129] These cases represent incompletely removed cysts and those with intramural invasion. Although conservative enucleation is the therapy of choice for those exhibiting no invasion, long-term follow-up remains mandatory.

Extraosseous Ameloblastoma

Since epithelial rests derived from dental lamina commonly are found within the gingiva, it is not surprising that peripheral odontogenic tumors are seen occasionally. Almost any odontogenic tumor that has been reported within bone also has been seen in the peripheral soft tissues overlying the tooth-bearing areas of the jaws.[150] Extraosseous ameloblastoma represents the most frequently encountered form of peripheral odontogenic tumor, representing slightly more than half of the documented cases.[151] Previous cases of intraoral basal cell carcinoma have been documented, but most authorities believe these should be included under the designation of peripheral ameloblastoma.[150]

The majority of extraosseous ameloblastomas most likely arise from rests of dental lamina, but rare cases have been reported in oral soft tissues not overlying bone.[152, 153] These examples lend support to the theory that some peripheral ameloblastomas arise from pluripotent basal-layer cells of the surface epithelium. In contrast, some investigators exclude all peripheral ameloblastomas that arise in soft tissue not overlying bone and believe that such tumors represent a variant of a salivary gland tumor or an adamantoid pattern of squamous cell carcinoma.[154]

Clinical Features. Clinically, most extraosseous ameloblastomas present as normal-colored, smooth-surfaced enlargements; but occasional tumors demonstrate an erythematous or papillary surface. Several clinical differences are noted between peripheral and intraosseous ameloblastomas.[155–157] The average age at diagnosis is 51 years, approximately 15 years later than its intrabony counterpart. Most tumors are smaller than 1.5 cm, but occasional tumors may be larger. Approximately 65% arise in the anterior regions of the jaws, and there is a mandibular predominance of 5 : 1.[129] Typically, no alterations are present radiographically except for occasional cupping or peripheral erosion of the underlying cortical bone. Rare multicentric cases are reported.[158]

Text continued on page 633

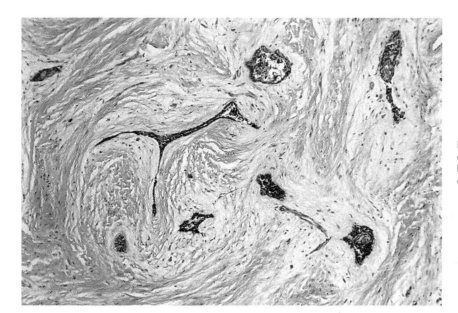

Figure 9–33. Desmoplastic ameloblastoma. Numerous small, widely scattered, and compressed islands of hyperchromatic odontogenic epithelium within hypocellular collagenous stroma.

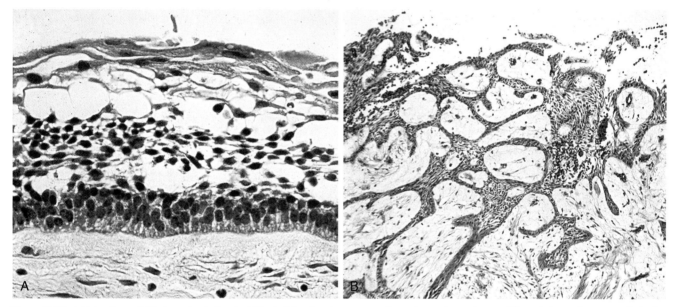

Figure 9–35. *A,* Unicystic ameloblastoma, luminal variant. Cystic lining that demonstrates hyperchromatism, columnar differentiation, and reverse polarization of the basal cell layer. Note the loose stratum spinosum and eosinophilic surface parakeratin. *B,* Unicystic ameloblastoma, plexiform variant. Interconnecting cords of odontogenic epithelium supported by a delicate and vascular connective tissue stroma.

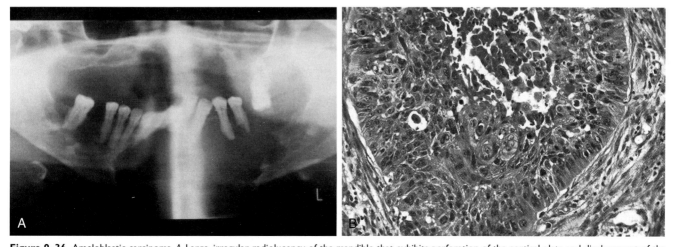

Figure 9–36. Ameloblastic carcinoma. *A,* Large, irregular radiolucency of the mandible that exhibits perforation of the cortical plate and displacement of the adjacent dentition. (From Neville BW, Damm DD, White DK, Waldron CA: *Color Atlas of Clinical Oral Pathology.* Philadelphia: Lea & Febiger, 1991.) *B,* The tumor cells demonstrate considerable pleomorphism and mitotic activity, but peripheral palisading can still be seen.

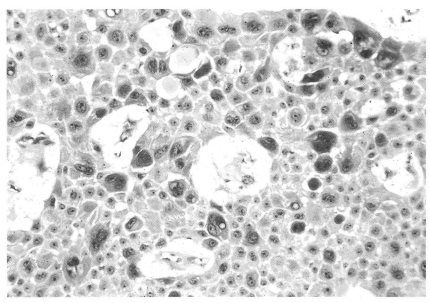

Figure 9–38. Calcifying epithelial odontogenic tumor. Sheet of large eosinophilic polyhedral epithelial cells that exhibit significant cellular and nuclear pleomorphism. Note pools of acellular eosinophilic amyloid.

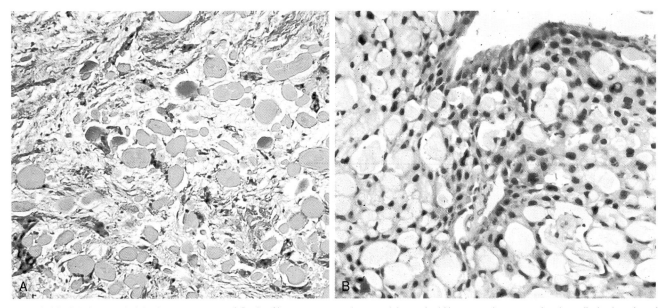

Figure 9–39. Calcifying epithelial odontogenic tumor. A, Pools of homogeneous and eosinophilic amyloid-like material intermixed with small islands and cords of odontogenic epithelium. B, Intraepithelial accumulation of amyloid-like material creating a cribriform appearance of the involved neoplastic island.

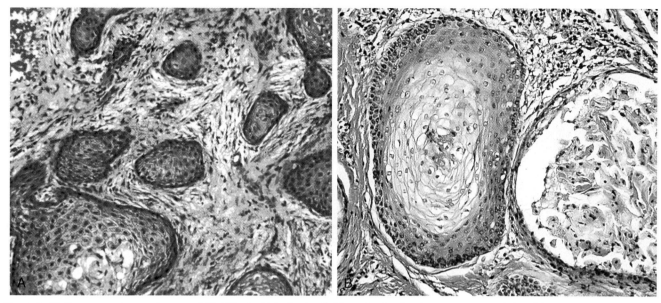

Figure 9–41. Squamous odontogenic tumor. A, Variable-sized islands of well-differentiated and uniform squamous epithelium. Note vacuolization of some of the islands. B, Vacuolization and microcyst formation of individual tumor islands.

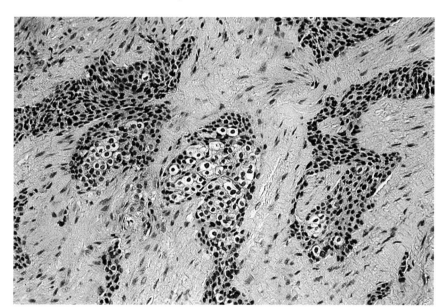

Figure 9–43. Clear cell odontogenic carcinoma. Islands of infiltrating odontogenic epithelium that are a mixture of clear cells and eosinophilic polygonal cells.

Figure 9–45. Intraosseous mucoepidermoid carcinoma. Sheet of neoplastic epithelium that exhibits a mixture of squamoid cells and mucous cells.

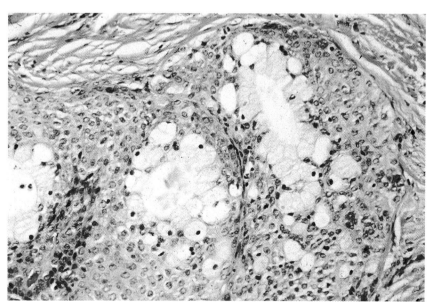

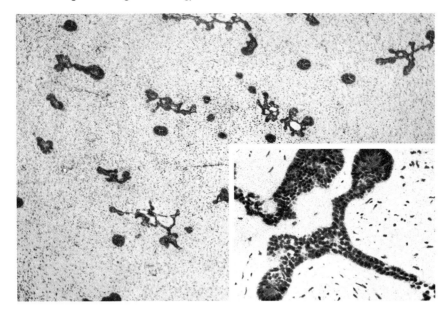

Figure 9–47. Ameloblastic fibroma. Low-power photomicrograph showing delicate strands of odontogenic epithelium set in a myxoid background. *Inset:* Medium-power photomicrograph showing bilayered strands of odontogenic epithelium and small islands of ameloblastoma-like epithelium. These are set in a background of myxoid connective tissue that resembles dental papilla.

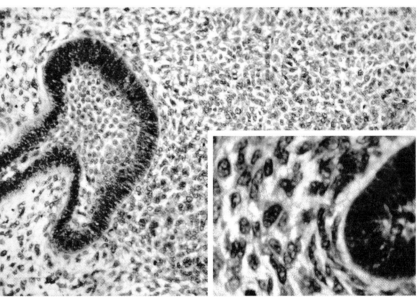

Figure 9–48. Ameloblastic fibrosarcoma. Medium-power photomicrograph showing a hypercellular proliferation of spindle-shaped cells with an island of odontogenic epithelium. *Inset:* High-power photomicrograph showing hyperchromatic and pleomorphic fibroblastic cells with evidence of mitotic activity. The odontogenic epithelial component appears relatively bland.

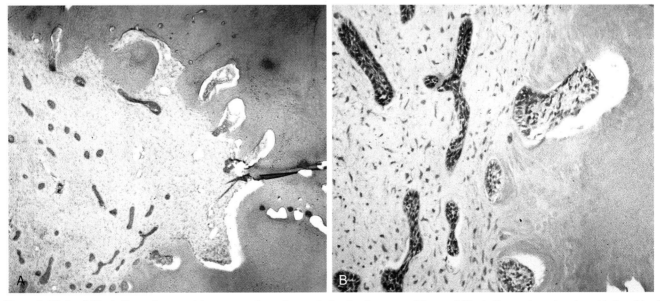

Figure 9–50. Ameloblastic fibro-odontoma. *A,* Low-power photomicrograph showing tissue resembling ameloblastic fibroma in conjunction with dental hard tissues. *B,* Medium-power photomicrograph showing dentin admixed with ameloblastic fibroma-like tissue.

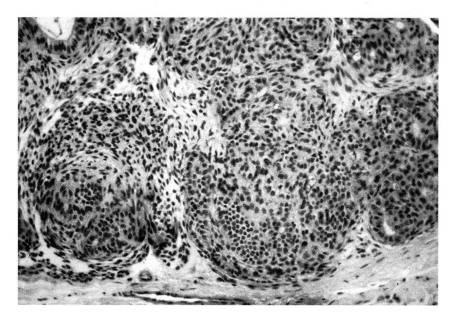

Figure 9–52. Adenomatoid odontogenic tumor. Medium-power photomicrograph showing an encapsulated proliferation of odontogenic lesional tissue characterized by solid, swirling zones of epithelial cells.

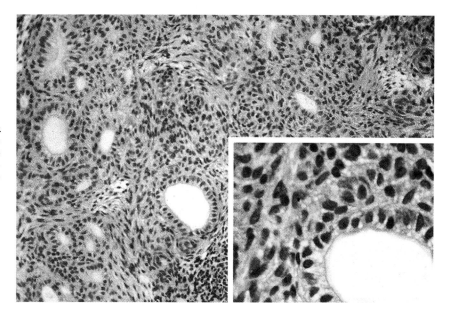

Figure 9–53. Adenomatoid odontogenic tumor. Medium-power photomicrograph showing solid areas composed of spindle-shaped cells as well as duct-like (adenomatoid) formations. *Inset:* High-power photomicrograph showing a duct-like structure composed of cuboidal to columnar epithelial cells.

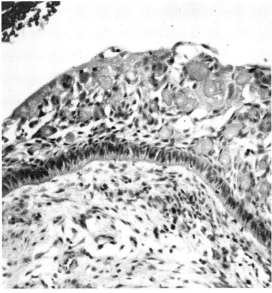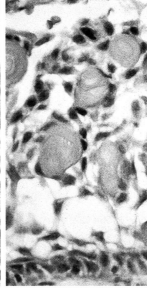

Figure 9–55. Calcifying odontogenic cyst. Medium-power photomicrograph showing a proliferation of odontogenic epithelial cells associated with a cystic lumen. *Inset:* High-power photomicrograph showing the palisaded basal cell layer of the lesional epithelium and the "ghost-cell" change that characterizes this process.

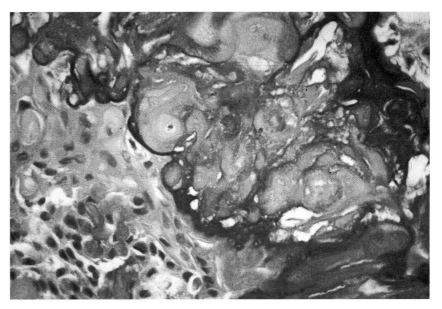

Figure 9–56. Calcifying odontogenic cyst. High-power photomicrograph showing "ghost-cell" change with areas of dystrophic calcification.

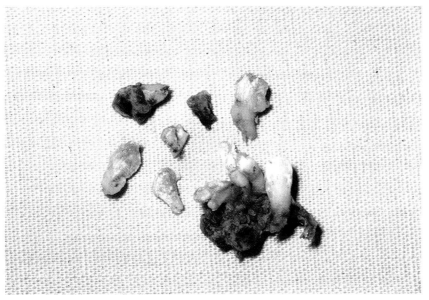

Figure 9–58. Compound odontoma. Gross examination reveals numerous small, malformed tooth-like structures.

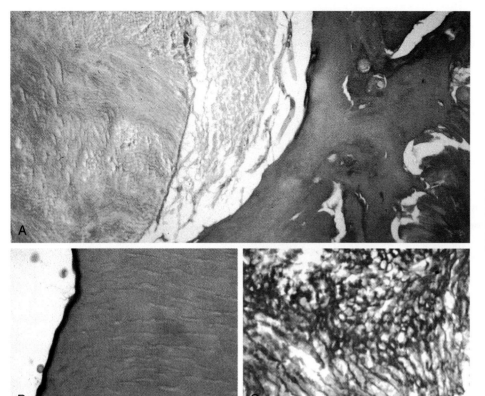

Figure 9–59. Complex odontoma. *A*, Medium-power photomicrograph showing enamel matrix (left) and dentin (right). *B & C*, High-power photomicrographs show the net-like pattern of enamel matrix *(B)* and the pattern of parallel tubules that characterizes dentin *(C)*.

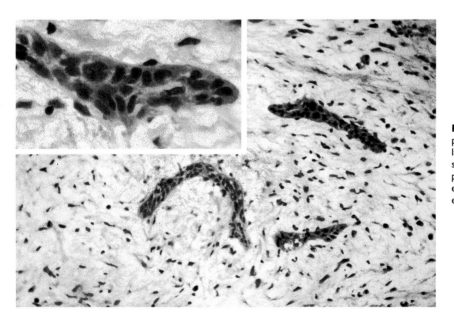

Figure 9–61. Central odontogenic fibroma. Low-power photomicrograph showing a moderately cellular fibroblastic proliferation associated with scattered strands of odontogenic epithelium. *Inset:* High-power photomicrograph showing a strand of odontogenic epithelium that has no cuboidal or columnar peripheral component, a characteristic feature of this lesion.

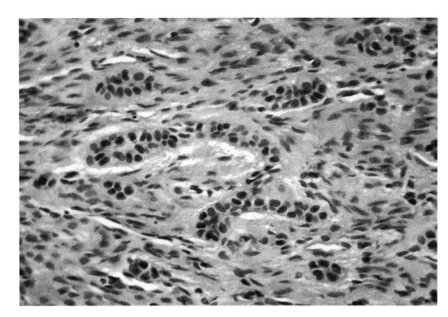

Figure 9–62. Central odontogenic fibroma. Medium-power photomicrograph showing a rather cellular proliferation of fibroblasts with abundant background collagen and strands of odontogenic epithelium.

Figure 9–64. Granular cell odontogenic tumor. Low-power photomicrograph showing a proliferation of lesional mesenchymal cells with abundant eosinophilic cytoplasm in association with strands of odontogenic epithelium. *Inset:* High-power photomicrograph showing the granular cytoplasm of the lesional cells as well as the bland appearance of the associated odontogenic epithelium.

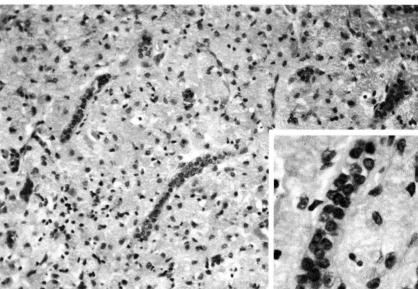

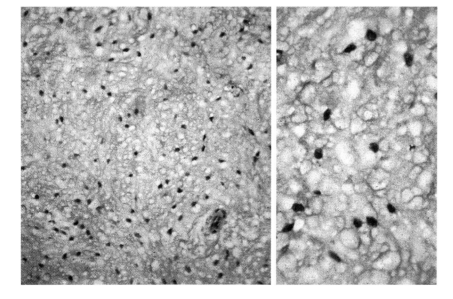

Figure 9–66. Odontogenic myxoma. Low-power photomicrograph showing a pale, myxomatous lesional cell proliferation. *Inset:* High-power photomicrograph showing stellate lesional cells set in a myxoid background with delicate collagen fibers.

Pathologic Features. Both plexiform and follicular patterns are seen within the tumor, which contains peripherally located columnar cells exhibiting reverse polarization. As expected, the extraosseous variant also demonstrates a histopathologic spectrum similar to that seen in conventional intraosseous ameloblastomas. In most cases, a mixed histopathologic pattern is noted; but, in contrast to those arising within bone, the second most common presentation is the acanthomatous variant.[129] Although in some cases the tumor is not contiguous with the surface epithelium, the majority are confluent with the overlying oral mucosa.

Treatment and Prognosis. Extraosseous ameloblastomas are not aggressive clinically, and permanent resolution usually is achieved with conservative excision. A recurrence rate of 8% has been reported, and local re-excision typically resolves the problem. Rare carcinomatous transformation does occur.[159–161]

Malignancy in Ameloblastoma

Tumors demonstrating ameloblastomatous differentiation and evidence of malignancy are separated into two categories.[162] *Malignant ameloblastoma* refers to a well-differentiated metastasizing ameloblastoma that cytopathologically is identical to its benign counterparts in both the primary site and in all metastatic deposits.[163–166] In contrast, *ameloblastic carcinoma* demonstrates cytopathologic features of malignancy in the primary tumor, in a recurrence, or in any metastatic foci.[167–170] Both types of malignancy are quite rare; as of this writing, only 44 cases of malignant ameloblastoma and 29 cases of ameloblastic carcinoma have been reported.

Malignant Ameloblastoma

Clinical Features. Factors associated with the development of malignant ameloblastoma include long duration of the tumor, extensive local disease, frequent surgical procedures, and radiation therapy. The primary tumors exhibit a mandibular predominance, with an 8:1 mandibular:maxillary ratio.[163] Most metastases are solitary rather than multiple. Pulmonary metastases are seen in 75% of cases, and the cervical lymph nodes and spine are the next most common locations. Liver, skull, diaphragm, brain, kidney, small bowel, and skin are affected less frequently. The average age at the time of initial surgery is 30.5 years, with a 1.5:1 male predominance.[163] A median time of 9 years elapses between the initial surgical intervention and the discovery of metastasis.[163]

Pathologic Features. In malignant ameloblastoma, the histopathologic features of both the primary and metastatic lesions do not differ significantly from conventional nonmetastasizing ameloblastomas. A significant majority of the tumors demonstrate a pure or mixed plexiform variant of ameloblastoma. In spite of this, the likelihood of metastasis cannot be predicted by morphologic criteria.

Treatment and Prognosis. The therapy of choice for malignant ameloblastoma is surgical resection of all tumor sites, with radiotherapy reserved for metastatic deposits not amenable to a surgical approach. Although no consistently effective chemotherapeutic regimen exists, rare positive responses are documented.[171, 172] Limited follow-up restricts accurate predictions, but the median survival time after metastasis is reported to be 2 years.[163]

Ameloblastic Carcinoma

Clinical Features. Ameloblastic carcinomas affect men slightly more often than women, and patients have a mean age of 33.5 years at initial surgery. The primary tumor exhibits a 5:1 mandibular predilection, and the lung represents the most common site of metastases. Clinically and radiographically, the lesions behave more aggressively than conventional ameloblastomas. Pain, swelling, rapid growth, trismus, and dysphonia are reported. Radiographically, the lesions are less defined; and perforation of the cortical bone with extension into surrounding soft tissue is not rare (Fig. 9–36A, see p. 625). Rare peripheral examples occur.[165, 173, 174]

Pathologic Features. Cytopathologically, ameloblastic carcinoma exhibits peripheral columnar differentiation and reverse nuclear polarization along with features of malignancy such as an increased nuclear:cytoplasmic ratio, cellular pleomorphism, and an increased mitotic index (Fig. 9–36B, see p. 625). The diagnosis can be made if these features are noted within the primary lesion; no metastatic focus is required. Definitive evidence of ameloblastic differentiation must be demonstrated to rule out primary intraosseous squamous cell carcinoma and metastasis from other sites.

Treatment and Prognosis. Owing to the small number of cases and insufficient follow-up, the therapy of choice for ameloblastic carcinoma remains rather indefinite. Complete surgical resection appears to be the most prudent. Although well-differentiated intraosseous ameloblastoma typically is resistant to radiotherapy, the response by ameloblastic carcinoma is not well documented. As is seen with malignant ameloblastoma, there is often a significant time span between the initial surgery and the appearance of metastatic disease. Once spread has been documented, death usually occurs within a year or so.

Calcifying Epithelial Odontogenic Tumor (Pindborg Tumor)

Also known as the Pindborg tumor, the calcifying epithelial odontogenic tumor is a most uncommon neoplasm that exhibits a prevalence 10 to 15 times less than ameloblastoma.[175–177] In a review of 2412 odontogenic tumors and hamartomas, this tumor accounted for only 1% of all cases. Although some investigators have suggested an origin from reduced enamel epithelium, histochemical evidence strongly suggests that this neoplasm arises from the stratum intermedium portion of the enamel organ.[178]

Clinical Features. As documented in a review of 113 cases, the calcifying epithelial odontogenic tumor arises over a wide age range that extends from the first to tenth decades.[176] Although the mean age at diagnosis is 40 years, the prevalence is spread rather evenly through the third to sixth decades. No sex predilection is seen.

The vast majority of the cases are intraosseous, but approximately 5% arise in peripheral locations.[176] A 2:1 mandibular:maxillary ratio is seen, with 90% of all tumors arising in the premolar/molar region; the molar region is the most common site by a ratio of close to 3:1 over other locations. In contrast, the few peripheral examples appear to prefer the anterior regions.

Clinically, most Pindborg tumors present as slowly enlarging and painless masses. Occasional patients report associated pain, nasal stuffiness, epistaxis, or headaches. Radiographically, the calcifying epithelial odontogenic tumor produces a radiolucency that may be well or poorly defined; and the majority are associated with impacted teeth (Fig. 9–37). As the lesion enlarges, there is a tendency for the area to develop a honeycomb-like multilocular pattern. Occasionally, radiopacities of variable size develop within the radiolucent areas. When the tumor is associated with an impacted tooth, the calcifications typically are most prominent adjacent to the crown of the tooth.

Pathologic Features. Although the histopathologic patterns are varied, the calcifying epithelial odontogenic tumor typically grows as islands or sheets of eosinophilic polyhedral epithelial cells that have well-defined cell borders and often distinct intercellular bridges. In other tumors, the cells are arranged in small nests or cords that are scattered widely through mature fibrous connective tissue. Rare examples are composed predominantly of cells with vacuolated cytoplasms, but these tumors also will demonstrate areas of typical eosinophilic cells.[179, 180]

The cytomorphology of the lesional cells may suggest a malignant process. Significant cellular and nuclear pleomorphism is not uncommon, and prominent nucleoli often are present (Fig. 9–38, see p. 626). Scattered multinucleated tumor giant cells may be seen. In spite of these findings, mitotic figures are very uncommon.

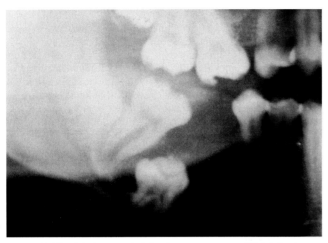

Figure 9–37. Calcifying epithelial odontogenic tumor. Well-defined pericoronal radiolucency associated with impacted first permanent mandibular molar on the right side. (Courtesy of Dr. Samuel McKenna.)

Extremely rare carcinomatous transformation has been documented[181]; but, in contrast, these cases reveal mitoses that are abnormal in both numbers and appearance.

Intermixed with the epithelial cells and present within the surrounding stroma are circular areas of a homogeneous, eosinophilic material that demonstrates an amyloid-like apple-green birefringence upon Congo-red staining (Fig. 9–39A, see p. 626). On occasion, intraepithelial accumulation creates a cribriform pattern of the neoplastic islands (Fig. 9–39B). The amyloid-like material may undergo Liesegang calcification, characterized by basophilic, concentric lamellar rings. As the material calcifies, the deposits change from periodic acid–Schiff (PAS) negative to strongly PAS positive.

Close examination of a number of adenomatoid odontogenic tumors will reveal cases that exhibit foci of calcifying epithelial odontogenic tumor. Since the adenomatoid odontogenic tumor contains pre-ameloblasts, stellate reticulum and stratum intermedium, it is not surprising that areas of calcifying epithelial odontogenic tumor can be seen arising from the stratum intermedium portion of the primary tumor.[182] Even though some examples are close to 90% Pindborg tumor, these combined tumors demonstrate an age distribution and clinical activity most consistent with an adenomatoid odontogenic tumor.

Differential Diagnosis. Primary intraosseous carcinoma, squamous odontogenic tumor, and metastatic squamous cell carcinoma may resemble calcifying epithelial odontogenic tumor, but the presence of amyloid-like material with concentric calcification aids in the differentiation. The WHO type of odontogenic fibroma closely resembles the pattern of Pindborg tumor that presents with widely scattered islands and cords of neoplastic epithelium within supporting collagenous stroma. In many of these cases, the amyloid-like material is not obvious and thorough examination is required for proper classification.

In those cases exhibiting clear cell differentiation, central mucoepidermoid carcinoma and metastatic renal cell carcinoma must be considered. Instead of amyloid-like material, mucoepidermoid carcinoma demonstrates scattered mucous cells, whereas the clear cells of renal cell carcinoma usually are glycogen- and lipid-positive. Clear cell odontogenic carcinoma also must be considered but lacks the amyloid-like material and typically exhibits distinctive malignant features such as poorly defined margins, perineural invasion, local recurrence, and lymph node metastasis.

Treatment and Prognosis. Because of the small number of reported cases and the lack of consistent follow-up, the true potential of the tumor has not been defined definitively. Initially, the tumor was thought to exhibit biologic activity similar to ameloblastoma, but more recent reviews reveal a recurrence rate less than 15%. The initial therapy in most reported recurrent cases was curettage, enucleation, or simple excision.

Although Pindborg tumors are expansile, they do not tend to demonstrate intramedullary spread as readily as conventional ameloblastoma. Marginal resection with a rim of normal tissue is the current therapy of choice. Wide resection appears unwarranted in typical examples. Although the number of cases is small, the clear cell variant has exhibited rare perineural invasion and a slightly increased recurrence rate of 22%.[180] In these clear cell cases, definitive resection of the entire mass with tumor-free margins is recommended. In all cases, long-term follow-up is mandatory. Extremely rare carcinomatous transformation with regional lymph node involvement has been documented in elderly patients.[181]

Squamous Odontogenic Tumor

The squamous odontogenic tumor is the most uncommon of all benign odontogenic neoplasms. In the last major review, 32 acceptable cases were discovered in the English-language literature.[183] Although many appear to be hamartomatous, others exhibit clinical activity that supports its classification as a neoplasm.

Although rests of Malassez are mentioned most frequently as the origin for these rare tumors, the histogenesis is unclear.[184–187] Rests of Malassez are highly differentiated epithelial islands that have participated in the formation of the adjacent dental root. No other odontogenic tumor is thought to arise from this quiescent source. Peripheral squamous odontogenic tumors are reported, and rests of Malassez do not reside in gingival soft tissues. In addition, pericoronal examples occur and exhibit no extension to areas inhabited by the rests of Malassez.

The basal cell layer of the surface oral mucosa has been mentioned as a possible origin, but immunohistochemical evaluations reveal differences in keratin proteins between the tumor and surface squamous epithelium. Primitive dental lamina also mentioned as a potential histogenetic source is present in all locations affected by squamous odontogenic tumors. Some investigators have suggested that these tumors may arise from more than one source that includes rests of Malassez, surface squamous epithelium, and rests of dental lamina (glands of Serres). Such variable heritage may help explain the differences in clinical activity.

Clinical Features. The squamous odontogenic tumor occurs over a wide age range, with cases documented from the second to eighth decades.[183] The prevalence peaks in the third decade with a mean age of occurrence of 40 years. A slight male and mandibular predominance is noted. In the maxilla, the anterior regions are affected most frequently, whereas the premolar/molar regions are most common in the mandible.

Classically, squamous odontogenic tumor presents as a semicircular or triangular (apex toward crest) radiolucency of the crestal portion of the alveolar ridge between roots of teeth (Fig. 9–40). Large tumors may extend into the mandibular body or involve the maxillary sinus. Occasional cases are associated with impacted teeth, and rare peripheral examples occur.[183]

Multiple sites are involved in approximately 25% of the cases.[188, 189] One report documents multicentric occurrence in three siblings, supporting a familial pattern in rare instances.[189] In another case, bilateral maxillary lesions were seen in association with a primary intraosseous squamous cell carcinoma of the mandible.[190]

Pathologic Features. Squamous odontogenic tumor presents with numerous variable-sized islands of well-differentiated and uniform squamous epithelium that does not exhibit any significant hyperchromatism, pleomorphism, or mitotic activity (Fig. 9–41A, see p. 627). Although many islands are irregular, a significant percentage exhibit smooth and rounded peripheral outlines. Even though occasional islands exhibit a peripheral, single-cell-thick layer of cuboidal cells, peripheral columnar differentiation and reverse polarization of the islands are absent. Vacuolization and microcyst formation is a constant feature (Fig. 9–41B). The islands are supported by a mature collagenous stroma.

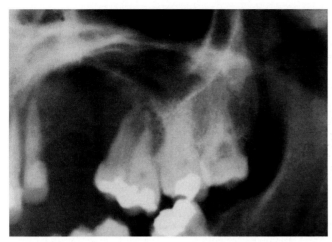

Figure 9–40. Squamous odontogenic tumor. Semicircular radiolucency of the maxilla on the left side. (Courtesy of Dr. Ed McGaha.)

Table 9–3. Primary Intraosseous Odontogenic Carcinomas (PIOC)

Type I	PIOC ex odontogenic cyst
Type II	Malignancies in ameloblastoma
	Malignant ameloblastoma
	Ameloblastic carcinoma
Type III	Clear cell odontogenic carcinoma
Type IV	Primary de novo intraosseous squamous cell carcinoma
Type V	Intraosseous mucoepidermoid carcinoma

origin is unknown, the tumor cells resemble clear-cell rests of primitive dental lamina that frequent the same locations.

Clinical Features. The mean age of occurrence of clear cell odontogenic carcinomas is 53 years with a peak in the fifth decade and only two instances below the age of 40 (14 and 17 years).[196] A marked female predominance is seen. The mandible is affected in 70%; but surprisingly, only 25% of these cases are located in the posterior regions. Similarly, 80% of maxillary tumors present in the anterior areas.

The most common clinical finding is jaw enlargement. Approximately 50% of patients present with mild pain or dull ache of the affected area. Radiographically, the tumors create an ill-defined lucency associated with extensive bone destruction (Fig. 9–42).

Pathologic Features. Two histopathologic patterns are seen. The first presents with large islands of clear epithelial cells with well-defined borders supported by mature cellular fibrous connective tissue. Usually, the tumors demonstrate a biphasic pattern created by a second population of eosinophilic polygonal cells. Frequently, individual islands exhibit a mixture of both cell types (Fig. 9–43, see p. 627). The clear cells reveal hyperchromatic or pyknotic nuclei but lack significant pleomorphism and mitotic activity. Individual tumors may contain predominantly clear cells or exhibit a small number of clear cells intermixed within the eosinophilic polygonal cells. Peripheral infiltrative margins are typical with permeation of the adjacent medullary bone.

The second pattern is less frequent and composed almost entirely of clear cells in which scattered islands demonstrate columnar differentiation and reverse polarization. Justifiably, such differentiation has led some investigators to classify this variant as a clear cell ameloblastic carcinoma. This latter pattern is encountered much less frequently than the biphasic variant that lacks ameloblastic differentiation. Interestingly, histochemical and ultrastructural evaluations of both variants closely approximate that seen in presecretory ameloblasts.

Typically, the clear cells stain positively with PAS and are diastase labile. In other cases, PAS positivity is not remarkable; and ul-

In many cases, the islands demonstrate intraepithelial globular, hyaline, or crystalloid structures. Upon histochemical evaluation, this eosinophilic material is incompatible with amyloid and thought to be prekeratin. In other examples, the islands demonstrate laminated calcified structures present intra-epithelially or in the surrounding connective tissue.

Differential Diagnosis. Occasionally, squamous odontogenic tumor has been misdiagnosed as squamous cell carcinoma or acanthomatous ameloblastoma. The reverse misdiagnoses also are not rare. The bland appearance of the islands, combined with microcyst formation and calcification, allows differentiation from squamous cell carcinoma. Acanthomatous ameloblastoma demonstrates obvious peripheral columnar differentiation with reverse polarization, important features not seen in squamous odontogenic tumors.

The greatest difficulty arises in distinguishing the squamous odontogenic tumor from the desmoplastic variant of ameloblastoma. In this pattern of ameloblastoma, peripheral columnar differentiation often is difficult to demonstrate but is seen with careful evaluation. In these cases, the islands typically are very irregular and exhibit hyperchromatic peripheral cells. This contrasts with the squamous odontogenic tumor that typically reveals numerous islands with smooth and rounded peripheral outlines. When extensive island irregularity is noted, an extensive search for peripheral columnar differentiation is warranted.

Several authors have documented squamous odontogenic tumor-like proliferations within the walls of odontogenic cysts.[191] These foci do not develop into solid tumor, and the associated cysts behave no differently than similar cysts without the tumor-like proliferations. These mural collections do not appear to be precursors of squamous odontogenic tumor and most likely represent a separate reactive process.

Treatment and Prognosis. Local excision and extraction of any involved teeth is the therapy of choice. With appropriate removal, recurrence is not expected. In rare, extensive cases, en bloc resection is necessary to eradicate the tumor. Only two recurrences are documented, and inability to control the tumor has not been reported.[183]

Clear Cell Odontogenic Carcinoma

In addition to the previously mentioned ameloblastic malignancies and carcinomas associated with odontogenic cysts, three additional patterns of primary intraosseous odontogenic carcinoma currently are known to exist (Table 9–3).[192] The most recently delineated form, the clear cell odontogenic carcinoma, was described initially in 1985.[193–195] To date, only 17 cases have been documented, but an associated clinical profile is beginning to emerge.[196] Although the

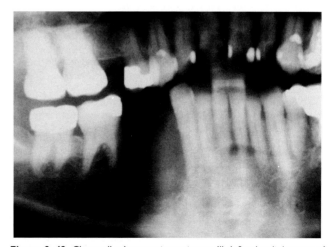

Figure 9–42. Clear cell odontogenic carcinoma. Ill-defined radiolucency of the body of the mandible on the right side. (Courtesy of Dr. Samuel McKenna.)

trastructural examination suggests that the clear cytoplasm is due to sparse organelles rather than enriched glycogen granules. The clear cells are negative with mucicarmine staining. Upon immunoperoxidase evaluation, the tumor reacts strongly to cytokeratin and weakly to epithelial membrane antigen. Variable reactivity to S-100 is noted.

Differential Diagnosis. The clear cell variant of calcifying epithelial odontogenic tumor may contain areas that resemble the clear cell odontogenic carcinoma. On closer evaluation, more typical eosinophilic polyhedral cells intermixed with amyloid-like material and concentric calcifications lead to the appropriate diagnosis.

Intraosseous mucoepidermoid carcinoma also may demonstrate clear cell areas, but these typically are not present in great numbers. In addition, scattered mucous cells in this lesion would distinguish it from clear cell odontogenic carcinoma.

Metastatic clear cell tumors to the jaws are most unusual. Histopathologically, differentiation from clear cell odontogenic carcinoma cannot be made with assurance unless areas with columnar differentiation and reverse polarization are observed. In equivocal cases, it is advisable to rule out a distant primary (especially renal cell carcinoma) before diagnosing a tumor as odontogenic in origin.

Treatment and Prognosis. Following conservative curettage, these tumors tend to recur and frequently become highly invasive, with direct extension far removed from the site of origin. Erosion through bone with widespread soft tissue invasion is common. Regional lymph node and hematogenous dissemination have been documented.[197–199]

With limited follow-up of the 17 reported cases, 4 patients have died of their disease. All patients alive and well 5 years after their initial therapy were treated by surgical resection. The aggressive nature of the tumor is obvious, necessitating wide surgical resection associated with long-term follow-up. If clinical lymphadenopathy is noted, lymph node dissection should be considered because of the propensity for regional lymph node involvement. The response to radiotherapy and chemotherapy have not been evaluated adequately.

Primary de Novo Intraosseous Squamous Cell Carcinoma

Primary de novo intraosseous squamous cell carcinoma arises within the jaws, exhibits no initial connection with the surface oral mucosa, and appears to develop from entrapped odontogenic epithelium, most likely rests of dental lamina. Since squamous cell carcinoma may appear within bone from other sources, the diagnosis is one of exclusion.

Clinical Features. Of the 39 cases currently documented, the patients' ages range from 4 to 76 years with a mean of 51 and a dramatic peak in the seventh decade.[200, 201] A male predominance of 2.3:1 is seen. Common clinical features include pain and swelling of the affected area. In many instances, the nonspecific clinical findings simulate inflammatory dental processes. In one series, 50% of affected patients had prior dental procedures (e.g., extractions, denture adjustments) attempting to resolve the symptoms associated with the neoplasm.[201] In these cases, the delay in diagnosis ranged from a few weeks to 18 months, with an average of 6.9 months.

Over 80% of the cases present in the mandible, with a striking predilection for the posterior regions.[202–204] Maxillary lesions have developed in the anterior portion of the jaw, but the absence of posterior examples may be due to difficulty in differentiating this tumor from antral carcinoma. Radiographically, de novo intraosseous carcinomas exhibit radiolucencies with a wide variation in size and shape. Slowly growing tumors often exhibit well-defined peripheries, whereas rapidly expanding lesions typically demonstrate poorly defined and ragged borders.

Pathologic Features. The histopathologic findings of de novo intraosseous squamous cell carcinoma vary from well-differentiated tumors exhibiting significant keratinization to nonkeratinizing, poorly differentiated carcinomas. In rare cases, spindle cell carcinoma is the predominant pattern. Although alveolar, plexiform, and palisading patterns are seen occasionally, no definitive ameloblastic differentiation (peripheral columnar cells with reverse polarization) is present.

Differential Diagnosis. The differential diagnosis includes acanthomatous ameloblastoma, squamous odontogenic tumor, ameloblastic carcinoma, mucoepidermoid carcinoma, antral carcinoma, squamous cell carcinoma of the surface oral mucosa, and metastatic carcinoma. Since many of the malignant neoplasms in the differential diagnosis may exhibit similar histopathologic features, the diagnosis is one of exclusion.

In an attempt to differentiate the tumor from surface squamous cell carcinoma, no surface ulceration must be present except that due to trauma or tooth extraction. The possibility of origin from another odontogenic cyst or tumor must be ruled out through thorough examination of the surgical specimen for evidence of a cystic component or other areas of differentiation (e.g., ghost cells, ameloblastic differentiation) consistent with another pattern of odontogenic neoplasia. Tumors of the posterior maxilla with antral extension cannot be diagnosed as odontogenic with any degree of certainty.

Squamous odontogenic tumor also may resemble well-differentiated de novo intraosseous carcinoma but lacks the hyperchromatism, pleomorphism, and mitotic index noted within carcinomas. In addition, de novo intraosseous carcinomas typically do not demonstrate central vacuolization and laminated calcifications. Intraosseous mucoepidermoid carcinoma can be ruled out easily by demonstrating negative mucicarmine staining.

The most common sites of origin for metastatic tumors to the jaws are the breast, lung, and kidney; less common sites include the thyroid, colon and rectum, prostate, and stomach.[201] The vast majority of metastatic squamous cell carcinomas to the jaws arise within the lungs. In all cases of suspected primary intraosseous carcinoma, affected patients should receive a thorough evaluation including chest radiographic studies with at least a 6-month follow-up in an attempt to detect any occult primary tumor.

Treatment and Prognosis. Currently, wide surgical resection is the therapy of choice. Although metastasis to regional lymph nodes occurs in 40%, no relationship is seen between nodal involvement and survival time.[200] In spite of this, ipsilateral regional lymph node dissection is recommended if there is clinical evidence of nodal involvement. Radiation therapy and chemotherapy occasionally are utilized following recurrences, but the effectiveness of these modalities is unclear because of the low number of cases and degree of documented follow-up. The prognosis is quite poor, with the 5-year survival rate judged to be between 30% and 40%.[201]

Intraosseous Mucoepidermoid Carcinoma

Less than 1% of mucoepidermoid carcinomas arise within the jaws, and they are classified most appropriately as odontogenic tumors, not as salivary gland neoplasms.[205–208] Mucous cell prosoplasia is a common finding in the epithelial lining of odontogenic cysts. In a review of 638 odontogenic cysts, mucous cells were noted in 42% of dentigerous cysts, 39.6% of apical periodontal cysts, 20% of lateral periodontal cysts, and 3.7% of odontogenic keratocysts.[209] No difference in mucous cell prevalence is seen in a comparison of maxillary and mandibular cysts, thus demonstrating that there is no relationship between the presence of mucous cells and the proximity of the cyst to the antrum or nasal cavity. In addition, 30% to 50% of intraosseous mucoepidermoid carcinomas are associated with impacted teeth, and histopathologic similarities are seen between these carcinomas and the recently described odontogenic cyst termed *glandular odontogenic cyst*. Intraosseous mucoepidermoid carcinomas most likely arise from odontogenic cysts exhibiting mucous cell differentiation or from primitive rests of dental lamina.

Clinical Features. Intraosseous mucoepidermoid carcinoma demonstrates a 2:1 female predominance, with the overwhelming majority arising within the fourth and fifth decades.[206] Some investigators suggest that the age of occurrence may be related to the marked hormonal effect on mucus-producing glands that begins at puberty.

Rare examples occur in patients under the age of 16 years, with a single case documented in the first decade.[210]

The tumor is two to three times more common in the mandible and patients typically present with swelling of the retromolar trigone.[211, 212] Pain also may be present. The number of maxillary lesions may be artificially low, since, to be acceptable, they must be embedded in maxillary bone without any sign of antral extension. The majority of intraosseous mucoepidermoid carcinomas arise in the third molar/ramus region of the mandible and typically present as well-defined radiolucencies that are multilocular in about half of the cases (Fig. 9–44).

Pathologic Features. Intraosseous mucoepidermoid carcinoma is similar to its salivary gland counterpart and may be predominantly cystic or solid. Cystic lesions are lined by squamous epithelium intermixed with scattered mucous-producing cells, often with intraluminal projections and areas of intramural solid tumor. Well-differentiated tumors exhibit a mixture of mucous cells, eosinophilic and polygonal squamous cells, and basaloid intermediate cells (Fig. 9–45, see p. 627).[213] Keratinization and clear cell differentiation are seen rarely. High-grade lesions demonstrate areas of solid tumor, exhibiting a mixture of squamous and intermediate cells with significant pleomorphism and mitotic activity. Although they may be infrequent, scattered mucous cells can be found.

Differential Diagnosis. Strict diagnostic criteria are required to eliminate the possibility of lesional origin outside the jaw bones. The involved jaw should exhibit intact cortical plates; and there should be radiographic evidence of bone destruction. Histopathologic confirmation of the tumor, positive mucin staining of lesional cells, absence of a histopathologically similar primary lesion of salivary glands or elsewhere, and exclusion of other forms of odontogenic tumors are mandatory prior to making this diagnosis. Maxillary lesions should be encased within the alveolar bone without antral extension. Since cortical bone may be destroyed by many primary intraosseous tumors, the requirement of an intact cortical plate can be waived if there is no overlying soft tissue tumefaction that would indicate a primary tumor arising in soft tissue.

A number of odontogenic tumors demonstrate features noted within mucoepidermoid carcinoma. Although occasionally growing in histopathologically similar patterns, squamous odontogenic tumor, clear cell odontogenic carcinoma, clear cell variant of calcifying epithelial odontogenic tumor, and primary intraosseous squamous cell carcinoma do not exhibit mucous cell differentiation. As mentioned previously, a large number of benign odontogenic cysts exhibit scattered mucous cells. In these cases, a diagnosis of mucoepidermoid carcinoma is inappropriate without evidence of an invasive, solid tumor–like growth or a significant intraluminal component.

Treatment and Prognosis. The treatment of choice is en bloc resection, with segmental mandibulectomy reserved for extensive lesions.[207] Neck dissection is indicated in cases with palpable cervical lymph nodes, and postoperative radiation is recommended for high-grade tumors.[206] Some investigators have suggested increased clinical aggressiveness associated with tumors that have perforated the cortical plate.[207] The histopathologic grading of intraosseous mucoepidermoid carcinoma does not appear to affect the prognosis.[207]

The overall recurrence rate appears to be 25%. Conservative therapy increases this percentage to 40%, while radical excision lowers the rate to 13%. Spread to regional lymph nodes occurs in 10% of patients, and only one distant metastasis to the clavicle has been documented.[214] Rare tumor-related deaths occur, and these have been associated with uncontrolled local recurrence or extension into the base of the brain.[213, 215]

Tumors of Odontogenic Epithelium With Odontogenic Ectomesenchyme With or Without Dental Hard Tissue Formation

Ameloblastic Fibroma

Even though it constitutes only about 2% of odontogenic tumors, the ameloblastic fibroma is significant because it can be mistaken for more aggressive lesions such as ameloblastoma. Both the mesenchymal and the epithelial components of this uncommon benign odontogenic lesion are thought to participate in the neoplastic process.[216]

Clinical Features. The ameloblastic fibroma is usually identified in younger individuals, with most series of cases reporting a mean age of 15 to 22 years; occasionally these tumors may be seen in middle-aged individuals, however. Approximately 70% to 80% of all cases are found in the posterior mandible, and a slight male predilection is usually reported.[216] Small lesions are typically asymptomatic, whereas larger ones may produce painless swelling. The tumor is characteristically unilocular when small, but as it enlarges, it tends to become multilocular (Fig. 9–46). The radiographic margins are either sharply demarcated or sclerotic, and the lesion is frequently associated with an impacted tooth.[216, 217]

Pathologic Features. The lesion is composed of a mixture of odontogenic epithelial and ectomesenchymal elements, both of which are neoplastic. The mesenchymal portion resembles dental papilla, a tissue characterized by plump, uniformly spaced fibroblastic cells set against a background of delicate collagen fibers and

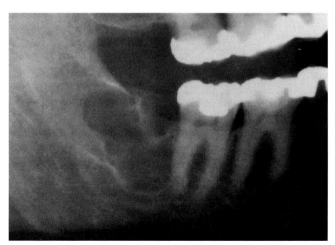

Figure 9–44. Intraosseous mucoepidermoid carcinoma. Multilocular radiolucency of the mandible immediately posterior to the permanent second molar. (Courtesy of Dr. Joseph Finelli.)

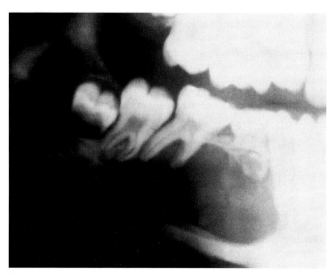

Figure 9–46. Ameloblastic fibroma. Large radiolucency involving the right posterior mandible. (Courtesy of Dr. Robert Owens.)

ground substance. This tissue is admixed with strands and islands of odontogenic epithelium, which resembles embryonic dental lamina (Fig. 9–47, see p. 628). Sometimes the odontogenic epithelial islands are large enough to vaguely resemble follicular ameloblastoma. The connective tissue component may also display varying degrees of hyalinization.

Differential Diagnosis. This lesion is most commonly mistaken for ameloblastoma because the characteristic background setting of the epithelial component is not taken into consideration by the pathologist. Ameloblastoma does not have a connective tissue background that resembles dental papilla, and the epithelial islands usually are larger and more complex than those of the ameloblastic fibroma. With increasing cellularity, mitotic activity, and atypia of the mesenchymal component, the possibility of ameloblastic fibrosarcoma must be addressed (see later discussion).

Treatment and Prognosis. The recommended treatment could range from aggressive curettage for a relatively small, unilocular lesion to wide local excision for a large, multilocular process. Simple curettage or enucleation may be inadequate for a significant percentage of these lesions. The prognosis is generally considered to be good, with a recurrence rate approximating 20% for those cases reported in the literature.[218]

Ameloblastic fibrosarcoma is a rare malignancy, with slightly more than 50 cases having been reported.[219] About one half of the cases appear to originate from recurrences of ameloblastic fibroma, and for this reason some authors have recommended that ameloblastic fibromas be treated more aggressively than has been advocated in the past.[219] The ameloblastic fibrosarcoma has been reported to occur somewhat more frequently in males than females, and they develop in an older age group compared with the ameloblastic fibroma, with a mean patient age of 27.5 years.[219] Approximately 80% affect the mandible, and clinical findings include pain and swelling. Radiographically, an expansile radiolucency with ragged margins is seen. Microscopically, the epithelial component appears essentially benign, while the mesenchymal component exhibits hypercellularity, nuclear hyperchromatism, mitotic activity, pleomorphism, and other features of malignancy (Fig. 9–48, see p. 628). With successive episodes of recurrence, the epithelial component has been reported to diminish in some cases. Treatment consists of radical surgical excision; however, an accurate prognosis is almost impossible to calculate owing to the rarity of this tumor. Nevertheless, several patients have died from either uncontrolled local disease or, less commonly, metastatic disease.[220]

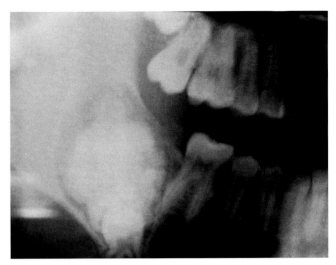

Figure 9–49. Ameloblastic fibro-odontoma. Well-demarcated radiolucency with prominent central radiopacity. This represents a late-stage lesion that consists mostly of complex odontoma with an area of ameloblastic fibroma in the superior portion. Note impacted molar tooth. (Courtesy of Dr. Bruce Wetmore.)

croscopically from ameloblastic fibroma, whereas the hard tissue component typically appears as a complex odontoma (Fig. 9–50, see p. 628). These two components may be present in varying proportions, depending on the particular lesion. As with several other odontogenic lesions, benign melanocytic colonization of the epithelial component has been reported in the ameloblastic fibro-odontoma.[223]

Differential Diagnosis. A developing odontoma may be mistaken for an ameloblastic fibro-odontoma, although a well-formed ameloblastic fibroma-like component is usually minimal or absent in the developing odontoma. The presence of odontogenic epithelium may cause the lesion to be confused with ameloblastoma or odontoameloblastoma, but the characteristic dental papilla-like setting for the epithelial component should argue against the diagnosis of ameloblastoma.

Treatment and Prognosis. The recommended treatment is conservative curettage, and the prognosis is considered to be excellent. Recurrence following conservative therapy is rarely seen.

Ameloblastic Fibro-odontoma

Ameloblastic fibro-odontoma is an uncommon odontogenic tumor that has histopathologic features of ameloblastic fibroma admixed with an odontoma.[221, 222] Although it was described as a distinct entity in the mid-1960s, some controversy persists as to whether the ameloblastic fibro-odontoma represents a distinct lesion or is merely a stage in the development of an odontoma. A significant proportion of ameloblastic fibro-odontomas seem to grow to a much larger size in comparison to the odontoma, suggesting that at least some of these tumors represent a separate and distinct lesion from the odontoma.

Clinical Features. This lesion is diagnosed during childhood in most instances. Slightly more than half of the cases are observed in the mandible. Unless there is failure of tooth eruption or a particularly large lesion causes swelling, the tumor is asymptomatic and may be detected on routine dental radiographic survey. A well-circumscribed unilocular radiolucency is typically seen, and the center of the lesion usually shows varying degrees of radiopacity, depending on the maturity of the odontogenic hard tissue structures (Fig. 9–49). Less commonly, the process may appear multilocular. The lesion often overlies an impacted tooth.

Pathologic Features. The ameloblastic fibro-odontoma is composed of an odontogenic soft tissue portion and an odontogenic hard tissue portion. The soft tissue portion is indistinguishable mi-

Odontoameloblastoma

Odontoameloblastoma is a very rare odontogenic tumor that represents an ameloblastoma arising in conjunction with an odontoma.[224]

Clinical Features. The few reported cases have occurred most often in the mandible of younger individuals, with an average age of approximately 12 years.[225] Clinical signs and symptoms include pain, delayed tooth eruption, and swelling. Radiographs show a unilocular or multilocular radiolucency with a variable amount of radiopaque material contained within the lesion.

Pathologic Features. Infiltrative ameloblastic epithelium is seen in conjunction with a histopathologically typical compound or complex odontoma.

Differential Diagnosis. A developing odontoma may have a fair amount of odontogenic epithelium associated with it. However, this is in a normal relation to the other developing dental tissues and shows no invasive properties. Ameloblastic fibro-odontoma could also be considered in the differential diagnosis, but the characteristic dental papilla-like stroma in which the ameloblastic epithelium resides should serve as a significant clue to the correct diagnosis.

Treatment and Prognosis. It is generally recommended that the lesion be treated like an ameloblastoma. Even though very few cases have been reported, the prognosis is thought to be similar to that of ameloblastoma.[225] Recurrences have been reported after simple curettage.

Adenomatoid Odontogenic Tumor

Adenomatoid odontogenic tumor is an uncommon benign odontogenic lesion, representing only 3% to 7% of all odontogenic tumors. The interesting and unique microscopic features have created a certain degree of controversy as to how to classify it. Older classification schemes have identified the adenomatoid odontogenic tumor as a lesion of odontogenic epithelial origin, and the term "adenoameloblastoma" was previously applied. Current evidence suggests that there may be dentin formed in some of these lesions. In the WHO classification of odontogenic tumors, the adenomatoid odontogenic tumor is placed in the category of "Tumors of odontogenic epithelium with odontogenic ectomesenchyme,"[226] and this is the classification used in this text.

Clinical Features. The adenomatoid odontogenic tumor usually is detected in younger patients,[227, 228] with a mean age of approximately 18 years being reported in most series. As many as 75% of these patients are under 20 years of age. A 2:1 female:male ratio is typically noted, and a 2:1 maxilla:mandible predilection is seen. About 75% of these lesions develop in the anterior jaws, and 75% are associated with an impacted tooth. Extraosseous tumors represent less than 3% of reported cases.[229, 230] Most adenomatoid odontogenic tumors are less than 3 cm in diameter, although occasionally much larger lesions are reported. Other than swelling, these tumors are characteristically asymptomatic. Radiographically the adenomatoid odontogenic tumor presents as a well-circumscribed, unilocular radiolucency which may contain radiopaque flecks (Fig. 9–51).[229] Separation of adjacent tooth roots or displacement of adjacent teeth occurs frequently. When associated with an impacted tooth, the lesion often surrounds the crown and includes a portion of the root of the affected tooth.[227, 231]

Pathologic Features. Grossly, the adenomatoid odontogenic tumor is encapsulated and, upon sectioning, may appear solid or show focal cystic areas. Histopathologic examination reveals a biphasic proliferation of odontogenic epithelial cells contained within a fibrous capsule (Fig. 9–52, see p. 629). The tumor cells form interlacing cords that blend into swirling spindle-cell nests and sheets. In these latter areas, scattered collections of columnar or cuboidal cells form characteristic duct-like structures of varying sizes, although the presence of these duct-like structures is not necessary for the diagnosis (Fig. 9–53, see p. 629). Mitoses are uncommon. Foci of basophilic, dystrophic-appearing calcified material may also be seen scattered throughout the tumor parenchyma, although this finding is variable. Globules of eosinophilic material that stains as amyloid can be demonstrated within the lumina of the duct-like structures of some lesions.

Differential Diagnosis. The microscopic features of this lesion are rather distinctive and usually do not present a diagnostic difficulty. The presence of the duct-like structures might suggest a lesion of salivary epithelial origin, an extremely rare event within the jaws. Adenomatoid odontogenic tumor may rarely be mistaken for an ameloblastoma by a pathologist unfamiliar with this lesion. Ameloblastoma, in contrast to adenomatoid odontogenic tumor, is not usually encapsulated. Furthermore, ameloblastoma shows columnar cells at the periphery of the tumor islands, rather than forming duct-like structures within the tumor.

Treatment and Prognosis. Enucleation with curettage is the treatment of choice, and the prognosis is considered to be excellent.[232] Recurrence is very rare. Of the approximately 500 reported cases of adenomatoid odontogenic tumor, only 1 acceptable case of recurrence has been documented.[229]

Calcifying Odontogenic Cyst

Calcifying odontogenic cyst was initially described by Gorlin et al. in 1962[233] as a possible oral analogue to the calcifying epithelioma of Malherbe (pilomatrixoma) of the skin, owing to the presence of ghost cell keratinization in both lesions. Although the condition is often described as being cystic (over 85% of the cases), a significant percentage of calcifying odontogenic cysts grow as more solid, seemingly neoplastic proliferations, and the term *dentinogenic ghost cell tumor* has been used to describe these lesions. For this reason, the calcifying odontogenic cyst is discussed in this section rather than with the odontogenic cysts.

Clinical Features. Most series of cases dealing with this lesion report no sex predilection, and an equal distribution between maxilla and mandible is typically seen.[234, 235] The calcifying odontogenic cyst may occur at any age, with a peak occurrence in the second and third decades (mean age, 33 years). The majority (65%) are found in the incisor/canine region. From 15% to 21% of these lesions have been reported peripherally within the gingival soft tissues, presenting as a sessile or pedunculated mass.[236, 237] Radiographs usually show a well-defined, unilocular radiolucency, but 10% to 25% of the cases are multilocular (Fig. 9–54A). Scattered radiopacities may be present within the lesion in one third to one half of cases (Fig. 9–54B).[238] Approximately one third of calcifying odontogenic cysts are associated with an impacted tooth, and resorption of adjacent tooth roots may be seen in about 50% of cases. The majority range between 2 and 4 cm in diameter, but lesions occasionally grow as large as 12 cm in greatest dimension.

Pathologic Features. In most instances, the calcifying odontogenic cyst is composed of a fibrous capsule that is lined by a proliferation of odontogenic epithelial cells (Fig. 9–55, see p. 630). These cells are loosely arranged and show a peripheral basal cell layer that has a cuboidal or columnar appearance, microscopic features similar to ameloblastoma. Unlike ameloblastoma, in the suprabasilar areas, variable numbers of the lesional epithelial cells undergo a process called *ghost cell change*. The involved cell becomes pale and eosinophilic, having a swollen cytoplasm with loss of the nucleus. A faint nuclear membrane outline can usually be discerned (Fig. 9–55*inset*). Traditionally this process has been described as keratinization, but some investigators have recently suggested that this process may represent coagulation necrosis.[235, 239] The ghost cell component frequently undergoes dystrophic calcification (Fig. 9–56, see p. 630), and an eosinophilic calcified matrix thought to represent dysplastic dentin may occasionally be found adjacent to the epithelial component.

At least two histopathologic classifications have been delineated for the calcifying odontogenic cyst. In one, four histopathologic subtypes were described,[240] whereas a more recent report subdivided the microscopic features into seven groups.[235] From a practical standpoint, it is important to understand that a spectrum of histopathologic patterns exists for this lesion, analogous to the histopathologic variations of ameloblastoma. As with ameloblastoma, there appears to be no evidence that significant differences in biologic behavior are associated with the various histopathologic sub-

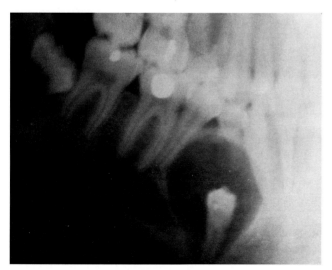

Figure 9–51. Adenomatoid odontogenic tumor. Well-demarcated unilocular radiolucency with fine radiopaque flecks, associated with the crown of an impacted right mandibular first premolar. (Courtesy of Dr. Tony Traynham.)

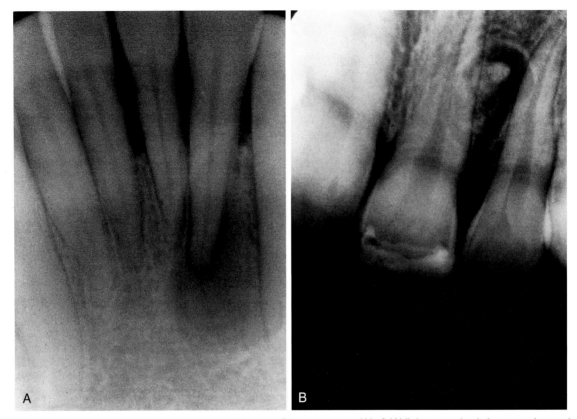

Figure 9–54. Calcifying odontogenic cyst. *A,* Well-demarcated radiolucency of the anterior mandible. *B,* Well-demarcated radiolucency with central radiopaque areas of the anterior maxilla.

types. Lesions with a cystic component represent 85% of the cases, while a solid pattern reminiscent of a neoplastic process is seen in 15%.[235] A summary of the basic features is presented below.

Cystic, Nonproliferative. In this predominantly cystic lesion, the epithelial lining may only be a few cells thick. Sparse dentinoid may be present, but no other hard tissues are seen. Such lesions constitute about 45% of all cystic calcifying odontogenic cysts.

Cystic, Proliferative/Ameloblastomatous. A prominent central cystic component is usually associated with various satellite cysts in the wall. Odontogenic epithelial proliferations that superficially resemble ameloblastoma extend into the lumen as well as the connective tissue wall of the lesion.

Odontoma-associated. Odontoma-like tissues are seen in the wall of the lesion.[241, 242]

Epithelial Odontogenic Ghost Cell Tumor. This form has a growth pattern that is most consistent with a neoplasm, characterized by ameloblastoma-like strands and islands of odontogenic epithelium that infiltrate the connective tissue. Varying amounts of an eosinophilic calcified material ("dentinoid") are typically present, thus this lesion has been termed *dentinogenic ghost cell tumor.*

Two cases of ameloblastoma arising in conjunction with a calcifying odontogenic cyst have been reported as well.[235] These lesions displayed prominent areas that showed invasion of the adjacent normal tissue by odontogenic epithelium that was characteristic of ameloblastoma. This appears to be a rare occurrence.

Differential Diagnosis. If the ghost cells are overlooked, this lesion could be confused with ameloblastoma. Interestingly, marked similarities exist between this lesion and the pituitary craniopharyngioma.[243, 244] Usually, distinguishing between these two lesions is not difficult because of the location of the craniopharyngioma intracranially or in a suprasellar location.[245] Fourteen cases of ectopic craniopharyngioma have been reported,[246] and these have typically shown a growth pattern consistent with origin in the subsellar region rather than in the maxilla. Ghost cells may also be seen in amelo-

blastic fibro-odontomas and odontomas, although in these lesions the ghost cells are not a prominent component.

Treatment and Prognosis. Enucleation and curettage are usually recommended as treatment, and the prognosis is considered to be good. Recurrences after rather conservative therapy appear to be uncommon. Rare examples of malignant transformation have been reported.[247, 248] The peripheral variant seems to have a prognosis similar to that of peripheral ameloblastoma, in that conservative surgical excision is typically curative.

Odontoma

Odontomas are the most frequently occurring odontogenic tumor, with a prevalence exceeding that of all other odontogenic tumors combined. This lesion is probably not a true neoplasm, but rather an odontogenic hamartoma. Odontomas generally present centrally within the jaws in either of two forms: *compound,* composed of multiple small tooth-like structures, or *complex,* consisting of irregular masses of dentin and enamel with no anatomic resemblance to a tooth. Rarely, peripheral odontomas have been reported in the gingival soft tissues.[249]

Clinical Features. Most odontomas are detected during childhood and adolescence.[250, 251] They are often associated with an unerupted tooth and usually are asymptomatic otherwise. Most are found when routine dental radiographs are obtained or when radiographs are taken to determine the reason for failure of a tooth to erupt. Odontomas are slightly more common in the maxilla compared with the mandible. Although both forms of odontoma occur with approximately equal frequency, compound odontomas are seen predominantly in the anterior maxilla, whereas complex odontomas usually present in the posterior portion of either the maxilla or mandible.[250] Radiographically, the compound odontoma presents as a collection of what appear to be small, malformed teeth contained within a unilocular, narrow radiolucent border (Fig. 9–57A). The

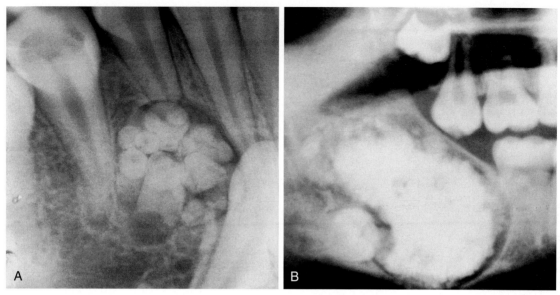

Figure 9–57. *A,* Compound odontoma. Well-demarcated unilocular radiolucency that contains several radiopaque structures resembling small malformed teeth. (Courtesy of Dr. Brent Bernard.) *B,* Complex odontoma. Well-demarcated unilocular radiolucency with central radiopacity involving the posterior mandible. Note impacted tooth at the inferior border of the lesion. (Courtesy of Dr. D.C. Wetmore.)

complex odontoma is also a unilocular lesion, but the central radiopaque component appears as an amorphous mass. This central area may have the density of tooth structure if the calcification process is well under way (Fig. 9–57*B*). A developing odontoma may simply appear as a well-circumscribed radiolucency if very little calcified product has been deposited. Many of these lesions overlie an impacted tooth. The majority of odontomas do not exceed the size of a tooth; however, occasionally these lesions may grow to 6 cm or more in diameter, resulting in jaw expansion.

Pathologic Features. The compound odontoma shows the formation of multiple small, malformed teeth (Fig. 9–58, see p. 630). The complex odontoma shows an admixture of dentin, enamel matrix, cementum, odontogenic epithelium, and dental papilla (Fig. 9–59, see p. 631). In more developed complex odontomas, the dentin component predominates. Foci of ghost cells may be found in as many as 20% of complex odontomas. Sometimes a dentigerous cyst may form from the dental follicle of an odontoma.

Differential Diagnosis. A developing odontoma can easily be mistaken for ameloblastoma or odontoameloblastoma because of the presence of a significant amount of odontogenic epithelium. The distinguishing feature is that this epithelium is in a normal relation to the developing odontogenic tissues, and no invasive component is seen.

Treatment and Prognosis. Treatment consists of conservative enucleation, and the prognosis is excellent. For large complex odontomas of the posterior mandible, careful consideration should be given to the surgical approach because of the thinning of the buccal or lingual plates of bone with resultant susceptibility to fracture.[252]

Tumors of Odontogenic Ectomesenchyme With or Without Included Odontogenic Epithelium

Central Odontogenic Fibroma

This relatively rare benign odontogenic neoplasm, with less than 50 reported cases, was separated into two variants, the so-called simple type and the WHO type, by Gardner in 1980.[253] In 1991, Handlers et al.[253] suggested that the distinction between the two lesions was often arbitrary and unclear, and they preferred one name, *central odontogenic fibroma,* since the behavior of the two variants appears

to be similar.[254] The 1992 WHO classification[255] describes the lesion as a proliferation of odontogenic ectomesenchyme, with or without included odontogenic epithelium, which is consistent with the definition by Handlers et al.

Clinical Features. The central odontogenic fibroma usually presents in an adult patient, with most series reporting a mean age of approximately 40 years (range, 9–80 years).[254] For reasons that are unknown, a female predilection is seen, with women outnumbering men by ratios ranging from 2:1 to 7:1, depending on the series reported.[254] Approximately 60% of reported cases have arisen in the maxilla. The majority of cases located in the maxilla affect the anterior segments of the jaw, whereas mandibular lesions tend to involve the posterior segments. The most common presenting clinical sign is swelling, but depression of the palatal mucosa has also been noted in some patients, as well as tooth mobility. Smaller odontogenic fibromas are usually asymptomatic. Radiographically, early lesions appear as well-defined unilocular radiolucencies (Fig. 9–60), but as the lesion enlarges it may become multilocular. In approximately 12% of cases, radiopaque flecks may be seen in the lesion.[256] Usually the central odontogenic fibroma arises between the roots of teeth, suggesting a periodontal ligament origin, and divergence of roots may be noted. Nearly one third of reported cases have involved the crown of an impacted tooth, although some of these simply may have been hyperplastic dental follicles. Resorption of adjacent tooth roots is also frequently observed.

Pathologic Features. A range of histopathologic patterns has been described, with the simple type of central odontogenic fibroma exhibiting evenly spaced, plump fibroblasts that are set against a background of delicate collagen fibers and variable amounts of ground substance (Fig. 9–61, see p. 631). Small nests of odontogenic epithelium may be present in minimal quantities or may be completely absent (Fig. 9–61*inset*). Rare foci of dystrophic calcification may be present. The WHO type, on the other hand, shows a cellular fibrous connective tissue with few to many islands of odontogenic epithelium (Fig. 9–62, see p. 632). Areas of myxoid change and hyalinization may be seen. The epithelium lacks palisading, reverse polarization, or stellate reticulum-like areas. Calcified material, sometimes referred to as dysplastic dentin, may be present. Infrequently, a giant cell granuloma-like component may accompany this lesion.[257, 258]

Differential Diagnosis. Those lesions with relatively sparse odontogenic epithelium may be mistaken for desmoplastic fibroma, a central fibromatosis that usually shows denser collagen production

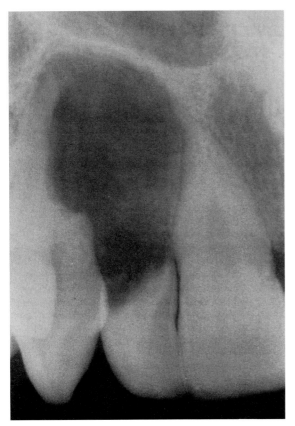

Figure 9–60. Central odontogenic fibroma. Radiolucency of the anterior maxilla showing significant root resorption of the lateral incisor and canine tooth. (Courtesy of Dr. Mark Bowden.)

and a more infiltrative growth pattern compared with central odontogenic fibroma. Furthermore, the desmoplastic fibroma shows a more fascicular pattern compared with central odontogenic fibroma. If a prominent amount of ground substance is produced, then the possibility of odontogenic myxoma should be entertained; however, focal myxoid zones in an otherwise fibrous lesion would be consistent with central odontogenic fibroma. With increasing amounts of the odontogenic epithelial component, one could mistake this lesion for ameloblastoma, although the classic reverse polarization of the nuclei associated with ameloblastoma is not seen. The calcifying epithelial odontogenic tumor might also enter the differential diagnosis if the lesion has abundant epithelium. Negative staining for amyloid, however, would tend to rule out the possibility of calcifying epithelial odontogenic tumor. An ameloblastic fibroma might be considered, but the mesenchymal component of the central odontogenic fibroma is generally more fibrous than would be expected for ameloblastic fibroma. Furthermore, the epithelial islands of the central odontogenic fibroma tend to form nests rather than the longer, ribbon-like strands seen in ameloblastic fibroma.

Treatment and Prognosis. Curettage generally is accepted as the treatment of choice, and the prognosis is good.[254] Approximately 14% of cases reported have recurred, but this figure may be high due to reporting bias.

Peripheral Odontogenic Fibroma

This uncommon lesion of the gingival soft tissues is histologically similar to the WHO type of odontogenic fibroma that occurs centrally within the jaws. Otherwise, there does not appear to be any connection between the two lesions. Previous reports of odontogenic gingival epithelial hamartoma and peripheral fibro-ameloblastic dentinoma probably represent examples of peripheral odontogenic fibroma.

Clinical Features. The peripheral odontogenic fibroma presents as a firm, slow-growing, sessile gingival mass and is most frequently encountered on the mandibular facial gingiva. Most of these lesions are less than 2 cm in diameter at the time of treatment, and a wide age range of affected patients has been reported.[259-262] Radiographically, no involvement of the underlying bone should be seen, although radiopaque flecks within the lesion may be detected in some cases.

Pathologic Features. The lesional tissue consists of a benign proliferation of cellular fibrous connective tissue interspersed with more myxoid fibrous connective tissue. Islands or strands of odontogenic epithelium are scattered throughout the connective tissue, particularly in the myxoid zones, but the amount of epithelium varies considerably from one lesion to the next. One may occasionally encounter dysplastic dentin, ovoid cementum-like calcifications, or spicules of osteoid within the lesional tissue.

Differential Diagnosis. Peripheral ossifying fibroma may also be seen on the gingiva, but this lesion does not have a significant amount of odontogenic epithelium associated with its fibroblastic proliferation. Peripheral ameloblastoma could be confused with peripheral odontogenic fibromas that have a significant amount of epithelium, although the reverse polarization of nuclei seen with ameloblastoma would be absent in the peripheral odontogenic fibroma.

Treatment and Prognosis. Conservative surgical excision is typically curative. The prognosis is considered to be excellent, and these lesions exhibit little tendency for recurrence.

Granular Cell Odontogenic Tumor (Granular Cell Odontogenic Fibroma)

Although the granular cell odontogenic tumor was initially reported as *granular cell ameloblastic fibroma*,[263, 264] the microscopic features of this rare lesion probably resemble those of a central odontogenic fibroma more than any other process. To date, only 14 examples have been reported.

Clinical Features. At the time of initial diagnosis, most affected patients are middle-aged (over 40 years of age) or older adults.[265, 266] The maxillary or mandibular posterior segments are most commonly involved. Most lesions are asymptomatic, but painless expansion of the affected area has been noted in some instances. Radiographs typically show a well-demarcated radiolucency (Fig. 9–63). Small intralesional calcifications have been described in some cases.

Pathologic Features. The tumor consists primarily of sheets of large cells with abundant, faintly eosinophilic granular cytoplasm

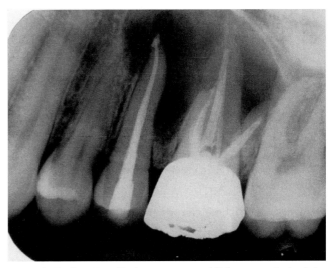

Figure 9–63. Granular cell odontogenic tumor. Well-circumscribed radiolucency in the left maxilla. (Courtesy of Dr. Steve Ferry.)

(Fig. 9–64, see p. 632), similar to the cells found in the granular cell tumor of the soft tissues. Interspersed strands of bland odontogenic epithelium showing no peripheral nuclear palisading are seen (Fig. 9–64*inset*). Sometimes calcified structures resembling cementum or foci of dystrophic calcification are detected. Immunohistochemical studies show that the granular cells in the granular cell odontogenic tumor are S-100–negative, in contrast to the positive S-100 reaction found in the granular cell tumor of the soft tissues.[267]

Differential Diagnosis. This lesion is so distinctive that the differential diagnosis would be quite limited, assuming the characteristic features were appropriately identified. The only other lesion with granular cells that would present in an intraosseous location would be the granular cell ameloblastoma, and that process is predominantly epithelial. In contrast, the granular cells of the granular cell odontogenic tumor represent the mesenchymal component of the lesion.

Treatment and Prognosis. Curettage seems to be curative, and the prognosis is excellent. Recurrence would not be anticipated with conservative therapy.

Odontogenic Myxoma

This benign neoplasm is assumed to be of odontogenic origin because it apparently affects only the jaw bones as a central lesion. No other bone in the body develops a central myxoma.

Clinical Features. Although the odontogenic myxoma may be diagnosed in patients from childhood through old age, most cases are detected in young adults (third decade of life).[268] Mandibular lesions are seen slightly more frequently than maxillary lesions. There is no apparent sex predilection. Radiographically, this tumor appears unilocular when small, and such lesions are typically found when routine dental radiographs are obtained. Although most of these tumors grow at a relatively slow pace, some may exhibit rapid growth. As the myxoma grows, a multilocular pattern develops (Fig. 9–65), and this is usually accompanied by painless swelling.[269] The larger lesions characteristically have a "soap-bubble" or "cob-web" radiographic appearance, similar to ameloblastoma.

Pathologic Features. On gross examination, the myxoma characteristically has a loose, gelatinous texture. Histologically, these lesions bear a striking resemblance to the mesenchymal portion of a developing tooth. Microscopic examination shows spindle-shaped or stellate-shaped fibroblastic cells set in a myxoid background with delicate, haphazardly arranged collagen fibers (Fig. 9–66, see p. 632).[270, 271] The lesional proliferation tends to infiltrate the adjacent bony trabeculae. Not infrequently, rests of odontogenic epithelium are seen within the tumor. A few myxomas may show a

little more collagen production in areas, and the term *fibro-myxoma* or *myxofibroma* has been used for this pattern.

Immunohistochemical studies of the odontogenic myxoma have generally shown the lesional cells to react with antibodies to vimentin and muscle-specific actin.[272] Conflicting descriptions of S-100 and glial fibrillary acidic protein positivity have been reported.

Differential Diagnosis. The structure that is most commonly mistaken histopathologically for odontogenic myxoma is the developing dental papilla, the immature mesenchymal tissue that becomes the dental pulp of a fully formed tooth.[273, 274] Dental papilla is composed of plump, stellate, and fusiform fibroblastic cells set in a myxoid matrix with delicate collagen fibers. This tissue, however, is always lined by a rim of odontoblasts along one margin. This feature, together with the radiographic appearance, should distinguish dental papilla from odontogenic myxoma. A dental follicle can also, at times, present with a myxoid appearance histopathologically. This tissue will be lined along one margin by reduced enamel epithelium, which again should differentiate this normal anatomic structure from the odontogenic neoplasm. The central myxoid neurofibroma also often enters into the differential diagnosis. Features of the myxoid neurofibroma include a prominent mast cell population, a positive S-100 immunohistochemical reaction, and zones that show parallel streaming with organization of the collagen and lesional cells into broad fascicles. Other central lesions that might show a significant myxoid component include chondromyxoid fibroma and myxoid chondrosarcoma. Both of these should show at least focal evidence of chondroid differentiation and, in the latter case, cellular atypia. The myxoid variant of desmoid fibromatosis would be distinguished from odontogenic myxoma by the presence of focal zones showing dense collagen bundles.

Treatment and Prognosis. For small lesions, aggressive curettage may be adequate. Large lesions may require en bloc or segmental resection, depending on the size and site. The prognosis is essentially good because these tumors do not metastasize. With conservative excision, recurrence can be anticipated for as much as one fourth of these tumors,[270] and this is most likely related to incomplete excision of the original lesion. Malignant transformation to myxosarcoma has been reported but appears to be a rare event.[275]

▌ REFERENCES

Introduction

1. Ten Cate AR: *Oral Histology: Development, Structure, and Function,* 4th ed. St. Louis: Mosby, 1994:58–80.
2. Bhaskar SN: *Orban's Oral Histology and Embryology,* 11th ed. St. Louis: Mosby–Year Book, 1991:28–48.
3. Kramer IRH, Pindborg JJ, Shear M: *Histological Typing of Odontogenic Tumours,* 2nd ed. New York: Springer-Verlag, 1992.
4. Waldron CA: Odontogenic cysts and tumors. In: Neville BW, Damm DD, Allen CM, Bouquot JE (eds): *Oral & Maxillofacial Pathology.* Philadelphia: WB Saunders, 1995:493–540.

Dentigerous Cyst

5. Ten Cate AR: *Oral Histology: Development, Structure, and Function,* 4th ed. St. Louis: Mosby, 1994:58–80.
6. Shear M: *Cysts of the Oral Regions,* 3rd ed. Boston: Wright, 1992:75–98.
7. Kreidler JF, Raubenheimer EJ, van Heerden WFP: A retrospective analysis of 367 cystic lesions of the jaw: The Ulm experience. *J Craniomaxillofac Surg* 1993;21:339–341.
8. Shear M: Developmental odontogenic cysts. An update. *J Oral Pathol Med* 1994;23:1–11.
9. Nakamura T, Ishida J, Nakano Y, et al.: A study of cysts in the oral region. Cysts of the jaws. *J Nihon Univ Sch Dent* 1995;37:33–40.
10. Waldron CA: Odontogenic cysts and tumors. In: Neville BW, Damm DD, Allen CM, Bouquot JE (eds): *Oral & Maxillofacial Pathology.* Philadelphia: WB Saunders, 1995:493–496.

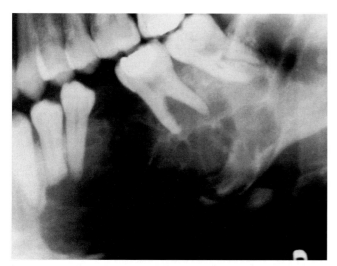

Figure 9–65. Odontogenic myxoma. Multilocular expansile radiolucency of the posterior mandible. (Courtesy of Dr. T.R. Kerley.)

11. Lustmann L, Bodner L: Dentigerous cysts associated with supernumerary teeth. *Int J Oral Maxillofac Surg* 1988;17:100–102.

12. Kusukawa J, Irie K, Morimatsu M, et al: Dentigerous cyst associated with a deciduous tooth: A case report. *Oral Surg Oral Med Oral Pathol* 1992;73:415–418.

13. Boyczuk MP, Berger JR: Identifying a deciduous dentigerous cyst. *JADA* 1995;126:643–644.

14. Kim J, Ellis GL: Dental follicular tissue: Misinterpretation as odontogenic tumors. *J Oral Maxillofac Surg* 1993;51:762–767.

15. Daley TD, Wysocki GP: The small dentigerous cyst: A diagnostic dilemma. *Oral Surg Oral Med Oral Pathol Oral Radiol Endod* 1995;79:77–81.

16. Gorlin RJ: Potentialities of oral epithelium manifest by mandibular dentigerous cysts. *Oral Surg Oral Med Oral Pathol* 1957;10:271–284.

17. Browand BC, Waldron CA: Central mucoepidermoid tumors of the jaws. *Oral Surg Oral Med Oral Pathol* 1975;40:631–643.

18. Waldron CA, Koh ML: Central mucoepidermoid carcinoma of the jaws: Report of four cases with analysis of the literature and discussion of the relationship to mucoepidermoid, sialodontogenic, and glandular odontogenic cysts. *J Oral Maxillofac Surg* 1990;48:871–877.

19. Knights EM, Brokaw WC, Kessler HP: The incidence of dentigerous cysts associated with a random sampling of unerupted third molars. *Gen Dent* 1991;39:96–98.

20. Sciubba JJ: Evaluating dentigerous cysts [letter]. *Gen Dent* 1991;39:313–314.

21. Knights EM: Evaluating dentigerous cysts [letter]. *Gen Dent* 1991;39:314–315.

22. Clauser C, Zuccati G, Barone R, et al: Simplified surgical-orthodontic treatment of a dentigerous cyst. *J Clin Orthod* 1994;28:103–106.

23. Leider AS, Eversole LR, Barkin ME: Cystic ameloblastoma. *Oral Surg Oral Med Oral Pathol* 1985;60:624–630.

24. Gardner AF: The odontogenic cyst as a potential carcinoma: A clinicopathologic appraisal. *JADA* 1969;78:746–755.

25. Maxymiw WG, Wood RE: Carcinoma arising in a dentigerous cyst: A case report and review of the literature. *J Oral Maxillofac Surg* 1991;49:639–643.

26. Johnson LM, Sapp JP, McIntire DN: Squamous cell carcinoma arising in a dentigerous cyst. *J Oral Maxillofac Surg* 1994;52:987–990.

Eruption Cyst

27. Shear M: *Cysts of the Oral Regions,* 3rd ed. Boston: Wright, 1992, pp 99–101.

28. Seward MH: Eruption cyst: An analysis of its clinical features. *J Oral Surg* 1973;31:31–35.

Odontogenic Keratocyst

29. Philipsen HP: Om keratocyster (kolesteatomer) i kaeberne. *Tandlaegebladet* 1956;60:963.

30. Shear M: *Cysts of the Oral Regions,* 3rd ed. Boston: Wright, 1992:4–45.

31. Browne RM: The odontogenic keratocyst. Clinical aspects. *Br Dent J* 1970;128:225–231.

32. Payne TF: An analysis of the clinical and histopathologic parameters of the odontogenic keratocyst. *Oral Surg Oral Med Oral Pathol* 1972;33:538–546.

33. Brannon RB: The odontogenic keratocyst: A clinicopathologic study of 312 cases: Part I: Clinical features. *Oral Surg Oral Med Oral Pathol* 1976;42:54–72.

34. Dayan D, Buchner A, Gorsky M, et al: The peripheral odontogenic keratocyst. *Int J Oral Maxillofac Surg* 1988;17:81–83.

35. Chehade A, Daley TD, Wysocki GP, et al: Peripheral odontogenic keratocyst. *Oral Surg Oral Med Oral Pathol* 1994;77:494–497.

36. Hodgkinson DJ, Woods JE, Dahlin DC, et al: Keratocysts of the jaw. Clinicopathologic study of 79 patients. *Cancer* 1978;41:803–813.

37. Ahlfors E, Larsson A, Sjögren S: The odontogenic keratocyst: A benign cystic tumor? *J Oral Maxillofac Surg* 1984;42:10–19.

38. Haring JI, Van Dis ML: Odontogenic keratocysts: A clinical, radiographic, and histopathologic study. *Oral Surg Oral Med Oral Pathol* 1988;66:145–153.

39. Kakarantza-Angelopoulou E, Nicolatou O: Odontogenic keratocysts: Clinicopathologic study of 87 cases. *J Oral Maxillofac Surg* 1990;48:593–599.

40. Anand VK, Arrowood JP Jr, Krolls SO: Odontogenic keratocysts: A study of 50 patients. *Laryngoscope* 1995;105:14–16.

41. Fantasia JE: Lateral periodontal cyst. An analysis of forty-six cases. *Oral Surg Oral Med Oral Pathol* 1979;48:237–243.

42. Neville BW, Mishkin DJ, Traynham RT: The laterally positioned odontogenic keratocyst. *J Periodontol* 1984;55:98–102.

43. Wright BA, Wysocki GP, Larder TC: Odontogenic keratocysts presenting as periapical disease. *Oral Surg Oral Med Oral Pathol* 1983;56:425–429.

44. Nohl FSA, Gulabivala K: Odontogenic keratocyst as periradicular radiolucency in the anterior mandible: Two case reports. *Oral Surg Oral Med Oral Pathol Oral Radiol Endod* 1996;81:103–109.

45. Woo S-B, Eisenbud L, Kleiman M, et al: Odontogenic keratocysts in the anterior maxilla: Report of two cases, one simulating a nasopalatine cyst. *Oral Surg Oral Med Oral Pathol* 1987;64:463–465.

46. Neville BW, Damm DD, Brock TR: Odontogenic keratocysts of the midline maxillary region. *J Oral Maxillofac Surg* 1997;55: 340–344.

47. Christ TF: The globulomaxillary cyst: An embryologic misconception. *Oral Surg Oral Med Oral Pathol* 1970;30:515–526.

48. Kanas RJ, DeBoom GW, Jensen JL: Inverted heart-shaped, interradicular radiolucent area of the anterior maxilla. *JADA* 1987;115:887–889.

49. Woolgar JA, Rippin JW, Browne RM: The odontogenic keratocyst and its occurrence in the nevoid basal cell carcinoma syndrome. *Oral Surg Oral Med Oral Pathol* 1987;64:727–730.

50. Robinson HBG: Classification of cysts of the jaws. *Am J Orthod Oral Surg* 1945;31:370–375.

51. Waldron CA: Odontogenic cysts and tumors. In: Neville BW, Damm DD, Allen CM, Bouquot JE (eds): *Oral & Maxillofacial Pathology.* Philadelphia: WB Saunders, 1995:496–500.

52. Browne RM: The odontogenic keratocyst: Histological features and their correlation with clinical behaviour. *Br Dent J* 1971;131:249–259.

53. Brannon RB: The odontogenic keratocyst: A clinicopathologic study of 312 cases: Part II: Histologic features. *Oral Surg Oral Med Oral Pathol* 1976;42:233–255.

54. Kratochvil FJ, Brannon RB: Cartilage in the walls of odontogenic keratocysts. *J Oral Pathol Med* 1993;22:282–285.

55. Rodu B, Tate AL, Martinez Jr MG: The implications of inflammation in odontogenic keratocysts. *J Oral Pathol Med* 1987;16:518–521.

56. Wright JM: The odontogenic keratocyst: orthokeratinized variant. *Oral Surg Oral Med Oral Pathol* 1981;51:609–618.

57. Crowley TE, Kaugars GE, Gunsolley JC: Odontogenic keratocysts: A clinical and histologic comparison of the parakeratin and orthokeratin variants. *J Oral Maxillofac Surg* 1992;50:22–26.

58. Vuahula E, Nikai H, Ijuhin N, et al: Jaw cysts with orthokeratinization: Analysis of 12 cases. *J Oral Pathol Med* 1993;22:35–40.

59. Meiselman F: Surgical management of the odontogenic keratocyst: Conservative approach. *J Oral Maxillofac Surg* 1994;52:960–963.

60. Williams TP, Connor FA Jr: Surgical management of the odontogenic keratocyst: Aggressive approach. *J Oral Maxillofac Surg* 1994;52:964–966.

61. Voorsmit RACA: The incredible keratocyst: A new approach to treatment. *Dtsch Zahnärztl Z* 1985;40:641–644.

62. Brøndum N, Jensen, VJ: Recurrence of keratocysts and decompression treatment. A long-term follow-up of forty-four cases. *Oral Surg Oral Med Oral Pathol* 1991;72:265–269.

63. Areen RG, McClatchey KD, Baker HL: Squamous cell carcinoma developing in an odontogenic keratocyst. *Arch Otolaryngol* 1981;107: 568–569.

64. Hennis HL, Stewart WC, Neville B, et al: Carcinoma arising in an odontogenic keratocyst with orbital invasion. *Documenta Ophthalmologica* 1991;77:73–79.

65. Foley WL, Terry BC, Jacoway JR: Malignant transformation of an odontogenic keratocyst: Report of a case. *J Oral Maxillofac Surg* 1991;49:768–771.

66. Anand VK, Arrowood JP Jr, Krolls SO: Malignant potential of the odontogenic keratocyst. *Otolaryngol Head Neck Surg* 1994;111:124–129.

67. Gorlin RJ: Nevoid basal cell carcinoma syndrome. *Medicine* 1987;66:98–113.

68. Gorlin RJ, Cohen MM Jr, Levin LS: Gorlin syndrome (nevoid basal cell carcinoma syndrome). In: Syndromes of the Head and Neck, 3rd ed. New York: Oxford University Press, 1990:372–380.

69. Woolgar JA, Rippin JW, Browne RM: A comparative histological study of odontogenic keratocysts in basal cell naevus syndrome and control patients. *J Oral Pathol* 1987;16:75–80.

Orthokeratinized Odontogenic Cyst

70. Wright JM: The odontogenic keratocyst: Orthokeratinized variant. *Oral Surg Oral Med Oral Pathol* 1981;51:609–618.
71. Crowley TE, Kaugars GE, Gunsolley JC: Odontogenic keratocysts: A clinical and histologic comparison of the parakeratin and orthokeratin variants. *J Oral Maxillofac Surg* 1992;50:22–26.
72. Vuhahula E, Nikai H, Ijuhin N, et al: Jaw cysts with orthokeratinization: Analysis of 12 cases. *J Oral Pathol Med* 1993;22:35–40.

Gingival (Alveolar) Cysts of the Newborn

73. Shear M: *Cysts of the Oral Regions,* 3rd ed. Boston: Wright, 1992:46–50.
74. Fromm A: Epstein's pearls, Bohn's nodules and inclusion cysts of the oral cavity. *J Dent Child* 1967;34:275–287.
75. Cataldo E, Berkman MD: Cysts of the oral mucosa in newborns. *Am J Dis Child* 1968;116:44–48.
76. Jorgenson RJ, Shapiro SD, Salinas CF, et al: Intraoral findings and anomalies in neonates. *Pediatrics* 1982;69:577–582.

Gingival Cyst of the Adult

77. Shear M: *Cysts of the Oral Regions,* 3rd ed. Boston: Wright, 1992:51–60.
78. Moskow BS, Siegel K, Zegarelli EV, et al: Gingival and lateral periodontal cysts. *J Periodontol* 1970;41:249–260.
79. Buchner A, Hansen LS: The histomorphologic spectrum of the gingival cyst in the adult. *Oral Surg Oral Med Oral Pathol* 1979;48:532–539.
80. Wysocki GP, Brannon RB, Gardner DG, et al: Histogenesis of the lateral periodontal cyst and the gingival cyst of the adult. *Oral Surg Oral Med Oral Pathol* 1980;50:327–334.
81. Nxumalo TN, Shear M: Gingival cyst in adults. *J Oral Pathol Med* 1992;21:309–313.
82. Waldron CA: Odontogenic cysts and tumors. In: Neville BW, Damm DD, Allen CM, Bouquot JE (eds): *Oral & Maxillofacial Pathology.* Philadelphia: WB Saunders, 1995:503–504.

Lateral Periodontal Cyst

83. Standish SM, Shafer WG: The lateral periodontal cyst. *J Periodontol* 1958;29:27–33.
84. Moskow BS, Siegel K, Zegarelli EV, et al: Gingival and lateral periodontal cysts. *J Periodontol* 1970;41:249–260.
85. Wysocki GP, Brannon RB, Gardner DG, et al: Histogenesis of the lateral periodontal cyst and the gingival cyst of the adult. *Oral Surg Oral Med Oral Pathol* 1980;50:327–334.
86. Waldron CA: Odontogenic cysts and tumors. In: Neville BW, Damm DD, Allen CM, Bouquot JE (eds): *Oral & Maxillofacial Pathology.* Philadelphia: WB Saunders, 1995:504–506.
87. Fantasia JE: Lateral periodontal cyst. An analysis of forty-six cases. *Oral Surg Oral Med Oral Pathol* 1979;48:237–243.
88. Cohen, D, Neville B, Damm D, et al: The lateral periodontal cyst: A report of 37 cases. *J Periodontol* 1984;55:230–234.
89. Rasmusson LG, Magnusson BC, Borrman H: The lateral periodontal cyst: A histopathological and radiographic study of 32 cases. *Br J Oral Maxillofac Surg* 1991;29:54–57.
90. Altini M, Shear M: The lateral periodontal cyst: An update. *J Oral Pathol Med* 1992;21:245–250.
91. Carter LC, Carney YL, Perez-Pudlewski D: Lateral periodontal cyst: Multifactorial analysis of a previously unreported series. *Oral Surg Oral Med Oral Pathol Oral Radiol Endod* 1996;81:210–216.
92. Weathers D, Waldron C: Unusual multilocular cysts of the jaw (botryoid odontogenic cysts). *Oral Surg Oral Med Oral Pathol* 1973;36:235–241.
93. Kaugars GE: Botryoid odontogenic cyst. *Oral Surg Oral Med Oral Pathol* 1986;62:555–559.
94. Greer RO, Johnson M: Botryoid odontogenic cyst: Clinicopathologic analysis of ten cases with three recurrences. *J Oral Maxillofac Surg* 1988;46:574–579.
95. Gurol M, Burkes EJ Jr, Jacoway J: Botryoid odontogenic cyst: Analysis of 33 cases. *J Periodontol* 1995;66:1069–1073.
96. Shear M, Pindborg JJ: Microscopic features of the lateral periodontal cyst. *Scand J Dent Res* 1975;83:103–110.

Glandular Odontogenic Cyst

97. International Association of Oral Pathologists: Proceedings of the slide seminar on odontogenic tumours and cysts. Case 4. Second meeting of the International Association of Oral Pathologists, Noordwijkerhout, The Netherlands, June 4th–7th, 1984.
98. Padayachee A, Van Wyk CW: Two cystic lesions with features of both the botryoid odontogenic cyst and the central mucoepidermoid tumour: Sialo-odontogenic cyst? *J Oral Pathol* 1987;16:499–504.
99. Gardner DG, Kessler HP, Morency R, et al: The glandular odontogenic cyst: An apparent entity. *J Oral Pathol* 1988;17:359–366.
100. High AS, Main DMG, Khoo SP, et al: The polymorphous odontogenic cyst. *J Oral Pathol Med* 1996;25:25–31.
101. Hussain K, Edmondson HD, Browne RM: Glandular odontogenic cysts. Diagnosis and treatment. *Oral Surg Oral Med Oral Pathol Oral Radiol Endod* 1995;79:593–602.
102. Economopoulou P, Patrikiou A: Glandular odontogenic cyst of the maxilla: Report of case. *J Oral Maxillofac Surg* 1995;53:834–837.
103. Waldron CA, Koh ML: Central mucoepidermoid carcinoma of the jaws: Report of four cases with analysis of the literature and discussion of the relationship to mucoepidermoid, sialodontogenic, and glandular odontogenic cysts. *J Oral Maxillofac Surg* 1990;48:871–877.

Periapical Cyst

104. Neville BW, Damm DD, Allen CM, Bouquot JE: *Oral & Maxillofacial Pathology.* Philadelphia: WB Saunders, 1995:105–109.
105. Kreidler JF, Raubenheimer EJ, van Heerden WFP: A retrospective analysis of 367 cystic lesions of the jaw: The Ulm experience. *J Craniomaxillofac Surg* 1993;21:339–341.
106. Nakamura T, Ishida J, Nakano Y, et al: A study of cysts in the oral region. Cysts of the jaws. *J Nihon Univ Sch Dent* 1995;37:33–40.
107. Shear M: *Cysts of the Oral Regions,* 3rd ed. Boston: Wright, 1992:136–162.
108. Stockdale CR, Chandler NP: The nature of the periapical lesion: A review of 1108 cases. *J Dent* 1988;16:123–129.
109. Spatafore CM, Griffin JA Jr, Keyes GG, et al: Periapical biopsy report: An analysis over a 10-year period. *J Endod* 1990;16:239–241.
110. Lustmann J, Shear M: Radicular cysts arising from deciduous teeth: Review of the literature and report of 23 cases. *Int J Oral Surg* 1985;14:153–161.
111. Mass E, Kaplan I, Hirshberg A: A clinical and histopathological study of radicular cysts associated with primary molars. *J Oral Pathol Med* 1995;24:458–461.
112. High AS, Hirschmann PN: Age changes in residual radicular cysts. *J Oral Pathol* 1986;15:524–528.
113. Shear M: Inflammation in dental cysts. *Oral Surg Oral Med Oral Pathol* 1964;17:756–767.
114. Browne RM: Metaplasia and degeneration in odontogenic cysts in man. *J Oral Pathol* 1972;1:145–158.
115. Rushton MA: Hyaline bodies in the epithelium of dental cysts. *Proc Royal Soc Med* 1955;48:407–409.
116. Shear M: The hyaline and granular bodies in dental cysts. *Br Dent J* 1961;110:301–307.
117. Sedano HO, Gorlin RJ: Hyaline bodies of Rushton. Some histochemical considerations concerning their etiology. *Oral Surg Oral Med Oral Pathol* 1968;26:198–201.

Carcinomas Arising in Odontogenic Cysts

118. Waldron CA: Odontogenic cysts and tumors. *In* Neville BW, Damm DD, Allen CM, Bouquot JE (eds): *Oral & Maxillofacial Pathology.* Philadelphia: WB Saunders, 1995:510–511.
119. Gardner AF: The odontogenic cyst as a potential carcinoma: A clinicopathologic appraisal. *JADA* 1969;78:746–755.
120. Waldron CA, Mustoe TA: Primary intraosseous carcinoma of the mandible with probable origin in an odontogenic cyst. *Oral Surg Oral Med Oral Pathol* 1989;67:716–724.
121. Eversole LR, Sabes WR, Rovin S: Aggressive growth and neoplastic potential of odontogenic cysts. *Cancer* 1975;35:270–282.
122. Browne RM, Gough NG: Malignant change in the epithelium lining odontogenic cysts. *Cancer* 1972;29:1199–1207.
123. van der Waal I, Rauhamaa R, van der Kwast AM, et al: Squamous cell carcinoma arising in the lining of odontogenic cysts. Report of 5 cases. *Int J Oral Surg* 1985;14:146–152.

124. Maxymiw WG, Wood RE: Carcinoma arising in a dentigerous cyst: A case report and review of the literature. *J Oral Maxillofac Surg* 1991;49:639–643.

125. Areen RG, McClatchey KD, Baker HL: Squamous cell carcinoma developing in an odontogenic keratocyst. *Arch Otolaryngol* 1981;107:568–569.

126. Hennis HL, Stewart WC, Neville B, et al: Carcinoma arising in an odontogenic keratocyst with orbital invasion. *Documenta Ophthalmologica* 1991;7:73–79.

127. Anand VK, Arrowood JP Jr, Krolls SO: Malignant potential of the odontogenic keratocyst. *Otolaryngol Head Neck Surg* 1994;111:124–129.

128. Siar CH, Ng KH: Squamous cell carcinoma in an orthokeratinised odontogenic keratocyst. *Int J Oral Maxillofac Surg* 1987;16:95–98.

Ameloblastoma

129. Reichart PA, Philipsen HP, Sonner S: Ameloblastoma: Biologic profile of 3677 cases. *Oral Oncol Eur J Cancer* 1995;31B:86–99.

130. Small IA, Waldron CA: Ameloblastomas of the jaws. *Oral Surg Oral Med Oral Pathol* 1955;8:281–297.

131. Nastri AL, Wiesenfeld D, Radden BG, et al: Maxillary ameloblastoma: A retrospective study of 13 cases. *Br J Oral Maxillofac Surg* 1995;33:28–32.

132. Vickers RA, Gorlin RJ: Ameloblastoma: Delineation of early histopathologic features of neoplasia. *Cancer* 1970;26:699–710.

133. Lurie R, Altini M, Shear M: A case report of kerato-ameloblastoma. *Int J Oral Surg* 1976;5:245–249.

134. Norval EJG, Thompson IOC, vanWyk CW: An unusual variant of keratoameloblastoma. *J Oral Pathol Med* 1994;23:465–467.

135. Hartman KS: Granular-cell ameloblastoma. A survey of twenty cases from the Armed Forces Institute of Pathology. *Oral Surg Oral Med Oral Pathol* 1974;38:241–253.

136. Waldron CA, El-Mofty SK: A histopathologic study of 116 ameloblastomas with special reference to the desmoplastic variant. *Oral Surg Oral Med Oral Pathol* 1987;63:441–451.

137. Eversole LR, Leider AS, Hansen LS: Ameloblastoma with pronounced desmoplasia. *J Oral Maxillofac Surg* 1984;42:735–740.

138. Philipsen HP, Ormiston IW, Reichart PA: The desmo- and osteoplastic ameloblastoma. Histologic variant or clinicopathologic entity? Case reports. *Int J Oral Maxillofac Surg* 1992;21:352–357.

139. Generson RM, Porter JM, Stratigos GT: Mural odontogenic epithelial proliferations within the wall of a dentigerous cyst: Their significance. *Oral Surg Oral Med Oral Pathol* 1976;42:717–721.

140. Müller H, Slootweg PJ: The ameloblastoma, the controversial approach to therapy. *J Maxillofac Surg* 1985;13:79–84.

141. Gold L: Biologic behavior of ameloblastoma. *Oral Maxillofac Clin N Am* 1991;3(1):21–71.

142. Williams TP: Management of ameloblastoma: A changing perspective. *J Oral Maxillofac Surg* 1993;51:1064–1070.

143. Robinson L, Martinez MG: Unicystic ameloblastoma: A prognostically distinct entity. *Cancer* 1977;40:2278–2285.

144. Gardner DG, Pecak AM: The treatment of ameloblastoma based on pathologic and anatomic principles. *Cancer* 1980;46:2514–2519.

145. Gardner DG: A pathologist's approach to the treatment of ameloblastoma. *J Oral Maxillofac Surg* 1984;42:161–166.

146. Gardner DG, Corio RL: The relationship of plexiform unicystic ameloblastoma to conventional ameloblastoma. *Oral Surg Oral Med Oral Pathol* 1983;56:54–60.

147. Leider AS, Eversole LR, Barkin ME: Cystic ameloblastoma: A clinicopathologic analysis. *Oral Surg Oral Med Oral Pathol* 1985;60:624–630.

148. Ackermann GL, Altini M, Shear M: The unicystic ameloblastoma: A clinicopathologic study of 57 cases. *J Oral Pathol* 1988;17:541–546.

149. Thompson IOC, Ferreira R, van Wyk CW: Recurrent unicystic ameloblastoma of the maxilla. *Br J Oral Maxillofac Surg* 1993;31:180–182.

150. Buchner A, Sciubba JJ: Peripheral epithelial odontogenic tumors: A review. *Oral Surg Oral Med Oral Pathol* 1987;63:688–697.

151. Batsakis JG, Hicks MJ, Flaitz CM: Pathology consultation. Peripheral epithelial odontogenic tumors. *Ann Otol Rhinol Laryngol* 1993;102:322–324.

152. Woo S-B, Smith-Williams JE, Sciubba JJ, et al: Peripheral ameloblastoma of the buccal mucosa: case report and review of the English literature. *Oral Surg Oral Med Oral Pathol* 1987;63:78–84.

153. Redman RS, Keegan BP, Spector CJ, et al: Peripheral ameloblastoma with unusual mitotic activity and conflicting evidence regarding histogenesis. *J Oral Maxillofac Surg* 1994;52:192–197.

154. Moskow BS, Baden E: The peripheral ameloblastoma of the gingiva. Case report and literature review. *J Periodontol* 1982;53:736–742.

155. Zhu EX, Okada N, Takagi M: Peripheral ameloblastoma: Case report and review of literature. *J Oral Maxillofac Surg* 1995;53:590–594.

156. El-Mofty S, Gerard NO, Farish SE, et al: Peripheral ameloblastoma: A clinical and histologic study of 11 cases. *J Oral Maxillofac Surg* 1991;49:970–974.

157. Gardner DG: Peripheral ameloblastoma: A study of 21 cases, including 5 reported as basal cell carcinoma of the gingiva. *Cancer* 1977;39:1625–1633.

158. Hernandez G, Sanchez G, Caballero T, et al: A rare case of a multicentric peripheral ameloblastoma of the gingiva: A light and electron microscopic study. *J Clin Periodontol* 1992;19:281–287.

159. Baden E, Doyle JL, Petriella V: Malignant transformation of peripheral ameloblastoma. *Oral Surg Oral Med Oral Pathol* 1993;75:214–219.

160. Lin SC, Lieu CM, Hahn LJ, et al: Peripheral ameloblastoma with metastasis. *Int J Oral Maxillofac Surg* 1987;16:202–204.

161. McClatchey KD, Sullivan MJ, Paugh DR: Peripheral ameloblastic carcinoma: A case report of a rare neoplasm. *J Otolaryngol* 1989;18:109–111.

Malignancy in Ameloblastoma

162. Elzay RP: Primary intraosseous carcinoma of the jaws. Review and update of odontogenic carcinomas. *Oral Surg Oral Med Oral Pathol* 1982;54:299–303.

163. Laughlin EH: Metastasizing ameloblastoma. *Cancer* 1989;64:776–780.

164. Houston G, Davenport W, Keaton W, et al: Malignant (metastatic) ameloblastoma: Report of a case. *J Oral Maxillofac Surg* 1993;51:1152–1155.

165. Baden E, Doyle JL, Petriella V: Malignant transformation of peripheral ameloblastoma. *Oral Surg Oral Med Oral Pathol* 1993;75:214–219.

166. Slootweg PJ, Müller H: Malignant ameloblastoma or ameloblastic carcinoma. *Oral Surg Oral Med Oral Pathol* 1984;57:168–176.

167. Corio RL, Goldblatt LI, Edwards PA, et al: Ameloblastic carcinoma: A clinicopathologic study and assessment of eight cases. *Oral Surg Oral Med Oral Pathol* 1987;64:570–576.

168. Nagai N, Takeshita N, Nagatsuka H, et al: Ameloblastic carcinoma: Case report and review. *J Oral Pathol Med* 1991;20:460–463.

169. Bruce RA, Jackson IT: Ameloblastic carcinoma. Report of an aggressive case and review of the literature. *J Craniomaxillofac Surg* 1991;19:267–271.

170. Lau SK, Tideman H, Wu PC: Ameloblastic carcinoma of the jaws: A report of two cases. *Oral Surg Oral Med Oral Pathol Oral Radiol Endod* 1998;85:78–81.

171. Lanham RJ: Chemotherapy of metastatic ameloblastoma: A case report and review of the literature. *Oncology* 1987;44:133–134.

172. Ramadas K, Jose CC, Subhashini J, et al: Pulmonary metastases from ameloblastoma of the mandible treated with cisplatin, adriamycin and cyclophosphamide. *Cancer* 1990;66:1475–1479.

173. Lin SC, Lieu CM, Hahn LJ, et al: Peripheral ameloblastoma with metastasis. *Int J Oral Maxillofac Surg* 1987;16:202–204.

174. McClatchey KD, Sullivan MJ, Paugh DR: Peripheral ameloblastic carcinoma: A case report of a rare neoplasm. *J Otolaryngol* 1989;18:109–111.

Calcifying Epithelial Odontogenic Tumor

175. Pindborg JJ, Vedtofte P, Reibel J, et al: The calcifying epithelial odontogenic tumor: A review of recent literature and report of a case. *APMIS* 1991;Suppl 23:152–157.

176. Franklin CD, Pindborg JJ: The calcifying epithelial odontogenic tumor: A review and analysis of 113 cases. *Oral Surg Oral Med Oral Pathol* 1976;42:735–765.

177. Pindborg JJ: A calcifying epithelial odontogenic tumor. *Cancer* 1958;11:838–843.

178. Matsumura T, Matsumura H, Mori M, et al: Calcifying epithelial odontogenic tumor (enzyme-histochemical findings). *J Jpn Stomatol Soc* 1971;20:274.

179. Krolls SO: Calcifying epithelial odontogenic tumor. A survey of 23

cases and discussion of histomorphologic variations. *Arch Pathol* 1974;98:206–210.

180. Hicks MJ, Flaitz CM, Wong MEK, et al: Clear cell variant of calcifying epithelial odontogenic tumor: Case report and review of the literature. *Head Neck* 1994;16:272–277.

181. Basu MK, Matthews JB, Sear AJ, et al: Calcifying epithelial odontogenic tumour: A case showing features of malignancy. *J Oral Pathol* 1984;13:310–319.

182. Damm DD, White DK, Drummond JF, et al: Combined epithelial odontogenic tumor: Adenomatoid odontogenic tumor and calcifying epithelial odontogenic tumor. *Oral Surg Oral Med Oral Pathol* 1983;55:487–496.

Squamous Odontogenic Tumor

183. Baden E, Doyle J, Mesa M, et al: Squamous odontogenic tumor: Report of three cases including the first extraosseous case. *Oral Surg Oral Med Oral Pathol* 1993;75:733–738.

184. Pullon PA, Shafer WG, Elzay RP, et al: Squamous odontogenic tumor: Report of six cases of a previously undescribed lesion. *Oral Surg Oral Med Oral Pathol* 1975;40:616–630.

185. Goldblatt LI, Brannon RB, Ellis GL: Squamous odontogenic tumor: Report of five cases and review of the literature. *Oral Surg Oral Med Oral Pathol* 1982;54:187–196.

186. Schwartz-Arad D, Lustman J, Ulmansky M: Squamous odontogenic tumor: Review of the literature and case report. *Int J Oral Maxillofac Surg* 1990;19:327–330.

187. Tatemoto Y, Okada Y, Mori M: Squamous odontogenic tumor: Immunohistochemical identification of keratins. *Oral Surg Oral Med Oral Pathol* 1989;67:63–67.

188. Mills WP, Davila MA, Beuttenmuller EA, et al: Squamous odontogenic tumor. Report of a case with lesions in three quadrants. *Oral Surg Oral Med Oral Pathol* 1986;61:557–563.

189. Leider AS, Jonker LA, Cook HE: Multicentric familial squamous odontogenic tumor. *Oral Surg Oral Med Oral Pathol* 1989;68:175–181.

190. Norris LH, Baghaei-Rad M, Malone PL, et al: Bilateral squamous odontogenic tumor and the malignant transformation of a mandibular radiolucent lesion. *J Oral Maxillofac Surg* 1988;42:827–834.

191. Wright JM: Squamous odontogenic tumorlike proliferations in odontogenic cysts. *Oral Surg Oral Med Oral Pathol* 1979;47:354–358.

Clear Cell Odontogenic Carcinoma

192. Waldron CA, Mustoe TA: Primary intraosseous carcinoma of the mandible with probable origin in an odontogenic cyst. *Oral Surg Oral Med Oral Pathol* 1989;67:716–724.

193. Waldron CA, Small IA, Silverman H: Clear cell ameloblastoma: An odontogenic carcinoma. *J Oral Maxillofac* 1985;43:707–717.

194. Hansen LS, Eversole LR, Green TL, et al: Clear cell odontogenic tumor: A new histologic variant with aggressive potential. *Head Neck Surg* 1985;8:115–123.

195. Eversole LR, Belton CM, Hansen LS: Clear cell odontogenic tumor: Histochemical and ultrastructural features. *J Oral Pathol* 1985;14:603–614.

196. Eversole LR, Duffey DC, Powell NB: Clear cell odontogenic carcinoma: A clinicopathologic analysis. *Arch Otolaryngol Head Neck Surg* 1995;121:685–689.

197. Fan J, Kubota E, Imamura H, et al: Clear cell odontogenic carcinoma: A case report with massive invasion of neighboring organs and lymph node metastasis. *Oral Surg Oral Med Oral Pathol* 1992;74:768–775.

198. Bang G, Koppang HS, Hansen LS, et al: Clear cell odontogenic carcinoma: Report of three cases with pulmonary and lymph node metastasis. *J Oral Pathol Med* 1989;18:113–118.

199. Milles M, Doyle JL, Mesa M, et al: Clear cell odontogenic carcinoma with lymph node metastasis. *Oral Surg Oral Med Oral Pathol* 1993;76:82–89.

Primary de Novo Intraosseous Squamous Cell Carcinoma

200. Suei Y, Tanimoto K, Taguchi A, et al: Primary intraosseous carcinoma: Review of the literature and diagnostic criteria. *J Oral Maxillofac Surg* 1994;52:580–583.

201. To EHW, Brown JS, Avery BS, et al: Primary intraosseous carcinoma of the jaws. Three new cases and a review of the literature. *Br J Oral Maxillofac Surg* 1991;29:19–25.

202. Müller S, Waldron CA: Primary intraosseous squamous carcinoma. Report of two cases. *Int J Oral Maxillofac Surg* 1991;20:362–365.

203. Lindqvist C, Teppo L: Primary intraosseous carcinoma of the mandible. *Int J Oral Maxillofac Surg* 1984;15:209–214.

204. Ruskin JD, Cohen DM, Davis LF: Primary intraosseous carcinoma: Report of two cases. *J Oral Maxillofac Surg* 1988;46:425–432.

Intraosseous Mucoepidermoid Carcinoma

205. Waldron CA, Mustoe TA: Primary intraosseous carcinoma of the mandible with probable origin in an odontogenic cyst. *Oral Surg Oral Med Oral Pathol* 1989;67:716–724.

206. Freije JE, Campbell BH, Yousif NJ, et al: Central mucoepidermoid carcinoma of the mandible. *Otolaryngol Head Neck Surg* 1995;112:453–456.

207. Brookstone MS, Huvos AG: Central salivary gland tumors of the maxilla and mandible: A clinicopathologic study of 11 cases with an analysis of the literature. *J Oral Maxillofac Surg* 1992;50:229–236.

208. Spiro RJ, Huvos AG, Berk R, et al: Mucoepidermoid carcinoma of salivary gland origin: A clinicopathologic study of 367 cases. *Am J Surg* 1978;136:461–468.

209. Browne RM: Metaplasia and degeneration in odontogenic cysts in man. *J Oral Pathol* 1992;1:145–158.

210. Ézsiás A, Sugar AW, Milling MAP, et al: Central mucoepidermoid carcinoma in a child. *J Oral Maxillofac Surg* 1994;52:512–515.

211. Browand BC, Waldron CA: Central mucoepidermoid tumors of the jaws: Report of nine cases and review of the literature. *Oral Surg Oral Med Oral Pathol* 1975;40:631–643.

212. Grubka JM, Wesley RK, Monaco F: Primary intraosseous mucoepidermoid carcinoma of the anterior part of the mandible. *J Oral Maxillofac Surg* 1983;41:389–394.

213. Waldron CA, Koh ML: Central mucoepidermoid carcinoma of the jaws: Report of four cases with analysis of the literature and discussion of the relationship to mucoepidermoid, sialodontogenic, and glandular odontogenic cysts. *J Oral Maxillofac Surg* 1990;48:871–877.

214. Lebsack JP, Marrogi AJ, Martin SA: Central mucoepidermoid carcinoma of the jaw with distant metastasis: A case report and review of the literature. *J Oral Maxillofac Surg* 1990;48:518–522.

215. Fredrickson C, Cherrick HM: Central mucoepidermoid carcinoma of the jaws. *J Oral Med* 1978;33:80–85.

Ameloblastic Fibroma and Ameloblastic Fibrosarcoma

216. Hansen LS, Ficarra G: Mixed odontogenic tumors: An analysis of 23 new cases. *Head Neck Surg* 1988;10:330–343.

217. Trodahl JN: Ameloblastic fibroma. A survey of cases from the Armed Forces Institute of Pathology. *Oral Surg Oral Med Oral Pathol* 1972;33:547–558.

218. Zallen R, Preskar M, McClary S: Ameloblastic fibroma. *J Oral Maxillofac Surg* 1982;40:513–517.

219. Müller S, Parker DC, Kapadia SB, et al: Ameloblastic fibrosarcoma of the jaws: A clinicopathologic and DNA analysis of five cases and review of the literature with discussion of its relationship to ameloblastic fibroma. *Oral Surg Oral Med Oral Pathol Oral Radiol Endod* 1995;79:469–477.

220. Park HR, Shin KB, Sol MY, et al: A highly malignant ameloblastic fibrosarcoma: Report of a case. *Oral Surg Oral Med Oral Pathol Oral Radiol Endod* 1995;79:478–481.

Ameloblastic Fibro-odontoma

221. Miller AS, Lopez CF, Pullon PA, et al: Ameloblastic fibro-odontoma. Report of seven cases. *Oral Surg Oral Med Oral Pathol* 1976;41:354–365.

222. Slootweg PJ: An analysis of the interrelationship of the mixed odontogenic tumors: Ameloblastic fibroma, ameloblastic fibro-odontoma, and the odontomas. *Oral Surg Oral Med Oral Pathol* 1981;51:266–276.

223. Kitano M, Tsuda-Yamada S, Semba I, et al: Pigmented ameloblastic fibro-odontoma with melanophages. *Oral Surg Oral Med Oral Pathol* 1994;77:271–275.

Odontoameloblastoma

224. Kramer IRH, Pindborg JJ, Shear M. The WHO histological typing of odontogenic tumors. Cancer 1992;70:2988–2994.
225. Thompson IOC, Phillips VM, Ferreira R, et al: Odontoameloblastoma: A case report. *Br J Oral Maxillofac Surg* 1990;28:347–349.

Adenomatoid Odontogenic Tumor

226. Kramer IRH, Pindborg JJ, Shear M. The WHO histological typing of odontogenic tumors. *Cancer* 1992;70:2988–2994.
227. Giansanti JS, Someren A, Waldron CA: Odontogenic adenomatoid tumor (adenoameloblastoma). Survey of 111 cases. *Oral Surg Oral Med Oral Pathol* 1970;30:69–86.
228. Courtney RM, Kerr DA: The odontogenic adenomatoid tumor. A comprehensive study of twenty new cases. *Oral Surg Oral Med Oral Pathol* 1975;39:424–435.
229. Philipsen HP, Reichart PA, Zhang KH, et al: Adenomatoid odontogenic tumor: biologic profile based on 499 cases. *J Oral Pathol Med* 1991;20:149–158.
230. Kearns GJ, Smith R: Adenomatoid odontogenic tumour: An unusual cause of gingival swelling in a 3-year-old patient. *Br Dent J* 1996;181:380–382.
231. Abrams AM, Melrose RJ, Howell FV: Adenoameloblastoma. A clinical pathologic study of ten new cases. *Cancer* 1968;22:175–185.
232. Geist S-MY, Mallon HL: Adenomatoid odontogenic tumor: Report of an unusually large lesion in the mandible. *J Oral Maxillofac Surg* 1995;53:714–717.

Calcifying Odontogenic Cyst

233. Gorlin RJ, Pindborg JJ, Clausen FP, et al: The calcifying odontogenic cyst: A possible analogue to the cutaneous calcifying epithelioma of Malherbe. An analysis of fifteen cases. *Oral Surg Oral Med Oral Pathol* 1962;15:1235–1243.
234. Buchner A: The central (intraosseous) calcifying odontogenic cyst: An analysis of 215 cases. *J Oral Maxillofac Surg* 1991;49:330–339.
235. Hong SP, Ellis GL, Hartman KS: Calcifying odontogenic cyst. A review of ninety-two cases with reevaluation of their nature as cysts or neoplasms, the nature of ghost cells, and subclassification. *Oral Surg Oral Med Oral Pathol* 1991;72:56–64.
236. Raubenheimer EJ, van Heerden WFP, Sitzman F, et al: Peripheral dentinogenic ghost cell tumor. *J Oral Pathol Med* 1992;21:93–95.
237. Buchner A, Merrell PW, Hansen LS, et al: Peripheral (extraosseous) calcfying odontogenic cyst. *Oral Surg Oral Med Oral Pathol* 1991;72:65–70.
238. Devlin H, Horner K. The radiological features of calcifying odontogenic cyst. *Br J Radiol* 1993;66(785):403–407.
239. Gunhan O, Celasun B, Can C, et al: The nature of ghost cells in calcifying odontogenic cyst: An immunohistochemical study. *Ann Dent* 1993;52(1):30–33.
240. Prætorius F, Hjørting-Hansen E, Gorlin RJ, et al: Calcifying odontogenic cyst. Range, variations and neoplastic potential. *Acta Odontol Scand* 1981;39:227–240.
241. Oliveira JA, da Silva CJ, Costa IM, et al: Calcifying odontogenic cyst in infancy: Report of case associated with compound odontoma. *ASDC J Dent Child* 1995;62(1):70–73.
242. Hirshberg A, Kaplan I, Buchner A: Calcifying odontogenic cyst associated with odontoma: a possible separate entity (odontocalcifying odontogenic cyst). *J Oral Maxillofac Surg* 1994;52:555–558.
243. Bernstein ML, Buchino JJ: The histologic similarity between craniopharyngioma and odontogenic lesions: A reappraisal. *Oral Surg Oral Med Oral Pathol* 1983;56:502–511.
244. Paulus W, Stöckel C, Krauss J, et al: Odontogenic classification of craniopharyngiomas: A clinicopathologic study of 54 cases. *Histopathology* 1997;30:172–176.
245. Miller DC: Pathology of craniopharyngiomas: clinical import of pathological findings. *Pediatr Neurosurg* 1994;21(suppl 1):11–17.
246. Graziani N, Donnet A, Bugha TN, et al: Ectopic basisphenoidal craniopharyngioma: Case report and review of the literature. *Neurosurgery* 1994;34:346–349.
247. Ellis GL, Shmookler BM: Aggressive (malignant?) epithelial odontogenic ghost cell tumor. *Oral Surg Oral Med Oral Pathol* 1986;61:471–478.
248. Tanaka N, Iwaki H, Yamada T, et al: Carcinoma after enucleation of a calcifying odontogenic cyst: a case report. *J Oral Maxillofac Surg* 1993;51:75–78.

Odontoma

249. Castro GW, Houston G, Weyrauch C: Peripheral odontoma: Report of case and review of literature. *ASDC J Dent Child* 1994;61(3):209–213.
250. Budnick SD: Compound and complex odontomas. *Oral Surg Oral Med Oral Pathol* 1976;42:501–506.
251. Kaugars GE, Miller ME, Abbey LM: Odontomas. *Oral Surg Oral Med Oral Pathol* 1989;67:172–176.
252. Blinder D, Peleg M, Taicher S: Surgical considerations in cases of large mandibular odontomas located in the mandibular angle. *Int J Oral Maxillofac Surg* 1993;22:163–165.

Central Odontogenic Fibroma

253. Gardner DG: The central odontogenic fibroma: An attempt at clarification. *Oral Surg Oral Med Oral Pathol* 1980;50:425–432.
254. Handlers JP, Abrams AM, Melrose RJ, et al: Central odontogenic fibroma: Clinicopathologic features of 19 cases and review of the literature. *J Oral Maxillofac Surg* 1991;49:46–54.
255. Kramer IRH, Pindborg JJ, Shear M. The WHO histological typing of odontogenic tumors. *Cancer* 1992;70:2988–2994.
256. Kaffe I, Buchner A: Radiologic features of central odontogenic fibroma. *Oral Surg Oral Med Oral Pathol* 1994;78:811–818.
257. Allen CM, Hammond HL, Stimson PG: Central odontogenic fibroma, WHO type. A report of three cases with an unusual associated giant cell reaction. *Oral Surg Oral Med Oral Pathol* 1992;73:62–66.
258. Odell EW, Lombardi T, Barrett AW, et al: Hybrid central giant cell granuloma and central odontogenic fibroma-like lesions of the jaws. *Histopathology* 1997;30:165–171.

Peripheral Odontogenic Fibroma

259. Buchner A, Ficarra G, Hansen LS: Peripheral odontogenic fibroma. *Oral Surg Oral Med Oral Pathol* 1987;64:432–438.
260. Kenney JN, Kaugars GE, Abbey LM: Comparison between the peripheral ossifying fibroma and peripheral odontogenic fibroma. *J Oral Maxillofac Surg* 1989;47:378–382.
261. Slabbert H, Altini M: Peripheral odontogenic fibroma: A clinicopathologic study. *Oral Surg Oral Med Oral Pathol* 1991;72:86–90.
262. Daley TD, Wysocki GP: Peripheral odontogenic fibroma. *Oral Surg Oral Med Oral Pathol* 1994;78:329–336.

Granular Cell Odontogenic Tumor

263. Waldron CA, Thompson CW, Conner WA: Granular-cell ameloblastic fibroma. *Oral Surg Oral Med Oral Pathol* 1963;16:1202–1213.
264. Takeda Y: Granular cell ameloblastic fibroma, ultrastructure and histogenesis. *Int J Oral Maxillofac Surg* 1986;15:190–195.
265. White DK, Chen S-Y, Hartman KS, et al: Central granular-cell tumor of the jaws (the so-called granular-cell ameloblastic fibroma). A clinical and ultrastructural study. *Oral Surg Oral Med Oral Pathol* 1978;45:396–405.
266. Vincent SD, Hammond HL, Ellis GL, et al: Central granular cell odontogenic fibroma. *Oral Surg Oral Med Oral Pathol* 1987;63:715–721.
267. Chen S-Y: Central granular cell tumor of the jaw. An electron microscopic and immunohistochemical study. *Oral Surg Oral Med Oral Pathol* 1991;72:75–81.

Odontogenic Myxoma

268. White DK, Chen S-Y, Mohnac AM, et al: Odontogenic myxoma. A clinical and ultrastructural study. *Oral Surg Oral Med Oral Pathol* 1975;39:901–917.
269. Moshiri S, Oda D, Worthington P, et al: Odontogenic myxoma: Histochemical and ultrastructural study. *J Oral Pathol Med* 1992;21:401–403.
270. Muzio LL, Nocini PF, Favia G, et al: Odontogenic myxoma of the jaws. A clinical, radiologic, immunohistochemical, and ultrastructural study. *Oral Surg Oral Med Oral Pathol Oral Radiol Endod* 1996;82:426–433.
271. Schmidt-Westhausen A, Becker J, Schuppan D, et al: Odontogenic

myxoma: Characterization of the extracellular matrix (ECM) of the tumour stroma. *Oral Oncol Eur J Cancer* 1994;30B:377–380.

272. Lombardi T, Lock C, Samson J, et al: S100, alpha-smooth muscle actin and cytokeratin 19 immunohistochemistry in odontogenic and soft tissue myxomas. *J Clin Pathol* 1995;48:759–762.

273. Kim J, Ellis G: Dental follicular tissue. Misinterpretation as odontogenic tumors. *J Oral Maxillofac Surg* 1993;51:762–767.

274. Suarez PA, Batsakis JG, El-Naggar AK: Don't confuse dental soft tissues with odontogenic tumors. *Ann Otol Rhinol Laryngol* 1996;105:490–494.

275. Lamberg MA, Calonius BP, Makinen JE, et al: A case of malignant myxoma (myxosarcoma) of the maxilla. *Scand J Dent Res* 1984;92:352–357.

10 : Cysts of the Neck, Unknown Primary Tumor, and Neck Dissection

■ *Mario A. Luna and Madeleine Pfaltz*

The occurrence of a cervical mass is a rather common event under a wide variety of conditions, including congenital, inflammatory, and neoplastic diseases. The disease process may be located within lymph nodes or in the soft tissues of the head and neck and it may appear as a cystic or solid tumor. Because of this diversity, a broad spectrum of possibilities must be considered in the differential diagnosis in patients who present with cervical masses. Although information obtained by routine history, physical examination, and radiologic techniques allows considerable narrowing of the diagnostic possibilities, a definitive diagnosis depends on histologic evaluation of the surgical specimen. The pathologic diagnosis of the disease and the treatment of these patients poses a challenge for both pathologists and head and neck surgeons.

▮ ANATOMY

Most descriptions of the neck divide the anatomy, for discussion purposes, into triangles. The use of triangles is simply an organizational device that parcels the volume of anatomic detail in the neck into reasonable study units.[1] The triangles of the neck aid in the localization of superficial mass lesions and define lymph node drainage patterns.

Triangles of the Head and Neck

Classically the neck has been divided into two major triangles, the anterior and the posterior triangles (Fig. 10–1). The anterior triangle is defined laterally by the sternocleidomastoid muscle, superiorly by the mandible, and anteriorly by the midline. The hyoid bone divides the anterior triangle into the suprahyoid region, containing the floor of the mouth, sublingual gland, submandibular gland, and lymph nodes, whereas the infrahyoid region contains the larynx, hypopharynx, cervical trachea, esophagus, thyroid gland, and parathyroid glands. The anterior triangle is subdivided by the superior belly of the omohyoid muscle into four smaller triangles: the submental, submandibular, carotid, and muscular triangles.

The single submental triangle is bounded laterally by the anterior belly of the digastric muscles, superiorly by the mandible, and inferiorly by the hyoid bone.

The submandibular triangle, also known as the digastric triangle, is bounded anteriorly by the anterior belly of the digastric muscle, posteriorly by the posterior belly of the digastric muscle, superiorly by the mandible, and inferiorly by the mylohyoid and hyoglossus muscles.

The carotid triangle is bounded by the superior belly of the omohyoid muscle, the posterior belly of the digastric muscle, and the sternocleidomastoid muscle and inferiorly by the inferior pharyngeal constrictor and thyrohyoid muscles.

The muscular triangle, or inferior carotid triangle, is bounded anteriorly by the midline of the neck, posteriorly and superiorly by the superior belly of the omohyoid muscle, and posteriorly and inferiorly by the sternocleidomastoid muscle.

The posterior triangle of the neck is bounded by the clavicle and the sternocleidomastoid and trapezius muscles. This triangle is divided by the inferior belly of the omohyoid muscle into the subclavian triangle inferiorly and the occipital triangle superiorly.

The occipital triangle is bounded by the sternocleidomastoid muscle, the inferior belly of the omohyoid muscle, and the trapezius muscle.

The subclavian triangle is bounded by the inferior belly of the omohyoid muscle, the sternocleidomastoid muscle, and the clavicle, and inferiorly by the scalene muscles. The components of each triangle are listed in Table 10–1.

Lymphatic Regions of the Neck

According to the anatomic studies of Rouviere[2] and the radiologic studies of Fisch[3] and Reede et al.,[4] the cervical lymphatic system is organized into three functional units: (1) Waldeyer's tonsillar ring, (2) the transitional lymph nodes located between the head and neck, and (3) the cervical lymph nodes, in their proper sense.

The Waldeyer's tonsillar ring consists of the palatine tonsils, lingual tonsil, adenoids, and adjacent submucosal lymphatics. The transitional nodes are arranged in a circular manner at the transition of the head and neck regions and include (1) submental lymph nodes, (2) submandibular lymph nodes, (3) parotid lymph nodes, (4) retroauricular lymph nodes, (5) occipital lymph nodes, (6) retropharyngeal nodes, and (7) sublingual lymph nodes.

The cervical lymph nodes can be divided into superficial and deep nodes, and each of these groups into lateral and medial. The deep lateral cervical lymph nodes are arranged in three chains: (1) the internal jugular vein chain, (2) the spinal accessory nerve chain, and (3) the supraclavicular lymph node chain. The internal jugular nodes and the spinal accessory lymph nodes are divided into upper, middle, and lower nodes. The deep medial cervical group consists of the prelaryngeal, prethyroidal, pretracheal, and paratracheal lymph nodes.

The superficial cervical lymph nodes are divided into a lateral and a medial group. The superficial medial lymph nodes of the neck are distributed around the anterior jugular vein. The superficial lateral cervical nodes are located along the external jugular vein.

Figure 10–2 shows the system for describing the location of lymph nodes in the neck using the levels recommended by the Committee for Head and Neck Surgery and Oncology of the American Academy for Otolaryngology–Head and Neck Surgery.[5, 6]

▮ CYSTS OF THE NECK

Cervical cysts are common occurrences. They are often congenital as a result of aberrations in the normal progression of the development of the head and neck. On other occasions, they may represent benign or malignant neoplastic diseases. In adults, an asymptomatic neck cyst should be considered a malignancy until proven otherwise.[7] With the exception of thyroid nodules and salivary gland tumors, neck masses in adults have the following characteristics: 80%

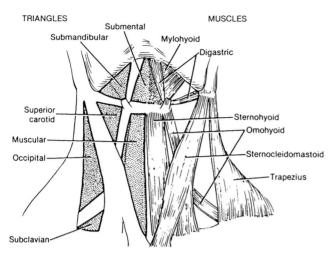

Figure 10–1. Muscles and triangles of the neck.

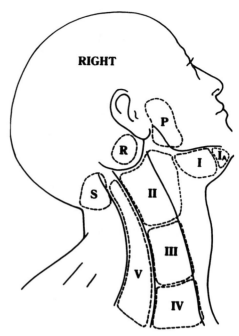

Figure 10–2. Level system for location of cervical lymph nodes. I_A, submental group; I, submandibular group; II, upper jugular group; III, middle jugular group; IV, lower jugular group; V, posterior triangle group. P, parotid, R, retroauricular; S, suboccipital.

of the masses are neoplastic, 80% of the neoplastic masses are malignant, 80% of these malignancies are metastatic, and in 80%, the primary tumor is located above the level of the clavicle.[7]

In contrast, 90% of the neck cysts in children represent benign conditions. In a review by Torsiglier et al.[8] of 445 children with neck masses, 55% of the masses were congenital cysts, 27% were inflammatory, 11% were malignant, and 7% were miscellaneous conditions. Table 10–2 lists the causes of neck masses in the order of frequency with which they occur, according to the age of the patient. Table 10–3 lists the anatomic site, histopathologic characteristics, and differential diagnoses of the most common benign cystic tumors in the neck.[7–12]

Developmental Cysts

Branchial Cleft Cysts, Sinuses, and Fistulas

Branchial apparatus anomalies are lateral cervical lesions that result from congenital developmental defects arising from the primitive branchial arches, clefts, and pouches.

Embryogenesis. The branchial apparatus consists of four pairs of arches separated externally by four paired grooves and internally by four paired pouches.[13] The external grooves are called branchial clefts, and the internal pouches are known as pharyngeal pouches; they are separated by their branchial plates. Each branchial arch is supplied by an artery and a nerve and develops into well-defined muscles, bone, and cartilage. The branchial apparatus undergoes this complex development and differentiation during the third through seventh embryonic weeks. Many anatomic structures develop completely or in part within the branchial apparatus (Table 10–4).[13]

A number of theories exist to explain the genesis of branchial cleft anomalies.[14] The most widely accepted theory is that the rem-

Table 10–1. Contents of Triangles of the Neck

Triangle	Contents
Submental	Submental lymph nodes
	Branches of facial artery and vein
Submandibular	Submandibular lymph nodes
	Submandibular gland and duct
	Hypoglossal and lingual nerves
Carotid	Superior and middle cervical lymph nodes
	Internal jugular vein, common carotid artery and its bifurcation, external carotid artery and superior thyroid, lingual, and its occipital branches
	Hypoglossal and vagus nerves
Subclavian	Inferior cervical lymph nodes
	Thoracic duct on left side, subclavian vein and artery
	Phrenic nerve
Occipital	Posterior superficial cervical lymph nodes
	Parts of the supraclavicular, transverse cervical, greater auricular, lesser occipital, and spinal accessory nerves
Muscular	Infrahyoid strap muscles
	Aerodigestive tract
	Thyroid gland complex

Data from Bielamowicz SA, Storper IS, Jabour BA, et al: Spaces and triangles of the head and neck. *Head Neck* 1994;164:383–388.

Table 10–2. Order of Frequency of Cystic Tumors of the Neck According to Age

Infants and Children	Adolescents	Adults
Thyroglossal ducts cyst	Thyroglossal duct cyst	Metastatic cystic carcinoma
Branchial cleft cyst	Branchial cleft cyst	Thyroglossal cyst
Lymphangioma	Cervical bronchial cyst	Cervical ranula
Hemangioma	Cervical thymic cyst	Branchial cleft cyst
Teratoma and dermoid	Teratoma and dermoid	Laryngocele
Cervical bronchial cyst	Metastatic thyroid carcinoma	Parathyroid cyst
Cervical thymic cyst		Cervical thymic cyst
Laryngocele		
Metastatic thyroid carcinoma		

Data from Maisel RH: When your patient complains of a neck mass. *Geriatrics* 1980;35:3–8; Torsiglier AJ Jr, et al: Pediatric neck masses: Guidelines for evaluation. *Int J Pediatr Otorhinolaryngol* 1988;16:199–210; Park JW: Evaluation of neck masses in children. *Am Fam Physician* 1995;51:1904–1912; Guarisco JL: Congenital head and neck masses in infants and children, part I. *Ear Nose Throat J* 1991;70:40–47; May M: Neck masses in children: Diagnosis and treatment. *Ear Nose Throat J* 1978;57:136–158; and Som PH, et al: Parenchymal cysts of the lower neck. *Radiology* 1985;157:399–406.

Table 10–3. Benign Cystic Neck Lesions

Lesion	Usual Location	Pathology	Main Differentials
Thyroglossal duct cyst	Midline, two thirds below hyoid bone, one fourth off midline, anterior-medial to CA and IJV	Lined by respiratory and/or squamous epithelium, 40% contain thyroid tissue	Dermoid; ranula if suprahyoid; cystic neuroma
First branchial cleft cyst	Medial inferior or posterior to concha and pinna	Type I lined by keratinized stratified squamous epithelium without adnexal structures; lymphoid tissue in majority; type II ectodermal and mesodermal elements	Parotid cyst; dermoid
Second branchial cleft cyst	Lateral neck, unrelated to hyoid, anterior to SCM and lateral to CA and IJV, most present near angle of mandible	Lined by stratified squamous epithelium (90%), respiratory epithelium (8%), or both (2%); lymphoid tissue nodular or diffuse (90%).	Metastatic cystic squamous carcinoma; lateral thyroglossal duct cyst; cystic neuroma
Third branchial cleft cyst	Region of laryngeal ventricle or deep to internal carotid, intimately associated to vagus nerve	Lined by stratified squamous epithelium	Laryngocele; saccular cyst
Cervical thymic cyst	Off midline, lower neck anterior to CA and IJV	Lined by cuboidal, columnar, or stratified squamous epithelium, thymic tissue in wall	Parathyroid cysts; cervical thymoma
Parathyroid cyst	95% near inferior thyroid border, off midline, anterior to CA and IJV	Lined by cuboidal epithelium, parathyroid tissue in wall	Cystic parathyroid adenoma; thyroid cyst; thyroglossal duct cyst
Subcutaneous bronchial cyst	Subcutaneous tissue or skin suprasternal notch, manubrium sterni, skin of lower neck (rarely)	Lined by ciliated, pseudostratified columnar epithelium; smooth muscle and mucous serous glands in wall; rarely, cartilage present.	Dermoid; teratoma; branchial cleft cyst; thyroglossal duct cyst
Dermoid cyst	Near midline, usually in upper neck	Lined by stratified squamous epithelium, numerous ectodermal derivatives	Thyroglossal duct cyst; ranula, if suprahyoid.
Cervical ranula	Off midline and suprahyoid in submental or submandibular triangles	Pseudocyst without epithelial lining; extravasated mucin, histiocytes and mucocytes	Dermoid cyst; thyroglossal duct cyst

CA, carotid artery; IJV, internal jugular vein; SCM, sternocleidomastoid muscle.

nants result from incomplete obliteration of the branchial clefts, arches, and pouches. Lesions may take the form of cysts, sinuses (internal or external), or fistulas. Cystic lesions presumably develop as the result of buried epithelial cell rests. Sinus anomalies have, by definition, a communication with either the external skin surface or the pharyngeal mucosa, and they end as a blind tubular or saccular anomaly within mesenchymal tissue. These anomalies likely arise from incomplete obliteration of part of a branchial groove. Fistulas

Table 10–4. Structures Derived from Branchial Apparatus

Branchial Apparatus	Structures Derived
First	Incus, malleus, sphenomandibular ligament, mandible, anterior two thirds of tongue, sublingual and submandibular glands, eustachian tube, tympanic cavity and membrane, mastoid air cells, and external auditory canal, and contributes to the pinna.
Second	Stapes, styloid process, stylohyoid ligament, part of hyoid bones, stapedius muscle, muscles of expression, part of the base of tongue, and a portion of the auricle, and contributes to the tonsils.
Third	Hyoid bone, tongue, inferior parathyroid glands, and thymus.
Fourth	Thyroid cartilage, epiglottis, muscles of the pharynx, and superior parathyroid glands.

Data from The pharynx and its derivatives. In: Gray SW, Skandalaris R (eds): *Embryology for Surgeons.* Philadelphia: WB Saunders, 1972:15–58; Work WP: Newer concepts of first branchial cleft defects. *Laryngoscope* 1972;82:1581–1593; and Proctor B, Proctor C: Congental lesions of the head and neck. *Otolaryngol Clin North Am* 1970;3:221–248.

suggest complete communication from the ectodermal surface to the endodermal surface and presumably relate to an incompletely closed branchial plate or its rupture.

Despite this seemingly simple concept concerning embryogenesis, a wholly acceptable hypothesis of the origin of branchial anomalies has not been agreed upon. Most theories center around the idea that they originate in salivary gland inclusions in lymph nodes, the branchial apparatus, or, to a lesser extent, the thymic duct.[14] However, most authorities still abide by the branchial duct theory.

Clinical and Pathologic Features. Branchial cleft cysts, fistulas, and sinuses occur with equal frequency in males and females. The precise location and course of these anomalies depend on the particular branchial pouch or cleft from which they are derived. They are bilateral in 2% to 10% of patients, and some may be familial, with the mode of inheritance being an autosomal dominant gene with reduced penetrance and variable expressivity.[15, 16] They generally exist as an isolated phenomenon but in rare instances may be associated with other defects such as patent ductus arteriosus, tear duct atresia, hearing abnormalities, preauricular pits, and malformed auricles.[17] The cysts are usually 2 to 6 cm in diameter and are lined by stratified squamous epithelium (90%), respiratory epithelium (8%), or both (2%).[18] Repeated infections cause the wall to become fibrotic, and the epithelium may then be partially replaced by granulation or fibrous tissue. Lymphoid tissue, either nodular or diffuse, occurs in the wall of 97% of the cysts and often contains germinal centers and subcapsular or medullary sinuses, or both (Fig. 10–3).[18] The contents of the cysts may be cheesey, mucoid, serous, or, if infected, purulent.

First Branchial Cleft Anomalies. The most comprehensive review of these anomalies was published by Olson et al.[19] They reviewed 460 branchial cleft anomalies at the Mayo Clinic; 38 (8%) were of first branchial cleft origin. Of these, 68% were cysts, 16%

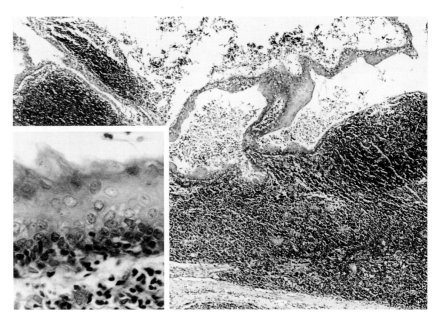

Figure 10–3. Branchial cleft cyst showing abundant lymphoid tissue with germinal centers. The cyst is lined by stratified squamous epithelium *(inset)*.

were sinuses, and 16% were fistulas. These anomalies occur predominantly in females and were found in newborn and geriatric patients. Clinically, they may masquerade as parotid tumors or as an otitis with ear drainage.[20–22]

First branchial cleft disorders are classified into two types.[23] Type I defects are those that embryologically duplicate the membranous external auditory canal and contain only ectodermal elements. Histologically, they are often confused with ordinary epidermoid cysts, as they are lined only by keratinized stratified squamous epithelium unassociated with adnexal structures (hair follicles, sweat glands, sebaceous glands) or cartilage (Fig. 10–4, see p. 655). Characteristically, they are located medially, inferiorly, or posteriorly to the concha and pinna. Drainage from the cyst or fistula may occur in any of these sites. The fistula (or sinus tract) often parallels the auditory canal and ends in a blind cul-de-sac at the level of the mesotympanum. In some instances, parotid tissue may be associated with the tract. The external auditory canal, both membranous and bony, is intact, and hearing is normal.

Type II deformities are composed of both ectodermal and mesodermal elements and therefore contain, in addition to skin, cutaneous appendages and cartilage (Fig. 10–5, see p. 655). This type of defect is thought to represent an embryologic duplication of both the auditory canal and the pinna.[23] Patients with type II defects usually present with an abscess or fistula at a point just below the angle of the mandible. The tract extends upward over the angle of the mandible through the parotid gland, toward the external auditory canal. The tract may end short of or drain into the auditory canal, usually along the anteroinferior border near the cartilaginous-bony junction.[20, 23] Communication of the tract with the middle ear is distinctly uncommon. Type II defects are therefore more intimately associated with the parotid gland than are type I defects.

In some instances, either because of the histology and/or location, a distinction between type I and II lesions cannot always be made. Olson and colleagues therefore suggested that first cleft abnormalities be classified only as to whether the lesion is a cyst, sinus, or fistula.[19] Pathologically, first branchial cleft abnormalities must be differentiated from epidermoid cysts (especially type I), dermoids (especially type II), and cystic sebaceous lymphadenoma.[20]

Second Branchial Cleft Anomalies. These are by far the most common anomalies, accounting for up to 90% of branchial cleft anomalies in some series.[24] The external opening, when present, is usually located along the anterior border of the sternocleidomastoid muscle at the junction of its middle and lower thirds. The tract, if there is one, follows the carotid sheath; it crosses over the hypoglos-

sal nerve, courses between the internal and external carotid arteries, and ends at the tonsillar fossa.[25, 26]

Cysts of the second cleft are three times more common than fistulas.[25, 26] There is no sex predominance. Most patients (75%) are 20 to 40 years old at the time of diagnosis. Because fewer than 3% of cysts are found in patients older than 50 years, pathologists must be careful in making such a diagnosis in this age group; a metastatic squamous cell carcinoma in a cervical lymph node with cystic degeneration may masquerade as a branchial cleft cyst.[27]

Third Branchial Cleft Anomalies. Disorders of this cleft are rare. Cysts, when they occur, present in the region of the laryngeal ventricle and are lined by stratified squamous epithelium.[24] Fistulas open externally along the anterior margin of the lower third of the sternocleidomastoid muscle. If complete, the tract should ascend in relation to the carotid sheath, pass superior to the hypoglossal nerve and inferior to the glossopharyngeal nerve, course behind the internal carotid artery, penetrate the thyrohyoid membrane, and open into the pyriform sinus.[24, 25, 28] Cysts lying deep to the internal carotid artery and intimately associated with the vagus nerve are probably remnants of the third cleft or pouch.[29]

Fourth Branchial Cleft Anomalies. These anomalies remain more of a theoretical possibility than a reality, although one or two cases have been reported. Anomalies would have to have external openings along the anterior border of the sternocleidomastoid muscle in the lower neck, and the tracts would have to descend along the carotid sheath into the chest, passing under either the arch of the aorta on the left or the subclavian artery on the right (both vessels are derived from the fourth branchial arch). They would then ascend in the neck, and their internal openings would be in the esophagus, a fourth branchial pouch derivative.[30–32] Anomalies in this area of the body might be confused with thymic cysts.

Treatment. Complete surgical excision is the only satisfactory method of treatment for these lesions. The lesions are prone to recurrent infection and scarring, rendering dissection tedious and difficult. Any infection should be treated with antibiotics and the area drained before surgical excision is attempted. Aspiration of an uninfected cyst is not indicated, because this may predispose the patient to infection and make dissection more hazardous. The wall of the cyst and the tract may be extremely adherent to adjacent nerves and vessels.

The surgical principles are similar regardless of whether one is dealing with a first, second, or third cleft remnant, although the approaches are different.[24–26]

Branchiogenic Carcinoma

Branchiogenic carcinoma, or primary cervical neoplastic cysts, are of interest mainly from an historical viewpoint. Few, if any, of the purported examples of this entity fulfill the four criteria that Martin[33] considered necessary to establish the diagnosis. These criteria are as follows:

1. The cervical tumor occurs along the line extending from a point just anterior to the tragus to the clavicle, along the anterior border of the sternocleidomastoid muscle.

2. The histologic appearance must be consistent with an origin from tissue known to be present in branchial vestigia.

3. No primary source of the carcinoma should be discovered after at least 5 years of follow-up.

4. There is histologic demonstration of cancer arising in the wall of an epithelial-lined cyst situated in the lateral aspect of the neck.

The fulfillment of these criteria is practically impossible, and the actual existence of the "branchiogenic carcinoma" must remain entirely hypothetical.[34] Batsakis and McBurney[35] have estimated that, even accepting tentative examples of branchiogenic carcinoma, its incidence would be minuscule (0.3% of all malignant supraclavicular neoplasms). There is no doubt that most, if not all, of these lesions are actually cervical node metastases with a cystic pattern. The tonsillar region, or more generally, the anatomic region of Waldeyer's tonsillar ring, is notorious for producing cystic solitary metastases that resemble the usual appearance of branchial cysts.[36] The most recent reviews of the cases published in the literature were made by Cecena et al.[37] and Suarez-Aleaga et al.[38] in 1995.

Thyroglossal Duct Cyst

Among the various developmental neck cysts, the thyroglossal duct cyst is the most common, accounting for up to 70% of such lesions.[9–11]

Embryogenesis. During the fourth week in utero, the thyroid anlage arises in an invagination of endodermal cells of the floor of the pharynx and quickly becomes bilobed as it descends into the neck. During migration, the gland remains connected to the floor of the pharynx (foramen cecum, at the tongue base) by means of a hollow canal, the thyroglossal duct.[39, 40] The thyroglossal tract usually atrophies and becomes obliterated between the fifth and tenth weeks. If involution fails to take place, cysts or sinuses may occur anywhere along the pathway of descent.

Clinical Features. Clinically, approximately 90% of the cysts occur in the midline of the neck,[40] although some may occur paramedianally, most often to the left.[41] Overall, 73.8% occur below the hyoid bone, 24.1% are suprahyoidal, and 2.1% occur intralingually.[40] In a series of 1316 thyroglossal cysts analyzed by Allard,[42] no sex predominance was found. Patients less than 10 years old accounted for 31.5% of the patients in the series. The cysts occurred in patients in their second decade 20.4% of the time. Patients in their 20s made up 13.5% of the total, and 34.6% of the cases occurred in patients older than 30 years. At the time of presentation, 60% of patients had cysts and 40% had sinuses or fistulas, or both.[42] Rarely, thyroglossal duct cysts may be familial.[43]

Cysts may fluctuate in size. Often there are no symptoms except the presence of the mass, unless the cyst becomes infected.[44] Intralingual cysts may cause choking spells, dysphagia, and cough. Fistulas may occur spontaneously or may be secondary to trauma, infection, drainage, or inadequate surgery. The incidence has been estimated at 15% to 34%.[44]

Thyroid scintiscans should probably be obtained on all patients undergoing surgical excision of thyroglossal duct cysts. Despite the fact that a small amount of functioning thyroid tissue is associated with the tract in 30% of cases, it rarely, if ever, represents the only functioning thyroid tissue, as is often true with lingual thyroid cysts.[45, 46]

Pathologic Features. Cysts are usually about 2.4 cm in diameter, but cysts 10 cm in diameter have been recorded.[47, 48] They are lined by respiratory or squamous epithelium, or both, or, if infection has occurred, by granulation tissue or scar tissue (Fig. 10–6, see p. 655).[40] Fistulas are almost invariably secondary to infection. Rare cysts may contain gastric epithelium.

The incidence of finding thyroid tissue in association with thyroglossal remnants varies according to the diligence with which it is sought. In routine sections, it is found in about 5% of cases. When serial sections are examined, thyroid tissue can be found in 40% of specimens.[40] Mucus glands have been identified in 60% of the cases studied by Sade and Rosen.[48] These authors believe the mucus glands to be part of the normal anatomy of the thyroglossal tract and not just glands normally found at the base of the tongue.

Treatment and Prognosis. The treatment of thyroglossal duct remnants, whether cyst, sinus, or fistula, is complete surgical excision using the Sistrunk operation.[49] This consists of a block excision of the entire thyroglossal tract to the foramen cecum, as well as removal of the central 1 to 2 cm of the hyoid bone. If this procedure is employed, the rate of disease recurrence is less than 5%.[40] If the central hyoid bone is not removed, a disease recurrence rate as high as 25% may be expected.[50]

Rare reports of malignancy in thyroglossal duct remnants are found in the literature. Eighty percent of neoplasms are papillary thyroid carcinomas; those remaining are predominantly follicular carcinomas or squamous carcinomas.[51–55] Criteria for diagnosis include, preferably by microscopic examination, the demonstration of a thyroglossal remnant and a normal thyroid gland. Because of the paucity of cases and the fact that the malignancy is not recognized until after complete pathologic examination of the remnant, it is difficult to delineate treatment and prognosis. Most researchers agree, however, that (1) total thyroidectomy is not routinely indicated as long as there are no palpable abnormalities in the gland and no significant scintiscan findings, and (2) the Sistrunk operation probably offers a reasonable chance of cure.[51–55]

Cervical Thymic Cyst

Cervical thymic cysts are morphologically identical to their mediastinal counterpart.[56] They are found in the anterior triangle of the neck along the normal path of descent of the thymus, with or without parathyroid glands, and they may have a fibrous band or a solid thymic cord connection to the pharynx or mediastinum.

Embryogenesis. The thymus originates from the third branchial pouches in the sixth week of development. Thymic tubules rapidly elongate and descend along the thymopharyngeal tracts until they fuse in the midline at 8 weeks. Migration continues inferiorly until the thymus rests in the superior mediastinum at 12 weeks.[57] It is believed that most cervical thymic cysts arise from remnants of the thymopharyngeal duct that failed to involute.[57, 58]

Clinical Features. Cervical thymic cysts are virtually never recognized as such clinically; most are confused with branchial cleft cysts and, less often, with thyroglossal cysts and laryngoceles. The most common presenting symptom is a slowly enlarging mass that may or may not be painful.

The cysts occur more often on the left side; males are affected twice as often as females.[58] Sixty-seven percent occur in patients in the first decade. The remainder occur in patients in their second and third decades.[56, 59, 60] Cervical thymic cysts characteristically occur adjacent to or within the carotid sheath and therefore present in or near the anterior cervical triangle. They can be found anywhere from the angle of the mandible to the sternum, paralleling the sternocleidomastoid muscle and the normal embryologic pathway of the thymus.[61] Cysts containing both thymus and parathyroid may be referred to as third pharyngeal pouch cysts.

Pathologic Features. Grossly, the cysts are round to tubular and can measure more than 7 cm in the greatest dimension. The epithelial lining may be composed of columnar, cuboidal, or stratified squamous cells (Fig. 10–7, see p. 656). In some areas, it may be re-

Text continued on page 663

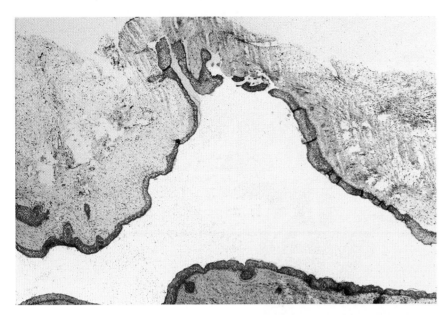

Figure 10–4. Type I first branchial cleft abnormality. Stratified squamous epithelium is lining the cavity. Note the absence of adnexal structures.

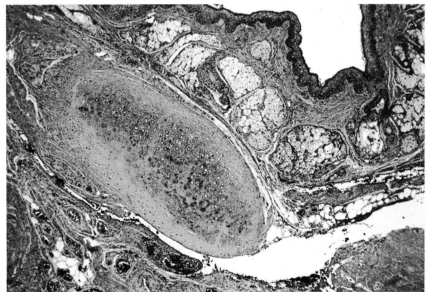

Figure 10–5. Type II first branchial cleft abnormality. Note the presence of skin adnexal structures and cartilage.

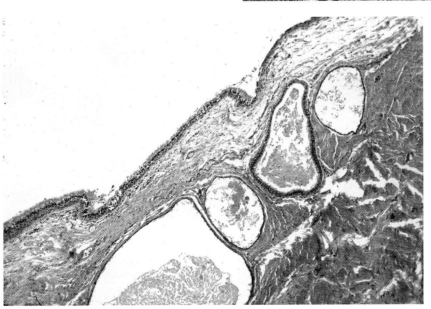

Figure 10–6. Thyroglossal duct cyst lined by ciliated columnar epithelium. Note mucous glands in the wall.

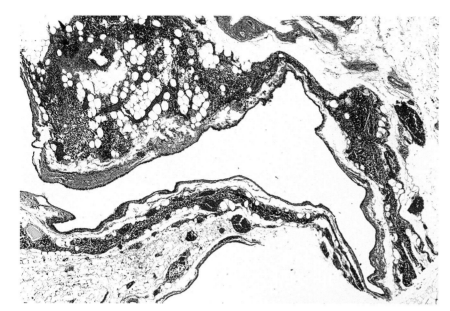

Figure 10–7. Cervical thymic cyst lined by cuboidal epithelium. Note thymic tissue in wall.

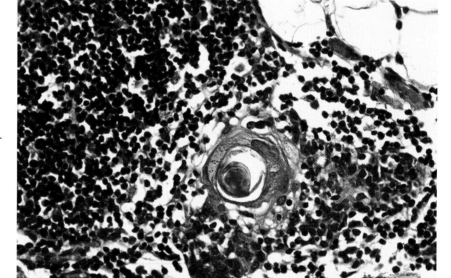

Figure 10–8. High-power view of a Hassall's corpuscle in the wall of a cervical thymic cyst.

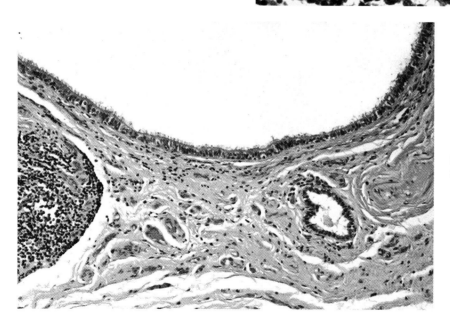

Figure 10–9. Cervical bronchial cyst. Respiratory epithelium lines the cyst.

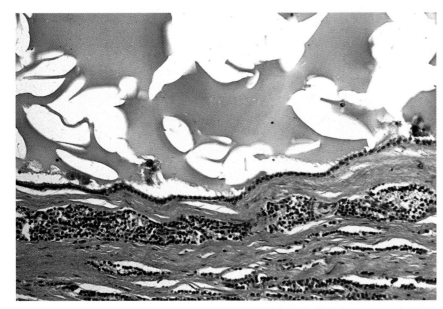

Figure 10–10. Parathyroid cyst. Cuboidal epithelium lines the cyst. Note parathyroid tissue in the wall.

Figure 10–11. Dermoid cyst. Note cavity lined by squamous epithelium and dermal adnexa in wall.

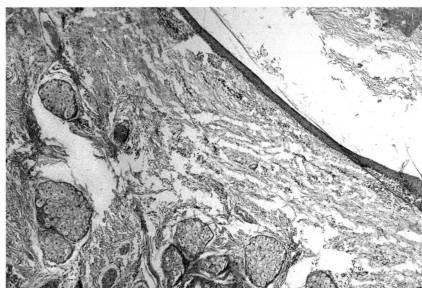

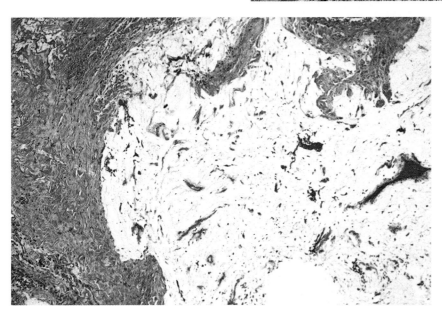

Figure 10–12. Plunging ranula exhibiting mucus in connective tissue.

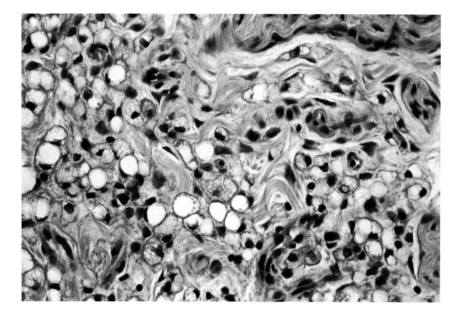

Figure 10–13. Plunging ranula. Note mucocytes in vascularized connective tissue.

Figure 10–14. Cavernous lymphangioma. Dilated lymphatic channels are present. Some of the channels have smooth muscle in their walls.

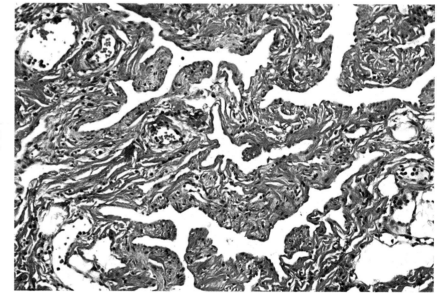

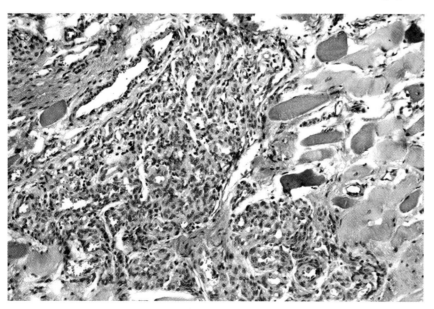

Figure 10–15. Intramuscular capillary hemangioma. Note capillary-sized vessels with plump endothelial cells lining small vascular spaces.

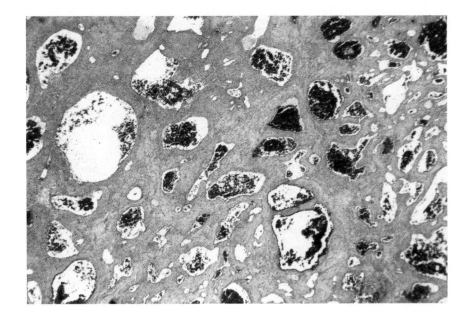

Figure 10–16. Cavernous hemangioma. Large vessels are lined by bland endothelium.

Figure 10–18. Mature teratoma showing mesodermal (cartilage), endodermal (respiratory glands), and ectodermal (skin) derivatives.

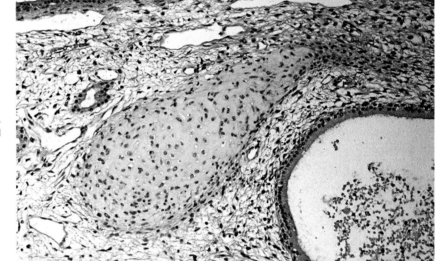

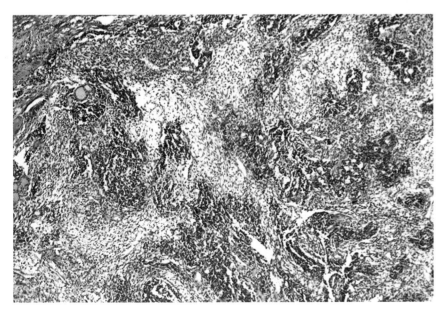

Figure 10–19. Immature teratoma composed of primitive neuroectodermal tissue.

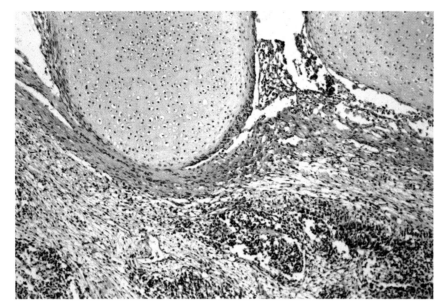

Figure 10–20. Malignant teratoma showing immature cartilage, clusters of neuroepithelium, and spindle cells.

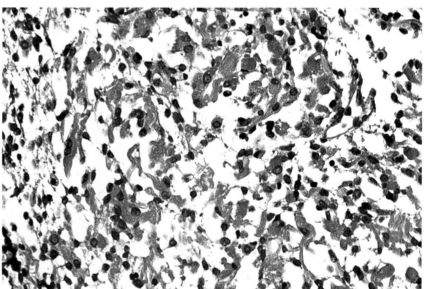

Figure 10–21. High-power view of myogenous elements (the spindle cells shown in Figure 10–20). Note cross-striations.

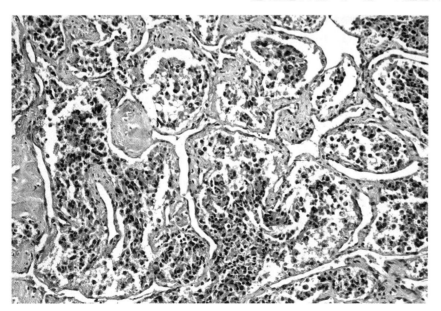

Figure 10–22. Carotid body paraganglioma showing prominent Zellballen pattern.

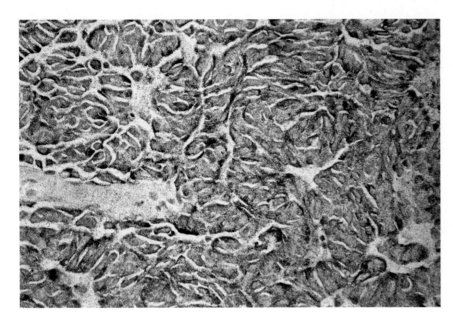

Figure 10–24. Vagal body paraganglioma with black argyrophil granules in cytoplasm of tumor cells (Gremelius stain).

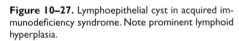

Figure 10–27. Lymphoepithelial cyst in acquired immunodeficiency syndrome. Note prominent lymphoid hyperplasia.

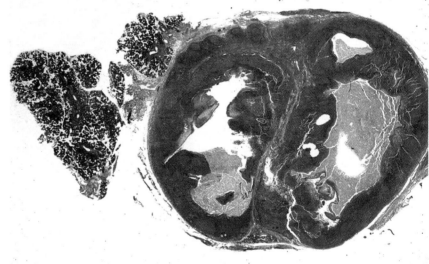

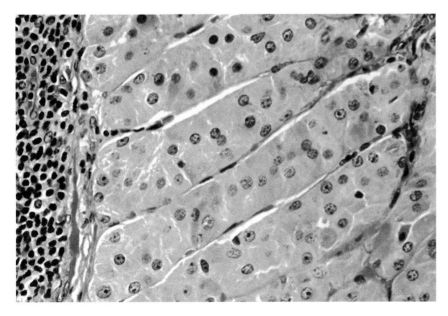

Figure 10–29. Oncocytoma in lymph node.

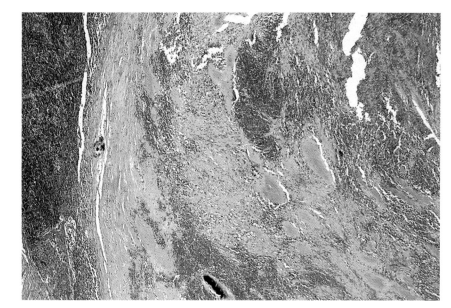

Figure 10–30. Low-power view of intranodal myofibroblastoma in submandibular lymph node.

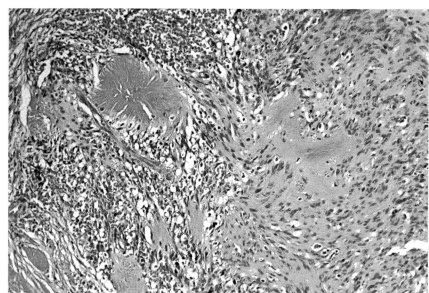

Figure 10–31. High-power view of intranodal myofibroblastoma in submandibular lymph node showing amianthoid fibers.

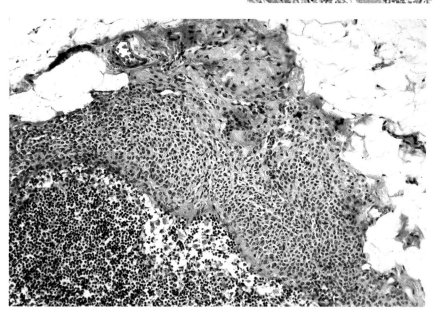

Figure 10–32. Benign nevus cells in capsule of submandibular lymph node.

placed by granulation or fibrous tissue, and on occasion, cholesterol clefts are present.[58] Thymic tissue found in the cyst wall will qualify the cyst as a thymic cyst. However, numerous sections may be required to identify the thymic tissue (Fig. 10–8, see p. 656). Parathyroid tissue may or may not be present. The cysts have no malignant potential, but a benign papillary adenoma has been described.[62]

Treatment. Complete surgical excision is the treatment of choice.

Cervical Bronchial Cyst

Bronchial cysts are uncommon congenital lesions found predominantly in the thoracic cavity, within the lung, or in the mediastinum. In some instances, they may present clinically in the neck.[63]

Embryogenesis. Bronchial cysts are derived from small buds of diverticula that separate from the foregut during the formation of the tracheobronchial tree. When they occur outside the thoracic cavity, the cysts presumably arise from erratic migration of sequestered primordial cells.[64]

Clinical Features. Most cervical bronchial cysts are present in the skin and the subcutaneous tissue of the suprasternal notch. Rarely, they are found in the lower anterior neck, the chin, or the shoulder.[63–65] They are more common in males than in females by a ratio of 3:1.[64] The cysts usually become clinically apparent at or soon after birth and appear as asymptomatic nodules that slowly increase in size. Draining sinuses that exude mucoid material are present in about one third of the cases.[63] The cysts become more conspicuous when Valsalva's maneuver is performed.

Pathologic Features. Noninfected cysts are grossly tubular rather than of an ovoid configuration, and they are filled with either clear serous or thick mucoid material. The cyst wall is thin, and the inner surface is smooth or trabeculated.

The bronchial cyst is lined by ciliated, pseudostratified, columnar epithelium (Fig. 10–9, see p. 656). Squamous stratified epithelium often makes up the lining of the sinus, but this epithelium rarely lines the cyst unless the cyst is infected. The cyst wall contains smooth muscle, elastic fibers, and mucoserous glands.[63, 64] Cartilage is seldom present in cervical cysts, although it is common in their intrathoracic counterparts. Lymphoid tissue, when present, is scanty and focal but never diffuse and excessive.

Differential Diagnosis. A bronchial cyst can be distinguished from a teratoma by the complete absence of tissues other than those that can be explained on the basis of a malformation of the respiratory tract. A dermoid cyst can be excluded by the lack of hair and skin appendages and the absence of squamous epithelium. The presence of smooth muscle, mucoserous glands, and cartilage (should it be found) and the paucity of lymphoid tissue eliminate the possibility of a branchial cleft cyst. A thyroglossal duct cyst can be differentiated from a bronchogenic cyst if thyroid follicles are found. Furthermore, a thyroglossal duct cyst does not contain smooth muscle or cartilage.[64] The lack of ciliated epithelium separates lateral cervical cysts containing gastric mucosa from cervical bronchogenic cysts.[66]

Treatment. Complete surgical excision along with its sinus tract is curative.[63, 64] Malignancies have not been described in cervical bronchial cysts.

Parathyroid Cysts

Parathyroid cysts are rare lesions that have a surgical incidence rate of 0.001% to 3% and that constitute 0.6% of all thyroid and parathyroid lesions.[67] The anterior cervical triangle is the site of most parathyroid cysts that present as neck masses.[67–69] The cysts may be functional, but the majority are nonfunctional.[67]

Embryogenesis. The cause of parathyroid cysts is not clear, and a variety of theories have been proposed. That the cysts are embryologic remnants of the third and fourth branchial clefts or result from coalescence of multiple microscopic cysts, degeneration of a parathyroid adenoma, or retention of glandular secretions have been

suggested. No single theory adequately explains all cases. It may be that those cysts with clear, colorless fluid are developmental in origin, whereas the cysts with bloody or straw-colored fluid may result from infarction or cystic degeneration of a parathyroid adenoma.[67] These latter lesions tend to be functioning cysts.[67]

Clinical Features. Most patients with parathyroid cysts present with asymptomatic low anterior neck masses. Tracheal and esophageal compression, hoarseness secondary to recurrent laryngeal nerve compression, and pain secondary to hemorrhage into the cyst have been reported.[67–69] About 95% of the cysts occur below the inferior thyroid border, and 65% are associated with the inferior parathyroid glands.[67] However, cysts have been identified from the angle of the mandible to the mediastinum, and they can occur in the thyroid lobe or posterior to it.[67]

There appear to be two distinct groups of parathyroid cysts: nonfunctioning and functioning.[67] The nonfunctioning cysts make up the majority of cases and are about two to three times more common in women than they are in men. The mean age of the patients is 43.3 years. Nonfunctioning cysts occur almost exclusively in the inferior parathyroid glands.[68] The functioning cysts account for 11.5% to 30% of the cases,[70] are more common in men by a ratio of 1.6:1, and tend to occur in sites other than the inferior parathyroid glands, from the angle of the mandible to the mediastinum.[70] The mean age of these patients is 51.9 years. Most patients with functioning cysts have signs and symptoms of hyperparathyroidism, but the disease can be clinically occult and may be discovered only by finding abnormal serum calcium and phosphorus levels or elevated serum parathyroid hormone (PTH) levels.[67] Multiple parathyroid cysts have been reported in patients with hyperparathyroidism, and rarely, a multiloculated cyst can occur.[70]

Fine-needle aspiration is the principal diagnostic tool. Aspiration of clear fluid with an elevated parathyroid hormone level is a definite indication of a parathyroid cyst. The C-terminal/midmolecule of the parathyroid hormone should be assayed, because the N-terminal-specific assay is frequently associated with false-negative results.[69]

Pathologic Features. The cysts vary from 1 to 10 cm in diameter. They are usually grayish-white, translucent, and unilocular with a thin membranous capsule. The inner surface is smooth and may contain small, light brown areas.

Histologic studies show that a parathyroid cyst's wall is usually formed by a solitary layer of compressed cuboidal or low columnar epithelium, with either chief cells or oxyphil cells present in the fibrous wall (Fig. 10–10, see p. 657). Some cysts may not have any identifiable parathyroid tissue. Even in these cases, however, a diagnosis can be established by testing the cyst fluid.[67, 69]

The presence of lymphoid tissue and the stratified squamous epithelium lining the cyst would help distinguish those unusual branchial cleft cysts with parathyroid tissue from parathyroid cysts.[71]

Treatment. Aspiration may be curative, but persistence or recurrence of the cyst is a sign that surgical removal is in order.[69] Functional cysts are associated with a high risk of other parathyroid gland abnormalities such as hyperplasia or adenoma.[67]

Dermoid Cysts

Histogenetically and histologically speaking, the term *dermoid cyst* should be reserved for a cystic neoplasm that originates from the ectoderm and mesoderm; endoderm is never found.[72] The head and neck area is a common site of occurrence for dermoid cysts; this area accounts for 34% of these cysts.[73–77] Other sites include the ovaries and the central nervous system. Dermoid cysts of the head and neck are located most often in the subcutaneous tissues.[76]

Embryogenesis. The positions of these dermoid cysts at the midline and along the lines of embryonic fusion of the facial processes are consistent with origin by inclusion of ectodermal tissue. Such inclusions would take place along lines of closure at junctions of bone, soft tissue, and embryonic membranes.

Clinical Features. Dermoid cysts of the head and neck may occur in people of almost any age. More than 50% are detected by the time a person is 6 years old, and approximately one third are present at birth.[74] The distribution between sexes is approximately equal. The cysts may range in size from a few millimeters to 12 cm in diameter. Dermoid cysts in the neck are rare but can account for close to one fourth (22%) of midline or near-midline neck lesions.[77] They have been reported in the upper neck, near the thyroid cartilage, and as low as the suprasternal notch. These cysts usually grow slowly and do not cause pain. On palpation, the cysts are soft to fluctuant.

Pathologic Features. Microscopically, this developmental cyst is lined by stratified squamous epithelium supported by a fibrous connective tissue wall. Numerous ectodermal derivatives may be seen, including dermal adnexa such as hair follicles, sebaceous glands, and sweat glands (Fig. 10–11, see p. 657).

Treatment. Complete surgical excision is required, after which there is little risk of recurrence.

Miscellaneous Cysts

Mucoceles, ranulas, and laryngoceles are considered miscellaneous cysts. Ranulas are actually pseudocysts: they lack an epithelial lining. However, because they mimic true cysts histopathologically as well as clinically or radiographically, it is reasonable and convenient to include them in a general discussion of cystic lesions. Mucoceles are discussed in the chapter on pathology of the salivary glands.

Ranula

A ranula can be defined as a mucous extravasation from a traumatized sublingual gland or duct; the lesion extends into the soft tissues of the floor of the mouth above the mylohyoid muscle. There are two types of ranula: simple (or intraoral) and deep (or plunging).[78] The latter are referred to as cervical ranulas because they invade downward into the tissues of the neck. Both variants affect males and females of any age, including neonates.[79] Although these pseudocysts are generally unilateral, isolated instances of bilateral simple or deep ranulas have been documented.[80, 81] Although similar, each type of ranula has a distinctive clinical appearance and behavior. The simple ranulas are more thoroughly discussed in the chapter dealing with the pathology of the oral cavity.

Plunging or Cervical Ranula

A plunging or cervical ranula appears as a soft, usually asymptomatic swelling in the submandibular or sublingual triangle, with or without evidence of a cystic lesion in the floor of the mouth.

Cervical ranulas invade the neck either posteriorly, in which case they lie lateral to the lingual nerve or to Wharton's duct and may displace the submandibular gland, or through the mylohyoid muscle.[82] One of every three people is thought to have discontinuities of the mylohyoid muscle. Thus, the ranula often has ready access to the neck through the floor of the mouth.[83]

Clinical Features. A painless, soft, ballotable neck mass is the most common clinical presentation of a ranula. Parapharyngeal extension may be present. Many sizes of cervical ranulas have been seen at the time of treatment. Usually located above the hyoid bone and in the submental or submandibular region, the lesions may extend deeply into the neck to the supraclavicular region and upper mediastinum or posteriorly to the skull base.

Pathologic Features. Most ranulas, whether oral or cervical, are pseudocysts with no epithelial lining. Mucus extravasated from the sublingual glands enters the soft tissues and dissects fascial planes. The histologic appearance of the ranula varies with time.[83] Ranulas with a short clinical history and without prior intervention manifest loose, vascularized connective tissue surrounding a collection of mucin; microscopically, a ranula resembles a bursa or even an angioma (Fig. 10–12, see p. 657). Histiocytes and so-called mu-

cocytes lie in the cyst walls and may be dominant in some areas, as seen in histologic sections. The extreme clarity of the cytoplasm of these cells may lead to a mistaken diagnosis of clear cell carcinoma (Fig. 10–13, see p. 658). Over time, the mucin, histiocytes, and mucocytes become less prominent, and the appearance of the ranula is that of a dense, well-vascularized, fibrous pseudocyst. Chronic or acute inflammatory cells are never conspicuous in any stage of the ranula's development.

Differential Diagnosis. The plunging ranula may mimic other cystic or glandular swellings, for example, dermoid and epidermoid cysts, thyroglossal duct cysts, or cystic hygromas.[81, 82] Quick and Lowell[84] have pointed out that no specific clinical diagnostic tests are available to distinguish between these lesions. Submandibular sialograms may show displacement of the gland by an intrinsic mass, whereas plain radiographs or xeroradiographs may demonstrate merely a soft tissue mass of undetermined nature. Consequently, a definitive diagnosis is dependent on postoperative histopathologic evaluation of the surgical specimen.

Treatment and Prognosis. The management of these lesions requires removal of the sublingual gland and excision of the ranula; thus, a 0% recurrence rate is achieved. Excision of only the ranula was followed by a 25% recurrence rate, whereas marsupialization had a 36% recurrence rate.[79, 85]

Laryngocele

A laryngocele is a dilatation of the laryngeal saccule, which is filled with air. It is a rare condition. Stell and Maran[86] calculated that laryngoceles occur in about 1 in 2,500,000 people per year in the United Kingdom. From the published literature, laryngoceles appear to be most common in white people, and far more common in men; the ratio of men to women with this lesion is about 7:1. The most common age incidence is in the fifties. Most laryngoceles are unilateral.[86–90]

Three types of laryngoceles have been described:

1. An internal laryngocele is confined to the interior of the larynx, extending into the paraglottic region of the false vocal cord and the aryepiglottic fold. Internal laryngoceles are discussed in the chapter dealing with the pathology of the larynx.

2. An external laryngocele extends and dissects superiorly through the thyrohyoid membrane and is intimately associated with the superior laryngeal nerve. This type of laryngocele is labeled external because it frequently presents as a mass lateral to the thyrohyoid membrane.

3. A combined internal-external laryngocele has both internal and external components existing simultaneously.

External or combined internal-external laryngoceles may present with a cervical mass adjacent to the thyrohyoid membrane. About half of all laryngoceles are represented by the mixed type. Stell and Maran[86] found the external type to be the second most common, but the work of Canalis et al.[87] shows the internal type to be the second most common.

Factors that increase intralaryngeal pressure, such as coughing, straining, or blowing wind instruments, are said to foster the development of laryngoceles. Presumably, the gradual weakening of the laryngeal tissues during aging is contributory. Laryngoceles are an occupational hazard of professional glassblowers. Whether the neck of the saccule acts as a one-way valve, allowing the entrance of air but preventing its egress, is controversial.[88] Clearly, such a mechanism might be operative when laryngoceles are associated with neoplastic or inflammatory processes that partially obstruct the ventricular opening.

Clinical Features. Many laryngoceles are discovered incidentally when radiographs of the neck or endolaryngeal examinations are done because related symptoms are present. Such symptoms include hoarseness, cough, and the sensation of a foreign body in the throat. An external or combined laryngocele may present as a cervical mass adjacent to the thyrohyoid membrane. If large enough, internal or combined laryngoceles may cause airway distress.[86, 87]

Diagnosis is most easily established by indirect laryngoscopy and soft-tissue radiography. Internal and combined laryngoceles appear as submucosal masses in the region of the false vocal cord and the aryepiglottic fold. With the use of a flexible fiberoptic laryngoscope, these masses may be seen to enlarge when Valsalva's maneuver is performed.

Pathologic Features. On gross examination of the undissected larynx, a laryngocele may appear as a bulge of the lateral supraglottic mucosa or as a bulge lateral to the aryepiglottic fold. When the larynx is sliced transversely, it is seen that the bulge represents an air-filled dilatation of the saccule, which communicates with the mucosal surface of the larynx via the ventricle. An internal laryngocele is confined to the interior of the larynx and extends posterosuperiorly toward the false vocal cord, into the aryepiglottic fold. An external laryngocele extends superiorly by bulging out above the thyrohyoid membrane; the "internal" portion of the saccule remains of normal size. The protrusion of the dilated saccule through the thyrohyoid membrane takes place where the superior laryngeal nerve, artery, and vein penetrate that membrane. The mixed type of laryngocele shows features of both external and internal types. Histologic studies of the laryngocele wall show the lining to be composed of respiratory epithelium in all cases. Like the normal saccule lining from which it is derived, this epithelial surface may be somewhat papillated, although many laryngoceles have lost this feature of the saccular epithelium, presumably because of distension and stretching. There is a variable degree of chronic inflammation beneath the epithelium and the fibrous lamina propria.

Should the communication between a laryngocele and the laryngeal lumen become obstructed, fluid may accumulate within the sac. If mucus is found, a more appropriate term for the anomaly is a *laryngomucocele;* and if pus is found, it is called a *laryngopyocele.*[91] Should a laryngocele become completely filled with fluid, it is difficult to distinguish from a saccular cyst.

Carcinoma of the larynx has been associated with unilateral laryngoceles.[92, 93] In autopsy series, the incidence varies from 2% to 18%. Laryngoceles may be bilateral in cases of carcinoma of the larynx as well. This association mandates a careful examination of the larynx to rule out the presence of a neoplasm in all cases of laryngoceles in adults.

Treatment. Many surgeons favor the external lateral neck approach in the surgical management of virtually all laryngoceles, citing the improved exposure, minimal morbidity, and reduced chance of recurrence associated with this approach.[94]

Cystic Neoplasms

Cystic Hygroma and Lymphangioma

Cystic hygroma and lymphangioma represent the two ends of the spectrum of histologic classification of lymphatic lesions.[95] Whether these are true neoplasms or represent malformations or hamartomas is still debated, but this issue is of no clinical consequence. These lymphatic lesions may be divided into three morphologic types: capillary (lymphangioma circumscriptum), cavernous (lymphangioma cavernosum), and cystic (cystic hygroma).[96]

Cystic hygroma and lymphangiomas are not common. Bill and Sumner[95] reported on 61 patients with these lesions seen at a children's hospital during a 25-year period. The frequency was an average of only five cases for every 3000 admissions per year. In a series of 152 benign tumors of the neck, only four (2.6%) lymphangiomas were found.[97]

Embryogenesis. These lesions are thought to arise from sequestration of portions of the primitive embryonic anlage or as areas of localized lymphatic stasis caused by congenital blockage of regional lymphatic drainage.[95]

Clinical Features. A review of several series indicates that about 50% of these cysts are present at birth and 75% to 90% are present by a child's third year.[97–103] In most series, there was either no significant sex difference or a very slight male prevalence.[97–99] In general, symptoms relate to pressure caused by the painless, enlarging mass. Cystic hygromas and cavernous lymphangioma may grow progressively at variable rates or remain static. They occasionally regress and sometimes even spontaneously disappear. Their size may vary considerably, at times being massive. Neck asymmetry is cosmetically disturbing. Most lesions are cystic or wormy upon palpation.

Capillary, or simple, lymphangioma (lymphangioma circumscriptum) is clinically the least significant of the three types. This type usually is confined to the superficial skin and less conspicuously in the deep dermis, where small vesicle-like lesions are formed.[100] These lesions are usually asymptomatic, but they may be seen in conjunction with the other two forms of neoplasm.

The separation of cavernous lymphangioma from cystic hygroma is valid only in the clinical sense, as histopathologically the lesions are similar.[95] On gross examination, the distinctive pattern that separates the two is primarily based on the location and the quality of the surrounding soft tissues. In the neck, these tissues are loose and permit expansion, and this lymphatic tumor will expand into the typical multicystic appearance of a hygroma.

Cystic hygroma is most common in the neck and is frequently found in the posterior triangle lying behind the sternocleidomastoid muscle. It is less common in the anterior cervical triangle.[97, 101–104] However, as a hygroma enlarges, it may extend into the anterior compartment, upward into the cheek or parotid region, or down into the mediastinum or axilla.[98]

Lymphangiomas occur in a variety of body locations, including the retroperitoneum, mesentery, inguinal region, extremities, mediastinum, and within viscera.[101] The head and neck region, however, accounts for between 40% and 70% of all lesions. Das Gupta[101] lists four series of cavernous lymphangiomas totaling 151 cases, with 61 (40.4%) involving the head and neck. Van Cauwelaert and Gruwez reviewed 453 reported cases of lymphangioma.[102] The neck was involved in 39% and the head in 20% of these cases.

Pathologic Features. Simple lymphangiomas, or lymphangioma simplex, are composed of capillary-like lymphatic vasculature. Cavernous lymphangiomas are composed of dilated lymphatic channels with or without an adventitial layer. Cystic hygromas or cystic lymphangiomas contain large multilocular cysts.

Cavernous lymphangioma and cystic hygroma are histologically very similar and consist of dilated, thin-walled sinuses that are filled with eosinophilic, acellular lymph fluid. These sinuses are lined by one or more layers of flat endothelial cells.[96] The spaces range in size from capillary to cavernous. The intervening stroma may be quite scanty, with closely packed channels, or it may be more abundant, with the spaces separated by stroma. The stroma varies from a loose, myxomatous, lace-like material to areas with dense hyalinization. When there has been previous infection, the amount of stroma is markedly increased. Scattered lymphoid aggregates are also found, occasionally in the form of germinal follicles, and wisps of smooth muscle fiber may also be present (Fig. 10–14, see p. 658). In 61 tumors described by Bill and Sumner,[95] 21 appeared without cystic spaces, 23 were composed of large cysts only, and 17 had a combination of small cavernous spaces and large cysts.

The form and structure of the lymphatic tumor is probably related to the anatomic location. Cystic hygromas arise in areas with defined fascial planes and loose connective tissue that allows for the expansion of individual cysts and their insinuation into surrounding structures. Lymphangiomas are found in regions with more compact anatomy, with muscle fibers or glandular tissue interlocking with superficial tissues, such as the parotid gland, tongue, or floor of the mouth.

Treatment and Prognosis. The best approach to these lesions is surgery in which as wide an excision as possible is made while preserving appearance and function.[102–104] They are radioresistant, and the use of radiation therapy in infants and young children is to be avoided whenever possible. Despite the benign nature of these lesions, surgical management is difficult, especially in cavernous lymphangioma, because of its tendency to spread along vital structures and the subsequent high incidence of recurrence. Harkins and

Sabiston[103] reported that 88 operations were required in 27 patients with cavernous lymphangioma. Watson and McCarthy[104] reported a 41% recurrence rate (17 of 41 patients) in their series of cases of cavernous lymphangioma, whereas only 1 (7%) of 14 patients with cystic hygromas experienced recurrence. De Serres et al.[105] recently proposed a staging system for lymphatic malformations of the head and neck to be used to predict the outcome of surgical treatment. Stage I patients had unilateral infrahyoid disease and a 17% incidence of complications overall. Stage II patients had unilateral suprahyoid disease and 41% incidence of complications. Stage III patients had unilateral suprahyoid and infrahyoid disease and a complication rate of 67%. Stage IV patients with bilateral suprahyoid disease had a complication rate of 80%, while stage V patients with bilateral suprahyoid and infrahyoid disease had a 100% incidence of complications.

Hemangioma

Hemangiomas of the face and neck are most often congenital. They are the most common tumors of infancy and early childhood. These lesions may be intracutaneous, subcutaneous, both intracutaneous and subcutaneous, or intramuscular. Visceral involvement may occur in the larynx, oral cavity, and salivary glands. In roughly three quarters of the patients, hemangiomas are present at birth, and in close to 90% of patients, the lesions have manifested by the first year of life. Most of these lesions involute spontaneously by the time a child is 7 years old.

Hemangiomas are classified histologically as capillary, cavernous, or mixed/cellular, based on the size of the proliferating vascular spaces.[96] Because infiltrative hemangiomas may assume any of these forms, no significant prognostication can be made for these patients on the basis of the tumor's histologic appearance alone.[106]

Embryogenesis. The exact nature of these vascular tumors is not known, but it is likely that the majority are hamartomas rather than neoplastic growths.

Clinical Features. The biologic behavior of particular hemangiomas varies according to the clinical presentation, and it is thus appropriate to discuss the clinical characteristics of these lesions. Edgerton and Hiebert's clinical classification of benign vascular tumors is the most widely accepted system (Table 10–5).[107]

The neonatal staining hemangioma is a blue or pink area of discoloration, generally located in the posterior midline of the scalp, neck, or sacrum. Present at birth, the lesion gradually disappears after several months.

According to Edgerton and Hiebert,[107] intradermal hemangiomas present two clinical variants. Frequently present at birth, these hemangiomas are pink to purple and tend to have a sensory nerve distribution, for instance, the trigeminal nerve. The salmon patch variety is faintly pink to rust in color, is flat on the skin surface, and

Table 10–5. Classification of Benign Vascular Lesions

I. Hemangioma
   A. Neonatal staining
   B. Intradermal capillary
      Salmon patch
      Port-wine stain
   C. Juvenile
      Strawberry mark
      Strawberry capillary
      Capillary cavernous
II. Arteriovenous fistula
   Congenital
   Traumatic or acquired
   Cirsoid
III. Angiomatous syndromes

Data from Edgerton MT, Hiebert JM: Vascular and lymphatic tumors in infancy, childhood, and adulthood. A challenge of diagnosis and treatment. *Curr Probl Cancer* 1978;2:4–43.

does not spontaneously regress. Location and size are the determinants for treatment, to which the salmon patch is notoriously resistant. Port-wine stains are darker in color, are present at birth, and do not expand significantly with time.

Juvenile capillary hemangiomas characteristically manifest a complete or partial spontaneous resolution. They may be present at birth or appear during the first few weeks of life. The three major clinical varieties are the strawberry mark, the strawberry capillary hemangioma, and the capillary-cavernous hemangioma.

The strawberry mark occurs approximately once in every 100 live births. It is generally present at birth and consists of a pale halo of depigmented skin (1 to 4 cm in diameter) surrounding a core of telangiectasis. Nearly all strawberry marks spontaneously disappear, but a few develop into strawberry mark en plaque.

The strawberry capillary hemangioma is also a common lesion and is often present at birth as a tiny red spot. Rapid growth during the next 3 to 6 months is common. This raised and circumscribed hemangioma usually involutes when a child is between 1 and 4 years old.

Capillary-cavernous hemangiomas are also usually present at birth and frequently extend to the deep dermis and subcutaneous tissues. Between the first and sixth months of age, the growth of these lesions often accelerates markedly. The lesions may become quite large, causing deformity of the involved part. Resolution can occur, but it is usually only partial.[108]

Pathologic Features. Hemangiomas vary greatly in their gross and microscopic appearances, depending on whether they are capillary, cavernous, or of mixed type, and in many cases it is not possible to conclusively classify these types because they are all part of the same histologic spectrum.[109–112] In general, hemangiomas of the capillary type, especially the juvenile subtype, are the most likely to be confused with a malignant tumor. They are composed of a myriad of capillary-sized vessels with plump endothelial cells lining vascular spaces that have small inconspicuous lumina (Fig. 10–15, see p. 658). In most areas, well-developed lumen formation is apparent, although occasionally the tumor may have a solid cellular appearance. In some cases, there may be mitotic activity, intraluminal papillary tufting, and a proliferation of vessels within perineural spaces. None of these features is indicative of malignancy in these neoplasms.[106, 109, 110]

The cavernous form of hemangioma is easily recognized as a benign vascular tumor. These tumors are composed of large vessels lined by bland, attenuated endothelium that seldom shows a significant degree of pleomorphism (Fig. 10–16, see p. 659).

Electron microscopy and immunohistochemistry studies can be helpful in defining the vascular nature of these tumors. Solid nests of endothelium are surrounded by basal lamina and are encircled by a cuff of pericytes. More mature areas, of course, display canalization of the vessels. Weibel-Palade bodies may be present but tend to be scarce in less mature areas (Fig. 10–17).

Factor VIII-associated protein, Ulex europaeus agglutinin, and CD31 can be identified within the cellular hemangiomas of infancy but are often not apparent in the solid or immature-appearing areas, and they only become significant in the well-canalized portions of the tumor.[113]

Differential Diagnosis. It is most important in the differential diagnosis to distinguish capillary hemangioma from angiosarcoma. Capillary hemangiomas, whether deep or superficial, do not develop the freely anastomosing sinusoidal pattern encountered in most well-differentiated angiosarcomas, nor do they possess nuclear pleomorphism and hyperchromatism. In addition, the location of the lesion is important. Most superficial angiosarcomas are located in the scalp of elderly patients, and angiosarcoma of the deep soft tissues is quite rare; therefore, a vascular tumor of skeletal muscle is statistically more likely to be benign than malignant.

Treatment and Prognosis. There is no consensus about the treatment of cutaneous hemangiomas and some mucosal hemangiomas of infants and children. According to Margileth,[114] "spontaneous involution of the juvenile hemangiomas was reported 82 years

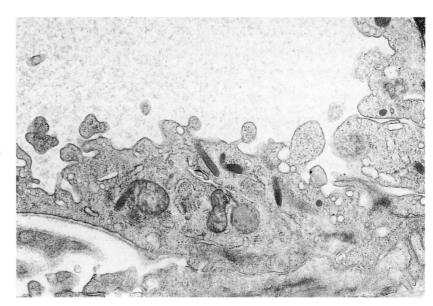

Figure 10–17. Weibel-Palade bodies may be present in mature areas of hemangiomas.

ago and has been documented in nearly 2500 children." Illing-worth[115] reports that very few (2%) of these hemangiomas require active therapy. It is also generally thought that hemangiomas that grow larger in the first few months of life and then cease to grow before the patient is 1 year old usually involute. In contrast, hemangiomas that do not actively enlarge early in the life of the patient usually do not involute, and flat hemangiomas are less likely to involute than raised ones.

Therapy is required in some cases of congenital hemangiomas, but in any treatment program, the frequency and extent of involution associated with that lesion should be taken into consideration. Conservation is the therapeutic mandate. Such management requires patience and perseverance on the part of both the physician and the parents of the patient, but will be justified by the ultimate results.[107, 114, 115]

Infiltrative Hemangiomas

Although a conservative approach is appropriate for the management of superficially located hemangiomas of the skin and soft tissues, the more deeply seated (subcutaneous, intramuscular, and deep fascial) hemangiomas manifest a locally infiltrative growth that poses therapeutic difficulties. These hemangiomas can occur in both children and adults, are usually either capillary or cavernous in type, and may be quite resistant to various modalities of treatment, as shown by the Mayo Clinic experience.[109] Intramuscular hemangiomas are a distinct type that presents in skeletal muscles (see Fig. 10–15). They constitute less than 1% of all hemangiomas and occur most often in the trunk and extremities. Approximately 14% of these lesions are found in the head and neck, and the masseter and trapezius muscles account for more than half of the reported cases.[109, 110] Capillary and cavernous types predominate, and approximately 20% of these lesions will recur after treatment.

Teratoma

Teratomas are neoplasms composed of elements from each of the three germ layers (ectoderm, mesoderm, and endoderm). These tumors may arise in a variety of sites. The most common location in infancy is the sacrococcygeal region, which accounts for nearly 40% of the total cases. Other sites include the gonads, head and neck, mediastinum, retroperitoneum, body wall, brain, spinal cord, and liver.[116] Cervical teratomas represent only about 3% of all teratomas.[117] In the head and neck region, lesions are also found in the central nervous system, orbit, temporal fossa, oropharynx, nasopharynx, nasal cavity, palate, and tonsil.[118]

Teratomas arising in the cervical region are rare. Although they were previously divided into those arising from the thyroid gland and those arising elsewhere, this distinction has not proved to be clinically useful. The most significant clinical marker divides the tumors presenting in infancy or early childhood from those presenting after the first decade of life. The former group primarily exhibits benign clinical behavior. However, such lesions are associated with a high mortality rate at the time of birth, generally because the airway and pulmonary function are compromised. The latter group is composed of tumors that are usually smaller and more likely to be malignant.[113]

Various systems of classification for teratomas have been advanced. The majority of these were considered by Gonzalez-Crussi,[119] who presented a tentative new classification system for all teratomas that does not rely on the primary site of occurrence of the tumor (Table 10–6). This classification system, which incorporates many of the guidelines brought forth by Norris et al.[120] for the grading of ovarian teratomas, appears to be an excellent compromise and has been recommended by most authors.

Embryogenesis. The exact origin of teratomas is not yet known, although numerous theories have been presented. These include the germ cell theory, the embryonic cell theory, the unifying hypothesis theory, the extraembryonic cell theory, the included-twin hypothesis, and the fetus-in-fetu theory. Gonzalez-Crussi[119] recently discussed these theories in considerable detail.

Clinical Features. Cervical teratoma presents clinically as a mass in the neck that is usually discovered at birth.[121–125] Live-born infants commonly experience acute respiratory distress, including stridor, apnea, and cyanosis, caused by compression of the trachea by the tumor mass. It is important to recognize teratomas of the neck early; surgery can often save the life of the infant, especially when esophageal and tracheal obstruction are present.

Most congenital cervical teratomas are diagnosed antenatally, often by ultrasonographic studies.[126, 127] The frequent practice of routine ultrasonographic examination has decreased the incidence of unexpected lesions at delivery. Polyhydramnios is associated with approximately 20% of all cases and is more likely to occur in larger lesions.[122, 127]

More than 90% of cervical teratomas occur in neonates or infants[116–118] and are rare in patients older than 1 year. These tumors appear with similar frequency in both males and females; and in the United States, cervical teratomas appear to have equal incidence among white and black populations.[121–124]

Cervical teratomas in adults are extremely rare. Fewer than 20 tumors, including tumors originating in the thyroid, have been described.[128, 129] In contrast to the pediatric cervical teratomas, a cer-

Table 10–6. Classification of Teratomas

I. Benign teratomas
  A. Mature teratoma
    Grade 0 (all component tissues appear well differentiated)
    Grade 1 (occasional microscopic foci contain incompletely differentiated tissues, not exceeding 10% of the sampled surface)
  B. Immature teratoma, benign
    Grade 2 (immature tissues make up 10% to 50% of the sampled tumor surface)
    Grade 3 (over half the surface examined is composed of undifferentiated tissues of uncertain metastatic potential; a benign course is still possible)
II. Malignant teratomas
  A. Areas of germ cell tumor
    Germinoma (seminoma, dysgerminoma)
    Embryonal carcinoma
    Choriocarcinoma
    Yolk sac tumor
    Mixed (any combination of the above)
  B. Nongerminal malignant tumor pattern
    Carcinoma
    Sarcoma
    Malignant embryonal tumor
    Mixed
  C. Immature teratoma, malignant
    Teratoma that would otherwise be classified as benign, immature teratoma, but which subsequently became metastatic

Data from Gonzalez-Crussi F: Extranodal teratomas. In: *Atlas of Tumor Pathology,* 2nd series, fascicle 18. Washington, DC: Armed Forces Institute of Pathology, 1982.

vical teratoma in an adult should be considered malignant until proven otherwise. These tumors have occurred in men and women whose ages ranged from 23 to 77 years.

Pathologic Features. Grossly, these tumors are usually cystic, but they can be solid or multiloculated. They are commonly encapsulated, lobulated masses that measure up to 15 cm in the greatest dimension.[119]

Microscopically, the teratomas occurring in the neck region are similar to those found in other anatomical regions. Skin, skin appendages, fat, glial tissue, smooth muscle, cartilage, bone, minor salivary glands, respiratory and gastrointestinal epithelium, and areas of more immature or embryonal tissue may be present (Fig. 10–18, see p. 659). It is exceedingly important to adequately sample all potentially teratomatous tumors. Specifically, solid areas with necrosis should be carefully examined. It is not unusual to find, in teratomas throughout the body, small foci of malignant germ-cell tumors, especially endodermal sinus tumor or choriocarcinoma. The presence of the latter two tissue types will adversely affect patient prognosis. Such tissue types are unusual in head and neck teratomas. It is also important for the pathologist to recognize that the more immature fetal tissues have malignant potential (Fig. 10–19, see p. 659).[130] Patients whose tumors have extensive areas of immature tissue require close clinical follow-up. Congenital teratomas at all sites in the body tend to follow benign clinical behavior, whereas those presenting after early childhood often follow a malignant course. Although most of the sacrococcygeal teratomas present at birth are benign, a significant percentage (25%) are malignant. Cervical teratomas in the neonate are almost always benign, whereas the few reported cases of cervical teratoma arising in adults were malignant (Figs. 10–20 and 10–21, see p. 660).[128, 129]

To the best of our knowledge, only seven cases of congenital cervical teratoma with metastasis have been reported.[131] Resection seems to offer the best control in cases with aggressive biologic behavior.

Treatment. Most authors strongly favor operative management of teratomas.[126, 131] As Gundry et al.[132] noted in their review, the mortality rate for surgical cases was 15%, compared with 80% for those cases managed without resection.

Paragangliomas

Paragangliomas are neoplasms of neural crest origin that arise in several extra-adrenal locations. In the head and neck, they may arise from the carotid body, vagal body, and jugulotympanic paraganglia. Less commonly, paragangliomas can involve the orbit, nose, nasopharynx, and larynx.[133] In this section, we discuss only neoplasms of the carotid body and intravagal paraganglia.

Carotid Body Paraganglioma

Carotid body paragangliomas are the most common tumors of the head and neck paraganglia, making up 60% to 70% of the tumors of this type.[133–138] They are uncommon neoplasms. Lack et al.[133] found 69 paragangliomas (0.12%) of the head and neck in more than 600,000 operations, and only 1 in 13,400 autopsies at Memorial Hospital in New York City.

Embryogenesis. Paraganglionic tissue of the head and neck is embryologically derived from the neural crest. It develops in the paravertebral region in association with the arterial vessels and cranial nerves of the ontogenetic gill arches and is associated with the autonomic nervous system.[134]

Clinical Features. A painless neck mass located beneath the anterior edge of the sternocleidomastoid muscle just lateral to the tip of the hyoid bone is the most common clinical manifestation of a carotid body tumor. Some series show the tumor to be more common in female patients, whereas others describe an almost equal incidence among males and females.[133–138] The mean age of patients is between 43 and 51 years, but this tumor can be found in people of any age.

The reported incidence of multicentric paragangliomas ranges from 10% in the nonfamilial type to as high as 50% in the familial variety.[139, 140] These tumors have been noted in association with medullary carcinoma of the thyroid and in patients with neurofibromatosis.[141]

On physical examination, it is possible to move the carotid body tumor from side to side, but not in a vertical direction, and the tumor may transmit the arterial pulse.[133–138] The diagnosis can almost always be established preoperatively by selective angiography, which shows a vascular mass at the carotid artery bifurcation.[136, 137]

Pathologic Features. Grossly, the tumors are partially encapsulated and firm. They are reddish gray to brown in a cut section. They vary in size from 2 to 9 cm in diameter, with an average diameter of 4 cm.

Shamblin and associates[142] have described three classes of carotid body tumors. Group I tumors are small and easily dissected from the adjacent vessels. Group II tumors are more adherent and partially surround the vessel. Group III tumors are large and adhere intimately to the entire circumference of the carotid bifurcation. In Group I tumors, small, often asymptomatic lesions can usually be resected without injury to the underlying vessel. Group II lesions are less easily dissected and occasionally produce symptoms. They are amenable to careful surgical excision, but the surgeon must be prepared for a bypass should resection be necessary. Group III lesions often produce symptoms, and these lesions can incarcerate the carotids and make resection and replacement of the artery necessary.

Microscopically, the prevailing histologic pattern is that of epithelioid cells arranged in distinct clusters (Zellballen) separated by a prominent capillary network (Fig. 10–22, see p. 660). The Zellballen are round to oval and vary slightly in size within each tumor. The cell nests are set off by reticulin fibers. In addition to a Zellballen pattern, the cells can be arranged in ribbons or cords that are divided and compressed by extensive fibrous bands.

Chief cells are the predominant cell type; they vary from ovoid to polyhedral with a moderate amount of pale eosinophilic granular cytoplasm. Areas of spindle cells with a sarcomatoid appearance may be found; other areas are highly vascular and resemble an angioma or hemangiopericytoma. Mitotic figures are uncommon. Most tumor cells have a bland appearance, but it is not uncommon to find scattered pleomorphic cells with hyperchromatic nuclei.

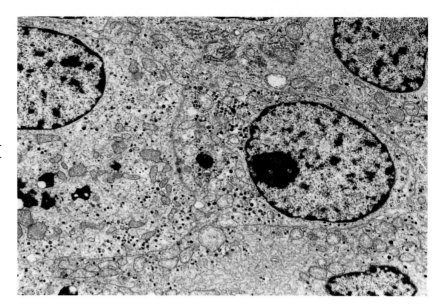

Figure 10–23. Carotid body paraganglioma with cytoplasmic processes showing electron-dense, membrane-bound neurosecretory granules.

Electron microscopy studies show the tumor cells to contain neurosecretory granules (Fig. 10–23).[134] Light microscopy studies reveal cells that are argyrophilic but argentaffin-negative by silver staining (Fig. 10–24, see p. 661).

In an immunohistochemical study of 29 paragangliomas of the head and neck, of which nine were carotid body tumors, Johnson et al.[143] found that all carotid body paragangliomas stained strongly for neuron-specific enolase, synaptophysin, and chromogranin A. Warren et al.[144] found that their nine carotid body tumors stained intensely for neuron-specific enolase and that some contained a variety of hormones including serotonin, leu-enkephalin, substance P, vasoactive intestinal peptide, gastrin, somatostatin, vasopressin, melanocyte-stimulating hormone (MSH), and calcitonin.

Fewer than 10% of carotid body paragangliomas are reported to be malignant.[145] The only reliable criterion for establishing the diagnosis of malignancy is the presence of local lymph node, distant metastases, or extensive local invasion.[133, 146] Locally aggressive tumor growth is probable if two or more of the following are present: central necrosis of the Zellballen, invasion of vascular or lymphatic spaces, or the presence of mitotic figures.[133]

Differential Diagnosis. Although histologic findings are generally quite distinctive, the differential diagnosis of paragangliomas of the head and neck may include endocrine neoplasms arising from the thyroid (medullary carcinoma) or parathyroid glands and other poorly differentiated carcinomas.[143] Less commonly, alveolar soft-part sarcoma, granular cell tumor, or melanoma are included in the differential diagnosis.[143]

Treatment and Prognosis. Surgical therapy is the essential method of treatment for carotid body paragangliomas.[136, 137] If the neoplasm is completely excised, recurrence is rare, occurring in about 10% of cases.[136–137] Radiation therapy may be useful as a palliative method for those rare carotid body paragangliomas that cannot be controlled by surgical means.[135]

Intravagal Paraganglioma

Intravagal paraganglioma is the third most common paraganglioma of the head and neck after the carotid body and glomus jugulare tumors.

Embryogenesis. These tumors arise from small dispersed collections of paraganglia that follow the cervical course of the vagus nerve, particularly at the level of the jugular and nodal ganglia. However, intravagal paragangliomas may be located at any point along the cervical path of the vagus nerve.[133]

Clinical Features. These lesions are more frequent in women than in men, and in about 10% to 15% of the cases, multiple tumors

have been noted. Patient ages parallel those for carotid body lesions, with the mean age being approximately 50 years old, with a range of 18 to 71 years old.[147, 148] The tumor usually manifests itself as a painless neck mass located behind the angle of the mandible. This type of tumor not infrequently bulges into the pharynx and produces dysphagia.

The tumor's closeness to the nerves at the base of the brain produces neurological symptoms including weakness of the tongue, vocal cord paralysis, hoarseness, and Horner's syndrome.

Intravagal paragangliomas can be clearly distinguished from carotid body tumors arteriographically because they usually lie above the carotid bifurcation and cause anterior displacement of the vessels without widening of the bifurcation point.

Pathologic Features. Grossly, intravagal paragangliomas appear well circumscribed, but they may extend upward into the base of the skull and range from 2.0 to 6.0 cm in diameter.

They are histologically similar to carotid body tumors, except that they are often traversed by dense fibrous bands that represent the residual vagal perineurium. The cells do not stain for chromaffin, but stains for argyrophilic granules are positive.[134] Ultrastructurally, the tumors contain chief cells that show a gradation in cytoplasmic density similar to the light and dark cells of the carotid body. The chief cells contain dense core neurosecretory granules, some of which have a more elongated or "pleomorphic" appearance than those of a carotid body tumor.[133, 147]

Treatment and Prognosis. Surgery is the treatment of choice for intravagal paragangliomas. Local infiltration of vagal body tumors and extension into the cranial vault represent significant problems in disease control. Vagal body tumors occasionally metastasize, with the rate of metastasis estimated at 16%.[148, 149]

In the review by Chaudhry,[147] 13 of 72 (18%) intravagal paragangliomas had metastasized (only 4 of these to distant sites), whereas the remainder involved only the regional lymph nodes.

Cervical Salivary Gland Neoplasms

Heterotopic salivary gland neoplasms arising in cervical lymph nodes may resemble cervical cysts. These are uncommon neoplasms, and the pathologist may confuse them with metastatic salivary gland tumors.[150, 151]

Embryogenesis. As early as the sixth week of intrauterine life, a complex anatomic relationship exists in the 16 mm embryo between the parotid analogue and the developing system of upper cervical lymph nodes. Proximity and contact of these anlagen explain both the entrapment of salivary tissue within lymph nodes and the development of lymph nodes within the parotid gland.[152] The role of these ectopic islands of salivary gland tissue within the lymph nodes in the pathogenesis of lymphoepithelial cysts and some neoplastic lesions has been considered by several authors.[152]

Clinical Features. This type of neoplasm presents as a painless mass, often cystic, located in the periparotid region, the upper neck, or the anterior cervical triangle. Occasionally, however, these tumors have been described in the lower neck.[153] In the series reported by Zajtchuk et al.[150] and Luna and Monheit,[151] the age of the patients ranged from 10 to 81 years old with a mean of 45 years. Females were affected more commonly than males in a ratio of 3:1.

Pathologic Features. The tumors that most often arise in ectopic salivary gland tissue in the lymph nodes are Warthin's tumor and sebaceous lymphadenoma, which are most often found within intraparotid lymph nodes and less often within extraglandular lymph nodes. Rarely, other types of salivary gland tumors arise within lymph nodes, including mixed tumors, membranous adenomas (dermal analogue tumors), acinic cell carcinomas, and mucoepidermoid carcinomas.[150-155] The morphology of the neoplasms is identical to their intrasalivary gland counterparts.

Treatment and Prognosis. Surgical excision is the treatment of choice. In malignant tumors, excision of the adjacent major salivary gland may appear to be the appropriate treatment to define the site of the primary tumor, because malignant salivary gland tumors located within lymph nodes suggest metastatic disease. Their prognosis is similar to tumors arising in the major salivary glands.

Miscellaneous Lesions

Other neoplasms that may appear as cervical cysts are cystic neuromas and cervical thymomas. Neuromas, especially when they are large, can undergo cystic degeneration. In the neck, the most common locations of those neuromas is along the course of the vagus nerve or the cervical sympathetic chain.[156]

Cervical thymomas are noteworthy principally for their unusual location, and this feature alone may cause difficulties in the pathologic assessment of the excised tissues.[157, 158] It has been postulated that these neoplasms arise either from ectopic thymus or remnants of branchial pouches that retain the potential to differentiate along the thymic line.[157] These rare tumors that occur in the soft tissues of the neck show complete or partial histologic resemblance to thymus tissue (fetal, mature, or involuted) and to mediastinal thymomas. They are classified as being of one of four types: ectopic hamartomatous thymoma; cervical thymoma; spindle epithelial tumor with thymus-like differentiation (SETTLE); or carcinoma showing thymus-like differentiation (CASTLE). Of these, the first is benign and the second can be locally aggressive.[157] The third and fourth types of neoplasm are malignant.

Infectious processes often simulate cervical cysts. Such infections can be bacterial,[159] fungal,[160] parasitic,[161] or viral[162] in nature. Cholesteatoma, amyloidosis, and carotid artery aneurysms have been reported to simulate cervical cystic masses.[163-165]

▮ UNKNOWN PRIMARY TUMOR

A cervical mass is frequently the first clinical manifestation of a tumor in the head and neck region. Cervical lymph node metastasis is the presenting symptom in almost 50% of all nasopharyngeal carcinomas, in 28% of carcinomas of the tonsils, in 23% of carcinomas of the base of the tongue, in 23% of thyroid carcinomas, and in 17% of carcinomas of the hypopharynx.[166-167] In 85% to 90% of patients presenting with metastatic disease in a cervical node, the primary tumor site will be found after a thorough physical, radiologic, and endoscopic examination.[168] However, in 10% to 15% of patients, a primary tumor will not be found despite a detailed examination. It is difficult to evaluate the frequency of these cervical metastases of unknown origin relative to the total number of patients with tumors of the upper respiratory and digestive tracts. It varies between 2.6% and 9% according to larger series.[166, 169-172]

Clinical Features

Metastatic cervical disease in the absence of a primary tumor is most frequently seen in patients who are between the fifth and sixth decades of life. The average patient is 60 years old. Disease is seen more commonly in men than in women by a ratio of 4:1.[173-180] The patients are usually consumers of alcohol or tobacco or both. Seventy percent of patients present with a unilateral, single affected lymph node measuring more than 3 cm in diameter. Twenty percent of patients have unilateral multiple affected lymph nodes, and 10% have bilateral multiple affected lymph nodes. The most common locations are the upper jugular lymph nodes, followed by midjugular and supraclavicular nodes.[176, 179, 180]

The site of adenopathy is important because the lymphatic drainage of an enlarged node may provide a clue to the location of the primary tumor (Table 10–7).[168, 173, 181–184] However, not all tumors will metastasize according to these rules, and the possibility of an unusual metastatic pathway has to be considered in the differential diagnosis.[182] Lymph nodes located in the supraclavicular fossa are the likely targets for metastases from tumors located below the clavicle; the most common sites of such a primary tumor are the lungs, the breast, the gastrointestinal tract, and the genitourinary tract.[168, 174, 181, 185]

The Search for a Primary Tumor

A careful and systematic clinical investigation that focuses on detecting the primary tumor site is mandatory in all patients who present with metastatic cervical adenopathy. The identification of the primary tumor is important for several reasons. Instead of irradiating all mucosal surfaces from nasopharynx to hypopharynx, radiation portals may be focused on the site of the primary tumor, and thus morbidity from radiation treatment can be significantly reduced. In addition, radiation will not control every occult primary tumor, and in fact, the late appearance of a primary tumor cannot be ruled out.[186]

A physical examination that includes a detailed medical history with information about possible skin cancers treated in the past and a complete otorhinolaryngologic examination must be done as the first step in the search for a primary tumor. If the primary tumor is found, a biopsy sample of the lesion should be obtained. Under the

Table 10–7. Probable Site of the Primary Tumor According to the Location of Cervical Metastases

Location of Nodes	Primary Tumor Site
Submental	Anterior floor of mouth, anterior tongue, lip
Submaxillary	Anterior floor of mouth, anterior tongue, retromolar trigone, glossopalatine pilar, skin lateral face
Jugulodigastric	Lateral and posterior tongue, epipharynx, nasopharynx, palate, tonsil, larynx
Midjugular	Epipharynx, oropharynx, base of tongue, larynx
Low jugular	Thyroid, epipharynx, base of tongue, larynx
Supraclavicular	Lung, thyroid, gastrointestinal, genitourinary
Upper posterior	Nasopharynx
Low posterior	Nasopharynx, thyroid

Data from Batsakis JG: The pathology of head and neck tumors: The occult primary and metastases to the head and neck, part 10. *Head Neck* 1981;3:409–423; de Braud F, et al: Metastatic squamous cell carcinoma of an unknown primary localized to the neck. Advantages of an aggressive treatment. *Cancer* 1989;64:510–515; Berg T, Torelmalm NG: Cervical and mediastinal lymph node as an otorhinolaryngeal problem. *Ann Otol Rhinol Laryngol* 1969;78:663–670; Coker DD, et al: Metastases to lymph nodes of the head and neck from an unknown primary site. *Am J Surg* 1977;134:517–522; Lindberg R: Distribution of cervical lymph node metastases from squamous cell carcinoma of the upper respiratory and digestive tract. *Cancer* 1972;29:1446–1449; and Molinari R, et al: A statistical approach to detection of the primary cancer based on the site of neck lymph node metastases. *Tumori* 1977;63:267–282.

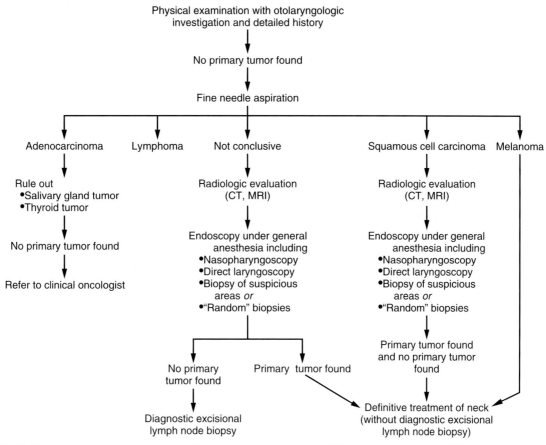

Figure 10–25. Algorithm for evaluation of patients with an unknown primary tumor. CT, computed tomography; MRI, magnetic resonance imaging.

assumption that a suspicious node is positive for disease, the surgeon may definitively treat the neck without performing an excisional node biopsy.

If no primary tumor is found, further investigations according to the algorithm (Fig. 10–25) are necessary. Fine-needle aspiration (FNA) biopsy is a rapid, inexpensive, and safe procedure that can be done at the time of the patient's first presentation and immediately after a regional physical examination.[187, 188] FNA usually gives a reliable diagnosis when squamous cell carcinoma is present, although for the diagnosis of malignant lymphoma or undifferentiated carcinoma the results will not be sufficient. In large series in which FNA biopsy specimens of cervical node tissue have been studied, the procedure has given reliable results with false-positive and false-negative rates of less than 1% and less than 3%, respectively.[189, 190] Computed tomographic (CT) or magnetic resonance imaging (MRI) studies are helpful not only with respect to the staging of the cervical adenopathy but also in detecting elusive primary tumors that spread submucosally.[191–195] In addition, CT and MRI scans may reveal suspicious areas, of which biopsy samples may then be selectively obtained under general anesthesia. Therefore, CT or MRI scans, or both, should be done before biopsies. If no suspicious lesions are detected, "random" biopsy samples have to be taken from the most probable sites of occult primary tumors, namely the nasopharynx, the base of the tongue, the piriform sinus, and the tonsils.[168] If no primary tumor is found after all of the procedures described in the algorithm (see Fig. 10–25), and the patient has squamous cell carcinoma cells in the FNA sample, the surgeon can proceed to treat the neck without excisional biopsy of the enlarged node. An excisional biopsy of an enlarged node for histologic diagnosis should only be done if the results of all examinations listed in Figure 10–25 are negative and the FNA biopsy has been inconclusive or if the patient is young and there is a high likelihood of lymphoma.

A physician's reluctance to perform an excisional biopsy is based on the fact that the procedure may increase the risk of inducing tumor spread.[184, 196] The high morbidity of the procedure[197] and the hindrance of subsequent therapy because of scarring or vascular impairment[184, 198, 199] are also reasons for caution. However, not all authors agree on the detrimental effect of pretreatment biopsy. In several studies, no differences in recurrence of neck disease or in survival time were found between patients who underwent pretreatment open biopsy and patients who had biopsies at the time of definitive treatment, but the results concerning distant metastases have been contradictory.[199–201] Finally, the physician must remember that the application of proper oncologic, radiotherapeutic, and surgical techniques is probably more important than the effect of a pretreatment biopsy.[180, 198, 201] Ancillary studies include chest and paranasal radiographs, barium given orally, mammography, and radioisotope scans of the thyroid gland. Fluorodeoxy-glucose-labeled positron emission tomography has given promising results with respect to localization of primary tumors, but this new modality is still under evaluation.[202]

Especially in patients with a diagnosis of nonkeratinizing or undifferentiated carcinoma in a lymph node, measurements of Epstein-Barr virus antibody titers may be beneficial in defining occult nasopharyngeal carcinoma. The most specific antibodies for this disease are IgA antibodies to viral capsid antigen and IgG antibodies to early antigen, which may be elevated in the presence of a small primary tumor.[203, 204]

Medullary carcinoma of the thyroid gland may cause elevated basal or post-provocative calcitonin levels, even if the lesion is microscopically small.[205–206]

Unilateral screening tonsillectomy has been recommended by Malissard and Forcard[207] and Righi and Sofferman[208] as a productive procedure in patients with neoplastic enlargement of upper jugular and midjugular nodes. These authors located a primary tumor in the tonsils in 30% of the patients with an occult primary tumor. The histologic findings in the tonsillectomy specimen have given additional credit to this procedure, because the tumors have been shown to arise from crypts and spread submucosally rather than along the surface. Thus, such tumors may remain undetected in biopsy specimens taken from the mucosal surface.[208]

Pathology

Gross and Microscopic Findings

The gross appearance of a metastasis is only important when present in a cystic node, because in cystic metastases, the primary tumor is most frequently located in the palatine tonsils or in Waldeyer's ring.[36, 177, 195]

Histologically, 80% to 85% of all cervical metastases from an unknown primary tumor are squamous cell carcinomas. In order of decreasing frequency, undifferentiated carcinoma, adenocarcinoma, thyroid carcinoma, melanoma, sarcoma, and salivary gland carcinoma make up the other metastatic types.[175, 176, 179, 182, 199] However, the frequency of each histologic type varies with the location of the involved nodes; in the low cervical and supraclavicular area, the percentage of adenocarcinomas increases.[179] Separate evaluations of supraclavicular lymph nodes have revealed 30% to 40% metastatic adenocarcinomas.[174, 184, 185, 209, 210] In this location, the primary adenocarcinoma is found (in order of decreasing frequency) in the lung, the breast, the stomach, the prostate, the ovary, or the colon and rectum.[181] In contrast, metastatic adenocarcinomas in the upper cervical region most likely originate from the paranasal sinuses, especially the ethmoid sinus.[168]

The histologic appearance of a given metastasis will usually not allow a conclusion concerning the origin of the occult primary tumor. Only in undifferentiated carcinoma of nasopharyngeal type and in thyroid carcinoma does the histologic appearance of the metastatic lesion suggest the location of the primary tumor. Histochemical stains are of limited value because glycogen and, to a lesser extent, mucin can be found in many tumors.

Electron Microscopy, Immunohistochemistry, Molecular, Cytogenetics, and Other Special Studies

More than 80% of all cases can be diagnosed using tissue sections stained with hematoxylin-eosin, which reliably indicate the presence of squamous cell carcinoma. In poorly differentiated or undifferentiated tumors, immunohistochemical studies should be used for further classification.[211, 212] The precise identification of tumor lineage is especially important with respect to chemotherapy-sensitive or even curable neoplasias such as malignant lymphomas, germ-cell tumors, sarcomas, or neuroendocrine tumors.[213, 214]

First, epithelial and nonepithelial tumors should be distinguished by application of antibodies to cytokeratin. Cytokeratin-negative cases should then be investigated with antibodies to leukocyte-common antigen to demonstrate or rule out malignant lymphoma. The importance of this reaction is reflected by the fact that 30% to 70% of all tumors diagnosed as poorly differentiated neoplasms were identified as malignant non-Hodgkin's lymphomas in retrospective immunohistochemical investigations.[215–217] If the reactions for both cytokeratin and leukocyte-common antigen are negative, staining for S100 protein and HMB-45 antigen can be applied for the diagnosis of malignant melanoma. Cytokeratin-positive cases should additionally be investigated with antibodies to S100 protein and actin to rule out a salivary gland tumor, and antibodies to thyroglobulin and calcitonin are needed for the diagnoses of follicular and medullary carcinoma of the thyroid.[206, 218] Carcinoma of the prostate, may present with cervical adenopathy, especially of the left side, and should be considered as a possible primary tumor in male patients with adenocarcinoma.[219, 220] The diagnosis can be confirmed by the use of antibodies to prostate-specific antigen (PSA). However, the physician should remember that positivity for PSA may occasionally be found when salivary gland tumor tissue is tested.[221] Chromogranin stains and punctate perinuclear keratin staining are helpful in identifying neuroendocrine tumor lineage.

In cases of undifferentiated and nonkeratinizing metastatic carcinoma, the presence of Epstein-Barr virus may be verified by either in situ hybridization or polymerase chain reaction studies. Both methods provide a very high degree of sensitivity and specificity when used to identify the virus in nasopharyngeal carcinomas and their metastases.[222–225]

Demonstration of estrogen receptors in a metastatic adenocarcinoma should not be interpreted as reliable evidence of a breast tumor or a gynecologic tumor as the primary tumor. Indeed, estrogen receptors may be found not only in adenocarcinoma from many other sites, including tumors of salivary gland and thyroid gland origin, but also in brain tumors, malignant melanomas, and sarcomas.[226] When immunohistochemical staining is inconclusive, demonstration of specific ultrastructural features such as neuroendocrine granules, premelanosomes, surface microvilli, intracellular lumina, or tonofilaments by electron microscopy may contribute to the correct classification.[227]

With advances in cytogenetic and molecular genetic analyses and increased availability of DNA hybridization and polymerase chain reaction, investigations focusing on the identification of specific genetic changes may gain importance, especially with respect to patients with an unknown primary tumor. Several tumor entities, including germ-cell tumors, Ewing's sarcoma, synovial sarcoma, alveolar rhabdomyosarcoma, neuroblastoma, neuroepithelial tumors, and non-Hodgkin's lymphoma may present clinically as a neck mass and can now be identified based on their specific cytogenetic abnormalities.[228] In cases of two primary squamous cell tumors—not uncommon in the upper aerodigestive tract—the primary tumor giving rise to the metastatic spread may be verified by comparing the types of *p53* mutations found in both primary tumors and in the metastatic tissue.[229, 230]

Differential Diagnosis

Differential diagnosis should focus on more than subclassification of malignant tumors as outlined in the previous section. In addition, the pathologist should be aware that benign lesions may be confused with metastatic disease.

The presence of a malignant squamous epithelium with a cystic appearance rules out a benign lymphoepithelial cyst, a branchial cleft cyst, or cystic lymphoid hyperplasia in acquired immunodeficiency syndrome. In all these entities, the bland appearance of the epithelium that lines the cysts will help to rule out metastatic squamous cell carcinoma (Fig. 10–26). In addition, the cysts seen in patients with acquired immunodeficiency syndrome are frequently multiple and bilateral, and the associated lymphoid tissue may exhibit features consistent with persistent generalized lymphadenopathy (Fig. 10–27, see p. 661).[231] (See the section on branchiogenic carcinoma.)

Another problem in differential diagnosis is the distinction of inclusions of benign glandular structures from adenocarcinoma. These inclusions are histologically benign; they lack dysplasia and atypia. In addition, no desmoplasia is present in the stroma as seen in metastatic adenocarcinoma. Heterotopic salivary gland tissue is frequently found in cervical nodes, especially in the periparotid tissue, and may be the origin of benign and malignant salivary gland tumors (Fig. 10–28). Histologic diagnoses in the cases published so far include benign mixed tumor,[150] salivary dermal analogue tumor,[154] oncocytoma,[150] mucoepidermoid carcinoma,[150, 155, 232] acinic cell carcinoma,[150, 233] adenoid cystic carcinoma,[234] and oncocytic carcinoma (Fig. 10–29, see p. 661).[150]

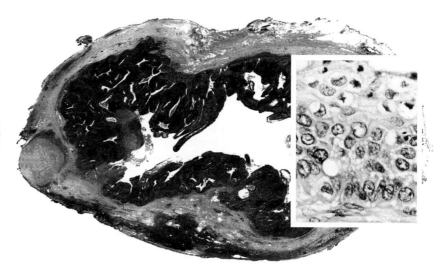

Figure 10–26. Metastatic cystic squamous carcinoma in lymph node. *Inset,* High-power view of malignant squamous epithelial lining. Compare with branchial cleft cyst shown in Figure 10–3.

The controversy concerning the existence of non-neoplastic thyroid follicles in cervical lymph nodes has not been completely resolved yet.[235–237] The demonstration of thyroid carcinoma in every case in which the whole gland was available for investigation strongly supports the neoplastic nature of thyroid follicles in lymph nodes, irrespective of their histology.[235, 236] In contrast, Meyer at al.[237] consider microscopic inclusions of benign-appearing thyroid follicles as benign, especially because they were not associated with the development of progressive carcinoma. The authors describe five autopsy cases in which cervical nodes contained thyroid tissue and serially sectioned the entire thyroid gland. Only one had a primary tumor and this was located in the contralateral lobe. Criteria to classify the thyroid tissue as benign need to be very stringent. Overlapping or water clear or ground glass nuclei, papillae, psammoma bodies, multiple involved nodes, or nodes with greater than one-third replacement by thyroid tissue should be regarded as metastatic papillary carcinoma. Although a benign course does not prove their non-neoplastic origin, thyroid follicles in lymph nodes are always an incidental finding; they are discovered in patients with another type of cancer of the head and neck. Hence, the diagnostic and therapeutic procedures should be suited to the lesser risk of a probably small thyroid cancer in the context of the life-threatening head and neck cancer for which the patient was originally evaluated.

Benign spindle cell neoplasms have been described in the lymph nodes of the submandibular region (Figs. 10–30 and 10–31, see p. 662).[238, 239] These intranodal myofibroblastomas have to be distinguished from metastatic spindle cell tumors (spindle cell carcinoma, malignant melanoma, or sarcoma) and from spindle cell tumors arising primarily in lymph nodes, such as Kaposi's sarcoma, and spindle cell tumors presumed to be of reticulum cell lineage.[240] Benign nevus cell aggregates have been found in the capsules of lymph nodes. This rare finding should not lead to an erroneous diagnosis of malignancy (Fig. 10–32, see p. 662).[241]

Another extremely rare lesion is cervical thymoma, which is noteworthy mainly for its unusual location. This feature alone may cause difficulties in both clinical management and pathologic evaluation.[242] Especially in small tissue samples, such as on frozen section material, epithelial structures may not be present, and the abundance of lymphocytes might raise the possibility of malignant lymphoma. On the other hand, the presence of epithelial structures within abundant lymphoid tissue should not be confused with metastatic carcinoma.

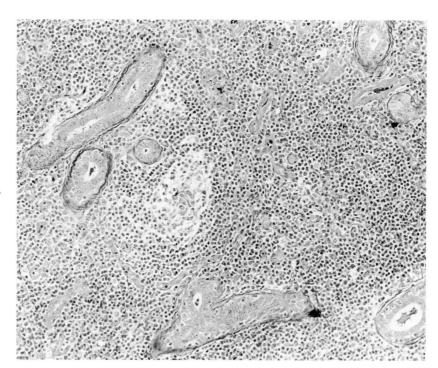

Figure 10–28. Salivary gland inclusions in lymph node.

Treatment and Prognosis

For optimum treatment results with a minimum of complications, careful patient selection is essential. The therapeutic strategy depends on different factors, including the stage of disease, the clinical presentation and location of the node or nodes,[243] histologic findings, and the age and general condition of the patient. Surgery and irradiation have been used to treat cervical metastases in the absence of a primary tumor, and in addition to the neck, presumed sites of occult primary tumors are usually covered by radiotherapy portals. The combination of surgery and radiotherapy has resulted in a considerable drop in the rate of disease recurrence above the clavicle. This improvement in locoregional control has led to changing patterns of recurrence: now distant metastases are more often the cause of death, and the long-term prognosis is worsened by the fact that approximately 6% of patients per year develop a second primary tumor, usually arising in the upper respiratory or gastrointestinal tracts.[244]

The most reliable indicator for prognosis in a patient with a cervical metastasis of unknown origin is the clinical stage of the neck. This is reflected by a decrease in 5-year survival rate from about 60% to 20% with progression from Stage N1 to N3.[186, 245, 246] The position of the node is also related to prognosis: patients with low cervical and supraclavicular nodes have a very poor prognosis. These patients usually have adenocarcinomas, with a primary tumor located below the clavicle. In the series by Fitzpatrick and Kotaik,[185] only 1 of 35 patients with supraclavicular nodes survived 5 years. In addition, histologic parameters are related to prognosis; as mentioned, adenocarcinomas, except those of thyroid origin, are associated with poor prognosis.[168, 179] The spread of metastatic carcinoma beyond the capsule of the lymph node is a prognostic factor for the rate of disease recurrence in the neck and overall survival rate.[247, 248] (See Microscopic Examination in Neck Dissection.) A desmoplastic stromal pattern within the metastatic lymph node has recently also been associated with an increased recurrence rate of neck disease.[249]

The proportion of patients in whom the primary tumor is detected within 5 years of initial treatment has dropped from 30% in studies published between 1957 and 1973[169, 175, 176, 250–253] to about 10% in studies published since 1990.[180, 186, 245, 246, 254, 255] This is probably the result of a more vigorous search for primary tumors, facilitated by improved diagnostic technologies. The majority of primary tumors are detected within 3 years after treatment of metastatic disease ends.[172, 175] Almost 50% of these primary tumors are located in the region of Waldeyer's tonsillar ring.[168, 169, 175, 176, 180, 250, 251] Below the clavicle, the largest numbers of primary tumors are found in the lungs and in the gastrointestinal tract.[250–252, 256–258] According to most authors, the incidence of primary tumors identified after initial treatment of neck nodes is lower in patients who undergo radiotherapy than in those who do not.[245, 258] However, remarkably low rates have also been found in studies including patients who have had surgery only or radiotherapy limited to the neck without inclusion of all potential mucosal primary tumor sites.[255, 259–262] If the tumor is not discovered, the physician must assume that the lesion was too small to be detected. Although spontaneous regression of a primary tumor could be another explanation, there are no cases in which such activity can be proven to have occurred.

▮ NECK DISSECTION

An important new classification system for neck dissections was recently put forth by The American Academy of Otolaryngology-Head and Neck Surgery, Inc., and the American Society of Head and Neck Surgery.[6] The new system has brought order to the confusion that existed in the late 1980s when diverse names were used to refer to the same operations.

Cervical Lymph Node Groups

The cervical lymph node groups routinely removed in the neck dissection procedures are submental and submandibular; upper, middle, and lower jugular; and the posterior triangle. It is also convenient to refer to groups of lymph nodes using the level system as described by the Sloan-Kettering Memorial Hospital Group (see Fig. 10–2).[5]

Lymph Node Group Boundaries

The following definitions are recommended for the boundaries of the lymph node groups removed in radical neck dissection.[6]

Level I: Submental group—Lymph nodes within the submental triangle. Submandibular group—Lymph nodes within the boundaries of the anterior and posterior bellies of the digastric muscle and the body of the mandible. The submandibular gland is included in the specimen when the lymph nodes within this triangle are removed.

Level II: Upper jugular group—Lymph nodes located around the upper third of the internal jugular vein and adjacent spinal accessory nerve extending inferiorly from the level of the carotid bifurcation (surgical landmark) or hyoid bone (clinical landmark) to the skull base. The posterior boundary is the posterior border of the sternocleidomastoid muscle, and the anterior boundary is the lateral border of the sternohyoid muscle.

Level III: Middle jugular group—Lymph nodes located around the middle third of the internal jugular vein extending from the carotid bifurcation superiorly to the omohyoid muscle (surgical landmark) or inferiorly to the cricothyroid notch (clinical landmark). The posterior boundary is the posterior border of the sternocleidomastoid muscle, and the anterior boundary is the lateral border of the sternohyoid muscle.

Level IV: Lower jugular group—Lymph nodes located around the lower third of the internal jugular vein extending from the omohyoid muscle superiorly to the clavicle inferiorly. The posterior boundary is the posterior border of the sternocleidomastoid muscle, and the anterior boundary is the lateral border of the sternohyoid muscle.

Level V: Posterior triangle group—This group comprises predominantly the lymph nodes located along the lower half of the spinal accessory nerve and along the transverse cervical artery. The supraclavicular nodes are also included in this group. The posterior boundary is the anterior border of the trapezius muscle, the anterior boundary is the posterior border of the sternocleidomastoid muscle, and the inferior boundary is the clavicle.

Level VI: Anterior compartment group—This group includes lymph nodes surrounding the midline visceral structures of the neck extending superiorly from the level of the hyoid bone to the suprasternal notch inferiorly. On each side, the lateral boundary is the medial border of the carotid sheath. Located within this compartment are the perithyroidal lymph nodes, paratracheal lymph nodes, lymph nodes along the recurrent laryngeal nerves, and precricoid lymph nodes.

Classification

Neck dissections are classified primarily based on the lymph node groups of the neck that are removed, and secondarily on the anatomic structures that may be preserved, such as the spinal accessory nerve, the sternocleidomastoid muscle, and the internal jugular vein. Neck dissections are divided into four categories: radical, modified radical, selective, and extended (Table 10–8).[6, 263]

The radical neck dissection consists of the removal of all five lymph node groups of one side of the neck (Level I–V). This includes the removal of the sternocleidomastoid muscle, the internal jugular vein, and the spinal accessory nerve. The modified radical neck dissection refers to excision of all lymph nodes routinely re-

Table 10–8. Classification of Neck Dissections

I. Radical
II. Modified radical
III. Selective
    A. Lateral
    B. Supraomohyoid
    C. Posterolateral
    D. Anterior
IV. Extended

Data from Robbins KT, et al: Standardizing neck dissection terminology: Official report of the academy's committee for head and neck surgery and oncology. *Arch Otolaryngol Head Neck Surg* 1991;117:601–605.

moved by radical neck dissection, with preservation of one or more of the nonlymphatic structures (i.e., spinal accessory nerve, internal jugular vein, and sternocleidomastoid muscle).

A selective neck dissection is any type of cervical lymphadenectomy in which there is preservation of one or more of the lymph node groups that are removed in a radical neck dissection. The four subtypes of selective neck dissection are supraomohyoid, posterolateral, lateral, and anterior neck dissection (see Table 10–8).[263, 264]

The term *extended radical neck dissection* refers to a given neck dissection that is extended to include either lymph node groups or nonlymphatic structures that are not routinely removed in a standard radical neck dissection.

Gross Examination of Specimens

The following procedure pertains to standard radical neck dissections and needs to be modified for the other three types. Because the main anatomic landmarks are lacking in a surgically removed tissue specimen, the orientation and labeling of the lymph node groups must be done by the surgeon. This is especially important in selective and extended neck dissections.

After the tissue specimen has been oriented and the platysma muscle has been removed, the first step in a gross examination is to measure the dimensions of the sternocleidomastoid muscle and the internal jugular vein and describe their involvement by the tumor. Next, the pathologist should dissect and divide the submandibular gland, sternocleidomastoid muscle, and internal jugular vein and separate the node-containing fat into the five levels: sublingual and submandibular, superior jugular, middle jugular, lower jugular, and posterior. The presence of tumor in soft tissues, submandibular gland, and muscle should be described. The number of lymph nodes (by level) should be noted, and if tumor tissue is present, the size of metastases and presence of extracapsular extension is likewise indicated. Tissue sections are then submitted for microscopic examination of all lymph nodes (separated by level), the submandibular gland, the sternocleidomastoid muscle, and the internal jugular vein. If the neck dissection is of the extended type, sections of all extra lymph node groups and nonlymphatic structures that were removed should be submitted for microscopic examination.

Microscopic Examination and Determinants of Prognosis

The aim of the microscopic examination is to discover the histologic features that are important in predicting patient outcome or that may determine whether the patient should be given adjuvant therapy. The five important parameters are the number of positive lymph nodes, the presence of metastasis in different groups of lymph nodes, the presence or absence of extracapsular spread (ECS), size of metastasis, and the presence of desmoplastic reaction in metastatic tissue.

Of these parameters, ECS has been increasingly identified as a major prognostic factor in terms of recurrent disease in the neck and overall survival.[247, 248] In a study by Johnson et al.,[248] histopatho-

logic evidence of ECS was associated with a statistically significant reduction in survival rate. In cases in which ECS was present, 39% of patients survived, compared with 75% of patients in cases without ECS. Patients with ECS had an increased risk of and shorter periods of time to disease recurrence. Local disease recurred in 42% and 18% of cases, respectively, in 6 months and distant metastases occurred in 14% and 4% of cases, respectively, in 18 months. Similar results were observed by Close et al.[265] and Carter et al.[247] Furthermore, the study by Carter et al. demonstrated a 10-fold difference in the risk of disease recurrence in the neck in patients with macroscopic ECS versus patients with only microscopic ECS or no ECS at all.[247] It should be noted, however, that not all authors view the prognostic significance of ECS with such gravity.[266] ECS should now be studied in a more rigorous manner with respect to quality and quantity, and it must be correlated with patient prognosis and treatment in a prospective manner before its true significance can be assessed.

Prognostic significance has often been attributed to the number of involved nodes and the number of involved nodal groups.[267] In a multivariate analysis performed by Carter et al.[247] using Cox regression methods, the important factors in predicting survival time were the number of involved nodes and the number of involved anatomic groups ($P = 0.005$).[247] Involvement of the lower jugular and posterior triangle nodes and noncontiguous or multiple disease sites were associated with poorer prognoses.[267] However, the relative importance of these parameters in predicting recurrent neck disease is still disputed.[268, 269]

As with other characteristics of metastases to cervical lymph nodes, absolute numbers of or percentages of positive nodes and node size are generally not useful prognostic indicators.[269] Schuller et al.[269] performed discriminate analysis on 12 characteristics of metastatic lymph nodes (e.g., number, percentage positive, size, anatomic position) and attempted to correlate these with length of survival. Although involvement of the posterior triangle and noncontiguous or multiple sites were associated with a more serious prognosis whether considered individually or collectively, there was no parameter accurate enough to be used by the clinician in prognostication. The size of a lymph node, however, does correlate with the presence of histologically proven metastasis.[270] Cachin[270] found that lymph nodes larger than 5 cm contained metastasis in 100% of the cases, in contrast to lymph nodes that measured 4 cm or less, in which only 66% contained metastatic deposits.

In a recent study by Olsen et al.,[249] a desmoplastic stromal pattern in a lymph node metastasis was associated with a nearly sevenfold increase in the risk of recurrent neck disease.

■ REFERENCES

Anatomy

1. Bielamowicz SA, Storper IS, Jabour BA, et al: Spaces and triangles of head and neck. *Head Neck* 1994;164:383–388.
2. Rouviere H: *Anatomy of the Human Lymphatic System.* Translated by MT Tobiar and JW Edwards. Ann Arbor, MI: Edward Bros. Inc., 1948.
3. Fisch V: *Lymphography of the Cervical Lymphatic System,* Philadelphia: WB Saunders Co, 1968.
4. Reede DL, Bergeron RT: The CT evaluation of the normal and diseased neck. *Semin Ultrasound CT MR* 1986;7:181–201.
5. Shah JP, Strang E, Spiro RH, et al: Neck dissection, current status and future possibilities. *Clin Bull* 1981;11:25–33.
6. Robbins KT, Medina JE, Wolfe GT, et al: Standardizing neck dissection terminology. Official report of the academy's committee for head and neck surgery and oncology. *Arch Otolaryngol Head Neck Surg* 1991; 117:601–605.

Cysts, General

7. Maisel RH: When your patient complains of a neck mass. *Geriatrics* 1980;35:3–8.
8. Torsiglier AJ Jr, Tom LW, Ross AJ, et al: Pediatric neck masses: Guide-

lines for evaluation. *Int J Pediatr Otorhinolaryngol* 1988;16:199–210.

9. Park JW: Evaluation of neck masses in children. *Am Fam Physician* 1995;51:1904–1912.

10. Guarisco JL: Congenital head and neck masses in infants and children, part I. *Ear Nose Throat J* 1991;70:40–47.

11. May M: Neck masses in children: Diagnosis and treatment. *Ear Nose Throat J* 1978;57:136–158.

12. Som PH, Sacher M, Lanzieri CF, et al: Parenchymal cysts of the lower neck. *Radiology* 1985;157:399–406.

Branchial Cleft Cysts

13. The pharynx and its derivatives. In: Gray SW, Skandalakis JE (eds): *Embryology for Surgeons.* Philadelphia: WB Saunders Co, 1972:15–61.

14. Colledge J, Ellis H: The aetiology of lateral cervical (branchial) cysts: Past and present theories. *J Laryngol Otol* 1994;108:653–659.

15. Gutierrez C, Bardajic, Bento L, et al: Branchio-oto-renal syndrome: Incidence in three generations of a family. *J Pedriatr Surg* 1993;28:1527–1529.

16. Coppage KB, Smith RJ: Branchio-oto-renal syndrome. *J Am Acad Audiol* 1995;6:103–110.

17. Hunter AGW: Inheritance of branchial sinuses and preauricular fistulas. *Teratology* 1974;9:225–228.

18. Bhaskar SN, Bernier JL: Histogenesis of branchial cysts: A report of 468 cases. *Am J Pathol* 1959;35:407–423.

19. Olson KD, Maragos NE, Weiland LH: First branchial cleft anomalies *Laryngoscope* 1980;90:423–436.

20. Belenky WM, Medina JE: First branchial cleft anomalies. *Laryngoscope* 1980;90:23–29.

21. Wetke R: First branchial cleft anomaly. *Ugeskr Laeger* 1993;155:1971–1972.

22. Mukherji SK, Tart RP, Slattery WH, et al: Evaluation of first branchial anomalies. *J Comput Assist Tomogr* 1993;17:576–581.

23. Work WP: Newer concepts of first branchial cleft defects. *Laryngoscope* 1972;82:1581–1593.

24. Proctor B, Proctor C: Congenital lesions of the head and neck. *Otolaryngol Clin North Am* 1970;3:221–248.

25. Liston SL, Siegel LG: Branchial cysts, sinuses and fistulas. *Ear Nose Throat J* 1967;58:504–509.

26. Verheire VM, Daele JJ: Second branchial cleft-pouch set fistulae, sinuses and cysts in children. *Acta Otorhinolaryngol Belg* 1991;45:437–442.

27. Flanagan PM, Roland NJ, Jones AS: Cervical node metastases presenting with features of branchial cysts. *J Laryngol Otol* 1994;108:1068–1071.

28. Himalstein MR: Branchial cysts and fistulas. *Ear Nose Throat J* 1980;59:47–54.

29. Vade A, Griffiths A, Hotaling A, et al: Thymopharyngeal duct cyst: MR imaging of a third branchial arch anomaly in a neonate. *J Magn Reson Imaging* 1994;4:614–616.

30. Al-Ghamdi S, Freedman A, Just N, et al: Fourth branchial cleft cyst. *J Otolaryngol* 1992;21:447–449.

31. Whitworth IH, Suvarna SK, Wight RG, et al: Fourth branchial arch anomaly: A rare incidental finding in an adult. *J Laryngol Otol* 1993;107:238–239.

32. Tanaka H, Igarashi T, Teramoto S, et al: Lymphoepithelial cyst in the mediastinum with an opening to the trachea. *Respiration* 1995;62:110–113.

33. Martin H, Morfit HM, Ehrlich H: The case for branchogenic cancer (malignant branchioma). *Ann Surg* 1950;132:867–887.

34. Compagno J, Hyams VJ, Safavian M. Does branchiogenic carcinoma really exist? *Arch Pathol Lab Med* 1976;100:341–314.

35. Batsakis JG, McBurney TA: Metastatic neoplasms to the head and neck. *Surg Gynecol Obstet* 1971;133:673–671.

36. Micheau C, Cachin Y, Caillou B: Cystic metastases in the neck revealing occult carcinoma of the tonsil. *Cancer* 1974;33:228–233.

37. Cecena-Falcon LA, Gomez G, Soto ZD, et al: Carcinoma branchogenic en un nino y revision de la literatura. *Patologia (Mex)* 1994;32:29–33.

38. Suarez B, Fernandez JA, Lopez G, et al: Carcinoma epidermoide sobre quiste branchial. *Pathologia (Esp)* 1995;28:55–57.

Thyroglossal Duct Cysts

39. Todd NW: Common congential anomalies of the neck. Embryology and surgical anatomy. *Surg Clin North Am* 1993;73:599–610.

40. Solomon JR, Rangecroft L: Thyroglossal duct lesions in children. *J Pediatr Surg* 1984; 19:555–561.

41. O'Hanlon DM, Walsh N, Lorry J, et al: Aberrant thyroglossal cyst. *J Laryngol Otol* 1994;108:1105–1107.

42. Allard RHB: The thyroglossal duct cyst. *Head Neck* 1982;1:134–136.

43. Klin B, Serous F, Fried K, et al: Familial thyroglossal duct cyst. *Clin Genet* 1993;43:101–103.

44. Liu TP, Jeng KS, Yang TL, et al: Thyroglossal duct cyst. An analysis of 92 cases. *Clin Med J* 1992;49:72–75.

45. Sturgis EM, Miller RH: Thyrogossal duct cysts. *J La State Med Soc* 1993;145:459–461.

46. Lim-Dunham JE, Feinstein KA, Yousefzadeh DK, et al: Sonographic demonstration of a normal thyroid gland excludes ectopic thyroid in patients with thyroglossal duct cyst. *AJR Am J Roentgenol* 1995;164:1489–1491.

47. Soucy P, Penning J: The clinical relevance of certain observations on the histology of the thyroglossal tract. *J Pediatr Sur* 1984;19:506–510.

48. Sade J, Rosen G: Thyroglossal cysts and tracts: A histological and histochemical study. *Ann Otol Rhinol Laryngol* 1968;77:139–145.

49. Sistrunk WE: The surgical treatment of cysts of the thyroglossal tract. *Ann Surg* 1920;71:121–122.

50. Ellis PDM, Van Nostrand AWP: The applied anatomy of thyroglossal tract remnants. *Laryngoscope* 1977;87:765–770.

51. Van Vuuren PA, Balm AJ, Gregor RT, et al: Carcinoma arising in thyroglossal remnants. *Clin Otolaryngol* 1994;19:506–515.

52. Yanagibawa K, Eisen RN, Sasaki CT: Squamous cell carcinoma arising in a thyroglossal duct cyst. *Arch Otolaryngol Head Neck Surg* 1992; 118:538–541.

53. Cote DN, Sturgis EM, Peterson T, et al: Thyroglossal duct cyst carcinoma: An unusual case of Hürthle cell carcinoma. *Otolaryngol Head Neck Surg* 1995;113:153–156.

54. Kresnik E, Gallowitsch HJ, Plob J, et al: Squamous cell carcinoma of the thyroid originating from a thyroglossal duct cyst. *Nuklearmedizin* 1995;34:76–78.

55. Mahnke CG, Jamig V, Wermer JA, et al: Primary papillary carcinoma of the thyroglossal duct: Case report and review of the literature. *Auris Nasus Larynx* 1994;21:258–263.

Thymic Cysts

56. Fahmy S: Cervical thymic cysts: Their pathogenesis and relationship to branchial cysts. *J Laryngol Otol* 1974;88:47–60.

57. Moore KL: *The Developing Human—Clinically Oriented Embryology,* 4th ed. Philadelphia: WB Saunders, 1988:179–184.

58. Miller MB, DeVito MA: Cervical thymic cyst. *Otolaryngol Head Neck Surg* 1995;112:586–589.

59. Ellis HA: Cervical thymic cysts. *J Surg* 1967;54:17–20.

60. Strome M, Eraklis A: Thymic cysts in the neck. *Laryngoscope* 1977;87:1645–1649.

61. Zarbo RJ, Areen RG, McClatchey KD, et al: Thyropharyngeal duct cyst. A form of cervical thymus. *Ann Otol Rhinol Laryngol* 1983;92:284–289.

62. Suzuki T: Papillary adenoma in a lateral cervical cyst. *Acta Pathol J* 1987;37:2019–2024.

Bronchogenic Cysts

63. Fraga S, Helwig EB, Rosen SH: Bronchogenic cysts in the skin and subcutaneous tissue. *Am J Clin Pathol* 1971;56:230–238.

64. Tresser NJ, Dahms B, Bermer JJ: Cutaneous bronchogenic cyst of the back: A case report and review of the literature. *Pediatr Pathol Lab Med* 1994;14:207–212.

65. Dolgin SE, Groisman GM, Shah K: Subcutaneous bronchogenic cysts and sinuses. *Otolaryngol Head Neck Surg* 1995;112:763–766.

66. Gosin AK, Wildes TO: Lateral cervical cyst containing gastric epithelium. *Arch Pathol Lab Med* 1988;112:96–98.

Parathyroid Cyst

67. Clark OH: Parathyroid cysts. *Am J Surg* 1978;35:395–402.

68. Turner A, Lampe HB, Cramer H: Parathyroid cysts. *J Otolaryngol* 1989;18:11–13.

69. Entwistle JWC, Pierce CV, Johnson DE, et al: Parathyroid cysts: Report of the sixth and youngest pediatric case. *J Pediatr Surg* 1994;29:1528–1529.

70. Wang CA, Vickery AL, Maloop F: Large parathyroid cysts mimicking thyroid nodules. *Ann Surg* 1972;175:448–451.

71. Redleaf MI, Walker WP, Alt LP: Parathyroid adenoma associated with a branchial cleft cyst. *Arch Otolaryngol Head Neck Surg* 1995; 121:113–115.

Dermoid

72. Ferlito A, Devaney KO: Developmental lesions of the head and neck. Terminology and biologic behavior. *Ann Otol Rhinol Laryngol* 1995;104:913–918.

73. Taylor BW, Erich JB, Dockerty MD: Dermoids of the head and neck. *Minn Med* 1966;49:1535–1540.

74. McAvoy JM, Zukerbraum L: Dermoid cysts of the head and neck in children. *Arch Otolaryngol Head Neck Surg* 1976;102:271–273.

75. Holt GR, Holt JE, Weaver RG: Dermoids and teratomas of the head and neck. *Ear Nose Throat J* 1979;58:37–41.

76. Brownstein MH, Helwig EB: Subcutaneous dermoid cysts. *Arch Dermatol* 1973;107:237–239.

77. Katz AD: Midline dermoid tumors of the neck. *Arch Surg* 1974;109:822–826.

Ranulas

78. Batsakis JG, McClatchey KD: Cervical ranulas. *Ann Otol Rhinol Laryngol* 1988;97:561–562.

79. Black RJ, Croft CB: Ranula: Pathogenesis and management. *Clin Otolaryngol* 1982;7:299–303.

80. Barnard NA: Plunging ranula: A bilateral presentation. *Br J Oral Maxillofac Surg* 1991;29:112–113.

81. Horiguchi H, Kakuta S, Nagumo M: Bilateral plunging ranula: A case report. *Int J Oral Maxillofac Surg* 1995;24:174–175.

82. Mizuno A, Yamaguchi K: The plunging ranula. *Int J Oral Maxillofac Surg* 1993;22:113–115.

83. Langlois NE, Kolhe P: Plunging ranula: A case report and a literature review. *Hum Pathol* 1992;11:1306–1308.

84. Quick CA, Lowell SH: Ranula and the sublingual salivary gland. *Arch Otolaryngol* 1977;103:397–400.

85. Yoshimura Y, Obara S, Kondoh T, et al: A comparison of three methods used for treatment of ranula. *J Oral Maxillofac Surg* 1995;53:280–282.

Laryngocele

86. Stell PM, Maran AGD: Laryngocele. *J Laryngol Otol* 1975;89:915–924.

87. Canalis RF, Maxwell DS, Hemenway WC: Laryngocele: An updated review. *J Otolaryngol* 1977;6:191–198.

88. De Santo LW: Laryngocele, laryngeal saccules and laryngeal saccular cysts: A developmental spectrum. *Laryngoscope* 1974;84:1291–1296.

89. Thomas DM, Madden GJ: Bilateral laryngoceles. *Ear Nose Throat J* 1993;72:819–821.

90. Chu L, Gassack GS, Orr JE, et al: Neonatal laryngoceles: A cause for airway obstruction. *Arch Otolaryngol Head Neck Surg* 1994;120:454–458.

91. Altamar-Rios J, Morales-Rozo O: Laryngocele and pyolaryngocele. *Ann Otorrinolaryngol Iber* 1992;19:393–394.

92. Micheau C, Luboinski B, Lamchi P, et al: Relationship between laryngoceles and laryngeal carcinoma. *Laryngoscope* 1978;88:680–685.

93. Brugel FJ, Grevers G, Vogl TJ: Coincidental appearance of laryngocele and laryngeal carcinoma. *Laryngo-Rhino-Otologie* 1991;70:511–514.

94. Yarington CT, Frazer JP: An approach to the internal laryngocele and other submucosal lesions of the larynx. *Ann Otol Rhinol Laryngol* 1966;75:956–963.

Lymphangioma

95. Bill AH, Sumner DS: A unified concept of lymphangiomas and cystic hygroma. *J Am Coll Surg* 1965;120:79–86.

96. Wassef, M: Cervicocephalic hemangiomas and vascular malformations. Histological appearance and classification. *J Mal Vasc* 1992;17:20–25.

97. Emery PJ, Bailey CM, Evans JNG: Cystic hygroma of the head and neck. A review of 37 cases. *J Laryngol Otol* 1984;98:613–619.

98. Glasson MJ, Taylor SF: Cervical, cervicomediastinal, and intrathoracic lymphangiomas. *Prog Pediatr Surg* 1991;27:63–83.

99. Ninh TN, Ninh TX: Cystic hygroma in children: A report of 126 cases. *J Pediatr Surg* 1974;9:191–198.

100. Peachy RDG, Whimster IW: Lymphangioma of skin. A review of 96 cases. *Br J Dermatol* 1970;83:519–524.

101. Das Gupta TK: Tumors of the Soft Tissues. Norwalk, CT: Appleton-Century-Crofts, 1983.

102. Van Cauwelaert PH, Gruwez JA: Experience with lymphangioma. *Lymphology* 1978;11:43–49.

103. Harkins GA, Sabiston DC: Lymphangioma in infancy and childhood. *Surgery* 1960;47:811–820.

104. Watson WL, McCarthy WD: Blood and lymph vessel tumors: A report of 1056 cases. *J Am Coll Surg* 1940;71:569–575.

105. De Serres LM, Sie KCY, Richardson MA: Lymphatic malformations of the head and neck: A proposal for staging. *Arch Otolaryngol Head Neck Surg* 1995;121:577–582.

Hemangiomas

106. Rossiter JL, Hendrix RA, Tom W, et al: Intramuscular hemangioma of the head and neck. *Otolaryngol Head Neck Surg* 1993;108:18–26.

107. Edgerton MT, Hiebert JM: Vascular and lymphatic tumors in infancy, childhood, and adulthood: A challenge of diagnosis and treatment. *Curr Probl Cancer* 1978;2:1–44.

108. Yuasa K, Shimizu T, Toyoda T: The giant cavernous hemangioma of the neck. *J Jap Assoc Thorac Surg* 1992;48:1274–1278.

109. Hoehn JG, Farrow GM, Devine KD, et al: Invasive hemangioma of the head and neck. *Am J Surg* 1970;120:497–500.

110. Clemis JD, Briggs DR, Changus GW: Intramuscular hemangiomas in the head and neck. *Can J Otolaryngol* 1975;4:339–347.

111. Premachandra DJ, Milton CM: Childhood hemangiomas of the head and neck. *Clin Otolaryngol* 1991;16:117–123.

112. Fitzpatrick EL, Cote DN: Hemangiomas of the head and neck. *J La State Med Soc* 1995;147:291–295.

113. DeYoung BR, Wick MR, Fitzgibbon JF, et al: CD 31: An immunospecific marker for endothelial differentiation in human neoplasms. *Appl Immunohistochem* 1993;1:97–100.

114. Margileth AM: Developmental vascular abnormalities. *Pediatr Clin North Am* 1971;18:773–785.

115. Illingworth RS: Thoughts on treatment of strawberry naevi. *Arch Dis Child* 1976;51:139–140.

Teratomas

116. Tapper D, Lack E: Teratomas in infancy and childhood. Arch Surg 1983;198:398–410.

117. Jordan RB, Gauderer MWL: Cervical teratoma: An analysis, literature review and proposed classification. *J Pediatr Surg* 1988;23:583–591.

118. Batsakis JG, El-Naggar AK, Luna M: Teratomas of the head and neck with emphasis on malignancy. *Ann Otol Rhinol Laryngol* 1995;104: 456–500.

119. Gonzalez-Crussi F: Extragonadal teratomas. In: *Atlas of Tumor Pathology*, 2nd series, fascicle 18. Washington, DC: Armed Forces Institute of Pathology, 1982.

120. Norris HJ, Zirkin HJ, Benson WL: Immature (malignant) teratomas of the ovary: A clinicopathologic study of 58 cases. *Cancer* 1976;37: 2359–2372.

121. Lack E: Extragonadal germ cell tumors of the head and neck region. Review of 16 cases. *Hum Pathol* 1985;16:56–64.

122. Silverman R, Mendelsohn IR: Teratoma of the neck: Report of two cases and review of the literature. *Arch Dis Child* 1960;35:159–170.

123. Watanatittan S, Othersen HB, Hughson MD: Cervical teratomas in children. *Progr Pediatr Surg* 1981;14:225–239.

124. Ward RF, April M: Teratomas of the head and neck. *Otolaryngol Clin North Am* 1989;22:621–629.

125. Nmadu PT: Cervical teratoma in later infancy: Report of 13 cases. *Ann Trop Pediatric* 1993;13:95–98.

126. Azizkhan RG, Haase GM, Applebaum H, et al: Diagnosis, management and outcome of cervico-facial teratomas in neonates: A Children Cancer Group Study. *J Pediatr Surg* 1995;30:312–316.

127. Thurkow AL, Visser GHA: Ultrasound observations of a malignant cervical teratoma of the fetus in a case of polyhydramnios: Case history and review. *Eur J Obstet Gynecol Reprod Biol* 1983;14:375–384.

128. Colton JJ, Batsakis JG, Work WP: Teratomas of the neck in adults. *Arch Otolaryngol* 1978;104:271–272.

129. Bowker CM, Whittaker RS: Malignant teratomas of the thyroid. Case report and literature review of thyroid teratomas in adults. *Histopathology* 1992;21:81–83.

130. Batsakis JG, Litter ER, Oberman HA: Teratomas of the neck. A clinicopathologic appraisal. *Arch Otolaryngol* 1964;79:619–624.
131. Rothschild MA, Catalano P, Urken M, et al: Evaluation and managment of congenital cervical teratoma. *Arch Otolaryngol Head Neck Surg* 1994;120:444–448.
132. Gundry SR, Wesley JR, Klein MD, et al: Cervical teratomas in the newborn. *J Pediatr Surg* 1983;18:382–386.

Paragangliomas

133. Lack E, Cubilla AZ, Woodruff JM: Paragangliomas of the head and neck region: A pathologic study of tumors from 71 patients. *Hum Pathol* 1979;10:191–218.
134. Grimley PM, Glemner GG: Histology and ultrastructure of carotid body paragangliomas: Comparison with normal gland. *Cancer* 1967;20:1473–1488.
135. Powell S, Peters N, Hermer C: Chemodectoma of the head and neck: Results of treatment in 84 patients. *Int J Radiat Oncol Biol Phys* 1992;22:919–924.
136. Hodge KM, Byers RM, Peters LJ: Paragangliomas of the head and neck. *Arch Otolaryngol Head Neck Surg* 1988;114:872–877.
137. Kraus DH, Sterman BM, Haraim AG, et al: Carotid body tumors. *Arch Otolaryngol Head Neck Surg* 1990;116:1384–1387.
138. Milewski C: Morphology and clinical aspects of paragangliomas in the areas of the head and neck. *HNO* 1993;4:526–531.
139. Borowy ZJ, Probst L, Deitel M, et al: A family exhibiting carotid body tumors. *Can J Surg* 1992;35:546–551.
140. McCaffrey TV, Meyer FB, Michels VV, et al: Familial paraganglioma of the head and neck. *Arch Otolaryngol Head Neck Surg* 1994;120:211–216.
141. Ali IM, Graham C, Sanalla B, et al: Carotid body tumor associated with hyperparathyroidism. *Ann Vasc Surg* 1994;8:595–598.
142. Shamblin WR, ReMine WH, Sheps SG, et al: Carotid body tumor: Clinicopathologic analysis of ninety cases. *Am J Surg* 1971;122:732–739.
143. Johnson TL, Zarbo RJ, Lloyd RV, et al: Paragangliomas of the head and neck: Immunohistochemical neuroendocrine and intermediate filament typing. *Mod Pathol* 1988;1:216–223.
144. Warren W, Inchul L, Gould VE, et al: Paragangliomas of the head and neck. Ultrastructural and immunohistochemical analysis. *Ultrastruct Pathol* 1985;8:333–343.
145. Merino MJ, Livolsi VA: Malignant carotid body tumor: Report of two cases and review of the literature. *Cancer* 1981;47:1403–1414.
146. Bhansali SA, Bojrab DI, Zarbo RJ: Malignant paragangliomas of the head and neck: Clinical and immunohistochemical characterization. *Otolaryngol Head Neck Surg* 1991;104:132–137.
147. Chaudhry AP, Haar JG, Koul A, et al: A non-functioning paraganglioma of vagus nerve: An ultrastructural study. *Cancer* 1979;43:1689–1695.
148. Hakin JP, Eisela DW: Vagal paraganglioma (review). *Arch Otolaryngol* 1993;119:466–468.
149. Irons GB, Weiland LH, Brown WL: Paragangliomas of the neck. Clinical and pathologic analysis of 116 cases. *Surg Clin North Am* 1977;57:575–583.

Salivary Gland Lesions

150. Zajtchuk JT, Paton CA, Hyams VJ: Cervical heterotopic salivary gland neoplasms: A diagnostic dilemma. *Otolaryngol Head Neck Surg* 1982;80:178–181.
151. Luna M, Monheit J: Salivary gland neoplasms arising in lymph nodes. A clinicopathologic analysis of 13 cases. *Lab Invest* 1988;58:58a.
152. Senger MI, Applebaum EL, Ley KD: Heterotopic salivary tissue in the neck. *Laryngoscope* 1979;89:1772–1778.
153. Fantozzi RD, Bone RC, Fox R: Extraglandular Warthin's tumors. *Laryngoscope* 1985;95:682–688.
154. Luna MA, Tortoledo ME, Allen M: Salivary dermal analogue tumor arising in lymph nodes. *Cancer* 1987;59:1165–1169.
155. Valdez-Gomez JJ, Abad-Collazo ME, Borrajero-Martinez I: Carcinoma mucoepidermoid originado en ganglio linfatico. *Patologia (Mex)* 1993;31:211–214.

Miscellaneous Lesions

156. Al-Ghandi S, Black MJ, Lafond G: Extracranial head and neck schwannomas. *J Otolaryngol* 1992;2:86–88.

157. Chan JK, Rosai J: Tumors of the neck showing thymic or related branchial pouch differentiation: A unifying concept. *Hum Pathol* 1991;22:349–367.
158. Martin JME, Randhawa G, Temple WJ: Cervical thymoma. *Arch Pathol Lab Med* 1986;110:354–357.
159. Saitz EW: Cervical lymphadenitis caused by atypical mycobacteria. *Pediatr Clin North Am* 1981;28:823–839.
160. Gruber B, Rippon J, Dayal VS: Phaeomycotic cyst (chromoblastomycosis) of the neck. *Arch Otolaryngol Head Neck Surg* 1988;114:1031–1032.
161. Soyla L, Aydogan LB, Kiroglu M, et al: Hydatic cyst in the head and neck area. *Am J Otolaryngol* 1995;16:123–125.
162. Cleary KR, Batsakis JG: Lymphoepithelial cyst of the parotid gland region. A new face on an old lesion. *Ann Otol Rhinol Laryngol* 1990;99:62–64.
163. Hughes GB, Damiani KA, Kinney SE, et al: Aural cholesteatoma presenting as a large neck mass. *Otolaryngol Head Neck Surg* 1980;88:34–36.
164. Endicott JN, Cohen JJ: Amyloidosis presenting as a mass in the neck. *Laryngoscope* 1979;89:1224–1228.
165. Cunningham MJ, Rueger RG, Rothfus WE: Extracranial carotid aneurysm: An unusual neck mass in a young adult. *Ann Otol Rhinol Laryngol* 1989;98:396–399.

Unknown Primary Tumors

166. Martin H, Morfit HM: Cervical lymph node metastasis as the first symptom of cancer. *Surg Gynecol Obstet* 1944;78:133–159.
167. Martin H, Romieu C: The diagnostic significance of a lump in the neck. *Postgrad Med* 1952;11:491–500.
168. Batsakis JG: The pathology of head and neck tumors: The occult primary and metastases to the head and neck, Part 10. *Head Neck* 1981;3:409–423.
169. Comess MS, Beahrs OH, Dockerty MB: Cervical metastases from occult carcinoma. *J Am Coll Surg* 1957;104:607–617.
170. Fried MP, Diehl WH, Brownson R Jr, et al: Cervical metastasis from an unknown primary. *Ann Otol Rhinol Laryngol* 1975;84:152–157.
171. Lefebvre JL, Coche-Dequenant B, Ton Van J, et al: Cervical lymph nodes from unknown primary tumor in 190 patients. *Am J Surg* 1990;160:443–446.
172. Richard JM, Micheau C: Malignant cervical adenopathies from carcinomas of unknown origin. *Tumori* 1977;63:249–258.

Clinical Features

173. de Braud F, Heilbrun LK, Ahmed K, et al: Metastatic squamous cell carcinoma of an unknown primary localized to the neck. Advantages of an aggressive treatment. *Cancer* 1989;64:510–515.
174. Feldmann PS: Pathologic and cytologic diagnosis of a lump in the neck. In: Chrettien PB, Johns ME, Shedded DP, et al (eds): *Head and Neck Cancer,* vol 1. Philadelphia: Decker, 1985:281–283.
175. Jesse RH, Neff LE: Metastatic carcinoma in cervical nodes with unknown primary lesion. *Am J Surg* 1966;112:547–553.
176. Jesse RH, Perez CA, Fletcher GH: Cervical lymph node metastasis: Unknown primary cancer. *Cancer* 1973;31:854–859.
177. Regauer S, Mannweller S, Anderhuber W, et al: Cystic lymph node metastases of squamous cell carcinoma of Waldeyer's ring origin. *Br J Cancer* 1999;79:1437–1442.
178. Nguyen C, Shenouda G, Black MJ, et al: Metastatic squamous cell carcinoma to cervical lymph nodes from unknown primary mucosal sites. *Head Neck* 1994;16:58–63.
179. Spiro RH, DeRose G, Strong EW: Cervical node metastasis of occult origin. *Am J Surg* 1983;146:441–446.
180. Wang RC, Goepfert H, Barber AE, et al: Unknown primary squamous cell carcinoma metastatic to the neck. *Arch Otolaryngol Head Neck Surg* 1990;116:1388–1393.
181. Berge T, Toremalm NG: Cervical and mediastinal lymph node as an otorhinolaryngeal problem. *Ann Otol Rhinol Laryngol* 1969;78:663–670.
182. Coker DD, Casterline PF, Chambers RG, et al: Metastases to lymph nodes of the head and neck from an unknown primary site. *Am J Surg* 1977;134:517–522.
183. Lindberg R: Distribution of cervical lymph node metastases from squamous cell carcinoma of the upper respiratory and digestive tract. *Cancer* 1972;29:1446–1449.

184. Molinari R, Cantu H, Chiesa F, et al: A statistical approach to detection of the primary cancer based on the site of neck lymph node metastases. *Tumori* 1977;63:267–282.
185. Fitzpatrick PJ, Kotalik JF: Cervical metastases from an unknown primary tumor. *Radiology* 1974;110:659–663.

Search for Primary Tumor

186. Maulard C, Housset M, Brunek P, et al: Postoperative radiation therapy for cervical lymph node metastases from an occult squamous cell carcinoma. *Laryngoscope* 1992;102:884–890.
187. Eisele DW, Shermann ME, Koch WM: Utility of immediate on-site cytopathologic procurement and evaluation in fine needle aspiration biopsy of head and neck masses. *Laryngoscope* 1992;102:1328–1330.
188. Tunkel DE, Baroody FM, Sherman ME: Fine-needle aspiration biopsy of cervicofacial masses in children. *Arch Otolaryngol Head Neck Surg* 1995;121:533–536.
189. Smith Frable MA, Frable WJ: Fine needle aspiration biopsy revisited. *Laryngoscope* 1982;92:1414–1418.
190. Schwarz R, Chan NH, MacFarlane JK: Fine needle aspiration cytology in the evaluation of head and neck masses. *Am J Surg* 1990;159:482–485.
191. Dillon WP, Harnsberger HR: The impact of radiologic imaging on staging of cancer of the head and neck. *Semin Oncol* 1991;18:64–79.
192. Mancuso AA, Hanafee WN: Elusive head and neck carcinomas beneath intact mucosa. *Laryngoscope* 1983;93:133–139.
193. Muraki AS, Mancuso AA, Harnsberger HR: Metastatic cervical adenopathy from tumors of unknown origin: The role of CT. *Radiology* 1984;152:749–753.
194. Tein RD, Hesselink JR, Chu PK, et al: Improved detection and delineation of head and neck lesions with fat-suppression spin-echo MR imaging. *AJNR* 1991;12:19–24.
195. Wensel JP, Talbot JM: Cystic squamous cell carcinoma metastatic to the neck from occult primary. *Ann Otol Rhinol Laryngol* 1992;101:1021–1023.
196. McGuirt WF: Neck mass: Patient examination and differential diagnosis. In: Cunnings CW, Krause CJ, Schuller DE, et al (eds): *Otolaryngology Head and Neck Surgery,* vol 2. St. Louis, Mosby, 1986:1587.
197. Gooder P, Palmer M: Cervical node biopsy: A study of its morbidity. *J Laryngol Otol* 1984;98:1031–1040.
198. Ellis ER, Mendenhall WM, Rao PV, et al: Incisional or excisional biopsy before definitive radiotherapy, alone or followed by neck dissection. *Head Neck* 1991;13:177–183.
199. McGuirt WF, McCabe BF: Significance of node biopsy before definitive treatment of cervical metastatic carcinoma. *Laryngoscope* 1978;88:594–597.
200. Razack MS, Sako K, Marchetta FC: Influence of initial neck biopsy on the incidence of recurrence in the neck and survival in patients who subsequently undergo curative resectional surgery. *J Surg Oncol* 1977;9:347–335.
201. Robbins KT, Cole R, Marvel J, et al: The violated neck: Cervical node biopsy prior to definitive treatment. *Otolaryngol Head Neck Surg* 1986;94:605–610.
202. Greven KM, Williams DW, Keyes JW, et al: Positron emission tomography of patients with head and neck carcinoma before and after high-dose irradiation. *Cancer* 1994;74:1355–1359.
203. Harwick RD: Cervical metastases from an occult primary site. *Semin Oncol* 1991;7:2–8.
204. Pearson GR, Weiland LH, Neel HB, et al: Application of Epstein-Barr virus (EBV) serology to the diagnosis of North American nasopharyngeal carcinoma. *Cancer* 1983;51:260–268.
205. Jacobs EL, Haskell CM: Clinical use of tumor markers in oncology. *Curr Probl Cancer* 1991;15:299–351.
206. Pearlman SJ, Sawson W, Biller HF: Occult medullary carcinoma of the thyroid presenting as neck and parapharyngeal metastases. *Otolaryngol Head Neck Surg* 1988;99:509–512.
207. Malissard L, Forcard JJ: Cervical lymph node metastases from squamous cell carcinoma with unknown primary tumor: Is tonsillectomy necessary for diagnosis of subclinical tumor? Paris: Proceedings of the 17th International Congress of Radiology, 1989:167.
208. Righi PD, Sofferman RA: Screening unilateral tonsillectomy in the unknown primary. *Laryngoscope* 1995;105(5 Pt):548–550.

Pathology

209. de Braud F, Al-Sarraf M: Diagnosis and management of squamous cell carcinoma of unknown primary tumor site of the neck. *Semin Oncol* 1993;20:273–278.
210. Neumann KH, Nystrom SJ: Metastatic cancer of unknown origin: Nonsquamous type. *Semin Oncol* 1982;9:427–434.
211. Hainsworth JD, Wright EP, Johnson DH, et al: Poorly differentiated carcinoma of unknown primary site: Clinical usefulness of immunoperoxidase staining. *J Clin Oncol* 1991;9:1931–1938.
212. Mackay B, Ordonez NG: Pathological evaluation of neoplasms with unknown primary site. *Semin Oncol* 1993;20:206–228.
213. Garrow GC, Greco FA, Hainsworth JD: Poorly differentiated neuroendocrine carcinoma of unknown primary tumor site. *Semin Oncol* 1993;20:287–291.
214. Horning SJ, Carrier EK, Rouse RV, et al: Lymphoma presenting as histologically unclassified neoplasms: Characteristics and response to treatment. *J Clin Oncol* 1989;7:1281–1287.
215. Azar HA, Espinoza CG, Richman AV, et al: "Undifferentiated large cell" malignancies: An ultrastructural and immunocytochemical study. *Hum Pathol* 1982;13:323–333.
216. Gatter KC, Alcock C, Heryet A, et al: Clinical importance of analysing malignant tumors of uncertain origin with immunohistochemical techniques. *Lancet* 1985;1:1302–1305.
217. Hales SA, Gatter KC, Heryet A: The value of immunocytochemistry in differentiating high-grade lymphoma from other anaplastic tumors from 1940–1960. *Leuk Lymphoma* 1989;1:59–63.
218. Homan MR, Gharib H, Goellner JR: Metastatic papillary cancer of the neck: A diagnostic dilemma. *Head Neck* 1992;14:113–118.
219. Cho KR, Epstein JI: Metastatic prostatic carcinoma to supradiaphragmatic lymph nodes. A clinicopathologic and immunohistochemical study. *Am J Surg Pathol* 1987;11:457–463.
220. Jones H, Antony PP: Metastatic prostatic carcinoma presenting as left-sided cervical adenopathy: A series of 11 cases. *Histopathology* 1992;21:149–154.
221. Van Kieken JHJM: Prostate marker immunoreactivity in salivary gland neoplasms: A rare pitfall in immunohistochemistry. *Am J Surg Pathol* 1993;17:410–414.
222. Feinmesser R, Feinmesser M, Freeman JL, et al: Detection of occult nasopharyngeal primary tumors by means of in situ hybridizytion. *J Laryngol Otol* 1992;106:345–348.
223. Feinmesser R, Miyazaki, Cheung R, et al: Diagnosis of nasopharyngeal carcinoma by DNA amplification of tissue obtained by fine-needle aspiration. *N Engl J Med* 1992;326:17–21.
224. Walter MA, Menaquez-Palanca J, Peiper SC: Epstein-Barr virus detection in neck metastases by polymerase chain reaction. *Laryngoscope* 1992;102:481–485.
225. Dictor M, Siven M, Tennvall J, et al: Determination of nonendemic nasopharyngeal carcinoma by in situ hybridization for Epstein-Barr virus EBR1 RNA: Sensitivity and specificity in cervical node metastases. *Laryngoscope* 1995;105(Pt 1):407–412.
226. Curtis CW, Ollayos MC, Riordan GP, et al: Estrogen receptor detection in paraffin sections of adenocarcinoma of the colon, pancreas and lung. *Arch Pathol Lab Med* 1994;118:630–632.
227. Hammar S, Bockus D, Remington F: Metastatic tumors of unknown origin: An ultrastructural analysis of 265 cases. *Ultrastruct Pathol* 1987;11:209–250.
228. Ilson DH, Motzer RJ, Rodriguez E, et al: Genetic analysis in the diagnosis of neoplasms of unknown primary tumor site. *Semin Oncol* 1993;20:229–237.
229. Chung KY, Mukhopadhyay T, Kim J, et al: Discordant p53 mutations in primary head and neck cancers and corresponding second primary cancers of the upper aerodigestive tract. *Cancer Res* 1993;53:1676–1683.
230. Zariwala M, Schmid S, Pfaltz M: p53 gene mutations in oropharyngeal carcinomas: A comparison of solitary and multiple primary tumors and lymph node metastases. *Int J Cancer* 1994;56:807–862.

Differential Diagnosis

231. Ryan JR, Ioachim HL, Marmer J, et al: Acquired immune deficiency syndrome-related lymphadenopathies presenting in the salivary gland lymph nodes. *Arch Otolaryngol* 1985;111:554–556.
232. Smith A, Winkler B, Perzin HK, et al: Mucoepidermoid carcinoma arising in ectopic salivary gland tissue. *Cancer* 1985;55:400–403.
233. Yacoub U, Carstens PH, Biscopink RJ, et al: Acinic cell tumor in ec-

topic salivary gland tissue (letter). *Arch Pathol Lab Med* 1981; 105:500–501.

234. Stell PM, Cruickshank AH, Stoney P: Adenoid cystic carcinoma presenting as a mass in the neck. *J Laryngol Otol* 1986;100:1203–1204.

235. Butler JJ, Tulinius H, Ibanez ML, et al: Significance of thyroid tissue in lymph nodes associated with carcinoma of the head and neck or lung. *Cancer* 1967;20:103–112.

236. Clark RL, Hickery RC, Butler JJ, et al: Thyroid cancer discovered incidentally during treatment for an unrelated head and neck cancer. *Ann Surg* 1966;163:665–671.

237. Meyer JS, Steinberg LS: Microscopically benign thyroid follicles in cervical lymph nodes. *Cancer* 1969;24:302–311.

238. Aguacil-Garcia A: Intranodal myofibroblastoma in a submandibular lymph node. A case report. *Am J Clin Pathol* 1992;97:69–72.

239. Fletcher CDM, Stirling RW: Intranodal myofibroblastoma presenting in the submandibular region: Evidence of a broader clinical and histological spectrum. *Histopathology* 1990;16:287–294.

240. Weiss IM, Berry GJ, Dorfmann RF, et al: Spindle cell neoplasms of lymph nodes of probable reticulum cell lineage. True reticulum cell sarcoma? *Am J Surg Pathol* 1990;14:405–414.

241. Jensen JL, Correll RW: Nevus cell aggregates in submandibular lymph nodes. *Oral Surg Oral Med Oral Pathol* 1980;50:552–556.

242. Martin JME, Randhawa G, Temple WJ: Cervical thymoma. *Arch Pathol Lab Med* 1986;110:354–357.

Treatment and Prognosis

243. Strasnick B, Moore CM, Abemayor E, et al: Occult primary tumors. The management of isolated submandibular lymph node metastases. *Arch Otolaryngol Head Neck Surg* 1990;116:173–176.

244. Vikram B: Changing patterns of failure in advanced head and neck cancer. *Arch Otolaryngol* 1984;110:564–565.

245. Davidson BJ, Spiro RH, Patel S, et al: Cervical metastases of occult origin: The impact of combined modality therapy. *Am J Surg* 1994;168:395–399.

246. Marcial-Vega VA, Cardenes H, Perez Ca, et al: Cervical metastases from unknown primaries: Radiotherapeutic management and appearance of subsequent primaries. *Int J Radiat Oncol Biol Phys* 1990;19:919–928.

247. Carter RL, Bliss JM, Soo KH, et al: Radical neck dissections for squamous carcinomas: Pathological findings and their clinical implications with particular reference to transcapsular spread. *Int J Radiat Oncol Biol Phys* 1987;13:825–832.

248. Johnson JT, Meyers EN, Bedetti CD, et al: Cervical lymph node metastasis: Incidence and implications of extracapsular carcinoma. *Arch Otolaryngol* 1985;111:534–537.

249. Olsen KD, Caruso M, Foote L: Primary head and neck cancer. Histologic predictors of recurrence after neck dissection in patients with lymph node involvement. *Arch Otolaryngol Head Neck Surg* 1994;120:1370–1374.

250. Aquarelli MJ, Matsunaga RS, Cruze K: Metastatic carcinoma of the neck of unknown primary origin. *Laryngoscope* 1961;71:962–964.

251. Barrie JR, Knapper WH, Strong EW: Cervical nodal metastases of unknown origin. *Am J Surg* 1970;120:466–470.

252. France CJ, Lucas R: The management and prognosis of metastatic neoplasm of the head and neck with an unknown primary. *Am J Surg* 1963;106:835–839.

253. Marchetta FC, Murphy WT, Kovaric JJ: Carcinoma of the neck. *Am J Surg* 1963;106:974–979.

254. Carlson LS, Fletcher GH, Oswald MJ: Guidelines for radiotherapeutic techniques for cervical metastases from an unknown primary. *Int J Radiat Oncol Biol Phys* 1986;12:2101–2110.

255. Coster JR, Foote RL, Olsen KD, et al: Cervical nodal metastasis of squamous cell carcinoma of unknown origin: Indications for withholding radiation therapy. *Int J Radiat Oncol Biol Phys* 1992;23:743–749.

256. Bridger GP, Reay-Young P: Metastatic neck tumor of unknown primary origin. *Med J Aust* 1978;2:49–51.

257. Nordstrom DG, Tewfik HH, Latourette HB: Cervical lymph node metastases from unknown primary. *Int J Radiat Oncol Biol Phys* 1979;5:73–76.

258. Harper CS, Mendall WM, Parsons JT, et al: Cancer in neck nodes with unknown primary site: Role of mucosal radiotherapy. *Head Neck* 1990;12:463–469.

259. Glynne-Jones RGT, Anand AK, Young TE, et al: Metastatic carcinoma in the cervical lymph nodes from occult primary. *Int J Radiat Oncol Biol Phys* 1990;118:289–294.

260. Jones AS, Cook JA, Phillips DE, et al: Squamous carcinoma presenting as an enlarged cervical lymph node. *Cancer* 1993;72:1756–1761.

261. Perez CA, Jesse RH, Fletcher GH: Metastatic carcinoma in cervical lymph nodes: Unknown primary site. In: Jesse RH (ed): *Neoplasia of the Head and Neck.* Chicago, Year Book Medical Publishers, 1974:289–302.

262. Silverman CL, Marks JE, Lee F, et al: Treatment of epidermoid and undifferentiated carcinomas from occult primaries presenting in cervical lymph nodes. *Laryngoscope* 1983;93:645–648.

Neck Dissection

263. Medina JE, Houck JR: Advances in neck dissection. *Arch Otolaryngol Head Neck Surg* 1995;9:183–196.

264. Byers RM: Modified neck dissection: A study of 967 cases from 1970 to 1980. *Am J Surg* 1985;150:414–421.

265. Close LB, Brown PM, Vuich MF, et al: Microvascular invasion and survival in cancer of the oral cavity and oropharynx. *Arch Otolaryngol Head Neck Surg* 1989;115:1304–1309.

266. Grandi C, Alloisio M, Moglia D, et al: Prognostic significance of lymphatic spread in head and neck carcinomas: Therapeutic implications. *Head Neck* 1985;8:67–73.

267. Leemans CR, Tiwari R, Navta JJP, et al: Regional lymph node involvement and its significance in the developement of distant metastases in head and neck carcinoma. *Cancer* 1993;71:452–456.

268. Snow GB, Annyas AA, Van Slotten EA, et al: Prognostic factors of neck node metastasis. *Clin Otolaryngol* 1982;7:185–192.

269. Schuller DE, McGuirt WF, McCabe BF, Young D: The prognostic significance of metastatic cervical lymph nodes. *Laryngoscope* 1980;90:557–570.

270. Cachin Y: Management of cervical nodes in head and neck cancer. In: Evans PHR, Robin PE, Fielding JWL (eds): *Head and Neck Cancer.* New York: Alan R. Liss, 1983:168–177.

11 ∷ Ear: External, Middle, and Temporal Bone

■ *Gustave L. Davis*

Lesions of the ear reflect the composition and environmental exposures of the ear's constituent parts: the skin, subcutaneous tissues, and cartilage of the external ear; the mucosa, ossicles and bone, nerves, muscles, and blood vessels of the middle ear and mastoid; and the specialized epithelium and nerves of the inner ear, which, encased within the temporal bone, transmute sound and position sensation to electrical impulses and produce and regulate the flow of endolymph.

Embryologically, the ear is formed by the intersection of three developmental embryonic layers "not causally connected in development but linked together only through the medium of their definitive functioning" (Yntema cited by Van De Water and Rubin[1]). The external ear, including the pinna or auricle, external auditory meatus, and canal to the squamous epithelial layer of the tympanum (eardrum), is formed by the ectoderm and mesoderm of the first branchial groove and adjacent first (mandibular) and second (hyoid) branchial arches. The middle ear epithelium, lining the auditory (eustachian) tube, middle ear, and mastoid cavities, is an endodermal derivative of the first pharyngeal pouch with mesodermal contributions lining the mastoid and epitympanic and hypotympanic cavities. The tympanic membrane is derived from both external and middle ear; the external squamous surface is contiguous with that of the external auditory canal, and an endodermally derived simple cuboidal, columnar, or flat epithelium lines the middle ear. A portion of the tympanum, the pars flaccida, lacks an intermediate mesenchyme. The middle ear ossicles and supporting tissues are first and second branchial arch mesenchyme derivatives. The inner ear develops, by mesodermal and neural induction, from the ectodermal otic placode rather than from the branchial apparatus. An appreciation of the embryologic origins of the ear is useful in interpreting the "origins" of tumors, the potential of cells for metaplastic change, and discussions of choristoma and origin of cholesteatoma.

The surgical anatomy of the ear is reviewed by Ross and Sasaki[2] in their discussion of radical temporal bone surgery for malignant tumors. Michaels' presentation of the histology of the ear[3] is comprehensive and well illustrated, as is his ear, nose, and throat pathology text.[4]

The vast majority of ear lesions submitted for pathologic examination (biopsy) are (1) from the skin[5, 6] of the external ear (pinna, meatus, or canal), (2) inflammatory (8:1 ratio of inflammatory:neoplastic lesions[7]), and (3) due to traumatic or actinic insults.

Analysis of tumors of the ear from major referral centers[7, 8] and community and university hospitals show similar frequencies of tumor types and location (Table 11–1). In the Barnes Hospital series,[7] the most common tumors, in order of frequency, are squamous cell and basal cell carcinomas, predominantly of the external ear (45%); paragangliomas of the middle ear (14%); adenomatous neoplasms (10%); osteoma of the external canal (7%); carcinoma, not otherwise specified (6%); nerve sheath tumors (3%); and nevi or melanoma of the external ear (3%). Remaining are miscellaneous benign and malignant mesenchymal tumors, including rhabdomyosarcoma (1%) in children. The community hospital (Bridgeport Hospital) files contain more common benign squamous cysts and keloids and fewer middle ear–temporal bone neoplasms.

Lesions of the internal auditory canal are under-represented in these series. The relative numbers of lesions of the external ear and nevi or melanoma and acoustic neuroma vary depending on the nature of the referring services—that is, otology, dermatology, or neurosurgery.

Recently published color atlases of head and neck pathology illustrate virtually all ear tumors, accompanied by accepted nomenclature.[9, 10]

Tumors of the ear are rare relative to inflammatory lesions. However, since they occur in the same age groups and have similar clinical presentations, biopsy differentiation between inflammatory and neoplastic (benign or malignant) is necessary and often difficult.

Lesions of the external ear are predominantly lumps and bumps of skin and cartilage origin in elderly individuals. Tumors of the external canal are often not visible and are manifested early by "fullness" and later by a mass, fluid drainage, or bloody discharge. Hearing loss and pain are symptoms of increasing size and invasion and are clinical manifestations of malignancy. Ulceration and superimposed inflammation can lead to an erroneous "inflammatory" diagnosis, but, except for otitis in diabetic patients, necrotic inflammatory masses are usually necrotic tumors. Evaluation of the site, size, and spread of neoplastic lesions with sophisticated imaging techniques is mandatory.

Middle ear lesions present with hearing loss, and, with an otoscope, a mass can be seen behind the normal or bulging eardrum. Chronic otitis media is a sequel of acute otitis media in children, but in adults, chronic otitis media is a sign of a systemic disease or neoplasm. Hearing loss occurs early in the course of middle ear disease owing to encroachment on the conductive chain of ossicles. Enlargement of the lesion can cause the drum to bulge into the external canal or destroy the drum. Both neoplasms and infection spread from the middle ear posteriorly into the mastoid, medially into the jugular fossa, and superiorly through the tegmen into the cranial cavity and laterally through the drum.

Lesions of the inner ear, located within the temporal bone, had been relatively inaccessible to biopsy, but with current imaging techniques, fine-needle aspiration biopsy, endoscopes, and recently developed base of the skull neuro-otologic techniques, no part of the ear is unreachable by skilled operators. Inner ear tumors are predominantly nerve sheath tumors, meningiomas, and rare lipomatous tumors of the eighth cranial nerve involving the internal auditory meatus. The newly identified papillary tumor of the endolymphatic sac, associated with von Hippel-Lindau disease, is a rare and controversial lesion.

∷ EXTERNAL EAR
Lumps and Bumps

With few exceptions, lesions of the external ear are similar to lesions of skin and soft tissues in other parts of the body but particularly reflect exposure of the skin and underlying cartilage to environmental actinic injury (Table 11–2).

Table 11-1. Frequency of Ear Neoplasms at Four Institutions (%)

Neoplasm	BH*	AFIP†	YNH‡	BPT§
Squamous	48	53	66	61
Benign	3	4	6	17
cysts			4	14
papilloma, etc			2	3
Squamous cell carcinoma	35	27	27	16
Basal cell carcinoma	10	22	26	11
Neuroepithelial/Neural	21	26	25	16
Nevi	2	6	12	8
Melanoma	1	2	9	2
Nerve sheath	3	12		4
Schwannoma		12		2
Neurofibroma		<1		1
Granular cell		1		<1
Paraganglioma	14	4	3	0
Merkel cell tumor			<1	<1
Meningioma		1		<1
Heterotopic brain		<1		
Neuroblastoma		<1		
Glandular	10	11	1	2
Adenoma	6	5	<1	<1
Auricle		<1		
External canal	3	2		<1
Middle ear	3	3	<1	<1
Adenocarcinoma	4	3	0	0
Carcinoma not otherwise specified	6			
Benign not otherwise specified	2			
Metastases	<1	2	2	<1
Malignant not otherwise specified			1	<1
Mesenchymal lesions	12	11	5	24
Fibrohistiocytic				
Benign		2	1	1
Malignant		<1		
Keloid				15
Leiomyoma		<1		
Leiomyosarcoma		<1		
Rhabdomyosarcoma	<1	2	<1	<1
Sarcoma not otherwise specified		1		
Vascular	2	<1	1	2
Kaposi's sarcoma		<1		
Lymphangioma		<1		
Hemangioma	2		1	2
Bone/cartilage	7	4	<1	1
Benign	7	4	<1	1
Malignant		<1		
Langerhans' cell granulomatoses	<1	<1	<1	
Lymphoproliferative	1	<1		
Congenital		<1		
Dermoid		<1		
Hamartoma		<1		
Choriostoma		<1		
Tragus				<1
TOTAL NUMBER	219	1781	235	293

*(BH) Barnes Hospital data derived from Table 13–1, Davis GL: Tumors and inflammatory conditions of the ear. In: Gnepp DR, ed: *Pathology of the Head and Neck.* New York: Churchill Livingstone, 1988:548.

†(AFIP) Armed Forces Institute of Pathology data derived from Table 25, Hyams VJ, Batsakis JG, Michaels L: Tumors of the upper respiratory tract and ear. *Atlas of Tumor Pathology,* 2nd series, fascicle 25. Washington, DC: Armed Forces Institute of Pathology, 1988:260–261.

‡(YNH) Yale and §(BPT) Bridgeport Hospital-Bridgeport Pathology Consultants, previously unpublished data.

Table 11-2. Differential Diagnosis of Nodules of the External Ear

Painful Nodules

Chondrodermatitis nodularis
If secondarily ulcerated and infected
    Basal cell carcinoma
    Squamous cell carcinoma
    Keratoacanthoma
    Actinic keratosis

Painless Nodules

Basal cell carcinoma	Any site; pearly edge with telangiectasia
Squamous cell carcinoma	Top surface of helix
Keratoacanthoma	Top surface of helix
Actinic keratosis	Top surface of helix, not discrete
Elastotic nodule	Bilateral pearly papules on anterior antihelix
Gouty tophi	Creamy papules on helix and antihelix, aspirate urate crystals
Cartilaginous pseudocyst	Fluctuant swelling in upper half of auricle, aspirate oily fluid
Pseudopyogenic granuloma	Multiple itchy nodules in concha

Painful Swollen Ear

Relapsing polychondritis	Entire ear but lobe is inflamed; other areas of cartilage affected
Subperichondral hematoma	Recent trauma with hemorrhage
Acute perichondritis	Infected ear, systemic symptoms

Ear Lobe Swelling

Local disease	Keloid, epidermal cyst, granuloma, viral wart, acne cyst
Systemic disease	Leukemia/lymphoma, sarcoid granulomas

Adapted from Lawrence CM: Chondrodermatitis nodularis. *In* Arndt KA, Le Boit PE, Robinson JK, et al., eds: *Cutaneous Medicine and Surgery.* Philadelphia: W.B. Saunders, 1996:509.

Congenital Developmental Anomalies

Congenital anomalies of the external ear include the deformed pinna and persistent tracts, pits, cysts, duplications, and anomalous (hamartomatous) glandular tissues in and around the external and middle ear, reflecting the complexities of embryologic branchial arch derivation.

Accessory Tragus

The most common congenital lesion in our Bridgeport Pathology files (see Table 11–1) is accessory tragus[11] located anterior to the tragus of the ear. It is removed from infants for cosmetic reasons and consists of a central core of cartilage surrounded by normal skin (Fig. 11–1).

Preauricular Cysts and Sinuses

Clinical Features. Preauricular cysts and fistulous tracts[12–14] above the hyoid bone associated with the parotid gland and external ear are derived from the first branchial arch. Cysts and tracts may persist into adulthood and become secondarily infected and drain, or they may be removed for cosmetic reasons. Congenital anomalies caused by incomplete closure of the first branchial cleft occur as clefts, cysts, and tracts in and about the ear. The anomalies have been classified as type I and type II depending on their location and composition. These lesions usually present in infancy and childhood but may first be diagnosed in adults.[13] They are found along the ex-

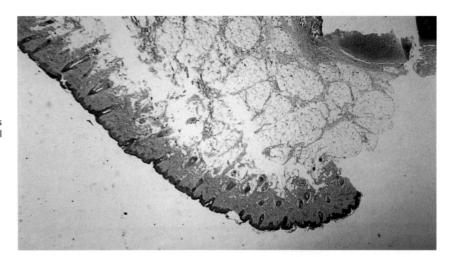

Figure 11–1. Accessory tragus. A subcutaneous "bar" of mature cartilage is surrounded by normal skin.

ternal auditory canal from the eardrum to the junction of the tragus and antitragus.

Pathologic Features. The cysts and tracts are lined predominantly by squamous epithelium with varying amounts of respiratory and mucinous epithelium. Type I anomalies are cystic and entirely ectodermal (Fig. 11–2) without skin adnexa or cartilage; type II anomalies are composed of skin with adnexal structures and cartilage and can involve the drum and middle ear.[14] The fistulas, cysts, and sinuses extend inferiorly into an area bounded by the hyoid bone, sternocleidomastoid muscle, and mandible and deeply to involve the parotid gland and facial nerve. These lesions are not usually associated with other facial malformations.

Differential Diagnosis. Differential diagnoses will vary with the age of the patient. In infants, *cystic hygromas* are not localized lesions. In adults, tumors of the parotid gland and adjacent lymph nodes can be cystic. The *lymphoepithelial cyst of the parotid gland or lymph node*[15] is a well-defined lesion in patients infected with human immunodeficiency virus 1 (HIV-1) (Fig. 11–3). The cysts are lined by nonkeratinizing squamous epithelium, not by the oncocytic lining epithelium characteristic of Warthin's tumor (cystadenoma lymphomatosum). Imaging studies are needed for the diagnosis of lesions of the parotid gland and temporomandibular joint, which can present as masses anterior or posterior to the tragus (see subsequent discussion).

Treatment and Prognosis. Type I anomalies can be simply excised but occasionally require superficial parotidectomy and facial

nerve dissection.[13, 14] Adequate treatment of type II anomalies requires surgical excision of the skin and surrounding cartilage of the external auditory canal with superficial parotidectomy and facial nerve dissection. These lesions should not recur if they are completely excised.

Epidermal Cysts of the Skin

Epidermal cysts of the pinna may be congenital (dermoid), acquired (traumatic keratinous epidermal inclusion), or cystic hair follicle tumors (Fig. 11–4). These are not sebaceous cysts; they contain keratin, not sebum.

Congenital dermoid cysts[16] of the skin are found in lines of closure near the ears, eyes, nose, and cheeks. The dermoid cyst is lined by epidermal squamous cells containing keratohyalin granules and surrounded by normal accessory hair follicles and glands.

Similar keratinous cysts lacking surrounding hair follicles and glands may be found anywhere on the pinna and are called *keratinous "epidermal" cysts* (see Fig. 11–4A).

The *pilar cyst* (wen) is a benign cystic neoplasm derived from the hair shaft epithelium characterized by a lining squamous epithelium that lacks keratohyalin (see Fig. 11–4B). Variants include *pilomatrixoma*[17] (calcifying epithelioma of Malherbe) (see Fig. 11–4C) and cystic *tricholemmoma* (see Fig. 11–4D). These hair shaft tumors are often located at or in the external meatus.

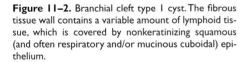

Figure 11–2. Branchial cleft type 1 cyst. The fibrous tissue wall contains a variable amount of lymphoid tissue, which is covered by nonkeratinizing squamous (and often respiratory and/or mucinous cuboidal) epithelium.

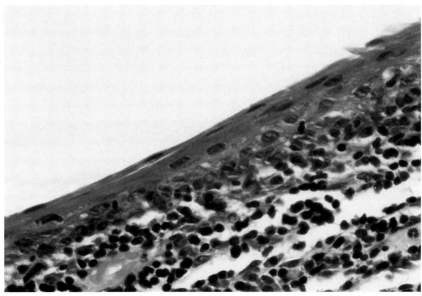

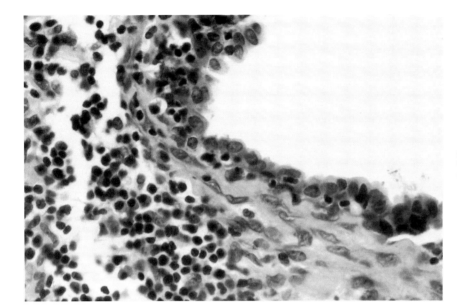

Figure 11–3. Lymphoepithelial cyst of the parotid gland related to human immunodeficiency virus infection. Nonkeratinizing squamous epithelium lines cysts in the lymphoid tissue within the parotid gland.

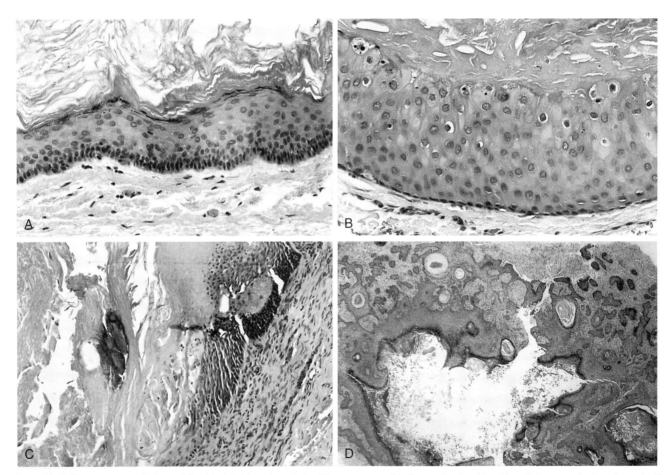

Figure 11–4. Keratinous cystic lesions of the skin. *A*, Epidermal cyst is lined by squamous epithelium replicating skin with a distinct granular layer, keratohyalin granules and hard keratin filling the cyst. No skin appendages are present. *B*, Pilar cyst (wen) is lined by squamous epithelium derived from the hair shaft, lacking distinct keratohyalin granules and maturing to make soft keratin, which fills the cyst. *C*, Pilomatrixoma (calcifying epithelioma of Malherbe) is a cystic tumor of the hair root matrix similar to the wen, but the squamous lining contains hair root matrix cells and the soft keratin within the cyst contains outlines of "ghost" cells and foci of calcification. *D*, Trichofolliculoma, a cystic tumor of the distal hair shaft is lined by keratinous squamous epithelium containing well-developed hairs. Small cystic hair shafts bud from the larger central cyst.

Treatment and Prognosis. Simple excision is curative, but ruptured cysts can incite an extensive foreign body granulomatous reaction to keratin squames and hair.

Cartilaginous Pseudocyst

Clinical Features. Cartilaginous pseudocyst, or idiopathic cystic chondromalacia, of the auricular cartilage[18, 19] presents as a painless diffuse mass in the concha of the upper half of the auricle. This is likely a heterogeneous group of lesions representing congenital dysplasia of cartilage in infants and tramatic pseudocysts in children and adults.

Pathologic Features. Biopsy is rarely performed but will yield fragments of cartilage lacking a cellular lining.

Differential Diagnosis. The clinical differential diagnoses of relapsing polychondritis, chondrodermatitis nodularis helicis, and traumatic perichondritis can be disregarded by the absence of pain and inflammation. Histologic examination eliminates vascular or cartilaginous neoplasms but clinical presentation and location are characteristic.[20]

Treatment and Prognosis. Treatment varies from aspiration of oily serous fluid to oral administration of steroids.

Traumatic Injury

Clinical Features. The auricle is the site of traumatic injury varying from direct physical damage resulting in extensive scarring (cauliflower ears[20]) of the pinna to *keloid* formation in the ear lobes.

The ear lobes produce most of the traumatic material removed and sent to the pathology service. Keloid, an overgrowth of broad bands of dense sclerotic scar tissue, commonly occurs in lobes following ear piercing (Fig. 11–5). Metallic pigmentation, argyria,[21] the deposition of silver, and foreign body granulomas also occur.

Granuloma (acanthoma) fissuratum, or *spectacle frame acanthoma,*[22] is a traumatic deformity of the pinna due to the pressure of tight eyeglass frames, which scar and groove the posterior aspect of the pinna. Histologically, there is a central hyperkeratotic plug that is driven down to cartilage, a pattern similar to chondrodermatitis helicis (see later discussion), but the location and history are specific.

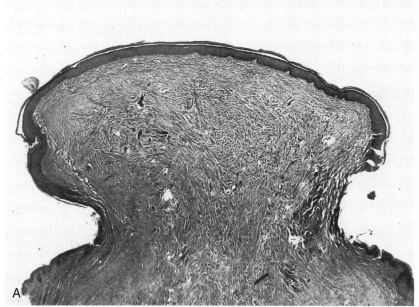
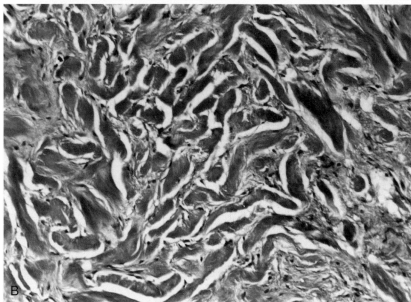

Figure 11–5. Keloid. *A,* Keloid projects from the skin surface. The epidermis is usually intact but may be ulcerated. *B,* The keloid is a hypertrophied scar composed of dense birefringent collagen bundles.

Xanthogranuloma

Clinical Features. Ear piercing and the stimulus of foreign material are also considered in the etiology of xanthogranuloma.[23–27] A Massachusetts General Hospital series of 34 cases had a male:female ratio of 4:1, with an age range from birth to 50 years and peaks at less than 1 year and between 20 and 30 years of age. Juvenile xanthogranuloma in infancy is more often multiple, with rare visceral involvement reported; most will involute by the end of the first year of life. The adult form, in adolescents and young adults, tends to be localized on the ear lobe.

Pathologic Features. Histologically, both types are composed of foamy histiocytes (xanthoma cells), multinucleated (Touton) giant cells, lymphocytes, and eosinophils (Fig. 11–6) organized in recognizable patterns (xanthogranulomatous, xanthomatous, fibrohistiocytic, and combinations), which have no relationship to clinical outcome. The xanthoma cells and Touton giant cells contain lysozyme but not S-100 protein, indicating that they are macrophage/monocyte, not dendritic cell, derivatives.

Differential Diagnosis. The differential diagnosis includes infections due to mycobacteria (leprosy[28] as well as tuberculosis and other related mycobacteria) and fungi (the diagnosis of which requires the use of acid-fast and fungus tissue stains and cultures), and granular cell tumor. Dendritic cell proliferations (Langerhans' cell granulomatosis) are CD1a and S-100 positive. Granular cell tumor[29] is a dermal tumor composed of infiltrating cells of Schwann cell origin, which have granular cytoplasm and benign central nuclei (Fig. 11–7, see p. 687). Unlike xanthogranuloma, there frequently is ex-

tensive pseudoepitheliomatous hyperplasia of the overlying epidermis (see later). Granular cell tumors may be found in multiple skin sites.

Treatment and Prognosis. Since xanthogranuloma can spontaneously involute by 1 year of age, no treatment is recommended in infants. For persistent childhood lesions and those in adults, local excision is appropriate for cosmesis, deformity, or loss of function. Children with both xanthogranuloma and neurofibromatosis are at risk for the development of chronic myelogenous leukemia.[30]

Inflammatory Lesions

The exposure of the helix of the pinna to both sun and cold results in a variety of inflammatory, reactive, and neoplastic lesions that are clinically similar and require biopsy for differentiation. Overwhelmingly, the most common pinna lesions seen in surgical pathology practice (see Tables 11–1 and 11–2) are basal cell carcinomas and squamous proliferative lesions of actinic etiology ranging from keratoses to squamous cell carcinoma. The inflammatory lesions discussed subsequently can mimic actinic malignancies clinically and often histologically, owing to pseudoepitheliomatous hyperplasia of the reactive squamous epithelium.

Chondrodermatitis Helicis (Nodularis)

Clinical Features. Chondrodermatitis helicis (nodularis)[31, 32] is a crusted, ulcerated painful nodule on the helix (less often the an-

Text continued on page 696

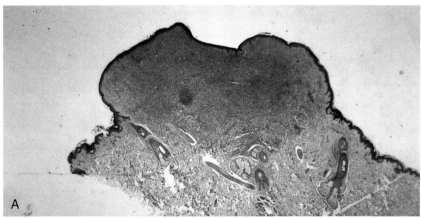

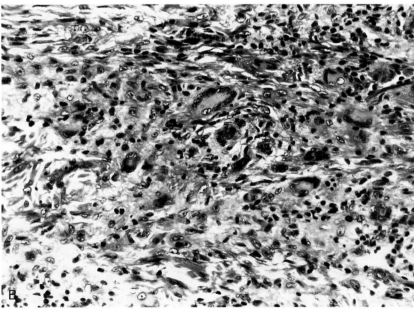

Figure 11–6. Xanthogranuloma. A, Xanthogranuloma forms a nodule that projects above the skin surface and may ulcerate. There is no pseudoepitheliomatous hyperplasia. B, The dermis contains a discrete nodular mixture of macrophages, Touton giant cells, lymphocytes, and eosinophils.

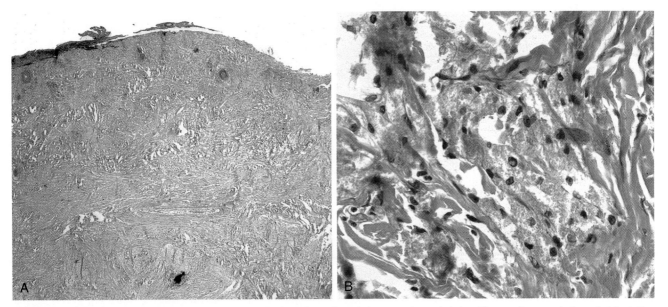

Figure 11–7. Diffusely infiltrating dermal granular cell tumor: Epidermal pseudoepitheliomatous hyperplasia (not illustrated) can mask the underlying infiltrating granular cell tumor. The dermis is infiltrated by indistinct pale granular cells that have small, centrally located nuclei.

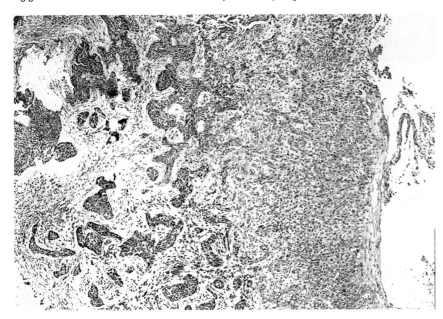

Figure 11–10. Basal-squamous carcinoma. This locally invasive, well-differentiated carcinoma has histologic features of both basal and squamous carcinoma: a palisading pattern of basal cells and distinct keratinization with keratin pearl formation.

Figure 11–11. Keratoacanthoma. Keratoacanthoma forms a cup-shaped projection from the skin surface with a collarette of well-differentiated proliferating squamous epithelium surrounding a central keratin core.

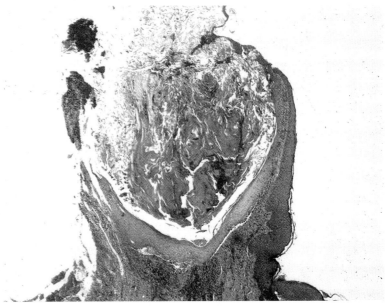

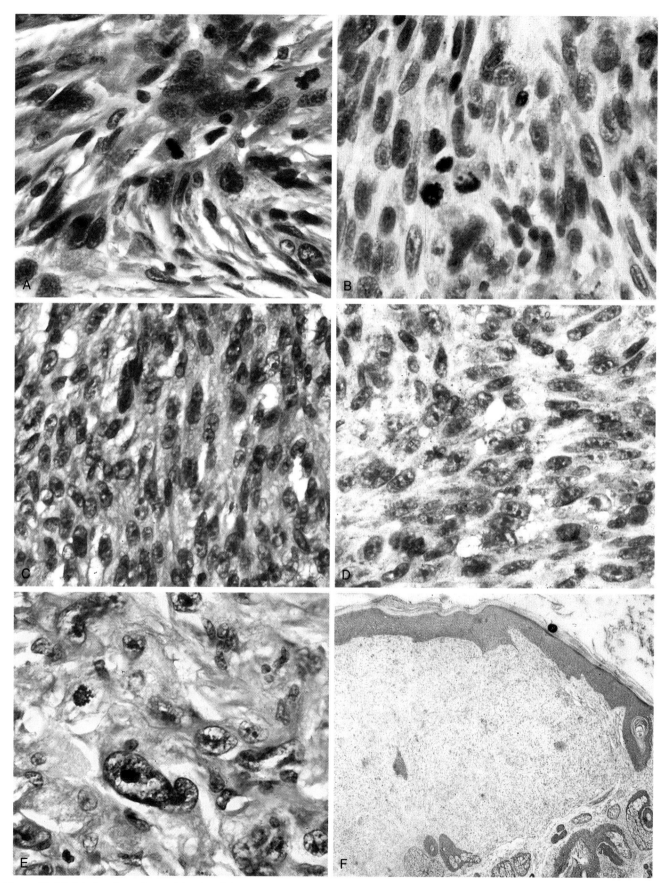

Figure 11–12. Spindle cell neoplasms of the skin of the pinna require immunoperoxidase studies for identification. Spindle cell (sarcomatoid) carcinoma *(A)*, spindle cell amelanotic melanoma *(C)*, and atypical fibroxanthoma *(E)* are virtually indistinguishable with hematoxylin-eosin stain. Spindle cell (sarcomatoid) carcinoma expresses cytoplasmic keratin CK-22 *(B)*; melanoma expresses HMB-45 *(D)*. Neither are expressed in atypical fibroxanthoma (CK-22 shown) *(F)*. (Immunoperoxidase with hematoxylin counterstain [B, D, F].)

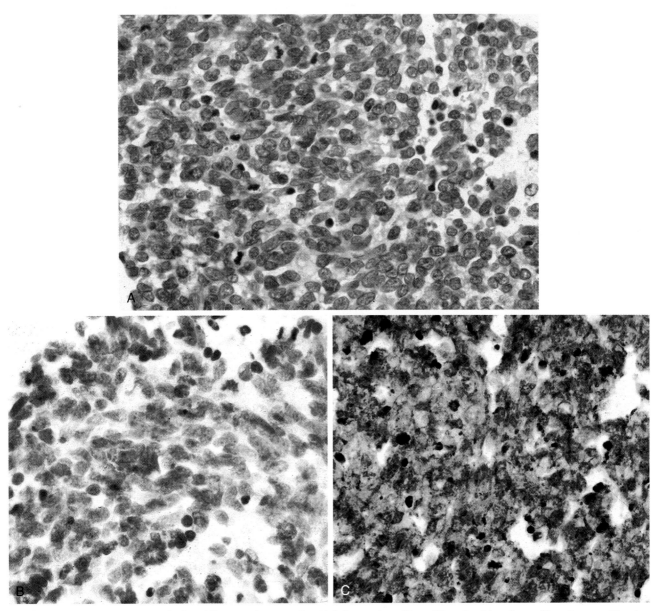

Figure 11–14. Merkel cell carcinoma. Small, undifferentiated tumor cells with little cytoplasm *(A)* are differentiated from "oat cell" carcinoma and lymphoma by perinuclear cytoplasmic expression of keratin AE1/AE3 *(B)* and cytoplasmic membrane expression of chromogranin A *(C)*. (Immunoperoxidase with hematoxylin counterstain [B, C].)

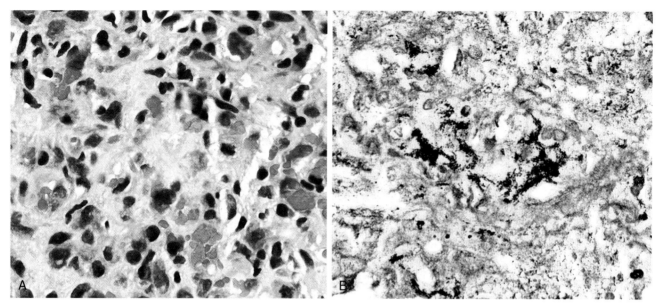

Figure 11–16. Bartonellosis (bacillary angiomatosis). Dermal bartonellosis can be differentiated from Kaposi's sarcoma by scattered stromal hematoxyphilic granular aggregates *(A)*, which are silver staining bacteria *(B)*. (Warthin-Starry stain.) (Courtesy of Dr. P. LeBoit, UCSF.)

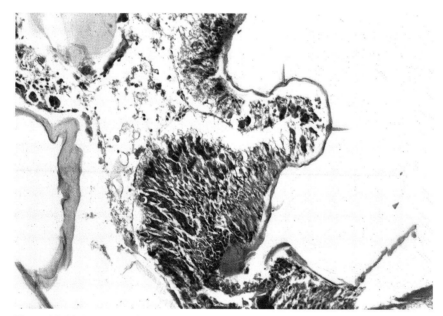

Figure 11–19. Insect parts. Surface bristles and internal organs identify a foreign body in the external auditory canal as insect larva.

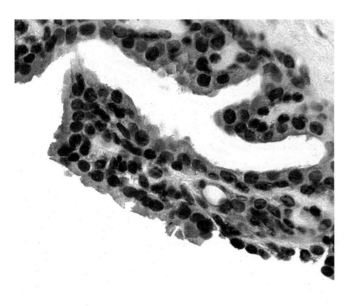

Figure 11–20. Ceruminoma. Ceruminous glands of the ear canal form cystic, solid, or papillary tumors formed by one to two layers of cuboidal cells with granular cytoplasm, basal nuclei, and cytoplasmic "snouts" of apocrine decapitation secretion. Basal myoepithelial cells are present.

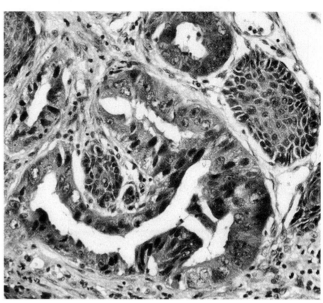

Figure 11–21. Low-grade adenocarcinoma of ceruminal gland origin. Low-grade adenocarcinomas maintain glandular pattern with cytologic atypia, mitotic activity, and tumor necrosis.

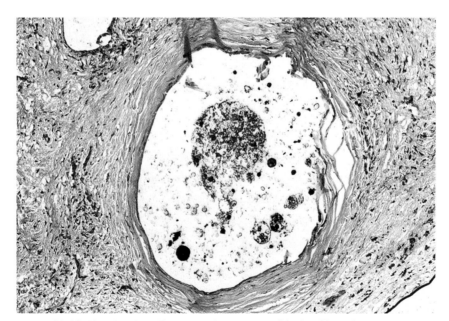

Figure 11–28. Myospherulosis: Erythrocyte-derived "parent" bodies, 20 to 120 μm in diameter, which contain smaller spherules 5 to 7 μm in diameter, are located within holes in inflamed fibrous tissue.

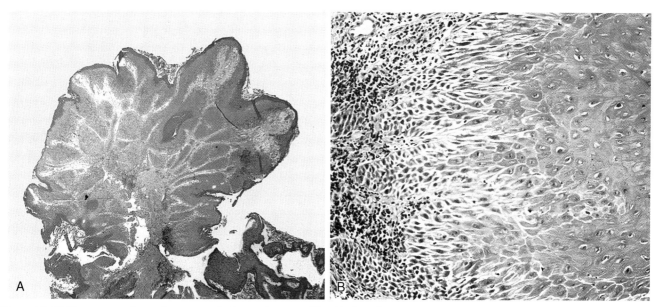

Figure 11–29. Verrucous carcinoma. A warty exophytic growth pattern *(A)* and bulbous but invasive rete pegs *(B)* distinguish verrucous squamous cell carcinoma from hyperplasia.

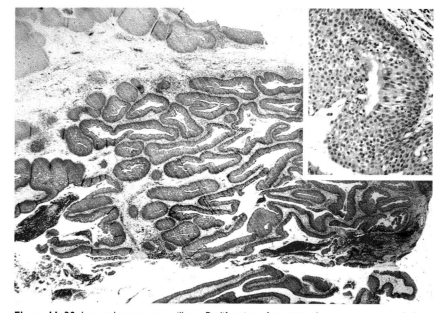

Figure 11–30. Inverted squamous papilloma. Proliferation of transitional-type squamous epithelium on the mucosal surface and subjacent ducts forming nodular masses. *Inset:* The hyperplastic transitional epithelium is not dysplastic and contains residual glandular epithelium.

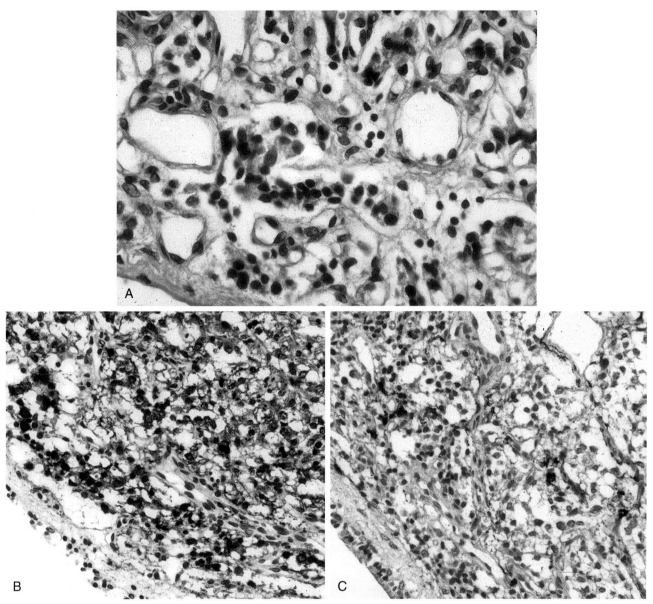

Figure 11–31. Paraganglioma. *A,* The histologic appearance of paraganglioma, nests of small neuroendocrine chief cells (Zellballen) in a vascularized stroma, can be obscured by the small size of the lesion, crush artifact, and hemorrhage. *B,* Chief cells variably express neuroendocrine markers. (Chromogranin immunoperoxidase with hematoxylin counterstain.) *C,* Sustentacular cells, peripheral to the chief cells, express S-100 protein and keratin. (S-100 protein immunoperoxidase with hematoxylin counterstain.)

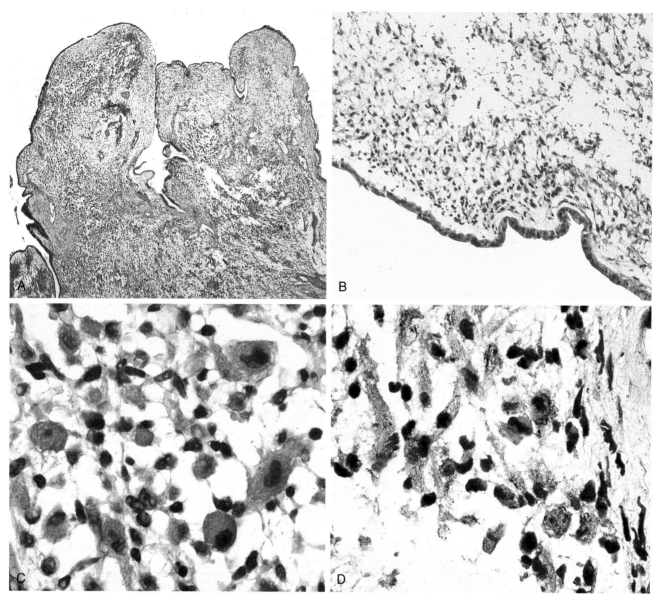

Figure 11–34. Rhabdomyosarcoma. *A,* Rhabdomyosarcoma simulates an "aural polyp" grossly. *B,* Histologic examination shows a condensed layer of small cells, a "cambium layer," immediately beneath the surface mucosa. *C,* Rhabdomyoblasts, eosinophilic cells with hyperchromatic, often pyknotic nuclei express desmin. Strap cells with cross striations are rarely evident. *D,* Immunoperoxidase stain for desmin counterstained with hematoxylin.

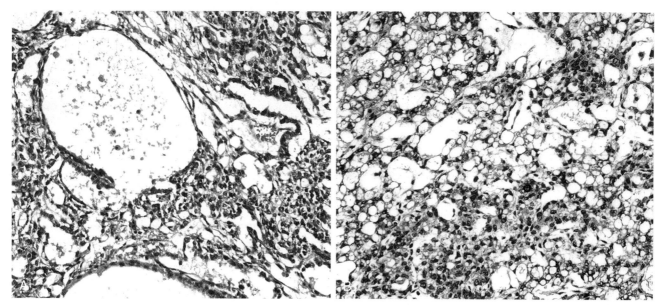

Figure 11–35. Yolk sac tumor. A, Yolk sac tumor is composed of small round blue cells arranged in a vacuolate pattern with formation of Schiller-Duval bodies (center and upper right) and expressing alpha fetoprotein. B, Immunoperoxidase stain to alpha fetoprotein with hematoxylin counterstain.

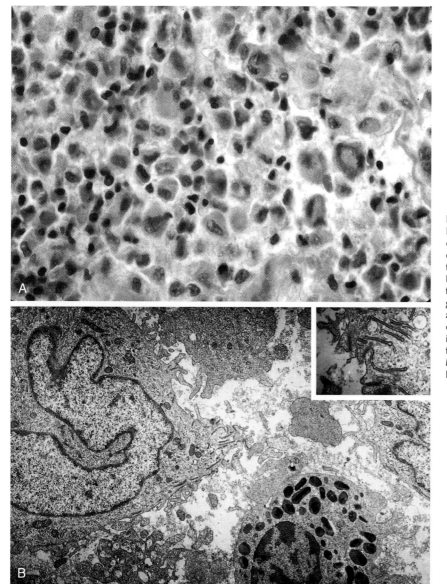

Figure 11–36. Langerhans' cell granulomatosis. A, Langerhans' cell granulomatosis is a mixture of eosinophils and 10 to 12 μm poorly outlined Langerhans' cells. The nuclei of the latter are characteristically reniform to oval and clefted with a nuclear groove. Multinucleated cells are present. B, Ultrastructurally, folded nuclei enclose cytoplasm, forming the nuclear groove of the Langerhans' cell. Birbeck granules (inset) are bilamellar tubules of variable length and average diameter of 34 nm. (Electron micrograph, 3000× mag; inset 30000× mag.) (From Davis GL: Tumors and inflammatory conditions of the ear. In Gnepp DR (ed): Pathology of the Head and Neck. New York: Churchill Livingstone, 1988:566.)

tihelix) of older men (mean age 60 years, range 31–82). It is twice as common in men as in women. Patients relate a long history (1 month to 25 years) of pain, often exacerbated by cold. The disease is attributed to pressure trauma, poor vascularization of the pinna, and collagen damage from the sun and cold. The size of the lesions is not recorded in the cited papers but lesions may be 1 cm in diameter in situ.

Pathologic Features. Histologically, there is skin ulceration with a benign reactive hyperplastic epidermis, with hyperkeratosis or parakeratosis or both, acute and chronic inflammation, dermal scarring with granulation tissue, and necrobiosis of collagen that extends to the subjacent cartilage (Fig. 11–8). The necrotic tissues are eliminated through the ulcerated skin surface, a process described as a *perforating dermatitis*.[33]

Differential Diagnosis. Clinical differential diagnosis includes ulcerating squamous or basal cell carcinoma, which occurs in the same age group and location. Other nodular lesions located on the helix such as *elastic* or *weathering nodules,*[34, 35] *dystrophic calcification,* and *calcified cartilage*[36–38] clinically resemble chondrodermatitis and are associated with trauma or actinic or cold exposure. There is usually no other associated disease of cartilage, but a similar lesion has been described in systemic sclerosis.[39]

Treatment and Prognosis. Irrespective of local therapy (excision, topical and injected steroids, laser, or electrocautery), up to 30% of lesions recur.[31]

Amyloid

Amyloid[40, 41] derived from actinically injured keratinocytes can accumulate as pink globular material (lichen amyloidosis) in the papillary dermis. Congo red stain, which imparts the characteristic orange hue to the amyloid, is apple green when viewed through polarizing filters.

Pernio (Chilblains)

Clinical Features. Localized painful, erythematous inflammatory nodules, known as *pernio*[42] or *chilblains,* result from exposure to a cold, but above freezing, humid environment, which exacerbates heat loss. Pernio occurs equally in men and women, with a mean age of 48 years (range, 10–75 years). It may be primary and idiopathic with a positive antinuclear antibody test and not associated with other concurrent disease. Pernio associated with other diseases and cold exposure can be considered to be "secondary." Pernio-like le-

sions ("mimics") also occur in other autoimmune diseases in the absence of cold exposure.

Pathologic Features. Histologically, pernio and its mimics are characterized by dermal angiocentric lymphocytosis, papillary edema, and lymphocytic exocytosis involving rete pegs and sweat glands.

Differential Diagnosis. Patients with systemic or extracutaneous autoimmune disease such as systemic lupus erythematosus, viral hepatitis, rheumatoid arthritis, cryofibrinogenemia, and hyperglobulinemia may present with secondary perniosis but show "frequent vascular fibrin deposition involving reticular dermal vessels."[42] In addition to the above histologic characteristics, histiocytic infiltrates and noncaseating granulomas signify secondary pernio and require appropriate cultures and tissue stains. Patients with iritis, rheumatoid arthritis, or Crohn's disease can show giant cell vasculitis and a granuloma annulare-like tissue reaction.[42]

Treatment and Prognosis. Protection from cold exposure and treatment of underlying disease are required in susceptible individuals.

Gout

Urate crystals deposit in the skin of the helical edge as gouty tophi (Fig. 11–9A). Both gout and pseudogout (calcium pyrophosphate) can affect the temporomandibular joint and present as a painful inflamed preauricular mass.[43]

Pathologic Features. The clinical diagnosis can be confirmed by needle aspiration of the lesion with demonstration of the characteristic needle-like urate crystals with polarizing filters (Fig. 11–9B). The aspirate and surgical specimen should be fixed in alcohol to preserve the water soluble urate crystals. The rhomboid pyrophosphate crystals of pseudogout are insoluble in aqueous fixatives and will remain in tissues.

Perichondritis

Perichondritis is a diffuse infiltrate of inflammatory or neoplastic leukocytes in the skin of the external ear. Acute *"malignant"* perichondritis in diabetics[44] due to pseudomonas is very destructive and infiltrative with rapid involvement of parotid gland and facial nerve, external auditory canal, and middle ear and thence temporal bone and brain invasion.

Neutrophilic eccrine hidradenitis,[45] an acute inflammatory infiltrate about eccrine glands in patients undergoing chemotherapy for malignancy, can present with swollen inflamed ears. *Acute my-*

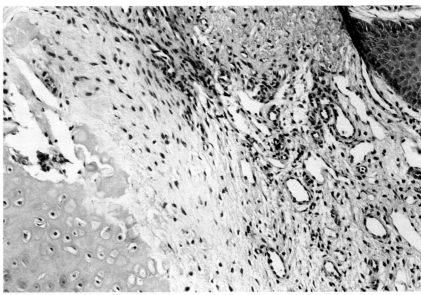

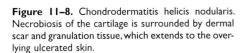
Figure 11–8. Chondrodermatitis helicis nodularis. Necrobiosis of the cartilage is surrounded by dermal scar and granulation tissue, which extends to the overlying ulcerated skin.

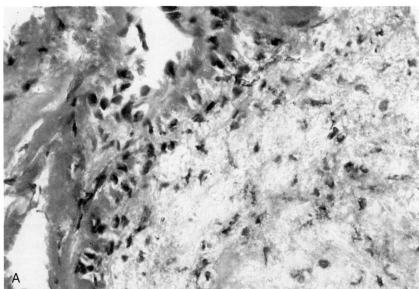

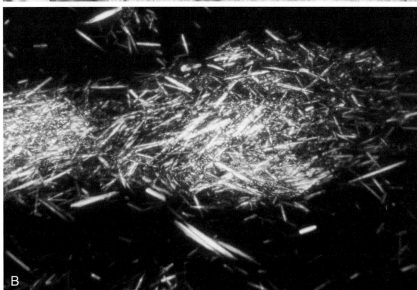

Figure 11–9. Gout. *A,* Urates deposit as tophi in the edge of the helical skin. *B,* Needle-aspirated tophus material smeared on a glass slide and alcohol fixed contains birefringent needle-shaped urate crystals. (Unstained, photographed with crossed polarizing filters. 20× mag.)

eloid leukemia,[46] *T-cell lymphoma,*[47] and *acquired immunodeficiency disease (AIDS)–related non-Hodgkins' lymphoma*[48, 49] can present as auricular perichondritis.

Relapsing Polychondritis

Clinical Features. Relapsing polychondritis[50–55] is a systemic autoimmune disease of type II collagen, occurring equally in affected men and women, with a median age of 47 years (range, 17–86 years). Floppy ears and saddle nose[50] are dramatic effects of cartilage destruction, and almost 50% of patients have hearing impairment due to inner ear damage. Disease of the eyes is common, and one fourth to one third of patients die of cardiovascular system or respiratory tract involvement. Bilateral recurrent auricular chondritis that undergoes spontaneous resolution is characteristic of the disease.

Pathologic Features. Acutely, patients have diffuse, bilateral, painful erythematous auricles. The cartilage and perichondrium are necrotic and inflamed and, with healing, are replaced by scar tissue with loss of structural support. The severity of the disease is directly related to levels of antibody to type II collagen and deposition of immune complexes and complement in cartilage.

The disease is associated with patients having HLA-DR4, and about one third of patients also have associated systemic lupus erythematosus or rheumatoid arthritis. Relapsing polychondritis can

be a paraneoplastic syndrome that precedes the onset of myelodysplasia.[56]

Treatment and Prognosis. Systemic steroid therapy modifies the acute disease and reduces the frequency and severity of recurrences but does not prevent progression of the disease.

Neoplasms

Neoplasms of the ear are rare: only 1 in 10,000 patients with ear complaints has an ear malignancy. Clinically, tumors present similarly,[57] either as actinic lesions on the helix or as a mass in the external auditory canal or middle ear; all require biopsy for differentiation. Squamous cell carcinoma and basal cell carcinoma, the most common ear neoplasms (80–90% of all ear tumors), are found in approximately equal numbers (see Table 11–1).[7]

Basal Cell Carcinoma

Clinical Features. Basal cell carcinoma[58, 59] is predominantly a lesion of the auricular helix. There is a male predominance with a mean age at diagnosis of 60 years.

Pathologic Features and Differential Diagnosis. Basal cell carcinomas, which do rarely occur at the external auditory meatus and extend into the canal, must be differentiated from adenoid cystic carcinoma. The basal cell carcinoma will invariably arise from the overlying skin and maintain areas of typical picket-fence basal epithelium with spindle cell or squamous differentiation (Fig. 11–10, see p. 687). Adenoid cystic carcinoma arises from below the surface squamous epithelium and is composed of organoid aggregates of uniformly small basaloid cells with little cytoplasm or differentiation and the characteristic cribriform pattern. Further aid in differentiation is the presence of acid and neutral mucopolysaccharides in the hyalin connective tissue surrounding the aggregates and within cribriform spaces and tubules of the adenoid cystic carcinoma.[9]

Treatment and Prognosis. Local excision suffices for auricular lesions. Metastases and death are uncommon.[59] Within the canal, delay in diagnosis and deep invasion by the tumor can require partial temporal bone resection for adequate removal.

Squamous Cell Carcinoma

Clinical Features. The origins, clinical manifestations, sex distribution, treatment, and prognosis of squamous cell carcinoma differ depending on the site of origin, the pinna or the external auditory canal.

Lesions of the pinna are associated with actinic injury and occur in men over 70 years of age who have had many actinic keratoses or squamous cell carcinomas removed from the exposed skin of the head and neck.[60, 61]

Squamous cell carcinoma of the external auditory canal[62] is more insidious in its presentation than that of the pinna. There is a female preponderance with a mean age of 60 years, a decade earlier than in patients with squamous cell carcinoma of the pinna. Symptoms, often present for less than a year, include drainage, pain, and hearing loss, indicating an extensive, invasive lesion.

Pathologic Features. Squamous cell carcinoma is characterized by proliferation of squamous cells with abnormal cytologic manifestations of malignancy and abnormal keratinization (dyskeratosis). Basal-squamous lesions, tumors with histologic characteristics of both basal cell and squamous cell carcinoma, are not unusual (see Fig. 11–10 p. 687).

Differential Diagnosis. Squamoproliferative lesions of the skin of the pinna include reactive pseudoepitheliomatous hyperplasia, fibroepithelial papillomas (skin tags), warts (verruca vulgaris), actinic (solar or senile) keratoses, in situ (Bowen's disease), and invasive squamous (epidermoid) carcinoma in all of its guises. Well-differentiated lesions mimic reactive hyperplasia (see later discussion).

Keratoacanthoma is a distinct clinicopathologic entity simulating well-differentiated squamous cell carcinoma. The proliferative lesion grows quickly, forming a cup shape with a central core of keratin (Fig. 11–11, see p. 687). The surrounding proliferating, well-differentiated squamous epithelium has an indistinct basement membrane and can seem to be invasive. These lesions will atrophy and expel the central keratin. It is important, however, to warn the surgeon that absolute histologic differentiation from squamous cell carcinoma is not ensured and that the lesion had best be completely excised.

Spindle cell (sarcomatoid) squamous cell carcinoma requires differentiation from other spindle cell neoplasms (melanoma, fibroxanthoma, and other mesenchymal tumors) with immunoperoxidase studies (Fig. 11–12A&B, see p. 687) (see later).

Treatment and Prognosis. Local excision of pinna lesions usually suffices for local control, but residual or recurrent disease still occurs in 25% of patients. Approximately 10% of invasive squamous cell carcinomas metastasize to regional lymph nodes; patients with such metastases can be treated with neck dissection.[62] Even with reported poor control and clinical persistence, death is usually due to other, intercurrent disease.[63]

In the external auditory canal, in response to chronic irritation, pseudoepitheliomatous hyperplasia can simulate a well-differentiated squamous cell carcinoma.[64] If the patient presents with symptoms and signs of pain and bloody ear discharge lasting longer than 2 months with an ulcerated ear mass, a diagnosis of car-

cinoma is likely. If there is no pain and the ear discharge has taken place over a period less than 2 months, the lesion should be treated conservatively with antibiotics. If, after 2 to 3 weeks, no resolution has occurred, the lesion should be excised with a border of normal tissue and a carcinoma should be sought by histopathologic examination.[64]

Spread of the external auditory canal tumors depends on the location within the canal: anteriorly, invasion through the cartilaginous canal extends to the parotid gland and lymph nodes; posteriorly, adjacent to the bony canal, spread is into the postauricular space and, medially, into the middle ear. Squamous cell carcinomas of the canal metastasize to regional nodes more frequently than do pinna lesions, but the 5-year tumor-related death rate of about 50% is due to local invasion rather than metastases.[65]

Treatment for invasive squamous cell carcinoma of the canal is temporal bone resection (partial, total, or piecemeal), depending on the extent of the tumor. The defect is covered with a skin or muscle flap and is postoperatively irradiated. This treatment is associated with a 50% 5-year survival rate in several series.[66, 67]

Malignant Melanoma

Clinical Features. Malignant melanoma, though relatively rare, is the third most common malignancy of the external ear, accounting for 7% to 16% of all head and neck melanomas.[68–72] As with the other actinically related neoplasms, squamous and basal cell carcinomas, there is a 2:1 male:female ratio with a mean age at diagnosis of 72 years.

Pathologic Features. Malignant melanoma is one of the great mimics among neoplastic lesions. It can be pigmented or amelanotic, ulcerate or form a nodule, and, histologically, simulate epithelial and mesenchymal neoplasms (Fig. 11–12C&D, see p. 687). When presented with a poorly differentiated epithelioid or sarcomatoid neoplasm one must always ask "could this be a melanoma?" and apply differential immunoperoxidase stains.

Melanoma arises in a pre-existing nevocellular lesion of the skin or mucous membrane, and junctional change should be identified to differentiate primary from metastatic melanoma. Excisional biopsies of previously biopsied skin nevocellular lesions may have hemosiderophages and myofibroblasts (scar) partially or completely replacing the original lesion. Iron and trichrome staining or vimentin or actin expression (reactive) and S-100 or HMB-45 expression (melanoma) distinguish between scar and spindle cell melanoma.

Treatment and Prognosis. Treatment varies depending on the location on the ear: peripheral pinna lesions undergo wide local excision or amputation; more central lesions, adjacent to or involving the external auditory meatus, require much more extensive surgery including partial temporal bone resection. Prognosis is related to depth of invasion. Seven of the 16 cases reported by Davidsson et al.[70] were nodular, and depth of invasion varied from 0.15 mm to 11.5 mm; 9 of the 16 were Clark level IV or V at diagnosis. All patients had wide excision, but of the four (25%) who died, three did so within 1 year of diagnosis. Prophylactic neck dissection, including superficial parotidectomy, is deemed appropriate only for Clark level IV or V lesions.

Fibrous Histiocytoma (Dermatofibroma)

Clinical Features. Fibrous histiocytomas[73] are benign polymorphous cutaneous tumors to which several names have been applied: subepidermal nodular fibrosis, dermatofibroma, fibroxanthoma, and sclerosing hemangioma. Dermatofibroma is probably a better term, since the predominating spindle cells are not clearly histiocytes. These painless lesions are typically found in the upper dermis of the extremities in adults.

Pathologic Features. They are poorly circumscribed usually with infiltrating margins and are composed of spindly mononuclear or multinuclear cells, with amphophilic cytoplasm, which are classically arranged in a storiform pattern. Epidermal hyperplasia frequently overlies the lesion. Variable numbers of foamy macrophages and Touton giant cells are present. Birefringent collagen is surrounded by spindle cells at the periphery of the lesion. Various descriptive modifying adjectives are applied to fibrous histiocytomas depending on the mixture of cell types, vascularity, and hemosiderin in the lesion: angiomatoid, epithelioid, giant cell, or cellular.

Differential Diagnosis. In 1964, Kempson and McGavran[74] described a "histologically 'malignant' but biologically benign lesion of the skin" to which they applied Helwig's term *atypical fibroxanthoma.* The well-circumscribed ulcerated nodular lesions occurred in the sun-exposed skin of 21 patients: 15 men, 6 women, mean age 67 years, range 52 to 86 years. Five of the lesions occurred on the ear.

The atypical fibroxanthomas are composed of intermixed cell types, fusiform to round cells with variable numbers of giant cells (Fig. 11–12*E&F*, see p. 687). There is remarkable variability in nuclear and nucleolar size and shape, but mitotic activity is low at 1 per 10 high-power fields. The cellular and nuclear pleomorphism resulted in the initial pathologic diagnoses in the 21 cases: sarcoma in 10, carcinoma in 4, melanoma in 1, and atypical fibroxanthoma in 6. However, the lesions do not recur when adequately locally excised and act in an otherwise benign fashion.

Recently three cases of an atypical fibroxanthoma variant were described in which osteoclast-like giant cells were dispersed within the tumor.[75] Twenty percent of 74 cases of another variant of fibroxanthoma, *benign cellular fibrous histiocytoma,* described by Calonje et al.,[76] occurred in the head and neck, including three cases in the external ear.[77] This lesion occurs in young men (2:1 male:female, mean age 33 years, range 9 months to 86 years) and has ill-defined margins with extension into the deep reticular dermis. Eosinophilic spindle cells with a mean mitotic rate of 3 per high-power field dominate, but there is an admixture of spindle cells, giant cells, and foam cells. The pleomorphism of the "atypical" fibroxanthoma is not present but focal storiform pattern, epidermal hyperplasia, and peripheral hyalinized collagen bundles found in dermatofibroma are present. Although 26% of these lesions recurred within 3 years following inadequate excision, none metastasized.

The atypical fibroxanthoma must be differentiated from the actinic malignancies that it mimics by its pleomorphism: spindle cell (sarcomatoid) epidermoid carcinoma, and melanoma. Each entity has unique ultrastructural characteristics. Squamous cell carcinoma has desmosomes and intracellular keratin; melanoma has melanosomes and premelanosomes; fibrous histiocytoma has myofilaments characteristic of myofibroblasts. A battery of immunocytochemical "stains" can aid in the differentiation of these spindle cell neoplasms (Table 11–3). Squamous cell carcinoma expresses cytokeratins; melanoma, S-100 protein, and human melanoma B-45; atypical fibroxanthoma expresses muscle-specific actin, vimentin, and α_1-antitrypsin/antichymotrypsin, and macrophage lineage markers such as KP-1 (see Fig. 11–12, p. 687). Fibrous histiocytomas are negative for desmin[78] (thus differentiating them from smooth muscle tumors,[79] which contain both smooth muscle actin and desmin) and are usually immunoreactive to macrophage-monocyte markers such as KP-1.[78] Strong LN-5 (CD74) immunoreactivity is reported in "malignant" fibrous histiocytomas and "large" atypical fibrous histiocytomas with subcutaneous extension, but not in superficial atypical fibroxanthoma,[80] and CD-34 expression in dermatofibrosarcoma

protuberans[73] may be useful in predicting the behavior of these confusing lesions.

Treatment and Prognosis. As clinicopathologic entities, these fibrous lesions differ in patient population, histologic appearance, and propensity for local recurrence. They do not recur if adequately surgically excised.

Nodular Fasciitis

Clinical Features. Nodular fasciitis[81, 82] is a benign reactive proliferation of myofibroblasts[83] in response to a traumatic insult, which is not documented in the vast majority of patients. Patients present with a rapidly growing mass lesion that can involve the skin adjacent to the ear, the pinna, or the external auditory canal. Most of the lesions seem to be well circumscribed. Half of the cases reported by Thompson et al.[82] were dermal; the remainder were subcutaneous or could not be separated between dermal and fascial. Nodular fasciitis in the ear canal is often ulcerated and bleeds. Patients are approximately equally divided between men and women, with a mean age of 27 years (range, 1–76 years), a population similar to that of fibrous histiocytoma described earlier.

Pathologic Features. Histologically, the lesion is characterized by spindle-shaped myofibroblasts loosely aggregated in a nodular storiform pattern with adjacent hypocellular myxoid areas, acellular keloid-like collagen, and rare giant cells. Not unexpectedly, spindle cells react with myofibroblast markers vimentin, actin, and KP-1. Mitotic figures are readily identifiable, reflecting the rapid growth noted clinically, but atypical forms are not seen.

Treatment and Prognosis. The preferred form of therapy is adequate local surgical excision of the lesion. This can be difficult in or around the ear with attempts to maintain cosmesis. Recurrence is infrequent, occurring in only 1% to 2% of patients.

Myxoma (Carney Complex)

Clinical Features. Myxomas of the external ear involve both the pinna and the canal in a rare familial autosomal dominant syndrome known as Carney's complex.[84] The patients have myxomas, spotty pigmentation, endocrine tumors, and schwannomas. They occur equally in males and females with ages ranging from birth to 41 years (mean 19.3 years).

Pathologic Features. Histologically, polypoid or sessile myxomas occurring on the pinna or in the canal are composed of bland myxomatous stroma and a proliferating, often basaloid, surface squamous epithelium (Fig. 11–13).

Differential Diagnosis. As a consequence of the latter, differential diagnoses based on superficial biopsies may range from squamous papilloma to epidermal inclusion cyst, trichoepithelioma, and basal cell carcinoma. Any myxomatous lesion on or in the ear of an infant or young child also requires consideration of rhadomyosarcoma (see later).[85]

Treatment and Prognosis. Myxomas are treated with wide local excision. Recurrences, which are frequent, can be re-excised; they do not metastasize. When myxoma is diagnosed, the clinician should be alerted to the possibility of Carney complex syndrome because of the occurrence of potentially fatal cardiac myxomas.

Table 11–3. Differential Immunocytochemical Staining of Spindle Cell Tumors of the Pinna

	KER	EMA	S-100	HMB45	KPI	αIAT	ACT	DES	VIM
Epidermoid carcinoma	+	+	−	−	−	−	−	−	−
Malignant melanoma	−	−	+	+	−	−	−	−	−
Fibrous histiocytoma	−	−	−	−	+	+	+	−	+
Nodular fasciitis	−	−	−	−	+	?	+	−	+
Leiomyoma	−	−	−	−	−	−	+	+	+

ACT, muscle specific actin; α1AT, α$_1$-antitrypsin and/or chymotrypsin; DES, desmin; EMA, epithelial membrane antigen; HMB45, human melanoma B-45 protein; KER, keratins; KP1, macrophage/monocyte lineage marker; S-100, S-100 protein; VIM, vimentin.

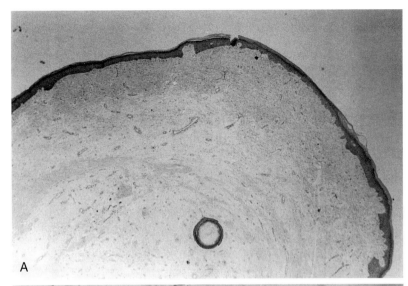

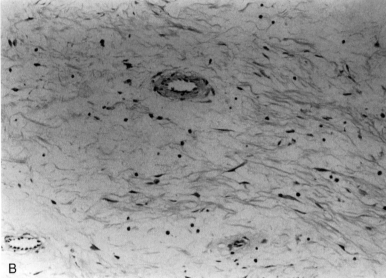

Figure 11–13. Myxoma. The myxoma is composed of loose myxomatous connective tissue containing thin-walled blood vessels and covered with attenuated epidermis. (Courtesy of Dr. JA Carney, Mayo Clinic.)

Merkel Cell Tumor

Clinical Features. Merkel cell tumor[86–90] is a malignant cutaneous neuroendocrine small cell tumor found in the skin of elderly individuals. It is derived from Merkel cells found in hair follicle mechanoreceptors and as isolated cells in oral mucosa, epidermis, and dermis.

Pathologic Features. The tumor is composed of sheets and aggregates of undifferentiated small cells that fill the dermis (Fig. 11–14A, see p. 689). Ultrastructurally, the cells are characterized by perinuclear keratin fibrils, peripheral cytoplasmic dense core granules, and zona adherens intercellular junctions.

Differential Diagnosis. Immunocytochemistry is a major aid in diagnosis with a dot-like perinuclear keratin staining pattern (Fig. 11–14B, see p. 689), cytoplasmic and membrane expression of chromogranin (Fig. 11–14C, see p. 689), and synaptophysin differentiating this tumor from lymphoma, poorly differentiated carcinoma, and melanoma.[88, 89] Cytokeratin-20 (a low molecular weight cytokeratin with restricted expression to gastrointestinal tract and urinary tract epithelium) positivity in the majority of tumor cells also strongly supports a diagnosis of Merkel cell carcinoma.[90]

Treatment and Prognosis. This is an aggressive malignant tumor acting more like oat cell carcinoma than carcinoid. Recurrences are common (26–44%) in spite of wide local excision. Metastases to regional lymph nodes (75%) and distant sites (33%) occur despite therapeutic lymph node resection, radiation, and chemotherapy. The reported 5-year survival rate ranges from 30% to 64% of patients.[89]

Kaposi's Sarcoma and Bacillary Angiomatosis-Peliosis (Bartonellosis)

Clinical Features. In the pre-AIDS era, Kaposi's sarcoma[91] was a rare indolent disease of older men of Eastern European and Mediterranean heritage, initially involving the skin of the extremities, not the head and neck. It now occurs as a common aggressive neoplasm (after lymphomas) in much younger (mean age 38 years, range 22 to 50 years), HIV-infected patients. Tumors involve not only the skin and mucosal surfaces of the head and neck but also lymph nodes and viscera. The widespread organ involvement by the sarcoma and concomitant opportunistic infections are manifestations of the marked suppression of cellular immunity and the poor prognosis for the AIDS patient.

Pathologic Features. Spindle cells dominate the histologic picture with interspersed extravasated erthrocytes suggesting a vascularized fibrous histiocytoma (Fig. 11–15). The spindle cells express immunocytochemical endothelial markers. A new, recently discovered γ-herpesvirus, Kaposi's sarcoma-associated herpesvirus or human herpesvirus-8, has been propagated from these lesions and may be an etiologic agent.[92]

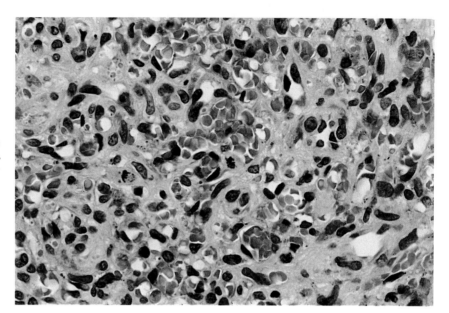

Figure 11–15. Kaposi's sarcoma. Small blood vessels with hyperplastic endothelium, a spindle cell stroma, and extravasated erythrocytes characterize the dermal lesion of Kaposi's sarcoma.

Differential Diagnosis. The skin lesions of Kaposi's sarcoma cannot be clinically differentiated from those of *bacillary angiomatosis-peliosis (Bartonellosis),*[93] which also occurs in HIV-infected individuals. Bartonellosis is a vasoproliferative response to infection by α_2 purple bacteria *Bartonella,* which consists of two species.[94, 95] The domestic house cat is the resevoir and the cat flea is the vector for *Bartonella henselae,* which causes *cat scratch disease* in immunologically intact individuals. *Bartonella quintana* transmitted through the bite of the body louse is the cause of *Trench fever.* In immunodepressed individuals, infection by either species of *Bartonella* results in disseminated angioproliferative lesions in the skin, bones, and viscera (especially in the liver and spleen), termed *bacillary angiomatosis-peliosis.* This lesion has been reported to have occurred at the site of a cat scratch in two apparently immunocompetent children.[96]

Histologically, *bacillary angiomatosis* is characterized by a well-demarcated, pyogenic granuloma-like area in the upper dermis composed of lobular aggregates of blood vessels with endothelial hyperplasia (Fig. 11–16, see p. 690).[96, 97] The overlying epidermis is thinned and may be ulcerated. Between and among the blood vessels are microabscesses with polymorphonuclear leukocytes and basophilic smudges, which Warthin-Starry or Steiner silver preparations show to be bacilli (Fig. 11–16*B*) and Brown and Hopps stain shows to be gram-negative.

Treatment and Prognosis. Differentiation between Kaposi's sarcoma and bacillary angiomatosis is extremely important, since the latter can be treated with macrolide (erythromycin) and tetracycline antibiotics and the former treated symptomatically by surgical excision as the need arises.

Angiolymphoid Hyperplasia with Eosinophilia

Clinical Features. Angiolymphoid hyperplasia with eosinophilia,[98–100] although rare, has a propensity for the skin of the ear in middle-aged men as single or multiple plum-colored, itchy intradermal nodules or plaques, which may bleed with mild trauma. There is no association with immunosuppression or HIV infection.

Pathologic Features. Proliferating capillaries are associated with dense lymphocytic inflammatory infiltrates, which also contain eosinophils and mast cells. Endothelial cell hyperplasia is prominent and there can be an arteriovenous "malformation" at the periphery of the capillary proliferation. The etiology of this lesion is not clear, and it has been described as an *epithelioid hemangioendothelioma.* A histologically similar lesion, which occurs in soft tissues and

lymph nodes, accompanied by peripheral eosinophilia, in younger Asian men is known as *Kimura's disease.*[100]

Differential Diagnosis. The differential diagnosis includes Kaposi's sarcoma, bacillary angiomatosis, low-grade angiosarcoma, Langerhans' cell granulomatosis (eosinophilic granuloma) (see later discussion), and lymphoma. Although the endothelial cells are large (epithelioid), often with mitotic activity, there is neither cytologic atypia, hyperchromasia, or papillations in the vascular lumens typical of angiosarcoma nor the spindle cell pattern with extravasated erythrocytes typical of Kaposi's sarcoma. Similarly, prominent vasculature with epithelioid endothelial cells together with immunohistochemical markers can separate angiolymphoid hyperplasia with eosinophilia from lymphoma.

Treatment and Prognosis. Angiolymphoid hyperplasia with eosinophilia has been successfully treated with many types of local therapy. Wide local excision is favored, but this lesion may spontaneously regress.

Cartilaginous Neoplasms

Clinical Findings. True cartilaginous neoplasms of the external ear are uniquely rare. The only report in a MEDLINE search, 1985 through 1998, that of bilateral chondromas in the pinnas,[101] is more likely bilateral cartilaginous pseudocysts (idiopathic cystic chondromalacia) than chondroma of the auricle as the authors contend.

Pleomorphic adenoma (benign mixed tumor) occurs in the pinna skin (chondroid syringoma)[102] but more often arises from the ceruminous glands in the external auditory canal. If the cartilaginous component is prominent and the epithelial component not adequately sampled, mixed tumor may be misdiagnosed as a chondroma.[103]

Similarly, synovial chondromatosis of the temporomandibular joint can present as a mass anterior to, or in, the external auditory meatus.[43, 103, 104] Synovial chondromatosis is a reactive synovial cartilaginous metaplasia in response to injury or trauma—a degenerative arthropathy.[43] It occurs in large joints of adults but has also been reported to occur in the temporomandibular joint.[43, 103, 104] The masses of cartilage can erode the joint capsule and invade surrounding soft tissue and skull base.

Pathologic Features. Synovial chondromatosis forms lobules of hyalin cartilage with enlarged, often multiple, active chondrocytes in chondrocytic lacunae (Fig. 11–17). The histologic appearance of proliferation suggests a diagnosis of chondrosarcoma, but

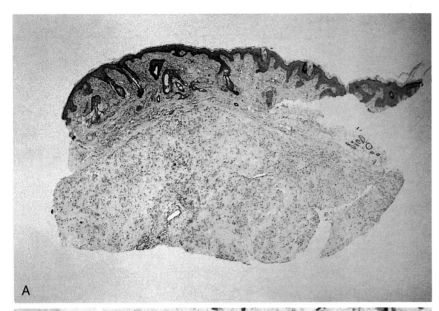

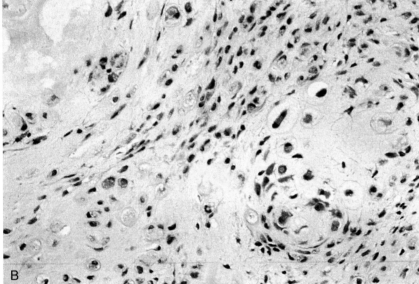

Figure 11–17. Synovial chondromatosis. *A,* Subcutaneous mass, *B,* High power detail. Multiple chondrocytes are found within lacunae. An orderly pattern of chondrocyte maturation is lacking but mitoses are inconspicuous.

mitoses are rarely found in spite of nuclear atypia. The proliferative nature of synovial chondromatosis compared to cartilage from a tragus or enchondroma is reflected by its low level of *C-erb* expression and a nondiploid DNA profile.[105] However, mitotic activity and Ki-67 protein expression, characteristic of chondrosarcoma, are not found in synovial chondromatosis or "benign" cartilage.[106, 107]

Treatment and Prognosis. The extent of the surgical procedure needed to extirpate the lesion depends on the results of imaging studies in defining the primary, parotid gland, or temporomandibular joint origin of the tumor. Wide local excision suffices for these lesions. Treatment of temporomandibular synovial chondromatosis can be as simple as arthroscopic shaving of the articular surfaces[108] or massive resection of lesions invading the skull base.[109]

EXTERNAL AUDITORY CANAL

Virtually all of the lesions described previously also occur in the external auditory canal.[110, 111] Owing to the enclosed nature of the canal, however, the clinical manifestations of these canal lesions differ and occur later in the course of the disease. The surgical pathologist is presented with small portions of polypoid, inflamed tissue ("aural polyp") obtained via an operating otoscope. Lesions may arise in the canal or be extensions "in" from the skin of the meatus or "out" from the middle ear.

Keratosis Obturans

Clinical Features. Complaints of fullness in the ear, decreased hearing, and discharge from the ear can yield, on otoscopic examination, a plug of inspissated cerumen and keratin[112] that fills and expands the canal and is known as *keratosis obturans.*[113] This occurs in "younger" patients, is often bilateral, and may be associated with sinusitis or bronchitis (suggesting a relationship to cystic fibrosis), but there is no association with middle ear or mastoid disease and the drum is intact. The keratin plug can irritate the squamous lining of the canal, but there is no ulceration, invasion, or destruction of the canal or bone.

Pathologic Features. Histologically, the plug is composed of alternating layers of cerumen and squames (Fig. 11–18).

Differential Diagnosis. Primary *external ear cholesteatoma*[114–116] can arise from the inferior aspect of the canal as an ulcer or diverticulum filled with keratin and squames. The lesion is lined with normally maturing squamous epithelium (which differentiates it from a squamous malignancy) and is surrounded by an inflamma-

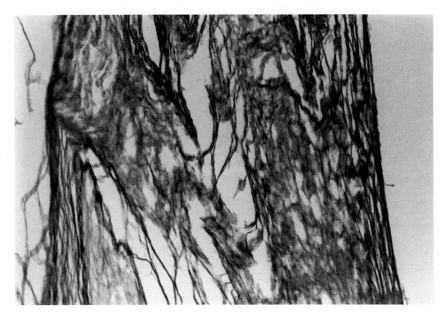

Figure 11–18. Keratosis obturans. The "wax" plug in the external auditory canal is composed of layers of anucleate squames.

tory stroma. There is no evidence of malignancy in these lesions, but histologic evaluation is necessary to separate them from invasive neoplastic lesions. The expanding lesion extends into the canal as a pearly cyst and erodes into the subjacent bone. The drum is intact and there is no association with middle ear or mastoid disease, unlike middle ear cholesteatoma. The ear canal cholesteatoma occurs in older patients than does keratosis obturans, with a mean age of 48 years and a range of 20 to 72 years, and equally in men and women. Lesions can be bilateral, and there is a variable history of previous infection or trauma to the ear.

Treatment and Prognosis. In keratosis obturans, removal of the plug is curative, although it may re-accumulate.

Surgical treatment of auditory canal cholesteatoma varies depending on the size and extention of the lesion. Lesions within the canal can be curettaged; larger lesions eroding or invading bone require more extensive but local surgery.

Foreign Bodies, Trauma, Otitis Externa

Complaints of fullness, hearing loss, and discharge from the ear can also yield, on otoscopic examination, foreign bodies such as hair pins, pencil erasers, and insect parts (Fig. 11–19, see p. 690).[117] Trauma to the epithelial lining of the ear canal of diabetic patients can cause a severe *Pseudomonas* infection known as "malignant" external otitis because of the difficulty in irradiation and its subsequent extension to the skull base and brain.[117–120] A more common infection is *swimmer's ear*[121, 122] or *otomycosis,* caused by superficial aspergillus infection in a chronically wet ear canal.

Neoplasms

Clinical Features. Squamous neoplasms were discussed previously in the context of actinic injury to the skin of the external ear. Primary neoplasms of the canal are predominantly glandular tumors derived from the adnexal glands of the external auditory canal skin. These tumors are (1) either benign adenomas with apocrine and ceruminous or salivary gland characteristics, (2) carcinomas (predominantly of the adenoid cystic variety), or (3) low- and high-grade carcinomas "not otherwise specified."[123–126] The benign and malignant tumors occur with equal frequency in men and women, with a mean age of 49 years (range 26–89 years). Pain, discharge, and facial nerve palsy are clinical predictors of malignancy.

Pathologic Features. The benign glandular tumors of the canal are commonly called *ceruminomas,*[127, 128] since most retain apo-

crine characteristics of the ceruminous glands of origin with granular cytoplasm, apocrine decapitation, cytoplasmic "snouts" on the luminal surface, and small, cytologically benign nuclei (Fig. 11–20, see p. 691). The glands are composed of one to two cell layers with demonstrable basal myoepithelial cells. The tumors can be solid, papillary, and cystic. In other locations with apocrine glands, similar tumors are known as *hidradenoma* or *syringocystadenoma.* If the name "ceruminoma" is to be of value,[128] it should be restricted to adenomas of the external canal that have apocrine differentiation. Other adnexal/salivary gland adenomas in the external canal include *pleomorphic adenoma (mixed tumor),*[129, 130] *eccrine cylindroma,*[131] and *hidradenoma papilliferum,*[132] which also can present as polypoid masses within the canal.

Low-Grade Carcinoma

Low-grade carcinomas that maintain distinct histologic patterns[133] are differentiated from adenomas by invasion and indistinct borders resulting in the presence of tumor at resection margins, mitotic activity, and tumor necrosis (Fig. 11–21, see p. 691). Adequate local excision cures these tumors.

Adenoid Cystic Carcinoma

An adenoid cystic pattern (Fig. 11–22), even if cytologically "benign," is diagnostic of adenoid cystic carcinoma. These adenoid cystic tumors are clinically and histologically[9] similar to those arising in salivary glands; they widely infiltrate tissues, invade nerve sheaths, and have an insidious, prolonged clinical course.[134] Death occurs in almost 50% of patients and is due to pulmonary metastases or intracranial extension. These tumors require wide radical resection since local recurrence is common, often at a long interval after resection. Poor prognostic findings are tumor at the resection margins, bone and nerve involvement, and local recurrence. Irradiation is palliative. But for the size of the tumor in the respective site, it may be impossible to separate tumors arising in the salivary gland and invading the ear canal from those arising in the canal and invading the parotid.

High-Grade Adenocarcinoma

High-grade carcinomas are a heterogeneous group of poorly differentiated neoplasms that are difficult to differentiate from metastatic neoplasms or those extending from the parotid gland or middle ear. They have a poor prognosis; the majority of patients die within 4 years following diagnosis.[124]

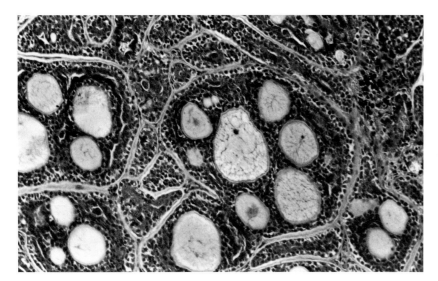

Figure 11–22. Adenoid cystic carcinoma. An adenoid cystic pattern of glandular proliferation predicts infiltration of tissue and prolonged insidious clinical course.

Bone Tumors

It is not clear whether the common, benign tumors of the bony portion of the canal are reactive or neoplastic. Virtually all of these are exostoses and osteomas,[134, 135] often associated with exposure to cold water (swimmers and surfers) and external otitis and conductive hearing loss due to canal obstruction. Osteoma is unilateral, single, and pedunculated; exostoses are bilateral, multiple, and broad-based.[134] Fenton et al.[134] were unable to differentiate between *exostosis* and *osteoma* by routine histologic examination (Fig. 11–23). Symptomatic patients who do not respond to medical treatment of the external otitis and have greater than 80% obstruction of the canal may require local transmeatal removal of the excess bone "with a specialized mallet and thin chisel technique."[135]

Neural Tumors

Nerve sheath tumors *(schwannoma* and *neurofibroma)* occur in the external ear canal as isolated tumors or as part of genetic peripheral neurofibromatosis type 1 (NF-1).[136, 137] Nerve sheath tumors in infants or children are almost always associated with NF-1 and have the potential for malignant change.[138] These nerve tumors should be differentiated from other spindle cell tumors, fibrous histiocytoma,[139] and leiomyoma[140] by characteristic histologic and immunoperoxidase staining patterns. Local excision suffices, but familial neurofibromatosis must be considered whenever a diagnosis of nerve sheath tumor is made (see later).

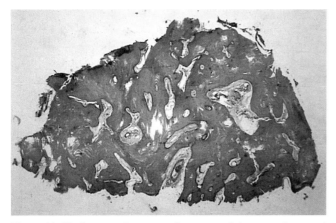

Figure 11–23. Osteoma. Osteoma and exostosis of the external ear canal are histologically identical; both are composed of dense mature bone with well-ordered osteons.

Miscellaneous Other Tumors

Paraganglioma rarely arises in the external auditory canal.[141] More frequently it is an extension of middle ear paraganglioma through a destroyed eardrum (see later discussion). Similarly, *rhabdomyosarcoma,* originating in the canal or middle ear, can present as an "aural polyp" in the canal.[142] *Yolk sac (endodermal sinus)* tumor of the external auditory canal of infants is similarly reported (see later).[143] *Meningioma* can occur rarely in sites outside of the central nervous system[144–146] separate from the meninges, including the ear, skin of the head and neck, nose and paranasal sinuses, and mediastinum and lungs. Meningiomas arising in the petrous bone can extend into the external auditory canal or middle ear, the latter presenting as otitis media with protrusion through the eardrum.[144]

Treatment and Prognosis. Imaging procedures must be used to evaluate the presumed site of origin and size and extent of the neoplasms in the external canal to plan appropriate therapy. Adequate surgical resection potentially involves parotid gland, neck lymph nodes, and middle ear and mastoid and base of the skull resection.

MIDDLE EAR

Products of inflammation are the most common otologic specimens submitted to the surgical pathology laboratory. These inflammatory tissues from the middle ear or mastoid may confuse the pathologist, since congenital, inflammatory, reactive, and neoplastic lesions in the middle ear can all present with similar symptoms (fullness, tinnitus, pain, hearing loss, discharge), imaging signs of a mass lesion with or without bone erosion, and, pathologically, as an inflamed or necrotic "mass." Differential diagnosis of the biopsy material requires sufficient knowledge of the clinical and imaging information so that a necrotic tumor will not be missed. This is particularly true in children in whom neoplasms are extremely rare and often initially misdiagnosed as inflammation.

Pathologic studies of temporal bones obtained at autopsy[147, 148] have provided basic information regarding etiology and spread of middle and inner ear disease. With the advent of modern imaging techniques, the temporal bone can be clinically "dissected" with localized disease accessible to biopsy by neurotologic techniques.

Congenital Anomalies and Choristoma

Hairy (Dermoid) Polyps and Dermoid Cysts

Clinical Features. Hairy polyps growing within the pharynx, eustachian tube, or middle ear of infants are congenital accessory auricles, similar to accessory tragus.[149-151] Based on a comparative analysis of eight pharyngeal dermoid polyps and four pharyngeal teratomas from the files of the Armed Forces Institute of Pathology with the histologic features of developing fetal auricles and a literature review, Heffner et al.[149] argue that these polyps are not teratomas in the neoplastic sense but are congenital anomalies of the first branchial cleft, choristomas, or malplaced, histologically normal tissue. They occur in newborn and infant children, causing recurrent otitis media that is not responsive to usual drainage and antibiotic therapy.

Pathologic Features. Biopsy will yield benign squamous epithelium from the polyp surface without necrosis or myxoid tissue suggestive of rhabdomyosarcoma. The "polyp" is composed of an elastic cartilage plate surrounded by submucosa and skin, similar to an auricle.

Treatment and Prognosis. Although lacking malignant or neoplastic potential, these lesions have been associated with congenital abnormalities of the ossicles and facial nerve but not of the external ears. Excision is curative.

Congenital Ectopia

Clinical Features. Congenital ectopic tissues (choristoma)[152, 153] are found in the middle ear either incidentally or as a symptomatic mass at any age. In spite of a theoretic possibility, there is no convincing evidence that middle ear glandular neoplasms originate in salivary gland choristomas. A unilateral conductive hearing deficit is typically the first manifestation of salivary gland choristoma, which is associated with deformed or absent ossicles.

Pathologic Features. Brain or meningeal tissue, or both, may be associated with congenital defects in the overlying bony roof of the middle ear,[154–156] but they more often herniate through inflammatory defects of bone secondary to longstanding chronic otitis media or cholesteatoma.

Treatment and Prognosis. Closure of the defect is imperative to prevent extension of infection and inflammation into the subdural space.

Chronic Otitis Media

Chronic Otitis Media in Children

Clinical Features. In children, middle ear inflammation is secondary to obstruction of the eustachian tube orifice by nasopharyngeal inflammation and edema, hyperplastic tonsillar lymphoid tissue, or tubal ciliary malfunction due to viral infection.

Pathologic Features. The inflamed edematous middle ear mucosa generates a serous effusion (acute serous otitis media). Continued infection or inflammation produces mucinous metaplasia with the formation of a tenacious mucinous effusion in the middle ear, "glue ear," and permanent change in middle ear environment and structure (chronic otitis media) including intraepithelial and subepithelial mucous glands and a predominantly chronic inflammatory cell population of lymphocytes, monocytes, and plasma cells.[157, 158]

Differential Diagnosis. Polypoid vascular granulation tissue in the middle ear—aural polyp[159] (Fig. 11–24), reactive foreign body-type giant cells containing lipid crystals—cholesterol granuloma[160] (Fig. 11–25), fibrous adhesions and scarring and calcification of the eardrum (tympanosclerosis[161]), and bone resorption[162] destroy the auditory function of the middle ear. Persistent infection can spread to the mastoid cavity and, with inflammatory mediated bone destruction, to the brain. Destruction of the thin tegmen, the bony roof of the middle ear, not only allows for spread of the infection or inflammation to the brain but can result in herniation of brain and membranes into the middle ear (encephalocele).[163, 164]

Treatment and Prognosis. The treatment of chronic otitis media at this stage requires curettage of the middle ear cavity and drainage. Histologic examination of the curettaged material can provide specific information regarding the etiology of otitis media that does not respond to drainage and antibiotic treatment.

Cholesteatoma

Clinical Features. Cholesteatoma is a peculiar lesion found predominantly in the middle ear in association with otitis media. One third to one half of patients with active chronic otitis media will develop cholesteatoma.[165]

Pathologic Features. It is not a "tumor of cholesterol" or lipid[160] but inflamed granulation tissue stroma surrounding or supporting the squamous epithelial that lines a cavity (Fig. 11–26) filled with anucleate squames.[160, 165] The cholesteatoma forms an expansile pearly cyst within the middle ear or mastoid cavity.

The specific site and mode of origin of cholesteatoma is controversial.[166–168] It can originate from the exterior squamous epithelial surface of the inflamed drum with migration of squamous epithelium as a retraction pocket into the middle ear or from squamous metaplasia of the inflamed middle ear mucosa. Some cholesteatomas are also of congenital origin, but the presumed origin from persistent "epidermoids"[166]—that is, squamous epithelium present in the fetus in middle ear mucosa adjacent to the tympanic membrane—is not resolved.[167, 168]

Differential Diagnosis. Since the cyst is rarely intact after surgical removal, direct communication between the surgeon and pathologist is helpful in identifying the nature of the lesion. In the absence of a cyst, or given a description of a warty or verrucous lesion or extensive necrosis, a diagnosis of verrucous or well-differentiated squamous carcinoma must be considered.

Cytokine-recruited monocytes and osteoclasts and the expansile pressure of the cholesteatoma cyst resorb bone,[169, 170] and the cyst can rupture, generating a foreign body inflammatory reaction (cholesterol granuloma).[160]

The pearly cystic in situ appearance is characteristic, but in an adult with longstanding chronic otitis media and extensive bone destruction, thought must be given to squamous cell carcinoma. Differential diagnosis is based on the orderly maturation of the squamous epithelium lying on an inflammatory stroma without cytologic malignant characteristics or evidence of tissue invasion.

Treatment and Prognosis. Cholesteatoma is removed by curettage of the middle ear and mastoid.

Otitis Media in Adults

The adult onset of chronic otitis media is invariably due to neoplasms of the nasopharynx or middle ear involvement by a systemic granulomatous infection or reactive process.

Pathologic Features and Differential Diagnosis

Tuberculosis

Tuberculosis occasionally occurs as chronic otitis media, lasting months to years.[171–173] Among patients with active pulmonary infection in a 22-year review of chronic otitis media at the Massachusetts Eye and Ear Infirmary,[172] only 2% had otitis media; 42% of tuberculosis patients with otitis media had no evidence of pulmonary infection.

When chronic or recurrent otitis media has not responded to conventional drainage and antibiotic therapy, all material biopsied from the middle ear must be cultured for mycobacteria and fungi as well as aerobic and anaerobic bacteria, since superinfection is common.[172] To be diagnostic of tuberculosis infection, the granulomas must be differentiated from foreign body type cholesterol granulomas (commonly found in biopsied chronic otitis media) and other granulomatous diseases such as sarcoid and Wegener's granulomatosis, by the use of appropriate tissue stains and cultures. We prefer acridine orange fluorescence over Ziehl-Neelsen type acid-fast stains for mycobacteria because of the ease of screening.

Sarcoidosis

Sarcoidosis is a systemic granulomatous disease response to an as yet unknown antigen stimulus, occurring predominantly in young adult black women. Sarcoid occurs in the middle ear most commonly secondary to active nasopharyngeal disease[174, 175] and rarely as a primary middle ear mass.

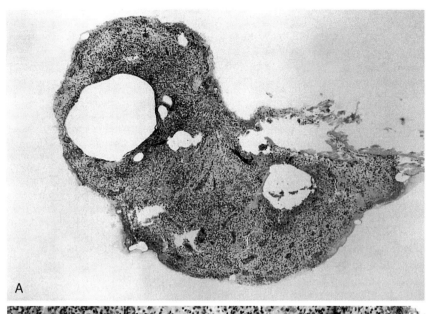

Figure 11–24. The aural polyp is a polypoid growth (A) of granulation tissue (B) present in the middle ear or external ear canal.

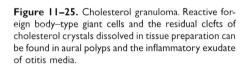

Figure 11–25. Cholesterol granuloma. Reactive foreign body–type giant cells and the residual clefts of cholesterol crystals dissolved in tissue preparation can be found in aural polyps and the inflammatory exudate of otitis media.

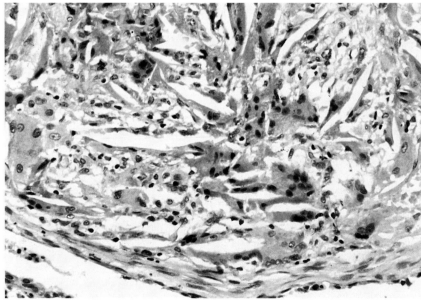

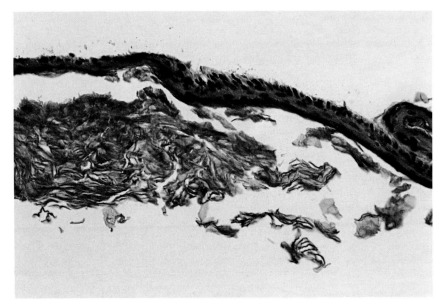

Figure 11–26. Cholesteatoma. This epidermal cyst is lined by squamous epithelium, which contains keratohyalin and matures to form squames, which fill the cyst.

Histologically, it is similar to sarcoid in other body sites (Fig. 11–27) with noncaseating granulomas in fibrous tissue and negative mycobacterial and fungal cultures and acid-fast and fungal tissue stains. Neurotologic sarcoid[175] affecting the meninges, brain, and cranial nerves can require biopsy of other, more accessible involved tissue, in conjunction with a characteristic chest radiograph and elevated serum angiotensin-converting enzyme (ACE) levels for diagnosis. The incidence of sarcoid otitis media is not known because of the scarcity of reports, but it likely does not occur in the middle ear, or as neurotologic disease, in the absence of obvious systemic disease with pulmonary or mediastinal lymphadenopathy. Sarcoid usually responds to corticosteroid therapy.

Acquired Immunodeficiency Syndrome

I could not find reports of clinically detected ear infections in AIDS patients due to *Mycobacterium avium intracellulare* or fungi other than *Pneumocystis carinii*.[176–178] In infection with *Pneumocystis carinii*, the biopsy shows the foamy exudate characteristically seen in pulmonary alveolar spaces, and organisms can be demonstrated with appropriate silver stains. Internal auditory canal gumma occurs in AIDS patients with neurosyphilis.[179]

Michaels et al.[180] found severe active otitis media in 4 of 16 temporal bones obtained from autopsies of AIDS patients; two cases revealed cryptococcosis, one case necrotizing acoustic neuritis with cytomegalovirus infection, and a fourth, Kaposi's sarcoma. Davis et al.[181] studied the temporal bones obtained from autopsies of 14 men with AIDS, none of whom had had deafness and 1 of whom had a history of vertigo. They found acute otitis media in 4, chronic otitis media in 2, and serous otitis media in 3 patients; inner ear findings were abnormal in 1 patient. They recovered adenovirus type 6, cytomegalovirus, and herpesvirus type 1 from the ears of 3 patients, a lower recovery than from either the eyes or the brains of the same patients, suggesting that asymptomatic viral ear infections in these AIDS patients are nonpathogenic and secondary to immunosuppression.

Other Exotic Infectious and Inflammatory Disorders

Histiocytes in the middle ear exudate may harbor exotic microorganisms such as *Klebsiella* from intranasal scleroma,[182] lepra bacilli from the nasopharynx, or granuloma donovani transmitted during vaginal delivery.[183]

Malakoplakia

Malakoplakia,[184] a disease caused by defective macrophage lysozymal response to ingested bacteria, is characterized by histiocytes that

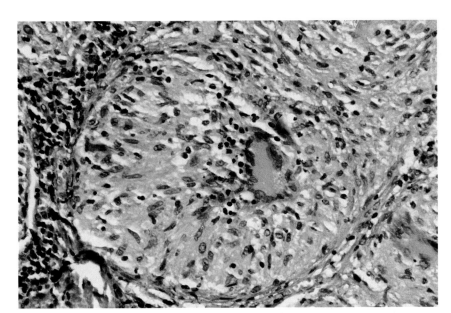

Figure 11–27. Sarcoidosis. Non-caseating granulomas, lacking microorganisms (mycobacteria, fungi) or a foreign body, are consistent with sarcoidosis.

contain periodic acid-Schiff–positive, diastase-resistant granules (von Hanseman cells) and Michaelis-Gutmann bodies, lamellated calcific bodies. Although most frequently found in the urinary tract secondary to coliform bacterial infections, malakoplakia can occur in the ear.[184]

Myospherulosis

Myospherulosis[185] is a rare iatrogenic sequel of chronic otitis media and upper respiratory tract and sinus infection associated with the use of petrolatum-based gauze packing. The middle ear biopsy is characterized by a "swiss-cheese" pattern of holes in the fibrous stroma, which is surrounded by numerous histiocytes, multinucleated giant cells, and varying degrees of acute and chronic inflammation (Fig. 11–28, see p. 691). Within the space are "parent bodies," sac-like structures measuring 20 to 120 μm in diameter, which contain smaller spherules measuring 5 to 7 μm in diameter. A variety of identities has been considered, including pollen, vegetable matter, algae, fungi, and parasites, but the lesions have been reproduced experimentally in rats with antibiotic ointment and in vitro by mixing red blood cells with ointments. Both peroxidase and immunostaining for hemoglobin support the erythrocyte origin of these structures; the usual fungal stains are not reactive.[186] A similar lesion, "ointment granuloma," without the spherular structures but containing lipogranulomas, is also attributed to petrolatum-based ointments.[187] Treatment centers on removal of the foreign and inflammatory material.

Wegener's Granulomatosis and Related Vasculitides

Clinical Features. Wegener's granulomatosis[188–195] is a clinicopathologic multisystem disease entity commonly occurring in the lungs, nasopharynx, nasal cavities, and kidneys. The disease occurs equally in men and women with a mean age of 36 years (range 13–74 years). Among the 126 head and neck disease biopsies in 70 Wegener's patients reported by Devaney et al.,[191] 4 were from the middle ear, 3 from the mastoid, and 2 from the external ear.

Pathologic Features. The disorder is characterized by the triad of (1) granulomatous inflammation, (2) extensive tissue necrosis, and (3) vasculitis, all of which may not be present in the biopsy. Cultures and special stains fail to demonstrate microorganisms. The diagnosis of Wegener's granulomatosis is supported by cytoplasmic staining with serum antineutrophil cytoplasmic antibody (cANCA), an antiprotease 3 with 85% to 98% specificity.[192, 193]

Differential Diagnosis. Chronic otitis media can also occur in patients with other immune-mediated vasculitis syndromes, including polyarteritis, rheumatoid arthritis, and leukocytoclastic vasculitis.[194, 195]

Treatment and Prognosis. Treatment is with corticosteroids and cytotoxic drugs; the prognosis is related to severity of the renal lesions.

Idiopathic Hypereosinophilic Syndrome

Clinical Features. Idiopathic hypereosinophilic syndrome[196] is a systemic disease of young adults that affects many organs, including heart, lung, skin, and nervous system, with a chronic inflammatory infiltrate dominated by eosinophils and a peripheral eosinophilia. In addition to pulmonary eosinophilic alveolitis, patients can have obliterative chronic otitis media with eosinophils and histocytes.

Pathologic Features and Differential Diagnosis. Histopathologic differential diagnosis includes Langerhans' cell (eosinophilic) granuloma of bone and Hodgkin's lymphoma. The absence of bone lesions and failure to characterize the histiocytes as Langerhans' cells with S-100 and CD1a immunohistochemistry rule out eosinophilic granuloma (see subsequent discussion). Hodgkin's lymphoma involving the middle ear can be ruled out by the absence of a heteromorphic cell population and Reed-Sternberg cells in the middle ear infiltrate and the lack of another definitive tissue diagnosis of Hodgkin's lymphoma in the patient.

Treatment. This apparently "allergic" disease responds to low doses of oral prednisone.

Otosclerosis

Clinical Features. Otosclerosis[197, 198] is a metabolic disorder of bone modeling of the inner ear otic capsule, which forms the medial wall of the middle ear. Patients experience bilateral conductive hearing loss in their third and fourth decades as new bone fixes the stapes footplate to the oval window. Otosclerosis becomes clinically manifest with conductive hearing loss in young adults, with a 2:1 female:male ratio and autosomal dominance with 40% penetrance. Studies of human leukocyte antigens suggest both familial and sporadic occurrence. The specific mechanism of disordered bone remodeling is unknown. Conductive hearing is restored by stapedectomy. The etiology of the sensorineural hearing loss rarely associated with otosclerosis is not known and is not attributable to bone encroachment in the inner ear. The disease comes to the attention of the pathologist when part of the stapes is removed from the oval window following replacement by a prosthesis used to restore conductive hearing. Only the uninvolved, histologically normal, U-shaped stapes crura and head are removed; the prosthesis is inserted through the fused footplate.

▪ NEOPLASMS OF THE MIDDLE EAR AND TEMPORAL BONE
Squamous Cell Carcinoma

Clinical Features. The role of chronic middle ear infection in the etiology of squamous cell carcinoma is controversial. Virtually all carcinoma patients have chronic otitis media, but Michaels and Wells[199] found only 28 cases of squamous carcinoma among 40,000 patients with chronic otitis media seen at London's Royal National Throat, Nose and Ear Hospital, 1962 through 1978. Kenyon et al.,[200] on the basis of their 25-year retrospective study of 21 patients with squamous cell carcinoma of the middle ear, postulated that "a history of chronic suppuration with or without cholesteatoma predisposes the patient to tumor development . . . ." In both series,[189, 190] the patient population is similar, with a total of 27 women and 22 men and a mean age of 62 years (range, 33–85 years). The most common initial complaints were pain and a bloody or fetid discharge, and all patients reported hearing impairment. Cholesteatoma occurred in only three of the patients reported by Kenyon et al.[200]

Pathologic Features. Histopathologic examination shows a multifocal origin of squamous cell carcinoma in metaplastic squamous mucosa in the chronically inflamed middle ear or mastoid with transition from carcinoma in situ to invasive carcinoma. The squamous mucosa of the external canal can also be involved. The tumor spreads intracranially by destroying the thin medial bony wall adjacent to the carotid canal or mastoid ear spaces. Histologically, squamous cell carcinoma can vary from well to poorly differentiated, the latter initially responding to radiation therapy.

Differential Diagnosis. *Verrucous carcinoma* can originate in the external auditory canal, middle ear, and mastoid. These well-differentiated carcinomas have the grossly characteristic warty or cauliflower appearance in situ which, with the presence of bone invasion, rules out cholesteatoma, in spite of the lack of dysplasia in superficial biopsies (Fig. 11–29, see p. 692).[201, 202] *Basaloid squamous* *cell carcinoma* of the base of the tongue, larynx, and hypopharynx/pyriform sinuses can also invade the middle ear via the eustachian tube. Cytokeratin positivity and the absence of neuroendocrine, desmin, and actin markers separate these basaloid squamous tumors from neuroendocrine and adenoid cystic carcinomas.[203, 204]

Treatment and Prognosis. Squamous cell carcinoma is treated primarily by mastoidectomy and radiation. After 5 years, only 39% of the 23 patients reported by Michaels and Wells[199] were alive; death was due to intracranial spread, but two patients also had metastases to the lungs and neck lymph nodes. The slow but insidious growth of the tumor with extensive bone invasion by the time it becomes symptomatic results in a poor prognosis despite attempts at radical surgery. The few verrucous carcinomas reported[201, 202] had favorable outcomes following wide surgical excision compared with squamous carcinoma.

Inverted Squamous Papilloma

Clinical Features. Inverted papilloma occurs in the middle ear either as a primary tumor or in association with other upper respiratory papillomas.[205–209] Wenig[205] reports five women, aged 19 to 57 years (median, 31 years) who complained of pain, hearing loss, and otorrhea predating the diagnosis from several months to 20 years. All had chronic otitis media; none had sinonasal or nasopharyngeal papillomas. Tumors were confined to the middle ear without bone destruction, although two women had perforated tympanic membranes. Middle ear inverted papillomas also occur in association with similar papillomas of the upper respiratory tract,[206] either by direct continuity or in a multicentric fashion. Malignant transformation to, or coexistence with, squamous cell carcinoma reportedly occurs in 3% to 24% of lesions.[206]

Pathologic Features. These tumors are polypoid, fill the middle ear cavity, and are histologically identical to sinonasal papillomas (Fig. 11–30, see p. 692).[207]

Differential Diagnosis. Immunohistochemistry may be useful in evaluating the development of invasive carcinoma in papillomas. Expression of CD44, a cell adhesion molecule, is increased in the papillary tumors but decreases with invasion.[210]

Human papillomaviruses (HPV) are associated with both benign and malignant proliferations of squamous mucosa in the genitalia and head and neck. HPV 6 E6/E7 has been detected with polymerase chain reaction (PCR) and reverse transcription PCR in a nasal inverted papilloma from a 36-year-old renal transplant recipient immunosuppressed with cyclosporin A,[211] but yet not found using PCR[205] or immunohistochemical[212] techniques in inverted papillomas from apparently immunocompetent individuals. Jin et al.,[213] using PCR analysis, found DNA to HPV in 11 of 14 cases of squamous cell carcinoma of the middle ear associated with longstanding otitis media (HPV-16 in 11 of 14 and both HPV-16 and HPV-18 in 5 of the 11).

Treatment and Prognosis. Local surgical excision appears to suffice, but common recurrence (or multiplicity) requires additional resection.[215]

Paraganglioma

Paraganglioma is the most common tumor of the middle ear and is the second most common tumor of the ear after basal and squamous tumors, accounting for 14% of all ear neoplasms in the Barnes Hospital series (see Table 11–1).[7] Although constituting only 3% of all Yale New Haven Hospital ear neoplasms, paragangliomas accounted for seven of the 12 middle ear tumors (58%) (two were adenomas, two rhabdomyosarcomas, and one a chondroid chordoma).

Clinical Features. Paraganglia in the ear are branchomeric members of the diffuse chemoreceptor neuroendocrine system associated with nerves and blood vessels.[214] The endocrine cells of the paraganglia, and their neoplastic counterparts, contain or secrete a variety of regulatory hormones, amines, and polypeptides, but signs and symptoms attributable to neuroendocrine function of the tumors (pheochromocytoma or carcinoid) are rarely of clinical significance.[215, 216]

Tumors of paraganglia, paragangliomas, have also been called glomus tumors, chemodectomas, and carotid body tumors (tumor of the largest paraganglion, the carotid body). In the ear, they are collectively known as jugulotympanic paraganglia after the paraganglia located in the adventitia of the jugular bulb below the middle ear, and those found in the middle ear with the tympanic branch and plexus of the ninth cranial nerve (Jacobsen's nerve) and the auricular branch of the 10th cranial nerve (Arnold's nerve).[214]

Jugulotympanic paragangliomas[214, 217–223] occur overwhelmingly in women (5:1 ratio), at an average age of 50 years (range, 21–80 years), and are bilateral in 10% to 16% of patients. They have been reported to occur in an infant[224] and an 11-year-old boy.[225] Jugular paragangliomas that arise in the lateral temporal bone can erode into the base of the skull and present as an intracranial tumor, extend into the internal jugular vein, or erode through the bony floor of the middle ear, filling the middle ear as an "aural polyp." Destruction of the bone about the jugular bulb is a characteristic imaging sign, but the jugular site of origin may not be obvious in large destructive lesions.

Tympanic paragangliomas[214] are smaller but, arising in the middle ear, present with early symptoms of conductive hearing loss and pulsatile tinnitus of long duration (1 month to 28 years, mean of 3 years) and, less commonly, otorrhea and local pain. A mass can be seen behind an intact eardrum, and the paraganglioma can perforate the drum as an aural polyp protruding into the external ear canal.

Ten percent of jugulotympanic paragangliomas occur in families[226] with an autosomal dominant mode of inheritance, at a younger age (average 34 years, range, 16–69 years) than sporadic tumors, equally among men and women, and in multiple head and neck sites (42%), most commonly the carotid body, followed by the glomus jugulare.

High-resolution computed tomography[227–229] is the primary imaging technique for identifying paragangliomas and is particularly useful in delineating bone erosion or destruction. Selective angiography identifies the characteristic "angiographic blush." Indium-111-octeotride scintigraphy can identify tumors that contain somatostatin or its analogues.[230]

Pathologic Features. The paraganglioma is composed of nests of "chief" cells that have small central hyperchromatic nuclei and pale, often clear cytoplasm (Fig. 11–31A, see p. 693).[214, 218] The nests are described as Zellballen (cell balls), the outline of which can be demonstrated with reticulin stains. Peripheral sustentacular support cells are poorly defined in hematoxylin-eosin stains. Some tumors show neuroblastic and fibrillar differentiation. In spite of the characteristic pattern, biopsy diagnosis may be difficult because of the small pieces of tissue obtained, sclerosis, and prebiopsy radiation or embolization therapy.[231, 232]

Electron microscopy[233] reveals chief cells with heterogeneous dense core neurosecretory granules. Neuron specific enolase (NSE), chromogranin A, synaptophysin, and serotonin are demonstrated most frequently in chief cells with immunoperoxidase preparations (Fig. 11–31B, see p. 693). Sustentacular cells are more readily demonstrated by S-100 (Fig. 11–31C) or, less frequently, glial fibrillary acidic protein (GFAP) positivity. Keratin is rarely demonstrated in either chief or sustentacular cells.

Differential Diagnosis. Clinically, lesions of the ear presenting with pulsatile tinnitus include arteriovenous malformations or fistulas, an ectatic carotid bulb, and middle ear aneurysm,[234] in addition to vascular lesions of the middle ear such as hemangioma,[235–238] meningioma,[239] aural (inflammatory) polyp, and metastatic carcinoma.[240, 241] High-resolution computed tomography, selective angiography, and somatostatin receptor scintigraphy clinically define paragangliomas.

Histologically, differential diagnosis is among paraganglioma, adenomatous tumors of the middle ear, and meningioma. Adenomas

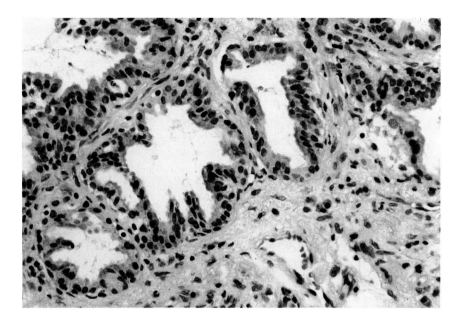

Figure 11–32. Middle ear adenoma. Cuboidal to columnar cells with small benign hyperchromatic nuclei lacking mitoses can form glands, pseudo-rosettes or sheets. Cytoplasm can contain mucin or neuroendocrine markers or both.

are composed of cells similar to those in paraganglioma but with larger more vesicular nuclei, abundant cytoplasm,[208] and cells arranged in sheets, cords, or glands, and, occasionally, mucin production. Immunoperoxidase studies are definitive, since the adenomatous tumor cells contain keratin, mucins, and lysozyme as well as various neuroendocrine products and since the S-100–positive sustentacular cells, characteristically found in paraganglioma, are not present. Meningioma can express epithelial membrane antigen.

Treatment and Prognosis. Rare paragangliomas show mitotic activity and necrosis and metastasize to regional lymph nodes, lungs, and liver. More commonly, aggressive, rapidly growing tumors invade locally. There are no consistent histologic, DNA, or oncoprotein studies that predict aggressive growth better than the extent of the tumor by imaging studies, and mitotic activity and tumor necrosis. Jugulotympanic paragangliomas spread by expansion and erosion of preformed channels in bone and tissue.

Local surgical excision usually suffices for tympanic tumors but recurrence is common (27–70%) following difficult local surgery for larger erosive jugular paragangliomas, particularly when patients have cranial neuropathies. Large and recurrent lesions have been treated successfully with radiation and embolization.[218–222, 241] Octeotride, a somatostatin analogue, has a growth inhibiting effect on paraganglioma and is useful as a therapeutic as well as diagnostic imaging agent.[230]

Glandular Neoplasms

Clinical Features. Glandular neoplasms of the middle ear are much less common than paragangliomas (by 1996 only about 100 cases had been reported[242]) but can easily be confused with them both clinically and pathologically. In 1976, Hyams and Michaels[243] reported 20 cases of a benign adenomatous neoplasm (adenoma) "with an apparent origin from the middle ear mucosal epithelium." Their findings were confirmed by subsequent case reports,[244–246] summarized by Mills.[247] The adenomas occur equally in men and women, with a mean age of 40 years (median 37; range, 14–80 years). Decreased hearing and tinnitus were the most common presenting symptoms, but one fourth of the patients were without symptoms. The eardrum was perforated in 24 tumors. Imaging studies aid in clinically separating adenoma from paraganglioma.[244, 247] Adenoma forms an avascular mass in the middle ear without bone erosion, which can involve the region of the eustachian tube, often encasing the ossicles.[245, 246]

Pathologic Features. Adenoma of the middle ear is composed of cuboidal to columnar cells with distinct cell borders and eosinophilic cytoplasm (Fig. 11–32). The small central hyperchromatic nuclei rarely contain nucleoli and are without mitotic activity. The cells can be arranged in a glandular configuration in a fibrous stroma, a back-to-back and pseudorosette pattern, or as disorganized sheets of cells that lack cohesion. Mucins can be demonstrated within the gland lumens. The cells contain argyrophilic granules and cytoplasmic lysozyme granules. Ultrastructural examination confirms the light microscopic characteristics, showing both mucigen and lysozyme granules, keratin intermediate filaments, and no dense core neurosecretory-type granules.[242–250]

Additional reports of middle ear adenomas demonstrated cells with trabecular growth patterns that had histologic and ultrastructural characteristics of carcinoid tumors[251–262]: perinuclear argyrophilic granules, cytoplasmic keratin, and, ultrastructurally, dense core neurosecretory and mucin granules. Immunoperoxidase studies demonstrated granules expressing NSE, serotonin, synaptophysin, pancreatic polypeptide-related peptides, glucagon-related peptides, and chromogranin A in the same or different cells.

Azzoni et al.[263] also demonstrated hindgut-type tumor antigens, prostatic acid phosphatase, and CAR-5 mucin in middle ear carcinoids. The presence of CAR-5 mucin in normal middle ear mucosa suggested a homology between middle ear (foregut) and rectal (hindgut) carcinoid tumors. However, neuroendocrine cells have not been demonstrated in normal middle ear mucosa.

Middle ear adenomatous tumors may therefore lack neuroendocrine characteristics and stain for lysozyme and mucin (adenoma), have combined mucin and neuroendocrine characteristics (mixed adenoma/carcinoid), or, lacking lysozyme and mucin, show only neuroendocrine markers (carcinoid). Although peptide hormones have been demonstrated, clinical carcinoid syndrome has not been reported in association with middle ear adenoma or carcinoid.[259]

Differential Diagnosis. Histologically, adenoma/carcinoid can be separated from paraganglioma by the use of a reticulin stain to demonstrate Zellballen phenomenon in the latter and with appropriate immunoperoxidase staining characteristics (Table 11–4). There are rare occurrences of metastases of known neoplasms from other sites to the middle ear and temporal bone that histologically simulate adenoma/carcinoid (see later discussion). Metastatic thyroid, prostate, and breast cancer can be separated out by characteristic tumor markers—thyroglobulin, prostatic specific antigen, and breast cystic disease protein and estrogen or progesterone receptor protein. A plasmacytoid middle ear adenoma[264] may be confused with plasma-

Table 11–4. Differential Staining Among Middle Ear Glandular Neoplasms

	NSE/CHR	KER	S-100	LYS	MUC	tTHY	PSA	TGB	VIM
Paraganglioma	+	–	+	–	–	–	–	–	–
Adenoma	–	+	–	+	+	–	–	–	–
Carcinoid	+	+	–	–	–	–	–	–	–
Adenocarcinoid	+	+	–	+	+	–	–	–	–
ELS tumor	±	+	±	–	–	–	–	–	±
Choroid plexus papilloma	–	+	+	–	–	+	–	–	–
Metastatic carcinoma									
Prostate	–	+	–	–	–	–	+	–	–
Thyroid	–	+	–	–	–	–	–	+	–
Renal cell	–	+	–	–	–	–	–	–	+

ELS, endolymphatic sac; KER, keratins; LYS, lysozyme; MUC, mucin; NSE/CHR, neuron specific enolase and/or chromogranin; PSA, prostate specific antigen; S-100, S-100 protein; TGB, thyroglobulin; tTHY, transthyretin (prealbumen); VIM, vimentin.

cytoma or chronic inflammation in a fibrous stroma. Isolated case reports of adenoid cystic[265] and mucoepidermoid[266] carcinomas hypothetically attribute their origin in the middle ear to salivary gland choristoma. However, no normal residual gland is described and origin in the external canal or parotid cannot be ruled out.

Treatment and Prognosis. The phenotype of the middle ear adenomatous tumors does not appear to influence treatment and prognosis. These are all benign tumors; adequate treatment involves complete surgical removal of the tumor including involved ossicles and any extension into the mastoid. There is no evidence of invasion or metastases by these well-differentiated tumors. Poorly differentiated neuroendocrine tumors, similar to those cited in the larynx and sinonasal region,[86] have not been reported in the middle ear and temporal bone.

Endolymphatic Sac Tumor (Low-Grade Adenocarcinoma, Aggressive Papillary Middle Ear Tumor)

Clinical Features. In 1988, Gaffey et al.[267] reported 10 cases (one of their own and nine cases from a literature review) of an *aggressive papillary middle ear tumor* (APMET) that was distinguishable from middle ear adenoma by its histologic papillarity and aggressive clinical behavior, with hypervascularity, bone destruction, and frequent intracranial invasion without metastasis. A subsequent review, by Benecke et al.,[268] of "adenomatous tumors of the middle ear and mastoid," discussed five patients with papillary tumors similar to case 1 reported by Gaffney et al.,[267] which destroyed bone with intracranial invasion. Combined, these two reviews yielded 15 cases of APMET (11 women and four men; mean age, 39; range, 21–57 years).

In retrospect, prior to the report of Gaffey et al.,[267] among 14 reported cases of adenomas and adenocarcinoma of the middle ear[269–274] are nine additional cases with tumors manifesting aggressive clinical behavior, massive petrous bone destruction, and a vascular tumor in the cerebellar pontine angle.[269–271] These nine tumors are histologically different from middle adenoma showing papillarity and cystic and glandular, thyroid-like follicles. One of the patients,[271] a 7-year-old girl, also had a cerebellar hemangioblastoma.

In his 1987 text, Michaels[275] mentioned two cases of a rare, apparently benign epithelial neoplasm of the inner ear endolymphatic system resembling choroid plexus, having a papillary appearance with an avascular stroma. He cited similar cases that had been observed previously in temporal bone studies by Gussen[276] and Schuknecht,[277] and in the endolymphatic sac, biopsied following decompression for Meniére's disease, by Hassard et al.[278] In 1989, Heffner[279] reported 20 cases of *low-grade adenocarcinoma of probable endolymphatic sac origin,* ascribing an endolymphatic sac origin to the aggressive papillary-follicular tumors (APMET) that de-

stroy the temporal bone and establishing them as entities separate from middle ear adenomas.[280–282]

Poe et al.[283] observed that aggressive papillary tumors of the temporal bone were associated with von Hippel-Lindau disease (VHL). VHL is an autosomal dominant, inherited disorder with variable penetrance, characterized by vascularized tumors and cysts, including central nervous system hemangioblastoma, retinal angioma, renal cell carcinoma, clear cell papillary cystadenoma of the epididymis, endolymphatic sac tumor, pheochromocytoma, and hepatic and pancreatic cysts.[284–288] It occurs in an estimated 1 in 36,000 live births. A tumor suppressor gene is located on chromosome 3p25,[284] and patients with VHL have one mutated allele and one wild-type allele. Loss of wild-type allele in VHL patients is associated with tumor development. VHL gene protein is expressed in both normal VHL target tissues and non-VHL–associated neoplastic tissues.[287]

Based on the co-occurrence of APMET and a benign adnexal papillary tumor of probable mesonephric origin (APMO) in a patient with VHL, together with a literature review showing that 7 of 46 (15%) reported APMETs and four APMOs occurred in patients with VHL, Gaffey et al.[288] concluded that these tumors are additional major visceral manifestations of VHL. Retrospective review of other reports of adenomas and adenocarcinoma[270, 291–295] of the middle ear and temporal bone include cases of papillary tumors with associated hemangioblastoma, which are, in retrospect, previously unrecognized manifestations of VHL.

Heffner's paper[279] generated additional case reports and further discussions[280–295] regarding middle ear versus endolymphatic sac origin of these "Heffner's tumors." However the increased number of reported cases (<70) summarized by Wenig and Heffner[296] and Roche et al.[297] and more sensitive imaging[298, 299] showing small tumors originating in the endolymphatic sac strongly supported an endolymphatic origin for all these aggressive papillary (ELS) tumors.

Pathologic Features. The ELS tumors show distinctive papillary, cystic, and follicular histologic patterns, which simulate choroid plexus, renal cell, and thyroid tumors (Fig. 11–33). The papillae and glands are covered or lined by a single layer of cuboidal to columnar clear cells with a vascular stroma. Since the central nuclei show little variability, pleomorphism, or mitoses, these tumors had all been considered to be low-grade based on histology but malignant based on aggressively invasive behavior.

Comparative ultrastructural and immunohistochemical studies of fresh biopsies and specimens grown in tissue culture[288, 289, 300–303] show ultrastructure and immunohistochemical staining patterns (consistent epithelial markers, variable staining with vimentin, S-100, and NSE) similar to normal endolymphatic sac epithelium.[303–304] Megerian et al.[305] note that transthyretin (prealbumin) is expressed in choroid plexus papillomas but not in papillary ELS tumors.

Differential Diagnosis. The clear cell papillary and follicular histologic patterns of endolymphatic sac tumors imitate metastatic carcinoma (Fig. 11–33B–D). Currently, consideration of metastases from thyroid and prostate tumors can be eliminated by immunohis-

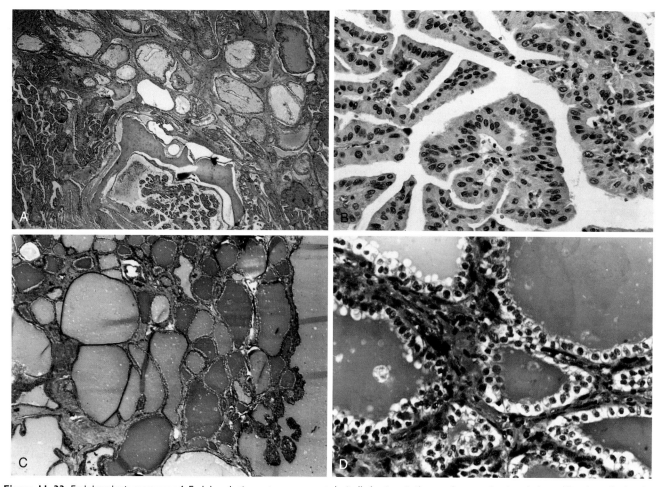

Figure 11–33. Endolymphatic sac tumor. *A*, Endolymphatic sac tumors are cytologically benign, similar to adenomas, but invade bone. Histologically they have papillary (*B*), follicular (*C,D*), and clear cell (*D*) patterns, which emulate metastatic thyroid, renal cell, or prostate carcinoma. (Courtesy of Dr. Bruce Wenig.)

tochemistry (negative prostatic specific antigen and thyroglobulin). Differentiating ELS tumor from metastasis from a coexisting renal cell carcinoma may be difficult. Renal cell carcinomas will show nuclear pleomorphism, eccentric nuclei, more than one cell layer lining follicles, glycogen and fat in tumor cells, and mitotic activity. Keratin and vimentin immunohistochemical markers are present in both tumors. Clear cell tumors of the epididymis and endolymphatic sac tumor, co-occurring with renal cell carcinoma in VHL patients, were initially considered to be metastases from the renal cell carcinoma. Inactivation of both wild-type alleles accounts for the apparently sporadic (unassociated with other manifestations of VHL disease) appearance of clear cell papillary cystadenoma of the epididymis, renal cell carcinoma, hemangioblastomas, and ELS tumors.[306, 307] Any temporal bone folliculopapillary tumor having nuclear pleomorphism and a high mitotic rate should be considered metastatic in origin. Choroid plexus papillomas, in spite of histologic similarity to ELS tumors at the cerebellopontine angle, arise in the ventricle and do not invade bone.[296]

Treatment and Prognosis. Although ELS tumors are large and locally aggressive, often involving the middle and posterior cranial fossae and bone at the time of diagnosis, they are biologically low-grade carcinomas and do not metastasize. Wide surgical excision with adequate margins cures small lesions; transpetrosal resection can be used when hearing is intact. When the tumor involves the labyrinth or cochlea, transcochlear or translabyrinthine temporal bone resection is necessary.[297] Radical temporal bone resection[279] has been successful, with 11 of the 12 patients so treated being free of disease for 2 to 12 years (mean, 5.7 years) following surgery. Pre-

operative embolization[308] has successfully "shrunk" a tumor prior to surgery.

A sensitive magnetic resonance imaging (MRI) screen of 121 VHL patients[309] detected 13 patients (10.7%) with ELS tumors. Sixty-five percent of unselected VHL patients had pure tone threshhold hearing abnormalities, 53% (23/43) of which were bilateral. Hearing loss, tinnitus, and vertigo were the most common symptoms in patients with ELS tumors. Early identification of ELS tumors in a VHL population with screening MRI of petrous bones and audiometry for bilateral disease can potentially find small tumors that are locally resectable without compromising hearing or vestibular function. There are insufficient data to determine whether there are sporadic ELS tumors or whether all such patients have VHL, but all patients with ELS tumors must be evaluated for VHL, bilaterality, and other tumors and cysts.

Rhabdomyosarcoma

Rhabdomyosarcoma (RMS) is the most common tumor of the ear in children,[310] accounting for 7% of ear tumors reported by Dehner and Chen.[311] It is next in frequency of occurence after squamobasal cell tumors, melanoma, and glomus tumors of the ear (see Table 11–1).[7, 8, 311] Thirty-five percent to 50% of childhood RMS occur in the head and neck, of which 7% to 13% arise in the ear.[310–312]

Aural RMS occurs equally in boys and girls, with an age range from 1 to 12 years and an average age at clinical onset between 4 and 5 years.[311] Less commonly, RMS occurs in the head and neck, including the ear, of young adults, ages 18 through 36 years, with a male to female ratio of $1:2$.[313]

Common presenting signs are a mass in the auditory canal with hearing loss and, in 50% of patients, a cranial nerve palsy at presentation. Imaging shows extensive bone destruction in the middle ear and mastoid with craniospinal spread.[311]

Pathologic Features. Biopsy of the auditory canal or middle ear mass often generates a diagnosis of aural polyp (Fig. 11–34A, see p. 694). A botryoid, or grape-like, growth pattern may not be evident, and extensive inflammation and necrosis can mask the histologic characteristics of the tumors.

In children under the age of 12 years, an embryonal pattern dominates. The malignant cells are small, dark, and slightly spindled in a loose myxoid background. If there is polypoid proliferation in a space (botryoid), a growth layer (cambium) of condensed tumor cells beneath the mucosal surface may be obvious (Fig. 11–34B, see p. 694). There is a mix of larger polygonal cells with acidophilic cytoplasm and compact stroma. Mitoses and striated strap cells are occasionally found (Fig. 11–34C). In adolescents, an alveolar pattern predominates.[312, 313] Immunohistochemically, the acidophilic cytoplasm of the larger cells stains with vimentin, desmin, and muscle specific actin (Fig. 11–34D). Electron microscopic studies are difficult because of the small size of the biopsy area, necrosis, and rarity of cells showing myocontractile fibrils.

Differential Diagnosis. The major differential diagnosis is with inflammation—chronic otitis media with aural polyp (see Fig. 11–24). The absence of previous otitis, hearing loss, and cranial nerve palsies alert both the clinician and pathologist to the possibility of a neoplasm in spite of the patient's age. Imaging will show extensive bone destruction.

Necrosis, hemorrhage, and inflammation can cause delay in pathologic diagnosis, but a high degree of suspicion and appropriate use of immunohistochemistry will differentiate RMS from inflammation and other childhood tumors such as yolk sac tumor,[314, 315] Langerhans' cell granulomatosis (see later discussion) or Ewing's sarcoma.[316] Yolk sac tumors may manifest, in addition to the characteristic Schiller-Duval body (Fig. 11–35A, see p. 695), a vacuolate microcystic pattern that could be confused with alveolar RMS. Yolk sac tumor cells contain keratin and alpha-fetoprotein (Fig. 11–35B).

Treatment and Prognosis. Twenty-five years of study[317–321] have established the primary role of chemotherapy in the treatment of childhood RMS with irradiation of meninges and central nervous system. There is no role for primary surgical resection of aural RMS, irrespective of the patient's age.

Prognosis is related to the site and depth of the tumor at the time of diagnosis, symptomatic bone destruction, and central nervous system spread. For treatment purposes, RMS is classified as (1) orbital, (2) nasal or nasopharyngeal–nonorbital nonparameningeal, and (3) aural–parameningeal.[318] The poor 5% to 10% 5-year overall survival rate for aural RMS achieved in the 1970s has improved to 70% with earlier diagnosis and improved chemotherapy and irradiation protocols.[321]

In juveniles, the high proportion of parameningeal tumors and the frequent alveolar pattern contribute to a more adverse outcome, with only 2 long-term survivors among 12 patients.[313] Regional lymph node and pulmonary metastases occur, but death is due to central nervous system spread.

Metastatic and Other Rare Tumors

Metastases to the temporal bone are infrequent, otologic symptoms are rare, and the patient invariably has a known primary tumor.[322] The metastases reflect the relative frequency of the primary tumors, with (in order of frequency) breast, lung, kidney, prostate, stomach, cervix and uterus, pharynx, nasopharynx, larynx, and thyroid accounting for more than half of cited primary sites. The diagnosis of metastatic carcinoma is based on knowledge of a primary site and histologic pattern confirmed with appropriate immunohistochemical

studies.[322–325] The clear cell papillary follicular pattern of ELS tumor is separated from metastatic prostatic and follicular carcinomas by negative prostate specific antigen (PSA) and thyroglobulin (TGB), respectively. In the absence of specific immunohistochemical tumor markers, the cytologic characteristics of malignancy and intracellular lipid material and glycogen present in renal cell carcinoma must be used to differentiate between renal cell carcinoma and ELS, both of which occur in VHL patients (see earlier).

Malignant Melanoma

More cases of melanoma metastatic to the temporal bone have been reported (five)[322] than primary malignant melanoma of the middle ear (two).[326, 327] Melanoma can originate in the middle ear, destroy the drum, and present as an aural polyp in the external auditory canal or, more commonly, originate in the external ear meatus or canal and invade the middle ear and temporal bone. Differentiation between primary and metastatic melanoma requires documentation of another site of origin or known primary tumor and histologic documentation of in situ melanoma in the presumed mucosal site of origin.[328]

Other Neoplasms

Poorly documented isolated case reports exist of leiomyosarcoma,[329] fibrosarcoma,[330] and "synovial" sarcoma.[331] All malignant spindle cell tumors require immunohistochemical studies to differentiate among sarcomatoid squamous cell carcinoma, mesenchymal tumors, and melanoma (see earlier). Meningioma can involve the middle ear by direct extension from the overlying meninges (meningocele), from "ectopic" arachnoidal cells in the temporal bone, or in association with cranial nerves (see earlier).[144–146, 239]

Lymphoproliferative disorders primarily involving the temporal bone can secondarily affect the middle ear, but primary involvement of the middle ear is exceptional; primary extramedullary plasmacytoma in the middle ear has been reported.[332, 333] Hodgkin's disease has been reported to occur in the middle ear secondary to upper cervical lymph node disease,[334] but Langerhans' cell granulomatosis is a much more likely diagnosis (see later). Knowledge of pre-existing disease, AIDS status, and specific immunohistochemical T-cell markers can assist in differentiating T-cell lymphoma[335] extending from the brain and bone marrow to the middle ear from otitis media.

Primary tumors of petrous bone are extremely rare. Chondrosarcoma of the skull base can erode into the temporal bone.[336–338]

Langerhans' (Dendritic) Cell Granulomatosis

Langerhans' cell granulomatosis is a proliferative disorder of dendritic (Langerhans') cells, which are ubiquitous in skin and lymphoid tissues and are involved in antigen presentation to T lymphocytes in the cell-mediated immune process.[339] Since the dendritic cells are neither histiocytes nor macrophages, the disease is best called Langerhans' (dendritic) cell granulomatosis[340] rather than histiocytosis.[341, 342] The variety of dendritic cell proliferations (focal, multifocal, or diffuse in bone and viscera, at all ages) previously resulted in the unifying clinical concept of histiocytosis X, encompassing eosinophilic granuloma, Hand-Schüller-Christian disease, and Letterer-Siwe disease.

Willman et al.[343] report clonality of a dendritic cell population, but additional genetic investigations are needed to differentiate reactive (dendritic cell hyperplasia) from neoplastic proliferations. Lieberman et al.[340] liken Langerhans' cell granulomatosis to sarcoid, another cellular immune proliferative disorder secondary to an unknown antigen.

Langerhans' cell granulomatosis is predominantly a disorder of childhood but occurs at all ages. Among 238 cases reported from Memorial Sloan-Kettering Hospital,[340] 65% were male and 35% female, with ages ranging from 1 month to 66 years (mean, 17.6 years; median, 11 years). Unifocal disease was present in 64.3% of patients, with skull involvement in 16%. Otitis externa, recurrent otitis media, and mastoiditis secondary to a local osseous lesion were not uncommon.

Radiographs show punched-out lytic bone lesions; the classic "onion skinning" is a parosteal reaction with involvement of cortical bone.[344]

Pathologic Features. Histologically, the lesion is a mixture of Langerhans' cells and eosinophils in varying proportions (Fig. 11–36A, see p. 695). The Langerhans' cell is 10 to 12 μm in diameter with poorly outlined, slightly eosinophilic cytoplasm. Nuclei are characteristically reniform to oval, irregularly clefted or lobated, with "nuclear grooves" or folds. Ultrastructurally (Fig. 11–36B), characteristic Birbeck's granules are rigid tubular structures of variable length and average diameter of 34 nm. There is a striated zipper-like core between two electron-dense bilamellar membranes. Folded or clefted nuclei encompass cytoplasm, forming the "nuclear grooves" seen with the light microscope.[339, 340]

The definitive diagnosis of Langerhans' cell granulomatosis requires either demonstration of Birbeck's granules by electron microscopy or immunohistochemical detection of CD1a.[345]

Differential Diagnosis. The differential diagnosis involves subacute and chronic inflammation, other eosinophilic infiltrates, and histiocytic or macrophage lesions including xanthogranuloma and Hodgkin's disease. CD1a expression is specific for dendritic cells, which lack macrophage markers, thus separating them from CD1a-negative, KP-1–positive histiocytes and macrophages, monocytes and giant cells, and granulocytes, which may be secondarily involved in the lesion.[345] S-100 protein is a sensitive but nonspecific marker for dendritic cells.

Treatment and Prognosis. Local excision or curettage is sufficient treatment for focal disease. Multifocal or disseminated disease requires chemotherapy (methotrexate and prednisone), radiation therapy, or a combination of both.[340, 346] Antimicrobials are needed for treatment of otitis media and mastoiditis. There were no deaths in the Memorial Sloan-Kettering series[340]; the six infants with disseminated disease were the only deaths among 28 children with histiocytosis X at Children's Hospital of Los Angeles.[346]

▌ INNER EAR

Tumors of the Internal Auditory Canal and Cerebellopontine Angle

Neurofibromatosis

Clinical Features. The majority of tumors in the internal auditory canal and cerebellopontine angle are derived from cranial nerve sheaths (neuroma), or are meningiomas, both of which are associated with neurofibromatosis.

A 1987 National Institutes of Health consensus conference defined the clinical criteria for the diagnosis of the neurofibromatoses (Table 11–5), two distinct diseases dominated by nerve sheath tumors and overlapping clinical findings.[347] Both neurofibromatoses are transmitted as autosomal dominant traits, but half of the cases occur sporadically as new mutations. They affect men and women equally.

Neurofibromatosis 1 (NF-1, von Recklinghausen's disease, or peripheral neurofibromatosis) occurs once in 4000 live births. The diagnosis is usually made before age 10 by the presence of café-au-lait spots and dermal neurofibromas. The NF-1 gene is found on chromosome 17.[136, 347]

In contrast, neurofibromatosis 2 (NF-2 or central neurofibromatosis) occurs in 1 of 50,000 live births, with acoustic (cranial nerve) neuromas (schwannomas) that are usually bilateral (90%), intracranial and paraspinal meningioma, and presenile lens opacities. Café-au-lait spots and neurofibromas are uncommon. The gene is lo-

Table 11–5. NIH Consensus Conference Clinical Criteria for the Diagnosis of Neurofibromatoses

A. Neurofibromatosis 1, NF-1 (von Recklinghausen's or peripheral neurofibromatosis): two or more of the following:
   1. Six or more café au lait macules over 5 mm in greatest diameter in prepubertal individuals and over 15 mm in greatest diameter in postpubertal individuals
   2. Two or more neurofibromas of any type or one plexiform neurofibroma
   3. Freckling in the axillary or inguinal regions
   4. Optic glioma
   5. Two or more Lisch nodules (iris hamartomas)
   6. A distinctive osseous lesion such as sphenoid dysplasia or thinning of the long bone cortex, with or without pseudoarthrosis
   7. A first degree relative (parent, sibling, or offspring) with NF-1 by the above criteria.
B. Neurofibromatosis 2, NF-2
   1. Bilateral eighth nerve masses seen with appropriate imaging techniques; *or*
   2. A first-degree relative with NF-2 and either unilateral eighth nerve mass, *or* two of the following: neurofibroma, meningioma, glioma, schwannoma, or juvenile posterior lenticular opacity.

From Neurofibromatosis Conference Statement. National Institutes of Health Consensus Development Conference. *Arch Neurol* 1988;45:575–578.

calized to chromosome 22q12 and encodes merlin/schwannomin, a family of proteins associated with plasma cytoskeleton functions.[348] Among unselected patients with vestibular schwanomma, 5.5% are reported as having NF-2.[349] Both sporadic and hereditary vestibular schwannomas will manifest loss of tumor suppressor protein, which will not be manifest in next of kin of sporadic cases.[349] The molecular genetics of NF-1 and NF-2 (as well as meningioma, paraganglioma, and von Hippel-Lindau disease) have most recently been reviewed by Irving.[350]

Among 440 pediatric patients in the Children's Hospital of Philadelphia neurofibromatosis clinic,[136] 434 had NF-1 and 6 had NF-2 with equal male:female distribution. Otologic manifestations of neurofibromatosis recorded in 6.4% of these patients were as follows: 22 of the 434 NF-1 patients had neurofibromas, 19 of the external ear and canal, 2 of the middle ear, and 1 of the eight cranial nerve; all six of the NF-2 patients had acoustic neuromas, bilateral in five and unilateral in one.

Schwannomas (neurilemmoma, acoustic/vestibular neuroma, NF-2) are derived from nerve sheaths of the cranial nerves, predominantly the vestibular division of the eighth nerve, and are commonly known as acoustic or vestibular neuromas. The tumors enlarge, expanding out of the internal auditory meatus and forming a cerebellopontine angle mass, which can erode the internal auditory meatus and canal. Compression by the tumor can cause fifth and other adjacent cranial nerve palsies and cerebellar dysfunction. Hearing loss, often bilateral, is the major clinical symptom.[136, 347]

Pathologic Features. NF-1 and NF-2 tumors are derived from nerve sheath Schwann cells but have different pathologic characteristics, growth patterns, and malignant potentials (Table 11–6).

NF-1 neurofibromas form solitary, occasionally plexiform, globular to fusiform masses in the skin of the ear pinna and external canal. They have been demonstrated in the middle ear in asymptomatic patients who underwent screening imaging studies.[136] The tumors are grossly fusiform and mucoid on cut section and incorporate nerve fibers. Microscopically, the tumors are composed of wavy, spindly, occasionally palisading (Fig. 11–37A) cells (S-100 protein–positive), in a myxoid stroma with axons variably scattered throughout the tumor.[351]

The schwannoma, in contrast, is grossly lobular and appears to be eccentrically encapsulated relative to the nerve; cross section is yellow and microcystic. Microscopically (Fig. 11–37B), the tumor has a biphasic degenerative appearance consisting of two characteristic histologic patterns: Antoni type A, palisading club-shaped nu-

Table 11–6. Clinical and Pathological Comparisons Between NF-1 and NF-2

	Neurofibromatosis (NF)-1	Neurofibromatosis (NF)-2
Gene	chromosome 17	chromosome 22
Incidence (live births)	1/4000	1/50,000
Age at diagnosis	<10 years	>20 years
Location	Peripheral: skin of ear	Central: 8th cranial nerve cerebellopontine angle (90% bilateral)
Signs/Symptoms	Wormy dermal mass Café au lait spots	Hearing/vestibular loss
Lesion	Neurofibroma	Neurilemmoma (schwannoma) (acoustic neuroma)
	Neurofibrosarcoma	Meningioma
Gross	Fusiform, plexiform Multiple White, solid, mucoid	Eccentric, lobular Bilateral Yellow, cystic
Histology	Wavy fusiform myxoid stroma	Antoni A Verocay bodies Antoni B microcystic stroma

clei lacking distinctive cytoplasm, forming Verocay bodies; and Antoni type B, small round cells with indistinct cytoplasm resembling lymphocytes, microcystic spaces in the stroma (cystic degeneration), fat-laden histocytes (xanthoma cells), hemosiderin, and hyalinized thick-walled blood vessels. A reticulin stain shows pericellular reticulin representing the Schwann cell lamellar basement membrane. The cells are regularly S-100 protein–positive.[351]

Differential Diagnosis. Neurofibromas can transform into *malignant peripheral nerve sheath tumors* (MPNST), large, fleshy, highly malignant tumors that are differentiated from cellular neurofibromas with increased cellular density, cellular atypia, and occasional mitoses by their high degree of anaplasia, mitotic activity (Fig. 11–38A), necrosis, higher p53 and Ki-67 labeling indices, and S-phase fraction and aneuploidy.[136, 351–356] MPNST most often are peripheral neurofibrosarcomas,[351, 353] but they rarely present in the skin and paranasal sinuses of the head and neck[354, 355] and may involve the acoustic nerve.[356, 357] Heterologous elements (Fig. 11–38B), including rhabdomyoblastic and epithelial differentiation, found in some of these neurogenic sarcomas provide the name *triton tumor* (three "prongs").[353–357]

Differentiating between schwannoma and neurofibroma is important, since the latter has the potential for malignant change. Schwannomas rarely occur sporadically and peripherally as plexiform lesions that do not have a malignant potential.[358, 359] In contrast, rare central neurofibrosarcomas[136] and triton tumors[356, 357] do occur.

Treatment and Prognosis. Neurofibromas are resected only when they become symptomatic due to size. Rapid growth may signal malignancy, but the highly malignant neurogenic sarcomas fail surgical and oncologic treatment regimens.

Small asymptomatic schwannomas identified in screening programs of NF-2 populations by the use of hearing and vestibular function tests and imaging[136] have been resected in attempts to preserve auditory and vestibular functions. The neuromas have "pseudocapsules," which permit "shelling out" procedures in attempts to save the nerve for hearing and vestibular function.[360] In spite of apparent incomplete excision, only 0.3% of these slow-growing tumors recur over an average time interval of 10 years.[361] Flow cytometric analysis of proliferation markers showed no "fundamental differences between the recurrent acoustic tumor group and a larger group of . . . acoustic tumors.[361]

Better hearing preservation can be achieved with small vestibular schwannomas (≤1.0 cm in size) via a middle fossa surgical approach than with a retrosigmoid approach.[362] The complete loss of hearing and vestibular function attendant upon complete removal of the nerve and tumor must be weighed against "watchful waiting" with repeat follow-up MRI and hearing and vestibular function tests and later decompression. Recently available gamma knife radiosurgery can reportedly "provide long-term control of acoustic neuromas while preserving neurologic function."[363]

The occurrence of neurofibrosarcoma is too rare to justify removal of asymptomatic inner ear tumors.

Meningioma

Clinical Findings. Meningioma is the second most common tumor in NF-2.[364] Ten percent of all meningiomas occur at the cerebellopontine angle. Meningioma can cause hearing loss, simulating acoustic neuroma, and can, by involvement of the dura overlying the endolymphatic sac, cause vestibular symptoms of Meniére's disease.[365]

Pathologic Features. Fibrous meningioma may be difficult to histologically differentiate from schwannoma (Fig. 11–37C), but it expresses epithelial membrane antigen and not S-100 protein. Meningotheliomatous meningioma is apparently formed by a molecular pathway independent of NF-2, distinct from fibroblastic and transitional meningiomas.[348] Meningioma at the cerebellopontine angle has also occurred in association with cutaneous meningioma of the external auditory canal.[366]

Differential Diagnosis. In addition to meningioma, *lipoma* of the eighth cranial nerve can occur in the internal auditory canal. These tumors usually arise in men in the third to fifth decade, causing unilateral hearing loss and tinnitus. Lipoma is extremely rare and is not associated with neurofibromatosis.[367–371] Lipoma cannot be clinically distinguished from acoustic neuroma or meningioma but is suggested by high signal density on a T1-weighted MRI scan. The nerve is symmetrically enlarged due to an admixture of mature fat cells, neurons, and ganglion cells, which are recognizable by frozen section at surgery.[367]

Primary *B-cell lymphoma*[372] and *cavernous hemangioma*[373] have been reported to occur at the internal auditory meatus, clinically simulating acoustic neuroma and meningioma.

Magnetic resonance imaging can be used to identify the site of origin of the tumor within the internal auditory canal with growth to the cerebellopontine angle or vice versa. MRI is sensitive for determination of tumor site but not specific for tumor type.

Meniére's Disease or Labyrinthitis

Clinical Features. Meniére's disease is a disorder of the cochlear labyrinth clinically characterized by tinnitus, episodic vertigo, and fluctuating sensorineural hearing loss.[374]

Pathologic Features. Dilation of the fluid-filled endolymphatic spaces, or endolymphatic hydrops, is associated with chronic inflammation (rarely, ESL tumors or metastatic neoplasms)[375] in the surrounding perilymphatic fibrous tissue, which interferes with either production or resorption of endolymphatic fluid. Light, electron, and immunohistochemical microscopic studies of the small pieces of endolymphatic sac and duct produced by surgical decompression suggest an immunologic function of the sac,[376, 377] in addition to secretion of endolymph.

Treatment and Prognosis. Episodic vertigo is the major clinical problem. Treatment of vertigo is based on decreasing fluid production with diuretic drugs, which alter fluid balance, or decreasing fluid accumulation with surgical endolymphatic sac shunts and fistulas. Unsuccessful alteration of fluid dynamics may require ablation of the end organ or neuronal pathway by surgical or aminoglycoside destruction of the vestibular nerve. Unfortunately, none of these procedures is found to be more effective at controlling episodic vertigo

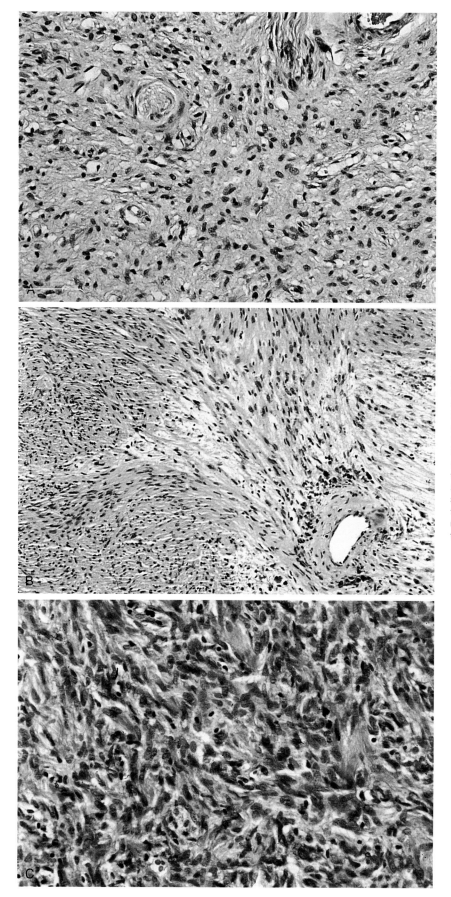

Figure 11–37. Spindle cell tumors of the cerebellar pontine angle. A, Neurofibroma is composed of wavy, spindly cells in a myxoid stroma; axons are variably scattered throughout the tumor. B, Schwannoma has a biphasic pattern: Antoni type A (left), palisading club-shaped nuclei with indistinct cytoplasm (Verocay bodies) and Antoni type B (right), small round cells with indistinct cytoplasm, microcystic spaces, xanthoma cells, hemosiderin, and hyalinized thick-walled blood vessels. C, Fibrous meningioma is also composed of spindle cells with indistinct cytoplasm, but the nuclei are larger and more ovoid than the neural tumors and the myxoid or microcystic stroma is absent. This tumor expresses vimentin and epithelial membrane antigen but not S-100 protein.

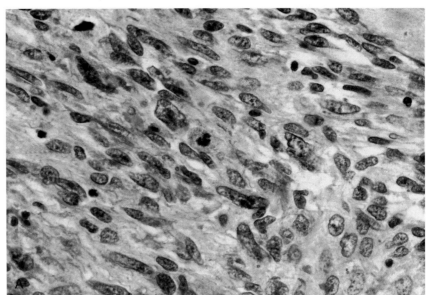
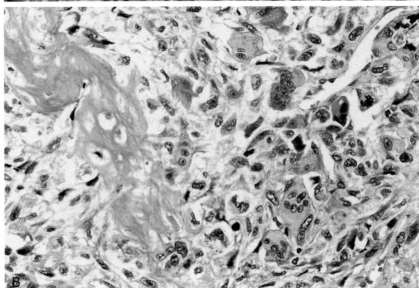

Figure 11–38. Malignant peripheral nerve sheath tumor (MPSNT). A spindle cell stromal sarcoma in a patient with neurofibromatosis-1 has pleomorphic nuclei and many mitotic figures *(A)* and focal giant cell differentiation with osteoid (osteosarcoma) *(B)*.

than is placebo therapy (60–80% effective), owing to poorly controlled clinical studies and poorly understood pathophysiology of the disorder.[374]

ACKNOWLEDGMENTS

This work was supported by The Dorothy and Harry Davis Memorial Pathology Education and Research Fund #080, Bridgeport Hospital Foundation.

I thank Katherine Stemmer Frumento, previously Director of the Bridgeport Hospital Medical Library, now at Sloan-Kettering Memorial Hospital, for her invaluable help in providing references, and Susan Davis for reviewing the manuscript to ensure its readability.

REFERENCES

1. Van De Water TR, Rubin RJ: Organogenesis of the ear. In: Hinchcliffe R, Harrison D, eds: *Scientific Foundations of Otolaryngology.* London: William Heineman Medical Books, 1976:173–184.
2. Ross DA, Sasaki CT: Cancer of the ear and temporal bone. In: Myers EN, Suen JY, eds: *Cancer of the Head and Neck.* Philadelphia: W.B. Saunders, 1996:586–588.
3. Michaels L: Ear. In: Sternberg SS, ed. *Histology for Pathologists.* New York: Raven Press, 1992:925–949.
4. Michaels L: *Ear, Nose and Throat Histopathology.* London: Springer-Verlag, 1987.
5. Lucente FE, Lawson W, Novick NL: *The External Ear.* Philadelphia: W.B. Saunders, 1995.
6. Arndt KA, Leboit PE, Robinson JK, et al., eds: *Cutaneous Medicine and Surgery: An Integrated Program in Dermatology.* Philadelphia: W.B. Saunders, 1995.
7. Davis GL: Tumors and inflammatory conditions of the ear. In: Gnepp D, ed: *Pathology of the Head and Neck.* New York: Churchill Livingstone, 1988:547–583.
8. Hyams VJ, Batsakis JG, Michaels L: Tumors of the upper respiratory tract and ear. In: *Atlas of Tumor Pathology,* 2nd series, fascicle 25. Washington DC: Armed Forces Institute of Pathology, 1988:258–330.
9. Shanmugaratnam K, ed: *Histological Typing of Tumours of the Upper Respiratory Tract and Ear,* 2nd ed. New York: Springer-Verlag, 1991.
10. Wenig BM: *Atlas of Head and Neck Pathology.* Philadelphia: W.B. Saunders, 1993.

Lumps and Bumps

11. Cohen PR: Pathological cases of the month. Accessory tragus. *Am J Dis Child* 1993;147:1123–1124.
12. Simpson RA: Lateral cysts and fistulas. *Laryngoscope* 1969;79:30–59.

13. Triglia J-M, Nicollas R, Ducroz V, et al.: First branchial cleft anomalies. A study of 39 cases and a review of the literature. *Arch Otolaryngol Head Neck Surg* 1998;124:291–295.
14. Nofsinger YC, Tom LWC, LaRossa D, et al.: Periauricular cysts and sinuses. *Laryngoscope* 1998;107:883–887.
15. Ihrler S, Zietz C, Riederer A, et al.: HIV-related parotid lymphoepithelial cysts. *Virchow Arch* 1996;429:139–147.
16. Ikeda M, Muto J, Omachi S: Dermoid cyst of the auricle: Report of two cases. *Auris Nasus Larynx* 1990;16:193–197.
17. Vinayak BC, Cox JG, Ashton-Key M: Pilomatrixoma of the external auditory meatus. *J Laryngol Otol* 1993;333–334.
18. Zhu L, Wang X: Histological examination of the auricular cartilage and pseudocyst of the auricle. *J Laryngol Otol* 1992;106:103–104.
19. Lee JA, Panarese A: Endochondral pseudocyst of the auricle. *J Clin Pathol* 1994;47:961–963.
20. Heffner DK, Hayms VJ: Cystic chondromalacia (endochondral pseudocyst) of the auricle. *Arch Pathol Lab Med* 1986;110:740–743.
21. Khalak R, Roberts JK: Images in clinical medicine. Cauliflower ear. *N Engl J Med* 1996;335:399.
22. Morton CA, Fallowfield M, Kemett D: Localized argyria caused by silver earrings. *Br J Dermatol* 1996;135:484–485.
23. Thomas MR, Sadiq HA, Raweily EA: Acanthoma fissuratum. *J Laryngol Otol* 1991;105:301–303.
24. Yoshida GY: Xanthogranuloma of the external auditory canal. *Otolaryngol Head Neck Surg* 1995;112:626–627.
25. Raimer SS, Sanchez RL: The histiocytoses of childhood. In: Arndt KA, Leboit P, Robinson J, et al, eds: *Cutaneous Medicine and Surgery: An Integrated Program in Dermatology.* Philadelphia: W.B. Saunders, 1995:1620–1625.
26. Tahan SR, Pastel- Levy C, Bhan AK, et al.: Juvenile xanthogranuloma. *Arch Pathol Lab Med* 1989;113:1057–1061.
27. Sueki H, Saito T, Iijima M, et al.: Adult-onset xanthogranuloma appearing symmetrically on the ear lobes. *J Am Acad Dermatol* 1995;32:372–374.
28. Pollack JD, Pincus RL, Lucente FE: Leprosy of the head and neck. *Otolaryngol Head Neck Surg* 1987;97:93–96.
29. Alidina R, Werschler P, Nigra T, et al.: A solitary tumor on the ear lobe. Granular cell tumor. *Arch Dermatol* 1994;130:913–916.
30. Zvulunov A, Barak Y, Metzker A: Juvenile xanthogranuloma, neurofibromatosis, and juvenile chronic myelogenous leukemia. *Arch Dermatol* 1995;131:904–908.

Inflammatory Lesions

31. Santa Cruz DJ: Chondrodermatitis nodularis helicis: A transepidermal perforating disorder. *J Cutan Pathol* 1980;7:70–76.
32. Lawrence CM: Chondrodermatitis nodularis. In: Arndt KA, Leboit P, Robinson J, et al., eds: *Cutaneous Medicine and Surgery: An Integrated Program in Dermatology.* Philadelphia: W.B. Saunders, 1995:507–511.
33. Millard PR, Young E, Harrison DE, et al.: Reactive perforating collagenosis: Light, ultrastructural and immunohistological studies. *Histopathology* 1986;10:1047–1056.
34. Requena L, Aguilar A, Sanchez YE: Elastotic nodules of the ears. *Cutis* 1989;44:452–454.
35. Kavanaugh GM, Bradfield JW, Collins CM, et al.: Weathering nodules of the ear: A clinicopathological study. *Br J Dermatol* 1996;135:550–554.
36. Paslin DA: Cartilaginous papule of the ear. *J Cut Pathol* 1991;18:60–63.
37. Azon-Masoliver A, Ferrando J, Mavarra E, et al.: Solitary congenital nodular calcification of Winer located on the ear: Report of two cases. *Pediatr Dermatol* 1989;6:191–193.
38. Larson PL, Weinstock MA, Welch RH: Calcification of the auricular cartilage: A case report and literature review. *Cutis* 1992;50:55–57.
39. Bottomley WW, Goodfield MDJ: Chondrodermatitis nodularis helicis occurring with systemic sclerosis: An under-reported association? *Clin Exp Dermatol* 1994;19:219–220.
40. Hicks BS, Weber PJ, Hashimoto K, et al.: Primary cutaneous amyloidosis of the auricular concha. *J Am Acad Dermatol* 1988;18:19–25.
41. Barnadas MA, Perez M, Esuius J, et al.: Papules in the auricular concha: Lichen amyloidosis in case of biphasic amyloidosis. *Dermatologica* 1990;181:149–151.
42. Crowson AN, Magro CM: Idiopathic pernio and its mimics: A clinical and histological study of 38 cases. *Hum Pathol* 1997;28:478–484.
43. Scully RE, Mark EJ, McNeely WF, et al.: Case records of the Massachusetts General Hospital. Weekly clinicopathological exercises. Case 29-1996. A 59-year-old man with gout and a painful preauricular mass. *N Engl J Med* 1996;335:876–881.
44. Oluwole M: Pyoderma gangrenosum: An unusual case of periaural ulceration. *Br J Clin Pract* 1995;49:330–331.
45. Ostlere LS, Wells J, Stevens HP, et al.: Neutrophilic eccrine hidradenitis with an unusual presentation. *Br J Dermatol* 1993;128:696–698.
46. Padmore RF, Bedard YC, Chapnick J: Relapse of acute myelogenous leukemia presenting as acute otitis externa: A case report. *Cancer* 1984;53:569–572.
47. Samuel LM, Matheson LM, Mac Dougall C, et al.: Massive cutaneous large cell T-cell non-Hodgkin's lymphoma of the pinna. *Clin Oncol (R Coll Radiol)* 1995;7:196–197.
48. Levin RJ, Henick DH, Cohen AR: Human immunodeficiency virus-associated non-Hodgkins lymphoma presenting as an auricular perichondritis. *Otolaryngol Head Neck Surg* 1995;112:493–495.
49. Kieserman SP, Finn DG: Non-Hodgkin's lymphoma of the external auditory canal in an HIV-positive patient. *J Laryngol Otol* 1995;109:751–754.
50. Zeuner M, Straub RH, Rauh G, et al: Relapsing polychondritis: Clinical and immunogenetic analysis of 62 patients. *J Rheumatol* 1997;24:96–101.
51. Trentham DE: Relapsing polychondritis. In: Arndt KA, Leboit P, Robinson J, et al., eds: *Cutaneous Medicine and Surgery: An Integrated Program in Dermatology.* Philadelphia: W.B. Saunders, 1995:512–514.
52. Valenzuela R, Cooperrider PA, Gogate P, et al.: Relapsing polychondritis. Immunomicroscopic findings in cartilage of ear biopsy specimens. *Hum Pathol* 1980;11:19–22.
53. McCune WJ, Schiller AJ, Dynesius-Trentham RA, et al.: Type II collagen-induced auricular chondritis. *Arthritis Rheum* 1982;25:266–273.
54. Yoo TJ, Lee M-K, Min YS, et al.: Epitope specificity and T cell receptor usage in type II collagen induced autoimmune ear disease. *Cell Immunol* 1994;157:249–262.
55. Piette J-C, Frances C: Images in clinical medicine: Relapsing polychondritis. *N Engl J Med* 1995;332:580.
56. Scully RE, Mark EJ, McNeely WF, et al., eds: Case records of the Massachusetts General Hospital. Weekly clinicopathological exercises Case 38-1997. Inflammation of the ears, anemia, and fever 21 years after treatment for Hodgkin's disease. *N Engl J Med* 1997;337:1753–1760.

Neoplasms

57. Nemchjek AJ, Amedee RG: Tumors of the external ear. *J La Med Soc* 1995;147:239–242.
58. Betti R, Inselvini E, Gualandri L, et al.: Basal cell carcinomas of the auricular region: A study of 23 cases. *J Dermatol* 1995;22:655–658.
59. Stell P: Basal cell carcinoma of the external auditory meatus. *Clin Otolaryngol* 1984;187–190.
60. Chen KTK, Dehner LP: Primary tumors of the external and middle ear. I. Introduction and clinico-pathologic study of squamous cell carcinoma. *Arch Otolaryngol* 1978;104:247–252.
61. Byers R, Kasler K, Redmon B, et al.: Squamous carcinoma of the external ear. *Am J Surg* 1983;146:447–450.
62. Austin JR, Stewart KL, Fawzi N: Squamous cell carcinoma of the external auditory canal. Therapeutic prognosis based on a proposed staging system. *Arch Otolaryngol Head Neck Surg* 1994;120:1228–1232.
63. Thomas SS, Matthews RN: Squamous cell carcinoma of the pinna: 6 year study. *Br J Plastic Surg* 1994;47:81–85.
64. Gacek MR, Gacek RR, Gantz B, et al.: Pseudo-epitheliomatous hyperplasia versus squamous cell carcinoma of the external auditory canal. *Laryngoscope* 1998;108:620–623.
65. Lee D, Nash M, Har-El G: Regional spread of auricular and periauricular cutaneous malignancies. *Laryngoscope* 1996;106:998–1001.
66. Kinney SE, Wood BG: Malignancies of the external ear canal and temporal bone: Surgical techniques and results. *Laryngoscope* 1987;97:158–164.
67. Ross DA, Sasaki CT: Cancer of the ear and temporal bone. In: Myers EN, Suen JY, eds: *Cancer of the Head and Neck.* Philadelphia: W.B. Saunders, 1995:586–588.
68. Byers RM, Smith JL, Russell N, et al.: Malignant melanoma of the external ear. Review of 102 cases. *Am J Surg* 1980;140:518–521.
69. Gussack GS, Reintgen D, Cox E, et al: Cutaneous melanoma of the head and neck: A review of 399 cases. *Arch Otolaryngol* 1983;109:803–808.
70. Davidsson A, Jellquist HB, Villamn K, Westman G: Malignant melanoma of the ear. *J Laryngol Otol* 1993;107:798–802.
71. Langman AW, Yarington CT, Patterson SD: Malignant melanoma of the

external auditory canal. *Otolaryngol Head Neck Surg* 1996;114:645–648.

72. Bono A, Bartoli C, Maurichi A, et al.: Melanoma of the external ear. *Tumori* 1997;83:814–818.

73. Hurt MA, Santa Cruz DJ: Tumors of the skin. In: Fletcher CDM, ed: *Diagnostic Histopathology of Tumors,* vol II. New York: Churchill Livingstone, 1995:1014–1023.

74. Kempson RL, McGavran MH: Atypical fibroxanthomas of the skin. *Cancer* 1964;17:1463–1471.

75. Tomascewski M-M, Lupton GP: Atypical fibroxanthoma: An unusual variant with osteoclast-like giant cells. *Am J Surg Pathol* 1997;21:213–218.

76. Calonje E, Mentzel T, Fletcher CDM: Cellular benign fibrous histiocytoma. *Am J Surg Pathol* 1994;18:668–676.

77. Morrissey G, Robinson AC, Stirling R: Cellular benign fibrous histiocytoma of the external auditory meatus. *J Laryngol Otol* 1996;119:98–100.

78. Longacre TA, Smoller BR, Rouse RV: Atypical fibroxanthoma: Multiple immunohistochemical profiles. *Am J Surg Pathol* 1993;17:1199–1203.

79. Inoue F, Matsumoto K: Vascular leiomyoma of the auricle. *Arch Dermatol* 1983;119:445–446.

80. Lazuva R, Moynes R, May D, et al.: LN-2 (CD74) A marker to distinguish atypical fibroxanthoma from malignant fibrous histiocytoma. *Cancer* 1997;79:115–124.

81. Katahashi T, Shimada F, Omura K, et al.: A case of nodular fasciitis arising in the auricle. *Auris Naris Larynx (Tokyo)* 1995;22:59–64.

82. Thompson LDR, Fanburg-Smith JC, Wenig BM: Nodular fasciitis (NF) of the external ear region: A clinico-pathologic study of 50 cases. *Lab Invest* 1998;78:124A.

83. Schurch W, Seemayer TA, Gabbiani G: The myofibroblast. A quarter century after its discovery. *Am J Surg Pathol* 1998;22:141–147.

84. Ferreiro JA, Carney JA: Myxomas of the external ear and their significance. *Am J Surg Pathol* 1994;18:274–280.

85. Burrows NP, Ratnavel RC, Grant JW, et al.: Auricular embryonal rhabdomyosarcoma. *Dermatol* 1994;189:301–303.

86. Sibley RK, Rosai J, Foucar E, et al.: Neuroendocrine (Merkel cell) carcinoma of the skin. *Am J Surg Pathol* 1980;4:211–221.

87. Weymuller EA Jr, Marks M, Ridge D: Merkel cell carcinoma of the ear. *Head Neck* 1991;13:68–71.

88. Mills SE: Neuroendocrine tumors of the head and neck: An elected review with emphasis on terminology. *Endocrine Pathol* 1996;7:229–243.

89. Haag ML, Glass LF, Fenske NA: Merkel cell carcinoma. Diagnosis and treatment. *Dermatol Surg* 1995;21:669–683.

90. Chan JKC, Suster S, Wenig BM, et al.: Cytokeratin 20 immunoreactivity distinguishes Merkel cell (primary cutaneous neuroendocrine) carcinomas and salivary gland small cell carcinomas of various sites. *Am J Surg Pathol* 1997;21:226–234.

91. Gnepp DR, Chandler W, Hyams V: Primary Kaposi's sarcoma of the head and neck. *Ann Intern Med* 1984;100:107–114.

92. Foreman KE, Friborg J, Kong W, et al.: Propagation of a human herpesvirus from AIDS-associated Kaposi's sarcoma. *N Engl J Med* 1997;336:163–171.

93. Tappero JW, Koehler JE: Bacillary angiomatosis or Kaposi's sarcoma? *N Engl J Med* 1997;337:1888.

94. Koehler JE, Sanchez MA, Garrido CS, et al.: Molecular epidemiology of *Bartonella* infections in patients with bacillary angiomatosis-peliosis. *N Engl J Med* 1997;337:1876–1883.

95. Tompkins LS: Of cats, humans and *Bartonella. N Engl J Med* 1997;337:1916–1917.

96. Smith KJ, Skelton HG, Tuur S, et al.: Bacillary angiomatosis in an immunocompetent child. *Am J Surg Pathol* 1997;18:597–600.

97. LeBoit PE, Berger TG, Egbert BM, et al.: Bacillary angiomatosis. The history and differential diagnosis of a pseudoneoplastic infection in patients with human immunodeficiency virus disease. *Am J Surg Pathol* 1989;13:909–920.

98. Vallis RC, Davies DG: Angiolymphoid hyperplasia of the head and neck. *J Laryngol Otol* 1988;102:100–101.

99. Murty GE, Cox NH: Angiolymphoid hyperplasia with eosinophilia: An uncommon tumor of the external auditory canal. *Ear Nose Throat J* 1990;69:102–103, 106–107.

100. Ferlito A, Caruso G: Angiolymphoid hyperplasia with eosinophilia of the external ear (Kimura's disease). *ORL J Otorhinolaryngol Relat Spec* 1985;47:139–144.

101. Quercetani R, Gelli R, Pimpinelli N, et al.: Bilateral chondroma of the auricle. *J Dermatol Surg Oncol* 1988;14:436–438.

102. Ito A, Nakashima T, Kitamura M: Pleomorphic adenoma of the auricle. *J Laryngol Otol* 1982;96:1137–1140.

103. Reinish EL, Feinberg SE, Devaney K: Primary synovial chondromatosis of the temporomandibular joint with suspected traumatic etiology. *Int J Maxillofac Oral Surg* 1997;76:419–421.

104. Thompson K, Schwartz HC: Synovial chondromatosis of the temporomandibular joint presenting as a parotid mass: Possibility of confusion with a benign mixed tumor. *Oral Surg Oral Med Oral Pathol* 1986;62:377–380.

105. Davis RI, Foster H, Biggart DJ: C-erb B-2 staining in primary synovial chondromatosis: A comparison with other cartilaginous tumours. *J Pathol* 1996;179:392–395.

106. Davis RT, Foster H, Arthur K, et al.: Cell proliferation studies in primary synovial chondromatosis. *J Pathol* 1998;184:18–23.

107. Mertens F, Jonsson K, Willen H, et al.: Chromosome rearrangements in synovial chondromatous lesions. *Br J Cancer* 1996;74:251–255.

108. Carls FR, von Hochstetter A, Engelke W, et al.: Loose bodies in the temporomandibular joint: The advantages of arthroscopy. *J Craniomaxillofac Surg* 1995;23:215–221.

109. Kessler P, Hardt N, Kuttenberger J: Synovial chondromatosis of the temporomandibular joint with invasion into the middle cranial fossa. *Mund Kiefer Gesichtschir* 1997;Nov;1(6):353–355.

External Auditory Canal

110. Friedmann I. Pathological lesions of the external auditory meatus: A review. *J R Soc Med* 1990;83:34–37.

111. Selesnick SH: Diseases of the external auditory canal. *Otolaryngol Clin North Am* 1996;29.

112. Naiberg JB, Robinson A, Kwok P, et al.: Swirls, wrinkles and the whole ball of wax (the source of keratin in cerumen). *J Otolaryngol* 1992;21:142–148.

113. Piepergerdes JC, Kramer BM, Behnke EE: Keratosis obturans and external auditory canal cholesteatoma. *Laryngoscope* 1980;90:383–391.

114. Sismanis A, Huang C-E, Abedi E, et al.: External ear canal cholesteatoma. *Am J Otol* 1986;7:126–129.

115. Garin P, Degols J-C, Delos M: External auditory canal cholesteatoma. *Arch Otol Head Neck Surg* 1997;123:62–65.

116. Sapci T, Ugur G, Kakavus A, et al.: Giant cholesteatoma of the external auditory canal. *Ann Otol Rhinol Laryngol* 1997;106:471–473.

117. Varledzides E, Tsilighiris E, Mougelas C: Ear myiasis: Case report. *Pan Minerva Med* 1981;23:43–46.

118. Brook I, Frazier EH, Thompson DH: Aerobic and anaerobic microbiology of external otitis. *Clin Infect Dis* 1991;15:955–958.

119. Doroghazi RM, Nadol JB, Hysolp NE, et al.: Invasive external otitis. *Am J Med* 1991;71:603–614.

120. Kohut RI, Lindsay JR: Necrotizing ("malignant") external otitis. Histopathologic processes. *Ann Otol* 1979;88:714–720.

121. Umeda Y, Nakajima M, Yoshioka H: Surfer's ear in Japan. *Laryngoscope* 1989;99(6 Pt 1):639–641.

122. Rinaldi MG: Invasive aspergillosis. *Rev Infect Dis* 1983;5:1061–1077.

Neoplasms

123. Wetli CV, Pardo V, Millard M, et al.: Tumors of ceruminous glands. *Cancer* 1972;29:1169–1178.

124. Dehner LP, Chen KTK: Primary tumors of the external and middle ear. Benign and malignant glandular neoplasms. *Arch Otolaryngol* 1980;106:13–19.

125. Lynde CW, McLean DI, Wood WS: Tumors of the ceruminous glands. *Am Acad Dermatol* 1984;11:841–847.

126. Lesser RW, Spector GJ, Devineni VR: Malignant tumors of the middle ear and external auditory canal: A 20 year review. *Otolaryngol Head Neck Surg* 1987;96:43–47.

127. Mansour P, George MK, Pahor AL: Ceruminous gland tumors: A reappraisal. *J Laryngol Otol* 1992;106:727–732.

128. Mills RG, Douglas-Jones T, Williams RG: 'Ceruminoma'—a defunct diagnosis. *J Laryngol Otol* 1995;109:180–188.

129. Tang X, Tamura Y, Tsutumi Y: Mixed tumor of the external auditory canal. *Pathol Int* 1994;44:80–83.

130. Haraguchi H, Hentona H, Tanaka H, et al.: Pleomorphic adenoma of the external auditory canal: A case report and review of the literature. *J Laryngol Otol* 1996;110:52–56.

131. Sharma HS, Meorkamal MZ, Zainol H, et al.: Eccrine cylindroma of the ear canal. Report of a case. *J Laryngol Otol* 1994;108:706–709.

132. Nissim F, Czernobilsky B, Ostfeld E: Hidradenoma papilliferum of the external auditory canal. *J Laryngol Otol* 1981;95:843–848.
133. Perzin KH, Gullane P, Conley J: Adenoid cystic carcinoma involving the external auditory canal. A clinicopathologic study of 16 cases. *Cancer* 1982;50:2873–2883.
134. Fenton JE, Turner J, Fagan PA: A histopathologic review of temporal bone exostoses and osteomata. *Laryngoscope* 1996;114:624–628.
135. Whitaker SR, Cordier A, Kosjak S, et al.: Treatment of external auditory canal exostoses. *Laryngoscope* 1998;108:195–199.
136. Smullen S, Willcox T, Wetmore R, et al.: Otologic manifestations of neurofibromatosis. *Laryngoscope* 1994;104:663–665.
137. Lustig LR, Jackler RK: Neurofibromatosis type I involving the external auditory canal. *Otolaryngol Head Neck Surg* 1996;114:299–307.
138. Behar PM, Myers LL, Hameer HR, et al.: Pathologic quiz case 2—Malignant peripheral nerve sheath tumor (PNST) of the greater auricular nerve. *Arch Otolaryngol Head Neck Surg* 1998;124:109–112.
139. Morrissey G, Robinson AC, Stirling R: Cellular benign fibrous histiocytoma of the external auditory meatus. *J Laryngol Otol* 1996;110:98–100.
140. Petshenik AJ, Linstrom CJ, MacCormick SA: Leiomyoma of the external auditory canal. *Am J Otol* 1996;17:133–136.
141. Singh KB, Hanna GS, Dinnen JS: Paraganglioma of the external auditory canal. *J Laryngol Otol* 1993;107:228–229.
142. Dehner LP, Chen KTK: Primary tumors of the external and middle ear. III. A clinicopathologic study of embryonal rhabdomyosarcoma. *Arch Otolaryngol* 1978;104:399–403.
143. Fukuingawa M, Miyazawa Y, Harada T, et al.: Yolk sac tumor of the ear. *Histopathol* 1995;27:563–567.
144. Keppes JJ: Meningiomas. *In Biology, Pathology, and Differential Diagnosis.* USA, New York: Masson Publishing, 1982:45.
145. Langford LA: Pathology of meningiomas. *J Neurooncol* 1996;29:17–21.
146. Hu B, Pant M, Cornford M, et al.: Association of primary intracranial meningioma and cutaneous meningioma of external auditory canal. *Arch Pathol Lab Med* 1998;122:97–99.

Middle Ear

147. Michaels L: Temporal bone histopathology in middle ear disease. *Clin Otolaryngol* 1980;5:225–226.
148. Michaels L: The temporal bone: An organ in search of a histopathology. *Histopathology* 1991;18:391–394.

Congenital Lesions and Choristoma

149. Heffner DK, Thompson LDR, Schall DG, et al.: Pharyngeal dermoids ("hairy polyps") as accessory auricles. *Ann Otol Rhinol Laryngol* 1996;10:819–824.
150. Parnes LS, Sun AH: Teratoma of the middle ear. *J Otolaryngol* 1995;24:165–167.
151. Navarro Cunchillos M, Bonachero MD, Navarro Cunchillos M, et al.: Middle ear teratoma in a newborn. *J Laryngol Otol* 1996;110:875–877.
152. Bottril ID, Chawla OP, Ransay AD: Salivary gland choristoma of the middle ear. *J Laryngol Otol* 1992;106:630–632.
153. Hinni ML, Beatty CW: Salivary gland choristoma of the middle ear: Report of a case with review of the literature. *Ear Nose Throat J* 1996;75:422–424.
154. Falconi M, Aristegui M, Landoffi M, et al.: Meningoencephalic herniation into the middle ear. *Acta Otorhinolaryngol Ital* 1995;15:305–311.
155. Gray BG, Willinsky RA, Rutka JA, et al.: Spontaneous meningocele, a rare middle ear mass. *AJNR* 1995;16:203–207.
156. Martin N, Sterkers D, Murat M, et al.: Brain herniation into the middle ear cavity: MR imaging. *Neuroradiol* 1989;31:184–186.

Chronic Otitis Media

157. Wright CG, Meyerhoff WL: Pathology of otitis media. *Ann Otol Laryngol* 1994;103:24–26.
158. Chao WY, Shen CL: Ultrastructure of the middle ear mucosa in patients with chronic otitis media with cholesteatoma. *Eur Arch Otorhinolaryngol* 1996;253:56–61.
159. Gaafar H, Maher A, Al-Ghazzawi E: Aural polypi: A histopathological and histochemical study. *ORL Otorhinolaryngol Relat Spec* 1982;44:108–115.
160. Ferlito A, Devaney KO, Rinaldo A, et al.: Ear cholesteatoma versus cholesterol granuloma. *Ann Otol Rhinol Laryngol* 1997;106:79–85.
161. Bhaya MH, Schachern PA, Morizono T: Pathogenesis of tympanosclerosis. *Otolaryngol Head Neck Surg* 1993;109:413–420.
162. Gantz BJ, Maynard J: Ultrastructural evaluation of biochemical events of bone resorption in human chronic otitis media. *Am J Otol* 1982;3:279–283.
163. Iurato B, Bux G, Colucci S, et al.: Histopathology of spontaneous brain herniation into the middle ear. *Acta Otolaryngol* 1992;112:328–333.
164. McGregor DH, Cherian R, Kepes JJ, et al.: Case reports: Heterotopic brain tissue of middle ear associated with cholesteatoma. *Am J Med Sci* 1994;308:180–183.

Cholesteatoma

165. Michaels L: Pathology of cholesteatoma: A review. *J Royal Soc Med* 1979;72:366–369.
166. Michaels L: *Ear, Nose and Throat Histopathology.* London: Springer-Verlag, 1987:47–51.
167. Kayhan FT, Mutlu C, Schachern PA, et al.: Significance of epidermoid formations in the middle ear in fetuses and children. *Arch Otolaryngol Head Neck Surg* 1997;123:1293–1297.
168. Levine JL, Wright CG, Powlowski KS, et al.: Postnatal persistence of epidermoid rests in the human middle ear. *Laryngoscope* 1998;108:70–73.
169. Swartz J: Cholesteatomas of the middle ear. Diagnosis, etiology, and complications. *Radiol Clin North Am* 1984;22:15–35.
170. Chole RA: Cellular and subcellular events of bone resorption in human and experimental cholesteatoma: The role of osteoclasts. *Laryngoscope* 1984;94:76–95.

Otitis Media in Adults

171. Ramages LJ, Gertler R: Aural tuberculosis: A series of 25 patients. *J Laryngol Otol* 1985;99:1073–1080.
172. Skolnik O, Nadol JB, Baker AS: Tuberculosis of the middle ear: Review of the literature with an instructive case report. *Rev Infect Dis* 1986;8:403–410.
173. Robertson K, Kumar A: Atypical presentations of aural tuberculosis. *Am J Otolaryngol* 1995;16:294–302.
174. Tyndel FJ, Davidson GS, Birman H, et al: Sarcoidosis of the middle ear. *Chest* 1994;105:182–183.
175. Shah UYK, White JA, Gooey JE, et al.: Otolaryngologic manifestation of sarcoidosis: Presentation and diagnosis. *Laryngoscope* 1997;107:67–75.
176. Quaranta A, Bartoli R, Resta L, et al.: Candida and stapedial otosclerosis: Histopathlogical findings. *ORL Otorhinolaryngol Relat Spec* 1992;54:334–336.
177. Schinella RA, Breda SD, Hammerschlag PE: Otic infection due to *Pneumocystis carinii* in an apparently healthy man with antibody to the human immunodeficiency virus. *Ann Intern Med* 1987;106:399–400.
178. Smith MA, Hirschfield L, Zahtz G, et al.: Pneumocystis carinii otitis media. *Am J Med* 1988;85:745–746.
179. Little JP, Gardner G, Acker JD, et al.: Otosyphilis in a patient with human immunodeficiency virus: Internal auditory canal gumma. *Otolaryngol Head Neck Surg* 1995;112:488–492.
180. Michaels L, Soucek S, Liang J: The ear in the acquired immunodeficiency syndrome: I. Temporal bone histopathologic study. *Am J Otol* 1994;15:515–522.
181. Davis LE, Rarey KE, McLaren LC: Clinical viral infections and temporal bone histologic studies of patients with AIDS. *Otolaryngol Head Neck Surg* 1995;113:695–701.
182. Soni NK, Hemani DD: Scleroma of the eustachian tube: Salpingoscleroma. *J Laryngol Otol* 1994;108:944–946.
183. Govender D, Naidoo K, Chetty R: Granuloma inguinale (Donovanosis). *Am J Clin Pathol* 1997;108:510–514.

Malakoplakia

184. Azadeh B, Ardehali S: Malakoplakia of middle ear: A case report. *Histopathol* 1983;7:129–134.

Myospherulosis

185. Kyriakos M: Myospherulosis of the paranasal sinuses, nose and middle ear. A possible iatrogenic disease. *Am J Clin Pathol* 1977;67:118–130.

186. Travis WD, Chin-Yang L, Weiland LH: Immunostaining for hemoglobin in two cases of myospherulosis. *Arch Pathol Lab Med* 1986; 110:763–765.

187. Corcoran ME, Chole RA, Sykes JM, et al.: Ointment granuloma complications after cosmetic and otologic surgery. *Otolaryngol Head Neck Surg* 1996;114:634–638.

Wegener's Granulomatosis

188. McCaffrey TV, McDonald TJ, Facer GW, et al.: Otologic manifestations of Wegener's granulomatosis. *Otolaryngol Head Neck Surg* 1980;88:586–593.

189. Kornblut AD, Wolff SM, deFries HO, et al.: Wegener's granulomatosis. *Otolaryngol Clin North Am* 1982;15:673–683.

190. McDonald TJ, DeRemee RA: Wegener's granulomatosis. *Laryngoscope* 1983;93:220–231.

191. Devaney KO, Travis WD, Hoffman G, et al.: Interpretation of head and neck biopsies in Wegener's granulomatosis. *Am J Surg Pathol* 1990;14:55–64.

192. Bajema IM, Hagen EC, van der Woude FJ, et al.: Wegener's granulomatosis: A meta-analysis of 349 literary case reports. *J Lab Clin Med* 1997;129:17–22.

193. Gaudin PB, Askin FB, Falk RJ, et al.: The pathologic spectrum of pulmonary lesions in patients with anti-neutrophil cytoplasmic autoantibodies specific for anti-protease 3 and anti-myeloperoxidase. *Am J Clin Pathol* 1995;104:7–16.

194. Hill JH, Graham MD, Gikas PW: Obliterative fibrotic middle ear disease in systemic vasculitis. *Ann Otol* 1980;89:162–164.

195. Allen NB, Bressler PB: Diagnosis and treatment of the systemic and cutaneous necrotizing vasculitis syndromes. *Med Clin North Am* 1997; 81:243–259.

Idiopathic Hypereosinophilic Syndrome

196. Takayama K, Yadohisa O, Furuno T, et al.: Case report: The first case of idiopathic hypereosinophilic syndrome involved with lung and middle ear. *Am J Med Sci* 1995;309:282–284.

Otosclerosis

197. Davis GL: Pathology of otosclerosis: A review. *Am J Otolaryngol* 1987;8:273–281.

198. Swartz J: Otosclerosis, diagnosis, and differential diagnosis. *Sem Ultrasound CT MR* 1989;10:251–261.

MIDDLE EAR NEOPLASMS

Squamous Cell Carcinoma

199. Michaels L, Wells M: Squamous cell carcinoma of the middle ear. *Clin Otolaryngol* 1980;5:235–248.

200. Kenyon GS, Marks PV, Scholtz CL, et al.: Squamous cell carcinoma of the middle ear. A 25 year retrospective study. *Ann Otol* 1985;94:273–277.

201. Woodson GE, Jurco S, Alford BR, McGavran MH: Verrucous carcinoma of the middle ear. *Arch Otolaryngol* 1981;107:63–65.

202. Edelstein DR, Smouha E, Sacks SH, et al.: Verrucous carcinoma of the temporal bone. *Ann Otol* 1986;95:447–453.

203. Morice W, Ferreiro JA: Distinction of basaloid squamous carcinoma from adenoid cystic and small cell undifferentiated carcinoma by immunohistochemistry. *Lab Invest* 1997;76:116A.

204. Wieneke JA, Thompson LDR, Wenig BM: Basaloid squamous cell carcinoma (BSCC) of the sinonasal tract. *Lab Invest* 1997;76:118A.

Inverted Papilloma

205. Wenig BM: Schneiderian-type mucosa papillomas of the middle ear and mastoid. *Ann Otol Rhinol Laryngol* 1996;105:226–233.

206. Raveh E, Feinmesser R, Shpitzer T, et al.: Inverted papilloma of the nose and paranasal sinuses: A study of 56 cases and review of the literature. *Isr J Med Sci* 1996;32:1163–1167.

207. Stone DM, Berktold RE, Ranganathan C, et al.: RJ: Inverted papilloma of the middle ear and mastoid. *Otolaryngol Head Neck Surg* 1987; 97:416–418.

208. Kaddour HS, Woodhead CJ: Transitional cell papilloma of the middle ear. *J Laryngol Otol* 1992;106:628–629.

209. Seshul MJ, Eby TL, Crowe DR, et al.: Nasal inverted papilloma with involvement of middle ear and mastoid. *Arch Otolaryngol Head Neck Surg* 1995;1045–1048.

210. Ingle R, Jennings TA, Goodman ML, et al.: CD44 expression in sinonasal inverted papillomas and associated squamous cell carcinoma. *Am J Clin Pathol* 1998;109:309–314.

211. Harris MO, Beck JC, Terrell JE, et al.: Expression of human papillomavirus 6 in inverted papilloma arising in a renal transplant recipient. *Laryngoscope* 1998;108:115–119.

212. Sarker FH, Visscher DW, Kintanar EB, et al.: Sinonasal schneiderian papillomas: Human papilloma virus typing by polymerase chain reaction. *Hum Pathol* 1992;5:329–409.

213. Jin Y-T, Tsai S-T, Li C, et al.: Prevalence of human papillomavirus in middle ear carcinoma associated with chronic otitis media. *Am J Pathol* 1997;150:1327–1333.

Paraganglioma

214. Lack EE: Tumors of the adrenal gland and extra-adrenal paraganglia. *Atlas of Tumor Pathology,* 3rd series, fascicle 19. Washington DC: Armed Forces Institute of Pathology, 1997:343–354, 395–409.

215. Farrior JB III, Hyams VJ, Benke RH, et al.: Carcinoid apudoma arising in a glomus jugulare tumor. Review of the endocrine activity in glomus jugulare tumors. *Laryngoscope* 1980;90:110–119.

216. Mandigers CM, van Gils AP, Derksen J, et al.: Carcinoid tumor of the jugulo-tympanic region. *J Nucl Med* 1996;37:270–272.

217. Spector GJ, Maisel RH, Ogura JH: Glomus tumors in the middle ear. I. Analysis of 46 patients. *Laryngoscope* 1973;83:162–171.

218. Chen KTK, Dehner LP: Primary tumors of the external and middle ear. II. A clinicopathologic study of 14 paragangliomas and three meningiomas. *Arch Otolaryngol* 1978;104:253–259.

219. Reddy EK, Mansfield CM, Hartmam GV: Chemodectoma of glomus jugulare. *Cancer* 1983;52:337–340.

220. Brown JS: Glomus jugulare tumors revisited. A ten year statistical follow-up of 231 cases. *Laryngoscope* 1985;95:284–248.

221. Watkins LD, Mendoza N, Cheesman AD, et al.: Glomus jugulare tumours: A review of 61 cases. *Acta Neurochir (Wien)* 1994;130:66–70.

222. Brammer RE, Graham MD, Kamink JL: Glomus tumors of the temporal bone: Contemporary evaluation and therapy. *Otol Clin North Am* 1984;17:499–513.

223. Spector GJ, Ciralsky R, Maisel RH, et al.: IV. Multiple glomus tumors in the head and neck. *Laryngoscope* 1975;85:1066–1075.

224. Busby DR: Glomus tympanicum tumor in infancy. *Arch Otol* 1974;99:377–378.

225. Yaniv E, Sade J: Glomus tympanicum in a child. *Int J Ped Otorhinolaryngol* 1983;5:93–97.

226. McCaffrey TV, Meyer FB, Michels VV, et al.: Familial paragangliomas of the head and neck. *Arch Otolaryngol Head Neck Surg* 1994;120:1211–1216.

227. Valavanis A, Shubiger O, Oguz M: High resolution CT investigation of nonchromaffin paragangliomas of the temporal bone. *AJNR* 1983;4:516–519.

228. Phelps PD, Lloyd GAS: Glomus tympanicum tumors: Demonstration by high resolution CT. *Clin Otolaryngol* 1983;8:15–20.

229. Swartz JD, Korsvik H: High-resolution computed tomography of the paragangliomas of the head and neck. *CT J Comp Tomogr* 1984;8:197–202.

230. Kau R, Arnold W: Somatostain receptor scintigraphy and therapy of neuroendocrine (APUD) tumors of the head and neck. *Acta Otolaryngol (Stockh)* 1996;116:345–349.

231. Elizade JM, Eizaguirre B, Florencio MR, et al.: Frozen section diagnosis in a jugulo-tympanic paraganglioma. *J Laryngol Otol* 1993;107:75–77.

232. Balli R, Dallari, Bergamini G, et al.: Avascular tympanojugular paraganglioma. *Laryngoscope* 1996;106:721–723.

233. Warren WH, Lee I, Gould VE, et al.: Paragangliomas of the head and neck: Ultrastructural and immunohistochemical analysis. *Ultrastruct Pathol* 1985;8:333–343.

234. Dayal VS, Lafond G, Van Nostrand AWP, et al.: Lesions simulating glomus tumors of the middle ear. *J Otolaryngol* 1983;12:175–179.

235. Rutka J, Hawke M: Cavernous hemangiomas of the incus (an incidental finding). *J Otolaryngol* 1989;18:94–95.

236. Mair IW, Roald B, Lilleas F, et al.: Cavernous hemangioma of the middle ear. *Am J Otol* 1994;15:254–256.

237. Manning SC, Culbertson MC, Vuitch F: Bilateral middle ear lobular capillary hemangiomas. *Otolaryngol Head Neck Surg* 1990;102:85–88.

238. Sutbeyez Y, Salimoglu E, Karrasen M, et al.: Haemangiopericytoma of the middle ear: Case report and literature review. *J Laryngol Otol* 1995;109:997–999.

239. Salama N, Stafford N: Meningiomas presenting in the middle ear. *Laryngoscope* 1982;92:92–97.

240. Hellier WPL, Crockard HA, Cheesman AD: Metastatic carcinoma of the temporal bone presenting as glomus jugulare and glomus tympanicum tumors: A description of two cases. *J Laryngol Otol* 1997;111:963–966.

241. Spector GJ, Maisel RH, Ogura JH: Glomus jugulare tumors: II. A clinicopathologic analysis of the effects of radiotherapy. *Ann Otol* 1974;83:26–32.

Glandular Neoplasms of the Middle Ear (Adenoma and Carcinoid Tumor)

242. Arnold B, Zeitz C, Muller-Hocker J, et al.: Adenoma of the middle ear mucosa. *Eur Arch Otorhinolaryngol* 1996;253:65–68.

243. Hyams VJ, Michaels L: Benign adenomatous neoplasm (adenoma) of the middle ear. *Clin Otolaryngol* 176;1:17–26.

244. Riches WG, Johnston WH: Primary adenomatous neoplasms of the middle ear. Light and electron microscopic features of a group distinct from the ceruminomas. *Am J Clin Pathol* 1982;77:153–161.

245. Jahrsdoerfer RA, Fechner RF, Moon CN Jr, et al.: Adenoma of the middle ear. *Laryngoscope* 1983;93:1041–1044.

246. Pallanch JF, McDonald TJ, Weiland LH, et al.: Adenocarcinoma and adenoma of the middle ear. *Laryngoscope* 1982;92:47–54.

247. Mills SE, Fechner RE: Middle ear adenoma. A cytologically uniform neoplasm displaying a variety of architectural patterns. *Am J Surg Pathol* 1984;8:677–685.

248. McNutt MA, Bolen JW: Adenomatous tumor of the middle ear. *Am J Clin Pathol* 1985;84:541–547.

249. Batsakis JG: Adenomatous tumors of the middle ear. *Ann Otol Rhinol Laryngol* 1990;98:749–752.

250. Hardingham M: Adenoma of the middle ear. *Arch Otolaryngol Head Neck Surg* 1995;121:342–344.

251. Murphy GF, Pilch BZ, Dickersin GR, et al.: Carcinoid tumor of the middle ear. *Am J Clin Pathol* 1980;73:816–823.

252. Inoue S, Tanaka K, Kannae S: Primary carcinoid tumor of the ear. *Virchows Arch* 1982;396:357–363.

253. Friedmann I, Galey FR, House WF, et al.: A mixed carcinoid tumor of the middle ear. *J Laryngol Otol* 1983;97:465–470.

254. Tange RA, Borden J, Schipper MEJ, et al.: A case of carcinoid tumor of the middle ear. *J Laryngol Otol* 1984;98:1021–1026.

255. Stanley MW, Horwitz CA, Levison RM, et al.: Carcinoid tumors of the middle ear. *Am J Clin Pathol* 1987;87:592–600.

256. Kambayashi J, Isidoya M, Urae T, et al.: A case of carcinoid tumor of the middle ear producing peptide hormones. *Auris Nasus Larynx* 1988;15:155–163.

257. Ruck P, Pfisterer EM, Kaiserling E: Carcinoid tumor of the middle ear. A morphological and immunohistochemical study with comments on histogenesis and differential diagnosis. *Pathol Pract* 1989;18:496–503.

258. Kodama H, Takezawa H, Suzuki T, et al.: Carcinoid of the middle ear. *J Laryngol Otol* 1989;103:86–91.

259. Krouse JH, Naldo KB Jr, Goodman ML: Carcinoid tumors of the middle ear. *Ann Otol Rhinol Laryngol* 1990;99:547–552.

260. Hale RJ, McMahon RF, Whittaler JS: Middle ear adenoma: Tumour of mixed mucinous and neuroendocrine differentiation. *J Clin Pathol* 1991;44:652–654.

261. Nyrop M, Guldhammerskov B, Katholm M, et al.: Carcinoid tumor of the middle ear. *Ear Nose Throat J* 1994;73:688–693.

262. Himi T, Saitoh H, Ohguro S, et al.: Carcinoid tumor of the middle ear. *Auris Nasus Larynx* 1995;22:128–133.

263. Azzoni C, Bonato M, D'Adda T, et al.: Well-differentiated tumours of the middle ear and of the hindgut have immunocytochemical and ultrastructural features in common. *Virchows Arch* 1995;426:411–418.

264. Ribe A, Fernandez PL, Ostertag H, et al.: Middle ear adenoma (MEA): A report of two cases, one with predominant "plasmacytoid" features. *Histopathology* 1997;30:359–364.

265. Soh KB, Tan HK, Sinniah R: Mucoepidermoid carcinoma of the middle ear: A case report. *J Laryngol Otol* 1996;110:249–251.

266. Cannon CR, McLean WC: Adenoid cystic carcinoma of the middle ear and temporal bone. *Otolaryngol Head Neck Surg* 1983;91:96–99.

Endolymphatic Sac Tumor (Low-Grade Adenocarcinoma, Aggressive Papillary Middle Ear Tumor)

267. Gaffey MJ, Mills SE, Fechner RE, et al.: Aggressive papillary middle ear tumor. A clinicopathologic entity distinct from middle-ear adenoma. *Am J Sur Pathol* 1988;12:790–797.

268. Benecke JE, Noel FL, Carberry JN, et al.: Adenomatous tumors of the middle ear and mastoid. *Am J Otol* 1990;11:20–26.

269. Cilluffo JM, Harner SG, Miller RH: Intracranial ceruminous gland adenocarcinoma. *J Neurosurg* 1981;55:952–956.

270. Pallanch JF, McDonald TJ, Weiland LH, et al.: Adenocarcinoma and adenoma of the middle ear. *Laryngoscope* 1982;92:47–54.

271. Schuller DE, Conley JJ, Goodman JH, et al.: Primary adenocarcinoma of the middle ear. *Otolaryngol Head Neck Surg* 1983;91:280–283.

272. Robson AK, Eveson JW, Smith IM, et al.: Papillary adenocarcinoma of the middle ear. *J Laryngol Otol* 1990;104:91–96.

273. Forrest AW, Turner JJ, Fagan: Aggressive papillary middle ear tumour. *J Laryngol Otol* 1991;105:950–953.

274. Morita M, Mori N, Takashima H, et al.: Primary poorly differentiated adenocarcinoma of the middle ear. *Auris Nasus Larynx* 1994;21:59–63.

275. Michaels L: *Ear, Nose and Throat Pathology.* London: Springer-Verlag, 1987:124.

276. Gussen R: Ménière's disease: New temporal bone findings in two cases. *Laryngoscope* 1971;81:1695–1707.

277. Schuknecht HF: *Pathology of the Ear.* Cambridge, MA: Harvard University Press, 1974:444.

278. Hassard AD, Boudreau SF, Cron CC: Adenoma of the endolymphatic sac. *J Otolaryngol* 1984;13:213–216.

279. Heffner DK: Low-grade adenocarcinoma of probable endolymphatic sac origin: A clinicopathologic study of 20 cases. *Cancer* 1990;64:292–302.

280. Batsakis JG, el-Naggar AK: Papillary neoplasms (Heffner's tumor) of the endolymphatic sac. *Ann Otol Rhinol Laryngol* 1993;102:648–651.

281. Lo WW, Applegate LJ, Carberry JH, et al.: Endolymphatic sac tumors: Radiologic appearance. *Radiology* 1993;189:199–204.

282. el-Naggar AK, Pflatz M, Ordonez NB, et al.: Tumors of the middle ear and endolymphatic sac. *Pathol Ann* 1994;29(Pt 2):199–231.

283. Poe DS, Tarlov EC, Thomas CB, et al.: Aggressive papillary tumors of temporal bone. *Otolaryngol Head Neck Surg* 1993;108:80–86.

284. Maher ER, Kaelin WG jr: von Hippel-Lindau Disease. *Medicine* 1997;76:381–391.

285. Los M, Jansen GH, Kaelin WG, et al.: Expression pattern of the von Hippel-Lindau protein in human tissues. *Lab Invest* 1997;75:231–238.

286. Gilcrease MZ, Schmidt L, Zbar B, et al: Somatic von Hippel-Lindau mutation in clear cell papillary cystadenoma of the epididymis. *Hum Pathol* 1995;26:1341–1346.

287. Corless CL, Kibel AS, Iliopoulos O, et al.: Immunostaining of the von Hippel-Lindau gene product in normal and neoplastic human tissues. *Hum Pathol* 1997;28:459–464.

288. Gaffey MJ, Mills SE, Boyd JC: Aggressive papillary tumor of middle ear/temporal bone and adnexal papillary cystadenoma. Manifestations of von Hippel-Lindau disease. *Am J Surg Pathol* 1994;18:1254–1260.

289. Megerian CA, McKenna MJ, Nuss RC, et al.: Endolymphatic sac tumors: Histologic confirmation, clinical characterization, and implication in von Hippel-Lindau disease. *Laryngoscope* 1995;105:801–808.

290. Castleman B, McNeely BU: Case records of the Massachusetts General Hospital. Weekly clinicopathological exercises. Case 47-1966. *N Engl J Med* 1966;275:950–959.

291. Schuknecht H: *Pathology of the Ear.* Cambridge, MA: Harvard University Press, 1974:443.

292. Lavoie M, Mornecy RM: Low-grade papillary adenomatous tumors of the temporal bone: Report of two cases and review of the literature. *Mod Pathol* 1995;8:603–608.

293. Pollak A, Bohmer A, Spycher M, et al.: Are papillary adenomas endolymphatic sac tumors? *Ann Otol Rhinol Laryngol* 1996;104:613–619.

294. Pollak A; In reply: Lavoie, Morency RM: Correspondence RE: Lavoie M, et al: Low-grade papillary adenomatous tumors of the temporal bone: Report of two cases and review of the literature. *Mod Pathol* 1996;9:460–461.

295. Schick B, Kahle G, Kronsbein H, et al.: Papillary tumor of the endolymphatic sac. *HNO* 1996;44:329–332.

296. Wenig BM, Heffner DK: Endolymphatic sac tumors: Fact or fiction? *Adv Anat Pathol* 1996;3:378–387.

297. Roche P-H, Dufour H, Figarella-Branger D, et al.: Endolymphatic sac tumors: Report of three cases. *J Neurosurg* 1998;88:927–932.

298. Ho VT, Rao VM, Doan HT, et al.: Low-grade adenocarcinoma of probable endolymphatic sac origin: CT and MR appearance. *AJNR* 1996; 17:168–170.

299. Kemperman G, Neumann HP, Scheremet R, et al.: Deafness due to bilateral endolymphatic sac tumours in a case of von-Hippel Lindau syndrome. *J Neurol Neurosurg Psychiatry* 1996;61:318–320.

300. Rouquette I, Delisle M-B, Cervera P, et al.: Adenocarcinome papillaire avec etude immunohisto-chimique. *Ann Pathol* 1996;16: 271–275.

301. Feghali JG, Levin RJ, Llena J, et al.: Aggressive papillary tumors of the endolymphatic sac: Clinical and tissue culture characteristics. *Am J Otol* 1995;16:778–782.

302. Levin RJ, Feghali JG, Morgenstern N, et al.: Aggressive papillary tumors of the temporal bone: An immunohistochemical analysis in tissue culture. *Laryngoscope* 1996;106:144–147.

303. Buie HT, Linthicum FH Jr, Hofman FM, et al.: An immunohistochemical study of the endolymphatic sac in patients with acoustic neuromas. *Laryngoscope* 1989;99:775–778.

304. Altermatt HJ, Gebbers J-O, Arnold W, et al.: The epithelium of the human endolymphatic sac: Immunohistochemical characterization. *ORL Otorhinolaryngol Relat Spec* 1990;52:113–120.

305. Megerian CA, Pilch BX, Bhan AK, et al.: Differential expression of transthyretin in papillary tumors of the endolymphatic sac and choroid plexus. *Laryngoscope* 1997;107:216–221.

306. Vortmeyer AO, Gnarra JR, Emmert-Buck MR, et al.: von Hippel-Lindau gene deletion detected in the stromal cell component of a cerebellar hemangioblastoma associated with von Hippel-Lindau disease. *Hum Pathol* 1997;28:540–543.

307. Vortmeyer AO, Choo D, Pack SD, et al.: Von Hippel-Lindau disease gene alterations associated with endolymphatic sac tumor. *J Nat Cancer Inst* 1997;89:970–972.

308. Mukherji SK, Castillo M: Adenocarcinoma of the endolymphatic sac: Imaging features and preoperative embolization. *Neuroradiology* 1996;38:179–180.

309. Manski TJ, Heffner DK, Glenn GM, et al.: Endolymphatic sac tumors. A source of morbid hearing loss in von Hippel-Lindau's disease. *JAMA* 1997;277:1461–1466.

Rhabdomyosarcoma

310. Wiener ES: Head and neck rhabdomyosarcoma. *Sem Pediatr Surg* 1994;3:203–206.

311. Dehner LP, Chen KT: Primary tumors of the external and middle ear. III. A clinicopathologic study of embryonal rhabdomyosarcoma. *Arch Otolaryngol* 1978;104:399–403.

312. Bale PM, Parsons RE, Stevens MM: Pathology and behavior of juvenile rhabdomyosarcoma. In: Bennington JL, ed. *Pathology of Neoplasms in Children and Adolescents.* Philadelphia: W.B. Saunders, 1986;196–222.

313. Nakleh RE, Swanson PE, Dehner LP: Juvenile (embryonal and alveolar) rhabdomyosarcoma of the head and neck. A clinical, pathologic, and immunohisto- chemical study of 12 cases. *Cancer* 1991;67:1019–1024.

314. Fukunaga M, Miyazawa Y, Harada T, et al.: Yolk sac tumor of the ear. *Histopathology* 1995;27:563–567.

315. Devaney KO, Ferlito A: Yolk sac tumors (endodermal sinus tumors) of the extracranial head and neck regions. *Ann Otol Rhinol Laryngol* 1997;106:254–260.

316. Triche TJ, Askin FB: Neuroblastoma and the differential diagnosis of small, round, blue cell tumors. *Hum Pathol* 1983;14:569–595.

317. Sessions DG, Ragab AH, Vieti TJ, et al.: Embryonal rhabdomyosarcoma of the head and neck in children. *Laryngoscope* 1973;83:890–897.

318. Sutow WW, Lindberg RD, Gehan EA, et al.: Three-year relapse-free survival rates in childhood rhabdomyosarcoma of the head and neck. Report from the Intergroup Rhabdomyosarcoma Study. *Cancer* 1982; 49:2217–2221.

319. Raney RB Jr, Lawrence W Jr, Maurer HM, et al.: Rhabdomyosarcoma of the ear in childhood. A report from the Intergroup Rhabdomyosarcoma Study-I. *Cancer* 1983;51:2356–2361.

320. Wiatrak BJ, Persak ML: Rhabdomyosarcoma of the ear and temporal bone. *Laryngoscope* 1989;99:1188–1192.

321. Flamant F, Rodary C, Rey A, et al.: Treatment of non-metastatic rhabdomyosarcomas in childhood and adolescence. Results of the International Society of Paediatric Oncology: MMT84. *Eur J Cancer* 1998; 34:1050–1067.

Metastastic Tumors

322. Nelson EG, Hinojosa R: Histopathology of metastatic temporal bone tumors. *Arch Otolaryngol Head Neck Surg* 1991;117:189–193.

323. Batsakis JG, McBurney TA: Metastatic neoplasms to the head and neck. *SGO* 1971;133:673–677.

324. Merrick Y: Metastatic colon adencarcinoma of the middle ear. *Arch Otorhinolaryngol* 1983;238:103–105.

325. Sahin AA, Ro JY, Ordonez NG, et al.: Temporal bone involvement by prostatic adenocarcinoma: Report of two cases and review of the literature. *Head Neck* 1991;134:349–354.

Malignant Melanoma

326. McKenna WEL, Holmes WF, Harwick R: Primary melanoma of the middle ear. *Laryngoscope* 1984;94:1459–1460.

327. Sherman IW, Swift AC, Haqqami MT: Primary mucosal malignant melanoma of the middle ear. *J Laryngol Otol* 1991;105:1061–1064.

328. Davis GL: Malignant melanoma arising in mature ovarian cystic teratoma (dermoid cyst). Report of two cases and literature analysis. *Int J Gynecol Pathol* 1996;15:356–362.

Other Neoplasms

329. Zbaren P: Leiomyosarcoma of the middle ear and temporal bone. *Ann Otol Rhinol Laryngol* 1994;103:537–541.

330. Singh PK, Singh RL, Agerwal A, et al.: Fibrosarcoma of the middle ear [letter]. *Ear Nose Throat J* 1989;68:479–480.

331. O'Keefe LJ, Ramesden RT, Berzgales AR: Primary synovial sarcoma of the middle ear. *J Laryngol Otol* 1993;107:1070–1072.

332. Landiloris DC, Nikolopoulos TP, Feredikis EA, et al.: Primary extramedullary plasmacytoma in the middle ear: Differential diagnosis and management. *J Laryngol Otol* 1994;108:868–870.

333. Panosian MS, Roberts JK: Plasmocytoma of the middle ear and mastoid. *Am J Otol* 1994;15:264–267.

334. Solanellas J, Esteban F, Soldado L, et al.: Hodgkin's disease of the middle ear and mastoid. *J Laryngol Otol* 1996;110:869–871.

335. Kobayashi K, Igarashji M, McBride RA, et al.: Temporal bone pathology of metastatic T-cell lymphoma. *Acta Otolaryngologica (Stockh)* 1988;Suppl 447:113–119.

336. LeMay DR, Sun JK, Mendel E, et al.: Chondromyxoid fibroma of the temporal bone. *Surg Neurol* 1997;48:148–152.

337. Harvey SA, Wiet RJ, Kazan R: Chondrosarcoma of the jugular foramen. *Am J Otol* 1994;15:257–263.

338. Kletzker GR, Smith PG, McIntire LD, et al.: Presentation and management of uncommon lesions of the middle ear. *Am J Otol* 1995;16:634–642.

Langerhans' Cell Granulomatosis

339. Hammar S, Bockus D, Remington F, et al.: The wide spread distribution of Langerhans cells in pathologic tissues: An ultrastructural and immunohistochemical study. *Hum Pathol* 1986;17:894–905.

340. Lieberman PH, Jones CR, Steinman RM, et al.: Langerhans cell (eosinophilic) granulomatosis. *Am J Surg Pathol* 1996;20:519–552.

341. Ladisch S, Gadner H, Elinder G: Langerhans cell granulomatosis [letter to the editor]. *Am J Surg Pathol* 1997;21:1523.

342. Lieberman PH: Langerhans cell granulomatosis [author's reply]. *Am J Surg Pathol* 1997;21:1523–1524.

343. Willman CL, Busque L, Griffith BB, et al: Langerhans'-cell histiocytosis (histiocytosis X): a clonal proliferative disease. *N Engl J Med* 1994;331:154–160.

344. Angeli SI, Luxford WM, Lo WWM: Magnetic resonance imaging in the evolution of Langerhans' cell histiocytosis of the temporal bone: Case report. *Otolaryngol Head Neck Surg* 1996;114:120–124.

345. Emile J-F, Wechsler J, Brousse N, et al.: Langerhans' cell histiocytosis. Definitive diagnosis with the use of monoclonal antibody O10 on routinely paraffin-embedded samples. *Am J Surg Pathol* 1995; 19:636–641.

346. Alessi DM: Histiocytosis X of the head and neck in a pediatric population. *Arch Otolaryngol Head Neck Surg* 1992;118:945–948.

INNER EAR

Internal Auditory Canal and Cerebellopontine Angle Tumors

347. National Institutes of Health Consensus Development Conference. Neurofibromatosis Conference Statement. *Arch Neurol* 1988;45:575–578.

348. Wellenreuther R, Waha A, Vogel Y, et al.: Quantitative analysis of neurofibromatosis type 2 gene transcripts in meningiomas supports the concept of distinct molecular variants. *Lab Invest* 1997;77:601–606.

349. Welling DB: Clinical manifestations of mutations in the neurofibromatosis type 2 gene in vestibular Schwannomas (acoustic neuromas). *Laryngoscope* 1998;108:178–189.

350. Irving RM: The molecular pathology of tumours of the ear and temporal bone. *J Laryngol Otol* 1998;112:1011–1018.

351. Burger PC, Scheithauer BW: Dysgenetic disorders: Tumors of the central nervous system. In: *Atlas of Tumor Pathology,* 3rd series, fascicle 10. Washington, DC: Armed Forces Institute of Pathology, 1994:379–390.

352. Lin BT-Y, Weiss LM, Medeiros LJ: Neurofibroma and cellular neurofibroma with atypia. *Am J Surg Pathol* 1997;21:1443–1449.

353. Ordonez NG, Tornos C: Malignant peripheral nerve sheath tumor of the pleura with epithelial and rhabdomyoblastic differentiation. *Am J Surg Pathol* 1997;21:1515–1521.

354. Bhatt S, Graeme-Cook F, Joseph MP, et al.: Malignant triton tumor of the head and neck. *Otolaryngol Head Neck Surg* 1991;105:738–742.

355. Heffner DK, Gnepp DR: Sinonasal fibrosarcomas, malignant schwannomas and "triton" tumors. *Cancer* 1992;70:1089–1101.

356. Best PV: Malignant triton tumour in the cerebellopontine angle: Report of a case. *Acta Neuropathol* 1987;74:92–96.

357. Han DH, Kim DG, Chi JG, et al.: Malignant triton tumor of the acoustic nerve. *J Neurosurg* 1992;76:874–877.

358. Hirose T, Scheithauer BW, et al.: Giant plexiform schwannoma: A report of two cases with soft tissue and visceral involvement. *Mod Pathol* 1997;10:1075–1081.

359. Lewis WB, Mattucci KF, Smilari T: Schwannoma of the external auditory canal: An unusual finding. *Int Surg* 1995;80:287–290.

360. Kuo TC, Jackler RE, Wong K, et al.: Are acoustic neuromas encapsulated tumors? *Otolaryngol Head Neck Surg* 1997;117:606–609.

361. Shelton C: Unilateral acoustic tumors: How often do they recur after translabyrinthine removal? *Laryngoscope* 1995;105(9 Pt 1):958–966.

362. Irving RM, Jackler RK, Pitts LH: Hearing preservation in patients undergoing vestibular schwannoma surgery: Comparison of middle fossa and retrosigmoid approaches. *J Neurosurg* 1998;88:840–845.

363. Kondziolka D, Lunsford LD, McLaughlin MR, et al.: Long-term outcomes after radiosurgery for acoustic neuromas. *N Engl J Med* 1998;339:1426–1433.

364. Zeitouni AG, Zagzag D, Cohen NL: Meningioma of the internal auditory canal. *Ann Otol Rhinol Laryngol* 1997;106:657–660.

365. Friedman RA, Nelson RA, Harris JP: Posterior fossa meningiomas intimately involved with the endolymphatic sac. *Am J Otol* 1996;17:612–616.

366. Hu B, Pant M, Cornford M, et al.: Association of primary intracranial meningioma and cutaneous meningioma of external auditory canal. *Arch Pathol Lab Med* 1998;122:97–99.

367. Christensen WN, Lang DM, Epstein J: Cerebellopontine angle lipoma. *Hum Pathol* 1986;17:739–743.

368. Singh SP, Cottingham SL, Slone W, et al.: Lipomas of the internal auditory canal. *Arch Pathol Lab Med* 1996;120:681–683.

369. Greinwald JH Jr, Lassen LF: Lipomas of the internal auditory canal. *Laryngoscope* 1997;107:364–368.

370. Murakami S, Yanagihara N, Takahashi H, et al.: Angiolipoma of internal auditory canal presenting repeated sudden hearing loss. *Otolaryngol Head Neck Surg* 1997;117:S80–S84.

371. Marie B, Baylac F, Coffinet L, et al.: Lipomes du conduit auditif interne. *Ann Pathol* 1998;18:52–54.

372. Angeli SI, Brackmann DE, Xenellis JE, et al.: Primary lymphoma of the internal auditory canal. *Ann Otol Rhinol Laryngol* 1998;107:17–21.

373. Omojola MF, al Hawashim NS, Zuwayed MA, et al.: CT and MRI features of cavernous haemangioma of internal auditory canal. *Br J Radiol* 1997;70:1184–1187.

Endolymphatic Sac—Meniere's Disease

374. Merchant SN, Rauach SD, Nadol JB Jr: Meniere's disease. *Eur Arch Otorhinoloaryngol* 1995;252:63–75.

375. Michaels L: Meniere's disease: Pathology of the vestibular system; presbycusis. In: Ear, Nose, and Throat Pathology. London: Springer-Verlag, 1987:102–112.

376. Danckwardt-Lilliestrom N, Rask-Andersen H, Linthicum FH, et al.: A technique to obtain and process surgical specimens of the human vestibular aqueduct for histopathologic studies of the endolymphatic duct and sac. *ORL Otorhinolaryngol Relat Spec* 1992;54:215–219.

377. Danckwardt-Lilliestrom N, Friberg U, Kennifors A, et al.: "Endolymphatic sacitis" in a case of active Meniere's disease. An ultrastructural histopathologic investigation. *Ann Otol Rhinol Laryngol* 1997;106:190–198.

12 Hematopoietic Lesions

Daniel A. Arber and L. Jeffrey Medeiros

BENIGN LESIONS

Histologic Patterns

Benign reaction patterns in lymph nodes can generally be divided into two groups: lymphadenitis and lymphoid hyperplasia. Lymphadenitis is usually caused by an infectious agent. However, there are other diseases that may cause extensive necrosis and can be classified as lymphadenitis, such as systemic lupus erythematosus or Kikuchi-Fujimoto disease. By contrast, lymphoid hyperplasia is a response to antigenic stimulation without actual lymph node infection. There are three general patterns of reactive lymphoid hyperplasia, although many diseases cause a mixture of these patterns: follicular hyperplasia, paracortical hyperplasia, and sinus histiocytosis.[1] Granulomatous disorders do not readily fit within this conceptual framework.

Follicular Hyperplasia

Follicular hyperplasia is the result of preferential stimulation of the B cell compartments of the lymph node. Histologically, there is marked enlargement of the lymphoid follicles, most of which are situated in the lymph node cortex. The follicles consist of reactive germinal centers surrounded by well-defined mantle zones. The germinal centers are composed of a mixture of small cleaved, large cleaved, small noncleaved, and large noncleaved lymphoid cells, histiocytes with tingible body macrophages, and follicular dendritic reticulum cells. Typically, the germinal centers exhibit polarization; at one pole many small noncleaved and large noncleaved cells are present with a relatively high nuclear: cytoplasmic ratio and, at the other pole, many large cleaved and small cleaved cells are present with a much lower nuclear: cytoplasmic ratio. At low power, this cellular distribution results in one pole staining darker (more blue) than the other when hematoxylin-eosin staining is used. The surrounding mantle zones are composed of small round lymphoid cells with condensed chromatin and minimal cytoplasm.

In reactive follicular hyperplasia, the follicles can become very large with bizarre shapes. Nevertheless, the follicles are situated predominantly in the cortex, are not back-to-back, and do not replace normal architecture. In contrast, in follicular lymphoma, the total number of follicles is greatly increased and the neoplastic follicles efface the normal architecture of both the cortex and the medulla.

Paracortical Hyperplasia

Paracortical hyperplasia is the result of preferential stimulation of the T-cell compartments. Histologically, the paracortical zones of the lymph node are greatly expanded and these regions have a "moth-eaten" or "starry-sky" appearance. This appearance results from the presence of histiocytes with tingible body macrophages in a sea of numerous small round lymphocytes and occasional interdigitating reticulum cells. As in all forms of hyperplasia, the normal architecture is not effaced nor do the lymphoid cells exhibit cytologic atypia.

Sinus Histiocytosis

Sinus histiocytosis is the result of preferential stimulation of sinus histiocytes. Histologically, the sinuses of the lymph node are widely distended by numerous cytologically normal histiocytes or macrophages. Lymph nodes draining the sites of malignant neoplasms or prostheses commonly exhibit sinus histiocytosis.

Progressive Transformation of Germinal Centers

Progressive transformation of germinal centers (PTGC) is a histologically distinctive form of follicular hyperplasia that is usually accompanied by typical follicular hyperplasia.[2, 3] There is no known specific etiology for PTGC.

Clinical Features. Patients with PTGC may be of all ages, although there is a predilection for children and adolescents. Males are more frequently affected.[3] Most patients present with a single enlarged lymph node without other symptoms. PTGC may be found in patients with nodular lymphocytic predominance Hodgkin's disease and initially was thought to occur with increased frequency in patients with this type of Hodgkin's disease, but closer scrutiny has not supported this view.[2, 3]

Pathologic Features. Histologically, lymph nodes involved by PTGC are recognized by the presence of large lymphoid follicles, up to four to five times normal size (Fig. 12–1, see p. 727).[2, 3] Closer inspection reveals that the large follicles represent the coalescence of two or more reactive lymphoid follicles. As the reaction pattern evolves, the separate secondary germinal centers appear to fuse into one large germinal center, and then begin to fragment as small lymphocytes infiltrate into the germinal centers (see Fig. 12–1). The latter stages of this process resemble follicle lysis, as originally described in benign lymph nodes infected with human immunodeficiency virus, with the exception being that there is usually little hemorrhage in PTGC. In the late stages of PTGC, the large follicles are devoid of germinal centers with few large lymphoid cells.

Immunohistochemical studies have shown that destruction of follicular dendritic reticulum cells is important in the pathogenesis of PTGC. In its early stages, the follicles are composed of germinal centers surrounded by mantle zone cells with an expanded and organized network of follicular dendritic reticulum cells. Later, the follicular dendritic reticulum cells are disrupted in the areas where small lymphoid cells infiltrate into the germinal centers.[2, 3]

Differential Diagnosis. The importance of PTGC lies in the recognition of this unusual reaction pattern and in distinguishing it from nodular lymphocytic predominance Hodgkin's disease. In the latter disease, numerous large, multilobated cells are present and the nodules fuse to replace normal architecture.

Treatment and Prognosis. There is no specific therapy for PTGC. These lesions usually resolve once the causative antigenic stimulation subsides.

Toxoplasma Lymphadenitis

Toxoplasma lymphadenitis is caused by infection with *Toxoplasma* species, usually *Toxoplasma gondii,* which humans are exposed to via contact with infected animal feces.

Clinical Features. Patients with *Toxoplasma* lymphadenitis most commonly present with one or a single group of enlarged lymph nodes, most commonly in the posterior cervical region. However, a subset of patients develop fever and generalized lymphadenopathy.[4, 5]

Pathologic Features. Histologically, *Toxoplasma* lymphadenitis can be reliably recognized if a triad of three histologic findings is identified: florid reactive follicular hyperplasia, clusters of epithelioid histiocytes found within the germinal centers of reactive lymphoid follicles, and a monocytoid B-cell reaction in the sinuses (Fig. 12–2, see p. 728).[4, 5] If all three findings are present, serologic studies are usually positive for Toxoplasma antibodies.[5] Toxoplasma cysts or intracellular trophozoites are rarely found in lymph node biopsy specimens.

Differential Diagnosis. A variety of other infectious disorders may cause histologic changes similar to Toxoplasma lymphadenitis. Most commonly, these disorders cause an extensive monocytoid B-cell reaction and reactive follicular hyperplasia.[6] Therefore, the presence of epithelioid histiocytes within the germinal centers of follicles is the most specific finding of the triad. Rarely, infections other than toxoplasmosis, such as human immunodeficiency virus (HIV) infection and leishmaniasis may cause reactive follicular hyperplasia, a sinusoidal monocytoid B-cell reaction, and the presence of paracortical epithelioid granulomas that can also be found in germinal centers.[6] Usually the granulomas are associated with necrosis and acute inflammatory cells. Granulomas and necrosis are not usual features of Toxoplasma lymphadenitis.

Although histologic findings can be very helpful in suggesting the presence of toxoplasmosis, serologic studies should be routinely recommended to definitively establish the diagnosis.

Treatment and Prognosis. The infection is usually self-limited in immunocompetent adults and older children, and no specific therapy is required. Immunodeficient patients require antibiotic therapy directed against the parasite.

Myoepithelial Sialadenitis, or Benign Lymphoepithelial Lesion

Clinical Features. Mikulicz's syndrome is defined as diffuse and bilateral enlargement of the salivary and lacrimal glands. A number of diseases may result in Mikulicz's syndrome, such as sarcoidosis, tuberculosis, and malignant lymphoma, but the most common cause is myoepithelial sialadenitis (MESA), also commonly referred to as benign lymphoepithelial lesion (BLEL), which is an autoimmune phenomenon. The term *Mikulicz's disease* has also been used as a synonym for MESA/BLEL.

The most common cause of MESA/BLEL is Sjögren's syndrome, but there are other causes, such as HIV infection.[7] Sjögren's syndrome is a systemic autoimmune disorder that causes Mikulicz's syndrome, keratoconjunctivitis, xerostomia, rheumatoid arthritis, and hypergammaglobulinemia.[7]

Pathologic Features. MESA/BLEL involving the major salivary glands is histologically characterized by two components: epimyoepithelial islands and extensive lymphoid infiltration (Fig. 12–3, see p. 729).[7] In the minor salivary glands, the changes are similar, although epimyoepithelial islands may be small or absent.

Epimyoepithelial islands are nests of epithelial cells that are extensively infiltrated by small lymphoid cells. Often abundant hyaline material accompanies the epithelial cells, which ultrastructurally has been proven to be basal lamina material. These findings indicate that epimyoepithelial islands originate as ducts that subsequently collapse. The ductal epithelium is infiltrated by small lymphoid cells of two types: small round and unremarkable lymphocytes and slightly larger lymphoid cells with mildly irregular nuclear contours and moderate pale or clear cytoplasm (see Fig. 12–3). Immunohistochemical studies have shown that the slightly irregular cells with clear or pale cytoplasm are predominantly B cells and the small round cells are T cells.

The lymphoid infiltrate progressively replaces the acinar tissue, resulting in atrophy. This infiltrate is composed of large reactive lymphoid follicles with secondary germinal centers and intervening areas of small lymphocytes and histiocytes. The lymphoid follicles are composed of polytypic B cells. The small lymphocytes surrounding and between the follicles are composed of normal T cells.

The MESA/BLEL condition and closely related lymphoepithelial cysts can occur in HIV-positive patients. Excluding the cystic component, the histologic findings in lymphoepithelial cysts are similar to those in MESA/BLEL.[8, 9] HIV has been identified within the follicular dendritic cells of these lesions.[9]

Treatment and Prognosis. Patients with MESA/BLEL as a result of Sjögren's syndrome have an incurable disease. There is no specific treatment, and the therapies used are designed to alleviate symptoms.

Patients with MESA/BLEL are at increased risk of developing non-Hodgkin's lymphoma, usually of B-cell lineage. The risk of malignant lymphoma in patients with MESA/BLEL and Sjögren's syndrome has been estimated to be 43.8 times that of the general population.[10, 11] B-cell non-Hodgkin's lymphomas can be generally divided into two groups: low-grade and high-grade. Rare cases of Hodgkin's disease and T-cell lymphoma also have been described, but the risk of these tumors in MESA/BLEL is significantly less than that of B-cell lymphomas.[10, 11]

Historically, high-grade B-cell non-Hodgkin's lymphomas arising in MESA/BLEL were the first to be recognized.[12] For example, in one study, 10 of 136 patients (7.4%) with Sjögren's syndrome developed non-Hodgkin's lymphoma.[13] Histologically, seven tumors were diffuse large cell or large cell immunoblastic lymphomas and three were cases of Waldenstrom's macroglobulinemia. Immunohistochemical studies, restricted at that time to polyclonal Ig light chain antibodies and fixed, paraffin-embedded sections, demonstrated monotypic Ig light chain and B-cell lineage in four tumors.

The increased risk of low-grade B-cell non-Hodgkin's lymphomas was recognized later, with the widespread availability of numerous antibodies, fresh frozen material, and improved immunohistochemical and molecular methods.[11, 13] Although the risk of low-grade B-cell lymphoma in MESA/BLEL is not well quantified, the risk is in addition to that of high-grade B-cell lymphoma.

The majority of low-grade B-cell lymphomas that arise in the setting of MESA/BLEL are lymphomas of mucosa-associated lymphoid tissue (MALT).[11] These tumors have been renamed *marginal zone B-cell lymphoma* in the Revised European-American Classification of Lymphoid Neoplasms (REAL) (discussed later).

The distinction between benign MESA/BLEL and low-grade B-cell MALT-lymphoma can be very difficult. In general, the larger the infiltrate, the greater the likelihood of lymphoma. However, this distinction may not possible without immunohistochemical studies in some cases and, in these lesions, most pathologists agree that low-grade B-cell lymphoma is present if a monotypic B-cell population can be detected.[11, 14] Since molecular methods used to detect Ig gene rearrangements are much more sensitive, particularly when using polymerase chain reaction–based methods, small monoclonal B-cell populations may be present in lesions that histologically and immunohistochemically meet the criteria for benign MESA/BLEL.[14] In this circumstance, we report the molecular finding and discuss its implications but do not unequivocally establish the diagnosis of lymphoma.

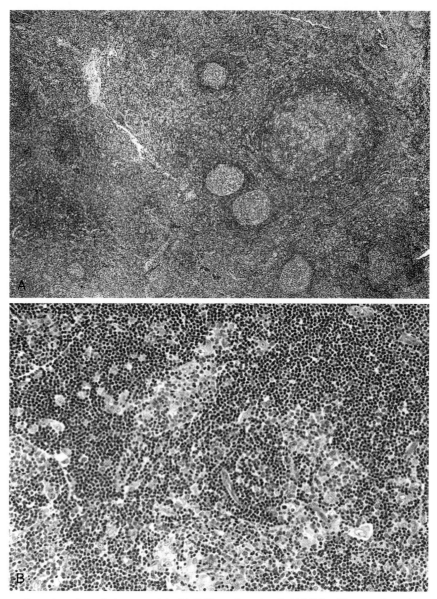

Figure 12–1. Progressive transformation of germinal centers. A, In this field, one large lymphoid follicle with a transformed germinal center (right) and four nearby normal follicles with reactive follicular hyperplasia are present. B, Transformed germinal centers have a mottled appearance, the pale cells being larger germinal center cells and the dark zones being small lymphocytes that infiltrate into the germinal center.

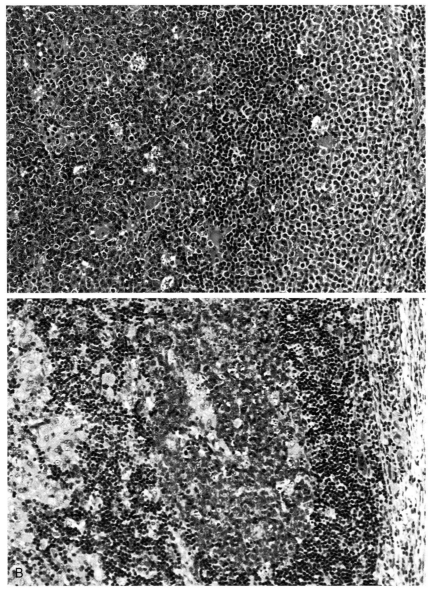

Figure 12–2. Toxoplasma lymphadenitis. *A,* In this field, a sinusoidal monocytoid B-cell reaction (right) and reactive follicular hyperplasia (left) are present. *B,* In this field, clusters of epithelioid histiocytes infiltrate into a hyperplastic lymphoid follicle.

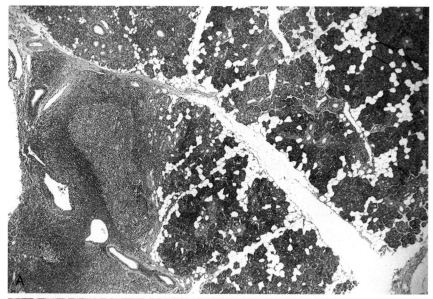

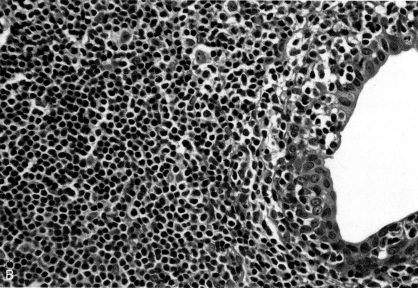

Figure 12–3. Myoepithelial sialadenitis/benign lymphoepithelial lesion. Immunohistochemical studies in this case revealed polytypic immunoglobulin light chain expression; polymerase chain reaction for immunoglobulin heavy chain gene rearrangements was negative. A, At low power, aggregates of lymphoid tissue surround parotid gland ducts. The lymphoid tissue is composed of reactive lymphoid follicles with follicular hyperplasia, T cells, and small lymphoid cells with pale cytoplasm immediately surrounding the ducts. B, The small lymphoid cells with pale cytoplasm infiltrate duct epithelium, forming lymphoepithelial lesions (right).

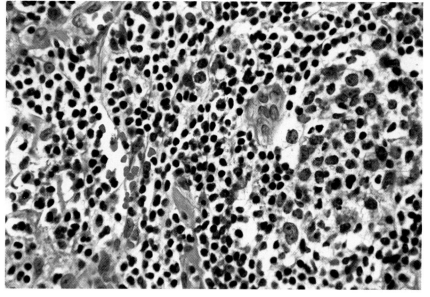

Figure 12–4. Kimura's disease showing a reactive follicle with interfollicular small vessels and eosinophils.

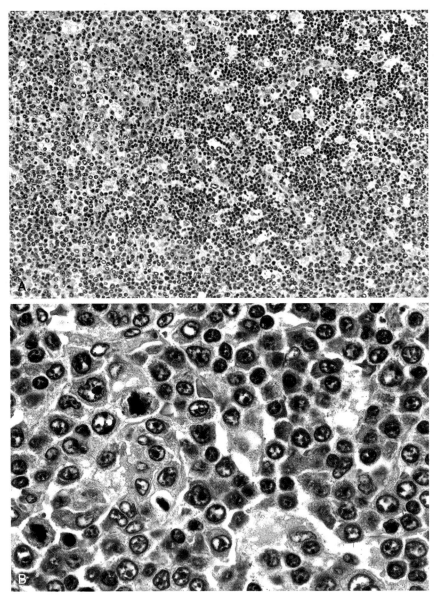

Figure 12–5. Infectious mononucleosis. *A,* At low power, the lymph node architecture is almost completely replaced. The darker nodule (right center) is the remnant of a lymphoid follicle. *B,* At high power, a range of cell types is present, including small lymphocytes, plasmacytoid lymphocytes, plasma cells, histiocytes, and immunoblasts.

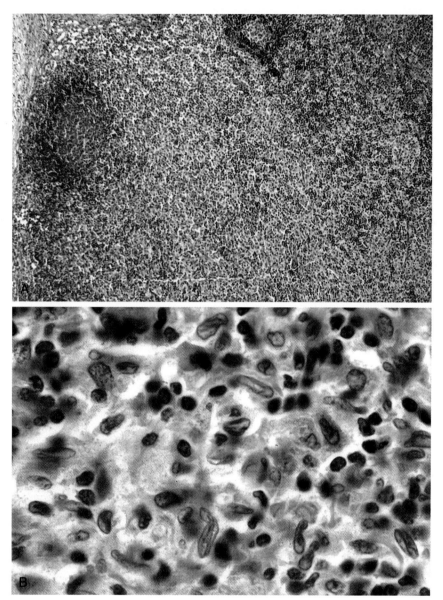

Figure 12–6. Dermatopathic lymphadenopathy. *A,* At low power the paracortical regions are expanded and are pale. *B,* Small lymphocytes are relatively decreased, and numerous interdigitating reticulum cells with twisted nuclei and linear grooves are present. Some histiocytes contain melanin pigment (right center).

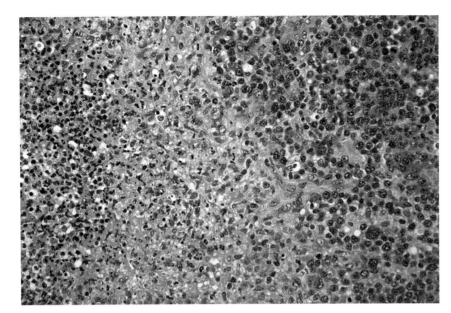

Figure 12–7. Cat scratch disease showing a zone of neutrophil-containing necrosis (left) surrounded by histiocytes and fibroblasts.

Figure 12–8. Lymph node from patient with human immunodeficiency virus and *Mycobacterium avium-intracellulare* infection. The lymph node is completely depleted of lymphocytes, and numerous histiocytes are present.

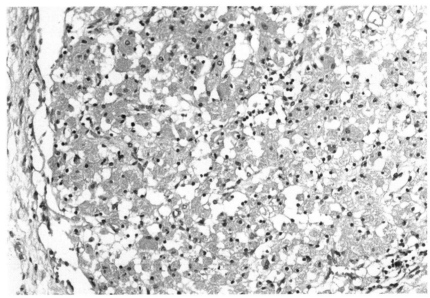

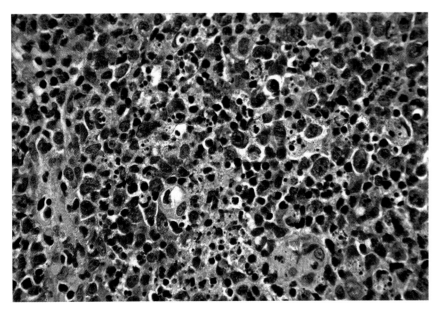

Figure 12–9. Kikuchi-Fujimoto disease showing a mixture of cells, including immunoblasts and histiocytes. There are characteristic foci of karyorrhexis without neutrophils.

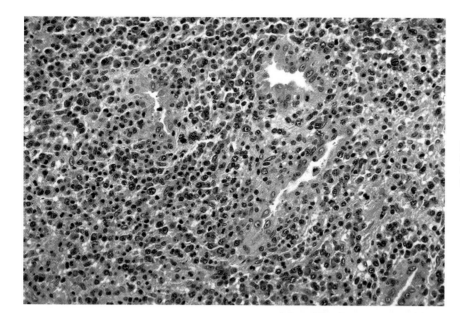

Figure 12–12. Angiolymphoid hyperplasia with eosinophilia. The endothelial cells are plump with abundant, eosinophilic cytoplasm. They are surrounded by a mixture of lymphoid cells and eosinophils.

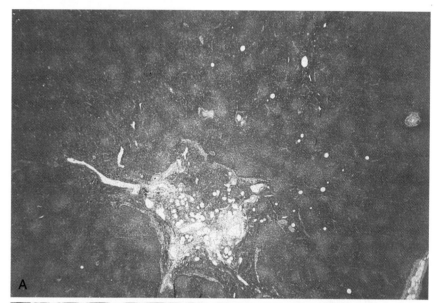

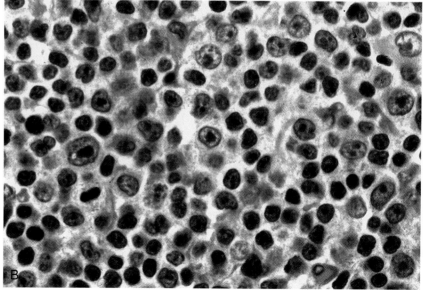

Figure 12–13. Chronic lymphocytic leukemia/small lymphocytic lymphoma. *A,* This neoplasm diffusely replaces lymph node architecture, and vaguely nodular pale zones, known as pseudofollicular growth centers, can be seen. *B,* A high-power view of the center of a pseudofollicular growth center showing a mixture of small lymphocytes, slightly larger and irregular prolymphocytes, and larger paraimmunoblasts with vesicular nuclei and central nucleoli.

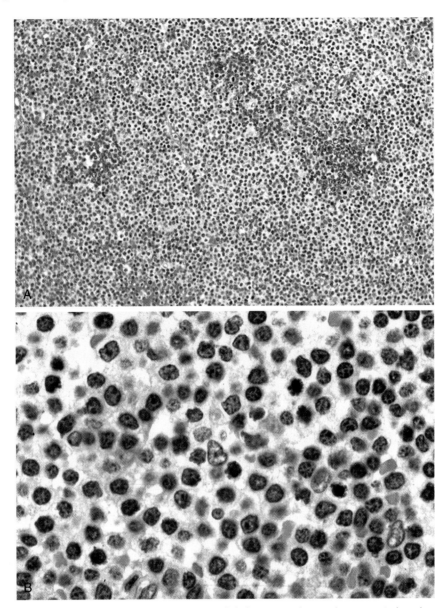

Figure 12–15. Marginal zone B-cell lymphoma/monocytoid B-cell lymphoma. *A,* At low power, this neoplasm extensively replaces the lymph node but spares residual germinal centers. *B,* The neoplastic cells have abundant pale cytoplasm and central round to slightly irregular nuclear contours.

Kimura's Disease

Clinical Features. Kimura's disease is a lymphadenopathy that usually involves the head and neck region with a predilection for young adult, Asian males.[15-18] Elevated serum IgE and peripheral blood eosinophilia are usually present. The proliferation forms large, multifocal masses that may involve subcutaneous tissue, salivary glands, and lymph nodes.

Pathologic Features. Microscopically, the lesion shows lymphoid tissue with reactive follicular hyperplasia and eosinophilic proteinaceous deposits within the germinal centers. The interfollicular areas contain numerous eosinophils with admixed small lymphocytes, plasma cells, and mast cells. In addition, postcapillary venules with low cuboidal to flat endothelium are increased in the interfollicular areas and encroach on the reactive germinal centers (Fig. 12-4, see p. 729). Eosinophils infiltrate the germinal centers in the areas of the vascular encroachment. Eosinophilic abscesses may be present. Immunohistochemical studies identify IgE deposition within the germinal centers as well as IgE-positive mast cells in the interfollicular areas.

Differential Diagnosis. The differential diagnosis of Kimura's disease and angiolymphoid hyperplasia with eosinophilia is discussed later. The mixed interfollicular cell composition of Kimura's disease may be suggestive of the background cells of Hodgkin's disease or of a T-cell lymphoma, but a neoplastic cell population is not identifiable in Kimura's disease.

Treatment and Prognosis. There is no specific therapy. The lymph node enlargement may persist for years, and the proliferation frequently recurs after biopsy; however, the overall prognosis is excellent. In some patients, Kimura's disease is associated with proteinuria.

Infectious Mononucleosis

Infectious mononucleosis is caused by Epstein-Barr virus (EBV) infection.

Clinical Features. Patients present with generalized lymphadenopathy, splenomegaly, and peripheral blood lymphocytosis. The diagnosis is most easily established by serologic studies.

Pathologic Features. Histologically, there is marked paracortical hyperplasia (Fig. 12-5, see p. 730), although a degree of follicular hyperplasia is present in the early stages of infection.[19, 20] The paracortical regions are markedly expanded by a polymorphous population of cells including small lymphocytes, plasmacytoid lymphocytes, immunoblasts, Reed-Sternberg-like cells, histiocytes, and plasma cells, and foci of coagulative necrosis may occur. As paracortical expansion becomes more marked, it overruns lymphoid follicles (see Fig. 12-5A). In the late stages of infection, the architecture can appear completely replaced, although usually there is some variable degree of residual follicles or patent sinuses.

Differential Diagnosis. Of all types of reactive lymphadenopathy, perhaps infectious mononucleosis is most likely to be misdiagnosed as non-Hodgkin's lymphoma.[19] Features that help prevent this error include the presence of any foci of residual normal architecture and the marked heterogeneity of the paracortical infiltrate (see Fig. 12-5B). Although non-Hodgkin's lymphomas and particularly T-cell lymphomas may be heterogeneous, these tumors are usually relatively more homogeneous than the changes of infectious mononucleosis.

Occasionally, a history of EBV infection is known when the lymph node or tonsil biopsy is examined. In this instance, we interpret the histologic findings cautiously, unless the histologic findings are unequivocally malignant.

Immunohistochemical studies for EBV latent membrane protein or in situ hybridization studies for EBV RNA can be very helpful in establishing the diagnosis.[20] Furthermore, immunohistochemical studies can be helpful if the differential diagnosis includes Hodgkin's disease. In infectious mononucleosis, the large lymphoid cells are CD45RB antigen–positive and CD15 antigen–negative. The reverse is true in Hodgkin's disease. The CD30 antigen is expressed by both immunoblasts in infectious mononucleosis and the Reed-Sternberg cells of Hodgkin's disease.

In the differential diagnosis of infectious mononucleosis and B-cell non-Hodgkin's lymphoma, immunohistochemical studies are also helpful, since B-cells are relatively infrequent in infectious mononucleosis. These studies are less helpful in distinguishing infectious mononucleosis from T-cell lymphoma. T-cell receptor gene rearrangement studies are a better means of making this distinction.

Treatment and Prognosis. Infectious mononucleosis is usually a self-limited infection that resolves in weeks or a few months. Antiviral agents, such as acyclovir or α-interferon have been used, but their benefit is not well established.

Dermatopathic Lymphadenopathy

Dermatopathic lymphadenopathy is a distinctive type of paracortical hyperplasia in which the interdigitating reticulum cells are greatly increased (Fig. 12-6, see p. 731).[21]

Clinical Features. Typically, dermatopathic lymphadenopathy occurs in lymph nodes draining sites of chronic cutaneous disease such as infections or cutaneous neoplasms.[22]

Pathologic Features. Interdigitating reticulum cells are large with relatively abundant pale cytoplasm and folded or twisted nuclei with thin nuclear membranes and small nucleoli. In advanced cases, other inflammatory cells such as plasma cells and eosinophils may be present and histiocytes contain melanin pigment.

Treatment and Prognosis. There is no specific therapy. The lymphadenopathy resolves if the antigenic stimulation subsides.

Cat Scratch Disease

The majority of cases of cat scratch disease are caused by *Rochalimaea henselae,* although some may also be caused by *Afipia felis.*[23, 24]

Clinical Features. The lymphadenopathy of cat scratch disease is usually unilateral and most commonly involves axillary or cervical lymph nodes.[25-27] Cat scratch disease usually affects children or young adults, resulting in an enlarged, slightly tender lymph node. The patient may have constitutional symptoms, including fever, malaise, and headache. Most cases are associated with a history of a cat scratch to the area drained by the lymph node 1 to 4 weeks prior to the development of adenopathy.

Pathologic Features. Morphologically, the lymph node is reactive with follicular hyperplasia, a mild interfollicular immunoblast proliferation, and foci of monocytoid B cells. Varying degrees of neutrophil-containing necrosis are also present, which range from granulomas with central necrosis to large areas of stellate abscesses with surrounding histiocytes and fibroblasts (Fig. 12-7, see p. 732). In many cases, rod-shaped bacilli are identifiable with Warthin-Starry or Dieterlé's stains within or adjacent to the areas of necrosis.[27-29]

Differential Diagnosis. The lymphadenopathy of tularemia as well as that of lymphogranuloma venereum are morphologically similar to that of cat scratch disease. Although lymphogranuloma venereum, a sexually transmitted disease caused by *Chlamydia,* usually involves inguinal lymph nodes, cervical lymph node involvement may occur. Tularemia usually involves axillary lymph nodes and is seen following exposure to rabbits. This morphologic pattern, therefore, is not pathognomonic for cat scratch disease. The presence of neutrophils in these diseases helps eliminate Kikuchi's disease from the differential diagnosis. Although microabscesses may be seen with Hodgkin's disease, the lack of Reed-Sternberg cells and their mononuclear variants would exclude such a diagnosis.

Treatment and Prognosis. Lymphadenitis as a result of cat scratch disease is a self-limited infection that does not require specific therapy.

Human Immunodeficiency Virus Infection

Persistent generalized lymphadenopathy is common in HIV-infected patients.[30, 31] Biopsies are most often performed in these patients to exclude treatable infections or malignant neoplasms such as Kaposi's sarcoma or malignant lymphoma. Intermediate and high-grade B-cell lymphomas are most common, but Hodgkin's disease and rarely T-cell lymphomas have been reported.[30]

Pathologic Features. Lymph node changes in benign HIV-infected lymph nodes may be arbitrarily divided into general stages.[30] Initially, there is marked reactive follicular hyperplasia. The secondary germinal centers are commonly very large with bizarre shapes, and, in some cases, the surrounding mantle zones may be absent. As in all forms of follicular hyperplasia, the germinal centers are composed of a heterogeneous mixture of cells, are polarized, and contain many tingible body macrophages. Evidence of follicle lysis may be found. In follicle lysis, small lymphocytes infiltrate into the germinal centers, often associated with hemorrhage.[31] Commonly there is also a marked monocytoid B-cell reaction in the sinuses. The paracortical regions are not prominent.

With time, the lymph node undergoes involution as manifested by lymphoid depletion. Initially there is a variable mixture of reactive follicular hyperplasia and lymphoid depletion, with subsequent progression to severe lymphoid depletion. The lymphoid follicles become smaller and depleted of lymphoid cells until only follicular dendritic cells remain. Some of these follicles may resemble the hyaline-vascular lesions of Castleman's disease. The paracortical regions become expanded as lymphoid cells are depleted, leaving plasma cells, histiocytes, and a prominent vascular network. The sinuses are widely patent.

Particularly in the later stages of HIV infection, infectious organisms are more likely to be found. For example, the presence of many histiocytes in the paracortical regions suggests *Mycobacterium avium-intracellulare* infection (Fig. 12–8, see p. 732). Similarly, the likelihood of malignant neoplasms is increased.[30]

Immunohistochemical studies parallel the histologic findings. In the early stages, lymphoid follicles are composed of polytypic B cells and follicular dendritic reticulum cells, and the paracortical regions are composed of both CD4$^+$/CD8$^-$ and CD4$^-$/CD8$^+$ cells, with the latter predominating.[32] Over time, the number of lymphoid cells is decreased and then absent. The plasma cells express polytypic Ig light chains.

Treatment and Prognosis. In patients with lymph node biopsy specimens without evidence of specific infection or neoplasm, prognosis is determined by the stage of HIV infection.

Kikuchi-Fujimoto Disease (Histiocytic Necrotizing Lymphadenitis)

Histiocytic necrotizing lymphadenitis was independently described by two different groups in Japan[32, 33] but is not localized to that geographic region.

Clinical Features. The patients are most often young adult females, and cervical lymph nodes are by far the most common site of involvement.[34–37] Patients usually present with a painless mass and may also have fever.

Pathologic Features. Microscopically, the nodal architecture is partially to completely effaced by a peculiar necrosis with an accompanying heterogeneous lymphohistiocytic proliferation (Fig. 12–9, see p. 732). The necrosis is well circumscribed and contains karyorrhectic debris without associated neutrophils. The lack of a neutrophilic infiltrate within the necrotic area is a helpful diagnostic

feature. The necrotic areas contain, and are surrounded by, a mixture of plasmacytoid monocytes, histiocytes with folded nuclei, and T immunoblasts. In some cases, presumably representing early involvement, the necrosis is not prominent, and only aggregates of histiocytes and immunoblasts with admixed karyorrhectic debris are present. The surrounding, uninvolved lymphoid tissue generally shows evidence of reactive follicular hyperplasia.

Differential Diagnosis. The lymphadenopathy of lupus is morphologically similar to that of Kikuchi-Fujimoto disease, except that the hematoxylin bodies of lupus may be seen in this disorder.[38] Because of the morphologic similarities between the two processes, as well as the similarity in age of presentation and female predominance, the possibility of lupus should be suggested and clinically excluded in patients with morphologic features of Kikuchi-Fujimoto disease. Other reactive lymphadenopathies, such as cat scratch disease, lymphogranuloma venereum, and *Yersinia enterocolitica* infection, can be excluded by the neutrophilic component of the necrosis in these diseases that is not seen in Kikuchi-Fujimoto disease. The heterogeneous cell population of this disease is helpful in excluding most malignant lymphomas, although failure to recognize the histiocytic component of the process may result in the mistaken diagnosis of an intermediate to high-grade malignant lymphoma.

Treatment and Prognosis. Kikuchi-Fujimoto disease is usually a self-limited condition that requires no specific therapy.

Inflammatory Pseudotumor

Inflammatory pseudotumor, also referred to as inflammatory myofibroblastic tumor or plasma cell granuloma, is an inflammatory and spindled cell proliferation that can occur at almost any site, including lymph nodes.[39–41] The cause is unknown.

Clinical Features. Patients often present with constitutional symptoms that include fever, weight loss, and a tumor mass or lymphadenopathy. Laboratory abnormalities such as anemia, hypergammaglobulinemia, and an elevated erythrocyte sedimentation rate are common. This tumor may occur at any age, with a median age of 32 to 33 years in lymph node cases.[39, 40] Extranodal cases, other than in the lung, apparently occur more commonly in children, with a median age of 9 years reported in a recent series.[41] In the head and neck region, these proliferations have been reported in the oropharynx, nasopharynx, major salivary glands, larynx, and trachea as well as in lymph nodes.

Pathologic Features. The tumors form firm tan or white circumscribed, but unencapsulated, masses and are histologically composed of spindled cells with admixed small vessels and inflammatory cells (Fig. 12–10). The spindled cells are fibroblasts or myofibroblasts, and the inflammatory cells include variable numbers of plasma cells, lymphocytes, neutrophils, eosinophils, and histiocytes. The spindled cells often have enlarged nuclei with nucleoli but do not demonstrate marked nuclear atypia. The lymphocyte component may include a spectrum of cells ranging from small lymphocytes to immunoblasts, and the histiocytes may form clusters of foamy cells.

Differential Diagnosis. The constitutional symptoms that frequently accompany inflammatory pseudotumor are suggestive of an infectious etiology, but a single etiologic agent has not been identified. Some cases have been reported to be associated with bacterial infections[42–44] and the Epstein-Barr virus,[45] and a similar proliferation occurs in association with mycobacterial infections in HIV-positive patients.[46] In addition to infectious proliferations, the differential diagnosis of inflammatory pseudotumor would include sarcomas, especially fibrosarcoma, leiomyosarcoma, and malignant fibrous histiocytoma. The lack of true cytologic atypia in the spindled cell component in inflammatory pseudotumor is the best clue that these proliferations do not represent a malignant process. Immunohistochemical studies are usually not helpful in this differential diagnosis, since the spindled cells of inflammatory pseudotumor are vimentin positive and may focally immunoreact for muscle

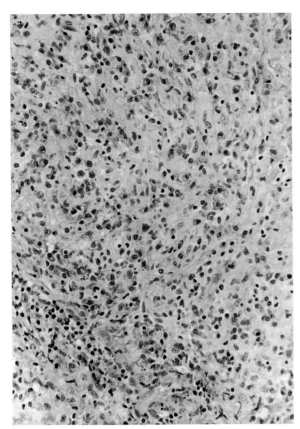

Figure 12–10. Inflammatory pseudotumor of lymph node showing a proliferation of relatively bland spindled cells with admixed lymphocytes and plasma cells.

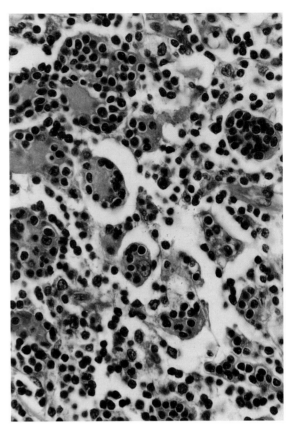

Figure 12–11. Sinus histiocytosis with massive lymphadenopathy with large lymphocytes expanding the lymph node sinuses. The histiocytes contain numerous small lymphocytes and the histiocyte nucleus near the center has a prominent nucleolus.

markers.[47] These special studies may be useful if the inflammatory infiltrate is intense, to exclude a malignant lymphoma. The lymphoid cells of inflammatory pseudotumor are predominantly of T lineage, including the larger immunoblastic cells. The plasma cell component is usually easily identifiable as polytypic using paraffin section immunohistochemistry for immunoglobulin light chains. The immunoblasts of inflammatory pseudotumor may superficially resemble Hodgkin's cells but do not have the characteristic CD45$^-$/CD15$^+$/CD30$^+$ phenotype of Reed-Sternberg cells and their variants.

Treatment and Prognosis. These are benign lesions that require no additional therapy following surgical excision, although they may recur.

Sinus Histiocytosis with Massive Lymphadenopathy (Rosai-Dorfman Disease)

Sinus histiocytosis with massive lymphadenopathy (SHML) is a rare histiocyte proliferation of unknown cause.

Clinical Features. SHML most often occurs in children but may be seen at any age.[48, 49] Cervical lymph nodes are involved in 87% of cases.[50] Multiple lymph nodes may be involved, and the enlarged lymph nodes are frequently matted, causing large tumor masses.

Pathologic Features. Grossly, the involved lymph nodes may have either a nodular or a diffuse yellow-white cut surface with capsular or pericapsular fibrosis. Histologically, the lymph node sinuses are massively expanded by peculiar histiocytes with round to oval, vesicular nuclei, and there is prominent capsular fibrosis. The histiocytic cells may have single or multiple nucleoli, which may be prominent (Fig. 12–11). Occasional multilobated nuclei may be

present, and the mitotic rate is usually low. The cells have abundant pink to eosinophilic cytoplasm and some cells may have foamy cytoplasm. Viable, intracytoplasmic lymphocytes are present within many of the histiocytic cells and this is a characteristic finding of SHML. These lymphocytes often form wreath-like rings within the cytoplasm. Less commonly, the histiocytes may contain intracytoplasmic plasma cells, neutrophils, or red blood cells. In addition to these histiocytic cells, the distended sinuses also contain plasma cells. The residual lymph node tissue is compressed, and marked reactive change of the germinal centers is usually not present.

In addition to cervical lymph node involvement, SHML may involve extranodal sites that frequently include tonsil, larynx, oral cavity, orbit, and nasal cavity.[51, 52] Although distended lymphoid sinuses are not present in these sites, the morphologic features are similar to those in lymph nodes. In some extranodal cases, however, the cellular infiltrate may have a more spindled appearance. In general, a lymphoid infiltrate is present, as well as aggregates of the characteristic histiocytes.

Differential Diagnosis. Although identification of the characteristic histiocytes with intracytoplasmic lymphocytes is often sufficient for diagnosis, immunohistochemical studies may also be useful in excluding other proliferations in the differential diagnosis of SHML.[53] The histiocytes of SHML are S100-positive in the vast majority of cases as well as expressing CD68. Although sinus histiocytosis cells are also CD68 positive, they are not diffusely S100-positive. In contrast to Langerhans' cell histiocytes, SHML histiocytes are CD1-negative and do not demonstrate Birbeck granules by electron microscopy. In addition, eosinophils are not a cellular component in SHML, as they are in most cases of Langerhans' cell histiocytosis. The sinusoidal pattern of the proliferation in SHML may suggest metastatic tumors or anaplastic large cell lymphoma. The cells in general do not demonstrate the cytologic atypia of most of these neoplasms, and the lack of keratin staining in SHML should exclude the diagnosis of carcinoma. The S100 protein expression may make differentiation from melanoma difficult, but the identification of cells with emperipolesis as well as the lack of HMB45 reactivity should aid in excluding melanoma. Up to half of cases of SHML have been reported to be CD30-positive, but this antigen is expressed only weakly and focally in SHML, as opposed to the strong expression seen in most cases of anaplastic large cell lymphoma. In addition, SHML does not demonstrate evidence of B or T cell gene rearrangement. The clinical presentation of matted lymph nodes as well as the capsular fibrosis may suggest Hodgkin's disease, but characteristic Reed-Sternberg cells are not seen in SHML and the histiocytes of SHML are CD15-negative. Finally, extranodal disease may morphologically mimic fibrohistiocytic tumors. The overtly malignant cells of malignant fibrous histiocytoma as well as the high mitotic rate of this tumor are not seen in SHML.

Treatment and Prognosis. In most cases of SHML, the lymphadenopathy eventually resolves without specific therapy.

Angiolymphoid Hyperplasia with Eosinophilia (Epithelioid Hemangioma)

Clinical Features. Angiolymphoid hyperplasia with eosinophilia (ALHE) is often confused with Kimura's disease but is a morphologically and clinically distinct entity.[15-18] Similar to Kimura's disease, the process frequently involves the head and neck region in young adult Asian males but may also affect non-Asians of both sexes. In contrast to Kimura's disease, ALHE is more often superficial, most frequently involving the dermis, and forms multiple, smaller papules or nodules. Lymph node involvement is uncommon and peripheral blood eosinophilia is less common in ALHE than in Kimura's disease.

Pathologic Features and Differential Diagnosis. Angiolymphoid hyperplasia with eosinophilia differs morphologically from Kimura's disease and is a vascular proliferation with a secondary lymphoid and eosinophilic infiltration. The predominant feature is the proliferation of small vessels with plump endothelial cells with abundant eosinophilic and vacuolated cytoplasm (Fig. 12–12, see p. 733). These proliferating small vessels often can be seen surrounding a damaged artery or vein. Scattered small lymphocytes and eosinophils may be present admixed with the vascular proliferation. The plump endothelial cells of ALHE differ from the flattened endothelium characteristic of Kimura's disease. Germinal center formation may be present but is not essential for a diagnosis of ALHE.

In addition to Kimura's disease, the differential diagnosis of ALHL includes vascular lesions of lymph nodes. The eosinophilic infiltrate as well as the lack of hyaline bodies is helpful in excluding Kaposi's sarcoma, and the endothelial atypia of angiosarcoma is not seen in ALHE.

Treatment and Prognosis. Angiolymphoid hyperplasia with eosinophilia is benign but may recur if excision is not complete.

Infarction

In some instances, a relatively large lymph node is biopsied and histologic sections reveal extensive necrosis, often with a surrounding rim of organizing granulation tissue. The finding of lymph node infarction is of concern because non-Hodgkin's lymphomas are a common cause, presumably via vascular compromise.[54, 55] These lymph nodes should be studied with a high index of suspicion.

Clinical Features. Patients present with lymphadenopathy, which may be painful, without apparent cause. A biopsy is done to exclude the possibility of a malignant neoplasm.

Pathologic Features and Differential Diagnosis. The predominant finding in the histologic sections is extensive necrosis. In many cases, a small area at the periphery of the biopsy specimen is

viable, allowing one to establish the correct diagnosis. If not found, it is important that the examiner carefully scrutinize the necrotic regions to distinguish coagulative from liquefactive necrosis. The latter is most often secondary to infection. In the former, one can often recognize eosinophilic ghosts of cells, which may suggest necrotic neoplasm.

Immunohistochemical studies can be helpful, as neoplastic cells may retain antigens despite having undergone necrosis. For example, the B-cell antibody L26 (CD20) may highlight most of the cell ghosts in the infarct, a finding highly suspicious for non-Hodgkin's lymphoma.[54] Furthermore, infarcted cell DNA may also be preserved and molecular studies may demonstrate a monoclonal population in cases of lymphoma.[55]

Treatment and Prognosis. The treatment is based on the cause of infarction. If the degree of infarction prevents definitive diagnosis, a repeat biopsy should be recommended, to be done either immediately or after a period of clinical follow-up.

▌ MALIGNANT LESIONS
Classification of Non-Hodgkin's Lymphomas

In 1956, Rappaport introduced the era of modern non-Hodgkin's lymphoma classification.[56] The approach of this classification was to first divide lymphomas by pattern, either nodular or diffuse, and then to further subclassify these neoplasms on the basis of cytologic features. Tumors composed of lymphocytes that closely resembled normal lymphocytes were termed well differentiated. Poorly differentiated non-Hodgkin's lymphomas were composed of relatively small lymphoid cells with irregular nuclear contours that less closely resembled normal lymphocytes. Lymphomas composed of large cells were designated histiocytic on the basis of their resemblance to normal histiocytes and were thought to be derived from these cells. Undifferentiated lymphomas were composed of cells of intermediate size that failed to demonstrate cytologic features resembling either lymphoid or histiocytic cells. Mixed lymphomas were composed of a mixture of poorly differentiated lymphocytes and histiocytes. Over time, additional categories, such as lymphoblastic lymphoma, were added.[57]

Although the Rappaport classification was popular with clinicians, as our understanding of the normal immune system improved, scientific inaccuracies in the Rappaport classification became apparent. In an attempt to address these inaccuracies, new classifications were proposed that attempted to relate lymphoid neoplasms more closely to their counterparts in the normal immune system. These classifications included the Lukes and Collins, British National Lymphoma Group, Dorfman, World Health Organization, and Kiel systems.[58] This number of classifications resulted in both confusion and controversy. In an attempt to resolve these differences, the National Cancer Institute funded an international study to test each of the major classifications on 1175 non-Hodgkin's lymphomas staged and treated in a relatively consistent manner.[58] On the basis of this study, published in 1982, it was concluded that each of the systems was useful in separating large numbers of patients with malignant lymphoma into subgroups with varying survival prospects and clinical features. Furthermore, no one scheme appeared to be superior to any other. The investigators then jointly developed a Working Formulation of non-Hodgkin's lymphomas, which they viewed not as an alternative classification but rather as a common language that might be used by all investigators to translate one classification scheme into another (Table 12–1). From a clinical viewpoint, the categories of lymphoma specified in the Working Formulation can be separated into three major groups: low grade, intermediate grade, and high grade, which are predictive of survival. However, it is important to emphasize that the Working Formulation was based purely on histologic data; immunologic and molecular data were not included.

With the application of immunologic and molecular methods to the study of non-Hodgkin's lymphomas, the deficiencies in the

Table 12–1. International Working Formulation

Low Grade

A. Malignant lymphoma, small lymphocytic
  Consistent with chronic lymphocytic leukemia
  Plasmacytoid
B. Malignant lymphoma, follicular, predominantly small cleaved cell
  Diffuse areas
  Sclerosis
C. Malignant lymphoma, follicular, mixed small cleaved and large cell
  Diffuse areas
  Sclerosis

Intermediate Grade

D. Malignant lymphoma, follicular, predominantly large cell
  Diffuse areas
  Sclerosis
E. Malignant lymphoma, diffuse, small cleaved cell
  Sclerosis
F. Malignant lymphoma, diffuse, mixed small and large cell
  Sclerosis
  Epithelioid cell component
G. Malignant lymphoma, diffuse, large cell
  Cleaved
  Noncleaved

High Grade

H. Malignant lymphoma, large cell immunoblastic
  Plasmacytoid
  Clear cell
  Polymorphous
  Epithelioid cell
I. Malignant lymphoma, lymphoblastic
  Convoluted cell
  Nonconvoluted cell
J. Malignant lymphoma, small noncleaved
  Burkitt's
  Non-Burkitt's

Miscellaneous

  Composite
  Mycosis fungoides
  Histiocytic
  Extramedullary plasmacytoma
  Unclassifiable

Table 12–2. Revised European-American Classification of Lymphoid Neoplasms

Non-Hodgkin's Lymphomas

B-Cell Lymphoma

I. Precursor B-cell neoplasm: Precursor B-lymphoblastic leukemia/lymphoma
II. Peripheral B-cell lymphomas
 1. B-cell chronic lymphocytic leukemia/small lymphocytic lymphoma
 2. Lymphoplasmacytoid lymphoma/immunocytoma
 3. Mantle cell lymphoma
 4. Follicle center lymphoma
 5. Marginal zone B-cell lymphoma
  Extranodal (mucosa-associated lymphoid tissue type ± monocytoid B cells)
  Provisional subtype: nodal (± monocytoid B cells)
 6. Provisional entity: splenic marginal zone lymphoma (± villous lymphocytes)
 7. Hairy cell leukemia
 8. Plasmacytoma/myeloma
 9. B-cell large cell lymphoma
  Subtype: primary mediastinal (thymic) B-cell lymphoma
 10. Burkitt's lymphoma
 11. Provisional entity: high-grade B-cell lymphoma, Burkitt-like

T-Cell and Putative Natural Killer (NK)–Cell Lymphomas

I. Precursor T-cell neoplasm: precursor T-lymphoblastic lymphoma/leukemia
II. Peripheral T-cell and NK-cell neoplasms
 1. T-cell chronic lymphocytic leukemia/prolymphocytic leukemia
 2. Large granular lymphocyte leukemia (LGL)
  T-cell type
  NK-cell type
 3. Mycosis fungoides/Sezary's syndrome
 4. Peripheral T-cell lymphomas, unspecified
  Provisional subtype: hepatosplenic γδ T-cell lymphoma
  Provisional subtype: subcutaneous T-cell lymphoma
 5. Angioimmunoblastic lymphoma
 6. Angiocentric lymphoma
 7. Intestinal T-cell lymphoma (± enteropathy-associated; ITCL)
 8. Adult T-cell lymphoma/leukemia (ATL/L)
 9. Anaplastic large cell lymphoma, CD30+, T- and null-cell types
 10. Provisional entity: anaplastic large-cell lymphoma, Hodgkin-like

Working Formulation have become more apparent. Working Formulation categories are heterogeneous and encompass more then one biologic entity. Furthermore, one disease can exhibit a morphologic spectrum and thus fit within more than one Working Formulation category. In 1994, a group of pathologists known as the International Lymphoma Study Group met and attempted to address many of the deficiencies in the Working Formulation by proposing a new classification, known as the Revised European-American Classification (Table 12–2).[59] In the remainder of this chapter, non-Hodgkin's lymphomas are referred to by the terms specified in this new classification. Working Formulation terms are also included where appropriate.

Treatment and Prognosis of Non-Hodgkin's Lymphomas

In spite of the many advantages of the Revised European-American Classification, it does not divide lesions into broad groups or grades that generally predict survival, as the Working Formulation did.[58] In particular, the clinical outcome of different types of non-Hodgkin's

lymphoma can be separated into three major groups: low grade, intermediate grade, and high grade. As a general rule, if non-Hodgkin's lymphomas were untreated, the survival of patients with low-grade neoplasms would be measured in years, in contrast with months for patients with intermediate-grade neoplasms and weeks for patients with high-grade tumors.

Low-grade non-Hodgkin's lymphomas are clinically indolent, and affected patients are usually adults with relatively long survival with or without aggressive therapy.[59] Systemic (B type) symptoms such as fever, night sweats, and weight loss occur in a minority of patients. These tumors involve sites where their normal counterparts are located. For example, follicular lymphomas derived from follicular center B-cells demonstrate a striking capacity to home to B-cell–dependent portions of the lymphoid system and have a nondestructive growth pattern. Like normal B cells in lymph node, neoplastic low-grade B cells commonly circulate and patients usually present with disseminated disease at presentation.[58, 59] Nevertheless, sanctuary sites such as the testis or central nervous system are rarely involved. Low-grade lymphomas may also respond to immunoregulation, related to either natural changes in host immunity or to therapeutic administration of immunomodulating drugs. Although low-grade lymphomas commonly respond to chemotherapy, the disease usually recurs and thus chemotherapy is often not curative.[60] Death comes either as a result of progressive growth with eventual replacement of normal hematopoietic and lymphoid tissues or via transformation to an intermediate or high-grade non-Hodgkin's lymphoma.

In contrast, intermediate- and high-grade non-Hodgkin's lymphomas have an aggressive natural history and patients have short survival, unless they are treated vigorously.[58] These tumors commonly involve extranodal regions and sanctuary sites such as the testis and central nervous system.[58, 59] Systemic (B) symptoms are more common. The normal counterparts of these cells in the immune system do not circulate, and thus a higher percentage of patients present with localized disease compared with low-grade neoplasms. Intermediate- and high-grade non-Hodgkin's lymphomas generally do not respond to immunoregulation. Aggressive chemotherapy is the treatment of choice, and commonly used regimens include a number of agents.[60] With appropriate treatment, long-term clinical remissions and probable cures have been obtained, with rates of success highest in patients with localized disease.

Chronic Lymphocytic Leukemia, or Small Lymphocytic Lymphoma

The tumor of chronic lymphocytic leukemia (CLL) is classified as malignant lymphoma, low-grade, small lymphocytic type in the Working Formulation.[58] Morphologically and immunophenotypically, the malignant cells of CLL are identical to those of nodal-based small lymphocytic lymphoma (SLL), and these two entities are thought to represent different manifestations of the same disease.[59, 61] Although patients with SLL may not present with leukemia, subclinical peripheral blood involvement is often present and progression to overt CLL is common.

Clinical Features. CLL/SLL occurs primarily in middle-aged and older patients with a peak incidence in the sixth to eighth decades.[59, 62] In most series, the ratio of male to female is approximately 1.5:1. Patients typically present with generalized lymphadenopathy, often with hepatosplenomegaly and bone marrow involvement with only vague symptoms such as weakness, anorexia, fever, and occasionally night sweats.[59, 62]

Pathologic Features. Lymph nodes involved by CLL/SLL are usually diffusely effaced (Fig. 12–13, see p. 733). Cytologically, the neoplastic cells are predominantly small round lymphocytes with inconspicuous nucleoli, clumped chromatin, scant cytoplasm, and infrequent mitoses. However, slightly larger lymphoid cells with irregular nuclear contours (known as prolymphocytes) and even larger cells with round vesicular nuclei and central nucleoli (called paraimmunoblasts) are also found.[62, 63] These cells may be scattered throughout the lesion or they may cluster into aggregates that have been referred to as pseudofollicular "growth centers" or "proliferation centers."[62, 63] These growth centers, examined under low power, may impart a vaguely nodular appearance (see Fig. 12–13).

A small subset of CLL/SLL cases exhibit mild plasmacytoid differentiation. Morphologically, the neoplastic cells in these cases have slightly more abundant cytoplasm and the nucleus may be eccentrically situated, thus resembling plasma cells. These cells contain cytoplasmic immunoglobulin, which may be secreted, producing a small monoclonal IgM paraprotein.[59] Since these tumors are immunophenotypically and molecularly indistinguishable from CLL/SLL, they are classified as such in the REAL classification.[59]

Immunophenotypically, CLL/SLL are B-cell tumors that express monotypic Ig light chains ($\kappa > \lambda$), IgM, usually IgD, and the pan-B-cell antigens CD19, CD20, and CD22.[59, 60] The B-cell–associated antigens CD21 and CD23 are usually positive and CD10 (CALLA) is usually negative. These tumors also express CD5 antigen, a T-cell antigen that is not expressed on the vast majority of normal B cells of adulthood but is expressed by CLL/SLL. Other T-cell antigens are negative. Using flow cytometry, the density of surface Ig or CD20 antigen expression by CLL/SLL cells is characteristically modest or "dim."[60]

Molecular studies of the antigen receptor genes in CLL/SLL have demonstrated rearrangements of the Ig heavy and light chain genes.[64] The *TCR* genes are usually in the germline configuration, although occasional cases may have *TCR* gene rearrangement (so-called lineage infidelity).[64] Approximately 50% of CLL/SLLs have chromosomal abnormalities as shown by conventional cytogenetics. Trisomy 12 and del(13q) are the two most common findings, in approximately 15% and 10% of cases, respectively.[65] The del(13q) usually occurs at the site of the retinoblastoma gene, at 13q14. Trisomy 12 and del(13q) are probably secondary events, present in a subclone of neoplastic cells.[65]

Differential Diagnosis. The differential diagnosis of CLL/SLL includes other types of low-grade B-cell lymphoma and mantle cell lymphoma. Unlike other low-grade B-cell lymphomas, CLL/SLL is composed of a mixture of small round cells, prolymphocytes, and paraimmunoblasts that commonly aggregate to form pseudofollicular growth centers. Furthermore, CLL/SLLs are CD5 antigen–positive whereas other low-grade B-cell tumors are almost always CD5 antigen–negative. Similar to CLL/SLL, mantle cell lymphomas are CD5 antigen–positive. However, in contrast with CLL/SLL, mantle cell lymphomas are composed of a monotonous population of small lymphoid cells without pseudofollicular growth centers, are usually negative for the CD23 antigen, commonly carry the t(11;14)(q13;q32) or *bcl*-1 gene rearrangements, and typically over-express BCL-1 protein.

Treatment and Prognosis. Particularly in its early stages, CLL is clinically indolent and patients have prolonged survival, for example, up to 20 years. These patients often do not need any specific therapy. However, with advancing clinical stage, patient survival is significantly shorter, more in keeping with other types of low-grade B-cell lymphoma of advanced stage. For these patients, systemic chemotherapy is indicated to improve peripheral blood counts or organ function, although it is usually not curative. Histologically, CLL/SLLs with a high mitotic rate (>30 mitoses per 20 high-power fields) and extensive necrosis are clinically more aggressive tumors.[66] Trisomy 12 also correlates with advanced stage disease and decreased survival and may correlate with atypical morphologic and immunologic features as well, such as an increased number of prolymphocytes and strong surface Ig expression by the neoplastic cells.[65]

Lymphoplasmacytoid Lymphoma/Immunocytoma

Lymphoplasmacytoid lymphoma/immunocytoma are tumors designated as malignant lymphoma, low-grade, small lymphocytic, plasmacytoid in the Working Formulation.[58] In the REAL classification, the term *lymphoplasmacytoid lymphoma/immunocytoma* (LPL/I) is reserved for tumors associated with a prominent monoclonal IgM paraprotein, often with the syndrome of Waldenström's macroglobulinemia.[59]

Clinical Features. Patients with LPL/I can present with a variety of symptoms and findings including mucous membrane bleeding, lymphadenopathy, hepatomegaly, peripheral neuropathy, and central nervous system abnormalities.[59, 67] Constitutional symptoms and anemia are common.[67] Most patients have a monoclonal IgM paraprotein in the serum, greater than 1 g/100 mL, and approximately one third of patients develop serum hyperviscosity and the clinical syndrome of Waldenström's macroglobulinemia. The lymphadenopathy is generalized but is usually modest relative to CLL/SLL. Hepatosplenomegaly is common. Involvement of peripheral blood and extranodal sites is relatively uncommon.[59, 67]

Pathologic Features. Lymph nodes involved by LPL/I retain their overall architecture. The neoplastic cells respect sinuses and tend to home to the medullary cords.[68] The capsule is extensively infiltrated, and perinodal adipose tissue is involved. Cytologically, the neoplastic cells are small lymphoid cells, many with slightly or more obviously increased cytoplasm characteristic of plasmacytoid differentiation. The tumor cells also may contain cytoplasmic globules (Russell's bodies) or intranuclear pseudoinclusions (Dutcher bodies) of IgM.[68] The evidence of plasmacytoid differentiation may be subtle or obvious in different cases of LPL/I. In the bone marrow, the neoplasm may focally or extensively involve the medullary space in a nodular (but not truly follicular) or diffuse pattern. Particularly in the bone marrow, cytologic evidence of plasmacytoid differentiation may not be easily appreciated.[69]

Immunophenotypic studies have shown that LPL/Is express monoclonal Ig light chain ($\kappa > \lambda$), IgM, and pan-B-cell antigens such as CD19, CD20, and CD22 and are negative for IgD and T-cell antigens including CD5.[59, 60] In cases with more extensive plasmacytoid differentiation, the CD20 antigen may not be expressed, similar to normal plasma cells that are typically CD20 negative.[60] The tumor cells also express plasma cell–associated antigens such as CD38.

Molecular analyses of LPL/I have shown Ig heavy and light chain gene rearrangements with the *TCR* genes, usually in the germline configuration.[63]

Differential Diagnosis. The differential diagnosis includes CLL and plasma cell neoplasms, such as plasmacytoma and plasma cell myeloma. Unlike CLL, LPL/I does not have pseudofollicular growth centers nor are the neoplastic cells positive for the CD5 antigen. Unlike plasma cell tumors, the neoplastic cells of LPL/I have lymphoid cytologic features with variable plasmacytoid differentiation. In addition, LPL/I almost always is positive for IgM; almost all plasma cell myelomas are positive for IgG or IgA or rarely IgD and are negative for IgM.

Prognosis. Patients with LPL/I have a low-grade neoplasm with a correspondingly indolent clinical course. Survival correlates with stage of disease.

Follicle Center Lymphoma, Follicular Lymphoma

Follicle center lymphomas (FCLs) as defined in the REAL classification[59] are better known as follicular lymphomas. The natural history of follicle center lymphomas is to become diffuse and accumulate large cells, with a correspondingly poorer prognosis. In the Working Formulation, these malignant lymphomas were arbitrarily subdivided, based on the numbers of small cleaved and large lymphoid cells, as low-grade follicular predominantly small cleaved cell, low-grade follicular mixed small cleaved and large cell, and intermediate grade follicular predominantly large cell groups.[58] Although useful prognostically, these groups are misleading in the sense that they convey the impression that these groups are distinct types of neoplasms. The recent REAL classification emphasizes that all FCLs are the same biologic entity, at different stages of disease evolution. The authors further suggested that grading FCLs as I, II, and III provides prognostic value while emphasizing the biologic similarity of all FCLs.[59] Whether this practice will be generally accepted is currently uncertain.

Clinical Features. Follicle center lymphoma is the most common type of non-Hodgkin's lymphoma in the United States, affecting approximately 20% of adults with malignant lymphoma.[59, 70] Predominantly older age groups are affected, with a peak incidence in the fifth and sixth decades; FCLs are rare in patients under the age of 20 years.[70] There is a slight male predominance and whites are affected more often than blacks.[58, 70] Most patients present with generalized disease involving lymph nodes, spleen, liver, and bone marrow.[58, 59] Some patients with FCL present with or develop obvious leukemia. The characteristic cell in the peripheral blood has a deeply clefted nucleus and is known as a "buttock cell." Leukemic involvement does not appear to influence prognosis.[71]

Pathologic Features. Histologically, the lymph node architecture is partially or completely effaced by neoplastic follicles, and a high absolute number of follicles is the best histologic criterion to establish the diagnosis of FCL (Fig. 12–14).[72] Unlike the lymphoid follicles in reactive hyperplasia, the follicles of FCL are of relatively uniform size, lack a well-defined lymphoid cuff, and do not show polarization of germinal centers.[72] Histiocytes are usually less frequent in neoplastic as compared with reactive follicles. Plasmacytoid differentiation is rare in all subtypes of FCL.[72]

Cytologically, in normal follicle germinal centers, lymphoid cells appear to undergo transformation in a sequence beginning as small noncleaved forms and progressing to large noncleaved, large cleaved, and finally to small cleaved forms.[73] The cells in neoplastic follicles mimic these normal cell types. The small cleaved lymphoid cells have irregular, cleaved nuclear contours and coarse, condensed chromatin. Large cleaved cells are similar but larger than small cleaved cells, with more open nuclear chromatin. Small noncleaved cells are intermediately sized with irregular chromatin and multiple distinct nucleoli. Large noncleaved lymphoid cells are approximately three times larger in diameter than small cleaved cells, with vesicular nuclei and one to three nucleoli. In these cells, usually one nucleolus is centrally located and one or two nucleoli are peripherally apposed to the nuclear membrane. Since the small noncleaved and large cells are the proliferating component, the number of mitotic figures present correlates with the number of small noncleaved and large cells.

The distinction between grade I, II, and III FCLs is based on arbitrary criteria that are not shared by all pathologists.[59] In one proposed system, the distinction between FCLs is made by counting the number of large lymphoid cells present.[74] In grade I (predominantly small cleaved cell) FCLs, large lymphoid cells are rare. Grade II (mixed small cleaved and large cell) FCLs contain five or more large lymphoid cells per 400X microscopic field (see Fig. 12–14). Grade III (predominantly large cell) FCLs are composed of 15 or more large noncleaved lymphoid cells per 400X field.

Immunophenotypic studies have shown that FCLs are B-cell neoplasms. The majority of grade I and II tumors express Ig, but up to 50% of grade III neoplasms may be Ig-negative.[59, 60] When Ig-positive, FCLs express monotypic Ig light chain ($\kappa > \lambda$). The majority of tumors express IgM, but approximately 25% of tumors express IgG or IgA, a not unexpected finding since normal follicular center cells can undergo Ig heavy chain switching following exposure to antigen. IgD is usually negative. All FCLs express pan-B-cell markers such as CD19, CD20, and CD22 and approximately 75% are positive for the CD10 antigen (CALLA).[59, 60] All T-cell antigens are negative. Using flow cytometry, FCLs express Ig and B-cell antigens at high density ("bright" immunofluorescence).[60]

Follicle center lymphomas have rearrangements of the Ig heavy and light chain genes and the *TCR* genes are usually in the germline configuration.[63] The molecular hallmark of FCLs is the t(14;18)(q32;q21).[75] Both cytogenetic and molecular analyses have demonstrated the t(14;18) in approximately 80% to 90% of cases.[75] In this translocation, the *bcl*-2 oncogene on chromosome 18q21 is juxtaposed with the Ig heavy chain gene joining region on chromosome 14q32. The *bcl*-2 gene is dysregulated, probably under the influence of Ig heavy chain gene regulatory elements.[76] The BCL-2 protein is a 25 kd molecule reported to be located on the inner mitochondrial membrane as well as other subcellular membranes.[77, 78] This protein is overexpressed in FCLs and appears to protect cells from programmed cell death (apoptosis). The inhibition of apoptosis prolongs B-cell life, resulting in an expanded compartment of cells at increased risk for additional molecular defects, presumably involved in neoplastic transformation.[78] However, BCL-2 protein expression is not limited to FCLs, as it is expressed by many subtypes of B-cell lymphoma without the t(14;18).[77] In addition, the presence of t(14;18) alone does not appear sufficient for neoplastic transformation, as this translocation has been identified in rare cells in the tonsils and lymph nodes of normal individuals, without clinical evidence of lymphoma.[79]

A small subset of cases of FCL have been reported that do not carry the t(14;18) but do carry other translocations, such as the

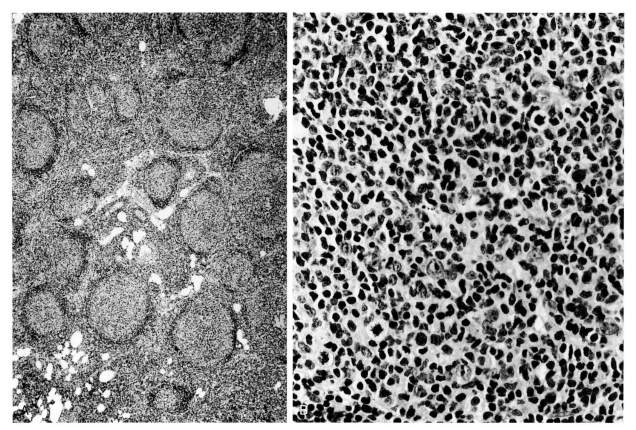

Figure 12–14. Follicular center lymphoma, follicular, grade 2 (mixed small cleaved and large cell). *A,* At low power, numerous neoplastic follicles are distributed throughout the cortex and medulla. *B,* A high-power view of one follicle shows many small cleaved cells with more than five large, noncleaved cells per microscopic field.

t(8;14) and t(2;18).[80, 81] Patients with these neoplasms usually have a clinically indolent course similar to t(14;18)-positive FCLs. This finding suggests that there are minor pathways of follicular lymphogenesis that are independent of the t(14;18).

Treatment and Prognosis. In spite of the presence of widespread disease, patients with FCL composed predominantly of small cleaved lymphoid cells (grade I) have relatively long survival.[58, 82] The median survival of patients with grade I FCL was 7.2 years in the Working Formulation study.[58] Progression from a purely follicular to a follicular and diffuse pattern is common, and the presence of a diffuse component without a significant increase of large lymphoid cells does not affect survival.[82] As the number of large lymphoid cells increases in FCLs, the tumor becomes a mixture of small cleaved and large cells (grade II) and then is composed of predominantly large lymphoid cells (grade III). A diffuse component usually accompanies the increased number of large cells.[82] Patients with mixed FCLs also have an indolent clinical course, although the large lymphoid cells are proliferating, and survival is less than that of patients with grade I neoplasms. In the Working Formulation study, the median survival of patients with grade II FCL was 5.1 years.[58] If the diffuse component in grade II tumors is less than 50%, it has a minimal effect on survival. However, when the diffuse component is greater than 50%, patients often have a more aggressive clinical course.[83] Grade III FCLs also commonly have a diffuse component and are clinically aggressive tumors that require chemotherapy.[58] The median survival of patients with grade III FCL in the Working Formulation study was 3 years.[58] Follicle center lymphomas may progress to a completely diffuse neoplasm, without any recognizable follicular architecture. In patients with multiple biopsy specimens, this progression can be documented.[84] It is also not uncommon for a patient with FCL with many sites of disease to have discordant histologic findings, with one biopsy site involved by a FCL composed of predominantly small cleaved cells or a mixture of small

cleaved and large cells, with a second site involved by a follicular or entirely diffuse lymphoma composed of large cells.[85]

Marginal Zone B-Cell Lymphoma

The category of marginal zone B-cell lymphoma in the REAL classification includes lymphomas that were originally designated as monocytoid B-cell lymphoma and low-grade B-cell lymphoma of the mucosa-associated lymphoid tissue (MALT). Both neoplasms are thought to represent different clinical presentations of a B-cell neoplasm believed to arise from normal marginal zone B-cells in the lymph node or their extranodal counterparts, respectively. Marginal zone B-cell lymphomas share distinctive histologic findings that are not easily or reproducibly classified and can fit within a number of Working Formulation categories.

Monocytoid B-Cell Lymphoma

Sheibani and colleagues originally recognized malignant lymphomas that morphologically resembled benign monocytoid B cells. They proposed the term *monocytoid B-cell lymphoma* (MBCL) for these neoplasms.[86]

Clinical Features. Patients with MBCL are usually elderly, and women are affected more often than men.[59, 86, 87] Most patients present with lymphadenopathy that is usually clinical stage I or II, involving lymph nodes of the head and neck regions. The parotid gland is involved in 10% to 20% of patients, and most of these patients have Sjögren's syndrome.[86, 88] In a small subset of cases, patients present with widespread disease. However, unlike other low-grade B-cell lymphomas with dissemination the liver, spleen, and bone marrow are uncommonly involved in MBCL. When patients with MBCL have concurrently involved nodal and extranodal sites, the neoplasm in extranodal sites closely resembles low-grade B-cell lymphoma of MALT.[59, 87]

Pathologic Features. Histologically, lymph nodes involved by MBCL have a pale appearance under low-power examination as a result of the abundant clear cytoplasm of the neoplastic cells (Fig. 12–15, see p. 734).[86–88] These tumors have a propensity to involve the marginal zones and surrounding sinuses in the lymph node. In a small subset of cases, MBCL is confined to the sinuses, and distinction from reactive monocytoid B cells is difficult without immunophenotypic or molecular studies. More often, MBCLs involve the marginal zones and sinuses and expand into the perifollicular compartments with sparing of germinal centers, or completely replace the lymph node architecture.

The cytologic features of MBCL are the most distinctive features of this neoplasm. The tumor cell cytoplasm is relatively abundant, pale eosinophilic or clear, with well-delineated cell borders (see Fig. 12–15). The tumor cell nuclei are small and cytologically bland, and mitotic figures are infrequent.[86–88]

Immunophenotypic studies have shown that MBCLs are mature B-cell neoplasms that express monotypic Ig light chain ($\kappa > \lambda$), usually IgM, and pan-B-cell antigens.[59, 60] These tumors usually do not express IgD and are negative for CD10, CD21, CD23, and T-cell antigens including CD5.

In a limited number of MBCL cases studied, the Ig genes have been rearranged and the TCR genes were usually in the germline configuration.[63] The *bcl*-2 gene has been in the germline configuration. Conventional cytogenetic studies have not revealed abnormalities common to most MBCLs.[89] Fluorescence in situ hybridization (FISH) studies have shown trisomy 3 in a subset of tumors.[90]

Differential Diagnosis. The differential diagnosis of MBCL includes benign monocytoid B-cell reactions and other types of low-grade lymphoma. Usually, benign monocytoid B-cell reactions are confined to the lymph node sinuses and are associated with other evidence of hyperplasia of the B-cell and/or T-cell compartments. Rarely, MBCL may be confined to the sinuses and, in this circumstance, immunohistochemical studies are needed to demonstrate a monoclonal B-cell population before the diagnosis of MBCL is established. Unlike most other low-grade lymphomas, which are composed of small lymphoid cells with minimal cytoplasm and therefore have a dark (blue) low-power appearance, MBCLs have cells with relatively abundant cytoplasm and appear pale at low power. Unlike CLL/SLL, MBCLs lack pseudofollicular growth centers. In contrast with mantle cell lymphoma, MBCLs have a subpopulation of large lymphoid cells. Furthermore, MBCLs are CD5-negative, unlike CLL/SLL and mantle cell lymphoma, and usually do not carry translocations, such as the t(11;14) in mantle cell lymphoma or the t(14;18) in FCL.

Treatment and Prognosis. Most patients reported with localized MBCL, many of whom were treated only by surgical excision or local irradiation, have responded well to therapy.[59, 86, 88] With prolonged clinical follow-up, more than 75% of these patients are alive, most without lymphoma.[88] Patients with generalized disease are usually treated with combination chemotherapy, often with a good response. However, a subset of patients may respond poorly to therapy, are at greater risk for transformation to higher grade lymphoma, and may develop composite lymphoma (i.e., MBCL coexistent with another type of non-Hodgkin's lymphoma).[88, 89, 91]

Extranodal Lymphoid Infiltrates

Prior to the advent of immunologic and gene rearrangement techniques, the diagnosis of extranodal low-grade B-cell lymphoma was infrequently made in patients without a history of nodal low-grade lymphoma. Instead, extranodal infiltrates composed of small round or slightly irregular lymphoid cells often admixed with plasma cells, histiocytes, and lymphoid follicles were classified as "pseudolymphomas," since clinical studies showed that in patients with these lesions, the disease pursued an indolent clinical course.[92] Immunophenotypic and gene rearrangement studies have since shown that

the majority of "pseudolymphomas" express monotypic Ig light chain and contain Ig gene rearrangements.[93] In at least one study, the presence of monotypic Ig light chain expression in extranodal "pseudolymphomas" correlated with an increased risk of systemic dissemination, providing further justification for their classification as malignant.[92] Thus, extranodal lymphoid infiltrates in which a monoclonal B-cell population is identified using immunohistochemical methods are now usually classified as low-grade B-cell lymphomas, and the majority of cases are examples of low-grade B-cell MALT-lymphomas.

Low-Grade B-Cell Lymphomas of Mucosa-Associated Lymphoid Tissue (MALT)

Low grade B-cell lymphomas of MALT were originally recognized by Isaacson and Wright as a subset of gastrointestinal lymphomas in European patients that resembled immunoproliferative small intestinal disease (also known as Mediterranean lymphoma).[94] Isaacson et al.[94, 95] initially suggested that these tumors arose from lymphoid tissue associated with mucosa. However, MALT-lymphomas have since been recognized in a number of different extranodal sites including the lung, thyroid gland (Fig. 12–16), salivary glands (Fig. 12–17, see p. 745), thymus, breast, conjunctiva (Fig. 12–18, see p. 746), gallbladder, liver, cervix, larynx, trachea, skin, soft tissue, and kidney.[95, 96] Thus, the term *MALT-lymphoma,* although it is still used, is misleading in the sense that not all MALT-lymphomas arise in sites involving mucosal surfaces.

Clinical Features. Low-grade B-cell lymphomas of MALT tend to be localized for prolonged intervals before disseminating and patients often present with a prolonged history that may be confused with an inflammatory process. For example, a patient with a MALT-lymphoma of the stomach may present with signs and symptoms suggestive of a benign gastric ulcer. Unlike nodal low-grade B-cell

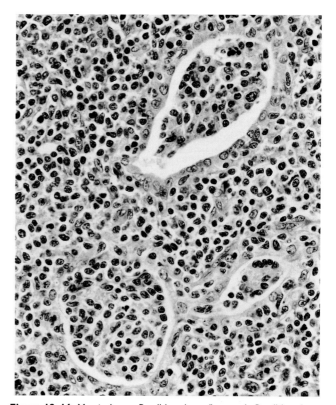

Figure 12–16. Marginal zone B-cell lymphoma/low-grade B-cell lymphoma of mucosa-associated lymphoid tissue of the thyroid gland. The neoplastic cells are small, with slightly to moderately irregular nuclear contours and abundant pale cytoplasm. Note extensive invasion of follicles. Some retraction artifact is also present.

lymphomas, MALT-lymphomas uncommonly involve the bone marrow, liver, spleen, or peripheral blood.[95, 96]

The pattern of dissemination of MALT lymphomas is also unlike that of nodal low-grade B-cell lymphomas. These tumors have a tendency to spread to other extranodal sites. For example, in one study MALT-lymphomas of the lung disseminated to other extranodal sites as often as they spread to lymph nodes.[97] When MALT-lymphomas involve lymph nodes, they resemble MBCL.

Pathologic Features. Four histologic findings are present in most low-grade B-cell lymphomas of MALT: a population of small and irregular lymphoid cells (originally named "centrocyte-like cells"), occasional neoplastic large lymphoid cells, lymphoepithelial lesions, and reactive lymphoid follicles (see Figs. 12–16, 12–17, and 12–18).[95]

The neoplastic small lymphoid cells exhibit a range of cytologic appearances. In many neoplasms, these cells have slightly irregular nuclear contours and relatively abundant clear cytoplasm resembling monocytoid B cells. In other cases, these cells are small and closely resemble small lymphocytes, often with plasmacytoid differentiation (see Fig. 12–18). In some neoplasms, the tumor cells appear biphasic, with one component being small lymphoid cells with minimal cytoplasm, while the other component exhibits extensive plasmacytoid differentiation with many cells resembling mature plasma cells. In yet other tumors, the neoplastic small cells have markedly irregular nuclear contours and resemble small cleaved lymphocytes.

In most low-grade MALT-lymphomas, large lymphoid cells are present, although they represent only a small minority of the tumor cells. However, in a small subset of cases, the large cells can be more numerous. When the large cells present are numerous and form aggregates, the neoplasm has progressed to a higher grade neoplasm.[95]

The neoplastic small cells have a marked tendency to invade epithelium, forming lymphoepithelial lesions, seen as small or larger aggregates of cells within the epithelium (see Figs. 12–16 and 12–17). Reactive lymphoid follicles are also usually present in MALT-lymphomas, usually surrounded by neoplastic cells. The tumor cells also may accumulate in the follicle centers (referred to as *colonization*) with the tumor then acquiring a nodular low power appearance.[98]

In addition to the clinical and histologic findings common to all low-grade B-cell MALT-lymphomas just described, there are also organ-specific differences. For example, lymphoid tissue is not normally present in the stomach. However, benign MALT is acquired and is commonly associated with *Helicobacter pylori* infection.[99] It seems likely that *H. pylori* induces benign MALT and predisposes to the development of low-grade B-cell lymphoma. Recent reports also have shown that benign MALT and low-grade B-cell lymphomas of gastric MALT may regress following antibiotic therapy appropriate for *H. pylori*.[100]

In the normal adult lung, MALT tissue is also poorly developed and inflammatory conditions usually precede the development of low-grade B-cell MALT-lymphoma of the lung. Two diseases frequently are associated with these tumors, Sjögren's syndrome and lymphoid interstitial pneumonia.[101] Similarly, low-grade B-cell MALT-lymphomas of the thyroid gland are usually associated with Hashimoto's thyroiditis.[102]

As described earlier in this chapter, low-grade B-cell MALT-lymphomas of the salivary gland are preceded by and arise in myoepithelial sialadenitis (MESA)/benign lymphoepithelial lesion (BLEL) and present most often as a result of Sjögren's syndrome (see Fig. 12–17).[9, 11] In general, low-grade MALT-lymphomas are more extensive than MESA/BLEL. In many cases, however, the distinction between MESA/BLEL and low-grade lymphoma is not possible without immunohistochemical methods.

Immunophenotypic studies have shown that low-grade B-cell lymphomas of MALT express monotypic Ig light chain ($\kappa > \lambda$), usually IgM, and pan-B-cell antigens.[59, 60] These tumors typically do not express IgD, the B cell–associated antigens CD10, CD21, or CD23, or T-cell antigens including CD5.

Molecular studies typically reveal Ig heavy and light chain gene rearrangements with *TCR* genes usually in the germline configuration.[63] Known B-cell oncogenes are not involved in MALT-lymphomas. There is limited information regarding the presence of chromosomal abnormalities. FISH studies have shown trisomy 3 in approximately half of low-grade B-cell MALT-lymphomas.[103] Rare MALT-lymphomas have been reported with a t(1;14)(p22;q32) or t(11;18)(q21;q21).[104, 105]

Treatment and Prognosis. Patients with localized low-grade B-cell lymphoma have a very indolent clinical course. Retrospective studies of patients with lesions interpreted as benign pseudolymphoma have identified cases of MALT-lymphoma treated only with surgical excision or localized radiation therapy with benign long-term follow-up.

However, patients with disseminated MALT-lymphoma behave similarly to patients with disseminated nodal low-grade B-cell lymphoma and are usually treated with chemotherapy.[91]

Both low-grade and high-grade lymphomas arising in MALT have been recognized. A low-grade component may be associated with a high-grade MALT-lymphoma, suggesting histologic progression.[96] Patients with high-grade large B-cell MALT-lymphoma have an aggressive neoplasm that behaves similarly to nodal diffuse large B-cell lymphoma and that requires chemotherapy.

Mantle Cell Lymphoma

The term *mantle cell lymphoma* (MCL) is now accepted as the most appropriate name for a tumor previously known as intermediate lymphocytic lymphoma, lymphocytic lymphoma of intermediate differentiation, centrocytic lymphoma, and mantle zone lymphoma.[59] In the Working Formulation, these tumors fit best within the diffuse small cleaved cell category.[58]

Clinical Features. Patients with MCL are usually elderly with generalized disease. In one study, the median age was 58 years and the male:female ratio was approximately 3:1.[106] Most patients have generalized lymphadenopathy (96%) and bone marrow involvement (87%) and the liver (55%) and spleen (57%) are commonly involved. An absolute peripheral blood lymphocytosis of more than 4000/mm^3 is uncommon, found in approximately 10% of patients.[106] Extranodal sites of involvement are common, found in 25% to 50% of patients, usually in association with nodal involvement. The extranodal sites most commonly involved are the gastrointestinal tract, Waldeyer's ring, and breast. Patients with gastrointestinal tract involvement may present with numerous polyps involving the stomach, small intestine, and colon. This presentation is referred to in the literature as multiple lymphomatous polyposis of the intestine.[107]

Pathologic Features. The diagnosis of MCL is most reliably made by examination of a lymph node biopsy specimen.[108–110] The lymph node architecture is replaced by a diffuse or vaguely nodular neoplasm (Figs. 12–19 and 12–20, see p. 746). In some cases, a mantle zone pattern results from the neoplasm selectively involving the follicle mantle zones surrounding central benign germinal centers (Fig. 12–21, see p. 747). Cytologically, MCL is composed of a monotonous population of small lymphoid cells with slightly to clearly irregular nuclear contours (Fig. 12–22, see p. 747). Although a group of MCLs includes tumor cells exhibiting a wide spectrum of nuclear irregularities, in an individual neoplasm, all of the tumor cells are remarkably similar. Large lymphoid cells are absent or rare. Other histologic findings common in MCLs include numerous eosinophilic epithelioid histiocytes (see Fig. 12–22) and germinal centers completely surrounded by tumor without a normal lymphoid cuff (so-called "naked" germinal centers). Pseudofollicular growth centers and plasmacytoid differentiation are not found in MCLs.[108–110]

A subset of MCLs are characterized by slightly larger lymphoid cells with finely dispersed nuclear chromatin and numerous mitotic figures (Fig. 12–23, see p. 747). These neoplasms are thought to

Text continued on page 753

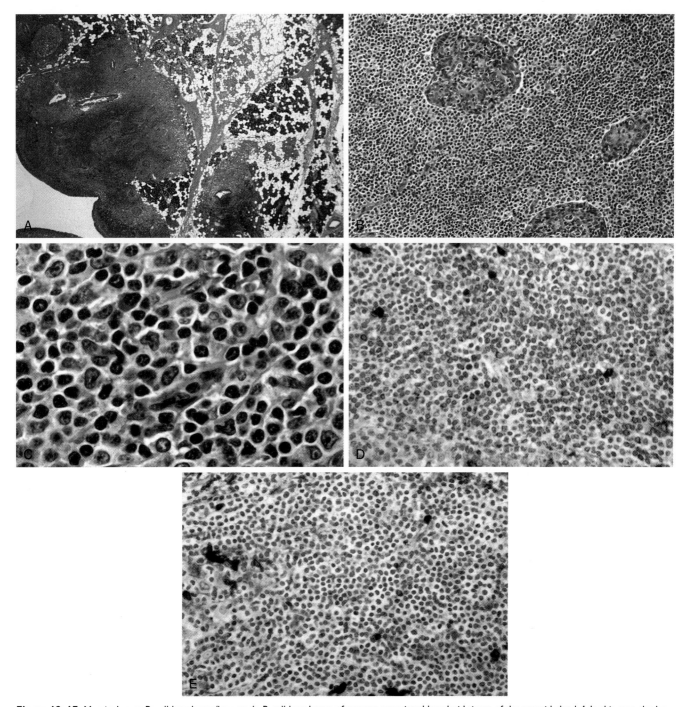

Figure 12–17. Marginal zone B-cell lymphoma/low-grade B-cell lymphoma of mucosa-associated lymphoid tissue of the parotid gland. *A,* In this case the lymphoid infiltrate forms a large mass replacing parotid gland parenchyma. *B,* Within the mass, lymphoepithelial lesions are present surrounded by an extensive infiltrate of small lymphoid cells with increased pale cytoplasm. *C,* The neoplastic cell population is heterogeneous and is composed of small lymphoid cells that are round, small lymphoid cells with slight plasmacytoid differentiation, small lymphoid cells with irregular nuclear contours, and occasional large lymphoid cells. The neoplastic cells expressed monotypic immunoglobulin κ light chain. *D,* Immunoglobulin κ light chain. *E,* Immunoglobulin λ light chain. (*D* and *E,* immunoperoxidase with hematoxylin counterstain.)

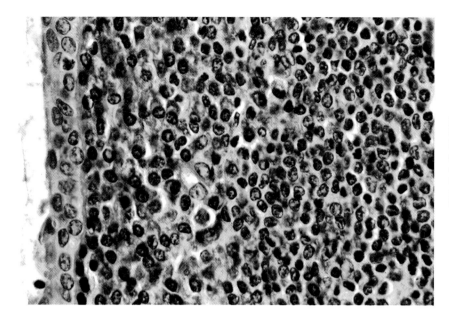

Figure 12–18. Marginal zone B-cell lymphoma/low-grade B-cell lymphoma of mucosa-associated lymphoid tissue of the conjunctiva. In this case, the subepithelial tumor cells exhibited extensive plasmacytoid differentiation, whereas the remainder of the tumor was composed of nonplasmacytoid small lymphoid cells. Both populations of cells expressed monotypic immunoglobulin κ light chain.

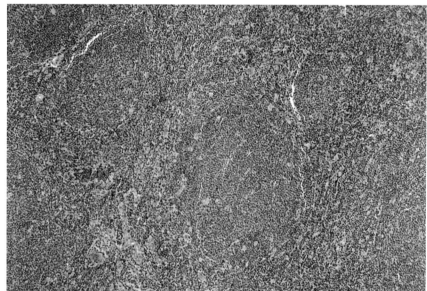

Figure 12–19. Mantle cell lymphoma, nodular pattern. The neoplasm is vaguely nodular at this power.

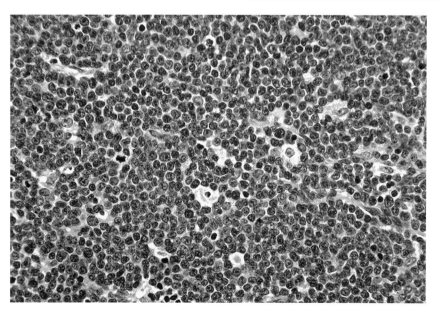

Figure 12–20. Mantle cell lymphoma, diffuse pattern. The neoplasm is diffuse, and, at this power, scattered "pink" histiocytes can be found. The tumor cell population is a monotonous population of small lymphoid cells with irregular nuclear contours, hyperchromatic nuclei, and small nucleoli.

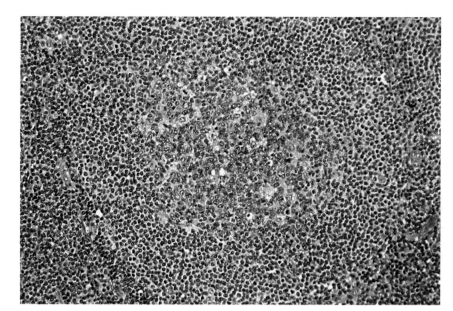

Figure 12–21. Mantle cell lymphoma, mantle zone pattern. In this case, the neoplasm involves the mantle zone, sparing a central reactive germinal center.

Figure 12–22. Mantle cell lymphoma. The neoplastic cells are monotonous with irregular nuclear contours. A benign histiocyte with eosinophilic cytoplasm (top center) is present.

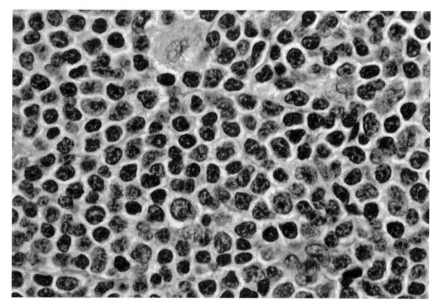

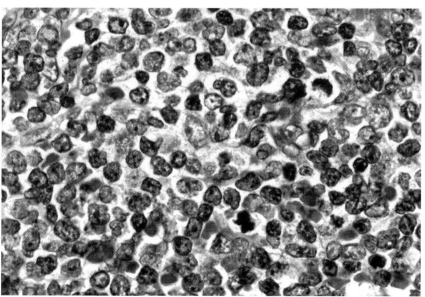

Figure 12–23. Mantle cell lymphoma, blastic variant. In this case, the neoplastic cells are slightly larger than those shown in Figure 12–22, with fine, blastic nuclear chromatin and an increased mitotic rate.

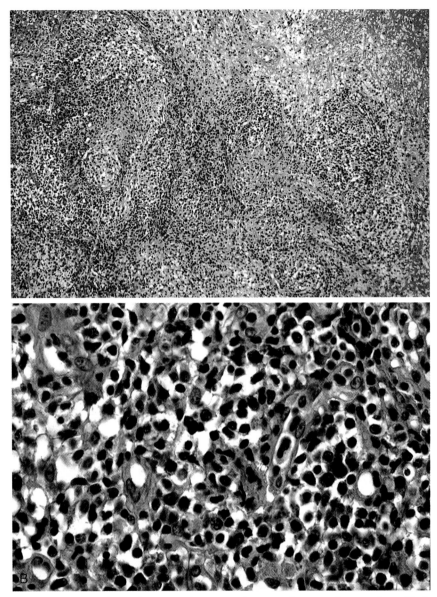

Figure 12–32. *A,* Nasal T cell/natural killer cell lymphoma showing zonal necrosis with tumor cells surrounding a small vessel in the upper portion of the figure. *B,* On higher magnification, the neoplastic infiltrate shows some variability in cell size with many cells having clear cytoplasm.

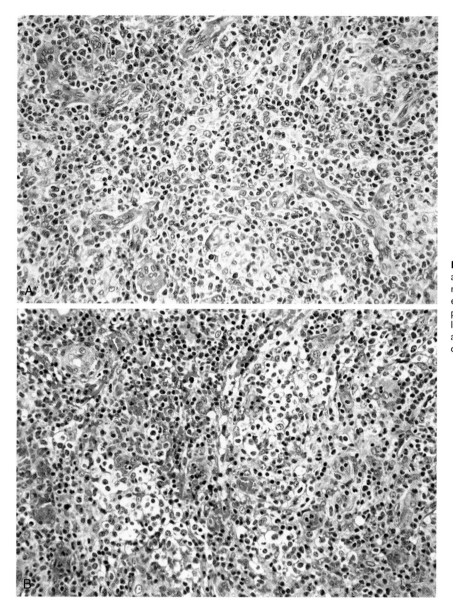

Figure 12–33. *A,* Angioimmunoblastic lymphadenopathy (AILD) showing effacement of the normal lymph node architecture. There is prominent vascular proliferation and a mixture of cells, including histiocytes, plasma cells, immunoblasts, and eosinophils. *B,* AILD-like T-cell lymphoma has similar cytologic features but also contains clusters of immunoblasts with abundant clear cytoplasm.

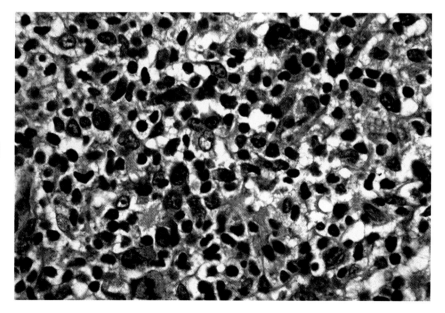

Figure 12–34. Adult T-cell lymphoma demonstrating great variation in nuclear size and shape of the tumor cells.

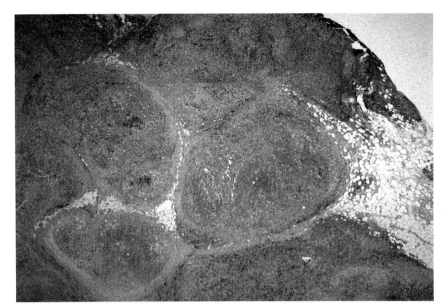

Figure 12–36. Nodular sclerosis Hodgkin's disease. At low magnification, broad bands of fibrosis are seen.

Figure 12–38. Mixed cellularity Hodgkin's disease. A, Scattered binucleate Reed-Sternberg cells and mononuclear variants of Reed-Sternberg cells are present with a background cellular population of lymphocytes, histiocytes, and eosinophils. B, The Hodgkin's cells express the CD30 antigen. (Immunoperoxidase with hematoxylin counterstain).

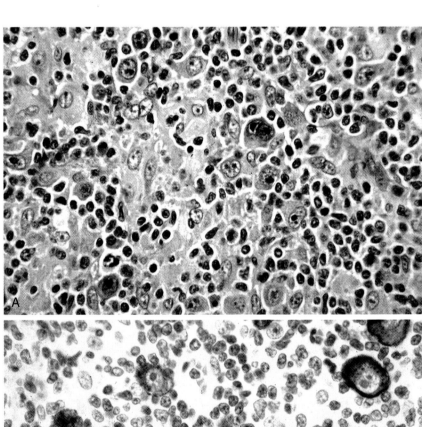

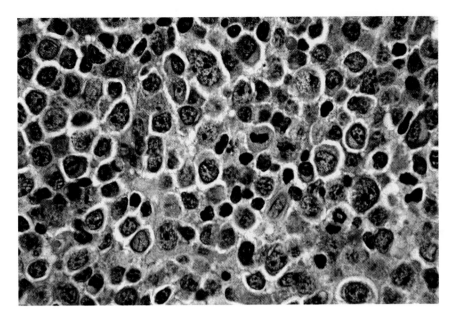

Figure 12–39. Plasmacytoma of the eyelid showing eccentric cytoplasm and moderately differentiated nuclear features.

Figure 12–41. Langerhans' cell histiocytosis in a patient with B-cell lymphoma. The cells have abundant eosinophilic cytoplasm with indented or grooved nuclei. Intermixed eosinophils are also present.

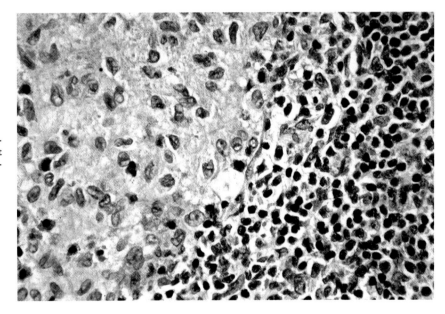

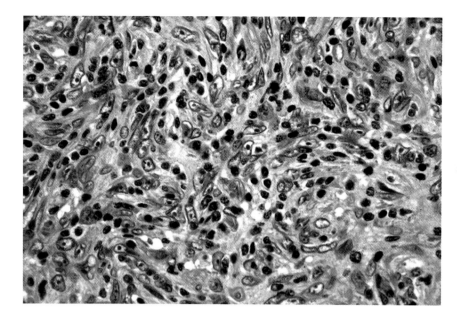

Figure 12–42. Follicular dendritic cell tumor with spindled tumor cells and scattered lymphocytes.

Figure 12–43. True histiocytic lymphoma. The tumors cells have eosinophilic cytoplasm and variably sized nuclei with nucleoli. The tumor demonstrated no evidence of B- or T-cell lineage.

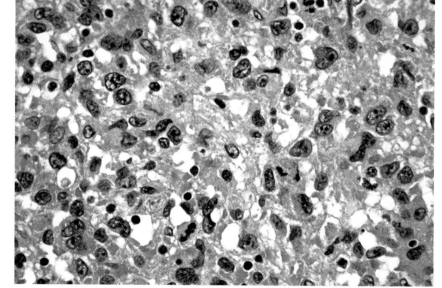

have a more aggressive clinical course, are most likely transformed from more typical MCL, and have been designated the blastic or blastoid variant of MCL.[109, 110] In one study of serially biopsied cases, blastic transformation occurred in 17% of patients.[111]

Immunophenotypic studies have demonstrated that MCLs express monotypic Ig light chain ($\kappa > \lambda$). The neoplastic cells also express IgM, IgD, pan-B-cell antigens, alkaline phosphatase, and the pan-T-cell antigen CD5.[59, 60] Mantle cell lymphomas are typically negative for the CD10 and CD23 antigens. This immunophenotype is very similar to the immunophenotype of normal mantle zone B lymphocytes. These tumors also express Ig and B-cell antigens with intermediate to high cell surface density.[60]

Mantle cell lymphomas have rearrangements of the Ig heavy and light chain genes, whereas the *TCR* genes are usually in the germline configuration.[63] The t(11;14)(q13;q32), as shown by conventional cytogenetic studies, is found more frequently in MCL than in other types of NHL.[112] Furthermore, rearrangements of the *bcl*-1 locus on chromosome 11q13, presumptive molecular evidence of the t(11;14), have been identified in over 75% of MCLs using Southern blot analysis.[113, 114] In this translocation, the *bcl*-1 gene (also known as *PRAD*-1 or *CCDNK*) is dysregulated. The *bcl*-1 gene is located 130 kb 5' of the breakpoint cluster region and encodes for cyclin D1.[115] Thus, the translocation results in overexpression of cyclin D1 that can be demonstrated using either Northern blot analysis or immunohistochemical methods.[115, 116] Cyclin D1 protein, via its interactions with other proteins such as cyclin-dependent kinases 4 and 6 and the retinoblastoma gene product, interact with the cell cycle at the transition from G1 to S phase.

Differential Diagnosis. The differential diagnosis of MCL includes other B-cell neoplasms composed of small lymphoid cells, in particular CLL/SLL and grade I FCL (predominantly small cleaved cell). Unlike CLL/SLL, MCLs lack pseudofollicular growth centers and are composed of a relatively monotonous population of small lymphoid cells. The characteristic mixture of small round cells, prolymphocytes, and paraimmunoblasts is absent in MCL. Immunophenotypic studies of CLL/SLL and MCL are similar, as both tumors express monotypic Ig, B-cell antigens, and CD5. However, MCL is usually CD23-negative, in contrast with approximately 75% of CLL/SLL. The t(11;14) is rare in CLL/SLL and common in MCL. Unlike FCLs, which always contain large noncleaved lymphoid cells, large cells are invariably absent in MCL. Follicular center lymphomas are also commonly CD10 positive and carry the t(14;18), uncommon findings in MCL.

Treatment and Prognosis. Currently, there is no optimal therapy for MCL. Recent studies have shown that MCLs combine the worst features of low-grade and intermediate-grade B-cell lymphomas. Patients present with generalized disease and their disease is incurable, similar to low-grade B-cell lymphomas. However, the median survival of patients with MCLs is much shorter than for other low-grade B-cell lymphoma types, more in keeping with intermediate-grade B-cell lymphomas.[91, 117] For example, in one study, the median survival of patients with MCL was 45 months.[117] Patient survival also correlates with the pattern of lymph node involvement.[108, 109, 118] Patients with a mantle zone pattern of lymph node involvement have significantly better survival than those patients with nodular or diffuse patterns of involvement in lymph nodes.

Diffuse Large B-Cell Lymphoma

The category of diffuse large B-cell lymphoma, as defined in the REAL classification, includes B-cell neoplasms previously designated as diffuse mixed small and large cell, diffuse large cleaved or noncleaved cell, and large cell immunoblastic in the Working Formulation.[59] Because these Working Formulation categories were heterogeneous and included B-cell and T-cell tumors with a variety of molecular abnormalities, the REAL classification separates B-cell and T-cell neoplasms, specifies a number of distinctive T-cell neo-

plasms (discussed subsequently), and collapses the B-cell tumors into one group termed *diffuse large B-cell lymphoma* (DLBCL).

Clinical Features. DLBCLs mainly occur in adults, with a median age in the sixth decade. Men are affected slightly more often than women.[58, 59] Although less common in children, DLBCLs also represent 15% to 20% of childhood non-Hodgkin's lymphomas. Patients often present with disease limited to one side of the diaphragm. Nodal presentation is most common, but these tumors frequently involve a variety of extranodal sites, in 40% to 50% of patients.[58] Approximately half of patients present with clinical stage III or IV disease. Diffuse large B-cell lymphomas, particularly in extranodal sites, commonly grow as large masses, often with extensive necrosis. Bone marrow involvement is uncommon, occurring in approximately 10% of patients. Diffuse large B-cell lymphomas not uncommonly involve privileged sites such as the testis and central nervous system.

Pathologic Features. Histologically, DLBCLs are composed of neoplastic cells with nuclei greater in size than the nuclei of benign macrophages; the latter are virtually always present admixed within lymphomas. Mitotic figures are usually numerous.[58, 59] Cytologically, the neoplastic cells can exhibit a spectrum of findings (Figs. 12–24, 12–25, and 12–26). Large cleaved cells range from 13 to 30 μm in size and have irregular or cleaved nuclear contours, relatively small nucleoli, and a thin rim of eosinophilic cytoplasm.[58, 59, 119] Sclerosis often accompanies tumors with many large cleaved cells, particularly in tumors involving extranodal sites. Large noncleaved lymphoid cells are 20 to 30 μm in size and have round or oval vesicular nuclei with two to three nucleoli and more abundant amphophilic cytoplasm. Often one nucleolus is centrally located and one or two nucleoli are peripherally apposed adjacent to the nuclear membrane. Mitotic figures are more common in large noncleaved cell as compared with large cleaved cell lymphomas. Immunoblasts are larger than large noncleaved cells with an eccentrically located vesicular round or oval nucleus containing a promi-

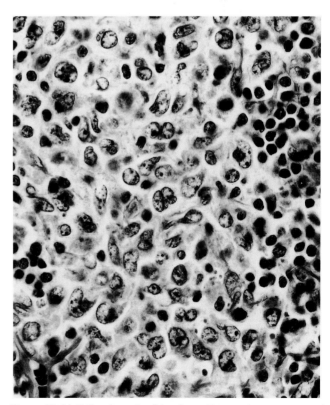

Figure 12–24. Diffuse large B-cell lymphoma. This neoplasm is composed predominantly of large cleaved cells with irregular nuclear contours and small nucleoli.

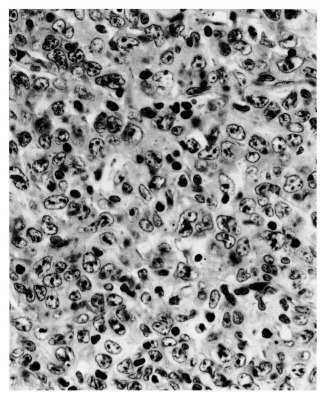

Figure 12–25. Diffuse large B-cell lymphoma. This neoplasm is composed of large noncleaved cells with vesicular nuclei with two or three small nucleoli. Occasional large cleaved cells and immunoblasts are present.

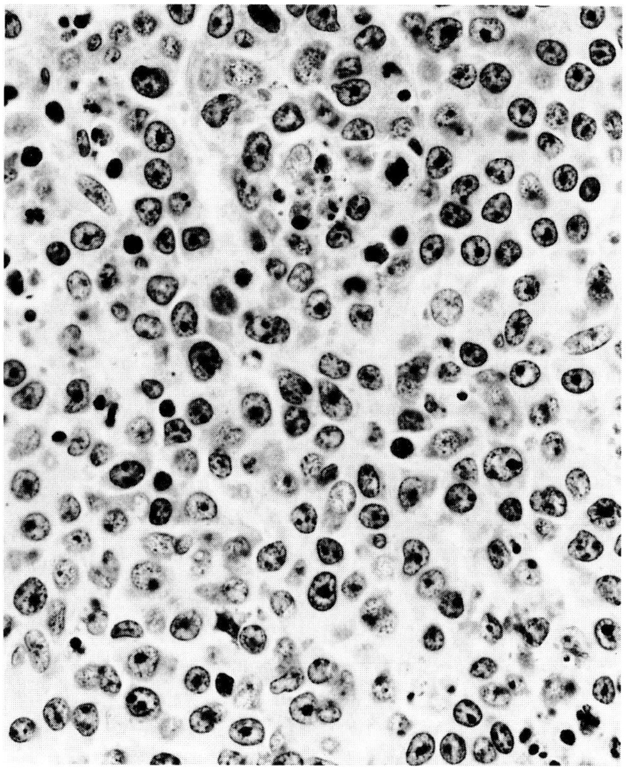

Figure 12–26. Diffuse large B-cell lymphoma. This neoplasm is composed predominantly of immunoblasts, each with a central prominent nucleolus.

nent, "target-like" central nucleolus and abundant amphophilic cytoplasm.

Although the descriptions of large cleaved and noncleaved cells and immunoblasts are distinctive, and many neoplastic large B cells fit within these descriptions, it is also true that neoplastic large cells exhibit a spectrum of differentiation and often have intermediate cytologic features. Furthermore, DLBCLs are commonly composed of a mixture of these cell types.[59]

Immunophenotypic studies have shown that these tumors are of mature B-cell lineage.[59, 60] Approximately two thirds of cases express monotypic Ig light chain ($\kappa > \lambda$), and IgM is the most common Ig heavy chain. However, a subset of cases express IgA or IgG; IgD is usually negative. Approximately one third of DLBCLs do not express surface or cytoplasmic immunoglobulins. Plasmacytoid lymphomas commonly express monotypic cytoplasmic Ig. These tumors express pan-B-cell antigens, a subset are CD10-positive, and they are negative for T-cell antigens. The majority of diffuse large B-cell lymphomas express activation markers and have a high rate of proliferation.

Diffuse large B-cell lymphomas have rearrangements of the Ig genes, and the *TCR* genes are usually in the germline configuration.[63] A subset of cases carry the t(14;18) as shown by conventional cytogenetic studies. Furthermore, the *bcl*-2 gene is rearranged in approximately 20% of cases. In these cases, the Ig heavy chain gene and *bcl*-2 gene rearrangements usually co-migrate, indicating the presence of the t(14;18)(q32;q21); these tumors may represent diffuse progression of an occult follicular lymphoma.[79, 120]

Another subset of DLBCLs have translocations or other abnormalities involving chromosome 3q27.[121, 122] This locus is the site of the *bcl*-6 gene, a zinc finger-encoding gene and candidate oncogene. The *bcl*-6 gene is rearranged in approximately 20% to 40% of these tumors, more often in extranodal neoplasms.[122]

Differential Diagnosis. Diffuse large B-cell lymphoma can be most easily confused with Burkitt's lymphoma, Burkitt-like lymphoma, and large cell lymphomas composed of T cells. Unlike DL-

BCL, Burkitt's lymphomas usually have a marked starry sky pattern and a cohesive low power appearance, and the tumors' cell nuclei are smaller, approximately the size of benign histiocyte nuclei. The nuclei of Burkitt's lymphoma cells are also distinctive, with coarsely clumped chromatin and two to five distinct nucleoli. The distinction between DLBCL and Burkitt-like high-grade B-cell lymphomas is more difficult. The nuclei in these diseases are similar. Burkitt-like lymphomas have smaller tumor cells, but there are cases of malignant lymphoma in which the tumor cells exhibit a spectrum of sizes, from small noncleaved (intermediate size) to large noncleaved, and this distinction can be arbitrary. A marked starry-sky pattern and a high mitotic rate favor the diagnosis of Burkitt-like high-grade B-cell lymphoma. Diffuse large-cell lymphomas of B-cell and T-cell lineage can be morphologically indistinguishable, and therefore immunophenotypic studies are recommended for this distinction. In general, T-cell large-cell lymphomas more often have a heterogeneous background inflammatory cell infiltrate, including eosinophils, plasma cells, and histiocytes, and exhibit vascular proliferation.

Treatment and Prognosis. If untreated, DLBCLs are invariably fatal, and most patients survive less than 2 years. However, these neoplasms are susceptible to chemotherapy with a significant chance for cure, particularly for patients with localized disease.[123] With newer chemotherapy regimens, complete response rates of over 80% have been reported.[123] Molecular studies have confirmed earlier suspicions that DLBCLs probably represent a number of different tumor types. For example, patients with de novo diffuse large B-cell lymphoma with *bcl*-2 gene rearrangement have an increased tendency to relapse than do patients with histologically similar tumors without *bcl*-2 rearrangement, more akin to the behavior of tumors of follicular center origin.[120] Diffuse large B-cell lymphomas that carry *bcl*-6 gene rearrangements appear to be a second subset. Patients with these tumors have improved survival and freedom from disease progression as compared with patients with DLBCLs that lack *bcl*-6 gene rearrangements.[122]

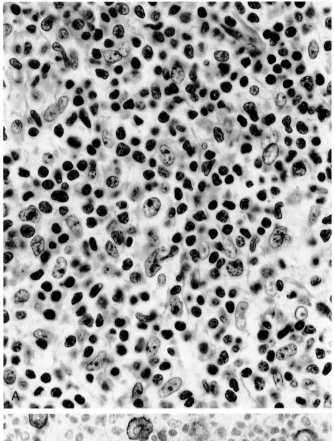

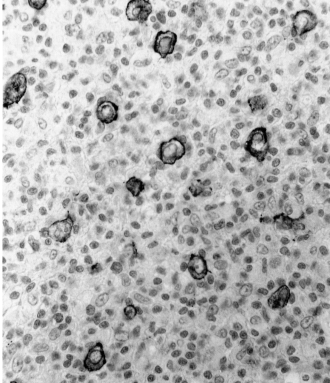

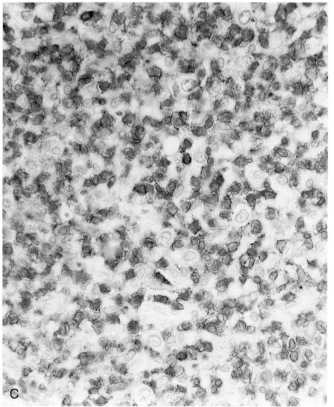

Figure 12–27. T-cell–rich B-cell lymphoma (diffuse large B-cell lymphoma). *A,* The architecture is replaced by a heterogeneous infiltrate composed of many small benign cells and a relatively small number of large tumors cells. *B* and *C,* The large cells are B cells positive for the CD20 antigen (*B,* L26), and the small cells are T cells positive for the CD45RO antigen (*C,* UCHL-1). (*B* and *C,* immunoperoxidase with hematoxylin counterstain.)

T-Cell–Rich B-Cell Lymphoma

T-cell–rich B-cell lymphomas (TCRBCLs) are malignant B-cell lymphomas in which the vast majority of cells found in the biopsy specimen are reactive T cells.[124–126] The predominance of T cells in these tumors may lead to an erroneous assessment of T-cell lineage,

and, in the past, many of these cases were classified as diffuse mixed small and large cell lymphomas of T-cell lineage.[125]

Clinical Features. Patients with TCRBCLs are similar to patients with DLBCLs. In one study, the median age was 53 years with a slight male predominance.[126] Splenomegaly and advanced clinical stage may be more common in TCRBCL patients than in DLBCL patients.[126]

Pathologic Features. T-cell–rich B-cell lymphomas are diffuse and are composed predominantly of small cytologically bland T cells (Fig. 12–27).[124–126] Numerous benign histiocytes may also be present. Within this infiltrate, often representing less than 5% to 10% of all cells, are scattered large, cytologically atypical lymphoid cells of B-cell lineage.

Owing to the small size of the neoplastic cell population, it is often difficult to demonstrate monotypic Ig light chain expression. However, the large cells are B cells that express a variety of pan-B-cell antigens. Southern blot hybridization and polymerase chain reaction studies have shown that these tumors contain Ig heavy and light chain gene rearrangements with TCR genes in the germline configuration. A subset of TCRBCLs have the t(14;18) or *bcl*-2 gene rearrangements.[124, 125]

Differential Diagnosis. The differential diagnosis of TCRBCL includes Hodgkin's disease and peripheral T-cell lymphoma. Unlike mixed cellularity Hodgkin's disease, the neoplastic large cells in TCRBCL usually resemble large noncleaved lymphoid cells. These cells are rarely binucleated or have large eosinophilic nucleoli, as occur in Reed-Sternberg cells.

Immunohistochemical studies are helpful. The neoplastic cells in TCRBCL are positive for CD45 and CD20 and are negative for CD15, CD30, and Epstein-Barr virus, as is common in mixed cellularity Hodgkin's disease. The distinction between TCRBCL and lymphocytic predominance Hodgkin's disease can be difficult. Since TCRBCLs are diffuse, the nodularity of nodular lymphocytic predominance Hodgkin's disease is very helpful. The distinction between TCRBCL and the diffuse form of lymphocytic predominance Hodgkin's disease can be impossible. Older age, widespread disease, and the presence of Ig gene rearrangements favors the diagnosis of TCRBCL. Unlike peripheral T-cell lymphoma, the large and cytologically atypical lymphoid cells in TCRBCL are B-cells. Large atypical B-cells are rare in peripheral T-cell lymphomas.

Treatment and Prognosis. It seems likely that TCRBCL is an unusual histologic manifestation of DLBCL rather than a distinct clinicopathologic entity.[124, 126, 127] Patients with TCRBCL respond to therapy in a manner similar to those with DLBCL.[126, 127] Furthermore, patients with TCRBCL may have a history of follicular lymphoma or, following treatment, may relapse with histologically typical follicular lymphoma or DLBCL.[124]

Malignant Lymphoma, Diffuse, Mixed Small and Large Cell

The category of malignant lymphoma, diffuse, mixed small and large cell, as described in the Working Formulation is particularly heterogeneous and is composed of a variety of neoplasms of mature B-cell and T-cell lineage.[58] Thus, in the REAL classification, the diffuse mixed small and large cell category is omitted and the neoplasms that would fit in this category are placed in other, more homogeneous categories.[59] Whether this proposal will be accepted is currently uncertain.

Burkitt's Lymphoma

The late British surgeon Denis Burkitt first described a form of lymphoma that he observed as a large jaw mass in children from Uganda. He was describing the endemic form of the disease. It is now known that Burkitt's lymphomas may be divided into three groups: endemic (African), sporadic (nonendemic), and HIV-associated.[128]

Clinical Features. Endemic Burkitt's lymphoma was first described in equatorial Africa, where it occurs in a region 15 degrees latitude north or south of the equator. Evidence of Epstein-Barr virus (EBV) infection is present in approximately 95% of patients. The

median age of patients with endemic Burkitt's lymphoma is 7 years, with a male:female ratio of 3:1. The jaw is the best known site of disease, involving the maxilla or mandible in 60% of patients, but large abdominal masses involving retroperitoneal structures, the gastrointestinal tract, or the gonads are also common.

Sporadic Burkitt's lymphomas occur in industrialized nations. EBV infection is present in a subset of patients, approximately 25%.[128] Patients affected are usually in the second or third decades of life, with a male:female ratio of 3:1. The jaw is infrequently involved and most patients present with large abdominal masses, frequently involving the ileocecal region of the bowel. Other sites commonly involved include abdominal and peripheral lymph nodes, pleura, and pharynx. Bone marrow and central nervous system involvement are uncommon at presentation. However, in approximately 10% to 20% of cases, the bone marrow and central nervous system are involved later in the clinical course. Leukemia may occur, usually as a terminal event. In addition, a small subset of patients who present with acute lymphoblastic leukemia, designated L3 in the French-American-British classification, have disease that is biologically similar to sporadic Burkitt's lymphoma.[59] HIV-associated Burkitt's lymphomas commonly involve extranodal and nodal sites.[129]

Pathologic Features. Endemic Burkitt's lymphoma, sporadic Burkitt's lymphoma, and Burkitt's lymphoma associated with acquired immunodeficiency syndrome are histologically indistinguishable (Fig. 12–28). The essential feature in these tumors is that neoplastic cells have nuclei equal to in size or smaller than the nuclei of benign macrophages.[130, 131] At low power, the neoplasms grow as expansile masses that diffusely infiltrate contiguous tissues. Reactive macrophages are almost always scattered throughout the tumor. The relatively clear cytoplasm of the histiocytes in a background of blue tumor cells imparts a starry-sky appearance. This pattern results from rapid cell turnover with individual cell necrosis and scavenging of debris by macrophages. The tumor cells are ovoid and of uniform shape with prominent nuclear membranes, coarse nuclear chromatin, and two to five basophilic nucleoli. Mitotic figures are numerous.

Immunophenotypic studies of the three types of Burkitt's lymphomas are similar. These tumors are of mature B-cell lineage and express monotypic Ig light chain ($\kappa > \lambda$), IgM, pan-B-cell antigens, and the CD10 antigen.[59, 60] Virtually all of the cells in Burkitt's lymphomas are proliferating. These tumors are negative for IgD, the CD21 and CD23 antigens, and T-cell antigens including CD5.

Burkitt's lymphomas have Ig heavy and light chain gene rearrangements; the TCR genes are usually in the germline configuration.[63] Approximately 75% of cases carry the t(8;14)(q24;q32), with the remaining cases having one of two variant translocations, the t(2;8)(p11;q24) or the t(8;22)(q24;q11).[132] Common to each of these translocations is the involvement of chromosome 8q24, the site of the c-*myc* oncogene. Via these translocations, the c-*myc* oncogene is juxtaposed with either the Ig heavy chain (14q32), Igκ (2p13), or the Igλ (22q11) gene loci, resulting in c-*myc* dysregulation. Increased C-MYC protein drives cell proliferation.[132]

Molecular studies have confirmed prior serologic studies that showed evidence of EBV infection. Approximately 90% to 95% of endemic, 50% of HIV-associated, and 25% of sporadic Burkitt's lymphomas contain EBV.[128] The EBV is episomal, consistent with latent infection. The virus is often present in multiple copies per cell and is monoclonal, indicating that the virus is present prior to neoplastic transformation.[128, 133] EBV alone, however, is not sufficient to cause Burkitt's lymphoma. Other cofactors are probably operative.[128]

Treatment and Prognosis. The high frequency of extranodal sites of disease in patients with Burkitt's lymphoma makes clinical or pathologic stage as determined using traditional staging systems of less prognostic value than schemes that assess either tumor burden or amenability to surgical excision.[134] Prognostic features in Burkitt's lymphoma generally correlate with tumor burden, such as high serum lactate dehydrogenase levels. Since the tumor is widely

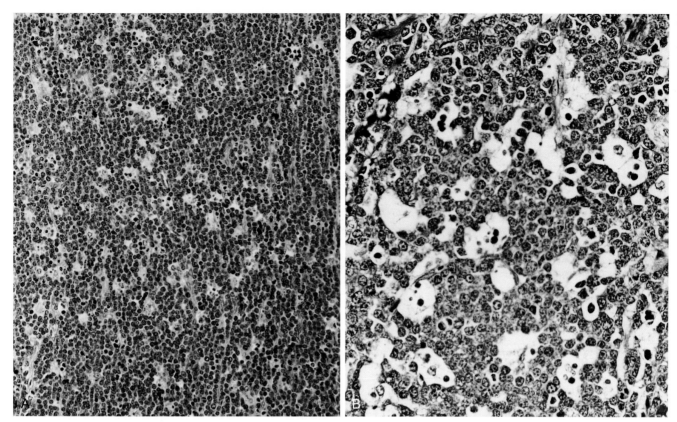

Figure 12–28. Burkitt's lymphoma. *A,* The neoplasm is diffuse with a prominent starry-sky pattern. *B,* The neoplastic cells are monotonous, approximately the size of benign histiocyte nuclei, and have clumped nuclear chromatin with two to five small nucleoli.

distributed at the time of initial presentation, the role of radiation therapy is limited.[128] Systemic chemotherapy is the treatment of choice, and Burkitt's lymphomas respond dramatically. With combination chemotherapy regimens, approximately 80% of patients including those with high-stage disease may respond completely and have long-term survival.[134, 135] Patients with HIV-associated Burkitt's lymphoma also respond well to combination chemotherapy, providing that their underlying immunodeficiency syndrome allows for adequate therapy.

High-Grade B-Cell Lymphoma, Burkitt-Like

High-grade B-cell Burkitt-like lymphomas are designated as small noncleaved cell, non-Burkitt's type in the Working Formulation.[58] Currently, this is a provisional category in the REAL classification.[60]

Clinical Features. Patients with high-grade B-cell Burkitt-like lymphoma are predominantly adults.[131, 136] The male:female ratio is approximately 2:1. Lymph nodes are involved more frequently than extranodal sites, although extranodal sites are involved commonly. Waldeyer's ring and the bone marrow are involved more often than in patients with Burkitt's lymphomas.[131, 136] In adults, these clinical features are more similar to those of DLBCLs than they are to those of Burkitt's lymphomas.

Pathologic Features and Differential Diagnosis. Burkitt-like lymphomas are diffuse, often have a starry-sky pattern, and have a high proliferation rate with numerous mitotic figures. However, the neoplastic cells cytologically have features intermediate between Burkitt's lymphoma cells and the cells of DLBCLs. In particular, the neoplastic cells are of intermediate size, as is the case in Burkitt' lymphomas, but there is greater nuclear pleomorphism and the nuclear chromatin is more vesicular with more prominent nucleoli, similar to DLBCLs.[59, 137–139]

Immunophenotypic studies have demonstrated that these tumors are of mature B-cell lineage and express monotypic Ig light chain ($\kappa > \lambda$), IgM, and pan-B-cell antigens.[59, 60] Molecular studies have shown Ig heavy and light chain gene rearrangements with germline *TCR* genes in most cases.[66, 133] The *bcl*-2 gene is rearranged in up to 30% of tumors, c-*myc* rearrangements are rare, and EBV may be present in a minority of tumors.[133] These immunophenotypic and molecular findings are similar to those of DLBCLs.

This group of tumors in the Revised European-American Classification may not represent a true biologic entity and may not be histologically reproducible.[59] A subset of these neoplasms may represent the most aggressive end of the spectrum of DLBCLs, whereas others may be more akin to Burkitt's lymphoma.

Treatment and Prognosis. Irrespective of origin, high-grade Burkitt-like B-cell lymphomas are responsive to combination chemotherapy with potential for cure.[136] Since the distinction between Burkitt's lymphoma and Burkitt-like lymphoma can be difficult, it is important to remember the patient's age. In adults, the difference between true Burkitt's lymphomas and Burkitt-like lymphomas is important for some chemotherapy protocols. In children, however, Burkitt's lymphomas and high-grade B-cell Burkitt-like lymphomas have similar biologic behavior.[137, 138]

Precursor Lymphoblastic Lymphoma/ Leukemia

The category of precursor lymphoblastic lymphoma/leukemia in the REAL classification includes neoplasms designated as malignant lymphoma, lymphoblastic in the Working Formulation as well as acute lymphoblastic leukemia (ALL).[58] Since lymphoblastic lymphoma shares many clinical, histologic, and immunologic features with ALL, these entities appear to represent different clinical manifestations of the same disease. These tumors can be further divided into precursor B-cell and precursor T-cell types. Approximately 10% to 20% of lymphoblastic lymphomas and 80% to 90% of ALLs are of B-cell lineage. By contrast, 80% to 90% of lymphoblastic lymphomas and 10% to 20% of ALLs are of T-cell type.[59, 139]

Precursor B-Cell

Clinical Features. The majority of patients with precursor B-cell lymphoblastic lymphoma/leukemia (LBL) are children who present with ALL. Lymphadenopathy may occur but is usually not prominent. A subset of patients may present with clinical findings more in keeping with lymphoma, and these patients may present with unusual sites of disease including subdiaphragmatic lymph nodes, skin (Fig. 12–29), and bones.[58] Rarely, patients with precursor B-cell LBL present with a mediastinal mass.[139]

Pathologic Features. The normal lymph node architecture is replaced by a diffuse, relatively uniform proliferation of small cells that often stream out into perinodal tissues. The neoplastic cells have scant cytoplasm and nuclei with fine nuclear chromatin that may be either convoluted or round (see Fig. 12–29). Mitotic figures are numerous. Owing to the high growth rate, a "starry-sky" pattern secondary to individual cell necrosis and scavenging by macrophages may be present in one third of cases. No histologic features correlate with immunophenotype.

Immunologic studies of precursor B-cell LBL best illustrate the concept that non-Hodgkin's lymphomas represent clonal expansions of cells frozen in a state of differentiation. This phenomenon allows one to deduce that a variety of antigens are acquired in sequence, most likely reflecting the sequence of expression by non-neoplastic lymphoid cells during development.

Precursor B-cell LBLs initially express the CD19 antigen, closely followed by the CD10 antigen (common acute lymphoblastic leukemia antigen). The CD22 and CD20 antigens are then acquired sequentially. These antigens are detectable in the cell cyto-plasm prior to expression on the cell surface. The tumor cells do not express surface Ig. "Pre-B-cell" LBLs express cytoplasmic IgM in addition to other B-cell antigens and originate from a B-cell precursor cell at a slightly later stage of development.[60] Prior to the availability of monoclonal antibodies, these neoplasms were referred to as having a "null cell" or "common" immunophenotype: Ig-negative and CD10-positive.

Gene rearrangement studies of precursor LBLs have contributed to our knowledge of gene rearrangements in neoplastic and (by inference) normal lymphocyte development.

Similar to surface antigen expression, the antigen receptor genes appear to rearrange sequentially, with a developmental hierarchy.[63] At the earliest stage of B-cell differentiation, the Ig heavy chain gene undergoes rearrangement. Then the Ig κ light chain gene rearranges. Only if neither Ig κ light chain gene allele is functionally rearranged, then the Ig λ light chain gene rearranges. This is the molecular mechanism that allows a given B cell to express only one Ig light chain (the principle of allelic exclusion).[140] Thus, precursor B-cell LBLs always contain Ig heavy chain gene rearrangements; more mature tumors also have Ig light chain gene rearrangements.[63, 141] Lineage infidelity (also known as lineage promiscuity) is also common in precursor B-cell LBLs. In other words, T-cell receptor (β, γ, or δ) gene rearrangements have been identified in up to 80% of precursor B-cell LBLs.[141]

Many translocations have been reported in precursor B-cell LBLs. The t(9;22), t(12;21), and t(1;19) and translocations involving 11q23 are most common.[142] The t(9;22)(q34;q11), also known as the Philadelphia chromosome, is one of the most common recurrent chromosomal translocations, detected in 5% of children and approximately 20% to 25% of adults with precursor B-cell ALL.[143] This translocation joins the c-*abl* gene at chromosome 9q34 with the *bcr* locus at 22q11. The result is a chimeric mRNA transcript that encodes a fusion gene with increased tyrosine kinase activity. Two types of the t(9;22) occur. In 25% to 50% of adults with ALL, the translocation is identical to that seen in chronic myeloid leukemia,

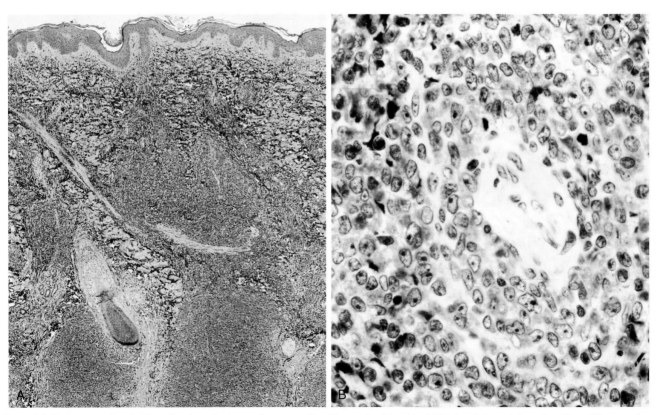

Figure 12–29. Precursor lymphoblastic lymphoma/leukemia of precursor B-cell lineage involving skin. *A*, The dermis is partially replaced by a diffuse neoplasm. *B*, The neoplasm is composed of small lymphoid cells with blastic nuclear chromatin and visible but inconspicuous nucleoli.

and the fusion protein is 210 kd, known as p210. In the remaining 50% to 75% of adults with ALL, the breakpoint on chromosome 22 occurs 100 kb 5' or upstream, resulting in a 190 kd fusion protein (p190) with higher tyrosine kinase activity and higher transforming capacity than p210.

Precursor B-cell LBL of "pre-B cell" (cytoplasmic IgM positive) type are commonly associated with the t(1;19) chromosomal translocation. In this translocation, the *E2A* gene on chromosome 1 is joined to the *PbxI* gene on chromosome 19.[144] A chimeric transcription factor is the result, postulated to deregulate genes involved in leukemogenesis.

Similarly, translocations involving 11q23 such as the t(4;11), t(9;11), and t(11;19) occur in infants with precursor B-cell lymphoblastic leukemia. This translocation involves the *MLL* gene on chromosome 11q23.[142]

Treatment and Prognosis. Patients with precursor B-cell LBLs have high-grade neoplasms that rapidly disseminate, may involve privileged sites such as the testis and central nervous system, and are fatal if untreated. These tumors respond favorably to chemotherapy regimens designed after those used for ALL, which differ from those used for other clinically high-grade non-Hodgkin's lymphoma.[145] The presence of the t(9;22) in ALL correlates with a poorer prognosis.[143]

Precursor T-Cell

Clinical Features. Patients with precursor T-cell LBLs tend to be adolescents and young adults with widespread, supradiaphragmatic lymphadenopathy.[58, 59, 139] Males outnumber females in a 2:1 ratio. The peak age incidence is in the second decade of life, and 50% to 80% of patients present with a mediastinal mass.[59, 139] Peripheral blood involvement is seen in at least one third of patients

with precursor T-cell LBLs at presentation, and sometime during the clinical course in 80% of those patients who die from the disease.

Pathologic Features. Precursor B-cell and T-cell LBLs are histologically identical (Fig. 12–30).[139] Immunophenotypic studies have shown that these tumors express T-cell antigens in patterns that closely correlate with the stages of normal thymocyte differentiation. The earliest precursor T-cell LBLs correlate with the prothymocyte stage and express the T-cell antigens CD7 and CD2. CD7 is the earliest T-cell antigen expressed. T-cell LBLs that correspond to the cortical thymocyte stage also express the CD1 and CD5 antigens and are either CD4−/CD8− or CD4+/CD8+. At this stage, cytoplasmic CD3 antigen is present, although this antigen may not be expressed on the cell surface. T-cell LBLs of the late cortical or medullary stage of thymic differentiation also express surface CD3, mature into either CD4+/CD8− or CD4−/CD8+, and lose the CD1 antigen.

An extremely useful marker in the diagnosis of precursor T-cell (and B-cell) LBL is terminal deoxynucleotidyl transferase (TdT), a distinct type of DNA polymerase normally present only in immature lymphocytes.[60] This enzyme is found in almost all cases of precursor T-cell and B-cell LBL and is negative in mature T-cell and B-cell lymphomas. Terminal deoxynucleotidyl transferase is involved in the process of gene rearrangement and is thought to add extra nucleotide bases between the variable, diversity, and joining regions of rearranging genes.[63]

Molecular studies of precursor T-cell LBLs have shown patterns of T-cell receptor (*TCR*) gene rearrangement, corresponding to the stage of differentiation of the neoplasm. In a small subset of cases of T-cell LBL with an early thymic immunophenotype, rearrangements of only the *TCRδ* gene, or both the *TCRδ* and *TCRγ* genes may be identified.[146] In the remaining early thymic and the middle and late thymic immunophenotype, all of the *TCR* genes are

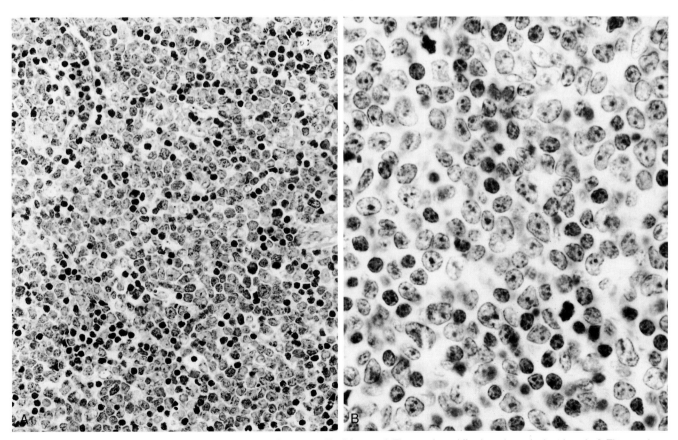

Figure 12–30. Precursor lymphoblastic lymphoma/leukemia of precursor T-cell lineage. *A,* The neoplasm diffusely replaces the lymph node. *B,* This neoplasm, cytologically similar to the cells shown in Figure 12–29, is composed of small lymphoid cells with blastic nuclear chromatin and inconspicuous nucleoli.

rearranged. (The *TCR*δ gene is rearranged and subsequently deleted.)[146] These findings have suggested a hierarchy of *TCR* gene rearrangement in developing T lymphocytes: the *TCR*δ gene rearranges first, followed by rearrangement of the *TCR*γ and the *TCR*β genes, lastly followed by rearrangement of the *TCR*α locus.

Lineage infidelity or promiscuity is common in precursor T-cell LBLs. Immunoglobulin heavy chain gene rearrangements occur in approximately 30% of precursor T-cell neoplasms.[63, 141]

A number of non-random chromosomal translocations have been identified in subsets of precursor T-cell LBLs.[142] Of these, cytogenetic and molecular studies have identified del 1p32 or the t(1;14)(p32;q11) most frequently, in up to 30% of cases.[147] Most commonly, a small interstitial deletion occurs in the *tal*-1 gene (also known as *SCL* and *tcl*-5). Less often, the t(1;14) results in the *tal*-1 and *SIL* genes being joined. Both mechanisms are thought to be the result of illegitimate recombination, mediated by the V(D)J recombinase mechanism using heptamer-nonamer-like sequences flanking each gene.[147] The *tal*-1 gene encodes for a nuclear transcription factor. Immunohistochemical studies have shown that TAL-1 protein can also be expressed in neoplasms without deletion or the t(1;14), indicating that other mechanisms are involved in TAL-1 expression.[148]

Treatment and Prognosis. Unless effectively treated, the disease progression of patients with precursor T-cell LBL is a rapidly downhill course with widespread dissemination. Bone marrow and central nervous system involvement at presentation are adverse prognostic signs. Patients with precursor T-cell LBLs respond favorably to chemotherapy regimens designed after those used for ALL, which differ from those used for other clinically high-grade non-Hodgkin's lymphoma.[145]

Peripheral T-Cell Lymphomas

Peripheral T-cell lymphomas are neoplasms of mature T lymphoid cells, in contrast to precursor T-cell lymphoblastic lymphoma/leukemia. In Western countries, these tumors are fairly uncommon, representing approximately 10% of all malignant lymphomas. The classification of these neoplasms has been historically inconsistent. Although many cases can be placed in the diffuse mixed small and large cell, diffuse large cell, and large cell immunoblastic lymphoma categories of the Working Formulation, many cases have unique features that are not included in this classification. Other detailed classifications of T-cell lymphomas have been proposed.[59, 149, 150] The REAL classification[59] lists 10 peripheral T-cell lymphoma entities or provisional entities but still includes the large category of "peripheral T-cell lymphoma, unspecified."

Clinical Features. Peripheral T-cell lymphomas may occur at any age and demonstrate a male predominance.[151–153] The patients often have a history of dermatologic or autoimmune disease, may have "B symptoms," and frequently present with extranodal sites involved by disease. In general, T-cell lymphomas present at higher stage (stage III or IV) than most B-cell lymphomas, and it has been traditionally felt that these tumors are more aggressive than B-cell lymphoma.[152, 154] Whether this is true is not clear, since some studies have shown a similar response to modern therapy strategies when T-cell and B-cell lymphomas are compared.[153, 155]

Pathologic Features. T-cell lymphoma may show focal intrafollicular lymph node involvement, or diffuse architectural distortion may be seen with complete loss of follicles or normal landmarks.[149, 151, 156] Vascular proliferation is frequently present, associated with the tumor cells, and background eosinophils, plasma cells, and histiocytes are commonly present. The tumor cell population may be quite variable with a spectrum of cells possible, ranging from small irregular lymphocytes to medium-sized lymphocytes, to large immunoblasts (Fig. 12–31). The small irregular lymphocytes may be morphologically similar to the small cleaved cells seen in follicular lymphomas, but the neoplastic small T cells are frequently more convoluted in appearance, and a true follicular pattern is not

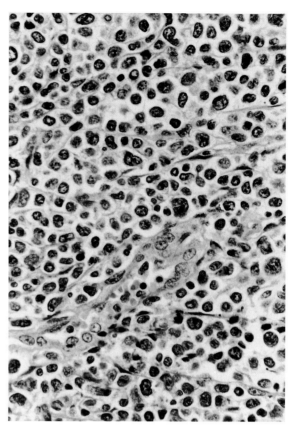

Figure 12–31. Peripheral T-cell lymphoma with an associated small vessel. The neoplastic lymphocytes have irregular nuclear contours and are variable in size. Many cells have abundant clear cytoplasm.

present. Despite the morphologic differences of T-cell lymphomas from most lymphomas of B-lineage, enough overlap exists between the morphology of B and T cell malignancies that one cannot reliably predict the lineage of a given lymphoma based solely on these features.[157] Immunophenotyping studies are essential for proper lineage determination.

The vast majority of T-cell lymphomas are CD45/CD45RB (leukocyte common antigen)–positive. T-lineage antigen expression can be identified on paraffin sections in most cases with immunoreactivity for CD3, CD43, or CD45RO antigens, or a combination of these, and negative reactions for CD20 and other B-lineage antigens. Frozen section or flow cytometric immunophenotyping is useful for the identification of other T-lineage–associated antigens, particularly CD2, CD4, CD5, CD7, and CD8. Most T-cell lymphomas are CD4-positive and CD8-negative, but CD4⁻/CD8⁺, CD4⁻/CD8⁻, and CD4⁺/CD8⁺ combinations are also possible. The loss of a T-lineage–associated antigen is helpful in the determination of neoplasia, with CD7 and CD5 being the most commonly lost.[158, 159] No immunohistochemical marker of T-cell clonality, such as immunoglobulin expression in B cells, is available; however, the combination of morphologic changes with the immunologic determination of a T-cell phenotype is often sufficient for diagnosis. If the morphologic impression includes a differential diagnosis of a reactive T-cell proliferation, molecular studies for the detection of rearrangements of the T-cell receptor (*TCR*) genes may be useful to identify the presence of clonality. Such studies are traditionally performed by Southern blotting for the *TCR* α and β chains using fresh or frozen tissue. More recently, the polymerase chain reaction has been used to detect *TCR* receptor rearrangements, often of *TCR* γ chain. This technique may be performed using formalin-fixed, paraffin-embedded tissues.

Ten percent to 15% of T-cell malignancies will not demonstrate evidence of *TCR* gene rearrangements.[160] These lymphomas generally lack surface CD3 and CD5 antigen expression and express one or more natural killer cell–associated antigens (particularly CD56).[161, 162] These cases are of probable natural killer cell origin and are usually CD43-, CD45RO-, and cytoplasmic CD3-positive on paraffin sections. This difference in CD3 expression is attributable to the tumor cells' expressing only the ε subunit of the CD3 antigen.[163] This subunit alone is not detected by the Leu4 or T3 monoclonal antibodies commonly used for frozen section or flow cytometric immunophenotyping, but is detectable with the polyclonal CD3 antibodies commonly used for paraffin-section immunohistochemistry. These *TCR*-negative, CD56-positive cases frequently present at extranodal sites and include the angiocentric or T-cell/natural killer cell lymphomas.[164] In addition to these cases, there are several other types of peripheral T-cell lymphoma that have distinct clinical and pathologic features and are separated from the "unspecified" group of the REAL classification. Those that particularly pertain to the head and neck region will be discussed in more detail.

T-Cell/Natural Killer Cell Lymphoma (Angiocentric T-Cell Lymphoma)

Clinical Features. Malignant lymphomas with features of both T-cells and natural killer (NK) cells are frequently encountered in Asia, Mexico, Central America, and South America, although they are relatively uncommon in North America and Europe.[165–168] These tumors often involve the upper respiratory tract, particularly the sinonasal area, and frequently secondarily involve other extranodal sites, including skin.[161, 162, 164, 169]

These T/NK-cell lymphomas are the most common type of lymphoma to involve the nose in some countries and are relatively more common in the sinonasal area in all geographic locations.[170, 171] However, in most studies the majority of sinonasal lymphomas in North American and European patients are of B-cell lineage.[165, 166, 172] Many of the B-cell lineage sinonasal lymphomas in these studies may represent secondary involvement.

Included under T/NK-cell lymphomas are cases that were previously interpreted as polymorphic reticulosis or lethal midline granuloma and are often difficult to differentiate from reactive lesions.[168, 173, 174] The tumors may present in various sites, including nasal or orbital masses or as destructive lesions of the palate.

Pathologic Features. T/NK-cell lymphomas usually show a spectrum of neoplastic cells, similar to other peripheral T-cell lymphomas, and are characteristically associated with an inflammatory infiltrate and necrosis (Fig. 12–32, see p. 748). Tumor cells may be concentrated around blood vessels and may be associated with destruction of the blood vessel wall. Although such angiocentricity is a common finding in these tumors, this feature may be absent in nasal lymphoma specimens and its presence is not required for the diagnosis.[175] For this reason, some hematopathologists do not use the term "angiocentric" diagnostically and prefer the term T/NK-cell lymphoma. In small specimens without obvious angiocentric lesions, it may be very difficult to distinguish a reactive cellular population from a neoplastic infiltrate. A high index of suspicion is necessary in such cases, as well as knowledge of the clinical features of the patient's case.

Paraffin section immunohistochemical studies demonstrate the irregular lymphoid cells, including large immunoblasts, to be positive for the T-cell lineage–associated antigens CD43 and CD45RO as well as demonstrating cytoplasmic CD3 using the available polyclonal antibodies. As mentioned previously, the cells may be CD3-negative, particularly by frozen section immunohistochemistry, are frequently CD56-positive, and usually do not demonstrate *TCR* gene rearrangements. In situ hybridization studies for Epstein-Barr virus (EBV) EBER-1 RNA is positive in the vast majority of cases,[171, 176] and this finding may be diagnostically useful in small biopsy specimens with only a few tumor cells present. Immunohistochemical staining for the EBV latent membrane protein-1 (LMP-1) may not be as sensitive for the detection of EBV as the in situ hybridization method in this disease.[176]

Differential Diagnosis. The differential diagnosis of nasal T/NK-cell lymphoma includes other non-Hodgkin's lymphomas, lymphomatoid granulomatosis, Wegener's granulomatosis, and infectious diseases with abundant necrosis. Most other non-Hodgkin's lymphomas of the sinonasal area represent B-cell lymphomas or lymphomas that secondarily involve the site. Immunohistochemical studies as well as knowledge of the clinical history will aid in identifying these cases. Lymphomatoid granulomatosis is an angiocentric lesion that involves the respiratory tract and is associated with EBV, similar to T/NK-cell lymphoma. A large number of T cells are present in lymphomatoid granulomatosis, similar to T/NK-cell lymphoma. However, the T cells are small and reactive, and the atypical, large, EBV-positive cells of this disorder are usually of B-cell lineage.[177] Such angiocentric large B cells are not usually seen in cases of T/NK-cell lymphoma. Wegener's granulomatosis may demonstrate extensive necrosis with an angiocentric pattern but will not have the atypical lymphoid cell population of a T/NK-cell nasal lymphoma. Also, the necrosis of Wegener's granulomatosis is usually in a geometric pattern, and giant cells may be seen, unlike T/NK-cell lymphoma. Similarly, an atypical lymphoid cell population will not be seen with infectious diseases; special stains for fungal organisms should be performed in all suspicious cases.

Angioimmunoblastic Lymphadenopathy and Angioimmunoblastic Lymphadenopathy–Like T-Cell Lymphoma

Angioimmunoblastic lymphadenopathy with dysproteinemia (AILD) and immunoblastic lymphadenopathy are similar or identical processes. Because of the high frequency of T-cell lymphoma in patients with this condition, some pathologists consider all cases of AILD to be T-cell lymphomas.[59] Other pathologists prefer to separate cases of AILD from AILD-like T-cell lymphoma, believing that these diseases represent a spectrum ranging from premalignant AILD that may be a reversible process to the frankly malignant AILD-like T-cell lymphoma.[178]

Clinical Features. AILD and AILD-like T-cell lymphoma usually occur in elderly persons with generalized lymphadenopathy, hepatosplenomegaly and cutaneous rashes.[179–181] The patients frequently have fevers, night sweats, and other constitutional symptoms as well as laboratory evidence of autoimmune hemolytic anemia and hypergammaglobulinemia. The disease course is variable, with some patients' symptoms resolving with corticosteroid therapy, some patients developing severe infections, and other patients' condition progressing to malignant lymphoma.[182] Most lymphomas developing in these patients are of T-cell lineage, although B-cell lymphomas may also occur.[181–183]

Pathologic Features. Both AILD and AILD-like T-cell lymphoma cause diffuse architectural distortion with loss or regression of germinal centers (Fig. 12–33, see p. 749). Marked, arborizing vascular proliferation is present. Periodic acid-Schiff–positive amorphous material may be deposited throughout the involved tissue. The cellular infiltrate consists of small lymphocytes, plasma cells, eosinophils, epithelioid histiocytes, large lymphocytes, and immunoblasts. In AILD-like T-cell lymphoma, the immunoblasts usually have abundant clear cytoplasm and form clusters, as compared with the individual immunoblasts seen typically in AILD.

Immunophenotypic studies identify the immunoblast clusters to be of T-cell lineage, usually with aberrant loss of one or more T-cell antigens in AILD-like T-cell lymphoma. In AILD, the immunoblasts may represent a mixture of T and B cells without aberrant loss of T-cell antigens.

In cases of AILD, *TCR* gene rearrangement clonal bands of weak intensity may be present by Southern blotting[184–186]; however, the presence of large, intense bands is highly suggestive of progression to AILD-like T-cell lymphoma.

Adult T-Cell Leukemia/Lymphoma

Adult T-cell leukemia/lymphoma (ATLL) is a systemic disease that represents a clinicopathologic entity caused by the human T-cell leukemia virus-1 (HTLV-1).[187–189]

Clinical Features. The disease affects adults with an average age of 50 years in specific regions of Southern Japan as well as the Caribbean, western Africa, and the southeastern United States. In most cases, this is an aggressive disease, with patients presenting with lymphadenopathy, hepatosplenomegaly, skin lesions, hypercalcemia, and leukemic involvement, although chronic, nonleukemic and smoldering cases have been described.[190]

Pathologic Features. The peripheral blood cells are a heterogeneous mix of atypical lymphoid cells that include polylobated or cloverleaf-shaped nuclei. The involved lymph nodes are diffusely effaced by a proliferation of medium to large cells with cerebriform to polylobated nuclei (Fig. 12–34, see p. 749). Although the pattern might vary from a diffuse, medium-sized cell to a mixed or large cell proliferation, these cytologic differences do not appear to have prognostic significance. The neoplastic cells are generally CD4-positive T cells that also express the CD25 antigen.

Cases of ATLL have presented with head and neck involvement,[188, 191, 192] but ATLL is a systemic disease with multiple sites involved in most cases. The differential diagnosis of ATLL frequently includes mycosis fungoides and Sezary syndrome because of the presence of skin lesions and circulating atypical lymphoid cells. Lymph node involvement by these diseases may not be differentiated solely on morphologic grounds. The presence of cloverleaf cells in tissue sections would be suggestive of ATLL, but this degree of cytologic atypia may not be present in all cases. Serologic evaluation for HTLV-1, correlation with the clinical features, and calcium levels are often necessary for proper diagnosis.

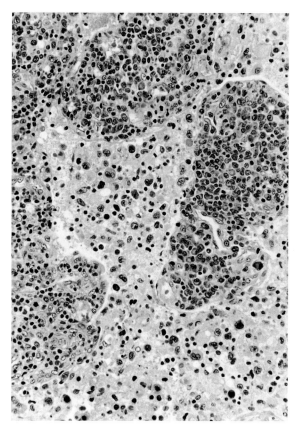

Figure 12–35. Anaplastic large-cell lymphoma. The lymph node sinuses are expanded by large pleomorphic cells that might be confused with metastatic carcinoma.

Anaplastic Large Cell Lymphoma

Clinical Features. Anaplastic large cell lymphoma (ALCL) is a neoplasm that may affect both children and adults in several different forms.[193–195] In adults, some cases present with only cutaneous involvement; these cases appear to be closely related to lymphomatoid papulosis and have a relatively good prognosis with only local therapy.[195] The remaining cases of ALCL may represent both nodal and extranodal disease or progression of another type of malignant lymphoma and may involve any anatomic site including the head and neck region.

Pathologic Features. Lymph node involvement by ALCL is characteristically partial with preferential involvement of sinuses, although diffuse involvement may occur (Fig. 12–35). The lymph node capsule may be thickened and parenchymal fibrosis may be present, but the nodular fibrosis of nodular sclerosis Hodgkin's disease is generally absent. Two cytologic forms of the tumor are described.[193, 196] The most common and characteristic form is one of markedly anaplastic large cells with a high mitotic rate and prominent nucleoli. Many of the cells are multinucleated in this form with "donut-like" cells. A more monomorphic form may also occur without the multinucleated cells. These cases have large lymphoid cells with abundant basophilic cytoplasm and round to oval nuclei and prominent nucleoli. Cases intermediate to these two forms may also occur. The background hematopoietic cell population in ALCL may be heterogeneous, consisting of small lymphocytes, plasma cells, histiocytes, eosinophils, neutrophils, or a combination of these. Cases with an abundance of histiocytes have been termed *lymphohistiocytic T-cell lymphomas.*[197] Although not specifically part of the Working Formulation,[58] ALCL would be classified as a high-grade, immunoblastic lymphoma, polymorphous type by many hematopathologists.

Approximately one third of cases of anaplastic large cell lymphoma are CD45-negative; therefore, the lack of expression of this marker alone should not be used to exclude hematopoietic origin of

an anaplastic malignant neoplasm. The majority of cases of ALCL are of T-cell lineage. Most studies have recognized cases of B-cell ALCL; 10% to 37% of cases with characteristic morphologic features have this immunophenotype.[193, 194, 196, 198–200] The REAL classification places such B-cell lineage cases in the broad category of diffuse large B-cell lymphoma.[59] The term *anaplastic large cell lymphoma* is reserved for cases of T-cell or null-cell lineage in this classification. The T-cell lineage tumors usually express CD3, CD43, or CD45RO by paraffin section immunohistochemistry, and aberrant loss of T-cell antigens as well as T-cell receptor gene rearrangements are usually identifiable using fresh and frozen tissues.[198, 200, 201] Null-cell ALCL lacks T-cell receptor gene rearrangements as well as T-cell lineage antigen expression but may still express the CD43 antigen. The tumors are also characteristically CD30-positive, showing diffuse and intense staining for this antigen with the Ki-1 and BerH2 antibodies.[196, 198] This CD30 expression led to earlier descriptions of these cases as "Ki-1 lymphoma" or "CD30-positive lymphoma." Since this entity is not defined solely by CD30 antigen expression, the use of these terms is discouraged. The tumor cells of ALCL are also positive for epithelial membrane antigen (EMA), and rare cases of keratin-positive and CD15-positive ALCL have been reported.[199, 202]

The t(2;5) cytogenetic translocation, involving the *alk* gene of chromosome 2p23 and the *npm* gene of chromosome 5q23, may be identified in many cases of ALCL.[203–205] This translocation is particularly common in childhood T-cell lineage and null-cell cases with systemic disease. The translocation is less common in adults, in cases of B-cell lineage ALCL, and in patients with only cutaneous disease. Immunohistochemical studies for alk protein expression reliably detect the t(2;5)-positive cases.[205a]

Differential Diagnosis. The differential diagnosis of ALCL includes other non-Hodgkin's lymphomas, Hodgkin's disease, metastatic tumors, and histiocytic neoplasms. Other non-Hodgkin's lymphomas may be CD30-positive but usually without the diffuse, intense expression seen in ALCL. Such cases are usually large-cell lymphomas without the unique morphologic features described earlier. The differential diagnosis of ALCL versus Hodgkin's disease may be very difficult in some cases, particularly in the very rare cases of CD15-positive ALCL. EMA expression may be useful, since this is commonly present in ALCL, and is absent in the classic types of Hodgkin's disease. In addition, the tumor cells of most head and neck cases of Hodgkin's disease are positive for the Epstein-Barr virus (EBV), whereas the vast majority of cases of ALCL are EBV-negative.[206, 207] Most investigators have failed to detect t(2;5) or alk protein expression in cases of Hodgkin's disease,[205, 208, 209] although one group has reported this to be a common finding[210] and t(2;5) has been identified in non-Hodgkin's lymphomas of B-cell lineage without features of ALCL.[211, 212] Metastatic lesions, particularly carcinoma and melanoma, can usually be excluded easily with an immunohistochemical panel that includes a keratin cocktail, S100, and HMB45. Since ALCL are commonly EMA-positive, EMA antibodies alone should not be used to support a diagnosis of carcinoma. Histiocytic neoplasms are rare but may have morphologic features similar to those of ALCL. In fact, many cases previously diagnosed as malignant histiocytosis probably represented examples of anaplastic large cell lymphoma.[213] For this reason, detailed immunophenotypic and gene rearrangement studies should be performed to exclude a T-cell lineage neoplasm before a diagnosis of malignant histiocytosis is made.

Hodgkin's Disease

Hodgkin's disease is a neoplastic proliferation of Reed-Sternberg cells and mononuclear variants of Reed-Sternberg cells (Hodgkin's cells). There is an overall male predominance and a bimodal age distribution involving young adults (15 to 40 years) and older adults (55 to 74 years). Particularly in developing countries, the disease also occurs in young children (less than 10 years old). The origin of the neoplastic cells is controversial, but recent evidence suggests a lymphoid origin. Lukes and Butler originally described six different types of Hodgkin's disease: nodular lymphocytic and histiocytic (L&H), diffuse L&H, nodular sclerosis, mixed cellularity, diffuse fibrosis, and reticular types (Table 12–3).[214] Subsequently, at the Rye conference the Lukes and Butler classification was narrowed into four categories.[215] The nodular and diffuse L&H types of Lukes and Butler were combined into lymphocyte predominance and the diffuse fibrosis and reticular types were combined into lymphocyte depleted. The categories of nodular sclerosis and mixed cellularity were unchanged. This nomenclature has remained relatively unchanged in the more recent REAL classification.[59] Because of the distinctive clinicopathologic features of nodular L&H lymphocyte predominant Hodgkin's disease, it is now commonly separated from the other types of Hodgkin's disease, often referred to in the literature as the "classic" types of Hodgkin's disease.

Clinical Features. Hodgkin's disease involves the cervical and supraclavicular lymph nodes in 60% to 80% of all patients,[216] although the frequency of neck node involvement may be lower in elderly patients when compared with the childhood and young adult groups.[217] At least half of all head and neck Hodgkin's disease cases are of the mixed cellularity type, with the remaining cases typed as nodular sclerosis, lymphocyte predominance, or unclassifiable in most studies.[218, 219] In contrast to lymph nodes of the lower neck, 2% or less of Hodgkin's disease cases present in the lymphoid tissues of Waldheyer's ring and the upper neck,[220–224] and this frequency is much less than that for non-Hodgkin's lymphomas of the same sites.[225] Nasopharyngeal and tonsil involvement, both rare, appear to occur with relatively equal frequency[218, 219] and often arise in patients who have a concurrent or previous history of lymph node involvement at a more typical site.[218] An even higher percentage of mixed cellularity type Hodgkin's disease has been reported to involve the tonsils and nasopharynx.[218] Involvement of the salivary glands and thyroid by Hodgkin's disease is also quite rare, with no special type appearing to predominate.[226–228] In the thyroid, the tumor may present clinically as a nodule and mimic a goiter or other primary thyroid disease. Other sites, including the palate, nasal septum, buccal mucosa, tongue, and eye, have been reported but are exceedingly rare.[222]

Pathologic Features. The diagnosis of classic Hodgkin's disease is dependent on the identification of Reed-Sternberg cells and mononuclear Hodgkin cells within the appropriate inflammatory background of cells. Hodgkin's cells have abundant cytoplasm and may have multilobated nuclei or may be multinucleated. The nucleus has a thickened nuclear envelope with vesicular chromatin. Chromatin clearing is present surrounding large eosinophilic nucleoli, which are characteristic of this neoplasm. Fixation and cellular degeneration may alter the appearance of the neoplastic cells in Hodgkin's disease. With formalin fixation, some cells may show prominent nuclear retraction, resulting in a clear zone surrounding the nucleus. Such cells are termed *lacunar* cells and may not be seen with other types of fixation, such as B5.

"Mummified" cells are Hodgkin's cells that have pyknotic nuclei, to the degree that nucleoli may not be identifiable, with contracted eosinophilic cytoplasm. The background cells of Hodgkin's disease are non-neoplastic and usually greatly outnumber the neoplastic cells. These background cells in Hodgkin's disease are a mixture of small lymphocytes, plasma cells, eosinophils, neutrophils, and fibroblasts, which vary in number and proportion in different individual cases.

The *nodular sclerosis* subtype of Hodgkin's disease is the most common type overall but is relatively less common in the head and neck region. In nodular sclerosis, the lymph node capsule is characteristically thickened, and broad bands of birefringent collagen are present within the lymph node surrounding nodules of tumor (Fig. 12–36, see p. 750). In the nodules, the background cells characteristically show an abundance of eosinophils, and lacunar cells are prominent. The "diagnostic" binucleated Reed-Sternberg cell can be difficult to identify in some cases. Zonal areas of necrosis may also be present. Although the characteristic fibrosis of nodular sclerosis may be only focal, its presence in any area is sufficient for the diagnosis of this subtype. A syncytial variant of nodular sclerosis has been described in which large syncytial sheets of lacunar cells are present.[229]

Two subtypes of nodular sclerosis Hodgkin's disease have been described by the British National Lymphoma Investigation[230] and are designated grades I and II. Grade II cases are associated with a poor response to initial therapy, an increased rate of relapse and decreased survival as compared to grade I cases. Cases are classified as grade II if (1) more than 25% of the cellular nodules show reticular

Table 12–3. Hodgkin's Disease: Comparison of Three Classifications

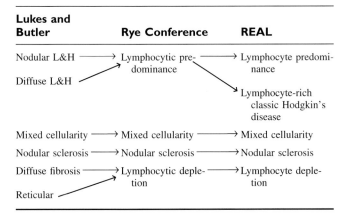

Lukes and Butler	Rye Conference	REAL
Nodular L&H	Lymphocytic predominance	Lymphocyte predominance
Diffuse L&H		Lymphocyte-rich classic Hodgkin's disease
Mixed cellularity	Mixed cellularity	Mixed cellularity
Nodular sclerosis	Nodular sclerosis	Nodular sclerosis
Diffuse fibrosis	Lymphocytic depletion	Lymphocyte depletion
Reticular		

L&H, lymphocytic and histiocytic.

or pleomorphic lymphocyte depletion; (2) greater than 80% of the cellular nodules show the fibrohistiocytic variant of lymphocyte depletion; or (3) more than 25% of the nodules contain numerous bizarre and highly anaplastic-appearing Hodgkin's cells without depletion of lymphocytes. All cases that did not fulfill these criteria would be designated as grade I. Cases of syncytial variant of nodular sclerosis Hodgkin's disease are generally considered as grade II.

The neoplastic Reed-Sternberg and lacunar (Hodgkin's) cells of nodular sclerosis Hodgkin's disease are typically negative or only weakly reactive for the leukocyte common antigen (LCA; CD45) while expressing the CD30 (Ki-1; BerH2) and CD15 (LeuM1) antigens.[231] Most cases are negative for B-cell and T-cell lineage associated antigens, although a subpopulation will express the CD20 antigen along with the typical CD45−/CD15+/CD30+ phenotype. In 25% to 40% of all nodular sclerosis cases, the neoplastic cells will express the Epstein-Barr virus latent membrane protein-1 (LMP-1). The background lymphocytes are predominantly CD4-positive helper T lymphocytes.

Lymphocyte predominance Hodgkin's disease appears to represent two distinct entities. The majority of cases correlate with the nodular L&H category of Lukes and Butler and are often referred to in the literature as either nodular lymphocyte predominance or nodular paragranuloma. In these cases, the lymph node is effaced by lymphoid nodules that are larger than reactive germinal centers or the nodules seen in follicular lymphomas. The low-power pattern is similar to that seen in progressive transformation of germinal centers, and progressive transformation of germinal centers as well as reactive follicular hyperplasia may be present within a lymph node that is also involved by nodular lymphocyte predominance Hodgkin's disease.[232] The large nodules are composed of small lymphocytes, epithelioid histiocytes, and L&H cells. L&H cells are large cells with very little cytoplasm. The enlarged nuclei have vesicular chromatin and may have irregular nuclear contours, which

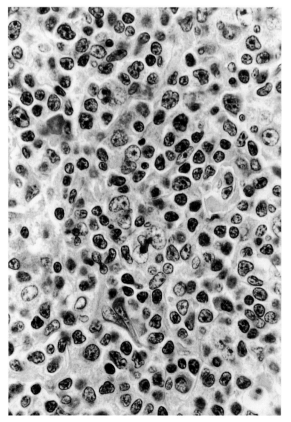

Figure 12–37. Lymphocyte predominance Hodgkin's disease. Lymphocytic and histiocytic (L & H) cells are present (center) and have irregular, lobulated nuclei with small nucleoli.

have led to their description as "popcorn" or "elephant ear" cells (Fig. 12–37). The L&H cells generally have one to multiple nucleoli that are smaller and less eosinophilic than the nucleoli of either Reed-Sternberg or Hodgkin's cells in the classic types of Hodgkin's disease. Classic Reed-Sternberg cells are uncommon to absent and background eosinophils are rare.

The L&H cells of nodular lymphocyte predominance also differ immunologically from the neoplastic cells of the other classic types of Hodgkin's disease. The L&H cells are usually positive for LCA, epithelial membrane antigen (EMA), and CD20 and are negative for CD15 and usually CD30.[218] The background cell population of nodular lymphocyte predominance Hodgkin's disease also differs immunophenotypically from those seen in the classic types of Hodgkin's disease, with an increased number of CD20-positive small B lymphocytes.[233, 234] In addition, CD57 (Leu-7) positive cells are present that may form rings or wreaths around the L&H cells of some cases.[235] The distinct B-cell immunophenotype, as well as the excellent prognosis of patients with low-stage disease, have led to the conclusion that nodular lymphocyte predominance is an entity distinct from the other classic types of Hodgkin's disease.[236]

What was once termed *diffuse L&H Hodgkin's disease* by Lukes and Butler is poorly defined. In some cases, the immunophenotype of the neoplastic cells is identical to that seen in nodular lymphocyte predominance. In addition, there is a second form in which rare Reed-Sternberg cells are present that are morphologically and immunophenotypically typical of the neoplastic cells in the classic types of Hodgkin's disease, with a background of predominantly small lymphocytes and no evidence of sclerosis. Background eosinophils are usually sparse. The designation *lymphocyte-rich classic Hodgkin's disease* has been used for such cases in the REAL classifcation.[59]

Lymphocyte depletion Hodgkin's disease represents less than 5% of all cases of Hodgkin's disease, and many cases previously diagnosed as this type probably represent non-Hodgkin's lymphomas.[237] There are two morphologic types of lymphocyte depletion Hodgkin's disease, the diffuse fibrosis type and the reticular type, as originally described by Lukes and Butler.[214] Both show diffuse replacement of the lymph node architecture by fibrous tissue and tumor cells with a decreased number of background lymphocytes. The diffuse fibrosis type shows replacement of the node by a proliferation of non-birefringent connective tissue without the broad collagen bands of nodular sclerosis. Hodgkin's and Reed-Sternberg cells are present with fibrosis surrounding individual tumor cells. With the reticular type of Hodgkin's disease, the Hodgkin's cells are numerous and extremely pleomorphic. Such a proliferation may impart a sarcomatous appearance, making the diagnosis of Hodgkin's disease difficult without immunohistochemical studies.

The neoplastic cells of lymphocyte depletion Hodgkin's disease are immunophenotypically similar to the neoplastic cells in the other classic types of Hodgkin's disease, as described for nodular sclerosis. In the majority of cases, the Reed-Sternberg and Hodgkin's cells are positive for Epstein-Barr latent membrane protein.

Mixed cellularity is the second most common type of Hodgkin's disease overall and is the most common type to involve the head and neck region. Many pathologists use this term for cases that do not fit the criteria for the other types of Hodgkin's disease. In most cases, the lymph node architecture is diffusely replaced by a mixture of background cells and Hodgkin's cells, including fairly numerous Reed-Sternberg cells (Fig. 12–38, see p. 750). Lacunar cells and mummified cells are generally not prominent. The lymph node capsule is intact and the fibrous bands of nodular sclerosis are not seen. Necrosis is not commonly present. Abundant background histiocytes and eosinophils are commonly seen as well as background small T lymphocytes.

The immunophenotype of the neoplastic cells in mixed cellularity Hodgkin's disease is similar to that of the Reed-Sternberg and Hodgkin's cells of nodular sclerosis (described previously) and lymphocyte depletion. Epstein-Barr virus latent membrane protein is present in the neoplastic cells of over two thirds of cases.

Other histologic types of Hodgkin's disease have been described. The term *cellular phase of nodular sclerosis* Hodgkin's disease is used for cases with a generally nodular pattern, but without the broad fibrous bands of typical nodular sclerosis.[214] These cases often have abundant lacunar and mummified cells more typical of nodular sclerosis. Others prefer to classify such cases as mixed cellularity.[238] *Interfollicular* Hodgkin's disease may occur in lymph nodes that otherwise show evidence of florid reactive follicular hyperplasia.[239] Such cases can be easily missed if the rare interfollicular Hodgkin's cells are not recognized. Since this type of Hodgkin's disease represents only partial involvement, it is often not possible to classify the type of disease further. Cases in which only partial node involvement is present or less than adequate material is available may be termed *unclassifiable.*

Epstein-Barr Virus and Hodgkin's Disease. Overall, in 40% to 50% of cases of Hodgkin's disease, the Reed-Sternberg and Hodgkin's cells exhibit evidence of Epstein-Barr virus (EBV) infection.[240] This percentage is even higher in cases of mixed cellularity Hodgkin's disease; up to 90% of cases have been reported to be EBV-positive in cervical lymph nodes.[241] Similarly, 67% of Hodgkin's disease cases of Waldeyer's ring have been recently shown to be EBV-positive.[230] This relatively high frequency of EBV infection is believed to be related to the role of Waldeyer's ring, as well as cervical lymph nodes, as reservoirs for the virus. The frequency of EBV infection in Hodgkin's disease is also higher in underdeveloped countries, where a higher frequency of childhood Hodgkin's disease is also present.[242]

Epstein-Barr virus is most reliably detected by in situ hybridization for EBER-1 RNA, small RNAs that are produced in the hundreds of thousands in the nucleus of cells with latent EBV infection. In Hodgkin's disease, however, latent membrane protein-1 (LMP-1) is virtually always expressed by the infected cells[242] and immunohistochemical analysis for LMP-1 is generally easier to perform than the in situ hybridization studies. When EBV-positive, virtually all of the Hodgkin's cells will demonstrate evidence of the virus in contrast to the negative background cells.

Molecular Biology of Hodgkin's Disease. With the exception of the detection of EBV EBER RNA, most molecular studies are of limited diagnostic utility in Hodgkin's disease. In general, immunoglobulin heavy and light chain as well as T cell receptor α, β, and γ chain gene rearrangements are not detectable by Southern blot hybridization in the majority of cases of Hodgkin's disease.[243, 244] This finding, however, may be related to the relatively low number of neoplastic cells in most cases in comparison to the background hematopoietic cells. A subpopulation of cases will demonstrate clonal gene rearrangements, particularly of immunoglobulin genes, when specimens with a high content of neoplastic cells are studied[243] or when more sensitive polymerase chain reaction (PCR) methods are employed.[245, 246]

Although the neoplastic cells of lymphocyte predominant Hodgkin's disease are of B-cell lineage by immunophenotyping, it is not yet clear whether they represent a monoclonal proliferation. Light chain restriction has been demonstrated by some authors by both immunohistochemistry and in situ hybridization,[247, 248] although one study using single cell microdissection of L&H cells reported the cells to be polyclonal using PCR.[249]

The detection of t(14;18) involving the *bcl-2* locus in Hodgkin's disease is controversial. Some groups have found evidence of this rearrangement, the translocation found in the majority of follicular lymphomas, in approximately one third of cases using PCR,[250, 251] whereas others have not duplicated these results.[247, 252] The translocation is not commonly identified by cytogenetics, although other clonal cytogenetic abnormalities have been reported,[251, 253] and *bcl-2* gene translocations are usually not identified by Southern blotting. One group has found a similar frequency of *bcl-2* gene rearrangements by PCR in cases of Hodgkin's disease and in reactive lymph nodes.[254] These findings have led to the suggestion that t(14;18)

translocations found by PCR may actually represent changes in the background lymphoid cells rather than in the neoplastic cells.[251, 254] The t(2;5), a common translocation in anaplastic large cell lymphomas, was identified in cases of Hodgkin's disease in one study,[210] but this finding has not been confirmed by others.[208, 209]

Differential Diagnosis. There is a wide differential diagnosis for Hodgkin's disease that includes metastatic tumors, non-Hodgkin's lymphomas, and reactive proliferations. Metastatic tumors,[255] particularly carcinoma, melanoma, and germ cell tumors, may have cells that simulate Reed-Sternberg cells, but the mixed inflammatory background of Hodgkin's disease is frequently absent.

In the head and neck region, nasopharyngeal carcinoma has been reported to closely mimic Hodgkin's disease.[256] Immunohistochemical studies for keratin and S100 are useful for identifying metastatic carcinoma and melanoma, respectively, in lymph nodes, and placental-like alkaline phosphatase reactivity is helpful in identifying germ cell tumors such as seminoma. Rare cases of lymphocyte-depleted Hodgkin's disease may have the appearance of sarcoma with spindled cells and neoplastic giant cells. In Hodgkin's disease, the spindled cell component is non-neoplastic and does not show the nuclear atypia expected in a sarcoma. Again, immunohistochemical analysis is helpful in these cases by demonstrating the classic immunophenotype of Reed-Sternberg and Hodgkin's cells, which is not seen in sarcomas.

Non-Hodgkin's lymphomas may also mimic Hodgkin's disease. Rare cases of small lymphocytic lymphoma/chronic lymphocytic leukemia (SLL/CLL) can have large cells that resemble Reed-Sternberg cells.[257] These cases, however, have a monotonous background of small B lymphocytes that typically co-express the T-cell–related antigens CD5 and CD43. The Reed-Sternberg–like cells may have a B-cell immunophenotype or may have a classic Hodgkin's cell phenotype. Those with the classic Hodgkin's cell immunophenotype may later develop classic HD. Peripheral T-cell lymphomas may also simulate Hodgkin's disease, since they frequently have a mixed cell composition that may include large lymphoid cells, histiocytes, and eosinophils. The neoplastic T cells may also resemble Reed-Sternberg and Hodgkin's cells, but they are usually accompanied by a broader morphologic spectrum of neoplastic cells that include small and medium-sized T cells. Although T-cell lymphomas may be CD30- and even CD15-positive, immunophenotyping studies usually reveal a leukocyte common antigen (LCA; CD45 or CD45RB)–positive T-cell lineage phenotype (CD3-, CD43-, or CD45RO-positive in paraffin sections). Frozen section immunophenotyping will frequently identify aberrant loss of one or more T-cell lineage associated antigens, and gene rearrangement studies will usually show a prominent T-cell receptor rearrangement by Southern blot analysis, consistent with a large monoclonal T-cell population. Anaplastic large cell lymphomas of T, B, or null cell lineage frequently have cells that resemble Reed-Sternberg and Hodgkin's cells, and these cells are characteristically CD30-positive and may be CD45-negative. A sinusoidal proliferation of neoplastic cells as well as a broad morphologic spectrum of tumor cells are clues suggestive of a non-Hodgkin's lymphoma. Anaplastic large cell lymphomas are usually EMA and alk-positive, whereas the cells of Hodgkin's disease are characteristically EMA and alk-negative. In addition, EBV infection is uncommon in anaplastic large cell lymphoma and its presence would be more suggestive of classic Hodgkin's disease.[206, 207] T-cell–rich B-cell lymphoma may be difficult to distinguish from cases of lymphocyte predominant Hodgkin's disease; however, the nodular pattern usually seen with nodular lymphocyte predominant Hodgkin's disease is not generally present in T-cell–rich B-cell lymphoma. In addition, the ring of CD57-positive lymphocytes seen in some cases of nodular lymphocyte predominant Hodgkin's disease is characteristically absent in T-cell–rich B-cell lymphoma.[221]

Necrotizing granulomatous lymphadenitis of cervical lymph nodes may simulate Hodgkin's disease, but the areas of necrosis are surrounded by relatively bland-appearing histiocytes without the neoplastic cells of Hodgkin's disease. Patients with chronic lymphadenitis may also present with enlarged lymph nodes with thickened capsules and fibrosis that is similar to the fibrous bands of Hodgkin's disease. Such specimens may have scattered immunoblasts, but typical Hodgkin's cells are absent or rare and the cells are generally scattered and do not cluster like Hodgkin's cells. In addition, the enlarged cells are generally CD45-positive, mark as a mixture of B and T lymphocytes, and generally do not have the immunophenotype of Hodgkin's cells. Viral lymphadenitis will also give an immunoblastic proliferation that is similar to interfollicular Hodgkin's disease. Viral inclusions, when present, may simulate the large eosinophilic nucleoli of Hodgkin's cells. Immunophenotyping studies may again be useful in these cases, as may in situ hybridization and immunohistochemical analysis for the specific viral agent, such as herpes simplex virus or cytomegalovirus. Infectious mononucleosis[20] may cause diffuse obliteration of the normal nodal architecture with areas of necrosis and cells morphologically identical to Reed-Sternberg and Hodgkin's cells. However, infectious mononucleosis also contains a wide spectrum of plasma cells, plasmacytoid cells, and immunoblasts that is not typical of the background cells of Hodgkin's disease. These cells, of course, are also EBV-positive and may express the CD30 antigen similar to Hodgkin's disease. Because of these similarities, great caution must be used in the interpretation of tonsilar biopsies and nasopharyngeal biopsy specimens, especially in children. Since Hodgkin's disease is rare in these sites and infectious mononucleosis is common, the pathologist should ensure that infectious mononucleosis is entirely excluded before entertaining a diagnosis of Hodgkin's disease, and even then the diagnosis must be made with caution and with an immunophenotypic work-up.

Treatment and Prognosis. For patients with localized disease, radiation therapy is curative if the neoplasm can be adequately treated. For patients with stage III or IV disease or for patients with high-risk localized disease (e.g., bulky mediastinal involvement), combined chemotherapy is recommended. Two chemotherapy regimens are most commonly used: ABVD (doxorubicin [Adriamycin], bleomycin, vinblastine, dacarbazine) and MOPP (nitrogen mustard [mustine], vincristine [Oncovin], procarbazine, prednisone). One or both of these regimens in alternating cycles may be used. Hodgkin's disease is a highly curable disease, independent of histologic findings. Response to therapy is determined by stage, the presence of B symptoms, and other risk factors such as disease bulk.

Extramedullary Plasmacytoma

Plasmacytomas are clonal, neoplastic plasma cell proliferations that are further subdivided into extramedullary plasmacytomas and solitary plasmacytomas of bone.[258] Although plasmacytomas of the head and neck region may partially involve bone, they are generally considered to be in the extramedullary group and are commonly not associated with multiple myeloma.

Clinical Features. Approximately 80% of all extramedullary plasmacytomas occur in the head and neck region,[258–260] and plasmacytomas represented 4% of all benign and malignant nonepithelial tumors of the nasal cavity, paranasal sinuses, and nasopharynx in one series.[261] The tumor occurs most commonly in males and most cases present in patients over 40 years of age, with the sixth decade of life being the most common age of occurrence. The nasopharynx, nose, sinus, and tonsil are the most common primary sites, with patients presenting with symptoms of nasal or other airway obstruction or epistaxis; although virtually any head and neck site may be a primary site of involvement. Plasmacytomas of the skin of the head and neck region as well as those of the orbit more frequently represent secondary involvement by tumor.[259] Primary plasmacytoma of the thyroid also occurs rarely and is reported to be associated with surrounding reactive germinal center formation, with changes of lymphocytic thyroiditis and fibrosis.[262]

Extramedullary plasmacytomas are not usually associated with systemic amyloidosis; however, local amyloid deposits may be seen associated with the tumor.[263]

Pathologic Features. Plasmacytomas may be well, moderately, or poorly differentiated based on histologic examination.[259, 260] Well-differentiated tumors may be difficult to distinguish from reactive proliferations and are composed of a uniform population of mature-appearing plasma cells with round, eccentric nuclei with clumped peripheral nuclear chromatin. Nucleoli are absent or inconspicuous in these cases, and a cytoplasmic perinuclear hof is usually present. Poorly differentiated plasmacytomas may be composed of cells that are not obviously of plasma cell origin with large, pleomorphic nuclei. The nuclear chromatin is more fine and immature, and prominent nucleoli are present and often multiple. The characteristic perinuclear hof of mature plasma cells is usually absent. Moderately differentiated tumors have intermediate features (Fig. 12–39, see p. 751).

Although plasmacytomas are B-cell lineage neoplasms, they usually lose many of the cell surface antigens that are typical of B lymphocytes, such as leukocyte common antigen (LCA/CD45), CD19, CD20, and CD22.[264] In addition, immunoglobulin light and heavy chains are frequently not present on the cell surface of these tumors and clonality cannot be assessed in many cases by routine frozen section of flow cytometric immunophenotyping for this reason. Cytoplasmic immunoglobulin, however, is easily detectable by routine paraffin-section immunohistochemistry.[265] In addition, clonality can be determined by flow cytometry performed following cell permeabilization. In addition to cytoplasmic immunoglobulin expression, neoplastic plasma cells also express CD138 and the activation antigen CD38. Evidence of Epstein-Barr virus is not present in the majority of cases.[265]

Differential Diagnosis. The differential diagnosis of well-differentiated plasmacytoma is with reactive plasma cell proliferations and lymphoplasmacytic lymphomas. It may not be possible to distinguish plasmacytoma from a reactive proliferation on hematoxylin-eosin–stained sections alone. In particular, the germinal center formation and fibrosis commonly seen with plasmacytoma of the thyroid might mimic inflammatory pseudotumor (plasma cell granuloma).

Immunohistochemical studies in paraffin section for immunoglobulin light chains will demonstrate a monotypic plasma cell population in the vast majority of plasmacytomas, whereas the plasma cells of inflammatory pseudotumor are polytypic. Lymphoplasmacytic lymphomas will show a spectrum of cells ranging from small lymphocytes to plasmacytoid lymphocytes and plasma cells, in contrast to the rather monotonous population of mature plasma cells seen with well-differentiated plasmacytoma.

Moderately and poorly differentiated plasmacytomas must be distinguished from metastatic tumors and high-grade malignant lymphomas. Malignant melanoma may have eccentric pleomorphic nuclei with prominent nucleoli, similar to a poorly differentiated plasmacytoma. The lack of immunoglobulin expression as well as detection of S100 protein and the melanoma-associated marker HMB-45 are all useful for the correct diagnosis of melanoma. Large-cell immunoblastic lymphoma with plasmacytoid features may be very difficult to differentiate from a poorly differentiated plasmacytoma. Most plasmacytomas express either IgA or IgG immunoglobulins, in contrast to IgM expression in most lymphomas.[266] However, sufficient numbers of IgG-positive malignant lymphomas exist to make this criterion alone insufficient for diagnosis. Additional immunophenotypic differences, however, do exist. As mentioned, plasmacytomas do not usually express CD20 or CD45 but are CD38-positive. In contrast, most immunoblastic lymphomas express B-cell or T-cell lineage associated antigens, are CD45-positive, and are CD38-negative.[264] Therefore, a combination of immunoglobulin studies as well as other marker studies can resolve this differential diagnosis in most cases. The clinical features of the patient may also aid in the differential diagnosis, since most extramedullary plasmacytomas of the head and neck represent a single localized disease process.

Treatment and Prognosis. In general, extramedullary plasmacytomas of the head and neck region are radiosensitive and can be cured, although a subgroup of patients have recurrence or develop systemic disease. The reason for a more favorable prognosis in this site is not clear, but it has been speculated that the response to therapy is related to the small size of the tumors at the time of diagnosis in comparison to plasmacytomas at other sites.[260] Several features, however, have been found to suggest a poor response to therapy and include the presence of bone infiltration, immature nuclear chromatin, and the presence of prominent nucleoli.[258, 267] Patients with these features are at increased risk of developing local recurrence or multiple myeloma.

Extramedullary Myeloid Cell Tumors

The neoplastic proliferation of myeloid cells outside of the bone marrow is known by a variety of names, including extramedullary myeloid cell tumor (EMCT), granulocytic sarcoma, and chloroma. The term *chloroma* relates to the green color of the cut section of the gross lesion. Such proliferations may occur de novo or may be seen in patients with a history of a chronic myeloproliferative disorder, myelodysplastic syndromes, or acute myeloid leukemia.[268–271] Patients with de novo EMCTs frequently will develop acute leukemia,[268, 271, 272] although a subgroup of patients may not.[272]

Clinical Features. EMCT may occur at any age and at essentially any site. The head and neck region is frequently involved, with the orbit, nose, nasopharynx, tonsil, and cervical lymph nodes all being relatively common sites of disease.[268, 270–273] In patients with a previous history of a chronic myeloproliferative disorder, the development of an EMCT is a poor prognostic indicator, with most patients developing bone marrow evidence of blast crisis within a few months of development of the lesion, frequently resulting in the rapid death of the patient.[268, 269] The tumors may be solitary or multiple at the time of presentation.[268] Orbital EMCTs occur in up to 16% of patients with acute myeloid leukemia of all types.[274, 275] Tumors at this site are virtually always in children and are usually bilateral with resultant proptosis.[276] Bilateral tonsillar involvement as well as nasal and nasopharyngeal tumors may be rapidly enlarging masses that result in acute respiratory distress.[273]

Pathologic Features. Grossly, the tumors form homogeneous masses. The characteristic green cut surface of the tumor may only be obvious at the time of sectioning, with the color fading upon exposure to air.[268] Well-differentiated, poorly differentiated, and blastic histologic types have been described.[270] All show a diffuse cellular proliferation. Well-differentiated tumors show evidence of myeloid maturation, with eosinophilic myelocytes frequently identifiable. These cases are usually cytochemically positive for chloroacetate esterase. Poorly differentiated tumors morphologically resemble large-cell lymphomas with irregular nuclei, prominent nucleoli, and somewhat vesicular chromatin. Cytoplasmic granules are not obvious but may be identified in rare cells. Blastic tumors have finer nuclear chromatin with a high mitotic rate and no obvious cytoplasmic granules (Fig. 12–40).

Traditionally, extramedullary myeloid cell tumors were identified cytochemically with chloroacetate esterase stains on paraffin sections; however, one third to one quarter of cases will be cytochemically negative.[270, 271] Paraffin section immunohistochemistry is useful and is now preferred over cytochemical studies alone.[270, 271, 277] Most cases of EMCTs will react for CD45, CD43, and myeloperoxidase by paraffin section immunohistochemistry, while being negative for the lymphoid antigens CD3, CD45RO, and CD20. CD43 antigen expression, detected by the Leu-22 antibody, is found in almost all cases and other CD43 antibodies also detect a high percentage of cases. Since CD43 is frequently used as T-cell lineage associated antibody in the evaluation of lymphomas, CD43-positive tumors should be further evaluated with additional T-cell lineage antibodies before a myeloid cell tumor is excluded in favor of a T-cell lymphoma.[278] EMCTs are generally negative for the other T-cell lineage antigens, such as CD3 and CD45RO, and most cases will immunoreact with myeloperoxidase to confirm the myeloid nature of the

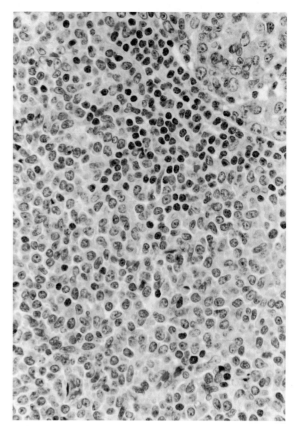

Figure 12–40. Extramedullary myeloid cell tumor involving a lymph node. A residual germinal center is present (top right). The tumor cells have fine, blast-like nuclear chromatin and indistinct cytoplasm.

proliferation. Frozen section immunohistochemistry or flow cytometric immunophenotyping of fresh tissue is useful to identify additional myeloid antigens, such as CD13 and CD33, as well as antigens associated with immaturity, such as CD34 and CD117. However, these tumors are rare and may not be suspected at the time of biopsy. For this reason, fresh or frozen tissue often is not available for study.

Differential Diagnosis. Extramedullary myeloid cell tumors, particularly the poorly differentiated and blastic types, are most often confused with malignant lymphomas.[270, 272] Poorly differentiated EMCTs may resemble large-cell lymphoma but usually do not have the characteristic two to three small nucleoli of most large-cell lymphomas and have more abundant and basophilic cytoplasm than the usual large-cell lymphoma. The monomorphic variant of anaplastic large-cell lymphoma may have cytoplasmic and nuclear features resembling EMCTs.[193, 196] The identification of a myeloperoxidase-negative tumor with a B-cell or T-cell lymphoma phenotype, with the exception of CD43 expression, is sufficient to exclude an EMCT, and CD30 expression is generally absent in these tumors. The blastic type of EMCT is most often confused with small noncleaved cell lymphoma (including Burkitt's lymphoma) and lymphoblastic lymphoma. Small noncleaved cell lymphomas are CD20-positive and myeloperoxidase-negative, whereas only up to 8% of EMCTs are CD20-positive.[270, 271, 277] The rare cases of CD20-positive EMCTs show weak and focal CD20 expression compared with usually strong and diffuse expression of malignant lymphomas. Lymphoblastic lymphomas or precursor B-cell or T-cell lineage may be CD43-positive; however, cytoplasmic CD3 expression can be detected by paraffin section immunohistochemistry in most cases of T-cell acute lymphoblastic leukemia/lymphoma, and the CD79a antibody will react with the majority of precursor B-cell tumors. The paraffin section identification of TdT expression is also quite useful in identifying cases of lymphoblastic leukemia/lymphoma, although a subpopulation of myeloid leukemias are TdT-positive.[279]

Treatment and Prognosis. Patients with EMCT are treated as they would be if they presented with acute myelogenous leukemia. Combination chemotherapy is indicated, with differences in regimens depending on the type of leukemia. Bone marrow transplantation may be indicated. The prognosis of patients with EMCT is essentially identical to that of patients with acute myeloid leukemia.

Langerhans' Cell Histiocytosis

Langerhans' cell histiocytosis (LCH) (histiocytosis X or Langerhans' cell granulomatosis)[280] is a clonal proliferation[281, 282] that affects males almost twice as often as females and consists of several quite variable clinical diseases that are morphologically identical. Historically, the disease entities were defined under the term *Histiocytosis X*[283] as eosinophilic granuloma (solitary disease), Hand-Schüller-Christian syndrome (triad of skull defects, exophthalmos, and diabetes insipidus) and Letterer-Siwe syndrome (systemic disease with fever, otitis media, hepatosplenomegaly, lymphadenopathy, anemia, bone lesions, and seborrheic cutaneous lesions). Since many cases do not fit well into these fairly rigid early categories, they may also be divided into the following: *unifocal disease* (eosinophilic granuloma), *multifocal unisystem disease* (including Hand-Schüller-Christian syndrome), and *multifocal multisystem disease* (including Letterer-Siwe syndrome).

Clinical Features. Langerhans' cell histiocytosis may occur at any age. and the median age of presentation varies with the different clinical syndromes. Unifocal disease occurs most often in older children and young adults, whereas multifocal unisystem disease and multifocal multisystem disease generally affect young children and infants.[284–287] The clinical course of LCH is variable, with some patients undergoing spontaneous regression while others progress with resultant infection and death. Patient survival is inversely related to the number of organs involved, with multifocal multisystem disease having the worst prognosis.

Virtually any anatomic location may be involved by LCH, but the head and neck region is the most frequently involved.[287–291] Specifically, the skull is most commonly involved by any type of LCH. The jaw is the second most common site involved in the head and neck region, and lymph nodes draining bone or skin lesions may be involved. In bone, clusters or individual cells are present and may surround or entrap portions of lamellar bone.

Pathologic Features. Cytologically, the Langerhans' cells have "coffee bean" oval nuclei that are folded or indented. The nuclei are characteristically grooved with small or absent nucleoli. Multinucleated cells are common. The cells have moderately abundant clear to eosinophilic cytoplasm. Mitotic activity is quite variable and may be absent, and atypical mitoses are usually not seen. Background eosinophils are usually numerous, often forming abscesses. Clusters of foamy histiocytes may also be present, and osteoclast-like giant cells are common. Background lymphocytes and neutrophils may be present. Involved lymph nodes may be diffusely replaced but are most often only focally involved with sinusoidal distention and frequent perinodal tissue extension. Lymph nodes draining bone or skin sites of involvement may not be enlarged but still show partial sinusoidal involvement. The eosinophilic abscesses and other background cells seen in bone lesions are less common within involved lymph nodes. Neither the category of disease nor the aggressiveness of the process can be reliably predicted based on histologic features alone.[292]

Langerhans' cell histiocytes are positive for vimentin, HLA-DR, S100, CD4, and CD1 and are variably positive for CD68 and placental alkaline phosphatase.[293–296] In general, the neoplastic cells are negative for B- and T-cell markers such as CD20, CD45RA, and CD45RO; however, they may express cytoplasmic CD2 and CD3. Although Langerhans' cells characteristically demonstrate Birbeck granules by electron microscopy, such study is not required for diagnosis.[280] The detection of CD1a expression by immunohistochemistry is sufficient for a definitive diagnosis, and antibodies are now available for the detection of this antigen in paraffin sections.[297]

CD1a expression is reportedly limited to Langerhans' cells, immature thymocytes, and T lymphoblastic malignancies.

In addition to the above-mentioned syndromes, LCH may be found incidentally associated with malignant neoplasms (Fig. 12–41, see p. 751).[298, 299] Although Hodgkin's disease is the most commonly associated neoplasm, non-Hodgkin's lymphomas, acute myeloid leukemias, and non-hematopoietic neoplasms have also been reported. The focus of LCH may be directly associated with the malignancy or may be at an unrelated site.

Differential Diagnosis. The differential diagnosis of LCH would include metastatic tumors, malignant lymphomas, and histiocytic proliferations. Metastatic tumors, such as carcinoma and melanoma, can be easily excluded by an immunohistochemical panel that includes keratin, S100, HMB-45, and CD1. Exclusion of CD1, however, may lead to the erroneous conclusion of an immunophenotype that is consistent with malignant melanoma (keratin-negative, S100-positive). Sinusoidal involvement by an anaplastic large cell lymphoma is usually not a diagnostic problem. Although the cells of LCH may be multinucleated, they do not show the nuclear anaplasia characteristic of this tumor. In addition, LCH cells do not express the CD30 antigen. Most histiocytic proliferations, such as reactive sinusoidal hyperplasia and sinus histiocytosis with massive lymphadenopathy (SHML), do not have the cleaved or grooved nuclei of LCH; and the vesicular nuclear chromatin and phagocytosis of SHML are not present in LCH. Dermatopathic lymphadenopathy characteristically contains Langerhans' cells, but they are located in the paracortical region of the lymph node rather than within sinuses. Also, the cells of dermatopathic lymphadenopathy are accompanied by many melanin-containing histiocytes that are not seen in LCH.

Treatment and Prognosis. For patients with unifocal involvement, surgical excision may be adequate for cure. Local lesions are also responsive to radiation therapy. For the smaller subset of patients with generalized disease, chemotherapy may be required. The prognosis depends on the extent of disease and the response to chemotherapy.

Dendritic Reticulum Cell Tumors and True Histiocytic Lymphoma

Follicular and interdigitating dendritic reticulum cell tumors are rare, related tumors that may occur within lymph nodes at virtually any anatomic site, although most cases present involving cervical or supraclavicular lymph nodes.[300–303] They differ from Langerhans' cell histiocytosis morphologically as well as by their lack of CD1 antigen and Birbeck granules.

Clinical Features. The rarity of these tumors precludes definitive statements about their clinical features.

Pathologic Features. *Follicular dendritic reticulum cell tumors* are composed of spindled cells with bland nuclei that may contain admixed small lymphocytes (Fig. 12–42, see p. 752). By electron microscopy, the tumors demonstrate long cytoplasmic processes connected by numerous desmosomes. Immunohistochemical studies demonstrate that the tumor cells are characteristically positive for the dendritic cell antigens CD21 and CD35. The tumor cells are also CD68-positive, but may be CD45- and S100-negative.

Interdigitating reticulum cell tumors may morphologically resemble non-Hodgkin's lymphoma or may have spindled cells similar to follicular dendritic reticulum cell tumors. Interdigitating cell processes without well-formed desmosomes are seen by electron microscopy, and the tumors are negative for B-cell and T-cell lineage antigens. Interdigitating tumors cells are positive for CD45, S100, and CD68.

True histiocytic lymphoma is a neoplastic proliferation of cells of histiocytic lineage that may present with node-based or extranodal, often cutaneous or subcutaneous, disease.[304–306] This term is preferred over malignant histiocytosis, since many of the cases historically termed malignant histiocytosis actually represented non-Hodgkin's lymphomas, including anaplastic large cell lymphoma, when further studied with immunologic and molecular biologic techniques.[213, 277, 307, 308] Lymph node involvement by true histiocytic lymphoma may be partial or diffuse and consists of a proliferation of malignant histiocyte-like cells (Fig. 12–43, see p. 752). The cells have prominent nucleoli and may be multinucleated with abundant eosinophilic cytoplasm. The cells should be CD68-positive and must be negative for all T-cell and B-cell lineage specific markers by immunohistochemistry as well as negative for CD30, keratin, S100, and HMB45. In addition, the tumor must lack both immunoglobulin and T-cell receptor gene rearrangements.

Differential Diagnosis. The differential diagnosis of follicular dendritic or interdigitating reticulum cell tumors includes metastatic sarcomas and spindle cell carcinomas. Immunohistochemical studies are essential to establish the diagnosis and to exclude other neoplasms. The CD35 antigen is expressed by follicular dendritic but not interdigitating reticulum cell tumors.

The differential diagnosis of true histiocytic lymphoma includes metastatic tumors and malignant lymphomas, all of which should be excluded by immunohistochemistry and molecular studies prior to diagnosis. The cytologically malignant features of the tumor cells in true histiocytic lymphoma is helpful in differentiating true histiocytic lymphoma from other histiocytic proliferations such as follicular dendritic cell tumors, sinus histiocytosis with massive lymphadenopathy, storage diseases, and hemophagocytic syndromes.

Treatment and Prognosis. The small number of cases reported precludes any statements regarding appropriate therapy. In general, follicular dendritic reticulum cell tumors have a tendency to recur, but overall patients have prolonged survival. Interdigitating reticulum cell tumors are much more aggressive, with some patients dying of generalized disease. Most patients reported with true histiocytic lymphoma have developed disseminated lymphoma with death from disease.

REFERENCES

Benign Lesions

1. Schnitzer B: Reactive lymphoid hyperplasia. In: Jaffe ES, ed. *Surgical Pathology of Lymph Nodes and Related Organs. Major Problems in Pathology Series,* volume 16, 2nd ed. Philadelphia: W.B. Saunders, 1994:98.

Progressive Transformation of Germinal Centers

2. Hansmann M-L, Fellbaum C, Hui PK, et al: Progressive transformation of germinal centers with and without association to Hodgkin's disease. *Am J Clin Pathol* 1990;93:219.
3. Ferry JA, Zukerberg LR, Harris NL: Florid progressive transformation of germinal centers: A syndrome affecting young men, without early progression to nodular lymphocyte predominance Hodgkin's disease. *Am J Surg Pathol* 1992;16:252.

Toxoplasma Lymphadenitis

4. Stansfeld AG: The histologic diagnosis of toxoplasmic lymphadenitis. *J Clin Pathol* 1961;14:565.
5. Dorfman RF, Remington JS: Value of lymph node biopsy in the diagnosis of toxoplasmosis. *N Engl J Med* 1973;289:878.
6. Sheibani K, Fritz RM, Winberg CD, et al: "Monocytoid" cells in reactive follicular hyperplasia with and without multifocal histiocytic reactions: An immunohistochemical study of 21 cases including suspected cases of toxoplasmosis lymphadenitis. *Am J Clin Pathol* 1984;81:453.

Myoepithelial Sialadentis/Benign Lymphoepithelial Lesion

7. Daniels TE: Benign lymphoepithelial lesion and Sjögren's syndrome. In: Ellis GL, Auclair PL, Gnepp DR, eds. *Surgical Pathology of the Salivary Glands. Major Problems in Pathology Series,* volume 25. Philadelphia: W.B. Saunders, 1991:83.

8. Kornstein MJ, Parker GA, Nottmils A: Immunohistology of the benign lymphoepithelial lesion in AIDS–related lymphadenopathy. *Hum Pathol* 1988;19:1359.
9. Labouyrie E, Merlio JPH, Beylot-Bory M, et al: Human immunodeficiency virus type 1 replication within cystic lymphoepithelial lesion of the salivary gland. *Am J Clin Pathol* 1993;100:41.
10. Sciubba JJ, Auclair PL, Ellis GL: Malignant lymphomas. In: Ellis GL, Auclair PL, Gnepp DR, eds. *Surgical Pathology of the Salivary Glands. Major Problems in Pathology Series,* volume 25. Philadelphia: W.B. Saunders, 1991:528.
11. Hyjek E, Smith WJ, Isaacson PG: Primary B-cell lymphoma of salivary glands and its relationship to myoepithelial sialadenitis. *Hum Pathol* 1988;19:766.
12. Zulman J, Jaffe R, Talal N: Evidence that the malignant lymphoma of Sjögren's syndrome is a monoclonal B-cell neoplasm. *N Engl J Med* 1978;299:1215.
13. Schmid U, Helbron D, Lennert K: Development of malignant lymphoma in myoepithelial sialadenitis (Sjögren's syndrome). *Virchows Arch A (Pathol Anat)* 1982;395:11.
14. Diss TC, Wotherspoon AC, Speight P, et al: B-cell monoclonality, Epstein-Barr virus, and t(14;18) in myoepithelial sialadenitis and low-grade B-cell MALT lymphoma of the parotid gland. *Am J Surg Pathol* 1995;19:531.

Kimura's Disease and Angiolymphoid Hyperplasia with Eosinophilia

15. Kung ITM, Gibson JB, Bannatyne PM: Kimura's disease: A clinicopathological study of 21 cases and its distinction from angiolymphoid hyperplasia with eosinophilia. *Pathology* 1984;16:39.
16. Kuo T, Shih L, Chan H: Kimura's disease. Involvement of regional lymph nodes and distinction from angiolymphoid hyperplasia with eosinophilia. *Am J Surg Pathol* 1988;12:843.
17. Chan JKC, Hui PK, Ng CS, et al: Epithelioid haemangioma (angiolymphoid hyperplasia with eosinophilia) and Kimura's disease in Chinese. *Histopathology* 1989;15:557.
18. Hui PK, Chan JKC, Ng CS, et al: Lymphadenopathy of Kimura's disease. *Am J Surg Pathol* 1989;13:177.

Infectious Mononucleosis

19. Childs CC, Parham DM, Berard CW: Infectious mononucleosis: The spectrum of morphologic changes simulating lymphoma in lymph nodes and tonsils. *Am J Clin Pathol* 1987;53:304.
20. Strickler JG, Fedeli F, Gorwitz CA, et al: Infectious mononucleosis in lymphoid tissue. Histopathology, in situ hybridization, and differential diagnosis. *Arch Pathol Lab Med* 1993;117:269.

Dermatopathic Lymphadenopathy

21. Gould E, Porto R, Albores-Saavedra J, et al: Dermatopathic lymphadenitis. The spectrum and significance of its morphologic features. *Arch Pathol Lab Med* 1988;112:1145.
22. Burke JS, Colby TV: Dermatopathic lymphadenopathy: Comparison of cases associated and unassociated with mycosis fungoides. *Am J Surg Pathol* 1981;5:343.

Cat Scratch Disease

23. Anderson B, Sims K, Regnery R, et al: Detection of *Rochalimaea henselae* DNA in specimens from cat scratch disease patients by PCR. *J Clin Microbiol* 1994;32:942.
24. Alkan S, Morgan MB, Sandin RL, et al: Dual role of *Afipia felis* and *Rochalimaea henselae* in cat-scratch disease. *Lancet* 1995;345:385.
25. Naji AF, Carbonell F, Barker HJ: Cat scratch disease. A report of three new cases, review of the literature, and classification of the pathologic changes in the lymph nodes during various stages of the disease. *Am J Clin Pathol* 1962;38:513.
26. Campbell JAH: Cat-scratch disease. *Pathol Annu* 1977;12:277.
27. Miller-Catchpole R, Variakojis D, Vardiman JW, et al: Cat scratch disease. Identification of bacteria in seven cases of lymphadenitis. *Am J Surg Pathol* 1986;10:276.
28. Wear DJ, Margileth AM, Hadfield TL, et al: Cat scratch disease: A bacterial infection. *Science* 1983;221:1403.

29. Korbi S, Toccanier M, Leyvraz G, et al: Use of silver staining (Dieterlé's stain) in the diagnosis of cat scratch disease. *Histopathology* 1986;10:1015.

Lymphadenopathy in Human Immunodeficiency Virus Infection

30. Ioachim HL, Cronin W, Roy M, et al: Persistent lymphadenopathies in people at high risk for HIV infection. Clinicopathologic correlations and long-term follow-up in 79 cases. *Am J Clin Pathol* 1990;93:208.
31. Wood GS, Garcia CF, Dorfman RF, et al: The immunohistology of follicle lysis in lymph node biopsies from homosexual men. *Blood* 1985;66:1092.

Kikuchi-Fujimoto Disease

32. Kikuchi M: Lymphadenitis showing focal reticulum cell hyperplasia with nuclear debris and phagocytes: A clinico-pathological study. *Nippon Ketsueki Gakkai Zasshi* 1972;35:379.
33. Fujimoto Y, Kozima Y, Yamaguchi K: Cervical subacute necrotizing lymphadenitis: A new clinicopathologic entity. *Naika* 1972;20:920.
34. Pileri S, Kikuchi M, Helbron D, et al: Histiocytic necrotizing lymphadenitis without granulocytic infiltration. *Virchows Archiv A Pathol Anat* 1982;395:257.
35. Turner RR, Martin J, Dorfman RF: Necrotizing lymphadenitis. A study of 30 cases. *Am J Surg Pathol* 1983;7:115.
36. Dorfman RF, Berry GJ: Kikuchi's histiocytic necrotizing lymphadenitis: An analysis of 108 cases with emphasis on differential diagnosis. *Semin Diagn Pathol* 1988;5:329.
37. Chamulak GA, Brynes RK, Nathwani BN: Kikuchi-Fujimoto disease mimicking malignant lymphoma. *Am J Surg Pathol* 1990;14:514.

Lymphadenopathy in Systemic Lupus Erythematosus

38. Medeiros LJ, Kaynor B, Harris NL: Lupus lymphadenitis: Report of a case with immunohistologic studies on frozen sections. *Hum Pathol* 1989;20:295.

Inflammatory Pseudotumor

39. Perrone T, De Wolf-Peeters C, Frizzera G: Inflammatory pseudotumor of lymph nodes. A distinctive pattern of nodal reaction. *Am J Surg Pathol* 1988;12:351.
40. Davis RE, Warnke RA, Dorfman RF: Inflammatory pseudotumor of lymph nodes: Additional observations and evidence for an inflammatory etiology. *Am J Surg Pathol* 1991;15:744.
41. Coffin CM, Watterson J, Priest JR, et al: Extrapulmonary inflammatory myofibroblastic tumor (inflammatory pseudotumor): A clinicopathologic and immunohistochemical study of 84 cases. *Am J Surg Pathol* 1995;19:859.
42. Janigan DT, Marrie TJ: An inflammatory pseudotumor of the lung in Q fever pneumonia. *N Engl J Med* 1983;308:86.
43. Matsubara O, Tan-Liu NS, Kenney RM, et al: Inflammatory pseudotumor of the lung: Progression from organizing pneumonia to fibrous histiocytoma or to plasma cell granuloma in 32 cases. *Hum Pathol* 1988;19:807.
44. Wiernik PH, Rader M, Becker NH, et al: Inflammatory pseudotumor of spleen. *Cancer* 1990;66:597.
45. Arber DA, Kamel OW, van de Rijn M, et al: Frequent presence of the Epstein-Barr virus in inflammatory pseudotumor. *Hum Pathol* 1995;26:1093.
46. Chen KTK: Mycobacterial spindle cell pseudotumor of lymph nodes. *Am J Surg Pathol* 1992;16:276.
47. Facchetti F, de Wolf Peeters C, De Wever I, et al: Inflammatory pseudotumor of lymph nodes. Immunohistochemical evidence for its fibrohistiocytic nature. *Am J Pathol* 1990;137:281.

Sinus Histiocytosis and Massive Lymphadenopathy

48. Rosai J, Dorfman RF: Sinus histiocytosis with massive lymphadenopathy: A newly recognized benign clinicopathological entity. *Arch Pathol* 1969;87:63.

49. Rosai J, Dorfman RF: Sinus histiocytosis with massive lymphadenopathy: A pseudolymphomatous benign disorder. Analysis of 34 cases. *Cancer* 1972;30:1174.
50. Foucar E, Rosai J, Dorfman RF: Sinus histiocytosis with massive lymphadenopathy (Rosai-Dorfman disease): Review of the entity. *Semin Diagn Pathol* 1990;7:19.
51. Montgomery EA, Meis JM, Frizzera G: Rosai-Dorfman disease of soft tissue. *Am J Surg Pathol* 1992;16:122.
52. Wenig BM, Abbondanzo SL, Childers EL, et al: Extranodal sinus histiocytosis with massive lymphadenopathy (Rosai-Dorfman disease) of the head and neck. *Hum Pathol* 1993;24:483.
53. Eisen RN, Buckley PJ, Rosai J: Immunophenotypic characterization of sinus histiocytosis with massive lymphadenopathy (Rosai-Dorfman disease). *Semin Diagn Pathol* 1990;7:74.

Lymph Node Infarction

54. Norton AJ, Ramsey AD, Isaacson PG: Antigen preservation in infarcted lymphoid tissue: A novel approach to the infarcted lymph node using monoclonal antibodies effective in routinely processed tissues. *Am J Surg Pathol* 1988;12:759.
55. Laszewski MJ, Belding PJ, Feddersen RM, et al: Clonal immunoglobulin gene rearrangement in the infarcted lymph node syndrome. *Am J Clin Pathol* 1991;96:116.

Classification of Non-Hodgkin's Lymphomas

56. Rappaport H, Winter WJ, Hicks EB: Follicular lymphoma: A reevaluation of its position in the scheme of malignant lymphoma, based on a survey of 253 cases. *Cancer* 1956;9:792.
57. Nathwani BN, Kim H, Rappaport H: Malignant lymphoma, lymphoblastic. *Cancer* 1976;38:964.
58. Rosenberg SA, Berard CW, Brown BW, et al: National Cancer Insitute sponsored study of classifications of non-Hodgkin's lymphomas: Summary and description of a working formulation for clinical usage. *Cancer* 1982;49:2112.
59. Harris NL, Jaffe ES, Stein H, et al: A revised European-American classification of lymphoid neoplasms: A proposal from the International Lymphoma Study Group. *Blood* 1994;84:1361.

Therapy of Non-Hodgkin's Lymphomas

60. Freedman AS, Nadler LM: Non-Hodgkin's Lymphomas. In: Holland JF, Bast RC, Morton DL, Frei E, Kufe DW, Weichelbaum RR, eds. *Cancer Medicine,* 4th ed. Baltimore: Williams & Wilkins, 1997:2757–2795.

Chronic Lymphocytic Leukemia/Small Lymphocytic Lymphoma

61. Stetler-Stevenson M, Medeiros LJ, Jaffe ES: Immunophenotypic methods and findings in the diagnosis of lymphoproliferative diseases. In: Jaffe ES, ed. *Surgical Pathology of Lymph Nodes and Related Organs. Major Problems in Pathology Series,* volume 16, 2nd ed. Philadelphia: W.B.Saunders, 1994:22.
62. Morrison WH, Hoppe RT, Weiss LM, et al: Small lymphocytic lymphoma. *J Clin Oncol* 1989;7:598.
63. Dick FR, Maca RD: The lymph node in chronic lymphocytic leukemia. *Cancer* 1978;41:283.
64. Medeiros LJ, Bagg A, Cossman J: Molecular genetics in the diagnosis and classification of lymphoid neoplasms. In: Jaffe ES, ed. *Surgical Pathology of Lymph Nodes and Related Organs. Major Problems in Pathology Series,* volume 16, 2nd ed. Philadelphia: W.B.Saunders, 1994:58.
65. Matutes E, Oscier D, Garcia Marco J, et al: Trisomy 12 defines a group of CLL with atypical morphology. Correlation between cytogenetic, clinical and laboratory features in 544 patients. *Br J Hematol* 1996;92:382.
66. Evans HL, Butler JJ, Youness EL: Malignant lymphoma, small lymphocytic type: A clinicopathologic study of 84 cases with suggested criteria for intermediate lymphocytic lymphoma. *Cancer* 1978; 41:1440.

Lymphoplasmacytoid Lymphoma/Immunocytoma

67. Heinz R, Stacher A, Giessen HP, et al: Lymphoplasmacytic/lymphoplasmacytoid lymphoma: A clinical entity distinct from chronic lymphocytic leukemia? *Blut* 1981;43:183.
68. Harrison CV: The morphology of the lymph node in the macroglobulinemia of Waldenstrom. *J Clin Pathol* 1972;25:12.
69. Rywlin AM, Civantos F, Ortega RS, et al: Bone marrow histology in monoclonal macroglobulinemia. *Am J Clin Pathol* 1975;63:769.

Follicular Lymphoma

70. Greiner TC, Medeiros LJ, Jaffe ES: Non-Hodgkin's lymphoma. *Cancer* 1995;75(Suppl): 370.
71. Melo JV, Robinson DS, de Oliveira MP, et al: Morphology and immunology of circulating cells in leukaemic phase of follicular lymphoma. *J Clin Pathol* 1988;41:951.
72. Nathwani BN, Winberg CD, Diamond LW, et al: Morphologic criteria for the differentiation of follicular lymphoma from florid reactive follicular hyperplasia: A study of 80 cases. *Cancer* 1981;48:1974.
73. Lukes RJ, Collins RD. Immunological characterization of human malignant lymphomas. *Cancer* 1974;34:1488.
74. Mann RB, Berard CW: Criteria for the cytologic subclassification of follicular lymphomas: A proposed alternative method. *Hematol Oncol* 1985;3:1183.
75. Weiss LM, Warnke RA, Sklar J, et al: Molecular analysis of the t(14;18) chromosomal translocation in malignant lymphomas. *N Engl J Med* 1987;317:1185.
76. Tsujimoto Y, Cossman J, Jaffe ES, et al: Involvement of the *bcl-2* gene in human follicular lymphoma. *Science* 1985;228:1440.
77. Zutter M, Hockenbery D, Silverman GA, et al: Immunolocalization of the *bcl-2* protein within hematopoietic neoplasms. *Blood* 1991;78:1062.
78. deJong D, Pring FA, Mason DY, et al: Subcellular localization of the bcl-2 protein in malignant and normal lymphoid cells. *Cancer Res* 1994;54:256.
79. Aster JC, Kobayashi Y, Shiota M, et al: Detection of the t(14;18) at similar frequencies in hyperplastic lymphoid tissues from American and Japanese patients. *Am J Pathol* 1992;141:291.
80. Ladanyi M, Offit K, Parsa NZ, et al: Follicular lymphoma with the t(8;14)(q24;q32): A distinct clinical and molecular subset of t(8;14)-bearing lymphomas. *Blood* 1992;79:2124.
81. Rimokh R, Gadoux M, Bertheas M-F, et al: *FVT*-1, a novel human transcription unit affected by variant translocation t(2;28)(p11;q21) of follicular lymphoma. *Blood* 1993;81:136.
82. Warnke RA, Kim H, Fuks Z, et al: The coexistence of nodular and diffuse patterns in nodular non-Hodgkin's lymphomas: Significance and clinicopathologic correlation. *Cancer* 1977;40:1229.
83. Hu E, Weiss LM, Hoppe RT, et al: Follicular and diffuse mixed small-cleaved and large-cell lymphoma: A clinicopathologic study. *J Clin Oncol* 1985;3:1183.
84. Jones R, Young RC, Berard CW, et al: Histologic progression in non-Hodgkin's lymphoma: Implications for survival and clinical trials. *Proc Am Soc Clin Oncol* 1979;20:353.
85. Fisher RI, Jones RB, DeVita VT, et al: Natural history of malignant lymphomas with divergent histologies at staging evaluation. *Cancer* 1981;47:2022.

Marginal Zone B-Cell Lymphoma

86. Sheibani K, Burke JS, Swartz WG, et al: Monocytoid B-cell lymphoma: Clinicopathologic study of 21 cases of a unique type of low-grade lymphoma. *Cancer* 1988;62:1531.
87. Nizze H, Cogliatti SB, Von Schilling C, et al: Monocytoid B-cell lymphoma: Morphological variants and relationship to low-grade B-cell lymphoma of the mucosa-associated lymphoid tissue. *Histopathology* 1991;18:403.
88. Ngan B-Y, Warnke RA, Wilson M, et al: Monocytoid B-cell lymphoma: A study of 36 cases. *Hum Pathol* 1991;22:409.
89. Slovak ML, Weiss LM, Nathwani BN, et al: Cytogenetic studies of composite lymphomas: Monocytoid B-cell lymphoma and other B-cell non-Hodgkin's lymphomas. *Hum Pathol* 1993;24:1086.
90. Brynes RK, Almaguer PD, Leathery KE, et al: Numerical cytogenetic abnormalities of chromosomes 3, 7, and 12 in marginal zone B-cell lymphomas. *Mod Pathol* 1996;9:995.

91. Fisher RI, Dahlberg S, Nathwani BN, et al: A clinical analysis of two indolent lymphoma entities: Mantle cell lymphoma and marginal zone lymphoma (including the mucosa-associated lymphoid tissue and monocytoid B-cell subcategories). A Southwest Oncology Group Study. *Blood* 1995;85:1075.
92. Medeiros LJ, Harmon DC, Linggood RM, et al: Immunohistologic features predict clinical behavior of orbital and conjunctival lymphoid infiltrates. *Blood* 1989;74:2121.
93. Knowles DM, Athan E, Ubriaco A, et al: Extranodal noncutaneous lymphoid hyperplasias represent a continuous spectrum of B-cell neoplasia: Demonstration by molecular genetic analysis. *Blood* 1989;73:1635.
94. Isaacson P, Wright DH: Malignant lymphoma of mucosa-associated lymphoid tissue: A distinctive type of B-cell lymphoma. *Cancer* 1983;52:1410.
95. Isaacson PG: Lymphomas of mucosa-associated lymphoid tissue (MALT). *Histopathology* 1990;16:617.
96. Harris NL: Extranodal lymphoid infiltrates and mucosa-associated lymphoid tissue (MALT): A unifying concept. *Am J Surg Pathol* 1991;15:879.
97. Li G, Hansmann M-L, Zwingers T, et al: Primary lymphomas of the lung: Morphological, immunohistochemical and clinical features. *Histopathology* 1990;16:519.
98. Isaacson PG, Wotherspoon AC, Diss T, et al: Follicular colonization in B-cell lymphoma of mucosa-associated lymphoid tissue. *Am J Surg Pathol* 1990;15:519.
99. Genta RM, Hamner HW, Graham DY: Gastric lymphoid follicles in *Helicobacter pylori* infection: Frequency, distribution, and response to triple antibiotic therapy. *Hum Pathol* 1993;24:577.
100. Wotherspoon AC, Doglioni C, Diss T, et al: Regression of primary low-grade B-cell gastric lymphoma of mucosa-associated lymphoid tissue type after eradication of *Helicobacter pylori*. *Lancet* 1993;342:575.
101. Addis BJ, Hyjek E, Isaacson PG: Primary pulmonary lymphoma: A reappraisal of its histogenesis and its relationship to pseudolymphoma and lymphoid interstitial pneumonia. *Histopathology* 1988;13:1.
102. Hyjek E, Isaacson PG: Primary B cell lymphoma of the thyroid and its relationship to Hashimoto's thyroiditis. *Hum Pathol* 1988;19:1315.
103. Wotherspoon AC, Finn TM, Isaacson PG: Trisomy 3 in low-grade B-cell lymphomas of mucosa associated lymphoid tissue. *Blood* 1995;85:2000.
104. Wotherspoon AC, Soosay GN, Diss TC, et al: Low-grade primary B-cell lymphoma of the lung: An immunohistochemical, molecular, and cytogenetic study of a single case. *Am J Clin Pathol* 1990;94:655.
105. Griffin CA, Zehnbauer BA, Beschorner WE, et al: t(11;18)(q21;q21) is a recurrent chromosome abnormality in small lymphocytic lymphoma. *Genes Chromosomes Cancer* 1992;4:153.

Mantle Cell Lymphoma

106. Bookman MA, Lardelli P, Jaffe ES, et al: Lymphocytic lymphoma of intermediate differentiation: Morphologic, immunophenotypic, and prognostic factors. *J Natl Cancer Inst* 1990;82:742.
107. O'Briain DS, Kennedy MJ, Daly PA, et al: Multiple lymphomatous polyposis of the gastrointestinal tract: A clinicopathologically distinctive form of non-Hodgkin's lymphoma of B-cell centrocytic type. *Am J Surg Pathol* 1989;13:691.
108. Weisenburger DD, Duggan MJ, Perry DA, et al: Non-Hodgkin's lymphomas of mantle zone origin. *Pathol Annu* 1991;26:139.
109. Lardelli P, Bookman MA, Sundeen J, et al: Lymphocytic lymphoma of intermediate differentiation: Morphologic and immunophenotypic spectrum and clinical correlations. *Am J Surg Pathol* 1990;14:752.
110. Pittaluga S, Wlodarska I, Stul MS, et al: Mantle cell lymphoma: A clinicopathologic study of 55 cases. *Histopathology* 1995;26:17.
111. Norton AJ, Matthews J, Pappa V, et al: Mantle cell lymphoma: Natural history defined in a serially biopsied population over a 20-year period. *Ann Oncol* 1995;6:249.
112. Leroux D, Le Marc'hadour F, Gressin R, et al: Non-Hodgkin's lymphomas with t(11;14)(q13;q32): A subset of mantle zone/intermediate lymphocytic lymphoma? *Br J Hematol* 1991;77:346.
113. Medeiros LJ, Van Krieken JH, Jaffe ES, et al: Association of *bcl-1* rearrangements with lymphocytic lymphoma of intermediate differentiation. *Blood* 1990;76:2086.
114. Williams ME, Swerdlow SH, Rosenberg CL, et al: Characterization of chromosome 11 translocation breakpoints at the bcl-1 and PRAD-1 loci in centrocytic lymphoma. *Cancer Res* 1992;52(Suppl):5541S.
115. Motokura T, Bloom T, Kim HG, et al: A novel cyclin encoded by a *bcl1*-linked candidate oncogene. *Nature* 1991;350:512.

116. deBoer CJ, Schuring E, Dreef E, et al: Cyclin D1 protein analysis in the diagnosis of mantle cell lymphoma. *Blood* 1995;86:2715.
117. Teodorovic I, Pittaluga S, Kluin-Nelemans JC, et al: Efficacy of four different regimens in 64 mantle-cell lymphoma cases: Clinicopathologic comparison with 498 other non-Hodgkin's lymphoma subtypes. *J Clin Oncol* 1995;13:2819.
118. Majilis A, Pugh W, Rodriguez MA, et al: Three histological variants of mantle cell lymphoma exhibit striking heterogeneity in clinical behavior and biological features (abstract). *Blood* 1993;82:388.

Diffuse Large B-Cell Lymphoma

119. Nathwani BN, Dixon DO, Jones SE, et al: The clinical significance of the morphological subdivision of diffuse "histiocytic" lymphoma: A study of 162 patients treated by the Souhtwest Oncology Group. *Blood* 1982;60:1068.
120. Jacobson JO, Wilkes BM, Kwiatkowski DJ, et al: *bcl-2* rearrangements in de novo diffuse large cell lymphoma: Association with distinctive clinical features. *Cancer* 1993;72:231.
121. Lo Coco F, Ye BH, Lista F, et al: Rearrangements of the *bcl*6 gene in diffuse large cell non-Hodgkin's lymphoma. *Blood* 1994;83:1757.
122. Offit K, Lo Coco F, Louie DC, et al: Rearrangement of the *bcl-6* gene as a prognostic marker in diffuse large-cell lymphoma. *N Engl J Med* 1994;331:74.
123. Straus DJ, Wong G, Yaholom J, et al: Diffuse large cell lymphoma. Prognostic factors with treatment. *Leukemia* 1991;5(Suppl 1):32.
124. Krishnan J, Walberg K, Frizzera G: T-cell-rich large B-cell lymphoma: A study of 30 cases, supporting its histologic heterogeneity and lack of clinical distinctiveness. *Am J Surg Pathol* 1994;18:455.
125. Medeiros LJ, Lardelli P, Stetler-Stevenson M, et al: Genotypic analysis of diffuse, mixed cell lymphomas: Comparison with morphologic and immunophenotypic findings. *Am J Clin Pathol* 1991;95:547.
126. Greer JP, Macon WR, Lamar RE, et al: T-cell-rich B-cell lymphomas: Diagnosis and response to therapy in 44 patients. *J Clin Oncol* 1995;13:1742.
127. Rodriguez J, Pugh WC, Cabanillas F: T-cell-rich B-cell lymphoma. *Blood* 1993;82:1586.

Burkitt's Lymphoma

128. Magrath IT: African Burkitt's lymphoma: History, biology, clinical features, and treatment. *Am J Pediatr Hematol Oncol* 1991;13:222.
129. Ioachim HL, Dorsett B, Cronin W, et al: Acquired immunodeficiency syndrome—associated lymphomas: Clinical, pathologic, immunologic, and viral characteristics of 111 cases. *Hum Pathol* 1991;22:659.
130. Berard CW, O'Conor GT, Thomas LB, et al: Histopathological definition of Burkitt's tumour. *Bull WHO* 1983;40:1393.
131. Miliauskas JR, Berard CW, Young RC, et al: Undifferentiated non-Hodgkin's lymphomas (Burkitt's and non-Burkitt's types): The relevance of making this histologic distinction. *Cancer* 1982;50:2115.
132. Haluska FG, Finger LR, Kagan J, et al: Molecular genetics of chromosomal translocations in B- and T-lymphoid malignancies. In: Cossman J, ed. *Molecular Genetics in Cancer Diagnosis.* New York: Elsevier, 1990:143.
133. Yano T, van Krieken JHJM, Magrath IT, et al: Histogenetic correlations between subcategories of small noncleaved cell lymphomas. *Blood* 1992;79:1282.
134. Murphy SB: Classification, staging and end results of treatment of childhood non-Hodgkin's lymphomas: Dissimilarities from lymphomas in adults. *Semin Oncol* 1980;7:332.
135. Murphy SB, Magrath IT: Workshop on pediatric lymphomas: Current results and prospects. *Ann Oncol* 1991;2(Suppl 2):219.

High-Grade B-Cell Lymphoma, Burkitt-Like

136. Levine AM, Pavlova Z, Pockros AW, et al: Small noncleaved follicular center cell (FCC) lymphoma: Burkitt and non-Burkitt variants in the United States. I. Clinical features. *Cancer* 1983;52:1073.
137. Wilson JF, Kjeldsberg CR, Sposto R, et al: The pathology of non-Hodgkin's lymphoma of childhood. II. Reproducibility and relevance of the histologic classification of "undifferentiated" lymphomas (Burkitt's versus non-Burkitt's). *Hum Pathol* 1987;18:1008.
138. Hutchison RE, Murphy SB, Fairclough DL, et al: Diffuse small non-cleaved cell lymphoma in children, Burkitt's versus non-Burkitt's types. Results from the Pediatric Oncology Group and St. Jude Children's Research Hospital. *Cancer* 1989;64:23.

Precursor Lymphoblastic Lymphoma/Leukemia, B-Cell and T-Cell

139. Medeiros LJ: Intermediate and high grade lymphomas in the working formulation. In: Jaffe ES, ed. *Surgical Pathology of Lymph Nodes and Related Organs. Major Problems in Pathology Series,* volume 16, 2nd ed. Philadelphia: W.B. Saunders, 1994:283.
140. Korsmeyer SJ, Hieter PA, Ravetch JV, et al: Developmental hierarchy of immunoglobulin gene rearrangements in human leukemic pre-B-cells. *Proc Natl Acad Sci USA* 1981;78:7096.
141. Felix CA, Poplack DG, Reaman GH, et al: Characterization of immunoglobulin and T-cell receptor gene patterns in B-cell precursor acute lymphoblastic leukemia of childhood. *J Clin Oncol* 1990;8:431.
142. Cline MJ: The molecular basis of leukemia. *N Engl J Med* 1994;330:328.
143. Preti H, O'Brien S, Giralt S, et al: Philadelphia-chromosome-positive adult acute lymphocytic leukemia: Characteristics, treatment results, and prognosis in 41 patients. *Am J Med* 1994;97:60.
144. Nourse J, Mellentin JD, Galili N, et al: Chromosomal translocation t(1;19) results in synthesis of a homeobox fusion mRNA that codes for a potential chimeric transcription factor. *Cell* 1990;60:535.
145. Reiter A, Schrappe M, Parwaresch R, et al: Non-Hodgkin's lymphoma of childhood and adolescence: Results of a treatment stratified for biologic subtypes and stage—a report of the Berlin-Frankfurt-Munster group. *J Clin Oncol* 1995;13:359.
146. deVillartay J-P, Pullman A, Andrade R, et al: γ/δ lineage relationship within a consecutive series of human precursor T-cell neoplasms. *Blood* 1989;74:2508.
147. Kikuchi A, Hayyashi Y, Kobayashi S, et al: Clinical significance of TAL1 gene alteration in childhood T-cell acute lymphoblastic leukemia and lymphoma. *Leukemia* 1993;7:933.
148. Chetty R, Pulford K, Jones M, et al: SCL/Tal-1 expression in T-acute lymphoblastic leukemia: An immunohistochemical study and genotypic study. *Hum Pathol* 1995;26:994.

Peripheral T-Cell Lymphoma, Unspecified

149. Suchi T, Lennert K, Tu L, et al: Histopathology and immunohistochemistry of peripheral T cell lymphomas: A proposal for their classification. *J Clin Pathol* 1987;40:995.
150. Stansfeld AG, Diebold J, Kapanci Y, et al: Updated Kiel classification for lymphomas (letter). *Lancet* 1988;1:292.
151. Knowles DM II, Halper JP: Human T-cell malignancies. Correlative clinical, histopathologic, immunologic, and cytochemical analysis of 23 cases. *Am J Pathol* 1982;106:187.
152. Greer JP, York JC, Cousar JB, et al: Peripheral T-cell lymphoma: A clinicopathologic study of 42 cases. *J Clin Oncol* 1984;2:788.
153. Horning SJ, Weiss LM, Crabtree GS, et al: Clinical and phenotypic diversity of T cell lymphomas. *Blood* 1986;67:1578.
154. Lippman SM, Miller TP, Spier CM, et al: The prognostic significance of the immunotype in diffuse large-cell lymphoma: A comparative study of the T-cell and B-cell phenotype. *Blood* 1988;72:436.
155. Kwak LW, Wilson M, Weiss LM, et al: Similar outcome of treatment of B-cell and T-cell diffuse large-cell lymphomas: The Stanford experience. *J Clin Oncol* 1991;9:1426.
156. Weis JW, Winter MW, Phyliky RL, et al: Peripheral T-cell lymphomas: Histologic, immunohistologic, and clinical characterization. *Mayo Clin Proc* 1986;61:411.
157. Jaffe ES, Strauchen JA, Berard CW: Predictability of immunologic phenotype by morphologic criteria in diffuse aggressive non-Hodgkin's lymphomas. *Am J Clin Pathol* 1982;77:46.
158. Borowitz MJ, Reichert TA, Brynes RK, et al: The phenotypic diversity of peripheral T-cell lymphomas: The Southeastern Cancer Study Group experience. *Hum Pathol* 1986;17:567.
159. Picker LJ, Weiss LM, Medeiros LJ, et al: Immunophenotypic criteria for the diagnosis of non-Hodgkin's lymphoma. *Am J Pathol* 1987;128:181.
160. Weiss LM, Picker LJ, Grogan TM, et al: Absence of clonal beta and gamma T-cell receptor gene rearrangements in a subset of peripheral T-cell lymphomas. *Am J Pathol* 1988;130:436.

T/NK-Cell Lymphoma

161. Jaffe ES: Classification of natural killer (NK) cell and NK-like T-cell malignancies. *Blood* 1996;87:1207.
162. Emile J, Boulland M, Haioun C, et al: CD5⁻ CD56⁺ T-cell receptor silent peripheral T-cell lymphomas are natural killer cell lymphomas. *Blood* 1996;87:1466.
163. Ohno T, Yamaguchi M, Oka K, et al: Frequent expression of CD3 in CD3 (Leu 4)-negative nasal T-cell lymphomas. *Leukemia* 1995;9:44.
164. Wong KF, Chan JKC, Ng CS, et al: CD56 (NKH1)-positive hematolymphoid malignancies. An aggressive neoplasm featuring frequent cutaneous/mucosal involvement, cytoplasmic azurophilic granules, and angiocentricity. *Hum Pathol* 1992;23:798.
165. Fellbaum C, Hansmann M, Lennert K: Malignant lymphomas of the nasal cavity and paranasal sinuses. *Virchows Archiv A Pathol Anat* 1989;414:399.
166. Weiss LM, Gaffey MJ, Chen Y, et al: Frequency of Epstein-Barr viral DNA in "western" sinonasal and Waldeyer's ring non-Hodgkin's lymphomas. *Am J Surg Pathol* 1992;16:156.
167. Kanavaros P, Lescs M, Brière J, et al: Nasal T-cell lymphoma: A clinicopathologic entity associated with peculiar phenotype and with Epstein-Barr virus. *Blood* 1993;10:2688.
168. Jaffe ES, Chan JKC, Su I, et al: Report of the workshop on nasal and related extranodal angiocentric T/natural killer cell lymphomas. Definitions, differential diagnosis, and epidemiology. *Am J Surg Pathol* 1996;20:103.
169. Macon WR, Williams ME, Greer JP, et al: Natural killer-like T-cell lymphomas: Aggressive lymphomas of T-large granular lymphocytes. *Blood* 1996;87:1474.
170. Chan JKC, Ng CS, Lau WH, et al: Most nasal/nasopharyngeal lymphomas are peripheral T-cell neoplasms. *Am J Surg Pathol* 1987;11:418.
171. Arber DA, Weiss LM, Albújar PF, et al: Nasal lymphomas in Peru. High incidence of T-cell immunophenotype and Epstein-Barr virus infection. *Am J Surg Pathol* 1993;17:392.
172. Abbondanzo SL, Wenig BM: Non-Hodgkin's lymphoma of the sinonasal tract. A clinicopathologic and immunophenotypic study of 120 cases. *Cancer* 1995;75:1281.
173. Ramsay AD, Rooney N: Lymphomas of the head and neck 1: Nasofacial T-cell lymphoma. *Oral Oncol Eur J Cancer* 1993;29B:99.
174. Strickler JG, Meneses MF, Habermann TM, et al: Polymorphic reticulosis: A reappraisal. *Hum Pathol* 1994;25:659.
175. Jaffe ES: Nasal and nasal-type T/NK cell lymphoma: A unique form of lymphoma associated with the Epstein-Barr virus. *Histopathology* 1995;27:581.
176. Chan JKC, Yip TTC, Tsang WYW, et al: Detection of Epstein-Barr viral RNA in malignant lymphomas of the upper aerodigestive tract. *Am J Surg Pathol* 1994;18:938.
177. Guinee D, Jaffe E, Kingma D, et al: Pulmonary lymphomatoid granulomatosis. Evidence for a proliferation of Epstein-Barr virus infected B-lymphocytes with a prominent T-cell component and vasculitis. *Am J Surg Pathol* 1994; 18:753.

Angioimmunoblastic Lymphadenopathy and Angioimmunoblastic Lymphadenopathy–Like T-Cell Lymphoma

178. Watanabe S, Sato Y, Shimoyama M, et al: Immunoblastic lymphadenopathy, angioimmunoblastic lymphadenopathy, and IBL-like T-cell lymphoma. A spectrum of T-cell neoplasia. *Cancer* 1986;58:2224.
179. Frizzera G, Moran EM, Rappaport H: Angio-immunoblastic lymphadenopathy with dysproteinaemia. *Lancet* 1974;1:1070.
180. Lukes RJ, Tindle BH: Immunoblastic lymphadenopathy. A hyperimmune entity resembling Hodgkin's disease. *N Engl J Med* 1975;292:1.
181. Frizzera G, Moran EM, Rappaport H: Angio-immunoblastic lymphadenopathy. Diagnosis and clinical course. *Am J Med* 1975;59:803.
182. Pangalis GA, Moran EM, Nathwani BN, et al: Angioimmunoblastic lymphadenopathy. Long-term follow-up study. *Cancer* 1983;52:318.
183. Nathwani BN, Rappaport H, Moran EM, et al: Malignant lymphoma arising in angioimmunoblastic lymphadenopathy. *Cancer* 1978;41:578.
184. Weiss LM, Strickler JG, Dorfman RF, et al: Clonal T-cell populations in angioimmunoblastic lymphadenopathy and angioimmunoblastic lymphadenopathy-like lymphoma. *Am J Pathol* 1986;122:392.
185. Lipford EH, Smith HR, Pittaluga S, et al: Clonality of angioimmunoblastic lymphadenopathy and implications for its evolution to malignant lymphoma. *J Clin Invest* 1987;79:637.
186. Feller AC, Griesser H, Schilling CV, et al: Clonal gene rearrangement patterns correlate with immunophenotype and clinical parameters in patients with angioimmunoblastic lymphadenopathy. *Am J Pathol* 1988;133:549.

Adult T-Cell Leukemia/Lymphoma

187. Bunn PA Jr, Schechter GP, Jaffe E, et al: Clinical course of retrovirus-associated adult T-cell lymphoma in the United States. *N Engl J Med* 1983;309:257.
188. Jaffe ES, Cossman J, Blattner WA, et al: The pathologic spectrum of adult T-cell leukemia/lymphoma in the United States. *Am J Surg Pathol* 1984;8:263.
189. Kikuchi M, Mitsui T, Takeshita M, et al: Virus associated adult T-cell leukemia (ATL) in Japan: Clinical, histological and immunological studies. *Hematol Oncol* 1986;4:67.
190. Yamaguchi K, Nishimura H, Kohrogi H, et al: A proposal for smoldering adult T-cell leukemia: A clinicopathologic study of five cases. *Blood* 1983;62:758.
191. Ohguro S, Himi T, Harabuchi Y, et al: Adult T-cell leukaemia-lymphoma in Waldeyer's ring: a report of three cases. *J Laryngol Otol* 1993;107:960.
192. Kohno T, Uchida H, Inomata H, et al: Ocular manifestations of adult T-cell leukemia/lymphoma: A clinicopathologic study. *Ophthalmology* 1993;100:1794.

Anaplastic Large-Cell Lymphoma

193. Chott A, Kaserer K, Augustin I, et al: Ki-1-positive large cell lymphoma. A clinicopathologic study of 41 cases. *Am J Surg Pathol* 1990;14:439.
194. Greer JP, Kinney MC, Collins RD, et al: Clinical features of 31 patients with Ki-1 anaplastic large-cell lymphoma. *J Clin Oncol* 1991; 9:539.
195. de Bruin PC, Beljaards RC, van Heerde P, et al: Differences in clinical behaviour and immunophenotype between primary cutaneous and primary nodal anaplastic large cell lymphoma of T-cell or null cell phenotype. *Histopathology* 1993;23:127.
196. Chan JKC, Ng CS, Hui PK, et al: Anaplastic large cell Ki-1 lymphoma. Delineation of two morphological types. *Histopathology* 1989;15:11.
197. Pileri S, Falini B, Delsol G, et al: Lymphohistiocytic T-cell lymphoma (anaplastic large cell lymphoma CD30+/Ki-1+ with a high content of reactive histiocytes). *Histopathology* 1990;16:383.
198. Stein H, Mason DY, Gerdes J, et al: The expression of the Hodgkin's disease associated antigen Ki-1 in reactive and neoplastic lymphoid tissue: Evidence that Reed-Sternberg cells and histiocytic malignancies are derived from activated lymphoid cells. *Blood* 1985;66:848.
199. Delsol G, Al Saati T, Gatter KC, et al: Coexpression of epithelial membrane antigen (EMA), Ki-1, and interleukin-2 receptor by anaplastic large cell lymphomas. Diagnostic value in so-called malignant histiocytosis. *Am J Pathol* 1988;130:59.
200. Hansmann M, Fellbaum C, Bohm A: Large cell anaplastic lymphoma: Evaluation of immunophenotype on paraffin and frozen sections in comparison with ultrastructural features. *Virchows Archiv A Pathol Anat* 1991;418:427.
201. O'Connor NTJ, Stein H, Gatter KC, et al: Genotypic analysis of large cell lymphomas which express the Ki-1 antigen. *Histopathology* 1987;11:733.
202. Frierson HF Jr, Bellafiore FJ, Gaffey MJ, et al: Cytokeratin in anaplastic large cell lymphoma. *Mod Pathol* 1994;7:317.
203. Morris SW, Kirstein MN, Valentine MB, et al: Fusion of a kinase gene, *ALK*, to a nucleolar protein gene, *NPM*, in non-Hodgkin's lymphoma. *Science* 1994;263:1281.
204. Lopategui JR, Sun L, Chan JKC, et al: Low frequency association of the t(2;5)(p23;q35) chromosomal translocation with CD30⁺ lymphomas from American and Asian patients. A reverse transcriptase-polymerase chain reaction study. *Am J Pathol* 1994;146:323.
205. Lamant L, Meggetto F, Al Saati T, et al: High incidence of t(2;5)(p23;q35) translocation in anaplastic large cell lymphoma and its lack of detection in Hodgkin's disease. Comparison of cytogenetic analysis, reverse transcriptase-polymerase chain reaction, and P-80 immunostaining. *Blood* 1996;87:284.
205a. Cataldo KA, Jalal SM, Law ME, et al: Detection of t(2;5) in anaplastic large cell lymphoma. Comparison of immunohistochemical studies, FISH, and RT-PCR in paraffin-embedded tissue. *Am J Surg Pathol* 1999;23:1386.

206. Brousset P, Rochaix P, Chittal S, et al: High incidence of Epstein-Barr virus detection in Hodgkin's disease and absence of detection in anaplastic large-cell lymphoma in children. *Histopathology* 1993; 23:189.

207. Lopategui JR, Gaffey MJ, Chan JKC, et al: Infrequent association of Epstein-Barr virus with CD30-positive anaplastic large cell lymphomas from American and Asian patients. *Am J Surg Pathol* 1995;19:42.

208. Ladanyi M, Cavalchire G, Morris SW, et al: Reverse transcriptase polymerase chain reaction for the Ki-1 anaplastic large cell lymphoma-associated t(2;5) translocation in Hodgkin's disease. *Am J Pathol* 1994; 145:1296.

209. Weiss LM, Lopategui JR, Sun L, et al: Absence of the t(2;5) in Hodgkin's disease. *Blood* 1995;85:2845.

210. Orscheschek K, Merz H, Hell J, et al: Large-cell anaplastic lymphoma-specific translocation (t[2;5][p23;q35]) in Hodgkin's disease: Indication of a common pathogenesis? *Lancet* 1995;345:87.

211. Downing JR, Shurtleff SA, Zielenska M, et al: Molecular detection of the (2;5) translocation of non-Hodgkin's lymphoma by reverse transcriptase-polymerase chain reaction. *Blood* 1995;85:3416.

212. Arber DA, Sun L, Weiss LM: Detection of the t(2;5)(p23;q35) chromosomal translocation in large B-cell lymphomas other than anaplastic large cell lymphoma. *Hum Pathol* 1996;27:290.

213. Bucsky P, Favara B, Feller AC, et al: Malignant histiocytosis and large cell anaplastic (Ki-1) lymphoma in childhood: Guidelines for differential diagnosis—report of the Histiocytic Society. *Med Pediatr Oncol* 1994;22:200.

Hodgkin's Disease

214. Lukes RJ, Butler JJ: The pathology and nomenclature of Hodgkin's disease. *Cancer Res* 1966;26:1063.

215. Lukes RJ, Carver LF, Hall TC, et al: Report of the nomenclature committee. *Cancer Res* 1966;26:1311.

216. Ultmann JE, Moran EM: Clinical course and complications in Hodgkin's disease. *Arch Intern Med* 1973;131:332.

217. Mir R, Anderson J, Strauchen J, et al: Hodgkin's disease in patients 60 years of age and older. Histologic and clinical features of advanced-stage disease. *Cancer* 1993;71:1857.

218. Todd GB, Michaels L: Hodgkin's disease involving Waldeyer's lymphoid ring. *Cancer* 1974;34:1769.

219. Kapadia SB, Roman LN, Kingma DW, et al: Hodgkin's disease of Waldeyer's ring. Clinical and histoimmunophenotypic findings and association with Epstein-Barr virus in 16 cases. *Am J Surg Pathol* 1995;19:1431.

220. McNelis FL, Pai VT: Malignant lymphoma of head and neck. *Laryngoscope* 1969;79:1076.

221. Kaplan HS, Dorfman RF, Nelsen TS, et al: Staging laparotomy and splenectomy in Hodgkin's disease: Analysis of indications and patterns of involvement in 285 consecutive, unselected patients. *Natl Cancer Inst Monogr* 1973;36:291.

222. Wood NL, Coltman CA: Localized primary extranodal Hodgkin's disease. *Ann Intern Med* 1973;78:113.

223. Saul SH, Kapadia SB: Primary lymphoma of Waldeyer's ring. Clinicopathologic study of 68 cases. *Cancer* 1985;56:157.

224. Mauch PM, Kalish LA, Kadin M, et al: Patterns of presentation of Hodgkin's disease: Implications for etiology and pathogenesis. *Cancer* 1993;71:2062.

225. Rowley H, McRae RD, Cook JA, et al: Lymphoma presenting to a head and neck clinic. *Clin Otolaryngol* 1995;20:139.

226. Compagno J, Oertel JE: Malignant lymphoma and other lymphoproliferative disorders of the thyroid gland: A clinicopathologic study of 245 cases. *Am J Clin Pathol* 1980;74:1.

227. Hyman GA, Wolff M: Malignant lymphomas of the salivary glands. Review of the literature and report of 33 new cases, including four cases associated with the lymphoepithelial lesion. *Am J Clin Pathol* 1976;65:421.

228. Schmid U, Helbron D, Lennert K: Primary malignant lymphomas localized in salivary glands. *Histopathology* 1982;6:673.

229. Strickler JG, Michie SA, Warnke RA, et al: The "syncytial variant" of nodular sclerosis Hodgkin's disease. *Am J Surg Pathol* 1986;10:470.

230. MacLennan KA, Bennett MH, Tu A, et al: Relationship of histopathologic features to survival and relapse in nodular sclerosing Hodgkin's disease. A study of 1659 patients. *Cancer* 1989;64:1686.

231. Chittal SM, Caverivière P, Schwarting R, et al: Monoclonal antibodies in the diagnosis of Hodgkin's disease: The search for a rational panel. *Am J Surg Pathol* 1988;12:9.

232. Burns BF, Colby TV, Dorfman RF: Differential diagnostic features of nodular L&H Hodgkin's disease, including progressive transformation of germinal centers. *Am J Surg Pathol* 1984;8:253.

233. Coles FB, Cartun RW, Pastuszak WT: Hodgkin's disease, lymphocyte predominant type: Immunoreactivity with B-cell antibodies. *Mod Pathol* 1988;1:274.

234. Poppema S, Kaiserling E, Lennert K: Nodular paragranuloma and progressively transformed germinal centers. Ultrastructural and immunohistologic findings. *Virchows Arch [Cell Pathol]* 1979;31:211.

235. Kamel OW, Gelb AB, Shibuya RB, et al: Leu7 (CD57) reactivity distinguishes nodular lymphocyte predominance Hodgkin's disease, T cell rich B cell lymphoma and follicular lymphoma. *Am J Pathol* 1993;142:541.

236. Mason DY, Banks PM, Chan J, et al: Nodular lymphocyte predominance Hodgkin's disease: A distinct clinicopathological entity. *Am J Surg Pathol* 1994;18:526.

237. Kant JA, Hubbard SM, Longo DL, et al: The pathologic and clinical heterogeneity of lymphocyte-depleted Hodgkin's disease. *J Clin Oncol* 1986;4:284.

238. Lukes RJ: Criteria for involvement of lymph node, bone marrow, spleen, and liver in Hodgkin's disease. *Cancer Res* 1971;31:1755.

239. Doggett RS, Colby TV, Dorfman RF: Interfollicular Hodgkin's disease. *Am J Surg Pathol* 1983;7:145.

240. Weiss LM, Chang KL: Molecular biologic studies in Hodgkin's disease. *Semin Diagn Pathol* 1992;9:272.

241. O'Grady J, Stewart S, Elton RA, et al: Epstein-Barr virus in Hodgkin's disease and site of origin of tumour. *Lancet* 1994;343:265.

242. Chang KL, Albújar PF, Chen YY, et al: High prevalence of Epstein-Barr virus in the Reed-Sternberg cells of Hodgkin's disease occurring in Peru. *Blood* 1993;83:496.

243. Weiss LM, Strickler JG, Hu E, et al: Immunoglobulin gene rearrangements in Hodgkin's disease. *Hum Pathol* 1986;17:1009.

244. Schmid C, Pan L, Diss T, et al: Expression of B-cell antigens by Hodgkin's and Reed-Sternberg cells. *Am J Pathol* 1991;139:701.

245. Manazanal A, Santon A, Oliva H, et al: Evaluation of clonal immunoglobulin heavy chain rearrangements in Hodgkin's disease using the polymerase chain reaction (PCR). *Histopathology* 1995;27:21.

246. Hummel M, Ziemann K, Lammert H, et al: Hodgkin's disease with monoclonal and polyclonal populations of Reed-Sternberg cells. *N Engl J Med* 1995;333:901.

247. Schmid C, Sargent C, Isaacson PG: L and H cells of nodular lymphocyte predominant Hodgkin's disease show immunoglobulin light chain restriction. *Am J Pathol* 1991;139:1281.

248. Stoler MH, Nichols GE, Symbula M, et al: Lymphocyte predominance Hodgkin's disease. Evidence for a κ light chain-restricted monotypic B-cell neoplasm. *Am J Pathol* 1995;146:812.

249. Delabie J, Tierens A, Wu G, et al: Lymphocyte predominance Hodgkin's disease: Lineage and clonality determination using a single-cell assay. *Blood* 1994;84:3291.

250. Stetler-Stevenson M, Crush-Stanton S, Cossman J: Involvement of the bcl-2 gene by Hodgkin's disease. *J Natl Cancer Inst* 1990; 82:855.

251. Poppema S, Kaleta J, Hepperle B: Chromosomal abnormalities in patients with Hodgkin's disease: Evidence for frequent involvement of the 14q chromosomal region but infrequent bcl-2 gene rearrangement in Reed-Sternberg cells. *J Natl Cancer Inst* 1992;84:1789.

252. Louie DC, Kant JA, Brooks JJ, et al: Absence of t(14;18) major and minor breakpoints and of *Bcl*-2 protein overproduction in Reed-Sternberg cells of Hodgkin's disease. *Am J Pathol* 1991;139:1231.

253. Tilly H, Bastard C, Delastre T, et al: Cytogenetic studies in untreated Hodgkin's disease. *Blood* 1991;77:1298.

254. Corbally N, Grogan L, Keane MM, et al: *Bcl*-2 rearrangement in Hodgkin's disease and reactive lymph nodes. *Am J Clin Pathol* 1994;101:756.

255. Strum SB, Park JK, Rappaport H: Observation of cells resembling Sternberg-Reed cells in conditions other than Hodgkin's disease. *Cancer* 1970;26:176.

256. Zarate-Osorno A, Jaffe ES, Medeiros LJ: Metastatic nasopharyngeal carcinoma initially presenting as cervical lymphadenopathy: A report of two cases that resembled Hodgkin's disease. *Arch Pathol Lab Med* 1992;116:862.

257. Momose H, Jaffe ES, Shin SS, et al: Chronic lymphocytic leukemia/small lymphocytic lymphoma with Reed-Sternberg-like cells and possible transformation to Hodgkin's disease: Mediation by Epstein-Barr virus. *Am J Surg Pathol* 1992;16:859.

258. Bataille R: Localized plasmacytomas. *Clin Haematol* 1982;11:113.

Extramedullary Plasmacytoma

259. Kapadia SB, Desai U, Cheng VS: Extramedullary plasmacytoma of the head and neck: A clinicopathologic study of 20 cases. *Medicine* 1982;61:317.
260. Woodruff RK, Whittle JM, Malpas JS: Solitary plasmacytoma. I: Extramedullary soft tissue plasmacytoma. *Cancer* 1979;43:2340.
261. Fu Y, Perzin KH: Nonepithelial tumors of the nasal cavity, paranasal sinuses and nasopharynx. A clinicopathologic study. IX. Plasmacytomas. *Cancer* 1978;42:2399.
262. Aozasa K, Inoue A, Yoshimura H, et al: Plasmacytoma of the thyroid gland. *Cancer* 1986;58:105.
263. Wiltshaw E: The natural history of extramedullary plasmacytoma and its relation to solitary myeloma of bone and myelomatosis. *Medicine* 1976;55:217.
264. Strickler JG, Audeh MW, Copenhaver CM, et al: Immunophenotypic differences between plasmacytoma/multiple myeloma and immunoblastic lymphoma. *Cancer* 1988;61:1782.
265. Aguilera NS, Kapadia SB, Nalesnik MA, et al: Extramedullary plasmacytoma of the head and neck: use of paraffin sections to assess clonality with *in situ* hybridization, growth fraction, and the presence of Epstein-Barr virus. *Mod Pathol* 1995;8:503.
266. Strand WR, Banks PM, Kyle RA: Anaplastic plasma cell myeloma and immunoblastic lymphoma. Clinical, pathologic, and immunologic comparison. *Am J Med* 1984;76:861.
267. Meis JM, Butler JJ, Osborne BM, et al: Solitary plasmacytomas of bone and extramedullary plasmacytomas. A clinicopathologic and immunohistochemical study. *Cancer* 1987;59:1475.

Extramedullary Myeloid Cell Tumors

268. Neiman RS, Barcos M, Berard C, et al: Granulocytic sarcoma: A clinicopathologic study of 61 biopsied cases. *Cancer* 1981;48:1426.
269. Terjanian T, Kantarjian H, Keating M, et al: Clinical and prognostic features of patients with Philadelphia chromosome-positive chronic myelogenous leukemia and extramedullary disease. *Cancer* 1987;59:297.
270. Traweek ST, Arber DA, Rappaport H, et al: Extramedullary myeloid cell tumors: An immunohistochemical and morphologic study of 28 cases. *Am J Surg Pathol* 1993;17:1011.
271. Roth MJ, Medeiros LJ, Elenitoba-Johnson K, et al: Extramedullary myeloid cell tumors: An immunohistochemical study of 29 cases using routinely fixed and processed paraffin-embedded tissue sections. *Arch Pathol Lab Med* 1995;119:790.
272. Meis JM, Butler JJ, Osborne BM, et al: Granulocytic sarcoma in nonleukemic patients. *Cancer* 1986;58:2697.
273. Muller S, Sangster G, Crocker J, et al: An immunohistochemical and clinicopathological study of granulocytic sarcoma ('chloroma'). *Hematol Oncol* 1986;4:101.
274. Banna M, Aur R, Akkad S: Orbital granulocytic sarcoma. *Am J Neuroradiol* 1991;12:255.
275. Shome DK, Gupta NK, Prajapati NC, et al: Orbital granulocytic sarcomas (myeloid sarcomas) in acute nonlymphocytic leukemia. *Cancer* 1992;70:2298.
276. Zimmerman LE, Font RL: Ophthalmologic manifestations of granulocytic sarcoma (myeloid sarcoma or chloroma). *Am J Ophthalmol* 1975;80:975.
277. Hudock J, Chatten J, Miettinen M: Immunohistochemical evaluation of myeloid leukemia infiltrates (granulocytic sarcomas) in formaldehyde-fixed, paraffin-embedded tissue. *Am J Clin Pathol* 1994;102:55.
278. Segal GH, Stoler MH, Tubbs RR: The "CD43 only" phenotype. An aberrant, nonspecific immunophenotype requiring comprehensive analysis for lineage resolution. *Am J Clin Pathol* 1992;97:861.
279. Chilosi M, Pizzolo G: Review of terminal deoxynucleotidyl transferase. Biological aspects, methods of detection, and selected diagnostic applications. *Appl Immunohistochem* 1995;3:209.

Langerhans' Cell Histiocytosis

280. The Writing Group of the Histiocyte Society. Histiocytosis syndromes in children. *Lancet* 1987;1:208.
281. Willman CL, Busque L, Griffith BB, et al: Langerhans'-cell histiocytosis (histiocytosis X): A clonal proliferative disease. *N Engl J Med* 1994;331:154.
282. Yu RC, Chu C, Buluwela L, et al: Clonal proliferation of Langerhans cells in Langerhans cell histiocytosis. *Lancet* 1994;343:767.

283. Lichtenstein L: Histiocytosis X. *Arch Pathol* 1953;56:84.
284. Williams JW, Dorfman RF: Lymphadenopathy as the initial manifestation of histiocytosis X. *Am J Surg Pathol* 1979;3:405.
285. Motoi M, Helbron D, Kaiserling E, et al: Eosinophilic granuloma of lymph nodes: A variant of histiocytosis X. *Histopathology* 1980;4:585.
286. Alessi DM, Maceri D: Histiocytosis X of the head and neck in a pediatric population. *Arch Otolaryngol Head Neck Surg* 1992;118:945.
287. Angeli SI, Alcalde J, Hoffman HT, et al: Langerhans' cell histiocytosis of the head and neck in children. *Ann Otol Rhinol Laryngol* 1995;104:173.
288. Hartman KS: Histiocytosis X: A review of 114 cases with oral involvement. *Oral Surg Oral Med Oral Pathol* 1980;49:38.
289. Irving RM, Broadbent V, Jones NS: Langerhans' cell histiocytosis in childhood: Management of head and neck manifestations. *Laryngoscope* 1994;104:64.
290. Quraishi MS, Blayney AW, Walker D, et al: Langerhans' cell histiocytosis: head and neck manifestations in children. *Head Neck* 1995;17:226.
291. Kilpatrick SE, Wenger DE, Gilchrist GS, et al: Langerhans' cell histiocytosis (histiocytosis X) of bone. A clinicopathologic analysis of 263 pediatric and adult cases. *Cancer* 1995;76:2471.
292. Risdall RJ, Dehner LP, Duray P, et al: Histiocytosis X (Langerhans' cell histiocytosis). Prognostic role of histopathology. *Arch Pathol Lab Med* 1983;107:59.
293. Azumi N, Sheibani K, Swartz WG, et al: Antigenic phenotype of Langerhans cell histiocytosis: An immunohistochemical study demonstrating the value of LN-2, LN-3, and vimentin. *Hum Pathol* 1988;19:1376.
294. Ruco LP, Pulford KAF, Mason DY, et al: Expression of macrophage-associated antigens in tissues involved by Langerhans' cell histiocytosis (histiocytosis X). *Am J Clin Pathol* 1989;92:273.
295. Ornvold K, Ralfkiaer E, Carstensen H: Immunohistochemical study of the abnormal cells in Langerhans' cell histiocytosis (histiocytosis X). *Virchows Archiv A Pathol Anat* 1990;416:403.
296. Hage C, Willman CL, Favara BE, et al: Langerhans' cell histiocytosis (histiocytosis X): Immunophenotype and growth fraction. *Hum Pathol* 1993;24:840.
297. Krenács L, Tiszalvicz L, Krenács T, et al: Immunohistochemical detection of CD1a antigen in formalin-fixed and paraffin-embedded tissue sections with monoclonal antibody 010. *J Pathol* 1993;171:99.
298. Burns BF, Colby TV, Dorfman RF: Langerhans' cell granulomatosis (histiocytosis X) associated with malignant lymphomas. *Am J Surg Pathol* 1983;7:529.
299. Egeler RM, Neglia JP, Puccetti DM, et al: Association of Langerhans' cell histiocytosis with malignant neoplasms. *Cancer* 1993;71:865.

Dendritic Reticulum Cell Tumors and True Histiocytic Lymphoma

300. Monda L, Warnke R, Rosai J: A primary lymph node malignancy with features suggestive of dendritic reticulum cell differentiation. A report of 4 cases. *Am J Pathol* 1986;122:562.
301. Nakamura S, Hara K, Suchi T, et al: Interdigitating cell sarcoma. A morphologic, immunohistologic, and enzyme-histochemical study. *Cancer* 1988;61:562.
302. Weiss LM, Berry GJ, Dorfman RF, et al: Spindle cell neoplasms of lymph nodes of probable reticulum cell lineage. True reticulum cell sarcoma? *Am J Surg Pathol* 1990;14:405.
303. Hollowood K, Pease C, MacKay AM, et al: Sarcomatoid tumours of lymph nodes showing follicular dendritic cell differentiation. *J Pathol* 1991;163:205.
304. Hanson CA, Jaszcz W, Kersey JH, et al: True histiocytic lymphoma: Histopathologic, immunophenotypic and genotypic analysis. *Br J Haematol* 1989;73:187.
305. Ralfkiaer E, Delsol G, O'Conner NTJ, et al: Malignant lymphomas of true histiocytic origin: A clinical, histological, immunophenotypic and genotypic study. *J Pathol* 1990;160:9.
306. Kamel OW, Gocke CD, Kell DL, et al: True histiocytic lymphoma: A study of 12 cases based on current definition. *Leuk Lymphoma* 1995;18:81.
307. Weiss LM, Trela MJ, Cleary ML, et al: Frequent immunoglobulin and T-cell receptor gene rearrangements in "histiocytic" neoplasms. *Am J Pathol* 1985;121:369.
308. Ornvold K, Carstensen H, Junge J, et al: Tumours classified as "malignant histiocytosis" in children are T-cell neoplasms. *APMIS* 1992;100:558.

13 ▪ Cutaneous Tumors and Pseudotumors of the Head and Neck

▪ *Mark R. Wick*

There are few, if any, cutaneous neoplasms of the head and neck that are unique to that topographic region. Accordingly, a consideration of skin tumors in this area of the body must be rather expansive. There are some dermatologic lesions that are so uncommon (or unknown) in otorhinolaryngologic practice, however, that discussion of their attributes is understandably omitted. The following chapter addresses those neoplastic skin lesions of the face, neck, and scalp that may be encountered by the pathologist with any degree of regularity. By force of spatial constraint, the morphologic features of those proliferations are the principal focus of this review; attendant clinical and epidemiologic details are largely left to the contents of other monographs.

▪ CUTANEOUS EPITHELIAL NEOPLASMS OF THE HEAD AND NECK

Benign Skin Tumors of Surface Epithelial Components

Benign neoplasms of the integument of the head and neck are relatively common, and malformative lesions that simulate neoplastic processes also occur in this body area. These are few in number and can be considered under the rubric of *epidermal nevi*.[1, 2]

Epidermal nevi typically assume gross and histologic appearances that mimic those of verruca vulgaris or seborrheic keratosis. Hence, all of these benign proliferations can be considered together. Verrucae and verruca-like nevi demonstrate regular papillomatosis with a "spiky" surface aspect, acanthosis, regional parakeratosis, and variable degrees of nuclear atypia. A particularly important form of verruciform nevus is the nevus sebaceus, which is found on the scalp and neck.[3, 4] Its microscopic appearance is somewhat variable, depending on the age of the lesion.[1, 4] However, it regularly features the presence of localized epidermal papillomatosis, with hyperkeratosis, hypergranulosis, and fusion of rete pegs. With time, varying degrees of adnexal hyperplasia are superimposed on this description, such that excess numbers of sebaceous glands and apocrine glands are observed (Fig. 13–1). Conversely, hair follicles are either lacking or embryonic in appearance within nevi sebacei. True verrucae differ from verruciform epidermal nevi in also demonstrating multifocal koilocytosis, coarse clumping of keratohyaline cytoplasmic material, and regional "ground glass" homogenization of nuclear chromatin.[1]

Seborrheic keratoses are characterized by a small polygonal-cell constituency, an interanastomosing trabecular substructure that is based on the rete ridge pattern of the skin, and the presence of intercellular accumulations of keratin (so-called "horn cysts"). There are several recognized microscopic variants of seborrheic keratosis, including acanthotic, hyperkeratotic, reticulated, clonal, and inflamed subtypes.[1, 5, 6] The nuances of those lesions are implicit in their names. A special comment is in order, however, in reference to inflamed seborrheic keratosis. That variant may demonstrate a rather alarming degree of nuclear atypia and mitotic activity, but, because such lesions still retain the basic attributes of seborrheic keratosis,

they should be labeled as such.[6] There are no convincing examples of true malignant transformation of seborrheic keratosis.

Warty dyskeratoma is another benign epidermal tumor with a distinctive histologic appearance. Clinically, however, it takes the form of a nondescript 3 to 10 mm nodule with a raised periphery and, often, a central pore-like opening (Fig. 13–2, see p. 779).[7] Keratinous debris may extrude from the latter structure, or the lesion may be pruritic. Under the microscope, one sees localized acanthosis of the infundibular portion of adjacent hair follicles, with acantholysis of the overlying epithelium and follicular keratin "plugs." The acantholytic keratinocytes may demonstrate focal cytoplasmic hypereosinophilia and the formation of "corps ronds," as seen in Darier's disease (a potentially systemic dermatosis). However, as noted by Kao,[1] the latter disease involves more than three adjacent hair follicles, whereas warty dyskeratoma does not.

Lichen planus–like keratosis is another benign proliferation that looks like the localized version of a disseminated dermatosis—namely, lichen planus.[8–10] As such, it has irregular sawtoothed acanthosis, hypergranulosis, hyperkeratosis, lichenoid lymphoid or lymphoplasmacytic inflammation, basal vacuolar change in keratinocytes, and the presence of cytoid or Civatte's bodies at the dermoepidermal junction. There are some subtle differences in the degrees of these changes between lichen planus–like keratosis and lichen planus,[9, 10] but the most pragmatic way of separating these two entities is to ask the clinician whether the lesion is solitary or not. The answer is "yes" in lichen planu–like keratosis and "no" in lichen planus.

Actinic keratosis is a premalignant alteration in the epidermis that clearly is related to actinic skin damage. It demonstrates disordered maturation of the epithelium, together with nuclear atypia, nucleomegaly, multifocal pyknosis, misplaced suprabasilar mitotic activity, and dyskeratosis.[11–13] There is typically marked actinic elastosis in the subjacent corium. Variations on this general histologic picture include acantholytic (adenoid) and hypertrophic forms of actinic keratosis.[13]

Malignant Skin Tumors of Surface Epithelial Components

Basal Cell Carcinoma

There is no question that basal cell carcinoma (BCC) is the most common cutaneous malignancy of the head and neck. Because of its relationship to actinic damage of the skin and the number of fair-skinned persons who are still refractory to wearing sun-blocking topical lotions during outside activities, the frequency with which BCC is seen in the general population is still increasing.

This tumor has a great number of clinical appearances, a description of which is beyond the scope of this discussion. However, it most commonly presents itself as a discrete ulcer with "rolled," heaped-up, pearly-white edges or as a gray-white or flesh-colored nodule in the skin of the face and neck.

Pathologic Features. As is true of many carcinomas, BCC displays a considerable diversity of appearances under the micro-

777

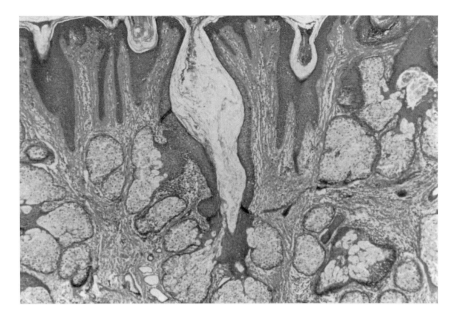

Figure 13–1. Nevus sebaceus of scalp, showing surface papillomatosis and sebaceous hyperplasia. This is one of the most common types of organoid nevus.

scope. These appearances can be divided into nodulocystic, superficial, adenoid, morpheaform, infiltrative, keratotic, and pigmented forms, as well as rarer variants.[14, 15]

Nodulocystic BCC is the most common (approximately 70% of cases) and is composed of rounded or bluntly branched lobules of small hyperchromatic cells, which are connected to the overlying epidermis by narrow cords or broad trabeculae (Fig. 13–3). These cellular clusters vary slightly to moderately in size and shape; however, they are typified by the roughly parallel alignment of peripheral nuclei at right angles to those in the center of the nodules—so-called "peripheral palisading." The tumor cells themselves are uniform in size and polygonal in shape, with generally oval nuclei and inconspicuous nucleoli. Exceptionally, spindled or "giant" dysplastic nuclear forms may be observed; these appear to have no prognostic significance.[16] Cytoplasm is scanty and amphophilic, and mitotic activity is variable. From 0 to 2 division figures are typically seen per high-power (×400) field, but up to 10 may be observed in selected neoplasms. The stroma in this form of BCC is fibromyxoid and, in specimens fixed in formalin, characteristically exhibits a retraction from tumor cell clusters. Peritumoral actinic elastosis is almost invariably seen in the surrounding dermis.

Not uncommonly, centrilobular necrosis in nodular BCCs accounts for their "cystic" quality, both clinically and microscopically. Necrotic areas in adjacent cellular lobules may become confluent, yielding broad areas of anucleated debris. The overlying epidermis may or may not be ulcerated. As stated, there are several distinctive histologic variants of BCC, including the superficial-multifocal, nodulocystic, adenoid, infiltrative, morpheaform, adamantinoid, clear-cell, signet ring–cell, pilar-keratotic, organotypic, eccrine, apocrine, fibroepitheliomatous, basosebaceous, pigmented (melanotic), basosquamous, metatypical, and dedifferentiated (carcinosarcomatous) forms. These are discussed in detail in other textbooks; however, it should be noted that the infiltrative, morpheaform, metatypical, and basosquamous variants of BCC do have an apparently greater propensity for local recurrence than other microscopic subtypes of the tumor.

Specialized Pathologic Features. Because of the prevalence of BCC and its corresponding familiarity to most pathologists and dermatologists, specialized pathologic studies are not usually necessary for diagnosis. Nevertheless, occasional cases of BCC may simulate adnexal carcinomas of the skin, such as adenoid cystic carcinoma of eccrine glands[17] and basaloid sebaceous carcinoma.[18] In such circumstances, conventional special stains, electron microscopy, or immunohistochemistry can be employed to resolve interpretative difficulties.

Conventional Special Stains. Basal cell carcinoma contains a negligible amount of glycogen, as demonstrated by relative nonreactivity with a periodic acid–Schiff stain. The mucicarmine reaction is seen focally in examples of apocrine BCC, as well as in tumors containing signet-ring cells; the same neoplasms display diastase-resistant positivity for periodic acid–Schiff stain. Similarly, the colloidal iron technique can be used to label the epithelium-related mucosubstance in adenoid BCC and will also stain the stroma of

Text continued on page 789

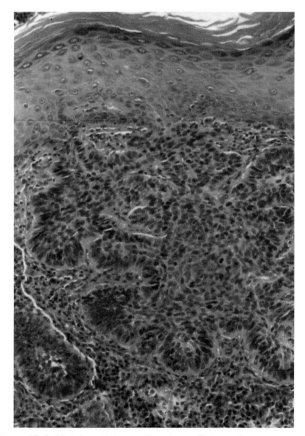

Figure 13–3. Nodulocystic basal cell carcinoma. This neoplasm is composed of solid nests of compact basaloid cells that demonstrate peripheral nuclear palisading.

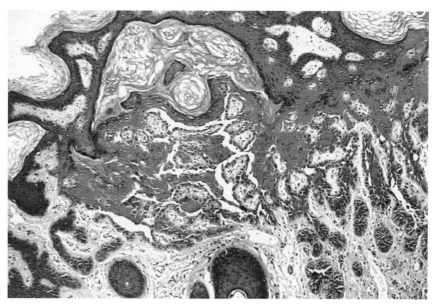

Figure 13–2. Warty dyskeratoma of the face. Dyscohesive, dyskeratotic cells in the epidermis create a peculiarly characteristic pseudopapillary image, with accompanying epidermal hyperplasia.

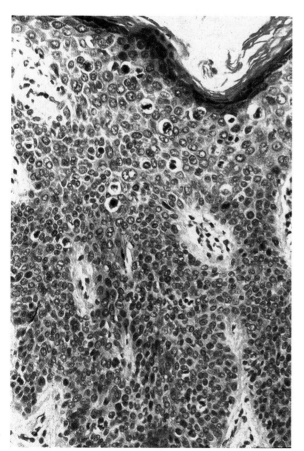

Figure 13–4. Bowen's disease (intraepidermal squamous cell carcinoma). The entire epidermis is replaced by a proliferation of cytologically atypical keratinocytes, with loss of maturation.

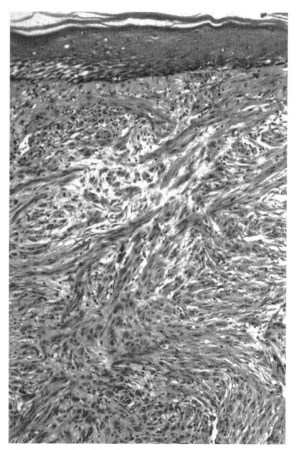

Figure 13–5. Spindle cell squamous carcinoma of the face. This neoplasm is composed of a uniform but anaplastic population of fusiform cells that appear to blend with the basal aspect of the overlying epidermis.

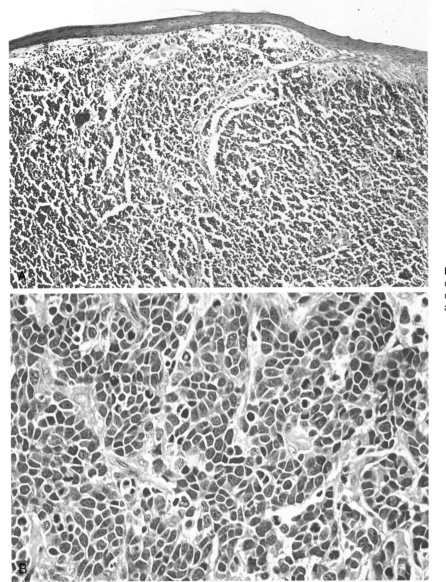

Figure 13–7. Merkel cell carcinoma of the face. A, A uniform population of small round tumor cells is separated from the epidermis by a Grenz zone. B, There is a suggestion of organoid growth.

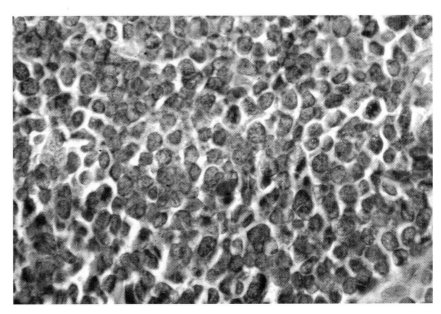

Figure 13–8. Cytologic appearance of Merkel cell carcinoma, showing nuclear homogeneity, dispersed chromatin, inconspicuous nucleoli, and a high mitotic rate.

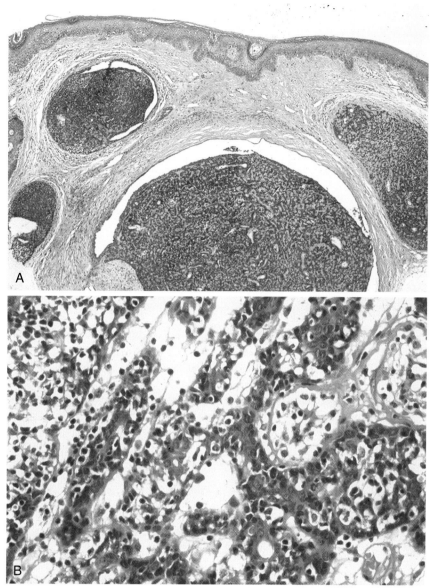

Figure 13–11. *A*, Eccrine spiradenoma, represented by a dermal mass composed of basaloid cells in cords and nests. *B*, Dilated stromal blood vessels and intratumoral lymphocytes are apparent in spiradenoma.

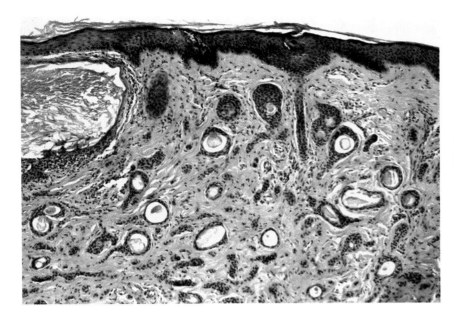

Figure 13–12. Dermal syringoma, showing circumscribed tubular and solid arrays of polygonal cells, some of which have central lumina and a comma-like configuration.

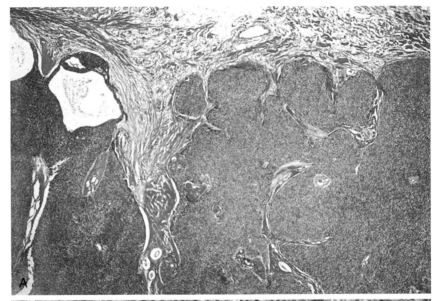

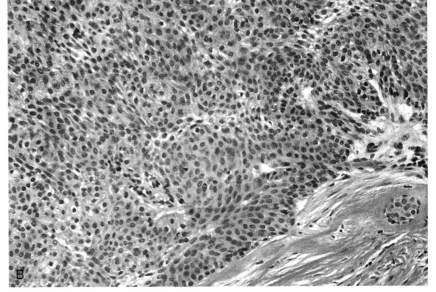

Figure 13–14. A, Eccrine acrospiroma of the neck, showing nested groups of polygonal tumor cells that are fairly sharply circumscribed with regard to the surrounding dermal connective tissue. Focal microcystic change is also apparent. B, The cytologic uniformity and sharp margination of acrospiroma are shown here.

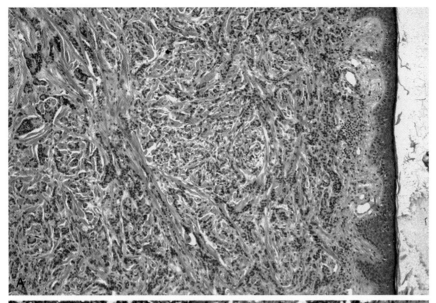

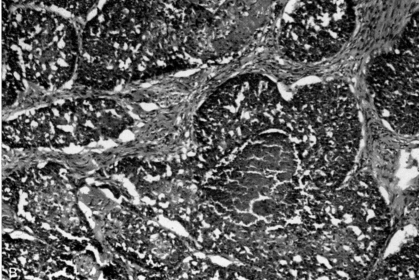

Figure 13–16. *A,* Ductal eccrine carcinoma of the face, showing a randomly invasive proliferation of solid tubules and gland-like arrays of tumor cells in the dermis. The resemblance to invasive ductal carcinoma of the breast is striking. *B,* Foci of spontaneous necrosis are evident in this ductal eccrine carcinoma.

Figure 13–17. Mucinous eccrine carcinoma, in which nests and cords of polygonal tumor cells are suspended in a voluminous mucoid matrix. The image resembles that of mucinous breast cancer.

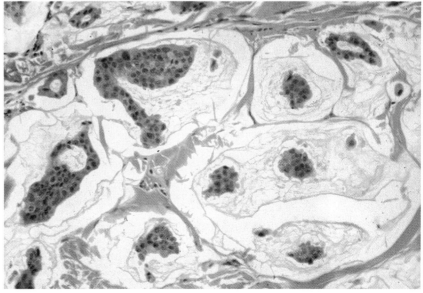

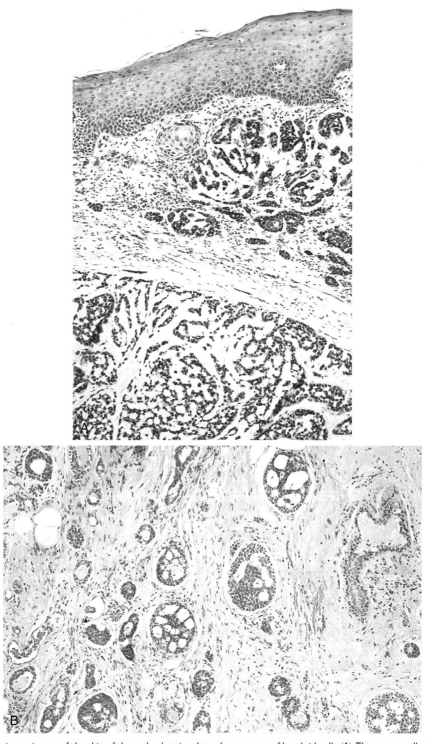

Figure 13–19. Adenoid cystic carcinoma of the skin of the scalp, showing dermal aggregates of basaloid cells *(A)*. The tumor cells are arranged in tubular profiles, cribriform arrays, and solid cords *(B)*.

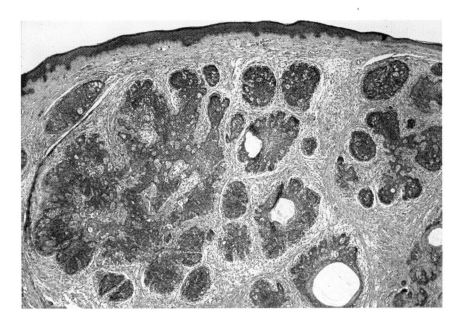

Figure 13–20. Classical trichoepithelioma, manifested by rounded aggregates of basaloid cells in the dermis with focal central production of pilar keratin. There is no mucomyxoid stroma or epithelial retraction, as seen in pilar-type basal cell carcinoma.

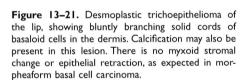

Figure 13–21. Desmoplastic trichoepithelioma of the lip, showing bluntly branching solid cords of basaloid cells in the dermis. Calcification may also be present in this lesion. There is no myxoid stromal change or epithelial retraction, as expected in morpheaform basal cell carcinoma.

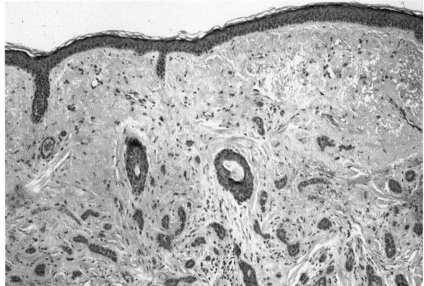

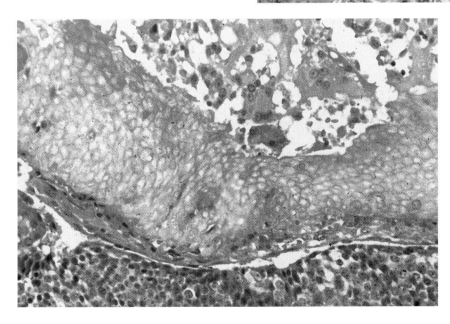

Figure 13–23. Pilomatrixoma of the neck, showing juxtaposition of compact basaloid tumor cells with zones of "ghost cell" keratinization.

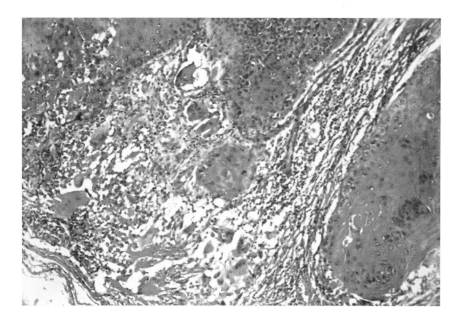

Figure 13–24. Proliferating pilar tumor, demonstrating circumscribed proliferation of cords and nests of overtly keratinocytic cells with foci of trichilemmal-type keratinization.

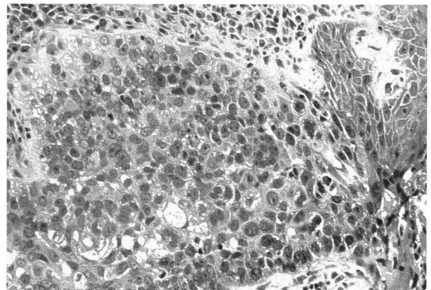

Figure 13–26. Focal pagetoid intraepidermal spread of sebaceous carcinoma of the dermis.

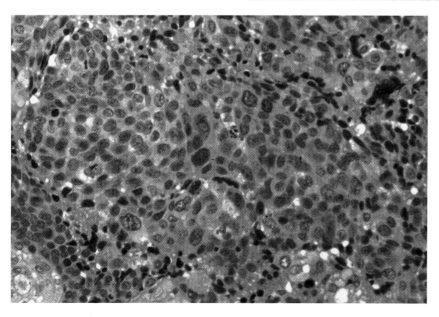

Figure 13–28. Pilomatrix carcinoma, showing nuclear enlargement, vesicular chromatin, and prominent nucleoli in the tumor cells. Areas of ghost cell keratinization were seen elsewhere in the lesion (compare with Figure 13–23).

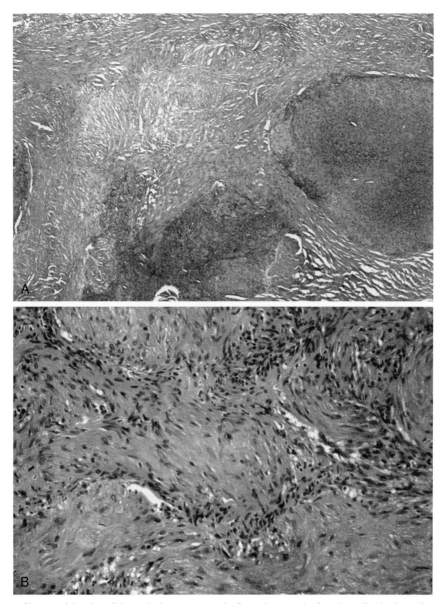

Figure 13–30. *A,* Solitary myofibroma of the skin of the neck, demonstrating the fascicular growth of cytologically bland spindle cells that are set in a variably fibrous stroma. *B,* The growth pattern and cellular details of the lesion are shown to better advantage here.

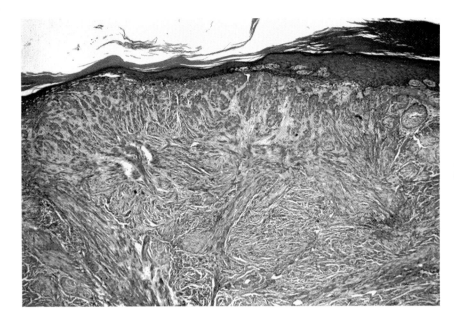

Figure 13–31. Dermatomyofibroma of the face, showing a plate-like proliferation of spindle cells with a fascicular substructure.

Figure 13–32. Glomus tumor of the skin of the face, represented by solid nests of bland polygonal cells that are centered on a neurovascular complex in the dermis.

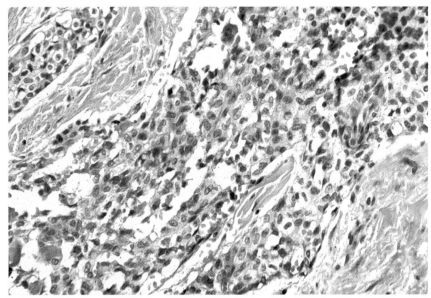

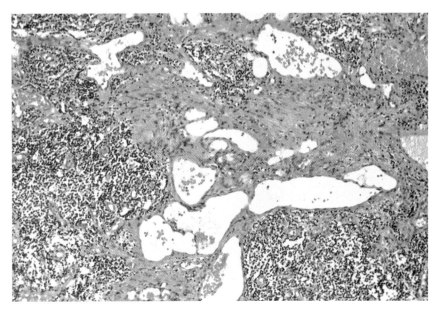

Figure 13–34. Deep lymphangioma of the neck (so-called "cystic hygroma"), showing dilated lymphatic vascular channels that are surrounded by lymphocytic aggregates.

most BCCs faintly. Hyaluronidase digestion will abolish the latter but not the former of these reactivities. The Movat stain also labels the contents of pseudoglandular profiles in adenoid neoplasms, but they are periodic acid–Schiff–negative. This constellation of results differs from that of true glandular tumors of the skin. Lipid stains (oil-red-O and Sudan IV) are nonreactive with conventional BCC, but amyloid can be detected by the Congo Red, Lieb's, or thioflavine-T techniques in up to 70% of such neoplasms.[19–21] The latter finding appears to be independent of histologic subtype and may be related to a relatively high degree of tumor cell apoptosis.

Immunohistochemistry. Among all malignant neoplasms of the skin, those showing cellular differentiation toward keratinocytes (BCC and squamous carcinoma) are immunohistochemical "have-nots." They lack most specialized determinants other than cytokeratin polypeptides (the basic cytoskeletal proteins of epithelial cells and neoplasms) and a restricted group of cell-membrane–related cell products. Specifically, epithelial membrane antigen, other human milk fat globule proteins, CD15, S100 protein, and carcinoembryonic antigen are not observed in BCCs.[22, 23]

Thomas et al.[24] demonstrated that normal epidermal basal cells and BCCs display selective immunoreactivity for low molecular weight (40 to 46 kd) keratin proteins. In contrast, other keratinocytes, pilar tumors, and squamous carcinomas exhibit staining for a broad spectrum of cytokeratins (45 to 65 kd). These observations may be useful in separating small-cell squamous carcinoma (see later discussion) from BCC. However, they do not allow for a similar distinction between BCCs and sudoriferous or sebaceous tumors, since these adnexal lesions also have a typically restricted (low molecular weight) keratin profile.[18, 25, 26] Immunostains for the other cell products listed in the previous paragraph attain their value in the latter differential diagnosis. Recent additions to the immunohistologic armamentarium of reagents include antibodies to BER-EP4 and the bcl-2 protein, both of which decorate BCCs (as well as various appendage tumors) but not squamous cell carcinomas.[27, 28] It also is of interest that the intratumoral amyloid seen in many cases of BCC is apparently of keratinaceous origin, as documented immunocytochemically.[29] This finding further supports the premise that BCC-amyloid is related to apoptosis and degeneration of cytoskeletal protein.

Additional cell-membrane determinants that have been detected in BCC are of little diagnostic use. These include markers of active cellular proliferation[30–32] and β_2-microglobulin, a component of human histocompatibility locus antigens.[33] A proposal has been made that malignant tumors lacking β_2-microglobulin are more likely to exhibit an aggressive clinical course.[33] In general, this premise has not proved to be valid; in specific reference to BCC, β_2-microglobulin has no relationship to biologic behavior.[34]

Eccrine BCC may express S100 protein in the tubular profiles corresponding to adnexal differentiation, but carcinoembryonic antigen is absent in such lesions. The presence of gross cystic disease fluid protein-15 (a marker for apocrine differentiation)[35, 36] has not yet been assessed in apocrine BCC.

As a final note on this topic, it is of interest that many BCCs incite an inflammatory response in the surrounding dermis. Reactive hematopoietic cells consist primarily of lymphocytes, which have been shown to manifest a predominance of T-cell immunopheno-types.[37]

Differential Diagnosis. Several other primary cutaneous neoplasms enter into differential diagnosis with basal cell carcinoma variants. These include conventional trichoepithelioma (which resembles keratotic BCC), desmoplastic trichoepithelioma (with similarities to morpheaform BCC),[38] small-cell squamous carcinoma[39] and basaloid sebaceous carcinoma[29] (which mimic nodulocystic BCC), and adenoid cystic eccrine carcinoma (simulating adenoid or eccrine BCC).[17, 23]

In general, classic trichoepitheliomas exhibit a much more organoid growth pattern than BCC, with more equally sized cellular lobules. Also, broad connections to the epidermis are rare in dermal hair sheath tumors (except via pilosebaceous units), whereas they are regularly observed in cases of BCC. Finally, the fibromyxoid

stroma of BCC is not recapitulated by the fibrous matrix in tricho-epithelioma, nor is cellular retraction as prominent a feature of the latter tumor. In difficult cases, immunohistochemical determinations of cytokeratin profiles may be employed diagnostically to separate these lesions, as described earlier.[26] Indeed, all of these points may fail to make the distinction under consideration here, for reasons to be discussed subsequently.

Desmoplastic trichoepithelioma (DTE) can be distinguished from morphea-like BCC by the uniform observation of horn cysts in the former, along with an absence of expansile cell nests and the nearly universal presence of epidermal hyperplasia. Also, DTE occurs in a younger patient population than typical cases of morphea-form BCC.[38]

Small-cell squamous carcinoma is devoid of nuclear palisading, as well as the fibromyxoid stroma of BCC. Moreover, tumor cell nuclei in small-cell squamous carcinoma are vesicular with prominent nucleoli, as opposed to the generally compact, non-nucleated forms seen in BCCs.[39] Basaloid sebaceous carcinoma must be distinguished from "basosebaceous" BCC. This separation is particularly difficult, since the distribution of obvious areas of sebaceous differentiation may be similar in both lesions, and each has the capacity for nuclear palisading.[18] Pagetoid involvement of the epidermis favors an interpretation of sebaceous carcinoma but is not invariably present. Diagnosis may be facilitated by lipophilic stains on frozen tissue, or immunostains for epithelial membrane antigen in difficult cases.[18] Sebaceous carcinomas display diffuse positivity with both of these techniques,[31, 40] whereas basosebaceous BCC is reactive only in areas of obvious sebaceous differentiation. Ultrastructural studies reveal the widespread presence of intracytoplasmic lipid droplets in only the first of these two lesions.[18]

Adenoid cystic sweat gland carcinoma lacks the epidermal connections of adenoid or eccrine BCC. Nonetheless, the distinction between these entities is extremely challenging, accounting for the fact that several reported examples of eccrine BCC actually appear to represent adenoid cystic carcinomas. The reverse of this situation holds true as well. Immunostains for carcinoembryonic and epithelial membrane antigens are extremely helpful in this context, since they are consistently positive in adenoid cystic carcinoma and negative in BCC.[23, 26] Rarely, adenoid cystic carcinomas of salivary gland origin may metastasize to the skin. Those tumors also lack an epidermal connection and have an immunohistochemical profile similar to that of their primary cutaneous counterparts. Obviously, these comments make it apparent that the diagnostic distinction between such lesions must be accomplished by careful clinicopathologic correlation rather than by special studies.

Treatment and Prognosis. There are several variants of cutaneous BCC that have a particular tendency for local recurrence. These include the morpheaform, metatypical (squamoid), and infiltrative subtypes. Formal surgical resection with the use of frozen sections to determine margin status is recommended for the latter lesions. Other forms of BCC can be managed with a variety of treatment modalities, including electrodesiccation, curettage, and conservative local excision.

Squamous Cell Carcinoma

Squamous cell carcinoma (SCC) of the skin is capable of assuming a diversity of clinical and histologic growth patterns, like BCC, but it typically presents itself as a non-healing ulcer or an irregular cutaneous nodule. From a morphologic perspective, these patterns include conventional, adenoid, spindled-pleomorphic, small-cell, clear-cell, and verrucous variants.[41–54] Also, this neoplasm can be graded according to its level of nucleocytoplasmic differentiation and depth of dermal invasion.[54, 55] Lastly, SCC in situ (Bowen's disease) has a distinctive clinicopathologic appearance but may be confused with a number of other dermatopathologic entities.[56]

Bowen's disease usually appears clinically in middle age or adulthood, as an irregular, reddish, and scaly thickening of the skin.[56] Both sun-exposed and protected cutaneous areas may be affected by this proliferation. When it occurs on the glans penis, Bowen's disease is traditionally referred to as *erythroplasia of Queyrat.*[57]

Histologically, Bowen's disease is characterized by global epidermal atypia, acanthosis, and elongation of the rete ridges (Fig. 13–4, see p. 779). There is little or no maturation of neoplastic keratinocytes within the epidermis, and their nuclear-to-cytoplasmic ratios are greatly increased. The basement membrane is intact, but the atypical proliferation may involve the follicular infundibula fairly deeply. Nuclear chromatin is either hyperchromatic and uniformly distributed, or vesicular; nucleoli are often prominent. Tumor cell size varies significantly from case to case, and even within the same lesion. One of the hallmarks of this lesion is the irregular dispersal of dyskeratotic cells throughout the epidermis; these often show an artifactual retraction from their "neighbors" and contain hypereosinophilic cytoplasm and pyknotic nuclei. Also, random mitoses are regularly observed, which are not uncommonly atypical in shape. The horny layer of the skin is moderately thickened and parakeratotic.[56]

Some cases of Bowen's disease show nests of atypical keratinocytes in an otherwise unremarkable epidermis, and still others manifest cytoplasmic clarity in the neoplastic cells.[56, 58] The first of these patterns was formerly included in the now-defunct concept of "intraepidermal epithelioma of Borst-Jadassohn."[59] Strayer and Santa Cruz[56] have also described atrophic, psoriasiform, verrucous, and metaplastic forms of Bowen's disease. The last of these variants features the presence of intraepidermal amyloid, mucinous cells, or foci of sebaceous differentiation.[60]

Invasive squamous cell carcinoma (SCC) has developed from Bowen's disease in less than 1% to 11% of cases, in various reports.[56, 61–63] When this occurs, the infiltrative component often manifests a more well-differentiated cytologic appearance than that present above the basement membrane. Foci of dermal fibrosis and chronic inflammation beneath apparently intra-epidermal SCC should prompt examination of step sections, to detect areas of microinvasion.

Conventional Squamous Cell Carcinoma

Conventional SCC features the interanastomosing growth of cords and nests of polygonal cells, with eosinophilic or amphophilic cytoplasm and enlarged nuclei. The latter contain generally vesicular chromatin and prominent nucleoli; mitotic activity is variable, and mitoses may be atypical in shape. Dyskeratotic cells are regularly present, along with parakeratosis of the horny layer.

Well-differentiated neoplasms (Broders' grade 1)[54] have abundantly keratinized, glassy eosinophilic cytoplasm and intercellular "bridges" on high-power microscopy. Tumor cells are often arranged focally in a concentric fashion, enclosing masses of anucleated keratin—so-called "keratin pearls." Invasive growth extends downward into the dermis in a jagged fashion and usually extends no deeper than the mid-reticular layer. Fibrosis and lymphoplasmacytic inflammation typically are evident at the interface between corium and tumor, but necrosis is unusual. The level of nucleocytoplasmic differentiation in these lesions roughly approximates that of the normal keratinocyte.

The lesion known as *keratoacanthoma* is, in my opinion, really a grade 1 SCC.[64–66] This tumor subtype is characterized by the potential for clinical regression; its low-power microscopic profile resembles a volcano, with a central keratin-filled crater and lateral, protuberant, epidermal "lips" composed of well-differentiated keratinocytes. The base of a keratoacanthoma often shows an irregular downward proliferation of rete ridges with subjacent fibrosis and inflammation. Small collections of neutrophils are scattered throughout the neoplastic epithelium, and perineural invasion can be observed in some examples. Keratoacanthoma may grow rapidly, a trait that, together with its characteristic macroscopic appearance, allows the clinician to recognize it before excision. When this history is obtained and the typical histologic image is seen, it is my

practice to diagnose the lesion as well-differentiated squamous cell carcinoma, with features of so-called "keratoacanthoma." This interpretation simultaneously confirms the attending physician's impression and conveys the truism that the pathologist cannot tell which keratoacanthomas will regress spontaneously (presumably through immunologic lysis) and which will not.

Moderately differentiated SCC (Broders' grades 2 and 3) shows less propensity for pearl formation, is more deeply invasive, has less eosinophilic cytoplasm, and manifests more nuclear hyperchromasia and mitotic activity. Regional necrosis within cell nests makes its appearance at this level of differentiation, and invasion of blood vessels and perineural sheaths may be appreciated. Tumoral lobules tend to be less uniform in shape and size than those of well-differentiated SCC and have a more irregular outline.

Poorly differentiated SCC (Broders' grade 4) commonly infiltrates the subcutis and has little if any obvious keratinization. Cytoplasm is amphophilic, nuclei are more pleomorphic and hyperchromatic, and mitoses are abundant. Necrosis is typically prominent, and cellular lobules often become confluent and have extremely irregular borders. Lymphatic and perineural invasion may be observed in roughly 50% of cases.

Surface ulceration becomes more likely as the level of differentiation lessens. Conversely, residual actinic keratosis-like changes in the surrounding epidermis are usually seen in well-differentiated tumors of sun-exposed skin areas. Regardless of grade, SCC in such locations is associated with prominent elastosis of the contiguous dermis.

A number of histologic variants of SCC have been described, again similar to BCC. These include adenoid (acantholytic-pseudoglandular), small-cell, spindle-cell/pleomorphic, hydropic (clear-cell), and verrucous forms. Of these, adenoid and spindle-cell squamous carcinomas seem to behave more aggressively than "conventional" tumors of this type, whereas verrucous carcinoma is an indolent lesion that seldom, if ever, spreads outside the skin. Spindle-cell (sarcomatoid) and verrucous SCC are overrepresented in the skin of the head and neck. Accordingly, those subtypes are discussed further here.

Spindled and Pleomorphic-Cell Squamous Cell Carcinoma

Some examples of grade 4 SCC are composed exclusively of fusiform and giant pleomorphic cells, with little or no keratinization (Fig. 13–5, see p. 779).[41, 55, 67, 68] Necrosis is variable, but mitotic activity is regularly evident and focally atypical. The surrounding dermis often shows edema rather than fibrosis, and peritumoral inflammation may or may not be apparent. Continuity between these neoplasms and an intact overlying epidermis is observed in a minority of cases; most manifest surface ulceration.

Spindle-cell and pleomorphic SCCs characteristically occur in sun-damaged skin. In common with other poorly differentiated cutaneous squamous neoplasms, deep infiltration of the dermis, subcutis, and underlying fascia is frequently observed.[55]

Verrucous Squamous Cell Carcinoma

Squamous carcinomas that grossly simulate giant condylomata or verrucae have been diversely described as giant condyloma of Buschke and Loewenstein,[69] carcinoma cuniculatum,[46] or verrucous carcinoma[42, 70] based on their anatomic locations. Basically, all of these lesions are identical and can be considered as a group. Verrucous SCC displays marked papillomatosis and acanthosis, with "church-spiring" of the neoplastic epidermis. As a rule, cytologic atypia is only slight in this neoplasm, mitotic activity is scant, and dyskeratosis is less marked than in other forms of SCC (Fig. 13–6). Infiltration of the dermis occurs in broad, blunt cellular tongues, rather than the jagged profiles seen in conventional squamous carcinoma. Reactive fibrosis and inflammation are minimal. Vascular and perineural invasion are seen only rarely.

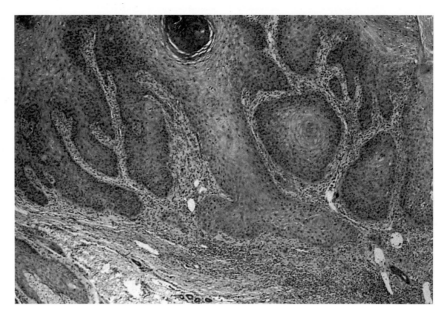

Figure 13–6. Verrucous carcinoma of the nose. This tumor demonstrates papilliform as well as bluntly invasive growth of minimally atypical keratinocytes.

The criteria just given should be rigorously met before a squamous carcinoma can be labeled as verrucous. This is so because other forms (such as conventional SCC) may occasionally demonstrate verrucous growth but do not behave as indolently as true verrucous carcinoma. In particular, tumors displaying marked cellular atypia and abnormal mitotic figures should not be classified as verrucous SCC.

Special Pathologic Studies

Conventional Special Stains. Conventional histochemical staining methods are of limited use in the diagnostic definition of SCC. The periodic acid–Schiff method yields variable reactivity with this neoplasm; however, if a clear-cell cutaneous tumor fails to contain glycogen, metastatic renal cell carcinoma and eccrine carcinoma may be excluded from consideration, and hydropic SCC assumes greater importance in the differential diagnosis.[47] Mucin stains are nonreactive with SCC, as are the alcian blue and colloidal iron techniques. These findings also may be of some assistance in discriminating between adenoid squamous carcinoma and sweat gland tumors.

Immunohistochemistry. As noted earlier in the section on BCC, squamous cell carcinoma of the skin demonstrates reactivity for medium and high molecular weight cytokeratins.[24] Poorly differentiated tumors typically express low molecular weight keratin as well.[23] Spindle-cell and pleomorphic squamous carcinomas manifest the facultative ability to re-express vimentin, the intermediate filament seen in virtually all embryonic cells and in mature mesenchymal tissues.[23, 26] Thus, reliance on vimentin immunostains alone is not a valid means of separating spindle-cell carcinomas from true sarcomas. Similarly, α_1-antichymotrypsin or CD68, which have been touted as markers for "fibrohistiocytic" neoplasms, are also present in pleomorphic SCC and should not be used exclusively in diagnosis in the absence of intermediate filament stains.

An interesting trend in immunoreactivity can be seen with antibodies to epithelial membrane antigen (EMA) in the analysis of SCC of varying grades. Well-differentiated cutaneous tumors lack EMA, moderately differentiated SCC expresses it patchily, and high-grade neoplasms are diffusely positive for this determinant.[23, 48] The significance of these findings is unclear at a molecular level, but it would appear that EMA immunostains may have some role in prognostication of the clinical behavior of SCC.

Other antigens of interest in dermatopathology, such as S100 protein, carcinoembryonic antigen, neuron-specific enolase, BER-EP4, and bcl-2 protein, are absent in squamous carcinoma of the skin regardless of grade.[23, 26] The differential diagnostic use of these reactants will be discussed subsequently. Also, some publications on

SCC have considered the expression of molecular moieties usually associated with normal keratinocytes. These include involucrin, filaggrin, and peptidylarginine deiminase.[71] As expected, such proteins are expressed in a progressively diminishing fashion, as tumor differentiation lessens. Also, they appear to have little utility in the diagnostic separation of pseudoepitheliomatous hyperplasia and keratoacanthoma from well-differentiated squamous carcinoma.

Differential Diagnosis. Because of its potential variability of appearance, SCC of the skin may be confused microscopically with several other cutaneous neoplasms and pseudoneoplastic proliferations, including extramammary Paget's disease, pseudoepitheliomatous hyperplasia, sweat gland carcinoma, epithelioid angiosarcoma, atypical fibroxanthoma, spindle-cell amelanotic melanoma, Merkel cell carcinoma, basal cell carcinoma, basaloid sebaceous carcinoma, and small-cell eccrine carcinoma. Among these lesions, melanomas are distinguishable by their positivity with the Fontana stain and their immunoreactivity for S100 protein in the absence of keratin. Sweat gland carcinoma morphotypes express carcinoembryonic antigen—with or without gross cystic disease fluid protein-15—and may be S100 protein–positive as well. Merkel cell carcinoma shows a characteristic keratin-staining pattern (see later), and may be reactive for chromogranin as well. Sarcomas typically lack keratin and instead express vimentin, and pseudoepitheliomatous hyperplasia does not demonstrate the degree of cytologic atypicality or disorganized basal growth that is observed in even well-differentiated squamous cell carcinoma.

Treatment and Prognosis. The treatment of cutaneous squamous cell carcinoma is generally quite similar to that applied to BCC. Potentially aggressive variants of SCC, however, such as the sarcomatoid, adenoid, and injury-associated forms, should be formally resected with frozen section–directed assurance of marginal status. Regional lymph node dissection is also a possibility if clinical examination demonstrates lymphadenopathy. The overall survival of patients who are managed with these precepts approximates 90% at 5 years' follow-up.

Primary Neuroendocrine Carcinoma of the Skin (Merkel Cell Carcinoma)

Primary neuroendocrine (Merkel cell) carcinoma of the skin (PNCS) characteristically is seen in middle-aged to elderly patients, with a predilection for sun-exposed skin areas.[72, 73] It usually takes the form of an erythematous to violaceous nodule but may occasionally demonstrate extensive ulceration and ill-defined borders.[73]

Pathologic Features. Typical PNCS is characterized by the medullary, organoid, or trabecular growth of small oval cells in the corium, with various degrees of intercellular cohesion. A Grenzzone is usually present between the tumor and the epidermis (Fig. 13–7, see p. 780); however, the latter structure may be involved focally in approximately 10% of cases. Dermal appendages are usually spared, but permeative growth into the subcutis is often apparent. Adipocytes may be entrapped by tumor cells, yielding an appearance simulating that of lymphoma cutis. Regional coagulative necrosis and apoptosis are common within PNCS. Nuclei are round to oval, with evenly dispersed chromatin, inconspicuous nucleoli, and abundant mitoses (up to 12 per high-power field) (Fig. 13–8, see p. 780). Cytoplasm is scanty and amphophilic, and cellular borders are indistinct. The stroma of PNCS may be sclerotic focally (sometimes mimicking the appearance of amyloid) and is richly endowed with capillary- or venule-sized vessels, which may be dilated. Lymphatic invasion is apparent in 20% of cases, and variably intense stromal lymphoplasmacytic inflammation is evident in most examples.[73]

Variations on the histopathologic description just given include lesions showing scattered uninucleated tumor "giant" cells, formation of Homer-Wright rosettes, myxoid stroma, spindle-cell growth, foci of squamous or glandular differentiation, and focal desmoplasia.[73, 74] Another subtype of PNCS is the "oat-cell" variant, displaying nests of small, hyperchromatic, partially crushed tumor cells with prominent nuclear molding. The microscopic similarities between the latter and metastatic pulmonary small-cell neuroendocrine carcinoma are obvious; however, I have only very rarely observed the Azzopardi phenomenon (DNA encrustation of intratumoral blood vessels) in PNCS, whereas it is common in metastatic oat-cell carcinoma of the lung. Gould et al.[75] documented a spectrum of differentiation in PNCS, including intermediate- and large-cell subtypes. It is probable that the cases of "primary cutaneous carcinoid" reported by other authors fall into the second of these categories.[73]

Primary Neuroendocrine Carcinoma of the Skin Associated with Other Skin Lesions

The association between PNCS and squamous carcinoma is now well recognized.[75, 76] Roughly 25% of patients with neuroendocrine skin cancer have had squamous carcinoma in the same cutaneous region, either metachronously or synchronously with the former lesion. Both invasive SCC and Bowen's disease have been documented in this context. In addition, Silva et al.[77] have described a case in which overt sweat gland carcinoma and PNCS were admixed. I have observed one example of cutaneous neuroendocrine carcinoma arising in a background of hypohidrotic ectodermal dysplasia; the patient also had multifocal basal cell carcinomas and trichoepitheliomas in the same skin field. Moreover, in the M.D. Anderson Hospital experience with this neoplasm, 9 of 67 cases showed the concurrence of PNCS and adjacent BCC.[77] Nevertheless, a histologic admixture of these two neoplasms has not been reported to date. Another example of PNCS in my files occurred in a large congenital nevus, and one patient mentioned by Silva and colleagues had had a noncontiguous malignant melanoma.[77]

Special Pathologic Studies

Conventional Special Stains. The periodic acid–Schiff method may demonstrate scanty glycogen in the cells of PNCS, but this reactivity is seen in less than 15% of cases. The mucicarmine stain is consistently negative, but alcian blue and colloidal iron techniques sometimes result in labeling of the tumoral stroma. Argyrophil stains (e.g., Grimelius, Churukian-Schenk) are positive in less than 10% of cutaneous neuroendocrine carcinomas that have been formalin-fixed, but preservation in Bouin's solution yields silver-reactivity in the majority of cases.[78] Argentaffin and amyloid stains are uniformly negative.

Immunohistochemistry. PNCS is typified by consistent reactivity for cytokeratin in one of two patterns, diffuse or globular/paranuclear. The second of these is diagnostic of neuroendocrine differentiation in a cutaneous small-cell tumor[79] but is seen in only 60% to 70% of cases. Concomitant positivity for neurofilament protein can be detected in 33%, with a similar cytoplasmic distribution. Additional evidence for the epithelial differentiation of cutaneous neuroendocrine carcinomas is represented by immunopositivity for epithelial membrane antigen. This determinant is less ubiquitous than cytokeratin in such tumors, but it is apparent in over 75% of cases. The most sensitive "endocrine" marker for PNCS is neuron-specific enolase, the gamma-gamma dimer of 2-D-phosphoglycerate hydrolase. Although neuron-specific enolase is seen in all tumors of this type, it is not specific for PNCS. As mentioned previously, occasional basal cell carcinomas express this protein as well, and I have also observed it in sweat gland carcinomas. The latter finding is not unexpected, since some studies have demonstrated neuron-specific enolase in normal eccrine glands. Chromogranin, a very specific indicator of neuroendocrine differentiation, is seen in 33% of PNCS cases[79]; in addition, 5% to 30% exhibit focal reactivity for vasoactive intestinal polypeptide, calcitonin, pancreatic polypeptide, adrenocorticotropic hormone, gastrin, insulin, or somatostatin.[80] S100 protein and carcinoembryonic antigen are consistently lacking in PNCS.

Differential Diagnosis. The differential diagnosis of small-cell neoplasms of the skin is extensive. Small-cell SCC, eccrine carcinoma, and malignant melanoma must be included in this group, as well as malignant lymphoma, metastatic neuroendocrine carcinoma from visceral sites (especially the lungs), peripheral neuroepithelioma (primitive neuroectodermal tumor), and Ewing's sarcoma.[72, 73] Immunohistochemical studies are extremely useful in this context (Fig. 13–9).

Treatment and Prognosis. Treatment of PNCS is predicated on complete surgical excision. Because of the aggressive nature of this tumor, heroic resections are sometimes necessary to gain local control and provide the best chance of cure. Regional lymph node dissection should be undertaken if the primary lesion is larger than 2 cm in maximum dimension; shows more than 10 mitoses per 10 400× microscopic fields; demonstrates extensive lymphatic or vascular invasion; has an oat-cell morphology; or is associated with obvious lymphadenopathy. Irradiation and chemotherapy have been utilized as adjunctive treatments for PNCS, but, in general, such interventions afford only palliative benefit. Roughly 75% of Merkel cell carcinomas recur locally or metastasize to local nodal chains, and approximately 65% of patients eventually succumb to their tumors because of additional visceral spread.

▪ ADNEXAL NEOPLASMS

Adnexal tumors of the skin are diverse, from either a nosologic or a histologic perspective. Indeed, entire textbooks have been devoted to the clinicopathologic aspects of such neoplasms.[81, 82] Accordingly, only brief summaries of those lesions that preferentially affect the head and neck are provided here.

Benign Tumors of Sweat Gland Origin

Several adnexal tumors with sweat glandular differentiation are observed with some regularity in the skin of the face, neck, and scalp. *Dermal cylindroma* may be observed as a solitary sporadic lesion or as a multifocal process in the context of the "turban tumor" (Ancell-Spiegler) syndrome.[83] In either of these contexts, the tumors are composed of two cell populations, one compact and basaloid and the other showing a polygonal shape with more abundant amphophilic cytoplasm. Nuclear chromatin is dispersed, without apparent nucleoli, and mitotic activity is sparse. There are two striking aspects of this neoplasm that allow for its ready recognition under low-power microscopy; these are represented by a "jigsaw puzzle" pattern of growth—with angular cell nests molding to one another in a fibrous stroma—and the regular disposition of brightly eosino-

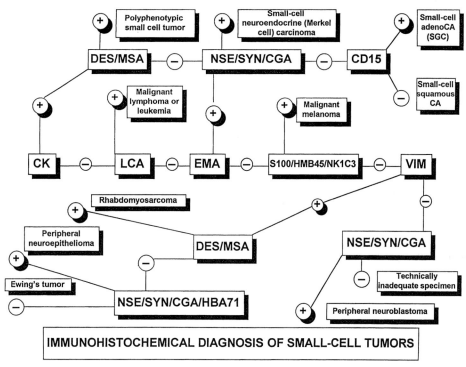

Figure 13–9. Algorithm for immunohistologic diagnosis of small-cell cutaneous neoplasms, beginning with cytokeratin staining (CK).

philic, hyaline basement membrane material throughout the cellular clusters and immediately around them in the dermal connective tissue (Fig. 13–10). Cylindroma quite often exhibits an irregular pattern of peripheral growth, with "buds" of tumor in the dermis or subcutis that are detached from the main mass. This finding has no

adverse prognostic importance and should not be used to label such lesions "malignant." Similarly, rare examples of cylindroma that demonstrate brisk mitotic activity show no untoward behavior if the nuclear features and overall architecture are characteristic of that entity. Occasional tumors in this category may be associated with cu-

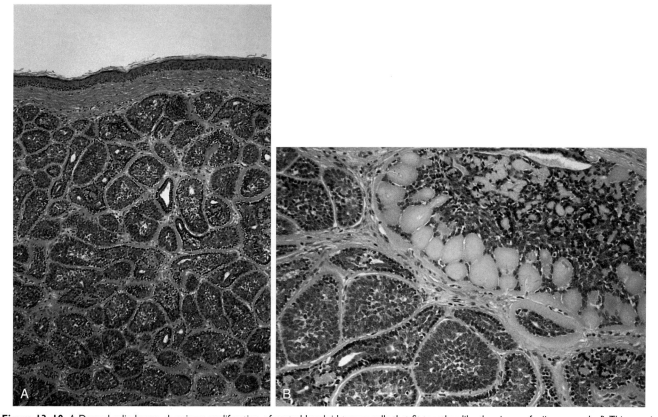

Figure 13–10. *A,* Dermal cylindroma, showing a proliferation of nested basaloid tumor cells that fit together like the pieces of a jigsaw puzzle. *B,* This area in a dermal cylindroma demonstrates the intratumoral eosinophilic deposits of basement membrane that are characteristic of this neoplasm.

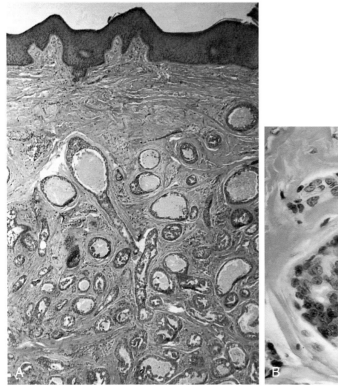
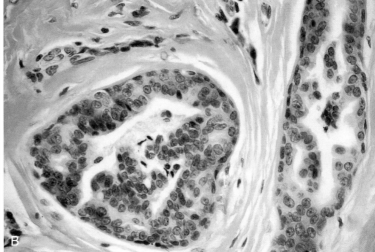

Figure 13–13. *A,* Papillary eccrine adenoma, a form of tubulopapillary hidradenoma that features the presence of tubular cell arrays in the dermis, each of which contains internal micropapillae. *B,* The resemblance between papillary eccrine adenoma and simple ductal hyperplasia of the female breast is readily apparent.

taneous trichoepitheliomas or spiradenomas in the same skin field, as well as basal cell adenomas or adenocarcinomas in major or minor salivary glands.

Eccrine spiradenoma differs in appearance only slightly from the description just given for cylindromas. The former of these two neoplasms lacks a jigsaw puzzle profile, and instead shows the presence of intralesional vascular channels that are often dilated and disposed toward the periphery of tumor cell clusters (Fig. 13–11, see p. 781).[84] Another characteristic of spiradenoma is the consistent dispersion of mature lymphocytes throughout the mass, much as one would expect in tumors of the thymic epithelium. Otherwise, the potential for basement membrane deposition and irregular, permeative, peripheral growth of the lesion is shared between spiradenoma and cylindroma. In occasional instances, it may, in fact, be difficult to distinguish between these two pathologic entities microscopically.

Eccrine and apocrine "hidrocystomas" are limited almost exclusively to the facial skin. In actuality, they are probably not neoplasms at all but rather localized dilatations of the eccrine and apocrine ducts that are occasioned by traumatic obstruction.[85, 86] Microscopically, such lesions manifest a saccular space that is lined with variably proliferative polyhedral epithelial cells that may, on occasion, form micropapillae; anywhere from one to more than 10 layers of epithelium may be observed. In the eccrine form, the cells are compact, with cuticle formation at the luminal aspect of the lesion. Apocrine hidrocystoma, on the other hand, exhibits a composition by large cells with granular eosinophilic cytoplasm and luminal decapitation secretion. Mitotic activity is absent.

Syringoma is another benign eccrine proliferation that is probably malformative rather than neoplastic in most cases. It commonly is multifocal and is relatively restricted to the skin of the upper face (particularly the lower eyelids) and the genital region.[87, 88] Small, comma-shaped tubules of cells—many of which contain central lumina and a luminal cuticle—are dispersed throughout a collagenous matrix in the dermis in this lesion. Syringomas are exquisitely circumscribed on low-power microscopy, and they are entirely devoid

of nuclear atypia, mitotic activity, and permeative growth (Fig. 13–12, see p. 782). Nevertheless, a small punch or shave biopsy through the center of such a tumor can provide an image that is maddeningly similar to that of a form of adnexal carcinoma (see later),[89] making primary excision the preferred approach to the management of this proliferation.

Hidradenomas of the eccrine and apocrine types are grouped together by many observers into two main categories: tubulopapillary hidradenomas[90, 91] and acrospiromas (Figs. 13–13 and 13–14, see p. 782).[92] Both of these clusters of tumors show a basic composition by uniform polygonal cells that are variably aggregated into solid nests—subdivided from one another by fibrovascular stroma of heterogeneous density—or that line the peripheral aspects of dermal microcysts or form intraductal tubulopapillary complexes. Both eccrine and apocrine cytologic features may be observed (see earlier discussion) in such lesions, and communication between cellular nests in the corium and similar aggregates in the epidermis may occur via penetrating columns of cells that resemble the normal acrosyringia. Some neoplasms showing the last-cited of these attributes have the histologic profile that is associated with classical eccrine "poroma" (Fig. 13–15).[93] Benign hidradenomas are circumscribed on low-power microscopy, and they are therefore not "allowed" to exhibit irregular "budding" into the adjacent stroma. The latter finding usually equates with low-grade malignancy. Similarly, zonal necrosis, extensive clear-cell change, and areas of obvious nuclear atypia (with increased nucleocytoplasmic ratios and nucleoli) are indicators of malignant acrospiromas.

Malignant Sweat Gland Tumors

There are basically six malignant sweat gland tumors that have some propensity to affect the head and neck. The first—*malignant acrospiroma*—has just been mentioned.

A second is *ductal eccrine carcinoma* (DEC), a lesion that bears a striking structural homology to ductal adenocarcinoma of the breast (Fig. 13–16, see p. 783).[94] As such, DEC is composed of epithelioid cells arranged in tubules or solid nests and cords, with at least modest nuclear atypia and randomly disposed growth throughout a fibrotic dermis. The peripheral borders of such tumors are irregular and permeative; abnormal mitotic figures and foci of spontaneous necrosis are often found as well. There are no immunohistochemical or ultrastructural features of DEC that may be used to separate it from metastatic mammary carcinoma. Thus, careful examination of the breasts and meticulous history-taking are paramount in resolving this differential diagnosis. Oddly, patients with DEC often state that a solitary skin lesion has been present for at least several months, and often for years. These are not the features of cutaneous metastases.

A third form of sweat gland carcinoma in this region is that of *mucinous eccrine (primary "colloid") carcinoma* (MEC).[95, 96, 97] This neoplasm shares the same relatedness to mammary tumors that was mentioned above in connection with DEC. Accordingly, MEC shows cords and nests of relatively uniform polygonal cells that are suspended in pools of epithelial mucin (Fig. 13–17, see p. 783). The latter material stains with the periodic acid–Schiff and mucicarmine methods and is resistant to diastase digestion. The tumor is further subdivided by fibrovascular stroma, which is variably collagenized. Nests of neoplastic cells usually infiltrate the dermis and subcutis irregularly at the advancing edges of MEC. The degree of nuclear atypia seen in the constituents of this tumor is typically slight, and mitotic figures are typically limited in scope. Regional necrosis is only exceptionally observed. Some examples of MEC contain an admixture of more solidly cellular tissue that resembles DEC. This type of "hybrid" tumor is also mirrored in the breast.

A fourth variety of adnexal carcinoma with at least partial eccrine differentiation is represented by *microcystic adnexal carcinoma* (MAC).[89, 98] This lesion manifests the haphazard proliferation of solid dermal cell nests—often with internal concentricity—or tubular dermal cellular profiles, some of which may resemble those seen in syringomas (Fig. 13–18). The tumor cells show surprisingly bland nuclear features and only rare mitotic activity; similarly, necrosis is uncommon. However, the clearly aggressive nature of this neoplasm is reflected in its propensity to infiltrate perineural sheaths and vascular adventitia, as well as common invasion of the subcutis or even underlying muscle and bone. The predominant architectural characteristics of MAC have led some observers to describe it using an alternate term, *sclerosing sweat duct carcinoma.*[99] Nevertheless, this tumor regularly contains dermal microcysts that contain pilar-type keratin, and occasional examples show sebaceous, multivacuolar cytoplasmic differentiation. Thus, the less committal nosologic designation of MAC is preferred for routine diagnostic use.

A fifth type of sweat gland carcinoma seen in the head and neck is *ductopapillary apocrine carcinoma.*[100] This neoplasm is largely confined to the eyelids, axillae, and genitoperineal region, where apocrine glands are found in the highest density. Its cytoarchitectural features are quite similar to those of DEC, with two salient modifications. Ductopapillary apocrine carcinoma additionally exhibits the possible formation of tumoral papillae, which are supported by delicate fibrovascular cores and mantled by several layers of tumor cells. Moreover, the cytoplasm in that tumor is relatively copious and obviously eosinophilic, often containing a fine granularity as well. In those areas of the lesion in which tubule formation or papillae are apparent, the neoplastic cells abutting glandular spaces commonly show decapitation secretion with the elaboration of luminal "snouts."

Last, one form of sweat gland carcinoma with special relevance to the head and neck is the primary dermal *adenoid cystic carcinoma* (ACC). The microscopic image of that lesion is identical to that of salivary glandular ACC (Fig. 13–19, see p. 784); hence, skin lesions arising near the major salivary glands may create diagnostic difficulty.[101] However, there have been no well-documented examples of salivary glandular ACC that have metastasized to the dermis in the absence of a known primary tumor. Thus, worries about such an event are probably unjustified. A more real concern is the distinction between cutaneous ACC and adenoid BCC,[102] which share many points of histologic similarity. Attention to the usual stromal changes seen in BCC can resolve this potential problem; in addition, immunostains for epithelial membrane antigen, carcinoembryonic antigen, and S100 protein are positive in ACC but not in BCC.

Treatment and Prognosis. All of the forms of sweat gland carcinoma just cited have the ability to recur locally and pursue an aggressive course of regional growth, even after seemingly complete initial excision. Consequently, it has been arbitrarily decided that the surgical approach to such lesions should be like that which would be employed for a similarly sized malignant melanoma. MEC seldom metastasizes distantly and MAC never does so, but DEC and ductopapillary apocrine carcinoma can spread to regional lymph nodes as well as internal viscera such as the lungs, liver, and bone. This behavior is realized in anywhere from 15% to 50% of cases, and, unfortunately, there are no reliable morphologic or adjunctive biologic markers that can be used to predict that eventuality.

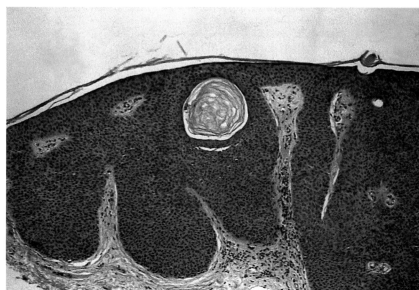

Figure 13–15. Eccrine poroma, represented by an intraepidermal proliferation of basaloid tumor cells that focally invade the dermis, recapitulating the eccrine acrosyringium.

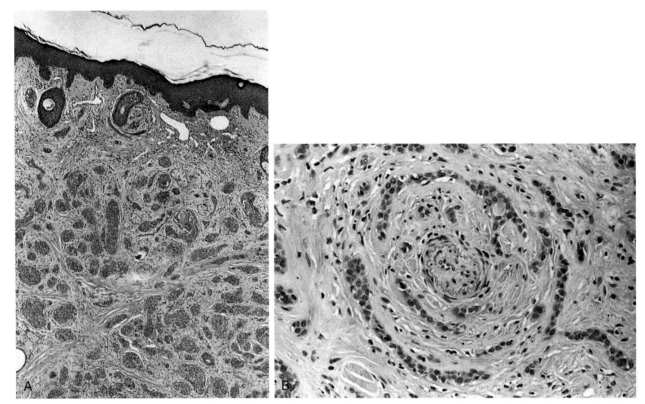

Figure 13–18. *A*, Microcystic adnexal carcinoma (MAC) of the skin, showing deeply invasive cords and rounded nests of polygonal tumor cells. *B*, The propensity for MAC to surround and invade blood vessels and perineurial sheaths is shown here.

Benign Pilosebaceous Neoplasms

Several tumors that show differentiation along sebaceous or follicular lineages show a preference to arise in the skin of the head and neck. These include sebaceous adenoma, trichofolliculoma, classic trichoepithelioma, desmoplastic trichoepithelioma, trichilemmoma, pilomatrixoma, proliferating pilar (trichilemmal) tumor, and tumor of the follicular infundibulum.

Sebaceous adenoma is composed of mature sebaceous cells with abundant, finely vacuolated cytoplasm and central ovoid nuclei. Chromatin is compact, with inconspicuous nucleoli and no mitoses. The overall profile of this lesion is that of a lobulated, sharply circumscribed, upper to mid-dermal mass without necrosis or budding of cellular nests into the adjacent corium.[103, 104] An arbitrary distinction from florid sebaceous hyperplasia (defined by three or more sebaceous lobules per pilosebaceous unit) is made in favor of adenoma if a confluence of sebaceous glands is seen that fills at least one low-power microscopic field. Some examples of sebaceous adenoma demonstrate a minor population of more basaloid cells that tend to be concentrated around the periphery of the constituent lobules, and they may be admixed with mature sebaceous cells as well. Such terms as "sebaceoma" and "Muir-Torre adenoma" have been used in reference to the latter designation. With regard to the latter designation, it should be remembered that *any* sebaceous cutaneous lesion (including basal cell carcinoma with sebaceous differentiation) may be linked to the Muir-Torre syndrome, which features malignancies in several visceral organs in concert with tumors of the skin.[105]

Trichofolliculoma has been described as a "caricature" of the normal hair follicle. It shows a constellation of several maturing keratinocytic projections that emanate from a central follicular lumen and often embrace a diminutive or aberrantly formed hair shaft.[106] The tumor cells are polyhedral rather than basaloid, and they contain relatively voluminous eosinophilic cytoplasm.

On the other hand, *trichoepithelioma* does not exhibit nearly as high a level of follicular differentiation. In classic form, it is a sharply delimited, dermal mass that is composed of islands and cords of uniformly basaloid cells that are punctuated by pilar microcysts.[107] In contrast to most basal cell carcinomas, trichoepitheliomas do not demonstrate retraction artifacts between cellular nests and the surrounding stroma, and the intratumoral dermal matrix is collagenized rather than mucomyxoid (Fig. 13–20, see p. 785). Lastly, there are no appreciable areas of apoptotic cell loss in the cell clusters of trichoepithelioma, again unlike basal cell carcinomas. "Immature" trichoepithelioma shares all of these attributes except for the presence of pilar microcysts, and it is particularly challenging to distinguish from BCC for that reason.[108] Recent immunohistochemical studies have suggested that bcl-2 protein is unique to BCC in this narrow context[109]; however, our laboratory has observed reactivity for the latter marker in both basal cell carcinomas and classic trichoepitheliomas. In light of that information and the highly differentiated nature of some BCCs—with multiple foci of obvious pilosebaceous differentiation—it may, in fact, be true that classic "trichoepitheliomas" are basal cell carcinomas in fully evolved form.

Desmoplastic trichoepithelioma differs substantially at a histologic level from the description just given. This neoplasm is a plate-like, sharply outlined growth in the upper dermis, composed of solid cords and tubules of mature keratinocytes (more like those seen in trichofolliculoma) that tend to interlock with one another.[110, 111] Dystrophic calcification is commonly superimposed on the contents of pilar microcysts, which are again randomly distributed throughout the lesion (Fig. 13–21, see p. 785). Differential diagnosis in small samples of desmoplastic trichoepithelioma primarily concerns trichofolliculoma and MAC. The last of these three tumors may be recognized by immunoreactivity for carcinoembryonic antigen, and desmoplastic trichoepithelioma does not contain hair shafts, as seen in trichofolliculoma.

The neoplastic nature of *trichilemmoma* has been called into serious question by some investigators, who prefer the interpretation that it instead represents a folliculocentric verruca vulgaris.[112] It is best to keep an open mind on this issue, and for that reason a discussion of this entity is included here. Trichilemmoma is a lobulated, clear-cell polygonal-cell proliferation that is indeed centered on hair follicles with extensions into the adjacent dermis. It manifests a zone of nuclear palisading at the peripheral aspects of constituent lobules and may demonstrate foci of pilar keratinization as well (Fig. 13–22).[113] Multiple trichilemmomas (sometimes termed *trichilemmomatous hamartomas*) have been found in some patients with Cowden's syndrome, another disease complex that potentially includes visceral carcinomas.[114] A desmoplastic form of trichilemmoma has also been described, in which narrow outgrowths of mitotically active tumor cells project from the lesional epicenter and are surrounded by fibroblastic stromal elements.[115] Fears over a diagnosis of malignancy in this context may be assuaged by attention to the low-power microscopic image of the tumor, which demonstrates its circumscription.

Pilomatrixoma (calcifying epithelioma of Malherbe) is a germinal neoplasm that shows an exclusively intradermal origin and a distinctive cellular composition. It is composed of multiple rounded or slightly irregular lobules of basaloid cells with slightly open chromatin, small nucleoli, and notable mitotic activity.[116, 117] The central aspects of the cell nests are variably replaced by "ghost cell" clusters, representing groups of effete keratinizing epithelium in which only the faint outlines of the nuclear contours are seen within a brightly eosinophilic cytoplasmic background (Fig. 13–23, see p. 785). The "ghost cell" foci often become dystrophically calcified and may even be metaplastically ossified, and they are rather commonly surrounded by foreign body–type giant cells. A particular danger in the interpretation of this lesion is presented by requests for frozen section examination. This procedure accentuates the nucleolar size and vesicular nature of the tumor cells of pilomatrixoma;

these features, together with the presence of keratinization and mitotic figures, have resulted in an erroneous interpretation of squamous cell carcinoma on more than one occasion. However, attention to the zonal nature of the tumor and the particular features of the "ghost cells" will avoid such errors. Locally infiltrative and "perforating" variants of pilomatrixoma also have been described.[117]

Proliferating pilar tumor (PPT) is a neoplasm that has been alternatively designated as "proliferating trichilemmal tumor" or "proliferating trichilemmal cyst."[118, 119] It typically forms a multilobulated nodular mass in the dermis that protrudes into the overlying epidermis and commonly elevates it, sometimes with ulceration. PPT is composed of mature keratinocytes with copious eosinophilic cytoplasm, vesicular nuclei, and discernible small nucleoli (Fig. 13–24, see p. 786). Mitotic activity is often brisk, mild nuclear pleomorphism is present, and zones of spontaneous degeneration and calcification in the lesion may be mistaken for necrosis. Thus, it is easy to understand why PPT is so often confused with squamous cell carcinoma. Nonetheless, the low-power architectural profile of PTTs is again reassuringly discrete. Rounded, pushing interfaces with the adjacent corium and subcutis are indicative of benignancy despite the above-cited atypicality of the tumor cells.

Tumor of the follicular infundibulum is a peculiar small upper dermal lesion that may be mistaken for superficial-multifocal basal cell carcinoma because it is composed of horizontally disposed plates of slightly basaloid epithelial cells that bud into the corium from the bases of the follicular ostia and are interconnected by vertically aligned bars of cells with similar cytologic features.[120] There is no stromal retraction surrounding such lesions, nor is the intratumoral matrix myxoid in character, as it is in BCC.

Malignant Pilosebaceous Neoplasms

Malignancies of the sebaceous glands and pilar apparatus are more limited in number. They include ocular and extraocular sebaceous carcinoma, trichilemmal carcinoma, pilomatrix carcinoma, malignant proliferating pilar tumor, and pilar carcinoma–not otherwise specified.

Sebaceous carcinomas are most common in the modified skin of the eyelids, where they often present in a manner that clinically simulates that of a chalazion.[121] Hence, surgical pathologists should react with alarm if the surgeon consigns excised "chalazions" to the waste bin without pathologic examination. Extraocular lesions of this type may arise in many skin fields, but they have a predilection for the central and upper facial skin. Histologically, sebaceous carcinomas show quite a range of differentiation, from obviously multivacuolated epithelium to basaloid or squamoid populations of cells with more occult cytoplasmic lipid content (Fig. 13–25).[122, 123] These are arranged in infiltrative cords and clusters in the dermis, but roughly 50% of cases also manifest the pagetoid spread of tumor cells into the surface epithelium, with or without regional in situ carcinoma in intact pilosebaceous units (Fig. 13–26, see p. 786).[124] Nuclei are much like those of squamous tumors—with common mitotic forms—but the cytoplasm of sebaceous carcinomas generally has a more amphophilic or basophilic quality than that seen in surface-keratinocytic neoplasms. Overt sebaceous differentiation—with complex, "bubbly" intracellular compartmentalization—is generally most obvious in the central aspects of dermal cell nests. Occasional examples of sebaceous carcinoma exhibit comedo-type central necrosis inside tumor cell aggregates, or they may display extensive formation of keratin "pearls." In reference to differential diagnosis with other clear-cell cutaneous neoplasms, it should be emphasized that sebaceous carcinoma shows a myriad of delicate cytoplasmic vacuoles within the tumor cells, whereas elements of clear-cell lesions with sweat glandular, pilar, surface-epithelial, or melanocytic derivation contain large, generally solitary intracytoplasmic zones of lucency. These patterns can often be accentuated using fat stains on wet tumor tissue or immunostains for epithelial membrane antigen if only paraffin-embedded specimens are avail-

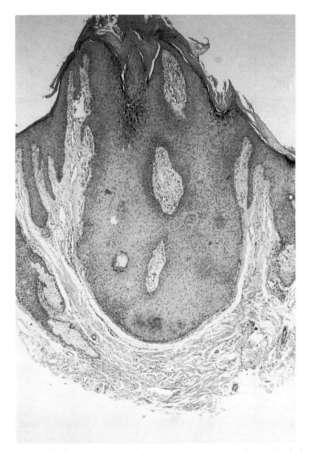

Figure 13–22. Trichilemmoma, demonstrating symmetrical growth of clear tumor cells around a central hair follicle. Palisading of nuclei is apparent in the peripheral aspects of the neoplasm.

able for further study. Differential diagnostic alternatives include basosebaceous basal cell carcinoma (see earlier discussion); malignant acrospiroma with clear-cell features; hydropic squamous cell carcinoma; trichilemmal carcinoma (vide infra), and "balloon cell" malignant melanoma. Application of selected immunostains and attention to histomorphologic nuances can separate these lesions from one another.

Trichilemmal carcinoma was first described by Headington in 1976[125]; however, this entity has received scant attention until recently.[126, 127] It is characterized by a lobulated proliferation of atypical clear cells that partially or completely replace pilosebaceous units, as well as adjacent segments of the surface epithelium (Fig. 13–27). Nuclear atypia is easily appreciated in this tumor; mitotic activity, multifocal pilar-type keratinization, and limited areas of necrosis are regularly observed as well. The lesion commonly exhibits nuclear palisading at the peripheral aspects of cellular lobules. Foci of dermal invasion may emanate from either the epidermal or follicle-based components of the tumor, and these are attended by stromal desmoplasia.

Pilomatrix carcinoma has the same general architectural features as described for pilomatrixoma. Overtly malignant pilomatrical tumors have a low-power microscopic image that is identical to that of invasive pilomatrixoma, with clusters and cords of cells budding from the main mass into the surrounding dermis and subcutis. However, it differs from the latter entity in showing obvious cytologic features of malignancy (Fig. 13–28, see p. 786).[128, 129] These include high nucleocytoplasmic ratios, vesicular chromatin, prominent eosinophilic nucleoli, brisk mitotic activity, and foci of spontaneous tumor necrosis. Indeed, many areas of pilomatrix carcinomas are reminiscent of primary lymphoepithelioma-like carcinoma of the skin,[130] which in turn strongly resembles nasopharyngeal carcinoma. The principal difference between these neoplasms is the regular presence of ghost cell clusters in pilomatrix carcinomas.

Malignant proliferating pilar tumor similarly may be separated from ordinary PPT based on established histologic criteria.[131] These primarily include a more uniformly high-grade cytologic appearance, and, most importantly, the presence of irregular invasion of the surrounding corium and hypodermis by tongues of tumor cells that "bud" from the main mass.

Pilar carcinoma, not otherwise specified (also called *high-grade proliferating pilar tumor*)[132] is extremely similar histologically to high-grade squamous cell carcinoma, except for two important points. The first difference is the presence of pilar-type ("abrupt") keratinization in the former of these two lesions, and the other is a lack of a broad connection between the dermal tumor mass and the surface epithelium, which may nonetheless be ulcerated.

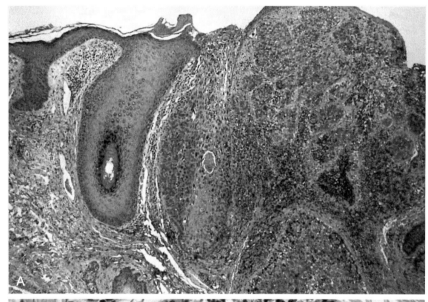
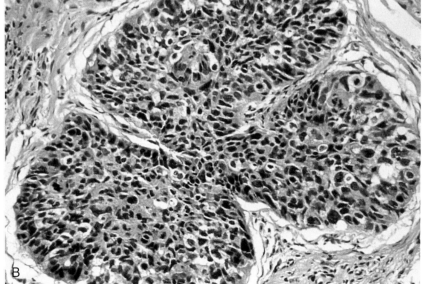

Figure 13–25. *A,* Sebaceous carcinoma of the face, showing a nodular invasive mass in the dermis that abuts the epidermal basement membrane. *B,* The obvious atypicality and focal cytoplasmic multivacuolation of sebaceous carcinoma cells are shown here.

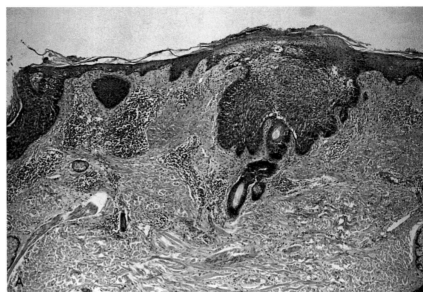

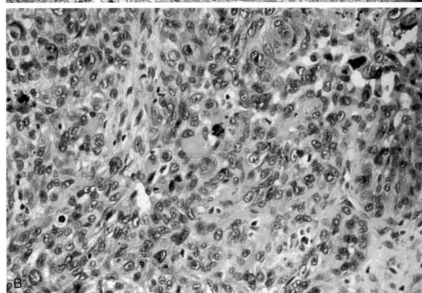

Figure 13–27. *A,* Trichilemmal carcinoma of the skin, showing the abruptly invasive nature of the tumor and its interposition between histologically normal segments of epidermis. *B,* Nuclear atypia and trichilemmal-type keratinization typify tricholemmal carcinoma and distinguish it from ordinary squamous carcinoma.

Some lesions with this appearance may arise in transition from PPTs; therefore, a proportion of cases of pilar carcinoma, not otherwise specified may be considered to represent a subtype of malignant proliferating pilar tumors.

MESENCHYMAL TUMORS AND PSEUDOTUMORS

With a few selected exceptions, mesenchymal neoplasms of the skin are generally uncommon. This fact, together with the wide histologic repertoire that such lesions may exhibit, often makes their accurate diagnosis challenging for the clinician and dermatopathologist. This chapter outlines a practical approach to the recognition and proper categorization of cutaneous benign and malignant mesenchymal neoplasms and tumor-like conditions. Inasmuch as entire textbooks have been devoted to this topic, I do not purport to provide an exhaustive, all-encompassing treatise on such lesions. Rather, those clinical and pathologic features that allow for reliable classification and management of mesenchymal proliferations are stressed.

Several morphotypes of sarcoma were formerly included inappropriately in textbooks on dermatopathology. For all practical purposes, synovial sarcoma, liposarcoma, extraskeletal chondrosar-coma, and fibrosarcoma are restricted to the deep soft tissues. Therefore, they are not discussed here.

General Clinical Features

The clinical characteristics of cutaneous mesenchymal neoplasms are rather nondescript in most instances. Such tumors may present as plaque-like or nodular lesions that are only uncommonly ulcerated and have generally been present for months or years. Some—such as the common dermatofibroma—are superficial, circumscribed, firm dermal lesions that are freely mobile on palpation. More deeply seated neoplasms are fixed to underlying structures and are more ill-defined on clinical examination.

The age of the patient is important in the formulation of a tenable clinical differential diagnosis in this context. Children under the age of 1 year virtually never develop sarcomas of the skin and superficial soft tissues. Likewise, malignant tumors of this type are uncommon in other pediatric patients as well.[133] On the other hand, de novo mesenchymal neoplasms in elderly individuals are biologically aggressive in a sizable proportion of cases.

The color and consistency of tumors in this category may contribute to clinical interpretation. For example, vascular neoplasms are red or violaceous, whereas others of a myofibroblastic nature commonly have a pale, white-tan, translucent appearance. Lymphangiomas and lipomas are often fluctuant, whereas sarcomas of various types may be "woody" on palpation. Even though the "dimple sign" (downward retraction of a lesion induced by lateral compression) is equated by many clinicians with a diagnosis of dermatofibroma, this finding is nonspecific and is observed in association with any tumor that forms a connection between the dermis and superficial subcutis. Similarly, overlying hyperpigmentation of the epidermis is seen as a reaction to many slow-growing and localized mesenchymal tumors of the corium, both benign and malignant in nature.

Multiplicity of such neoplasms offers another clue to proper diagnosis in some instances. Von Recklinghausen's disease may feature the presence of multiple cutaneous lesions, and this potential is shared by tumors with myofibroblastic, smooth muscular, and endothelial differentiation.

Pain on palpation or after minor trauma is a characteristic that is peculiar to a relatively limited set of cutaneous mesenchymal tumors. These are included among the lesions represented by the acronym ANGEL—*a*ngiolipoma, post-traumatic *n*euroma, *g*lomus tumor, *e*ccrine spiradenoma, and *l*eiomyoma cutis.[134]

Finally, the topographic location of such proliferations is sometimes a helpful point of differential diagnosis. For example, sporadic angiosarcomas and atypical fibroxanthomas are largely confined to the skin of the face and scalp, whereas other mesenchymal neoplasms are extremely rare in those sites.

Conditions that Predispose to Cutaneous Mesenchymal Neoplasia

Several heritable conditions may predispose individuals to cutaneous mesenchymal neoplasia. These include von Recklinghausen's disease (neurofibromas, vascular proliferations, neurilemmomas, and striated muscle tumors); tuberous sclerosis (angiofibromas, lipomas, connective tissue hamartomas); the Klippel-Trenauney-Weber, "blue rubber bleb," Sturge-Weber, and Maffuci's syndromes (vascular neoplasms); Gardner's syndrome (fibromatoses, lipomas); Bannayan's syndrome (hemangiomas and lipomas); the basal cell nevus syndrome (fetal rhabdomyomas and rhabdomyosarcomas); and familial lipomatosis. All of these afflictions are autosomal dominant traits.[133]

Ambient conditions also can play a role in the genesis of mesenchymal tumors or tumor-like conditions. For example, exposure to megavoltage irradiation—occupational or otherwise—is linked to the potential development of malignant fibrous histiocytoma, nerve sheath sarcoma, and angiosarcoma in the affected field of skin and soft tissue.[135–137]

Lastly, experience over the past decade has witnessed the association between a particular infectious agent—the human immunodeficiency virus (HIV)—and mesenchymal neoplasia of the skin. The relationship among HIV infection, the resulting acquired immunodeficiency syndrome (AIDS), and the development of mucocutaneous Kaposi's sarcoma[138] is now all too familiar to physicians everywhere.

Immunohistologic Findings in Cutaneous Mesenchymal Neoplasms

Paraffin section immunohistochemistry represents a useful tool in the distinction between mesenchymal proliferations. The detection of keratin proteins with this technique can be equated with the presence of epithelial differentiation, in like manner to the observation of cell membrane–based immunoreactivity for epithelial membrane antigen (EMA). Muscle-specific actin, desmin, and "smooth-muscle" (α-isoform) actin are expected in myogenous lesions. S100 protein, the CD57 antigen, and myelin basic protein may be expressed by

schwannian neoplasms, although a final interpretation of the significance of these markers is dependent on the histologic context and an absence of the other antigens mentioned thus far.[139] The latter caveats also apply to "endothelial" determinants, which potentially include von Willebrand factor, receptors for *Ulex europaeus* I agglutinin, and the CD31 and CD34 antigens.[140, 141]

"Neuroectodermal" lineage markers are represented by neuron-specific (gamma dimer) enolase, CD57, chromogranin, and synaptophysin, as interpreted in the context of a small round-cell proliferation. Only the last two of these four indicators are truly specific for neuroectodermal differentiation, but the others serve a useful screening role or contribute to ultimate diagnosis in combination with other determinants.[139]

Vimentin is ubiquitous among mesenchymal proliferations of all types, because it represents the "primordial" intermediate filament class of such lesions. Nevertheless, this marker is indeed useful as a sort of "internal control" for tissue antigenicity in general.[142] Also, if it represents the *only* determinant seen in a mesenchymal proliferation, a diagnosis of fibroblastic or "fibrohistiocytic" neoplasia is indicated.[143] With these points of submicroscopic information in mind, a directed discussion of such lesions is undertaken in the remainder of this chapter.

Biologically benign and "borderline" cutaneous mesenchymal neoplasms are sufficiently distinctive on clinicopathologic grounds that they can be considered individually as distinctive entities. However, overtly malignant tumors in this category have a propensity to demonstrate overlapping microscopic features. Therefore, they shall be grouped together in four generic categories: small round-cell tumors, spindle-cell neoplasms, epithelioid lesions, and pleomorphic tumors.

Specific Findings in Cutaneous Mesenchymal Tumors and Pseudotumors

Benign Neoplasms

Fibrous Papule

Fibrous papules are common lesions that occur in the mid-facial skin of adults, the majority of whom are white. These tumors are small, firm, tan or light brown papules that are largely cosmetic nuisances.[144] Simple excision is curative.

Whether fibrous papules are truly neoplastic is an unresolved question at present and has remained so since the original description of these lesions.[145] They are characterized by a localized proliferation of bland fusiform fibroblasts in the reticular and papillary dermis, often forming concentric densities around hair follicles.[146] This feature accounts for one of the synonyms for fibrous papule—perifollicular fibroma.[147] Stellate cells, which often contain melanin pigment, are also interspersed throughout these proliferations; the surrounding skin demonstrates a proliferation of telangiectatic capillaries and venules and may contain melanophages as well. Guitart et al.[148] have reported two examples in which small foci of epithelioid granular cells were apparent.

Some authors prefer the view that fibrous papule is merely a form of regressed intradermal nevus.[149] Based on results of immunostaining for factor XIIIa (a putative marker for "dermal dendrocytes") in such lesions, others have advanced the premise that they represent unique dermal mesenchymal neoplasms.[150] However, because of experience with the wide distribution of factor XIIIa in a variety of soft tissue neoplasms from different anatomic locations, I do not share the latter opinion.

Angiofibroma ("Adenoma Sebaceum" of Pringle)

Patients who have tuberous sclerosis (an autosomal-dominant phakomatosis including intracerebral glial nodules, connective tissue nevi of the dermis, and rhabdomyomas of the viscera) may also develop facial or periungual papular lesions that are virtually indistinguishable clinically from fibrous papules on an individual basis.[151] However, the tumefactions of tuberous sclerosis arise earlier in life and do not show the topographic restriction or unifocality of the latter proliferations. Similar lesions also may be seen sporadically as solitary growths in acral skin sites. Although they were described initially as "adenomata sebaceum" by Pringle[152] because they have a yellow-tan appearance and were thought to be adnexal in nature, it is now clear that such proliferations are best categorized as angiofibromas.

The microscopic profile of angiofibromas is essentially the same as that just described for fibrous papules. There is, perhaps, a bit more telangiectasia in the former of these lesions, and melanin-containing cells are not as notable. Nevertheless, this separation is artificial at best. Indeed, I believe that fibrous papule, angiofibroma, "pearly penile papule," acquired digital fibrokeratoma, and oral mucosal "fibroma" all form part of the same spectrum, the basic nature of which is fibroblastic with secondary reactive vascular ectasia.[153]

Myofibroblastic Proliferations

Myofibroblastic neoplasms in the skin of the head and neck may be solitary or multifocal, and they are classically placed into one of several discrete clinicopathologic categories. *Infantile (congenital) myofibromatosis* is a condition affecting newborn children and those under the age of 1 year. They present with firm, tan-pink nodular lesions of the dermis and superficial subcutis, with no particular topographic predilection. The lesions are often multiple and may be associated with similar proliferations in the viscera and bones.[154–157] If the latter are present (disseminated myofibromatosis), the prognosis is guarded because multi-organ failure may supervene as a result of the growing tumefactions.[154] On the other hand, restricted cutaneous infantile myofibromatosis is a relatively innocuous condition.

Hyaline fibromatosis primarily affects children, who have masses in the scalp and the mucosal surfaces. It is often observed as firm tan-pink plaques in the gingiva and may have a familial distribution.[158, 159] Multifocality of the lesions is common, and therefore surgical removal may be followed by development of new masses in contiguous sites.[158]

Desmoid-type (aggressive) fibromatosis typically involves the skin only secondarily, because it is centered in the aponeuroses of deep muscle groups.[160] This lesion develops during pregnancy or the immediate postpartum period in some women, in whom it characteristically arises in the abdominal wall. Extra-abdominal examples of desmoid-type fibromatosis can be seen in patients of all ages[161] and both sexes, with a predilection for the extremities.[160] The condition

is typified by firm, ill-defined, slowly growing nodular masses that may be multifocal and slightly painful on palpation.[162] It can attain a maximum size of several centimeters and has a stubborn tendency to recur after surgical removal. Rare cases are fatal because of their location in a vital but relatively inaccessible body site, with recalcitrant local growth.[160, 163]

Solitary adult myofibromas are micronodular masses that are virtually identical to the individual lesions of infantile myofibromatosis, except that they appear in post-pubertal patients.[164, 165] Conservative surgical removal constitutes sufficient treatment, with only rare examples of recurrence.[166] Kamino et al.[167] recently reported a lesion dubbed "dermatomyofibroma," which has many clinical similarities to solitary myofibromatosis. It shows a striking tendency to arise only in the proximal extremities, however, and is more plaque-like grossly and microscopically.

With minor alterations, the appearance of the fibromatoses is a consistent one. It features the presence of interweaving fascicles of cytologically bland spindle cells with slightly fibrillar cytoplasm, set in a collagenous matrix and punctuated by a distinctive vascular network (Fig. 13–29). The latter is composed of venule-sized blood vessels with thick pericytic cuffs. Despite the fact that the stroma of the fibromatoses is often sclerotic, the lesional vascular lumina are typically open and slightly branched.[154–157, 161, 164–166]

These characteristics may lead to confusion with hemangiopericytomas (see subsequent discussion), particularly in infantile myofibromatosis cases.[168] In fact, it is my belief that most, if not all, reported examples of "congenital hemangiopericytoma"[169, 170] actually represented myofibroblastic proliferations.

Myxoid change is also common in the matrix around intralesional vessels, and these areas typically contain cells that are more stellate than fusiform.[171] Cellularity is variable in the myofibromatoses; hypodense zones with abundant collagenous or myxoid stroma are admixed with others that manifest closely apposed spindle cells, which may assume rounded contours.[154, 164] Peripheral interfaces between these tumors and surrounding tissues are indistinct, and the lesions typically blend imperceptibly with the surrounding dermis or deeper soft tissue.[161] Mitotic activity in the myofibromatoses is characteristically limited, and observation of more than 1 to 2 mitoses per 10 high-power (40×) microscopic fields should therefore lead one to consider an alternative diagnosis.

Specialized histologic findings typify selected members of this lesional category. Infantile myofibromatosis and solitary myofibroma of adults are characterized by multinodular or fascicular plaque–like proliferations of spindle cells, set in a variably myxoid stroma (Fig. 13–30, see p. 787). Alternation between hypocellular and densely cellular zones in such lesions yields a distinctively di-

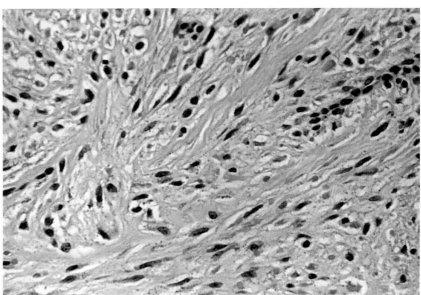

Figure 13–29. Desmoid fibromatosis of the neck, showing the fascicular growth of relatively bland spindle cells, punctuated by small but thick-walled blood vessels.

morphic appearance, and supporting blood vessels may be staghorn-shaped. Hyaline fibromatosis manifests cytoplasmic lucency in proliferating myofibroblasts and zones of extreme paucicellularity, where the stroma takes on a glassy, eosinophilic, hyaline character.

Dermatomyofibroma is also a unique member of this group on histologic grounds, in that it has a more diffuse growth pattern in the dermis, with entrapment of cutaneous adnexa and extension into the subcutis via fibrous septa (Fig. 13–31, see p. 788).[167] Parallel fascicles of fusiform cells in this plaque-like lesion are arranged in parallel with the skin surface, and the individual cells are invested by delicate cuffs of collagen. The cytoplasm is delicately fibrillar, and the tumor cells often assume a serpiginous contour. However, dermatomyofibroma does not appear to have the tendency toward nodular growth or alternation in cellular density that characterizes solitary adult myofibromatosis.[164, 167]

Glomus Tumors

Glomus tumors typically have an acral distribution topographically, and they are papulonodular lesions that may be tan-pink, red, or blue. These neoplasms are often extremely painful with even slight compression and can occur in both children and adults.[172] They may be multifocal and inherited as an autosomal dominant condition.[173]

Sheets and rounded nests of ovoid or polyhedral cells with bland oval nuclei and a moderate amount of amphophilic cytoplasm are typical of the glomus tumor, which may be located in the dermis or subcutis and is a circumscribed lesion.[172] The cells of glomus tumors may focally be arranged in cords or festoons, and they also may enclose vascular "lakes" of variable size (Fig. 13–32, see p. 788).[174] When the latter formations are prominent, the term *glomangioma* is sometimes employed diagnostically. Mitotic activity is variable in glomus tumors, but it has little significance when present. Necrosis and nuclear pleomorphism are absent.

There is a passing similarity between glomus tumor and deep hemangiopericytoma on cytologic grounds, but the distinctively branching stromal vessels of the latter neoplasm[175] are not observed in the former lesion. Other, more pertinent differential diagnostic considerations include angiomatoid intradermal nevus and solid eccrine hidradenoma (acrospiroma) or spiradenoma.[174] The last three tumors are described elsewhere in this chapter, and careful attention to microscopic nuances usually allows them to be distinguished from glomus tumor or glomangioma. Interpretive difficulties may also be resolved with the use of immunostains for S100 protein, keratin, and muscle-specific actin, only the last of which is seen in glomus tumors.[26, 174]

Rhabdomyomas and Rhabdomyomatous Mesenchmal Hamartomas

Rhabdomyomas are benign proliferations of striated muscle cells that may be seen in patients of all ages, although children are typically favored. Three types are recognized, known as the adult, fetal, and juvenile forms.[176–179] The first of these does not occur in the skin but is confined to mucosal surfaces.[177, 180] Fetal rhabdomyomas show a propensity to affect the superficial soft tissues of the proximal trunk, particularly at the base of the neck.[178] The juvenile variant has most often been observed on the extremities.[179] All of these lesions are tan-brown, firm, smooth nodules. They are cured by conservative excision.

Rhabdomyomatous mesenchymal hamartomas are polypoid lesions that appear to be confined to the facial skin of infants. Only a few examples have been reported, as pedunculated, soft, flesh-colored excrescences.[181–183] As their name implies, such proliferations are thought to be malformative rather than neoplastic.

Rhabdomyomas, in each of their variant forms, are basically characterized by a proliferation of large, plump, eosinophilic cells that demonstrate the cytoplasmic cross-striations that are typical of striated muscle. These constitute the entire neoplastic population in adult rhabdomyoma,[176–177] whereas the fetal subtype also contains more nondescript spindle cells and compact hyperchromatic round cells in admixture (Fig. 13–33).[178] Juvenile rhabdomyoma has a distinctly fascicular growth pattern and is likewise composed of overtly striated muscle cells and fusiform cells with serpiginous contours.[179] The nuclei of all cellular variants are hyperchromatic and bland, with no mitotic activity or significant pleomorphism. Unlike malignant striated muscle tumors, rhabdomyomas are typically well circumscribed and may be surrounded by a fibrous pseudocapsule.

Rhabdomyomatous mesenchymal hamartoma demonstrates the haphazard interposition of variably sized fascicles or single fibers of mature striated muscle in the dermis and superficial subcutis.[181–183] The muscular bands mold themselves to cutaneous adnexa and may be associated with neural branches. A polypoid configuration is reproducible in these cases. The bases of the excrescences are narrower than their distal aspects, yielding a club-shaped image.

Benign Vascular (Endothelial) Neoplasms

There are basically only two types of benign cutaneous vascular neoplasms, lymphangiomas and hemangiomas. Lymphangiomas have two potential clinical presentations. *Superficial circumscribed lymphangiomas* usually arise early in life, as multifocal papules or verrucoid lesions. *Deep lymphangiomas* may be seen at any age. These take the form of large, ill-defined, fluctuant nodules or plaques and are still called "cystic hygromas" by many observers. Both variants tend to affect the head and neck and the skin of the axillae, but other topographic sites may be involved as well.[184–187]

Regardless of their particular histologic appearances, hemangiomas may be observed throughout life and assume relatively uniform macroscopic characteristics.[188–190] They are bluish-red, nonulcerated, relatively well-circumscribed, variably fluctuant masses that may be macular, plaque-like, or protuberant in nature and commonly blanch when manually compressed by the examiner. The sizes of hemangiomas vary considerably, from 1 to 2 mm to more than 20 cm in greatest dimension. Large areas of the skin surface may be affected by those lesions that are part of the Sturge-Weber syndrome, and these also tend to be confined to one side of the body. Hemangiomas are commonly congenital proliferations, and, if so, they may regress spontaneously with maturation of the host.[188–190] Patients with Kimura's disease (generally included as a form of cutaneous hemangiomatosis) have multifocal nodular and violaceous lesions of the skin, peripheral eosinophilia, and enlargement of those lymph nodes draining the affected cutaneous area.[191] Another distinctive subtype—targetoid hemosiderotic hemangioma—is named for its characteristic clinical appearance, simulating that of an archery target at some stage of lesional evolution.[192]

Despite the fact that all cutaneous hemangiomas are benign, some variants, such as lobular capillary hemangioma and infiltrating hemangioma, may be floridly multifocal and difficult to approach surgically.[193] Recurrence of such lesions therefore does not necessarily indicate progression to a biologically aggressive neoplasm.

Superficial circumscribed lymphangiomas are typified by a proliferation of small, thin-walled vessels in the superficial papillary dermis, lined by attenuated endothelial cells. They have no discernible pericytic cuff and are filled with slightly eosinophilic luminal material. The overlying epidermis commonly forms "collarettes" around the lymphatic vascular channels, and acanthosis or hyperkeratosis may also be apparent. Accompanying inflammation in the surrounding corium is scant or absent.[187, 194]

Deep lymphangiomas are composed of larger vascular spaces that are centered in the deep reticular dermis and subcutis, with no epidermal reaction to them. Luminal proteinaceous lymphatic fluid is abundant, and it characteristically assumes a "scalloped" appearance in conventional paraffin sections. Surrounding connective tissue is usually sclerotic; numerous lymphoid cells may be admixed with the lymphatic channels and are often present within them as well (Fig. 13–34, see p. 788). Lesional endothelial cells are again

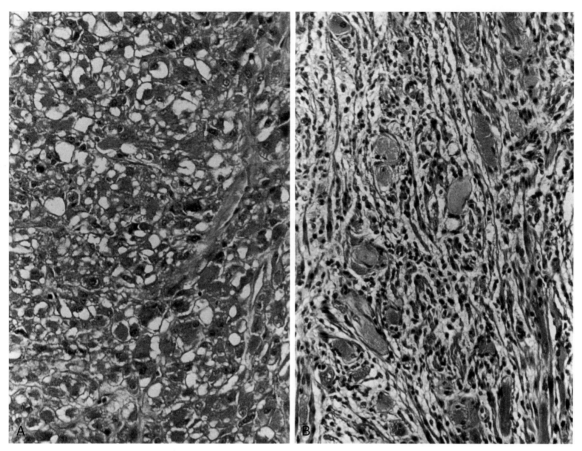

Figure 13–33. *A,* Adult rhabdomyoma of the lip, showing sheets of polygonal cells with brightly eosinophilic cytoplasm and intracellular vacuolization. *B,* Fetal rhabdomyoma of the neck, containing a tripartite cellular population. Spindle cells, small basaloid round cells, and maturing eosinophilic rhabdomyocytes are evident in admixture with one another.

flattened and inconspicuous.[184–186] Erythrocytes are scarce in both forms of cutaneous lymphangioma. The abnormal lymphatic vessels in deep lymphangiomas commonly extend into the deep dermis and subcutis. Therefore, it is important to excise them adequately to prevent recurrence, which, in the best of circumstances, is still seen in 15% to 20% of cases.

In the past few years, several microscopic variants of hemangioma of the skin have been recognized. These include the well-known capillary and cavernous subtypes, composed of small-bore and large ectatic vascular spaces, respectively, as well as mixed capillary-cavernous/venous hemangiomas,[188] lobular capillary hemangiomas (pyogenic granulomas),[195] cellular capillary hemangiomas,[195] acquired tufted hemangiomas,[196] glomeruloid hemangiomas,[197] verrucous hemangiomas,[198] infiltrating hemangiomas,[199] targetoid hemangiomas (see earlier discussion),[200] epithelioid (histiocytoid) hemangiomas,[201, 202] and Kimura's tumor or disease.[191, 202]

The basic structure of all of these proliferations is that *of organized formation of complete intercellular lumina,* mantled by pericytic cuffs of variable thickness and lined by bland endothelial cells with a spectrum of appearances.[203] Another feature common to all the hemangiomas (possibly excepting "infiltrating" and "targetoid" lesions) is a *lobular* configuration.[195, 203] Discrete groups of lesional blood vessels and investing pericytes are separated from one another by fibrous stroma, and they contain a central "feeder" vessel in each lobule.[194] Indeed, the lobular capillary hemangioma is the prototypical example of this morphologic arrangement (Fig. 13–35). Although the latter tumor is most commonly superficial and polypoid—often with overlying ulceration—it also may be seen deep in the dermis or subcutis.[204] Examples of lobular capillary hemangioma that are traumatized may show regenerative nuclear atypia and

mitotic activity in constituent endothelial cells[194]; indeed, I have seen lesions such as this that were misdiagnosed as vascular sarcomas because of these features. However, attention to the fact that the lobular character of the tumor is retained in these circumstances should help avoid erroneous interpretations.

Cellular capillary hemangioma is simply regarded as a variant form of lobular capillary hemangioma in which the boundaries between adjacent lobules are indistinct, and the lumina formed by constituent endothelial cells are extremely small. In my opinion, this lesion is synonymous with the "angioblastoma" of Nakagawa.[205] Another alternative designation—"juvenile hemangioendothelioma"—is unacceptable for diagnostic use, because hemangioendotheliomas in general are regarded as potentially malignant neoplasms.

Verrucous hemangioma is a variant of cavernous hemangioma that is typified by overlying epidermal papillomatosis, parakeratosis, and hyperkeratosis.[198] Keratinocytic rete ridges extend downward in this tumor to "embrace" or surround lesional blood vessels, much like angiokeratoma (see later discussion).

Acquired tufted hemangioma is another subtype of LCH, in which the lobules of tumor cells project into ectatic but pre-existing dermal veins and lymphatics (Fig. 13–36, see p. 805).[196, 206] This arrangement yields a low-power appearance that has been likened to "cannon balls in the dermis" by Wilson-Jones and Orkin.[206] In light of this description, it is likely that some examples of "intravenous pyogenic granuloma" documented by Cooper et al.[207] would now be regarded as acquired tufted hemangiomas.

Glomeruloid hemangioma is a variant in which proliferating vascular channels take on the size of dermal venules and are grouped together in discrete clusters such that they passingly resemble glomeruli of the kidney under low-power microscopy.[208] The significance of such tumors resides in their association with the POEMS syndrome, a constellation of disorders (*p*olyneuropathy, *o*rgano-megaly, *e*ndocrinopathies, *m*onoclonal gammopathies, and *s*kin lesions) that is usually linked to an underlying lymphoproliferative disease or plasma cell dyscrasia.[197, 208]

Infiltrating hemangioma is again composed of venule-sized channels, but this lesion differs from the others described thus far in that it shows no circumscription. A disorganized proliferation of randomly arranged (but complete) luminal profiles is seen throughout the dermis and subcutis in this variant, and it may involve underlying fascia and muscle as well. Viscera, bones, and multiple soft tissue sites are affected in some cases, justifying diagnostic use of the term *angiomatosis.*[199]

The *targetoid hemosiderotic hemangioma* and another closely allied variant, *microvenular hemangioma,* are probably related to the infiltrating variant just cited.[192, 200, 209] Nonetheless, the first two of these lesions show a greater penchant for formation of incomplete and interanastomosing vascular spaces that "dissect" through dermal collagen and subcuticular tissue (Fig. 13–37, see p. 805).[192] Small papillary projections of bland endothelial cells also may project into the lumina of targetoid hemangiomas.[193, 200] These histologic features often cause considerable concern regarding the potential diagnosis of a vascular sarcoma. Nonetheless, the advancing boundaries of targetoid hemangiomas are relatively well defined (unlike those of

endothelial malignancies), and an organized rim of dense hemosiderin deposition is often apparent peripherally.[200] Other lesions with closely similar microscopic features include the so-called benign lymphangioendothelioma[210] and multinucleate angioreticulo-histiocytoma.[211] These tumors do differ from targetoid hemangioma, however. Benign lymphangioendothelioma contains proteinaceous lymphatic fluid rather than luminal erythrocytes, lacks stromal hemosiderin deposits, has a more regimented superficial constituency by vertically aligned vascular spaces, and may be invested by lymphoid infiltrates. Angioreticulohistiocytoma contains multinucleated stromal cells that border vascular spaces and, in some foci, may appear to line them.

The lesion now known as *epithelioid hemangioma*[202] has been the subject of considerable terminologic debate in recent years. Alternative designations for this tumor include angiolymphoid hyperplasia with eosinophilia[212] and histiocytoid hemangioma.[202] The salient feature of epithelioid hemangiomas is the plump, cuboidal appearance of the endothelial cells that line constituent blood vessels (Fig. 13–38). The latter channels have the dimensions of capillaries or venules, and their lumina are indistinct because the space occupied by proliferating endothelia. Nuclear contours in the tumor cells are round or slightly indented, chromatin is dispersed, and nucleoli are indistinct.[202] These characteristics led Rosai et al.[201] to

Text continued on page 821

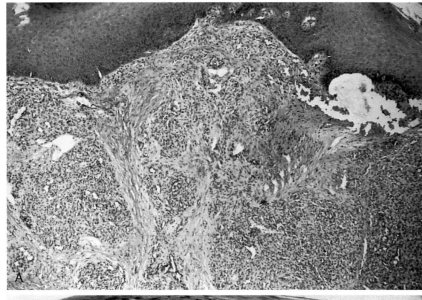

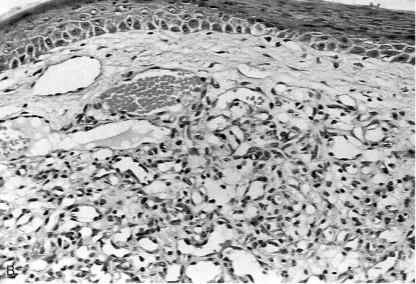

Figure 13–35. *A,* Lobular capillary hemangioma (so-called "pyogenic granuloma") of the scalp, demonstrating discrete lobules of proliferating blood vessels. *B,* The substructure of each lobule features large central "feeder" vessels and smaller, arborizing peripheral vessels.

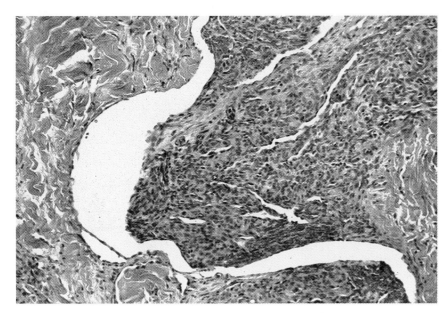

Figure 13–36. Tufted angioma of the neck, showing projection (tufting) of a lobule of proliferating blood vessels into a pre-existing dermal vein.

Figure 13–37. A, Targetoid hemosiderotic hemangioma (THH) of the dermis, demonstrating an ill-defined low-power profile in the dermis. B, High-power view of THH showing "dissecting" growth of new vascular channels in the dermis. This image may cause confusion with low-grade angiosarcoma or patch-stage Kaposi's sarcoma.

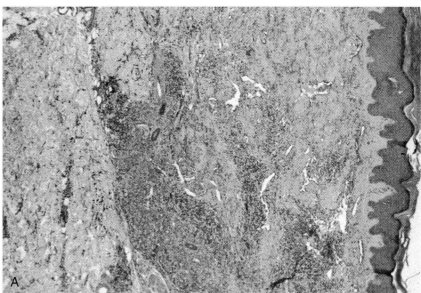

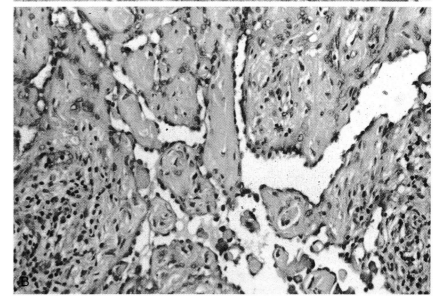

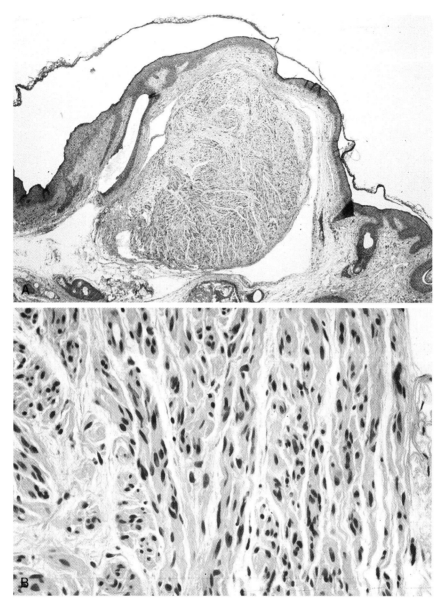

Figure 13–39. *A*, Palisading neuroma of the dermis, exhibiting sharply circumscribed growth of spindle cells in the dermis. *B*, The serpiginous profiles and focal palisading of tumor cell nuclei are shown here.

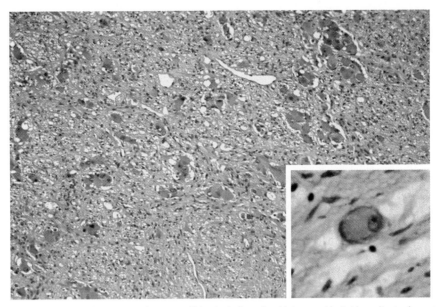

Figure 13–40. Ganglioneuroma of the dermis, showing an admixture of bland spindle cells with large epithelioid ganglionic elements having prominent nucleoli and abundant eosinophilic cytoplasm. *Inset,* The aforementioned features are shown here at higher magnification.

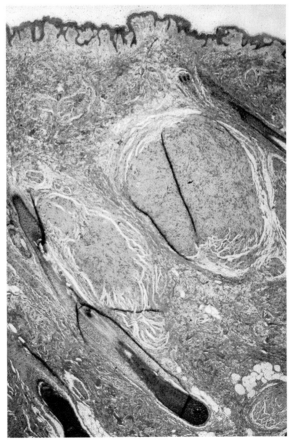

Figure 13–41. Plexiform neurofibroma of the neck, represented by discrete fascicles of spindle cells that resemble a miniature neural plexus.

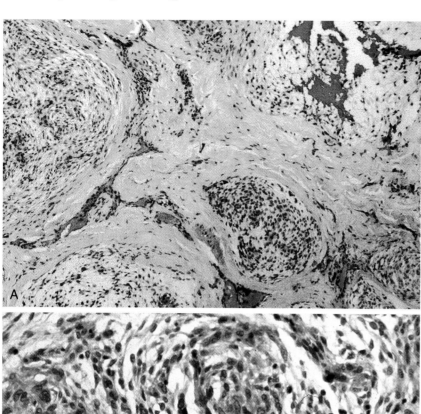

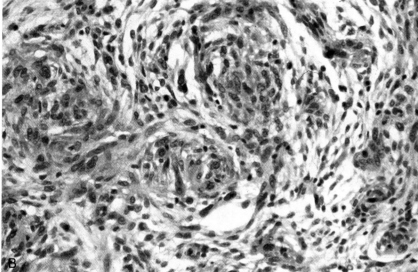

Figure 13–43. *A,* Neurothekeoma of the face, showing relatively tight clusters of polygonal and fusiform tumor cells in the dermis. These focally assume a concentric interrelationship. *B,* Slight nuclear hyperchromasia and modest pleomorphism are apparent in this neurothekeoma.

Figure 13–45. Spindle cell lipoma of the cervical subcutis, showing an admixture of ordinary adipocytes, bland spindle cells, and myxoid matrix.

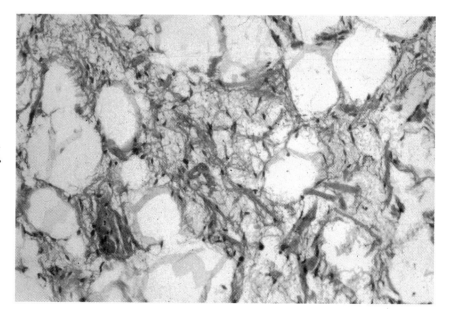

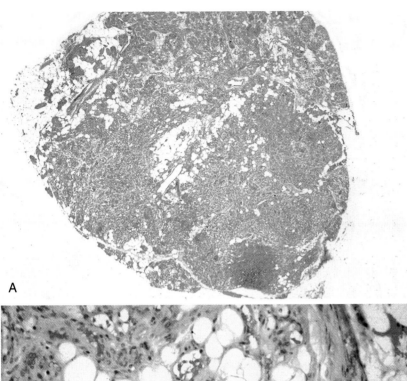

A

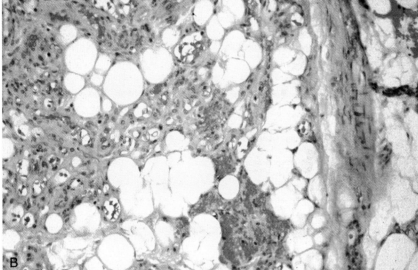

B

Figure 13–46. *A,* Cellular angiolipoma, represented by a sharply circumscribed dermal mass that appears largely solid on low power microscopy. *B,* Higher power examination demonstrates entrapment of adipocytes by proliferating blood vessels that are concentrated at the periphery of intratumoral lobules.

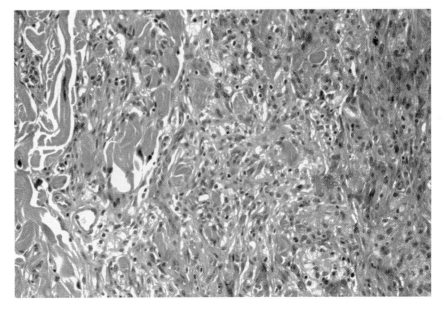

Figure 13–48. Dissection of dermal collagen into rounded or fragmented masses is evident at the periphery of this dermatofibroma of the neck.

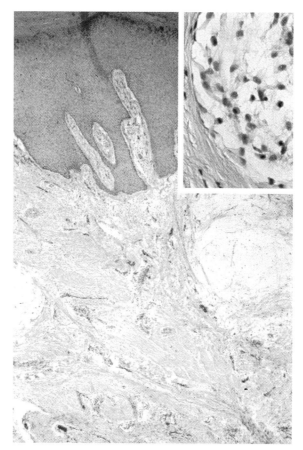

Figure 13–50. Cutaneous myxoma, showing the nodular proliferation of bland spindle cells in the dermis, which are separated by abundantly myxoid stroma. *Inset,* The innocuous appearance of dermal myxoma is seen well here.

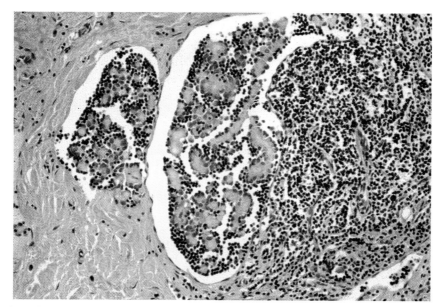

Figure 13–51. Intratumoral globular deposits of eosinophilic basement membrane material are typical of the Dabska tumor (endovascular angioendothelioma) of the dermis. Aggregates of polygonal endothelial tumor cells project into large vascular spaces and are associated with small lymphocytes.

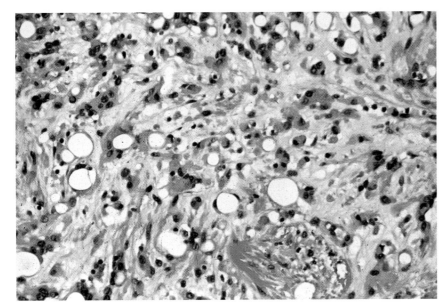

Figure 13–52. Epithelioid hemangioendothelioma of the subcutis of the scalp. Small nests and cords of polygonal tumor cells are disposed randomly throughout the soft tissue, and some contain small intracytoplasmic lumina.

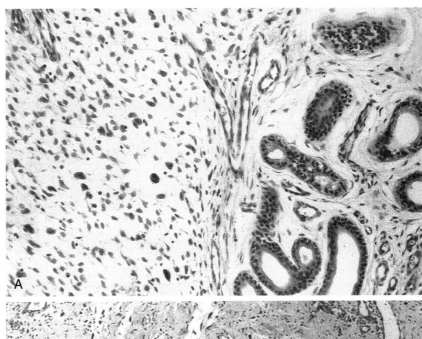

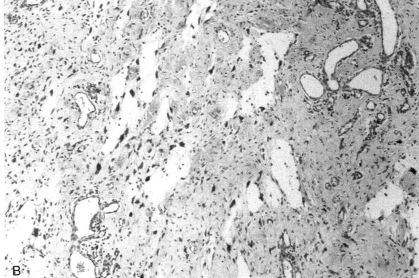

Figure 13–55. *A,* Giant cell fibroblastoma of the neck in an adolescent. The superficial aspect of this tumor shows relatively bland spindle cells that are set in a slightly myxoid stroma. *B,* Deeper portions of the neoplasm demonstrate pseudovascular spaces that are mantled by floret-type giant cells.

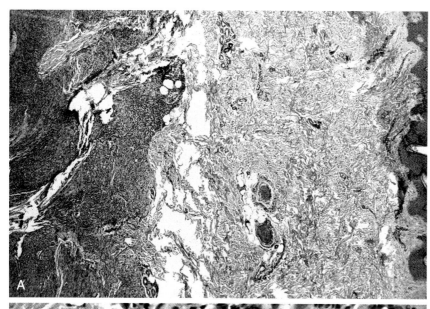

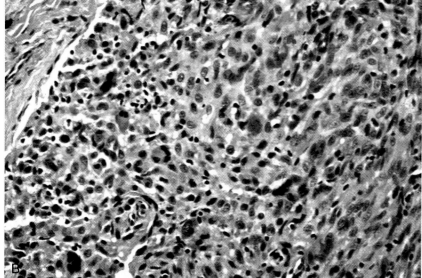

Figure 13–56. *A*, Plexiform fibrous histiocytoma of the skin of the neck. Densely cellular fascicles of spindle cells are apparent in the deep dermis. *B*, Scattered multinucleated cells, some of which may have the characteristics of osteoclasts, also typify this neoplasm.

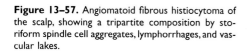

Figure 13–57. Angiomatoid fibrous histiocytoma of the scalp, showing a tripartite composition by storiform spindle cell aggregates, lymphorrhages, and vascular lakes.

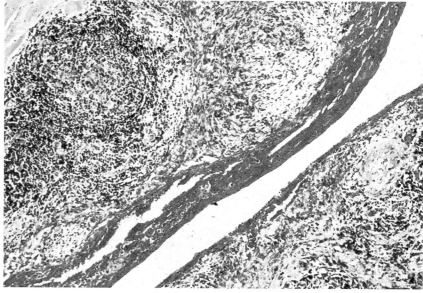

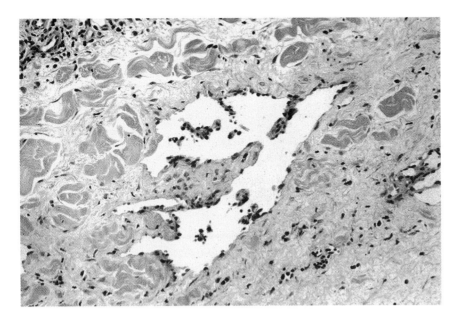

Figure 13–61. The "promontory" sign in patch-stage Kaposi's sarcoma of the facial skin, wherein new vascular channels surround and isolate pre-existing venules.

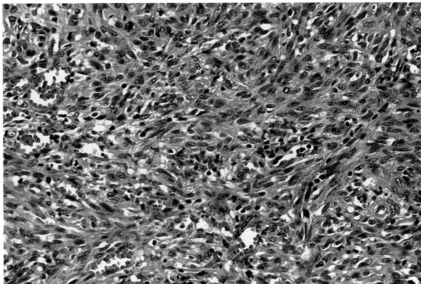

Figure 13–62. Cytoplasmic vacuolization is apparent in the proliferating spindle cells of nodular-stage Kaposi's sarcoma.

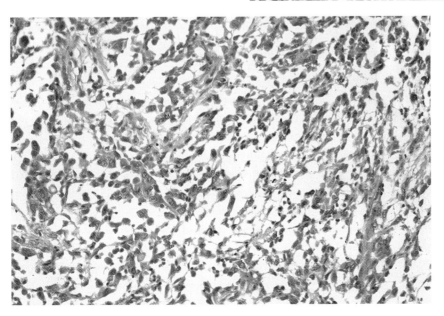

Figure 13–63. Epithelioid malignant peripheral nerve sheath tumor, showing cords of polygonal tumor cells set in a myxoid stroma.

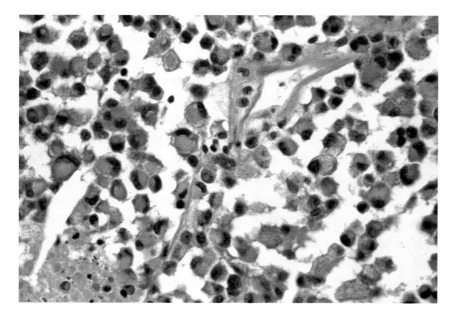

Figure 13–64. Rhabdoid tumor of the skin, demonstrating dyscohesive sheets of polygonal neoplastic cells with densely eosinophilic globular cytoplasm and eccentric nuclei with prominent nucleoli.

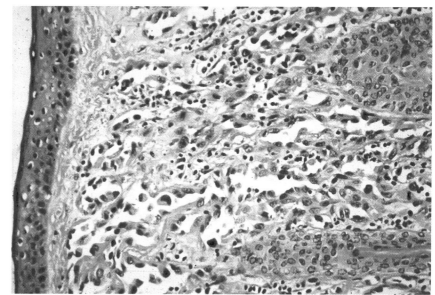

Figure 13–65. Dermal angiosarcoma of the facial skin, exhibiting the random proliferation of inter-anastomosing vascular channels in the corium and subcutis.

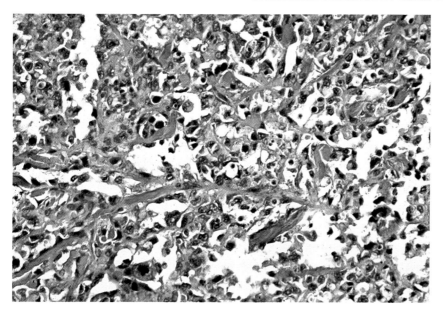

Figure 13–66. The formation of new vascular channels in angiosarcoma "dissects" through dermal collagen, subcutaneous fat, and subjacent muscle.

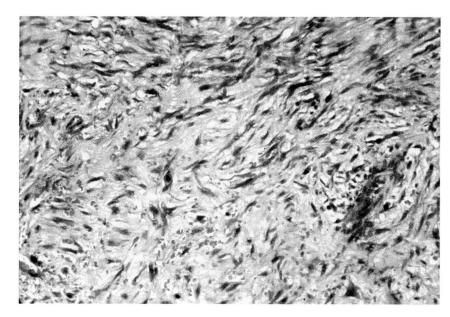

Figure 13–70. Nodular fasciitis of the lip, showing a proliferation of bland spindle cells with tenuous apposition to one another. This yields a so-called "tissue culture" appearance. Prominent vascularity, extravasation of erythrocytes into the stroma, and mitotic activity are common.

Figure 13–71. An admixture of proliferating bland spindle cells and lymphocytes characterizes this inflammatory pseudotumor of the skin of the neck.

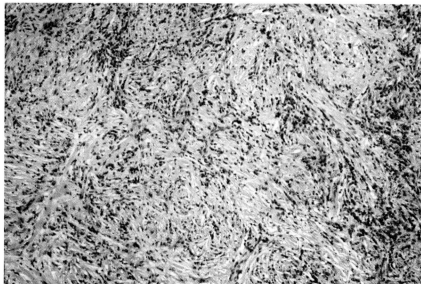

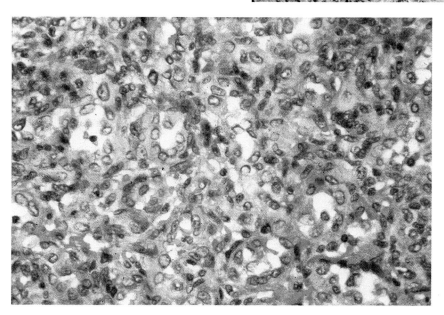

Figure 13–73. Bacillary angiomatosis, showing a proliferation of venule- or capillary-sized blood vessels in the dermis. The constituent endothelial cells are similar to those of epithelioid hemangiomas (see Figure 13–38), but they also contain granular cytoplasmic inclusions that represent bacterial organisms.

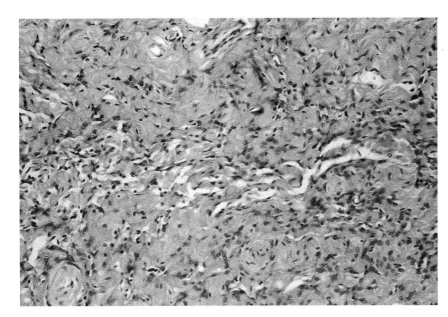

Figure 13–75. Cutaneous meningocele, exhibiting "dissection" of dermal collagen in the scalp by racemose arrays of bland polygonal cells. There is a passing resemblance to the deep components of giant cell fibroblastomas (see Figure 13–55B).

Figure 13–76. "Top-heavy" permeation of the dermis by mature lymphocytes, in a Jessner lesion (benign lymphoid infiltrate) of the facial skin.

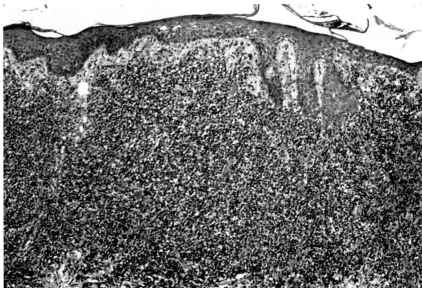

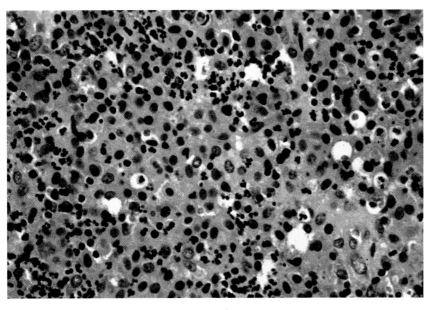

Figure 13–79. An admixture of atypical large lymphoid cells and neutrophils is seen in cutaneous Kikuchi's disease.

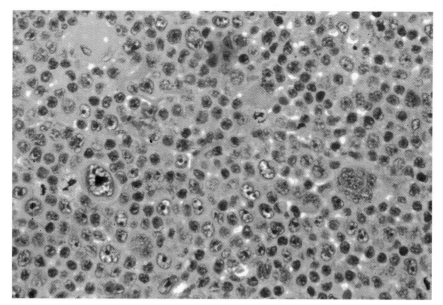

Figure 13–80. Pleomorphism is striking among the nuclei of the large polygonal cells that make up this anaplastic large-cell lymphoma of the subcutis of the scalp.

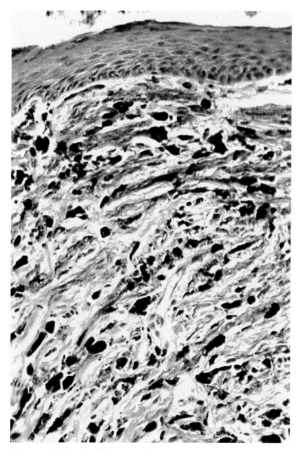

Figure 13–82. Proliferation of densely pigmented bland dermal spindle cells is apparent in this blue nevus.

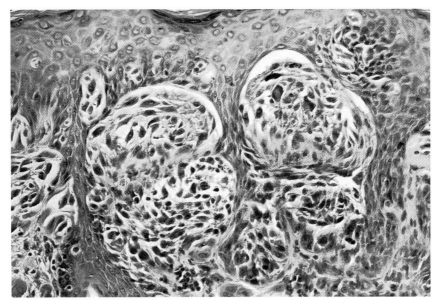

Figure 13–84. Spitz nevus of the face in a child, showing characteristic "clefting" of the dermal melanocytic theques away from the epidermal basement membrane zone.

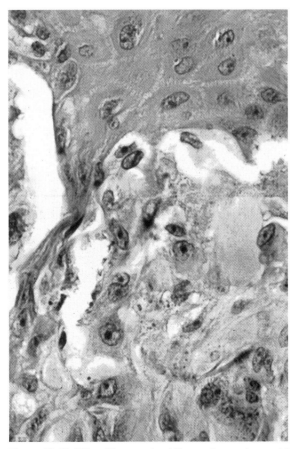

Figure 13–85. "Glassy," hypereosinophilic cytoplasm and potential intranuclear pseudoinclusions are additional features of Spitz nevus.

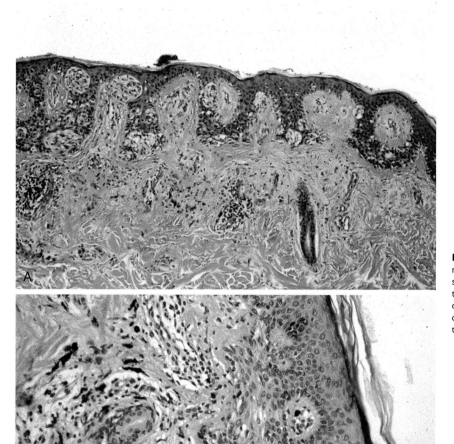

Figure 13–87. Architecturally disordered junctional nevus, in which nests of melanocytes are irregular in size and shape (A). They bud from the sides as well as the tips of rete ridges and are accompanied by upper dermal lamellar fibrosis (B). Lateral bridging of adjacent melanocytic theques is another typical finding in this tumor.

Figure 13–88. Atypical intraepidermal melanocytic proliferation (AIMP), not further specified. This lesion shows variably dyscohesive groups of atypical melanocytes, primarily at the basal aspect of the epidermis but also, to a lesser degree, in more superficial layers. All of the criteria for a diagnosis of malignant melanoma in situ are not satisfied in such cases, but AIMP is regarded as a definite precursor of that lesion.

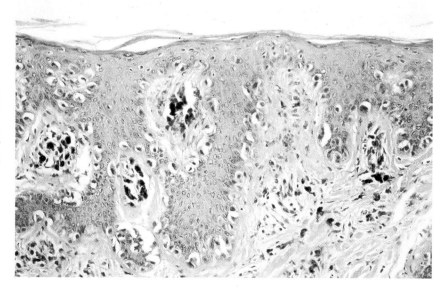

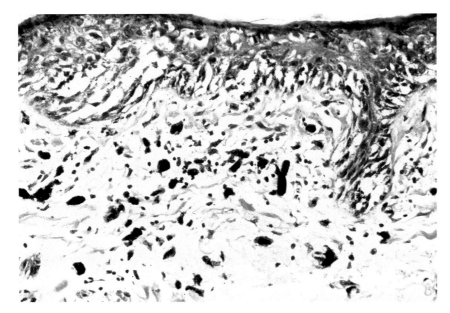

Figure 13–89. Lentigo maligna (a clinically special form of in situ melanoma) of the face, showing epidermal atrophy, continuous and dyscohesive proliferation of atypical melanocytes at the base of the epidermis, prominent dermal actinic elastosis, and dermal melanophages.

Figure 13–90. Higher power view of lentigo maligna, better illustrating the nuclear atypia of constituent melanocytes as well as involvement of cutaneous appendages by the proliferation.

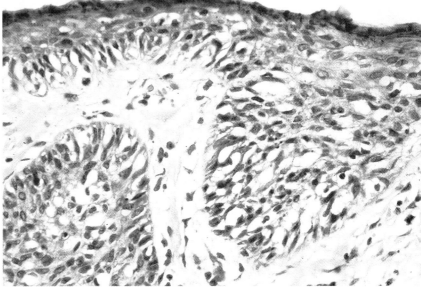

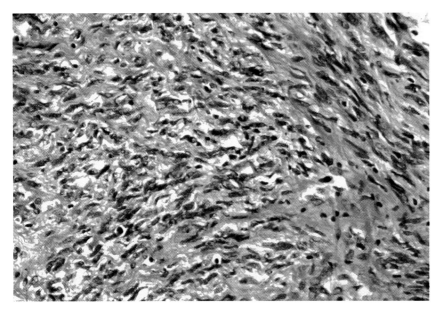

Figure 13–92. Neuroid ("neurotropic") melanoma of the facial skin, showing a virtually indistinguishable image to that of cutaneous malignant peripheral nerve sheath tumor (see Figure 13–60A).

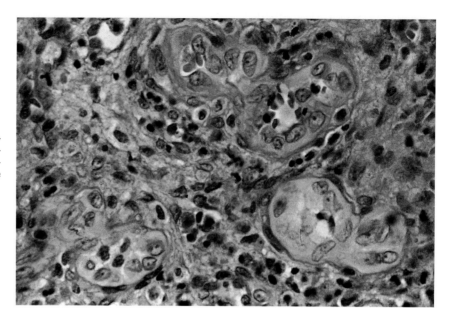

Figure 13–38. Epithelioid ("histiocytoid") hemangioma, showing the close apposition of tubular, capillary-sized blood vessels in the dermis. Each of the neoplastic cells contains a plump nucleus that recalls the attributes of histiocytes.

focus on a morphologic similarity between the nuclei of such neoplasms and those of histiocytes. Angiolymphoid hyperplasia with eosinophilia is nothing more than an inflamed version of epithelioid hemangioma, in which the stroma between constituent dermal blood vessels is rich in lymphocytes and eosinophils.[212]

Like other morphologic variants of hemangioma, a basically lobular substructure is observed in epithelioid hemangiomas as well. Nevertheless, a unique finding in the latter neoplasms is their potential association with large arteries or veins in the skin, such that the tumoral blood vessels appear to "spin off" of pre-existing vascular adventitia like a swarm of bees.

Considerable attention has also been given to the possible synonymity between epithelioid hemangioma and Kimura's disease or tumor.[191] Points of convincing clinicopathologic dissimilarity do exist between these two neoplasms, however. Kimura's tumor features a striking stromal lymphoid infiltrate—complete with germinal centers—and is centered more deeply in the skin. Moreover, constituent vessels are more elongated than those of epithelioid hemangioma, and tumor cell nuclei do not have the complex contours of those in the latter lesion. As already mentioned, Kimura's disease often includes the presence of regional lymphadenopathy and eosinophilia in the peripheral blood, whereas epithelioid hemangiomas are unassociated with these findings.[202]

Benign Neural Tumors

Neuromas and Ganglioneuromas

Only one type of cutaneous neuroma is recognized in the head and neck at present. *Post-traumatic neuromas*[213, 214] are seen almost exclusively on the digits, but *palisading neuroma*[215, 216] is typically a facial lesion. The latter usually presents as a small, nodular, tan-pink tumor. It favors adult patients, with no predilection for gender.

Ganglioneuromas rarely arise in the skin as such[217] but rather are typically found in modified mucosal surfaces such as the lips and genital skin. They are largely restricted to patients with the multiple endocrine neoplasia syndrome, type 2b (Gorlin's syndrome),[218] in which medullary thyroid carcinoma, pheochromocytoma, parathyroid hyperplasia, and a marfanoid habitus are also seen. Mucosal ganglioneuromas are typically multiple and take the form of irregular nodules of variable size.[217] However, a case of solitary ganglioneuroma of the skin has been reported under the rubric of "ganglion cell choristoma."[219]

Palisading neuromas, on the other hand, are indeed actual neoplasms. They are centered in the mid-dermis and often show a pe-

ripheral fibrous capsule. Fascicles of bland, amitotic spindle cells are internally intertwined around one another, and tumor cell nuclei manifest a tendency to align themselves in registers or palisades within each fascicle (Fig. 13–39, see p. 806).[215, 216] Nuclear contours are sometimes serpiginous, as the individual cell profiles themselves may be. The cytoplasm is slightly eosinophilic. However, it lacks the fibrillation that would be expected in a smooth muscle tumor, which represents the most likely histopathologic diagnostic alternative. Similarly, fascicles cut in cross section do not exhibit the zones of perinuclear cytoplasmic clarity that are seen in leiomyomas.

Ganglioneuromas differ only slightly from the description just given. The points of dissimilarity between these tumors and palisaded neuromas include a lack of encapsulation in ganglioneuroma and, more importantly, the presence of well-formed ganglion cells that are interspersed throughout.[217, 219] The latter elements are variable in number, but they are easily recognized by their polyhedral shape, vesicular nuclei, and prominent nucleoli (Fig. 13–40, see p. 807).

Neurofibromas

Neurofibromas of the skin are not uncommon as sporadic neoplasms, in which case they are nondescript soft papules or nodules measuring up to 3 cm in greatest dimension. Any skin field may be affected by solitary neurofibromas (including modified mucosae), and they are likewise seen at all ages.[220, 221]

Multiple neurofibromas—particularly if they are accompanied by "cafe au lait" lesions and are seen in patients under the age of 10 years—strongly suggest a diagnosis of von Recklinghausen's disease (VRD).[222–224] The plexiform variant of these neoplasms, which is pathognomonic of VRD even if solitary,[222, 225] may attain a size of more than 20 cm. It can greatly distort the superficial soft tissue, so that the affected skin acquires a pendulous appearance ("elephantiasis neuromatosa").[222] The cut surface of plexiform neurofibromas has been likened to a "bag of worms."

Neurofibromas are spindle cell tumors with a bland cytologic appearance, serpiginous nucleocytoplasmic contours, and infiltrative, poorly delimited boundaries with surrounding dermis or soft tissue. These lesions are microscopically uniform throughout and may be restricted to the corium or extend deeply into the subcutis. Myxoid stromal change is relatively common, but a tendency toward nuclear palisading is generally not appreciated in neurofibromas. The tumor cells are arranged haphazardly, in thin fascicles, or in a

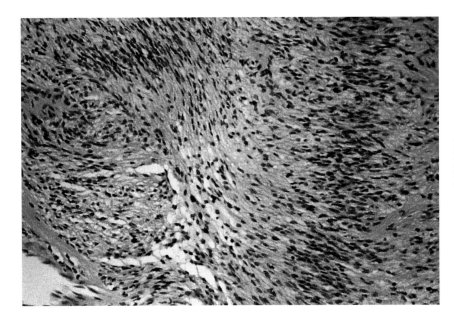

Figure 13–42. Neurilemmoma of the dermis, showing focal palisading of nuclei and serpiginous nuclear profiles. This tumor differs from palisading neuroma in that it usually also contains hypocellular areas with a distinctly myxoid stroma.

vaguely storiform pattern in sporadic neurofibromas, with entrapment of dermal collagen and appendages.[222] Intralesional mast cells are often numerous.

On the other hand, plexiform neurofibroma has a distinctive configuration that recalls a distorted neural plexus. Irregular fascicles of proliferating but banal Schwann cells are separated from one another by myxofibrous stroma or adipose tissue in this neoplasm, such that each grouping of spindle cells resembles a miniature nerve trunk (Fig. 13–41, see p. 807). Occasionally, melanin-containing cells or structures resembling meissnerian or pacinian corpuscles may punctuate these proliferations.[222, 226] To reiterate, making the histologic interpretation of plexiform neurofibroma is tantamount to assigning a diagnosis of VRD to the patient; hence, one should require that the above-cited microscopic features are all present before taking this step.

Mitotic activity, local hypercellularity, necrosis, and nuclear atypia are worrisome features in lesions thought to be neurofibromas. It is well known that great difficulty may be encountered in distinguishing such neoplasms from selected malignant peripheral nerve sheath tumors (see subsequent discussion) of low histologic grade, particularly if they are several centimeters in size.[227] Therefore, reports on lesions with the alarming features just cited should make special note of them, and the preferred diagnostic terminology in such instances is *peripheral nerve sheath tumor of indeterminate biologic potential.*

Another problem concerning neurofibromas is their distinction from ordinary but extensively "neurotized" melanocytic intradermal nevi. Serial sections are often required to search for small foci of residual melanocytes in the latter lesions, and it is admittedly impossible to make the distinction just cited in some cases.

Neurilemmomas

Neurilemmomas (schwannomas) are essentially identical to sporadic neurofibromas on clinical grounds. There is a potential association between cutaneous variants of the former neoplasms and VRD if the lesions are multifocal; this is a rare occurrence.[222]

Neurilemmomas differ from neurofibromas in two respects. First, they demonstrate a biphasic cellular growth pattern; second, they are often encapsulated and contain internal thick-walled stromal blood vessels.[221]

The two major microscopic patterns in neurilemmoma are known as the Antoni A and Antoni B configurations. These feature the presence of dense spindle-cell foci with potential nuclear palisading (Verocay bodies) and myxoid or edematous, paucicellular ar-

eas composed of bland myxoid or stellate tumor cells, respectively (Fig. 13–42).[222, 228] Intratumoral mast cells are again numerous. Nuclear characteristics are usually bland, although traumatized, long-standing superficial ("ancient") neurilemmomas may show nuclear enlargement and hyperchromasia as secondary changes. Mitotic activity is scant, but unlike the case with neurofibroma, some division figures may be "tolerated" without alarm regarding possible malignancy.

Neurilemmoma is much more versatile than other peripheral nerve sheath tumors, with respect to its modes of microscopic differentiation. Variants of this neoplasm include one containing small groups of epithelium, with or without mucin production (glandular neurilemmoma)[229]; another showing an admixture of melaninized cells (melanotic neurilemmoma)[230, 231]; a plexiform subtype in which the macroscopic appearance of the tumor simulates that of plexiform neurofibroma (but linkage with VRD is lacking)[232, 233]; a variant dominated by plump epithelioid tumor cells (epithelioid neurilemmoma)[234]; and a form in which both melaninization and psammomatous calcification are apparent (psammomatous-melanotic neurilemmoma).[235] Some authors have used the term *cellular schwannoma* in describing some cutaneous tumors with extremely dense Antoni A areas. However, this designation is most properly applied to a cellular and mitotic subset of encapsulated neurilemmomas that occur in the deep soft tissues of the midline.[236] Therefore, I do not endorse its application in the context of dermatopathology.

Neurothekeomas

Neurothekeoma is an unusual benign peripheral nerve sheath tumor that shows a reproducible tendency to arise in the skin of the head, neck, and arms in patients under 30 years of age. It presents as a nondescript, soft, tan nodule or plaque measuring up to 3 cm and is non-tender. The cut surfaces of such lesions are often myxoid or "slimy."[237]

It should be mentioned that the term *neurothekeoma* has several diagnostic synonyms. These include *pacinian neurofibroma*[238] and *dermal nerve sheath myxoma.*[222, 239] Because it is most apt in describing the histologic features of the tumor, however, I prefer the first of these three designations.

Neurothekeomas are circumscribed neoplasms that are composed of distinctive theques of spindled and stellate cells in an internally concentric arrangement, and with a generally bland cytologic appearance. The background stroma is variably myxoid or myxofibrous, and the tumor is centered in the deep dermis or superficial subcutis. Limited mitotic activity may be observed but is of no prognostic consequence in neurothekeoma, and focal but modest nuclear hyperchromasia of epithelioid or multinucleated cells also may be evident in some cases (Fig. 13–43, see p. 808).[238] Although the great majority of other benign peripheral nerve sheath tumors are immunoreactive for S100 protein and the CD57 antigen, these markers are lacking in neurothekeomas.[240] Such results have prompted the suggestion that these neoplasms may pursue perineural cell differentiation.

Still other reports have appeared on cellular neurothekeoma. This variant is more superficially located in the dermis and has a more vaguely theque-like growth pattern. Moreover, constituent cells may be polygonal, with "glassy" eosinophilic cytoplasm and nuclei that resemble those of ordinary nevocytes.[241] Indeed, the major differential diagnostic problem in cases of cellular neurothekeoma lies in excluding epithelioid or Spitz nevi. Immunostains may contribute to resolving such uncertainties; the latter proliferations are uniformly positive for S100 protein, whereas cellular neurothekeomas are not.[241]

Granular Cell Tumors

Granular cell tumors are tan, dome-shaped nodules with smooth surfaces, measuring up to 3 cm in greatest dimension. They occur at all ages and all topographic locations, with no preference for either gender,[242–244] and they may be multifocal.

The hallmark of granular cell tumor is its exclusive composition by polyhedral cells with eccentric oval nuclei, dispersed nuclear chromatin, and overtly granular eosinophilic cytoplasm (Fig. 13–44).[242] The neoplastic cells permeate the dermis irregularly, entrapping collagen bundles and cutaneous adnexa, and may extend into the superficial subcutis. The low-power appearance of this lesion is accordingly circumscribed but not encapsulated.[244, 245] Rare mitotic figures may be seen in benign granular cell tumors; however, atypical division figures, necrosis, vascular permeation, and overlying ul-

ceration should prompt one to consider an alternative diagnosis (see subsequent section on malignant peripheral nerve sheath tumors).[246]

The justification for including granular cell tumor in this section on nerve sheath tumors is obtained from data on its ultrastructural features and immunohistologic attributes.[247, 248] Most neoplasms of this type (approximately 85%) show electron microscopic evidence of schwannian differentiation[247, 249]; likewise, immunoreactivity for S100 protein, CD57 antigen, and myelin basic protein links such lesions to neurofibromas and neurilemmomas nosologically.[247, 248] Nevertheless, in a minority of cases, it must be conceded that granular cell change may simply be a nonspecific degenerative alteration (reflecting an abundance of secondary cytoplasmic phagolysosomes) in other neoplasms that are not neural in nature. For example, it has been reported in myogenous and epithelial proliferations as well.[247, 250] Granular cell variants of the latter lesions do not show any idiosyncrasies of behavior when compared with their "conventional" forms.

Benign Tumors of Adipose Tissue

Lipomas

Lipomas are almost ubiquitous in the adult population, and these "lumps" and "bumps" are generally part of the normal variation in human physiognomy that I have come to accept. Nonetheless, when they arise in cosmetically unacceptable locations or in patients who are naturally anxious about "growths," the dermatologist or surgeon provides the pathologist with examples to study histologically. On macroscopic grounds, lipomas are easily compressible, mobile, irregularly nodular lesions that may be located in the deep soft tissues or the subcutis and can attain an impressive size.[251] The fatty nature of such tumors on cut section is usually obvious.

Particular clinical variants of lipoma with which one must be familiar include the spindle-cell, pleomorphic, and vascular (angiolipomatous) subtypes.[252–255] The first of these is most often seen on

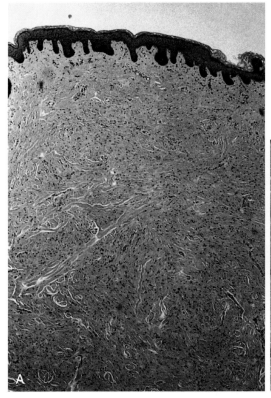
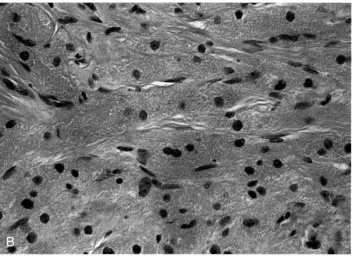

Figure 13–44. A, Granular cell tumor of the lip, showing replacement of the dermis by a uniform population of polygonal tumor cells. B, The neoplastic cells have compact, central nuclei and abundantly granular eosinophilic cytoplasm.

the upper trunk in elderly patients, with a male predominance. The base of the neck and the interscapular region are particularly common sites of origin for spindle cell lipomas.[252, 253, 256] These lesions are firmer and more fixed to surrounding tissue than the usual lipoma and therefore may engender some concern. Pleomorphic lipomas likewise may have a firm consistency and are observed on the extremities or the head and neck.[257] Angiolipomas have a broader anatomic distribution but are distinguished from other lipoma variants by their tendency to be painful when traumatized or palpated.[258]

Rare patients manifest the syndrome of familial lipomatosis, wherein hundreds of fatty lesions appear throughout adult life in all topographic sites.[259, 260] As mentioned at the outset of this chapter, lipomas also may be components of Gardner's syndrome (with familial adenomatous polyposis of the colon).[251]

In regard to microscopic findings, usual banal lipomas represent localized overgrowths of mature adipocytes that are bounded by thin fibrous capsules. Internal stroma is delicate and inconspicuous, and there is no tendency for matrical sclerosis with increasing size.[260, 261]

Spindle cell lipoma is a triphasic neoplasm in which lobules of mature fat cells are interposed with dense zones of bland spindle cell growth and other areas of prominent myxoid stromal change (Fig. 13–45, see p. 808).[252, 253] In some cases, the latter two components may be dominant, leading to diagnostic consideration of a neural or fibroblastic proliferation; in rare examples, metaplastic osteoid or cartilage is seen in such tumors as well.[252, 256]

Pleomorphic lipoma differs from the usual type by its content of "floret" cells.[254, 257] These are multinucleated and atypical but cytologically bland elements that are interspersed throughout the background population of mature adipocytes. A modest increase in stromal fibrous tissue also may be apparent within such masses, recalling the image of well-differentiated sclerosing liposarcomas of deep soft tissue. Nonetheless, the overall configuration of the mass—including sharp circumscription, a superficial location, and a lack of mitotic activity and lipoblasts—serves to allay any concern over a diagnosis of malignancy.[257] As stated previously, liposarcoma virtually never arises in the subcutis.

Angiolipoma is typified by the proliferation of small groups of capillary- or venule-sized blood vessels in the setting of otherwise typical lipoma.[255, 258] The vascular clusters tend to be disposed toward the periphery of adipocytic lobules and may also be associated with small collections of nondescript spindle cells.[255] One form of this neoplasm features a prominent overgrowth of vascular elements containing fibrin microthrombi, such that they actually dominate the mass. Such tumors—known as "cellular" angiolipomas[262]—can be confused with angioleiomyomas and other lesions that are basically spindle-cell proliferations (Fig. 13–46, see p. 809). Nonetheless, the consistent presence of lobulated aggregates of fat cells, microthrombi in stromal blood vessels, and foci of myxoid stromal change serve to separate angiolipomas from these other possibilities.

Hibernomas

Hibernomas are exceedingly rare tumors that demonstrate differentiation toward brown (fetal) fat.[263, 264] They may be observed in patients of all ages; the subcuticular soft tissues of the head and neck, upper trunk, and axillae are the favored cutaneous sites of origin. The clinical appearance of such tumors is identical to that of conventional lipomas, but hibernomas are tan-brown rather than yellow on cut section.[263] One may regard them simply as fetal lipomas because of these attributes.

Hibernomas closely recapitulate the appearance of banal lipomas microscopically, except for the detailed features of the tumor cells. In contrast to a composition by mature adipocytes with uniformly lucent single vacuoles, the cells of hibernomas are multivacuolated with eosinophilic cytoplasm (Fig. 13–47) and internal lipofuscin granules. These lesions are usually well circumscribed or encapsulated, lobulated, and devoid of mitoses.[263, 264]

Benign Fibrohistiocytic Tumors

Dermatofibromas

Dermatofibromas are frequently seen by all physicians, probably representing the most common mesenchymal tumors of the skin. These lesions are firm papules or nodules measuring less than 1 cm with slightly irregular borders; they may be multiple or familial; and they dimple when laterally compressed.[265–269] Any skin field may be affected, but the extremities are favored; patients are generally postpubertal.[266] Overlying epidermal hyperpigmentation is often present and may be so prominent that a diagnosis of melanoma is considered by the clinician. Similarly, pseudoepitheliomatous hyperplasia over dermatofibromas may simulate basal cell carcinoma or squamous cell carcinoma macroscopically.[270] It is my belief that dermatofibroma is merely the endpoint in a spectrum of maturation exhibited by benign fibrohistiocytic lesions of the skin in general. As such, it is closely related to juvenile xanthogranuloma, nodular histiocytoma, fibrous histiocytoma (not otherwise specified), and subepidermal fibroma, and it probably represents a relatively mature member of this group that reflects a long period of clinical evolution.[271]

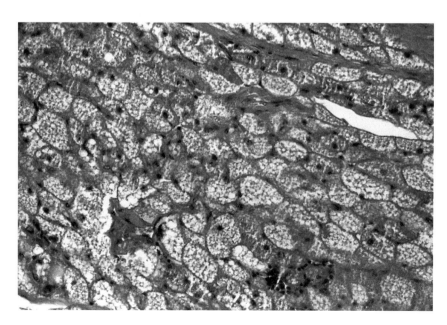

Figure 13–47. Hibernoma of the neck, demonstrating a uniform composition by "brown fat" cells like those seen in fetal adipose tissue.

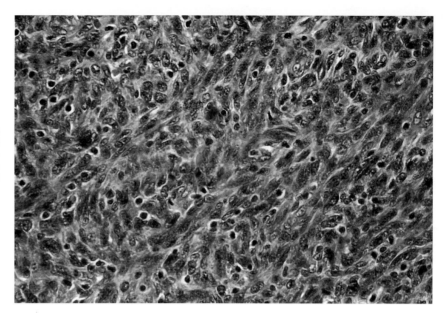

Figure 13–49. Atypical fibrous histiocytoma of the facial skin, showing a storiform proliferation of spindle cells and foam cells in the deep dermis. Based on lesional cellularity and size alone, confusion with dermatofibrosarcoma (see Figure 13–54) may occur in evaluating these tumors.

Microscopically, dermatofibromas are circumscribed lesions; they show a variably dense composition by compact spindle cells in the dermis, admixed with an abundantly collagenous matrix and scattered foamy histiocytes. As in "fibrohistiocytic" tumors in general, a storiform pattern of cellular growth is often seen.[266] Multinucleated cells of the Touton or floret types are also commonly interspersed throughout these lesions.[271] Their peripheral aspects blend gradually with the surrounding connective tissue, often isolating rounded, sclerotic bundles of collagen (Fig. 13–48, see p. 809); when subcutaneous involvement is present, it is limited in scope and confined to extension into interlobular fibrous septa of the hypodermis.[266, 267, 271, 272] Stromal vascularity in this neoplasm is represented by delicately arborizing capillaries that may assume a "chicken-wire" configuration. Mitotic activity is variable, as is the presence of focal nuclear hyperchromasia and pleomorphism in proliferating cells. Extremes in the latter characteristics have resulted in such terms as *pleomorphic fibroma, atypical fibrous histiocytoma,* and *dermatofibroma with monster cells* in reference to variations in the general microscopic attributes of dermatofibromas.[273–275] Nevertheless, there is no reliable evidence to suggest that these neoplasms ever undergo aggressive transformation, providing that they have the overall histopathologic attributes of the lesions under discussion here.

One special subtype of dermatofibroma contains vascular lakes that are mantled by giant cells, fibroblasts, and macrophages, surrounded by zones of intratumoral hemorrhage and hemosiderin deposition. This lesion is known as *aneurysmal fibrous histiocytoma* and arises principally in middle-aged adults as a slowly growing papule or nodule with a long evolution.[276, 277] It should not be confused with *angiomatoid* fibrous histiocytoma, as described later, or with examples of dermatofibroma that show pseudoangiomatous features because of artifactual (fixation- or processing-related) clefts between groups of the proliferating cells. Other variants of dermatofibroma include lesions with abundant reactive lymphoid infiltration, entrapped and proliferating epithelium, nuclear palisading, marked hemosiderosis, and divergent smooth muscular or granular cell components (personal unpublished observations).[266–281]

Benign Recurring Fibrous Histiocytomas

Over the past several years, it has been recognized that a set of cutaneous fibrohistiocytic tumors exists that is not easily reconciled with those having the prototypical features of conventional dermatofibroma. The former lesions may occur at any age, with a wider topographic distribution than that of usual dermatofibromas. More-

over, they are more deeply based in the dermis and subcutis and have a multinodular appearance. Recurrence after seemingly adequate excision is observed in up to 40% of cases. In light of all of these attributes, the terms *benign fibrous histiocytoma with potential for local recurrence* (BFHPR) or *atypical fibrous histiocytoma* have been appended to such proliferations.[282, 283]

In parallel with the aforementioned points of clinical dissimilarity between BFHPR and dermatofibroma, the microscopic appearances of these tumors are also reproducibly divergent. BFHPR is composed entirely of fusiform or stellate cells in short fascicles or storiform arrays, without any multinucleated elements or nuclear pleomorphism and only a few foam cells (Fig. 13–49).[282] It shows a multinodular profile on low-power microscopy and often involves the subcutis, in contrast to the uninodular, irregularly expansile, and almost purely dermal nature of dermatofibroma.[283] Hyalinized, keloidal-type stromal collagen is commonly entrapped by the tumor cells in BFHPR, and a delicately branching vascular matrix is routinely apparent.[283] Mitotic activity can almost always be found, but pathologic division figures are absent.[282, 283]

Other Benign Neoplasms

Myxomas

Myxomas of the skin are extremely uncommon, and most lesions labeled as such in the past represent dermal mucous cysts of the digits rather than actual neoplasms.[284] True myxomas are most often seen in patients who have the NAME syndrome (*n*evi, *a*trial myxomas, *m*yxomas of skin and mammary glands, and *e*phelides). These individuals are adolescents and young adults who also manifest endocrine hyperactivity (particularly Cushing's syndrome) as part of a complex disorder with autosomal dominant inheritance.[285]

Cutaneous myxomas in this setting are papules or nodules that average approximately 1 to 2 cm in maximal diameter and occur on the face and trunk. The lesions are soft, compressible, and tan or pink. Although cutaneous tumors in the NAME syndrome represent only a cosmetic nuisance, they may be an invaluable clue to the existence of this complex. Such a realization may be life-saving for the patient, inasmuch as either the atrial myxomas or endocrinopathies that constitute additional parts of the syndrome may prove fatal if left untreated.[285]

Histologically, cutaneous myxomas are centered in the dermis or superficial subcutis. They are extremely paucicellular on low-power microscopy, appearing mainly as circumscribed, lightly basophilic balls of mucus. Within the abundant myxoid stroma, one finds scant numbers of bland, fusiform or stellate fibroblast-like cells, which are widely separated and admixed with inconspicuous fibrovascular stromal elements (Fig. 13–50, see p. 810). Occasional vacuolated polygonal cells may be apparent as well, potentially simulating adipocytes or lipoblasts. However, colloidal iron or alcian blue stains show that their cytoplasmic vacuoles contain stromal mucin rather than fat. Myxomas never demonstrate mitotic activity or nuclear atypia in the proliferating cells.[286] Cutaneous mucinosis may also enter differential diagnostic consideration in this context. However, that condition is typified by virtually acellular, diffuse accumulation of stromal mucin in the interstices of the dermis, with irregular peripheral contours. Moreover, a clinical association with collagen vascular diseases or a thyroidopathy is often present in cases of mucinosis of the skin.

Solitary Fibrous Tumors

Over the last decade, it has become apparent that solitary fibrous tumor—called *subpleural fibroma* when seen in the thorax—may arise over a wide range of anatomic locations, including (but not limited to) the pleura, peritoneum, pericardium, testicular tunic, subcutis, soft tissue, mediastinum, thyroid, meninges, orbit, nasal cavity, and paranasal sinuses.[286] When it is seen in the head and neck, this lesion usually presents as a nondescript space-occupying mass, with secondary symptoms and signs that are related to size and compression of local structures. Rare examples also apparently may synthesize an insulin-like peptide and are associated with paraneoplastic hypoglycemia.

Pathologically, solitary fibrous tumors are unencapsulated and are composed of dense aggregates of bland spindle cells that are enmeshed in hyalinized fibrous stroma. The cells do not assume any particular growth configuration, and the image of solitary fibrous tumor is therefore often described as "patternless." Mitotic figures are variable in number, but they are usually easily seen. Occasionally, foci with relative nuclear atypia and heightened cellularity are observed; these do not, in and of themselves, connote malignancy in solitary fibrous tumor; in fact, the criteria for sarcoma arising in this setting are rather vague. My personal requirement is that spontaneous necrosis, infiltrative growth, overt nuclear atypia, and mitotic activity all need to be present concurrently to render a diagnosis of malignant solitary fibrous tumor.

The behavior of uncomplicated solitary fibrous tumor is typically that of an indolent lesion. It is curable with complete but conservative excision, and only uncommon examples with local recurrence are seen.

BIOLOGICALLY BORDERLINE CUTANEOUS MESENCHYMAL TUMORS

Borderline tumors may be defined as those that have a substantial tendency to recur—often with significant morbidity—and, in rare circumstances, metastasize to distant sites as well. In the skin, three particular classes of neoplasms include such lesions: endothelial proliferations, myogenous tumors, and others of a fibrohistiocytic character.

Borderline Endothelial Tumors

Papillary Endovascular Angioendotheliomas

Papillary endovascular angioendotheliomas (PEA) were first described by Dabska in 1969[287] and have become known as Dabska's tumors. They are apparently seen only in children and adolescents as fluctuant, ill-defined reddish plaques or nodules that range in size up to 5 cm. A zone of dermal edema may surround such neoplasms.[287, 288] "Metastases" of PEA to regional lymph nodes were reported in the seminal series of cases, but other authors have since suggested the alternative interpretation that the nodal implants actually represented tumor "satellites" as part of a field neoplasia phenomenon.[289] Nevertheless, PEA does have a marked propensity to recur locally after surgical excision, justifying its inclusion as a "borderline" proliferation.[287, 290]

The microscopic features of PEA are distinctive. As its name suggests, this tumor is confined to pre-existing vascular spaces in the corium, most of which have the properties of dilated lymphatic channels. Also, similar to deep lymphangiomas of the skin, PEA features contiguous dermal fibrosis and intralesional aggregates of lymphocytes. The latter cells are also evident in intimate admixture with plump endothelial cell clusters inside of the affected vessels.[194, 287, 290]

The papillae of PEA are composed of polyhedral cells with round nuclei, dispersed chromatin, and small nucleoli. As just mentioned, mature lymphocytes commonly mantle the peripheral aspects of the papillary formations, and they contain internal, globular, intercellular eosinophilic deposits of basement membrane material (Fig. 13–51, see p. 810). These inclusions may be labeled with the periodic acid–Schiff stain or with immunostains for laminin and collagen type IV.[194]

Adjacent blood vessels in PEA that do not contain papillae are nonetheless lined with atypical endothelial cells, with hyperchromatic nuclei. Small areas of racemose vascular proliferation also may be apparent in the dermis, as seen in well-differentiated angiosarcomas. Mitotic activity is present but limited in scope.[194, 287]

Epithelioid Hemangioendotheliomas

Epithelioid hemangioendotheliomas are subcutaneous lesions that only uncommonly involve the dermis. As such, they present as firm tan-pink nodules and plaques measuring several centimeters in maximum diameter. These lesions primarily arise in adult patients with a slight predilection for women. The trunk and extremities are the usual sites of origin,[194, 291] but the head and neck may be affected as well. Some patients with epithelioid hemangioendotheliomas of the skin will concurrently have histologically identical tumors in the lung (where they were known in the past as intravascular bronchoalveolar tumors) and the liver.[292] Under these conditions, it is impossible to determine whether the visceral and cutaneous lesions are independent primary neoplasms, or whether they represent metastases of one another. Epithelioid hemangioendotheliomas recur in up to 40% of cases, and approximately 15% metastasize to distant extracutaneous locations.[291, 292]

Epithelioid hemangioendothelioma is typified by disorganized sheets and cords of large polyhedral tumor cells with amphophilic cytoplasm, prominent cytoplasmic vacuoles, and round but eccentric nuclei. Chromatin is vesicular and small nucleoli are often seen (Fig. 13–52, see p. 811).[291] The neoplastic cells make no attempt to form complete intercellular vascular lumina, as seen in epithelioid hemangiomas.[194] However, like epithelioid hemangiomas, epithelioid hemangioendotheliomas have a proclivity for growth around pre-existing large blood vessels. Mitotic activity and necrosis may be apparent, but they are relatively inconspicuous when present. The background stroma is variably fibrous or myxoid in character.[292]

Two diagnostic errors are common in the evaluation of epithelioid hemangioendotheliomas. First, one may focus on the cord-like arrays of polygonal cells in some cases, leading to a misinterpretation of metastatic carcinoma. Second, those lesions with extensive cytoplasmic vacuolization may erroneously be labeled as adipocytic in nature. The application of electron microscopy or immunohistochemical studies for epithelial and endothelial determinants (see earlier) is useful in resolving such uncertainties.[194]

Superficial Hemangiopericytoma

Hemangiopericytoma only uncommonly arises in the subcutis, and most examples of this tumor are situated in the deep soft tissues.[175]

"Hemangiopericytoma" has become an overused diagnosis over the past 30 years, in apparent disdain of its originators' admonitions.[293] It is likely that some examples of fibromatosis, poorly differentiated carcinoma, and leiomyosarcoma have been included under this rubric.

Bona fide examples of subcuticular hemangiopericytoma are nodular, firm, reddish lesions that may attain a maximum size of 5 to 6 cm. They may be slightly tender to palpation, similar to smooth muscle tumors.[294] Adults are affected almost exclusively, with a peak during middle life, and the extremities are the favored sites of origin for these neoplasms.

Biologically, hemangiopericytoma of the subcutis has the potential to recur in up to 50% of cases. However, examples that metastasize distantly are rare (<1%).[175]

Hemangiopericytoma is a cytologically monotonous, unencapsulated neoplasm that is composed of bluntly fusiform or polyhedral cells. These are arranged in large clusters or sheets, punctuated by numerous blood vessels with the caliber of venules or capillaries (Fig. 13–53). Vascular lumina in most examples focally demonstrate a staghorn-like configuration, branching like the antlers of a deer.[293] It should be noted, however, that this histologic finding has been overstressed as a criterion for the diagnosis of hemangiopericytoma; staghorn vessels also may be observed in tumors of epithelial, car-

tilaginous, and leiomyomatous or leiomyosarcomatous types,[246] and they conversely can be inconspicuous in occasional hemangiopericytomas.

Nuclear chromatin in the tumor cells of hemangiopericytoma is compact and hyperchromatic; accordingly, nucleoli are difficult to discern. Cytoplasm is modest in amount and amphophilic.

Several microscopic features are worrisome in regard to the potential for superficial hemangiopericytoma to metastasize. These include a mitotic count of 4 or more per 10 high-power (40X) fields, spontaneous necrosis, and focally marked nuclear pleomorphism and atypia.[175] If such findings are observed, a note should be made in the pathology report that the neoplasm may have the ability to spread distantly, and close follow-up should be urged.

Differential diagnosis between hemangiopericytoma and lesions simulating it may be extremely difficult (if not impossible) on conventional microscopy. Immunostains are extremely useful in this regard. Although it putatively shows modified myogenous differentiation, hemangiopericytoma is reactive only for vimentin and does not express actin isoforms or desmin, in contrast to leiomyoma and leiomyosarcoma. It similarly lacks epithelial markers, unlike carcinomas and sarcomas that represent histologic mimics of hemangiopericytoma.[295]

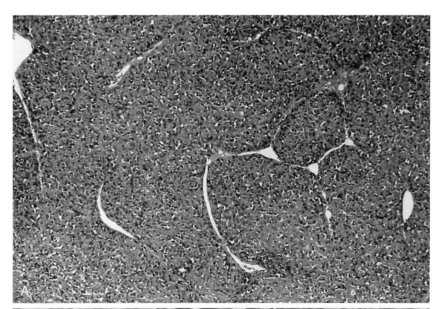
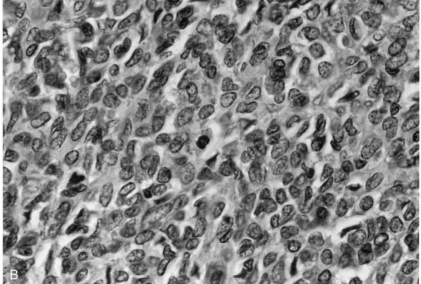

Figure 13–53. *A,* Subcutaneous hemangiopericytoma of the neck, showing solid expanses of epithelioid tumor cells that are supported by branching stromal blood vessels. Some of them resemble moose antlers. *B,* Dense apposition of polygonal cells is typical of hemangiopericytoma; nuclear atypia is slight.

Borderline "Fibrohistiocytic" Neoplasms

Dermatofibrosarcoma Protuberans

Dermatofibrosarcoma protuberans (DFSP) is typically a slowly growing, firm, reddish plaque or nodule that tends to arise on the proximal extremities and trunk.[246] Most patients are adults,[296] but cases in children have also been well documented.[297] The overlying skin is attenuated in almost all instances, and it may be ulcerated.[296–300]

Dermatofibrosarcoma protuberans shows a reproducible tendency to recur after simple surgical excision and does so in approximately 50% of cases. With repeated regrowth of this tumor, it may assume a multinodular appearance, and the development of regional satellite lesions is also possible.[246] The latter eventuality is worrisome, because metastasizing variants of this tumor have usually recurred many times before distant spread occurs[298]; the disease-free interval between successive recurrences typically shortens each time.

As its name implies, DFSP is a tumor that by definition protrudes above the surface of the contiguous, uninvolved skin. Accordingly, neoplastic cells are typically seen throughout the dermis, and many lesions lack a Grenz zone between the tumor and the epidermal basement membrane. DFSP is the archetypal storiform lesion, in which short spindle cells are arranged in a "pinwheel" fashion throughout the mass (Fig. 13–54).[296] Nuclei show only modest pleomorphism and dispersed chromatin, and mitoses are generally scarce. The giant cells that are so common in benign cutaneous fibrohistiocytic neoplasms are absent in DFSP[246]; therefore, observation of such elements should lead the pathologist to another diagnostic interpretation.

In its deep aspects, DFSP tends to infiltrate the subcuticular fat in a permeative fashion, rather than using interlobular fibrous septa as scaffolds for downward growth as seen in unusually large dermatofibromas.[272] A time-honored adage for some dermatopathologists has been that DFSP and dermatofibroma differ only in their vertical extent of growth.[272] However, careful scrutiny of each neoplasm shows additional points of dissimilarity. The abundant collagenous stroma, xanthoma cells, and multinucleated giant cells of dermatofibroma are not seen in DFSP; conversely, storiform growth is much more pronounced in the latter tumor. However, the lesions do share a tendency to induce hyperpigmentation and acanthosis in the overlying epidermis.[272, 299]

Several microscopic variants of DFSP have now been recognized. The myxoid subtype demonstrates a stromal mucin-rich matrix in which small capillaries are regularly interspersed; storiform growth is only vaguely represented in this lesion.[301] Pigmented DFSP is also known as the Bednar tumor. It is virtually identical to conventional dermatofibrosarcoma, except that pigmented stellate and spindle cells are regularly interspersed throughout the mass.[302] These have been shown convincingly to contain melanin, and I have seen examples of Bednar tumor that were misdiagnosed as melanomas as a consequence of this finding. Still other variants of DFSP show a partial composition by granular cells, or densely cellular, fibrosarcoma-like zones, in which the degree of nuclear atypia and mitotic activity is greater and a herringbone pattern of cell growth is observed.[303–305] Smooth muscle differentiation also may be observed in DFSP in this particular context.[306] Lastly, evolution of DFSP into a high-grade pleomorphic tumor (with the features of malignant fibrous histiocytoma) has been reported.[307, 308] I consider the latter form to represent "dedifferentiated" DFSP. It is tempting to speculate that metastasis of dermatofibrosarcomas will not occur until dedifferentiation supervenes, but I know of no systematic evaluation of this premise in the literature. A study by Connelly and Evans[305] failed to document an association between fibrosarcoma-like growth in DFSP and heightened aggressiveness.

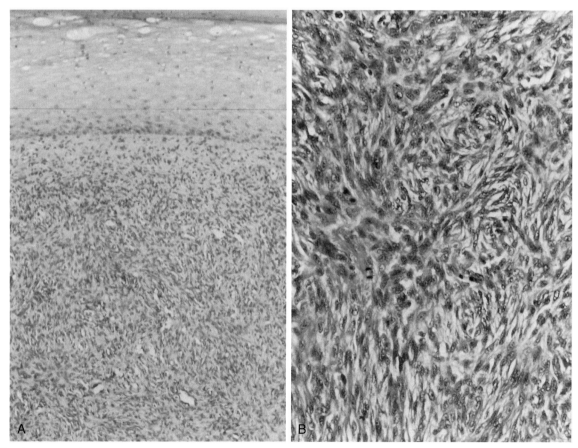

Figure 13–54. A, Dermatofibrosarcoma protuberans (DFSP) of the scalp, showing a prototypically storiform proliferation of spindle cells that abuts and elevates the epidermis. B, The cellular monotypism and storiform growth of DFSP are shown here.

Some may consider the distinction between DFSP and benign fibrous histiocytoma with potential for recurrence to represent a fine point of academia. I do not share this view because of differences in histology[283] and the documented metastatic potential of some recurring dermatofibrosarcomas.[298] To reiterate, distant spread has never been reported in reference to BFHPR.[282, 283] In those cases in which the separation of dermatofibroma and DFSP is deemed difficult on the basis of morphologic criteria, immunostains for CD34 (the human hematopoietic progenitor cell antigen) and factor XIIIa are often helpful. DFSP is diffusely CD34-positive and factor XIIIa-negative, whereas dermatofibromas (and additional fibrohistiocytic tumor types other than DFSP) show the converse of this profile or only limited CD34 reactivity at the advancing edge of the lesion.[309]

Giant Cell Fibroblastoma and Giant Cell Angiofibroma

In 1983, Shmookler and Enzinger[310] reported a peculiar tumor of childhood that they designated as *giant cell fibroblastoma* (GCF). Patients with this lesion are less than 20 years old, and it typically takes the form of an ill-defined flesh-colored nodule on the neck, trunk, or extremities. The cut surfaces of GCF are commonly described as "gelatinous."[311–314]

Giant cell fibroblastoma recurs in up to 50% of cases after excision; however, there have been no examples of distant metastasis to date.[311, 314] This neoplasm is grouped with the fibrohistiocytic proliferations because of the observation that recurrent GCF may be indistinguishable from DFSP (either in classic or variant forms) microscopically[311]; moreover, de novo DFSP may contain GCF-like foci.[315]

A biphasic pattern of growth typifies GCF. Superficial elements of the neoplasm in the papillary and reticular dermis are represented by bland stellate cells that are set in a fibromxyoid stroma, punctuated by floret-type multinucleated giant cells (Fig. 13–55, see p. 811).[311] Deeper components assume an angiectoid appearance, in which interconnecting pseudovascular spaces are observed. The latter channels are lined in part by floret cells and do not contain erythrocytes.[313] Peripheral aspects of the proliferation blend with the surrounding dermis, but the deep interface with subjacent subcutaneous fat is usually more distinct. Mitotic figures are rare in GCF, and storiform growth is lacking in de novo examples.

As mentioned, recurrent lesions may retain the histologic profile just described, or they may acquire nearly all of the microscopic features of conventional DFSP. Cases of GCF that regrew as Bednar tumors have been documented.[316]

Differential diagnosis primarily centers on giant cell angiofibroma, angiosarcoma, and rudimentary meningocele (see subsequent discussion). The latter two lesions are easily excluded from consideration by attention to clinical data, because angiosarcoma virtually never occurs in children or adolescents, and rudimentary meningocele is often congenital and may be associated with an underlying defect in the cranial bones.[317]

Giant cell angiofibroma (GCA) was described by Dei Tos et al. in 1995.[318] It is closely similar to GCF except for a few select points. GCA prefers the head and neck (particularly the orbit)[318, 319] and is at least partially encapsulated, in contrast to the infiltrative growth of GCF. Moreover, GCA contains larger vascular spaces—sometimes resembling dilated lymphatics—and does not exhibit a relationship to DFSP. The immunophenotype of the two tumors is virtually identical, featuring reactivity for CD34 in stromal and multinucleated cells alike. Interestingly, DFSP is uniformly CD34-positive as well, and it is plausible to group it with GCF, GCA, and solitary fibrous tumor conceptually, as a neoplastic "family."

Plexiform Fibrous Histiocytomas

Plexiform fibrous histiocytoma (PFH) was first described by Enzinger and Zhang in 1988.[320] In that series, 65 patients were de-

scribed, all of whom were children, adolescents, or young adults. They had nodular lesions that most often arose in the subcutaneous tissues of the extremities and measured up to several centimeters at diagnosis. There were no particularly distinguishing macroscopic characteristics of such tumors.

Since that time, several other examples of PFH have been documented.[321] It has become increasingly clear that this neoplasm has a marked proclivity for local recurrence (in up to 67% of cases), but there have been only two instances of metastasis to regional lymph nodes. No patient with PFH has died of the tumor.[320, 321]

On low power microscopy, PFH has an appearance that closely imitates that of plexiform neural tumors and causes differential diagnostic difficulty in regard to the latter neoplasms. One observes fascicles of spindle cells in the corium and subcutis, separated from one another by unremarkable dermal fibrous or subcuticular adipose tissue. The aggregates of tumor cells are arranged in such a manner that they recapitulate the image of a miniature nerve plexus.[320] However, closer inspection shows several points of difference between PFH and peripheral nerve sheath neoplasms. The former lesion is composed of relatively nondescript spindle cells with enlarged, minimally pleomorphic, slightly hyperchromatic nuclei, and notable mitotic activity. Focal storiform growth within each fascicle is often seen, and the tumor cells also may mantle small pseudovascular spaces or myxoid foci. A key finding is the presence of osteoclast-like giant cells, which are interspersed among the fusiform elements (Fig. 13–56, see p. 812).[320, 321] These are essentially never observed in nerve sheath tumors.

The margins of PFH are indistinct, and one cannot always be certain that the lesion has been excised completely in limited resection specimens. This feature probably contributes to the high incidence of local recurrence reported in most series.

Angiomatoid Fibrous Histiocytoma

Among all superficial mesenchymal neoplasms, the angiomatoid fibrous histiocytoma (AFH) is unusual in many respects. Patients tend to be adolescents—with a mean age of 17 years—but occasional examples also arise in elderly adults.[322–324] The extremities, trunk, and head and neck region are the preferred sites of origin for AFH, the sizes of which range from 0.5 to 12 cm. On cut section, the tumor has an obviously cystic and hemorrhagic quality and is composed of dense white-grey tissue.[324]

Most notably, this lesion may be associated with systemic symptoms and signs, even though the tumor mass may be relatively small and localized. Distant effects of AFH include hypochromic-microcytic anemia, extreme fatigue, weight loss, and fever. All of these problems resolve after resection of the neoplasm.[322]

Costa and Weiss[324] recently evaluated 108 examples of AFH, with attention to its behavior. Local recurrence was observed in 12% of cases, 4.7% developed metastases, and only one patient died of disease. It would appear, therefore, that a biologically borderline status is appropriate for this neoplasm.

There are three basic microscopic constituents to AFH. These include solid sheets of spindled or bluntly fusiform tumor cells, focally assuming a storiform growth pattern; central erythrocytic pools that are not mantled by endothelial cells; and surrounding lymphoid inflammation (often with germinal center formation) with or without a fibrous pseudocapsule (Fig. 13–57, see p. 812).[322–324]

The degree of nuclear atypia in the cells of AFH is modest; chromatin is vesicular, with small nucleoli and mitotic activity. Scattered pleomorphic giant cells may be dispersed throughout the neoplastic population in some cases; myxoid stromal change and deposition of hemosiderin also may be seen.[324]

An important diagnostic error in reference to AFH is to mistake the tumor for an organizing hematoma. It should be remembered that broad, compact sheets of spindle cells are never observed in the latter lesion but are regularly seen in AFH. Negative results of immunostains for endothelial markers also assist in excluding true vascular neoplasms.

⁝ OVERTLY MALIGNANT MESENCHYMAL NEOPLASMS

Those mesenchymal neoplasms that demonstrate a reproducible tendency for recurrence *and* distant metastasis are rightly considered to be overtly malignant. These tumors manifest a variety of cellular lineages, as detailed subsequently. As mentioned at the outset of this chapter, they are grouped together by generic histologic appearance because many malignant lesions have the capacity to manifest an undifferentiated image on conventional microscopy. Accordingly, differential diagnostic considerations are broader and will receive more attention than those presented heretofore.

Small-Cell Malignant Neoplasms

Among small round-cell neoplasms of the skin and superficial soft tissue, peripheral neuroepithelioma[325] (PNE; also known as *primitive neuroectodermal tumor*)[326, 327] is considered to be closely allied, if not identical, to extraskeletal Ewing's sarcoma.[328–330] Both lesions are rare in the superficial subcutis and dermis, where they present as nodular, red-violet, ill-defined tumefactions.[325, 328, 329] Patients with PNE are usually children, adolescents, or young adults, but older individuals are occasionally affected as well. The neoplasms may attain a maximum dimension of 10 cm and are rapidly growing. The trunk and extremities are favored locations for PNE.[325]

The clinical behavior of this tumor is an aggressive one. Even with prompt diagnosis and therapy, PNE is attended by a 5-year mortality rate of approximately 50%; distant metastases to lungs, liver, bones, and brain are common.[331]

Peripheral neuroepithelioma represents one of the quintessential small round-cell tumors. One observes sheets, vague nests, and occasional cords of closely apposed monomorphic neoplastic cells that are approximately twice to three times the size of mature lymphocytes. These aggregates are separated from one another by a delicate but complex fibrovascular stromal network. Mitotic activity is variable but may be surprisingly sparse; similarly, cellular apoptosis and regional necrosis may or may not be present (Fig. 13–58).[332]

The nuclear detail of PNE is the most helpful clue to its recognition. Chromatin is typically evenly distributed, and nucleoli, if present, are small. Cytoplasm is modest in amount and amphophilic.[325]

A minority of PNE cases exhibit the presence of intercellular rosettes, betraying the primitive neural nature of this neoplasm.[325]

However, the fibrillary intercellular meshwork seen in many examples of metastatic neuroblastoma—an important differential diagnostic alternative—is lacking in PNE.[332] Similarly, focal nuclear pleomorphism or multinucleation are uniformly absent, in contrast to the characteristics of small round-cell (embryonal or alveolar) rhabdomyosarcoma (which would also be extremely unusual as a primary cutaneous tumor).[332] Lastly, Merkel cell carcinoma enters into diagnostic consideration in this context, because the latter tumor may arise deep in the skin without any intervening dermal component. Because it is somewhat related to PNE in terms of cellular differentiation, electron microscopy or immunohistology are often necessary to obtain a final distinction between these lesions.[332] Merkel cell carcinoma is diffusely reactive for keratin, whereas PNE shows only scattered positivity or, far more commonly, none at all for this marker. Conversely, PNE regularly expresses vimentin and the MIC-2 gene product but Merkel cell tumors do not.

Finally, malignant lymphoma of the subcutis may simulate any of the other small cell neoplasms, including PNE.[73] The nuclei of lymphoid cells differ from those of other alternatives, because they are more irregular in contour and have a greater tendency to overlap one another. Nevertheless, the most certain indicator of hematopoietic differentiation is the CD45 immunostain, which is absolutely specific and also has a high level of sensitivity.[333]

Spindle-Cell Neoplasms

Leiomyosarcoma

The clinical features of cutaneous leiomyosarcoma are similar regardless of whether it is based in the dermis or in the subcutis, except that the latter lesions tend to be larger and, obviously, more deep seated.[334–336] Subcutaneous leiomyosarcoma recurs approximately twice as often as dermal leiomyosarcoma does (50% vs 25%), and distant metastasis is observed to the lungs, other soft tissue sites, and the liver in 30% to 40% of cases originating in the subcutis.[246] Visceral spread from dermal leiomyosarcoma, on the other hand, is extremely rare.

Subcutaneous leiomyosarcoma is basically similar microscopically to dermal leiomyosarcoma, but it commonly demonstrates a greater degree of cellular pleomorphism, nuclear atypia, and mitotic activity (Fig. 13–59). Fascicles of fusiform cells in this tumor extend deeply into the hypodermal adipose tissue and often involve underlying fascia and striated muscle as well.[334, 335] Prominent stromal vascularity is also more common in the subcutaneous variant of

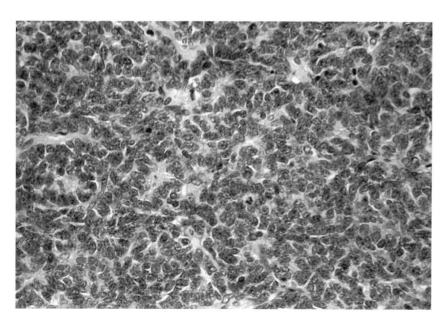

Figure 13–58. Peripheral neuroepithelioma (primitive neuroectodermal tumor) of the subcutis of the scalp in a child. Uniform small round tumor cells focally aggregate into rosettes.

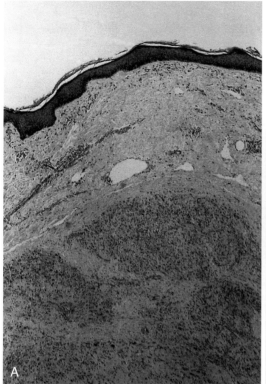
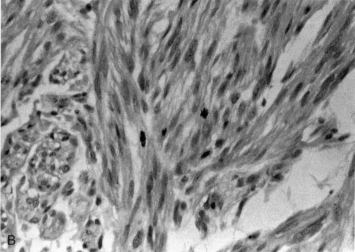

Figure 13–59. *A,* Subcutaneous leiomyosarcoma of the neck, showing the fascicular growth of spindle cells. *B,* High-power examination demonstrates modest nuclear atypia and mitotic activity.

leiomyosarcoma, yielding the designations of *angioleiomyosarcoma* or *vascular leiomyosarcoma.* In fact, based on the results of immunohistologic analysis—showing frequent reactivity for the CD57 antigen (a potential marker of vascular medial smooth muscle) in subcutaneous leiomyosarcoma—a proposal has been made that this subtype pursues specialized vascular myogenous differentiation.[336]

Malignant Peripheral Nerve Sheath Tumors

Outside the setting of von Recklinghausen's disease (VRD), the existence of cutaneous malignant peripheral nerve sheath tumors (MPNST) has been questioned in the past. It is well recognized that approximately 1% to 3% of patients with VRD—both children and adults—will develop malignant transformation in superficial neurofibromas, in which cases the latter lesions rapidly expand in size and often become painful.[337]

Sporadic cutaneous MPNST have been accepted as bona fide entities increasingly over the last few years. These lesions are nodules or plaques with variable growth rates, and they have a propensity to arise on the neck, trunk, or extremities of adults.[338, 339] Ulceration may supervene, and local paresthesias or dysesthesias are sometimes observed if the masses are associated with major nerves.

The behavior of MPNST is generally predicated upon its size, location, and surgical resectability. However, those tumors arising in the skin more often demonstrate local recurrence (in approximately 80% of cases) than distant metastasis (15% to 20%).[338]

The microscopic features of MPNST are variable; indeed, this neoplasm is one of the great "chameleons" of pathology. In most cases, one observes a modestly pleomorphic proliferation of spindle cells in the dermis and subcutis, in which cellularity is highly variable from region to region. The tumors cells are randomly arranged or configured in fascicles that may intersect one another at acute angles (the so-called herringbone growth pattern) and many contain wavy or serpiginous nuclei (Fig. 13–60).[338–340] Myxoid stromal change is evident in approximately one third of all cases, and a fo-

cally storiform arrangement of tumor cells is often observed as well.[339]

These lesions entrap cutaneous appendages rather than destroying them, but the peripheral margins of growth are indistinct. Permeation into the subcutis and underlying soft tissue is common. Nuclear atypia is modest to moderate, and mitotic activity is present but not striking.

Occasional examples of cutaneous MPNST—particularly those occurring in patients with VRD—manifest divergent mesenchymal differentiation. Tumors showing an admixture of rhabdomyosarcomatous elements (see previous discussion) with the spindle-cell population are known as *malignant triton tumors.*[341] Although de novo rhabdomyosarcoma is a highly aggressive neoplasm, triton tumors are paradoxically no different biologically than conventional MPNST. Other divergent elements that have been reported in such lesions include those resembling osteosarcoma, pigmented malignant melanoma (melanotic MPNST), chondrosarcoma, adenocarcinoma (glandular MPNST), and angiosarcoma.[342]

Electron microscopic evaluation demonstrates elongated, overlapping cytoplasmic processes in the spindle cells of MPNST. Focal formation of pericellular basal lamina is also common, as are primitive appositional plaques between adjacent tumor cells.[246]

Immunohistologic studies show reactivity for S100 protein in approximately 50% of cases, CD57 in 33%, and myelin basic protein in 15% to 20%.[343] When used as a panel, one or more of these markers is present in 70% of all lesions. Divergent tumors also may express desmin or muscle-specific actin, keratin, or von Willebrand factor and the CD31 or CD34 antigens. In light of this heterogeneity in the immunophenotype of MPNST, it may be safely said that ultrastructural assessments are usually more definitive in resolving diagnostic difficulties.[139]

Differential diagnosis includes leiomyosarcoma, as well as spindle-cell squamous carcinoma, dermatofibrosarcoma protuberans, atypical fibroxanthoma, and desmoplastic or neurotropic melanoma.[338] All but the last of these possibilities are adequately

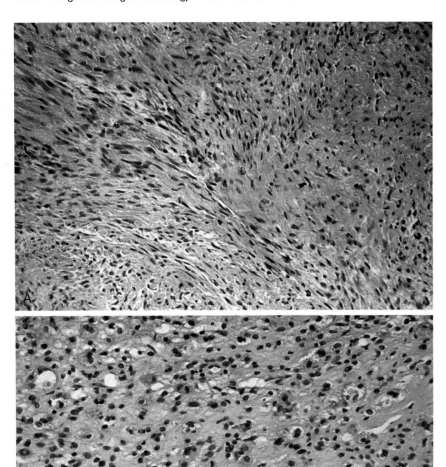

Figure 13–60. A, Low-grade malignant peripheral nerve sheath tumor (MPNST) of the dermis, showing heightened cellularity and mitotic activity when compared with Figures 13–41 and 13–42. B, Slightly more plump neoplastic cells are evident in this dermal "triton tumor" variant of MPNST.

distinguished from MPNST by electron microscopy and immunohistology.[246] It must be acknowledged that neuroid spindle-cell melanomas and true nerve sheath tumors share many points of synonymity.[344] Ultrastructural features of the two groups are virtually identical, inasmuch as spindle-cell melanomas often lose their synthesis of cytoplasmic premelanosomes.[345] Similarly, the HMB-45 antigen—a specific determinant of melanocytic cells—is absent in almost all neuroid melanomas and is not seen in MPNST.[346] Thus, one may not be able to make this distinction with certainty, in the absence of a concurrent or previous intra-epidermal melanocytic proliferation at the same anatomic site. However, whether separation of the two tumors is *necessary* is also a contentious point, because of similarities in their biologic potential and behavior.[340]

Pending resolution of this issue, I demand that a diagnosis of sporadic cutaneous MPNST should be made only under the following circumstances: an epidermal melanocytic lesion must be absent; electron microscopy and immunohistology must be performed, and the results should not demonstrate apparent melanocytic differentiation.

Kaposi's Sarcoma

The clinical characteristics of Kaposi's sarcoma (KS) are by now all too familiar to most physicians, because of the tremendous increase in the incidence of this tumor occasioned by the advent of the AIDS epidemic in the 1980s. Prior to that time, KS was relatively rarely encountered outside of the Mediterranean basin and Africa.[347]

This neoplasm occurs in four well-defined clinical settings.[347-349] *Classic Kaposi's sarcoma* is a disease that predominantly affects elderly men of Middle-Eastern or Italian heritage and manifests itself as multiple, coalescent, red-brown macules and plaques on the distal lower extremities. A subset of patients has lesions that resemble deep lymphangiomas, accompanied by lymphedema of the extremities. Nodular, sometimes ulcerated tumors of the skin and viscera eventually supervene in this variant, but only after a prolonged period of time. *African KS* is seen in young black patients from restricted portions of the African continent. Women are almost as frequently afflicted as men, and their mean age is less than that of classic KS patients by two to three decades. The disorder is more rapidly progressive in African KS, with relatively early appearance of nodular lesions and involvement of lymph nodes and internal organs. *KS associated with iatrogenic immunosuppression* shares clinical features with both the classic and the African subtype and primarily affects recipients of allogeneic organ transplants. *AIDS-related KS* is precipitated by infection with HIV. At the outset of the AIDS pandemic, it was first noted in young homosexual men,[350] with lesser numbers of cases in intravenous drug abusers and recipients of infected blood products.

Although the other manifestations of AIDS have become more evenly distributed among all infected patient populations, KS has remained largely confined to homosexual males. In fact, its incidence has already begun to decline, even though the number of HIV-infected individuals continues to rise on a worldwide scale. The reasons for these epidemiologic peculiarities are unknown at present.[351]

AIDS-related KS has a deceptively innocuous appearance at its onset, taking the form of ill-defined macular "patches" that often resemble ecchymoses.[352] In contrast to the topographic confinement of the classic variant, KS in AIDS patients may affect virtually any skin field and also is seen in the mucosae.[350] Visceral involvement also appears rapidly, similar to that seen in the African form.

Interestingly, three common threads have emerged that bind all of the variants of KS together. One factor is the HLA-DR5 allele, which is greatly overrepresented in KS patients when compared with the population at large.[353] The others are seropositivity for the cytomegalovirus[354] and molecular evidence for integration of a herpesvirus-related nucleic acid sequence in the tumor cells.[355] Indeed, some authors have advanced the hypothesis that KS is not a neoplasm at all but instead represents an unusual tissue reaction to the latter infectious agent.[356] I do not subscribe to this view. It has been shown that KS cells express an activated oncogene, termed *K-FGF.*[357] Moreover, the features of this proliferation in transfection studies are most consistent with those of a true neoplasm,[357] and the pattern of visceral involvement seen in advanced cases[347] is unlike that of any known viral disease.

This is not to say that cytomegalovirus and Herpesvirus play no role whatever in the genesis of KS. As mentioned earlier, genomic segments of these agents have been localized to the nuclei of KS cells.[358] It would therefore appear tenable to conclude that KS may result from the effects of coinfection with HIV, cytomegalovirus, and Herpesvirus in susceptible (HLA-DR5-positive?) individuals, allowing some or all of these viruses to express a latent potential for cellular transformation and oncogenesis.

Whereas classic KS is an indolent process that only infrequently causes death of the patient directly, African, transplant-associated, and HIV-related variants evolve more rapidly and are often fatal.[347] Chemotherapy with vinca alkaloids has proven successful in controlling the first of these subtypes, and, with withdrawal of immunosuppressive medications, it also often suffices to control the transplant-associated form.[359] However, there is currently no effective treatment for African and AIDS-related KS.

The reason that KS was included in this section is that its histologic spindle-cell pattern is most well known to pathologists. Nevertheless, all subtypes of the tumor will be described here for the sake of convenience.

Clinically "early" KS most often takes a macular or patch form.[352] Microscopically, this variant is extremely subtle. One often sees only a limited proliferation of small, attenuated, interanastomosing but bland blood vessels in the periappendageal reticular corium, together with an excess of nondescript spindle cells throughout the dermal connective tissue. In addition, small pre-existing blood vessels are often invested by a lymphoplasmacytic infiltrate. The "promontory" sign, wherein neovascular channels are formed around native vessels—yielding profiles that simulate the promontory of a cliff—is a helpful diagnostic finding (Fig. 13–61, see p. 813).[194, 348, 352] Small groupings of venule-like blood vessels are also interspersed randomly throughout the dermis in some cases, and extravasated erythrocytes are inconspicuous if present at all.[348] McNutt et al.[360] have also called attention to the fact that endothelia within "new" (neoplastic) blood vessels of KS are often apoptotic in the patch-stage. This observation is unique and would not be expected in benign vascular proliferations.

Plaque-stage KS features the appearance of more organized aggregates of spindle cells, forming small fascicles in admixture with capillary-sized neovascular channels, extravasated erythrocytes, hemosiderin, and stromal hemosiderin granules.[194, 347, 348, 361] The groupings of neoplastic cells are most often diffusely dispersed throughout the dermis, but they sometimes assume a pseudolobular

configuration.[348] Another useful diagnostic clue that appears at this phase of tumor evolution is the presence of hyaline globules in the neoplastic endothelial cells. These represent phagocytosed erythrocytes, as documented by the peroxidase reaction, and they also may be stained with the periodic acid–Schiff–diastase method.[347] Hyaline globules are not sufficient unto themselves for a diagnosis of KS, because they can rarely be seen in non-neoplastic vascular proliferations of the skin.[348, 361] However, they are helpful when interpreted in the proper context. Finally, small papillary projections of tumor cells may be observed within ectatic neovascular spaces in this stage of KS, together with racemose, "dissecting" luminal profiles throughout the dermis.[361]

The truly spindle-cell stage of KS is its "nodular" phase, in which fusiform elements constitute the bulk of the proliferating cell population. Their nuclei are only modestly hyperchromatic, with indistinct nucleoli, and cytoplasm is scant and amphophilic. A notable diagnostic feature is the presence of cytoplasmic vacuoles in the spindle cells, probably representing a primitive attempt at vascular lumen formation (Fig. 13–62, see p. 813).[362] Another helpful microscopic finding is that the fusiform cells of KS appear to spare dermal zones that surround pre-existing vessels, leaving hypocellular cuffs around the latter structures.[363] Extravasated erythrocytes and stromal hemosiderin deposition are maximal in scope in the nodular stage of KS, and hyaline globules often are numerous in the neoplastic cells.

Another continuing controversy regarding KS focuses on the nature of the proliferating elements in its spindle-cell form. There is no question that patch-stage and plaque-stage disease features reproducible immunoreactivity for endothelial markers, but these determinants are only occasionally detected in the spindle cell variant. Some authors contend that KS is a modified lymphatic endothelial tumor,[364] whereas others have concluded that it is not endothelial at all.[365] I prefer the premise that KS begins as a vascular endothelial neoplasm that undergoes reproducible clonal evolution to yield a cellular population resembling myofibroblasts.[347]

Differential diagnosis includes leiomyosarcoma, spindle-cell melanoma, spindle-cell squamous carcinoma, MPNST, and spindle-cell angiosarcoma. All but the last of these possibilities are easily excludable by attention to histologic detail or application of special studies.[348, 361, 362]

Spindle-cell angiosarcoma is a rare lesion, the microscopic attributes of which are nearly identical to those of nodular KS.[194, 362] Nevertheless, the clinical features of the two conditions usually differ substantially, as detailed subsequently. Spindle-cell angiosarcoma also exhibits a much higher degree of nuclear atypia and mitotic activity. Moreover, immunostains for *Ulex europaeus* I lectin binding sites, CD31, and CD34 are typically positive in spindle-cell angiosarcoma but not in spindle-cell KS.[347]

Epithelioid (Polygonal-Cell) Neoplasms

Epithelioid Leiomyosarcoma

There are no appreciable differences in the clinical presentation or behavior of epithelioid cutaneous leiomyosarcoma, compared with the features of the usual forms of this neoplasm.[366, 367] The latter have already been discussed.

Epithelioid leiomyosarcoma differs considerably in microscopic appearance from that of conventional spindle-cell smooth muscle tumors. The former lesion is composed predominantly of polygonal cells arranged in sheets or clusters. Nuclei are vesicular with variably prominent nucleoli, and the cytoplasm is lightly eosinophilic and homogeneous. Mitotic activity is routinely observed.[366]

Epithelioid leiomyosarcoma provides few histologic clues to its myogenous nature. This is appreciated only by electron microscopy—showing pinocytosis, plasmalemma-associated dense plaques, cytoplasmic microfilaments and dense bodies, and pericellular basal lamina—or through immunohistologic studies demonstrating reactivity for desmin and muscle-specific actin.[139] Differential diagnosis includes virtually all other epithelioid malignancies of the skin.

Epithelioid Malignant Peripheral Nerve Sheath Tumors

The clinical features of epithelioid malignant peripheral nerve sheath tumor (MPNST) are identical to those of the spindle-cell form of this tumor, and the reader is referred back to the discussion of the latter variant for details.

Epithelioid MPNST is dissimilar to spindle-cell nerve sheath sarcomas microscopically. It is composed solely of polyhedral cells that are arranged in cords, clusters, and sheets, often separated by myxoid or mucinous stromal material (Fig. 13–63, see p. 813). Nuclei are vesicular with prominent nucleoli, mitotic activity is brisk, and cytoplasm is amphophilic or eosinophilic and modest in quantity.[368, 369] Interpretation of this relatively nondescript image (vis-a-vis other epithelioid cell sarcomas) is aided in some cases by an obvious association between the tumor and a large cutaneous or subcutaneous nerve. However, it is complicated in other instances by the fact that epithelioid MPNST may show obvious melanin production by the neoplastic cells, in mimicry of melanotic neurilemmomas. The latter eventuality may produce great consternation in differential diagnosis with metastatic melanoma (particularly with its myxoid variant).[370] This problem is soluble only with electron microscopy or immunohistology. The first of these studies shows the generic ultrastructural features of MPNST (see earlier) but may indeed demonstrate premelanosomes in the pigmented elements. Immunohistologically, HMB-45 is not observed in epithelioid MPNST, as expected in truly melanocytic neoplasms.[139]

Malignant Granular Cell Tumors

Malignant cutaneous granular cell tumors (MGCT) are exceedingly uncommon, and fewer than 30 well-documented examples have been reported.[371–374] They have an average size of 4 cm and are seemingly restricted to adult patients, with a predominance in women.[246] Although no anatomic location is unknown as a site of origin for MGCT of the skin, the majority have occurred on the proximal extremities or trunk as subcuticular nodules or ill-defined plaques.

Recurrence after adequate surgical excision is the usual indicator that a granular cell tumor of the skin has aggressive biologic potential.[250] Metastases of MGCT have been seen in over 50% of reported cases, involving the regional lymph nodes, lungs, liver, bones, and brain. Mortality approximates 80%.[246]

The microscopic features of MGCT are closely similar to those of its benign counterpart, as described earlier. However, putative histologic signs of malignancy in such lesions include broad zones of spontaneous necrosis, obvious invasion of stromal blood vessels, and numerous mitotic figures with atypical forms.[246]

It is also likely that the gross size of the tumor plays a role in determining the biology of MGCT. Those tumors that are larger than 3 cm are at principal risk for recurrence or metastasis, providing that they also demonstrate the above-cited atypical microscopic features.[246]

Although most MGCT—like their benign counterparts—demonstrate a schwannian phenotype by electron microscopy and immunohistologic analysis,[375] a subset of granular cell tumors exists that is microscopically atypical and has an "uncommitted" immunophenotype.[250] These lesions are usually polypoid, with a maximum size of 2 cm or less. They may recur, but metastasis is unreported to date.

The differential diagnosis of MGCT of the skin includes other primary cutaneous neoplasms and also metastatic tumors with a granular-cell appearance. Leiomyosarcoma of the skin may have a predominantly granular cell phenotype, as may basal cell carcinoma.[250] Likewise, selected examples of metastatic renal cell carcinoma or mammary adenocarcinoma with granular cell change may simulate the appearance of primary MGCT of the skin.[376]

Malignant Rhabdoid Tumor of the Skin

Malignant rhabdoid tumor of the skin is another rare lesion, few cases of which have been reported.[377, 378] Therefore, its "typical" macroscopic features are uncertain at this time. Those examples that have been documented to date have taken the form of ill-defined nodules in the scalp or genital skin of adults, measuring several centimeters in greatest dimension.

In a generic sense, this neoplasm is extremely aggressive and often metastasizes widely. This feature characterizes the behavior of rhabdoid tumors of the viscera, which have been documented in the kidney, liver, uterus, oral cavity, urinary bladder, deep soft tissues, heart, and central nervous system.[379]

Malignant rhabdoid tumors are characterized by sheets and clusters of neoplastic cells with distinctive cytologic features. Nuclei are oval or round with vesicular chromatin and prominent nucleoli. The cytoplasm is amphophilic or eosinophilic and contains a characteristic "hyaline mass" of brightly eosinophilic, homogeneous material that displaces nuclei to eccentric positions within the cell (Fig. 13–64, see p. 814).[380]

In cutaneous sites, malignant rhabdoid tumor of the skin has been seen as a dermal or subcuticular proliferation. Cutaneous appendages were effaced in the former setting, and the lesions were ill-defined peripherally with irregular permeation of surrounding connective tissue.[377, 378] Mitotic activity is abundant in rhabdoid tumors, and atypical division figures are not uncommon.

Ultrastructurally, malignant rhabdoid tumors consistently show tight perinuclear aggregates of intermediate filaments, corresponding to the "hyaline masses" seen at a light microscopic level.[379, 380] Intercellular junctional complexes may be present as well. On the other hand, immunopathologic characteristics of these neoplasms have varied considerably, according to their topographic origins. In the skin, reactivity with antibodies to keratin, epithelial membrane antigen, vimentin, and carcinoembryonic antigen has been documented.[356, 378] In other anatomic locations, malignant rhabdoid tumors may also express glial fibrillary acidic protein, S100 protein, desmin, and muscle-specific actin. These attributes have led some authors to conclude that rhabdoid tumors do not represent a unified group of neoplasms with regard to cellular lineage.[379, 380] Instead, they propose that the rhabdoid phenotype is a "final common morphologic pathway" assumed by poorly differentiated tumors with dissimilar patterns of differentiation.[380] Indeed, in particular reference to the skin, it should also be remembered that malignant melanoma is also capable of assuming a "rhabdoid" appearance in primary or metastatic lesions.[380] Thus, an unqualified diagnosis of MRTS must follow the exclusion of melanocytic differentiation through appropriate special studies.

Angiosarcoma

Angiosarcoma of the skin is characteristically seen in one of several well-defined clinical contexts. These encompass idiopathic proliferations on the scalp or face of elderly patients; occurrence in a field of prior therapeutic irradiation after a lag period of 5 or more years; and development in an area of chronic cutaneous lymphedema (the so-called Stewart-Treves syndrome).[381] An exceedingly small minority of tumors do arise outside of the situations just cited, as lesions of the extremities or trunk in individuals with no apparent predisposing conditions.

Angiosarcomas likewise show a variety of macroscopic presentations. They may be large, multinodular, ill-defined, violaceous, bloody, and sometimes ulcerated masses; vague ecchymosis-like macular lesions; ligneous, "brawny" alterations in the skin that simulate erysipelas; and multifocal, seemingly discrete bluish-red nodules that imitate cavernous hemangiomas.[194]

The behavior of angiosarcoma is uniformly aggressive. Those patients whose neoplasms are less than 10 cm in maximum dimension may derive some benefit from radical surgical excision and postoperative irradiation, but almost all affected individuals will eventually die of unmanageable local tumor growth or distant metastases.[382]

In classic form, angiosarcoma is a disorganized proliferation of polyhedral atypical endothelial cells with hyperchromatic nuclei and scant amphophilic cytoplasm. The tumor cells mantle racemose, interconnecting, sieve-like vascular channels in the skin that dissect through dermal collagen and deeper tissues and contain luminal red blood cells (Fig. 13–65, see p. 814).[383–386] Cutaneous appendages are variably entrapped or destroyed by the proliferation; hemosiderin and chronic inflammatory cells may be interspersed throughout the lesion. Large tumors may ulcerate the overlying epidermis multifocally. Micropapillae of neoplastic cells are frequently seen projecting into the neovascular channels of angiosarcomas, and the supporting (stromal) blood vessels may also show nuclear atypia in endothelial cells. Mitotic activity is variable in scope but always present. Necrosis may or may not be observed.[384–386]

Several well-documented microscopic variants of angiosarcoma have been recognized. These include the spindle-cell subtype (as described earlier),[194, 362] a solid epithelioid form,[387] minimal-deviation (hemangioma-like) angiosarcoma,[388] a granular-cell variant,[389] and a pleomorphic subtype with the potential to simulate atypical fibroxanthoma or malignant fibrous histiocytoma.[381] Akiyama et al.[390] also reported two cases in which benign melanocytes and melanophages were intermixed with the neoplastic endothelial cells in the dermis.

Among these histologic forms, several merit further comment because they may be the sources of diagnostic error. Minimal-deviation angiosarcoma shows minimal cytologic atypia of constituent endothelial cells and forms more complete (tubular) vascular lumina in the upper dermis than those seen in other variants.[388] Nonetheless, specimens including the deep dermis and subcutis inevitably reveal the racemose dissecting endothelial profiles that are characteristic (Fig. 13–66, see p. 814). The danger here is in the interpretation of shallow punch biopsies or shave biopsies, such that minimal-deviation angiosarcomas may be mistaken for targetoid or microvenular hemangiomas. As described earlier, the latter hemangioma subtypes have a permeative pattern of growth in the dermis that mimics the superficial aspect of MDAS. Thus, all tumors demonstrating an atypical, disorganized pattern of neovasogenesis should be excised totally.

Epithelioid angiosarcoma is composed entirely or predominantly of plump polyhedral cells that imitate true epithelia.[381, 387] These occupy much of the lumen in vascular spaces formed by such lesions, and therefore the latter channels often contain few discernible erythrocytes and are not readily recognized as endothelial in nature.

Simulants of spindle-cell angiosarcoma were discussed earlier in connection with KS. Epithelioid vascular tumors may simulate true epithelial neoplasms (particularly "pseudovascular" or "angiomatoid" squamous carcinomas),[53, 391, 392] melanoma and clear-cell sarcoma, epithelioid sarcoma, epithelioid leiomyosarcoma, and large-cell lymphoma.[194] Pleomorphic variants of angiosarcoma can be confused with atypical fibroxanthoma, primary or metastatic undifferentiated carcinomas, melanoma, and malignant fibrous histiocytoma.[194] In these contexts, immunohistologic analysis is the most useful diagnostic tool. Endothelial tumors are reactive for vimentin, von Willebrand factor, CD31 and CD34 antigens, and *Ulex europaeus* I agglutinin receptors; they lack cytokeratin, epithelial membrane antigen, desmin, muscle-specific actin, and S100 protein, as seen in the alternatives just cited.[392, 393]

Pleomorphic Malignant Mesenchymal Tumors of the Skin

Atypical Fibroxanthoma

Atypical fibroxanthoma (AFX) of the skin was recognized and designated as such by Helwig in 1963.[394] It is seen principally in the sun-exposed skin areas of elderly patients, although 25% arise in ar-

eas of the trunk or extremities that are covered by clothing.[246] The ears, nose, and cheeks are the most frequent sites of origin. There is a male predominance of 2:1. Examples of AFX have been reported after previous therapeutic irradiation to the affected skin field.[365] In all cases, it is a nodular, protuberant, red-pink lesion with an average size of 2 cm and potential ulceration.[395–397] Some examples of AFX may attain a maximum size of up to 5 cm.

Even though it was initially considered to be a "pseudosarcoma" of the skin,[398] it is now apparent that AFX is a true neoplasm. Examples with repeated recurrence have been documented, as well as others that have metastasized to distant sites.[399, 400] The latter behaviors are admittedly rare, and most cases of AFX are cured by adequate surgical excision.[246] It may therefore be argued that discussion of this tumor entity would have been more appropriate in the section on borderline cutaneous neoplasms. Nevertheless, because of its many similarities to an indisputably malignant lesion—malignant fibrous histiocytoma,[401] as seen in deeper soft tissue sites—the decision was made to include AFX in this category.

Atypical fibroxanthoma is a dermally centered proliferation that usually abuts the epidermal basement membrane or is separated from it by only a narrow Grenz zone.[395] The lesion typically extends downward into the superficial subcutis or deeper; its peripheral borders are indistinct. Surrounding dermal actinic elastosis is usually striking.[395–397] The tumor cells are spindle-shaped, stellate, or multinucleated and pleomorphic, with hyperchromatic or vesicular chromatin, prominent nucleoli, and amphophilic cytoplasm (Fig. 13–67).[395, 397, 398, 402] They are arranged haphazardly or in vaguely storiform configurations. Mitotic activity is always brisk, and atypical division figures are usually present.[246] Small areas of spontaneous necrosis are observed in approximately 50% of cases, and foamy histiocytes may be admixed with the tumor cells surrounding these foci.

Rare examples of AFX have been reported in which "divergent" mesenchymal differentiation was apparent. For example, cases have been documented in which atypical chondro-osseous and osteoclast-like foci were evident.[403, 404] Extensively mxyoid stroma also may be seen. However, such findings do not seem to alter the behavior of these tumors.

Helwig and May[399] have shown that deep invasion by AFX into the subcutaneous fat or obvious permeation of blood vessels by the tumor is associated with the potential for recurrence and possible metastasis. Thus, lesions showing these attributes should be excised widely, with close patient monitoring thereafter.

Differential diagnosis of AFX is principally centered on the exclusion of two other tumors that may imitate this lesion to perfection: pleomorphic and spindle-cell ("sarcomatoid") squamous carcinoma of the skin[55, 65] and sarcomatoid malignant melanoma.[405] The presence of small foci with overt squamous differentiation or pigmentation in the latter neoplasms sometimes allows for their recognition by conventional microscopy. Nevertheless, this eventuality is uncommon. Hence, most pathologists now make the distinction among AFX, squamous carcinoma of the skin, and sarcomatoid malignant melanoma through the application of immunohistologic stains. Keratin reactivity separates squamous carcinomas from the other two possibilities, and a similar association exists between sarcomatoid malignant melanoma and positivity for S100 protein. AFX lacks both of these markers. All three neoplasms consistently express vimentin.[143, 405–408]

Summary of Immunohistochemical Findings in Malignant Mesenchymal Neoplasms of the Skin

To provide a synopsized reference on the immunopathologic features of malignant cutaneous mesenchymal tumors, algorithms pertaining to the generic categories presented above are shown in Figures 13–9, 13–68, and 13–69.

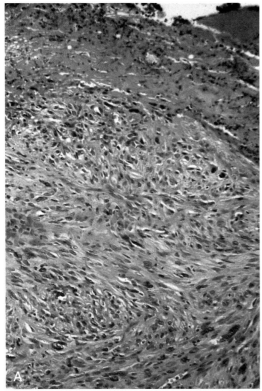

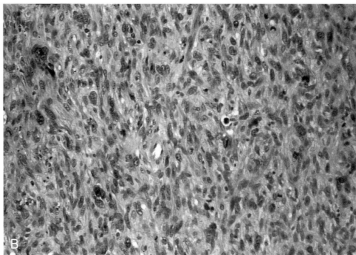

Figure 13–67. Atypical fibroxanthoma (AFX) of the facial skin showing surface ulceration (A) and a highly cellular proliferation of fusiform and pleomorphic elements in the dermis (B). The differential diagnosis centers around spindle cell squamous carcinoma and sarcomatous malignant melanoma.

▌ PSEUDONEOPLASTIC CUTANEOUS MESENCHYMAL PROLIFERATIONS

There are several reactive proliferations of mesenchymal cells in the skin and subcutis that may cause diagnostic consternation or be confused with true neoplasms. These are outlined in the following sections.

Nodular Fasciitis

Nodular fasciitis represents an idiosyncratic response to minor injury that is seen in the superficial soft tissues, primarily those of the distal extremities in children, adolescents, and young adults.[409] However, it has also been observed in other locations, including the oral cavity, salivary glands, and deep soft tissues, and may rarely oc-

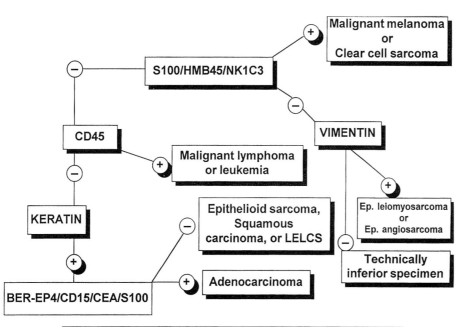

Figure 13–68. Algorithm for immunohistologic diagnosis of epithelioid malignancies of the skin beginning with keratin staining.

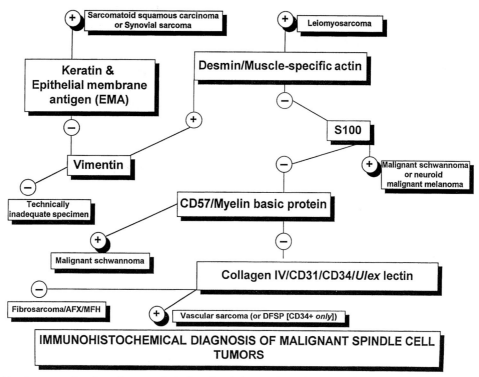

Figure 13–69. Algorithm for immunohistologic diagnosis of spindle-cell and pleomorphic malignancies of the skin beginning with keratin and epithelial membrane antigen staining.

cur in elderly individuals as well.[410] The typical clinical history is that of a very rapidly evolving mass that is slightly tender. The patient may or may not remember an episode of trauma to the area, because in some cases this is so minor that it escapes notice.[411] Differences in the clinical presentation of several clinical variants of the process are also determined by the site of the proliferation. Hence, *cranial fasciitis, intravascular fasciitis,* and *parosteal fasciitis*[412–414] may all be regarded as variations on the same pathologic theme.

Microscopically, nodular fasciitis is typified by a loosely fascicular, disorganized, or storiform proliferation of "activated" but cytologically bland fibroblasts and myofibroblasts; these contain ample amphophilic cytoplasm and oval nuclei with dispersed chromatin. The cells are separated from one another by variably edematous stroma with a myxoid aura, and acute and chronic inflammatory cells are often interspersed throughout (Fig. 13–70, see p. 815).[411] The proliferation has been said to exhibit a "tissue culture" appearance because of its dyshesive cellular nature.[409, 415] Supporting blood vessels are numerous, thin-walled, and capillary-sized, and zones of spontaneous erythrocytic extravasation are numerous.[410] Foci of keloidal-type matrical collagen are often seen in these lesions as well.

Small nucleoli may be seen in the proliferating cells of nodular fasciitis, and mitotic activity is characteristically brisk.[410, 416] The latter features largely account for the histopathologic confusion of this lesion with true sarcomas (primarily leiomyosarcoma or malignant fibrous histiocytoma). Nonetheless, the latter neoplasms are cytologically atypical, uncommonly contain inflammatory cells, and virtually never show prominent stromal erythrocyte extravasation as seen in nodular fasciitis.

Attention to these distinguishing microscopic features and characteristic clinical information will allow for the confident recognition of nodular fasciitis in the vast majority of cases. It may then be excised conservatively, and the patient may be reassured as to the reactive nature of the proliferation.

However, examples of nodular fasciitis do exist wherein organization (maturation) of the lesion obscures many of its salient fea-

tures and heightens a similarity to a true mesenchymal neoplasm. In these instances, it may truthfully be impossible to exclude the possibility of a low-grade sarcoma. Immunohistochemical analysis is of no assistance, because the myofibroblasts in nodular fasciitis share many points of antigenic similarity with tumor cells in leiomyosarcoma[336] (including reactivity for smooth-muscle actin, desmin, and vimentin). A practical solution to this dilemma is to recommend complete but conservative excision, with subsequent follow-up of the patient. Nodular fasciitis essentially never recurs, and lesional regrowth should be considered tantamount to an exclusion of this diagnosis.[416] In the circumstances just described, the pathologic interpretation of "myofibroblastic proliferation of uncertain biologic potential" is a prudent one.

Keloids and Hypertrophic Scars

Some individuals react to trauma idiosyncratically by the formation of other lesions that differ from nodular fasciitis. These are known as keloids and hypertrophic scars, and they are most often seen in non-white patients.[417] Minor abrasions, punctures, or lacerations may serve as the impetus for development of these proliferations, as may prior surgical procedures.[418] Clinically, one observes hard, variably sized nodules and plaques that attenuate the overlying epidermis and have a shiny red-pink appearance.[419]

The histologic appearance of hypertrophic scars and keloids is that of a continuum, wherein there are dense aggregates of dermal fibroblasts and the collagenous matrix that they produce. Cutaneous appendages and overlying rete ridges are usually effaced, and there is commonly a peripheral zone of capillary proliferation and scant chronic inflammation at the border of the lesion.[417] As hypertrophic scars mature, their high level of cellularity gives way to the accumulation of hyalinized, brightly eosinophilic collagen that is arranged haphazardly in broad bands in the dermis and superficial subcutis. The latter stage typifies the fully formed keloid.[418]

Inflammatory Pseudotumors of the Skin

Several examples have been described of an unusual dermal proliferation designated *inflammatory pseudotumor of the skin.*[420] Patients
with this condition were all adults, who presented with nodular, nontender, flesh-colored or pink tumefactions on the neck or extremities.
There was no history of trauma or other possibly predisposing conditions, and the lesional sizes ranged from 0.8 to 1.3 cm. Microscopically, pseudoencapsulated uninodular proliferations of bland fibroblasts and stromal venule- or capillary-sized blood vessels were
apparent in the deep dermis and subcutis, admixed with abundant
mature collagen fibers (Fig. 13–71, see p. 815). Numerous lymphocytes and plasma cells were interspersed throughout, with lesser
numbers of neutrophils and eosinophils. In 50% of cases, well-
formed germinal centers were evident at the lesional peripheries.[420]
Many of the supporting blood vessels in inflammatory pseudotumor
of the skin showed a concentric adventitial cuff of hyalinized
collagen, yielding a "targetoid" configuration. Immunostaining for
S100 protein demonstrated many intralesional Langerhans' cells as
well.

The major differential diagnostic considerations in cases of inflammatory pseudotumor of the skin include nodular fasciitis, angiolymphoid hyperplasia with eosinophilia, Kimura's disease, and
lymphocyte-rich dermatofibromas. The unique conjunction of com-
pactly proliferating fibroblasts and well-organized lymphoplasmacytic infiltrates serves to distinguish inflammatory pseudotumors
from other pathologic entities.

Malformations

A heritable condition, *Cowden's disease* (an autosomal-dominant
syndrome typified by facial trichilemmomas, hamartomatous or gan-
glioneuromatous intestinal polyposis, oral papillomatosis, and an increased risk of visceral carcinomas [see section on trichilemmo-
mas]), is associated with peculiar hamartomatous fibrous cutaneous
proliferations. They have been termed *storiform collagenoma* or
sclerotic fibroma[421] and present as nondescript, firm, single or
grouped nodules or papules, usually in the facial skin. Multifocality
constitutes strong evidence favoring the presence of the syndromic
complex.[421] This dermal lesion is sharply circumscribed histologically; it is characterized by hyalinized hypocellular fascicles of collagen that "spin" around one another like the blades of a pinwheel
(Fig. 13–72). Similar to the shagreen patch, isolated storiform collagenoma may also occur in patients with no familial or personal
evidence of syndromic disease.[422]

Common *acrochordons* ("skin tags") are almost ubiquitous
mesenchymal nevi that may affect any skin field at any age; they are
soft, polypoid, papillomatous lesions with a narrow stalk.[423] Some
acrochordons undoubtedly represent intradermal melanocytic nevi
that are undergoing resolution by extrusion, as supported by the occasional observation of small nests of nevocytes in these proliferations. Others may be regressing seborrheic keratoses.[424] The usual
case shows only a bland fibrovascular connective tissue core that is
mantled by slightly papillomatous epidermis[423]; however, rare cases
show an alarming degree of cytologic atypia in their mesenchymal
constituents (presumably due to repeated trauma). These lesions
have been termed *pseudosarcomatous polyps* by Williams et al.[425]

One vascular connective tissue nevus—*nevus flammeus* ("port
wine stain")—is relatively common in the general population,[426, 427]
but it is most well-known for its association with other pathologic
elements of the Sturge-Weber, Klippel-Trenauney-Weber, or Parkes-
Weber syndromes.[194, 427, 428] Clinically, nevus flammeus takes the
form of a variably prominent red-violet patch or plaque that is usually confined to one side of the body. It may be relatively inconspicuous or involve a large portion of the skin surface; the latter
eventuality is most often observed in syndromic rather than sporadic
cases.[427]

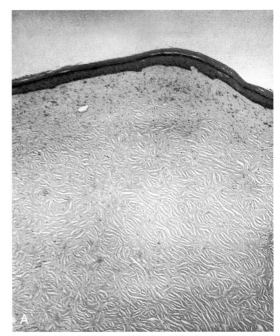

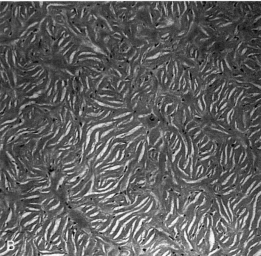

Figure 13–72. *A*, Storiform collagenoma (sclerotic fibroma), represented by
a circumscribed, hypocellular, nodular lesion of the dermis. *B*, The pinwheel-
like arrangement of the matrical collagen is obvious in this photograph.

The histologic appearance of this lesion is that of dermal telangiectasia, rather than a true hemangioma. Dilated vascular spaces of
varying sizes are dispersed throughout the corium, separated by relatively normal connective tissue and cutaneous appendages.[426] With
advancing age of the patient, the telangiectatic vessels may increase
in caliber so that they resemble large veins. In children, however,
this vascular malformation is often subtle, being composed of attenuated capillaries in the superficial dermis.[427]

Cutaneous telangiectasias are also part of the Osler-Weber-
Rendu syndrome, in association with vascular abnormalities of the
mucosae, ears, and nail beds. This autosomal dominant complex presents itself in adolescence or young adulthood as a generalized profusion of tiny macular or papular red lesions. Hemorrhage from the
nose and gut is potentially life-threatening in the Osler-Weber-
Rendu syndrome. The microscopic characteristics of the disease are
analogous to those of early-stage nevus flammeus, being represented
by numerous small-caliber, thin-walled blood vessels that are randomly distributed throughout the corium or the submucosa of the
oral cavity.[429] Similar lesions may appear sporadically during preg-

nancy in young women, or as acquired dermatomal eruptions in middle adulthood.[430, 431]

Lesions that Simulate Kaposi's Sarcoma

As a byproduct of the AIDS pandemic and consequently increased interest in vascular lesions of the skin, several non-neoplastic proliferations have been identified that may simulate Kaposi's sarcoma. In head and neck sites, these include proliferating dermal scars and reactions to the application of Monsel's solution.

Not uncommonly, biopsies of proliferating scars (following episodes of injury that the patient may not remember) are performed under the impression that these lesions represent cutaneous neoplasms. The resulting histologic profile is essentially that of organizing granulation tissue, featuring a regimented proliferation of capillaries and venules that are typically oriented vertically within the dermis.[361] Proliferation of intervening fibroblasts and myofibroblasts is frequent, with variable edema or dense collagen deposition in the surrounding dermal stroma. If the scar has been traumatized, red cell leakage and hemosiderin deposition may again be observed. Nonetheless, the overall image of this lesion is only superficially like that of KS, and diagnostic separation of the two conditions is typically straightforward.

The characteristics of reactions to the application of Monsel's solution (a dermatologic surgical styptic) are also closely similar to those of proliferating scars. Because this pharmaceutical includes iron salts, large irregular or rhomboidal clusters of iron pigment are also observed in tissue reactions to Monsel's preparation.[432]

An extremely interesting condition that has been recognized for only a few years is that known as *bacillary (epithelioid) angiomatosis*.[433–435] It is observed in patients who are infected with HIV, leading to particular concern that they have KS. Red-violet cutaneous nodules and plaques of variable sizes are seen in this disorder, without topographic predilections. The viscera also may be involved, heightening the mimicry of KS.[436]

Nevertheless, the histologic features of bacillary angiomatosis differ substantially from those of KS and are instead more similar to those of epithelioid hemangioma. Organized sheets or clusters of completely formed vascular channels are observed in the dermis, with indistinctly lobular profiles; an epidermal collarette is rather frequently seen at the lateral borders of the proliferation. Constituent endothelial cells are plump with abundant cytoplasm and bland nuclear features (Fig. 13–73, see p. 815), although mitotic activity and limited foci of necrosis may be apparent.[433–435] Intralesional

neutrophilia is a distinctive finding.[348] Close examination of the cells shows granular cytoplasmic inclusions that represent clusters of bacilliform organisms.[433–435] These have been shown to bear a taxonomic relationship to the cat-scratch agent (genus *Bartonella*), and they may be highlighted with the Warthin-Starry stain.[433, 435] Virtually identical cutaneous lesions are also seen in association with infection by another species of *Bartonella* in South American patients with Carrion's disease (verruga peruana, or bartonellosis).[437, 438]

Treatment of bacillary angiomatosis with appropriate antibiotics results in resolution of the disease.[433] Thus, pathologic confusion of this process with KS is a particularly egregious error.

A related but histologically dissimilar cutaneous proliferation is seen in patients with AIDS who are infected with atypical mycobacteria. In this context, spindle-cell lesions of the skin may be observed that emulate nodular KS.[439] They are composed of dermal fibroblast-like cells arranged in whorling fascicles, admixed with bands of sclerotic collagen, lymphocytes, and plasma cells. Careful scrutiny of the cytoplasm in the fusiform elements reveals granular inclusions that represent clumps of mycobacteria. These may be further delineated with Ziehl-Nielsen or Fite stains.[439] Appropriate antibiotic treatment of such spindle-cell reactions to mycobacteria results in only variable resolution of the lesions, but they clearly should not be confused with KS.

Potential Simulators of Angiosarcoma

There are two non-neoplastic cutaneous proliferations that may be mistaken for angiosarcoma by the unwary pathologist: papillary intravascular endothelial hyperplasia (PIEH; Masson's vegetant intravascular hemangioendothelioma)[440, 441] and rudimentary or true meningoceles (see earlier discussion).[317, 442, 443] Both lesions occur in well-defined clinical settings that differ markedly from those attending angiosarcomas. PIEH is seen as a consequence of trauma and thrombosis within pre-existing hematomas, hemangiomas, varices, or otherwise dilated blood vessels, usually on the distal extremities.[440] Meningoceles are dysraphic dermal or subcuticular malformations of infants and children that are situated near the midline of the body.[442, 443]

Microscopic examination of PIEH shows a racemose proliferation of bland endothelial cells that mantles hyalinized pseudopapillary cores of organized fibrinous thrombotic material (Fig. 13–74).[440, 441] Low-power assessment clearly demonstrates sharp confinement of the lesion to the lumen of a thrombosed hematoma

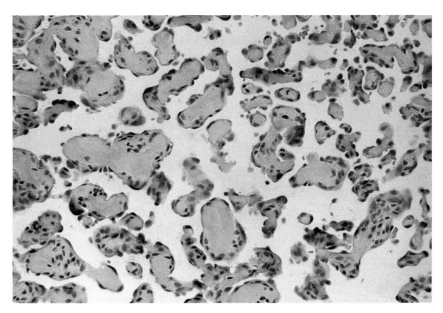

Figure 13–74. Intravascular papillary endothelial hyperplasia, showing the mantling of a recanalizing fibrin-rich endovascular thrombus by endothelial cells.

or a large vein or artery. The latter point is crucial to correct interpretation, because the internal aspects of PIEH may otherwise easily be mistaken for those of a low-grade angiosarcoma.[441]

Meningoceles are composed of flattened or low-cuboidal polyhedral cells that permeate the dermis in a "dissecting" fashion, with formation of internal pseudovascular spaces (Fig. 13–75, see p. 816). Focal aggregates of lesional cells may have a concentrically lamellated appearance, and microcalcifications of the psammomatous type also may be identified.[317, 442, 443] Rudimentary meningoceles arise almost exclusively in the skin of the scalp or posterior neck,[442] whereas true meningoceles of the skin may be encountered anywhere along the neuraxis.[443] The former of these malformations lacks histologic components other than those just described, but true meningoceles also may exhibit the presence of admixed glia, choroid plexus, fetal muscle, and embryonic vascular proliferations.[443] Meningeal lesions are uniformly immunoreactive for epithelial membrane antigen (EMA), but they lack endothelial markers.[317, 442] The converse of this profile is expected in true vascular neoplasms.

LYMPHOID LESIONS OF THE HEAD AND NECK

Benign Lymphoid Infiltrates

One of the most difficult differential diagnostic problems in cutaneous pathology is the separation of exuberant lymphoid hyperplasias—formerly given such names as lymphadenoma benigna cutis, Jessner's infiltrate, lymphocytoma cutis, and Spiegler-Fendt lesions—from malignant lymphomas arising in or affecting the scalp and facial skin.[444–449] Other benign lymphoreticular disorders that may be particularly troublesome for the pathologist include actinic reticuloid, drug-induced pseudolymphomas, Kikuchi's disease, and florid reactions to arthropod bites.[445, 448, 450, 451] As outlined by Banks,[444] there are several histologic features that one may cite to justify categorizing a cutaneous lymphoid infiltrate as benign or malignant. These include such findings as extensive epidermal damage, heterogeneity of the cellular infiltrate, and the presence of a "top-heavy" lymphoid population (Fig. 13–76, see p. 816) containing tingible-body macrophages on the benign side. Conversely, cellular monotony, a lack of epidermal reaction, extensive "dissection" of dermal collagen (Fig. 13–77), and a "bottom-heavy" profile argue for an interpretation of lymphoma. All of the various grades and recognized groups of lymphoreticular malignancies do indeed affect the

skin fields under discussion here,[445, 449, 452] and these can be discussed in three main categories as detailed subsequently.

Immunohistologic evaluation is often effective at resolving problems in this context, in cases in which "conventional" morphologic studies are nondiagnostic; hence, the results of this procedure are reviewed in some detail in the ensuing text, as applied in the context of histologic indeterminacy in lymphoid lesions of the skin. If immunophenotyping likewise proves to be indecisive, analysis of the infiltrate for immunoglobulin heavy-chain gene rearrangement or aberrations in the δ or γ T-cell-receptor genes may be undertaken by Southern blot technology or the polymerase chain reaction.[453–456]

Epidermotropic Infiltrates with the Pattern of Mycosis Fungoides

Selected drug-induced pseudolymphomatous infiltrates, chronic lichenoid and spongiotic dermatitides, and actinic reticuloid are those conditions that principally have the capacity to mimic mycosis fungoides (MF) histologically.[452] This is so because they may feature the presence of grouped lymphocytes in the epidermis as well as the dermal interstitium, and such cells commonly demonstrate at least a modest degree of "activation" and nuclear atypia. Nearly universally, these elements are also T cells, as are the proliferating cells of MF.[450, 452]

If it is available, frozen tissue can be studied immunohistologically to assess the presence or absence of an aberrant T-cell phenotype. Its absence is said to be defined by the loss of one or more pan-T-cell determinants (CD2, CD3, CD5, and CD7), or by the coexpression of antigens that are usually mutually exclusive (e.g., both CD4 and CD8 in the same cell population).[453, 454] CD7 is the pan-T-cell antigen cluster that is most often lost in MF, which is characteristically a proliferation of CD4+ cells.[453, 454] Nonetheless, this is not a universal finding in cutaneous T-cell lymphoma, and it has been reported in benign inflammatory conditions as well.[454] On the other hand, actinic reticuloid and most other chronic dermatitides do usually retain pan-T-cell markers and, with rare exceptions,[448] are composed predominantly of CD8+ lymphocytes.[451] Drug-induced pseudo-MF may have an immunophenotype like that of chronic spongiotic dermatitis, or it may simulate the profile of MF perfectly.[450] If the latter fact is disheartening, it is made more so by the knowledge that even genotyping studies may show T-cell receptor gene rearrangements in drug-related pseudolymphomas that are

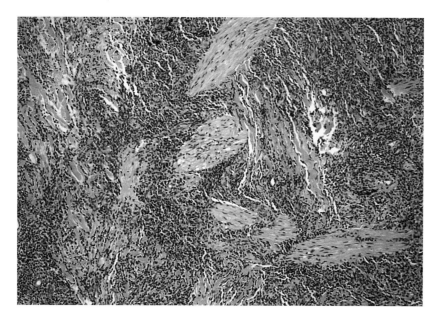

Figure 13–77. Effacement of the dermis by a peripheral T-cell lymphoma of the facial skin.

like those observed in MF.[455] In the final analysis, withdrawal of all medications—within feasible boundaries—and continued clinical surveillance over time may be the only means whereby pseudo-MF and true cutaneous T-cell lymphoma (CTCL) can be distinguished from one another in selected cases.

Paraffin sections are much less suitable substrates for the immunohistologic separation of benign and malignant T-cell infiltrates of the skin. This is so because the pan-T-cell antibodies that can be applied to fixed tissues (e.g., anti-CD3; Leu22/L60/MT-1 [the CD43 cluster]; and UCHL-1 [CD45R0]) are not as sensitive or specific as those used with frozen sections[456]; moreover, potential paraffin section markers of T-cell subsets were, until very recently, limited to one reagent—OPD4.[457] This antibody is putatively specific for CD4+ cells, but even this claim has been seriously questioned.[458] In any event, I have found in preliminary pilot studies that OPD4-positive intra-epidermal lymphoid infiltrates that also show concurrent negativity for CD3, CD43, or CD45R0 are more often seen in MF than in benign T-cell infiltrates of the skin. Nevertheless, these observations will require further validation before they can be applied confidently in a diagnostic setting. Currently, another monoclonal antibody with putative CD8-specificity[459] is also available commercially (clone C8/144B), but it has not undergone rigorous sensitivity and specificity testing as yet in the context under discussion.

Deep Lymphoid Infiltrates with the Pattern of Small-Cell or Mixed B-Cell Lymphomas

Generally speaking, "bulky" deep lymphoid infiltrates of the dermis and subcutis (Fig. 13–78) raise the specter of a B-cell lymphoma, rather than one of CTCL or peripheral T-cell lymphoma.[445, 448, 460, 461] Some of the former conditions are relatively easy to dispatch in short order as benign disorders, because they are composed principally of T-lymphocytes or show an admixture of B and T cells. Such lesions include Jessner's infiltrates, active cutaneous lupus erythematosus, and inflammatory cutaneous "pseudotumors."[416, 420, 446] However, other infiltrates such as lymphadenoma benigna cutis, lymphocytoma cutis, and follicular variants of cutaneous lymphoid hyperplasia (CLH) do, in fact, contain a large number of B lymphocytes and are capable of causing substantial diagnostic consternation.[445, 448, 460, 462]

Frozen section studies are helpful if they show restriction of λ or κ light chain immunoglobulin expression by the constituent B

cells.[463] By convention, this profile must demonstrate a ratio of at least 10:1 with respect to one light chain over the other.

Unfortunately, light chain immunostains are among the most difficult to perform technically, and they are often uninterpretable in even the best of laboratories. For that reason, our laboratory recently undertook an analysis of other determinants that might be used successfully in separating B-cell lymphomas from variants of CLH. In particular, attention was directed at the preferential use of paraffin sections, because these still constitute the substrates with which most pathologists deal on a daily basis. Results of this evaluation showed that B-cell lymphoma was the likely diagnosis when CD20 (detected by the antibody L26) and CD43 were coexpressed by the same population of lymphocytes; when 75% or more of the infiltrate marked as B cells; and when more than 30% of the cells were positive for proliferating cell nuclear antigen (PCNA).[464] The diagnostic standard for such conclusions was the clinical outcome of the study cases after long-term surveillance. These results parallel others obtained by Ngan et al.[465] in an analysis of extracutaneous lymphoid lesions.

The utility of another currently popular marker—the bcl-2 protein—has been analyzed in several recent studies of cutaneous lymphoid infiltrates. This moiety is an inhibitor of apoptosis, and it is overexpressed in malignant lymphoid cells that demonstrate a t(14;18) chromosomal translocation.[466] The latter is most characteristically seen in follicular small-cleaved-cell lymphomas. However, it would appear that bcl-2 protein has very limited differential diagnostic usefulness in the context of cutaneous lymphoproliferations. Many examples of CLH, CTCL, and various B-cell lymphomas of the skin are positive for bcl-2 protein, and one must restrict attention to only overtly follicular proliferations to realize any benefit from this marker.[467] As expected, follicular CLH is negative for bcl-2 protein, whereas follicular lymphomas are nearly universally positive.[466]

Cutaneous Large-Cell Lymphoproliferations

Occasional examples of follicular CLH may contain such a strikingly high number of reactive immunoblasts that they mimic the microscopic appearance of a nodular B-cell lymphoma of the large-cell type.[445, 448] Similarly, Kikuchi's disease—a rare benign lymphoproliferative disorder that is much more often seen in Asia than in the United States—is also composed of large atypical lymphoid elements that may cause confusion with a malignant process.[468]

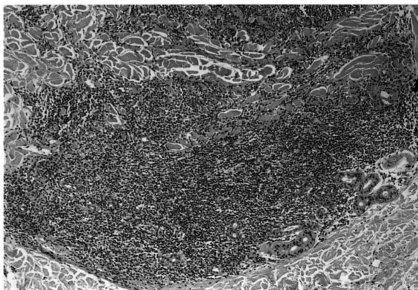

Figure 13–78. Deep infiltration of the dermis by vaguely follicular aggregates of neoplastic lymphoid cells in B-cell lymphoma cutis of the scalp.

In the first of these scenarios, that of florid follicular CLH, a correct diagnosis is greatly aided by routinely applying a broad panel of immunostains. These demonstrate a large number of B cells among the large cell population, but they also show the presence of normal follicular mantles, interfollicular zones rich in T cells, and accentuation of PCNA- or Ki-67-reactivity in the central aspects of the follicular aggregates. In other words, the results mirror those seen in lymph nodal hyperplasia. It should also be remembered with caution that CD30—a marker that may be associated with some large-cell lymphomas[469–471]—is also potentially seen in benign immunoblastic proliferations in the skin and elsewhere.[470] Therefore, the presence of this determinant should never be used as sole support for a diagnosis of lymphoid malignancy.

Kikuchi's disease features the presence of large, atypical mononuclear cells in the dermis, admixed with neutrophils and zones of necrosis (Fig. 13–79, see p. 816); as such, it is a potential imitator of a subtype of anaplastic large-cell lymphoma.[472] However, Kikuchi's disease is apparently a true histiocytic proliferation; it is correspondingly labeled by the monoclonal antibody MAC-387 and those in the CD68 group (e.g., KP-1), but not by CD20 or pan-T-cell reagents. Inasmuch as examples of cutaneous "malignant histiocytosis" have essentially vanished in the wake of nosologic reclassification occasioned by new technologies,[469] the latter findings constitute strong evidence for the presence of a benign disorder.

Cutaneous Large-Cell Lymphomas with Distinctive Histologic Features

Two forms of cutaneous large-cell lymphoma have unusual microscopic appearances that set them apart from other tumors in the same category. These lesions are represented by anaplastic large-cell (CD30+) lymphoma (ALCL)[469, 471, 473] and intravascular lymphomatosis (IVL; angiotropic large-cell lymphoma), which was formerly termed *malignant angioendotheliomatosis*.[474–476]

Anaplastic large-cell lymphoma encompasses the clinicopathologic entities that were once called "malignant histiocytosis" and "regressing atypical histiocytosis." Clinically, primary disease in the skin is often indolent, with lesions that may regress spontaneously. Otherwise, the appearance of ALCL is typical of malignant hematopoietic diseases of the skin, with violaceous or reddish plaques and nodules that may ulcerate. Histologically, one observes a markedly pleomorphic population of large polygonal or round cells with greatly heterogeneous nuclear shapes (Fig. 13–80, see p. 817). Mitoses are numerous and can be pathologically shaped; unlike other forms of lymphoma, ALCL also may exhibit large zones of geographic necrosis. Variants with myxoid stroma and spindle-cell change also have been documented.[471]

Immunohistologic peculiarities also distinguish ALCL from other non-Hodgkin's lymphomas of the skin. Up to 15% of cases may lack CD45 antigens; this feature, together with potential immunoreactivity for EMA (and even rarely for keratin)[477] make ALCL particularly prone to misdiagnosis as an anaplastic carcinoma.[471] Thus, inclusion of antibodies against CD30 is especially important in the evaluation of poorly differentiated cutaneous tumors. Another singular attribute of ALCL is its manifestation of a t(2;5) chromosomal translocation.[478] Although this tumor may be difficult to distinguish from Hodgkin's disease in lymph nodal sites, the extreme rarity of the latter disorder in the skin greatly lessens the importance of this problem in regard to cutaneous lesions. Lineage-related markers show that ALCL is composed of a mixture of T-cell, B-lymphocytic, and null-cell proliferations,[471, 473] but this does not appear to affect tumor behavior.

Intravascular lymphomatosis similarly assumes the clinical appearance that characterizes all cutaneous lymphomas.[474, 475] Nevertheless, there are several potential findings in this systemic disease that do distinguish it from other hematopoietic proliferations. The random intravascular growth of tumor cells in IVL may produce infarctive lesions in many viscera, yielding such manifestations as unusual dementia, multifocal sensorimotor deficits, pulmonary hypertension, Addison's disease, and renal failure.[476]

Microscopically, IVL usually demonstrates strict endovascular confinement of large, dyshesive, obviously malignant polygonal cells with irregular nuclear contours (Fig. 13–81). All types of dermal and subcutaneous blood vessels are potentially affected. Fibrin thrombi may be admixed with the malignant cells. Extravascular "seepage" of the neoplastic elements is observed in a small proportion of cases; when this occurs in the subcutis, the resulting histologic image is that of "stromal dissection" as seen in virtually all soft tissue lymphomas.

Intravascular lymphomatosis is predominantly a B-cell disease, although occasional examples have instead expressed T-lymphocytic phenotypes.[479, 480] This difference again plays no apparent role in the determination of tumor biology.

Clinicopathologic Correlations

One of the particularly irksome attributes of lymphoid lesions of the skin in the head and neck is that they appear to evolve differently than morphologically identical proliferations in other cutaneous fields. For example, patients with obvious primary follicular large-

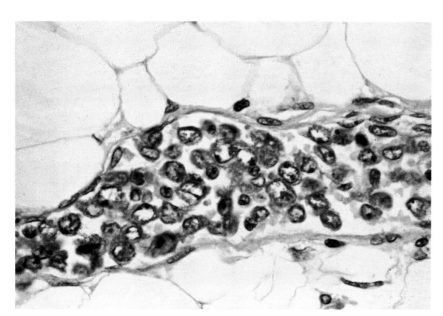

Figure 13–81. Strict confinement of malignant cells to the vascular lumina is typical of intravascular lymphomatosis, as seen in this facial lesion.

cell, mixed-cell, or large-cell anaplastic non-Hodgkin's lymphomas of the head and neck often pursue an indolent course that differs little from the course of lymphoid hyperplasias, despite administration of relatively unaggressive therapy.[445] Why this phenomenon occurs is unclear at present, and it is disheartening that there are no reliable evaluations that can identify those lymphomas in this subgroup that will instead become disseminated and ultimately prove fatal. On the other hand, patients with IVL do suffer from rapid progression of the tumor unless treated promptly and assiduously with multiagent chemotherapy.

▪ MELANOCYTIC PROLIFERATIONS

Because of the undoubted influence of solar skin damage on the development of melanocytic proliferations, these lesions are particularly common in the head and neck. Banal and variant nevi, lentigines, and malignant melanomas are all encountered in this topographic area.

Conventional Melanocytic Lesions

Ordinary nevi arising in the skin of the head and neck do not differ appreciably from those seen in other anatomic sites. Intradermal and compound melanocytic lesions demonstrate minor thematic variations, such as neurotization, papillomatous extrusion, fatty metaplasia, and immunologic lysis (the so-called halo phenomenon).[481] Junctional nevi may assume an extensively lentiginous appearance—potentially causing concern over a diagnosis of lentigo maligna[482] (melanoma-in-situ; see later)—but, if these proliferations retain their usual degree of intercellular cohesion and nuclear typicality, their recognition as innocuous lesions should be straightforward. Lentigines of the solar and "simple" types differ from one another mainly by the presence or absence (respectively) of dermal actinic elastosis and hyperplasia of the epidermal rete.[483] Otherwise, both forms of lentigo demonstrate a non-nested basal proliferation of bland melanocytes that contain an increased amount of cytoplasmic pigment.

Giant Congenital Nevi

Any form of melanocytic nevus may occur as a congenital tumor, demonstrating a tendency to grow into or along dermal appendages or neurovascular structures. However, a few of these lesions assume giant proportions and, as such, are removed for cosmetic or putatively prophylactic reasons.[484] In regard to the latter of these indications, it has been stated that approximately 4% to 10% of giant congenital nevi undergo malignant transformation, and, therefore, all of these lesions should be removed.[485] Although this phenomenon undoubtedly does occur, my experience has shown it to apply to fewer than 1% of giant congenital nevi. Many of the proliferations that were formerly interpreted as melanomas in this context probably represented the cellular atypia that so commonly characterizes congenital nevi in young children.[486, 487] This includes slight cellular dyshesion, modest nuclear hyperchromasia, and the placement of occasional nevocytes above the epidermal basal layer. Such observations have no importance in prepubertal patients.

Some congenital nevi are complex, including other elements besides melanocytes. The most well known of these is Becker's nevus,[488] which is an amalgam of smooth muscular, melanocytic, and, to some degree, epidermal-keratinocytic elements.

Blue Nevi

Blue nevi only uncommonly arise in the skin of the head and neck. These tumors are composed of elongated, densely pigmented, fusiform melanocytes that are arranged in fascicles or haphazard configurations in the middle to deep dermis and subcutis (Fig. 13–82, see p. 817).[489] Because of these characteristics and the Tindall effect on reflected light, blue nevi have a blue-black appearance clinically. The nuclear features of the proliferating cells are bland, with few if any mitoses. Occasionally, a more densely cellular appearance is present, with areas of "shoulder-to-shoulder" growth of the nevocytes, more sparse pigmentation, and modest nuclear enlargement. Such attributes serve to define cellular blue nevi,[490] which are nonetheless harmless biologically. Only if a significant element of deeply seated mitotic activity, marked nuclear atypia, or regional necrosis is seen should a diagnosis of malignant blue nevus be entertained.[491]

Nevi of Ota and Ito

So-called nevi of Ota and Ito are basically misdirected migration products of melanocytic (neural crest) maldevelopment rather than true nevi.[492] These lesions are, for unknown reasons, largely confined to patients of color, in whom they present as vaguely defined blue-black or gray patches on the face, the base of the neck, or the trunk. Microscopically, one sees heavily pigmented, stellate or fusiform melanocytes and melanophages that are randomly scattered in a fibrous background in the dermis or hypodermis. Nuclei are compact and mitoses are never present.

Deep Penetrating Nevi

Deep penetrating nevi are relatively recently characterized melanocytic tumors that are capable of assuming worrisome clinical or pathologic appearances. They measure between 1 and 3 cm macroscopically and are variably melaninized. Histologically, the hallmarks of deep penetrating nevi include a wedge-shaped dermal configuration (with the widest aspect being at the dermoepidermal interface); a composition by compact polygonal or bluntly spindled cells; irregular pigmentation; the occasional presence of small nucleoli; and, as its name suggests, permeating and plexiform growth into the lower reticular dermis or subcutaneous tissue (Fig. 13–83).[493–495] Again, obvious nuclear atypia, necrosis, or deeply placed mitoses should call a diagnosis of deep penetrating nevi into serious question and instead suggest the possibility of malignant melanoma.

Spitz (Spindled and Epithelioid Cell) Nevi

Spitz nevi occur predominantly in children, adolescents, and young adults, accounting for the unfortunate and now obsolete synonym of "juvenile melanoma" that was applied in the seminal works on these tumors.[496, 497] Clinically, Spitz nevi are papulonodular, well-circumscribed lesions that often have a pink-red appearance rather than a pigmented one. They usually measure less than 1 cm in greatest dimension. At a microscopic level, there are several distinctive features of such neoplasms. The tumor cells have a fusiform or plump epithelioid configuration, usually with moderately abundant eosinophilic cytoplasm that may have a granular or "hyaline" nature. Nuclei are vesicular or show dispersed chromatin; however, it is important to remember that discernible nucleoli and mitotic activity near the dermoepidermal junction are expected elements in Spitz nevi.[486, 498] Additional hallmarks include the presence of complex overlying epidermal hyperplasia—which "embraces" the melanocytic nests in the dermis—clefting of dermal melanocytic theques away from the basal epidermis, and the possible observation of intranuclear cytoplasmic invaginations or eosinophilic globules (Kamino bodies) at the epidermal basement membrane zone (Figs. 13–84 and 13–85, see p. 818).[499]

Spitz nevi are quintessentially symmetrical tumors. When they are composed solely of fusiform cells, they are often oriented vertically in groups, yielding a "raining down" image. Occasional variants have a densely sclerotic collagenous tumoral matrix.[500]

Some caveats must be borne in mind regarding the diagnosis of Spitz nevus. Because it shows such a predilection for young patients, extreme caution should be exercised before assigning this diagnostic label to an acquired lesion in a middle-aged or elderly adult. Indeed most "spitzoid" melanocytic tumors in such individuals also demonstrate asymmetry, deep mitoses, and focally marked nuclear atypia, and instead represent nevus-like melanomas[491] (see later discussion). The latter points touch upon a body of literature on "malignant" or "metastasizing" Spitz nevi.[501] In my view, those terms are oxymoronic and confusing to clinicians and should not be used. Similarly, "atypical Spitz nevus" is a designation that should rarely, if ever, be employed. When some—but not all—of the features of Spitz nevus are seen in a melanocytic proliferation, another more appropriate label (e.g., intradermal nevus, nevoid melanoma, or melanocytic proliferation of indeterminate biology) should be chosen, and the other microscopic peculiarities of the case can be included in a written comment.

Some junctional nevi have the cytologic attributes of Spitz nevi, but they show no intradermal elements and tend to exhibit a greater degree of melanin pigmentation. Such lesions are also known as *pigmented spindle cell nevi of Reed* (Fig. 13–86).[502]

Incompletely Excised Nevi

A practice that has increased with disturbing magnitude over the past several years is the incomplete removal of pigmented lesions by clinicians, often using punch or "shave" biopsies.[503] This is a deplorable approach to such tumors, for two reasons. First, it is well known that melanocytic proliferations may exhibit substantial regional variability in histology, such that a malignant melanoma may indeed exist focally therein but is missed through sampling error. Second, "recurrent" (actually *persistent and regrowing*) nevi often show atypical and confusing microscopic patterns that are occasioned by tissue repair in the wake of the prior surgical insult.[504–506] This response incurs the potential to either underestimate or overestimate the biologic potential of the proliferation (usually the latter). Therefore, excisional biopsy of all pigmented tumors should be strongly encouraged, and it may well be necessary to include a disclaimer regarding sampling artifact in reports on incompletely removed nevi.

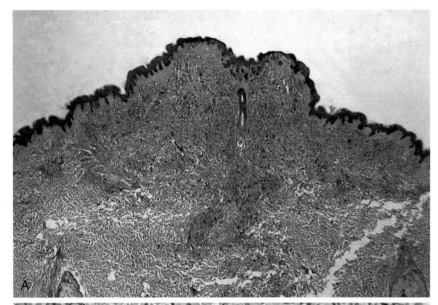

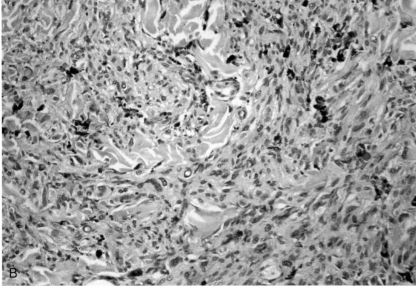

Figure 13–83. Deep penetrating nevus of the scalp, showing a wedge-shaped lesion with its base at the epidermal basement membrane *(A)*. Fascicular and plexiform arrangement of bland spindled melanocytes with variable melaninization is apparent in this lesion *(B)*.

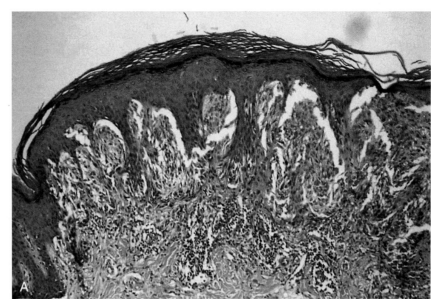

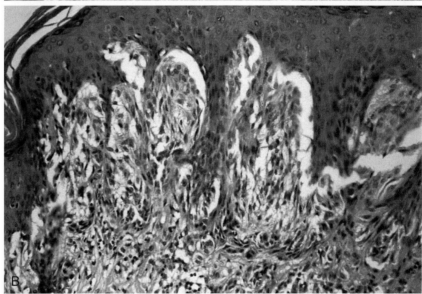

Figure 13–86. Pigmented spindle cell (Reed's) nevus, demonstrating numerous architectural similarities to Spitz nevi *(A)* but confinement to the dermoepidermal zone *(B)*.

Architecturally Disordered Nevi and Other Atypical Melanocytic Proliferations

Some examples of virtually all melanocytic nevus subtypes—intradermal, junctional, and compound—show atypical histologic or cytologic features, or both. When a predefined constellation of microscopic findings is observed, the term *architecturally disordered nevus* may be rightly applied. Criteria for this entity include a proliferative lentiginous or junctional melanocytic component, often with horizontal orientation of fusiform melanocytes; at least focal confluence of junctional melanocytic theques; lop-sidedness of pigmented cell nests, such that some bud laterally from rete ridges while others are located at the rete tips; and lamellar fibrosis in the papillary dermis beneath the nevocytic theques (Fig. 13–87, see p. 819).[507] Other helpful but more inconstant attributes include a junctional component that extends laterally past the dermal constituents of compound lesions (the so-called nevus "shoulder") and nuclear atypia in proliferating melanocytes in the lesion.

Until a few years ago, nevi with these characteristics were called "dysplastic."[508] However, because that appellation led to more and more unnecessarily aggressive surgical removal of "dysplastic" nevi, a Consensus Conference convened at the U.S. National Institutes of Health in 1992 recommended a change in official terminology to that of "architecturally disordered nevus" (ADN).[509] When ADNs are multifocally present in any given individual, they may be markers of the so-called BK-mole syndrome,[510] or other familial conditions that predispose to malignant melanoma. Nevertheless, sporadic solitary ADN is usually not a behavioral worry and should not be treated any differently than banal melanocytic nevi are. In particular, there is no need to widely excise ADN.[507] However, in light of the fact that some examples have, in fact, been reported that were complicated by the secondary development of melanomas, complete excision of ADNs is again a prudent goal, as it is for nevi in general.

After ADNs are discounted from further consideration, some other melanocytic lesions besides ordinary nevi and melanomas do remain. These most often show either an atypical lentiginous quality—with or without nuclear atypia in the proliferating cells—or limited upward "migration" (dyshesion) of melanocytes in the epidermis. Providing that the aggregate criteria for melanoma-in-situ are not fulfilled, one can utilize the term *atypical lentiginous melanocytic hyperplasia* or *atypical intraepidermal melanocytic proliferation* to describe such lesions in diagnostic reports (Fig. 13–88, see p. 819).[509, 511] Their biologic features are probably heterogeneous and have been incompletely chronicled, but they likely do not need more aggressive treatment beyond simple but complete surgical removal.

Malignant Melanomas of the Head and Neck

All of the major subtypes of malignant melanoma occur in the skin of the head and neck, with the exception of the acral-lentiginous variant, which is confined to the extremities. Among the others, including superficial spreading, nodular, lentigo maligna, and desmoplastic-neurotropic forms, the last two are relatively overrepresented in this topographic locale.

An exhaustive discussion of the criteria used to define malignant melanoma[486] clearly exceeds the scope of this chapter. However, asymmetry, cellular dyshesion, "migration" of atypical melanocytes through the epidermis, nuclear hyperchromasia and nucleolation, and aberrant mitotic activity are several of the cornerstones on which the histologic diagnosis is based. The microscopic characteristics of "conventional" superficial spreading and nodular melanoma have been well described elsewhere.[491] However, it is worth recalling that the cytologic and architectural features of such neoplasms may yield myxoid, signet ring–cell, hemangiopericytoid, adenoid-pseudopapillary, small-cell, "balloon-cell," pleomorphic, and rhabdoid appearances, all of which may additionally include the absence of melanin pigment in the tumor cells.[359, 491, 512]

Lentigo Maligna and Lentigo Maligna Melanoma

Melanomas with lentiginous features—that is, an essentially confluent proliferation of atypical melanocytes in the basilar portion of the epidermis—are most common in sun-exposed skin areas. However, several additional histologic criteria must be met before a diagnosis of lentigo maligna can be made. These include epidermal atrophy, extensive dermal actinic elastosis, and the presence of atypical melanocytes within the superficial aspects of skin appendages (e.g., pilosebaceous units) that are present in the biopsy specimens (Figs. 13–89 and 13–90, see p. 820).[513] If, in addition to this image, there is also an invasive tumor component in the corium, the term *lentigo maligna melanoma* may be applied.[491, 513] Particular cytologic features of lentigo maligna melanomas are similar to those of invasive melanomas in general, although spindle-cell differentiation is overrepresented in this specific context (see later).

Desmoplastic-Neuroid Malignant Melanoma

Melanomas that are composed predominantly or exclusively of relatively bland spindle cells are more common in the head and neck than in other anatomic areas,[514–520] as mentioned earlier. These tumors may or may not be associated with a concomitantly seen lentiginous component at the dermoepidermal junction, or with a history of previous lentigo maligna or lentigo maligna melanoma at the same site.

Desmoplastic melanomas show the elaboration of abundant stromal collagen—in which the tumor cells are randomly enmeshed—as well as potentially deep infiltration of the subcutis and even subjacent fascia and muscle (Fig. 13–91). Nuclear atypia in the proliferating spindle cells may be difficult to document because of its focality, and mitotic activity is similarly sparse.[521, 522] The overall image of desmoplastic melanomas is frighteningly similar to that of proliferating scar tissue; indeed, the distinction between these two possibilities is often impossible if frozen section examination of surgical margins is requested after an initial biopsy has established the diagnosis. Immunostains for S100 protein may be necessary to identify the neoplastic spindle cells in desmoplastic melanoma with certainty.[344]

Neuroid melanomas exhibit a striking resemblance to de novo peripheral nerve sheath tumors,[340, 344, 517, 519] but they again share the potential association with lentigo maligna or lentigo maligna melanoma that was cited in reference to desmoplastic variants. Serpiginous nuclear contours, nuclear palisading, myxoid stromal change, and the formation of neural tactoids are all common findings in neuroid melanoma (Fig. 13–92, see p. 820). Its propensity to invade pre-existing nerves in the skin accounts for another popular designation, that of *neurotropic melanoma*.[344] This feature also underscores the wisdom behind the examination of nerve margins in surgical resections of such tumors.

The separation of neuroid melanoma and nerve sheath sarcomas of the skin is subject to a certain arbitrariness, as previously discussed, in the absence of an obviously melanomatous component in the epidermis.[340] The regular loss of HMB45-immunoreactivity—as seen in most non-spindle cell melanomas—heightens this problem. Collagen type IV deposition also may be seen around the tumor cells of neuroid melanomas as well as nerve sheath tumors, and the latter marker therefore does not appear to have much differential diagnostic use in this setting.

The usually long-standing clinical character of desmoplastic and neuroid melanomas no doubt accounts for their common thick-

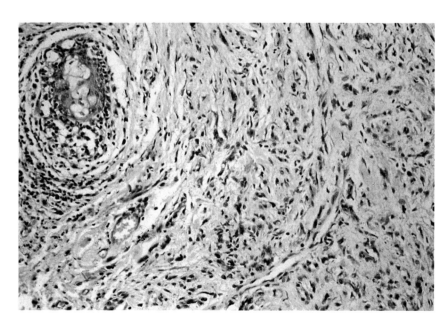

Figure 13–91. Desmoplastic malignant melanoma, showing the deeply infiltrative growth of fibroblast-like tumor cells in the dermis.

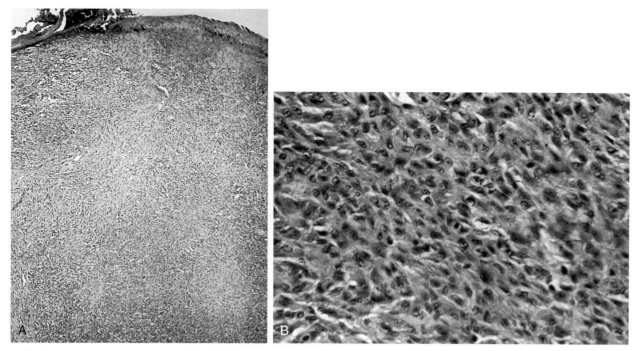

Figure 13–93. Nevoid melanoma of the skin of the neck. An asymmetrical proliferation of compact epithelioid nevoid tumor cells *(A)* is betrayed as malignant through recognition of mitotic figures at the base of the lesion *(B)*.

ness (up to several millimeters) at diagnosis. Nevertheless, the biologic evolution of these variants is more indolent than that of other melanomatous morphotypes, and overall fatality is not realized in full until 15 years or more after initial treatment has been given.[344, 521, 522]

Nevoid Melanomas

A small subset of cutaneous malignant melanomas of the head and neck does not differ drastically from selected intradermal or compound nevi upon low-power microscopic examination or even cytologic analysis. That is true because those tumors are minimally asymmetrical and are composed of uniform, compact, polygonal cells with dispersed chromatin and only small or indiscernible nucleoli. Such neoplasms have been designated as minimal deviation or borderline malignant melanomas,[523, 524] but I prefer the more descriptive term of *nevoid* melanomas.[525, 526]

The key points in the pathologic recognition of these lesions are their lack of cytologic "maturation" in comparing superficial and deep dermal aspects of the tumors and the presence of mitoses that are situated deep within the mass (Fig. 13–93). A proportion of nevoid melanomas show cytologic images that recall those of Spitz nevi (see earlier discussion) and have been termed *spitzoid* malignant melanomas by some authors.[527] If, in addition, a nevoid melanoma is asymmetrical, that finding would lend even more credence to a diagnosis of malignancy. In contrast to the contentions of other investigators,[528] I do not believe that nevoid melanomas differ in their biologic properties when compared with more usual melanomatous histotypes.

CONCLUSIONS

It should be obvious from the scope of this chapter that very few cutaneous tumors are unique to the skin of the head and neck, or, conversely, occur only outside that restricted topographic region. Thus, pathologists with a special interest in otorhinolaryngologic diseases must also be proficient at general dermatopathology. Likewise, head and neck surgeons also should have considerable familiarity with

dermatology in a broad sense to be effective practitioners. It is the author's hope that the foregoing discussion has contributed positively toward such goals.

REFERENCES

Benign Tumors of the Epidermis

1. Kao GF: Benign tumors of the epidermis. In: Farmer ER, Hood AF, eds. *Pathology of the Skin.* Norwalk, CT: Appleton & Lange, 1990:533–549.
2. Hurwitz S: Epidermal nevi and tumors of epidermal origin. *Pediatr Clin North Am* 1983;30:483–494.
3. De Lopez RMES, Hernandez-Perez E: Jadassohn's sebaceous nevus. *J Dermatol Surg Oncol* 1985;11:68–72.
4. Morioka S: The natural history of nevus sebaceus. *J Dermatol Surg Oncol* 1985;12:200–213.
5. Rowe L: Seborrheic keratosis. *J Invest Dermatol* 1957;29:165–176.
6. Sanderson KF: The structure of seborrheic keratoses. *Br J Dermatol* 1968;80:588–599.
7. Tanay A, Mehregan AH: Warty dyskeratoma. *Dermatologica* 1969;138:155–164.
8. Lumpkin LR, Helwig EB: Solitary lichen planus. *Arch Dermatol* 1966;93:54–55.
9. Prieto VG, Casal M, McNutt NS: Lichen planus–like keratosis: A clinical and histological reexamination. *Am J Surg Pathol* 1993;17:259–263.
10. Frigy AF, Cooper PH: Benign lichenoid keratosis. *Am J Clin Pathol* 1985;83:439–443.
11. Brownstein MH, Rabinowitz AD: The precursors of cutaneous squamous cell carcinoma. *Int J Dermatol* 1979;18:1–16.
12. Kao GF, Graham JH: Premalignant cutaneous disorders of the head and neck. In: England GM, ed. *Otolaryngology,* volume 5. Philadelphia: Harper & Row, 1986:1–20.
13. Wade TR, Ackerman AB: The many faces of solar keratoses. *J Dermatol Surg Oncol* 1978;14:730–734.

Malignant Tumors of the Epidermis

14. McGibbon DH: Malignant epidermal tumors. *J Cutan Pathol* 1985;12:224–238.

15. Wade TR, Ackerman AB: The many faces of basal cell carcinoma. *J Derm Surg Oncol* 1978;4:23–28.

16. Okun MR, Blumenthal G: Basal cell epithelioma with giant cells and nuclear atypicality. *Arch Dermatol* 1964;89:598–602.

17. Wick MR, Swanson PE: Primary adenoid cystic carcinoma of the skin. *Am J Dermatopathol* 1986;8:2–13.

18. Wolfe JT III, Wick MR, Campbell RJ: Sebaceous carcinomas of the oculocutaneous adnexa and extraocular skin. In: Wick MR, ed. *Pathology of Unusual Malignant Cutaneous Tumors*. New York: Marcel Dekker, 1985:77–106.

19. Hashimoto K, Brownstein MH: Localized amyloidosis in basal cell epitheliomas. *Acta Dermatol* 1973;53:331–339.

20. Looi LM: Localized amyloidosis in basal cell carcinomas: A pathologic study. *Cancer* 1983;52:1833–1836.

21. Masu S, Hosokawa M, Seiji M: Amyloid in localized cutaneous amyloidosis: Immunofluorescence studies with anti-keratin antiserum, especially concerning the difference between systemic and localized cutaneous amyloidosis. *Acta Dermatol* 1981;61:381–384.

22. Gatter KC, Pulford KAF, Van Stapel MJ, et al.: An immunohistological study of benign and malignant skin tumours: Epithelial aspects. *Histopathology* 1984;8:209–227.

23. Wick MR, Swanson PE: Immunohistochemical findings in tumors of the skin. In: DeLellis RA, ed. *Advances in Immunohistochemistry*. New York:Raven Press, 1988:395–429.

24. Thomas P, Said JW, Nash G, Banks-Schlegel S: Profiles of keratin proteins in basal and squamous cell carcinomas of the skin: A immunohistochemical study. *Lab Invest* 1984;50:36–41.

25. Miettinen M, Lehto VP, Virtanen I: Antibodies to intermediate filament proteins: The differential diagnosis of cutaneous tumors. *Arch Dermatol* 1985;121:736–741.

26. Wick MR, Kaye VN: The role of diagnostic immunohistochemistry in dermatology. *Semin Dermatol* 1987;5:136–147.

27. Jimenez FJ, Burchette JL Jr, Grichnik JM, Hitchcock MG: BER-EP4 immunoreactivity in normal skin and cutaneous neoplasms. *Mod Pathol* 1995;8:854–858.

28. Morales-Ducret CR, Van de Rijn M, LeBrun DP, Smoller BR: bcl-2 expression in primary malignancies of the skin. *Arch Dermatol* 1995;131:909–912.

29. Olsen KE, Westermark P: Amyloid in basal cell carcinoma and seborrheic keratosis. *Acta Dermatol Venereol* 1994;74:273–275.

30. Geary WA, Cooper PH: Proliferating cell nuclear antigen (PCNA) in common epidermal lesions. *J Cutan Pathol* 1992;19:458–468.

31. Furukawa F, Imamura S, Fujita M, et al.: Immunohistochemical localization of proliferating cell nuclear antigen/cyclin in human skin. *Arch Dermatol Res* 1992;284:86–91.

32. Healy E, Angus B, Lawrence CM, Rees JL: Prognostic value of Ki67 antigen in basal cell carcinomas. *Br J Dermatol* 1995;133:737–741.

33. Dahl M: Beta-2-microglobulin in skin cancer. *J Am Acad Dermatol* 1981;5:698–699.

34. Kallioinen M, Dammert K: Beta-2-microglobulin in benign and malignant adnexal skin tumours and metastasizing basocellular carcinomas. *J Cutan Pathol* 1984;11:27–34.

35. Mazoujian G, Pinkus GS, Haagensen DE Jr: Extramammary Paget's disease—evidence for an apocrine origin. An immunoperoxidase study of gross cystic disease fluid protein-15, carcinoembryonic antigen, and keratin proteins. *Am J Surg Pathol* 1984;8:43–50.

36. Ormsby AH, Snow JL, Su WPD, Goellner JR: Diagnostic immunohistochemistry of cutaneous metastatic breast carcinoma: A statistical analysis of the utility of gross cystic disease fluid protein-15 and estrogen receptor protein. *J Am Acad Dermatol* 1995;32:711–716.

37. Claudy AL, Viac J, Schmitt D, et al.: Identification of mononuclear cells infiltrating basal cell carcinomas. *Acta Derm (Stockholm)* 1976;56:361–365.

38. Brownstein MH, Shapiro L: Desmoplastic trichoepithelioma. *Cancer* 1977;40:2979–2986.

39. Wick MR, Manivel JC, Millns JL: Histopathologic considerations in the management of skin cancer. In: Schwartz RA, ed. *Skin Cancer: Recognition and Management*. New York: Springer–Verlag, 1988:246–275.

40. Rulon DB, Helwig EB: Cutaneous sebaceous neoplasms. *Cancer* 1974;33:82–102.

41. Battifora H: Spindle-cell carcinoma: Ultrastructural evidence of squamous origin and collagen production by the tumor cells. *Cancer* 1976;37:2275–2282.

42. Brownstein MH, Shapiro L: Verrucous carcinoma of skin: Epithelioma cuniculatum plantare. *Cancer* 1976;38:1710–1716.

43. Eusebi V, Ceccarelli C, Piscioli F, et al.: Spindle-cell tumours of the skin of debatable origin: An immunocytochemical study. *J Pathol* 1984;144:189–199.

44. Feldman PS, Barr RJ: Ultrastructure of spindle-cell squamous carcinoma. *J Cutan Pathol* 1976;3:17–24.

45. Johnson WC, Helwig EB: Adenoid squamous cell carcinoma. *Cancer* 1966;19:1639–1650.

46. Kao GF, Graham JH, Helwig EB: Carcinoma cuniculatum (verrucous carcinoma of the skin): A clinicopathologic study of 46 cases with ultrastructural observations. *Cancer* 1982;49:2395–2403.

47. Kuo TT: Clear-cell carcinoma of the skin: A variant of the squamous cell carcinoma that simulates sebaceous carcinoma. *Am J Surg Pathol* 1980;4:573–583.

48. Kuwano H, Hashimoto H, Enjoji M: Atypical fibroxanthoma distinguishable from spindle-cell carcinoma in sarcoma-like skin lesions. *Cancer* 1985;55:172–180.

49. Lever WF: Adenoacanthoma of sweat glands. *Arch Dermatol Syphilol* 1947;56:157–171.

50. Lichtiger B, Mackay B, Tessmer CF: Spindle-cell variant of squamous cell carcinoma. A light and electron microscopic study of 13 cases. *Cancer* 1970;26:1311–1320.

51. Ritter JH, Mills SE, Nappi O, Wick MR: Angiosarcoma-like neoplasms of epithelial organs: True endothelial tumors or variants of carcinoma? *Semin Diagn Pathol* 1995;12:270–282.

52. McKee PH, Wilkinson JD, Corbett MF, et al.: Carcinoma cuniculatum: A case metastasizing to skin and lymph nodes. *Clin Exp Dermatol* 1981;6:613–618.

53. Nappi O, Wick MR, Pettinato G, et al.: Pseudovascular adenoid squamous cell carcinoma of the skin: A neoplasm that may be mistaken for angiosarcoma. *Am J Surg Pathol* 1992;16:429–438.

54. Broders AC: Squamous cell epithelioma of the skin. *Ann Surg* 1921;73:141–160.

55. Evans HL, Smith JL: spindle-cell squamous carcinomas and sarcoma-like tumors of the skin: A comparative study of 38 cases. *Cancer* 1980;45:2687–2697.

56. Strayer DS, Santa Cruz DJ: Carcinoma in situ of the skin: A review of histopathology. *J Cutan Pathol* 1980;7:244–259.

57. Graham JH, Helwig EB: Erythroplasia of Queyrat. In: Graham JH, Johnson WC, Helwig EB, eds. *Dermal Pathology*. Hagerstown, MD: Harper and Row, 1972:597–606.

58. Jones RE Jr, Austin C, Ackerman AB: Extramammary Paget's disease: A critical reexamination. *Am J Dermatopathol* 1979;1:101–132.

59. Steffen C, Ackerman AB: Intraepidermal epithelioma of Borst–Jadassohn. *Am J Dermatopathol* 1985;7:5–24.

60. Fulling KH, Strayer DS, Santa Cruz DJ: Adnexal metaplasia in carcinoma in situ of the skin. *J Cutan Pathol* 1981;8:79–88.

61. Callen JP, Headington JT: Bowen's disease and non-Bowen's squamous intraepidermal neoplasia of the skin. *Arch Dermatol* 1980;116:422–426.

62. Graham JH, Helwig EB: Bowen's disease and its relationship to systemic cancer. *Arch Dermatol* 1959;80:133–159.

63. Szekeres G, De Giacomoni P: Ki67 and p53 expression in cutaneous Bowen's disease. *Acta Dermatol Venereol* 1994;74:272–278.

64. Hodak E, Jones RE, Ackerman AB: Solitary keratoacanthoma is a squamous cell carcinoma: Three examples with metastases. *Am J Dermatopathol* 1993;15:332–352.

65. Chalet MD, Connors RC, Ackerman AB: Squamous cell carcinoma vs. keratoacanthoma: Criteria for histologic differentiation. *J Derm Surg* 1975;1:16–17.

66. Kern WH, McCray MK: The histopathologic differentiation of keratoacanthoma and squamous cell carcinoma of the skin. *J Cutan Pathol* 1980;7:318–325.

67. Wick MR, Fitzgibbon JF, Swanson PE: Cutaneous sarcomas and sarcomatoid carcinomas of the skin. *Semin Diagn Pathol* 1993;10:148–158.

68. Izaki S, Hirai A, Yoshizawa Y, et al.: Carcinosarcoma of the skin: Immunohistochemical and electron microscopic observations. *J Cutan Pathol* 1993;20:272–278.

69. Balazs M: Buschke-Loewenstein tumour: A histologic and ultrastructural study of six cases. *Virchows Arch Pathol Anat* 1986;410:83–92.

70. Perez-Mesa CA, Kraus FT, Evans JC, Powers WE: Anaplastic transformation in verrucous carcinoma of the oral cavity after radiation therapy. *Radiology* 1966;86:108–115.

71. Kvedar JC, Fewkes J, Baden HP: Immunologic detection of markers of keratinocyte differentiation in neoplastic and preneoplastic lesions of skin. *Arch Pathol Lab Med* 1986;110:183–188.

72. Matsuo K, Sakamoto A, Kawai K, et al.: Small cell carcinoma of the skin: "Non-Merkel cell type." *Acta Pathol Jpn* 1985;35:1029–1036.

Primary Neuroendocrine (Merkel Cell) Carcinoma of the Skin

73. Wick MR, Scheithauer BW: Primary neuroendocrine carcinoma of the skin. In: Wick MR, ed. *Pathology of Unusual Malignant Cutaneous Tumors.* New York: Marcel Dekker, 1985:107–180.
74. Kossard S, Wittal R, Killingsworth M: Merkel cell carcinoma with a desmoplastic portion. *Am J Dermatopathol* 1995;17:517–522.
75. Gould VE, Moll R, Moll I, et al.: Neuroendocrine (Merkel) cells of the skin: Hyperplasias, dysplasias, and neoplasms. *Lab Invest* 1985;52:334–349.
76. Gould E, Albores-Saavedra J, Smith W, Payne CM: Eccrine and squamous differentiation in Merkel cell carcinoma: An immunohistochemical study. *Am J Surg Pathol* 1988;12:768–772.
77. Silva EG, Mackay B, Goepfert H, et al.: Endocrine carcinoma of the skin (Merkel cell carcinoma). *Pathol Annu* 1984;19(2):1–30.
78. Frigerio B, Capella C, Eusebi V, Tenti P, Azzopardi JG: Merkel cell carcinoma of the skin. *Histopathology* 1983;7:229–249.
79. Battifora H, Silva EG: The use of antikeratin antibodies in the immunohistochemical distinction between neuroendocrine (Merkel cell) carcinoma of the skin, lymphoma, and oat-cell carcinoma. *Cancer* 1986;58:1040–1046.
80. Sibley RK, Dahl D: Neuroendocrine (Merkel cell?) carcinoma of the skin. II. An immunohistochemical study of 21 cases. *Am J Surg Pathol* 1985;9:109–116.

Benign Sweat Gland Tumors

81. Wick MR, Swanson PE: *Cutaneous Adnexal Tumors: A Guide to Pathologic Diagnosis.* Chicago: ASCP Press, 1991.
82. Hashimoto K, Mehregan AH, Kumakiri M: *Tumors of the Skin Appendages,* Butterworths, Boston, 1987.
83. Crain RC, Helwig EB: Dermal cylindroma (dermal eccrine cylindroma). *Am J Clin Pathol* 1961;35:504–515.
84. Mambo NC: Eccrine spiradenoma: Clinical and pathologic study of 49 tumors. *J Cutan Pathol* 1983;10:312–320.
85. Ebner H, Erlach E: Ekkrine hidrozystome. *Dermatol Monatsschr* 1975;161:739–745.
86. Smith JD, Chernosky ME: Apocrine hidrocystoma (cystadenoma). *Arch Dermatol* 1974;109:700–702.
87. Pruzam DL, Esterly NB, Prose NS: Eruptive syringoma. *Arch Dermatol* 1989;125:1119–1120.
88. Isaacson D, Turner ML: Localized vulvar syringomas. *J Am Acad Dermatol* 1979;1:352–356.
89. Henner MS, Shapiro PE, Ritter JH, et al.: Solitary syringoma: A report of five cases and comparison with microcystic adnexal carcinoma. *Am J Dermatopathol* 1995;17:465–470.
90. Falck VG, Jordaan HF: Papillary eccrine adenoma: A tubulopapillary hidradenoma with eccrine differentiation. *Am J Dermatopathol* 1986;8:64–72.
91. Tellechea O, Reis JP, Marques C, Baptista AP: Tubular apocrine adenoma with eccrine and apocrine immunophenotypes or papillary tubular adenoma? *Am J Dermatopathol* 1995;17:499–505.
92. Johnson BL Jr, Helwig EB: Eccrine acrospiroma. *Cancer* 1969;23:641–657.
93. Pylyser K, DeWolf-Peeters C, Marien K: The histology of eccrine poroma. *Dermatologica* 1983;167:243–249.

Sweat Gland Carcinomas

94. Wick MR, Goellner JR, Wolfe JT III, Su WPD: Adnexal carcinomas of the skin. I: Eccrine carcinomas. *Cancer* 1985;56:1147–1162.
95. Mendoza S, Helwig EB: Mucinous (adenocystic) carcinoma of the skin. *Arch Dermatol* 1971;103:68–78.
96. Rodriguez MM, Lubowitz RM, Shannon GM: Mucinous (adenocystic) carcinoma of the eyelid. *Arch Ophthalmol* 1973;89:493–494.
97. Carson HJ, Gattuso P, Raslan WF, Reddy V: Mucinous carcinoma of the eyelid: an immunohistochemical study. *Am J Dermatopathol* 1995;17:494–498.
98. Goldstein DJ, Barr RJ, Santa Cruz DJ: Microcystic adnexal carcinoma: a distinct clinicopathologic entity. *Cancer* 1982;50:566–572.

99. Cooper PH: Sclerosing carcinomas of sweat ducts (microcystic adnexal carcinoma). *Arch Dermatol* 1986;122:261–264.
100. Aurora AL, Luxenberg MN: Case report of adenocarcinoma of glands of Moll. *Am J Ophthalmol* 1970;70:984–990.
101. Seab JA, Graham JH: Primary cutaneous adenoid cystic carcinoma. *J Am Acad Dermatol* 1987;17:113–118.
102. Cooper PH: Carcinomas of sweat glands. *Pathol Annu* 1987;22:83–124.

Benign Tumors and Tumor-Like Conditions of the Sebaceous Glands

103. Warren S, Warvi WN: Tumors of sebaceous glands. *Am J Pathol* 1943;19:441–460.
104. Lever WF: Sebaceous adenoma. *Arch Dermatol* 1948;57:102–111.
105. Fahmy A, Burgdorf WHC, Schosser RH, Pitha J: Muir-Torre syndrome: reevaluation of the dermatological features and consideration of its relationship to the family cancer syndrome. *Cancer* 1983;49:1898–1903.
106. Bhawan J, Calhoun J: Premature sebaceous gland hyperplasia. *J Am Acad Dermatol* 1983;8:136.
107. Fernandez N, Torres A: Hyperplasia of sebaceous glands in a linear pattern of papules: Report of four cases. *Am J Dermatopathol* 1984;6:237–244.

Benign Hair Follicle Tumors

108. Long SA, Hurt MA, Santa Cruz DJ: Immature trichoepithelioma: Report of six cases. *J Cutan Pathol* 1988;15:353–358.
109. Smoller BR, Van de Rijn M, Lebrun D, Warnke RA: *Bcl-2* expression reliably distinguishes trichoepitheliomas from basal cell carcinomas. *Br J Dermatol* 1993;131:28–33.
110. Brownstein MH, Shapiro L: Desmoplastic trichoepithelioma. *Cancer* 1977;40:2979–2986.
111. Kallionen M, Tuomi ML, Dammert K, Autio-Harmainen H: Desmoplastic trichoepithelioma. *Br J Dermatol* 1984;111:571–577.
112. Brownstein MH: Trichilemmoma: Benign follicular tumor or viral wart? *Am J Dermatopathol* 1980;2:229–231.
113. Ackerman AB, Wade TR: Tricholemmoma. *Am J Dermatopathol* 1980;2:207–224.
114. Brownstein MH, Mehregan AH, Bikowski JB: Trichilemmoma in Cowden's disease. *JAMA* 1977;238:26.
115. Hunt SJ, Kilzer B, Santa Cruz DJ: Desmoplastic trichilemmoma: histologic variant resembling invasive carcinoma. *J Cutan Pathol* 1990;17:45–52.
116. Colver GB, Buxton PK: Pilomatrixoma: An elusive diagnosis. *Int J Dermatol* 1988;27:176–178.
117. Marrogi AJ, Wick MR, Dehner LP: Pilomatrical tumors in children and young adults. *Am J Dermatopathol* 1992;14:87–94.
118. Janitz J, Wiedersberg H: Proliferating tricholemmal tumors. *Cancer* 1980;45:1594–1597.
119. Baptista AP, Garcia E, Silva L, Born MC: Proliferating trichilemmal cyst. *J Cutan Pathol* 1983;10:178–187.
120. Mehregan AH: Infundibular tumors of the skin. *J Cutan Pathol* 1984;11:387–395.

Sebaceous Carcinomas of the Skin

121. Ni C, Kuo PK: Meibomian gland carcinoma. *Jpn J Ophthalmol* 1979;23:388–401.
122. Wick MR, Goellner JR, Wolfe JT III, Su WPD: Adnexal carcinomas of the skin. II: Extraocular sebaceous carcinomas. *Cancer* 1985;56:1163–1172.
123. Rao NA, Hidayat AA, McLean IW, Zimmerman LE: Sebaceous carcinomas of the ocular adnexa. *Hum Pathol* 1982;13:113–122.

Malignant Tumors Showing Hair Follicle Differentiation

124. Russell WB, Page DL, Hough AJ, Lodgers LW: Sebaceous carcinoma of meibomian gland origin: The diagnostic importance of pagetoid spread of neoplastic cells. *Am J Clin Pathol* 1980;73:504–511.
125. Headington JT: Tumors of the hair follicle: A review. *Am J Pathol* 1976;85:480–505.

126. Boscaino A, Terracciano LM, Donofrio V, et al.: Tricholemmal carcinoma: A study of seven cases. *J Cutan Pathol* 1992;19:94–99.

127. Swanson PE, Marrogi AJ, Williams DJ, et al.: Tricholemmal carcinoma: Clinicopathologic study of ten cases. *J Cutan Pathol* 1992;19:100–109.

128. Gould E, Kurzon R, Kowalczyk AP, Saldana M: Pilomatrix carcinoma with pulmonary metastases. *Cancer* 1984;54:370–372.

129. Van der Walt JD, Rohlova B: Carcinomatous transformation in a pilomatrixoma. *Am J Dermatopathol* 1984;6:63–69.

130. Swanson SA, Cooper PH, Mills SE, Wick MR: Lymphoepithelioma-like carcinoma of the skin. *Mod Pathol* 1988;1:359–365.

131. Mehregan AH, Lee KC: Malignant proliferating trichilemmal tumors: Report of three cases. *J Dermatol Surg Oncol* 1987;13:1339–1342.

132. Batman PA, Evans HJR: Metastasizing pilar tumor of the scalp. *J Clin Pathol* 1986;39:757–760.

Mesenchymal Tumors of the Skin: General Features & Immunohistology

133. Dehner LP: *Pediatric Surgical Pathology,* 2nd ed. Baltimore: Williams & Wilkins, 1987:1–103.

134. Lendrum AC: Painful tumors of the skin. *Ann R Coll Surg Engl* 1947;1:62–67.

135. Laskin WB, Silverman TA, Enzinger FM: Postradiation soft tissue sarcomas. *Cancer* 1988;62:2330–2340.

136. Ducatman BS, Scheithauer BW: Postirradiation neurofibrosarcoma. *Cancer* 1983;51:1028–1033.

137. Goette DK, Detlefs RL: Postirradiation angiosarcoma. *J Am Acad Dermatol* 1985;12:922–926.

138. Muggia FM, Lonberg M: Kaposi's sarcoma and AIDS. *Med Clin North Am* 1986;70:109–138.

139. Wick MR, Swanson PE, Manivel JC: Immunohistochemical analysis of soft tissue sarcomas: Comparisons with electron microscopy. *Appl Pathol* 1988;6:169–196.

140. Ordonez NG, Batsakis JG: Comparison of *Ulex europaeus* I lectin and factor VIII-related antigen in vascular lesions. *Arch Pathol Lab Med* 1984;108:129–132.

141. Traweek ST, Kandalaft PL, Mehta P, Battifora H: The human hematopoietic progenitor cell antigen (CD34) in vascular neoplasia. *Am J Clin Pathol* 1991;96:25–31.

142. Battifora H: Assessment of antigen damage in immunohistochemistry: the vimentin internal control. *Am J Clin Pathol* 1991;96:669–671.

143. Wick MR, Kaye VN: The role of diagnostic immunohistochemistry in dermatology. *Semin Dermatol* 1986;5:346–358.

Benign Mesenchymal Tumors of the Skin

144. Graham JH, Sanders JB, Johnson WC, Helwig EB: Fibrous papule of the nose: A clinicopathological study. *J Invest Dermatol* 1965;45:194–205.

145. Rosen LB, Suster S: Fibrous papules: A light microscopic and immunohistochemical study. *Am J Dermatopathol* 1988;10:109–116.

146. Saylan T, Marks R, Wilson-Jones E: Fibrous papule of the nose. *Br J Dermatol* 1971;85:111–116.

147. Zackheim MS, Pinkus H: Perifollicular fibromas. *Arch Dermatol* 1960;82:913–919.

148. Guitart J, Bergfeld WF, Tuthill RJ: Fibrous papule of the nose with granular cells: Two cases. *J Cutan Pathol* 1991;18:284–287.

149. McGibbon DH, Wilson-Jones E: Fibrous papule of the face (nose): Fibrosing melanocytic nevus. *Am J Dermatopathol* 1979;1:345–351.

150. Cerio R, Rao BK, Spaull J, Wilson-Jones E: An immunohistochemical study of fibrous papule of the nose: 25 cases. *J Cutan Pathol* 1989;16:194–198.

151. Nickel WR, Reed WB: Tuberous sclerosis: Special reference to the microscopic alterations in the cutaneous hamartomas. *Arch Dermatol* 1962;85:209–224.

152. Pringle JJ: A case of congenital adenoma sebaceum. *Br J Dermatol* 1890;2:1–14.

153. Sanchez NP, Wick MR, Perry HO: Adenoma sebaceum of Pringle: A clinicopathologic review, with a discussion of related pathologic entities. *J Cutan Pathol* 1981;8:395–403.

154. Chung EB, Enzinger FM: Infantile myofibromatosis. *Cancer* 1981;48:1807–1818.

155. Allen PW: The fibromatoses: A clinicopathologic classification based on 140 cases (Part I). *Am J Surg Pathol* 1977;1:255–270.

156. Allen PW: The fibromatoses: A clinicopathologic classification based on 140 cases (Part II). *Am J Surg Pathol* 1977;1:305–321.

157. Coffin CM, Dehner LP: Soft tissue tumors in the first year of life: A report of 190 cases. *Ped Pathol* 1990;10:509–526.

158. Fayad MN, Tacoub A, Salman S, et al.: Juvenile hyalin fibromatosis: Two new patients and review of the literature. *Am J Med Genet* 1987;26:123–131.

159. Ramberger K, Krieg T, Kunze D, et al.: Fibromatosis hyalinica multiplex (juvenile hyalin fibromatosis). *Cancer* 1985;56:614–624.

160. Taylor LJ: Musculoaponeurotic fibromatosis: A report of 28 cases and review of the literature. *Clin Orthop Rel Res* 1987;224:294–302.

161. Ayala AG, Ro JY, Goepfert H, et al.: Desmoid fibromatosis: A clinicopathologic study of 25 children. *Semin Diagn Pathol* 1986;3:138–150.

162. Sundaram M, Duffrin H, McGuire MH, Vas W: Synchronous multicentric desmoid tumors (aggressive fibromatosis) of the extremities. *Skeletal Radiol* 1988;17:16–19.

163. Posner MC, Shiu MH, Newsome JL, et al.: The desmoid tumor: Not a benign disease. *Arch Surg* 1989;124:191–196.

164. Daimaru Y, Hashimoto H, Enjoji M: Myofibromatosis in adults (adult counterpart of infantile myofibromatosis). *Am J Surg Pathol* 1989;13:859–865.

165. Smith KJ, Skelton HG, Barnett TL, et al.: Cutaneous myofibroma. *Mod Pathol* 1989;2:603–609.

166. Hogan SF, Salassa JR: Recurrent adult myofibromatosis: A case report. *Am J Clin Pathol* 1992;97:810–814.

167. Kamino H, Reddy VB, Gero M, Greco MA: Dermatomyofibroma. *J Cutan Pathol* 1992;19:85–93.

168. Briselli MF, Soule EH, Gilchrist GS: Congenital fibromatosis: Report of 18 cases of solitary and 4 cases of multiple tumors. *Mayo Clin Proc* 1980;55:554–562.

169. Seibert JJ, Seibert RW, Weisenburger DS, et al.: Multiple congenital hemangiopericytomas of head and neck. *Laryngoscope* 1978;88:1006–1010.

170. Mentzel T, Calonje E, Nascimento AG, Fletcher CD: Infantile hemangiopericytoma versus infantile myofibromatosis. Study of a series suggesting a continuous spectrum of infantile myofibroblastic lesions. *Am J Surg Pathol* 1994;18:922–930.

171. Yokoyama R, Tsuneyoshi M, Enjoji M, et al.: Extra-abdominal desmoid tumors: Correlations between histologic features and biologic behavior. *Surg Pathol* 1989;2:29–42.

172. Shugart RR, Soule EH, Johnson EW: Glomus tumors. *Surg Gynecol Obstet* 1963;117:334–345.

173. Conant MA, Wiesenfeld SL: Multiple glomus tumors of the skin. *Arch Dermatol* 1971;103:481–486.

174. Kaye VN, Dehner LP: Cutaneous glomus tumor. *Am J Dermatopathol* 1991;13:2–6.

175. Enzinger FM, Smith BH: Hemangiopericytoma: An analysis of 106 cases. *Hum Pathol* 1976;7:61–72.

176. Czernobilsky B, Cornog JL Jr, Enterline HT: Rhabdomyoma: Report of cases with ultrastructural and histochemical studies. *Am J Clin Pathol* 1968;49:782–787.

177. Hajdu SI: *Pathology of Soft Tissue Tumors.* Philadelphia: Lea & Febiger, 1979:324–325.

178. Dehner LP, Enzinger FM, Font RL: Fetal rhabdomyoma: an analysis of nine cases. Cancer 1972;30:160–166.

179. Crotty PL, Nakhleh RE, Dehner LP: Juvenile rhabdomyoma: An intermediate form of skeletal muscle tumor in children. *Arch Pathol Lab Med* 1993;117:43–47.

180. Sangueza O, Sangueza P, Jordan J, White CR Jr: Rhabdomyoma of the tongue. *Am J Dermatopathol* 1990;12:492–495.

181. Sahn EE, Garen PD, Pai GS, et al.: Multiple rhabdomyomatous mesenchymal hamartomas of skin. *Am J Dermatopathol* 1990;12:485–491.

182. Mills AE: Rhabdomyomatous mesenchymal hamartoma of skin. *Am J Dermatopathol* 1989;11:58–63.

183. Ashfaq R, Timmons CF: Rhabdomyomatous mesenchymal hamartoma of skin. *Pediatr Pathol* 1992;12:731–735.

184. Flanagan BP, Helwig EB: Cutaneous lymphangioma. *Arch Dermatol* 1977;113:24–29.

185. Fisher I, Orkin M: Acquired lymphangioma (lymphangiectasis). *Arch Dermatol* 1970;101:230–234.

186. Peachy RO, Limm CC, Whimster IW: Lymphangioma of skin: A review of 65 cases. *Br J Dermatol* 1970;83:519–526.

187. Whimster IW: The pathology of lymphangioma circumscriptum. *Br J Dermatol* 1974;10:35–45.

188. Margileth AM: Cutaneous vascular tumors. *Med Probl Pediatr* 1975;17:101–110.

189. Donsky HJ: Vascular tumors of the skin. *Can Med Assoc J* 1968;99:993–1000.

190. Simpson JR: Natural history of cavernous hemangiomata. *Lancet* 1959;2:1057–1063.

191. Iizuka S: Eosinophilic lymphadenitis and granulomatosis: Kimura's disease. *Nihon Univ Med J* 1959;18:900–908.

192. Santa Cruz DJ, Aronberg J: Targetoid hemosiderotic hemangioma. *J Am Acad Dermatol* 1988;19:550–558.

193. Dekaminsky AR, Otero AC, Kaminsky CA, et al.: Multiple disseminated pyogenic granulomas. *Br J Dermatol* 1978;98:461–464.

194. Wick MR, Manivel JC: Vascular neoplasms of the skin: A current perspective. *Adv Dermatol* 1989;4:185–254.

195. Mills SE, Cooper PH, Fechner RE: Lobular capillary hemangioma: the underlying lesion of pyogenic granuloma. *Am J Surg Pathol* 1980;4:471–479.

196. Padilla RS, Orkin M, Rosai J: Acquired "tufted" hemangioma (progressive capillary hemangioma). *Am J Dermatopathol* 1987;9:292–300.

197. Bardwick PA, Zvaifler NJ, Gill GN, et al.: Plasma cell dyscrasia with polyneuropathy, organomegaly, endocrinopathy, M protein, and skin changes: the POEMS syndrome. *Medicine* 1980;59:311–322.

198. Imperial R, Helwig EB: Verrucous hemangioma: A clinicopathologic study of 21 cases. *Arch Dermatol* 1967;96:247–253.

199. Rao VK, Weiss SW: Angiomatosis of soft tissue: An analysis of the histologic features and clinical outcome in 51 cases. *Am J Surg Pathol* 1992;16:764–771.

200. Rapini RP, Golitz LE: Targetoid hemosiderotic hemangioma. *J Cutan Pathol* 1990;17:233–235.

201. Rosai J, Gold J, Landy R: The histiocytoid hemangiomas: A unifying concept embracing several previously described entities of skin, soft tissue, large vessels, bone, and heart. *Hum Pathol* 1979;10:707–730.

202. Urabe A, Tsuneyoshi M, Enjoji M: Epithelioid hemangioma versus Kimura's disease: A comparative clinicopathologic study. *Am J Surg Pathol* 1987;11:758–766.

203. Nichols GE, Gaffey MJ, Mills SE, Weiss LM: Lobular capillary hemangioma: An immunohistochemical study including steroid hormone receptor status. *Am J Clin Pathol* 1992;97:770–775.

204. Cooper PH, Mills SE: Subcutaneous granuloma pyogenicum: Lobular capillary hemangioma. *Arch Dermatol* 1982;118:30–33.

205. Satomi I, Tanaka Y, Murata J, et al.: A case of angioblastoma (Nakagawa). *Rinsho Dermatol* 1981;23:703–709.

206. Wilson-Jones E, Orkin M: Tufted angioma (angioblastoma): A benign progressive angioma, not to be confused with Kaposi's sarcoma or low-grade angiosarcoma. *J Am Acad Dermatol* 1989;20:214–225.

207. Cooper PH, McAllister HA, Helwig EB: Intravenous pyogenic granuloma: A study of 18 cases. *Am J Surg Pathol* 1979;3:221–228.

208. Chan JKC, Fletcher CDM, Hicklin GA, Rosai J: Glomeruloid hemangioma: a distinctive cutaneous lesion of multicentric Castleman's disease associated with POEMS syndrome. *Am J Surg Pathol* 1990;14:1036–1046.

209. Hunt SJ, Santa Cruz DJ, Barr RJ: Microvenular hemangioma. *J Cutan Pathol* 1991;18:235–240.

210. Wilson-Jones E, Winkelmann RK, Zachary CB, Reda AM: Benign lymphangioendothelioma. *J Am Acad Dermatol* 1990;23:229–238.

211. Smith T: Histiocytic diseases and tumors of the skin. In: Maize J, ed. *Cutaneous Pathology.* New York: Churchill-Livingstone, 1999.

212. Mehregan AH, Shapiro L: Angiolymphoid hyperplasia with eosinophilia. *Arch Dermatol* 1971;103:50–57.

213. Reed RJ, Bliss BO: Morton's neuroma: Regressive and productive intermetatarsal elastofibrositis. *Arch Pathol* 1973;95:123–129.

214. Scotti TM: The lesion of Morton's metatarsalgia (Morton's toe). *Arch Pathol* 1957;63:91–102.

215. Reed RJ, Fine RM, Meltzer HD: Palisaded encapsulated neuromas of the skin. *Arch Dermatol* 1972;106:865–870.

216. Dover JS, From L, Lewis A: Clinicopathologic findings in palisaded encapsulated neuromas. *J Cutan Pathol* 1986;13:77–82.

217. Geffner RE: Ganglioneuroma of the skin. *Arch Dermatol* 1986;122:377.

218. Carney JA, Sizemore GW, Lovestedt SA: Mucosal ganglioneuromatosis, medullary thyroid carcinoma, and pheochromocytoma: Multiple endocrine neoplasia, type 2b. *Oral Surg* 1976;41:739–752.

219. Rios JJ, Siaz-Cano SJ, Rivera-Hueto F, Willar JL: Cutaneous ganglion cell choristoma. *J Cutan Pathol* 1991;18:469–473.

220. Oshman RG, Phelps RG, Kantor I: A solitary neurofibroma on the finger. *Arch Dermatol* 1988;122:1185–1186.

221. Stout AP: Neurofibroma and neurilemoma. *Clin Proc* 1946;5:1–12.

222. Harkin JC, Reed RJ: Tumors of the peripheral nervous system. In: *Atlas of Tumor Pathology,* series 2, fascicle 3. Washington, DC: Armed Forces Institute of Pathology, 1969:29–96.

223. McCarroll HR: Clinical manifestations of congenital neurofibromatosis. *J Bone Joint Surg* 1950;32a:601–617.

224. Preston FW, Walsh WS, Clarke TH: Cutaneous neurofibromatosis (von Recklinghausen's disease): Clinical manifestations and incidence of sarcoma in 61 male patients. *Arch Surg* 1952;64:813–827.

225. Ross DE: Skin manifestations of von Recklinghausen's disease and associated tumors (neurofibromatosis). *Am Surg* 1965;31:729–740.

226. Saxen E: Tumours of tactile end-organs. *Acta Pathol Microbiol Scand* 1948;25:66–79.

227. Daimaru Y, Hashimoto H, Enjoji M: Malignant peripheral nerve sheath tumors (malignant schwannomas). *Am J Surg Pathol* 1985;9:434–444.

228. Saxen E: Tumors of the sheaths of the peripheral nerves (studies on their structure). *Acta Pathol Microbiol Scand* 1948;79(suppl):1–135.

229. Woodruff JM: Peripheral nerve tumors showing glandular differentiation (glandular schwannomas). *Cancer* 1976;37:2399–2413.

230. Font RL, Truong LD: Melanotic schwannoma of soft tissues. *Am J Surg Pathol* 1984;8:129–138.

231. Mennemeyer RP, Hammar SP, Titus JS, et al.: Melanotic schwannoma. *Am J Surg Pathol* 1979;3:3–10.

232. Fletcher CDM: Benign plexiform (multinodular) schwannoma: a rare tumor unassociated with neurofibromatosis. *Histopathology* 1986;10:971–980.

233. Iwashita T, Enjoji M: Plexiform neurilemmoma. *Virchows Arch A* 1987;411:305–309.

234. Taxy JB, Battifora H: Epithelioid schwannoma: Diagnosis by electron microscopy. *Ultrastruct Pathol* 1981;2:19–24.

235. Carney JA: Psammomatous melanotic schwannoma. *Am J Surg Pathol* 1990;14:206–222.

236. Fletcher CDM, Davies SE, McKee PH: Cellular schwannoma: A distinct pseudosarcomatous entity. *Histopathology* 1987;11:21–35.

237. Gallager RL, Helwig EB: Neurothekeoma: A benign cutaneous tumor of neural origin. *Am J Clin Pathol* 1980;74:759–764.

238. MacDonald DM, Wilson-Jones E: Pacinian neurofibroma. *Histopathology* 1977;1:247–255.

239. Fletcher CDM, Chan JKC, McKee PH: Dermal nerve sheath myxoma: A study of 3 cases. *Histopathology* 1986;10:135–145.

240. Aronson PJ, Fretzin DF, Potter BS: Neurothekeoma of Gallager and Helwig (dermal nerve sheath myxoma variant): Report of a case with electron microscopic and immunohistochemical studies. *J Cutan Pathol* 1985;12:506–519.

241. Barnhill RL, Mihm MC Jr: Cellular neurothekeoma: A distinctive variant of neurothekeoma mimicking nevomelanocytic tumors. *Am J Surg Pathol* 1990;14:113–120.

242. Lack EE, Worsham GF, Callihan MD, et al.: Granular cell tumor: A clinicopathologic study of 110 patients. *J Surg Oncol* 1980;13:301–316.

243. Sobel HJ, Churg J: Granular cells and granular cell lesions. *Arch Pathol* 1964;77:132–141.

244. Sobel HJ, Marquet E: Granular cells and granular cell lesions. *Pathol Annu* 1974;9:43–79.

245. Apisarnthanarax P: Granular cell tumor: An analysis of 16 cases and review of the literature. *J Am Acad Dermatol* 1981;5:171–183.

246. Manivel JC, Dehner LP, Wick MR: Nonvascular sarcomas of the skin. In: Wick MR, ed. *Pathology of Unusual Malignant Cutaneous Tumors.* New York: Marcel Dekker, 1985:211–279.

247. Abenoza P, Sibley RK: Granular cell myoblastoma and schwannoma: A fine structural and immunohistochemical study. *Ultrastruct Pathol* 1987;11:19–28.

248. Penneys NS, Adachi K, Ziegels-Weissman J, Nadji M: Granular cell tumors of the skin contain myelin basic protein. *Arch Pathol Lab Med* 1983;107:302–303.

249. Sobel HJ, Schwartz R, Marquet E: Light and electron microscopic study of the origin of granular cell myoblastoma. *J Pathol* 1973;109:101–111.

250. LeBoit PE, Barr RJ, Burall S, et al.: Primitive polypoid granular cell tumor and other cutaneous granular cell neoplasms of apparent non-neural origin. *Am J Surg Pathol* 1991;15:48–58.

251. Arnold HL, Odom RB, James WD (Eds): *Andrews' Diseases of the Skin: Clinical Dermatology,* 8th ed. Philadelphia: W.B. Saunders, 1990:682–744.

252. Fletcher CDM, Martin-Bates E: Spindle-cell lipoma: A clinicopathological study with some original observations. *Histopathology* 1987;11:803–817.

253. Duve SR, Muller-Hocker J, Worret WI: Spindle-cell lipoma of the skin. *Am J Dermatopathol* 1995;17:529–533.

254. Griffin TD, Goldstein J, Johnson WC: Pleomorphic lipoma. *J Cutan Pathol* 1992;19:330–333.

255. Dixon AY, McGregor DH, Lee SH: Angiolipomas: An ultrastructural and clinicopathologic study. *Hum Pathol* 1981;12:739–747.

256. Enzinger FM, Harvey DJ: Spindle-cell lipoma. *Cancer* 1975;36:1852–1859.

257. Shmookler BM, Enzinger FM: Pleomorphic lipoma: A benign tumor simulating liposarcoma. A clinicopathologic analysis of 48 cases. *Cancer* 1981;47:126–133.

258. Howard WR, Helwig EB: Angiolipoma. *Arch Dermatol* 1960;82:924–931.

259. Kurzweg FT, Spencer R: Familial multiple lipomatosis. *Am J Surg* 1951;82:762–765.

260. Osment LS: Cutaneous lipomas and lipomatosis. *Surg Gynecol Obstet* 1968;127:129–132.

261. Sahl WJ Jr: Mobile encapsulated lipomas. *Arch Dermatol* 1978;114:1684–1686.

262. Hunt SJ, Santa Cruz DJ, Barr RJ: Cellular angiolipoma. *Am J Surg Pathol* 1990;14:75–81.

263. Rigor VU, Goldstone SE: Hibernoma: A case report and discussion of a rare tumor. *Cancer* 1986;57:2207–2211.

264. Dardick I: Hibernoma: A possible model of brown fat histogenesis. *Hum Pathol* 1978;9:321–329.

265. Fitzpatrick TB, Gilchrist BA: Dimple sign to differentiate benign from malignant cutaneous lesions. *N Engl J Med* 1977;296:1518.

266. Gonzalez S, Duarte I: Benign fibrous histiocytoma of the skin: a morphologic study of 290 cases. *Pathol Res Pract* 1982;174:379–391.

267. Niemi KM: The benign fibrohistiocytic tumors of the skin. *Acta Dermatol Venereol* 1970;50(suppl):1–66.

268. Baraf CS, Shapiro L: Multiple histiocytomas. *Arch Dermatol* 1970;101:588–590.

269. Roberts JT, Byrne EH, Rosenthal D: Familial variant of dermatofibroma with malignancy in the proband. *Arch Dermatol* 1981;117:12–15.

270. Schoenfeld RJ: Epidermal proliferations overlying histiocytomas. *Arch Dermatol* 1964;90:266–270.

271. Marrogi AJ, Dehner LP, Coffin CM, Wick MR: Benign cutaneous histiocytic tumors in childhood and adolescence, excluding Langerhans' cell proliferations: A clinicopathologic and immunohistochemical analysis. *Am J Dermatopathol* 1992;14:8–18.

272. Kamino H, Jacobson M: Dermatofibroma extending into the subcutaneous tissue: Differential diagnosis from dermatofibrosarcoma protuberans. *Am J Surg Pathol* 1990;14:1156–1165.

273. Fukamizu H, Oku T, Inoue K, et al.: Atypical (pseudosarcomatous) cutaneous histiocytoma. *J Cutan Pathol* 1983;10:327–333.

274. Leyva WH, Santa Cruz DJ: Atypical cutaneous fibrous histiocytoma. *Am J Dermatopathol* 1986;8:467–471.

275. Tamada S, Ackerman AB: Dermatofibroma with monster cells. *Am J Dermatopathol* 1987;9:380–387.

276. Santa Cruz DJ, Kyriakos M: Aneurysmal (angiomatoid) fibrous histiocytoma of the skin. *Cancer* 1981;47:2053–2061.

277. Sood U, Mehregan AH: Aneurysmal (angiomatoid) fibrous histiocytoma. *J Cutan Pathol* 1985;12:157–167.

278. Barker SM, Winkelmann RK: Inflammatory lymphadenoid reactions with dermatofibroma/histiocytoma. *J Cutan Pathol* 1986;13:222–226.

279. Goette DK, Helwig EB: Basal cell carcinomas and basal cell carcinoma-like changes overlying dermatofibromas. *Arch Dermatol* 1975;111:589–592.

280. Schwob VS, Santa Cruz DJ: Palisading cutaneous fibrous histiocytoma. *J Cutan Pathol* 1986;13:403–407.

281. Bernstein JC: Hemosiderin histiocytoma of the skin. *Arch Dermatol* 1939;40:390–396.

282. Franquemont DW, Cooper PH, Shmookler BM, Wick MR: Benign fibrous histiocytoma of the skin with potential for local recurrence. *Mod Pathol* 1990;3:158–163.

283. Marrogi AJ, Dehner LP, Coffin CM, Wick MR: Atypical fibrous histiocytoma of the skin in childhood and adolescence. *J Cutan Pathol* 1992;19:268–277.

284. Johnson WC, Graham JH, Helwig EB: Cutaneous myxoid cyst. *JAMA* 1965;191:15–20.

285. Carney JA, Gordon H, Carpenter PC, et al.: The complex of myxomas, spotty pigmentation, and endocrine overactivity. *Medicine* 1985;64:270–283.

286. Hanau CA, Miettinen M: Solitary fibrous tumor: Histological and immunohistochemical spectrum of benign and malignant variants presenting at different sites. *Hum Pathol* 1995;26:440–449.

Mesenchymal Cutaneous Tumors with "Borderline" Malignant Potential

287. Dabska M: Malignant endovascular papillary angioendothelioma of the skin in childhood: Clinicopathologic study of 6 cases. *Cancer* 1969;24:503–510.

288. DeDulanto F, Armijo-Moreno M: Malignant endovascular papillary hemangioendothelioma of the skin: The nosological situation. *Acta Dermatol Venereol* 1973;53:403–408.

289. Manivel JC, Wick MR, Swanson PE, et al.: Endovascular papillary angioendothelioma of childhood: A vascular tumor possibly characterized by "high" endothelial differentiation. *Hum Pathol* 1986;17:1240–1244.

290. Patterson K, Chandler RS: Malignant endovascular papillary angioendothelioma: Cutaneous borderline tumor. *Arch Pathol Lab Med* 1985;109:671–673.

291. Weiss SW, Enzinger FM: Epithelioid hemangioendothelioma: a vascular tumor often mistaken for a carcinoma. *Cancer* 1982;50:970–981.

292. Weiss SW, Ishak KG, Dail DH, et al.: Epithelioid hemangioendothelioma and related lesions. *Semin Diagn Pathol* 1986;3:259–287, 279–287.

293. Stout AP, Murray MR: Hemangiopericytoma. *Am J Surg* 1942;116:26–33.

294. Saunders TS, Fitzpatrick TB: Multiple hemangiopericytomas: Their distinction from glomangiomas (glomus tumors). *Arch Dermatol* 1957;76:731–734.

295. D'Amore ESG, Manivel JC, Sung JH: Soft tissue and meningeal hemangiopericytomas: An immunohistochemical and ultrastructural study. *Hum Pathol* 1990;21:414–423.

296. Burkhardt BR, Soule EH, Winkelmann RK, Ivins JC: Dermatofibrosarcoma protuberans: A study of fifty-six cases. *Am J Surg* 1966;111:638–644.

297. McKee PH, Fletcher CDM: Dermatofibrosarcoma protuberans presenting in infancy and childhood. *J Cutan Pathol* 1991;18:241–246.

298. McPeak CJ, Cruz T, Nicastri AD: Dermatofibrosarcoma: An analysis of 86 cases—five with metastases. *Ann Surg* 1967;166:803–816.

299. Taylor HB, Helwig EB: Dermatofibrosarcoma protuberans: A study of 115 cases. *Cancer* 1962;15:717–725.

300. Fletcher CDM, Evans BJ, Macartney JC, et al.: Dermatofibrosarcoma protuberans: A clinicopathological and immunohistochemical study with a review of the literature. *Histopathology* 1985;9:921–938.

301. Frierson HF Jr, Cooper PH: Myxoid variant of dermatofibrosarcoma protuberans. *Am J Surg Pathol* 1983;7:445–450.

302. Dupree WB, Langloss JM, Weiss SW: Pigmented dermatofibrosarcoma protuberans (Bednar tumor): A pathologic, ultrastructural, and immunohistochemical study. *Am J Surg Pathol* 1985;9:630–639.

303. Wrotnowski U, Cooper PH, Shmookler BM: Fibrosarcomatous change in dermatofibrosarcoma protuberans. *Am J Surg Pathol* 1988;12:287–293.

304. Ding J, Hashimoto H, Enjoji M: Dermatofibrosarcoma protuberans with fibrosarcomatous areas: A clinicopathologic study of nine cases and a comparison with allied tumors. *Cancer* 1989;64:721–729.

305. Connelly JH, Evans HL: Dermatofibrosarcoma protuberans: A clinicopathologic review with emphasis on fibrosarcomatous areas. *Am J Surg Pathol* 1992;16:921–925.

306. Calonje E, Fletcher CDM: Myoid differentiation in dermatofibrosarcoma protuberans and its fibrosarcomatous variant: Clinicopathologic analysis of 5 cases. *J Cutan Pathol* 1996;23:30–36.

307. Volpe R, Carbone A: Dermatofibrosarcoma protuberans metastatic to lymph nodes and showing a dominant histiocytic component. *Am J Dermatopathol* 1983;5:327–334.

308. O'Dowd J, Laidler P: Progression of dermatofibrosarcoma protuberans to malignant fibrous histiocytoma: Report of a case with implications for tumor histogenesis. *Hum Pathol* 1988;19:368–370.

309. Cohen PR, Rapini RP, Farhood AI: Dermatofibroma and dermatofibrosarcoma protuberans: Differential expression of CD34 and factor XIIIa. *Am J Dermatopathol* 1994;16:573–574.

310. Shmookler BM, Enzinger FM: Giant cell fibroblastoma: a peculiar childhood tumor (abstract). *Lab Invest* 1983;46:7a.

311. Shmookler BM, Enzinger FM, Weiss SW: Giant cell fibroblastoma. *Cancer* 1989;64:2154–2161.

312. Abdul-Karim W, Evans HL, Silva EG: Giant cell fibroblastoma: A report of three cases. *Am J Clin Pathol* 1985;83:165–170.

313. Dymock RB, Allen PW, Stirling JW, et al.: Giant cell fibroblastoma: A

distinctive recurrent tumor of childhood. *Am J Surg Pathol* 1987;11:263–271.

314. Fletcher CDM: Giant cell fibroblastoma of soft tissue: A clinicopathological and immunohistochemical study. *Histopathology* 1988;13:499–508.

315. Beham A, Fletcher CDM: Dermatofibrosarcoma protuberans resembling giant cell fibroblastoma: Report of two cases. *Histopathology* 1990;17:165–167.

316. DeChadarevian JP, Coppola D, Billmire DF: Bednar tumor pattern in recurring giant cell fibroblastoma. *Am J Clin Pathol* 1993;100:164–166.

317. Marrogi AJ, Swanson PE, Kyriakos M, Wick MR: Rudimentary meningocele: clinicopathologic features and differential diagnosis. *J Cutan Pathol* 1991;18:178–188.

318. Dei Tos AP, Seregard S, Calonje E, Chan JKC, Fletcher CDM: Giant cell angiofibroma: A distinctive orbital tumor in adults. *Am J Surg Pathol* 1995;19:1286–1293.

319. Mikami Y, Shimizu M, Hirokawa M, Manabe T: Extraorbital giant cell angiofibromas. *Mod Pathol* 1997;10:1082–1087.

320. Enzinger FM, Zhang R: Plexiform fibrohistiocytic tumor presenting in children and young adults: An analysis of 65 cases. *Am J Surg Pathol* 1988;12:818–826.

321. Hollowood K, Holley MP, Fletcher CDM: Plexiform fibrohistiocytic tumour: Clinicopathological, immunohistochemical, and ultrastructural analysis in favor of a myofibroblastic lesion. *Histopathology* 1991;19:503–513.

322. Enzinger FM: Angiomatoid malignant fibrous histiocytoma: A distinct fibrohistiocytic tumor of children and young adults, simulating a vascular neoplasm. *Cancer* 1979;44:2146–2157.

323. Kay S: Angiomatoid malignant fibrous histiocytoma: Report of two cases with ultrastructural observations of one case. *Arch Pathol Lab Med* 1985;109:934–937.

324. Costa MJ, Weiss SW: Angiomatoid malignant fibrous histiocytoma: A followup study of 108 cases with evaluation of possible histologic predictors of outcome. *Am J Surg Pathol* 1990;14:1126–1132.

Overtly Malignant Mesenchymal Tumors of the Skin

325. Hashimoto H, Enjoji M, Nakajima T, et al.: Malignant neuroepithelioma (peripheral neuroblastoma): A clinicopathologic study of 15 cases. *Am J Surg* Pathol 1983;7:309–318.

326. Dehner, LP: Primitive neuroectodermal tumor and Ewing's sarcoma. *Am J Surg* Pathol. 1993;17:1–13.

327. Jacinto CM, Grant-Kels JM, Knibbs DR, et al.: Malignant peripheral neuroectodermal tumor presenting as a scalp nodule. *Am J Dermatopathol* 1991;13:63–70.

328. Patterson JW, Maygarden SJ: Extraskeletal Ewing's sarcoma with cutaneous involvement. *J Cutan Pathol* 1986;13:46–58.

329. Peters MS, Reiman HM Jr, Muller SA: Cutaneous extraskeletal Ewing's sarcoma. *J Cutan Pathol* 1985;12:476–485.

330. Mierau GW: Extraskeletal Ewing's sarcoma (peripheral neuroepithelioma). *Ultrastruct Pathol* 1985;9:91–98.

331. Jurgens H, Bier V, Harms D, et al.: Malignant peripheral neuroectodermal tumors. *Cancer* 1988;61:349–357.

332. Triche TJ, Askin F: Neuroblastoma and the differential diagnosis of small-, round-, blue-cell tumors. *Hum Pathol* 1983;14:569–595.

333. Michels S, Swanson PE, Frizzera G, Wick MR.: Immunostaining for leukocyte common antigen using an amplified avidin-biotin-peroxidase complex method and paraffin sections. *Arch Pathol Lab Med* 1987;111:1035–1039.

334. Dahl I, Angervall L: Cutaneous and subcutaneous leiomyosarcoma: a clinicopathologic study of 47 patients. *Pathol Europ* 1974;9:307–315.

335. Fields JP, Helwig EB: Leiomyosarcoma of the skin and subcutaneous tissue. *Cancer* 1981;47:156–169.

336. Swanson PE, Stanley MW, Scheithauer BW, Wick MR: Primary cutaneous leiomyosarcoma. *J Cutan Pathol* 1988;15:129–141.

337. George E, Swanson PE, Wick MR: Malignant peripheral nerve sheath tumors of the skin. *Am J Dermatopathol* 1989;11:213–221.

338. Dabski C, Reiman HM Jr, Muller SA: Neurofibrosarcoma of skin and subcutaneous tissues. *Mayo Clin Proc* 1990;65:164–172.

339. Misago N, Ishii Y, Kohda M: Malignant peripheral nerve sheath tumor of the skin: A superficial form of this tumor. *J Cutan Pathol* 1996;23:182–188.

340. Wick MR: Malignant peripheral nerve sheath tumors of the skin. *Mayo Clin Proc* 1990;65:279–282.

341. Daimaru Y, Hashimoto H, Enjoji M: Malignant "triton" tumors. *Hum Pathol* 1984;15:768–778.

342. Ducatman BS, Scheithauer BW, Piepgras DG, et al.: Malignant peripheral nerve sheath tumors: A clinicopathologic study of 120 cases. *Cancer* 1986;57:2006–2021.

343. Wick MR, Swanson PE, Scheithauer BW, Manivel JC: Malignant peripheral nerve sheath tumor: An immunohistochemical study of 62 cases. *Am J Clin Pathol* 1987;87:425–433.

344. Kossard S, Doherty E, Murray E: Neurotropic melanoma: A variant of desmoplastic melanoma. *Arch Dermatol* 1987;123:907–912.

345. DiMaio SM, Mackay B, Smith JL, et al.: Neurosarcomatous transformation in malignant melanoma: An ultrastructural study. *Cancer* 1982;50:2345–2354.

346. Gown AM, Vogel AM, Hoak D, et al.: Monoclonal antibodies specific for melanocytic tumors distinguish subpopulations of melanocytes. *Am J Pathol* 1986;123:195–203.

347. Wick MR: Kaposi's sarcoma unrelated to the acquired immunodeficiency syndrome. *Curr Opin Oncol* 1991;3:377–383.

348. Chor PJ, Santa Cruz DJ: Kaposi's sarcoma: A clinicopathologic review and differential diagnosis. *J Cutan Pathol* 1992;19:6–20.

349. Gottlieb GJ, Ackerman AB (Eds): *Kaposi's Sarcoma: A Text and Atlas.* Philadelphia: Lea & Febiger, 1988:73–112.

350. Gottlieb GJ, Ackerman AB: Kaposi's sarcoma: An extensively disseminated form in young homosexual men. *Hum Pathol* 1982;13:882–892.

351. Jaffe HW: Acquired immune deficiency syndrome: Epidemiologic features. *J Am Acad Dermatol* 1990;22:1167–1171.

352. Ackerman AB: The patch stage of Kaposi's sarcoma. *Am J Dermatopathol* 1979;1:165–172.

353. Pollack MS, Safai B, Myskowski PL, et al.: Frequencies of HLA and Gm immunogenetic markers in Kaposi's sarcoma. *Tissue Antigens* 1983;21:1–8.

354. Boldogh I, Beth E, Huang ES, et al.: Kaposi's sarcoma: IV. Detection of CMV-DNA, CMV-RNA, and CMNA in tumor biopsies. *Int J Cancer* 1981;28:469–474.

355. Jin YT, Tsai ST, Yan JJ, et al.: Detection of Kaposi's sarcoma–associated herpes virus–like DNA sequence in vascular lesions: A reliable diagnostic marker for Kaposi's sarcoma. *Am J Clin Pathol* 1996;105:360–363.

356. Costa J, Rabson AS: Generalized Kaposi's sarcoma is not a neoplasm. *Lancet* 1983;1:58.

357. Delli-Bovi P, Basilico C: Isolation of a rearranged human transforming gene following transfection of Kaposi's sarcoma DNA. *Proc Natl Acad Sci USA* 1987;84:5660–5664.

358. Fenoglio CM, Oster M, LoGerfo P, et al.: Kaposi's sarcoma following chemotherapy for testicular cancer in a homosexual man: Demonstration of cytomegalovirus DNA in sarcoma cells. *Hum Pathol* 1982;13:955–959.

359. Dantzig PE: Chemotherapy for Kaposi's sarcoma. *Arch Dermatol* 1976;112:1179.

360. McNutt NS, Fletcher V, Conant MA: Early lesions of Kaposi's sarcoma in homosexual men: An ultrastructural comparison with other vascular proliferations in skin. *Am J Dermatopathol* 1983;3:62–73.

361. Blumenfeld W, Egbert BM, Sagebiel RW: Differential diagnosis of Kaposi's sarcoma. *Arch Pathol Lab Med* 1985;109:123–127.

362. Snover DC, Rosai J: Vascular sarcomas of the skin. In: Wick MR, ed. *Pathology of Unusual Malignant Cutaneous Tumors.* New York: Marcel Dekker,, 1985:181–209.

363. Templeton AC: Kaposi's sarcoma. *Pathol Annu* 1981;17:315–336.

364. Beckstead JH, Wood GS, Fletcher V: Evidence for the origin of Kaposi's sarcoma from lymphatic endothelium. *Am J Pathol* 1985;119:294–300.

365. Harrison AC, Kahn LB: Myogenic cells in Kaposi's sarcoma: An ultrastructural study. *J Pathol* 1978;124:157–160.

366. Suster S: Epithelioid leiomyosarcoma of the skin and subcutaneous tissue. *Am J Surg Pathol* 1994;18:232–240.

367. Chung EB: Current classification of soft tissue tumors. In: Fletcher CDM, McKee PH, eds. *Pathobiology of Soft Tissue Tumors.* New York: Churchill-Livingstone, 1990:43–82.

368. Morgan KG, Gray C: Malignant epithelioid schwannoma of superficial soft tissue? A case report with immunohistology and electron microscopy. *Histopathology* 1985;9:765–775.

369. DiCarlo EF, Woodruff JM, Bansal M, Erlandson RA: The purely epithelioid malignant peripheral nerve sheath tumor. *Am J Surg Pathol* 1986;10:478–490.

370. Bhuta S, Mirra JM, Cochran AJ: Myxoid malignant melanoma. *Am J Surg Pathol* 1986;10:203–211.

371. Cadotte M: Malignant granular cell myoblastoma. *Cancer* 1974; 33:1417–1422.

372. Al-Sarraf M, Loud A, Vaitkevicius V: Malignant granular cell tumor. *Arch Pathol* 1971;91:550–558.

373. MacKenzie DH: Malignant granular cell myoblastoma. *J Clin Pathol* 1967;20:739–742.

374. Simsir A, Osborne BM, Greenebaum E: Malignant granular cell tumor: A case report and review of the recent literature. *Hum Pathol* 1996;27:853–858.

375. Shimamura K, Osamura RY, Ueyama Y, et al.: Malignant granular cell tumor of the right sciatic nerve. *Cancer* 1984;53:524–529.

376. Franzblau MJ, Manwaring J, Plumhof C, et al.: Metastatic breast carcinoma mimicking granular cell tumor. *J Cutan Pathol* 1989;16:218–222.

377. Dabbs DJ, Park HK: Malignant rhabdoid skin tumor: An uncommon primary skin neoplasm. *J Cutan Pathol* 1988;15:109–115.

378. Perrone T, Swanson PE, Twiggs L, et al.: Malignant rhabdoid tumor of the vulva. *Am J Surg Pathol* 1989;13:848–858.

379. Tsokos M, Kouraklis G, Chandra RS, et al.: Malignant rhabdoid tumor of the kidney and soft tissues: Evidence for a diverse morphological and immunocytochemical phenotype. *Arch Pathol Lab Med* 1989;113:115–120.

380. Wick MR, Ritter JR, Dehner LP: Malignant rhabdoid tumors: clinico-pathologic review and conceptual discussion. *Semin Diagn Pathol* 1995;12:233–248.

381. Cooper PH: Angiosarcomas of the skin. *Semin Diagn Pathol* 1987;4:2–17.

382. Holden CA, Spittle MF, Wilson-Jones E: Angiosarcoma of the face and scalp: Prognosis and treatment. *Cancer* 1987;59:1046–1057.

383. Wilson-Jones E: Malignant angioendothelioma of the skin. *Br J Dermatol* 1964;76:21–39.

384. Girard C, Johnson WC, Graham JH: Cutaneous angiosarcoma. *Cancer* 1970;26:868–883.

385. Hodgkinson DJ, Soule EH, Woods JE: Cutaneous angiosarcoma of the head and neck. *Cancer* 1979;44:1106–1113.

386. Maddox JC, Evans HL: Angiosarcoma of skin and soft tissue: A study of forty-four cases. *Cancer* 1981;48:1907–1921.

387. Perez-Atayde AR, Achenbach H, Lack EE: High-grade epithelioid angiosarcoma of the scalp: An immunohistochemical and ultrastructural study. *Am J Dermatopathol* 1986;8:411–418.

388. Miyachi Y, Imamura S: Very low-grade angiosarcoma. *Dermatologica* 1981;162:206–208.

389. McWilliam LJ, Harris M: Granular cell angiosarcoma of the skin: Histology, electron microscopy, and immunohistochemistry of a newly recognized tumor. *Histopathology* 1985;9:1205–1216.

390. Akiyama M, Naka W, Harada T, Nishikawa T: Angiosarcoma with dermal melanocytosis. *J Cutan Pathol* 1989;16:149–153.

391. Bancrjcc SS, Eyden BP, Wells S, et al.: Pseudoangiosarcomatous carcinoma: A clinicopathological study of seven cases. *Histopathology* 1992;21:13–23.

392. Ritter JH, Mills S, Nappi O, Wick MR: Angiosarcoma-like neoplasms of epithelial organs: True endothelial tumors or variants of carcinoma? *Semin Diagn Pathol* 1995;12:270–282.

393. Swanson PE, Wick MR: Immunohistochemical evaluation of cutaneous vascular neoplasms. *Clin Dermatol* 1991;9:243–254.

394. Helwig EB: Atypical fibroxanthoma. *Texas J Med* 1963;59:664–667.

395. Fretzin DF, Helwig EB: Atypical fibroxanthoma of the skin: A clinicopathologic study of 140 cases. *Cancer* 1973;31:1541–1552.

396. Alguacil-Garcia A, Unni KK, Goellner JR: Atypical fibroxanthoma of the skin. *Cancer* 1977;40:1471–1480.

397. Dahl I: Atypical fibroxanthoma of the skin: A clinicopathological study of 57 cases. *Acta Pathol Microbiol Scand* 1976;84:183–197.

398. Beham A, Fletcher CD: Atypical 'pseudosarcomatous' variant of cutaneous benign fibrous histiocytoma: Report of eight cases. *Histopathol* 1990;17:167–169.

399. Helwig EB, May D: Atypical fibroxanthoma of the skin with metastasis. *Cancer* 1986;57:368–376.

400. Grosso M, Lentini M, Carrozza G., Catalano A: Metastatic atypical fibroxanthoma of skin. *Pathol Res Pract* 1987;182:443–447.

401. Oshiro Y, Fukuda T, Tsuneyoshi M: Atypical fibroxanthoma versus benign and malignant fibrous histiocytoma. A comparative study of their proliferative activity using MIB-1, DNA flow cytometry, and p53 immunostaining. *Cancer* 1995;75:1128–1134.

402. Calonje E, Wadden C, Wilson-Jones E, Fletcher CD: Spindle-cell non-pleomorphic atypical fibroxanthoma: Analysis of a series and delineation of a distinctive variant. *Histopathol* 1993;22:247–254.

403. Val-Vernal JF, Corral J, Fernandez F, Gomez-Bellvert C: Atypical fibroxanthoma with osteoclast-like giant cells. *Acta Dermato-Venereologica* 1994;74:467–470.

404. Wilson PR, Strutton GM, Stewart MR: Atypical fibroxanthoma: Two unusual variants. *J Cutan Pathol* 1989;16:93–98.

405. Leong ASY, Wick MR, Swanson PE: Immunohistology and electron microscopy of anaplastic and pleomorphic tumors. Cambridge, U.K.: Cambridge Press, 1997;59–108.

406. Ma CK, Zarbo RJ, Gown AM: Immunohistochemical characterization of atypical fibroxanthoma and dermatofibrosarcoma protuberans. *Am J Clin Pathol* 1992;97:487–493.

407. Longacre TA, Smoller BR, Rouse RV: Atypical fibroxanthoma. Multiple immunohistologic profiles. *Am J Surg Pathol* 1993;17:1199–1209.

408. Eckert F, Burg G, Braun-Falco O, Schmid U, Gloor F: Immunostaining in atypical fibroxanthoma of the skin. *Pathol Res Pract* 1988;184:27–34.

Pseudoneoplastic Mesenchymal Proliferations of the Skin

409. Price EB Jr, Silliphant WM, Shuman R: Nodular fasciitis: A clinicopathologic analysis of 65 cases. *Am J Clin Pathol* 1961;35:122–136.

410. Meister P, Buckmann FW, Konrad E: Extent and level of fascial involvement in 100 cases with nodular fasciitis. *Virchows Arch A Pathol Anat Histol* 1978;380:177–185.

411. Shimizu S, Hashimoto H, Enjoji M: Nodular fasciitis: An analysis of 250 patients. *Pathology* 1984;16:161–166.

412. Lauer DH, Enzinger FM: Cranial fasciitis of childhood. *Cancer* 1980;45:401–406.

413. Price SK, Kahn LB, Saxe N: Dermal and intravascular fasciitis. Unusual variants of nodular fasciitis. *Am J Dermatopathol* 1993;15:539–543.

414. Hutter RV, Foote FW, Francis KC, et al.: Parosteal fasciitis. *Am J Surg* 1962;104:800–807.

415. Lai FM, Lam WY: Nodular fasciitis of the dermis. *J Cutan Pathol* 1993;20:66–69.

416. Bernstein KE, Lattes R: Nodular (pseudosarcomatous) fasciitis: A non-recurrent lesion. Clinicopathologic study of 134 cases. Cancer 1982; 49:1668–1678.

417. Murray JC, Pollack SV, Pinnell SR: Keloids and hypertrophic scars. *Clin Dermatol* 1984;2:121–133.

418. Ketchum LD, Cohen IK, Masters FW: Hypertrophic scars and keloids: A collective review. *Plast Reconstr Surg* 1974;53:140–154.

419. Murray JC, Pollack SV, Pinnell SR: Keloids: A review. *J Am Acad Dermatol* 1981;4:461–470.

420. Hurt MA, Santa Cruz DJ: Cutaneous inflammatory pseudotumor. *Am J Surg Pathol* 1988;14:764–773.

421. Requena L, Gutierrez J, Sanchez-Yus E: Multiple sclerotic fibromas of the skin: A cutaneous marker of Cowden's disease. *J Cutan Pathol* 1991;19:346–351.

422. Metcalf JS, Maize JC, LeBoit PE: Circumscribed storiform collagenoma (sclerotic fibroma). *Am J Dermatopathol* 1992;13:122–129.

423. Templeton HJ: Cutaneous tags of the neck. *Arch Dermatol* 1936;33:495–505.

424. Waisman M: Cutaneous papillomas of the neck: Papillomatous seborrheic keratoses. *South Med J* 1957;50:725–731.

425. Williams BT, Barr RJ, Barrett TL, et al.: Cutaneous pseudosarcomatous polyps: A histological and immunohistochemical study. *J Cutan Pathol* 1996;23:189–193.

426. Barsky SH, Rosen S, Geer DE, et al.: The nature and evolution of port wine stains: A computer-assisted study. *J Invest Dermatol* 1980;74:154–157.

427. Finley JL, Noe JM, Arndt KA, et al.: Port-wine stains: Morphologic variations and developmental lesions. *Arch Dermatol* 1984;120:1453–1455.

428. Lindenauer SM: The Klippel-Trenaunay syndrome. *Ann Surg* 1965; 162:303–314.

429. Hashimoto K, Pritzker MS: Hereditary hemorrhagic telangiectasia: An electron microscopic study. *Oral Surg Oral Med Oral Pathol* 1972; 34:751–768.

430. McGrae JD Jr, Winkelmann RK: Generalized essential telangiectasia. *JAMA* 1963;185:909–913.

431. Wilkin JK, Smith JG Jr, Cullison DA, et al.: Unilateral dermatomal superficial telangiectasia. *J Am Acad Dermatol* 1983;8:468–477.

432. Amazon K, Robinson MD, Rywlin AM: Ferrugination caused by Monsel's solution: Clinical observations and experimentations. *Am J Dermatopathol* 1980;2:197–205.

433. LeBoit PE, Berger TG, Egbert BM, et al.: Bacillary angiomatosis. *Am J Surg Pathol* 1989;13:909–920.

434. Tappero JW, Perkins BA, Wenger JD, Berger TG: Cutaneous manifestations of opportunistic infections in patients infected with human immunodeficiency virus. *Clin Microbiol Rev* 1995;8:440–450.

435. LeBoit PE: Bacillary angiomatosis. *Mod Pathol* 1995;8:218–222.

436. Cockerell CJ, Webster GF, Whitlow MA, Friedman-Kien AE: Epithelioid angiomatosis: a distinct vascular disorder in patients with the acquired immunodeficiency syndrome or AIDS-related complex. *Lancet* 1987;2:654–656.

437. Arias-Stella J, Lieberman PH, Erlandson RA, Arias-Stella J Jr: Histology, immunochemistry, and ultrastructure of the verruga in Carrion's disease. *Am J Surg Pathol* 1986;10:595–610.

438. Arias-Stella J, Lieberman PH, Garcia-Carceres U, et al.: Verruga peruana mimicking malignant neoplasms. *Am J Dermatopathol* 1987; 9:279–291.

439. Brandwein M, Choi HSH, Strauchen J, et al.: Spindle-cell reaction to nontuberculous mycobacteriosis in AIDS, mimicking a spindle-cell neoplasm. *Virchows Arch A* 1990;416:281–286.

440. Hashimoto H, Daimaru Y, Enjoji M: Intravascular papillary endothelial hyperplasia: A clinicopathologic study of 91 cases. *Am J Dermatopathol* 1983;5:539–546.

441. Kuo TT, Sayers CP, Rosai J: Masson's "vegetant intravascular hemangioendothelioma": A lesion often mistaken for angiosarcoma. *Cancer* 1976;38:1227–1236.

442. Sibley DA, Cooper PH: Rudimentary meningocele. *J Cutan Pathol* 1989;16:72–80.

443. Berry AD III, Patterson JW: Meningoceles, meningomyeloceles, and encephaloceles: A neurodermatopathologic study of 132 cases. *J Cutan Pathol* 1991;18:164–177.

Cutaneous Lymphoproliferative Lesions

444. Banks PM: Lymphoid neoplasms of the skin. In: Wick MR, ed. *Pathology of Unusual Malignant Cutaneous Tumors.* New York: Marcel Dekker, 1985:299–356.

445. Burke J: Malignant lymphomas of the skin: Their differentiation from lymphoid and non-lymphoid cutaneous infiltrates that simulate lymphoma. *Semin Diagn Pathol* 1985;2:169–182.

446. Akasu R, Kahn HJ, From L: Lymphocyte markers on formalin-fixed tissue in Jessner's lymphocytic infiltrate and lupus erythematosus. *J Cutan Pathol* 1992;19:59–65.

447. Smolle J, Torne R, Soyer HP, Kerl H: Immunohistochemical classification of cutaneous pseudolymphomas: Delineation of distinct patterns. *J Cutan Pathol* 1990;17:149–159.

448. Smoller BR, Glusac EJ: Histologic mimics of cutaneous lymphoma. *Pathol Annu* 1995; 30(1):123–141.

449. Slater DN: Diagnostic difficulties in "non-mycotic" cutaneous lymphoproliferative diseases. *Histopathology* 1992;21:203–213.

450. Rijlaarsdam U, Willemze R: Cutaneous pseudo-T-cell lymphomas. *Semin Diagn Pathol* 1991;8:102–108.

451. Toonstra J: Actinic reticuloid. *Semin Diagn Pathol* 1991;8:109–116.

452. LeBoit PE: Variants of mycosis fungoides and related cutaneous T-cell lymphomas. *Semin Diagn Pathol* 1991;8:73–81.

453. Wood GS, Abel EA, Hoppe RT, et al.: Leu-8 and Leu-9 antigen phenotypes: Immunological criteria for the distinction of mycosis fungoides from cutaneous inflammation. *J Am Acad Dermatol* 1986;14:1006–1013.

454. Ralfkiaer E: Immunological markers for the diagnosis of cutaneous lymphomas. *Semin Diagn Pathol* 1991;8:62–72.

455. Bignon YJ, Souteyrand P: Genotyping of cutaneous T-cell lymphomas and pseudolymphomas. *Curr Prob Dermatol* 1990;19:114–123.

456. Perkins SL, Kjeldsberg CR: Immunophenotyping of lymphomas and leukemias in paraffin-embedded tissues. *Am J Clin Pathol* 1993; 99:362–373.

457. Yoshino T, Mukuzono H, Aoki H, et al.: A novel monoclonal antibody (OPD4) recognizing a helper/inducer T-cell subset. Its application to paraffin-embedded tissues. *Am J Pathol* 1989;134:1339–1346.

458. Chadburn A, Husain S, Knowles DM: Monoclonal antibody OPD4 detects neoplastic T cells but does not distinguish between CD4 and CD8 neoplastic T cells in paraffin tissue sections. *Hum Pathol* 1992;23:940–947.

459. Mason DY, Cordell JL, Gaulard P, et al.: Immunohistological detection of human cytotoxic/suppressor T-cells using antibodies to a CD8 peptide sequence. *J Clin Pathol* 1992;45:1084–1088.

460. Kerl H, Smolle J: Classification of cutaneous pseudolymphomas. *Curr Prob Dermatol* 1989;19:167–176.

461. Berti E, Alessi E, Caputo R: Reticulohistiocytoma of the dorsum (Crosti's disease) and other B-cell lymphomas. *Semin Diagn Pathol* 1991;8:82–90.

462. Toyota N, Matsuo S, Iizuka H: Immunohistochemical differential diagnosis between lymphocytoma cutis and malignant lymphoma in paraffin-embedded sections. *J Dermatol* 1991;18:586–591.

463. Picker LJ, Weiss LM, Medeiros LJ, et al.: Immunophenotypic criteria for the diagnosis of non-Hodgkin's lymphoma. *Am J Pathol* 1987;128:181–201.

464. Ritter JH, Adesokan PN, Fitzgibbon JF, Wick MR: Paraffin section immunohistochemistry as an adjunct to morphologic analysis in the diagnosis of cutaneous lymphoid infiltrates. *J Cutan Pathol* 1994;21:481–493.

465. Ngan BY, Picker LJ, Medeiros LJ, Warnke RA: Immunophenotypic diagnosis of non-Hodgkin's lymphoma in paraffin sections: Coexpression of L60 (Leu 22) and L26 antigens correlates with malignant histologic findings. *Am J Clin Pathol* 1989;91:579–583.

466. Utz GL, Swerdlow SH: Distinction of follicular hyperplasia from follicular lymphoma in B5-fixed tissues: Comparison of MT2 and *bcl*-2 antibodies. *Hum Pathol* 1993;24:1155–1158.

467. Triscott JA, Ritter JH, Swanson PE, Wick MR: Immunoreactivity for *bcl*-2 protein in cutaneous lymphomas and lymphoid hyperplasias. *J Cutan Pathol* 1995;22:2–10.

468. Kuo TT: Cutaneous manifestations of Kikuchi's histiocytic necrotizing lymphadenitis. *Am J Surg Pathol* 1990;14:872–879.

469. Kaudewitz P, Burg G: Lymphomatoid papulosis and Ki-1 (CD30)-positive cutaneous large cell lymphomas. *Semin Diagn Pathol* 1991; 8:117–124.

470. Stein H, Mason DY, Gerdes J, et al.: The expression of the Hodgkin's disease-associated antigen Ki-1 in reactive and neoplastic tissue. *Blood* 1985;66:848–858.

471. Menestrina F, Chilosi M, Scarpa A: Nodular lymphocyte predominant Hodgkin's disease and anaplastic large-cell lymphoma: Distinct entities or nonspecific patterns? *Semin Diagn Pathol* 1995;12:256–269.

472. Kuo TT: Kikuchi's disease (histiocytic necrotizing lymphadenitis): A clinicopathologic study of 79 cases with an analysis of histologic subtypes, immunohistology, and DNA ploidy. *Am J Surg Pathol* 1995; 19:798–809.

473. Banerjee SS, Heald J, Harris M: Twelve cases of Ki-1-positive anaplastic large cell lymphoma of skin. *J Clin Pathol* 1991;44:119–125.

474. Bhawan J, Wolff SM, Ucci AA, et al.: Malignant lymphoma and malignant angioendotheliomatosis: One disease. *Cancer* 1985;55:570–576.

475. Wrotnowski U, Mills SE, Cooper PH: Malignant angioendotheliomatosis: An angiotropic lymphoma. *Am J Clin Pathol* 1985;83:244–248.

476. Wick MR, Mills SE: Intravascular lymphomatosis: Clinicopathologic features and differential diagnosis. *Semin Diagn Pathol* 1991;8:91–101.

477. Frierson HF Jr, Bellafiore FJ, Gaffey MJ, et al.: Cytokeratin in anaplastic large cell lymphoma. *Mod Pathol* 1994;7:317–321.

478. Kinney MC, Greer JP, Glick AD, et al.: Anaplastic large cell Ki-1 malignant lymphomas: Recognition, biological and clinical implications. *Pathol Annu* 1991; 26(1):1–24.

479. Sepp N, Schuler G, Romani N, et al.: Intravascular lymphomatosis (angioendotheliomatosis): Evidence for a T-cell origin in two cases. *Hum Pathol* 1990;21:1051–1058.

480. Sheibani K, Battifora H, Winberg CD, et al.: Further evidence that "malignant angioendotheliomatosis" is an angiotropic large-cell lymphoma. *N Engl J Med* 1986;314:943–948.

Melanocytic Neoplasms of the Skin

481. Imber MJ, Mihm MC: Benign melanocytic tumors. In: Farmer ER, Hood AF, eds. *Pathology of the Skin.* Norwalk, CT: Appleton & Lange, 1990:663–683.

482. Wolinsky S, Silvers DN: The small lentiginous nevus. *Am J Dermatopathol* 1985;7(suppl):5–12.

483. Mehregan AH: Lentigo senilis and its evolution. *J Invest Dermatol* 1975;65:429–433.

484. Silvers DN, Helwig EB: Melanocytic nevi in neonates. *J Am Acad Dermatol* 1981;4:166–175.

485. Rhodes AR: Pigmented birthmarks and precursor melanocytic lesions

of cutaneous melanoma identifiable in childhood. *Pediatr Clin North Am* 1983;30:435–463.

486. LeBoit PE: Simulants of malignant melanoma: A rogue's gallery of melanocytic and nonmelanocytic imposters. In: LeBoit PE, ed. *Malignant Melanoma & Melanocytic Neoplasms*. Philadelphia: Hanley & Belfus, 1994:195–258.

487. Manciati ML, Clark WH, Hayes FA, Herlyn M: Malignant melanoma simulants arising in congenital melanocytic nevi do not show experimental evidence for a malignant phenotype. *Am J Pathol* 1990; 136:817–829.

488. Urbanek WR, Johnson WC: Smooth muscle hamartoma associated with Becker's nevus. *Arch Dermatol* 1978;114:104–106.

489. Dorsey CS, Montgomery H: Blue nevus and its distinction from Mongolian spot and the nevus of Ota. *J Invest Dermatol* 1954;22:225–236.

490. Rodriguez HA, Ackerman AB: Cellular blue nevus: Clinicopathologic study of forty-five cases. *Cancer* 1968;21:393–405.

491. Perkocha LA: Classification of melanoma in adults and children. In: LeBoit PE, ed. *Malignant Melanoma & Melanocytic Neoplasms*. Philadelphia: Hanley & Belfus, 1994:299–338.

492. Mishima Y, Mevorah B: Nevus Ota and nevus Ito in American negroes. *J Invest Dermatol* 1961;36:133–154.

493. Seab JA, Graham JH, Helwig EB: Deep penetrating nevus. *Am J Surg Pathol* 1989;13:39–44.

494. Cooper PH: Deep penetrating (plexiform spindle cell) nevus. *J Cutan Pathol* 1992;19:172–180.

495. Mehregan DA, Mehregan AH: Deep penetrating nevus. *Arch Dermatol* 1993;129:328–331.

496. Spitz S: Melanomas of childhood. *Am J Pathol* 1948;24:591–609.

497. Allen AC: Juvenile melanomas of children and adults and melanocarcinomas of children. *Arch Dermatol* 1960;82:325–335.

498. Weedon D, Little JH: Spindle and epithelioid cell nevi in children and adults: A review of 211 cases of the Spitz cell nevus. *Cancer* 1977;40:217–225.

499. Kamino H, Misheloff E, Ackerman AB, et al.: Eosinophilic globules in Spitz's nevi: New findings and a diagnostic sign. *Am J Dermatopathol* 1979;1:319–324.

500. Barr RJ, Morales RV, Graham JH: Desmoplastic nevus: A distinct histologic variant of mixed spindle cell and epithelioid cell nevus. *Cancer* 1980;46:557–564.

501. Smith KJ, Barrett TL, Skelton HG, et al.: Spindle cell and epithelioid cell nevi with atypia and metastasis (malignant Spitz nevus). *Am J Surg Pathol* 1989;13:931–939.

502. Smith NP: The pigmented spindle cell tumor of Reed: an underdiagnosed lesion. *Semin Diagn Pathol* 1987;4:75–87.

503. Geisse JK: Biopsy techniques for pigmented lesions of the skin. In: LeBoit PE, ed. *Malignant Melanoma & Melanocytic Neoplasms*. Philadelphia: Hanley & Belfus, 1994:181–193.

504. Kornberg R, Ackerman AB: Pseudomelanoma: Recurrent melanocytic nevus following partial surgical removal. *Arch Dermatol* 1975; 111:1588–1590.

505. Park HK, Leonard DD, Arrington JH, et al.: Recurrent melanocytic nevi: Clinical and histologic review of 175 cases. *J Am Acad Dermatol* 1987;17:285–292.

506. Sexton M, Sexton CW: Recurrent pigmented melanocytic nevus: A benign lesion, not to be mistaken for malignant melanoma. *Arch Pathol Lab Med* 1991;115:122–126.

507. Piepkorn MW: A perspective on the dysplastic nevus controversy. In: LeBoit PE, ed. *Malignant Melanoma & Melanocytic Neoplasms*. Philadelphia: Hanley & Belfus, 1994:259–279.

508. Sagebiel RW: The dysplastic melanocytic nevus. *J Am Acad Dermatol* 1989;20:496–501.

509. National Institutes of Health Consensus Conference: Diagnosis and treatment of early melanoma. *JAMA* 1992;268:1314–1319.

510. Clark WH Jr, Reimer RR, Greene M, et al.: Origin of familial malignant melanoma from heritable melanocytic lesions: The B-K mole syndrome. *Arch Dermatol* 1978;114:732–738.

511. Clark WH Jr, Evans HL, Everett MA, et al.: Early melanoma: Histologic terms. *Am J Dermatopathol* 1991;13:579–582.

512. Nahkleh RE, Wick MR, Rocamora A, et al.: Morphologic diversity in malignant melanomas. *Am J Clin Pathol* 1990;93:731–740.

513. Clark WH Jr, Mihm MC: Lentigo maligna and lentigo maligna melanoma. *Am J Pathol* 1969;55:39–53.

514. Conley J, Lattes R, Orr W: Desmoplastic malignant melanoma (a rare variant of spindle cell melanoma). *Cancer* 1971;28:914–936.

515. Frolow GR, Shapiro L, Brownstein MH: Desmoplastic malignant melanoma. *Arch Dermatol* 1975;111:753–754.

516. Batsakis JG, Bauer R, Regezi JA, Campbell T: Desmoplastic melanoma of the maxillary alveolus. *J Oral Surg* 1979;37:107–109.

517. Gentile R, Donovan D: Neurotropic melanoma of the head and neck. *Laryngoscope* 1985;95:1161–1166.

518. Shields JA, Elder D, Arbizo V, et al.: Orbital involvement with desmoplastic melanoma. *Br J Ophthalmol* 1987;71:279–284.

519. Schroeder WH, Hosler MW, Martin RA: Neurotropic melanoma of the head and neck. *Missouri Med* 1987;84:242–246.

520. Anstey A, Wilkinson JD, Black MM: Facial desmoplastic malignant melanoma. *J Royal Soc Med* 1991; 84(1):47–48.

521. Egbert B, Kempson R, Sagebiel R: Desmoplastic malignant melanoma: A clinicopathologic study of 25 cases. *Cancer* 1988;62:2033–2041.

522. Jain S, Allen PW: Desmoplastic malignant melanoma and its variants: A study of 45 cases. *Am J Surg Pathol* 1989;13:358–373.

523. Reed RJ: Minimal deviation melanoma. *Hum Pathol* 1990;21:1206–1211.

524. Reed RJ, Ichinose H, Clark WH Jr, Mihm MC: Common and uncommon melanocytic nevi and borderline melanomas. *Semin Oncol* 1975;2:119–147.

525. Schmoeckel C, Castro CE, Braun-Falco O: Nevoid malignant melanoma. *Arch Dermatol Res* 1985;277:362–369.

526. Wong TY, Duncan LM, Mihm MC: Melanoma mimicking dermal and Spitz's nevus ("nevoid melanoma"). *Semin Surg Oncol* 1993;9:188–193.

527. Okun MR: Melanoma resembling spindle and epithelioid cell nevus. *Arch Dermatol* 1979;115:1416–1420.

528. Phillips ME, Margolis RJ, Merot Y, et al.: The spectrum of minimal deviation melanoma: A clinicopathologic study of 21 cases. *Hum Pathol* 1986;17:796–806.

14 ∶ Molecular Biology and Genetics of Head and Neck Tumors

Stephen P. Naber and Hubert J. Wolfe

Progress in genetics and molecular biology has resulted in the emergence of new concepts to explain the etiology and pathogenesis of many human disease processes, including neoplasia. Technologic advances in molecular biology have provided tools that make it possible for medical scientists to study alterations in gene structure that are associated with a particular disease. The rapidity of these advances has been a result of progress made in the Human Genome Project, which, upon completion, will provide the genetic code for the approximately 100,000 human genes and their regulatory elements. This information, coupled with the ability to analyze nucleic acids rapidly and inexpensively, has already spawned an era of diagnostic testing in which detection of specific genetic alterations in diseased tissues refines the morphologic diagnosis and, in many cases, provides useful information for treatment and prognosis. Indeed, there has been a progressive development of our knowledge base from the description of gross chromosomal changes to the identification of specific alterations in the deoxyribonucleic acid (DNA). This has seen the greatest clinical utility in some hematopoietic malignancies in which detection of the presence of specific cytogenetic and molecular alterations provides a specific diagnosis and predicts which chemotherapeutic agents may be more effective.

The molecular pathology of solid tumors has been more difficult to analyze, and the discovery of tumor-specific genetic alterations, which can provide definitive diagnostic or therapeutic guidance, has progressed more slowly. Much of this is a result of the morphologic complexity of solid tumors and the more diverse spectrum of genetic changes that are usually present. Solid tumors are the most common neoplasms that head and neck pathologists encounter, and considerable research activity has been focused on molecular carcinogenesis and neoplastic progression. At present, there are only a few examples of solid tumors in which the determination of a specific genetic alteration helps to make a diagnosis or a therapeutic decision, but technologic advances promise to change that in the near future.

▮ OVERVIEW OF GENETIC ANALYSIS IN PATHOLOGY

The human genome contains an orderly sequence of over 3 billion nucleotides in each cell, which are arranged into 23 pairs of chromosomes in the nucleus of somatic cells. An alteration in the structure of the DNA that is heritable in the progeny of a cell is termed a mutation. These may be somatic or germinal mutations. Somatic mutations are confined to a particular tissue or tumor within an individual and cannot be passed to succeeding generations of offspring. Germ line, or germinal, mutations occur in the gametes of an individual and may not affect the individual but are then transmitted to successive generations. In human disease, genetic alterations may be large enough to be observed microscopically, such as the gain or loss of portions of, or entire, chromosomes or gross rearrangement of their structure. Some of these changes result in disease or death, whereas others may cause no detectable disorder and be discovered only incidentally. On the other hand, a submicroscopic alteration of the DNA as small as a point mutation, which alters only a single nucleotide out of the 3 billion, may result in a lethal disorder. In either case, there is structural alteration of the DNA, and the size of the DNA fragment involved may differ by orders of magnitude. Therefore, the techniques required to detect genetic alterations vary depending on the nature of the structural change of the DNA (Fig. 14–1).

Cytogenetics

Traditional cytogenetics evaluates by direct microscopic observation the numerical and morphologic status of fixed and stained chromosomes prepared from cultured cells arrested in metaphase. The chromosome constitution of a tissue, also termed the karyotype, includes the number of autosomal chromosomes and the number and type of sex chromosomes. The normal diploid human karyotype has 22 pairs of autosomes and two sex chromosomes and is designated 46,XX for females and 46,XY for males. Chromosomal abnormalities may be numerical or structural in nature. If the chromosome number is abnormal, but is an exact multiple of the haploid chromosome number, it is termed euploid, such as the common triploid 69,XXY karyotype observed in partial hydatidiform molar gestations. Any chromosome number other than an exact multiple of the haploid number is termed aneuploid. For example, loss of one chromosome 5 in a tissue would result in a karyotype of 45,XX,−5 and is termed monosomy of chromosome 5. Abnormalities of chromosome structure occur as a result of chromosomal breakage followed by abnormal reconstitution. The most common type of structural abnormality is a translocation in which there has been a rearrangement of genetic material following chromosomal breakage and reconstitution. These may be either balanced (termed reciprocal or robertsonian), if there has been no alteration in the total complement of genetic material, or unbalanced, if there has been a net gain or loss of genetic material. There is standard cytogenetic nomenclature for designating human chromosomes and their changes[1,2] and only the essentials are introduced here. The chromosome is identified by its number with the long arm designated q and the short arm p, for example, 12q would represent the long arm of chromosome 12. There are distinct morphologic regions on each chromosome, and the various regions and bands are numbered consecutively from the centromere outward along each chromosome arm. For example, 9q34 identifies chromosome 9, the long arm, region 3, band 4. A translocation is abbreviated t, and the designation t(9;22)(q34;q11) describes a translocation between chromosomes 9 and 22 with the breakpoint in chromosome 9 at band q34 and in chromosome 22 at band q11.

The genetic profile of tumors may be assessed at different levels of resolution, depending on the methodology used. Karyotype analysis is a screening method that looks at the gross composition and structure of the entire genetic complement. This technique requires culture of the tumor cells, and analysis is restricted to cells that are dividing. Since solid tumors are composed of a mixture of neoplastic cells as well as other cells, it may be difficult to identify the cell types in culture. Karyotypes of cells from solid tumors are generally complex but often reveal nonrandom chromosomal changes, which help focus the search for submicroscopic changes of

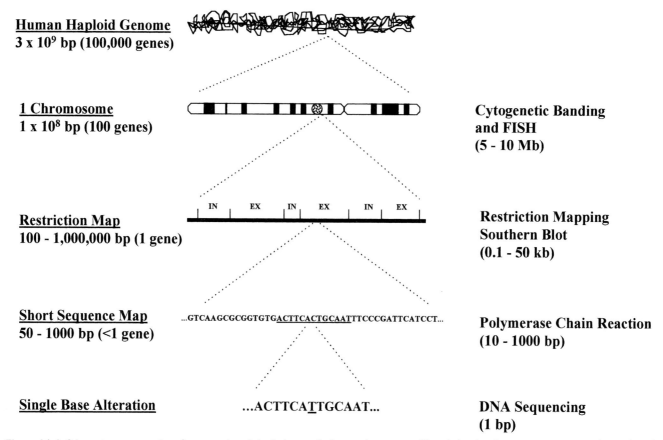

Human Haploid Genome
3×10^9 bp (100,000 genes)

1 Chromosome
1×10^8 bp (100 genes)

Cytogenetic Banding
and FISH
(5 - 10 Mb)

Restriction Map
100 - 1,000,000 bp (1 gene)

IN   EX   IN   EX   IN   EX

Restriction Mapping
Southern Blot
(0.1 - 50 kb)

Short Sequence Map
50 - 1000 bp (<1 gene)

...GTCAAGCGCGGTGTG<u>ACTTCACTGCAA</u>TTTCCCGATTCATCCT...

Polymerase Chain Reaction
(10 - 1000 bp)

Single Base Alteration

...ACTTCA<u>T</u>TGCAAT...

DNA Sequencing
(1 bp)

Figure 14–1. Schematic representation of cytogenetic and physical maps of a human chromosome. The relative sizes in genome mapping are shown along the left side and the techniques used to assess genetic changes and their levels of resolution are indicated on the right. A cytogenetic map provides a framework for developing a physical map of a specific region of a chromosome. The restriction map depicts a gene or portion of a gene composed of introns (IN) and exons (EX). More precise mapping to the level of single base pair changes may be determined. bp, base pair; kb, kilobase; Mb, megabase.

pathogenetic importance. The techniques of molecular biology work in concert with cytogenetics and operate at a higher level of resolution to allow characterization of structural changes at the level of genes or alterations of the primary DNA base pair sequence.

Techniques of Molecular Genetics

Most of the information obtained regarding the genetic changes in solid tumors is derived from molecular analysis of tumor tissue. By analyzing DNA extracted from tumor tissue using Southern blot and polymerase chain reaction–based techniques, one can detect alterations in gene structure as small as point mutations. Since these techniques look at minute portions of the entire genome, the areas to be studied have often been selected based on the location of nonrandom chromosomal changes observed by cytogenetics.

The entire discipline of molecular biology rests on the chemical property of DNA to form a double-stranded molecule in which one strand will bind, or hybridize, to the opposite, complementary strand in a precise fashion dictated by the order of the purine and pyrimidine bases. Several seminal advances in nucleic acid technology have allowed the discipline of molecular biology to flourish and the structure of the genome to be elucidated. The first of these was the discovery of restriction enzymes, a class of molecules that can digest DNA at enzyme-specific recognition sites and thereby allow the large DNA molecule to be mapped according to the location of the restriction enzyme digestion sites. After digestion with a restriction enzyme or enzymes, the DNA is cleaved into a mixture of specific fragments of various sizes, which can be easily manipulated following size separation by gel electrophoresis. After transfer by blotting of the DNA fragments from the gel onto a substrate such as a nylon filter, they are irreversibly bound in the position they occupied in the gel. This is the basis of the Southern blot technique in which a DNA probe is used to identify a specific target sequence on DNA fragments that have been sorted by size within a mixture of genomic DNA. Alterations in gene size within a DNA fragment created between two restriction enzyme sites, or the creation or destruction of restriction enzyme recognition sites by mutation, changes the size of the restriction fragment identified by a particular probe and hence reflects a change in gene structure. Since some of these specific genetic alterations are known to be related to a particular disease or pathologic state and can be clearly separated from the normal condition, the Southern blot technique may be used diagnostically. Another critical technical advance in molecular biology was the implementation of rapid methods for determining the sequence of bases in the DNA molecule. These techniques have become highly automated so that specific mutations in primary DNA structure can be determined directly and inexpensively.

Analysis of gene expression can also be accomplished by membrane hybridization. The Northern blot assay has been used extensively to assess the level of messenger ribonucleic acid (mRNA) expression in extracts of total RNA from cells and tissues. In this case, the various species of RNA are separated according to size by gel electrophoresis and then transferred to a membrane for hybridization with either a DNA or complementary RNA probe. Analysis of protein expression can be conducted by a similar technique termed Western blotting, in which precipitated proteins from a cellular or tissue extract are separated by electrophoresis and then probed with a labeled antibody targeted to a specific protein.

The technique that has most revolutionized molecular diagnostics is the polymerase chain reaction (PCR). Essentially, this is an in vitro enzymatic synthesis that amplifies short (up to 3000 base pairs) but specific DNA sequences, which are delimited by a pair of oligonucleotide primers used to initiate the synthesis. The power of this technique is its extraordinary sensitivity, which can amplify only a few copies of template DNA into an analyzable amount of DNA (microgram quantities) within hours. The amplified PCR product can be analyzed by size and by sequence determination, or the amount of product amplified can be quantitated. Levels of mRNA expression or the presence of RNA viral sequences can also be estimated by PCR by first converting the RNA into complementary DNA (cDNA) copies by the use of reverse transcriptase. Specific primers are then hybridized to specific targets in the cDNA and amplified by the usual PCR reactions. The amount of amplified product can then be quantitated and, within certain limits, is directly proportional to the starting amount of cDNA, which, in turn, was dependent on the amount of RNA in the original sample. Consequently, the PCR has numerous applications and is used widely in diagnostic procedures for inherited disorders, infectious diseases, neoplasia, and identity testing.

All of the techniques described thus far are limited to detecting changes at specific genetic loci or in measuring the levels of a particular mRNA present in a tissue sample. Furthermore, they do not permit the easy evaluation of large numbers of genetic loci or mRNAs and thereby limit the amount of information that can be obtained readily. One of the key concepts of neoplasia is that it is a result of the accumulation of numerous genetic changes over time and involves the alteration of numerous genes involved in the control of cell growth and differentiation. Therefore, the detection of only single genetic alterations is likely to be of little diagnostic or predictive value in the evaluation of a tumor, since it will not necessarily reflect the functional state of the neoplastic tissue nor be specific for the tumor type. There are important exceptions to this generalization, but these are limited chiefly to hematopoietic and lymphoid neoplasms and to certain uncommon mesenchymal and primitive small, round, blue-cell tumors in which certain genetic alterations characterize a type of tumor or predict its behavior or response to certain therapies. For the common epithelial tumors that constitute the preponderance of neoplasms in the head and neck and elsewhere, limited genetic analysis has been of little practical help in this regard. With the development of cDNA microarrays or "gene chips," there is now promise that genetic analysis of tumor tissue will yield useful information concerning gene activity.

This technology allows thousands of genes to be monitored simultaneously by measuring their transcriptional activity and obtaining a profile of the differential expression of genes that are responsible for certain cellular functions.[3] Such profiles of gene activity may assess those involved in signal transduction, cell cycle and proliferation, angiogenesis, cytoskeletal reorganization, and other critical physiologic functions, since these demonstrate distinctive patterns of regulation.[4] This approach is being used to elucidate and compare tumor-specific gene expression profiles in human tumors and in normal tissues[5–7] and is providing useful information on the genetic changes underlying tumor behavior.

Role of the Surgical Pathologist in Molecular Diagnosis

These technical advances in molecular biology are creating new strategies by which traditional nonmolecular diagnostic methods are becoming new tools for genetic analysis. The era of molecular cytogenetics has been introduced by fluorescent in situ hybridization (FISH), which makes it possible to localize the chromosomal position of particular DNA sequences by hybridizing a DNA probe labeled with a fluorescent dye to intact metaphase chromosomes or to interphase nuclei immobilized on a microscope slide.[8] Consequently, FISH is a useful molecular biologic adjunct to routine karyotyping and is now becoming a powerful new technique in sur-

gical pathology, since it can detect minute chromosomal additions, deletions, and complex translocations in the nuclei of fixed cells obtained by touch preparations from fresh tissue or in paraffin-embedded tissue sections.

Two recent advances in molecular cytogenetics demonstrate how visualization and localization of target DNA sequences at the chromosomal and cellular levels are becoming valuable tools for the cytogenetic assessment of tumors.[9] One of these, comparative genomic hybridization, can be applied to archival tumor DNA to produce a visual map for localizing changes in DNA copy number that may be present in a tumor. A second technique, spectral karyotyping, utilizes differentially labeled chromosome painting probes to display all human chromosomes in different colors to facilitate the characterization of numerical and structural chromosome aberrations. Findings from these molecular cytogenetic screening techniques help focus the search for specific, tumor-associated molecular alterations to regions of the chromosomes, which reveal recurrent and highly consistent changes. These technical advances now enable surgical pathologists to perform certain rapid, specific, genetic tests on the same routine surgical pathologic specimens on which a morphologic diagnosis is being made.

Surgical pathologists now need to be aware of special procedures that will ensure that samples of tumors and other tissues are properly prepared and stored for appropriate molecular analysis. Certain analyses that employ either high molecular weight genomic DNA or intact RNA may require that samples of tissue be frozen as soon as possible after excision of a tumor. Procedures for sampling and storing fresh tumor tissue in the frozen state are simple and easily implemented in most laboratories.[10] However, technologic developments now allow the application of PCR-based testing and FISH to paraffin-embedded tissues and to cytologic preparations, which has transformed archival tissue collections into DNA and RNA banks suitable for diagnostic and research applications. As a result, the anatomic pathologist has become the custodian of this nucleic acid bank and is now a central participant working to solve the numerous legal and ethical questions that have arisen in the realm of genetic analysis.

One of the shortcomings of molecular analysis performed on whole tumor tissues is the dilution of DNA from the neoplastic cells by that from stromal, inflammatory, or other non-neoplastic components of the tumor. This uncertainty has been greatly reduced by the use of microdissection techniques, in which minute, precise areas of tumor can be excised from paraffin sections on a microscope slide and removed from adjacent tissue, and the nucleic acids extracted and used in PCR-based analyses (Fig. 14–2).[11, 12] This allows the area of tissue being sampled to be examined by the pathologist to verify that the lesion is present and that appropriately preserved cells are being used for analysis. Sampling by microdissection can be performed by hand under microscopic guidance or by sophisticated instrumentation using laser technology to excise the desired area of tissue.[13] Updated information regarding tissue microdissection and related techniques is available from the National Cancer Institute Cancer Genome Anatomy Project (see Methodology section at http://www.ncbi.nlm.nih.gov//ncicgap/).

Rapid analysis of chromosomal enumeration, detection of chromosomal translocations, and detection of oncogene amplification can be obtained within hours of excision of a specimen by performing FISH on touch preparations from the cut surface of a solid tumor. The clinical utility of this technique has been demonstrated in neuroblastoma, in which the level of N-*myc* oncogene amplification correlates with prognosis.[14] Amplification of the *HER2/neu* oncogene in infiltrating breast carcinoma has been used as an indicator for tailoring chemotherapy.[15] Paraffin-embedded archival tissue is also suitable as starting material for FISH analysis. Nuclei can be obtained by enzymatic disaggregation of tissue from 50-μm thick paraffin sections and then applied to microscope slides as a monolayer for FISH. If preservation of tissue architecture is essential, FISH can be carried out on slides with routine 5-μm thick paraffin sections.

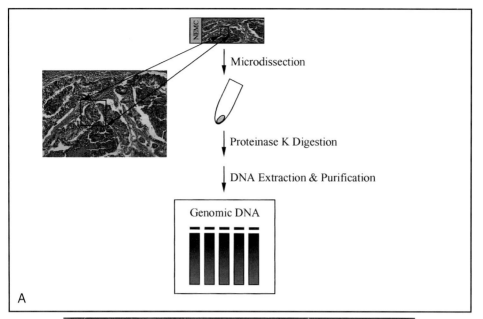

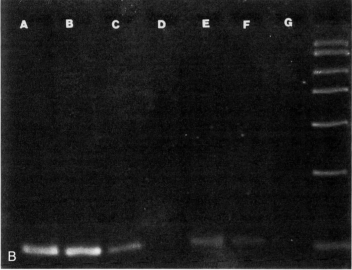

Figure 14–2. Tissue microdissection and DNA analysis in archival tissue. *A,* Cells of interest can be microdissected from an intact tissue section and then the minute quantities of extracted nucleic acids are amplified by polymerase chain reaction for detailed analysis. *B,* Detection of Epstein-Barr virus (EBV)–related sequences in nucleic acid extracted from formalin-fixed, paraffin-embedded tissue excised by microdissection from three cases of nasopharyngeal carcinoma. The results are shown using an ethidium bromide–stained agarose gel. Lanes A, B, and C contain the products of reverse transcriptase–polymerase chain reactions. Lane D is the negative control and lanes E and F are positive EBV controls. Molecular size markers ranging from 50 to 2000 base pairs are shown on the far right.

CONCEPTS OF CANCER AND MOLECULAR DIAGNOSIS

Nucleic acid–based methods for the detection of cancer-related genetic changes are powerful by virtue of their exquisite specificity and sensitivity, and many tests for neoplasia-related genetic changes are becoming routine in pathology laboratories. For the pathologist, the greatest difficulty lies in interpreting such test results in light of other laboratory and clinical findings and in helping the clinician understand the significance of the test result in any particular case. Malignancy arises through the accumulation of inherited (germline) or acquired (somatic) mutations in critical genes (proto-oncogenes and tumor supressor genes), which regulate cell growth and differentiation. Sporadic cancers account for approximately 90% of all cancers, and the associated mutations are somatic and are confined to the cancer cells themselves. Therefore, it is especially important to establish whether the genetic test involves the detection of germinal or somatic mutation because in germinal mutation, the interpretation may influence the assessment of a patient's risk for a particular cancer; whereas with somatic mutation, it may help refine the diagnosis or influence the therapeutic strategy in a patient with cancer. In either case, it must be remembered that a complex array of genetic changes underlies the initiation and progression of a cancer, and, with a few notable exceptions, the detection of only one or two of these may be of limited value in the diagnosis and management of the malignancy.

In the approximately 10% of cancers in which the individual has a hereditary cancer syndrome and carries a specific germline susceptibility mutation in all cells of the body, it is likely that this mutation is present in a tumor suppressor gene involved in the cellular signaling pathways regulating growth and differentiation. Identification of individuals and families who are likely to be affected by an inherited cancer syndrome requires recognition of certain clues. The development of cancer at a young age or the presence of multiple primary tumors, even with common cancers, should raise the suspicion of an inherited cancer syndrome. Family genetic studies have a greater potential for success if there is a history of multiple affected and unaffected members and if more than two generations are available for study. These types of studies may not be possible if the family size is small or if there is poor documentation of cancer in the family history. A major confounding feature in the pursuit of a mutation associated with an inherited cancer is the phenomenon of incomplete penetrance of the gene. In this case, family members who carry the mutant allele do not develop cancer because of the influence of other genetic or environmental factors.

The gene mutation associated with a specific inherited cancer may not be identified and the nucleotide sequence of the gene associated with the tumor not known. In this case, indirect DNA diagnosis, termed linkage analysis, may be used to map a particular gene associated with a tumor and follow its segregation through a kindred by virtue of its close physical proximity, that is, linkage, to a known genetic marker. Such maps determine the relative locations of genetic markers within a segment of DNA. Since this type of analysis does not identify the mutant gene itself, it requires testing of affected and relevant unaffected family members in at least two generations to have predictive value. It is still the preferred method of analysis in diseases that may be caused by any of a number of mutations in a single gene.

The basis of this indirect testing lies in the probability that two genetic loci that are close to one another will tend to remain together during random assortment of genetic material during meiosis. Since cells contain two sets of homologous chromosomes (one paternally and one maternally inherited), a particular DNA segment has two alleles, one on each of the two homologous chromosomes. Discrimination between homologous chromosomes can be accomplished by the use of DNA sequence-based genetic markers, which have a high likelihood of being able to discriminate between the two alleles. These consist of small, tandemly repeated DNA sequences termed minisatellites (10 to 50 base pairs per repeat) and microsatellites (2 to 4 base pairs repeated from 5 to 25 times), which are highly polymorphic and can be used to identify individuals. There are approximately 30,000 microsatellite loci scattered throughout the genome, and the number of repeats that an individual has at any particular locus is inherited from the parents in a stable fashion such that one allele may, for example, have four repeats and the homologous allele seven. The segregation of a marker throughout two or more generations of a family in multiple individuals affected with a tumor serves to localize a region of DNA that may contain a mutation related to the development of that particular cancer. Cytogenetic and molecular approaches may then be used in a strategy known as positional cloning to refine the genetic map of the putative disease region and, ultimately, identify the gene sequence and the specific disease mutation. The pathologist has a critical role in this process, since discrepancies between an individual's phenotype and genotype can result from an incorrect diagnosis.

Another potential marker for assessing cellular potential for neoplastic growth may be linked to the genetic changes that are associated with cellular aging. After a finite number of divisions, cells become arrested in a nondividing state of cellular senescence. Recent evidence indicates that the incomplete replication of chromosomal ends, or telomeres, results in telomeric shortening, which is a signal for the cell to become senescent.[16] This is a property of normal somatic cells as opposed to germ cells and stem cells, which contain telomerase, an enzyme that stabilizes telomere length and permits their proliferative capacity. There is evidence that telomerase is reactivated in immortal cancer cells, thereby preventing telomere shortening and playing a role in tumor formation.[17]

Various mechanisms of genetic alteration are relevant to human cancer, and understanding of these mechanisms is essential for proper interpretation of genetic tests. This chapter does not attempt to discuss these mechanisms in detail, but provides an overview for conceptual purposes. As the sequence information for more human genes becomes known, more opportunities for direct gene diagnosis will be available. Once a normal gene sequence has been identified, then detection of a mutation can be accomplished by techniques that focus specifically on the area of abnormality. Since mutations cause a structural alteration in the DNA, detection and recognition of these is essentially "surgical pathology" of the gene. Mutations can destroy existing restriction enzyme recognition sites or can create new ones, thereby providing a strategy for their detection based on the different patterns of DNA fragments, which would be obtained upon digestion of a defined segment of either normal or mutated DNA. Even if a mutation does not alter or create restriction enzyme recognition sites, its presence can be detected by allele-specific hybridization. A short (oligonucleotide) probe for the normal allele will hybridize to a mutant allele with less affinity, which enables discrimination between DNA that is normal and DNA that carries one or two mutant alleles. A third opportunity for direct DNA diagnosis is to detect mutations that alter the length of a specific segment of DNA by deletion or expansion.

In neoplasia, there are examples of characteristic genetic alterations associated with certain tumors; however, the process of neoplastic progression and tumor formation is considered to be the result of an accumulation of numerous genetic insults. One target of genetic mutation in cancer is a diverse array of genes termed oncogenes. These are altered forms of proto-oncogenes, which are classes of normal cell regulatory factors that function to promote normal cell growth and differentiation. When a proto-oncogene encoding such a regulatory molecule undergoes mutation into an oncogene, the end result is an overexpression of its growth-promoting activity. The alterations leading to these changes include point mutations, such as those that activate the *ras* family of membrane-associated G proteins; amplification of gene copy number, as in the tyrosine kinase growth factor receptors, such as *neu*; and chromosomal translocations as characterized by the familiar Philadelphia translocation of chromosomes 9 and 22 to activate the *abl* gene in chronic myelogenous leukemia.

The proto-oncogenes, which have a dominant, growth-promoting role in their regulation of the cell cycle, act in concert with other genes that normally function to constrain cell growth. These are the tumor supressor genes whose products function to inhibit cell growth. In contrast to the overactivity resulting from an oncogene mutation, a mutation in a tumor supressor gene, such as *p53*, results in a loss of its function and contributes directly to the altered phenotype of malignant cells. This is a recessive phenomenon that led to the "two-hit hypothesis" of Knudson, which states that both alleles of such a gene must be inactivated for tumor development to occur. In the classic model of tumor supressor gene function as depicted by the retinoblastoma (*Rb*) gene, an individual with one normal allele and one mutated or absent one is normal but is at increased risk for developing retinoblastoma and certain other cancers. Development of cancer in this case is associated with mutation or loss of both normal alleles. This type of allelic loss provides a strategy for identifying genetic loci, which may be putative tumor supressor genes.

Since every gene has two alleles, one inherited from each parent, an individual is therefore heterozygous for the normal allele at any given locus. When mutation affects one or both of the alleles, the individual is no longer heterozygous for the normal gene, and loss of heterozygosity (LOH) is said to have occurred. If an individual inherits one mutated allele, he or she is phenotypically normal because the normal product of the gene is still encoded by the remaining normal allele. However, the person is at a greater risk of developing a malignancy, since an additional somatic mutation in the remaining allele will remove the function of the tumor suppressor gene. Development of a sporadic tumor is a much less likely event, since both alleles of the tumor suppressor gene must be inactivated by somatic mutations. The accumulation of genetic lesions that activate oncogenes and inactivate tumor supressor genes results in deregulated cell growth. Increasingly, evidence supports a central genetic concept that malignant tumors evolve as the result of the acquisition of multiple, sequential genetic alterations, which are responsible for the neoplastic progression from a normal cell to immortal ones with a malignant phenotype. The evolution of subclones with additional nonrandom genetic changes occurs during the life of a tumor and is the means by which tumors acquire the capacity to invade tissues and to metastasize. These genetic changes are nonrandom and are clonal, implying that all cells of a tumor possess some common genetic alterations that confer a malignant phenotype. It is the ability to detect these genetic alterations that has led to the development of cytogenetic and molecular diagnostic tests that have become part of the standard of care for many patients with hematopoietic malignancies. Solid tumors tend to have more complex patterns of chromosomal and molecular alterations. Even though solid tumors are far more common than leukemia and lymphoma, far less is known about their genetic changes and the implications they might have in the tumor's biologic behavior and clinical course. The pathologist plays an important role in the study of tumor genetics, as it is essential to correlate these abnormalities in the context of tumor histopathology. Familiarity with several basic concepts of genetic analysis will make this task easier.

Approaches to the Genetic Analysis of Tumors

The general concepts and techniques of genetic analysis, including the limitations and strengths of the methods, have been introduced. The following discussion outlines the general approaches that have been taken to elucidate genetic changes that are specifically associated with tumors.

Cytogenetics

Frequently, the first step in the genetic analysis of tumors has been to characterize the chromosomal abnormalities of the tumor cells using routine cytogenetics. At the level of microscopic chromosome analysis, detection of whole chromosome gain or loss and rearrangements such as additions, deletions, and translocations is accomplished. In common solid tumors of the head and neck, as well as in other anatomic sites, consistent chromosomal abnormalities that are common to a specific type of tumor have not been identified. Instead, a recurrent clustering of aberrations has been observed in several chromosomal regions[18] including regions that are frequently deleted or duplicated.[19] These are regions that may contain possible oncogenes or tumor supressor genes and are then targeted for analysis at the molecular genetic level.

Loss of Heterozygosity Studies

The tumor suppressor genes are thought to be the most common sites of genetic damage contributing to the development of tumors, so the first molecular studies of a suspect region are often to determine whether there is LOH or allelic imbalance. If this is present at a specific genetic locus, it may imply the presence of a tumor suppressor gene. However, most models of neoplastic progression,[20] including those for head and neck tumors,[21] focus on the emergence of clonal populations of cells. These then undergo additional genetic alterations, which confer a selective growth advantage on these cells and result in a malignant phenotype with the potential for tumor formation, invasion, and metastasis. This process is the result of accumulated genetic alterations, and it is generally found that multiple genomic sites have undergone LOH. These allelic losses represent irreversible changes in the DNA, which will be inherited by succeeding generations of cells as the tumor proliferates. Therefore, evaluating tumor DNA by allelotype analysis may provide a useful correlation between a molecular genetic lesion and aspects of tumor behavior.

Microsatellite Instability

Errors in DNA replication are a common event. The cell has evolved mechanisms that correct these errors and maintain the stability of the genome. These genes are highly conserved throughout evolution and are responsible for reading the fidelity of the new DNA strand following replication and making enzymatic repairs when errors are detected.[22] If these surveillance and repair systems are defective, as first noted in certain familial tumors, additional mutations accumulate in succeeding generations of tumor cells.[23] This results in further genetic heterogeneity in the tumor and forms the basis for the

phenotypic changes that are responsible for neoplastic progression. Evidence of this genetic instability in a tumor can be obtained by detecting changes in the number of tandem repeats in the alleles at various loci of microsatellite DNA. Comparison of microsatellite size in tumor DNA with that in the individual's normal tissues can be used to assess the degree of microsatellite instability in the tumor. When sufficient numbers of microsatellite loci are assessed, a molecular identification, or fingerprint, of the tumor is obtained and provides evidence for genetic destabilization due to functional loss of DNA mismatch repair activity. Microsatellite instability in sporadic cancers may occur at various stages, depending on the type of tumor. In head and neck squamous cell carcinomas, detection of these changes in microsatellites may provide a means of identifying the origin of metastatic tumors and mapping areas of epithelial cell populations that may contain clonal genetic changes predisposing a tissue to tumor development.

MOLECULAR BIOLOGY OF HEAD AND NECK TUMORS

A wide range of head and neck tumors have been evaluated for cytogenetic and molecular genetic changes, and the spectrum of applications of these techniques parallels that seen in other solid tumors. Ultimately, the objective of these analyses is to provide useful tools that will improve the methods for screening, diagnosing, staging, and treating tumors. The following sections discuss the concepts and major advances that have resulted from molecular analysis of tumors of the lining of the upper aerodigestive tract, salivary glands, and selected soft tissues.

Squamous Cell Carcinoma of the Head and Neck

Squamous cell tumors are among the most common malignancies worldwide[24] and the most studied of head and neck tumors with regard to genetic alterations. Molecular analysis is providing insights into the pathogenesis of head and neck cancer, and models for the molecular progression of the genetic changes associated with histopathologic features have been proposed.[25] Field cancerization is a major concept underlying the susceptibility and development of head and neck squamous cell carcinoma. This hypothesis has proposed that carcinogens induce genetic changes throughout the mucosa of the upper aerodigestive tract[26] and that these accumulate with age.[27] The first general step in elucidating this mechanism has been to determine whether areas of chromosomal deletion are present in tumor DNA and, if so, to ascertain whether these are responsible for loss or inactivation of critical tumor supressor genes. This has been approached by using routine cytogenetic analysis, comparative genomic hybridization,[28] and chromosomal in situ hybridization, all of which have demonstrated progressive genetic changes in head and neck squamous cell carcinomas. More precise localization of these changes is determined by analyses of microsatellite DNA sequences, which have shown numerous allelic losses in head and neck squamous cell carcinomas. The most commonly deleted region is reported to be on chromosome 9p21[29] in an area that contains a *p53*-dependent cell cycle regulatory gene. Further investigation revealed that allelic losses in this region were detected in the precursor lesions of squamous dysplasia and carcinoma in situ, implying that chromosome 9p21 deletions are an early event in the progression of squamous cell carcinoma of the head and neck.[30] Although the precise mechanism of putative tumor suppressor gene inactivation and its functional significance cannot always be determined with certainty, it is clearly understood that the progressive accumulation of mutations that activate proto-oncogenes and inactivate tumor supressor genes leads to a clonal expansion of cells that are genetically identical throughout much of their genome. Even though no consistent tumor-specific genetic markers are known for head and neck squamous cell carcinoma, the extreme sensitivity of the PCR makes it possible to detect gene mutations that may serve as molecular markers of cancer in both screening and diagnostic applications.

The major difficulty is dissecting which of the genetic changes, which are now easily detectable, are significant for diagnostic and therapeutic use. The potential for using molecular screening methods for gene mutations in saliva as a means for detecting tumor cells shed from upper aerodigestive squamous cell carcinomas has been demonstrated.[31] Point mutations in the *p53* tumor supressor gene were used as markers for squamous cell carcinoma, because it is considered to be the most common gene mutation known in this tumor.[32] Although these were patient-specific mutations obtained by cloning *p53* gene segments from saliva samples and then screening them with probes for *p53* gene mutations identified in the patient's primary tumor, the potential for clinical application of molecular screening techniques to identify cancer cells in a large population of normal cells was established. Similarly, the use of sensitive molecular techniques to assess histologically negative surgical margins and lymph nodes following primary surgical resection of head and neck squamous cell carcinomas identified clonal tumor cells in nearly three quarters of the surgical margins and one quarter of the lymph nodes deemed negative by light microscopy.[33] Disease-free survival was increased in patients who were negative by molecular analysis. This approach may be helpful in identifying patients who might benefit from additional surgical or adjuvant therapy and spare those with negative molecular results.

Another major problem in head and neck pathology that is being addressed by molecular analysis is the determination of the primary tumor site upon presentation of a cervical lymph node metastasis without an obvious mucosal lesion. Microsatellite analysis of directed mucosal biopsies has demonstrated that genetic alterations associated with potential clonal neoplastic growth of cells can occur in histologically normal epithelium and that these populations of cells can be genetically related to those resulting in the metastasis.[34] These studies raised the possibility of clinical utility regarding the use of genetic analysis in the management of patients with head and neck squamous cell carcinomas. The confirmation that some patients harbored mucosal genetic alterations identical to those that appeared in primary tumors years later implies that a protocol for systematic mucosal biopsies may be useful for increasing the likelihood of obtaining a diagnostic specimen in patients at risk for these tumors. Furthermore, in patients with metastatic disease, these directed biopsies may be used to map mucosal sites with the same genetic alterations as in the metastasis to direct radiation therapy when a primary tumor cannot be identified.

The detection of genetic lesions that are signals for potential tumor development would be very useful in individuals who are at increased risk for developing upper aerodigestive tract carcinomas. Even though genetic alterations such as an association between cigarette smoking and mutation of the *p53* gene have been found in head and neck squamous cell carcinoma,[35] this is not a specific marker for this tumor, but only suggests a role for tobacco in molecular progression. However, molecular surveillance of the upper aerodigestive epithelium may eventually become practical, particularly if precursor mucosal lesions are present. Risk of malignancy has been predicted from LOH analysis at multiple microsatellite loci that are known to be frequently lost in oral squamous cell carcinomas. A study by Rosin et al.[35a] used tissue microdissection in biopsy specimens to obtain areas of oral dysplasia and from which LOH profiles were used to estimate the risk of progression to invasive carcinoma. Lesions that progressed to carcinoma had significantly different LOH profiles from those that did not progress. Specifically, patients with LOH at 3p and/or 9p were at risk for progression and the relative risk was increased when this was coupled with LOH at other sites (4q, 8p, 11q, 13q, and 17p). Another study[35b] used the same approach to evaluate archival tissue from serial biopsies in patients with recurrent dysplasia in the upper aerodigestive tract and found that accumulation of specific allelic losses associated with head and neck squamous carcinoma was associated with histopathologic progression. These important observations show how genetic analysis of biopsy and archival tissues may be a useful adjunct to histopathologic evaluation for improving classification of oral premalignant lesions.[35c] Conventional biopsies for risk assessment must be limited in number and are random if no clinical precursor lesion is evident. Since it is known that tumors can develop at a distance from visible suspicious lesions,[36] alternative strategies may be useful to improve methods of risk assessment. One molecular approach is based on the concept that the entire target tissue acquires genetic damage over time, and a measure of that accumulated genetic damage may provide a means for estimating the risk for tumor development. The challenge is to obtain representative sampling of the tissue at risk and to detect a genetic alteration that would be highly predictive of future tumor development. The requirement for such a tumor-specific marker is still elusive; however, the potential for molecular screening techniques in head and neck cancer is promising. A study using chromosomal in situ hybridization demonstrated that the degree of chromosomal instability increased with the histologic progression toward carcinoma and confirmed that the process extended to histologically normal tissue adjacent to tumors.[37] At the cytologic level, the feasibility for using molecular diagnostic techniques in screening for head and neck cancers has been supported by the ability to detect clonal chromosomal abnormalities in exfoliated cells from the saliva of patients with head and neck squamous cell carcinoma.[31] Additionally, sensitive molecular analysis may have a role in monitoring a patient's tumor burden or metastatic status by detecting circulating DNA shed from senescent tumor cells. This was elegantly demonstrated by the detection of serum DNA microsatellite alterations, which were specific to the primary tumors in a series of head and neck cancer patients with advanced disease.[38] Another potential source of tumor-specific genetic alterations may be found in mitochondrial DNA where such mutations have been detected in saliva samples from patients with primary head and neck tumors. The mutation-containing mitochondrial DNA was over 200 times as abundant as mutated nuclear p53 in these samples.[38a] Because of their clonal nature and abundant copy number, mitochondrial mutations may provide a powerful molecular marker for cancer that can be easily obtained by noninvasive screening procedures.

The methodology and the strategies for molecular screening are essentially available, but their implementation awaits the discovery of genetic alterations that are specific to the development of any given tumor type. To achieve this, a more complete understanding of the genetic and cellular mechanisms of tumorigenesis is essential.

Salivary Gland Tumors

Salivary gland neoplasms are relatively uncommon and represent less than 2% of tumors in humans but possess a wide variety of histologic appearances and biologic behaviors. Because of the small numbers of tumors examined, attempts to correlate studies of genetic alterations with tumor progression have been mostly inconclusive. Series combining benign and malignant salivary gland tumors have employed DNA ploidy analysis, cytogenetics, fluorescent in situ hybridization, and molecular genetic characterization. Benign neoplasms have been shown to lack DNA aneuploidy and numeric chromosomal abnormalities, whereas low-grade malignant tumors tended to have small gains and losses of chromosomal material and were generally diploid or nearly diploid. High-grade tumors had extensive chromosomal aneusomy and were DNA aneuploid.[39] The heterogeneity of genetic changes observed, both between tumors of the same histologic type and within an individual tumor, supports the concept of clonal evolution within tumors in which subpopulations of cells acquire additional genetic mutations, resulting in progression of tumor growth.

Benign Tumors

Pleomorphic adenomas constitute the bulk of benign tumors examined for chromosomal and genetic change and have been the only ones in which common alterations have been observed. Considerable numbers of cytogenetic analyses have been conducted on benign salivary gland tumors, and hundreds of cases with clonal karyotypic abnormalities have been reported. More than two thirds of salivary gland adenomas possess nonrandom structural chromosomal changes, and tumor subgroups have been separated on the basis of karyotypic patterns. The most common karyotypic abnormalities involve either the long arm of chromosome 8 (8q12) or the long arm of chromosome 12 (12q13-15). Results of molecular genetic studies of pleomorphic adenomas revealed LOH at multiple 8q loci as a common finding, and another allelotype study demonstrated few areas of loss with the exception of 12q.[40, 41] Frequent LOH at 8q, a site of documented translocations in pleomorphic adenomas, did not correlate with clinical and pathologic features of these tumors.[42] Overall, microsatellite instability was detected at a low frequency and suggests that replication error may be an early genetic event in some of these tumors.[40]

These findings suggest that an important growth regulatory gene may exist in the 8q and 12q regions of pleomorphic adenomas. Studies of a developmentally regulated zinc finger gene termed pleomorphic adenoma gene 1 (*PLAG1*) indicate that it is a target in tumors with t(3;8)(p21;q12) translocations resulting in activation of its expression.[43] Two thirds of pleomorphic adenomas examined in one study overexpressed *PLAG1*, and this was observed not only in tumors with abnormalities in the 12q13-15 region, but also in those tumors with normal karyotypes.[44] This implies that *PLAG1* activation is a common event in these tumors and that the mechanism of activation may result from minute, cryptic genetic rearrangements in this region as well as possible alterations in the gene itself (*SG6*). Other regulatory genes observed to be involved in genetic alterations of the 12q13-15 region in pleomorphic adenomas include the *HMGIC* gene, which has been identified in fusions of sequences from the *NFIB* gene from chromosome 9p12-24.[45]

Malignant Tumors

Malignant tumors make up an even smaller category of salivary neoplasms, and investigation of chromosomal and genetic changes has been limited primarily to examination of a small series of tumors and to case reports. Nevertheless, the information supports the existence of some common patterns of genetic change. In one group of malignant salivary gland neoplasms, a wide spectrum of chromosomal changes was observed, with gain or loss of whole chromosomes being the most common abnormality. Translocations were detected in mucoepidermoid, adenoid cystic, and ductal carcinomas.[46] To display allelic loss patterns in a group of salivary gland tumors, all autosomal arms of the chromosomes were evaluated using microsatellite markers. Mucoepidermoid carcinomas revealed significant allelic losses at 2q, 5p, 12p, and 16q, whereas adenoid cystic carcinomas exhibited losses at 1p, 2p, 17p, 19p, and 20p.[41] Amplifications of the oncogenes *myc* and *mdm2* have been reported at 8q23-24 and 12q13-15, respectively, in a case of malignant mixed tumor.[47] To date, there are no consistent patterns of genetic change available that provide diagnostic utility.

Soft Tissue

One uncommon tumor that may occur in the head and neck and present diagnostic difficulty is the synovial sarcoma. This tumor contains a highly characteristic translocation, t(X;18)(p11;q11), in over 90% of cases, frequently as the sole cytogenetic abnormality.[48] The translocation can be detected by routine cytogenetic analysis, as well as by FISH, providing an opportunity to detect this abnormality either from cultured fresh tumor tissue or by interphase cytogenetics on touch preparations or fixed tissue. The translocation results in an *SYT/SSX* fusion gene, which encodes a novel mRNA and protein that is detectable by PCR, in situ hybridization, or immunohistochemistry.

Multiple Endocrine Neoplasia

The purpose of the discussion thus far has been to present the concepts of molecular diagnostics as they may be applied to head and neck neoplasms. Clearly, in the common epithelial tumors of the head and neck, the state of knowledge of their molecular genetic characteristics remains at the level of elucidating mechanisms of tumorigenesis and neoplastic progression. Currently, no applicable diagnostic tests are in routine practice that employ genetic analysis of these tumors for the purpose of making decisions regarding clinical management, but there is little doubt that these will emerge. The exception to this is the case of medullary thyroid carcinoma (MTC) associated with the multiple endocrine neoplasia (MEN) syndrome, type II, in which specific mutations of the *ret* proto-oncogene predict, with virtually 100% certainty, the development of familial medullary thyroid carcinoma. It is the first example in which definitive prophylactic surgical therapy for ablation of an organ is undertaken on the basis of the results of a genetic test in the absence of the disease phenotype.

In this case, the clinical material was key to understanding the molecular defect, which, in turn, has allowed for the prenatal or perinatal diagnosis of the diseases MEN IIa and b. These inherited disorders are associated with proliferative lesions in multiple endocrine systems, including the thyroidal C-cell (MTC), the parathyroid (parathyroid hyperplasia), and the adrenal medulla (pheochromocytoma). MEN IIb differs from MEN IIa by also having other distinctive phenotypic features, including multiple mucosal neuromata, megacolon, and marfanoid features. These clinicopathologic correlations were established in the 1960s and, initially, these entities were viewed as medical curiosities. However, with the development of sensitive laboratory assays for serum calcitonin levels, the early detection of MTC was possible and multiple kindreds were identified that carried the trait. In 1969, a large kindred was identified at the New England Medical Center at the same time that a highly sensitive assay for serum calcitonin was developed, allowing prospective study and early detection of MTC. This program began 8 years after Sipple's first description of the disease.[49] Currently, this kindred has over 160 members, representing four generations. They were studied on an annual basis for basal and stimulated calcitonin levels. When abnormally high, they reflected either clinically occult MTC or the preinvasive precursor of MTC, C-cell hyperplasia.[50, 51] These patients were treated with total thyroidectomy and central node dissection. To date, on the basis of serum calcitonin levels alone, 48 family members have undergone surgery with only one false-positive finding on pathologic review. The majority of members have had a small MTC, usually less than 5 mm in diameter, arising in a background of C-cell hyperplasia.

This family proved very important in the early genetic linkage analysis that allowed the localization of the genetic defect to the pericentromeric region of chromosome 10.[52] Detection of the *ret* proto-oncogene as the responsible candidate gene was first reported in 1993, virtually simultaneously by two groups, one relying heavily on this kindred for molecular analysis. They found the mutation at codon 634 changing a highly conserved cysteine to an arginine.[53] In other kindreds with MEN IIa, mutations have been found at other exons. In contrast, MEN IIb had its mutations in the region coding for the intracellular rather than the extracellular domain of the oncogene product.

A *ret* molecular assay now allows for the detection in the perinatal period of family members with the molecular defect who are at risk for developing MTC. Waiting up to 20 years for the development of hypercalcitoninemia is no longer required. Now the chief clinical issue is deciding at what age surgery should be performed. In our kindred, 3 years of age has been arbitrarily set as the lower limit, but in other affected groups surgery has been performed at 1 year of age.

With MEN I, it took considerably longer to discover its genetic basis (1997) than MEN IIa and b. MEN I is characterized by the development of proliferative endocrine lesions of the anterior pituitary, parathyroid, and gastroenteropancreatic axis but not medullary thyroid carcinoma. Other tumors that may occur are adrenal and thyroid follicular adenomas, paragangliomas, and lipomata. The MEN I gene is on chromosome 11 and consists of 10 exons, which code for a 2.9 kb transcript and a 610 amino acid gene product called menin. Multiple different point mutations have been found, but most of the mutations produce a loss of function of the gene product, and, in contrast to MEN IIa and IIb, the gene appears to be a tumor suppressor gene rather than a proto-oncogene.[54] It is now possible not only to detect affected kindreds but also to identify individual family members at risk for the development of disease. However, since over 145 different mutation sites have already been recorded, there appears to be no "hot spots" in the gene, as in *ret* proto-oncogene. This requires extensive molecular analysis of the gene in clinically suspect patients. Once the mutation site for a specific kindred is known, it only requires analysis of that specific gene sequence to determine whether a given family member is at risk.

The discovery of the genetic basis of MEN II and the resultant applicability of a molecular genetic test to determine definitive surgical therapy is a splendid example of the progress that led from biochemical testing to genetic linkage analysis and, finally, to a specific molecular biologic test. In other solid tumors, the main conclusion that emerges from the modern study of cancer genetics and molecular biology is that increasing numbers of specific genetic abnormalities are associated with particular tumors, and many of these are now being correlated with stages of neoplastic progression. Cytogenetically, some of these alterations may be considered a primary aberration found as the sole karyotypic abnormality in a particular tumor type. Even if these may have diagnostic utility and are considered to have a causal role in tumorigenesis, it is likely that they are early changes and it is doubtful that a sole genetic change is responsible for the progressive biologic disturbances that characterize a neoplasm. Numerous studies support the concept that there is a molecular evolution required for tumorigenesis and that these multiple genetic alterations involve the activation of oncogenes and loss of tumor suppressor genes. Cytogeneticists have long been aware of the multiple secondary aberrations that develop in tumor cells carrying a primary aberration and recognized this as a visible manifestation of clonal evolution of tumor cell populations.[55] It is now well understood that cells have the ability to repair DNA damage or errors in replication. If there are inherited or acquired defects in the genes encoding the proteins involved in DNA repair, mutations in other genes, such as those involved in cell cycle regulation, may then occur during the process of normal cell division. Cells with these types of defects in the DNA repair system are then poised to acquire new phenotypic properties via selective pressure, and the process of neoplastic progression is enhanced.

Two major developments will likely facilitate our understanding of the genetic changes in cancer and how these relate to the biologic behavior of tumors. First, the ability to microdissect purified cell populations from sections of tumor tissue is now available and allows investigators to select cells from specific regions of a tumor that may characterize such behavior as lymphatic invasion. The capability of amplifying nucleic acid sequences from the DNA and RNA in these preserved cells provides sufficient amounts of material for analysis with cDNA microarray technology.[56, 57] With this type of approach, the study of patterns of gene expression in tumor cells with distinct phenotypic characteristics will be possible and new diagnostic and prognostic information will emerge. This information will prove of use to the pathologist and oncologist and will ensure the pathologist an expanding role in the field of oncology.

REFERENCES

Overview of Genetic Analysis

1. ISCN: An international system for human cytogenetic nomenclature. In: Harnden DG, Klinger HP, eds. *Birth Defects: Original Article Series*, Vol 21, No.1. New York: March of Dimes Birth Defects Foundation, 1985.
2. ISCN: Guidelines for cancer cytogenetics. In: Mitelman F, ed. *Supplement to an International System for Human Cytogenetic Nomenclature.* Basel: S Karger, 1991.
3. Bowtell DD: Options available—-from start to finish—-for obtaining expression data by microarray. *Nat Genet* 1999;21(1 Suppl):25–32.
4. Iyer VR, Eisen MB, Ross DT, et al: The transcriptional program in the response of human fibroblasts to serum. *Science* 1999;283:83–87.
5. Bubendorf L, Kononen J, Koivisto P, et al: Survey of gene amplifications during prostate cancer progression by high-throughput fluorescence in situ hybridization on tissue microarrays. *Cancer Res* 1999;59:803–806.
6. Khan J, Saal LH, Bittner ML, et al: Expression profiling in cancer using cDNA microarrays. *Electrophoresis* 1999;20:223–229.
7. Khan J, Simon R, Bittner M, et al: Gene expression profiling of alveolar rhabdomyosarcoma with cDNA microarrays. *Cancer Res* 1998;58:5009–5013.
8. Wolman SR: Fluorescence in situ hybridization: A new tool for the pathologist. *Hum Pathol* 1994;25:586–590.
9. Reid T, Liyanage M, du Manoir S, et al: Tumor cytogenetics revisited: Comparative genomic hybridization and spectral karyotyping. *J Mol Med* 1997;75:801–814.
10. Naber SP: Continuing role of a frozen tissue bank in molecular pathology. *Diagn Mol Pathol* 1996;5:253–259.
11. Diaz-Cano SJ, Brady SP: DNA extraction from formalin-fixed, paraffin embedded tissues. Protein digestion as a limiting step for retrieval of high quality DNA. *Diag Mol Pathol* 1997;6:342–346.
12. Syvanen AC, Peltonen L: Accurate quantitation of mRNA species by polymerase chain reaction and solid phase minisequencing. In: Celis J, ed. *Cell Biology: A Laboratory Handbook.* New York: Academic Press, 1994.
13. Emmet-Buck MR, Bonner RF, Smith PD, et al: Laser capture microdissection. *Science* 1996;274:998–1001.
14. Shapiro DN, Valentine MB, Rowe ST, et al: Detection of N-*myc* gene amplification by fluorescence in situ hybridization. Diagnostic utility for neuroblastoma. *Am J Pathol* 1993;142:1339–1346.
15. Ross JS, Fletcher JA: The *HER-2/neu* oncogene in breast cancer: Prognostic factor, predictive factor, and target for therapy. *Stem Cells* 1998;16:413–428.

Concepts of Cancer and Molecular Diagnosis

16. van Steensel B, de Lange T: Control of telomere length by the human telomeric protein TRF1. *Nature* 1997;385:740–743.
17. Holt SE, Shay JW, Wright WE: Refining the telomere-telomerase hypothesis of aging and cancer. *Nat Biotechnol* 1996;14:836–839.
18. Scholes AGM, Field JK: Genomic instability in head and neck cancer. *Curr Top Pathol* 1996;90:201–222.
19. Cowan JM: Cytogenetics in head and neck cancer. *Otolaryngol Clin North Am* 1992;25:1073–1087.
20. Vogelstein B, Fearon ER, Hamilton SR, et al: Genetic alterations during colorectal-tumor development. *N Engl J Med* 1988;319:525–532.
21. Hart TC: Applications of molecular epidemiology to head and neck cancer. *Otolaryngol Clin North Am* 1997;30:21–34.
22. Jiricny J: Eukaryotic mismatch repair: An update. *Mutat Res* 1998;409:107–121.
23. Jiricny J: Replication errors: Challenging the genome. *EMBO J* 1998;17:6427–6436.

Molecular Biology of Head and Neck Tumors

24. Vokes EE, Weichselbaum RR, Lipman SM, Hong WK: Head and neck cancer. *N Engl J Med* 1993;328:184–194.
25. Sidransky D: Molecular genetics of head and neck cancer. *Curr Opin Oncol* 1995;7:229–233.
26. Papadimitrakopoulou VA, Shin DM, Hong WK: Molecular and cellular biomarkers for field cancerization and multistep process in head and neck tumorigenesis. *Cancer Metastasis Rev* 1996;15:53–76.
27. Jin C, Jin Y, Wennerberg J, et al: Clonal chromosomal aberrations accu-

mulate with age in the upper aerodigestive tract mucosa. *Mutat Res* 1997;374:63–72.

28. Bockmühl U, Wolf G, Schmidt S, et al: Genomic alterations associated with malignancy in head and neck cancer. *Head Neck* 1998;20:145–151.

29. Nawroz H, van der Riet P, Hruban RH, et al: Allelotype of head and neck squamous cell carcinoma. *Cancer Res* 1994;54:1152–1155.

30. van der Riet P, Nawroz H, Hruban RH, et al: Frequent loss of chromosome 9p21-22 early in head and neck cancer progression. *Cancer Res* 1994;54:1156–1158.

31. Boyle JO, Mao L, Brennan JA, et al: Gene mutations in saliva as molecular markers for head and neck squamous cell carcinomas. *Am J Surg* 1994;168:429–432.

32. Boyle JO, Hakim J, Koch WM, et al: The incidence of p53 mutations increases with the progression of head and neck cancer. *Cancer Res* 1993;53:4477–4480.

33. Brennan JA, Mao L, Hruban RH, et al: Molecular assessment of histopathologic staging in squamous-cell carcinoma of the head and neck. *N Engl J Med* 1995;332:429–435.

34. Califano J, Westra WH, Koch W, et al: Unknown primary head and neck squamous cell carcinoma: Molecular identification of the site of origin. *J Natl Cancer Inst* 1999;91:599–604.

35. Brennan JA, Boyle JO, Koch WM, et al: Association between cigarette smoking and mutation of the p53 gene in squamous-cell carcinoma of the head and neck. *N Engl J Med* 1995;332:712–717.

35a. Rosin MP, Cheng X, Poh C, et al: Use of allelic loss to predict malignant risk for low-grade oral epithelial dysplasia. *Clin Cancer Res* 2000;6:357–362.

35b. Califano J, Westra WH, Meininger G, et al: Genetic progression and clonal relationship of recurrent premalignant head and neck lesions. *Clin Cancer Res* 2000;6:347–352.

35c. Mao L: Can molecular assessment improve classification of head and neck premalignancy. *Clin Cancer Res* 2000;6:321–322.

36. Silverman SJ, Gorsky M, Lozada F: Oral leukoplakia and malignant transformation. *Cancer* 1984;53:563–568.

37. Hittelman WN, Kim HJ, Lee JS, et al: Detection of chromosome instability of tissue fields at risk: In situ hybridization. *J Cell Biochem* 1996;25S:57–62.

38. Nawroz H, Koch W, Anker P, et al: Microsatellite alterations in serum DNA of head and neck cancer patients. *Nature Med* 1996;2:1035–1037.

38a. Fliss MS, Usadel H, Caballero OL, et al: Facile detection of mitochondrial DNA mutations in tumors and bodily fluids. *Science* 2000;287:2017–2019.

39. El-Naggar AK, Dinh M, Tucker SL, et al: Chromosomal and DNA ploidy characterization of salivary gland neoplasms by combined FISH and flow cytometry. *Hum Pathol* 1997;28:881–886.

40. El-Naggar AK, Hurr K, Kagan J, et al: Genotypic alterations in benign and malignant salivary gland tumors: Histogenetic and clinical implications. *Am J Surg Pathol* 1997;21:691–697.

41. Johns MM, Westra WH, Califano JA, et al: Allelotype of salivary gland tumors. *Cancer Res* 1996;56:1151–1154.

42. Gillenwater A, Hurr K, Wolf P, et al: Microsatellite alterations at chromosome 8q loci in pleomorphic adenoma. *Otolaryngol Head Neck Surg* 1997;117:448–452.

43. Kas K, Voz ML, Roijer E, et al: Promotor swapping between the genes for a novel zinc finger protein and beta-catenin in pleomorphic adenomas with t(3;8)(p21;q12) translocations. *Nat Genet* 1997;15:170–174.

44. Astrom AK, Voz ML, Kas K, et al: Conserved mechanism of PLAG1 activation in salivary gland tumors with and without chromosome 8q12 abnormalities: Identification of SII as a new fusion partner gene. *Cancer Res* 1999;59:918–923.

45. Geurts JM, Schoenmakers EF, Roijer E, et al: Identification of NFIB as recurrent translocation partner gene of HMGIC in pleomorphic adenomas. *Oncogene* 1998;16:865–878.

46. Martins C, Fonseca I, Roque L, et al: Malignant salivary gland neoplasms: A cytogenetic study of 19 cases. *Eur J Cancer B Oral Oncol* 1996;2:128–132.

47. Rao PH, Murty VV, Louie DC, Chaganti RS: Nonsyntenic amplification of MYC with CDK4 and MDM2 in a malignant mixed tumor of salivary gland. *Cancer Genet Cytogenet* 1998;105:160–163.

48. Kawai A, Woodruff J, Healey JH, et al: SYT-SSX gene fusion as a determinant of morphology and prognosis in synovial sarcoma. *N Engl J Med* 1998;338:153–160.

49. Sipple JH: The association of pheochromocytoma with carcinoma of the thyroid gland. *Am J Med* 1961;3:163–166.

50. Wolfe HJ, Melvin KEW, Cervi-Skinner SJ, et al: C-cell hyperplasia preceding medullary thyroid carcinoma. *N Engl J Med* 1973;289:437–441.

51. Gagel RF, Tashjian AH, Cummings T, et al: The clinical outcome of prospective screening for multiple endocrine neoplasia type 2a. An 18-year experience. *N Engl J Med* 1998;318:478–484.

52. Mathew CGP, Smith BA, Thorp K, et al: Deletion of genes in chromosome 10 in endocrine neoplasia. *Nature* 1987;328:524–526.

53. Mulligan LM, Gardner E, Smith BA, et al: Genetic events in tumor initiation and progression in multiple endocrine neoplasia type 2 genes. *Chrom Cancer* 1993;6:166–177.

54. Martin-Campos JM, Catasus L, Chico A, et al: Molecular pathology of multiple endocrine neoplasia type I: Two novel germline mutations and updated classification of mutations affecting MEN1 gene. *Diagn Mol Pathol* 1999;8:195–204.

55. Nowell PC: The clonal evolution of tumor cell populations. Acquired genetic lability permits stepwise selection of variant sublines and underlies tumor progression. *Science* 1976;194:23–28.

56. Fend F, Emmert-Buck MR, Chuaquo R, et al: Immuno-LCM: Laser capture microdissection of immunostained frozen sections for mRNA analysis. *Am J Pathol* 1999;154:61–66.

57. Luo L, Salunga RC, Guo H, et al: Gene expression profiles of laser-captured adjacent neuronal subtypes. *Nat Med* 1999;5:117–122.

Head and Neck Tumors: TNM Staging*

Lip and Oral Cavity
Pharynx: Nasopharynx, Oropharynx, Hypopharynx
Larynx
Paranasal Sinuses
Salivary Glands
Thyroid Gland
Soft Tissues
Lacrimal Gland

LIP AND ORAL CAVITY

Rules for Classification

The classification applies only to carcinomas of the vermilion surfaces of the lips and of the oral cavity, including those of minor salivary glands. There should be histologic confirmation of the disease.

The following are the procedures for assessing T, N, and M categories:

T categories	Physical examination and imaging
N categories	Physical examination and imaging
M categories	Physical examination and imaging

Definition of TNM

Primary Tumor (T)

TX	Primary tumor cannot be assessed
T0	No evidence of primary tumor
Tis	Carcinoma in situ
T1	Tumor 2 cm or less in greatest dimension
T2	Tumor more than 2 cm but not more than 4 cm in greatest dimension
T3	Tumor more than 4 cm in greatest dimension
T4 (lip)	Tumor invades adjacent structures (e.g., through cortical bone, inferior alveolar nerve, floor of mouth, skin of face)
T4 (oral cavity)	Tumor invades adjacent structures (e.g., through cortical bone, into deep [extrinsic] muscle of tongue, maxillary sinus, skin; superficial erosion alone of bone/tooth socket by gingival primary is not sufficient to classify as T4)

Regional Lymph Nodes (N)

NX	Regional lymph nodes cannot be assessed
N0	No regional lymph node metastasis
N1	Metastasis in a single ipsilateral lymph node, 3 cm or less in greatest dimension
N2	Metastasis in a single ipsilateral lymph node, more than 3 cm but not more than 6 cm in greatest dimension; or in multiple ipsilateral lymph nodes, none more than 6 cm in greatest dimension; or in bilateral or contralateral lymph nodes, none more than 6 cm in greatest dimension:
	N2a Metastasis in single ipsilateral lymph node more than 3 cm but not more than 6 cm in greatest dimension
	N2b Metastasis in multiple ipsilateral lymph nodes, none more than 6 cm in greatest dimension
	N2c Metastasis in bilateral or contralateral lymph nodes, none more than 6 cm in greatest dimension
N3	Metastasis in a lymph node more than 6 cm in greatest dimension

Distant Metastasis (M)

MX	Distant metastasis cannot be assessed
M0	No distant metastasis
M1	Distant metastasis

Stage Grouping

Stage 0	Tis	N0	M0
Stage I	T1	N0	M0
Stage II	T2	N0	M0
Stage III	T3	N0	M0
	T1	N1	M0
	T2	N1	M0
	T3	N1	M0
Stage IVA	T4	N0	M0
	T4	N1	M0
	Any T	N2	M0
Stage IVB	Any T	N3	M0
Stage IVC	Any T	Any N	M1

PHARYNX (INCLUDING BASE OF TONGUE, SOFT PALATE, AND UVULA)

Rules for Classification

The classification applies only to carcinomas. There should be histologic confirmation of the disease.

The following are the procedures for assessing T, N, and M categories:

T categories	Physical examination, endoscopy, and imaging
N categories	Physical examination and imaging
M categories	Physical examination and imaging

*Used with the permission of the American Joint Committee on Cancer (AJCC®), Chicago, IL. The original source for this material is the AJCC® Cancer Staging Manual, 5th ed. (1997) published by Lippincott-Raven Publishers, Philadelphia, PA.

Definition of TNM

Primary Tumor (T)

TX	Primary tumor cannot be assessed
T0	No evidence of primary tumor
Tis	Carcinoma in situ

Nasopharynx

T1	Tumor confined to the nasopharynx
T2	Tumor extends to soft tissues of oropharynx and/or nasal fossa:
	T2a Without parapharyngeal extension
	T2b With parapharyngeal extension
T3	Tumor invades bony structures and/or paranasal sinuses
T4	Tumor with intracranial extension and/or involvement of cranial nerves, infratemporal fossa, hypopharynx, or orbit

Oropharynx

T1	Tumor 2 cm or less in greatest dimension
T2	Tumor more than 2 cm but not more than 4 cm in greatest dimension
T3	Tumor more than 4 cm in greatest dimension
T4	Tumor invades adjacent structures (e.g., pterygoid muscles, mandible, hard palate, deep muscle of tongue, larynx)

Hypopharynx

T1	Tumor limited to one subsite of hypopharynx and 2 cm or less in greatest dimension
T2	Tumor involves more than one subsite of hypopharynx or an adjacent site, or measures more than 2 cm but not more than 4 cm in greatest diameter without fixation of hemilarynx
T3	Tumor measures more than 4 cm in greatest dimension or with fixation of hemilarynx
T4	Tumor invades adjacent structures (e.g., thyroid/cricoid cartilage, carotid artery, soft tissues of neck, prevertebral fascia/muscles, thyroid and/or esophagus)

Regional Lymph Nodes (N): Nasopharynx

The distribution and the prognostic impact of regional lymph node spread from nasopharynx cancer, particularly of the undifferentiated type, is different from that of other head and neck mucosal cancers and justifies the use of a different N classification scheme.

NX	Regional lymph nodes cannot be assessed
N0	No regional lymph node metastasis
N1	Unilateral metastasis in lymph node(s), 6 cm or less in greatest dimension, above the supraclavicular fossa†
N2	Bilateral metastasis in lymph node(s), 6 cm or less in greatest dimension, above the supraclavicular fossa†
N3	Metastasis in a lymph node(s):
	N3a Greater than 6 cm in dimension
	N3b Extension to the supraclavicular fossa

†*Supraclavicular zone or fossa/definition.* This is relevant to the staging of nasopharyngeal carcinoma and is the triangular region originally described by Ho.* It is defined by three points:

(1) the superior margin of the sternal end of the clavicle;
(2) the superior margin of the lateral end of the clavicle;
(3) the point where the neck meets the shoulder.

---

*Ho JHC: An epidemiologic and clinical study of nasopharyngeal carcinoma. Int J Radiat Oncol Biol Phys 1978;4:183–197.

Note that this would include caudal portions of levels IV and V lymph node groups. All cases with lymph nodes (whole or part) in the fossa are considered N3b.

Regional Lymph Nodes (N): Oropharynx and Hypopharynx

NX	Regional lymph nodes cannot be assessed
N0	No regional lymph node metastasis
N1	Metastasis in a single ipsilateral lymph node, 3 cm or less in greatest dimension
N2	Metastasis in a single ipsilateral lymph node, more than 3 cm but not more than 6 cm in greatest dimension, or in multiple ipsilateral lymph nodes, none more than 6 cm in greatest dimension, or in bilateral or contralateral lymph nodes, none more than 6 cm in greatest dimension:
	Na2 Metastasis in a single ipsilateral lymph node more than 3 cm but not more than 6 cm in greatest dimension
	Nab Metastasis in multiple ipsilateral lymph nodes, none more than 6 cm in greatest dimension
	N2c Metastasis in bilateral or contralateral lymph nodes, none more than 6 cm in greatest dimension
N3	Metastasis in a lymph node more than 6 cm in greatest dimension

Distant Metastasis (M)

MX	Distant metastasis cannot be assessed
M0	No distant metastasis
M1	Distant metastasis

Stage Grouping: Nasopharynx

Stage 0	Tis	N0	M0
Stage I	T1	N0	M0
Stage IIA	T2a	N0	M0
Stage IIB	T1	N1	M0
	T2	N1	M0
	T2a	N1	M0
	T2b	N0	M0
	T2b	N1	M0
Stage III	T1	N2	M0
	T2a	N2	M0
	T2b	N2	M0
	T3	N0	M0
	T3	N1	M0
	T3	N2	M0
Stage IVA	T4	N0	M0
	T4	N1	M0
	T4	N2	M0
Stage IVB	Any T	N3	M0
Stage IVC	Any T	Any N	M1

Stage Grouping: Oropharynx, Hypopharynx

Stage 0	Tis	N0	M0
Stage I	T1	N0	M0
Stage II	T2	N0	M0
Stage III	T3	N0	M0
	T1	N1	M0
	T2	N1	M0
	T3	N1	M0
Stage IVA	T4	N0	M0
	T4	N1	M0
	Any T	N2	M0
Stage IVB	Any T	N3	M0
Stage IVC	Any T	Any N	M1

LARYNX
Rules for Classification

The classification applies only to carcinomas. There should be histologic confirmation of the disease.

The following are the procedures for assessing T, N, and M categories:

T categories	Physical examination, laryngoscopy, and imaging
N categories	Physical examination and imaging
M categories	Physical examination and imaging

Definition of TNM

Primary Tumor (T)

TX	Primary tumor cannot be assessed
T0	No evidence of primary tumor
Tis	Carcinoma in situ

Supraglottis

T1   Tumor limited to one subsite of supraglottis with normal vocal cord mobility

T2   Tumor invades mucosa of more than one adjacent subsite of supraglottis or glottis or region outside the supraglottis (e.g., mucosa of base of tongue, vallecula, medial wall of pyriform sinus) without fixation of the larynx

T3   Tumor limited to larynx with vocal cord fixation and/or invades any of the following: postcricoid area, pre-epiglottic tissues

T4   Tumor invades through the thyroid cartilage, and/or extends into soft tissue of the neck, thyroid, and/or esophagus

Glottis

T1   Tumor limited to the true vocal cords (may involve anterior or posterior commissure) with normal mobility:

    T1a   Tumor limited to one true vocal cord
    T1b   Tumor involves both true vocal cords

T2   Tumor extends to supraglottis and/or subglottis, and/or with impaired true vocal cord mobility

T3   Tumor limited to the larynx with true vocal cord fixation

T4   Tumor invades through the thyroid cartilage and/or to other tissues beyond the larynx (e.g., trachea, soft tissues of neck, including thyroid, pharynx)

Subglottis

T1   Tumor limited to the subglottis

T2   Tumor extends to vocal cords with normal or impaired mobility

T3   Tumor limited to larynx with vocal cord fixation

T4   Tumor invades through cricoid or thyroid cartilage and/or extends to other tissues beyond the larynx (e.g., trachea, soft tissues of neck, including thyroid, esophagus)

Regional Lymph Nodes (N)

NX	Regional lymph nodes cannot be assessed
N0	No regional lymph node metastasis
N1	Metastasis in a single ipsilateral lymph node, 3 cm or less in greatest dimension
N2	Metastasis in a single ipsilateral lymph node, more than 3 cm but not more than 6 cm in greatest dimension, or in multiple ipsilateral lymph nodes, none more than 6 cm in greatest dimension, or in bilateral or contralateral lymph nodes, none more than 6 cm in greatest dimension:
N2a	Metastasis in a single ipsilateral lymph node more than 3 cm but not more than 6 cm in greatest dimension
N2b	Metastasis in multiple ipsilateral lymph nodes, none more than 6 cm in greatest dimension
N2c	Metastasis in bilateral or contralateral lymph nodes, none more than 6 cm in greatest dimension
N3	Metastasis in a lymph node more than 6 cm in greatest dimension

Distant Metastasis (M)

MX	Distant metastasis cannot be assessed
M0	No distant metastasis
M1	Distant metastasis

Stage Grouping

Stage 0	Tis	N0	M0
Stage I	T1	N0	M0
Stage II	T2	N0	M0
Stage III	T3	N0	M0
	T1	N1	M0
	T2	N1	M0
	T3	N1	M0
Stage IVA	T4	N0	M0
	T4	N1	M0
	Any T	N2	M0
Stage IVB	Any T	N3	M0
Stage IVC	Any T	Any N	M1

PARANASAL SINUSES
Rules for Classification

The classification applies only to carcinomas. There should be histologic confirmation of the disease.

The following are the procedures for assessing T, N, and M categories:

T categories	Physical examination and imaging
N categories	Physical examination and imaging
M categories	Physical examination and imaging

Definition of TNM

MAXILLARY SINUS

Primary Tumor (T)

TX	Primary tumor cannot be assessed
T0	No evidence of primary tumor
Tis	Carcinoma in situ
T1	Tumor limited to the antral mucosa with no erosion or destruction of bone
T2	Tumor causing bone erosion or destruction, except for the posterior antral wall, including extension into the hard palate and/or the middle nasal meatus
T3	Tumor invades any of the following: bone of the posterior wall of maxillary sinus, subcutaneous tissues, skin of cheek, floor or medial wall of orbit, infratemporal fossa, pterygoid plates, ethmoid sinuses

T4   Tumor invades orbital contents beyond the floor or medial wall including any of the following: the orbital apex, cribriform plate, base of skull, nasopharynx, sphenoid, frontal sinuses

ETHMOID SINUS

Primary Tumor (T)

T1   Tumor confined to the ethmoid with or without bone erosion
T2   Tumor extends into the nasal cavity
T3   Tumor extends to the anterior orbit and/or maxillary sinus
T4   Tumor with intracranial extension, orbital extension including apex, involving sphenoid, and/or frontal sinus and/or skin of external nose

Regional Lymph Nodes (N)

NX   Regional lymph nodes cannot be assessed
N0   No regional lymph node metastasis
N1   Metastasis in a single ipsilateral lymph node, 3 cm or less in greatest dimension
N2   Metastasis in a single ipsilateral lymph node, more than 3 cm but not more than 6 cm in greatest dimension, or in multiple ipsilateral lymph nodes, none more than 6 cm in greatest dimension, or in bilateral or contralateral lymph nodes, none more than 6 cm in greatest dimension:
    N2a   Metastasis in a single ipsilateral lymph node more than 3 cm but not more than 6 cm in greatest dimension
    N2b   Metastasis in multiple ipsilateral lymph nodes, none more than 6 cm in greatest dimension
    N2c   Metastasis in bilateral or contralateral lymph nodes, none more than 6 cm in greatest dimension
N3   Metastasis in a lymph node more than 6 cm in greatest dimension

Distant Metastasis (M)

MX   Distant metastasis cannot be assessed
M0   No distant metastasis
M1   Distant metastasis

Stage Grouping

Stage 0	Tis	N0	M0
Stage I	T1	N0	M0
Stage II	T2	N0	M0
Stage III	T3	N0	M0
	T1	N1	M0
	T2	N1	M0
	T3	N1	M0
Stage IVA	T4	N0	M0
	T4	N1	M0
Stage IVB	Any T	N2	M0
	Any T	N3	M0
Stage IVC	Any T	Any N	M1

▪ MAJOR SALIVARY GLANDS (PAROTID, SUBMANDIBULAR, AND SUBLINGUAL)
Rules for Classification

The classification applies only to carcinomas of the major salivary glands. Tumors arising in minor salivary glands (seromucinous glands in the lining membrane of the upper aerodigestive tract) are not included in this classification but at their anatomic site of origin, e.g., lip. There should be histologic confirmation of the disease.

The following are procedures for assessing T, N, and M categories:

T categories	Physical examination and imaging
N categories	Physical examination and imaging
M categories	Physical examination and imaging

Definition of TNM

Primary Tumor (T)

TX   Primary tumor cannot be assessed
T0   No evidence of primary tumor
T1   Tumor 2 cm or less in greatest dimension without extraparenchymal extension
T2   Tumor more than 2 cm but not more than 4 cm in greatest dimension without extraparenchymal extension
T3   Tumor having extraparenchymal extension without seventh nerve involvement and/or more than 4 cm but not more than 6 cm in greatest dimension
T4   Tumor invades base of skull, seventh nerve, and/or exceeds 6 cm in greatest dimension

Regional Lymph Nodes (N)

NX   Regional lymph nodes cannot be assessed
N0   No regional lymph node metastasis
N1   Metastasis in a single ipsilateral lymph node, 3 cm or less in greatest dimension
N2   Metastasis in a single ipsilateral lymph node, more than 3 cm but not more than 6 cm in greatest dimension, or in multiple ipsilateral lymph nodes, none more than 6 cm in greatest dimension, or in bilateral or contralateral lymph nodes, none more than 6 cm in greatest dimension:
    N2a   Metastasis in a single ipsilateral lymph node more than 3 cm but not more than 6 cm in greatest dimension
    N2b   Metastasis in multiple ipsilateral lymph nodes, none more than 6 cm in greatest dimension
    N2c   Metastasis in bilateral or contralateral lymph nodes, none more than 6 cm in greatest dimension
N3   Metastasis in a lymph node more than 6 cm in greatest dimension

Distant Metastasis (M)

MX   Distant metastasis cannot be assessed
M0   No distant metastases
M1   Distant metastasis

Stage Grouping

Stage I	T1	N0	M0
	T2	N0	M0
Stage II	T3	N0	M0
Stage III	T1	N1	M0
	T2	N1	M0
Stage IV	T4	N0	M0
	T3	N1	M0
	T4	N1	M0
	Any T	N2	M0
	Any T	N3	M0
	Any T	Any N	M1

THYROID GLAND

Rules for Classification

The classification applies only to carcinomas. There should be microscopic confirmation of the disease and division of cases by histologic type.

The following are the procedures for assessing T, N, and M categories:

T categories	Physical examination, endoscopy, and imaging
N categories	Physical examination and imaging
M categories	Physical examination and imaging

Definition of TNM

Primary Tumor (T)

Note: All categories may be subdivided: (a) solitary tumor, (b) multifocal tumor (the largest determines the classification).

TX	Primary tumor cannot be assessed
T0	No evidence of primary tumor
T1	Tumor 1 cm or less in greatest dimension limited to the thyroid
T2	Tumor more than 1 cm but not more than 4 cm in greatest dimension limited to the thyroid
T3	Tumor more than 4 cm in greatest dimension limited to the thyroid
T4	Tumor of any size extending beyond the thyroid capsule

Regional Lymph Nodes (N)

Regional lymph nodes are the cervical and upper mediastinal lymph nodes.

NX	Regional lymph nodes cannot be assessed
N0	No regional lymph node metastasis
N1	Regional lymph node metastasis:
	N1a Metastasis in ipsilateral cervical lymph node(s)
	N1b Metastasis in bilateral, midline, or contralateral cervical or mediastinal lymph node(s)

Distant Metastasis (M)

MX	Distant metastasis cannot be assessed
M0	No distant metastasis
M1	Distant metastasis

Stage Grouping

Separate stage groupings are recommended for papillary, follicular, medullary, or undifferentiated (anaplastic carcinomas).

PAPILLARY OR FOLLICULAR

	Under 45 years	45 years and older
Stage I	Any T, Any N, M0	T1, N0, M0
Stage II	Any T, Any N, M1	T2, N0, M0
		T3, N0, M0
Stage III		T4, N0, M0
		Any T, N1, M0
Stage IV		Any T, Any N, M1

MEDULLARY

Stage I	T1	N0	M0
Stage II	T2	N0	M0
	T3	N0	M0
	T4	N0	M0
Stage III	Any T	N1	M0
Stage IV	Any T	Any N	M1

UNDIFFERENTIATED (ANAPLASTIC)

All cases are stage IV.

Stage IV	Any T	Any N	Any M

SOFT TISSUE SARCOMA

Rules for Classification

There should be histologic confirmation of the disease and division of cases by histologic type and grade.

The following are the procedures for assessing T, N, and M categories:

T categories	Physical examination and imaging
N categories	Physical examination and imaging
M categories	Physical examination and imaging

Definition of TNM

Primary Tumor (T)

TX	Primary tumor cannot be assessed
T0	No evidence of primary tumor
T1	Tumor 5 cm or less in greatest dimension:
	T1a superficial tumor
	T1b deep tumor
T2	Tumor more than 5 cm in greatest dimension:
	T2a superficial tumor
	T2b deep tumor

Note: Superficial tumor is located exclusively above the superficial fascia without invasion of the fascia; deep tumor is located either exclusively beneath the superficial fascia, or superficial to the fascia with invasion of or through the fascia, or superficial and beneath the fascia. Retroperitoneal, mediastinal, and pelvic sarcomas are classified as deep tumors.

Regional Lymph Nodes (N)

NX	Regional lymph nodes cannot be assessed
N0	No regional lymph node metastasis
N1	Regional lymph node metastasis

Distant Metastasis (M)

MX	Distant metastasis cannot be assessed
M0	No distant metastasis
M1	Distant metastasis

Histopathologic Grade

GX	Grade cannot be assessed
G1	Well differentiated
G2	Moderately differentiated
G3	Poorly differentiated
G4	Undifferentiated

Stage Grouping

Stage I

A (low grade, small, superficial and deep)	G1–2,	T1a–1b,	N0,	M0
B (low grade, large, superficial)	G1–2,	T2a,	N0,	M0

Stage II

A (low grade, large, deep)	G1–2,	T2b,	N0,	M0
B (high grade, small, superficial, deep)	G3–4,	T1a–1b,	N0,	M0
C (high grade, large, superficial)	G3–4,	T2a,	N0,	M0

Stage III

(high grade, large, deep)	G3–4,	T2b,	N0	M0

Stage IV

(any metastasis)	any G,	any T,	N1	M0
	any G,	any T,	N0	M1

CARCINOMA OF THE LACRIMAL GLAND

Rules for Classification

There should be histologic confirmation of the disease and division of cases by histologic type.

The following are the procedures for assessing T, N, and M categories:

T categories	Physical examination and imaging
N categories	Physical examination
M categories	Physical examination and imaging

Definition of TNM

Primary Tumor (T)

TX	Primary tumor cannot be assessed
T0	No evidence of primary tumor

T1	Tumor 2.5 cm or less in greatest dimension limited to the lacrimal gland
T2	Tumor 2.5 cm or less in greatest dimension invading the periosteum of the fossa of the lacrimal gland
T3	Tumor more than 2.5 cm but not more than 5 cm in greatest dimension:
	T3a Tumor limited to the lacrimal gland
	T3b Tumor invades the periosteum of the fossa of the lacrimal gland
T4	Tumor more than 5 cm in greatest dimension:
	T4a Tumor invades the orbital soft tissues, optic nerve, or globe without bone invasion
	T4b Tumor invades the orbital soft tissues, optic nerve, or globe with bone invasion

Regional Lymph Nodes (N)

NX	Regional lymph nodes cannot be assessed
N0	No regional lymph node metastasis
N1	Regional lymph node metastasis

Distant Metastasis (M)

MX	Distant metastasis cannot be assessed
M0	No distant metastasis
M1	Distant metastasis

Stage Grouping

No stage grouping is presently recommended.

Index ■
■
■

Note: Page numbers in **bold** refer to color figures, page numbers in *italics* refer to illustrations, and page numbers followed by t refer to tables.